PINNACLE

PAIN MANAGEMENT & REHABILITATION
Mark A. Banks MD

BOARD CERTIFIED PM&R, PAIN MGMT.

422 N. Columbus Street | Lancaster, Ohio 43130
Phone (740) 687-2700 | Fax (740) 687-2701

PHYSICAL MEDICINE

& REHABILITATION

RANDALL L. BRADDOM, M.D., M.S.

Chairman, Physical Medicine and Rehabilitation
Indiana University Medical Center
Community Hospitals Indianapolis
Indianapolis, Indiana

PHYSICAL MEDICINE & REHABILITATION

W.B. SAUNDERS COMPANY
A Division of Harcourt Brace & Company
Philadelphia   London   Toronto   Montreal   Sydney   Tokyo

W.B. SAUNDERS COMPANY
A Division of Harcourt Brace & Company

The Curtis Center
Independence Square West
Philadelphia, Pennsylvania 19106

Library of Congress Cataloging-in-Publication Data

Physical medicine & rehabilitation / [edited by] Randall L. Braddom;
  associate editors, Ralph M. Buschbacher . . . [et al.].—1st ed.
    p.   cm.

ISBN 0–7216–5243–3

1. Physical therapy.   2. Medical rehabilitation.   I. Braddom,
  Randall L.   [DNLM: 1. Physical Medicine.
  2. Rehabilitation.   WB 460 P5774 1996]   RM700.P465 1996

615.8′2—dc20

DNLM/DLC   95–11493

Physical Medicine & Rehabilitation   ISBN 0–7216–5243–3

Printed in the United States of America

Last digit is the print number: 9   8   7   6   5   4   3   2

This book is dedicated to my wife Carolyn
(the love of my life),
to my children Eric, Steven, and Karen
(the joys of my life),
to my parents Audy and Ruth Braddom
(who always believed in me),
to my partners in practice,
Janine Sheppard, Ralph and Lois Buschbacher, Paul Kern, and Marc Duerden
(who have put up with me),
and to my teachers and mentors, especially Ernest W. Johnson.
Without their support,
this book could not have been completed.

Associate Editors

Contributors

JUDY ADKINS, O.T.R.
Occupational Therapy, Indiana University Medical Center, Indianapolis, Indiana.
Prescription of Wheelchairs and Seating Systems

JAMES C. AGRE, M.D., PH.D.
Professor and Chairperson, Department of Rehabilitation Medicine, University of Wisconsin–Madison Medical School, Madison, Wisconsin.
Rehabilitation Concepts in Motor Neuron Diseases

AUGUSTA S. ALBA, M.D.
Associate Professor, Clinical Rehabilitation Medicine, New York University Medical Center, New York City; Director, Department of Rehabilitation Medicine, Medical Director, Nursing Facility, Goldwater Memorial Hospital, Roosevelt Island, New York.
Concepts in Pulmonary Rehabilitation

KAREN L. ANDREWS, M.D.
Consultant, Department of Physical Medicine and Rehabilitation, Mayo Clinic and Mayo Foundation; Assistant Professor of Physical Medicine and Rehabilitation, Mayo Medical School, Rochester, Minnesota.
Rehabilitation in Vascular Diseases

JAMES W. ATCHISON, D.O.
Assistant Professor, Residency Program Director, University of Kentucky, Lexington, Kentucky.
Manipulation, Traction, and Massage

MATTHEW N. BARTELS, M.D., M.P.H.
Chief Resident, Department of Rehabilitation Medicine, Columbia–Presbyterian Medical Center, New York, New York.
Cardiac Rehabilitation

CLAIRE E. BENDER, M.D.
Consultant, Department of Diagnostic Radiology, Mayo Clinic and Mayo Foundation; Associate Professor of Radiology, Mayo Medical School, Rochester, Minnesota.
Rehabilitation of Patients With Swallowing Disorders

DONNA JO BLAKE, M.D.
Assistant Professor, Department of Rehabilitation Medicine, University of Colorado Health Sciences Center; Staff Physiatrist, Denver Veterans Affairs Medical Center, Denver, Colorado.
Employment of Persons With Disabilities

CORWIN BOAKE, PH.D.
Assistant Professor, Department of Physical Medicine and Rehabilitation, University of Texas–Houston Medical School; Neuropsychologist, The Institute for Rehabilitation and Research, Houston, Texas.
Principles of Brain Injury Rehabilitation

CATHERINE F. BONTKE, M.D.
System Medical Director, Rehabilitation Services, The Rehabilitation Hospital of Connecticut, Hartford, Connecticut.
Principles of Brain Injury Rehabilitation

RANDALL L. BRADDOM, M.D., M.S.
Chairman, Physical Medicine and Rehabilitation, Indiana University Medical Center; Community Hospitals Indianapolis, Indianapolis, Indiana.
Prescription of Wheelchairs and Seating Systems

SUSAN L. BRAUN, M.L.S., O.T.R.
Director of WeeFim Services, Uniform Data System for Medical Rehabilitation, State University of New York at Buffalo, New York.
Quality and Outcome Measures for Medical Rehabilitation

ALLEN W. BROWN, M.D.
Senior Associate Consultant, Department of Physical Medicine and Rehabilitation, Mayo Clinic, Rochester, Minnesota.
Physical Agent Modalities

LOIS BUSCHBACHER, M.D.
Clinical Assistant Professor, Indiana University School of Medicine, Rehabilitation Associates, Indianapolis, Indiana.
Rehabilitation of Patients With Peripheral Neuropathics

RALPH M. BUSCHBACHER, M.D.
Clinical Assistant Professor, Department of Physical Medicine and Rehabilitation, Indiana University Hospital, Indianapolis, Indiana.
Prescription of Wheelchairs and Seating Systems; Deconditioning, Conditioning, and the Benefits of Exercise

DENISE I. CAMPAGNOLO, M.D., M.S.
Instructor, Department of Physical Medicine and Rehabilitation, UMDNJ, New Jersey Medical School, Newark, New Jersey.
Research in Physical Medicine and Rehabilitation

DIANA D. CARDENAS, M.D.
Professor, Department of Rehabilitation Medicine, University of Washington; Director, Rehabilitation Medicine Clinic, University of Washington Medical Center; Attending Physiatrist, University of Washington Medical Center; Project Director, Northwest Regional Spinal Cord Injury System, University of Washington, Seattle, Washington.
Urinary Tract and Bowel Management in the Rehabilitation Setting

KEVIN M. CAVES, B.S.M.E.
The Center for Applied Rehabilitation, Rancho Los Amigos Medical Center, Downey, California.
Computer Assistive Devices and Environmental Controls

DAVID CHEN, M.D.
Assistant Professor, Department of Physical Medicine and Rehabilitation, Northwestern University Medical School; Director, Spinal Cord Injury Rehabilitation, Midwest Regional Spinal Cord Injury Care System, Chicago, Illinois.
Rehabilitation of Patients With Spinal Cord Injuries

SAM C. COLACHIS III, M.D.
Associate Professor, Department of Physical Medicine and Rehabilitation, The Ohio State University; Director, Spinal Cord Injury Rehabilitation Services, The Ohio State University, Columbus, Ohio.
Osteoporosis: Its Prevention and Treatment

ANDREW J. COLE, M.D.
Clinical Assistant Professor, Departments of Physical Medicine and Rehabilitation, Department of Physical Therapy, University of Texas Southwestern Medical Center; Director, Spine Rehabilitation Services, Department of Physical Medicine and Rehabilitation, Baylor University Medical Center, Dallas, Texas.
Imaging Studies for the Physiatrist

BARBARA J. DE LATEUR, M.D., M.S.
Professor, Director and Lawrence Cardinal Sheehan Chair, Department of Physical Medicine and Rehabilitation, Johns Hopkins School of Medicine, Baltimore, Maryland.
Therapeutic Exercise

ANNE DEUTSCH, M.S., R.N., C.R.R.N.
Adjunct Instructor, School of Nursing, State University of New York at Buffalo; Consultant, Uniform Data System for Medical Rehabilitation, State University of New York at Buffalo, Buffalo, New York.
Quality and Outcome Measures for Rehabilitation

MARY E. DILLON, M.D.
Assistant Professor, Clinical Physical Medicine and Rehabilitation, Department of Physical Medicine and Rehabilitation, University of Cincinnati College of Medicine; Co-director, Drake Center, Inc., Cincinnati, Ohio.
Rehabilitation Management in Persons With AIDS and HIV Infection

MARY L. DOMBOVY, M.D.
Assistant Professor, Neurology and Orthopedics (Rehabilitation), University of Rochester; Chair, Department of Physical Medicine and Rehabilitation, St. Mary's Hospital, Rochester, New York.
Rehabilitation Concerns in Degenerative Movement Disorders of the Central Nervous System

DANIEL DUMITRU, M.D.
Professor and Deputy Chairman, Department of Rehabilitation Medicine, University of Texas Health Science Center at San Antonio, San Antonio, Texas.
Electrodiagnostic Medicine I: Basic Aspects

ALBERTO ESQUENAZI, M.D.
Associate Professor, Department of Physical Medicine and Rehabilitation, Temple University; Director, Moss Regional Amputee Center and Gait and Motion Analysis Laboratory, Moss Rehabilitation Hospital, Philadelphia, Pennsylvania.
Upper Limb Amputee Rehabilitation and Prosthetic Restoration

FRANK J. E. FALCO, M.D.
Medical Director, Comprehensive Spine and Sportscare PA, Lester, Pennsylvania.
Assessment and Treatment of Cervical Spine Disorders

VIRGIL W. FAULKNER, C.P.O.
Associate Professor, Department of Rehabilitation Medicine, The University of Texas Health Science Center at San Antonio; Director, Rehabilitation Engineering Laboratory (REL), The University of Texas Health Science Center at San Antonio, San Antonio, Texas.
Lower Limb Prostheses

GERALD FELSENTHAL, M.D.
Associate Professor, Department of Physical Medicine and Rehabilitation, Johns Hopkins University School of Medicine; Clinical Professor, Department of Epidemiology and Preventive Medicine, University of Maryland School of Medicine; Chief, Department of Rehabilitation Medicine, Sinai Hospital of Baltimore; Head, Division of Rehabilitation Medicine, Levindale Hebrew Geriatric Center and Hospital, Baltimore, Maryland.
Principles of Geriatric Rehabilitation

ROGER C. FIEDLER, PH.D.
Research Assistant Professor, Department of Rehabilitation Medicine, School of Medicine and Biomedical Sciences, State University of New York at Buffalo; Director of Research, Uniform Data System for Medical Rehabilitation, Center for Functional Assessment Research, State University of New York at Buffalo, Buffalo, New York.
Quality and Outcome Measures for Medical Rehabilitation

STEVEN V. FISHER, M.D.
Associate Professor, University of Minnesota Medical School, Department of Physical Medicine and Rehabilitation University of Minnesota Medical School; Chief, Department of Physical Medicine and Rehabilitation, Medical Director, Miland Knapp Rehabilitation Center, Hennepin County Medical Center, Minneapolis, Minnesota.
Spinal Orthoses in Rehabilitation

DAVID J. FORDYCE, PH.D.
Neuropsychology and Rehabilitation Psychology, Section of Physical Medicine and Rehabilitation, Virginia Mason Medical Center, Seattle, Washington.
Psychological Perspectives on Rehabilitation: Contemporary Assessment and Intervention Strategies

DEBORAH GAEBLER-SPIRA, M.D.
Assistant Professor, Northwestern University, Northwestern University Medical School; Director, Cerebral Palsy Program, Rehabilitation Institute of Chicago, Chicago, Illinois.
Rehabilitation of Children and Adults With Cerebral Palsy

JAN C. GALVIN, B.A.
The Galvin Group, Ltd., Tucson, Arizona.
Computer Assistive Devices and Environmental Controls

FAE H. GARDEN, M.D.
Assistant Professor, Baylor College of Medicine; Assistant Chief, Physical Medicine and Rehabilitation, St. Luke's Episcopal Hospital, Houston, Texas.
Principles of Cancer Rehabilitation

DIANE M.-L. GILBERT, M.D.
Assistant Professor, University of Texas Health Science
Center at San Antonio; Medical Director, Rehabilitation
Medicine Department, University Hospital, San Antonio,
Texas.
Sexuality Issues in Persons With Disabilities

WOLFGANG G. GILLIAR, D.O.
Physiatrist, San Mateo, California.
Manipulation, Traction, and Massage

THERESA A. GILLIS, M.D.
Assistant Professor, Department of Physical Medicine and
Rehabilitation, Baylor College of Medicine; Medical
Director, Rehabilitation Services, University of Texas, M.D.
Anderson Cancer Center, Houston, Texas.
Principles of Cancer Rehabilitation

GARY GOLDBERG, M.D.
Associate Professor, Department of Physical Medicine and
Rehabilitation, Temple University; Director,
Electrodiagnostic Laboratory, Moss Rehabilitation Hospital,
Philadelphia, Pennsylvania.
Research in Physical Medicine and Rehabilitation

MARTIN GRABOIS, M.D.
Professor, Departments of Physical Medicine and
Rehabilitation, Anesthesiology, and Restorative Neurology
and Human Neurobiology, Baylor College of Medicine,
Houston, Texas.
Chronic Pain Syndromes: Evaluation and Treatment

CARL V. GRANGER, M.D.
Professor, Rehabilitation Medicine, State University of New
York at Buffalo; Director, Center for Functional Assessment
Research, Department of Rehabilitation Medicine, State
University of New York at Buffalo, Buffalo, New York.
Quality and Outcome Measures for Medical Rehabilitation

DENNIS HART, M.D.
Chief Resident, Department of Physical Medicine and
Rehabilitation, University of Kentucky, Lexington, Kentucky.
The Prevention and Management of Pressure Ulcers

RICHARD L. HARVEY, M.D.
Instructor, Department of Physical Medicine and
Rehabilitation, Northwestern University Medical School;
Attending Physician, Center for Stroke Rehabilitation,
Rehabilitation Institute of Chicago, Chicago, Illinois.
Rehabilitation of Stroke Syndromes

ROSS M. HAYS, M.D.
Associate Professor, University of Washington School of
Medicine; Associate Director, Department of Rehabilitation
Medicine, Children's Hospital and Medical Center, Seattle,
Washington.
Rehabilitation Concepts in Myelomeningocele

PHALA A. HELM, M.D.
Chair and Professor, University of Texas Health Sciences
Center, Dallas, Texas.
Rehabilitation in Vascular Diseases

WILLIAM J. HENNESSEY, M.D.
Resident and Clinical Instructor, Department of Physical
Medicine and Rehabilitation, The Ohio State University
College of Medicine, Columbus, Ohio.
Lower Limb Orthoses

CHARLES P. HO, PH.D., M.D.
Clinical Assistant Professor of Radiology, Stanford
University School of Medicine Stanford; Medical Director,
Sand Hill Imaging Center, Menlo Park; Bayside Imaging
Center, Redwood City, California.
Imaging Studies for the Physiatrist

BETSY A. HOLLAND, M.D.
Medical Director, Marin Magnetic Imaging, Greenbrae;
Clinical Assistant Professor of Radiology, University of
California, San Francisco, California.
Imaging Studies for the Physiatrist

JASMINKA Z. ILICH, PH.D., R.D.
Clinical Assistant Professor, Department of Physical
Medicine and Rehabilitation and Department of Human
Nutrition, The Ohio State University; Senior Research
Associate, The Ohio State University School of Medicine,
Columbus, Ohio.
Osteoporosis: Its Prevention and Treatment

KATIE D. IRANI, M.B.B.S.
Assistant Professor, Department of Physical Medicine and
Rehabilitation, Baylor College of Medicine; Chief,
Department of Physical Medicine and Rehabilitation, Harris
County Hospital District, Houston, Texas.
Upper Limb Orthoses

REBECCA D. JACKSON, M.D.
Associate Professor, Department of Internal Medicine,
Division of Endocrinology and Metabolism, Department of
Physical Medicine and Rehabilitation, The Ohio State
University, Columbus, Ohio.
Electrical Stimulation

ERNEST W. JOHNSON, M.D.
Associate Dean, Ohio State University College of
Medicine, Columbus, Ohio.
*Lower Limb Orthoses; Upper Limb Musculoskeletal Pain
Syndromes*

MARK JOHNSTON, PH.D.
Assistant Professor, Physical Medicine and Rehabilitation,
UMDNJ/New Jersey Medical School, Newark; Director of
Outcome Research, Kessler Institute for Rehabilitation,
East Orange, New Jersey.
Quality and Outcome Measures for Medical Rehabilitation

RICHARD T. KATZ, M.D.
Associate Professor of Clinical Medicine (PM&R), St. Louis
University School of Medicine, Vice-President of Medical
Affairs, SSM Rehabilitation Institute, St. Louis, Missouri.
*Research in Physical Medicine and Rehabilitation;
Management of Spasticity*

MARGARET KELLY-HAYES, ED.D., R.N., C.R.R.N.
Associate Clinical Professor of Neurology (Neurological
Nursing), Department of Neurology, Boston University
School of Medicine, Boston; Investigator, Framingham
Study, Framingham, Massachusetts.
Quality and Outcome Measures for Medical Rehabilitation

JOHN C. KING, M.D.
Associate Professor, Department of Rehabilitation
Medicine, The University of Texas Health Science Center
at San Antonio; Attending Physician, Physical Medicine

and Rehabilitation Service, Audie L. Murphy Memorial Veterans Hospital, San Antonio, Texas.
Urinary Tract and Bowel Management in the Rehabilitation Setting

FRANCIS P. LAGATTUTA, M.D.
Assistant Clinical Professor, Loyola University, Maywood; Medical Director, GlenOaks Medical Center, Glendale Heights, Illinois.
Assessment and Treatment of Cervical Spine Disorders

EDWARD R. LASKOWSKI, M.D.
Consultant, Department of Physical Medicine and Rehabilitation, Co-Chair, Sports Medicine Center, Mayo Clinic and Mayo Foundation; Assistant Professor of Physical Medicine and Rehabilitation, Mayo Medical School; Rochester, Minnesota.
Concepts in Sports Medicine

BRIAN LAY
Consultant in Wheelchairs, Revco, Inc., Indianapolis, Indiana.
Prescription of Wheelchairs and Seating Systems

STEPHEN LEBDUSKA, M.D.
Clinical Assistant Professor, State University of New York Health Science Center at Syracuse; Chief, Rehabilitation Services, Veterans Administration Medical Center, Syracuse, New York.
Rehabilitation Issues in Plexopathies

TERESA L. MASSAGLI, M.D.
Assistant Professor, Departments of Rehabilitation Medicine and Pediatrics, University of Washington School of Medicine; Attending Physician, Department of Rehabilitation Medicine, Children's Hospital and Medical Center and University of Washington Affiliated Medical Centers, Seattle, Washington.
Rehabilitation Concepts in Myelomeningocele

VELIMIR MATKOVIC, M.D., PH.D.
Associate Professor, Department of Physical Medicine and Rehabilitation, Medicine and Nutrition, Director, Bone and Mineral Metabolism Laboratory, The Ohio State University; Director, Bone and Mineral Metabolism Laboratory, The Ohio State University College of Medicine, Columbus, Ohio.
Osteoporosis: Its Prevention and Treatment

DENNIS J. MATTHEWS, M.D.
Associate Clinical Professor, Department of Rehabilitation Medicine, Children's Hospital, University of Colorado, Denver, Colorado.
Examination of the Pediatric Patient; Rehabilitation Concepts in Motor Neuron Diseases

MICHAEL E. MAYO, M.B.B.S., F.R.C.S.
Professor of Urology, University of Washington; Attending Urologist, University of Washington Medical Center, Children's Hospital and Medical Center, Veterans Affairs Medical Center, Harborview Medical Center, University of Washington, Seattle, Washington.
Urinary Tract and Bowel Management in the Rehabilitation Setting

ROBERT D. McANELLY, M.D.
Assistant Professor, Department of Rehabilitation Medicine, The University of Texas Health Science Center

at San Antonio; Director of Resident Education and Medical Director of the Motion Analysis Laboratory, Warm Springs and Baptist Rehabilitation Network, Staff Physician, Rehabilitation Medicine Service, South Texas Veterans Healthcare System, Audie L. Murphy Division, San Antonio, Texas.
Lower Limb Prostheses

MICHAEL T. McCANN, M.D.
Assistant Professor, Departments of Anesthesiology and Physical Medicine and Rehabilitation, Baylor College of Medicine, Houston, Texas.
Chronic Pain Syndromes: Evaluation and Treatment

LISA A. McPEAK, M.D.
Assistant Professor, Department of Physical Medicine and Rehabilitation, University of Arkansas for Medical Sciences, Little Rock, Arkansas.
Physiatric History and Examination

CRISTINA M. MIX, B.S., O.T.R.
Occupational Therapist, The Children's Hospital, Denver, Colorado.
Achieving Functional Independence

BAHRAM MOKRI, M.D.
Consultant, Department of Neurology, Mayo Clinic and Mayo Foundation; Professor of Neurology, Mayo Medical School, Rochester, Minnesota.
Low Back Pain and Disorders of the Lumbar Spine

JONATHAN R. MOLDOVER, M.D.
Director, Outreach and Satellite Operations, Kessler Institute for Rehabilitation, West Orange, New Jersey.
Cardiac Rehabilitation

W. JERRY MYSIW, M.D.
Associate Professor, Department of Physical Medicine and Rehabilitation, The Ohio State University College of Medicine, Columbus, Ohio.
Electrical Stimulation

MARGE C. NELSON, O.T.
Occupational Therapist, Department of Physical Medicine and Rehabilitation, Mayo Clinic and Mayo Foundation, Rochester, Minnesota.
Rehabilitation of Patients With Swallowing Disorders

MAUREEN R. NELSON, M.D.
Assistant Professor, Department of Physical Medicine and Rehabilitation: Pediatrics, Baylor College of Medicine; Chief, Physical Medicine and Rehabilitation, Texas Children's Hospital, Houston, Texas.
Rehabilitation Concerns in Myopathies

JOHN J. NICHOLAS, M.D.
Professor, Chairman, Department of Physical Medicine and Rehabilitation, Residency Program Director, Rush Medical College, Rush University, Rush–Presbyterian–St. Luke's Medical Center, Chicago; Member, Board of Directors, Rehabilitation Medicine Clinics Inc., Wheaton, Illinois.
Joint and Soft Tissue Injection Techniques; Rehabilitation of Patients with Rheumatic Disorders

STEPHEN F. NOLL, M.D.
Consultant, Department of Physical Medicine and Rehabilitation, Mayo Clinic and Mayo Foundation; Assistant Professor of Physical Medicine and

Rehabilitation, Mayo Medical School, Rochester, Minnesota.
Rehabilitation of Patients With Swallowing Disorders

MICHAEL W. O'DELL, M.D.
Associate Professor of Physical Medicine and Rehabilitation, University of Cincinnati College of Medicine; Director, Brain Injury Rehabilitation Programs, Drake Center, Inc., Cincinnati, Ohio.
Rehabilitation Management in Persons With AIDS and HIV Infection

NICHOLAS K. OLSEN, D.O.
Rehabilitation Associates of Colorado; Staff Physician, Corporate Health Services, Denver, Colorado.
Musculoskeletal Disorders of the Lower Limbs

JERRY C. PARKER, PH.D.
Clinical Associate Professor of Internal Medicine, University of Missouri—Columbia; Chief, Psychology Service, Harry S. Truman Memorial Veterans Hospital, Columbia, Missouri.
Research in Physical Medicine and Rehabilitation

WILLIAM S. PEASE, M.D.
Associate Professor and Chairperson, Director, Residency Training Program, Department of Physical Medicine and Rehabilitation, The Ohio State University; Medical Director, Rehabilitation Services, Associate Medical Director, Gait Analysis Laboratory, The Ohio State University Medical Center, Columbus, Ohio.
Kinematics and Kinetics of Gait

ZACHARY M. PINE, M.D.
Assistant Professor of Rehabilitation Medicine, College of Physicians and Surgeons of Columbia University, New York, New York.
Research in Physical Medicine and Rehabilitation

JOEL M. PRESS, M.D.
Clinical Assistant Professor, Department of Physical Medicine and Rehabilitation, Northwestern University Medical School; Director, Sports Rehabilitations Program, Medical Director, Center for Spine, Sports and Occupational Rehabilitation, Rehabilitation Institute of Chicago, Chicago, Illinois.
Musculoskeletal Disorders of the Lower Limbs

PETER M. QUESADA, PH.D.
Assistant Professor, Division of Orthopaedics, Biomedical Engineering Center, The Ohio State University; Associate Director, Gait Analysis Laboratory, Ohio State University Hospital, Columbus, Ohio.
Kinematics and Kinetics of Gait

PAUL R. RAO, PH.D.
Adjunct Professor, Loyola College, Baltimore; Adjunct Professor, Gallaudet University; Director, Quality Improvement, Co-director, Stroke Recovery Program, Director, Speech Language Pathology Service, National Rehabilitation Hospital, Washington, D.C.
Adult Communication Disorders

LAWRENCE ROBINSON, M.D.
Associate Professor, Department of Rehabilitation Medicine, University of Washington School of Medicine;

Physiatrist-in-Chief, Harborview Medical Center, Seattle, Washington.
Electrodiagnostic Medicine II: Clinical Evaluation and Findings

ROBERT D. RONDINELLI, M.D., PH.D.
Associate Professor and Chairman, University of Kansas Medical Center, Kansas City, Kansas; Medical Director for Rehabilitation Services, Health Midwest, Kansas City, Missouri.
Practical Aspects of Impairment Rating and Disability Determination

THOM W. ROOKE, M.D.
Consultant, Division of Cardiovascular Diseases and Internal Medicine, Mayo Clinic and Mayo Foundation; Associate Professor of Medicine, Mayo Medical School, Rochester, Minnesota.
Rehabilitation in Vascular Diseases

ELLIOT J. ROTH, M.D.
Professor and Chairman, Department of Physical Medicine and Rehabilitation, Northwestern University Medical School; Medical Director, Rehabilitation Institute of Chicago, Chicago, Illinois.
Rehabilitation of Stroke Syndromes

DAMON C. SACCO, M.D.
Medical Director, California Advanced Imaging, San Francisco, California.
Imaging Studies for the Physiatrist

RICHARD SALCIDO, M.D.
Associate Professor and Chair, Department of Physical Medicine and Rehabilitation, Associate, Sanders-Brown Center on Aging, Associate, Department of Biomedical Engineering, University of Kentucky; University of Kentucky Hospital, Lexington, Cardinal Hill Rehabilitation Hospital, Lexington, Appalachian Regional Healthcare System, Lexington, Highlands Regional Medical Center, Paintsville, Kentucky.
The Prevention and Management of Pressure Ulcers

DONNA SCHRAMM, M.D.
Assistant Professor, Departments of Physical Medicine and Rehabilitation and Anesthesiology, Baylor College of Medicine, Houston, Texas.
Chronic Pain Syndromes: Evaluation and Treatment

JOHN A. SCHUCHMANN, M.D.
Associate Professor, Physical Medicine and Rehabilitation, Texas A&M University College of Medicine, Temple Campus; Chairman, Department of Physical Medicine and Rehabilitation, Scott and White Clinic, Temple, Texas.
Occupational Rehabilitation

DAN D. SCOTT, M.D.
Assistant Professor, Department of Rehabilitation Medicine, University of Colorado Health Science Center; Staff Physiatrist, Denver Veterans Affairs Medical Center, Denver, Colorado.
Employment of Persons With Disabilities

MEHRSHEED SINAKI, M.D., M.S.
Consultant, Department of Physical Medicine and Rehabilitation, Mayo Clinic and Mayo Foundation; Professor of Physical Medicine and Rehabilitation, Mayo Medical School, Rochester, Minnesota.
Low Back Pain and Disorders of the Lumbar Spine

ANN MARIE SMITH, Ph.D., R.N., C.R.R.N.
Staff Nurse, The Ohio State University Medical Center, Columbus, Ohio.
The Prevention and Management of Pressure Ulcers

KEVIN SMITH, M.D.
Assistant Professor, Anesthesiology and Physical Medicine and Rehabilitation, Baylor College of Medicine, Houston, Texas.
Chronic Pain Syndromes: Evaluation and Treatment

DONNA PIEPER SPECHT, P.T.
Physical Therapy Supervisor for Rehabilitation and Burns, The Children's Hospital, Denver, Colorado.
Achieving Functional Independence

M. CATHERINE SPIRES, M.D.
Instructor, University of Michigan School of Medicine; Director, Physical Medicine and Rehabilitation Residency Program, University of Michigan Hospitals, Ann Arbor, Michigan.
Rehabilitation of Patients With Burns

BARRY D. STEIN, M.D.
Clinical Assistant Professor, Department of Epidemiology and Preventive Medicine, University of Maryland School of Medicine; Attending Physiatrist, Sinai Hospital of Baltimore, Levindale Hebrew Geriatric Center and Hospital, Baltimore, Maryland.
Principles of Geriatric Rehabilitation

LYNNE M. STEMPIEN, M.D.
Assistant Clinical Professor, Department of Rehabilitation Medicine, University of Colorado; Assistant Medical Director, The Children's Hospital Rehabilitation Center, Denver, Colorado.
Rehabilitation of Children and Adults With Cerebral Palsy

SCOTT STOLL, D.O.
Resident, Department of Physical Medicine and Rehabilitation, University of Kentucky College of Medicine, Lexington, Kentucky.
Manipulation, Traction, and Massage

KATHRYN A. STOLP-SMITH, M.D., M.S.
Assistant Professor, Mayo Medical School; Consultant, Mayo Foundation, Rochester, Minnesota.
Electrodiagnostic Medicine III: Case Studies

ALEXANDER STRAJA, M.D.
Clinical Associate Professor, Departments of Anesthesiology and Physical Medicine and Rehabilitation, Baylor College of Medicine, Houston, Texas.
Chronic Pain Syndromes: Evaluation and Treatment

JEFFREY A. STRAKOWSKI, M.D.
Assistant Clinical Professor, The Ohio State University; Staff Physician, Riverside Methodist Hospital, Columbus, Ohio.
Upper Limb Musculoskeletal Pain Syndromes

RONALD S. TAYLOR, M.D.
Clinical Instructor, Department of Physical Medicine, Wayne State University, Detroit; Co-Residency Director,

Department of Physical Medicine, William Beaumont Hospital, Royal Oak, Michigan.
Rehabilitation of Persons With Multiple Sclerosis

JEFFREY M. THOMPSON, M.D.
Assistant Professor, Physical Medicine and Rehabilitation, Mayo Medical School; Consultant, Department of Physical Medicine and Rehabilitation, Mayo Clinic and Mayo Foundation, Rochester, Minnesota.
The Diagnosis and Treatment of Muscle Pain Syndromes

LANCE E. TREXLER, Ph.D.
Clinical Assistant Professor, Department of Physical Medicine and Rehabilitation, Indiana University School of Medicine; Clinical Director, Center for Neuropsychological Rehabilitation, Indianapolis, Indiana.
Psychological Perspectives on Rehabilitation: Contemporary Assessment and Intervention Strategies

DAVID C. WEBER, M.D.
Senior Associate Consultant, Department of Physical Medicine and Rehabilitation, Mayo Clinic, Rochester, Minnesota.
Physical Agent Modalities

ROBERT J. WEBER, M.D.
Professor, Chairman, Department of Physical Medicine and Rehabilitation, State University of New York Health Science Center, Syracuse, New York.
Rehabilitation Issues in Plexopathies

JOHN WHYTE, M.D., Ph.D.
Associate Professor, Department of Physical Medicine and Rehabilitation, Temple University, Philadelphia, Pennsylvania.
Research in Physical Medicine and Rehabilitation

J. WILLIAM WIAND, D.O.
Clinical Associate, Ohio University, Athens; Director, Musculoskeletal Imaging, Riverside Methodist Hospital, Columbus, Ohio.
Upper Limb Musculoskeletal Pain Syndromes.

ROBERT B. WINTER, M.D.
Clinical Professor, Orthopedic Surgery Department, University of Minnesota Medical School; Chief, Spine Service, Gillette Children's Hospital, St. Paul; Staff Surgeon, Twin Cities Spine Surgeons, Minneapolis, Minnesota.
Spinal Orthoses in Rehabilitation

GARY M. YARKONY, M.D.
Clinical Professor, Section of Orthopaedic Surgery and Rehabilitation Medicine, Department of Surgery, University of Chicago Medical Center; Vice President, Clinical Program Development, Schwab Rehabilitation Hospital, Chief of Rehabilitation Services, The University of Chicago Hospitals Rehabilitation Center, Chicago, Illinois.
Rehabilitation of Patients With Spinal Cord Injuries

JEFFREY L. YOUNG, M.D., M.A.
Assistant Professor, Department of Physical Medicine and Rehabilitation, Northwestern University Medical School; Co-director, Sports Rehabilitation Program, Director, Spine and Sports Fellowship Program, Rehabilitation Institute of Chicago, Chicago, Illinois.
Musculoskeletal Disorders of the Lower Limbs

Preface

Publication of this textbook marks both an end and a new beginning in the field of physical medicine and rehabilitation. It represents the end of an earlier series of textbooks begun by Dr. Frank Krusen in 1945. This textbook is a new beginning, designed by its editors to meet the needs of the modern practitioner.

When I was first approached by Lisette Bralow of the W.B. Saunders Company to consider editing a new textbook, I was overwhelmed with the complexity of the undertaking. By the time I gained sufficient confidence to accept the editorial duties, I had already decided on some of the basic tenets of the overall effort. When the editorial group met in Chicago in the summer of 1993, the remainder of the basic characteristics of the book were set. These characteristics include the following:

• The book is edited rather than authored by one person. The field of physical medicine and rehabilitation has grown so dramatically over the past few decades that there is no single practitioner who could reasonably write the book, especially one that contained information at the requisite cutting edge of quality.

• The book covers the breadth of physical medicine and rehabilitation. The number of pages allotted to each chapter reflects not only the available knowledge in that area, but also the editors' opinion of its current relative importance to practitioners of physical medicine and rehabilitation.

• The book is practical and clinically useful. Material carried in previous physical medicine and rehabilitation textbooks that was no longer clinically relevant was intentionally omitted.

• The book is user-friendly and features many tables and illustrations to speed the learning of the reader.

The 60 chapters of the book were ultimately written by 114 authors from 17 states. The authors, chosen strictly for their expertise and writing ability, included 37 women, members of many ethnic groups, and some persons who are themselves physically challenged. The authors range in age from residents to those with considerable gray hair, and they represent many disciplines other than physiatry (including neurology, orthopedics, urology, psychology, nursing, physical therapy, occupational therapy, and speech pathology, among others).

The chapters are arranged into four broad sections. Section I (Chapters 1 to 13) deals with the evaluation of the patients typically seen in the field of physical medicine and rehabilitation. Section II (Chapters 14 to 26) deals with the treatment techniques and special equipment used in physical medicine and rehabilitation. Section III (Chapters 27 to 34) deals with therapeutic problems that occur across many diagnoses in physiatric practice. Section IV (Chapters 35 to 60) deals with physiatric evaluation and treatment of specific diagnoses.

One problem often seen in edited books is a lack of evenness in the various chapters, both in writing style and in quality. The editors employed a number of techniques to help prevent such inconsistency. The authors submitted an outline before writing the text. The text of each chapter was then reviewed by an associate editor and by the editor-in-chief. The excellent staff at Saunders then performed their magic in redacting each chapter. Finally, the editors again reviewed each chapter, twice. It is rare indeed for such rigorous quality control to be carried out on any book, and we hope the resulting text reflects this care.

The textbook is designed to be read either in sections as a reference text or from cover to cover. It contains state-of-the-art knowledge that is designed to provide practical help for many different types of practitioners. Those readers needing even more in-depth knowledge will appreciate the list of selected references at the end of each chapter, most of which can be readily obtained from a medical library.

One of my personal goals for the book was for each chapter to be the best single textbook chapter ever written on the subject. Although I cannot claim that result was fulfilled for every chapter, I believe this book has achieved this goal for most. I extend congratulations to the authors and the associate editors for such an outstanding job.

For the reader, this book represents a smorgasbord of physiatric knowledge. Whether you use the book for a quick snack or a full meal of that knowledge, bon appétit!

RANDALL L. BRADDOM, M.D., M.S.

Acknowledgment

Sincere appreciation is extended to all those who helped assemble this book, especially Susan Johnson, Edna Swartzlander, Jane Baker, and Dolores Meloni.

Contents

Evaluation

Physiatric History and Examination

LISA A. McPEAK, M.D.

The physiatric history and physical examination are the basis for all therapeutic decision making. Although many physicians are aware of the conventional history and physical examination, outlined in familiar medical reference texts such as DeGowin and DeGowin's *Bedside Diagnostic Examination* (New York, Macmillan, 1994) and Bates' *A Guide to Physical Examination* (Philadelphia, JB Lippincott, 1991), the physiatric history and physical examination are quite different and are in many respects unique. The purpose of this chapter is both to outline and to highlight these differences.

The conventional history and physical examination is the basis on which the physiatric history and examination are built. The physiatrist tailors the procedures of the conventional history and physical process to outline best the problems of the physiatric patient population. Each section in this chapter focuses on the specific concerns that a physiatrist should emphasize during the history and examination.

The physiatric history and examination emphasize functional capacity in both the home and the community. The physiatrist determines not only physical deficits but also the functional impact of these deficits. The identification of functional problems allows for the assignment of functional goals that become the basis for development of the therapeutic management plan.

The physiatric history and physical examination should identify an individual's impairments, disabilities, and handicaps as defined by the World Health Organization (Table 1–1).[31] Although an individual can have multiple impairments, the impairments might not cause a disability or handicap unless they affect function in the home or community. For example, an impairment such as a 20 degree flexion contracture of the right arm might cause no disability or handicap in an individual with the ability to walk. This same impairment can cause considerable disability in an individual with complete paraplegia who must fully extend the elbow to accomplish a wheelchair transfer. To define an impairment as a disability or handicap, the physiatrist must assess the patient's function based on the physiatric history and examination.

Table 1–2 lists the major categories involved in the physiatric history and examination. Note that this table, if copied, will fit in a coat pocket and then can be used during each physiatric history and examination.

PHYSIATRIC HISTORY

Introduction

Most of a patient's problems can be identified with a thorough history. The physiatric history should be obtained in an organized manner so that no important items are missed.

Proper history taking involves listening carefully to the patient or caregiver, as he or she can best relate how the disease or injury results in functional problems. Try to use the patient's own words and avoid the temptation to reframe them into your own words. The patient is often unable to identify the problem directly, especially if a cognitive or psychosocial component of the problem exists.

TABLE 1–1 Definition of Impairment, Disability, and Handicap

Impairment: Any loss or abnormality of psychological, physiological, or anatomical structure or function.
Disability: Any restriction or lack resulting from an impairment of the ability to perform an activity in the manner or within the range considered normal for a human being.
Handicap: A disadvantage for a given individual, resulting from an impairment or a disability, that limits or prevents the fulfillment of a role that is normal for that individual.

From World Health Organization: Classification of Impairments, Disabilities, and Handicaps. Geneva, Switzerland, WHO, 1980.

TABLE 1–2 Outline of the Physiatric History and Examination

Physiatric history	Physiatric examination
Chief complaint	Functional examination
History of present problem	Mobility activities
Functional history	Activities of daily living
Mobility activities	Household activities
Activities of daily living	Driving
Household activities	Musculoskeletal examination
Community activities	Inspection
Cognition	Palpation
Communication	Joint stability
Vocation	Range of motion
Assistive devices	Contractures
Psychosocial history	Manual muscle testing
Substance abuse	Neurological examination
Family/friend support	Level of consciousness
Living situation	Mental status
Vocational history	Communication
Avocational history	Cranial nerves
Psychiatric history	Sensation
Sexual history	Motor control
Finances	Reflexes
Medications/allergies	General medical examination
Diet	**Summary**
Past medical/surgical history	**Problem list**
Family history	**Management plan**
Review of systems	**Goals**

In these situations, the examiner must closely observe the patient during the interview for any implied indication of problems. This involves careful scrutiny of body language, attitude, cooperativeness, and social awareness. A good physiatric history often includes identification of both implied and stated problems.

Obtaining a complete history requires the physiatrist to develop a rapport with the patient: Collect the history in a professional but caring and empathic manner. Shake hands with the patient (or use another greeting gesture if the patient is unable to shake hands), give an appropriate introduction, and address the patient by the last name. Introduction of the physician to any family or friends present is also important. Be aware of any signs of social or physical discomfort due to either the topic of discussion or pain. Both types of discomfort tend to decrease the patient's participation and accuracy during the interview process.

The physician should act as a facilitator, allowing the patient to speak freely, and should only occasionally ask a question to clarify the topic of discussion. The physician has to ask some specific questions to obtain all the necessary information, but the patient should be allowed to answer these questions freely. Without development of verbal rapport, the patient often feels uncomfortable, and problems can be missed or inadequately discussed.

The sources of the information for the physiatric history can be varied. The patient is the obvious source for most of the physiatric history, but due to communication or cognitive difficulties, the history might also need to be taken or confirmed through interviews with family and friends. Technical information about the patient's medical or physical problems can be obtained by questioning the patient's therapists, nurses, aides, and other physicians. It is not unusual for an examiner to find that individuals who deal with a patient have varied opinions as to the patient's

problems and functional skills. If this occurs, the physiatric examination should be tailored to help identify which opinions are the most factual.

Chief Complaint

The chief complaint in a physiatric history, as in a conventional history, should be transcribed from the patient's own words, whenever possible, and is usually only one or two sentences in length. Unlike the conventional history, it should focus on the functional loss or the reason for the functional loss. For example, on transfer to an inpatient rehabilitation facility, a patient who has had a cerebrovascular accident often complains of inability to walk or to dress, due to stroke-induced weakness. The chief complaint of the outpatient with low back pain might be the inability to perform a job because of decreased capability to stand and walk. Focusing on functional losses is a unique aspect of the physiatric history. Table 1–3 lists common presenting chief complaints of patients with physiatric problems and the corresponding discharge diagnoses.[28]

History of Present Problem

In a physiatric setting, identifying the problem is not only discovering an illness but also uncovering the functional implications. For this reason, the "history of the present illness" might be more appropriately labeled "history of the present problem." The problem should be described in a clear, chronological narrative that lists all of the patient's functional, medical, surgical, physical, and cognitive deficits. The date of onset of the illness or injury, subsequent problems, treatment provided, and complications since the onset should be documented. The history of the present problem should include the functional losses or restrictions that have occurred due to the illness or injury.

TABLE 1–3 Common Chief Complaints With Corresponding Diagnoses

Chief Complaint	Discharge Diagnosis
"Pain in calves after *walking* several blocks"	Peripheral vascular disease
"Can't *control* right leg"	Stroke
"Right-sided *clumsiness*, trouble with *balance*"	Multiple sclerosis
"Inability to *use* legs well"	Multiple sclerosis
"Can't *walk* or *talk* well"	Parkinsonism
"Leg weakness, unable to *stand* alone"	Transverse myelitis
"Pain in back and left leg. The more I *do physically*, the more I hurt"	Herniated disc
"*Walking* and *bladder trouble*"	Parkinsonism
"Low back pain increased by *walking* and *sitting*"	Lumbar disc disease
"Difficulty *walking*"	Musculoskeletal trauma
"Unable to *stand* up"	Stroke
"Aching wrist aggravated by *activity*"	Degenerative joint disease
"Difficulty with *ambulation* control"	Brain trauma

Used by permission from Stolov WC, Hays RM: Evaluation of the patient. *In* Kottke FJ, Lehmann JF (eds): Krusen's Handbook of Physical Medicine and Rehabilitation, ed 4. Philadelphia, WB Saunders, 1990, p 3.

Table 1–4 lists common questions that are asked in developing the history of the present problem.[22]

Functional History

Functional losses and restrictions should be well documented, as they are key items in the physiatric history. Patients should be specifically questioned about their ability to perform all necessary activities to function at home and in the community. List both the functional skills prior to and since the recent illness or injury. Each functional activity should be described as accurately as possible and the specific assistance levels required from a caregiver should be included. The Functional Independence Measure (Table 1–5) is a scale that describes the assistive levels commonly used for documentation purposes.[28] Physicians and others reading the functional history should be able to develop a clear picture of the patient's lifestyle both before and after the injury or illness. Functional activities usually discussed in the functional history are listed in Table 1–6.

Mobility Activities

Mobility is the capability of movement. Many times, an impairment resulting from an injury or an illness results in decreased independence in mobility. Each patient should be questioned about the ability to perform all the mobility activities, ranging from bed mobility to ambulation, both at home and in the community. Often an individual with an impairment requires assistive devices to improve function. Table 1–7 is a list of commonly used mobility assistive devices. Based on the functional history, the physiatrist should develop a good understanding of the patient's safety and independence in all mobility activities.

Bed mobility activities include rolling from one side of the bed to the other, and rolling from a supine to a prone position and back. Inability to do these activities places a patient at high risk for skin pressure ulcers. Patients with poor bed mobility skills require the help of a caregiver. Frequently, an individual with a new impairment is mobile in the hospital bed, with the use of side rails, but is unable to move in a regular bed. A bed with a soft mattress or a waterbed tends to make bed mobility skills more difficult. Individuals with leg weakness should be questioned as to the ability to move their legs in bed.

Transitional movements allow the individual to change from one level of mobility to another. For example, transitional movements include going from a supine to a sitting position and from a sitting to a standing position and back

again. Patients with an impairment might not have difficulty with either sitting or standing, but might be unable to perform the transitional movements required to move from one position to the other.

Sitting is an important functional skill. Sitting balance

TABLE 1–5 Description of the Levels of Function and Their Scores: Modified From the Functional Independence Measure (FIM)

Level of Function	Score	Definition
Independent		Another person is not required for the activity (NO HELPER).
	7	*Complete independence*—All of the tasks described as making up the activity are performed safely; without modification, assistive devices, or aids; and within a reasonable amount of time.
	6	*Modified independence*—One or more of the following may be true: The activity requires an assistive device, the activity takes more than reasonable time, or there are safety considerations.
Dependent		The patient requires another person for either supervision or physical assistance for the activity to be performed (REQUIRES HELPER).
	5	*Supervision or setup*—Patient requires no more help than standby or cueing without physical contact, or the helper sets up needed items.
	4	*Minimal contact assistance*—Patient requires no more help than touching and expends 75% or more of the effort.
	3	*Moderate assistance*—Patient requires more help than touching and expends 50% to 75% of the effort.
	2	*Maximal assistance*—Patient expends 25% to 50% of the effort.
	1	*Total assistance*—Patient expends less than 25% of the effort.

Adapted from the Guide for the Uniform Data Set for Medical Rehabilitation (Adult FIM), version 4.0. Buffalo, NY, State University of New York, 1993.

TABLE 1–4 Items Necessary to Develop the History of the Present Problem

1. Date of onset.
2. Character and severity (especially pain problems).
3. Location of problem (and radiation for pain problems).
4. Associated complaints.
5. Aggravating and alleviating factors (especially pain problems).
6. Previous medical and rehabilitation treatment plans and outcomes.

Adapted from Members of the Department of Neurology, Mayo Clinic and Mayo Clinic Foundation for Medical Education and Research: Clinical Examination in Neurology, ed 6. Philadelphia, WB Saunders, 1991.

TABLE 1–6 Functional Activities That Should Be Discussed in the Functional History

Mobility activities	Household activities
Bed mobility	Cooking
Transitional movements	Cleaning
Supine to sitting	Lawnwork
Sitting to standing	Community activities
Sitting	Driving
Standing	Shopping
Ambulation	Social outings
Stair climbing	Cognition
Wheelchair activities	Communication
Propulsion	Vocational activities
Parts management	
Transfer activities	
Activities of daily living	
Feeding	
Grooming	
Dressing	
Bathing	
Toileting	

TABLE 1–7 Commonly Used Mobility Assistive Devices

Crutches
    Axillary crutches
    Forearm crutches
    Platform crutches
Canes
    Straight cane
    Wide- or narrow-based quad cane
    Hemi-walker or pyramid cane
Walkers
    Standard or pick-up walker
    Rolling walker
    Platform walker
Wheelchairs
    Types
        Manual
        Powered
    Common modifications/specifications
        Lightweight
        Folding or solid frame
        Elevated or removable legrests
        Removable armrests
        Reclining
Off-the-shelf ankle foot orthoses
Common custom orthoses
    Plastic ankle-foot orthosis
    Metal ankle-foot orthosis
    Knee orthosis
    Knee-ankle-foot orthosis

requires adequate trunk and neck stability or strength and appropriate midline orientation. Midline orientation enables the patient to recognize normal upright body position. Midline orientation in patients with sensory-perceptual or muscular impairments is often poor. An individual with a new impairment may be unable to sit without support from one or both arms or without back support.

Good standing skills are required prior to functional ambulation. Independent standing requires adequate midline orientation, trunk stability, strength, and balance. Standing also requires adequate bilateral leg stability and strength. Standing is often only achieved through arm support in an individual with impairments. Individuals with sitting difficulties are usually unable to stand without assistance. This support can be supplied by assistive devices (Table 1–7) such as a straight cane or walker.

Walking involves several physical skills such as balance, strength, coordination, and midline orientation. As in standing, support for walking activities is also often required. Table 1–7 lists the devices commonly used to improve ambulation activities. As walking is usually more difficult on carpeted or uneven surfaces, the individual should be questioned as to the ability to walk on different surfaces.

Climbing or descending stairs is often an essential activity for an individual whose home has a few entry steps, or if the bedroom is on the second floor. Stair mobility should also be investigated because many community buildings are still only accessible by stairs. The level of assistance and devices required for stair mobility activities should be noted. The number of stairs an individual can or might need to ascend or descend is valuable functional information.

Many patients with impairments can be functional within the home and the community using a wheelchair as the primary mode of mobility. Transfer activities, lower limb management in the wheelchair, wheelchair parts management, and wheelchair propulsion skills are important functional activities. The patient should be questioned specifically as to the ability to do all these activities. Transfers are performed in different ways to differing surfaces, with or without assistance. The most common types of transfers are the stand pivot or the half-stand pivot transfer, the sliding board transfer, and the lateral lift transfer. Both types of stand pivot transfers require that the patient stand either partially or fully and pivot around toward a new surface. The sliding board transfer utilizes a wooden or a plastic board between two surfaces. The patient uses the upper extremities to lift and move the body along the board with each lift, until the new surface is reached. The lateral lift transfer requires that the patient lift the body in a lateral direction from one surface to another. Floor to wheelchair transfer ability is also investigated, because any patient using a wheelchair for mobility is at risk for falling out of the wheelchair. A patient who is unable to assist in the transfer activities is considered dependent for this skill, and requires the assistance of one or more caregivers for transfers. Specifics as to the transfer style and assistive devices utilized by the caregivers should be documented in the history.

Lower limb management in the wheelchair is an important factor in transfer activities. Patients with severe lower limb weakness must be able to manipulate their legs so the transfer can proceed without injury. They should also be able to place the legs correctly on the wheelchair legrest to prevent injuries during wheelchair propulsion. Wheelchair parts management includes the individual's ability to remove and replace armrests and legrests, and appropriate use of the wheelchair brakes. Improper use of the parts can make wheelchair transfer and propulsion activities unsafe.

More difficult wheelchair activities are important for the patient who is active within the community. This patient is questioned about wheelchair propulsion activities on carpets, up and down inclined surfaces, on uneven surfaces, and over curbs. Information concerning driving and the required assistive devices for driving is useful. The patient should be able to relate how to maneuver the wheelchair in and out of the car. Also, knowing how an individual who uses the wheelchair for mobility is able to go up and down a few stairs, if necessary, is important. Although this type of activity is not often recommended, it is occasionally done if the patient must go into a building with entry steps.

Activities of Daily Living

The history should assess activities of daily living (ADL) including feeding, grooming, dressing, bathing, and toileting activities. All of these tasks can require the use of assistive devices. Table 1–8 lists the assistive devices commonly used to improve ADL functional skills (see Chapters 24 and 26 for a more detailed discussion of ADL and assistive devices).

Feeding activities are often quite difficult for an impaired individual. Independent feeding requires the ability to open food packages before eating and the ability to use utensils correctly. The patient must also have the muscle strength, joint range, and coordination to bring the food or drink to the mouth. The patient also needs the endurance necessary

TABLE 1–8 Common Activities of Daily Living and Household Assistive Devices

Arm orthoses	Devices for dressing
Utilized to hold equipment	Reacher
Adapted hand orthosis	Button hook
Adapted wrist hand	Zipper pull
orthosis	Long-handled shoehorn
Universal cuff	Sock aid
Utilized to assist movement	Devices for bathing
Balanced forearm	Bath mitt
orthosis	Long-handled sponge
Arm sling suspension	Devices for cooking
orthosis	Suction scrub brush
Devices for feeding	Rocker knife
Adapted utensils	Adapted cooking utensils
Plate guard	Suction cutting board
Rocker knife	Suction bowl holder
Adapted cup or cup holder	One-handed jar opener
Straw	Reacher
Devices for grooming	Devices for cleaning
Adapted brush and comb	Dust mitt
Wash mitt	Adapted handles for cleaning
Adapted manual razor	equipment
Electric razor	Reacher
Adapted toothbrush	
Suction cup denture brush	

to complete a full meal. A loss of the ability to do any of these activities prevents independence in feeding.

Grooming includes all of the hygiene activities done each morning, including face and body bathing at the sink, brushing of teeth or dentures, applying antiperspirant or cologne, shaving, and hair combing or brushing. These activities require strength, coordination, endurance, and adequate limb range of motion to complete.

Dressing skills require both fine and gross motor coordination, balance, strength, and adequate limb range of motion. Upper body dressing includes donning underwear and a shirt or a dress. Pullover items are easier to don if the patient has adequate over-head shoulder range of motion. Buttoned items do not require the over-head shoulder range of motion but require fine motor coordination to manipulate the buttons. Independence in lower body dressing requires enough range of motion to reach the feet to don shoes and socks. The patient must have adequate balance and strength to pull up underwear, pants, or skirt. Those items can be donned while the patient is in bed, but he or she must have the ability to lift the buttocks to allow items to be pulled to the waist. The history should include specific information concerning whether the patient dresses in bed, from a chair, or in a standing position.

Bathing requires the ability to get in and out of the bathtub or shower safely, to sit or stand for the activity, and to do the cleansing activity itself. Several assistive devices can help the patient to safely perform bathing mobility skills. Items such as a transfer tub bench, a bath chair, and a hand-held shower head can improve the individual's independence for bathing activities. The actual cleansing activity during bathing requires strength, coordination, and range of motion to bathe every part of the body. Assistive devices, such as a long-handled sponge, can help the individual to reach all parts of the body.

Toileting skills include mobility activities such as transferring on and off the toilet, sitting on the toilet, and

standing. Assistive devices such as grab bars, elevated toilet seats, and bedside commodes are often used by the individual with an impairment to make such mobility activities easier and safer. Clothing management and hygiene at the toilet are also important components in toileting activities. The individual requires good coordination, balance, and range of motion to complete these clothing and hygiene activities.

Household Activities

Many individuals consider household activities such as cooking, cleaning, and lawn work essential to their daily routine. For individuals who walk, these activities require good standing balance and endurance. Usually, these household activities require the use of both upper limbs. If an individual uses an assistive device such as a cane or a walker, household activities can be quite difficult. Household activities can also be performed from a wheelchair. Individuals who use the wheelchair as their primary mode of mobility are often able to perform fairly difficult household activities if the necessary household items are placed within reach. An individual who does not have the balance or endurance to do the household activities while standing can utilize either a stationary chair or a wheelchair to do the activities. Individuals often use assistive devices to help with household tasks; Table 1–8 lists some common household assistive devices.

Community Activities

Community activities such as driving, shopping, going to church, or participating in social outings are very important to many individuals. Assessing the community activities that patients consider important helps to delineate their lifestyle. It is important to know if new impairments are preventing individuals from performing their usual community activities. The individual should be specifically asked about desires to return to all or some of these activities.

Cognition

Cognition is the act or process of knowing. It includes adequate orientation to person, place, time, and situation, good memory skills, judgment, and capacity for abstract thought. Frequently, an individual with poor cognition is unable to recognize cognitive deficits and might not indicate cognition as a problem. When cognitive deficits are suspected, it is helpful to question family, friends, or healthcare workers who have come in contact with the patient. At other times, the patient can have some awareness of problems but might be unable to accurately describe the deficits. The history in this case should reflect the difficulties described by the caregivers or patient.

Communication

Communication is a process by which information is exchanged among individuals. Communication is primarily accomplished verbally, but nonverbal gestural and written communication are also important. It is important to learn if the patient or family members have identified a new communication problem. The individual might report decreased speech quality or dysarthria. Aphasia is a deficit in communication resulting from a central nervous system problem. If the patient or family is aware of a problem in speech or in written or gestural communication, this might represent aphasia. Both nonverbal gestural and written communication can be impaired when a neuromuscular problem affecting limb movement is present. Good communication skills also rely on adequate hearing and sight. It is important to note if the patient has a problem with hearing or sight, and if hearing aids or glasses are required to correct the problem (see Chapters 3 and 50 for further information on communication and aphasia).

Vocational Activities

For many individuals, return to vocational activities is a reasonable goal. The history should assess the vocation of the individual just prior to the recent injury or illness, some specific information as to the physical and cognitive job requirements, and the individual's ability to perform the job since the injury or illness (see Chapters 9 and 44 for further information).

Patient's Own Functional Goals

It is tempting to set goals without inquiring about the patient's specific goals. Goal attainment depends on patient motivation and cooperation. The history should document the specific wishes or goals of the patient. If the physician fails to ask the patient about goals, it might not be noted that the patient has unrealistic goals. These problems can be avoided with careful assessment of the patient's personal goals or wishes.

List of Functional Devices

During the functional history, many patients report having or needing multiple assistive devices or equipment items. These devices are usually used to improve either mobility skills or ADL and homemaking skills. There are actually hundreds of such assistive devices, but the most common are listed in Tables 1–7 and 1–8 (see also Chapter 26).

Psychosocial History

The psychosocial history provides vital information. The individual with a new impairment often has psychosocial problems related to the impairment and decreased functional skills. If the patient can no longer work, the loss of income places stress on the whole family. If a previously independent individual requires physical assistance from family members, the role of both the patient and family member within the home can be changed, leading to a stressful situation. It is important to understand the psychosocial situation so that the treatment plan addresses the patient's lifestyle and expected discharge options (see Chapter 4 for further information).

Substance Abuse

Knowledge of past substance abuse helps the physiatrist to understand possible future medical problems, to recommend counseling for the patient to prevent future problems, and to understand possible difficulties in the recovery process. The patient's history of smoking, alcohol abuse, and illegal drug abuse should be assessed. The patient must be made aware that truthfulness about past abuse of these items is important because continued abuse may slow recovery from the new injury or illness.

Chronic alcohol or illegal drug abuse typically decreases a patient's ability to participate in a rehabilitation program. Due to close patient supervision, abuse is rare during an inpatient rehabilitation program. The inpatient with a history of substance abuse should receive counseling to prevent a return to the abuse after discharge. Disabled individuals who are unable to return to their prior lifestyle are more likely to consider either alcohol or drug abuse after discharge, as a result of boredom and increased free time. The physiatrist should be able to recognize an individual at risk for such problems in the initial psychosocial history, so that counseling can begin early.

Smoking often leads to serious cardiopulmonary difficulties and interferes with a therapeutic exercise program. Smoking cessation should be aggressively encouraged and pursued.

Family/Friend Support

After an illness or injury, many individuals require assistance with functional skills. This assistance is usually obtained from family members and occasionally obtained from friends. At the time of admission, a possible primary caregiver should be identified. The patient should also identify any other family or friends who will be available to help periodically. The physical status of these potential caregivers should be known to identify possible problems with the patient's plan. If the patient has cognitive deficits that prevent safe decision making, the individual who is the primary decision maker should be identified.

Living Situation

It is important to document the patient's premorbid living situation. This involves such questions as whether the patient lived alone or with family members, the location of the bedroom, the number of steps into the home and into the bedroom, the size of the bathroom, and the type of floor covering. Early knowledge of restrictions to mobility within the home might prompt a home evaluation or the use of home modifications and special equipment items. Whether the home is owned or rented can be important if the patient cannot return to the previous home, or if extensive modifications are needed.

Vocational History

The patient's present job description was obtained in the functional history. Documentation of educational level and all previous job positions is necessary for the psychosocial history. The physiatrist must ensure that the rehabilitation program is appropriate to an individual's educational level. Information concerning prior job experience is also helpful if the patient will be unable to return to the previous job placement.

Avocational History

Avocational activities are frequently as important to the individual as vocational activities. Restrictions in the ability to participate in previous hobbies and social activities can be very stressful for the patient. A short summary of previously enjoyed leisure activities will help all members of the rehabilitation team to understand the patient's previous lifestyle and possible future goals.

Psychiatric History

Patient motivation and cooperation are imperative for a successful rehabilitation program. Psychiatric problems such as depression, anxiety, and suicidal or homicidal ideation can have a major influence on an individual's ability to cooperate. Depression is common immediately after a disabling injury, and patients should be questioned as to whether they have noted any feelings of sadness or depression since they developed the new problem. The stress of a new illness or injury can trigger a recurrence of a previous psychiatric problem. Instituting preventive measures such as supportive psychotherapy or psychiatric medications can prevent problems that could interfere with accomplishing the patient's goals for the program.

Sexual History

Questions concerning sexuality are often avoided by health practitioners. Sexuality and sexual activity are very important aspects of an individual's lifestyle. Questions concerning sexuality should be presented in such a manner that the patient or caregiver remains sufficiently comfortable to provide accurate answers. Past sexuality problems can become worse after a new illness or injury. Some diagnoses treated by physiatrists are associated with hypersexuality, and any premorbid sexual problems can be compounded. Erectile dysfunction, ejaculation difficulties, and decreased libido are common in male patients after an injury or illness. Likewise, female patients may commonly have problems with irregular menses, dysmenorrhea, dyspareunia, or decreased libido. Identification of sexual problems and consideration of counseling or medical management in the initial physiatric management plan can be very helpful (see Chapter 30 for further information).

Finances

Loss of income due to a new illness or injury can cause stress-related problems in the patient and the family. Early recognition of this problem can help decrease stress by allowing family members to work with the social worker and other physiatric team members to solve some of the financial difficulties.

Medications and Allergies

A complete list of medications and allergies should be obtained during the history. Any prescription or over-the-counter medications, and "home remedies" that the patient takes should be documented. Patients will omit mention of the over-the-counter medications and "home remedies" unless carefully questioned. The medication list should be reviewed for each medication's indication, side effects, and interactions. Many medications have unwanted cognitive and physical side effects, and reduction or avoidance of such medications is recommended.

Diet

Evaluation of the present diet is necessary to see if it is appropriate for the patient's current condition. The individual's medical problems should be reviewed to ensure that the diet will not present a risk of further complications. Bowel problems are very common in patients with new impairments. After a review of the patient's physical status and a gastrointestinal examination, a dietary change might be appropriate. If the patient complains of swallowing or chewing difficulties, a diet modification could be necessary.

Past Medical and Surgical History

Many medical and surgical problems can affect the patient's present function. Often individuals have learned to compensate effectively for a previous illness or injury, but when a new problem or impairment occurs, the ability to compensate for the previous problem might be lost. Many problems are progressive and are likely to cause further functional deficits as the patient ages.

Previous problems in any of the major body systems can affect the physiatric patient's performance in a therapeutic program. The physiatrist should follow the conventional history format to inquire about problems in all systems. The patient's cardiac, pulmonary, rheumatologic, neurological, and musculoskeletal system history is particularly pertinent information. As motivation to participate in the prescribed program is critical, the questions already outlined in the psychiatric history are of major importance as well.

Cardiovascular

Adequate cardiac function and stability are necessary for improvement in a physiatric program. Many patients have histories of congestive heart failure, myocardial infarction, arrhythmias, and severe coronary artery disease. Previous surgical procedures, such as pacemaker placement and coronary artery bypass surgery, are common as well. These problems at times need to be discussed in detail with the patient's cardiologist or primary physician. Further cardiac testing might be necessary prior to exercise prescription. Only with accurate information can the exercise prescription include specific cardiac precautions and exercise intensity to allow the patient the maximal safe exercise level (see Chapter 32 for further information).

Notation of symptoms of intermittent claudication and peripheral vascular disease, as well as the history of old amputations or gangrenous areas, is important. Individuals with serious vascular problems might need exercise restrictions that should be identified and followed strictly to prevent further vascular compromise. Periodic monitoring of vascular signs and symptoms during exercise is often warranted.

Pulmonary

Both obstructive and restrictive pulmonary problems can interfere with a patient's exercise tolerance. Investigation of previous pulmonary testing and discussion of the present physical status with the patient's primary medical physician can aid in exercise prescription. If there are questions concerning present pulmonary problems, pulmonary function tests might be necessary prior to any therapeutic activity. Attention should be paid to any airway problems, especially if an individual has a tracheostomy for airway protection. Oxygen requirements and stability on present oxygen level are important to assess (see Chapter 33 for further information).

Rheumatologic

Rheumatic disorders are common in the physiatric patient population. An exercise program can exacerbate rheumatologic symptoms. The history should include information concerning the rheumatologic disorder, previous sites of joint involvement, and the present level of disease activity. Information from the primary physician concerning the patient's course to date can be helpful (see Chapter 35 for further information).

Neurological

Chronic and progressive neurological problems can have a major effect on the patient's ability to improve or to tolerate the program. Specific history questions should include information about congenital neurological problems, seizure disorders, peripheral neuropathies, progressive neurological diseases, spinal cord and other central nervous system diseases, or trauma. Questions concentrating on such symptoms as muscular weakness, sensory loss, balance, and coordination are also helpful in assessing the patient's neurological status.

Specific questions concerning past cognitive and communication problems are important, as is information concerning previously effective communication techniques. Information about devices that improve communication, including hearing aids or eyeglasses, is valuable.

Musculoskeletal

Chronic or progressive musculoskeletal disorders can have a major impact on the physiatric therapeutic program. It is important to document disorders such as congenital muscular problems, progressive muscular diseases, amputations, joint contractures, traumatic injuries, osteoporosis, and previous bone fractures. Past musculoskeletal problems can medically restrict the patient from certain activities. The patient and, if necessary, the physicians who were managing these problems previously, should be questioned concerning any activity restrictions.

Individuals with previous neurological and musculoskeletal problems can have slow progress in a rehabilitation program. This should be considered when determining the goals and estimating the length of time needed to obtain the goals. Some of these patients return to their previous functional levels, but they need a longer period to do so. Others are not able to return to previous functional levels, and the program goals should reflect this.

Family History

The physiatrist should ask specific questions concerning family members known to have the same disease as the patient. This helps with overall disease prognostication for the patient. It is essential to learn if any other family members have signs and symptoms similar to the patient's, as this can help identify family members with an as-yet-undiagnosed genetic problem.

Other questions concerning cardiac, pulmonary, rheumatologic, neurological, and psychiatric illnesses in family members may help to determine the patient's risk for such medical problems in the future.

Review of Systems

A comprehensive review of systems often uncovers problems not previously noted that can affect the patient's clinical course. The physician should follow a conventional history taking format to inquire about problems in all systems of the body. The following discussion highlights common problems identified in the physiatric patient population. Table 1–9 provides sample review of systems questions that are specific to the physiatric history. Some systems, such as the pulmonary and cardiovascular systems, were discussed in other sections of this chapter and will not be addressed again.

Skin

Skin problems are common in patients with loss of mobility or sensation. Questions concerning rashes and skin pressure areas can help to identify these problems (see Table 1–9). Notation of any open surgical wounds or drains is important, as these can require specific care and precautions during therapeutic activities.

Gastrointestinal Status

Trouble swallowing and complaints of coughing during eating activities or the sensation of food "getting stuck" while swallowing can indicate significant problems that need further investigation. Symptoms of gas, heartburn, mild stomach pain, poor digestion, nausea, occasional vomiting, hemoptysis, and darkened stools can indicate subacute gastric problems, including gastrointestinal bleeding that could lead to anemia. Diarrhea, constipation, and bowel incontinence not only interfere with an individual's ability to participate in a physiatric program, but can also indicate a neurogenic bowel that requires management. Many individuals require a specific bowel program, including dietary modification and oral and rectal medications. The individual with a colostomy should be questioned as to the frequency and consistency of bowel movements through the colostomy and necessary colostomy care (see Chapter 28 for further information).

Genitourinary Status

Complaints of urinary frequency, polyuria, nocturia, dysuria, hematuria, urgency, and hesitancy can all indicate significant problems such as urinary tract infection, bladder outlet obstruction, kidney stones, and neurogenic bladder. Past surgical urinary tract procedures, such as nephrostomy, ileostomy, or suprapubic catheter placement, should be documented. Inquire about nonsurgical bladder management programs, including indwelling catheter or intermit-

TABLE 1–9   Review of Systems: Sample Questions Specific to the Physiatric History

System	Questions
Skin	1. Do you have any rashes?
	2. Can you tell me the size and location of open skin areas, if present?
	3. Do you have problems changing your position in bed?
	4. How long do you stay in one position in bed?
	5. How long do you sit up in the same chair?
	6. What are you using to treat your skin problem?
	7. Do you have any special cushions or a special mattress to prevent skin problems?
Gastrointestinal	1. Do you have any problems swallowing? Do you note the sensation of food "getting stuck," or do you cough while eating?
	2. Do you have problems with gas, heartburn, stomach pain, poor digestion, nausea, vomiting, diarrhea, constipation, or darkened stools?
	3. Are you on a bowel program? What is your bowel program?
Genitourinary	1. Do you have problems with frequency, burning with urination, dark or bloody-appearing urine, urgency, or hesitancy?
	2. Are you on a bladder program? What is your bladder program?
Nutritional	1. Do you have swallowing problems?
	2. Do you have appetite problems?
	3. Do you think you are eating and drinking enough?
	4. Do you eat or drink any nutritional supplements?
Neuromuscular	1. Do you have headaches often?
	2. Do you have any neurological problems such as weakness or sensory, visual, coordination, balance, or memory deficits that we have not yet discussed?
	3. Do you have any endurance problems?
	4. Do you have any musculoskeletal problems such as joint or muscle pain, abnormal joint motion, muscle atrophy, and muscle spasticity that we have not yet discussed?

tent catheter programs (see Chapter 28 for further information).

Nutritional Status

Without adequate nutrition it is often difficult for a patient to participate effectively in a physiatric program. Poor nutrition can be secondary to many different problems, ranging from swallowing dysfunction to decreased appetite. Individuals might be taking medication that decreases appetite or changes taste sensation. Depression also often leads to poor appetite and inadequate nutrition.

Questions concerning recent food and fluid intake help the physician to identify if the patient is at risk for an overall poor nutritional and hydration status. Documentation of the need for either caloric or protein supplementation is essential. Specifics concerning type of supplementation and the mode of supplementation (oral intake or nasogastric or gastrostomy tube) are important.

Neuromuscular Status

Specific neurological questions concerning headaches, weakness, numbness, tingling, visual problems, incoordination, disorientation, and memory problems should be asked if they have not been covered earlier in the history. Specific musculoskeletal questions about overall muscular endurance, joint and muscular pain or stiffness, abnormal joint motion, muscle atrophy, fasciculation, and spasticity are important.

Physiatric Examination

The main purpose of the physiatric examination is to confirm or disprove the diagnostic impression formed after obtaining the physiatric history and to identify other impairment or disabilities. The basis for the physiatric examination is the conventional physical examination as outlined in such texts as DeGowin and DeGowin,[8] and Bates.[3] The physiatrist uses all of the basic evaluation methods of inspection, palpation, percussion, and auscultation along with additional methods that assess impairment and disability.

As with the physiatric history, functional skills are emphasized in the physiatric examination. Special attention is paid to the ability to perform activities on request. This type of examination helps to assess the individual's physical impairments as well as cognitive and communication skills. If the individual is unable to follow commands, the physiatrist must use inventive techniques to increase the patient's ability to participate in the evaluation process. Basic knowledge of different cognitive and communicative deficits and utilization of techniques to decrease the deficits improve the physiatrist's ability to evaluate such patients.

The physiatrist must also use inventive means to evaluate an individual's functional skills. The physical examination should actually begin at the time of initial patient contact and continue throughout the physiatric history and examination. During this time the patient can demonstrate functional skills without the need for formal testing. At times the patient and the family have an inaccurate perception of functional capabilities and limitations. Careful observation might provide a more accurate estimate of the patient's skills.

The physiatric examination also includes a detailed evaluation of the musculoskeletal and neurological systems. The specific impairments that led to the patient's functional deficits should be identified. Since both physical impairments and disability are addressed in a physiatric therapeutic program, the physiatric examination must evaluate both types of problems. Specific attention is paid to impairments that might prevent the patient from safely participating in a physiatric program, or that can slow the patient's progress in a prescribed program.

Functional Examination

The functional examination includes evaluation of mobility skills, ADL, household activities, and community activities. Evaluation of cognitive and communication skills is also performed but is described later in the section on the neurological examination.

The examiner should determine the functional skills, the required level of assistance, and the need for assistive devices. Of the many methods for describing functional level, one that is becoming more commonly used is the Functional Independence Measure[13] (see Table 1–5).

For an accurate patient evaluation, it is helpful to have the appropriate assistive device available. This is not always possible, especially if the patient uses a unique or custom-fabricated device that was not brought to the examination. In these cases it might be necessary to provide the most appropriate replacement item or to re-examine the patient at a later date when the equipment is available.

A full patient assessment during the initial physiatric examination is not always possible due to safety issues and time limitations. The patient can have physical deficits that make it difficult for one person to perform safely the functional mobility examination of the patient. If there is no one available for assistance, it is better that the activity not be attempted, for the safety of both the patient and the examiner. With experience, most physiatrists develop an efficient examination technique that minimizes the time necessary for the formal functional examination.

Mobility Activities

The examination of mobility should proceed methodically, initially evaluating the most basic mobility skills and proceeding to increasingly difficult activities. Documentation of the assistance needed for each activity is important. Note whether the patient utilizes good body mechanics during mobility skills.

The most basic mobility activity is bed mobility. Examine whether the patient can roll from side to side, roll from supine to prone, and roll from prone to supine. This can be performed on an examination table or mat, but mobility is more difficult on a softer surface, such as a bed. Note if the patient must use the side rails of the bed or examination table for assistance. If the patient has weakness in one or more limbs, his or her limb management ability in the bed should also be noted.

The ability to move from supine to sitting should be observed; it is the most basic transitional movement. This movement is difficult if the individual is unable to roll onto one side or the other. Patients usually find it easier to first roll from the supine to the side-lying position, and then to push up with the upper limbs into a seated position while simultaneously swinging the legs down to the floor. This activity uses proper body mechanics to complete the task. To go directly from supine to sitting and then turning the body to swing the legs down to the floor not only requires

a higher energy expenditure but requires significant abdominal and trunk muscle strength.

When examining an individual's ability to sit, it should be noted if the individual is able to sit up straight in the midline (adequate midline orientation), and if he or she can sit without back support. The patient might need to use one or both arms to maintain the seated position. If the patient is able to sit in the midline, with or without support, then the sitting balance should be physically challenged. This is commonly done by applying a mild or moderate pressure or push in all directions to see if the individual is able to maintain the seated position. The push is done such that the patient can be prevented from falling if loss of balance occurs.

The next transitional movement examined is the act of going from the seated to the standing position. Observe if the patient can safely bend forward to bring the upper body weight anterior to and over the lower legs. The patient must then be able to lift the body into a standing position. Going from sitting to standing requires at least 100 degrees of knee flexion in one lower limb. The patient may or may not use the upper limbs initially to help push out of the seated position. Individuals with adequate lower limb strength should be able to go from sitting to standing without upper limb assistance.

With the patient in the standing position, evaluate midline orientation. The need for upper limb support and type of the assistive device utilized is documented. Standing balance is evaluated similarly to sitting balance, by providing the physical challenge of a pressure or push in all directions (within limits of safety).

Walking requires adequate standing skills, either with or without an assistive device, and should not be attempted unless the patient is able to demonstrate the required standing skills. Basic aspects of gait should be assessed, such as the individual's ability to maintain midline during walking, with or without an assistive device; the size of the base of stance; the fluidity of lower limb movements throughout all phases of the gait cycle; abnormal lower limb movements; appropriate use of an assistive device, if needed; and upper limb movements. Observe the patient's gait from the anterior, posterior, and both lateral positions if necessary. (For further information on gait analysis, see Chapter 5.)

If the patient can walk safely, the ability to descend and ascend stairs is tested. The number of stairs, the need for either one or two hand rails, the ability to use an assistive device if required, and the safety of ascending and descending stair technique is assessed. In an individual with an impairment in one leg, the stronger or normal leg should lead in ascending and the impaired leg should lead in descending.

Individuals using a wheelchair for mobility should be assessed for transfer and wheelchair propulsion skills. Patients should identify by name or description the type of transfer they intend to demonstrate. This knowledge helps in the event the examiner must provide assistance. It should be noted whether the patient uses the stand pivot transfer, the half-stand pivot transfer, the sliding board transfer, or the lateral lift transfer. Assess whether the patient can appropriately place and set up the wheelchair for the type of transfer performed. The transfer activity should be monitored for both safety and correct body mechanics. Observation of the patient's ability to transfer to different surface heights is also important, as most individuals are required to transfer to different surface levels during their daily routine. Some patients require either partial or total assistance for a transfer activity. If the caregiver who assists with the transfer is present, the caregiver and the patient should demonstrate the transfer technique.

Wheelchair propulsion activities on level surfaces can be observed on initial presentation to the clinic or hospital. If an individual is required to propel the wheelchair on different surfaces, try to test wheelchair skills on such surfaces. It is also helpful to examine the patient's ability to propel the wheelchair up and down ramps, onto and off of curbs, and on uneven surfaces if possible. In many cases, one should assess the patient's ability to get back into the wheelchair from the floor or ground.

Activities of Daily Living

Observation of ADL might not be possible if the patient requires some assistive devices that are not present during the examination. Many different types of each assistive device are available, and each brand usually has a variation that might aid one patient but not another. Common items should be available for the patient to demonstrate functional abilities (see Table 1–8). If a patient's equipment requirements are very specific, the patient should provide the equipment.

Feeding skills include the ability to set up a meal, use utensils or hold finger foods, and use upper limb movement to bring food to the mouth. Grooming activities usually include toothbrushing or denture care, washing the face and body at the sink, shaving, and hair-brushing. Patients are observed to see if they can use the equipment appropriately and to see how they use upper limb movement to complete the activity.

A full bathing and toileting evaluation is difficult to observe during the functional examination process due to patient modesty issues. Observing the individual perform the movement activities required for the transfer and the upper limb and body motions required for the activities is helpful. Dressing skills should be assessed. Patients should demonstrate their ability to open and close different fasteners, such as buttons, zippers, and shoelaces. Observing patients as they don and doff a coat or shirt is helpful.

Household Activities

During the functional evaluation the physiatrist is unable to test household activities in an environment similar to the home. Asking patients to demonstrate as closely as possible some of these activities might be the best option available to the examiner. Patients can easily demonstrate the ability to reach overhead items or items at their feet. They can also demonstrate sweeping or vacuuming activities. Cooking skills are hard to demonstrate outside of a kitchen, but they can use eating utensils to demonstrate such simple activities as cutting food for meal preparation.

Driving

Although driving skills cannot be fully assessed without driving a vehicle, demonstration of how the skill is per-

formed (including proper upper and lower limb use) can be done in the clinic or hospital. If a patient uses a wheelchair for mobility activities, an assessment can include observing the transfer technique into the car, and assessing the ability to place the wheelchair in the car.

Musculoskeletal Examination

The musculoskeletal examination is a major portion of the total physiatric examination. It requires inspection and palpation as well as unique tests, such as range of motion and manual muscle testing.[3, 5, 8, 15]

Inspection

All muscles, bones, and joints are closely inspected for any outward appearance of abnormality. Individual muscle shape, size, atrophy, and symmetry are inspected. If a difference is seen in side-to-side muscle symmetry or an abnormality noted in one muscle or muscle group, then objective measures such as limb circumference measurements are appropriate for documentation purposes. Joints and bones are inspected for deformities, swelling, redness, and abnormal positions. If present, note amputation levels, lengths, and shape.

Palpation

Patients often exhibit signs of muscle tenderness during this part of the examination. Note the activity that produces the tenderness and the site of the tenderness, and whether referred pain symptoms are present. The muscles are palpated to identify any abnormal swelling, warmth, and tight muscle bands. The exact position of a tight muscle band or area of tenderness within a muscle should be noted. Muscle tone is examined both during the range of motion and muscle palpation. The examiner should note whether the muscle palpated appears to have normal, increased, or decreased tone. During the bone and joint examination, each area should be palpated to identify the extent of any deformities, warmth, swelling, and pain with palpation.

Range of Motion

Adequate joint and limb range of motion (ROM) is essential for functional activities. Loss of joint ROM in the lower limbs can cause gait abnormalities or increased energy expenditure with walking, or it can prevent walking. Poor ROM in the upper limbs can prevent the performance of simple ADL.

The evaluation includes assessment of both active and passive ROM. Passive ROM is performed by the examiner while the patient is relaxed. Each joint is moved through all planes of motion by the examiner and is measured for the extent of its range. Active ROM is performed by the patient without the assistance of the examiner. It should be noted if the ROM activity produces pain.

Exact measurement of ROM activities is most often performed using a universal goniometer (Fig. 1–1). The universal goniometer consists of two movable arms that pivot around one point. Portable goniometers with arms 6 in. in length are commonly used, but depending on the joint measured, larger or smaller sizes are available. The measurement scale is in one degree intervals, 0 to 180

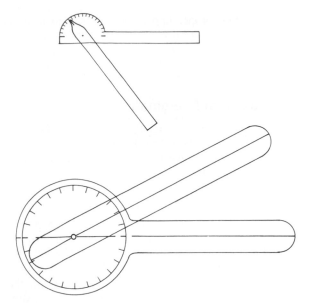

FIGURE 1-1 Two examples of universal goniometers commonly used by the clinician. (From Cole TM, Barry DT, Tobis JS: Measurement of musculoskeletal function. *In* Kottke FJ, Lehman JF (eds): Krusen's Handbook of Physical Medicine and Rehabilitation, ed 4. Philadelphia, WB Saunders, 1990, p 21.)

degrees in half-circle scales and 0 to 180 or 0 to 360 degrees in full-circle scales.

Goniometry is a relatively reliable method of ROM measurement.[14, 24] The clinician should utilize a systematic technique during each ROM examination to ensure reliability of the measurement. Accurate goniometry evaluation depends on standardized techniques that have been well described in reference texts.[2, 15, 24] The joint is initially placed in the anatomical position. The goniometer is placed lateral to the joint, except in the cases of a few joint motions (e.g., forearm supination and pronation). The examiner carefully instructs the patient in the motion required and the plane of movement necessary. Figure 1-2 depicts the three planes of movement. For measuring ROM, the

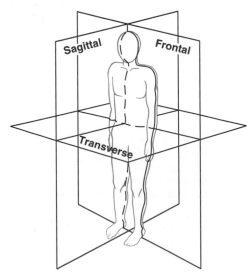

FIGURE 1-2 Three planes of motion.

patient moves the joint according to the instructions provided. The stationary arm of the goniometer remains in the anatomical joint position while the other goniometer arm is fixed carefully at the end of the patient's motion. The examiner reads the scale to obtain the active ROM. Passive ROM measurements require the same technique, except that the examiner moves the joints through the desired motions.

Several systems of measurements have been described in the past. The two most common include the 360-degree system proposed by Knapp and West[19, 20] and the 180-degree system proposed by Norkin and White.[26] In the 360-degree system, the patient is placed in anatomical position with the 0-degree point located over the patient's head and the 180-degree point below the patient's feet. In the sagittal plane, 0 to 180 degrees is anterior to the body, and 180 to 360 degrees is posterior to the body. The 180-degree system identifies the anatomical position as 0 degrees and movement away from the anatomical position in any of the three planes of motion is described by a positive number between 0 and 180 degrees. For example Figure 1-3 shows normal shoulder flexion and extension in both systems. The normal range from flexion to extension is 0 to 240 degrees in the 360-degree system. In the 180-degree system, flexion is from 0 to 180 degrees, and extension is measured separately as 0 to 60 degrees.[4, 24]

Review of the recent literature shows that most reference textbooks utilize the 180-degree system in an attempt to standardize measurement techniques.[2, 10, 18, 24, 26] Figures 1-4 through 1-19 describe the ROM examination on commonly evaluated joints utilizing the 180-degree system. Each figure outlines patient positioning, plane of motion, and goniometer placement. The shaded areas indicate normal ROM.

Spinal ROM is more difficult to measure, and techniques utilizing goniometers, plumb lines, and measuring tapes have been described. The reliability of these differing techniques is questionable.[10, 24] Inclinometers have also been suggested for accurate measuring of spinal ROM.[2, 11] The inclinometer is a fluid-filled instrument with either a 180- or 360-degree scale. It is placed on the patient's spine and utilizes the principle of gravity to determine a change in spinal position after movement. For example, the examiner places the inclinometer on a vertebral spinous process with the initial fluid level at 0 degrees and asks the patient to flex the spine. The examiner reads the measurement change produced when the instrument moves with the spine, but the fluid line remains stable due to the force of gravity. Cervical, thoracic, and lumbar spine movements in all planes can be measured utilizing inclinometers. Measurements are done with either one or two inclinometers.

The reader should refer to either the American Medical Association's *Guides to the Evaluation of Permanent Impairment*[2] or Gerhard's *Documentation of Joint Motion*[11] for specific inclinometer techniques to be used for each spinal segment range of motion. As examples, cervical flexion and extension are illustrated using a two-inclinometer technique (Fig. 1-20) and the one-inclinometer technique (Fig. 1-21).[2]

Joint Stability

The stability inherent in each joint depends on its bone integrity, ligamentous and joint capsule connections, and

Text continued on page 19

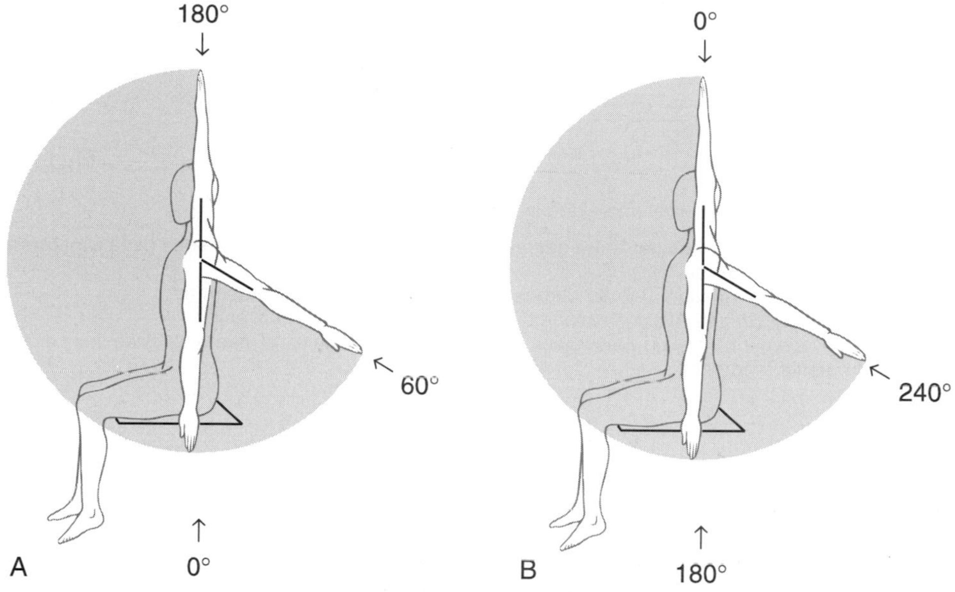

FIGURE 1–3 Shoulder flexion and extension. *A,* 180-degree system. *B,* 360-degree system.

180°
↓
60°
A   0°

0°
↓
240°
B   180°

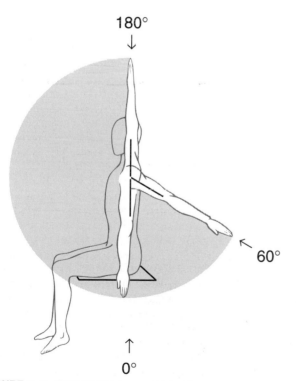

180°
↓
60°
0°

FIGURE 1–4 Shoulder flexion and extension.

Patient Position: Supine or sitting, arm at side, elbow extended.
Plane of Motion: Sagittal.
Normal ROM: Flexion, 0 to 180 degrees; extension, 0 to 60 degrees.
Movements Patient Should Avoid: Arching back, trunk rotation.
Goniometer Placement: Axis is centered on the lateral shoulder, stationary arm remains on 0 degrees, movement arm remains parallel to humerus.

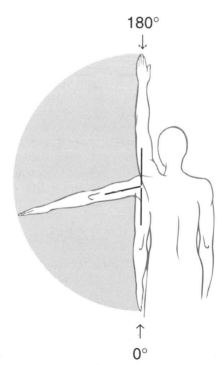

180°
↓
0°

FIGURE 1–5 Shoulder abduction.

Patient Position: Supine or sitting, arm at side, elbow extended.
Plane of Motion: Frontal.
Normal ROM: 0 to 180 degrees.
Movements Patient Should Avoid: Trunk rotation or lateral movement.
Goniometer Placement: Axis is centered on posterior or anterior shoulder, stationary arm remains at 0 degrees, movement arm remains parallel to humerus.

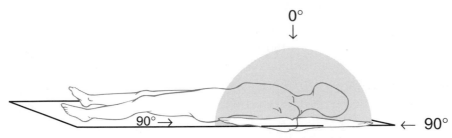

FIGURE 1–6   Shoulder internal and external rotation.

Patient Position: Supine, shoulder at 90 degrees of abduction, elbow at 90 degrees of flexion, forearm pronated.
Plane of Motion: Transverse.
Normal ROM: Internal rotation, 0 to 90 degrees; external rotation, 0 to 90 degrees.
Movements Patient Should Avoid: Arching back, trunk rotation, elbow movement.
Goniometer Placement: Axis on elbow joint through longitudinal axis of humerus, stationary arm remains at 0 degrees, movement arm remains parallel to forearm.

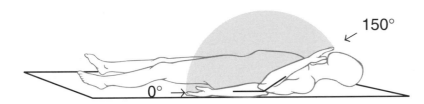

FIGURE 1–7   Elbow flexion.

Patient Position: Supine or sitting, forearm supinated.
Plane of Motion: Sagittal.
Normal ROM: 0 to 150 degrees.
Goniometer Placement: Axis is centered on lateral elbow, stationary arm remains on 0 degrees, movement arm remains parallel to forearm.

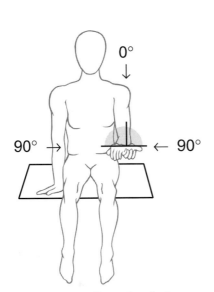

FIGURE 1–8   Forearm pronation and supination.

Patient Position: Sitting or standing, elbow at 90 degrees, wrist in neutral, pencil held in palm of hand.
Plane of Motion: Transverse.
Normal ROM: Pronation, 0 to 90 degrees; supination, 0 to 90 degrees.
Movements Patient Should Avoid: Arm, elbow, and wrist movements.
Goniometer Placement: Axis through longitudinal axis of forearm, stationary arm remains at 0 degrees, movement arm remains parallel to pencil held in patient's hand.

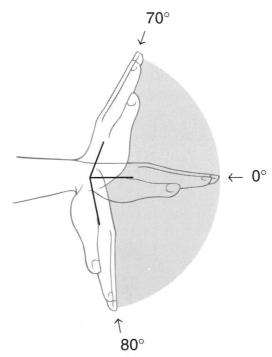

FIGURE 1–9   Wrist flexion and extension.

Patient Position: Elbow flexed, forearm pronated.
Plane of Motion: Sagittal.
Normal ROM: Flexion, 0 to 80 degrees; extension, 0 to 70 degrees.
Goniometer Placement: Axis is centered on lateral wrist over ulnar styloid, stationary arm remains on 0 degrees, movement arm remains parallel to fifth metacarpal.

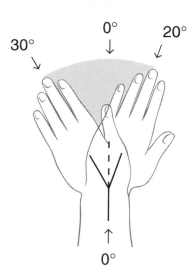

FIGURE 1–10   Wrist radial and ulnar deviation.

Patient Position: Elbow flexed, forearm pronated, wrist in neutral flexion and extension.
Plane of Motion: Frontal.
Normal ROM: Radial, 0 to 20 degrees; ulnar, 0 to 30 degrees.
Goniometer Placement: Axis is centered over dorsal wrist midway between distal radius and ulna,
   stationary arm remains on 0 degrees, movement arm remains parallel to third metacarpal.

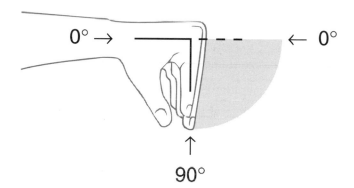

FIGURE 1–11   Second to fifth metacarpophalangeal flexion.

Patient Position: Elbow flexed, forearm pronated, wrist in neutral,
   fingers extended.
Plane of Motion: Sagittal.
Normal ROM: 0 to 90 degrees.
Goniometer Placement. Axis on dorsum of each metacarpophalangeal joint, stationary arm remains at 0 degrees, movement
   arm remains on dorsum of each proximal phalanx.

FIGURE 1–12   Second to fifth proximal interphalangeal flexion.

Patient Position: Elbow flexed, forearm pronated, wrist in neutral,
   metacarpophalangeal joints in slight flexion.
Plane of Motion: Sagittal.
Normal ROM: 0 to 100 degrees.
Goniometer Placement: Axis on dorsum of each interphalangeal
   joint, stationary arm remains on 0 degrees, movement arm remains on dorsum of each middle phalanx.

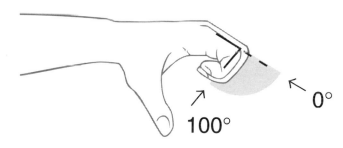

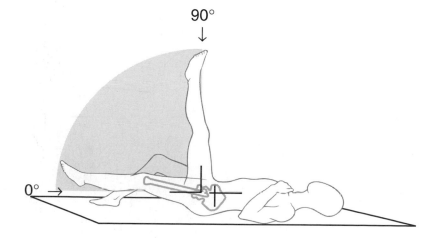

FIGURE 1–13   Hip flexion, knee extension.

Patient Position: Supine or lying on side, knee extended.
Plane of Motion: Sagittal.
Normal ROM: 0 to 90 degrees.
Movements Patient Should Avoid: Arching back.
Goniometer Placement: Axis is centered on lateral
   leg over greater trochanter, stationary arm remains at 0 degrees. (This is found by drawing a
   line from the anterior superior iliac spine to the
   posterior superior iliac spine, and then drawing
   another line, perpendicular to the first, that goes
   through the greater trochanter. The last line is
   0 degrees.) Movement arm remains parallel to
   lateral femur.

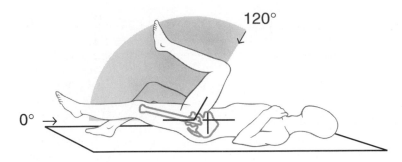

FIGURE 1–14 Hip flexion, knee flexion.

Patient Position: Supine or lying on side, knee flexed.
Plane of Motion: Sagittal.
Normal ROM: 0 to 120 degrees.
Movements Patient Should Avoid: Arching back.
Goniometer Placement: Same as in Figure 1–13.

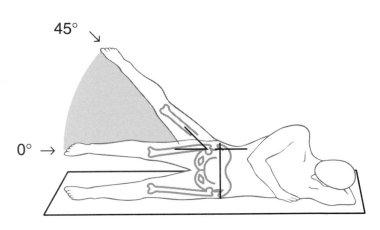

FIGURE 1–15 Hip abduction.

Patient Position: Supine or lying on side, knee extended.
Plane of Motion: Frontal.
Normal ROM: 0 to 45 degrees.
Movements Patient Should Avoid: Trunk rotation.
Goniometer Placement: Axis centered over greater trochanter, stationary arm is parallel to and below a line on patient drawn through both anterior superior iliac spines (this is perpendicular to 0 degrees), movement arm remains parallel to anterior femur.

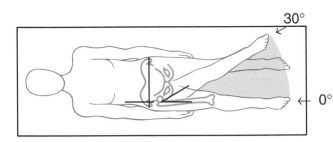

FIGURE 1–16 Hip adduction.

Patient Position: Supine, knee extended.
Plane of Motion: Frontal.
Normal ROM: 0 to 30 degrees.
Movements Patient Should Avoid: Trunk rotation.
Goniometer Placement: Same as in Figure 1–15.

FIGURE 1–17 Hip internal and external rotation.

Patient Position: Supine or sitting, hip at 90 degrees flexion, knee at 90 degrees flexion.
Plane of Motion: Transverse.
Normal ROM: Internal, 0 to 35 degrees; external, 0 to 45 degrees.
Movements Patient Should Avoid: Hip flexion movement, knee movement.
Goniometer Placement: Axis over knee joint through longitudinal axis of femur, stationary arm remains at 0 degrees, movement arm remains parallel to anterior tibia.

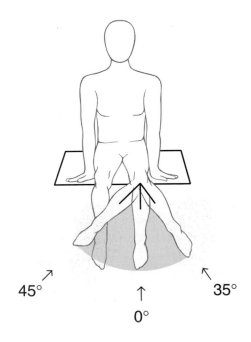

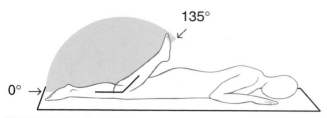

FIGURE 1–18   Knee flexion.

Patient Position: Prone or sitting, hip in neutral.
Plane of Motion: Sagittal.
Normal ROM: 0 to 135 degrees.
Goniometer Placement: Axis on lateral knee joint, stationary arm remains at 0 degrees, movement arm remains parallel to fibula laterally.

muscle activity. Each joint anatomically achieves stability differently. For example, shoulder joint stability depends mostly on muscle activity of the rotator cuff, whereas the hip joint depends on the ligamentous structures to provide much of the joint's stability. Basic knowledge of the joint anatomy is important for the clinician to be able to accurately diagnose joint instability problems.

Joint stability is evaluated by providing stress to all ranges of motion. If joint instability is noted, then a more specific examination of that joint using specialized tests is warranted, such as Lachman's test for ankle stability or McMurray's test for meniscus tear, which are well described in physical diagnosis texts.[3, 8, 15]

Contracture

A contracture causes the inability to perform full-joint ROM. It results from decreased tissue extensibility of soft tissues and muscle or from bony abnormalities.

Each contracture is evaluated for its possible cause.

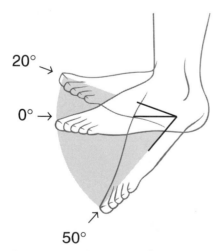

FIGURE 1–19   Ankle dorsiflexion and plantar flexion.

Patient Position: Sitting or supine with knee flexed to 90 degrees.
Plane of Motion: Sagittal.
Normal ROM: Dorsiflexion, 0 to 20 degrees; plantar flexion, 0 to 50 degrees.
Goniometer Placement: Axis is on sole of foot below lateral malleolus, stationary arm remains along shaft of fibula (this is perpendicular to 0 degrees), movement arm remains parallel to fifth metatarsal.

Significant joint contracture is often obvious just on visual inspection. Providing a gentle, prolonged passive stretch to the joint, soft tissues, and muscles can indicate whether the abnormality is caused by abnormalities in bone, muscle, or soft tissue. Both soft tissue and muscle contractures often decrease after prolonged stretch is applied. Contractures due to bony abnormalities do not change with prolonged stretch.

Shortening of muscles that cross two or more joints is not a joint contracture, but is often noted during an examination for contractures, as shortening of these muscles can lead to ROM abnormalities. Muscles that cross two joints are normally at a length disadvantage, and even a mild loss of extensibility can lead to problems in gait and other movements.

An example of a joint motion that involves both one- and two-joint muscles is hip flexion, involving the action of the illiopsoas, tensor fascia lata, rectus femoris, pectineus, and the adductor muscle group. This joint is specifically tested for shortness of both types of muscles using the Thomas test (Fig. 1–22). The patient is asked to lie supine with one leg dropped over the edge of the table so the knee is free to flex. The other limb is lifted and pulled to the chest by the patient. The examiner notes whether the back flattens on the table. (The examiner should have one hand behind the patient's back to palpate for this.) Normal muscle length of both the one- and two-joint muscles allows the posterior thigh of the first leg to lay flat on the table with approximately 80 degrees of knee flexion (see Figure 1–22A). Shortened one-joint muscles (illiopsoas, pectineus, adductors) are noted when knee flexion ability is good, but the thigh rises up off the examination table (see Fig. 1–22B). Shortened two-joint muscles (rectus femoris, tensor fascia lata) are diagnosed when the leg is able to maintain contact with the table but the knee cannot flex past 70 degrees (see Fig. 1–22C). If both the one- and two-joint muscles are shortened, the thigh rises off the table and the knee is unable to flex past 70 degrees (see Fig. 1–22D). Tensor fascia lata shortness can also cause abduction of the extended leg when this test is performed.[18]

Manual Muscle Testing

Manual muscle testing (MMT) is the technique physiatrists use to document muscle strength. MMT involves the actual test performance as well as muscle strength grading.

Prior to formal MMT, screening tests for muscle weakness can help to identify areas requiring specific evaluation. Upper limb strength is screened by having the patient grasp two of the examiner's fingers while the examiner attempts to free the fingers by pulling in all directions. A deep knee bend (squat and rise) screens proximal lower limb strength. Distal lower limb strength is evaluated by having the patient walk on the heels and then the toes, which tests ankle dorsiflexion and plantar flexion strength, respectively. Increased walking cadence often increases gait abnormalities, causing them to be more evident. Abdominal strength is screened by observing a patient's ability to go from supine to sitting while the hips and knees are flexed. If the same activity is performed with the hips and knees extended, both abdominal and illiopsoas strength is evaluated.

Formal MMT requires that the examiner be proficient in

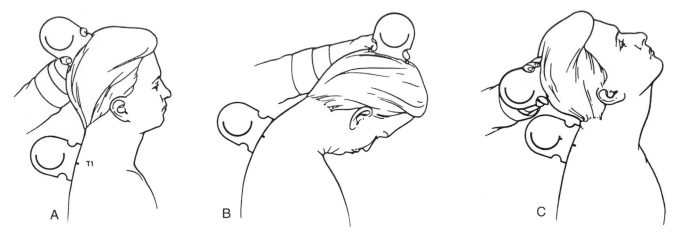

FIGURE 1–20 Two-inclinometer measurement technique for cervical flexion and extension.

1. With the patient seated, place the first inclinometer, aligned in the sagittal plane, over the T1 spinous process while holding the second inclinometer over the occiput. The head remains in neutral position while the inclinometers are set at 0 degrees *(A)*.
2. Ask the patient to flex maximally and record both angles. Subtract the T1 angle from the occipital angle to obtain the cervical flexion angle. *B,* Ask the patient to return the head to the neutral position so that both inclinometers read 0 degrees again.
3. Ask the patient to extend the neck as far as possible, again recording both inclinometer angles. Subtract the T1 angle from the occipital angle to obtain the cervical extension angle *(C)*.

(Adapted from Guide to the Evaluation of Permanent Impairment, ed 4. Chicago, American Medical Association, 1994, p 116.)

the test procedures required to assess each muscle or muscle group. This proficiency requires a working knowledge of muscle function and of the techniques described in MMT reference texts such as *Muscles: Testing and Function*[18] or *Muscle Testing: Techniques of Manual Examination.*[6] Proficiency also depends on developing expert manual skills that typically come from practice in MMT.

The test procedure should generally be performed using

the axiom "make and break." The patient is asked to "make" the muscle(s) being tested contract and to hold a specific position. The examiner then tries to "break" that muscle contraction by applying pressure at the distal end of the muscle or muscle tendon. The patient "makes" the muscle, contracting it into a set position, and the examiner attempts to "break" the muscle contraction.

MMT requires patient cooperation. Poor patient under-

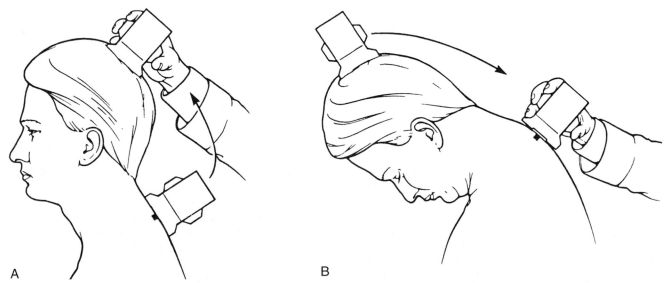

FIGURE 1–21 One-inclinometer measurement technique for cervical flexion and extension.

1. With the patient in the seated position, place the inclinometer, aligned in the sagittal plane, over the T1 spinous process and set the first 0 degree reading *(A,* position 1). Move the inclinometer to the occiput and set the second 0 degree reading *(A,* position 2).
2. Ask the patient to flex the head maximally and record the occipital flexion angle *(B,* position 3). Move the inclinometer to the T1 spinous process and record the angle while the subject maintains the head in flexion *(B,* position 4). Ask the patient to move the head back to the neutral position. Subtract the T1 reading from the occipital reading to obtain the cervical flexion angle.
3. After obtaining 0 degree readings, first from the T1 and then over the occiput, ask the patient to carry out full cervical extension. Record the angles first at the occiput and then over the T1 spinous process and subtract to obtain the cervical extension angles.

(From Guide to the Evaluation of Permanent Impairment, ed 4. Chicago, American Medical Association, 1994, p 117.)

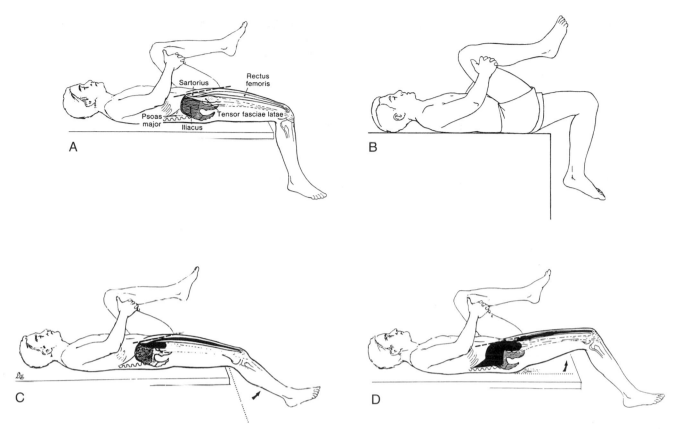

FIGURE 1–22 The Thomas test for hip flexor muscle tightness. *A,* Normal length of hip flexors. *B,* Shortness in one joint muscle only. *C,* Shortness in two joint muscles only. *D,* Shortness of both one and two joint muscles. (Adapted from Kendall FP, McCreary EK, Provance PG: Muscles Testing and Function, ed 4. Baltimore, Williams & Wilkins, 1993, pp 34–36.)

standing of the test procedure or poor motivation to participate causes inaccuracies. Pain often prevents a full muscle contraction or causes the patient to release the contraction suddenly when resistance is provided. This is called *break-away weakness,* and it should not be interpreted as true weakness. Documentation should reflect that pain prevented accurate MMT. A patient can also either consciously or subconsciously attempt to appear weak by a "ratchety" or inconsistent response to the resistance provided. Age, gender, pain, level of muscle conditioning, contractures, and joint stability are all factors that can lead to an inaccurate evaluation of normal muscle strength.

A few technique errors in MMT are important for the examiner to avoid. The examiner will generally want to place one hand above and below the joint being affected by the muscle contraction. Avoid placing the hands so that pressure is applied across more than one joint (if possible). Often, patients try to use other muscles to assist a weak muscle or muscle group. This is called *substitution,* and, if observed, the patient should be counseled on how to avoid contaminating the MMT with substitution. At times it is necessary to intentionally place a muscle at a mechanical disadvantage to show a minor degree of weakness. For example, testing elbow extension with the elbow in 90 degrees of flexion rather than full extension can show minor weakness, especially when comparing the muscle on one side to the same muscle on the other side of the body.

MMT can also be quantified by the use of strain gauges, dynamometers, and other apparatus. Dynamometers record the force being resisted by the patient's muscles during testing. Inexpensive commercial versions are available and are commonly used, for example, to measure pinch or grip strength.

Muscle strength grading was developed to document the results of MMT. The two most common systems of muscle grading, which are listed and defined in Table 1–10, utilize numbers and words to document the test. A third type of muscle strength grading, also listed in Table 1–10, uses percentages to describe muscle strength deficit, and is used clinically for impairment rating.[2, 27] The examiner should do each test in a simple but standardized manner so that the results can be used for future comparisons.

When describing a muscle or muscle group that has weakness, the examiner should systematically proceed through the different grades. The patient is asked to contract the muscle while the examiner palpates it. If no movement is palpable in the muscle, it is graded 0 (zero). If muscle contraction is palpable but no joint movement is noted, the muscle is at least grade 1 (trace). Next, the examiner asks the patient to contract the muscle in a gravity-eliminated position. If the patient is able to move the body part through the full ROM then the muscle has at least grade 2 (poor) strength. The patient is asked to contract the muscle to move the body part against gravity. If the patient can move the body part through the full range of motion against gravity, there is at least grade 3 strength (fair). The examiner then provides resistance to the muscle activity, and if the patient is able to resist a moderate

TABLE 1–10   Systems of Muscle Strength Grading

Number	Work	Motor Deficit (%)	Definition
5	Normal	0	Complete joint range of motion against gravity with full resistance
4	Good	1–25	Complete joint range of motion against gravity with moderate resistance
3	Fair	26–50	Full joint range of motion against gravity
2	Poor	51–75	Full joint range of motion with gravity eliminated
1	Trace	76–99	Visible palpable or muscle contraction; no joint motion produced
0	Zero	100	No visible or palpable muscle contraction

Adapted from Stillwell GK, deLateur BJ, Fordyce WE, et al: Physiatric Therapeutics in Self-Directed Medical Knowledge Program in Physical Medicine and Rehabilitation, ed 2. Chicago, American Academy of Physical Medicine and Rehabilitation, 1986, p A1.

amount of pressure, the muscle strength is a grade 4 (good). If the patient is able to provide full resistance, the muscle is grade 5 strength (normal). Grades 0 to 3 (zero to fair) are fairly objective, but both grades 4 and 5 (good to normal) depend on the examiner's subjective interpretation of the amount of resistance.[18, 27]

The actual MMT procedure is an evaluation of the individual's ability to perform a motion against resistance, and is not the ability of one muscle to contract separately from all other muscles. The physiological explanation is that the cortical cells in the motor cortex of the brain represent movements and not individual muscles.[1] When an individual is asked to do a specific movement to isolate the activity of one muscle, it is usually not possible for the patient to isolate the muscle. Several other muscles that also perform the movement are usually active at the same time. For example, when biceps strength is tested by elbow flexion, both the brachialis and brachioradialis assist the biceps with this activity. Often the examiner positions the patient's joint so as to isolate one muscle as much as possible. For example, if the patient's forearm pronation is tested with the elbow at 90 degrees of flexion, this tends to isolate the pronator teres; but if pronation is tested with the elbow in full flexion (150 degrees), the pronator quadratus is preferentially isolated.

In the following sections, MMT of multiple muscles is described in a manner that emphasizes function. Functional muscle groups are discussed, with some muscles included in more than one category. The primary muscles involved in the movements are emphasized. Each muscle's peripheral and root level innervation is listed. The innervation listed is the most frequently described innervation, but anatomical variations are common. Functional anatomy reference texts such as *Hollinshead's Functional Anatomy of the Limbs and Back*[16] should be reviewed to learn the primary muscles involved in the movements. MMT references are recommended for learning the proper positioning and techniques for muscle testing.[6, 18]

SHOULDER MOVEMENTS

Flexion (Fig. 1–23)
Deltoid, anterior portion (axillary nerve from posterior cord, C5, C6)

Pectoralis major, clavicular portion (medial and lateral pectoral nerve, C5 to T1)

Biceps brachii (musculocutaneous nerve from lateral cord, C5, C6)

Coracobrachialis (musculocutaneous nerve from lateral cord, C5, C6, C7)

Test. The shoulder is placed in approximately 90 degrees of flexion with the elbow flexed. The examiner should attempt to force the arm into extension, applying pressure over the distal humeral area. The anterior deltoid mainly produces this motion, although it is assisted by the other muscles.

Extension (Fig. 1–24)
Deltoid, posterior portion (axillary nerve from posterior cord, C5, C6)

Latissimus dorsi (thoracodorsal nerve from posterior cord, C6, C7, C8)

Teres major (lower subscapular nerve from posterior cord, C5, C6)

Test. The shoulder is placed in approximately 45 degrees of extension with the elbow extended. The examiner attempts to force the arm into flexion, applying pressure over the distal humeral area.

Abduction (Fig. 1–25)
Deltoid, middle portion (axillary nerve from posterior cord, C5, C6)

Supraspinatus (suprascapular nerve from upper trunk, C5, C6)

Test. The shoulder is placed in approximately 90 degrees of abduction. The examiner attempts to force the shoulder into adduction, applying pressure over the distal humeral area.

Adduction (Fig. 1–26)
Pectoralis major (medial and lateral pectoral nerve, C5 to T1)

Latissimus dorsi (thoracodorsal nerve from posterior cord, C6, C7, C8)

Teres major (lower subscapular nerve from posterior cord, C5, C6)

Test. The shoulder is placed at the side. The examiner attempts to pull the arm away from the side, applying pressure over the distal humeral area.

Internal Rotation (Fig. 1–27)
Subscapularis (upper and lower subscapular nerve from posterior cord, C5, C6)

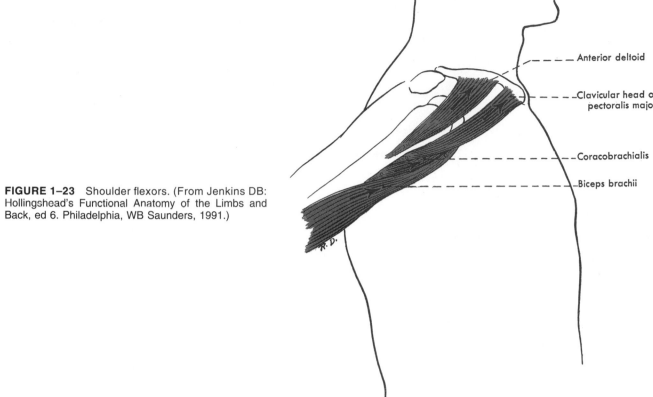

FIGURE 1–23 Shoulder flexors. (From Jenkins DB: Hollingshead's Functional Anatomy of the Limbs and Back, ed 6. Philadelphia, WB Saunders, 1991.)

- Anterior deltoid
- Clavicular head of pectoralis major
- Coracobrachialis
- Biceps brachii

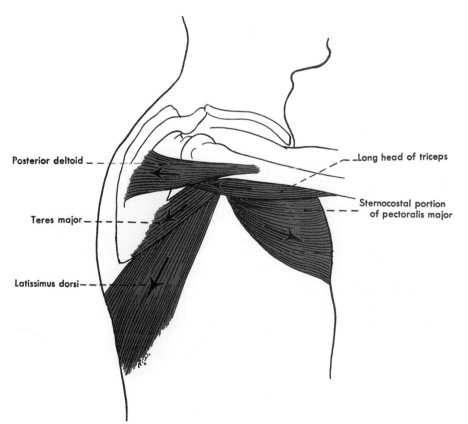

- Posterior deltoid
- Teres major
- Latissimus dorsi
- Long head of triceps
- Sternocostal portion of pectoralis major

FIGURE 1–24 Shoulder extensors. (From Jenkins DB: Hollingshead's Functional Anatomy of the Limbs and Back, ed 6. Philadelphia, WB Saunders, 1991.)

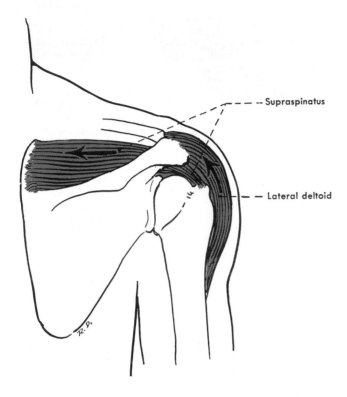

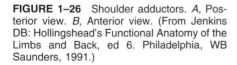

FIGURE 1–25 Shoulder abductors. (From Jenkins DB: Hollingshead's Functional Anatomy of the Limbs and Back, ed 6. Philadelphia, WB Saunders, 1991.)

FIGURE 1–26 Shoulder adductors. A, Posterior view. B, Anterior view. (From Jenkins DB: Hollingshead's Functional Anatomy of the Limbs and Back, ed 6. Philadelphia, WB Saunders, 1991.)

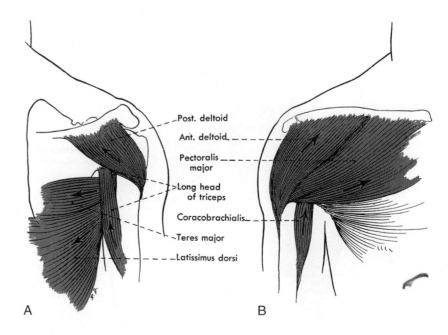

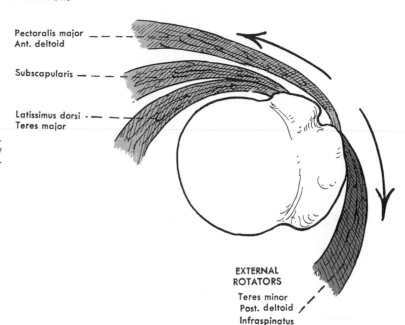

INTERNAL
ROTATORS

Pectoralis major
Ant. deltoid

Subscapularis

Latissimus dorsi
Teres major

EXTERNAL
ROTATORS
Teres minor
Post. deltoid
Infraspinatus

FIGURE 1–27 Shoulder internal and external rotators. (From Jenkins DB: Hollingshead's Functional Anatomy of the Limbs and Back, ed 6. Philadelphia, WB Saunders, 1991.)

Pectoralis major (medial and lateral pectoral nerve, C5 to T1)

Latissimus dorsi (thoracodorsal nerve from posterior cord, C6, C7, C8)

Deltoid, anterior portion (axillary nerve from posterior cord, C5, C6)

Teres major (lower subscapular nerve from posterior cord, C5, C6)

Test. The shoulder is placed in 90 degrees of abduction with full internal rotation and 90 degrees of elbow flexion. The examiner attempts to force the arm into external rotation, applying pressure over the distal forearm.

External Rotation (see Fig. 1–27)
Infraspinatus (suprascapular nerve from upper trunk, C5, C6)

Teres minor (axillary nerve from posterior cord, C5, C6)

Deltoid, posterior portion (axillary nerve from posterior cord, C5, C6)

Test. The shoulder is placed in 90 degrees of abduction with full external rotation and 90 degrees of elbow flexion. The examiner attempts to force the arm into internal rotation, applying pressure over the distal forearm.

ELBOW MOVEMENTS
Flexion (Fig. 1–28)
Biceps brachii (musculocutaneous nerve from lateral cord, C5, C6)

Brachialis (musculocutaneous nerve from lateral cord, C5, C6)

Brachioradialis (radial nerve from posterior cord, C5, C6)

Test. The elbow is placed in approximately 90 degrees of flexion. The examiner attempts to force the elbow into extension, applying pressure over the distal forearm. Depending on the forearm position, the examiner is able to more specifically test each of the three muscles. In full forearm supination, the biceps muscle is the primary elbow flexor, whereas in full forearm pronation, the brachialis is the primary flexor. If the forearm is held in 0 degrees or neutral between pronation and supination ("thumbs-up" position), the main muscle of elbow flexion is the brachioradialis.

Extension (Fig. 1–29)
Triceps (radial nerve from posterior cord, C6, C7, C8)

Test. The elbow is placed in a few degrees of elbow flexion. (The number of degrees of elbow flexion can vary from 30 to almost full extension. The elbow is never in a fully extended position, because in that position the patient may be able to stabilize it, and a subtle elbow extension weakness might be missed.) The examiner attempts to force the elbow into flexion, applying pressure over the distal forearm.

FOREARM MOVEMENTS
Pronation (Fig. 1–30)
Pronator quadratus (anterior interosseous branch of the median nerve, C7, C8, T1)

Pronator teres (median nerve from lateral cord, C6, C7)

Test. The elbow is placed in a position of full pronation. The examiner attempts to force the forearm into supination, applying pressure at the distal forearm. If the elbow is partially flexed (90 degrees) the pronator teres is primarily tested. If the elbow is held in a position of full flexion, the pronator quadratus is the main pronator muscle.

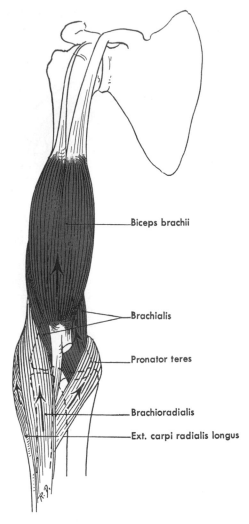

FIGURE 1–28   Elbow flexors. (From Jenkins DB: Hollingshead's Functional Anatomy of the Limbs and Back, ed 6. Philadelphia, WB Saunders, 1991.)

Supination (Fig. 1–31)
Supinator (radial nerve from posterior cord, C5, C6)

Biceps brachii (musculocutaneous nerve from lateral cord, C5, C6)

Test.   Because the biceps is tested by elbow flexion (see preceding section Elbow Movements: Flexion), the arm should be placed in a position to favor the supinator muscle strength. To do this, the elbow is placed in full flexion with the forearm in full supination. In this position the biceps is unable to assist in the act of supination. The examiner attempts to force the forearm into pronation, applying pressure at the distal forearm.

WRIST MOVEMENTS
Flexion (Fig. 1–32)
Flexor carpi radialis (median nerve from lateral cord, C6, C7)

Flexor carpi ulnaris (ulnar nerve from medial cord, C8, T1)

Test.   The wrist is placed in a neutral position between

radial and ulnar deviation and in full flexion, with the fingers extended. The examiner attempts to force the wrist into extension, applying pressure at the midpalm level. To more selectively test the flexor carpi radialis, the patient's wrist is placed in a position of radial deviation and full flexion. The examiner attempts to force the wrist into extension and ulnar deviation. To more selectively test the flexor carpi ulnaris, the patient's wrist is placed in a position of ulnar deviation and full flexion. The examiner attempts to force the wrist into extension and radial deviation.

Extension (Fig. 1–33)
Extensor carpi radialis longus (radial nerve from posterior cord, C6, C7)

Extensor carpi radialis brevis (radial nerve from posterior cord, C6, C7)

Extensor carpi ulnaris (radial nerve from posterior cord, C6, C7, C8)

Test.   The wrist is placed in a neutral position between radial and ulnar deviation and in full extension, with the fingers extended. The examiner attempts to force the wrist into flexion, applying pressure over the dorsum of the hand. To more selectively test the extensor carpi radialis longus, the patient's wrist is placed in a position of radial deviation

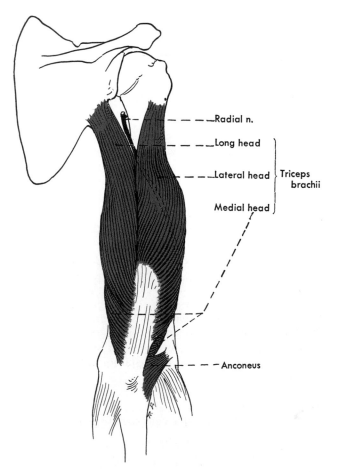

FIGURE 1–29   Elbow extensors. (From Jenkins DB: Hollingshead's Functional Anatomy of the Limbs and Back, ed 6. Philadelphia, WB Saunders, 1991.)

force the thumb into adduction (toward the palm), applying pressure just above the first metacarpophalangeal joint.

Thumb Opposition (see Fig. 1–34)

Opponens pollicis (median nerve, C8, T1)

Flexor pollicis brevis (superficial head: median nerve; deep head: ulnar nerve, C8, T1)

Abductor pollicis brevis (median nerve, C8, T1)

Test. The thumb is placed in opposition. The examiner attempts to force the thumb back into anatomical position, applying pressure just above the first metacarpophalangeal joint.

Second to Fifth Digit Flexion (see Fig. 1–34)

Flexor digitorum superficialis (median nerve, C7, C8, T1)

Flexor digitorum profundus (lateral portion: median nerve, medial portion: ulnar nerve, C8, T1)

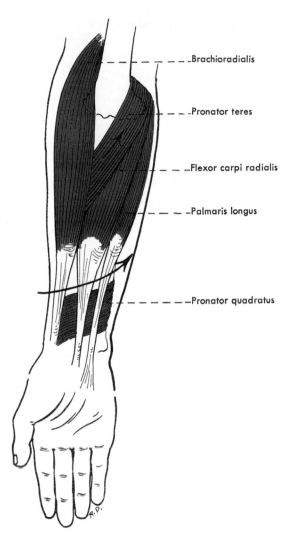

FIGURE 1–30 Forearm pronators. (From Jenkins DB: Hollingshead's Functional Anatomy of the Limbs and Back, ed 6. Philadelphia, WB Saunders, 1991.)

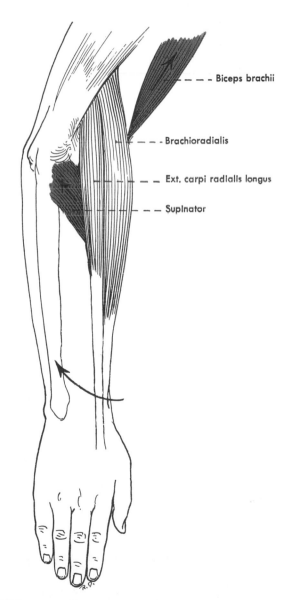

FIGURE 1–31 Forearm supinators. (From Jenkins DB: Hollingshead's Functional Anatomy of the Limbs and Back, ed 6. Philadelphia, WB Saunders, 1991.)

and full extension. The examiner attempts to force the wrist into flexion and ulnar deviation. To more selectively test the extensor carpi ulnaris, the patient's wrist is placed in a position of ulnar deviation and full extension. The examiner attempts to force the wrist into flexion and radial deviation. It is difficult to position the hand to isolate the extensor carpi radialis brevis because of the midline position of its tendon insertion in the wrist.

THUMB AND DIGIT MOVEMENTS. Only a few important strength testing movements are discussed; the reader should review reference texts for additional thumb and digit tests.

Thumb Abduction (Fig. 1–34)

Abductor pollicis brevis (median nerve, C8, T1)

Abductor pollicis longus (radial nerve, C6, C7)

Extensor pollicis brevis (radial nerve, C6, C7)

Test. The thumb is placed in abduction and perpendicular to the plane of the palm. The examiner attempts to

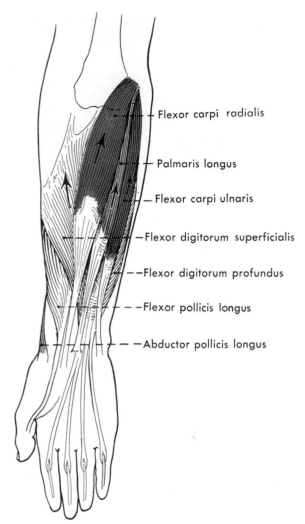

FIGURE 1–32 Wrist flexors. (From Jenkins DB: Hollingshead's Functional Anatomy of the Limbs and Back, ed 6. Philadelphia, WB Saunders, 1991.)

Lumbricals (lateral two: median nerve; medial two: ulnar nerve, C8, T1)

Interossei (ulnar nerve, C8, T1)

Test. Because the tendons of the flexor digitorum profundus extend to the distal phalanges, the examiner tests the strength of this muscle by attempting to force each distal phalangeal joint into extension after it is placed in a position of flexion. The tendons of the flexor digitorum superficialis extend to the middle phalanx. The examiner tests both the superficialis and the profundus by attempting to force each middle phalangeal joint into extension after each is placed in a position of flexion. The primary flexors of the metacarpophalangeal joints of the second to fourth digits are the lumbricals and the interossei. The examiner tests these muscles by attempting to force each metacarpophalangeal joint into extension after each is placed in a position of flexion. The primary flexors of the fifth digit metacarpophalangeal joint are the flexor and abductor digiti minimi muscles and MMT of flexion of this joint evaluates their strength.

Second to Fifth Digit Extension (see Fig. 1–34)
Extensor digitorum (radial nerve, C6, C7, C8)

Extensor indicis (radial nerve, C7, C8)

Extensor digiti minimi (radial nerve, C6, C7, C8)

Test. The second to fifth digits are placed in extension with the wrist in neutral position between flexion and extension (0 degrees). The examiner attempts to force each finger into flexion by applying a force over each proximal phalanx.

Second to Fourth Digit Abduction, First to Fifth Digit Adduction (see Fig. 1–34)
Dorsal interossei (ulnar nerve, C8, T1)

Palmar interossei (ulnar nerve, C8, T1)

Test. One method of testing adduction of these digits is to attempt to withdraw a piece of paper that has been placed between the patient's fingers while the patient attempts to retain the paper. Abduction is tested by placing each digit in abduction and attempting to force the digit into adduction. Note that the third digit cannot adduct, as movement of this digit to either side is abduction.

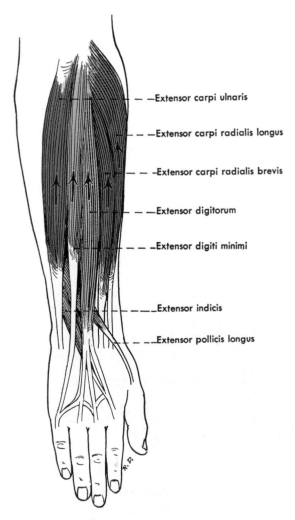

FIGURE 1–33 Wrist extensors. (From Jenkins DB: Hollingshead's Functional Anatomy of the Limbs and Back, ed 6. Philadelphia, WB Saunders, 1991.)

Fifth Digit Abduction (see Fig. 1–34)

Abductor digiti minimi (ulnar nerve, C8, T1)

Flexor digiti minimi (ulnar nerve, C8, T1)

Test. The patient's fifth digit is placed in abduction. The examiner attempts to force the digit into adduction by applying pressure just above the metacarpophalangeal joint.

HIP MOVEMENT

Flexion (Fig. 1–35)

Iliacus (femoral nerve, L2, L3, L4)

Psoas (lumbar plexus, L2, L3, L4)

Tensor fascia lata (superior gluteal nerve, L4, L5, S1)

Rectus femoris (femoral nerve, L2, L3, L4)

Pectineus (femoral or obturator nerve, L2, L3)

Adductor longus, brevis, anterior portion of magnus (obturator nerve, L2, L3, L4)

Test. Hip flexion is tested with the patient in both seated and supine positions. With the patient in a sitting position, the hip is placed in flexion by raising the knee. The examiner attempts to force the hip into extension, applying pressure over the distal anterior thigh. With the patient supine, the patient's hip is placed in flexion with the knee extended. The examiner attempts to force the hip into extension, applying pressure over the distal anterior thigh. The primary muscle of flexion is the iliopsoas, especially when resistance is applied.

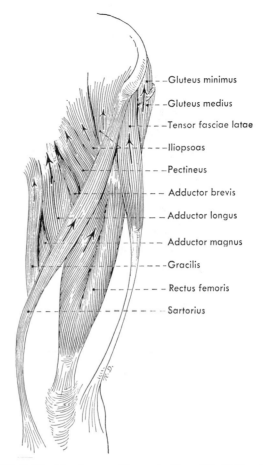

FIGURE 1–35 Hip flexors. (From Jenkins DB: Hollingshead's Functional Anatomy of the Limbs and Back, ed 6. Philadelphia, WB Saunders, 1991.)

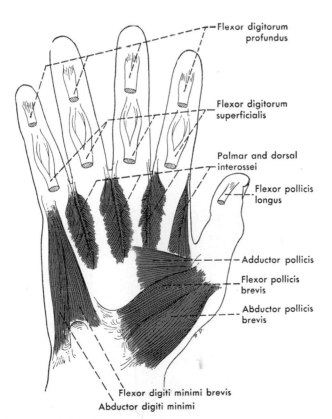

FIGURE 1–34 Muscles of the hand. (From Jenkins DB: Hollingshead's Functional Anatomy of the Limbs and Back, ed 6. Philadelphia, WB Saunders, 1991.)

Extension (Fig. 1–36)

Gluteus maximus (inferior gluteal nerve, L5, S1, S2)

Test. With the patient in a prone position, the hip is placed in extension with the knee flexed to 90 degrees. The examiner attempts to force the hip into flexion, applying pressure over the distal posterior thigh.

Abduction (Fig. 1–37)

Gluteus medius (superior gluteal nerve, L4, L5, S1)

Gluteus minimus (superior gluteal nerve, L4, L5, S1)

Tensor fascia lata (superior gluteal nerve, L4, L5, S1)

Test. With the patient in a side-lying position, the hip is placed in abduction. The examiner attempts to force the hip into adduction, applying pressure over the distal lateral thigh. An easier but less accurate test is performed with the patient seated. With the patient in a sitting position, the hips are placed in abduction (knees separated). The examiner attempts to force the hips into adduction, applying pressure over the distal lateral thighs.

Adduction (Fig. 1–38)

Adductor brevis (obturator nerve, L2, L3, L4)

Adductor longus (obturator nerve, L2, L3)

Adductor magnus, anterior portion (obturator nerve, L3, L4)

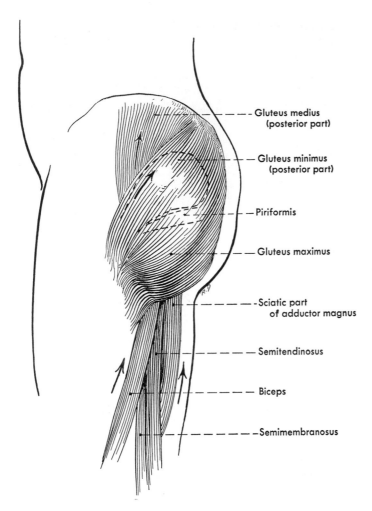

FIGURE 1–36 Hip extensors. Primary extensor is gluteus maximus. (From Jenkins DB: Hollingshead's Functional Anatomy of the Limbs and Back, ed 6. Philadelphia, WB Saunders, 1991.)

FIGURE 1–37 Hip abductors. (From Jenkins DB: Hollingshead's Functional Anatomy of the Limbs and Back, ed 6. Philadelphia, WB Saunders, 1991.)

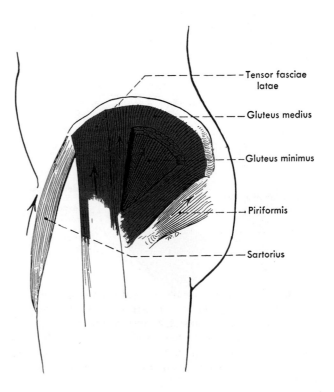

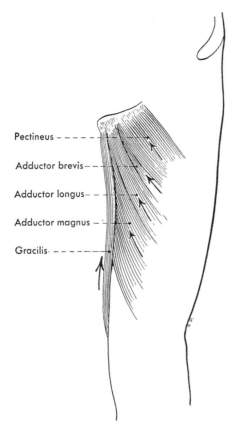

FIGURE 1–38 Hip adductors. (From Jenkins DB: Hollingshead's Functional Anatomy of the Limbs and Back, ed 6, Philadelphia, WB Saunders, 1991.)

Pectineus (femoral or obturator nerve, L2, L3)

Test. The most accurate method requires the patient to assume a side-lying position. With the patient in a side-lying position, the examiner positions the top leg in abduction and the patient is asked to bring the bottom leg up into adduction to meet the top leg. The examiner attempts to force the bottom leg down into abduction, applying pressure over the distal medial thigh. An easier but less accurate test is performed with the patient in a sitting position. The hips are placed in adduction (knees together). The examiner attempts to force the hips into abduction, applying pressure over the distal medial thigh.

Internal Rotation (Fig. 1–39)
Tensor fasciae latae (superior gluteal nerve, L4, L5, S1)

Pectineus (femoral or obturator nerve, L2, L3)

Gluteus minimus, anterior portion (superior gluteal nerve, L4, L5, S1)

Test. The patient is either seated with both knees bent at 90 degrees or prone with one knee bent at 90 degrees. In either position, the tested hip is placed in internal rotation. The examiner uses one hand to attempt to force the leg into external rotation, applying lateral pressure just above the ankle, while stabilizing the knee with the other hand.

External Rotation (Fig. 1–40)
Gluteus maximus (inferior gluteal nerve, L5, S1, S2)

Piriformis (nerve to piriformis, S1, S2)

Superior gemelli and obturator internus (nerve to obturator internus, L5, S1, S2)

Inferior gemelli and quadratus femoris (nerve to quadratus femoris, L4, L5, S1)

Test. The patient is either seated with both knees bent at 90 degrees or prone with one knee bent at 90 degrees. In either position, the tested hip is placed in external rotation. The examiner uses one hand to attempt to force the leg into internal rotation, applying pressure medially just above the ankle, while stabilizing the knee with the other hand.

KNEE MOVEMENTS
Flexion (Fig. 1–41)
Semitendinosus (tibial portion of sciatic nerve, L5, S1)

Semimembranosus (tibial portion of sciatic nerve, L5, S1)

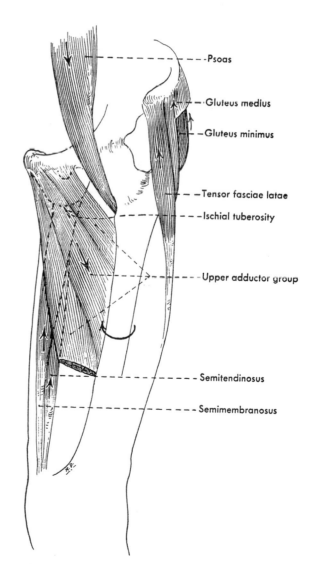

FIGURE 1–39 Hip internal rotators. Primary internal rotators are tensor fasciae latae, pectineus, and anterior portion of gluteus minimus. (From Jenkins DB: Hollingshead's Functional Anatomy of the Limbs and Back, ed 6. Philadelphia, WB Saunders, 1991.)

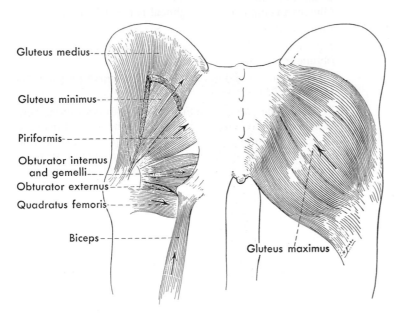

Gluteus medius

Gluteus minimus

Piriformis

Obturator internus
and gemelli

Obturator externus

Quadratus femoris

Biceps

Gluteus maximus

FIGURE 1–40 Hip external rotators. (From Jenkins DB: Hollingshead's Functional Anatomy of the Limbs and Back, ed 6. Philadelphia, WB Saunders, 1991.)

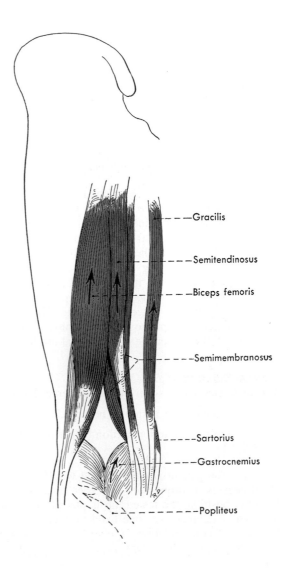

Gracilis

Semitendinosus

Biceps femoris

Semimembranosus

Sartorius

Gastrocnemius

Popliteus

FIGURE 1–41 Knee flexors. (From Jenkins DB: Hollingshead's Functional Anatomy of the Limbs and Back, ed 6. Philadelphia, WB Saunders, 1991.)

Biceps femoris (tibial portion of sciatic nerve, L5, S1, S2)

Test. The patient's knee is placed in 90 degrees of flexion while the patient is in a seated or prone position. The examiner attempts to force the leg into extension, applying pressure over the posterior tibial surface.

Extension (Fig. 1–42)
Quadriceps femoris (femoral nerve, L2, L3, L4)

Test. The knee is placed in approximately 30 degrees of flexion while the patient is in a seated or supine position. Full knee extension is avoided because the patient is able to stabilize the knee in that position, and minor quadriceps weakness may be missed. The examiner attempts to force the leg into flexion, applying pressure over the anterior tibial surface.

ANKLE MOVEMENTS
Dorsiflexion (Fig. 1–43)
Tibialis anterior (deep peroneal nerve, L4, L5, S1)

Extensor digitorum longus (deep peroneal nerve, L4, L5, S1)

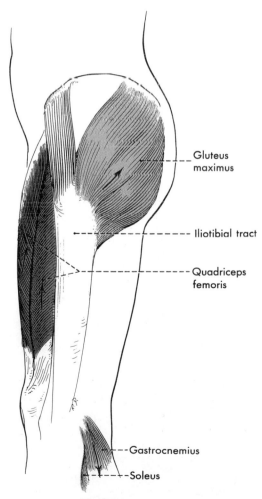

FIGURE 1–42 Knee extensors. Primary knee extensor is the quadriceps femoris. (From Jenkins DB: Hollingshead's Functional Anatomy of the Limbs and Back, ed 6. Philadelphia, WB Saunders, 1991.)

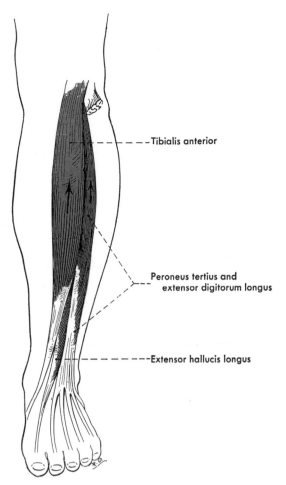

FIGURE 1–43 Ankle dorsiflexors. (From Jenkins DB: Hollingshead's Functional Anatomy of the Limbs and Back, ed 6. Philadelphia, WB Saunders, 1991.)

Extensor hallucis longus (deep peroneal nerve, L4, L5, S1)

Test. All of these muscles work together to produce dorsiflexion when the foot is in a neutral position between inversion and eversion. The ankle is placed in dorsiflexion. The examiner attempts to force the ankle into plantar flexion, applying pressure over the dorsum of the foot. To more selectively test the tibialis anterior, the ankle is placed in a position of inversion and full dorsiflexion. The examiner attempts to force the ankle into plantar flexion and eversion. To more selectively test the extensor digitorum longus, the ankle is placed in a position of eversion and full dorsiflexion. The examiner attempts to force the ankle into plantar flexion and inversion.

Plantar Flexion (Fig. 1–44)
Gastrocnemius (tibial nerve, S1, S2)

Soleus (tibial nerve, S1, S2)

Test. The ankle is placed in plantar flexion. The examiner attempts to force the foot into dorsiflexion, applying pressure over the plantar surface of the foot. To selectively test the gastrocnemius, the knee is extended. To more selectively test the soleus, the knee is flexed to 90 degrees.

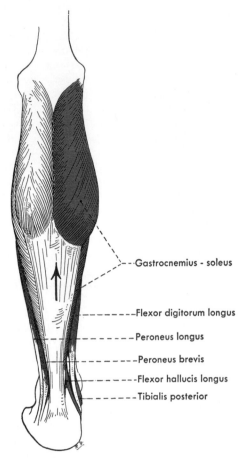

FIGURE 1–44 Ankle plantar flexors. (From Jenkins DB: Hollingshead's Functional Anatomy of the Limbs and Back, ed 6. Philadelphia, WB Saunders, 1991.)

These muscles are so strong that more functional tests such as standing or walking on toes may show weakness missed during MMT.

Inversion (Fig. 1–45)

Tibialis anterior (deep peroneal nerve, L4, L5, S1)

Tibialis posterior (tibial nerve, L5, S1)

Flexor digitorum longus (tibial nerve, L5, S1)

Flexor hallucis longus (tibial nerve, L5, S1, S2)

   Test. The tibialis anterior is more selectively tested in a position of inversion and dorsiflexion. The examiner attempts to force the foot into eversion and plantar flexion, applying pressure on the medial surface of the foot. The other three muscles produce plantar flexion and inversion. They are more selectively tested with placement of the foot in inversion and plantar flexion. The examiner attempts to force the foot into eversion and dorsiflexion, applying pressure on the medial surface of the foot.

Eversion (Fig. 1–46)

Extensor digitorum longus (deep peroneal nerve, L4, L5, S1)

Peroneus longus (superficial peroneal nerve, L4, L5, S1)

Peroneus brevis (superficial peroneal nerve, L4, L5, S1)

   Test. The extensor digitorum longus is more selectively tested in the position of eversion and dorsiflexion. The examiner attempts to force the foot into inversion and plantar flexion, applying pressure over the lateral surface of the foot. The peroneus longus and brevis produce plantar flexion and eversion. They are more selectively tested with placement of the foot in eversion and plantar flexion. The examiner attempts to force the foot into inversion and dorsiflexion, applying pressure over the lateral surface of the foot.

FOOT MOVEMENTS
First Digit Extension

Extensor hallucis longus (deep peroneal nerve, L4, L5, S1)

   Test. The first toe is placed in full extension. The examiner attempts to force it into flexion, applying pressure over the dorsum of the first toe.

Second to Fifth Digit Extension

Extensor digitorum longus (deep peroneal nerve, L4, L5, S1)

Extensor digitorum brevis (deep peroneal nerve, L5, S1)

   Test. The second to fifth toes are placed in full exten-

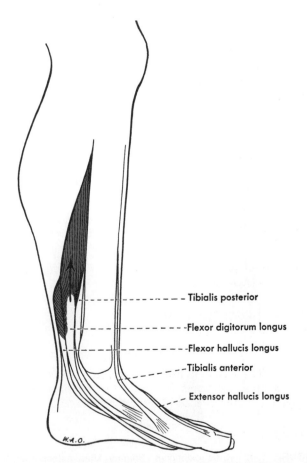

FIGURE 1–45 Ankle invertors. (From Jenkins DB: Hollingshead's Functional Anatomy of the Limbs and Back, ed 6. Philadelphia, WB Saunders, 1991.)

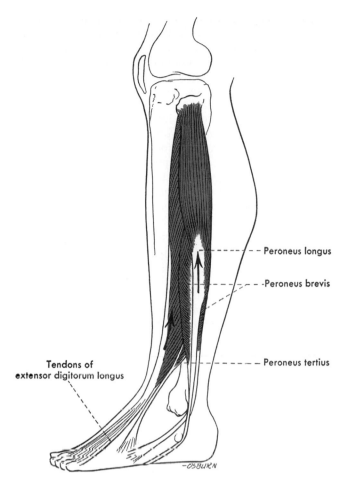

Tendons of
extensor digitorum longus

- - - - - Peroneus longus

- - - Peroneus brevis

- - - - Peroneus tertius

—OSBURN

FIGURE 1–46 Ankle evertors. (From Jenkins DB: Hollingshead's Functional Anatomy of the Limbs and Back, ed 6. Philadelphia, WB Saunders, 1991.)

sion. The examiner attempts to force them into flexion, applying pressure over the dorsum of the toes.

First Digit Flexion
Flexor hallucis longus (tibial nerve, L5, S1, S2)

Flexor hallucis brevis (medial plantar nerve, L5, S1)

Test. The first toe is placed in full flexion. The examiner attempts to force it into extension, applying pressure over the plantar surface of the first toe.

Second to Fifth Digit Flexion
Flexor digitorum longus (tibial nerve, L5, S1)

Flexor digitorum brevis (medial plantar nerve, L5, S1)

Test. The second to fifth toes are placed in full flexion. The examiner attempts to force them into extension, applying pressure over the plantar surface of the toes.

Neurological

Like the musculoskeletal examination, a complete neurological examination is essential to identify other impairments that may help to clarify or confirm a diagnosis.

Level of Consciousness

A decreased level of consciousness can prevent or seriously limit a patient from participation in a physiatric therapeutic program. Descriptive statements, including such adjectives as *lethargic,* are helpful, but are often misinterpreted by others due to the subjectivity of the information. Other subjective but sometimes helpful information includes the length of time and consistency with which an individual is able to attend to a task or to follow commands of the examiner before being unable to respond due to lethargy. This information is not only an indication of an individual's level of consciousness but also of endurance of attentiveness. A commonly used objective scale for an individual with impaired consciousness is the Glasgow coma scale (Table 1–11) which assigns a numeric value based on the best eye, motor, and verbal response. The scale ranges from 3 to 15, with 15 being the best score.[17] Patients with the diagnosis of a brain injury are initially evaluated utilizing a consciousness scale such as the Glasgow coma scale, and then periodically monitored for changes in their score. Note that the Glasgow coma scale does not include a measurement of functional capacity and should not be utilized by the practitioner to monitor function.

Mental Status

Many mental status examinations are commonly utilized to document cognitive ability. A simple, short evaluation is important to assess the patient's ability to participate in a therapeutic program. Usually this type of evaluation can be done in a few minutes. In-depth cognitive assessments and testing procedures often take several hours and should be completed under the direction of a practitioner who is familiar with the specific testing procedures. A referral for such an in-depth evaluation is often helpful to assist the physiatrist in tailoring the treatment program.

The following tests can be performed in a short cognitive evaluation at the bedside or in a clinic. Table 1–12 lists items that can be included in such a short cognitive evalua-

TABLE 1–11   Glasgow Coma Scale

Eye opening	
Spontaneous	E 4
To speech	3
To pain	2
Nil	1
Best motor response	
Obeys	M 6
Localizes	5
Withdraws	4
Abnormal flexion	3
Extensor response	2
Nil	1
Verbal response	
Oriented	V 5
Confused conversation	4
Inappropriate words	3
Incomprehensible sounds	2
Nil	1
Coma score (E + M + V) = 3 to 15	

From Jennett B, Teasdale G: Assessment of impaired consciousness. Contemp Neurol Series 1981; 20:78.

TABLE 1–12   Brief Bedside Mental Status Evaluation

1. Orientation
   Person, place, time, situation
2. Attention span
   Digit retention
3. Memory
   Immediate recall
   Recall at 5- and 10-minute intervals
4. General information
   Remote memory
   Basic intellect
5. Calculation
   Serial 7s
   Simple mathematics
6. Abstract thinking
   Proverb explanation
7. Judgment
   Societal norms

Adapted from Mancall EL: Alpers and Mancall's Essentials of the Neurologic Examination, ed 2. Philadelphia, FA Davis, 1981.

tion.[21, 22, 29] Adequate communication skills are necessary for participation in this type of evaluation. Patients with communication deficits might perform poorly or be unable to participate. If the patient is unable to answer the evaluation questions, it is appropriate to provide the patient with verbal cues to help with better understanding of the questions. This evaluates the individual's ability to respond appropriately to cues.

Orientation is a basic cognitive skill, and severe disorientation often indicates severe cognitive impairments. Orientation is easily tested by asking patients their name, the place, the time and date, and the present situation or reason for the physiatric evaluation.

Attention span, as discussed previously, can be subjectively documented by noting whether the patient is able to attend to tasks consistently during the history and examination. Digit retention is a more objective test. The examiner asks the patient to recall a series of single-digit numbers immediately, both forward and backward. The patient with an adequate attention span is usually able to recall at least five or six numbers forward and four to five numbers backward.[21]

Memory depends on the ability of an individual both to store and to retrieve information provided. The examiner provides the patient with three items to remember and asks the patient to immediately recall the items. The patient without immediate recall ability has difficulty with information storage and is unable to remember all three items after a short period of time, with or without cues. The patient with adequate immediate recall is asked to recall the items at a later time, usually after 5 and 10 minutes. The patient with good storage and retrieval of information is able to recall the items without difficulty. The patient with good storage but poor retrieval of information might require cues to recall some or all of the items. A patient who is unable to recall the items with cues might have information storage difficulties. Documentation of memory ability should include the number of items recalled and if cues were required.

Evaluation of general information helps assess the individual's remote memory and basic intellectual skills. The examiner should always take into account the patient's premorbid education and experience level and ask questions that the patient should be able to answer. Questions concerning common elected officials' names, such as that of the current President and those of recent past Presidents, state senators, and governors, are often appropriate. Well-known locations, such as state capitals and local tourist attractions, are common questions. Current events questions are appropriate for an individual who normally follows local or national news. Very simple questions concerning holidays are appropriate for the patient who is having difficulty with the preceding questions.

Calculation is tested by requesting that the patient serially subtract 7 from 100. Other simple addition, subtraction, multiplication, or division problems are appropriate. Problems with increasing difficulty can be presented if the patient is able to answer simple problems correctly. These questions are inappropriate for the patient who has not had formal mathematics education. If this patient normally purchases items without problems, then testing using monetary examples is appropriate.

Proverb explanation is commonly used to assess abstract thinking. A patient who has lost abstract thought ability will provide a concrete explanation, missing the basic principle of the proverb. Many individuals' educational backgrounds did not involve the use of proverbs, which can affect the patients' ability to answer correctly.

Judgment, like many of the other mental status activities, depends on the patient's background experience, but simple questions that reflect societal norms are often acceptable. Examples of such questions include what is done if a person smells smoke in a crowded theater, why it is inappropriate to yell "fire" in a theater, or what to do if a stamped and addressed envelope is found on the ground. (See Chapter 4 for further information.)

Communication

Communication deficits are often noted after an injury or illness. Specific in-depth evaluation of communication is necessary for any such individual, but a short examination at the hospital bedside or in the clinic can help guide the physiatrist in prescribing a more accurate treatment plan. Items often tested in a short communication examination are listed in Table 1–13.[7, 22] It is inappropriate to make

TABLE 1–13   Brief Bedside Communication Evaluation

1. Comprehension
   Verbal, tactile, and gestural commands
   One- and two-step commands
2. Verbal communication
   Name items
   Repeat words or phrases
   Fluency
   Quality
3. Reading
   Written commands
   Matching item with written word
   Reading comprehension
4. Writing
   Personal items
   Write names of items
5. Gestural communication
   Observation

a specific communication diagnosis after completing only this short examination, but difficulties with the items identify impairments that need to be treated prior to or during the physiatric therapeutic program.

Comprehension is evaluated by asking the patient to follow commands. Initially, these commands should be presented only verbally, thus assessing only auditory comprehension. If no response is obtained, then other gestural or tactile cues are added and the patient is monitored for a response. For example, the examiner might ask the patient to raise an arm. If no response is elicited initially, then the examiner might repeat the command while touching the patient's arm, thus providing a tactile cue. If there is still no response, a gestural cue might be added by repeating the question and touching the patient's arm while the examiner also raises an arm. Document the cues required for the patient to perform the activity. This assessment allows the examiner to evaluate the patient's ability to comprehend by utilizing different types of stimulation. It also provides the examiner with insight concerning the most effective way to present information.

The patient is also examined as to the level of command comprehension. The initial commands presented should be simple one-step commands such as "raise your arm," "open your mouth," "touch your nose." If the patient is able to do several of these commands without difficulty, then try two-step commands, such as "raise your arm, then open your mouth," which combine two activities that must be done in sequential order. If the patient is able to perform the two-step commands, the examiner might choose to evaluate the patient's ability to do more complex commands.

Verbal skills can be assessed by asking the patient to name simple, common items presented and to repeat simple words or phrases. The examiner should closely monitor the patient's verbal responses throughout the physiatric history and examination as to the appropriateness, the fluency of word utilization, and inappropriate speech repetition. Close monitoring often identifies common verbal problems such as anomias, inability to repeat, jargon, perseveration, and tangential speech. Documentation of decreased or absent verbalization is essential. If close monitoring of the individual with fluency problems is performed, the examiner can often identify the type of word (i.e., verb or noun) that the patient is having difficulty producing. The exact words that are spoken are documented in the individual with a very constricted vocabulary. Speech quality can be documented subjectively by a notation as to the articulation ability, phonation, pitch, tone, or prosody (see Chapter 3 for further information).

Reading and writing can be assessed in a patient with an adequate educational background. The patient's reading comprehension ability is assessed by writing a simple command and then asking the patient to read the command and perform it. The patient's ability to follow both one- and two-step written commands can be assessed in this way. Another common technique to help identify reading or communication problems is to ask the patient to match actual items with the written word. To assess both reading skills and comprehension, the patient is asked to read a sentence or paragraph and to verbally provide the examiner with a short synopsis. The examiner also can ask specific questions about either the same or another paragraph. Writing is evaluated by requesting that the individual write down simple personal data, such as name and address. If he or she is unable to do this, the patient should be asked to copy these items. Requesting that the patient write the names of specific items also helps to identify writing difficulties.

Patients who have difficulty with communication in both the verbal or the written form often use gestures to attempt to communicate. Documentation of appropriate use of gestures by an individual with otherwise poor communication skills helps other involved staff or family to improve communication. Gestural communication in the individual with adequate verbal skills is often utilized as a secondary form of communication. The observation of a patient's use of gestures and whether the gestures appropriately correspond to the verbal communication is important.

Cranial Nerve Examination

Evaluation of cranial nerve function is an essential part of the neurological evaluation. A good cranial nerve evaluation can help to identify the lesion site if an individual has a brainstem problem. (See Table 1–14 for a list of the cranial nerves, their function, and common evaluation procedures.[1, 21, 22])

Sensory Examination

Many clinicians believe that the sensory examination is the most difficult part of the neurological examination. The sensory evaluation can be extensive in the patient with a large number of sensory complaints. It also requires a significant degree of cooperation and subjective response from the patient. All of these facts can make the sensory examination difficult to interpret at times, but if the examination is performed in a systematic manner, valuable information is usually obtained.

The examiner should be aware of the normal dermatomal and peripheral nerve distribution to ensure completeness of the evaluation (Fig. 1–47). It is usually best to evaluate a normal area first, to ensure that the patient understands the sensory examination process. The sensory examination is also organized to evaluate both superficial and deep somatic sensations along with discriminative sensory functions.[1, 21]

The three superficial somatic sensations are touch, superficial pain, and thermal sensations. Touch is easily tested with a wisp of cotton. Superficial pain is assessed by a careful pinprick evaluation, because harshly applied stimuli can draw blood. Usually, the patient is asked to tell the examiner where and when each type of stimulus (cotton wisp or pinprick) is applied. The patient can also be asked to compare each stimulus applied with the sensation felt when the same stimulus is applied to an area of known normal sensation. Thermal sensation is commonly evaluated by the use of test tubes, one with hot water and another with cold water or chipped ice. The patient is asked to relate which test tube is touching a specific skin area. Also, the examiner can test just one thermal sensation (either hot or cold) and request that the patient relate any abnormal sensation it produces in the different areas of the body.

TABLE 1–14   Cranial Nerve Examination Techniques

Cranial Nerve	Test
I. Olfactory	Ask patient to smell common substances such as coffee, lemon, vinegar, peppermint, and rose water.
II. Optic	Perform funduscopic evaluation of optic nerve. Acuity testing can be done using standardized acuity charts if available. If charts are not available, then less accurate testing can be done by having the patient read different size newsprint. Visual field testing using the finger confrontation technique can reveal large visual field deficits. Small field deficits may require formal visual testing for diagnosis.
III. Oculomotor IV. Trochlear VI. Abducens	All three nerves are best tested together by checking ocular motility and pupillary reactions. The oculomotor nerve provides innervation to the superior rectus, the inferior rectus, the medial rectus, and the inferior oblique muscles of the eye. The trochlear nerve provides innervation to the superior oblique muscle whereas the abducens provides innervation to the last eye muscle, lateral rectus. The pupillary response is checked by flashing light in each eye and looking for an equal and contralateral pupillary contraction.
V. Trigeminal	This provides motor innervation to the masseter and temporal muscles, which are evaluated by asking the patient to clench his teeth; the examiner then palpates the cheek to feel the muscle contraction. The trigeminal nerve also supplies sensory innervation to the face and is easily evaluated using pinprick, thermal or light touch sensations. The trigeminal nerve is also evaluated by the corneal reflex (see Table 1–17).
VII. Facial	This provides motor innervation to the muscles of facial expression and taste sensation of the anterior two-thirds of the tongue. The examiner evaluates facial muscle movement by forehead wrinkling, eye closure, lip pursing, smiling, or grimacing. Upper motor neuron lesions do not manifest forehead weakness because this muscle is innervated by both sides of the cortex. A lower motor neuron lesion manifests weakness of all facial muscles. Taste of the anterior tongue can be tested using sugar or salt.
VIII. Auditory	The cochlear division is tested by using a tuning fork and performing the Rinne and Weber tests. Formal auditory testing is appropriate for the patient with auditory acuity problems. The vestibular portion is evaluated by observing for nystagmus. Caloric testing is appropriate in the patient with impaired consciousness.
IX. Glossopharyngeal	This supplies taste sensation to the posterior two-thirds of the tongue; it can be tested with either salt or sugar. It also supplies sensation to the pharynx and is tested along with the vagus nerve (next).
X. Vagus	This is the principal motor nerve to the pharynx and larynx. It is examined by watching the patient's soft palate and uvula move when saying "Ah." Gag reflex is tested by stimulating the back of the pharynx. The vagus nerve also provides motor innervation to the diaphragm muscle. Abnormal motion of the diaphragm indicates vagus nerve abnormality.
XI. Spinal accessory	This innervates the trapezius and sternocleidomastoid muscles. It is tested by resisting a shoulder shrug (trapezius) or by resisted head turning to one side (sternocleidomastoid).
XII. Hypoglossal	This innervates the tongue muscles. It is evaluated by tongue protrusion and observation for abnormal tongue movements.

Proprioception, vibration sense, and deep pain or pressure are all considered to be deep somatic sensations. Proprioception or joint position sensation is evaluated by testing the patient's perception of a distal joint position and motion. Often, the great toe in the lower limb and the small joints of the hand in the upper limb are used. If the patient has abnormal position sensation in the distal joints, then more proximal joints are tested to identify the level at which the patient's position sense is preserved. When moving the body part, it is important that the sides of the body part are grasped rather than the top or the bottom, as the patient may be able to perceive pressure in those areas, which would make the test less accurate. Distal to proximal vibratory sensation is also tested in the limbs with a tuning fork with a low frequency and long duration of vibration (128 dv). Usually the patient is asked to state when the vibration of the fork touching a bony prominence has disappeared. The fork is then immediately placed over a normal bony sensory area and the examiner asks the patient if the vibration is still perceived. As an alternative, after the patient's sense of vibration has disappeared, the fork can be placed on the same area of the examiner's body to compare the patient's sense with the examiner's vibratory sense. Deep pain or pressure is evaluated in each limb by deep palpation of a muscle group or by a firm pinch applied to a muscle tendon.

Discriminative sensory functions are called *cortical* or *integrative sensations,* because an abnormality in these functions usually results from a lesion in the sensory cortex or thalamocortical pathways.[1] These functions include two-point discrimination, cutaneous tactile localization, graphesthesia, and stereognosis. All three of these sensory functions depend on adequate superficial and deep somatic sensations. Poor somatic sensation prevents accurate testing of the discriminative functions.

Two-point discrimination is only accurately tested with a calibrated compass, with both compass points applied simultaneously. A less accurate but often more practical technique uses a paper clip with the two ends separated and measured so the distance between them is known. The examiner asks the patient if one or two stimulation points are felt. The normal distance at which two separate points are distinguished varies depending on the body area being tested. Common areas for such evaluation include the fingertips (normal separation, 3 to 5 mm), the dorsal surface of the hands and feet (normal separation, 20 to 30 mm), and the body surface (normal separation, 4 to 7 cm).[21] Cutaneous tactile localization is evaluated by asking the patient to close the eyes and to indicate the area that is touched or stimulated with a pinprick by the examiner. The patient should be able to indicate the area accurately over the hands and fingers, and within a few millimeters over the rest of the body. Graphesthesia is the ability to recognize numbers or letters traced on the body, often on the palm of the hand. Stereognosis is the ability to recognize familiar objects, such as a coin or safety pin, that are

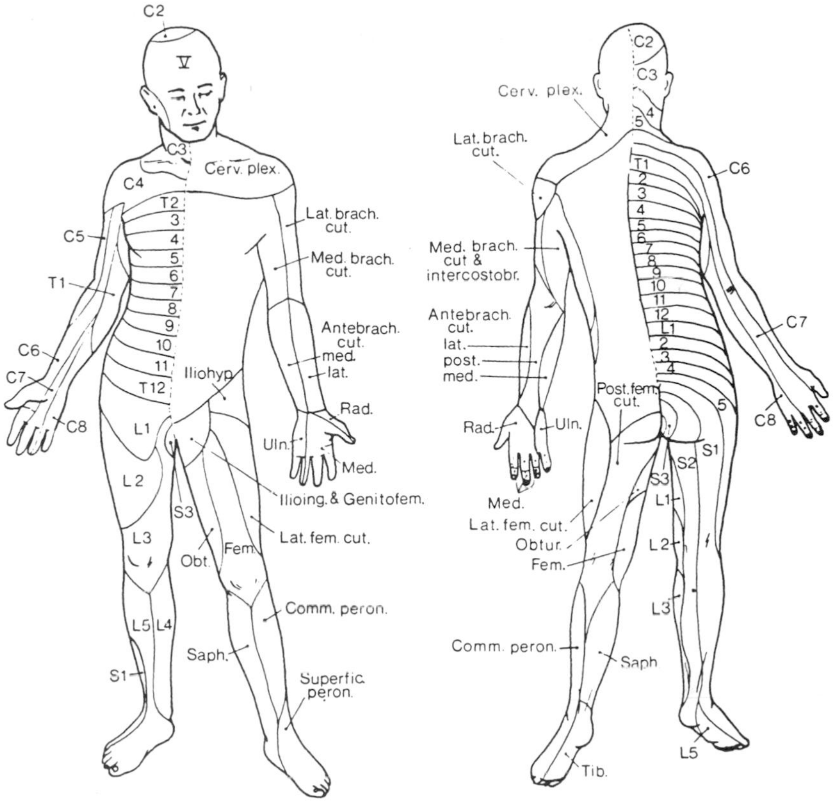

FIGURE 1–47 Distribution of peripheral nerves and dermatomes. (From Gilroy J, Holliday PT: Basic Neurology. New York, Macmillan, 1982.)

placed in the hand. The patient should be able to indicate the type of coin (e.g., nickel or quarter) placed in the hand.[1]

The phenomenon of sensory extinction or inattention is a discriminative sensation abnormality. It is revealed by simultaneous bilateral presentation of cutaneous stimuli to one area of the body. Extinction is diagnosed if the stimulus on only one side of the body is perceived. This phenomenon is most often seen in patients with a right parietal cortical lesion in which the left stimulus is neglected or extinguished.[1]

Motor Control

Motor control depends on adequate muscle strength, balance, coordination, and adequate motor planning of an activity. The presence of involuntary muscle movements can also prevent functional abilities.

Manual muscle testing, already discussed, is performed to evaluate muscle strength. Sitting and standing balance is often tested by applying a mild to moderate pressure or push in all directions to a patient who is in one of those positions. This activity has been discussed in the section on functional examination. Higher-level dynamic balance activities, such as tandem walking or braiding activities, can be tested in a patient who appears to have good standing balance.

Poor coordination can prevent independence in many functional skills. Gross motor coordination of the upper limb is evaluated by the finger-to-nose test. The patient should fully extend the limb to prevent inaccurate test results due to upper arm stabilization by the trunk muscles. Lower limb gross motor coordination is evaluated by the heel, knee-to-shin test. Fine motor coordination is best tested by rapid alternating movements. Hand movements such as hand tapping, rapid pronation and supination of the forearm along with hand tapping, and thumb to sequential finger movements evaluate upper extremity fine motor coordination. (The patient should be directed to touch the thumb to each fingertip in sequence, as quickly as possible.) Foot tapping evaluates fine motor movement in the lower limb. Asking the patient to rapidly repeat "ta" and "pa" evaluates tongue and mouth coordination.

The documentation of involuntary motor movements such as spasticity, tremors, chorea, athetosis, ballismus, and dystonia is important. Definitions of these involuntary movements are given in Table 1–15.

Apraxia is a loss or impairment in executing complex coordinated movements or in motor planning. An individual with apraxia can have difficulty with multiple functional skills, and the apraxia is often not noted until functional activities are evaluated. The examiner should observe the patient for motor planning problems during the functional examination. The patient is often unable to appropriately sequence the motor skills required to perform mobility activities, but has adequate strength on formal MMT. Other patients might have difficulty with appropriate object use, such as inappropriate use of feeding utensils and clothing management during dressing skills.

Motor Reflex Examination

Muscle stretch reflex (MSR) evaluation is essential. Each reflex is evaluated for symmetry as compared with the reflex on the opposite side, for hyporeflexic or hyperreflexic activity, and for spreading (reflex contraction noted not only in the muscle tested, but also in adjacent muscles).

TABLE 1–15 Definitions of Involuntary Motor Movements

Type	Definition
Spasticity	A state of hypertonicity associated with involuntary quick muscle contraction, increased muscle tone, and increased muscle stretch reflexes.
Tremors	Involuntary repetitive movements of a body part or parts, most often in a distal limb. The activity may resemble quivering or trembling. May be seen at rest or in association with movement.
Chorea	Involuntary arrhythmic movements that are forcible, rapid, and jerky in quality. Most often the movements are seen in the proximal limbs. They are often incorporated into voluntary movements in an attempt to make them less noticeable.
Ballisimus	These are unusually violent and flinging motions of the limbs.
Athetosis	A condition characterized by the inability to sustain a body part or parts in one position. Most often the distal limbs (fingers, hands, toes) are affected. The movements are relatively slow and fluid in nature.
Dystonia	A persistent posturing in one or more of the extremities, trunk, neck, or face.

From Adams RD, Victor M: Principles of Neurology, ed 5. New York, McGraw-Hill, 1993.

The MSRs should be observed to make certain that the appropriate response is obtained. Sometimes the opposite response occurs: the so-called *inverted reflex response.* See Table 1–16 for commonly evaluated MSRs.

Superficial reflex abnormality is noted in many individuals with neurological impairments (Table 1–17). Corneal, pharyngeal, and palatal reflexes are important in the patient with a suspected brainstem lesion. The other listed reflexes are very important in the diagnosis and level of spinal cord dysfunction.

Many abnormal reflexes can be observed after an illness or injury. The Babinski reflex or abnormal plantar response

TABLE 1–16 Muscle Stretch Reflexes

Reflex	Segmental Level
Biceps	C5, C6
Pronator teres	C6, C7
Triceps	C7, C8
Flexor digitorum profundus	C7, C8
Patellar	L2, L3, L4
Medial hamstrings	L5, S1
Achilles	S1, S2

is common. The reflex is elicited by stroking from the heel to the great toe on the base of the foot. The normal plantar reflex is flexion of the toes. The Babinski reflex is described as the abnormal extension and fanning of the toes. The Hoffman reflex is noted in the hand. It is elicited by very quick flexion of the third digit distal interphalangeal joint. The abnormal motion observed is a quick flexion movement of the ipsilateral thumb. Both of these reflexes can be indicative of an upper motor neuron lesion. The Hoffman reflex is normal in some individuals, especially in young women.

Primitive reflexes are abnormal adult reflexes that represent a return to a more infantile level of reflex activity. These often result from injury to the frontal cortex, but they are also seen in other disease processes. The *snout, rooting, palmomental,* and *reflex grasp reflexes* are all considered to be primitive reflexes.[21] The snout reflex is a lip-pursing response to a tap either just above or below the mouth. The rooting reflex is a quick contraction of the ipsilateral periorbital muscles toward a brushing tactile stimulus presented to the side of the mouth. A palmomental reflex is ipsilateral contraction of the chin facial muscles produced by a brisk tactile stimulation to the palm or brisk rotation motion of the thumb. Tactile stimulation to the palm can also produce a reflex grasp. The reflex grasp becomes stronger as the examiner attempts to remove his or her hand, which distinguishes the reflex from a voluntary grasp.

TABLE 1–17 Important Normal Superficial Reflexes

	Elicited By	Response	Segmental Level
Corneal	Touching cornea with hair	Contraction of orbicularis oculi	Pons
Pharyngeal	Touching posterior wall of pharynx	Contraction of pharynx	Medulla
Palatal	Touching soft palate	Elevation of palate	Medulla
Scapular	Stroking skin between scapulae	Contraction of scapular muscles	C5–T1
Epigastric	Stroking downward from nipples	Dimpling of epigastrium ipsilaterally	T7–T9
Abdominal	Stroking beneath costal margins and above inguinal ligament	Contraction of abdominal muscles in quadrant stimulated	T8–T12
Cremasteric	Stroking medial surface of upper thigh	Ipsilateral elevation of testicle	L1 and L2
Gluteal	Stroking skin of buttock	Contraction of glutei	L4 and L5
Bulbocavernous (male)	Pinching dorsum of glans	Insert gloved finger to palpate anal contraction	S3 and S4
Clitorocavernous (female)	Pinching clitoris	Insert gloved finger to palpate anal contraction	S3 and S4
Superficial anal	Pricking perineum	Contraction of rectal sphincters	S5 and coccygeal

Adapted from Mancall EL: Examination of the nervous system. *In* Alpers and Mancall's Essentials of the Neurologic Examination, ed 2. Philadelphia, FA Davis, 1993, p 25.

TABLE 1–18   Rehabilitation Plan

L.R. is a 32-year-old right-handed black woman, previously an independent homemaker, with a history of sickle cell disease and left hip fracture treated with open reduction and internal fixation 1 year ago; she is presenting for rehabilitation for paraplegia due to an acute T12 spinal cord injury and compression fracture after a fall 1 week ago. The spine is stable if she wears a thoracic lumbar orthosis when out of bed and when the head of the bed is elevated more than 30 degrees. Physical impairments on examination include flaccid paralysis of the lower limbs, L1 sensory level, poor endurance with upper limb activities, left hip flexion and abduction contracture of 10 degrees each, no clitorocavernous reflex, and no rectal tone. Historically, the patient relates that she has had no bowel movement in 4 days; a Foley catheter is in place, and the only activity she is able to do without assistance is feed herself. Socially, she lives in a second-floor apartment (accessible only by stair climbing) with her husband, who works during the day.

PROBLEM LIST

Rehabilitation problems

1. Functional deficits: Inability to perform any mobility activity, most activities of daily living, or household tasks, and to drive without assistance or assistive devices.
2. Flaccid paralysis bilateral lower limbs: poor lower limb management skills.
3. Poor endurance for upper limb activities.
4. Absent sensation below L1 level: High risk for skin pressure areas.
5. Left hip flexion and abduction contracture: possible positioning problem, high risk for left lower limb skin areas due to positioning problems, possible difficulty with limb management.
6. Flaccid neurogenic bowel: Poor bowel regulation at present.
7. Neurogenic bladder: Needs evaluation for appropriate bladder management.
8. Patient and family adjustment to disability.
9. Sexuality concerns.
10. Discharge planning/living situation: Apartment not wheelchair accessible, equipment needs.

Medical/surgical problems

1. T12 compression fracture: Stable with appropriate wearing of thoracic lumbar orthosis.
2. Sickle cell disease: Stable at present, but will require monitoring.
3. Left hip fracture with surgical repair 1 year ago: Surgically healed, but patient has a residual flexion and abduction contracture.

MANAGEMENT PLAN

1. Physical therapy (PT) to address mobility deficits concentrating on wheelchair activities, transfer skills, upper extremity endurance for these activities, sitting balance, and tolerance. The physical therapist will instruct patient on lower limb range of motion and management, concentrating on decreasing the left lower limb contractures. All team members will reinforce the skills once patient has received basic instructions from the PT.
2. Occupational therapy (OT) will concentrate on upper limb strengthening and endurance, activities of daily living, and, when it is appropriate, have patient begin homemaking and driving with assistive devices. All team members will reinforce the skills once patient has received basic instructions from the OT.
3. Nursing (RN) to monitor skin and assist patient with bowel and bladder management.
4. The management team (physician, PT, OT, RN, recreational therapist, psychologist, social worker, etc.) presents a patient-specific rehabilitation education program concentrating on prevention of future problems related to accessibility, mobility, skin, bowel, bladder, sexuality, and psychosocial and medical/surgical problems.
5. Community issues such as accessibility, driving, social activities, and difficult psychosocial situations are addressed by the team.
6. Management team emphasis is placed on helping patient identify appropriate discharge placement, including accessible living arrangement, home modifications if needed, special equipment needs, and support systems for financial and psychosocial issues.
7. Management team continues to monitor for lower limb strength and sensory improvements.
8. Management team continues to monitor for emergence of muscle tone in rectal and lower limb muscles.
9. Spinal stability maintained by patient's wearing of the spinal orthosis. Periodic spinal radiographs taken when necessary.
10. Maintain stability of the sickle cell disease with close monitoring of blood count and symptoms. Provide blood transfusions or other treatments as necessary.

Therapeutic precautions: Patient to wear spinal orthosis when out of bed and when head of bed is elevated more than 30 degrees.

Therapeutic setting: Inpatient rehabilitation setting necessary because patient is not safe or able to return to her previous living arrangement.

GOALS

1. Independence with wheelchair mobility skills.
2. Independence with activities of daily living.
3. Independence with household tasks at a wheelchair level.
4. Independence with driving with assistive devices.
5. Supervision or independence for community reentry activities.
6. Independence with lower limb management and range of motion program.
7. Independence with the bladder management program.
8. Independence with the bowel management program, or if patient unable to provide own bowel care due to trunk range of motion limit from the spinal orthosis, then independence with ability to instruct another to perform the bowel management program.
9. Independence with skin management program.
10. Knowledge of sexuality related issues.
11. Independence in knowledge about future medical/surgical problems related to spinal cord injury.
12. Identify a safe, accessible living situation.
13. Obtain necessary equipment.
14. Maintain stability of the sickle cell disease.
15. Maintain spinal stability.

Estimated time of goal attainment: 3 to 4 weeks.

Obstacles to goal attainment:

1. Decreased trunk range of motion due to spinal orthosis, which might prevent independence in some activities.
2. Left hip contractures might cause positioning and skin and limb management difficulties.
3. Poor upper limb endurance might prevent good progress in the rehabilitation program.

Time of reassessment of patient's status: 1 week.

General Medical Examination

A general medical examination is completed for all patients to rule out problems that might have an impact on progress in a physiatric therapeutic program. The examiner should be familiar with the general medical examination techniques as described in such reference texts as DeGowin and DeGowin,[8] and Bates.[3]

SUMMARY, PROBLEM LIST, PLAN, AND GOALS

After the physiatrist collects baseline patient data by history and examination, the information should be organized into a problem-oriented medical record.[9, 12, 30] This organization provides easy understanding of the data and allows other healthcare professionals quick access to information regarding the patient's status and treatment plans.

A summary of no more than a few sentences identifies the patient's major problems in a narrative form. The summary includes pertinent impairments, functional deficits, and medical and surgical problems. From the summary, the physician formulates a problem list. A recommended modification of the problems list separates the rehabilitation problems from the medical and surgical problems.[30] The separate problem lists help to further organize and simplify the problem list.

From this type of problem list the physiatrist develops a management plan, including treatment options for both the rehabilitation and medical or surgical problems. The management plan should be interdisciplinary and should address functional deficits, physical impairments, and psychosocial, medical, and surgical problems. The treatment plan addressing physical, occupational, or speech therapy options should identify specific recommendations for both exercise and treatment modalities. The physiatrist documents both therapeutic precautions and the treatment setting (either inpatient or outpatient).

In the rehabilitation setting, identification of treatment goals is necessary. The physiatrist identifies goals based on a realistic appraisal of rehabilitation and medical status, attainable after completion of the treatment plan. Obstacles to the goals and the estimated time of goal attainment are documented. Documentation of the time of patient reassessment is important. Periodic re-evaluation of the patient's progress in the treatment program allows the physiatrist to identify problems that require a readjustment of the plan and goals.

Table 1–18 is an example of a problem-oriented medical record that includes summary, problem list, management plan, and treatment goals.

References

1. Adams RD, Victor M: Principles of Neurology, ed 5. New York, McGraw-Hill, 1993.
2. American Medical Association: Guides to the Evaluation of Permanent Impairment, ed 4. Chicago, American Medical Association, 1994.
3. Bates B: A Guide to Physical Examination, ed 6. Philadelphia, JB Lippincott, 1991.
4. Cole TM, Tobis JS: Measurement of musculoskeletal function. In Kottke FJ, Lehmann JF (eds): Krusen's Handbook of Physical Medicine and Rehabilitation, ed 4. Philadelphia, WB Saunders, 1990, pp 20–71.
5. D'Ambrosia RD: Musculoskeletal Disorders: Regional Examination and Differential Diagnosis, ed 2. Philadelphia, JB Lippincott, 1986.
6. Daniels L, Worthingham C: Muscle Testing: Techniques of Manual Examination, ed 5. Philadelphia, WB Saunders, 1986.
7. Darley FL: Treatment of acquired aphasia. Adv Neurol 1975; 7:111–145.
8. DeGowin EL, DeGowin RL: Bedside Diagnostic Examination, ed 6. New York, Macmillan, 1994.
9. Dinsdale SM, Massman PL, Gullickson G, et al: The problem-oriented medical record in rehabilitation. Arch Phys Med Rehabil 1970; 51:488–492.
10. Erickson RP, McPhee MC: Clinical evaluation. In Delisa JA, Gans BM (eds): Rehabilitation Medicine: Principles and Practice, ed 2. Philadelphia, JB Lippincott, 1993, pp 51–95.
11. Gerhard JJ: Documentation of Joint Motion, rev ed 3. Portland, Oregon Medical Association, 1992.
12. Grabois M: The problem-oriented medical record: Modification and simplification for rehabilitation medicine. South Med J 1977; 70:1383–1385.
13. Guide for the Uniform Data Set for Medical Rehabilitation (Adult FIM), version 4.0. Buffalo, NY, State University of New York, 1993.
14. Hellebrandt FA, Duvall EN, Moore ML: The measurement of joint motion: III. Reliability of goniometry. Phys Ther Rev 1949; 29:302–307.
15. Hoppenfeld S: Physical Examination of the Spine and Extremities. New York, Appleton-Century-Crofts, 1976.
16. Jenkins DB: Hollingshead's Functional Anatomy of the Limbs and Back, ed 6. Philadelphia, WB Saunders, 1991.
17. Jennett B, Teasdale G: Assessment of impaired consciousness. Contemp Neurol 1981; 20:77–93.
18. Kendall FP, McCreary EK, Provance PG: Muscles: Testing and Function, ed 4. Baltimore, Williams & Wilkins, 1993.
19. Knapp ME, West CC: Measurement of joint motion. Univ Minn Med Bull 1944; 15:405–412.
20. Knapp ME: Measuring range of motion. Postgrad Med 1967; 42:A123–A127.
21. Mancall EL: Examination of the nervous system. In Mancall EL (ed): Alpers and Mancall's Essentials of the Neurologic Examination, ed 2. Philadelphia, FA Davis, 1993, pp 1–33.
22. Members of the Department of Neurology, Mayo Clinic and Mayo Foundation for Medical Education and Research: Clinical Examination in Neurology, ed 6. Philadelphia, WB Saunders, 1991.
23. Moll J, Wright V: Measurement of spinal movement. In Jayson MIV (ed): The Lumbar Spine and Back Pain, ed 3. London, Churchill Livingstone, 1987, pp 215–234.
24. Moore ML: Clinical assessment of joint motion. In Basmajian JV (ed): Therapeutic Exercise, ed 4. Baltimore, Williams & Wilkins, 1984, pp 192–224.
25. Moore ML: The measurement of joint motion: II. The technic of goniometry. Phys Ther Rev 1949; 29:256–264.
26. Norkin CC, White DJ: Measurement of Joint Motion: A Guide to Goniometry. Philadelphia, FA Davis, 1985.
27. Stillwell GK, deLateur BJ, Fordyce WE, et al: Physiatric Therapeutics, ed 2. Chicago, American Academy of Physical Medicine and Rehabilitation, 1986.
28. Stolov WC, Hays RM: Evaluation of the patient. In Kottke FJ, Lehmann JF (ed): Krusen's Handbook of Physical Medicine and Rehabilitation, ed 4. Philadelphia, WB Saunders, 1990, pp 1–19.
29. Strub RL, Black FW: The Mental Status Examination in Neurology, ed 3. Philadelphia, FA Davis, 1993.
30. Weed LL: Medical Records, Medical Education, and Patient Care: The Problem-Oriented Record As A Basic Tool. Cleveland, The Press of Case Western Reserve University, 1971.
31. World Health Organization: International Classification of Impairments, Disabilities and Handicaps. Geneva, Switzerland, WHO, 1980.

2

Examination of the Pediatric Patient

DENNIS J. MATTHEWS, M.D.

Examination of the child with suspected functional impairment requires not only assessment of the dysfunction but also understanding of the variations of normal childhood development. It requires an understanding of the interaction of organic pathological processes, normal development, and the psychosocial environment. Establishment of a diagnostic label is important, but determination of the the child's functional status ensures the proper rehabilitation management strategies. While the evaluation of the child has many similarities with that of the adult (see Chapter 1), there are many unique features.

DIAGNOSTIC EVALUATIONS

History

The clinical and developmental history is the basis of an accurate medical and rehabilitation diagnosis. The history is generally obtained from the parent or caretaker. With increasing age, children of school age and older are generally able to participate in the diagnostic interview. It is important to make both the child and parents comfortable. With younger children, long history taking may be facilitated by having the caregiver fill out a new patient questionnaire prior to the clinical examination.

Since cooperation and time are frequently problematic, it is important to quickly identify the chief complaint. This focuses the history and the physical examination. It is important to develop a functional inventory with emphasis on development and daily life, and the impact of the disability or impairment on the child's daily activities. Equally important is noting a child's abilities, limitations, and compensatory functional solutions.

Many childhood disabilities are caused by prenatal and perinatal problems. Maternal disease, acute illnesses, pregnancy and labor abnormalities, and family histories will arouse and guide the diagnostic examination and investigational studies. The time and type of movements of the fetus should be determined. It is important to get the history of duration of the pregnancy, ease or difficulty of labor, and complications of labor and delivery.

History of the newborn period provides many insights. It is important to note Apgar scores, any unusual cyanosis or respiratory distress, seizures, and other physical symptoms such as jaundice, anemia, and dysmorphic features. The parents' description of muscle tone and movement frequently provides insight into primary neuromuscular weakness.

Feeding history may provide warning signs of potential neurological abnormality. It is important to note any difficulties with sucking or swallowing; whether the baby was breast- or bottle-fed, and the volume and frequency of feedings. If feeding difficulties are present, determine the onset of the problems, method of feeding, reasons for changes, interval between feedings, amount taken at each feeding, and crying and weight changes.

Examination of the physical growth rate is important. These data can be plotted on physical growth charts which are readily available.[2, 3, 19, 26, 27, 32] Any sudden gain or loss in physical growth should be noted, particularly because its onset may correspond with the onset of organic or psychosocial illness. It also may be helpful to compare the child's growth with the rate of growth of the siblings or parents.

Determine the ages at which major developmental milestones were met, as this aids in assessing deviations from normal (Table 2-1). Accomplishments of major landmarks in gross motor, fine motor, and adaptive skills; language; and personal and social behavior should clarify whether the disability is confined primarily to the neuromuscular system or involves deficits in other areas as well. The coexistence of multiple problems will influence the rehabilitation program, interventional methods, and ultimate outcome.

Familiarity with the normal landmarks of early childhood development helps in the assessment of the infant

TABLE 2–1   Developmental Milestones

Age (mo)	Milestones
1	Lifts head (prone), vocalizes
3	Follows, laughs, smiles, good head control
5	Plays with feet, reaches for and grasps objects
6	Sits with support
8	Sits without support; equilibrium reflexes present; looks for objects
9	Plays peekaboo, gets to sitting position; parachute reflex; stranger anxiety
10	Pulls to stand, cruises, babbles
12–14	First words; walks
18	Multiple single words; uses spoon, removes clothes
24	Two-word phrases; throws overhand; "terrible 2s"
30	Knows full name, puts on clothing
36	Jumps, pedals tricycle, learns nursery rhymes
48	Hops, plays with others

and toddler.[5, 9, 18–20, 26, 30, 31, 38] A more formal assessment of the child's development can be made with the use of standardized developmental evaluations (Table 2–2). Most of these tests are easy to administer but they require some test familiarity and the cooperation of the child. Most important is the appropriate interpretation of the information obtained. Most of the infant tests rely heavily on motor responses to assess the child's interest in learning.[10] If children have major physical disabilities, drawing inferences about the child's current or future intellectual abilities has limitations.[10, 11, 28]

A psychosocial evaluation contributes to the understanding and management of the handicapped child. It assesses the child's learning style, probable impediments to learning, and the extent to which the child has built upon previous learning experiences. It describes the behavioral and cognitive strengths and weaknesses so that specific programming can be addressed both at home and in the school setting. A frequently valuable strategy is to get a description of the typical day's schedule. This provides insight into the functional impact of the disability.

A family history of similar or related problems is helpful. A formal pedigree often helps delineate inherited or congenital problems. Formal genetic counseling and evaluation is mandatory whenever a familial disease is suspected or known to exist.

Physical Examination

There is no routine or standard physical examination of children.[1, 5, 18, 19, 24] Each examination is individualized.

There are many physical differences which an examiner accustomed to adults might mistakenly consider abnormal in a child. There is a broad spectrum included in the term "normal." A single examination is valuable for determining current and acute illnesses, but the rate of change observed in serial examinations is frequently more important in the pediatric setting.

Every physician develops some "tricks" of examination with experience. The examination is generally performed with the parents present. The examination room should be comfortable and have an assortment of toys, games, and books to help put the child at ease. The examiner must create a relaxed atmosphere and devote sufficient time to establish a relationship of trust. Friendly advances during the history taking will allay some of the child's fear in preparation for the actual examination.

Observation is the first and frequently the most informative part of the examination. Many observations can actually be made as the child is brought into or walks into the examination room. Let the child sit on the parent's lap, or play with toys and games at a low table. A great deal of information about the child can be obtained by observing spontaneous play and interaction with the parent and the physician or examiner. The selection of toys and games may also indicate developmental level.

Begin the physical examination without instruments and gradually introduce the various necessary examining equipment. Physical examinations are performed on children by taking full advantage of opportunities that present themselves. The order of examination is more or less determined by the child rather than by the physician. Most examinations are performed with the child in the sitting position, although there are some children that prefer to stand or assume a variety of unusual positions.

The child is gradually undressed. Gentle touching, tickling, or funny sounds may make the child much more interactive. It is important to observe the child's general appearance. Through inspection, you are frequently able to detect physical anomalies, asymmetries, and weak or involuntary muscle movements. The skin is evaluated for lesions or abnormalities. Calluses, scars, bruises, and abrasions may indicate abnormalities in motor development and weightbearing.

Development of the skeletal musculature can be assessed by observing the present location and distribution of any atrophy or anomalies. Range of motion and contractures are observed through movement and spontaneous play.

Palpation of the skin and muscles may indicate abnormalities in the subcutaneous or underlying structures. Muscles are palpated to indicate size, bulk, and tone. Localized pain and swelling around joints need to be approached

TABLE 2–2   Developmental Evaluation and Screening Tests

Test	Age Range	Scope and Value
Denver Developmental Screening Test[15]	Birth–6 yr	Quick screen for deviations from normal development of normal and near-normal children; pattern of functional deviations guides further evaluation
Bayley Scale of Infant Development[3]	Birth–30 mo	Separate mental and motor scales; well-standardized; heavily weighted with motor-based items which limits predictive value in physically handicapped children
Gesell Developmental Schedule[17]	4 wk–6 yr	Indicator of current developmental level

carefully. Before anything frightening or painful is contemplated, it is important that the child and his or her parents be informed of what to expect. Generally, the use of instruments and potentially painful examination activities should be delayed until near the end of the examination (e.g., examination of the ears and throat). The complete physical examination should typically take the experienced physician no longer than 5 to 10 minutes. Rapid assessment is necessary to avoid exhausting the patient and his or her ability to provide limited cooperation. Regardless of the chief complaint or reason for a visit, a complete systematic examination should be performed and any abnormalities noted. Misdiagnosis is most frequently caused by careless omissions of simple procedures. Physiatrists should perform a complete general physical examination, even though the general primary healthcare of the handicapped child usually remains the responsibility of the primary pediatrician.

Examination of the neuromuscular system includes testing of reflexes, tone, active motion, coordination, and strength.[22] During the pediatric examination, most of these are assessed simultaneously rather than sequentially.

For the physiatrist, perhaps the most intimidating portion of the examination of the infant and toddler is interpretation of abnormal developmental reflexes (Table 2–3). The infantile developmental reflexes are related to various complex functions of the brainstem and spinal cord.[8, 9, 18, 20, 24, 31, 34] As higher, often cortical, control develops with age, these reflexes tend to disappear or change form. Failure to develop these reflexes, continuation of them past the usual age of disappearance, or asymmetrical expression of the reflexes are often important clues to the developmental status of the infant's nervous system.

As the child's central nervous system matures, proprioceptive patterns of movement become more important. These are generally stereotypical motor responses and spontaneous patterns of movement. They frequently depend upon trunk, head, neck, and limb positions. As the nervous system matures, there is more influence of the vestibular and visual system. Observations are made in regard to persistence of the patterns, frequency of movement, interference with functional activities, and asymmetries in presentations. Frequently, this leads to an assessment of the abnormalities in the development of the child's central and neuromuscular systems.

Muscle tone in newborns and young infants shows a great deal of variation, depending on their state of activity, alertness, and comfort. Flexor tone generally dominates in the first few months. Injuries to the central nervous system can present either as hypertonicity with damage to the cortical spinal or basal ganglia system, or as an initial period of hypotonicity that gradually evolves into hypertonicity. True hypotonia in the infant is generally a manifestation of anterior horn cell disease, myopathy, or neuropathy.

Muscle tightness can frequently assist in the diagnosis of possible muscle weakness. It usually occurs in the muscle group opposite or antagonistic to the paralyzed or weaker muscle group. It is important to routinely and quickly assess range of motion and muscle tightness in children. Children under the age of 4 to 5 years generally do not cooperate with formal muscle testing. Observation of their active motion most frequently provides information in regard to muscle strength. Infants need to be positioned so that the muscle group being tested can lift the appropriate part of the body against gravity. Specific muscle groups can be tested with withdrawal from stroking or tickling and, on some occasions, with noxious stimuli.

Young children should be observed to see which compensatory movement methods they have developed. Children generally move any way they can and they show great inventiveness in developing their own functional solutions. It is important to observe the child rolling, pulling to sitting, sitting without support, crawling, pulling to stand, and walking. The movement pattern frequently demonstrates a potential muscle weakness. A child's gait pattern is typically not stabilized until about the age of 7 years.[22] One must know what gait to expect of children of different ages. A child of 2 is starting to learn to run. By 3 years of age children can run very well. A 3-year-old is also able to walk on tiptoes, squat, and rise to a standing position without using the arms for help. A 4-year-old is able to hop and walk on heels and toes with adequate balance.

Routine manual muscle testing can be applied from school age on. The scoring system is similar to that used for adults, although compensation is made for body size and movement against gravity. Quantitative measurements are generally not required unless specific therapeutic interventions are contemplated.[29] Detection of incoordinated movements is based mostly on observing gross and fine motor activities. Since the impaired coordination is a common sign of central movement disorders, specific examinations can be more directed as the child gets older. Most children are able to walk a straight line unsteadily by placing one foot in front of the other around age 3, but tandem walking is usually not done well until age 5. With school-age children, formal evaluations of coordination and balance can be utilized. Other subtle symptoms include clumsiness of handwriting, drawing difficulties, problems with physical education and sporting activities, and on some occasions, avoiding particular motor activities.

The sensory examination also needs to be age-adjusted. Withdrawal to touch or pinprick in early infancy, along with crying and squirming, demonstrates that sensation is perceived. Withdrawal with isolated spinal reflex activity can be confused with volitional response, and knowledge of infant movement patterns will be helpful. Frequently, contrasting the infant's reaction to stimuli on the arms and face may help assess sensory abnormalities. Generally, by school age, children are able to cooperate with the sensory evaluation used in adults.

Examination of vision also has to be adapted based on

TABLE 2–3 Developmental Reflexes

Reflex	Present At	Disappears By
Root	Birth	3 mo
Moro	Birth	4–6 mo
Asymmetrical tonic neck	Birth	6–7 mo
Symmetrical tonic neck	2 mo	6–7 mo
Protective reactions		
Forward	5–6 mo	Persists
Lateral	6–7 mo	Persists
Posterior	9–10 mo	Persists

the child's ability to cooperate. The infant is able to follow a stimulus with the eyes to midline by 1 month and through 180 degrees by 3 months. Central nervous system dysfunction frequently presents with ocular motor imbalance.

Developmental Diagnosis

Assessment

Familiarity with the normal landmarks of early child development is essential to the assessment of the infant and toddler. The assessment should include a description of the child's gross motor and fine motor responses, verbal and nonverbal language, personal and social behavior, emotional characteristics, and adaptive skills. A formal assessment of the child's developmental status requires the use of a standardized examination. A multidisciplinary evaluation is particularly helpful when the initial diagnosis is being established and interventions are planned for a young child. It also can be used for periodic assessment of developmental progress throughout childhood and adolescence, especially for appropriate educational planning. It provides an assessment of overall development and its rate relative to other children. Diagnostic assessment relies on normed reference instruments that convey the child's developmental standing relative to a normal peer group. It provides valuable information on the assessment and formulation of the child's strengths and weaknesses for the purpose of individual program planning.

The results of infant tests are best interpreted as a measure of the infant's current developmental status relative to a normal peer group. Infant tests rely heavily on motor responses to assess the child's interest and learning. It can be difficult to draw inferences about the child's current or future intellectual ability in the presence of known physical limitations. Repeated studies have found low correlation between abilities measured on infant tests and later childhood intelligence quotients (IQs).[3, 10, 11] It is essential that infant test results be considered provisional and followed by periodic re-evaluation for further diagnostic and prognostic clarification.

The assessment of preschool and school-age children includes both physical and intellectual abilities. The strength of intelligence tests lies in their correlation with school performance (Table 2–4). Appropriately interpreted, they reflect the probability of standard academic achievement. It is important to note both overall score and the subscores to assess whether the child's abilities are evenly developed or whether there are patterns of strengths and weaknesses that are relevant to learning and general adaption.[10]

Most of the standardized intelligence tests rely heavily on language and motor performance. For some disabled children, (e.g., those with central language impairments, significant motor difficulties, and sensory deficits), alternative nonverbal and motor-eliminated assessments may be needed (Table 2–5). Vocabulary tests typically show the strongest correlation with overall intellectual ability and school success.

The test composite scores, or full-scale scores (IQs), are used to designate a child's overall level of intellectual functioning.[10] This is derived by comparing an individual child's performance with the performance of hundreds of children in a representative age-stratified norm group. On most tests, the mean score is 100, which represents average or normal intelligence. Classifications as superior or subaverage typically refer to scores that fall 2 SD above or below the mean. A definition of mental retardation, then, includes three components: (1) subaverage general intelligence, (2) concurrent deficits in adaptive behavior, and (3) developmental delay. Generally, all three criteria must be present to formally diagnose mental retardation.

The classification of mild mental retardation (IQ 55–69) encompasses the largest number of children with mental retardation. Generally they show delayed language development as a toddler and weaknesses in the acquisition of pre-academic writing skills. These children generally reach the third- to fifth-grade level academically. If the associated physical handicaps are mild enough, they may be independent in activities of daily living and achieve relative independence in adulthood.

Children with moderate mental retardation (IQ 40–54) have a slower rate of developmental attainment. There is also a higher incidence of neurological and physical disabilities. These children are frequently in special classes and are taught primarily self-care and practical daily living skills. As adults, many are able to achieve some independence in self-care skills, but usually continue to require supervision either at home or in group homes, and vocationally function primarily in sheltered workshops or protected employment.

The children with severe mental retardation (IQ 25–39) develop some functional language skills but no formal academic skills. They require intensive programming to master independence in activities of daily living. They require close supervision and supportive care as an adult. Profoundly retarded children (IQ <25) have limited language ability and limited potential for acquiring self-care skills. They also have a very high association with severe motor handicaps.

Several tests have been designed to evaluate visual-

TABLE 2–4   Intellectual Evaluations

Test	Age Range	Scope and Value
Stanford-Binet Intelligence Scale[37]	2 yr–adult	Detailed diagnostic assessment mental age and IQ; guidelines for hearing, visual, and motor handicaps
Wechsler Preschool and Primary Scale of Intelligence–Revised (WPPSI-R)[40]	3 yr–6½ yr	Verbal, performance, and full-scale scores; delineates strengths and weaknesses; not appropriate with severe developmental delays
Wechsler Intelligence Scale for Children–Revised (WISC-R)[39]	6–16 years	Verbal, performance, and full-scale scores; subtests point to specific areas of strength or dysfunction
Kaufman Assessment Battery for Children[23]	2½–12 yr	Measures mental processes independent of the content of acquired knowledge; useful for disadvantaged backgrounds

TABLE 2–5   Alternative Nonverbal and Motor-Eliminated Tests

Test	Age Range	Scope and Value
Peabody Picture Vocabulary Test (PPVT)[14]	2½–18 yr	Effective test of language, especially in children with speech and motor impairment
Leiter International Performance Scale[25]	2–18 yr	Measures nonverbal problem-solving abilities in deaf and speech- and motor-handicapped
Pictorial Test of Intelligence[16]	3–8 yr	Measures intellectual ability of multiply handicapped children; requires receptive language
Raven's Progressive Matrices[35]	6 yr–adult	Measures nonverbal intelligence and concept formation

TABLE 2–6   Perceptual Evaluations

Test	Age Range	Scope and Value
Beery-Buktenica Development Test of Visual-Motor Integration[4]	2–16 yr	Assesses visual-motor performance; ability to copy geometric shapes; age equivalence
Bender Visual-Motor Gestalt Test[7]	5 yr–adult	Assesses visual-motor performance; easy to administer; nine geometric designs

TABLE 2–7   Academic Achievement Tests

Test	Grade Level/Age Range	Scope and Value
Wide-Range Achievement Test: Revised (WRAT)[21]	Kindergarten–12th grade	Yields academic achievement level in reading, spelling, arithmetic; can measure programs
Woodcock-Johnson Psychoeducational Battery: Test of Achievement[41]	3 yr–adult	Yields age and grade level, percentiles, and standard scores in reading, mathematics, written language, and general tasks
Peabody Individual Achievement Test[13]	Kindergarten–12th grade	Only pointing response for overview of achievement; useful for handicapped

TABLE 2–8   Social and Adaptive Skills

Test	Age Range	Scope and Value
Vineland Adaptive Behavior Scale[36]	1 mo–adult	Questionnaire of social competence in communication, socialization, daily living skills, and motor skills; adjusted for handicapped
AAMD Adaptive Behavior Scale[33]	3 yr–adult	Activities of daily living; adaptive and maladaptive behaviors; assists in program planning

TABLE 2–9   Emotional Adjustment

Test	Age Range	Scope and Value
Manual Children's Apperception Test[6]	3–10 yr	Pictures of animals and humans in various situations; assesses adjustment patterns
Figure drawings[12]	4 yr–adult	Self-image and interpersonal relationships

motor maturity in children, and to detect delays or impairment in visual-perceptual skills and eye-hand coordination (Table 2–6). Children with neurological and developmental disabilities sometimes exhibit difficulties in visual-perceptual, perceptual-motor, auditory, kinesthetic, and tactile functioning. A wide variety of instruments are available to test for these impairments. Achievement tests are designed specifically to evaluate the child's performance in school subject areas (e.g., reading and mathematics) (Table 2–7). Scores are typically given in terms of school-grade equivalence, which can provide an estimate of the child's level of academic skill, as well as standard scores based on age norms. Many are paper-and-pencil tests that penalize handicapped children for their slower pace, poor attention, or difficulty keeping track of their place on the page. It is important that a skilled observer administer the test since observation of task approach can be used to adjust quantitative results.

A complete assessment of the disabled child must include a description of social and adaptive abilities (Table 2–8). It is important to establish the level of achievement in locomotor, communication, and self-care areas such as feeding, dressing, and toileting. It is also important to assess the mode and methods of interaction with family members, peers, and the child's ability to assume increasing levels of responsibility. A number of social adaptive scales have been developed to look at the ages at which children usually achieve such competencies, along with emotional adjustment (Table 2–9).

Care must be taken when arriving at a specific diagnosis on the basis of developmental testing performed early in a patient's life. In addition, central nervous system dysfunction is not incompatible with normal intelligence, and the degree to which a child can be intellectually impaired cannot be predicted solely on the basis of physical or motor deficits. Familiarity with the tests being utilized is essential when interpreting this information.

CONCLUSION

The pediatric examination shares a common purpose with all physiatric examinations: to ascertain the nature and cause of dysfunction. All the biologic, environmental, and developmental factors should be identified. The physiatrist working with the child, family, and rehabilitation team then seeks to foster an optimal developmental course to achieve each child's maximal functional potential.[10]

References

1. Barness CA: Manual of Pediatric Physical Diagnosis. St Louis, Mosby–Year Book, 1991.
2. Barness CA: Principles and Practice of Pediatrics. Philadelphia, JB Lippincott, 1994, pp 29–34.
3. Bayley N: Bayley Scale of Infant Development. New York, Psychological Corp, 1969.
4. Beery K, Buktenica N: Developmental Test of Visual-Motor Integration. Chicago, Follett, 1967.
5. Behrman RE, Vaughan VC (eds): Nelson's Textbook of Pediatrics. Philadelphia, WB Saunders, 1987.
6. Bellak L: Manual Children's Apperception Test. New York, Grune & Stratton, 1961.
7. Bender L: The Bender Visual-Motor Gestalt Test. New York, American Orthopsychiatric Association, 1946.
8. Bobath B: Abnormal Postural Reflex Activity Caused by Brain Lesions. London, Heinemann, 1971.
9. Capute AJ, Accardo PF, Vining EPG, et al: Primitive Reflex Profile. Baltimore, University Park Press, 1977.
10. Chinitz SP, Feder CZ: Psychological assessment. In Molnar GE (ed): Pediatric Rehabilitation. Baltimore, Williams & Wilkins, 1992.
11. DiBose R: Predictive value of infant intelligence scales with multiply handicapped children. Am J Ment Defic 1977; 81:388–390.
12. DiLeo J: Children's Drawings as Diagnostic Aides. New York, Brunner/Mazel, 1973.
13. Dunn L, Markwardt F: Manual: Peabody Individual Achievement Test. Circle Pines, Minn, American Guidance Service, 1970.
14. Dunn LM: Peabody Picture Vocabulary Test–Revised. Circle Pines, Minn, American Guidance Service, 1970.
15. Frakenburg WC, Dodds J, Archer P, et al: Denver II Technical Manual. Denver, Denver Developmental Materials, 1990.
16. French J: Manual: Pictorial Test of Intelligence. Boston, Houghton Mifflin, 1964.
17. Gesell A: Gesell Developmental Schedule. New York, Psychological Corp, 1940.
18. Green M: Pediatric Diagnosis: Interpretation of Symptoms and Signs in Different Age Periods. Philadelphia, WB Saunders, 1985.
19. Gundy JH: The pediatric physical examination. In Hoekelman RA (ed): Primary Pediatric Care. St Louis, Mosby–Year Book, 1992.
20. Illingworth RS: Development of the Infant and Young Child: Normal and Abnormal. New York, Churchill Livingstone, 1980.
21. Jastak S, Wilkinson GS: The Wide Range Achievement Test: Revised. Wilmington, Del, Jastak Associates, 1984.
22. Johnson EW: Examination for Muscle Weakness in Infants and Small Children. JAMA 1958;16:1306–1313.
23. Kaufman A, Kaufman N: Kaufman Assessment Battery for Children. Circle Pines, Minn, American Guidance Service, 1983.
24. Kottke FJ, Lehman JF (eds): Krusen's Handbook of Physical Medicine and Rehabilitation. Philadelphia, WB Saunders, 1990.
25. Leiter R: The Leiter International Performance Scale. Chicago, Stoelting, 1969.
26. Lowery GH: Growth and Development of Children. St Louis, Mosby–Year Book, 1986.
27. Lustig JV: Growth and Development. In Hathaway WE, Hay WW, Groothuis JR, Paisley JW (eds): Current Pediatric Diagnosis and Treatment. Norwalk, Conn, Appleton & Lange, 1993.
28. Molnar GE: A developmental perspective for the rehabilitation of children with physical disabilities. Pediatr Ann 1988; 17:766–776.
29. Molnar GE, Alexander J, Gatfeld N: Reliability of quantitative strength measurements in children. Arch Phys Med Rehabil 1979; 60:218–221.
30. Molnar GE, Kellerman WC: History and examination. In Molnar GE (ed): Pediatric Rehabilitation. Baltimore, Williams & Wilkins, 1992.
31. Molnar GE, Kellermann WC: Growth and development. In Molnar GE (ed): Pediatric Rehabilitation. Baltimore, Williams & Wilkins, 1992.
32. Nellhaus G: Head circumference from birth to eighteen years. Pediatrics 1968; 41:106–114.
33. Nihira K, Foster R, Shellhaas M, Leland N: AAMD Adaptive Behavior Scales. Washington, DC, American Association of Mental Deficiency, 1974.
34. Paine RS, Brazelton TB, Donovan DE, et al: Evolution of postural reflexes in normal infants and in the presence of chronic brain syndromes. Neurology 1964; 14:1036–1048.
35. Raven J: Raven's Progressive Matrices. Dumfries, Scotland, Crichton Royal, 1958.
36. Sparrow SS, Balla DA, Cicchetti DV: Vineland Adaptive Behavior Scale. Circle Pines, Minn, American Guidance Service, 1984.
37. Thorndike RL, Hagen EP, Sattler JM: The Stanford-Binet Intelligence Scale, ed 4. Chicago, Riverside, 1986.
38. Twitchell TE: Normal motor development. Phys Ther 1965; 45:419–423.
39. Wechsler D: Wechsler Intelligence Scale for Children–Revised. New York, Psychological Corp, 1974.
40. Wechsler D: Wechsler Preschool and Primary Scales of Intelligence–Revised. San Antonio, Psychological Corp, 1989.
41. Woodcock R, Johnson MD: Woodcock-Johnson Psychoeducational Battery: Tests of Achievement. Allen, Tex, DLM Teaching Resources, 1989.

3

Adult Communication Disorders

PAUL R. RAO, Ph.D.

If all my possessions were taken from me with one exception,
I would choose to keep the power of communication, for by it,
I would soon regain the rest.

Daniel Webster

OVERVIEW OF NORMAL COMMUNICATION PROCESSES

The ongoing dynamics of giving and getting information in our everyday lives is so routine that we often take for granted the gift of communication. Human communication is complex and multifaceted. Speech is just one component in one's repertoire of getting a message across. We use facial expression, gesture, tone of voice, writing, singing—many modes—to communicate a variety of intents. Besides strict information exchange, we communicate to describe events, converse, problem-solve, play, persuade, punish, pray or pun, and to participate in a host of other simple and sublime processes.

This chapter intends to provide a brief overview of normal communication processes followed by a discussion of adult communication disorders. What happens when you speak? Expression always begins with a thought. If it is to be spoken, it must first be organized by the language networks of the brain, according to certain linguistic rules. Only after the intended message is arranged in a certain sequence will your brain be ready to select the sequence of sounds to be spoken. Once the nervous system has encoded the message, the communication process commences with a symphony of synergy:

> . . . the *respiratory* muscles of the chest wall must be able to generate sufficient air pressure to drive the sound generator. The *phonatory* muscles of the larynx must generate enough vibrating energy for speech to be easily heard at a distance. The *articulatory* muscles of the vocal tract . . . must expand and contract this vibrating energy rapidly so that various sounds of speech that are shaped will fade

quickly and not blur into each other. The *auditory* system of the ear must transform the acoustic waves of speech sounds into neural signals so that speakers can monitor their own performance and listeners can focus on the speaker of interest. Finally coming full circle, the auditory system, as it extends from the ear to the brain, must respond selectively to the special features of speech by which it is decoded so that the meaning of the message can be understood.[46]

As Figure 3–1 illustrates, speech is a circular process, whether a person is attending to oneself or to another. The circularity of the speech process is seen in much greater detail in Figure 3–2, which shows that the process begins and ends with the brain.

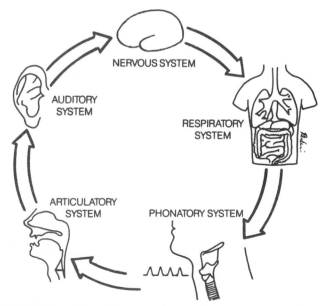

NERVOUS SYSTEM

AUDITORY SYSTEM

RESPIRATORY SYSTEM

ARTICULATORY SYSTEM

PHONATORY SYSTEM

FIGURE 3–1 The circle of communication. (From Perkins WH, Kent RD: Functional Anatomy of Speech, Language, and Hearing: A Primer. San Diego, College Hill Press, 1986.)

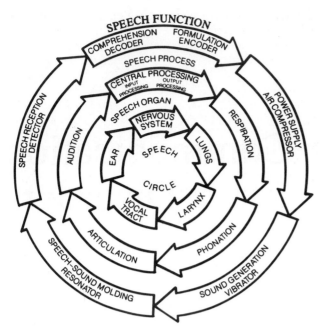

FIGURE 3–2 The processes of speech. (From Perkins WH, Kent RD: Functional Anatomy of Speech, Language, and Hearing: A Primer. San Diego, College Hill Press, 1986.)

HEARING

The human auditory mechanism analyzes sound according to changes in frequency (pitch) and intensity (loudness) over time. An audiologist uses an audiometer to measure hearing. Frequencies heard can be tested between 250 and 8000 hertz (Hz). Intensity is measured in decibels (dB) of sound pressure levels (SPLs), and can be tested from 0 to approximately 120 dB (the threshold for pain is around 125 dB). The most important part of the frequency spectrum is the range of frequencies critical for the understanding of speech. The human ear as a sensory receptor is remarkably responsive to the speech sounds that humans produce. The "speech range" extends roughly from 400 to 4000 Hz (4 kHz). Speech contains frequencies lower than 400 and greater than 4 kHz, but they are not necessary for nearly perfect intelligibility of routine conversational speech.

The mechanism of human hearing is simply one of transference of energy. The outer ear detects the sound pressure waves of speech in the air. These sound pressure waves are converted to mechanical vibrations, first by the tympanic membrane, and thereafter in the middle ear, a series of tiny bones (the ossicular chain) that leads to the cochlea of the inner ear. The cochlea is a fluid-filled, snail-shaped cavity within the temporal bone of the skull in which the mechanical vibrations are transformed into vibrations in fluid. The nerve endings in the cochlea act to transform the hydraulic vibration into nerve impulses that are then sent to the brain via the eighth cranial nerve.[11]

VOICE

Voice is the audible sound produced by phonation, but is only one component of the total speech act. Phonation has been defined as "sound generated by rapid vocal fold movement excited by exhaled airstream."[4] The "airstream" refers to respiration, the power source for voice and speech. Normal voice and speech are produced during the exhalation phase of respiration wherein the vocal folds adduct to constrict the glottis. This momentary interruption of the flow of air from the trachea through the larynx is repeated hundreds of times per second, resulting in phonation. The terms most commonly used in the context of discussing phonation may be found in Table 3–1. There are two types of phonation that occur during speech: voicing and whispering. In English there are approximately 40 phonemes (sounds), which are created by making exhaled air audible. Most speech sounds are voiced, but some are voiceless. Examples of voiced and voiceless sounds of American English are:

Voiced	**Voiceless**
All vowels	Aspirated *h*
b,d,g,z,v	*p,t,k,s,f*

The difference between voiced and voiceless speech can be easily heard and felt, for example, the production of *b* and *p* are made the same way, yet the larynx vibrates on *b* and is silent on *p*. Feel the Adam's apple on "bay" and "pay" and one will feel a vibration on *b* and not on *p*.

The outcome of speech has three phonological characteristics that are used to describe "voice"—pitch, quality, and loudness (see Table 3–1). Fundamental frequency (pitch) and intensity (loudness) are two elements of voice and speech that are controlled primarily by the interaction of the respiratory and laryngeal systems. Vocal intensity increases as (1) subglottic air pressure and the (2) closed phase of the vocal folds increase. Essentially we turn the volume up or down by manipulating both air pressure beneath the glottis as well as glottal resistance. Frequency increases as (1) subglottic pressure increases; (2) the larynx rises in the neck, shortening the pharyngeal dimensions; and (3) vocal fold length and tension increase.[4] The average

TABLE 3–1   Definitions of Terms Related to Phonation

Voice Audible sound produced by phonation.
Vocal parameters The elements of voice: pitch, loudness, quality, and flexibility.
  Pitch The perceptual correlate of frequency.
  Loudness The perceptual correlate of intensity.
  Quality The perceptual correlate of complexity.
  Flexibility The perceptual correlate of frequency, intensity, and complexity variations.
Dysphonia Abnormal voice, as judged by the listener, involving either pitch, loudness, quality, flexibility, or combinations thereof.
Aphonia Absence of a definable laryngeal tone. The voice is either severely breathy or whispered.
Mute Unable to phonate and articulate.
Vocal folds Synonymous with vocal cords—shelves of thyroarytenoid muscle covered with mucous membrane and fibroelastic tissue which project into the laryngeal airway.
Glottis The space between and bordered by the vocal folds when the latter are partially or fully abducted.
Adduction (of vocal fold) Movement of the vocal folds medially, toward the midline of the laryngeal airway.
Abduction (of vocal fold) Movement of the vocal folds laterally, away from the midline of the laryngeal airway.

Adapted with permission from Aronson AE: Clinical Voice Disorders. New York, Thieme, 1985, p 5.

fundamental frequency (pitch) for men is around 125 Hz; for women, around 200 Hz.

What is normal voice? Voices vary by age and sex, yet according to Moore,[42] they are judged as "normal" on the basis of cultural standards, education, environment, and other similar factors. Only general standards for normal voice can be stated[26]:

1. Quality must be pleasant.
2. Pitch level must be appropriate.
3. Loudness must be adequate.
4. Flexibility must be adequate.

Just as beauty is in the eye of the beholder, the "normal" voice is in the ear of the listener.

SPEECH

Speech is the motor activity by which the respiratory, laryngeal, and oral structures produce the sound patterns (phonemes) to communicate. Table 3–2 lists selected speech mechanisms and muscles and their motor innervations that relate to the dynamically interactive systems of respiration, phonation, and articulation. The speech production mechanism can be likened to a peculiar instrument with a variable resonator, capable of producing sounds that

TABLE 3–2   Selected Muscles of Speech Mechanism With Motor Innervation

Muscles	Motor Innervation
RESPIRATION	
Diaphragm	Phrenic
Sternomastoid	Accessory (XI)
External intercostal	Intercostals T2–12
Internal intercostal	Intercostals T2–12
External and internal oblique	Intercostals T6–12
Transversus abdominis	Intercostals T7–12
PHONATION	
Interarytenoid	Vagus (X), inferior
Lateral cricoarytenoid	Vagus (X), recurrent branch
Posterior cricoarytenoid	Vagus (X), recurrent branch
Thyroarytenoid	Vagus (X), recurrent branch
Cricothyroid	Vagus (X), recurrent branch
ARTICULATION	
Tongue	
Superior longitudinal	Hypoglossal (XII)
Inferior longitudinal	Hypoglossal (XII)
Transversus	Hypoglossal (XII)
Styloglossus	Hypoglossal (XII)
Palatoglossus	Accessory (XI)
Hypoglossus	Hypoglossal (XII)
Genioglossus	Hypoglossal (XII)
Mandible	
Masseter	Trigeminal (V), anterior
Temporalis	Trunk of mandibular branch
Internal, external, and pterygoid	Trunk of mandibular branch
Velopharyngeal mechanism	
Levator palatini	Vagus (X)
Tensor palatini	Trigeminal (V)
Palatoglossus	Accessory (XI)
Pharyngeal constrictor	Vagus (X)

From Zemlin W: Speech and Hearing Sciences: Anatomy and Physiology, ed 3. Englewood Cliffs, NJ, Prentice-Hall, 1968, pp 403–405. Used by permission.

are at one moment based on oscillation and at the next on turbulence. The entire system is powered by the air from the lungs.[11] The entire vocal tract is a dynamic series of cavities beginning at the vocal folds and ending at the lips. The primary articulatory structures along the vocal tract are the soft and hard palate, pharynx, tongue, teeth, lips, cheeks, and mandible. As air, voiced and voiceless, moves from the vocal folds along the vocal tract, the sequenced stream of sound evolves from the various modifications to the product that is finally heard. The vocal tract, with either voiced or voiceless sound, can function simultaneously as a sound filter (with various cavities such as the nares) and sound source (with various muscles and structures set in vibration by air such as the "raspberry" made by vibrating tongue and lips). For example, the resultant acoustic event for the speech sound /s/ begins as subglottal air puffs that are eventually expelled through the narrowed tongue, over the edges of the teeth and slightly parted lips, with an audible hissing sound.

Speech sounds are divided into vowels and consonants. Vowels are produced with a relatively open vocal tract, with the sound source beginning at the level of the larynx with the differentiation of one vowel from another, determined primarily by tongue posture and degree of lip opening. During the classic throat examination, the tongue is down and the mouth is wide open to say "aah," the vowel sound produced in the word "caught." Consonants are produced at varying points along the vocal tract and at varying degrees of constriction, from completely closed for plosive sounds to closely constricted, as in the earlier example, for the /s/ sound. In this context the role of the velopharyngeal (V/P) port should be mentioned: when the V/P port is open and sound is being resonated through the nasal cavity, the nasal consonants /m/, /n/, and /ng/ are produced. This aspect of speech is termed *resonance*, and relates to the degree of nasality in one's speech, the amount of resonance. In summary, the physiology of producing turbulence and pulse characteristics of consonants can be summed up under manner of articulation (e.g., plosive or fricative), place of articulation (e.g., lips-teeth or velum-tongue), and whether a voiced or voiceless airstream is being produced. Table 3–3 illustrates a variety of consonants charted by manner, place, and voice.

FLUENCY AND PROSODY

Fluency is the smoothness with which sounds, syllables, words, and phrases are joined together during oral language with lack of hesitations or repetitions.[10] Rate of speech has a fairly broad range given the dialectical differences seen throughout the country, for example, the "Southern drawl." The average number of words per minute (wpm), or speaking rate, is 125 and yet extremes of normal are seen in relation to a given person's educational, intellectual, and regional status. The concept of prosody may also be discussed in the context of rate. Prosody encompasses the rate, rhythm, loudness, and pitch contours that signal stress and therefore carry additional meaning beyond individual speech sounds, words, or sequences of words.[69] Although we are unable to ascribe prosody to any given mechanism in the speech chain, prosody can have a dramatic impact

TABLE 3–3   Articulation of Consonants by Manner, Place, and Voice

Manner of Articulation	Place of Articulation							
	Both Lips		Lips and Teeth		Tongue and Gum Ridge		Tongue and Velum	
	−V	V	−V	V	−V	V	−V	V
Stops	p	b			t	d	k	g
Fricatives			f	v	s	z		
Nasals		m				n		ng

Abbreviations: V, voiced; − V, voiceless.

on communication. Simply varying one's prosodics (e.g., vocal stress) can convey virtually any emotion or counter any verbal message, such as the sarcastic remark, "I am so happy my mother-in-law is visiting." Clearly, fluency and prosody are integral components in getting a message across.

LANGUAGE

For the purposes of this chapter, the way one defines language directly influences who will be classified as language-disordered. In the adult population language can be affected secondary to a host of neurological injuries, including stroke and brain injury. Current definitions of language are very broad and comprehensive. An example of such a definition was developed by the American Speech-Language and Hearing Association's Committee on Language.

Language is a complex and dynamic system of conventional symbols that is used in various modes for thought and communication. Contemporary views of language hold that: a) language evolves within specific historical, social, and cultural contexts; b) language, as rule governed behavior, is described by at least 5 parameters—phonologic, morphologic, syntactic, semantic, and pragmatic; c) language learning and use are determined by the interaction of biological, cognitive, psychosocial, and environmental factors; and d) effective use of language for communication requires a broad understanding of human interaction including such associated factors as non-verbal cues, motivation and sociocultural roles.[7]

Table 3–4 includes definitions and examples of the five aspects of language included in the definition. To establish a context to discuss language disorders such as aphasia, it is important to emphasize several issues that are not explicitly dealt with in the definition of language. The first

concept is that language is *arbitrary* (that the word "drink" is a sign that the community arbitrarily assigned meaning to) and that arbitrariness has implications for the rehabilitation of persons with a language impairment. Therapists may have to consider using *nonarbitrary* signals that have a direct relationship to the referent such as using iconic pictures or gestures for drink that do not employ the arbitrary signs of language (i.e., the spoken or written word "drink"). The second concept is that there are *levels of language* usage. Adults possess automatic speech such as counting or reflexive language (e.g., profanity) which may not be used to convey a message and may be termed the *automatic* level of language usage. The next level of language usage is *imitation*—simply repeating what is heard. This level is also not typically at the level needed to get a need met. The highest level of language usage and the one that gets at the functional nature of communication is the *propositional* level of language. I may be able to recite the days of the week (automatic), and repeat what is said to me (imitative), but neither of these two levels will assist me in getting a need met. The core of communication is to *propositionalize*—to convey a message, a want or need, a joke, etc.

In summary, verbal language may be divided into phonology (sound), semantics (meaning), syntax (order), and pragmatics (use of language in context). Two underlying concepts that are emphasized for further reference are the arbitrariness of language and the levels of language usage, including automatic, imitative, and propositional. The essence of what humans must do is make propositions—to intend to give or get a message across to others.

ADULT COMMUNICATION DISORDERS
Hearing Impairment

Hearing-impaired is a generic term that refers both to persons who are hard of hearing and those who are deaf.

TABLE 3–4   Definitions and Examples of the Five Dimensions of Language

Dimension	Definition	Example
Phonology	Rules governing the way the sounds of a language are organized	/ks/ sound in English can occur in the middle of a word (boxer) or the end (books), but never at the beginning
Semantics	Rules governing the meaning of words and word combinations	Pen = an instrument consisting of ink and used for writing
Morphology	Rules governing how words are formed	Grammatical morphemes may change the tense and aspect of sentences, e.g., plays, playing, played
Syntax	Rules governing how words are combined into larger meaningful units of phrases, clauses, and sentences	"Off the boat got" is not a well-formed grammatical sentence
Pragmatics	Rules governing the use of language in context	A speaker must be appropriate in initiating a conversation or changing a topic

Hard of hearing refers to partial impairment in the sense of hearing sufficient to cause difficulty with the comprehension of speech. *Deafness* refers to a degree of hearing loss sufficiently secure that hearing is nonfunctional for the ordinary purposes of daily life.[45] *Hearing loss* refers to the measured extent, or severity, to which the hearing is impaired. As was mentioned earlier, hearing acuity is measured in decibels and the terms generally used to describe the extent of the hearing loss are the following[32]:

Level of Loss	dB Level
Normal	0–20
Mild loss	20–40
Moderate loss	41–55
Moderately severe loss	56–70
Severe loss	71–90
Profound deafness	90 +

In addition, hearing impairment can be categorized as unilateral or bilateral, and the impairment can be temporary, permanent, or progressive. Types of hearing impairment can be related to the site of structural damage or blockage, and are termed *conductive, sensorineural, mixed,* and *central* (Table 3–5).

Voice Disorders

Normal voice falls within a wide range of acceptability, making it easier to define the disordered voice. A voice disorder is said to exist when the quality, pitch, or loudness of the voice, individually or severally, differs from that of other persons of similar age, sex, cultural background, and geographic location.[4, 42, 60] A common defining feature of a voice disorder is when a given voice draws attention to the speaker. The person who is usually the most critical of the voice is the owner of the voice.[61]

Laryngeal disorders have traditionally been classified as either functional or organic depending on their specific causes. Disorders range from aphonia (no voice) to various dysphonias (disorders of sound quality). Four specific causes of voice problems will be discussed: (1) increased vocal fold or laryngeal mass, or both; (2) neurological; (3) psychosocial; and (4) surgical.

The person with a voice complaint should initially be seen by an otolaryngologist (ear, nose, and throat [*ENT*] specialist). The otolaryngologist typically examines the patient using indirect laryngoscopy, fiberoptic laryngoscopy, or videostroboscopy to rule out any life-threatening disease or to determine if further medical intervention is indicated (e.g., surgical removal of a vocal cord polyp). The voice evaluation should (1) attempt to determine the cause, (2) describe the current vocal status, and (3) arrive at a communication diagnosis, prognosis, and plan. The diagnostic workup typically includes an extensive interview, oral peripheral examination, voice analysis (including respiration, phonation, resonance, and prosody), as well as an objective voice analysis using instrumentation. This assessment is key to uncovering the factors contributing to the vocal problem, to determining the patient's stimulability to achieve an improved vocal cord approximation, to gauge the degree of the patient's understanding of the disorder, and finally to assess willingness to participate in a remediation program.

Adult dysphonias that are due to a mass effect are often caused by a faulty phonatory attack (voice misuse or abuse) or substance abuse (smoking and alcohol). The interruption of the smooth approximation of the vocal folds results in a dysphonia. Dysphonias include *vocal nodules*—a callus formation at the anterior middle third of the vocal folds; *laryngitis*—an inflammation of the vocal fold mucosa; *vocal polyps*—fluid-filled sacs that may occur anywhere along the median edge of one or both vocal folds; and *contact ulcers*—occur around the area of the arytenoid cartilages. Intervention for these dysphonias typically involves a systematic step-by-step patient education and implementation regimen attempting to:

1. Identify misuse or abuse
2. Describe the effects of the patterns of misuse or abuse
3. Define the specific instances or circumstances of abuse or misuse
4. Modify the behavior
5. Monitor vocal change

The regimen may include periods of voice rest and often includes counseling to reduce or eliminate substance abuse.

TABLE 3–5   Definitions of Hearing Impairment and Various Causes

Hearing Impairment	Definition	Possible Cause
Conductive	Hearing impairment that results from involvement of the outer/middle ear systems	External blockage Perforated ear drum Otitis media Otosclerosis
Sensorineural	Hearing impairment that stems from damage to the inner ear, or neural fibers of the eighth cranial	Presbycusis Hereditary hearing loss Trauma Tumors Noise-induced Viral/bacterial illness Meniere's disease
Mixed	Hearing impairment that comprises both conductive and sensorineural components	See Sensorineural
Central	Hearing impairment that influences one's ability to comprehend spoken language and is related to damage to the auditory pathways in the brain	Trauma Tumors Vascular damage

Management of the vocal components basically involves re-establishing the proper coordination of respiration, phonation, resonance, and prosody and determining appropriate pitch, quality, and intensity.

Adult dysphonia of neurological origin (excluding dysarthria, which is discussed later) may be seen in the case of unilateral or bilateral vocal cord paralysis. The folds may be paralyzed in adduction (closed, a life-threatening condition), or in varying stages of abduction (opening). For a thorough discussion of the cause and treatment of vocal fold paralysis, the reader is referred to the text by Aronson.[4] Patients with cords fixed in an adducted position usually require a tracheostomy to maintain a functional airway. Phonation may be attained in these patients by occluding the stoma and exhaling for speech. In persistent closure due to abductor paralysis, surgical intervention may be indicated to reposition a cord laterally to provide sufficient opening for air. The surgical result, however, often leaves the patient with a breathy voice, as the cords are unable to fully approximate. In the case of adductor paralysis (folds in the open position), surgical intervention typically involves either injecting material into a fold to create a mass effect or surgically repositioning a cord to bring it closer to midline. The speech-language pathologist (SLP) typically is involved pre- and postsurgically in an effort to optimize the patient's efforts at producing the most functional voice possible given the physical condition of the laryngeal mechanism.[69]

Voice disorders of psychosocial origin may require psychological intervention in concert with the SLP voice regimen. As with all voice disorders, it is essential that a medical condition (especially a treatable one) be ruled out prior to initiation of therapy. The symptoms can range from a variety of dysphonias to complete aphonia.

A case of chronic hysterical aphonia (Case 1) was referred for SLP evaluation and treatment.

In another case (Case 2) the dysphonia resembled that due to an organic condition.

These cases illustrate the psychodynamics of voice, the potential for swift resolution, and the crucial role listening plays in the therapeutic process.

A voice disorder can also be one of the first symptoms of laryngeal cancer (CA). Patients with CA may be candidates for a laryngectomy, which is a total or partial surgical removal of the larynx. A partial laryngectomy may or may not affect vocal quality, depending on whether vocal fold tissue had been excised. A total laryngectomy results in a sudden and complete loss of voice. The postlaryngectomy patient has at least three speaking and several nonspeaking options:

Speaking Options

1. *Tracheoesophageal shunt.* A one-way valve prosthesis is inserted and air is permitted to pass from the trachea into the esophagus. "Esophageal sound" is produced by aerodynamics within the esophagus.

2. *Esophageal voice* is produced by oral injection of air into the esophagus followed by a rapid vibrating expulsion.

3. *Artificial larynx* is used by the speaker to generate sound for speech production purposes. The electrolarynx prosthesis may be a neck type or intraoral type and must be coordinated in placement and timing with articulated speech.

Nonspeaking Options

1. Writing
2. Complex and simple gestures
3. Communication board
4. Portable personal computer

Further detailed information on laryngectomee rehabilitation can be found in Keith and Darley.[28]

Speech Disorders

Apraxia of Speech

Two adult neurogenic communication disorders that fall under the generic term "speech" are apraxia of speech and dysarthria. *Apraxia of speech* (AOS) is a sensorimotor disorder of articulation and prosody that frequently accompanies Broca's aphasia and may also coexist with dysarthria. Just as the person with limb apraxia has difficulty programming the exact sequence of movements to complete a gesture, so too does the person with AOS present with a volitional programming problem in "saying" what is meant. The four salient characteristics of AOS are as follows[65]:

1. Effortful, trial-and-error, groping articulatory movements, and attempts at self-correction.
2. Dysprosody unrelieved by extended periods of normal rhythm, stress, and intonation.
3. Articulatory inconsistency on repeated productions of the same utterance.
4. Obvious difficulty initiating an utterance.

CASE 1

A.R. was a 15-year-old boy who had not voiced in months. The ENT examination was unremarkable and the family rejected psychiatric consultation. By using vegetative, nonspeech approaches (e.g., lifting, sighing, etc.), voice was attained after several sessions. Normal phonation slowly evolved from aphonia to falsetto to functional voice as the patient progressed in his ability to talk about his dissatisfaction with his "strict parochial school" and "strict" parents. Once the family became involved in treatment, and other school options and parenting strategies were explored, normal voice was regained and maintained at follow-up 1 year later.

CASE 2

A 26-year-old female schoolteacher was referred for chronic (1 year) severe dysphonia with normal ENT findings. The evaluation and treatment attempted to address the voice from an organic perspective (e.g., as would be employed to treat vocal nodules due to voice misuse) with training on the physiology and psychology of voice. No significant change was noted in the voice after a trial regimen of eight sessions in 1 month. At the conclusion of the trial regimen, the lack of results and the options remaining were discussed.

It was at this point, when it appeared that the dysphonia was permanent, that the patient broke down and reported that she had been raped over a year ago and had been unable to report it, even to her doctor. She felt certain that her "stressed voice" condition was due to that trauma. She was referred to a rape crisis center for counseling and voice therapy was planned to continue. The patient's voice returned to normal in weeks and she enrolled in a course of psychotherapy to work through her trauma.

AOS is believed by most experts to not be due to a language disorder, nor is it due to paralysis, weakness, or incoordination of the speech musculature.[18, 64] However, this "separate phenomenon" is a controversial issue since a number of experts are not convinced AOS exists in isolation.[3, 36] Patients with suspected AOS typically have left frontal lesions adjacent to Broca's area. The discriminating behaviors that differentiate AOS from aphasia and dysarthria are the following: relatively spared automatic speech; the absence of any significant motor control problems; and other language modalities that are superior to speech. The assessment of AOS should include a language screen and an extensive battery of speech production tests that elicit simple to complex volitional utterances under varying conditions (imitation, oral reading, spontaneous speech) (Case 3).[50]

Treatment of AOS typically moves from automatic speech, such as counting and opposites (e.g., yes and no), to progressive meaningful speech sound sequencing. Rosenbek[54] suggests the use of an eight-step task continuum ranging from maximal cuing from the clinician to initiating responses in a role-playing situation. Dabul and Bollier[14] suggest a phonetic approach where the patient practices repetitive, volitional control of simple syllables (e.g., me, may, my, mow, moo). Finally, melodic intonation therapy (MIT)[59] has been suggested as a right hemisphere ("musical brain") facilitative approach to speech. MIT is a four-step program in which natural melody patterns are used to facilitate speech. Ideal candidates for MIT have good comprehension and are verbally nonfluent. The treatment is painstaking and requires patience. In the Veterans' Administration (VA) cooperative study in which 19 AOS patients received treatment, 14 patients (74%) improved with treatment.[65] Even the patient with severe AOS can generally establish some core functional verbal repertoire. Based on the cardinal signs of the disorder, therapy is designed to enhance the opportunity of speech being initiated to improve volitional control of the oral musculature for speech purposes and to teach communication strategies that get the message across in the most efficient and effective manner possible.

Dysarthria

Dysarthria is a collective name for a group of motor speech disorders associated with disturbed neuromuscular control of speech due to central or peripheral nervous system damage.[18] Considering the systems involved in normal speech, neurological damage may affect respiration, phonation, articulation, resonance, and prosody.[43] It is important to point out that, unless a concomitant language disorder exists, language is *not* involved. Thus, the person with dysarthria is able to understand spoken language, read, write, and use a communication board, book, or device.

CASE 3

H.B., a patient with suspected global aphasia, was a 72-year-old woman who was mute with no hemiplegia. She had a history of unproductive home care for several months and was finally referred to a rehabilitation facility for a "more extensive speech workup." Presenting symptoms were no speech, little or no speech initiation, no reported reading or writing skills, and no use of gestures or of her simple communication book. Evaluation of speech and language revealed a person who had nearly intact listening comprehension, functional reading and writing at the sentence level, and no useful speech.

The resultant revised communication diagnosis was severe apraxia of speech, since the other three language modalities (listening, reading, and writing) were relatively spared and speech initiation and oral motor control for speech were severely compromised. Treatment began with the elicitation of automatic speech and monosyllabic words relevant to her activities of daily living (ADLs). Following 1 year of biweekly treatment, H.B. was able to telegraphically and intelligibly get her basic ADL messages across. Her listening, reading, and writing skills were near normal at the time of discharge.

DIFFERENTIAL DIAGNOSIS. A Mayo Clinic study[15] demonstrated that six types of dysarthria can be distinguished on the basis of perceptual characteristics: (1) flaccid, (2) spastic, (3) ataxic, (4) hypokinetic, (5) hyperkinetic, and (6) mixed (Table 3–6). Each type of dysarthria has *different auditory perceptual* characteristics which can be distinguished clinically, and accurate identification has implications for localization (e.g., spastic dysarthria in upper motor neuron disease).

ASSESSMENT. Assessment of motor speech disorders may be accomplished by both perceptual and physiological approaches. A basic clinical protocol for assessment of dysarthria begins with a detailed history. The clinician then screens hearing and vision and conducts an oral peripheral examination that includes testing alternating motion rates (e.g., rapid repetition of puh, tuh, kuh) and sequential motor rates (e.g., rapid repetition of puh, puh, puh), and prolongation of "ah." The speech evaluation proper should involve contextual speech, stress testing (varying prosodic emphasis), and contrasting stress tasks (e.g., *I* am going home vs. I am going *home*). Finally an informal and formal speech intelligibility test should be considered as part of the evaluation, such as the Tikofsky word list (an unpublished list of 50 phonetically balanced words) or Assessing Intelligibility of Dysarthric Speech.[68] The latter test is used to assess speech intelligibility at the word and sentence level. It also provides an overall intelligibility quotient as well as a measure of speaking rate.

TREATMENT. The overall goal of dysarthria treatment is enhanced functional communication.[55] In the case of anarthria (no speech), a nonverbal communication system may be developed that permits the patient to reliably communicate basic daily living needs. In the case of a person with severe dysarthria who has the potential for verbal communication, treatment attempts to address three overriding goals, namely, maximization of (1) speech intelligibility, (2) speech efficiency, and (3) functional independence. Clinicians may focus on the perceptual symptoms of the patient by attending to the most distinctive perceptual characteristics,[15] on the speech systems by employing a "physiological" approach,[43] or pragmatically and productively combine both approaches.[50] Figure 3–3 illustrates the vocal tract and the 10 functional components that generate or valve speech airstreams, as well as the aerodynamic variables that allow diagnostic inferences. For example, malfunction of a given component could be due to variations in muscle strength and tone or to abnormalities in timing the onset, duration, and offset of muscle contractions.[43] The clinician must be judicious in selecting what variable to manipulate to obtain the greatest "speech" payoff. The general prioritized dysarthria hierarchy of treatment moves through three stages: (1) early, to establish functional verbal skills; (2) middle, to maximize speech intelligibility; and (3) final, to increase the naturalness of speech. The equipment that might be necessary at various stages of treatment includes an alphabet board to signal the first letter of each spoken word in the early stage, a palatal lift to reduce hypernasality and nasal emission in the middle stage, and a pacing board to control speech rate in the final stage.

A caveat to all of the above is that the approaches described are applicable only to the patient with dysarthria who is recovering, for example, post stroke or traumatic brain injury (TBI). The treatment hierarchy for persons with dysarthria secondary to progressive diseases such as Parkinson's disease or multiple sclerosis (MS) is nearly the reverse. For example, in the latter stages of MS, the focus is on augmentative or alternative means of communication that can be used to get ADLs met.

Fluency Disorders

Stuttering is defined as the phenomenon of gaps, prolongations, or involuntary repetitions of a sound or syllable that occur during speech production. The most common type of stuttering is developmental dysfluency. Acquired stuttering is fairly rare (only 2% of cases of stuttering begin after the age of 10 years[35]). Since acquired stuttering is primarily due to brain injury, it has been termed *cortical* or *neurogenic* stuttering. An additional variety of acquired stuttering that does not fit the above description except for its relative rarity is psychogenic stuttering of adult onset. Adult-onset dysfluency is consequently either neurogenic or psychogenic.

DIFFERENTIAL DIAGNOSIS. When conducting a differential diagnostic evaluation of a patient with a presumed adult-onset dysfluency disorder, it is critical that the clinician consider all possibilities in the clinical environment[57]:

1. Neurogenic stuttering vs. *Palilalia*—"repetitions of words or phrases in which each repetition gets faster and faster and it may or may not become more unintelligible."[56]

2. Neurogenic stuttering vs. *Multiple self-corrections*—primarily seen in persons with left hemisphere injury that affects language.[50]

3. Neurogenic stuttering vs. *Psychogenic stuttering*—"stuttering begun in adulthood as a result of emotional trauma."[35]

4. Neurogenic stuttering vs. *Malingering*—"stuttering that is feigned for some ulterior gain."[53]

At a minimum, the dysfluency assessment should include a detailed history relating to the onset of the dysfluency; an oral peripheral examination; a voice, speech, language, and cognitive screen; and an extensive speech sample that includes singing, imitation, oral reading, narrative discourse, and conversation.

NEUROGENIC STUTTERING. Canter[13] classified neurogenic stuttering into three subgroups: the (1) dysarthric, (2) dyspraxic, and (3) dysnomic. Patients exhibit a fluency disorder that is predominantly either a disruption of motor speech, motor programming, or language, respectively. Rao[49] described Case 4.

This case illustrates an acquired dysfluency that appeared to be due to a combination of neurogenic dyspraxia (vocal control), dysarthria (motor control), and dysnomia (word

TABLE 3–6 Mayo Clinic Perceptual Classification of Dysarthrias

Type	Perceptual Characteristics	Localization	Causes	Neuromuscular Condition
Flaccid dysarthria	Breathy voice quality, hypernasality, consonant imprecision	Lower motor neuron	Viral infection (e.g., poliomyelitis), tumor, cerebrovascular accident (CVA), congenital conditions, disease (e.g., myasthenia gravis), palsies (e.g., bulbar, facial), trauma	Flaccid paralysis, weakness, hypotonia, muscle atrophy, fasciculation
Spastic dysarthria	Strained/strangled/harsh voice quality, hypernasality, slow rate, consonant imprecision	Upper motor neuron	CVA, tumor, infections (e.g., encephalitis), trauma, congenital conditions (e.g., spastic cerebral palsy)	Spastic paralysis, weakness, limited range of movement, slowness of movement
Ataxic dysarthria	Imprecise consonants, excess and equal stress, irregular articulatory breakdown	Cerebellar system	CVA, tumor, trauma, congenital condition (e.g., ataxic cerebral palsy, Friedreich's ataxia), infection, toxic effects (e.g., alcohol)	Inaccurate movement, slow movement, hypotonia
Hypokinetic dysarthria	Monopitch, monoloudness, reduced stress, imprecise consonants, inappropriate silences, short rushes	Extrapyramidal system	Parkinson's disease, drug-induced (e.g., reserpine or phenothiazine)	Slow movements, limited range of movement, immobility, paucity of movement, rigidity, loss of automatic aspects of movement, resting tremor
Hyperkinetic dysarthrias Predominantly quick	Imprecise consonants, prolonged intervals, variable rate, monopitch, harsh voice quality, inappropriate silences, distorted vowels, excess loudness variation	Extrapyramidal system	Chorea, infection, Gilles de la Tourette's syndrome, ballism	Quick involuntary movements (e.g., myoclonic jerks, tics, etc.), variable muscle tone
Predominantly slow	Imprecise consonants, strained/strangled/harsh voice quality, irregular articulatory breakdown, monopitch, monoloudness	Extrapyramidal system	Athetosis (e.g., acquired or congenital), infection, CVA, tumor, dystonia, drug-induced (e.g., tranquilizers), dyskinesia (e.g., torticollis, tardive dyskinesia)	Twisting and writhing movements, slow movements, involuntary movements, hypertonia
Mixed dysarthria Spastic-flaccid	Imprecise consonants, hypernasality, harsh voice quality, slow rate, monopitch, short phrases, distorted vowels, low pitch, monoloudness, excess and equal stress, prolonged intervals	Upper and lower motor neurons	Amyotrophic lateral sclerosis, trauma, CVA	Weakness, slow movement, limited range of movement
Spastic-ataxic-hypokinetic	Reduced stress, monopitch, monoloudness, imprecise consonants, slow rate, excess and equal stress, low pitch, irregular articulatory breakdown	Upper motor neuron, cerebellar, extrapyramidal	Wilson's disease	Intention tremor, rigidity, spasticity, slow movement
Variable (spastic-ataxic-flaccid)	Variable (e.g., slow rate, harsh voice quality, irregular articulatory breakdown)	Variable (e.g., upper motor neuron, cerebellar, lower motor neuron)	Multiple sclerosis	Variable (e.g., spasticity, weakness, slow movement, limited range of movement, inaccurate movement)
Others	Variable	Multiple CVAs, tumor, trauma, disease, etc.	Variable	

Adapted with permission from Darley FL, Aronson AE, Brown JR: Motor Speech Disorders. Philadelphia, WB Saunders, 1975, pp 76–77.

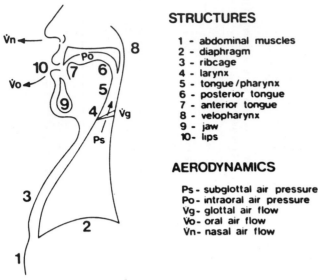

STRUCTURES

1 - abdominal muscles
2 - diaphragm
3 - ribcage
4 - larynx
5 - tongue/pharynx
6 - posterior tongue
7 - anterior tongue
8 - velopharynx
9 - jaw
10- lips

AERODYNAMICS

Ps - subglottal air pressure
Po - intraoral air pressure
Vg - glottal air flow
Vo - oral air flow
Vn - nasal air flow

FIGURE 3–3 The vocal tract and designation of 10 functional components that generate or valve the speech airstream, and the aerodynamic variables that allow inferences as to malfunction of the various components. (From Netsell R, Daniel B: Dysarthria in adults: Physiologic approach to rehabilitation. Arch Phys Med Rehabil 1979; 60:502–508.)

finding). This dysfluency responded to treatment in all three subclasses of the disorder. The treatment approaches employed in acquired stuttering mirror the traditional approaches employed with developmental dysfluency[10]:

- Bibliotherapy and patient education and counseling
- Easy onset
- Breathing exercises to control phonation
- Use of masking noise to distract speakers from their own speech
- Use of delayed auditory feedback forcing the speaker to reduce speech rate
- Use of pacing strategies such as finger tapping

Aphasia

Aphasia has been defined as an "acquired impairment of language processes underlying receptive and expressive modalities; caused by damage to areas of the brain that are primarily responsible for the language function."[16] The

communication problems most common after a left hemisphere stroke are aphasia, AOS, and dysarthria. The *volitional programming* aspects of AOS and the *motor speech* aspects of dysarthria that have already been discussed can be easily contrasted with the devastating *language* disorder of aphasia. Once related adult neurogenic communication disorders have been ruled out and aphasia has been diagnosed, the clinician should classify the type of aphasia. There are at least six existing classification systems in aphasiology ranging from the simplistic severity system to the more complex syndrome approach (Table 3–7). Although syndromes seem to be the preferred approach in today's practice,[50] many experts contest the usefulness or even the existence of syndromes.[17] See Rao[52] for a comprehensive, current review of the controversies surrounding classification and localization in aphasia. Kertesz[29] summarized the issue in favor of syndromes: "Most clinicians will agree that although aphasic disability is complex, many patients are clinically similar and will fall into recurring identifiable groups . . . There are many classifications, indicating that none is altogether satisfactory, but also that this effort is useful and even necessary to diagnose and treat aphasics or to understand the phenomena."

Syndromes of aphasia are *not* hard neurological signs but simply suggestive of the presence of brain damage in a particular location of the brain. When a patient with a lesion in the third left frontal convolution is hemiplegic and has nonfluent speech with good comprehension, the patient is almost universally referred to as having a Broca's aphasia. Table 3–8 summarizes the various aphasia syndromes and suggested localization following a left cerebrovascular accident. Few cases are reported in the current literature using any grouping in aphasia other than syndromes.

Three particular discriminating binary language behaviors helpful in classifying aphasia by syndrome are (1) fluency, (2) comprehension, and (3) repetion. *Fluency* suggests a binary anteroposterior view of the left cortex since nonfluent patients typically have anterior (frontal lobe) lesions, whereas fluent patients typically have posterior (temporal, parietal, or occipital lobe) lesions. *Comprehension* is another binary dimension wherein patients who have suffered strokes in the distribution of the left middle cerebral artery (MCA) can exhibit some degree of deficit in listening comprehension, whereas patients who have

CASE 4

A 52-year-old man developed severe neurogenic stuttering 1 hour after a motor vehicle accident in which he sustained no detectable trauma. He was referred for an SLP consultation to determine the nature of his fluency disorder, whether treatment would be beneficial, and whether resumption of his pre-trauma vocational status was feasible. The differential diagnostic dilemma was whether his dysfluency was neurogenic, psychogenic, or malingering. Once the acquired stuttering was deemed to be due to a sus-

pected, small, focal hemisphere lesion, a 5-month treatment program was undertaken that used a novel prosthetic approach to restore fluency. Once fluency was restored with the use of an artificial larynx (an application of Netsell and Daniel's[43] physiological approach for dysarthria in which a substitution is made for the phonatory component) with immediate and dramatic results, a residual dysnomic difficulty was discovered and treated.

TABLE 3–7   Classification Systems and Associated Tests for Aphasia

Criterion	Example(s)	Associated Tests	Proponent(s)
Severity	Mild, moderate, severe	Aphasia Language Performance Scales (ALPS)	Keenan & Brassell[27] (1975)
Modality	Receptive vs. expressive	Examining for Aphasia (EA)	Eisenson[20] (1954)
Behavioral	Simple aphasia, aphasia with visual involvement	Minnesota Test for the Differential Diagnosis of Aphasia (MTDDA)	Schuell[58] (1965)
Statistical	PICA 40%-ile PICA 75%-ile	Porch Index of Communicative Ability (PICA)	Porch[48] (1981)
Linguistic	Semantic aphasia Syntactic aphasia	Language Modalities Test (LMT)	Wepman & Jones[63] (1961)
Syndrome	Broca's aphasia Global aphasia	Boston Diagnostic Aphasia Examination (BDAE)	Goodglass & Kaplan[23] (1972)

From Rao P: The aphasia syndromes: localization and classification. *In* Topics in Stroke Rehabilitation. Rockville, Md, Aspen, 1994.

suffered strokes in the left posterior cerebral artery (PCA) exhibit some degree of deficit in reading comprehension. *repetion* distinguishes patients with MCA infarcts from those with lesions outside the MCA distribution. A left CVA patient who cannot repeat is this suspected of having Broca's, Wernicke's, a conduction, or a global aphasia. The following is a brief summary of the aphasia syndromes listed in Table 3–8.

BROCA'S APHASIA.   Persons with Broca's aphasia are *nonfluent* with telegraphic speech (like a telegram with the connecting words left out) and reduced verbal content. Phrase length is generaly less than four words and the verbal repertoire is almost exclusively composed of content words (e.g., nouns and verbs) with notable absence of function words (prepositions and conjunctions). Patients with Broca-type aphasia typically have functional comprehension, but have trouble following complex grammatical statements.

WERNICKE'S APHASIA.   Persons with Wernicke's aphasia are fluent with what is termed paragrammatism—speech running on with some semblance of grammatical structure. Phrase length is generally greater than five words and verbal productions are punctuated with paraphasic errors (words substitutions, e.g., pen for pencil) and poor repetition. Listening comprehension difficulty is a cardinal sign. In addition, the secondary language skills of reading and writing are typically also impaired.

ANOMIC APHASIA.   Persons with anomic aphasia are most striking in their "loss of words" both orally and in writing. They tend to circumlocute (talk around a word) and generally have functional reading and listening skills. Their fluency and repetition skills are also unremarkable.

GLOBAL APHASIA.   Persons with global aphasia are severely impaired in all language modalities, which results in an almost total inability to communicate orally. Fluency, repetition, and comprehension are all seriously compromised.

CONDUCTION APHASIA.   Persons with conduction aphasia have difficulty repeating a word or phrase back to the examiner. Spontaneous speech is relatively fluent with functional comprehension.

TRANSCORTICAL MOTOR APHASIA.   The patient with transcortical motor aphasia resembles the fluency and comprehension of a person with Broca's aphasia but has spared repetition skills. A hallmark of this syndrome is an adynamia (difficulty initiating speech).

TRANSCORTICAL SENSORY APHASIA.   This relatively rare syndrome is similar to Wernicke's, save for the retained ability to repeat.

ISOLATION SYNDROME.   Persons with this rare syndrome are severely impaired in all language-processing abilities except for the oasis of being able to repeat.

For additional elaboration of the various language profiles and the presumed sites of lesions for the various syndromes, see Albert et al.[3]

ASSESSMENT.   In the area of language assessment, the SLP is charged with conducting a differential diagnosis, establishing a prognosis, and determining whether or not treatment is indicated. Table 3–7 lists six tests for evaluation of a person with aphasia. Currently the two most frequently employed standardized aphasia examinations are the Boston Diagnostic Aphasia Examination (BDAE)[24] and the Western Aphasia Battery (WAB).[30] The tests are quite similar, employing the syndrome approach and systemati-

TABLE 3–8   Decision Tree for Classifying and Localizing Aphasia After a Left-Sided Cerebrovascular Accident

Impairment and Symptoms	Classification	Localization
Language impairment affecting linguistic components of semantics, syntax, phonology, or pragmatics, or any combination of these	Broca's	MCA, frontal lobe
	Wernicke's	MCA, temporal lobe
	Conduction	MCA, arcuate fasciculus
	Anomic	MCA, angular gyrus
	Global	MCA, multilobes
	Transcortical motor	ACA, prefrontal
	Transcortical sensory	PCA, parieto-occipital
	Isolation	ACA/PCA, watershed area
	Subcortical	Thalamus and basal ganglia
	Alexia with agraphia	PCA, angular gyrus
	Alexia without agraphia	PCA, medial-occipital and splenium of corpus callosum

Abbreviations: MCA, middle cerebral artery; ACA, anterior cerebral artery; PCA, posterior cerebral artery.

TABLE 3–9   Stimulus Response Matrix in a Language Assessment

	Stimulus		Response	
	Point	*Say*	*Write*	*Do*
SEE OBJECT	Visual matching	Naming	Written naming	Pantomime (praxis)
HEAR WORDS (SENTENCES)	Word discrimination Sentence comprehension	Word repetition Sentence repetition or answering questions	Writing from dictation	Follow commands
SEE WORDS (SENTENCES)	Word-object matching	Oral reading	Copy	Follow written commands
FEEL OBJECTS	Visual-tactile matching (stereognosis)	Tactile naming	Tactile-written naming	

From Albert ML, Goodglass H, Helm N, et al: Clinical Aspects of Dysphagia. New York, Springer-Verlag, 1981. Used by permission.

cally and comprehensively looking at spontaneous speech (content and fluency), auditory verbal comprehension, repetition, naming, reading, and writing.[31] An inventory of language input and output modalities is a general language assessment. Table 3–9 is a 4 × 4 matrix with 16 subtests that can easily serve as the basis for an inventory of language functions. Table 3–10 summarizes the components of a general language assessment.[47]

Functional communication assessment is an area that is increasingly coming under intense scrutiny. The rehabilitation clients (payers, patients, employers) are extremely interested in outcomes, and the optimal means to a functional outcome is a functional assessment. A useful definition for functional assessment of communication is as follows: "Assess the extent of the ability to communicate with others in a variety of contexts, considering environmental modifications, adaptive equipment, time required to communicate, and listener familiarity with the client. Special accommodations of the communicative partner to either receive or enhance reception must be considered."[6]

A functional communication assessment tool that is show-

TABLE 3–10   Components of the General Language Assessment

Auditory comprehension	Word identification/discrimination Yes/no reliability for personal/general questions Ability to follow commands, length and complexity Sentence/paragraph level retention and understanding
Visual comprehension	Ability to match symbols/letters Word identification skills Sentence/paragraph retention and comprehension Oral reading Functional reading skills
Speech	Social/automatic speech Word/sentence repetition Confrontation/responsive naming Verbal agility, mean length of utterance, fluency rating Analysis of form and content
Writing	Biographical information Letters, numbers: copying/dictation Word/sentence level Spontaneous sample

From Porcelli J: Aphasia assessment and treatment. Phys Med Rehabil Clin North Am 1991; 2:487–500. Used by permission.

ing real promise in eliciting consumer input and measuring outcomes is the Communication Effectiveness Index (CETI).[33] The CETI focuses on communicative need and assesses communication for social need, life skill, basic need, and health threat. It is based on direct observation by the patient's significant other of the patient's ability to perform 16 communicative skills relative to premorbid abilities in those skill areas. A sample of CETI items is as follows[33]:

Not at all able	**As able as before stroke**

Getting someone's attention

Communicating his or her emotions

Understanding writing

When patients are at a high enough communication level, they can also be involved in rating their communication skills using the CETI.

PROGNOSIS.   The prognostic variable approach is the most common one used to project ultimate communication status. Table 3–11 summarizes the research on prognostic variables important in aphasia and related neurogenic communication disorders following stroke. According to Rao,[50] the medical and speech language variables are more potent than the subject or other variables. In formulating a prognosis, the team asks the following three questions:

1. Prognosis for what?
2. Which factors are positive?
3. Which factors are negative?

Although the correspondence is not one to one, the practitioner is able to make a best "guestimate" about the odds of recovery based on the answers to these questions. Once an overall prognosis is made for return of functional communication, the clinician must estimate the patient's response to treatment:

1. Will treatment help?
2. If so, what modalities should be treated and in what order?
3. What type of treatment should be used?

Four caveats that may rule out one's candidacy for aphasia treatment are found in Davis.[17]

TABLE 3–11   Prognostic Variables Important to Aphasia and Related Neurogenic Communication Disorders Following Stroke

Patient Variables	Medical Variables	Speech and Language Variables	Other Variables
Age at onset, education, intelligence, handedness, monolingual or multilingual	Etiologic factors, site of lesion; extent of lesion, coexisting medical problems	Severity of disorder, classification and type of disorder, coexisting communicative impairment, memory and attentional deficits, sensorimotor and perceptual deficits, history of earlier treatment	Months after onset, motivation, stimulability, environment

Modified with permission from LaPointe L: Aphasia therapy: some principles and strategies for treatment. *In* Johns D (ed): Clinical Management of Neurogenic Communication Disorders, ed 2. Boston, Little, Brown, 1985, p 297.

- Perseveration and severe auditory comprehension deficit
- Inability to match objects
- Unreliable yes/no responses
- Jargon and empty speech without self-correction

TREATMENT. Today the focus of treatment is on function! One way to operationalize the "functional issues" with regard to aphasia treatment is to place the discussion in the context of the World Health Organization model of consequences of pathology[66]: "Impairment (dysfunction at the organ level), disability (functional consequences of impairment that affect performance of daily tasks), and handicap (social disadvantages resulting from an impairment or a disability)." With respect to aphasia, it is a result of a stroke that results in a language disability and a consequent communication handicap.

A simple definition of *handicap* is that it represents "a limitation of choice." It is precisely in this area of "choice" that the aphasiologist must attempt to minimize the handicap in aphasia by maximizing communication options. The following three macro approaches to aphasia rehabilitation may be employed to meet this challenge[51]:

1. Enhance functional capacity by assisting the person with aphasia to change behavior through functional communication treatment.

2. Reduce demands of the environment by removing noise in the system (e.g., turning off the TV) and optimizing transmission of signals (e.g., having action pictures in a communication book available).

3. Provide assistive devices and alternative methods by determining the menu of core needs and abilities, then training the person with aphasia in the use of alternative communication options to convey wants and needs (the use of Amer-Ind Code is an example of this approach). (See Rao[51] for a comprehensive review of the use of Amer-Ind Code.)

Specific popular approaches to aphasia treatment that may be employed are the following:

- *Melodic intonation therapy*[59] utilizes the intact musical right brain to "talk." Persons with good comprehension, poor fluency, and little available speech are thought to be ideal candidates.
- *Amer-Ind Code treatment*.[51] A form of gestural communication that employs nearly 250 iconic gestural signals to get a message across.
- *Functional communication treatment*.[8] Any therapeutic endeavor that seeks to improve the patient's reception, processing, and use of information germane to daily living.
- *Stimulation approach*.[19] The approach espoused by Hildred Schuell[58] that places primary emphasis on the stimulation presented to the person with aphasia; for example, the patient is asked to point to X and the patient responds.

An approach that is applicable to most functional methods is PACE therapy,[16] an acronym formed from "promoting aphasics' communicative effectiveness." PACE is based on the following four principles: (1) the clinician and patient participate equally as senders and receivers of messages; (2) there is an exchange of new information between the clinician and patient; (3) the patient has a free choice as to which communication channels are used to convey new information; and (4) feedback is provided by the clinician, as a receiver, in response to the patient's success in conveying the message. This pragmatic approach to aphasia typifies the thrust of today's treatment, which involves getting a message across by any means possible, whether it be via language, drawing, gesture, tone of voice, or any of a variety of other expressive methods.

EFFICACY. In an open letter to aphasiologists, Metter (a neurologist) charged that: "A greater emphasis is needed on approaching each case with the most realistic long term expectations and being able to specify these clearly and how they will benefit the patient in his day to day life."[38] Medical rehabilitation care providers in this era of health system reform are increasingly called upon to "show me your data" and to "prove that it works." Wertz et al.[65] reported on a tightly controlled VA cooperative study on aphasia that indicated that individual and group treatment was effective: "If the traditional belief is correct, that significant spontaneous recovery is completed by three to six months post onset, significant improvement in both groups beyond 26 weeks post onset indicates both individual and group treatment are efficacious methods for managing aphasic patients." In a recent study, Nicholas et al.[44] recently examined the evolution of severe aphasia in the first 2 years post onset and found that significant improvements in communicative functions were noted for up to 18 months, but the greatest improvement occurred in the first 6 months. Rao[50] reported on two patients who made dramatic progress in treatment: one patient returned home to enjoy a quality of life not experienced in 5 years post stroke and the other progressed from severe jargon aphasia to return to work in the customer service division of a major airline.

Right Hemisphere Communication Disorder

Until 20 years ago, persons with right hemisphere damage were not typically enrolled in a communication treatment program unless they exhibited a severe motor speech impairment (dysarthria). In the mid 1970s, however, with aphasiology beginning to explore pragmatics, attention was also being directed to persons with right hemisphere damage. These "right CVAs [cerebrovascular accidents]" sounded all right—they could talk in complete sentences and did not appear to have any difficulty finding the right word. The physician, the family, and the patient did not refer them to the SLP because "speech wasn't the problem." The problem, as Myers[39] discovered, was with communication. The communication impairment secondary to right hemisphere stroke has been defined as: "A breakdown in the expression and reception of complex, contextually based communicative events resulting from a disturbance of the attentional and perceptual mechanisms underlying nonsymbolic, experiential processing."[40] The key words in the definition are "context" and "attentional and perceptual mechanisms." In an isolated speech and language task, persons with right hemisphere stroke will typically exhibit no difficulty in laboratory language and speech tasks. The patient will break down "in context," however, when required to appreciate the emotion in another's voice, the words on the left side of a newspaper, or the face of a friend or family member. These are the symptoms of a problem that has as its basis the visual-attentional processing mechanism of the right hemisphere. The assessment and treatment of persons with right hemisphere communication impairments (RHCIs) is still in its infancy compared to the 125 years of literature on aphasiology. Despite this, we now have a clearer picture of what the classic RHCI profile is (Case 5).

According to Myers and Mackisack,[41] the communication deficits associated with RHCI can be divided into three broad categories:

Category	Examples of Problems
Linguistic	Confrontation naming and word fluency
Nonlinguistic	Left-sided neglect and visuospatial processing
Extralinguistic	Facial recognition and impulsivity of response

Although Myers and Mackisack use linguistic descriptions for the RHCI categories, it is important to restate that the "problem" is communication and the visual-attentional processing mechanism is the underlying basis for the disorder. It is certainly not surprising that a person with RHCI can have difficulty "getting the message in context" when left-sided neglect and impulsivity interfere with the reception and expression of a message.

Rao et al.[53] presented an RHCI case that contrasted two approaches to SLP rehabilitation, favoring interdisciplinary cotreatment as a preferred approach. Table 3–12 compares a multidisciplinary vs. an interdisciplinary approach to RHCI.

In summary, according to Tonkovich,[62] right hemisphere lesions give rise to a number of communication disorders and associated deficits that may interfere with normal communicative interactions. The classification and treatment approaches employed with persons with RHCI continue to evolve. There is a clear need for efficacy data with respect to the types of interventions with RHCI in order for clinicians to make informed decisions on whether to treat or not treat, and what approaches to employ. At present, treatment tasks tend to focus on the "behaviors" that cause problems communicating in context and not typically on the underlying process. An exciting exception to the compensation approach to RHCI is the approach of "edgeness," espoused by Myers and Mackisack.[41] This seven-stage technique appears to aid in the recovery of directed attention by presenting patients with a task that requires them to detect the boundaries of relevant space and perform tasks within that space. "Edgeness" readily translates into a reading technique called "bookness" wherein the patient must use the hand to outline the "edges" of the book and then proceed to scan, then read edge to edge. We are really just on the edge of the literature that is exploring communication in RHCI.

TABLE 3–12 Two Contrasting Approaches to Right-Sided Cerebrovascular Accident Rehabilitation in Speech-Language Pathology

Traditional Multidisciplinary Treatment	Interdisciplinary Cotreatment
Increase abstraction in all language modalities	Listing step by step the approach to accomplishing each ADL
Decrease impulsivity in treatment tasks via reminders, cues, etc.	Coaching with OT/nursing in shaving, bushing teeth, etc.
Increase left-sided awareness by introducing border concept, visual reminders, verbal cues	Coaching patient with PT stepwise in standing in parallel bars, transferring, wheelchair ambulation
Writing drills requiring print to remain within a highlighted border and cues and self-monitoring drills to decrease letter repetitions; reading from left to right with cues	Participating with therapeutic recreation in games—cueing patient in turn-taking, providing strategic and tactical advice, reminding of left-sided awareness
Reality orientation drills with log books	Log completion by each therapist after each activity, with patient reviewing same

Abbreviations: ADL, activities of daily living; OT, occupational therapy; PT, physical therapy.

E.R. was a 75-year-old man who suffered a right hemisphere stroke with resultant left hemiparesis, left homonymous hemianopsia, left-sided neglect, and a moderate to severe RHCI. On admission and after 1 month of inpatient rehabilitation, the patient was rated as completely dependent in ADLs. In team conference at 4 weeks' length of stay (LOS) the team recommended a daily regimen of SLP cotreatment of the patient, with occupational therapy (OT) and physical therapy (PT) to improve ADL skill development and carryover. At discharge, after 1 month of interdisciplinary cotreatment, E.R. was rated as moderately independent in ambulation, dressing and hygiene, and leisure activity. At 1-month follow-up in a nursing home setting, the patient had maintained his level of independence in ADLs and communication skills.

TRAUMATIC BRAIN INJURY. Fifteen years ago, TBI left few survivors. With the advent of better emergency techniques and the proliferation of trauma centers, persons who sustain a TBI are surviving in greater numbers than ever before. According to Ylvisaker and Szekeres,[67] the number of designated head injury rehabilitation programs in the United States increased from fewer than 50 in 1980 to nearly 1000 in 1994. Today, large numbers of rehabilitation professionals work exclusively with patients with TBI in a variety of clinical settings. Patients who suffer TBI may experience a variety of communication disorders that have been discussed: aphasia, anarthria, dysarthria, AOS, and cortical stuttering. The communication problem that is most commonly associated with TBI, however, is not based on language, speech, or fluency, but on cognition.

Cognitive communication impairments[6] is the generic term used to refer to the cognitively based communication disorders resulting from deficits in both linguistic and nonlinguistic cognitive processes. This population differs from the language-impaired patients following stroke in that they are typically younger, have lesions that are more diffuse, have a longer recovery period, and frequently have academic and vocational reentry as significant functional goals. According to Adamovich,[1] specific cognitive skills that may be impaired in TBI are perception, discrimination, organization, recall, and reasoning/problem solving. Persons with TBI may experience impairments in any or all stages of memory from attention and immediate recall to short and long term memory. Disturbances in executive functioning can occur even following a mild head injury with normal neuroradiological findings (see Chapter 49).

STAGES OF RECOVERY. The Rancho Los Amigos (RLA) Hospital Levels of Cognitive Recovery[25] is an eight-stage recovery scale that is widely used to rate the level of cognitive functioning. Ylvisaker and Szekeres[67] group RLA levels into three very broad stages: early, middle, and late.

Early Stages (RLA 2–3). Moves from generalized response to the environment to localized responses to specific stimuli, for example, pain, sound, visual tracking.

Middle Stages (RLA 4–6). Moves from the status where the patient is confused and agitated to the point where the patient is less confused, more appropriate in interaction, and, in a familiar environment, goal-directed.

Late Stage (RLA 7–8). Moves from the status where the patient is adequately oriented to the important aspects of life, is appropriate in interaction, and is goal-oriented, to the final stage where the patient's ultimate neurological improvement may continue to include cognitive-communication impairments that may compromise community, academic, or vocational reentry.

TREATMENT. There are little efficacy data available to suggest what works and doesn't work in cognitive-communicative remediation. Ylvizaker and Szekeres[67] provide some general principles of treatment that they believe are critical in designing treatment programs. A brief summary of those seven principles of treatment is as follows:

1. Success facilitates progress while building a positive self-concept.

2. Systematic gradation of activities carefully adjusted to meet individual needs facilitates improvement.

3. Generalization to real-world settings and activities must be a controlled component of intervention.

4. Sensitivity to executive system themes must be part of therapy sessions and the rehabilitation environment in general.

5. Integration of treatment among all staff and family members facilitates the individual's orientation, learning, and generalization of learned skills.

6. Whenever possible, personally meaningful activities and natural settings should be selected for cognitive-communicative treatment.

7. As much as possible, tasks should be designed that are consistent with the individual's pretraumatic personality, interests, and educational or vocational background as well as goals for the future.

Adamovich[1] summarizes the TBI treatment issue of today:

> The treatment of patients with TBI extends from the intensive care and rehabilitation units to outpatient programs, including day treatment and transitional living. . . . If successful home, community, school, and work re-entry is to occur, clinicians must address executive or pragmatic skills in real life situations. Finally, our ultimate treatment goals should be to empower our patients to make as many decisions as they are capable of making throughout the process of rehabilitation.[1]

Dementia

Dementia is an organic syndrome characterized by decline of memory and other intellectual functions in comparison with the patient's previous level of function. Conditions that can resemble dementia but are clearly distinguishable from dementia are delirium, psychiatric states, depression, and hearing loss. Dementia is a syndrome that can be due to numerous diseases, infections, toxins, and trauma.[9] Since many of the causes of dementia are treatable or reversible, a comprehensive case history and diagnostic medical workup is crucial. The Maryland Department of Aging[37] reports that the most common form of irreversible dementia is Alzheimer's disease (AD), which accounts for over half of all dementia cases. The second most common form is vascular dementia, accounting for approximately 25% of cases in the elderly. Some patients show the clinical and pathological features of both AD and vascular dementia. The rehabilitation team is charged with managing the patient and the family, with each discipline contributing a complementing component of care.

DIFFERENTIAL DIAGNOSIS. The communication problems commonly seen in dementia can be differentiated from those seen in single, left or right hemisphere strokes. According to Bayles,[9] there are at least six phenomena common but distinguishable between aphasia and dementia:

1. Memory deficits
2. Anomia
3. Perseveration
4. Dysfluency
5. Jargon
6. Circumlocution

Dementia is differentiated from aphasia and the other adult communication disorders that have already been reviewed by their cause (AD or multiple infarcts), course (decline), and constellation of symptoms (decrements in judgment, affect, memory, cognition, and orientation).

ASSESSMENT. Perhaps the most important portion of the assessment is the comprehensive case history obtained from the significant other to determine the type of onset, symptoms, and dysfunctional status of the person with dementia. The clinician must be sensitive to the "reversible problems" such as drugs and depression, but also be eclectic in administering a battery of tests. A frequently used tool to screen for dementia is the Mini-Mental Status Examination (MMSE),[21] a 30-point screen that examines the patient's orientation, registration, calculation, memory, language, praxis, ability to follow commands, and level of consciousness. In addition, the SLP might administer the entire WAB[30] obtaining an aphasia, language, and cortical quotient. The results of the interview, the MMSE, and the WAB should provide sufficient data, in concert with the medical and laboratory findings, to determine if an intellectual impairment exists and what stage the patient might be in. Dementia is often classified as being in the early, middle, or late stages of cognitive decline. Thus, the highest level or least level of impairment in dementia is the *early stage*. In this stage, the person with dementia is just beginning to falter in the area of pragmatics, having difficulty with orientation and difficulty with words (e.g., semantic level of language). The syntax and phonology of language is generally unimpaired. In the *middle stage* there is further deterioration of pragmatic, orientation, and semantic functions, and gradual disruption of grammar (e.g., syntax) is now evident. In the *late stage*, the patient has deteriorated

into global impairment, with no component of language being spared. Language sounds, words, grammar, and use all display severe levels of decrement. The patient at this level is oblivious to the environment and fairly nonresponsive. *The Thirty-Six Hour Day*[34] is a particularly useful book for family members as they cope with the staged, steady decline of dementia. Several recent articles on communication treatment for adults with dementia provide some degree of optimism in regard to slowing the intellectual decline.[12, 22]

References

1. Adamovich BB: The role of the speech-language pathologist in the evolution and treatment of adolescents and adults with traumatic brain injury. Special Interest Division July 1992, vol. 2, no. 1, pp. 1–6.
2. Adamovich BB, Henderson JA, Auerbach S: Cognitive Rehabilitation of Closed Head Injury Patients. San Diego, College-Hill Press, 1985.
3. Albert ML, Goodglass H, Helm N, et al: Clinical Aspects of Dysphasia. New York: Springer-Verlag, 1981.
4. Aronson AE: Clinical Voice Disorders. New York, Thieme, 1985.
5. ASHA: The role of speech-language pathologists in the identification, diagnosis, and treatment of individuals with cognitive-communicative impairments. ASHA 1988.
6. ASHA: Functional Communication Scales for Adults Project: Advisory Report. Rockville, Md, American Speech, Language and Hearing Association, 1990.
7. ASHA Committee on Language: Definition of language. ASHA 1983; 25:44.
8. Aten JL: Functional communication treatment. *In* Chapey R (ed): Language Intervention Strategies in Adult Aphasia, ed 3. Baltimore, Williams & Wilkins, 1994.
9. Bayles KA: Management of neurogenic communication disorders associated with dementia. *In* Chapey R (ed): Language Intervention Strategies in Adult Aphasia, ed 3. Baltimore, Williams & Wilkins, 1994.
10. Bloodstein O: A Handbook of Stuttering. Chicago: National Easter Seal Society, 1981.
11. Borden GJ, Harris KS: Speech Science Primer. Baltimore, Williams & Wilkins, 1980.
12. Bourgeois MS: Communication treatment for adults with dementia. J Speech Hear Res 1991; 34:831–844.
13. Canter GJ: Observations on neurogenic stuttering: a contribution to differential diagnosis. Br J Disord Commun 1971; 6:139–143.
14. Dabul B, Bollier B: Therapeutic approaches to apraxia. J Speech Hear Disord 1976; 41:268–276.
15. Darley FL, Aronson AE, Brown JR: Motor Speech Disorders. Philadelphia, WB Saunders, 1975.
16. Davis GA: A Survey of Adult Aphasia. Englewood Cliffs, NJ, Prentice-Hall, 1983.
17. Davis GA: A Survey of Adult Aphasia and Related Language Disorders, ed 2. Englewood Cliffs, NJ, Prentice-Hall, 1993.
18. Duffy JR: Differential diagnosis of acquired motor and psychogenic speech disorders, Course presented to Riverside Rehabilitation Institute, Norfolk, Va, August 1991.
19. Duffy JR: Schuell's stimulation approach to rehabilitation. *In* Chapey R (ed): Language Intervention Strategies in Adult Aphasia, ed 3. Baltimore, Williams & Wilkins, 1994.
20. Eisenson J: Examining for Aphasia. New York, Psychological Corp, 1954.
21. Folstein MF, Folstein SE, McHugh PR: "Mini-mental state": a practical method for grading the mental state of patients for the clinician. J Psychiatr Res 1975; 12:189–198.
22. Fromm D, Holland A: Functional communication in Alzheimer's disease. J Speech Hear Disord 1989; 54:535–540.
23. Goodglass H, Kaplan E: The Assessment of Aphasia and Related Disorders. Philadelphia, Lea & Febiger, 1972.
24. Goodglass H, Kaplan E: The Assessment of Aphasia and Related Disorders, ed 2. Philadelphia, Lea & Febiger, 1983.
25. Hagen C: Language disorders in head trauma. *In* Holland AL (ed): Language Disorders in Adults. San Diego, College-Hill Press, 1984.
26. Johnson W, Brown SF, Curtis JF, et al: Speech Handicapped School Children. New York, Harper, 1965.

27. Keenan JS, Brassell EG: Aphasia Language Performance Scales. Murfreesboro, Tenn, Pinnacle Press, 1975.

28. Keith RL, Darley FL: Laryngectomee Rehabilitation. Houston, College-Hill Press, 1986.

29. Kertesz A: Aphasia and Associated Disorders: Taxonomy, Localization, and Recovery. New York, Grune & Stratton, 1979.

30. Kertesz A: Western Aphasia Battery. New York, Grune & Stratton, 1982.

31. Kirk A, Kertesz A: Assessment of aphasia. *In* Hansen S, Tucker DM (eds): Neuropsychological Assessment. Physical Medicine and Rehabilitation: State of the Art Reviews. Philadelphia, Hanley & Belfus, October 1992.

32. Knauf VH: Communication training. *In* Katz J (ed): Handbook of Clinical Audiology. Baltimore, Williams & Wilkins, 1978.

33. Lomas J, Pickard L, Bester SR, et al: The Communication Effectiveness Index: Development and psychometric evaluation of a functional communication measure for adult aphasia. J Speech Hear Disord 1989; 54:113.

34. Mace NL, Rabins PV: The Thirty-Six Hour Day, ed 2. Baltimore, Johns Hopkins University Press, 1991.

35. Mahr G, Leith W: Psychogenic stuttering of adult onset. J Speech Hear Res 1992; 35:283–286.

36. Martin AD: Some objections to the term "apraxia of speech." J Speech Hear Disord 1974; 39:53.

37. Maryland Department of Aging: Definition of dementia. *In* Annual Report on Aging. Baltimore, Department of Health and Mental Hygiene, 1984.

38. Metter J: An open letter to ASHA. ASHA 1985; 27:43.

39. Myers PS: Profiles of communication deficits in patients with right cerebral hemisphere damage. *In* Brookshire R (ed): Clinical Aphasiology: Conference Proceedings. Minneapolis, BRK, 1979.

40. Myers PS: Right hemisphere communication impairment. *In* Chapey R (ed): Language Intervention Strategies in Adult Aphasia. Baltimore, Williams & Wilkins, 1986.

41. Myers PS, Mackisack EL: Right hemisphere syndrome. *In* LaPointe LL (ed): Aphasia and Related Neurogenic Language Disorders. New York, Thieme, 1990.

42. Moore GP: Organic Voice Disorders. Englewood Cliffs, NJ, Prentice-Hall, 1971.

43. Netsell R, Daniel B: Dysarthria in adults: Physiologic approach to rehabilitation. Arch Phys Med Rehabil 1979; 60:502–508.

44. Nicholas ML, Helm-Estabrooks N, Ward-Lonergan J, et al: Evolution of severe aphasia in the first two years post onset. Arch Phys Med Rehabil 1993; 74:830–836.

45. National Institute of Neurological Disease and Stroke (NINDS). National Institutes of Health, US Department of Health, Education, and Welfare: Human Communication and Its Disorders: An Overview. Bethesda, Md, NINDS Monograph no. 10, 1969.

46. Perkins WH, Kent RD: Functional Anatomy of Speech, Language, and Hearing: A Primer. San Diego, College Hill Press, 1986.

47. Porcelli J: Aphasia assessment and treatment. *In* Goldberg G (ed): Stroke Rehabilitation. Phys Med Rehabil Clin North Am 1991; 2:487–500.

48. Porch BE: Porch Index of Communicative Abilities, ed 3. Palo Alto, Calif, Consulting Psychologists Press, 1981.

49. Rao P: Neurogenic stuttering as a manifestation of stroke and a mask of dysnomia. Clin Commun Disord 1991; 1:31–37.

50. Rao P: Communication disorders. *In* Ozer M, Materson RS, Caplan LR (eds): Management of Persons with Stroke. St. Louis, Mosby–Year Book, 1994.

51. Rao P: Use of Amer-Ind Code by persons with aphasia. *In* Chapey R (ed): Language Intervention Strategies in Adult Aphasia, ed 3. Baltimore: Williams & Wilkins, 1994.

52. Rao P: The aphasia syndromes: localization and classification. *In* Topics in Stroke Rehabilitation. Rockville, Md, Aspen, 1994.

53. Rao P, Mackisack EL, Perr A, Moran L: An interdisciplinary approach to right CVA rehabilitation. Presented to the American Congress of Rehabilitation Medicine, Orlando, Fla, October 12, 1987.

54. Rosenbek J: Treatment of apraxia of speech in adults. *In* Perkins WH (ed): Dysarthria and Apraxia. New York, Thieme, 1983.

55. Rosenbek JC, LaPointe LL: The dysarthrias: description, diagnosis, and treatment. In Johns DF (ed): Clinical Management of Neurogenic Communication Disorders. Boston, Little, Brown, 1985.

56. Rosenbek J, Messert B, Collins M, Wertz RT: Stuttering following brain damage. Brain Language 1978; 6:82–96.

57. Roth CR, Aronson AE, Davis LJ: Clinical studies in psychogenic stuttering of adult onset. J Speech Hear Disord 1989; 54:634–646.

58. Schuell H: The Minnesota Test for Differential Diagnosis of Aphasia. Minneapolis, University of Minnesota Press, 1965.

59. Sparks RW, Deck JW: Melodic intonation therapy. *In* Chapey R (ed): Language Intervention Strategies in Adult Aphasia, ed 3. Baltimore, Williams & Wilkins, 1984.

60. Stemple J: Clinical Voice Pathology: Theory and Management. Columbus, Ohio, Charles E Merrill, 1984.

61. Stemple J: Voice disorders in adults. *In* Leahy MM (ed): Disorders of Communication: The Science of Intervention. New York, Taylor & Francis, 1989.

62. Tonkovich J: Communication disorders in the elderly. *In* Shadden B (ed): Communication Behavior and Aging: A Sourcebook. Baltimore, Williams & Wilkins, 1988.

63. Wepman J, Jones L: The Language Modalities Test for Aphasia. Chicago, University of Chicago Education Industry Service, 1961.

64. Wertz RT: Neuropathologies of speech and language: an introduction to patient management. In Johns DF (ed): Clinical Management of Neurogenic Communication Disorders. Boston, Little, Brown, 1985.

65. Wertz RT, La Pointe LL, Rosenbek JC: Apraxia of Speech in Adults. New York, Grune & Stratton, 1984.

66. World Health Organization: International Classification of Impairments, Disabilities, and Handicaps. Geneva, World Health Organization, 1990.

67. Ylvisaker M, Szekeres SF: Communication disorders associated with closed head injury. *In* Chapey R (ed): Language Intervention Strategies in Adult Aphasia, ed 3. Baltimore, Williams & Wilkins, 1984.

68. Yorkston KM, Beukelman DR: Assessment of Intelligibility of Dysarthric Speech. Austin, Tex, ProEd, 1981.

69. Yorkston KM, Beukelman DR: Speech and language disorders. *In* Kottke F, Stillwell G, Lehmann J (eds): Krusen's Handbook of Physical Medicine and Rehabilitation, ed 4. Philadelphia, WB Saunders, 1990.

4

Psychological Perspectives on Rehabilitation: Contemporary Assessment and Intervention Strategies

LANCE E. TREXLER, Ph.D., AND
DAVID J. FORDYCE, Ph.D.

CONCEPTUALIZING PSYCHOLOGICAL ASPECTS OF REHABILITATION

Psychological variables significantly influence the rehabilitation process and outcome. Psychological variables often moderate the expression of a medical disability or determine the extent to which the disability has an impact on functional adaptation. Moreover, in the case of acquired brain damage, psychological disorders are often primary impairments toward which rehabilitation efforts are directed (e.g., disorders of mnestic functions or states of unawareness). For these reasons, rehabilitation psychologists and neuropsychologists often play a significant role in determining not only the goals of rehabilitation but also, more importantly, the psychological aspects of rehabilitation. Psychologists in rehabilitation have subspecialized, especially since the mid-1970s, toward specific areas of rehabilitation, including rehabilitation of chronic pain, inpatient medical rehabilitation, vocational and industrial rehabilitation, and brain injury rehabilitation. A corresponding increase has occurred in theoretical and empirical literature in these areas since the 1970s as well.

An Overview of Psychological Approaches to Rehabilitation

Current formulations of human learning and emotional functioning provide a foundation for understanding the wide spectrum of recovery outcomes seen following injury, illness, or the onset of permanent impairment. This foundation also serves as a starting point for maximizing

adjustment and rehabilitation effectiveness. Premorbid intellectual skills or endowments; premorbid personality (including coping, social, and emotional skills); and familial, social, and economic contingencies all influence ultimate levels of disability. It is clear that for virtually all medical conditions (diseases, injuries, or impairments) a one-to-one correspondence does not exist between the simple presence or magnitude of such a condition and associated functional disability. Similarly, the disease model of traditional medicine, consistent with Cartesian mind-body dualism, does not serve the rehabilitation enterprise well.[61] For example, different individuals report widely varying experiences of back pain or discomfort (or the lack thereof) despite quite similar "objective" indices of tissue damage or pathological conditions. In this context, psychological assessment and intervention are not based on an illness model, and they are also not synonymous with, or a substitute for, psychiatric intervention. Rather, psychological services are best viewed as an integral component of medical rehabilitation. This is particularly true when psychological resources need to be incorporated into a rehabilitation intervention or when the patient's psychological limitations require treatment to prevent the compromising of the overall benefit from rehabilitation.

Classification and Terminology in Rehabilitation: Implications for Psychological Assessment and Rehabilitation

The National Center for Medical Rehabilitation and Research (NCMRR)[121] has provided a new classification for terminology in rehabilitation that expands that provided by the World Health Organization.[189] The NCMRR model provides a much more usable model for conceptualizing psychological assessment and intervention in rehabilitation (Table 4–1).

Missing from the NCMRR model is a variety of pre-existing individual psychological variables, such as coping skills or level of intellectual functioning. These types of pre-existing characteristics can have a significant impact on reaction and adaptation to disability. Moreover, these types of individual factors can have a significant influence on how pathophysiological limitations affect adaptation. Certainly psychological assessment seeks to provide insights as to the individual characteristics of the patient. For example, the extent to which patients believe or perceive that they have some control over their behavior and that what happens to them is not merely the consequence of luck or fate (referred to as "locus of control" in the psychological literature) has been demonstrated to influence the length of hospitalization and/or outcome in many different medical conditions. This has been demonstrated in coronary bypass patients,[101] with rate of recovery from stroke-induced hemiplegia,[126] and with significantly better levels of adaptation following traumatic head injury,[98, 119, 118] even when severity of injury was controlled.

Psychological assessment and intervention can target different levels in the NCMRR model. Neuropsychological assessment has its historical antecedents in making inferences about the pathophysiology of brain lesions, with special reference to the following: (1) the presence or absence of brain damage, and (2) the location of damage, if present.[38] A variety of psychological tests have been designed to assess emotional "impairments" and functional limitations that have directly resulted from pathophysiological sources or are a reaction to the resulting neurological impairments. Psychological assessments have not historically emphasized the description of functional limitations or disability. Advances in brain injury rehabilitation have promulgated the development of tests designed to measure such outcomes as psychosocial adaptation[97] and community integration.[185] These instruments were developed to directly measure disability associated with acquired brain damage for the following reasons: (1) the reasons for disability were unique to the type of pathophysiology (brain damage), and (2) the ability of neuropsychological tests to predict functional adaptation on a case-by-case basis is unclear.[2]

The impairments that result from a lesion and the attendant functional limitations and disabilities all interact dynamically in a manner that either facilitates or compromises adaptation. The quality of the interaction is largely determined by psychological and environmental variables. The model provided by the NCMRR provides a useful framework for determining the level at which, on a case-by-case basis, psychological assessment and interventions can be targeted.

PSYCHOLOGICAL ASSESSMENT

The psychological evaluation provides for the following: (1) the study of individual differences, such as personality and intellectual and cognitive factors, which moderate the expression of physiological function; (2) some determination of how individual differences might influence rehabilitation processes; and (3) evaluation of the presence and magnitude of certain "psychological impairments," such as depression, disinhibition, or short-term memory loss. Psychological assessment also strives to identify the factors that contribute to the propensity to report symptoms and the factors that influence participation in rehabilitation and ultimate outcome levels in impairment and disability.

Purposes of Psychological Assessment

Psychological assessment is not just the administration of psychological tests and the reporting of psychometric test scores. Psychological assessment is a clinical endeavor directed at theory-driven testing of hypotheses about human behavior. Psychological tests are generally constructed to provide objective, reliable, and valid observations about human behavior. However, the results of psychological tests must, by necessity, be integrated with clinical and subjective data, from which clinical interpretation can be provided. Psychological theories and constructs provide a framework from which certain tests are administered. Some of the theories and constructs are discussed in the following section.

The Nature and Extent of Higher Cortical Impairment

The rehabilitation of persons with either congenital or acquired brain dysfunction necessitates a distinctly unique approach to rehabilitation, by virtue of the fact that the person with brain damage presents with an altered capacity and style of learning. Certain approaches to rehabilitation and/or certain environmental conditions can impede or enhance learning in persons with brain damage. Some patients are able to learn through certain sensory modalities, but not through others. Patients with brain damage also often have difficulty generalizing what they learn in one situation to the next. Therefore, despite learning of a skill in a rehabilitation environment, the brain-damaged patient can mistakenly appear "unmotivated" simply because he

TABLE 4–1   Terminology in Disability Classification: The National Center for Medical Rehabilitation and Research Model (1993)

Pathophysiology	Interruption or interference with normal physiological and developmental processes or structures
Impairment	Loss or abnormality of cognitive, emotional, physiological, or anatomical structure or function
Functional limitation	Restriction or lack of ability to perform an action in the manner or within the range consistent with the purpose of the organ or organ system
Disability	Inability or limitation in performing tasks, activities, and roles to levels expected within physical and social contexts
Societal limitation	Restriction, attributable to social policy or barriers (structural or attitudinal), which limits fulfillment of roles or denies access to services and opportunities that are associated with full participation in society

TABLE 4–2 Determinants of Heterogeneity in Behavioral Effects of Brain Lesions

Premorbid factors	Intellect, psychosocial adjustment, coping skills
Age at onset	Children often "grow into" deficits; young adults recover better than older adults
Type of lesion	Diffuse lesions typically affect attention, memory, and metacognitive functions; focal lesions result in more specific syndromes; rapid-onset lesions result in more behavioral impairment than slow-onset lesions
Location of lesion	Cortical vs. subcortical, left vs. right hemisphere, anterior vs. posterior are relevant dimensions
Chronicity of lesion	Acute focal lesions present more immediate diffuse picture and resolve to more specific syndrome; diffuse lesions resolve in a more linear (severity) dimension

or she is not able to generalize the strategy used. For example, a brain-injured patient might not complete a wheelchair transfer at home because the same cues are not available as in the clinic, or because the patient has a different type of wheelchair at home. Rehabilitation of the person with brain injury is also unique because reorganization or compensation for neuropsychological impairments is often the goal of the rehabilitation. Persons with brain damage also often present with alterations in behavior and unique neurobehavioral syndromes that require medical and neuropsychological management. For these reasons, assessment of higher cortical functions has become an integral component of medical rehabilitation of persons with brain damage.

Persons with brain damage present enormous heterogeneity in terms of the type of neuropsychological impairment, the reasons for which are summarized in Table 4–2.[83, 96, 163] Determining localization of the lesion and evolution of the lesion, in both the acute and the chronic stages of brain injury, through neuroimaging and neuropsychological studies can be of assistance in choosing appropriate rehabilitation strategies.[14, 173, 187] For example, the size and location of a lesion on neuroimaging has been demonstrated to predict recovery from aphasia.[120] Patients with left hemisphere occipital asymmetry (advantage), as demonstrated on computerized tomography (CT), had better recoveries from aphasia.[23]

Langfitt and co-workers[87] suggested that the variety of neuroimaging strategies now available provides for the analysis of ". . . morphology → metabolism and biochemistry → neural conduction and transmission → neurological and behavioral function." This perspective, on a case-by-case basis, provides for the study of recovery in persons with brain injury and can be of some value in guiding both rehabilitative and pharmacological interventions.

It should also be noted, however, that contemporary research suggests that the best predictors of benefit from postacute brain injury neuropsychological rehabilitation are measures of insight, awareness, and acceptance.[10, 131] This suggests that pathophysiological factors (location, size, and type of lesion), as measured through neuroimaging techniques, and neuropsychological studies both describe rehabilitation-relevant individual factors. The individual factors

determine not only the prognosis for recovery but also the type of brain injury rehabilitation strategies that should be employed.[165–167] Neuropsychological assessment is no longer solely a diagnostic endeavor, but now can be used to establish a framework for *interventive*[71] or *ecological*[169] *neuropsychology.*

It is important to note that any brain lesion can influence the patient's ability to learn from rehabilitation. The neuropsychological examination should provide information as to not only what impairments might exist, but even as to how the rehabilitation staff should address or compensate for the impairments. Table 4–3 provides a gross classification of the types of disturbances of higher cortical functions that are evaluated in neuropsychological assessment.

Brain injury can also result in organic-based changes in emotional behavior secondary to subtle alterations in stability of temporolimbic functions.[150] Social interaction and integration are also often impaired secondary to neurobehavioral disorders (Table 4–4), which result from brain lesions.[16, 17, 96, 114, 150, 155] Patients are all different, and it is rare when a "pure" neurobehavioral syndrome is seen. Despite this, it is crucial in patient management that organic neurobehavioral changes following brain injury from posttraumatic emotional reactions be recognized and differentiated.

Cognitive, neurobehavioral, and emotional reactions to brain injury can interact, if not properly managed, and lead to a spiral of deterioration (Fig. 4–1). Goldstein[66] and Prigatano and co-workers[130] described a catastrophic reaction, usually precipitated by unexpected or unanticipated

TABLE 4–3 Disturbances of Higher Cortical Functions

Functions	Disturbances/Impairments
Motor and sensory	Hemiparesis Dyscoordination Dyspraxias Visual field defects Tactile, auditory, and visual sensitivity
Arousal and attention	Cognitive fatigue and poor endurance/sustained attention Distractability Modality-specific and global attention
Memory	Modality-specific (i.e., auditory, visual) memory Short-term working memory Prospective memory Autobiographical memory Episodic-semantic memory Procedural-declarative memory
Language and language-related	Dysphasias Dysgraphias Dyslexias Dyscalculias
Perceptual, visuospatial, and visuoconstructive	Agnosias Visual and auditory analysis and discrimination Hemispatial inattention and neglect Visuoconstructive disorders Dysprosodias

Executive and metacognitive	Problem-solving and abstraction
	Goal-directed behaviors
	  Self-regulation
	  Organization
	  Monitoring

TABLE 4–4   Partial Taxonomy of Neurobehavioral Disorders and Syndromes

DISORDERS OF AWARENESS

Anosognosia: Unawareness or denial of illness or consequences of brain lesion

Anosodiaphoria: Lack of emotional reaction to a deficit caused by a brain lesion

FRONTAL SYNDROMES

Dorsolateral convexity: Indifference, cognitive slowness, inertia, "pseudo-depression"

Orbitofrontal: Euphoria, hyperkinesia, disinhibition, "pseudo-psychopathic" behavior

TEMPOROLIMBIC SYNDROME

Intensification of affect/ethical/religious feelings, spontaneous episodes of rage, hypergraphia, hypersexuality, and hyposexuality

---

failure on tasks that had been easily accomplished before brain injury. Obviously, the patient's awareness of the failure or difficulty in performing the task is a requisite for the catastrophic reaction. The catastrophic reaction is characterized by angry outbursts, agitation, anxiety, and depression. Patients who are experiencing a catastrophic reaction often deteriorate in their approach to tasks and are unable to tolerate variability or a lack of rigid structure in the environment. Left undiagnosed and unmanaged, the overall adaptation of these patients typically deteriorates.

Research has demonstrated that cognitive and neurobehavioral impairments following brain injury, and not physical disability, impair long-term adjustment and social integration.[20, 21, 79, 160] The assessment, differential diagnosis, pharmacological management (the reader is referred to Gualtieri[72] for an excellent review), rehabilitation, and long-term case management of these disorders are essential.

Emotional Adjustment and Permanent Impairment

DEVELOPMENTAL STAGES. Emotional responses to acutely disabling conditions, such as spinal cord injury (SCI) or stroke, or to the onset of a potentially disfiguring or fatal disease, such as cancer, have traditionally been

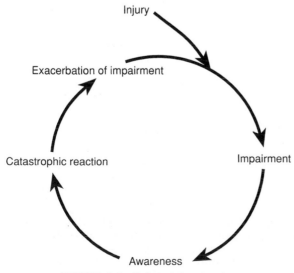

FIGURE 4–1   Spiral of deterioration.

thought to follow a natural course of evolution. The models essentially posit an initial state of significant distress or depression, which—over time and as a result of some active process of "working through"—resolves to a condition of acceptance and relative emotional harmony. It is now clear that such models reflect entrenched biases that are not well supported by empirical findings. Neither patients nor victims of loss[190] nor relatives[133] demonstrate consistent sequential trends in emotional adjustment. As reflected in group means, some general tendency for early distress to dissipate with time may exist,[52, 127, 145] but variability in emotional outcomes predominates. Most individuals never manifest a clinically significant depression, whereas in others such a state can develop and never resolve.[190]

Depression and Disability. Methodological problems or variations in experimental methods contribute to variable estimates of clinical depression in disabling conditions. Evaluating the presence of psychological distress in medical or disabled populations is not easy. Disturbances in sleep, appetite, arousal, motivation, communication, and affective modulation are common direct consequences of illness and effects of medications. This can lead to either the overdiagnosis or the underdiagnosis of depression in medical populations.[146] Problems in evaluating the presence of depression are especially apparent in brain injury, in which alterations in language, arousal, attention, or emotional expressiveness can cloud the diagnostic picture.[143]

In general, it appears that major psychological reactions occur in a *minority* of acutely impaired individuals. For example, in cross-sectional research, fewer than 30% of those surviving SCI evidence major emotional distress either in the acute stages of recovery[22, 41] or over longer periods of adaptation.[75] Rates of depression similar to those noted for SCI have been reported for rheumatoid arthritis,[62] multiple sclerosis,[45] type I diabetes mellitus,[153] burns,[127] and stroke.[68] Interestingly, these rates of depression are fairly typical of those found in a variety of general outpatient and inpatient medical settings.[122, 139, 146] They exceed base rates for major depressive symptoms in the general population,[140] which confirms that illness and impairment are not emotionally benign events; it is a finding that can also be derived from surveys of individuals with disabilities who live in the community.[111, 171] The majority of individuals living with chronically disabling conditions, however, do not appear to warrant formal psychiatric diagnosis. Signs of distress during rehabilitation or in later adjustment might well reflect normal human emotional experience.[73, 127]

Human Resilience and Coping. Humans appear to be typically fairly resilient in the face of difficult losses or the acquisition of permanent impairments, but significant depression is felt to be an understandable and natural response to loss. The fact that healthcare professionals frequently overestimate the degree of psychological distress in their patients might reflect this expectation.[39] More recent conceptualizations of normal human emotional functioning[28, 88] provide a framework for understanding responses to illness or impairment. Cassel's[28] formulation of emotional "suffering" is a useful example. It suggests that significant emotional distress is a *common* response to medical conditions that are perceived as threatening the future viability of the person. Such distress may last until the *perceived* threat has diminished. Within this context, it is not surprising that a variety of negative emotional states might occur during the course of adjusting to a chronic impairment. Their presence does not necessarily signify the presence of a pathological emotional process.

An examination of models of human emotional experience also helps to explain the frequent absence of clinically significant depression after injury or loss. For example, Lazarus and Folkman note that a particular emotional response arises out of a unique personal appraisal process.[88, 90] This process represents the product of assessments of personal meaningfulness, the level of possible control, the expectations for future change, and the potential to influence adjustment through coping. A particular emotional response flows from the *appraisal* of the event, not from the event itself. Appraisals are dependent on the personality, the experiences, the native endowment, the integrity of higher cortical functions, and the sociocultural context of the individual. Lazarus[89] has suggested that coping appraisals attempt to modulate emotional distress and that they can be roughly divided into problem-focused and emotion-focused domains (Table 4–5). Problem-focused coping typically refers to direct attempts to modify the stressor, avoid it, or develop some sense of control over its impact. Emotion-focused coping represents more avoidant-cognitive actions, such as denial or wishful thinking.

Recent research has attempted to understand the variability in emotional adjustment to impairment or loss through an analysis of individual differences in coping processes. A thorough understanding of the relationships between personality, coping skills, and emotional adjustment remains unclear. The following points appear to be generally supported by the findings to date: (1) Various studies have defined very specific types of coping skills or strategies. Although these may eventually prove to have clinical utility in understanding emotional responses to impairment, this body of research remains to be fully developed. The general dichotomy between problem-focused and emotion-focused coping has been sufficiently validated to be of some help.[4] (2) Some evidence exists that the degree to which a particular illness or impairment interferes with daily function is positively related to resultant emotional distress.[45, 55] (3) Although it has been hypothesized that emotion-focused coping skills might be more likely employed in situations in which actual control of illness or impairment are impossible or limited,[88] the highly dynamic nature of coping processes has made it difficult to validate such a relationship. (4) Although there is some correlation between the types of coping skills an individual employs at two different periods,[75] it is clear that these processes are highly dynamic. The nature of appraisal, coping, and adjustment reflects the particular interaction of person, illness, and circumstance at a given point.[4, 75, 84] (5) Evidence exists that *some* avoidant emotion-focused coping strategies might be negatively correlated with emotional well-being.[136, 174] As is reviewed in the next section, some avoidant strategies such as denial might be adaptive.

Denial. Those working in medical settings are familiar with the tendency for some disabled individuals and relatives to deny the existence (or ramifications) of acquired impairments. Denial is a highly dynamic, multifaceted coping process[26] and can be manifest through direct verbal report or inferred from behavior or the absence of overt expressions of emotional distress. In the case of certain types of brain injury (e.g., nondominant stroke or traumatic head injury), apparent denial is likely to be reflective of impairments in information processing, emotional arousal, or emotional expression.[59, 106, 143, 183] Denial and related phenomena are clearly evident in a variety of other nonneurological situations of loss. In addition, in brain injury patients it is often very difficult to locate the boundary between psychological denial and neurological anosognosia.[59, 178]

Optimal mental health has historically been thought to depend on a generally realistic appraisal of self and the world. Denial was considered maladaptive and a target for psychotherapeutic intervention (see Taylor and Brown[158] for a discussion). Depression was similarly thought to be a natural response to loss, and its absence a matter of psychological concern. As previously noted, however, significant depression is not the modal response to impairment. In fact, it appears that emotion-focused coping is frequently employed after loss.[157, 190] Denial, in all of its forms, appears to be related phenomenologically to the generally positive illusory perceptual biases often found in cognitive psychological research of normal, nondepressed individuals. For example, we evidence a tendency to view ourselves more positively than others, accept more credit for positive personal outcomes (compared with more negative ones), predict control over chance events, and harbor a generally optimistic outlook about the future.[158] In contrast, mildly depressed individuals are more balanced in self-perceptions and evidence more accurate predictions of control and future outcomes. More severe depression often yields quite negative appraisal tendencies.[9] If mental health is defined normatively, then the tendency to engage in positive illusory thinking might be reflective of optimal psychological function.[158]

Many avoidant strategies that disabled individuals employ for coping might be adaptive. In addition to problems of disturbed sleep and appetite, depression often has a negative impact on initiative, motivation, and, perhaps most significantly, social relationships. As emotional distress in reaction to loss is not always resolved,[190] strong confrontations of denial might be counterproductive.[59] Seemingly unrealistic expressions of hope can actually reinforce progress through rehabilitation. If denial is determined to increase the probability of safety risk or psychosocial failure, then it should be sensitively confronted. At various times

TABLE 4–5   Some Examples of Coping Skills or Coping-Relevant Personality Traits

Problem-Focused	Emotion-Focused
Information seeking	Avoidance
Seeking social	Denial
support	Threat minimization

Mixed	Traits
Cognitive restructuring	Locus of control
Selective ignoring	Learned resourcefulness
Blame self	Monitoring
Blame others	Blunting

in adjusting to loss or chronic disability, however, avoidant emotion-focused coping strategies might well be quite adaptive and promote psychological well-being.

Psychological Forces That Have an Impact on Impairment and Disability. We often believe that we are aware of our actual internal physiological state, but the correlations between physiological activity and reported physical sensations are small. Physical and emotional symptom reporting is subject to a number of psychological processes. Major findings from recent research in the field of cognitive psychology (see Cioffi[33] or Pennebaker[128] for reviews) can be summarized as follows: (1) Whereas the encoding of information (stimuli) from both the internal and external environments occurs continuously, awareness of such stimulation is highly selective. (2) Attention and awareness are dependent on the relative strengths and numbers of competing stimuli. Awareness is also driven by perceptual biases, expectancies, and beliefs. (3) The subsequent interpretation and labeling of a physiological stimulus reflects the product of a complex psychological process. This process is dependent on prior experience, current circumstances, and associated cues, goals, and perceived or anticipated consequences. (4) The report of physical symptoms, or the manifestation of behaviors or actions reflective of an illness state, is a human behavior like all others. It is, as a result, subject to the laws of learning and, perhaps most importantly, to the effects of environmental consequences.[61]

Following a medical event, such psychological forces begin to play an increasingly important role in overall level of disability. They can parallel the effects of physiological healing and rehabilitation, and therefore promote a reduction in overall disability. Such forces can also impede recovery and contribute to more severe and prolonged disability. The more negative outcomes can be particularly prevalent in situations of less severe initial injury or in situations in which physiological healing is nearly always complete. Prototypical conditions are back injury and concussion, in which a minority of individuals become chronically disabled.[15, 61]

Sensations related to such secondary effects as depression, anxiety, and physical disuse can, over the course of time, become associated with sensations related to injury or impairment. After healing or recovery has progressed, the conditioned associations can lead to attributions of continued impairment that reinforce prolonged disability. Symptoms or sensations reflective of normal human function can, following injury, subsequently be attributed to the injury.[109] Base rates for sensations that comprise part of either the chronic pain or postconcussion syndromes (e.g., back pain, headache, inattention, word-finding problems, forgetfulness) are surprisingly frequent in the general population, particularly among nonneurologically impaired disability groups.[69, 91, 92, 128] Secondary conditions such as emotional distress, fatigue, and physiological changes associated with prolonged convalescence and disuse can generate internal sensations that become confused with the continuing effects of injury or tissue damage.[61, 172] Coincident and independent sources of distress from family or vocational settings can also become incorporated into the experience of suffering that accompanies the impairment. Note

that these attributional phenomena often occur relatively unconsciously and automatically.

Social Factors and Rehabilitation. Alterations in social functioning following the onset of impairment can play a major role in concurrent and future adjustment. Social reinforcers can also exert a powerful influence on all aspects of recovery from injury. Illness and impairments are manifest in behaviors that are subject to influence by social consequences. Some symptoms such as pain are knowable only through behavioral expressions.[61] Although social support can ameliorate depression, perhaps by buffering the stresses associated with disability,[35] inappropriate social attention can accentuate suffering or enhance disability, pain, or dependency behaviors.[60, 170] Several studies of chronic pain patients have shown a positive relationship between a solicitous spouse responding to pain behavior and patient reports of pain and ratings of disability.[58, 141, 170] Entitlement systems such as Worker's Compensation insurance and Social Security disability insurance, and the compensatory forces associated with third-party lawsuits, can also influence symptom reporting and general levels of disability.[36, 70, 91, 107, 179, 180] Intervention with patients and families must sort out and selectively guide attributions and interactions that serve to maintain disability.

The origins of social isolation associated with disability are multifactorial and complex. Isolation can naturally follow loss in mobility skills or capacities for independent transportation. Brain injuries can alter communication skills through formal language impairments or through more subtle impairments of pragmatic communication. Nondisabled individuals experience a number of more negative psychosocial biases during their interactions with the disabled. These include heightened anxiety and devaluing beliefs that might well tend to decrease the likelihood of future contact.[47, 57] In disabled individuals, depression can also contribute to social isolation as well as be a consequence of reduced social contact. Depression and the quality and quantity of social relationships or interactions tend to covary in a negative fashion in nonmedical populations (see Barnett and Gotlib[5] for a review). Disability is often associated with a reduction in social contacts. Reduced socialization has been shown to be correlated with increased incidence of mortality in SCI,[85, 86] and depression in several disability groups.[52, 123, 137] Elliot, Frank, and others have shown how disabled individuals are viewed less favorably if they are depressed.[50, 51, 53]

The burden of the patient's altered social behavior on families can be substantial. This can be particularly true for the spouses or caregivers of brain-injured individuals,[20, 142, 152] for whom changes in the affected individuals' emotional and social behavior can have devastating consequences.

Types of Psychological Assessment

Psychological assessment is the integration of personal and medical history and behavioral observations with objectively derived test scores.[105] Psychological testing is therefore one component of a diagnostic process. The interpretation of objectively derived psychological test scores should, at a minimum, consider the following: (1) premorbid individual differences that might influence the patient's performance, (2) the circumstances in which the patient took the test and the medical condition, (3) the psychometric properties of the test (e.g., error of measurement, reliability, distribution of normative data), and (4) available research on ecological validity or predictive validity of the test. In this context, psychological tests are tools (albeit objective tools) that assist the psychologist with differential diagnosis and treatment planning.

The Clinical Interview and Behavioral Observations

Rehabilitation is intended to be a humanistically oriented enterprise. Meltzer,[113] a psychologist who suffered hypoxic encephalopathy, provided a particularly insightful series of recommendations to both patients and rehabilitation providers. After extensive inpatient and outpatient therapies, this author/patient concluded that no matter what particular intervention he received, it was the quality of the relationship between him and the therapist that determined the extent to which he benefited from therapy. The initial examiner, irrespective of his or her rehabilitation discipline, should consider these insights and their relevance for assessment in rehabilitation. Toward these ends, Strub and Black[154] have provided a very useful format for the mental status examination, which is a significant component of initial clinical interview. Table 4–6 provides an overall format for the initial examination, much of which comes

TABLE 4–6   Major Components of the Initial Examination

HISTORY
1. Description of present illness: Nature of onset, duration of illness, behavioral changes
2. Other relevant organic behavioral symptoms: Social judgment, attention and concentration, memory, orientation, language, reading, writing, and calculations
3. Previous neurological, psychiatric, and psychological symptoms: Previous neurological disease or psychiatric illnesses, seizures, head injuries, or concussion, drug and alcohol use and misuse, toxic exposures, paranoia, hallucinations, delusions, depression or anxiety disorders, previous treatment, coping strategies
4. Birth and developmental history: Birth trauma, developmental delays in motor, language, intellectual, academic, and emotional/social domains
5. Educational and vocational history: Highest grade, level of performance, achievement scores, types of jobs, stability of jobs
6. Family history: Neurological or psychiatric illness, family predilection for disease process that may involve central nervous system (e.g., hypertension), family support, family coping strategies, family stability, family awareness, and goals

BEHAVIORAL OBSERVATIONS, MOOD, AND NEUROBEHAVIORAL STATUS
1. General appearance: Age, height, weight, appearance for chronological age, posture, facial expression, eye contact
2. Personal cleanliness: Skin, hair, teeth
3. Habits of dress: Type of clothing, cleanliness and order of clothing, indications of neglect
4. Motor activity: Level of activity: placid-tense, hypokinetic-hyperkinetic, posturing
5. Mood: Appropriate to situation, sadness-euphoria, apathy-concern, stable or fluctuating
6. Emotional status: Anxiety, depression, agitation, anger, reality testing (delusions, hallucinations)
7. Neurobehavioral status: Orientation; awareness; motor, verbal, or affective impulsivity; other organic signs

from Strub and Black.[154] The initial interview provides an understanding of the individual patient as well as the framework or context in which a disability might exist. As previously discussed, the individual factors greatly influence the manifestation of the underlying impairment.

Based on the initial interview and review of the medical records, the psychologist determines which tests are clinically appropriate to administer, depending on the nature of the referral question and the needs of the individual. The following are general categories of some of the tests that can be utilized in the rehabilitation setting.

Measures of Cognitive, Emotional, and Personality Functioning

LOCUS OF CONTROL SCALES. As previously discussed, the extent to which the patient believes that he or she has some control over the impact of illness or disease can significantly influence outcome. Locus of control is easily measured with a brief questionnaire. The original scale was developed by Rotter,[144] but the most applicable version to rehabilitation is the Multidimensional Health Locus of Control Scale.[176] This Likert-type rating scale has three six-item subscales that include Internal Health Locus of Control, Chance Health Locus of Control, and Powerful Others Externality. This scale has been well researched with respect to reliability and validity, and adequate normative data exist.

SICKNESS IMPACT PROFILE. The Sickness Impact Profile (SIP) is another behaviorally oriented measure of health status, and it is frequently used not only to measure the patient's perception of the effects of a given illness on everyday behavior, but also to measure the effectiveness of a specific health care program. The SIP consists of 136 items that load into three overall dimensions, which comprise 12 categories of behavior. The types of everyday activities measured by the SIP are summarized in Table 4–7.[12] The SIP has been modified to make it more specific to head injury–related issues, but the results did not support a significant advantage of the modified SIP over the standard SIP.[159] The SIP has also been used in a variety of illnesses, including myocardial infarction and cardiac arrest, chronic obstructive pulmonary disease, low back pain, cancer, and end-stage renal disease.[11, 46, 76, 108, 125, 156] Its reliability and validity have also been well documented.[13, 129]

TABLE 4–7   Behaviors Measured by the Sickness Impact Profile

Dimension	Category of Behavior
Independent categories	Sleep and rest
	Eating
	Work
	Home management
	Recreation and pastimes
Physical	Ambulation
	Mobility
	Body care and movement
Psychosocial	Social interaction
	Alertness behavior
	Emotional behavior
	Communication

DEPRESSION INVENTORIES. There are a number of self-report screening measures of depression, including the Beck Depression Inventory,[6] the Zung Depression Scale,[191] and the Hamilton Rating Scale.[74] The Beck Depression Inventory is perhaps the best researched of these instruments. The primary disadvantage of these scales is that their intent is obvious, which makes dissimulation quite easy. Moreover, depression is not a unitary disorder and has physical or somatic symptoms, psychomotor retardation, mental slowness, and cognitive and affective components. Other approaches to the assessment of depression (e.g., the Minnesota Multiphasic Personality Inventory [MMPI]) allow for the psychometric separation of components of depression but are much longer than the Beck, Hamilton, and Zung scales.

MINNESOTA MULTIPHASIC PERSONALITY INVENTORY. The MMPI is probably the most widely used objective test of personality functioning, although there are some advantages to the more recent Millon Clinical Multiaxial Inventory-II.[116] The latter instrument is designed around Millon's theory of personality,[117] which has certain heuristic value. The original MMPI was developed by Hathaway and McKinley in 1943 and is composed of 566 true/false questions that comprise 14 clinical scales. *The MMPI Handbook*[40] described more than 550 possible scales that can be derived from the MMPI. More recently, the MMPI-2 has been developed,[24] which has some clinically important differences from the MMPI. Administration of the MMPI-2 usually requires about 60 to 90 minutes. Patients must have a sixth grade reading level to comprehend the questions and normative data begin at age 15 years. The 14 scales have descriptors, which have been summarized[44] and are provided in Table 4–8.

Taking the MMPI can be a trying experience for patients, and the rationale should be explained. It is very important that the psychologist explain the results to the patient, as failure to do so can lead to considerable anxiety and unfortunate misperceptions. The MMPI can be a very useful diagnostic tool, but can be interpreted *only* by a psychologist with specific training in the MMPI. Like any other psychological test, the results require clinical correlation. Elevations on certain scales can occur for a variety of reasons, and misinterpretations can obviously lead to misdiagnosis.

Intelligence and Achievement Tests

Intelligence tests are useful in rehabilitation for a variety of reasons, but are principally given either to assist with vocational or academic planning or as part of a neuropsychological examination for persons with known or suspected brain damage. The most commonly used test is the Wechsler Adult Intelligence Scale—Revised (WAIS-R).[177] The WAIS-R has also been revised by Kaplan and co-workers[81] to provide more useful information to neuropsychologists. The WAIS-R can be administered to persons 16 to 74 years of age. Administration of the WAIS-R typically takes 60 to 120 minutes. It is composed of 11 subtests, 6 of which statistically contribute to the Verbal Intelligence Quotient and 5 of which contribute to the Performance Intelligence Quotient. The scores are also combined in a way to yield a Full Scale Intelligence Quotient.

TABLE 4–8 Descriptors for High Scores on Validity and Clinical Scales of the Minnesota Multiphasic Personality Inventory

Scale	Name	Descriptor
VALIDITY SCALES		
L	L Scale	Conventional, rigid, self-controlled
F	F Scale	Restless, changeable, dissatisfied, opinionated
K	K Scale	Defensive, inhibited
CLINICAL SCALES		
1	Hypochondriasis	Immature, self-centered, demanding, complaining
2	Depression	Pessimistic, withdrawn, slow, timid, shy
3	Hysteria	Immature, egotistical, suggestible, friendly
4	Psychopathic deviate	Rebellious, resentful, impulsive, energetic, irresponsible
5	Masculine/ feminine	Aggressive, dominant, masculine
6	Paranoia	Suspicious, hostile, rigid, distrustful
7	Psychasthenia	Worrying, anxious, dissatisfied, sensitive, rigid
8	Schizophrenia	Confused, imaginative, individualistic, impulsive
9	Hypomania	Energetic, enthusiastic, active, sociable, impulsive
0	Social introversion	Aloof, sensitive, inhibited, timid

Adapted from DeMendonca M, Elliot L, Goldstein M, et al: An MMPI-based behavior descriptor/personality trait list. J Personal Assess 1984; 48:483–485.

A great variety of cognitive and intellectual functions are measured by the WAIS-R, and each subtest can be multifactorial. For example, the Digit Span subtest is rather simple and requires the patient to repeat spoken numeric digits. The first part of the subtest requires the patient to repeat the digits. Then the patient is asked to repeat the digits backward. This task principally requires auditory attention, concentration, and mental control. The Picture Arrangement subtest, in comparison, requires that the patient put in order a series of pictures that tell a story, not unlike a cartoon sequence. This task requires a variety of cognitive functions, including visual scanning, identification of visual detail, sequencing, foresight, and planning. The patient also typically verbalizes, either overtly or covertly, through the task as a means to help solve the problem, adding a verbal and linguistic component to the task. As a consequence, patients can succeed or fail on these tasks for many reasons. A sizable body of literature exists about the WAIS-R, and the reader is referred to Lezak[96] and Spreen and Strauss[151] for detailed reviews.

Measures of academic achievement are routinely given, such as intelligence tests, as part of neuropsychological testing or when questions regarding academic and vocational placement arise. The most comprehensive of the achievement tests is the Woodcock-Johnson Psychoeducational Battery—Revised.[188] This test provides a wide range of academic achievement information through nine subtests as follows: Letter-Word Identification, Calculation, Applied Problems, Dictation, Writing Samples, Science, Social Studies, and Humanities. This test can be administered to persons as young as 2 years and requires approximately 60 minutes to administer. If clinically appropriate, portions of the battery can be administered. The Woodcock-Johnson has been well researched and has excellent psychometric properties.

Another commonly used achievement test is the Peabody Individual Achievement Test—Revised (PIAT-R).[103] This test is not as comprehensive as the Woodcock-Johnson, but is better suited for patients with low verbal abilities.[151] The PIAT-R provides, in addition to a composite score, subtest scores for mathematics, reading recognition, reading comprehension, spelling, and general comprehension.

Neuropsychological Tests

BATTERY VS. INDIVIDUALIZED APPROACHES. The primary impetus for the development of neuropsychological assessment in the United States was to assist in neurological diagnosis. Prior to the development of CT, neuropsychological assessment was targeted at determining whether a brain lesion was present, and, if present, discerning its location and type. This diagnostic approach supported the development of the Halstead-Reitan Neuropsychological Test Battery.[134, 135] The Halstead-Reitan Neuropsychological Test Battery (HRNTB) comprises five core tests, which were originally developed by Halstead, in addition to other tests that are referred to as "Allied Procedures." The Allied Procedures were developed by Reitan and associates.[18] The HRNTB typically requires an entire day to administer, particularly when done with other neuropsychological tests. All of the HRNTB tests are administered in a very standardized manner, irrespective of individual differences. The HRNTB provides an objective, statistical, and quantitative evaluation of neuropsychological functions. It was developed to detect the presence or absence of brain damage, but in a rehabilitation setting this is now of less obvious practical benefit.

As the HRNTB was being developed in the United States, a different approach to neuropsychological assessment was simultaneously being constructed in the former Soviet Union. Luria[99, 100] contributed the first organized neuropsychological theory of brain functions and developed examination procedures that emphasize individual differences. Luria's approach to the examination of patients with cerebral lesions was later organized and articulated by Christensen.[30] Although a core set of tests is administered in the Luria Neuropsychological Investigation, each evaluation proceeds differently according to the patient's responses. In this approach to neuropsychological assessment, the examiner seeks to discover *how* the patient goes about performing the task, and whether or not the strategy the patient utilizes results in a successful outcome. When deficits in performance are noted, the examiner can manipulate the requirements of the test to determine the underlying (neuropsychological) reason for failure on the task. In this approach, the examiner can also manipulate the task to help determine what modifications are necessary to enable the patient to perform the task. This approach has obvious benefit from a rehabilitation perspective. The Luria Neuropsychological Investigation is wholly qualitative and yields no quantitative results, however.

Other approaches to neuropsychological assessment have been developing rapidly, including that of Kaplan, Milberg, and co-workers.[80, 115] Kaplan has developed a "process

approach" to neuropsychological assessment that in many ways bridges the advantages of the quantitative approach with those of the qualitative approach. The tests revised and developed by Kaplan emphasize (and quantify) the process (i.e., the strategies) that the patient uses while attempting to solve the problem. This approach still retains the achievement score, that is, the final score that reflects the extent to which the task was performed in a manner consistent with normative expectations. As previously mentioned, Kaplan and co-workers have revised the WAIS-R to enhance its utility in neuropsychological assessment and other new tests have been developed that are of certain utility in rehabilitation setting.[42] The interested reader is referred to Trexler and others[165] for further information on contemporary approaches to neuropsychological assessment in rehabilitation.

PURPOSE-SPECIFIC   NEUROPSYCHOLOGICAL TESTS. In the case of brain injury, sequential monitoring of patients' overall orientation can be quite useful in determining rate of progress and response to neuropharmacological treatment and in documenting evolution out of posttraumatic or anterograde amnesia. Too often patients are unknowingly discharged from the hospital in a state of post-traumatic or anterograde amnesia, often with disastrous results. The Galveston Orientation and Amnesia Scale[94] is a quick and objective measure that is invaluable. The Neurobehavioral Rating Scale[93] is also useful for rating the behavioral changes seen in brain injury. A variety of functions such as insight, emotional reactions, and disinhibition are rated on a seven-point scale. The Neurobehavioral Rating Scale is also helpful for tracking patient progress, and its reliability and validity have been studied in an inpatient rehabilitation setting.[37]

A variety of scales have been developed for measuring psychosocial and functional adaptation following brain injury and are sometimes used as part of neuropsychological assessment. The most useful include the Katz Adjustment Scale,[67, 82, 130] the Portland Adaptability Inventory[97] and a recent modification of this instrument,[102] and the Community Integration Questionnaire.[184, 185] These instruments provide valuable information about the patient's functional and psychosocial status, which is just as important as are neuropsychological data in the rehabilitation setting. When combined, the neuropsychological and functional-psychosocial data provide a more complete perspective from which to plan brain injury rehabilitation.

PSYCHOLOGICAL INTERVENTION

In rehabilitation settings, psychological interventions are typically divided into two broad areas: (1) maximizing general rehabilitation progress, and (2) teaching specific skills to facilitate ultimate psychosocial adjustment. Psychological goals and interventions are compatible with, and often support, the goals of other rehabilitation disciplines. Although traditional counseling sessions with rehabilitation clients or relatives might be employed, interventions are as likely to take the form of more frequent treatments of shorter duration. These can occur as "co-treatments" with other disciplines to reinforce general rehabilitation progress. Psychologists often also act in a consultation role with rehabilitation staff to assist in designing intervention strategies. Group interventions can be employed when issues of psychosocial adjustment or social skills are addressed. Psychologists are often also asked to assist with resistive patients, as well as to help staff manage their own reactions to the rehabilitation process.

Depressive Symptoms

Clinical depression or some subclinical depressive symptoms can have a negative impact on participation in rehabilitation and ultimate adjustment. Alterations in sleep or arousal secondary to significant depression can diminish the patient's energy available for rehabilitation. More importantly, the negative cognitive biases accompanying depression can have an impact on motivation, general activity level, socialization, and reactions to positive feedback.

Cognitive interventions for depression are based on the reasonably well-validated finding[5, 73, 147] that depressed individuals *tend* to view themselves, their environments, and the future with a negative bias[7] and/or expect future negative or adverse occurrences to be largely uncontrollable.[1] These biases are fueled by such underlying information processing styles as the tendencies to overgeneralize, think dichotomously, abstract selectively, personalize, excessively employ "should" statements, catastrophize negative events, and minimize the importance of positive occurrences.[138] Although the onset of disability can precipitate depressive symptoms, these negative cognitive biases act to sustain them. From a behavioral perspective, prolonged hospitalization and permanent impairment with associated depression can lead to a decrease in the capacity to access pleasurable events[95] or reinforcers, effectively producing a condition of punishment.[61]

Cognitive therapy for depression strives to help the patient become aware of irrational negative perceptual biases and to modify associated information processing styles. In nonmedical populations, cognitive therapy for depression has been shown to be as effective as pharmacological interventions in the amelioration of depressive symptoms and to be possibly superior in preventing future depressive episodes.[78, 182] Cognitive therapy for depression can be an effective approach for the depressive symptoms of rehabilitation patients, although normal mood variations associated with loss should be distinguished from more psychologically serious conditions. "Supportive counseling" can have a role, but care must be taken not to generate or promote sadness for its own sake. A sense of progress or the reinforcement of effort or skill acquisition should be supported. Note also the importance of not necessarily confronting apparent illusory positive beliefs (or at least self-reports) if such beliefs appear unrelated or nondetrimental to rehabilitation outcome or ultimate psychosocial adjustment.

Various behavioral strategies can also be employed to intervene in depressive symptoms. In fact, most psychological interventions for depression employ a mixture of cognitive and behavioral strategies. Use of these can help to alleviate the depressive forces normally stimulated by the rehabilitation process. During rehabilitation, patients can confront firsthand the magnitude of their disability. Both past reinforcing and current pleasurable experiences are typically lacking in inpatient settings. The rapid pace of delivery of rehabilitation services, especially now with shortened lengths of hospital stay, can produce fatigue and compound feelings of uncontrollability. Rehabilitation staffing, scheduling, and goal-setting decisions are often inappropriately made with little or no input from the patient. Individual therapies emphasize component or foundation skills in preparation for (or in lieu of) more functional and personally meaningful behaviors. Patients can have difficulty appreciating the relevance of these for their more important functional goals. Effective rehabilitation facilitates adjustment by actively including the patient in goal-setting and treatment planning discussions. Documentation or charting of progress in therapies, allowing some personal control in the daily schedule or choice of therapists, and promoting access to pleasurable activities are all interventions that can help reduce suffering and increase participation in rehabilitation. Facilitating generalization from the rehabilitation environment to more personally meaningful settings and establishing a specific outpatient program prior to discharge can assist the transition home and help alleviate associated concerns.

Psychological Treatment of Anxiety

The onset of serious illness or injury can set the stage for the development of anxiety symptoms. Hemiplegia, amputation, or other impairments affecting physical stability or balance can generate notable fears of falling. Some conditions such as chronic obstructive pulmonary disease (COPD) or certain cardiac impairments can create chronic anxiety related to doubts about future survival. These interact with the underlying medical state to further compromise function. Amputation, ostomy procedures, or other conditions altering physical appearance can induce a set of social avoidance behaviors that can compromise ultimate adjustment. Social anxiety and associated withdrawal can accompany awareness of alterations in interactional or communicative skill secondary to brain injury. A similar situation can arise over fear of incontinence from several conditions affecting bowel or bladder control.

Treatment of anxiety disorders is based on controlled exposure to the feared event or circumstance under conditions that optimize successful function. Anxiety nearly always leads to avoidance, perpetuating the emotional foundation and beliefs that continue to promote the anxiety. In addition to skill development during rehabilitation, several psychological interventions can promote easier exposure to the feared situation. Like depression, anxiety can be maintained by a set of irrational cognitive biases.[8, 29] Specific cognitive interventions designed to correct these beliefs facilitate recovery. Anxiety also generates a particular constellation of physiological responses, typically characterized by excessive sympathetic arousal. Teaching skills that modulate the magnitude of such arousal have served as a cornerstone for desensitization strategies. A variety of relaxation techniques are available (see Anderson[3] for a recent review) that, in combination with cognitive intervention and specific skill building, offer the anxious individual some sense of mastery and self control.

Interventions With Excessive Chronic Disability

Specific interventions are required in cases in which excessive disability seems related to faulty attributions or psychosocial contingencies. For example, the foundation for effective intervention in chronic pain is physical reactivation and the eroding of reinforcement contingencies that serve to maintain pain and related disability behaviors.[56, 60] Supervised progressive physical activity occurs *despite the presence of pain behaviors or reports of pain.* Rest, analgesics, and social attention are programmed to occur at times that are not pain reinforcing. Attempts are made to intervene in family and vocational arenas to maximize the probability that social forces reinforce independence and function rather than disability (see Chapter 41).

To accomplish these goals an attempt must be made to alter the attributions and beliefs of the patient. Cognitions about the meaning of pain must be altered or "reframed." Through teaching, patients learn about the complex, multifactorial nature of the perception of pain, and that chronic pain does not, in most cases, signify harm or danger. Similar strategies can be effective for other conditions in which misattribution and social contingencies reinforce excessive disability. Individuals experiencing prolonged postconcussive symptoms can benefit from progressive cognitive rehabilitation activities designed to underline their skills and progress in problem areas. Education about the natural course of recovery from concussion can facilitate the recasting of attributions of neuropsychological impairment into more reasonable directions that include the role of conditioning and the influence of emotional distress associated with early impairments. It is crucial to intervene in social or vocational domains that continue to promote disability.

Social Skills Training

Social skills training can assist ultimate psychosocial adjustment and minimize the relationship between disability and social isolation.[47] The nature of social interaction in traditional rehabilitation settings frequently offers little preparation for the disabled individual to deal with more natural social environments. In addition to the work on communication skills and social appropriateness that is typically included in brain injury rehabilitation activities, disabled individuals benefit from consideration of, and practice in, managing the more difficult social circumstances that they might have to confront. These can include the social ramifications of disability-specific issues (e.g., incontinence, wheelchair mobility, forgetfulness), but also present methods of minimizing uncomfortableness on the part of nondisabled interactional partners. Practice in statements that reduce disability-related uncertainty and anxiety in a communication partner can promote more successful social interactions.[124]

Resistive or "Unmotivated" Patients

Seemingly unmotivated, resistive, manipulative, or angry patients are not uncommon to the rehabilitation setting and can serve as a significant source of stress and frustration for staff. Not uncommonly, such behaviors are labeled as reflective of a personality flaw and lead to decisions to terminate services. They frequently reflect understandable responses to internal and external events (Table 4–9), however, and often offer opportunities for intervention.[19, 27] An analysis and discussion of which of these forces might be

TABLE 4–9   Common Sources of Resistance or Poor Motivation in Rehabilitation

Medical/Physical Factors	Psychological Factors
1. Effects of acute illness	1. Depression, anxiety, fear effects
2. Effects of acute pain	2. Lack of reinforcement/ pleasure
3. Lack of sleep/fatigue	3. Denial
4. Medicine effects	4. Efforts at sustaining control
5. Brain injury/delirium effects	5. Limited input into established program/goals
a. Anosognosia	6. Poor understanding of rehabilitation rationale
b. Disorientation/confusion	7. Poor appreciation of progress/ gains
c. Agitation	8. Personality conflict with therapist/physician
d. Memory impairment	9. Characterological traits of patient

operating can lead to interventions that maximize participation, as well as to alleviation of negative staff reactions. The shorter hospitalizations that are secondary to the pressures of recent healthcare changes have unfortunately made it easier to inappropriately dismiss the "resistive or unmotivated" patient as an inappropriate candidate for rehabilitation.

Neuropsychological Rehabilitation

The literature on neuropsychological approaches to brain injury rehabilitation has flourished since the early 1980s. A variety of types of interventions have been developed. In general, neuropsychological treatment of cognitive impairments either employs a theoretical-clinical or a psychometric approach.[161] Interventions that are driven by a *theoretical-clinical* approach utilize principles of brain function and the effects of brain lesions on cognitive function for the individual patient. In contrast, the *psychometric* approach bases the intervention on the results of tests of cognitive function.

Trexler and Thomas[164] provided a taxonomy of neuropsychological interventions, which describes essentially two levels of intervention. The first type of intervention is targeted at specific cognitive deficits that occur secondary to acquired brain injury (e.g., memory impairment, hemispatial inattention). Interventions that aim for the amelioration of specific cognitive deficits can be categorized into *cognitive remediation* and *compensatory* strategies. Remediation strategies largely seek to restore human abilities, whereas compensatory strategies involve the performance of an integrated set of performances. Cognitive remediation strategies are targeted at either restoration of the lost ability or at reorganizing the lost ability through incorporating intact or spared functions. Compensatory strategies employ either a task reorganization or a task substitution approach. *Task reorganization* refers to adding to or modifying the inputs, stages, or outputs of a task in a manner that can be performed by the patient and incorporated into daily life with practice. Task substitution refers to the training of entirely new skills that replace the impaired function (e.g., memory notebook).

A great variety of studies have addressed the efficacy of

interventions for specific cognitive disorders, and the available research provides support for neuropsychological interventions that seek to compensate for residual cognitive impairments. As an example, Sohlberg and Mateer[149] developed a systematic training procedure for utilizing a memory notebook. Some clinicians have naively attempted to encourage brain-damaged patients with memory deficits to compensate by using a notebook, but these investigators demonstrated that without rigorous and systematic training, patients did not learn to incorporate new behaviors into their daily life. The reader is encouraged to review the plethora of recent contributions for more specific information about specific neuropsychological interventions.[32, 54, 112, 148, 175]

Another neuropsychological intervention can be best described as an organized program of specialized rehabilitation, referred to as "holistic" neuropsychological rehabilitation.[10] The efficacy of postacute neuropsychological rehabilitation that employs a "holistic" approach has been demonstrated in a variety of studies.[10, 31, 102, 131, 132] A holistic approach to the rehabilitation of the person with acquired brain damage employs a therapeutic milieu with a variety of group therapies emphasizing awareness and emotional acceptance of residual deficits and compensation or remediation of cognitive impairments. Families are required to be quite involved, particularly from a psychotherapeutic standpoint, and these programs all emphasize a gradual and structured re-entry into a target discharge environment, such as a vocational placement. The length of treatment is sometimes fixed; that is, all patients are admitted and discharged at the same time, or it is individually determined by time of referral, and patients are admitted and discharged continuously. These programs are typically provided within a day treatment framework 4 to 5 days a week, and the average length of stay is typically 3 to 6 months, depending on the program and the patient. Two of the studies of outcome have been controlled,[131, 132] and the others have examined patients who were considerably past the period of spontaneous recovery with a pre-post methodology. When considered collectively, these studies demonstrate significant gains in psychosocial adaptation, independent living, employment status, reductions in health care utilization and costs, and cost savings[110] when persons with acquired brain damage are provided holistic neuropsychological rehabilitation.

PSYCHOLOGICAL ASPECTS OF REHABILITATION STAFF FUNCTIONING

The evaluation and treatment of rehabilitation patients is a social/psychological enterprise that involves the particular expertise of staff, which is displayed or shared through their own particular personality characteristics. Durgin[48] addressed the attitudes, knowledge, and skills that are integral to staff training. The rehabilitation environment paradoxically tends to use relatively young professionals, and yet with economic constraints, staff development and education resources are frequently reduced. Environments such as rehabilitation settings can also easily catalyze the personality conflicts and interpersonal dynamics among patients and staff. Professional, social, psychological, and economic forces all serve to magnify these conflicts and dynamics.

Several areas of importance have been considered, including the expectations that staff bring to the rehabilitation process and their impact on evaluation and intervention as well as issues of staff burnout and facilitation. It is often our general belief that an individual should be depressed following major loss or hardship. Each of us has his or her own unique expectations, however, about what should occur after such events. For example, correlations between patient and staff ratings of mood[25] or behavioral competency[43, 59] have been found to be modest. It has been noted that professionals can overestimate both the presence of depression among SCI patients relative to staff[168] and the degree of clinically significant depressive disorder in a general inpatient rehabilitation setting.[64] Similar tendencies have been noted in ratings of social impairment among brain-injured patients.[59] Caplan[25] has noted that different disciplines can systematically vary in tendencies to assign depressive symptoms to patients within a rehabilitation setting, and that to some extent members of a discipline selectively attend to different aspects of depressive phenomena. The obtained interprofessional differences might fit within the context for more general response biases, suggesting a tendency for professional helpers to overestimate the degree of psychopathology in their patients, particularly those who are more resistive.[186]

The relationships between rehabilitation patients and staff reflect a complex set of interactions based on the psychological makeup of both parties. The highly stressful and emotionally laden rehabilitation environment offers a rich opportunity for a variety of transference forces to flow freely between patient and staff. In addition to the patient's own emotional responses, rehabilitation staff frequently develop strong emotional reactions to their work in general (burnout) or to particular patients (countertransference). Trexler[162] suggested that the inherent stress in rehabilitation environments and the tendency to project blame on others often lead rehabilitation staff to be more territorial with respect to the roles of specific disciplines, to set unrealistic expectations for patients, or to blame the patient and family for either not making enough progress or not complying with therapy. Moreover, patients often incorporate rehabilitation staff into their own struggles of coping with life and their impairments.

We have discussed how staff can overestimate the degree of depression among rehabilitation populations. Gans[65] reviewed a variety of psychological transferences between staff and patients with obvious implications for patient and staff health. In addition to the already discussed tendency for staff to overestimate (or expect) some patients to be depressed, the opposite can also occur.[64] This could, in part, reflect the staff's struggles in accepting a patient's disability and their own general level of emotional exhaustion, leading to a minimization of the patient's emotional distress.[65] Staff members appear to carry to the rehabilitation setting expectations and biases of how the patient should respond, as well as of their own roles in facilitating cooperation and recovery. For example, particular diagnoses can yield particular expectations of the degree of expected psychological reactions,[65, 181] with violations of these expectations being likely to color patient/staff interactions.

Gans[65] perceptively described certain recurrent themes and offered possible methods of dealing with them. Patients can develop negative reactions to rehabilitation or to particular staff members because of their relative intactness, their constant scrutiny of the patients in difficult and sometimes embarrassing situations, their position of control, their self-confidence, or their perceived responsibility in any lack of progress that the patient experiences during rehabilitation. Staff can also develop negative feelings toward patients as they cope with feelings when patients don't improve, or as a consequence of dealing with the variety of resistive, splitting, manipulative, or blaming behaviors of their patients.

Dealing with staff reactions to the rehabilitation process is crucial, both with respect to the care of particular patients and to the prevention of burnout and staff turnover. Recent theoretical accounts of rehabilitation staff burnout have focused on components of emotional exhaustion, depersonalization of the patient, and a reduced sense of personal accomplishment.[104] The component of emotional exhaustion has been shown to be most powerfully linked to such factors as size of caseload, opportunities for job advancement, and general job satisfaction[104] and might, in part, be related to individual differences in coping skills of rehabilitation staff.[34] Gans[65] notes that rehabilitation staff rarely have sufficient training in psychology to adequately deal with the emotions and conflicts that they experience at work. He emphasizes active intervention in all cases in which conflicts arise, often involving a psychological evaluation with other rehabilitation team members present. The purpose of these meetings is to help staff understand the patient better so that they might be better able to *modify their own behavior*. He noted the importance of staff appreciating (1) that conflict in rehabilitation is inevitable (and sometimes desirable), (2) that premorbid emotional and personality problems are frequently the cause of conflictual patient behaviors in rehabilitation, and (3) that understanding these facts and basic themes of psychological defense can help staff not to personalize or tend to resist the more negative emotional and behavioral characteristics of their patients. Careful attention to issues of staff tension and burnout by supervisors and rehabilitation managers provides another tool for supporting staff. Helping staff develop new tools for coping with difficult patients can minimize burnout. Ensuring opportunities for advancement, promotion, continuing education, and wage increases can also offset the inherent strains of doing rehabilitation work. The reader is also referred to the work of Durgin and co-workers,[49] which is a very useful text that addresses staff development and training in brain injury rehabilitation.

CONCLUSION

Psychological assessment and treatment are increasingly valuable in all types of physical rehabilitation, from occupational rehabilitation to brain injury rehabilitation. Rehabilitation teams should include, or at least have access to, a psychologist. Rehabilitation clinicians also need to have at least a superficial understanding of the use and limitations of current psychological tests.

References

1. Abramson LY, Seligman MEP, Teasdale J: Learned helplessness in humans: Critique and reformulation. J Abnorm Psychol 1978; 87:49–74.
2. Acker MB: A review of the ecological validity of neuropsychological tests. In Tupper DE, Cicerone KD (eds): The Neuropsychology of Everyday Life: Assessment and Basic Competencies. Boston, Kluwer Academic Publishers, 1990, pp 19–56.
3. Anderson JP: Relaxation training and relaxation-related procedures. In Doleys DM, Meredith RL, Ciminero AR (eds): Behavioral Medicine: Assessment and Treatment Strategies. New York, Plenum Press, 1982, pp 69–82.
4. Auerbach SM: Stress management and coping research in the health care setting: An overview and methodological commentary. J Consult Clin Psychol 1989; 57:388–395.
5. Barnett PA, Gotlib IH: Psychosocial functioning and depression: Distinguishing among antecedents, concomitants, and consequences. Psychol Bull 1988; 104:97–126.
6. Beck AT: Beck Depression Inventory: Manual. San Antonio, Psychological Corporation, 1987.
7. Beck AT: Cognitive Therapy and Emotional Disorders. New York, International Universities Press, 1976.
8. Beck AT: Cognitive therapy: Past, present, and future. J Consult Clin Psychol 1993; 61:194–198.
9. Beck AT, Rush AJ, Shaw BF, Emery G: Cognitive Therapy of Depression. New York, Guilford Press, 1979.
10. Ben-Yishay Y, Silver SM, Piasetsky E, Rattock J: Relationship between employability and vocational outcome after intensive holistic cognitive rehabilitation. J Head Trauma Rehabil 1987; 2:35–48.
11. Bergner L, Bergner M, Hallstrom AP, et al: Health status of survivors of out-of-hospital cardiac arrest six months later. Am J Public Health 1984; 74:508–510.
12. Bergner M, Bobbitt RA, Carter WB, Gilson BS: The Sickness Impact Profile: Development and final revision of a health status measure. Med Care 1981; 14:787–805.
13. Bergner M, Bobbitt RA, Pollard WE, et al: The Sickness Impact Profile: Validation of a health status measure. Med Care 1976; 14:57–67.
14. Bigler ED, Kurth S, Blatter D, Abildskov T: Day-of-injury CT as an index to pre-injury morphology: Degree of post-injury degenerative changes identified by CT and MR neuroimaging. Brain Inj 1993; 7:125–134.
15. Binder L: Persisting symptoms after mild head injury: A review of the postconcussive syndrome. J Clin Exp Neuropsychol 1986; 8:323–346.
16. Bisiach E, Geminiani G: Glossary. In Prigatano GP, Schacter DL (eds): Awareness of Deficit after Brain Injury: Clinical and Theoretical Issues. New York, Oxford, 1991, pp 263–264.
17. Blumer D, Benson DF: Personality changes with frontal and temporal lobe lesions. In Benson DF, Blumer D (eds): Psychiatric Aspects of Neurologic Disease. New York, Grune & Stratton, 1975, pp 151–170.
18. Boll TJ: The Halstead-Reitan neuropsychology battery. In Filskov SB, Boll TJ (eds): Handbook of Clinical Neuropsychology. New York, John Wiley & Sons, 1981, pp 577–607.
19. Brockway JA, Fordyce WE: Psychological assessment and management. In Kottke FJ, Lehmann JF (eds): Krusen's Handbook of Physical Medicine and Rehabilitation. Philadelphia, WB Saunders, 1990, pp 153–170.
20. Brooks N, McKinlay W: Personality and behavior change after severe blunt head injury—a relative's view. J Neurol Neurosurg Psychiatry 1983; 46:336–344.
21. Brooks N, McKinlay W, Symington C, et al: Return to work within seven years of severe head injury. Brain Inj 1987; 1:5–19.
22. Buckelew SP, Baumstark KE, Frank RG, Hewet JE: Adjustment following spinal cord injury. Rehabil Psychol 1990; 35:101–110.
23. Burke HL, Yeo RA, Delaney HD, Conner L: CT scan cerebral hemispheric asymmetries: Predictors of recovery from aphasia. J Clin Exp Neuropsychol 1993; 15:191–204.
24. Butcher JN, Dahlstrom WG, Graham JR, et al: MMPI-2: Minnesota Personality Inventory-2: Manual for Administration and Scoring. Minneapolis, University of Minnesota Press, 1989.
25. Caplan B: Staff and patient perception of patient mood. Rehabil Psychol 1983; 28:67–78.

26. Caplan B, Shechter J: Denial and depression in disabling illness. *In* Caplan B (ed): Rehabilitation Psychology Desk Reference. Rockville Md, Aspen, 1987, pp 345–364.

27. Caplan B, Shechter J: Reflections on the "depressed," "unrealistic," "inappropriate," "manipulative," "noncompliant," "denying," "maladjusted," "regressed," etc. patient. Arch Phys Med Rehabil 1993; 74:1123–1124.

28. Cassel EJ: The nature of suffering and the goals of medicine. N Engl J Med 1982; 306:639–645.

29. Chambless DL, Gillis MM: Cognitive therapy of anxiety disorders. J Consult Clin Psychol 1993; 61:248–260.

30. Christensen A-L: Luria's Neuropsychological Investigation Test. Copenhagen, Munksgaard, 1974.

31. Christensen A-L, Pinner EM, Moller Pedersen P, et al: Psychosocial outcome following individualized neuropsychological rehabilitation of brain damage. Acta Neurol Scand 1992; 85:32–38.

32. Christensen A-L, Uzzell BP (eds): Brain Injury and Neuropsychological Rehabilitation: International Perspectives. Hillsdale, NJ, Lawrence Erlbaum, 1994.

33. Cioffi D: Beyond attentional strategies: A cognitive-perceptual model of somatic interpretation. Psychol Bull 1991; 109:25–41.

34. Clanton LD, Rude SS, Taylor C: Learned resourcefulness as a moderator of burnout in a sample of rehabilitation providers. Rehabil Psychol 1992; 37:131–140.

35. Cohen S, Wills TA: Stress, social support, and the buffering hypothesis. Psychol Bull 1985; 2:310–357.

36. Cook JB: The post-concussional syndrome and factors influencing recovery after minor head injury admitted to hospital. Scand J Rehabil Med 1972; 4:27–30.

37. Corrigan JD, Dickerson J, Fisher E, Meyer P: The Neurobehavioral Rating Scale: Replication in an acute, inpatient rehabilitation setting. Brain Inj 1990; 4:215–222.

38. Crockett D, Clark C, Klonoff H: Introduction—An overview of neuropsychology. *In* Filskov SB, Boll TJ (eds): Handbook of Clinical Neuropsychology. New York, John Wiley & Sons, 1981, pp 1–37.

39. Cushman LA, Dijkers MP: Depressed mood in spinal cord injured patients: Staff perceptions and patient realities. Arch Phys Med Rehabil 1990; 71:191–196.

40. Dahlstrom WG, Welsch GS: An MMPI Handbook: A Guide to Use in Clinical Practice and Research, vol 1 and 2. Minneapolis, University of Minnesota Press, 1960, 1975.

41. Davidoff G, Roth E, Thomas P, et al: Depression among acute spinal cord injury patients: A study utilizing the Zung self-rating depression scale. Rehabil Psychol 1990; 35:171–180.

42. Delis DC, Kramer JH, Friedlund AJ, Kaplan E: A cognitive science approach to neuropsychological assessment. *In* McReynolds P, Rosen JC, Chelune GJ (eds): Advances in Psychological Assessment. New York, Plenum Press, 1990, pp 101–132.

43. Dellario D, Anthony W, Rogers S: Client-practitioner agreement in the assessment of severely psychiatrically disabled persons' functional skills. Rehabil Psychol 1983; 28:243–248.

44. DeMendonca M, Elliott L, Goldstein M, et al: An MMPI-based behavior descriptor/personality trait list. J Personal Assess 1984; 48:483–485.

45. Devins GM, Seland TP, Klein G, et al: Stability and determinants of psychosocial well-being in multiple sclerosis. Rehabil Psychol 1993; 38:11–26.

46. Deyo RA, Diehl AK, Rosenthal M: How many days of bed rest for acute low back pain? A randomized clinical trial. N Engl J Med 1986; 315:1064–1070.

47. Dunn M: Social skills and rehabilitation. *In* Caplan B (ed): Rehabilitation Psychology Desk Reference. Rockville, Md, Aspen, 1987, pp 345–364.

48. Durgin CJ: Preparing staff to provide quality rehabilitation services: Problems and proposed solutions. *In* Dugin C, Schmidt ND, Fryer LJ (eds): Staff Development and Clinical Intervention in Brain Injury Rehabilitation. Gaithersburg, Md, Aspen, 1993, pp 3–22.

49. Durgin CJ, Schmidt ND, Fryer LJ (eds): Staff Development and Clinical Intervention in Brain Injury Rehabilitation. Gaithersburg, Md, Aspen, 1993.

50. Elliot TR, Frank RG: Social and interpersonal reactions to depression and disability. Rehabil Psychol 1990; 35:135–148.

51. Elliot TR, Frank RG, Corcoran J, et al: Previous personal experience and reactions to depression and physical disability. Rehabil Psychol 1990; 35:111–120.

52. Elliot TR, Herrick SM, Witty TE, et al: Social support and depression following spinal cord injury. Rehabil Psychol 1992; 37:37–48.

53. Elliot TR, Yoder B, Umlauf R: Nurse and patient reactions to social displays of depression. Rehabil Psychol 1990; 35:195–204.

54. Ellis DW, Christensen A-L (eds): Neuropsychological Treatment after Brain Injury. Boston, Kluwer Academic Publishers, 1989.

55. Felton BJ, Revenson TA: Coping with chronic illness: A study of controllability and the influence of coping strategies on psychological adjustment. J Consult Clin Psychol 1984; 52:343–353.

56. Fey SG, Williamson-Kirkland TE: Chronic pain: Psychology and rehabilitation. *In* Caplan B (ed): Rehabilitation Psychology Desk Reference. Rockville, Md, Aspen, 1987, pp 101–130.

57. Fichten CS, Robillard K, Judd D, Amsel R: College students with physical disabilities: Myths and realities. Rehabil Psychol 1989; 34:243–258.

58. Flor H, Kerns RD, Turk DC: The role of spouse reinforcement, perceived pain, and activity levels of chronic pain patients. J Psychosom Res 1987; 31:251–259.

59. Fordyce DJ, Roueche JR: Changes in perspectives of disability among patients, staff, and relatives during rehabilitation of brain injury. Rehabil Psychol 1986; 31:217–229.

60. Fordyce WE: Behavioral Methods for Chronic Pain and Illness. St. Louis, Mosby–Year Book, 1976.

61. Fordyce WE: Pain and suffering: A reappraisal. Am Psychol 1988; 43:276–283.

62. Frank RG, Chaney JM, Clay DL, Kay DR: Depression in rheumatoid arthritis: A re-evaluation. Rehabil Psychol 1991; 36:219–230.

63. Fuhrer MJ, Rintala DH, Hart KA, et al: Depressive symptomatology in persons with spinal cord injury who reside in the community. Arch Phys Med Rehabil 1993; 74:255–260.

64. Gans JS: Depression diagnosis in a rehabilitation hospital. Arch Phys Med Rehabil 1981; 64:386–389.

65. Gans JS: Facilitating staff interaction in rehabilitation. *In* Caplan B (ed): Rehabilitation Psychology Desk Reference. Rockville Md, Aspen, 1987, pp 185–218.

66. Goldstein K: The effects of brain damage on the personality. Psychiatry 1952; 15:245–260.

67. Goran DA, Fabiano RJ: The scaling of the Katz adjustment scale in a traumatic brain injury rehabilitation sample. Brain Inj 1993; 7:219–229.

68. Gordon WA, Hibbard MR, Egelko S, et al: Issues in the diagnosis of post stroke depression. Rehabil Psychol 1991; 36:71–88.

69. Gouvier WD, Cubic B, Jones G, et al: Postconcussion symptoms and daily stress in normal and head-injured college populations. J Clin Exp Neuropsychol 1992; 7:193–211.

70. Greenough CG, Fraser RD: The effects of compensation on recovery from low-back injury. Spine 198; 14:947–955.

71. Gross Y: A conceptual framework for interventive cognitive neuropsychology. *In* Trexler LE (ed): Cognitive Rehabilitation: Conceptualization and Intervention. New York, Plenum Press, 1982, pp 99–114.

72. Gualtieri CT: Neuropsychiatry and Behavioral Pharmacology. New York, Springer, 1991.

73. Haaga DAF, Dyck MJ, Ernst D: Empirical status of cognitive theory of depression. Psychol Bull 1991; 11:215–236.

74. Hamilton M: Development of a rating scale for primary depressive illness. Br J Soc Clin Psychol 1967; 6:278–296.

75. Hanson S, Buckelew SP, Hewett XX, O'Neal G: The relationship between coping and adjustment after spinal cord injury: 5-year follow-up study. Rehabil Psychol 1993; 38:41–52.

76. Hart LG, Evans RW: The functional status of ESRD patients as measured by the Sickness Impact Profile. J Chron Dis 1987; 40:1175–1305.

77. Hathaway SR, McKinley JC: Booklet for the Minnesota Multiphasic Personality Inventory. New York, Psychological Corporation, 1943.

78. Hollon SD, Shelton RC, Davis DD: Cognitive therapy for depression: Conceptual issues and clinical efficacy. J Consult Clin Psychol 1993; 61:270–275.

79. Jacobs H: The Los Angeles Head Injury Survey: Procedures and initial findings. Arch Phys Med Rehabil 1988; 69:425–431.

80. Kaplan E: Process and achievement revisited. *In* Wapner S, Kaplan B (eds): Toward a Holistic Developmental Psychology. Hillsdale, NJ, Lawrence Erlbaum, 1983.

81. Kaplan E, Fine D, Morris R, Dellis D: WAIS-R as a Neuropsychological Instrument. San Antonio, The Psychological Corporation, 1991.

82. Katz MM, Lyerly SB: Methods for measuring adjustment and social behavior in the community: I. Rationale, description, discriminative validity and scale development. Psychol Rep 1963; 13:503–535.

83. Kertesz A (ed): Localization and Neuroimaging in Neuropsychology. San Diego, Academic Press, 1994.

84. Kleinke CL: How chronic pain patients cope with depression: Relation to treatment outcome in a multidisciplinary pain clinic. Rehabil Psychol 1991; 36:207–218.

85. Krause JS: Survival following spinal cord injury: A 15-year prospective study. Rehabil Psychol 1991; 36:89–98.

86. Krause JS, Crewe NM: Prediction of long-term survival of persons with spinal cord injury. Rehabil Psychol 1987; 32:205–214.

87. Langfitt TW, Obrist WD, Alavi A, et al: Regional structure and function in head-injured patients: Correlation of CT, MRI, PET, CBF, and neuropsychological assessment. In Levin HS, Grafman J, Eisenberg, HM (eds): Neurobehavioral Recovery from Head Injury. New York, Oxford, 1987, pp 30–42.

88. Lazarus RS: Cognition and motivation in emotion. Am Psychol 1991; 46:352–367.

89. Lazarus RS: Progress on a cognitive-motivational-relational theory of emotion. Am Psychol 1991; 46:819–834.

90. Lazarus RS, Folkman S: Stress, Appraisal, and Coping. New York, Springer, 1986.

91. Lees-Haley PR, Brown RS: Neuropsychological complaint base rates of 170 personal injury claimants. Arch Clin Neuropsychol 1993; 8:203–209.

92. Lees-Haley PR, Fox DD: Neuropsychological false positives in litigation: Trail Making Test findings. Percept Mot Skills 1990; 70:1379–1382.

93. Levin HS, High WM, Goethe KE, et al: The Neurobehavioral Rating Scale: Assessment of the behavioral sequelae of head injury by the clinician. J Neurol Neurosurg Psychiatry 1987; 50:183–193.

94. Levin HS, O'Donnell VM, Grossman RG: The Galveston orientation and amnesia test: A practical scale to assess cognition after head injury. J Nerv Ment Dis 1979; 167:675–684.

95. Lewinsohn PM, Graff M: Pleasant activities and depression. J Consult Clin Psychol 1978; 41:271–278.

96. Lezak MD: Neuropsychological Assessment, ed 2. New York, Oxford, 1983.

97. Lezak MD: Relationships between personality disorders, social disturbances, and physical disability following traumatic brain injury. J Head Trauma Rehabil 1987; 2:57–69.

98. Lubuski AA, Moore AD, Stambrook M, Gill DD: Cognitive beliefs following severe traumatic brain injury: Association with post injury employment. Brain Inj 1994; 8:65–70.

99. Luria AR: Higher Cortical Functions in Man. New York, Basic Books, 1980.

100. Luria AR: The Working Brain. New York, Basic Books, 1973.

101. Mahler HI, Kulik JA: Preferences for health care involvement, perceived control and surgical recovery: A prospective study. Soc Sci Med 1990; 31:743–751.

102. Malec JF, Smigielski JS, DePompolo RW, Thompson JM: Outcome evaluation and prediction in a comprehensive-integrated post-acute outpatient brain injury rehabilitation programme. Brain Inj 1993; 7:15–29.

103. Markwardt FC: Peabody Individual Achievement Test—Revised. Circle Pines, Minn, American Guidance Service, 1989.

104. Maslach C, Florian V: Burnout, job setting, and self-evaluation among rehabilitation counselors. Rehabil Psychol 1988; 33:85–94.

105. Matarazzo JD: Psychological assessment versus psychological testing: Validation from Binet to the school, clinic, and courtroom. Am Psychol 1990; 45:999–1017.

106. McGlynn SM, Schacter DL: Unawareness of deficits in neuropsychological syndromes. J Clin Exp Neuropsychol 1989; 11:143–205.

107. McKinlay WW, Brooks DN, Bond MR: Post-concussional symptoms, financial compensation, and outcome of severe blunt head injury. J Neurol Neurosurg Psychiatry 1983; 46:1084–1091.

108. McSweeney AJ, Grant I, Heaton RK, et al: Life quality of patients with chronic obstructive pulmonary disease. Arch Intern Med 1982; 142:473–478.

109. Mechanic D: Social psychologic factors affecting the presentation of bodily complaints. N Engl J Med 1972; 286:1132–1139.

110. Mehlbye J, Larsen A: Social and economic consequences of brain damage in Denmark: A case study. In Christensen A-L, Uzzell B (eds): Brain Injury and Neuropsychological Rehabilitation: International Perspectives. Hillsdale, NJ, Lawrence Erlbaum, 1994, pp 257–268.

111. Mehnert T, Krauss HH, Nadler R, Boyd M: Correlates of life satisfaction in those with disabling conditions. Rehabil Psychol 1990; 35:3–18.

112. Meier MJ, Benton AL, Diller L (eds): Neuropsychological Rehabilitation. London, Churchill Livingstone, 1987.

113. Meltzer ML: Poor memory: A case report. J Clin Psychol 1983; 39:3–10.

114. Mesulam, M-M (ed): Principles of Behavioral Neurology. Philadelphia, FA Davis, 1985.

115. Milberg WP, Hebben N, Kaplan E: The Boston process approach to neuropsychological assessment. In Grant I, Adams KM (eds): Neuropsychological Assessment in Neuropsychiatric Disorders. New York, Oxford, 1986.

116. Millon T: Millon Clinical Multiaxial Inventory II Manual. Minneapolis, National Computer Systems, 1987.

117. Millon T: A theoretical derivation of pathological personalities. In Millon T, Klerman GL (eds): Contemporary Directions in Psychopathology: Toward the DSM-IV. New York, Guilford, 1986.

118. Moore AD, Stambrook M: Coping strategies and locus of control following traumatic brain injury: Relationship to long-term outcome. Brain Inj 1992; 6:89–94.

119. Moore AD, Stambrook M, Wilson KG: Cognitive moderators in adjustment to chronic illness: Locus of control beliefs following traumatic brain injury. Neuropsychol Rehabil 1991; 1:185–198.

120. Naeser MA: Neuroimaging and recovery of auditory comprehension and spontaneous speech in aphasia with some implications for treatment in severe aphasia. In Kertesz A (ed): Localization and Neuroimaging in Neuropsychology. New York, Academic Press, 1994, pp 245–296.

121. National Center for Medical Rehabilitation Research: Research Plan for the National Center for Medical Rehabilitation Research, NIH publication No. 93–3509. Washington, DC, U.S. Department of Health and Human Services, National Institutes of Health, 1993.

122. Nielsen AC, Williams TA: Depression in ambulatory medical patients. Arch Gen Psychiatry 1980; 37:999–1004.

123. Oades-Souther D, Olbrisch ME: Psychological adjustment to ostomy surgery. Rehabil Psychol 1984; 29:221–238.

124. Orr E, Aronson E: Relationships between orthopedic disability and perceived social support: Four theoretical hypotheses. Rehabil Psychol 1990; 35:29–42.

125. Ott CR, Sivarajan ES, Newton KM, et al: A controlled randomized study of early cardiac rehabilitation: The Sickness Impact Profile as an assessment tool. Heart Lung 1983; 12:162–170.

126. Partridge C, Johnston M: Perceived control of recovery from physical disability: Measurement and prediction. Br J Clin Psychol 1989; 28:53–59.

127. Patterson DR, Everett JL, Bombardier CH, et al: Psychological effects of severe burn injuries. Psychol Bull 1993; 113:362–378.

128. Pennebaker JW: The Psychology of Physical Symptoms. New York, Springer-Verlag, 1982.

129. Pollard WE, Bobbitt RA, Bergner M, et al: The Sickness Impact Profile: Reliability of a health status measure. Med Care 1976; 14:146–155.

130. Prigatano GP, Fordyce DJ, Zeiner HK, et al: Neuropsychological Rehabilitation after Brain Injury. Baltimore, Johns Hopkins, 1986, p 35.

131. Prigatano GP, Fordyce DJ, Zeiner HK, et al: Neuropsychological rehabilitation after closed head injury in young adults. J Neurol Neurosurg Psychiatry 1984; 47:505–513.

132. Prigatano GP, Klonoff PS, O'Brien KP, et al: Productivity after neuropsychologically oriented milieu rehabilitation. J Head Trauma Rehabil 1994; 9:91–102.

133. Rape RN, Bush JP, Slavin LA: Toward a conceptualization of the family's adaptation to a member's head injury: A critique of developmental stage models. Rehabil Psychol 1992; 37:3–22.

134. Reitan RM: Theoretical and methodological bases of the Halstead-Reitan neuropsychological test battery. In Grant I, Adams KM (eds): Neuropsychological Assessment of Neuropsychiatric Disorders. New York, Oxford, 1986, pp 3–30.

135. Reitan RM, Wolfson D: The Halstead-Reitan Neuropsychological Test Battery: Theory and Clinical Interpretation. Tucson, Neuropsychology Press, 1985.

136. Revenson T, Felton BA: Disability and coping as predictors of psychological adjustment to rheumatoid arthritis. J Clin Consult Psychol 1989; 57:344–348.

137. Rintala DH, Young ME, Hart KA, et al: Social support and the

well-being of persons with spinal cord injury living in the community. Rehabil Psychol 1992; 37:155–164.

138. Robins CJ, Hayes AM: An appraisal of cognitive therapy. J Consult Clin Psychol 1993; 61:205–214.

139. Rodin G, Voshart K: Depression in the medically ill: An overview. Am J Psychiatry 1986; 143:696–705.

140. Romano JM, Turner JA: Chronic pain and depression: Does the evidence support a relationship? Psychol Bull 1985; 97:18–34.

141. Romano JM, Turner JA, Friedman LS, et al: Observational assessment of chronic pain patient-spouse behavioral interactions. Behav Ther 1991; 22:549–567.

142. Rosenbaum M, Najenson T: Changes in life patterns and symptoms of low mood as reported by wives of severely brain-injured soldiers. J Consult Clin Psychol 1976; 44:881–888.

143. Ross ED, Rush AJ: Diagnosis and neuroanatomical correlates of depression in brain-damaged patients. Arch Gen Psychiatry 1981; 38:1344–1354.

144. Rotter JB: Generalized expectancies for internal versus external control of reinforcement. Psychol Monogr 1966, p 80.

145. Rubonis AV, Bickman L: Psychological impairment in the wake of disaster: The disaster-psychopathology relationship. Psychol Bull 1991; 109:384–399.

146. Schulberg HC, Saul M, McClellan M, et al: Assessing depression in primary medical and psychiatric practices. Arch Gen Psychiatry 1985; 42:1164–1170.

147. Segal ZV: Appraisal of the self-schema construct in cognitive models of depression. Psychol Bull 1988; 103:147–162.

148. Sohlberg MM, Mateer CA: Introduction to Cognitive Rehabilitation: Theory and Practice. New York, Guilford, 1989.

149. Sohlberg MM, Mateer CA: Training use of compensatory memory books: A three-stage behavioral. J Clin Exper Neuropsychol 1989; 11:871–891.

150. Spiers PA, Schomer DL, Blume HW, Mesulam M-M: Temporolimbic epilepsy and behavior. In Mesulam M-M (ed): Principles of Behavioral Neurology. Philadelphia, FA Davis, 1985, pp 289–326.

151. Spreen O, Strauss E: A Compendium of Neuropsychological Tests: Administration, Norms, and Commentary. New York, Oxford, 1991.

152. Stein PN, Gordon WA, Hibbard MR, Sliwinski M: An examination of depression in the spouses of stroke patients. Rehabil Psychol 1992; 37:121–130.

153. Stone JB, Bluhm HP, White MI: Correlates of depression among long-term insulin-dependent diabetics. Rehabil Psychol 1984; 29:85–94.

154. Strub R, Black FW: The Mental Status Examination in Neurology, ed 2. Philadelphia, FA Davis, 1985.

155. Stuss DT, Gow CA, Hetherington CR: "No longer Gage": Frontal lobe dysfunction and emotional changes. J Consult Clin Psychol 1992; 60:349–359.

156. Sugarbaker PH, Barofsky I, Rosenberg SA, Gianola FJ: Quality of life assessment of patients in extremity sarcoma clinical trials. Surgery 1982; 1:17–23.

157. Taylor SE: Adjustment to threatening events: A theory of cognitive adaptation. Am Psychol 1983; 38:1161–1173.

158. Taylor SE, Brown JD: Illusion and well-being: A social psychological perspective on mental health. Psychol Bull 1988; 103:193–210.

159. Temkin N, McLean A, Dikman S, et al: Development and evaluation of modifications to the Sickness Impact Profile for head injury. J Clin Epidemiol 1988; 41:47–57.

160. Thomsen IV: Late outcome of very severe blunt head trauma: A 10–15 year follow-up. J Neurol Neurosurg Psychiatry 1984; 47:260–268.

161. Trexler LE: Neuropsychological rehabilitation in the United States. In Meier MJ, Benton AL, Diller L (eds): Neuropsychological Rehabilitation. London, Churchill Livingstone, 1987, pp 473–480.

162. Trexler LE: Professional issues in neuropsychological rehabilitation. In Ellis DW, Christensen A-L (eds): Neuropsychological Treatment After Brain Injury. Boston, Kluwer Academic Publishers, 1989, pp 363–378.

163. Trexler LE, Thomas JD: Behavioral and cognitive deficits in cerebrovascular accident and closed head injury: Implications for cognitive rehabilitation. In Trexler LE (ed): Cognitive Rehabilitation: Conceptualization and Intervention. New York, Plenum Press, 1983, pp 27–62.

164. Trexler LE, Thomas JD: Research design in neuropsychological rehabilitation. In von Steinbuchel N, von Cramon DY, Poppel E

(eds): Neuropsychological Rehabilitation. Berlin, Springer-Verlag, 1992, pp 79–87.

165. Trexler LE, Webb PM, Zappala G: Strategic aspects of neuropsychological rehabilitation. In Christensen A-L, Uzzell BP (eds): Brain Injury and Neuropsychological Rehabilitation: International Perspectives. Hillsdale, NJ, Lawrence Erlbaum, 1994, pp 99–123.

166. Trexler LE, Zappala G: Neuropathological determinants of acquired attention disorders in traumatic brain injury. Brain Cogn 1988; 8:291–302.

167. Trexler LE, Zappala G: Re-examining the determinants of recovery and rehabilitation of memory defects following traumatic brain injury. Brain Inj 1988; 2:187–203.

168. Trieschmann RB: Spinal Cord Injuries: Psychological, Social, and Vocational Adjustment. New York, Pergamon Press, 1980.

169. Tupper DE, Cicerone KD: Introduction to the neuropsychology of everyday life. In Tupper DE, Cicerone KD (eds): The Neuropsychology of Everyday Life: Assessment and Basic Competencies. Boston, Kluwer Academic Publishers, 1990, pp 3–18.

170. Turk DC, Kerns RD, Rosenberg R: Effects of marital interaction on chronic pain and disability: Examining the down side of social support. Rehabil Psychol 1992; 37:259–274.

171. Turner RJ, McLean PD: Physical disability and psychological distress. Rehabil Psychol 1989; 34:225–242.

172. Uomoto JM, Esselman PC: Traumatic brain injury and chronic pain: Differential types and rates by head injury severity. Arch Phys Med Rehabil 1993; 74:61–64.

173. Uzzell BP, Dolinskas CA, Wiser RF, Langfitt TW: Influence of lesions detected by computed tomography on outcome and neuropsychological recovery after severe head injury. Neurosurgery 1987; 20:396–402.

174. Vitaliano PP, Katon W, Maiuro RD, Russo J: Coping in chest pain patients with and without psychiatric disorders. J Consult Clin Psychol 1989; 57:338–343.

175. von Steinbuchel N, Von Cramon DY, Poppel E: Neuropsychological Rehabilitation. Berlin, Springer-Verlag, 1992.

176. Wallston KA, Wallston BS, Devellis R: Development of the Multidimensional Health Locus of Control (MHLC) scales. Health Educ Monogr 1978; 6:160.

177. Wechsler D: Wechsler Adult Intelligence Scale—Revised: Manual. San Antonio, Psychological Corporation, 1981.

178. Weinstein EA, Kahn RL: Denial of Illness. Springfield, Ill, Charles C. Thomas, 1955.

179. Weissman HN: Distortions and deceptions in self presentation: Effects of protracted litigation in personal injury cases. Behav Sci Law 1990; 8:67–74.

180. Weissman HN: Forensic psychological assessment and the effects of protracted litigation on impairment in personal injury litigation. Forensic Rep 1991; 4:417–429.

181. Westbrook MT, Nordholm LA: Effects of diagnosis on reactions to patient optimism and depression. Rehabil Psychol 1986; 31:79–94.

182. Whisman MA: Mediators and moderators of change in cognitive therapy of depression. Psychol Bull 1993; 114:248–265.

183. Willanger R, Danielsen UT, Ankerhus J: Denial and neglect of hemiparesis in right-sided apoplectic lesions. Acta Neurol Scand 1981; 64:310–326.

184. Willer B, Ottenbacher KJ, Coad ML: The Community Integration Questionnaire: A comparative examination. Am J Phys Med Rehabil 1994; 73:103–111.

185. Willer B, Rosenthal M, Kreutzer JS, et al: Assessment of community integration following rehabilitation for traumatic brain injury. J Head Trauma Rehabil 1993; 8:75–87.

186. Wills TA: Perceptions of clients by professional helpers. Psychol Bull 1978; 85:968–1000.

187. Wilson JTL: Review: The relationship between neropsycological function and brain damage detected by neuroimaging after closed head injury. Brain Inj 1990; 4:349–363.

188. Woodcock RW, Mather N: Woodcock-Johnson Tests of Achievement. Allen, Tex, DLM Teaching Resources, 1989.

189. World Health Organization: International Classification of Impairments, Disabilities, and Handicaps: A Manual of Classification Relating to the Consequences of Disease. Geneva, WHO, 1980.

190. Wortman CB, Silver RC: The myths of coping with loss. J Consult Clin Psychol 1989; 57:349–357.

191. Zung WWK: A self-rating depression scale. Arch Gen Psychiatry 1965; 12:63–770.

5

Kinematics and Kinetics of Gait

WILLIAM S. PEASE, M.D., and
PETER M. QUESADA, PH.D.

Clinical observation of walking is a vital fundamental skill for the physiatrist. A computerized laboratory will never replace this clinical ability in association with the personal interaction with a patient. A gait analysis laboratory can provide a valuable service by quantifying gait observations made during the practice of physical medicine and rehabilitation. Accurate recording of joint movement and muscle actions expands the teaching of complex gait movements. Clinical care and research also are enhanced through quantitative assessment. Serial measurement of changes in walking patterns that occur as the outcome of treatment or with the use of adaptive aids can be quantified with a gait analysis laboratory.

Human walking is a fascinating, complex dynamic activity which varies subtly from one individual to another. A knowledgeable observer of gait always has "material" to study, and waiting at the airport need no longer be boring. A few cultural conventions affect gait around the world, but walking is remarkably constant among peoples of different cultures and behavioral styles.

NORMAL WALKING

The gait pattern is a rhythmic cycle of events which repeat in a coordinated manner[26] (Figs. 5–1 to 5–3). Understanding a single cycle is extrapolated easily to walking any distance. Initiating and stopping walking movement are complicated processes that will not be discussed in detail here. Learning to start and stop seems to be accomplished readily as an inherent part of learning to walk.

The gait cycle conventionally begins with a "heel-strike" contact with the floor initiating *stance phase*. Stance phase continues until the limb leaves the ground, entering *swing phase*. Swing phase allows the foot to step forward and one repetition of the cycle is compete as heel-strike reoccurs for the same leg. In normal walking, stance phase and swing phase are approximately 60% and 40% of gait cycle, respectively. Stance phase is subdivided into *single-limb stance* (40% of cycle; when the opposite limb is swinging), and two *double-limb stance* periods of about 10% each. During double-limb stance, support of body weight must be shifted from one leg to the other. Double limb stance is the defining feature that separates walking from running, the latter lacking double-limb support.

The initial period of double-limb stance follows foot-strike, during which time both feet are in contact with the ground until opposite *toe-off*. During double-limb stance, the trunk weight must be shifted from the opposite foot to prepare for single-limb stance. During single-limb stance the opposite leg advances forward (steps) and prepares to make its foot-strike. The single-limb stance leg must both balance and propel the body.

During a leg's second double-limb support period the leg pushes the body forward and transfers weight back to the opposite leg which is now beginning its stance phase. Swing phase begins when the foot no longer contacts the ground. Limb advancement during swing phase defines *step length*. An efficient swing phase ends with the swinging knee at or near full extension in order to maximize step length. Two successive step lengths equal *stride length*, which is the distance covered during one gait cycle (i.e., 2 steps = 1 stride). *Cadence* is the number of steps per minute. Gait velocity, *v*, is calculated as

$$v = \frac{SL \times C}{2},$$

where *SL* is stride length, *C* is cadence (gait velocity generally is converted into useful units, such as miles per hour or meters per second).

The Determinants of Gait

The basic mechanisms of human gait have been well understood through the "determinants" of gait, attributed

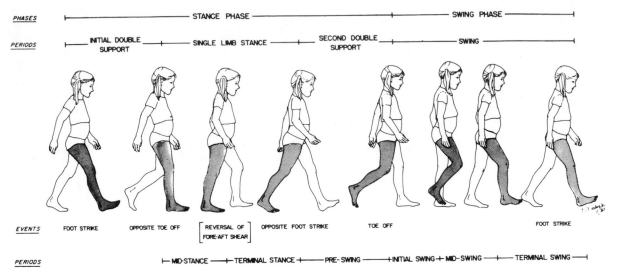

FIGURE 5–1   Sagittal view of gait events for shaded lower limb. (From Sutherland DH: Gait Disorders in Childhood and Adolescence. Baltimore, Williams & Wilkins, 1984.)

to Inman et al.[12] Knowledge of these six elements of motion of the lower limbs during walking has direct application in understanding the function and efficiency of walking. At its simplest, gait efficiency is understood by the movement of the body's center of gravity, located just anterior to the S1 vertebral body. These elements can be individually affected by disabling injuries and the effect of loss of individual elements can be easily understood if their functions are appreciated. Physiatric and surgical treatment of gait problems is often directed at restoring or compensating for the loss of one or more determinants or elements. The six determinants (elements) of gait are:

1. Pelvic rotation
2. Pelvic list (Trendelenburg)
3. Knee flexion in stance
4. Ankle flexion/extension mechanisms
5. Knee, ankle, and foot rotation
6. Lateral displacement of the pelvis

Each of these elements contributes to the efficiency of gait by smoothing the path of the center of gravity of the body. Optimal motion in walking would be the center of mass following a linear path (which only occurs with a rolling wheel). Deflections of the line of motion occur as

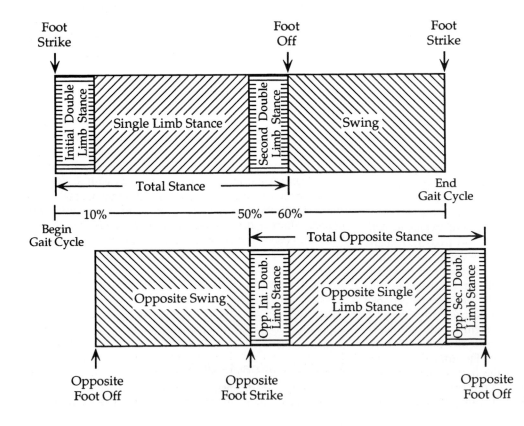

FIGURE 5–2 Time line representation of timing of each lower limb's gait events and periods, with approximate percentages of cycle indicated.

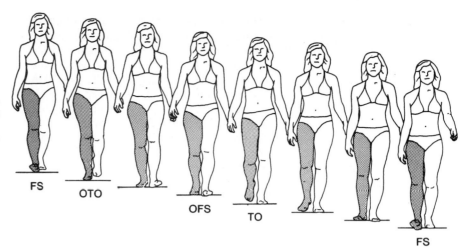

FIGURE 5–3 Frontal view of walking cycle (note that pelvic Trendelenburg gait is appreciated more readily in frontal plane). (From Sutherland DH: Gait Disorders in Childhood and Adolescence, Baltimore, Williams & Wilkins, 1984.)

the trunk rises above and laterally shifts over each foot during single stance. As these sinusoidal deflections from the line of travel diminish in amplitude, the mechanical work of walking is reduced.

Pelvic rotation occurs with each step; the side of the body in swing phase rotates forward. The first effect of pelvic rotation is to reduce the vertical drop of the center of gravity during double-stance phase. The second effect is to increase the length of the step by forward movement of the hip joint.

Pelvic list, or Trendelenburg, is the lowering of the pelvis on the swinging leg side (see Fig. 5–3). This drop of the pelvis reduces the vertical rise of the center of gravity as it passes over the stance leg. This pelvic drop must be compensated for by increased knee and ankle flexion so that the swinging leg can pass under the lowered hemipelvis.

Knee flexion occurs following heel-strike in gait and also serves efficiency of movement (see Fig. 5–1). The bending of the knee reduces the vertical elevation of the body at midstance by shortening the hip-to-ankle distance. A second effect is to absorb the shock of impact at heel-strike by lengthening contraction of the quadriceps. This impact control reduces the work needed to control the inertia of the trunk (the tendency of the body to continue forward when the leg stops).

Knee, ankle, and foot mechanisms work together to control movement of the center of gravity and to develop forward propulsion. At heel-strike ankle plantar flexion smoothes the curve of the falling pelvis. After midstance the knee extends as the ankle plantar-flexes and the foot supinates to restore length to the leg and diminish the fall of the pelvis at opposite heel-strike. The added effect of this is to increase the step length by moving the pivot point forward from the ankle to the metatarsophalangeal joints. In swing phase, the leg length is shortened by dorsiflexion and knee flexion which reduces the lever arm for leg swing, and allows foot clearance.

The last of Inman's elements is lateral displacement of the body. The net center of gravity of the body must lie above the base of support (stance foot). The trunk moves laterally to achieve this so that the step width and lateral displacement of the pelvis are both normally 4 to 5 cm. This adds a lateral sinusoidal wave of one period per stride

to the vertical motion of two periods per stride (rising over the foot on each step).

Rotation of the legs and of the trunk are also important components of the gait cycle and efficiency. This is most easily seen in rotation of the shoulder which proceeds opposite to rotation of the pelvis. The trunk and arm swing controls the inertial movements of their segment's center of mass. Rotation of the thigh, leg, and foot generally is opposite to pelvic rotation and maintains the foot in the forward direction.

Knowledge of these six determinants of gait allows one to begin to study the complex control system which brings about these elemental movements. Coordinated muscle contractions with concentric, isometric, and eccentric forces are necessary at key moments of the gait cycle.

In order to appreciate these interrelated control mechanisms the components of the gait cycle are reviewed in the following section as segments of time. During each phase of the gait cycle the interactions of muscle actions and elements of movement are systematically studied.

Normal Kinematics

Stance phase begins with a period of *initial double-limb stance* lasting from foot-strike until contralateral toe-off. This time period also is referred to as loading or weight acceptance, and represents 10% to 12% of the gait cycle time. During this interval the stance side of the pelvis is rotated forward. This forward pelvic rotation reaches its maximum angular excursion at the end of double-limb support. External hip rotation (characterized, though not necessarily quantified, by a decreasing angle between a pelvic posterior-to-anterior axis and a femoral lateral-to-medial axis) is occurring during this period, and it also peaks at opposite toe-off. Typically, hip Trendelenburg (i.e., lowering of the swing side of the pelvis relative to the stance side of the pelvis) begins at the onset of single-limb support, with the stance side of the pelvis elevating relative to the contralateral side. The hip is flexed maximally at foot-strike (Fig. 5–4, *top*) and begins to extend as the pelvis continues forward while the foot is stationary on the ground.

Knee and ankle movements are important components

of the loading period, or initial double-limb stance. The knee is nearly fully extended at foot-strike. Following foot-strike, the knee demonstrates a "flexion wave" which reaches a peak of about 20 degrees (Fig. 5–4, *center*). During this knee flexion, the quadriceps muscles contract eccentrically to absorb some of the body's energy at foot-strike, which reduces the burden of impact with the ground on other structures (e.g., heel pad, joint articular cartilage). The knee flexion wave also functions to reduce mechanical energy expenditure by diminishing the center of gravity's vertical rise as the body proceeds toward the stance foot. At the same time, additional impact energy is absorbed by eccentric activity of the dorsiflexor muscles, as the ankle plantar-flexes after foot-strike (Fig. 5–4, *bottom*) owing to ground reaction forces that have a line of action running posterior to the ankle. Initial double-limb stance ends with the foot in full contact with the floor and the knee at 20 degrees of flexion. The limb is prepared now to support the entire body weight during single-limb stance.

Single-limb stance is the gait cycle's "working phase," during which the trunk segment of the body is propelled past the stance foot. This period from opposite toe-off through opposite foot-strike occupies 38% to 40% of the gait cycle. (*Note*: Opposite foot-strike must occur at 50% of the gait cycle in a symmetrical gait.) During single-limb stance the pelvis rotates posteriorly from the view of the stance leg (i.e., the swing side of the pelvis progresses forward more rapidly than the stance side), and the pelvis reaches the neutral position just prior to opposite foot strike. Pelvic Trendelenburg (i.e., the stance side of the pelvis elevated relative to the swing side; see Fig. 5–3) peaks in the middle of this phase, with the pelvis tilted about 10 degrees in the frontal plane. Hip internal rotation progresses during this stage, and also passes neutral. The hip is the "pivot point" for the trunk above and extends to 0 degrees as the trunk passes over the foot.

The knee extends fully during single-limb stance phase. During this time of knee extension, the tibia is rotating around the ankle joint while the foot is flat on the floor. Heel rise occurs shortly before opposite foot-strike. At heel

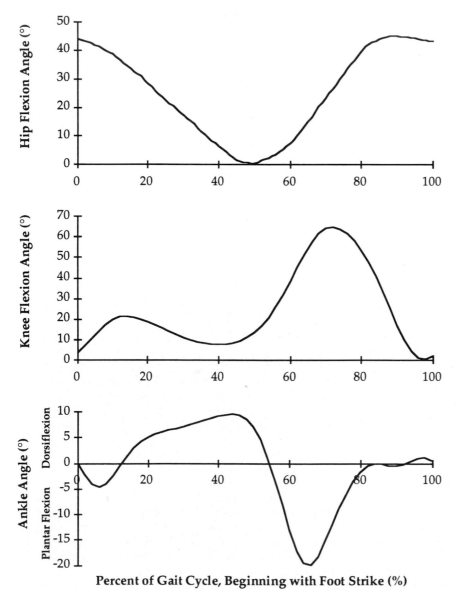

FIGURE 5–4 Normal (i.e., nonpathological) hip *(top)*, knee *(center)*, and ankle *(bottom)* joint angles in the sagittal plane for one gait cycle. The cycle is marked from 0% to 100% of the cycle time. The reader should use a vertical straight-edge in order to appreciate the simultaneous joint angles at any instant in the cycle.

Percent of Gait Cycle, Beginning with Foot Strike (%)

rise, the ankle angle reverses direction and plantar-flexes toward neutral and the knee begins to flex.

Second double-limb stance begins at opposite foot-strike and continues until ipsilateral toe-off. This time period, in symmetrical gait, is the same 10% to 12% of the gait cycle as was initial double-limb stance. During this time the pelvis continues to rotate posteriorly (the contralateral side of the pelvis is still progressing forward more rapidly than the stance side). Hip internal rotation continues to neutral. The stance side of the pelvis begins to lower in preparation for swing. Hip flexion begins during this period as knee flexion increases in preparation for swing. The ankle plantar-flexes rapidly as the limb is unloaded with the triceps surae still contracting. The ankle joint angle passes the neutral position and reaches maximum plantar flexion at the time of toe-off.

Swing phase can be thought of in two halves, which have distinct functional activities. Initial swing is a lower limb *acceleration* period in which active hip flexion advances the thigh. Terminal swing is a limb *deceleration* period, in which inertia is generally sufficient to maintain forward body progression, and the hip joint angle is maintained at its maximum excursion. These two periods are divided by "ankle crossing," which is the moment when the swing limb's ankle passes the stance ankle.

The pelvis rotates forward to the neutral position during initial swing phase. Abduction of the pelvis (Trendelenburg) maximizes late in initial swing, and lowers the pelvis on the swing side. This action reduces vertical body displacement and mechanical energy expenditure. Initial swing phase hip flexion proceeds more rapidly than in late double stance, and maximum angular excursion of the hip (40 degrees) occurs at ankle crossing. Hip rotation is external since limb alignment is forward as the pelvis rotates on the pivot of the contralateral hip. Flexion of the knee proceeds in linkage with that of the hip. Maximum knee flexion (about 60 degrees) is reached at the end of initial swing. During this time the ankle dorsiflexes rapidly from full plantar flexion to neutral.

Terminal swing begins with a complete change from acceleration to deceleration of the lower limb. Some of the momentum generated during initial swing must be dissipated before foot-strike to ensure stability. Pelvic rotation continues to advance the swing side forward, although pelvic rotation is not yet maximal at foot-strike. Consistent with this pelvic rotation, the hip is rotating externally. Hip flexion peaks early in terminal swing as some of the thigh's momentum is dissipated. Hip flexion then stabilizes, and knee joint motion reverses into extension due to the remaining forward momentum of the shank (lower leg). The knee then reaches full extension as dissipation of much of the shank's momentum is completed. With the ankle's task of toe clearance accomplished, the ankle joint angle remains stable in its neutral position during terminal swing.

Dynamic Electromyography

Muscle contractions during gait are studied most often by the recording of electromyographic (EMG) signals, representing depolarization of muscle fibers. Recording EMG signals with surface electrodes placed on the skin over a muscle is the most convenient method of EMG data collec-

tion, although it obviously is limited to superficial muscles. Data collection from deep-lying muscles (e.g., the posterior tibial and iliac muscles) or more selective recording of a smaller muscle near a larger one (e.g., the rectus femoris adjacent to the vastus muscles) often requires use of "fine-wire" electrodes, which are fashioned from extremely thin, flexible wire. Preamplified EMG signals can be transmitted by cables or broadcast by radio-wave telemetry to a receiver which can then be sampled by a computer system. Comparison of simultaneously recorded EMG signals, joint and limb movement, and ground reaction forces allows appreciation of the muscle activity that produces or restrains movement. Force of the muscle contractions is related to the amplitude of the EMG signal; however, the muscle force can be estimated only qualitatively.

Surface EMG is recorded easily with disposable, gelled electrodes which have minimal mass and attach securely (Fig. 5–5). Muscle movement relative to the skin causes uncontrollable variation in the signal, but in isometric contraction the EMG amplitude and force are linearly correlated. Electrode positions for a given muscle are chosen to minimize recording of other nearby muscles so as to avoid contamination. Typically bipolar electrode placements are used in which two electrodes are placed over the muscle belly. In such an arrangement, the signal recorded is the potential difference between the two electrodes.

Fine-wire recording of EMG signals also is performed widely. A typical bipolar fine-wire electrode configuration consists of two thin wires placed through the shaft of a 25-gauge syringe needle (Fig. 5–6). The ends of the wires are exposed (insulation removed) and the wires are aligned in an offset manner so as to avoid contact between the exposed portions of the two wires. With small amounts of insulated wire beyond the needle tip (one wire extended farther than the other to avoid bare wire contact, as mentioned above), the wire ends are bent over the needle edge to provide a means for the wires to "catch" in the muscle belly. The needle is inserted smoothly into the muscle and

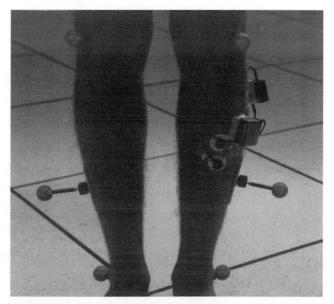

FIGURE 5–5 Disposable surface electrodes placed in a bipolar arrangement over the anterior tibialis muscle.

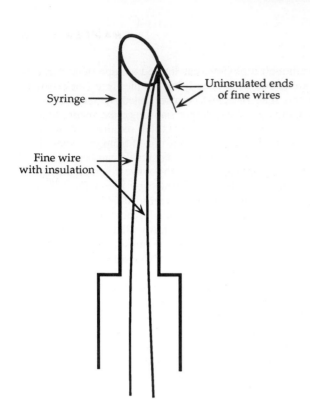

Syringe →

Uninsulated ends
of fine wires

Fine wire
with insulation

FIGURE 5–6 Schematic drawing of a bipolar fine-wire electrode preparation (note that wires extend unequal lengths beyond needle tip, such that exposed ends of wires do not contact one another).

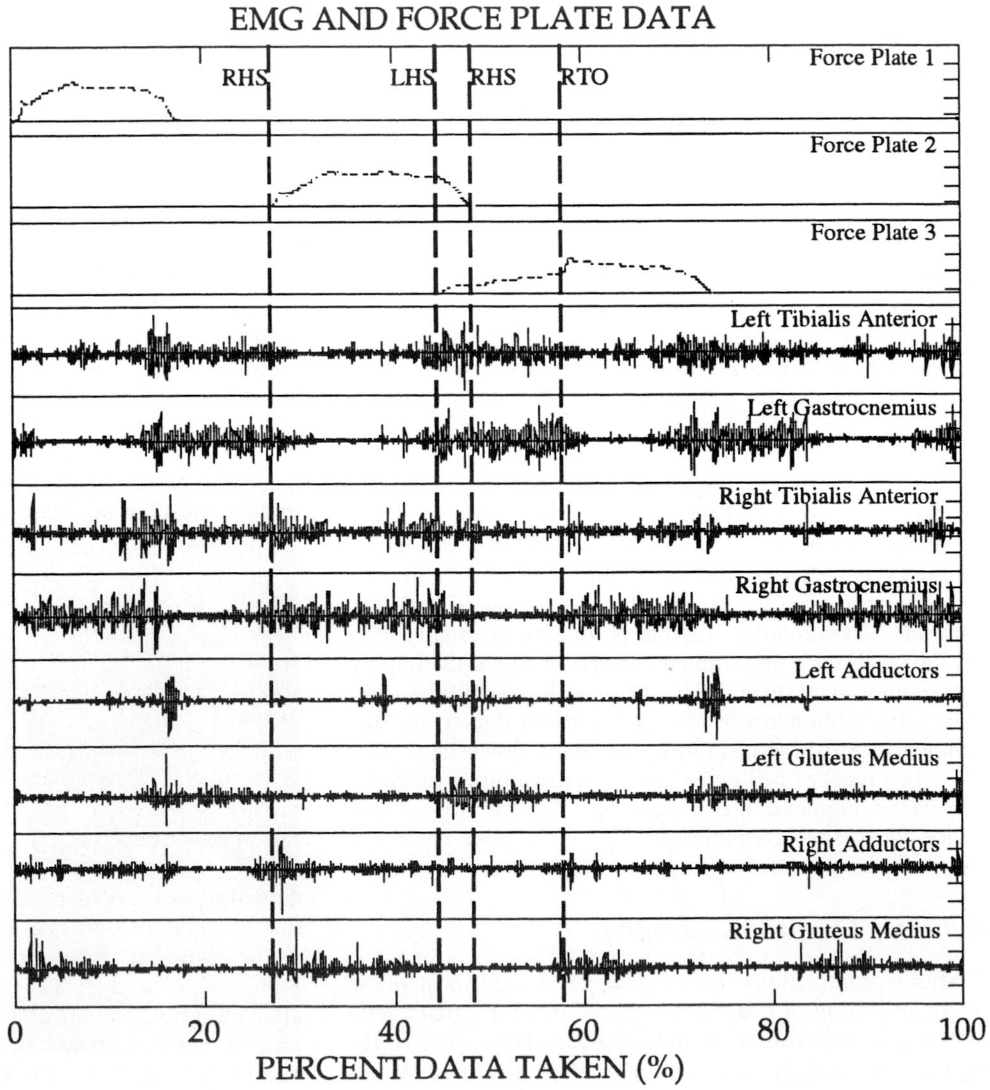

EMG AND FORCE PLATE DATA

FIGURE 5–7 Filtered electromyographic (EMG) outputs from Ohio State University Gait Analysis Laboratory (note that vertical force plate output at *top* of figure can be used in determining timing of gait events).

Force Plate 1

RHS   LHS RHS RTO

Force Plate 2

Force Plate 3

Left Tibialis Anterior

Left Gastrocnemius

Right Tibialis Anterior

Right Gastrocnemius

Left Adductors

Left Gluteus Medius

Right Adductors

Right Gluteus Medius

0   20   40   60   80   100

PERCENT DATA TAKEN (%)

removed, leaving the bent-back wires in position.[2] The wires are then attached to a preamplifier. After the laboratory session is completed, the wires are removed, with little trauma, by a gentle, firm pull.

Once collected, EMG signals generally are filtered (mechanical movement artifacts must be eliminated) and displayed in a convenient arrangement with gait cycle events identified (Fig. 5–7). The EMG signals then are related to the movements seen in kinematic analysis during the same phase of the gait cycle. In some laboratories EMG signals are rectified and smoothed by convention as well.

QUANTIFICATION OF JOINT MOTION

The joint motions described previously can be conceptualized easily with respect to the sagittal plane. One can obtain a simple approximation of a sagittal plane joint angle from estimates of the position of the joint, and the positions of one location on each of the two segments which meet at the joint.[2] For example, using the positions of markers placed at the lateral femoral epicondyle, greater trochanter, and lateral malleolus (Fig. 5–8), one can approximate a knee joint flexion-extension angle with a simple trigonometric relationship, such as

$$\theta_k = \cos^{-1}\left(\frac{\overline{HK}^2 + \overline{KA}^2 - \overline{HA}^2}{2\,\overline{HK}\,\overline{KA}}\right),$$

where θ_k is knee joint angle, $\overline{HA}$ is the distance from the

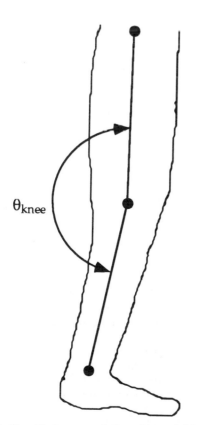

FIGURE 5–8 Simplified representation of knee joint angle using basic trigonometry.

greater trochanter to the lateral malleolus, $\overline{HK}$ is the distance from the greater trochanter to the lateral epicondyle, and $\overline{KA}$ is the distance from the lateral epicondyle to the lateral malleolus. These distances can be determined as

$$\overline{HA} = \sqrt{(x_H - x_A)^2 + (y_H - y_A)^2 + (z_H - z_A)^2},$$

$$\overline{HK} = \sqrt{(x_H - x_K)^2 + (y_H - y_K)^2 + (z_H - z_K)^2}, \text{ and}$$

$$\overline{KA} = \sqrt{(x_K - x_A)^2 + (y_K - y_A)^2 + (z_K - z_A)^2},$$

where x_H, y_H, z_H, x_K, y_K, z_K, and x_A, y_A, z_A are the Cartesian coordinates of the greater trochanter, lateral epicondyle, and lateral malleolus, respectively. An approach such as this one essentially models body segments as vectors. Although these vectors can lie anywhere in space, such methods account for joint motion in only one plane (i.e., joint motion about an axis perpendicular to the plane passing through the three points).

A majority of motion biomechanics laboratories (both research and clinical) determine joint angle trajectories about multiple axes of rotation (most often three axes). Lower limb joint motions generally are computed about axes of flexion-extension, internal-external rotation, and abduction-adduction. Although joint angles can be measured directly with electrogoniometers, estimation of joint angle trajectories from video-based marker position measurements is a more common means of obtaining joint motions (particularly in clinical settings and where joint kinetics are estimated).

Computation of joint motion about multiple axes requires that a minimum of three locations on each body segment be identified at each sampling interval for which multiaxis joint motions are desired. Mutual exclusivity of identified locations for each segment, typically, is not necessary. For example, one can include a knee joint center location as part of a thigh segment and as part of a shank segment. Marker locations often are chosen in order to facilitate approximation of joint center-of-rotation positions. Estimated joint centers commonly are used to define segments instead of measured positions of markers placed on the body surface in the vicinity of the corresponding joint.

With three locations measured (or estimated) for each body segment, the representation of each segment can take the form of an embedded local coordinate system (LCS) whose orientation is determined with respect to a global coordinate system (GCS). Algorithms for determining a segment's LCS orientation generally begin by forming an initial vector, $\vec{v}_1$, which connects two of the known (or estimated) locations (Fig. 5–9). A second vector, $\vec{v}_2$, is chosen to be perpendicular to the plane that passes through all three points. The third vector, $\vec{v}_3$, is formed to lie mutually perpendicular to the first two axes. After normalizing each of these vectors by its respective magnitude (i.e., length), one obtains three mutually perpendicular unit vectors (defined in the GCS) which fully describe the LCS orientation (i.e., the orientation of the LCS axes).

Several mathematical techniques exist for calculating joint angle trajectories from segment LCS information. A widely used method models joint rotations to occur about

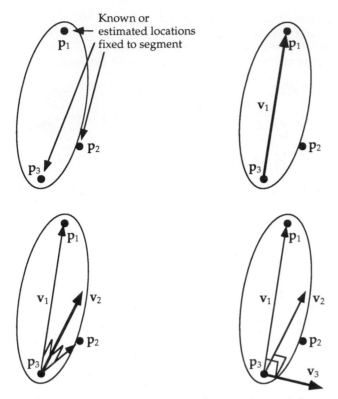

Known or estimated locations fixed to segment

FIGURE 5–9 Generalized sequence of steps taken to define an orthogonal local coordinate system for a given segment from three points assumed to be rigidly attached to the segment.

three specified axes[11] (Fig. 5–10). These axes of rotation include one axis chosen to be parallel to a proximal-segment LCS axis, and a second axis chosen to be parallel to a distal-segment LCS axis. The third axis of rotation is created to be mutually perpendicular to the first two selected axes, and is described mathematically as a unit vector in the axis direction. This third axis commonly is referred to as a "floating axis" since it is not selected from either segment. For lower limb applications (e.g., walking), an anatomical mediolateral axis typically is selected from the more proximal-segment LCS and is considered to be a joint flexion-extension axis. A longitudinal axis, chosen from the distal-segment LCS, then represents an internal-external rotation axis. An axis formed mutually perpendicular to these two axes functions as an abduction-adduction axis.

Applying the axes selection convention, described above, to the knee joint (Fig. 5–11) results in flexion-extension computed about a thigh mediolateral axis, internal-external rotation determined about a shank longitudinal axis, and abduction-adduction evaluated about a "floating axis," mutually perpendicular to the other two axes. The knee joint flexion-extension angle is computed as the angle that the floating axis needs to rotate about the flexion-extension axis to be parallel with the thigh-segment longitudinal axis. The internal-external rotation angle is the angle that the floating axis rotates about the internal-external rotation axis to be parallel with the shank-segment mediolateral axis. The abduction-adduction angle is the angle that the flexion-extension axis rotates about the floating axis to be parallel with the internal-external rotation axis. The angles de-

scribed here are approximately 90 degrees for a normal subject in an anatomically neutral position. Given the convention of reporting the neutral position values of (a) flexion-extension, (b) internal-external rotation, and (c) abduction-adduction to be zero, one generally reports the difference between a particular rotation and 90 degrees as the angle of interest (Fig. 5–11).

JOINT KINETICS

The term *kinetics* generally refers to the relationships between loads applied to bodies and the motions caused by such loads. Forces and moments are vector quantity loads which tend to move bodies translationally and rotationally, respectively (Fig. 5–12). With respect to lower limb joints, we often are interested in computing resultant joint moments,[3, 7, 25, 31, 33] since musculotendinous and ligamentous forces acting on lower limb segments are typically too numerous to determine from basic kinetic relationships. Some investigators have attempted to estimate musculotendinous and ligamentous forces by introducing assumptions that provide sufficient information to compute such forces.[5, 15, 21–23, 25] Such approximation techniques, however, are not used widely in clinical applications.

Several investigators, particularly those interested in lower limb prosthetics, have evaluated energy associated with lower limb joints during walking.[6, 20, 31, 33] In general terms, energy equals the integral of the dot product* of load and infinitesimal displacement, or

$$E = \int \vec{f} \cdot \vec{ds},$$

where E is energy, $\vec{f}$ is load, and $\vec{ds}$ is infinitesimal displacement. Subsequently, joint energy about a given axis can be computed as the area under a plot of joint moment about the axis of interest vs. joint angular displacement about the same axis.

Joint power has been another kinetic parameter of considerable interest to many investigators. *Power* is defined as the time rate of change of energy, or

$$P = \frac{d}{dt} E.$$

Given the previous relationship for energy, power can also be expressed as

$$P = \vec{f} \cdot \frac{\vec{ds}}{dt}.$$

Lower limb joint power at a given instant subsequently can be computed as either the slope of the joint energy time curve, or the dot product of joint moment and joint angular velocity at that instant.

Kinetic analysis, in many traditional engineering settings (e.g., robotics), involves input of known loading conditions and estimation of output motions. In human motion analy-

---

*The dot product of two vectors, $\vec{a}$ and $\vec{b}$, is the product of the magnitude of $\vec{a}$ and the projection of $\vec{b}$ in the direction of $\vec{a}$.

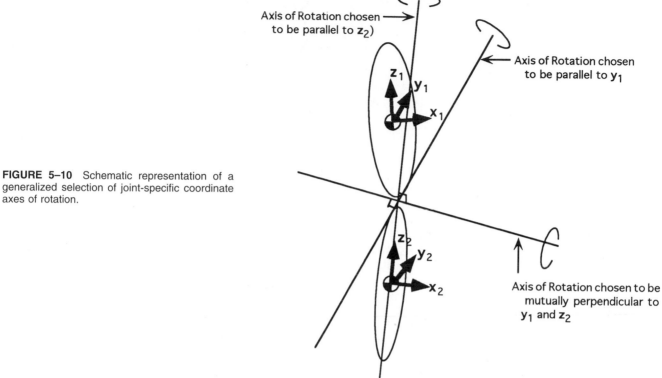

FIGURE 5–10 Schematic representation of a generalized selection of joint-specific coordinate axes of rotation.

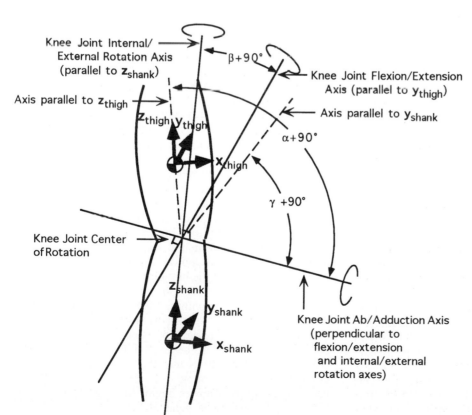

FIGURE 5–11 Diagram demonstrating a typical selection of joint coordinate axes of rotation for the knee joint.

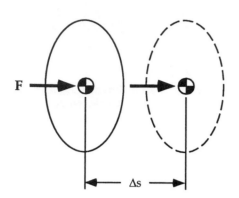

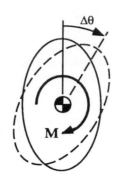

FIGURE 5–12 Generalized pictoral description of force (F) and linear displacement, Δs *(left)* and moment (M) and angular displacement, Δθ *(right).*

sis, measured body motions, typically, are known, and joint kinetics are computed using so-called inverse dynamics. Inverse dynamics approximation for lower limb joints involves segmenting feet, shanks, thighs, and pelvis into separate links. All relevant ground reaction, gravitational, and inertial loads are applied to each foot, and the resultant reaction force and moment are computed at each ankle joint. Ankle joint resultant loads are inverted and applied to each shank, along with shank gravitational and inertial loads, and knee joint resultant loads are approximated. Finally, inverted knee joint resultant loads and thigh gravitational and inertial loads are applied to each thigh, and the resultant loads at the hip joints are estimated.

NORMAL JOINT KINETICS

This discussion of joint kinetics during comfortable walking for normal subjects proceeds from the ankle to the knee and finally to the hip. This approach is consistent with the previously described inverse dynamics process of computing lower limb kinetics from the ground up to the hip.[32]

The external moment at the ankle joint acts initially at foot-strike to plantar-flex the foot (Fig. 5–13). With initial ankle joint plantar flexion at foot-strike, positive power from the external moment flows into the body and energy is absorbed at the ankle joint (Fig. 5–14) by active muscular forces and passive ligamentous and capsular restraints. Early stance phase EMG activity in the anterior tibial muscle is consistent with this accompanying external loading pattern. Dorsiflexion motion begins near the point in time when the external ankle joint moment switches to dorsiflexion. Power subsequently continues to flow into the body and the ankle continues to absorb energy.

Toward the end of stance phase, an external ankle joint dorsiflexion moment persists as the ankle begins to plantar-flex. Power then flows out of the body as the ankle joint generates a burst of energy. Such late stance energy generation at the ankle is frequently associated with the so-called push-off phase of gait. Midstance activity of the gastrocnemius-soleus complex is consistent with external dorsiflexion moments during this portion of the gait cycle. Debate regarding the true existence of push-off at terminal stance continues, however, due largely to the typical terminations of posterior calf muscle activity prior to foot-off.[8]

Many persons exhibit an external extension moment at the knee of very short duration at heel-strike. Regardless of the existence of this initial extension moment, nearly all normal subjects demonstrate the ensuing external flexion moment, lasting approximately one third of stance phase (see Fig. 5–13). The first portion of this external flexion is associated with power flow into the body and energy absorption at the knee joint, as the knee flexes (see Fig. 5–14). This "flexion wave" portion of stance phase has been associated with "shock attenuation" function. Power then flows from the body and energy is generated at the knee joint as the knee extends during the latter portion of the external flexion moment. This knee extension activity prevents a drop in the center of mass. Muscle activity is generally present in the exclusive knee-extending quadriceps muscles (i.e., vastus muscles), as might be anticipated from an external knee flexion moment. The external moment then reverts back to extension as the knee flexes in a controlled manner prior to swing phase. Power subsequently flows into the body during this external extension moment and energy is absorbed at the knee joint. This knee joint energy absorption period appears to coincide with a short period of activity in the rectus femoris muscle. Another reversal of the external moment into flexion occurs during latter swing as knee extension motion is decelerated. The knee joint again absorbs energy during this latter portion of swing, as power flows into the body and the vastus muscles again exhibit activity.

Persons without abnormalities begin stance phase with an external flexion moment at the hip (see Fig. 5–13), coincident with the hip moving toward extension from its most flexed position. This hip extension activity maintains forward progression as power flows from the body and energy is generated at the hip joint (see Fig. 5–14). Several hip extensor muscles (e.g., the semimembranosus, semitendinosus, gluteus maximus, biceps femoris–long head) are active during this initial period of hip extension. The external hip moment reverts to extension at approximately 20% of the gait cycle, as the hip continues to extend during stance. Power then flows into the body during the latter portion of stance, and energy is absorbed at the hip. During late stance, hip joint power begins flowing from the body and hip joint energy is generated, as hip flexion begins with the external hip joint moment in extension. Hip flexor muscles, such as the adductor longus and rectus femoris, are active during this period of the gait cycle.

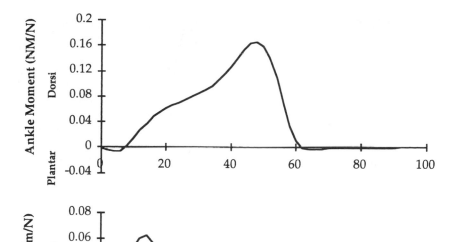

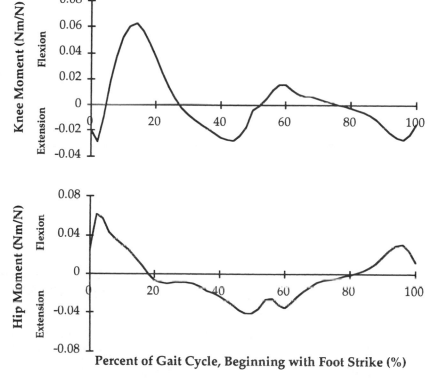

FIGURE 5–13 Normal (i.e., nonpathological) ankle *(top)*, knee *(center)*, and hip *(bottom)* joint moments in the sagittal plane for one gait cycle, normalized to body weight. The cycle is marked from 0% to 100% of the cycle time.

Percent of Gait Cycle, Beginning with Foot Strike (%)

USE AND ABUSE OF GAIT LABORATORIES

Gait analysis laboratories now can be found around the world being used for research, clinical care, and education. These laboratories provide valuable information for patient care in situations where complex gait abnormalities can frustrate attempts to improve walking. The need for advanced computer equipment, sophisticated software, and technical support places these laboratories under considerable financial pressure. The greatest abuse of these laboratories is performing analyses of abnormal gaits when there is little hope that the patient will benefit. As with any clinical research situation, lines between research and patient care must be drawn clearly enough so that patients are not charged professional fees for an evaluation for which advancement of research knowledge is the principal benefit.

CLINICAL PITFALLS OF GAIT ANALYSIS

Measurements obtained in the gait laboratory share a common failing with all other measurements of natural systems. A measurement contains artifacts produced by interaction between the measurement device and the system being measured. Subjective influences on interpretation of measurements can compound these errors greatly.

The most common pitfall in gait assessment is associated with the effect of walking velocity on gait patterns. Abnormal gait patterns are typically slower than normal. Interpretation of pathologic gait patterns requires an understanding of changes in these patterns that are produced when otherwise healthy persons walk at slower paces, with varying cadences and stride lengths. During slow walking, gait cycle percentages of double-limb stance periods lengthen, and gait cycle percentages of swing phase shorten. In some cases, absolute swing phase time remains fairly constant while total gait cycle time increases, resulting in a reduced ratio of swing/stance time.

Reduction of walking speed alters the roles of momentum, kinetic energy, and concentric muscular activity upon lower limb joint motion.[12, 13, 30] For example, when walking speed is reduced, early swing knee flexion and late swing knee extension often require active concentric muscle activ-

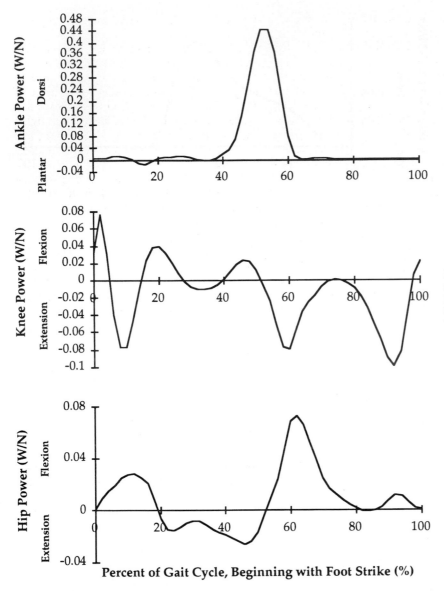

FIGURE 5–14 Normal (i.e., nonpathological) ankle *(top)*, knee *(center)*, and hip *(bottom)* joint powers in the sagittal plane for one gait cycle, normalized to body weight. The cycle is marked from 0 to 100% of the cycle time.

ity. Such need for active muscle contraction is generally absent at normal speeds where momentum and kinetic energy are sufficient to provide for these motions. Cocontraction of lower extremity muscles also is common at slower-paced walking, and probably results from increased need for stability rather than propulsion. Additionally, when walking is slowed, ground reaction forces typically do not display the two vertical reaction peaks associated with early stance impact and late stance push-off. In a stroke patient's gait, the nonhemiplegic side often displays altered stance phase parameters and muscle cocontractions which can vary with velocity,[24, 30] and laboratory control or reference data on slower velocities should be available. Such gait alterations are not necessarily primary deviations.

Cultural influences generally have a limited effect on gait patterns, but should be considered when evaluating causes of unusual gait patterns. Prosthetic specialists are well aware of the difficulty associated with training amputees to refrain from ill-advised habits developed while wearing a previous prosthesis. Similarly, learned behaviors of various types of persons can affect gait if they are continually repeated. Most altered gait patterns are associated with altered cadence or step length. Additionally, altered movement of the head-arms-trunk segment also can influence lower limb movement.

Clinical Examples

Rupture of Posterior Tibial Muscle Tendon

Analysis of gait in a patient with abnormal movement patterns requires an ability to separate primary from secondary gait deviations (i.e., compensation for the primary abnormality). Evaluation of a relatively simple case with a single lesion allows observation of primary and secondary effects of such a lesion on gait. Rupture of a posterior calf tendon (posterior tibial muscle) is one case in which loss of a force generator for gait results in widespread gait pattern abnormalities.

Primary deviations following rupture of a posterior tibial tendon are obviously at the ankle. Loss of tension force with a line of action posterior to the ankle greatly reduces plantar flexion force. A delay in heel rise in single-limb stance is demonstrated in sagittal plane ankle joint motion (Fig. 5–15). Such prolonged stance phase dorsiflexion often is referred to as a "calcaneal" gait pattern.

Delay in heel rise is associated with lower peak concentric ankle joint movement. Lower energy generation at the ankle is also observed.[8, 18] These changes result directly from reduced posterior calf muscle force generation. Secondary deviations of such injury are seen readily at the knee, hip, and pelvis. These deviations are more noticeable at faster walking speeds since posterior calf muscles are an important component of late stance phase propulsive force.[8]

Onset of knee flexion is delayed by reduced heel propulsion. Lack of ankle plantar flexion restrains forward movement of the lower limb. A delay in hip flexion initiation also is evident. Similarly, pelvic rotation is increased in amplitude as the weaker side of the pelvis fails to progress forward with the trunk (i.e., the contralateral side of the pelvis has increased pelvic rotation).

The secondary effect on hip rotation is to increase internal rotation of the ipsilateral hip at late stance. At the same time, the contralateral hip shows increased external rotation.

The pelvis tilts down on the ipsilateral side, again related to the lack of power generation to lift the heel. Swing is then initiated from this disadvantaged position of a lowered and retracted hemipelvis, and without the normal degree of knee and hip flexion. Compensation using active knee and hip flexion to produce forward movement of the swing phase occurs depending on the desired walking speed and step length. Walking efficiency and comfortable walking speed are both reduced.

The overall effect of this loss of a single power generator for gait is alteration of the ankle and knee of the affected side and both hips. The patient could present with foot pain due to increased dorsiflexion in late stance, or hip pain resulting from the greater range of internal rotation of the ipsilateral hip during the loading of late stance. This would be similar to, although less severe than, a rupture of the Achilles tendon. Awareness of the secondary effects of an injury allows the physiatrist to anticipate complications and formulate plans for prevention or early intervention.

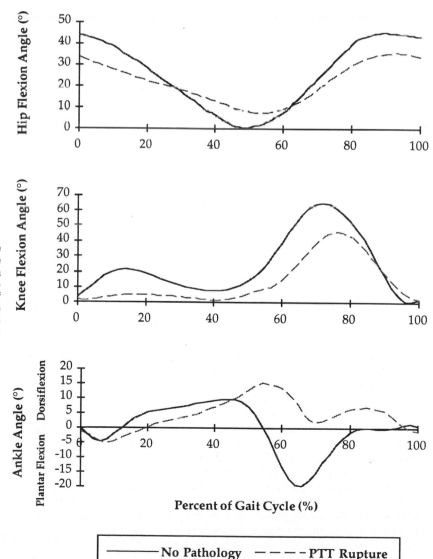

FIGURE 5–15 Sagittal plane hip *(top)*, knee *(center)*, and ankle *(bottom)* joint angles, for one gait cycle, of a person without pathology and a patient with a posterior tibial tendon (PTT) rupture. The cycle is marked from 0% to 100% of the cycle time. The reader is encouraged to place a vertical straight-edge on the page to appreciate the simultaneous joint angle positions at each instant of the gait cycle.

Severe Peroneal Neuropathy (Drop Foot)

Peroneal nerve injury results in weakness of the principal dorsiflexion and eversion muscles of the ankle, as well as diminished sensation on the dorsum of the foot. The principal kinematic effect is decreased dorsiflexion of the affected ankle during swing and loss of controlled plantar flexion following normal heel contact.[17] The result is a swing phase notable for maintained plantar flexion, flatfoot initial contact, and a "foot slap." Secondary deviation relates to the failure of these actions and the basic need for foot clearance in swing and for ankle stability at loading.

Hip and knee flexion in swing increases, improving foot clearance by effectively shortening the distance from hip to ankle at midswing. This can require active work of the knee flexors, which are usually passive in initial swing. Increased force generation of the hip flexors must also be opposed at the pelvis and lumbar (psoas) area. Extension of the knee must also be actively controlled and this precedes extension of the hip to prevent dragging the toe.[12]

To compensate for the ankle instability the step length is reduced, which diminishes momentum and the impact loading at foot-strike. Hip flexion at foot contact is less than normal in the short step, so the hip extends from its (greater than normal) peak flexion before foot-strike. The loss of normal energy absorption of the anterior tibial muscle at loading also limits the ability of the ankle to remain stable at impact.

The ankle-foot orthosis (AFO) is commonly prescribed for the patient with peroneal neuropathy. This device assists in dorsiflexion of the ankle to correct the principal gait deviation and to assist with mediolateral stability. The brace maintains dorsiflexion in swing, and reduces the need for exaggerated knee and hip flexion. The ankle is now dorsiflexed at initial foot contact; however, it cannot replicate the eccentric muscle activity which produces controlled plantar flexion during loading. The ankle is more stable for loading and the step length can increase, although typically not to normal.[17]

The AFO induces new secondary gait deviations of its own.[17] These are related to the restraint placed upon foot and ankle movement in rotation, as well as plantar flexion. A rigid brace produces early heel rise as the tibia pivots forward during stance phase. This effect delays the onset of knee flexion and impedes the initiation of swing. Foot and ankle rotation mechanisms during stance phase rotate to accommodate the ground reaction forces, and are coupled with hip and knee rotations. The AFO's restraint on the foot and ankle increases the amplitude of the knee and hip rotational movements.

Above-Knee Amputee

Gait deviations of an above-knee amputee are much more dramatic than the simple cases above.[12, 13] The loss of all neuromuscular control of the knee and ankle results in multiple primary deviations, and secondary deviations affecting the rest of the gait mechanism.

The primary deviations include abnormal motion at both the knee and ankle in the prosthetic limb (Fig. 5–16). At loading, the ankle of a typical solid-ankle, cushioned-heel (SACH) foot, incorporated in the majority of lower limb prostheses in the United States,[14] remains in its set position (generally about 90 degrees with respect to the shank, or with some slight plantar flexion if deemed desirable by the prosthetist) and absorbs some impact by cushion or spring at the heel. The knee does not flex during the loading response, since without the quadriceps it is unstable in flexion. The rigid ankle restrains the forward movement of the tibial component and assists in maintaining a rigid (stable) knee, although at a cost of forward momentum.

The forefoot, ankle, and knee are aligned to produce an external extensor moment at the knee as long as stance phase is maintained (Fig. 5–17). Knee flexion in late stance is delayed, by design, until toe-off occurs. Forward propulsion for swing of the prosthetic limb must be generated at a site other than the calf. Swing phase knee flexion is usually passive at comfortable walking speed. In this respect, the prosthesis is not at a great disadvantage. However, control of flexion and extension of the knee is important as walking speed varies. A damper on the knee mechanism (hydraulic control) provides improved control of the calf momentum at faster speeds, and prevents excessive angular movement.

At terminal swing, the amputee carefully maneuvers the prosthesis in preparation for loading. Active hip extension occurs, restraining the forward movement of the thigh. This movement of the thigh assists with knee extension, but shortens the step length. The shorter step length and reduced forward momentum at foot contact also affect the angle of the ground reaction force vector. This vector must be maintained at the knee joint center, or anterior to it, in order to maintain an extensor moment at the knee (see Fig. 5–17).

The hip on the prosthetic side is first affected, resulting in secondary deviation. These effects include the extensor movement in late swing, which has already been mentioned, and reduced rotation of the hip and pelvis. The pelvis drops in late stance on the prosthetic side owing to lack of propulsion from the calf. This is partly overcome by the contralateral abductor muscles and internal rotation at the hip. These increased muscle forces (gluteus medius, tensor fascia lata) produce more compressive loading on the hip during stance phase of the sound limb. In some persons, the affected pelvis is elevated to improve foot clearance through even greater force generation by the abductor muscles. Higher muscle forces here correlate with higher compressive forces in the acetabulum.

When foot clearance is a problem on the prosthetic side, it usually results from inefficient hip or knee flexion. A short residual limb could contribute to this, as would a poor socket fit. In addition to the pelvis elevation due to active abduction at the sound hip, the knee and ankle also assist foot clearance. The sound knee limits its stance phase flexion and maintains limb length. The ankle actively plantar-flexes in midstance, or produces "vaulting" in severe cases of this type of compensation.

The typical above-knee prosthesis user has a reduced velocity of comfortable walking, with similar reduction of both stride and cadence. Step lengths are usually symmetrical. The maximum knee flexion angles in swing are also equal since both are passively dependent upon velocity.

Stroke and Hemiplegia

Cerebral infarction or hemorrhage can radically change the motor control system for walking. Gait analysis typi-

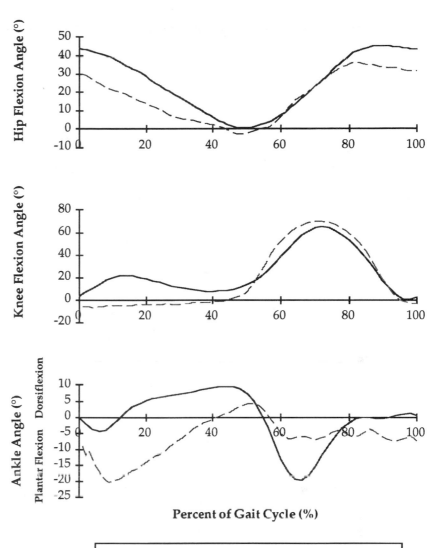

FIGURE 5-16 Sagittal plane hip *(top)*, knee *(center)*, and ankle *(bottom)* joint angles, for one gait cycle, of a person without pathology and a patient walking with an above-knee (AK) prosthesis. The cycle is marked from 0% to 100% of the cycle time.

cally records abnormal motion in essentially all body segments as multiple primary deviations lead to multiple secondary deviations. Many researchers believe, in fact, that severe cerebral infarction results in primary motor control problems in both lower limbs although, obviously, they are more pronounced on the side of hemiplegia.[24, 30]

Problems observed in the gait of the stroke patient include failure of power generation for propulsion, impaired coordinated muscle movement or delayed activation of muscles, antagonistic cocontraction or spastic tone, and reliance on passive means for stance stability.[20, 24, 28] Early in the course of recovery, muscle tone is low, and weakness and proprioceptive deficits are the primary problem (unpublished data). EMG signals are sometimes recorded from muscles which are not producing a useful contraction. Stability is the chief concern and the step-to-gait pattern with cane (weak leg first) is commonly taught to the patient.

The two problems of stability and muscle activation are particularly evident during double-limb stance phase. Swing phase (toe-off) is delayed on the hemiplegic side. This delay in initiation correlates well with the slowed

gait velocity (unpublished data). Since all of the primary initiation of swing (plantar flexion, hip flexion, and pelvic rotation) can be impaired in stroke, it is not surprising that there is a delay in toe-off.

During stance phase the hemiplegic leg is maintained with the knee in extension or slightly flexed. The predominant problem is the lack of variation in joint angles during stance phase. Alignment of the body over the joint lines allows passive stability without the need for variable muscle control. Muscle cocontraction is common at the joints which further limits angular movement. With forward movement, there is some passive dorsiflexion of the ankle, but the hip and knee fail to extend in late stance.

Swing phase is initiated by a combination of hip flexion and pelvic elevation. Pelvic elevation, or hip-hiking, is related to contralateral trunk leaning and abduction of the contralateral hip. Active hip flexion is often accompanied by active knee flexion as toe-off develops. In some cases, the forward momentum of the thigh results in posterior movement of the pelvis, a reversal of normal pelvic advancement (unpublished data) (Fig. 5-18).

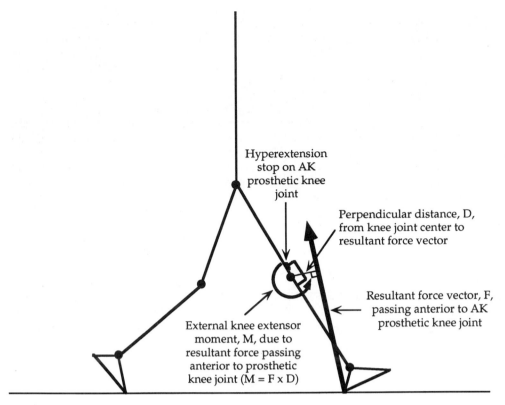

FIGURE 5-17 Schematic diagram of resultant ground reaction force in above-knee (AK) amputee producing external knee extensor moment about the knee flexion/extension axis (moment [M] = resultant force [F] × perpendicular distance [D] from knee joint to resultant force).

Through swing phase the ankle is in plantar flexion, which increases the need for hip and knee flexion to produce foot clearance. Late swing usually brings active hip extension with knee extension. Both initiation and termination of swing are inefficient with pelvic retraction at toe-off and hip extension before foot-strike, resulting in a shorter step.

Recovery of the ability to walk following a stroke is, of course, quite variable. Some persons with an initially severe impairment of walking are able to develop normal walking even under gait analysis scrutiny. The development of significant abnormal tone is a negative prognostic indicator and hemispasticity can result in a severe, permanent impairment of gait.

The patient with spasticity demonstrates a number of differences in the gait pattern. Foot-strike occurs with the foot actively plantar-flexed and inverted due to the action of the soleus and posterior tibial muscles. When this muscle force is sufficiently strong, body weight is not adequate to dorsiflex and produce heel contact.

Knee extension during stance is encouraged as a result of the moment produced at the ankle, knee, and hip. The plantar-flexed ankle position results in a ground reaction force anterior to the knee, causing an extension moment about the knee. The primary knee extensors (quadriceps) actively maintain the knee in extension with active extensor torque, which also serves to maintain the knee center posterior to the ground reaction force line. Active hip extensor muscles also produce an extensor moment which is resisted only by trunk inertia. Hamstring muscles cocontract with the quadriceps, but have a short lever arm at the knee and so produce little flexion moment.

Extensor tone usually requires a hip-hike to initiate swing phase. The rectus femoris, while serving as a hip flexor, also resists knee flexion in swing. Circumduction is sometimes needed to advance the limb. The adductor muscles can be active in early swing, limiting abduction and circumduction, as well as narrowing the step width, which can impair stability.

Correction of gait deviation in stroke is multifactorial, and is also addressed in Chapter 50. An AFO, which prevents the passive or active plantar flexion in swing and stance phases, can greatly improve gait mechanics and efficiency. By eliminating the drop-foot position in swing,

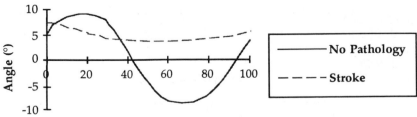

FIGURE 5-18 Typical transverse pelvic rotation following a stroke (compared with that for a person with no pathology) affecting the left side of the body (positive angle indicates right side of pelvis forward, relative to left side of pelvis).

there is less need for hip and knee flexion and pelvic elevation to gain foot clearance.[19] The improved foot-to-tibia alignment can also lessen the knee extensor torque in stance phase. Swing initiation is facilitated in some cases by the preflexed position of the ankle. During the period of decreased muscle tone, an orthosis to assist knee extension (usually temporary) improves stance stability.

Advanced gait skills require recovery of coordinated neuromuscular control at all joints. Physical therapy and gait training usually focus on (1) normalization of joint range of motion, (2) normalization of muscle tone, (3) strengthening of flexors, and (4) gait stability and confidence. Neuromuscular stimulation and biofeedback have both been demonstrated to have a beneficial effect upon gait.[4] Tone reduction by surgery or motor point or nerve block is also used to alter severe gait deviations.

Spastic Diplegia Due to Cerebral Palsy

Children with diplegia present with a variety of specific gait deviations. Poor motor control, spastic tone, bone growth, and joint and muscle contractures all contribute to these gait patterns. Treatment of the abnormal patterns by physical therapy,[28] adaptive equipment,[10] nerve block or neurolysis,[1, 29] or orthopedic surgery[9, 16, 27] depends on an accurate clinical evaluation of the child's gait problem. Ablative or reconstruction surgery requires special attention to the primary gait deviation, and prediction of the kinematic consequences of the anatomical changes.

One gait pattern that is common in spastic cerebral palsy (CP) is frequently referred to as "crouched." This apt description is of a child who stands and walks on the toes with the knees and hips flexed, and usually with adduction (scissoring) and internal rotation of the hips. However, the combination of asymmetry, muscle tone, contracture, and growth result in different specific gait patterns in individual children.

Foot contact and loading are typically with the toe first in CP, but *not* with the ankle in plantar flexion (Fig. 5–19). The knee flexion of 30 degrees and 40 degrees, at that time, causes the tibia to tilt forward, and the toe contact is made with the ankle in a neutral position. During loading, ankle dorsiflexion and knee flexion increase as a result of ground reaction forces which have a larger moment. Hip

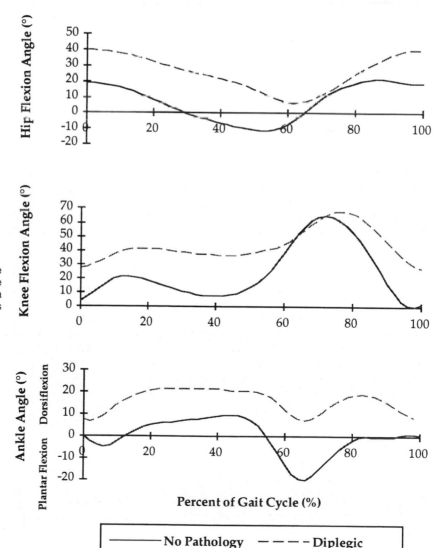

FIGURE 5–19 Sagittal plane hip *(top)*, knee *(center)*, and ankle *(bottom)* joint angles, for one gait cycle, of a person without pathology and a patient with diplegic cerebral palsy. The cycle is marked from 0% to 100% of the cycle time.

Percent of Gait Cycle (%)

——— No Pathology   – – – – Diplegic

flexion is maximal at foot contact and gradually extends from 40 degrees to 20 degrees of flexion during stance phase.

The ankle angle returns toward neutral in late stance, especially in double stance, with decreased loading in preparation for swing. At the same time, knee flexion gradually increases and hip extension reaches its maximum at -20 degrees. The hip is internally rotated more than normal at this stage. The tibia is also typically internally rotated, as is the foot. Careful evaluation of the position of the limb at this preswing phase is very important in planning treatment, since effective treatment usually depends on increasing step length.

During swing phase, the joint angular excursions are all reduced from normal and this moment results in shortened step length. The ankle, hip, and knee all flex in synergy in early swing, but the knee fails to extend in late swing. EMG recording often shows medial hamstring muscle activity in early swing but not in late swing, which is a reversal of the common pattern. The gastrocnemius EMG signal is recorded in late swing along with contraction of the quadriceps and lateral hamstrings (extensor synergy) in preparation for loading.

Gait analysis has been useful as a measurement device in evaluating the response to treatment of children with spastic CP. Studies have shown improved gait with posterior facing vs. standard anterior walkers. AFOs can effectively improve the gait of some children, and improve their gait efficiency. Treatment of range-of-motion deficiencies also can improve gait when there is a demonstrated problem. Dorsal rhizotomy has resulted in improved gait patterns and velocity. Various tendon lengthening and transfer

operations may be recommended to correct specific gait deviations with outcomes documented by gait analysis.[9, 27]

An example of the difficulty in assessment and treatment is the study by Thometz et al.[27] of the effects of medial hamstring lengthening in children with CP. These children demonstrated greater knee extension in stance and swing following the procedure. However, the angular excursion of the knee did not improve (i.e., it was also more extended in midswing). The step length was not improved, nor was the gait velocity. Performing the hamstring lengthening with additional transfer of the rectus femoris and the hamstring tendon is more effective for some children with spastic CP.[9]

Equipment Issues

Motion biomechanics laboratories vary considerably with respect to measurement equipment contained within them. Laboratories that function clinically typically contain equipment for measuring some common data categories, including joint motion, ground reaction forces, and EMG. Many laboratories also possess equipment for measuring contact normal stress (i.e., "pressure") at the foot-ground or foot-shoe interface. Footswitches, which monitor timing of gait events, are used widely as well.

Motion Data Collection

The substantial majority of motion biomechanics laboratories that function clinically use video-based systems to record raw kinematic data (Fig. 5–20). Video-based kinematic measurement involves recording, in camera-based two-dimensional coordinate systems, the locations of mark-

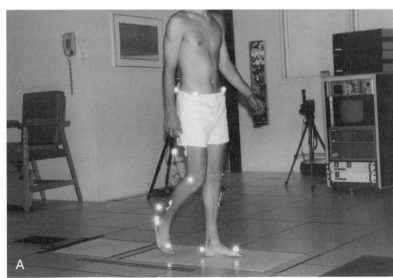

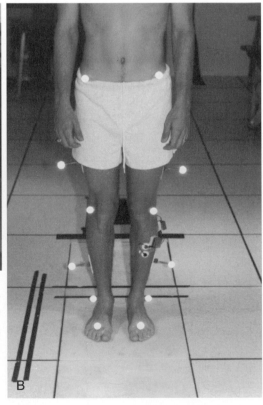

FIGURE 5–20 *A,* Gait analysis laboratory at Ohio State University using a VICON video-based motion analysis system (Oxford Metrics, Inc., Baton Rouge, La). *B,* Frontal view of lower extremity markers placed on the body. (Note: video-based systems require placement of markers on body segments to define local coordinate systems at the segments.)

ers placed on the body. At a given sampling frame, one can obtain the three-dimensional position (in a global or laboratory coordinate system) of any marker that is visible to at least two cameras.

Accuracy of video-based marker position measurement depends on several interrelated factors, including camera spatial resolution, lens distortion correction, object volume dimensions, calibration frame measurement, and marker size. Some of these factors (e.g., camera spatial resolution and lens distortion correction) are related primarily to the system used, while other factors are controllable by the user. Systems with higher-resolution cameras and more sophisticated lens distortion correction procedures typically produce more accurate and precise marker position data. Such systems also tend to generate three-dimensional marker position data from raw camera data more quickly; however, they are generally more expensive as well. Companies that produce commercially available systems for collecting video-based motion data include Oxford Metrics, Ltd. (Oxford, England); Motion Analysis Corp. (Santa Rosa, Calif); BTS Technology & Systems (Milan, Italy); and Peak Performance (Englewood, Colo). With respect to user-related factors, smaller object volumes and more sophisticated calibration frame measurement can increase marker position measurement accuracy, but also can reduce the number of walking cycles recorded and increase data collection time.

Many laboratories that are without sufficient financial resources to obtain video-based kinematic measurement systems collect relative joint angular motion data using electrogoniometers. Electrogoniometers are exoskeletal devices that are placed directly at the joint and generate electrical outputs that are related directly to relative joint angular position. Although not used widely in clinical laboratories, electrogoniometers can be particularly useful for remote data collection protocols, where use of a video-based system might be impractical. Electrogoniometers do not generate raw segment position information, and can be difficult to coordinate with ground reaction force data to compute joint kinetic information. Electrogoniometers also can be a substantial encumbrance to some patients.

Ground Reaction Force Measurement

Most motion biomechanics laboratories contain one or more force platforms for collecting raw kinetic data (Fig. 5–21). Force platforms measure one component of the ground reaction force perpendicular to the platform (i.e., vertical force), and two orthogonal components in the plane of the platform (i.e., horizontal forces, typically mediolateral and fore-and-aft forces). Force platforms measure one vertical and two horizontal components of the ground reaction force, and ground reaction moments about the platforms' vertical and horizontal axes. Force platforms generally utilize either strain gauges or piezoelectric sensors to measure ground reaction loads. Piezoelectric-based platforms typically are attributed with having higher natural frequencies and less crosstalk between load channels. Strain gauge–based platforms, however, are subject to less signal drift and are often less expensive.

Electromyography Measurement

Electromyography measurement systems, used clinically in motion biomechanics laboratories, can be classified broadly as either telemetered or hard-wired systems. Telemetered EMG systems encode and transmit EMG signals over radio waves to a receiver, and then decode the signals for visual display, electronic storage, or data processing. Hard-wired systems transmit EMG signals directly via cables. Telemetered and hard-wired systems can vary with respect to the number of EMG channels transmitted per radio frequency or per cable, respectively. Telemetered systems often are clinically desirable because the lack of a cable permits less restricted motion of the patient. Hard-wired systems, however, are less expensive and do not require tuning (i.e., adjusting) transmitters to the proper radio frequency.

Both telemetered and hard-wired systems generally can utilize either surface or fine-wire electrodes. Surface electrodes are often attractive because they are not invasive. Fine-wire electrodes, however, are more capable of recording isolated signals from a specific muscle without crosstalk contamination from adjacent muscle activity.

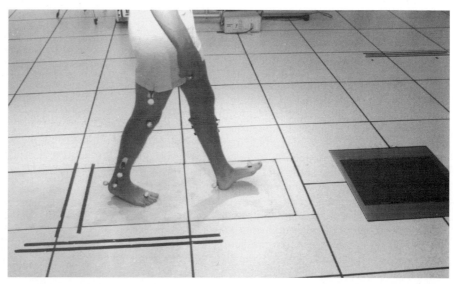

FIGURE 5–21 Strain gauge force platforms (Advanced Mechanical Technology, Inc., Watertown, Mass) at Ohio State University.

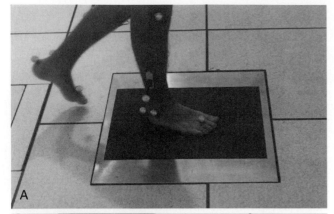

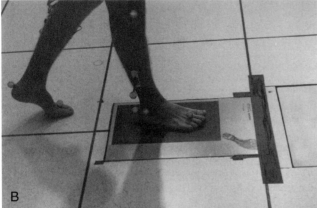

FIGURE 5–22 EMED-SF (Novell Electronics, Inc., Minneapolis) *(A)* and BTE (Baltimore Therapeutics Equipment, Co., Baltimore) *(B)* foot pressure platforms at Ohio State University.

Other issues to be considered with either telemetered or hard-wired systems used with either surface or fine-wire electrodes include preamplification of signals prior to transmission, preprocessing of raw data prior to data storage, and postprocessing of collected data. These issues can affect data collection complexity, system cost, data-processing time, and signal interpretation.

Foot Pressure Measurement

Foot pressure measurement devices can be categorized as either platform- (Fig. 5–22) or foot-based devices. Pressure platforms measure pressures at the foot-ground interface, and record direct plantar surface pressures only under barefoot conditions. Foot-based pressure measurement devices are typically either shoe insoles with embedded load sensor arrays, or individual load sensors, which must be applied to the specific foot surface regions of interest. Platform devices cannot record successive footsteps and cannot measure pressure at the foot-shoe interface. Pressure platforms, however, often have greater spatial resolution and durability than foot-based devices. In foot-based devices, individual sensors require a priori knowledge of regions where pressure measurements are desired. Insole pressure arrays can measure foot pressure across the entire plantar surface; however, they are typically more expensive than individual sensors.

References

1. Arendzen J, VanDuijin H, Beckmann M, et al: Diagnostic blocks of the tibial nerve in spastic hemiparesis: Effects on clinical, electrophysiological and gait parameters. Arch Phys Med Rehabil 1992; 24:75–81.
2. Basmajiam J, DeLuca C: Muscles Alive: Their Functions Revealed by Electromyography, ed 5. Baltimore, Williams & Wilkins, 1985.
3. Berchuck M, Andriacchi T, Bach B, Reider B: Gait adaptations by patients who have a deficient anterior cruciate ligament. J Bone Joint Surg [Am] 1990; 72A:871–877.
4. Cozean CD, Pease WS, Hubbell SL: Biofeedback and functional electric stimulation in stroke rehabilitation. Arch Phys Med Rehabil 1988; 6:401–405.
5. Crowninshield RD, Brand RA: A physiologically based criterion of muscle force prediction in locomotion. J Biomech 1981; 14:793–801.
6. Czerniecki JM, Gitter A, Munro C: Joint moment and muscle power output characteristics of below knee amputees during running: the influence of energy storing prosthetic feet. J Biomech 1991; 24:63–75.
7. Delp SL, Zajac FE: Force- and moment-generating capacity of lower-extremity muscles before and after tendon lengthening. Clin Orthop 1992; 284:247–259.
8. Dillingham T, Lehmann J, Price R: Effect of lower limb on body propulsion. Arch Phys Med Rehabil 1992; 73:647–651.
9. Gage J: Surgical treatment of knee dysfunction in cerebral palsy. Clin Orthop 1990; 253:45–54.
10. Greiner B, Czernieck J, Deitz J: Gait parameters of children with spastic diplegia: a comparison of effects of posterior and anterior walkers. Arch Phys Med Rehabil 1993; 74:381–385.
11. Grood ES, Suntay WJ: A joint coordinate system for the clinical description of three-dimensional motions: application to the knee. J Biomech Eng 1983; 105:136–144.
12. Inman VT, Ralston HJ, Todd F: Human Walking. Baltimore, Williams & Wilkins, 1981.
13. Jaegers S, Vos L, Rispens P, Hof A: The relationship between comfortable and most metabolically efficient walking speed in persons with unilateral above-knee amputation. Arch Phys Med Rehabil 1993; 74:521–525.
14. James KB, Stein RB: Improved ankle-foot system for above-knee amputees. Am J Phys Med 1986; 65:301–314.
15. Kaufman KR, An KW, Litchy WJ, Chao EY: Physiological prediction of muscle forces—I. Theoretical formulation. Neuroscience 1991; 40:781–792.
16. Lee E, Goh J, Bose K: Value of gait analysis in the assessment of surgery in cerebral palsy. Arch Phys Med Rehabil 1992; 73:642–646.
17. Lehman J, Condon S, deLateur B, Price R: Gait abnormalities in peroneal nerve paralysis and their correction by orthoses. Arch Phys Med Rehabil 1986; 67:380–386.
18. Lehman J, Condon S, deLateur B, Smith J: Gait abnormalities in tibial nerve paralysis: a biomechanical study. Arch Phys Med Rehabil 1985; 66:80–85.
19. Lehman J, Condon S, Price R, deLateur B: Gait abnormalities in hemiplegia: their correction by ankle foot orthoses. Arch Phys Med Rehabil 1987; 68:763–771.
20. Olney S, Griffin M, Morgan T, McBride I: Work and power in gait of stroke patients. Arch Phys Med Rehabil 1991; 72:309–314.
21. Patriarco AG, Mann RW, Simon SR, Mansour JM: An evaluation of the approaches of optimization models in the prediction of muscle forces during human gait. J Biomech 1981; 14:513–525.
22. Pedersen DR, Brand RA, Cheng C, Arora JS: Direct comparison of muscle force predictions using linear and nonlinear programming. J Biomech Eng 1987; 109:192–199.
23. Seirig A, Arvikar RJ: The prediction of muscular load sharing and joint forces in the lower extremities during walking. J Biomech 1975; 8:89–102.
24. Shiavi R, Bugle HJ, Limbird T: Electromyographic gait assessment, Part 2: Preliminary assessment hemiparetic synergy patterns. J Rehabil Res Dev 1987; 24:24–30.
25. Spoor CW, van Leeuwen JL, de Windt FH, Huson A: A model study of muscle forces and joint-force direction in normal and dysplastic neonatal hips. J Biomech 1989; 22:873–884.
26. Sutherland D, Olshen R, Biden E, Wyatt M: The Development of Mature Walking. London, MacKeith Press, 1988.
27. Thometz J, Simon S, Rosenthal R: The effect on gait of lengthening of the medial hamstrings in cerebral palsy. J Bone Joint Surg [Am] 1989; 71:345–353.

28. Trueblood P, Walker J, Perry J, Cronley J: Pelvic exercise and gait in hemiplegia. Phys Ther 1989; 69:18–26.

29. Vaughan C, Berman B, Peacock W: Cerebral palsy and rhizotomy: a 3-year follow-up with gait analysis. J Neurosurg 1991; 74:178–184.

30. Wagenaar R, Beek W: Hemiplegic gait: a kinematic analysis using walking speed as a basis. J Biomech 1992; 25:1007–1015.

31. Winter D: Energy generation and absorption at the ankle and knee during fast, natural, and slow cadences. Clin Orthop 1983; 175:147–154.

32. Winter DA: Biomechanics of human movement with applications to the study of human locomotion. Crit Rev Biomed Eng 1984; 9:287–314.

33. Winter DA, Sienko SE: Biomechanics of below-knee amputee gait. J Biomech 1988; 21:361–367.

6

Electrodiagnostic Medicine I: Basic Aspects

DANIEL DUMITRU, M.D.

The electrodiagnostic medicine consultation is the practice of medicine and as such is predicated upon a thorough understanding of the basic science and clinical aspects of nerve and muscle physiology. In addition to the normal physiologic functioning of these two primary tissues, the physician must also comprehend the manner in which nerve and muscle tissues react to various diseases. The practitioner must be aware of how the instrument detects and displays the recorded physiological potentials. Once these basic principles are mastered, the practitioner has taken the first step toward being able to perform an electrodiagnostic medicine consultation.

ACTION POTENTIAL GENERATION

The two basic excitable tissues in the human body are nerve and muscle. For our purposes, the basic principles of action potential generation in nerve and skeletal muscle are relatively similar, with the primary difference being that the length of action potential duration is considerably longer in muscle compared to nerve.

Resting Membrane Potential

All living cells have a potential difference across their cell membranes with the intracellular region negative compared to the extracellular environment.[26] When an action potential is not present, the cell is said to be in the resting state and the potential difference across the cell membrane is referred to as the resting membrane potential. The development and maintenance of the resting membrane potential can be conceptualized by a simple membrane model.

Suppose that a beaker is divided into left and right halves by an impermeable barrier or membrane with two different concentrations of aqueous potassium chloride solution[15] (left, 10 mM KCl; right, 100 mM KCl; Fig. 6–1). In solution, the KCl exists as positive potassium (K^+) ions (cations) and negative chloride (Cl^-) ions (anions). If a voltmeter (a device that measures potential differences) is placed across the two solutions, it will not measure a potential difference because there is a lack of physical continuity between the left and right halves of the beaker. There is no pathway for current to flow and without current flow there can be no potential difference. If the barrier has the ability for us to open only potassium channels, we can anticipate a flow of K^+ cations "down" the concentration gradient from the high (100 mM) to low (10 mM) ion concentration side of the beaker (see Fig. 6–1). The potassium ions will flow into the low concentration side of the container until there is a balance between the forces of the physical concentration gradient difference driving potassium to the lower concentration region, and the electrical gradient opposing this directional ion flow. Recall that the negative chloride ions cannot pass through the membrane and remain on the high concentration side of the beaker. As more and more positive potassium ions leave one side of the beaker, there begins to develop an unbalanced or "excess" amount of negative charges (Cl^-) on the high concentration side of the beaker with an equal buildup of excess positive charges (K^+) on the other side of the beaker. The increasing net negative charge of the beaker half with the remaining chloride ions begins to make it increasingly difficult for the positive potassium charges to leave the high concentration side of the beaker, while at the same time an increasing amount of positive potassium ions on the low concentration side of the beaker begin to repel newly entering potassium ions.

At some point, the opposing electrical charges on the two sides of the beaker prevent any more potassium from leaving the high concentration side of the beaker, even though there is still a higher potassium concentration on one side compared to the other. A balance exists, therefore, between the concentration forces driving potassium from the high to low concentration regions, and the electrical forces tending to keep potassium in the more concentrated portion of the beaker. Any potassium ions that randomly

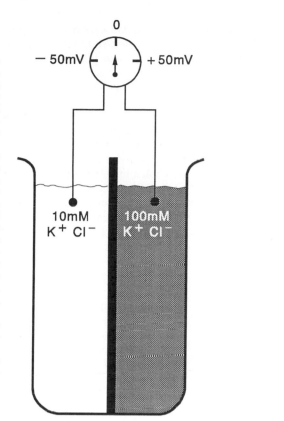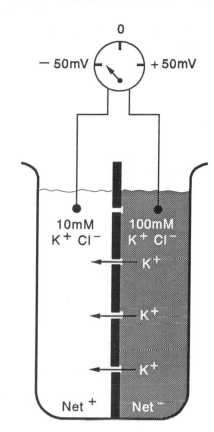

FIGURE 6-1 A beaker containing two different concentrations (10 mM and 100 mM) of a potassium chloride solution (KCl) existing as potassium (K⁺) and chloride (Cl⁻) ions. An impermeable partition separates the two different concentration solutions. A voltmeter placed across the partition fails to register any voltage difference. If the partition is made selectively permeable to just the potassium ions, the concentration gradient difference will drive potassium ions into the lower concentration side of the beaker until the electrical attraction from the accumulating negatively charged chloride ions prevents any further net K⁺ ion movement, thus establishing a dynamic equilibrium. At this point, a potential difference exists across the partition and represents the equilibrium potential. (From Dumitru D: Electrodiagnostic Medicine. Philadelphia, Hanley & Belfus, 1995.)

enter the lower concentration side of the beaker are balanced by potassium ions similarly crossing in the opposite direction. The situation where balance between electrical and concentration forces exists is said to be a dynamic equilibrium. Placing a voltmeter across the partition now measures a negative potential difference as electrical continuity is now present between the two halves of the beaker through the open potassium channels.

The above simple example can be applied to all cells in the body and in particular to nerve and muscle cells. We now use the nerve cell's axon as our example, although the same principles apply to muscle cells. The nerve cell is known to have a specialized cell membrane or plasmalemma permeable primarily to potassium and chloride ions in the resting state because of intramembranous potassium and chloride channels. It is said to be selectively permeable, or semipermeable.[29] These potassium channels are passive because they are always open and permit the free flow of these ions. Contained within the axon but incapable of crossing the cell membrane are large negatively charged protein molecules. This negative charge attracts potassium ions to cross the cell membrane through the passive potassium channels and accumulate within the axon. This process continues until there is so much potassium within the axon that the continued entry of more potassium ions is prevented by the high intracellular potassium concentration, even though all of the negative charges have not been balanced. This is because the potassium concentration gradient force now attempting to drive potassium out of the cell is just balanced by the negative electrical attraction force of anions pulling potassium ions into the cell. Similar to the above beaker

example, a dynamic equilibrium develops between the intracellular negative charges pulling potassium in and the high intracellular potassium concentration attempting to push potassium out. This dynamic equilibrium occurs at a point when the large intracellular negative potential is reduced by the inflowing potassium ions to a value of a transmembrane potential difference approximating a negative 80 to 90 mV compared to the extracellular environment.

Nernst Equation

The above examples of beakers and cells can be expressed mathematically by simply saying that the work or energy of developing the concentration gradient (W_{con}) is balanced by, or equal but opposite to that developed by the electrical gradient (W_{elec}) during the resting state: $W_{elec} = -W_{con}$. The negative sign is present to denote the "opposite" or balanced aspect of the work. The electrical work is expressed as $W_{elec} = Z_i FE_m$. The symbols designate specific aspects of defining electrical ion work: Z_i is the ion's charge, F is Faraday's constant, and E_m is the transmembrane potential. The work required to move ions across the membrane can be expressed as the natural logarithm of the ionic concentration differences between the intracellular ($[I]_i$) and extracellular ($[I]_e$) ions. Universal gas (R) and temperature (T) constants are conversion factors necessary to balance units between all of the variables. Substituting the above-noted variables into the balanced work equation results in:

$$W_{elec} = -W_{con}$$
$$Z_i FE_m = -RT \{Ln [I]_i - Ln [I]_e\}$$

This formula can be rearranged to find the potential at which the electrical work just balances the concentration work, that is, the dynamic equilibrium or resting membrane potential, by solving the above equation for E_m.

$$E_m = \frac{-RT}{Z_iF} \ln \frac{[I]_i}{[I]_e}$$

The above equation is more commonly known as the *Nernst equation* and is a mathematical statement of the potential at which all of the electrical and concentration forces are balanced in the resting state, which is the resting membrane potential.[26, 29] By substituting the actual values for the different variables and using the more familiar base 10 logarithm, the equation converts to the more recognizable form. Also, the approximate concentration ratio of intracellular to extracellular potassium is 20:1 (Table 6–1). The Nernst equation then becomes:

$$E_m = -(26 \text{ mV}) \, 2.3 \log_{10} [20 \div 1]$$
$$E_m = -75 \text{ mV}$$

The concept of -75 mV representing the equilibrium potential essentially means that at this voltage (intracellular 75 mV more negative than the extracellular region), the electrical and concentration forces are balanced and the cell will attempt to maintain this state. Injecting a small amount of positive charge into the cell with a microelectrode will depolarize (make the intracellular region less negative) to about -70 mV. A less negative intracellular potential means that it is now relatively more positive with excess positive charges compared to the resting state. This situation results in potassium ions exiting the cell because of excess positive charge repelling the ions and potassium ions flowing "down" their concentration gradient from high intracellular to low extracellular concentrations. The potassium continues to exit the cell until -75 mV is again achieved and all forces are in balance. Injecting small amounts of negative charge into the cell results in a similar but opposite situation with potassium entering the cell to again maintain the resting membrane potential.

Sodium Pump

Experimentation has shown that the Nernst equation predicts the resting membrane potential quite well with different extracellular potassium concentrations as long as the potassium concentration is relatively high. At low extracellular potassium concentrations there is a deviation of the resting membrane potential from that predicted with a less negative potential achieved. This finding suggests that at low potassium ion concentrations another ion (sodium or Na^+) has some influence on the resting membrane potential. It turns out that sodium has a very high extracellular compared to intracellular ion concentration, which results in small quantities of sodium ions leaking into the membrane through a few passive sodium channels in the cell's membrane. This relative impermeability of positive sodium ions, combined with a high extracellular but low intracellular concentration and resulting electrical drive to enter the cell (negative inside), would tend to "run down" the cell's resting membrane potential over time. Fortunately, the cell has developed a mechanism whereby this "run down" is prevented. Located within the cell membrane is an energy-dependent sodium-potassium pump, which pumps in potassium ions and pumps out sodium ions in just the right ratio of the sodium ions entering and the compensatory potassium ions exiting the cell. This ratio is two sodium ions being extruded for every three potassium ions taken into the cell. This pump maintains the exact ionic balance necessary to maintain the resting membrane potential.

Goldman-Hodgkin-Katz Equation

An important modification of the Nernst equation is the inclusion of ion permeability as being the primary influence on the cell's transmembrane voltage. Specifically, the greater an ion's permeability, the more likely it is to influence the transmembrane potential, because the equilibrium potential of the most permeable ion in effect becomes the cell's membrane potential. The equation accounting for the different permeability (designated as p in the equation below) factors is known as the Goldman-Hodgkin-Katz equation[26, 28, 29]:

$$E_m = \left(\frac{-RT}{F}\right) \left(2.3 \log_{10} \frac{pK[K^+]_i + pNa[Na^+]_i + pCl[Cl^-]_e}{pK[K^+]_e + pNa[Na^+]_e + pCl[Cl^-]_i}\right)$$

In this equation it can be seen that the cell's transmembrane voltage (E_m) is primarily dependent upon which ion has the greatest permeability. For example, in the resting state, we know that the permeability of potassium is relatively high owing to nonvoltage-gated passive-leak potassium channels, while that of sodium is very low. Chloride is passively distributed through nonvoltage-gated chloride channels, and thus adjusts to whichever ion's permeability predominates between potassium and sodium as dictated by the net transmembrane potential. With a high potassium and low sodium permeability, the above equation simplifies to the Nernst equation, that is, potassium is the predominant ionic species and E_m becomes -75 mV. If sodium permeability were to increase dramatically, then E_m would approach the sodium ion equilibrium potential of $+55$ mV. It would not quite reach this value because potassium continues to have some influence and would hold the maximum potential to a less positive (more negative) value of about $+40$ mV.

TABLE 6–1   Cellular Ionic Concentrations*

	Squid Axon		Mammalian Muscle	
	Intracellular	*Extracellular*	*Intracellular*	*Extracellular*
Na^+	50	440	10	145
K^+	400	20	160	4
Cl^-	52	560	3	114
A^-*	385	—	163	34

*The ionic concentrations are in millimoles per liter. A^- refers to the intracellular organic anions.

Data from Hille B: Introduction to physiology of excitable cells. *In* Patton HD, Fuchs AF, Hille B, et al (eds): Textbook of Physiology, ed 21. Philadelphia, WB Saunders, 1989; Jewett DL, Rayner MD: Basic Concepts of Neuronal Function. Boston, Little, Brown, 1984; Katz B: Nerve, Muscle, and Synapse. New York, McGraw-Hill, 1966; and Koester J: Resting membrane potential and acting potential. *In* Kandel ER, Schwartz JH (eds): Principles of Neural Science, ed 2. New York, Elsevier, 1985, pp 49–57.

Action Potential Generation

In addition to the passive (always open) potassium channels and relatively few passive sodium channels, there is also a second set of sodium and potassium channels within nerve and muscle cell membrane modulated by transmembrane voltage differences. They are voltage-gated because they open and close depending upon the voltage across the membrane.[23] Muscle and unmyelinated nerve contain both sodium and potassium voltage-gated channels (which are located at the nodes of Ranvier). The voltage-gated sodium and potassium ion channels are closed at the resting membrane potential. If the transmembrane voltage changes in the depolarization direction (less negative) and reaches about 15 to 20 mV less negative than the resting membrane potential, the voltage-gated sodium channels open. This results in an increased permeability of the sodium ion, a process known as sodium activation. As noted above, the Goldman-Hodgkin-Katz equation predicts that the transmembrane potential shifts toward the sodium ion equilibrium potential. This massive shift in transmembrane potential is referred to as depolarization. After staying open for a short period of time, the sodium gates automatically close (sodium inactivation) with a return of the resting membrane potential again dictated by the resting state ion permeabilities (repolarization). In muscle and unmyelinated nerve membranes, a delayed opening of potassium voltage-gated channels occurs secondary to the depolarization following sodium activation and occurring during sodium inactivation. This delayed potassium ion shift helps to dissipate any capacitive charge about the membrane and essentially assists repolarization.

It should be recognized that very few ions have to physically cross the membrane, either for sodium induced depolarization or the potassium-mediated repolarization assist. The important factor is the increase in permeability which drives the transmembrane shifts in both the depolarization and repolarization direction. The region of membrane where there are large numbers of voltage-gated sodium channels in the open position acts as a current sink for sodium ions to "sink" into the cell's interior. This implies that a nearby source for the sodium ions must be present. The surrounding membrane acts as the current source, thus in effect causing a current flow from the region about the current sink. Sodium ions are thereby removed from the outside of the membrane surrounding the sink (making this region relatively more negative) and deposited on the inside of the cell (Fig. 6–2). The ions within the cell migrate within it to help neutralize some of the interior's negative charge. This flow of current or charge transfer from extracellular to intracellular is referred to as a "local circuit current." The net effect of this charge transfer is to make the cell's interior less negative and the exterior more negative, thus acting to shift the transmembrane voltage in the depolarized direction about the current sink. If the charge transfer is sufficient to depolarize the cell by 15 to 20 mV, the membrane surrounding the sink is induced to permit sodium activation and hence undergo depolarization. This process can then continue along the length of the cell.

The above process creates an action potential spike at the original site of sodium activation. A mechanical, chemi-

cal, or electrical stimulus that causes the membrane potential to reach threshold over a localized region is all that is required to serve as the initiating stimulus of action potential generation. Once the process begins, it is self-sustaining as long as there are sufficient ion channels to repeat the process of depolarization. The intracellular action potential is essentially a monophasic positive spike: -75 mV resting potential; $+40$ mV spike; return to resting -75 mV with sodium inactivation and potassium activation (see Fig. 6–2). The membrane's threshold value must be reached in order to generate the self-sustaining action potential that is the same at all regions of the membrane. This concept is referred to as an "all-or-none phenomenon." Since in a good volume conductor like the body there are many ions to sustain passive current flows, the local circuit currents spread out in all directions.[13] It is the voltage generated by the depolarization-induced current flows that generates all of the potentials we observe on the instrument's cathode ray tube (CRT) screen.

Of note, in myelinated nerve, the nodes of Ranvier lack voltage-gated potassium channels and contain voltage-gated sodium channels.[43, 44] The action potential, therefore, "jumps" from one node to the next creating an efficient means of action potential propagation which is referred to as saltatory conduction. Repolarization in myelinated nerve, therefore, does not require a delayed potassium current for repolarization. As noted above, the resting membrane potential is restored once the permeability of sodium is reduced. Passive "back-leak" sodium and potassium currents are believed to mediate the discharge of the membrane's capacitance which accumulates over time with multiple action potential discharges.

PHYSIOLOGICAL FACTORS AFFECTING ACTION POTENTIAL PROPAGATION

There are a number of physiological factors which have a direct effect on action potential propagation. These physiological factors can be divided into those which can be altered by the practitioner and those intrinsic to the subject and beyond control. The most important factor readily amenable to change is an extremity's surface temperature. Physiological variables beyond the control of the clinician include gender, age, height, and digit circumference.

GENDER. Only a few studies have attempted to investigate the difference in nerve conduction studies between males and females.[3] There is noted to be a slight increase in the antidromic sensory nerve amplitudes for both the median and ulnar nerves recorded from the digits in women. Also, women demonstrate a greater nerve conduction velocity for upper and lower extremity nerves compared to men. Both of these differences, however, are eliminated when one considers limb length and digit circumference (see below).[36]

AGING. Several generalizations can be made regarding peripheral evoked sensory nerve action potentials (SNAPs) and aging. The conduction velocity demonstrates a consistent decline approximating 1 to 2 m/sec per decade.[33] The SNAP's duration is about 10% to 15% longer in 40- to 60-year-olds, and 20% longer in 70- to 88-year-old persons compared to persons 18 to 25 years old.[8] Compared to the

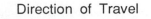

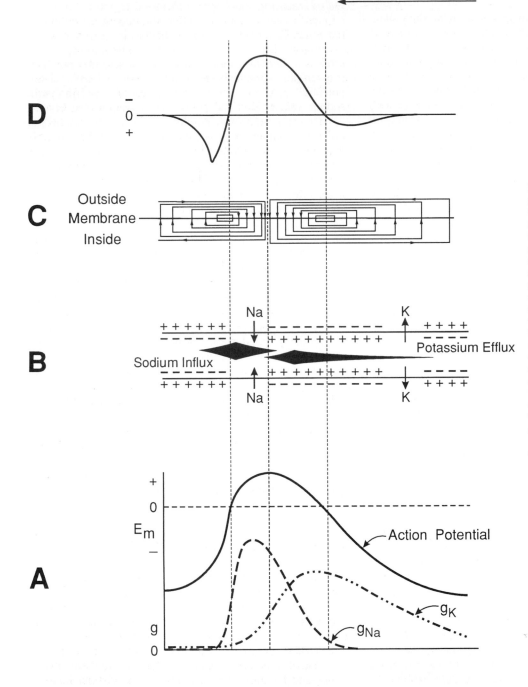

FIGURE 6–2 *A*, Sodium (g_{Na}) and potassium (g_K) ion conductances are depicted over time, resulting in an alteration of the transmembrane potential and creating an action potential. *B*, The spatial relationship of the sodium and potassium ion influx during an action potential is schematically depicted. Note the alteration of the transmembrane ionic potential differences corresponding to the depolarization and repolarization. *C*, Local circuit currents described the pathways of extracellular sodium ions entering the cell and then migrating longitudinally within the cell. *D*, Triphasic extracellular waveform associated with the intracellular monophasic action potential. (From Dumitru D: Electrodiagnostic Medicine. Philadelphia, Hanley & Belfus, 1995.)

18- to 25-year-old group, the SNAPs amplitude is one half and one third, respectively, for the 40- to 60- and 70- to 88-year-old groups. The distal sensory latencies reveal a similar prolongation with age. There is a suggestion that the median and radial nerves do not demonstrate considerable alteration with age.[17] At present there is disagreement as to the magnitude of change in SNAP parameters induced by the aging process.

The results of aging on conduction velocity have been examined in a number of upper and lower extremity nerves. Motor nerve conduction velocities reveal similar changes to sensory nerves. The newborn's motor nerve conduction velocities are about half of adult values, which are reached by 3 to 5 years of age.[2] After the age of 50 years, there is a progressive decline in the conduction velocity of the fastest motor fibers, approximating 1 to 2 m/sec per decade. There is a concurrent increase in the distal motor latency and decrease in the motor response's amplitude with advancing age. H-reflex latency demonstrates little alteration with aging in the healthy elderly.[18] The decrease in amplitude is difficult to ascertain clinically as there is a wide range of normal H-reflex amplitudes.

DIGIT CIRCUMFERENCE. Females consistently demonstrate significantly higher antidromic SNAP amplitudes for the median and ulnar nerves recorded from the second and fifth digits.[3] A negative linear correlation exists between finger circumference and amplitude for these two nerves. It is known that as the distance between the recording electrode and neural generator increases, the amplitude precipitously declines. Increasing the circumference of the finger displaces the electrode farther from the nerve. Since men have significantly larger finger circumferences than women, this appears to explain the difference in SNAP amplitudes. There is no evidence that this difference is due to an intrinsic neural difference between male and female nerves.

HEIGHT. Several investigations have documented slower nerve conduction velocities in taller compared with shorter persons with respect to lower limb nerve conductions.[9, 30] This difference is found to be independent of the limb's temperature or subject's age. The cause is unknown but distal nerve tapering or an abrupt change in axon diameter has been speculated to account for this finding.[13]

TEMPERATURE. Temperature is one of the most profound factors influencing nerve conduction studies. As the temperature of the nerve is lowered, the amount of current required to generate an action potential increases. Neural excitability is lowered with a reduction in temperature. This decreased excitability is a direct temperature effect on the nerve's action potential–generating mechanism at the nodes of Ranvier, and not a result of membrane resistance changes, that is, the transmembrane resistance is not increased by a drop in temperature.[24, 25] In addition to excitability, the morphology of an action potential is profoundly affected by a drop in temperature.

The action potential's amplitude, rise time, and fall time all increase as the nerve's temperature declines. The time required for the action potential of a cold nerve to reach its peak depolarization from the resting membrane level increases approximately 33%.[34] The time necessary for the action potential to return to its resting level is also increased, but much more so than the rise time (69%). Because both the duration and spike height increase, the area of the action potential increases dramatically at lower temperatures.

The compound muscle action potential (CMAP) arising from cooled muscle tissue demonstrates similar changes as those noted for SNAPs. The CMAP amplitude, duration, rise time, and area all increase as the muscle's temperature is reduced. Intramuscular recordings also reveal that those motor units in close proximity to the recording electrode are also increased in the same variables noted above.

Temperature also has an impact on nerve conduction velocities (NCVs). Based on the prolongation of the rise and fall time noted above, we should be able to infer the nerve's response to cooling with respect to NCV. Since propagation is saltatory in myelinated nerves, decreased temperature results in an increase in the amount of time necessary to reach the action potential's peak at each node of Ranvier. As cooling increases the time required at each node, slower conduction velocity results.

The first detailed investigation of temperature effects on NCV in human nerves revealed an NCV-to-temperature correlation of 2.4 m/sec/°C for median and ulnar motor conduction.[22] With every 1°C drop in temperature, there was a 2.4-m/sec decrease in the conduction velocity. Reductions in conduction velocity for upper extremity motor nerve fibers have also been found to approximate a decrease of 4% or 5%/°C.[10, 27] Correction factors utilizing subcutaneous and intramuscular readings are equally correct, but it is more convenient and less painful to use surface measurements.[20]

In the upper extremity, the relationship between temperature and NCV has been investigated for the surface temperature range of 26° to 33°C, measured at the midline of the distal wrist crease. Calculations reveal that for median motor and sensory nerves, NCV is altered 1.5 and 1.4 m/sec/°C respectively, while the distal latency for both changes 0.2 ms/°C.[19-21] The ulnar nerve demonstrated motor and sensory temperature relationships of 2.1 and 1.6 m/sec/°C respectively and a distal motor and sensory latency correlation of 0.2 ms/°C.[19-21]

Because of the profound effects of temperature on NCV, it is clear that reliable nerve studies require temperature control. A cool extremity, irrespective of the ambient room temperature, can result in latencies, NCVs, and amplitudes that are not in the "normal" range. A normal limb study can yield results that are spuriously thought to be abnormal, but which are only due to the low temperature. This is an especially important issue when an abnormal nerve is being studied. Correction factors are well known for normal nerve, but serious questions remain about how abnormal nerves respond to temperature variations. Although applying a correction factor is less time-consuming than heating the patient, it is questionable how accurately correction factors for temperature in normal nerves can be applied to abnormal nerves. Until more data are available regarding the best correction factor for diseased nerves, warming of the limb should be considered to be superior to using correction factors. It is recommended that the practitioner use at least a surface temperature between the stimulating and recording electrodes of 32°C for upper limbs, and 30°C for lower limbs. In persons with ischemic limbs or with altered sensation, great care must be exercised with respect to increasing the tissue's metabolic demand and injuring the patient.

WAVEFORM MORPHOLOGY GENERATION

As noted above, the current flow created by a depolarization sink is associated with a specific pattern of voltages known as isopotential lines[13] (Figs. 6–2 and 6–3). Recording a voltage at any point in space along this line results in the same voltage being recorded. As one moves farther from the current sink, the corresponding voltages decline as the current density also decreases. The pattern of isopotential lines in space create three distinct regions of voltage. The current sink is associated with a negative voltage while the two surrounding (leading and trailing) current sources are considered zones of positive voltage. Separating the current sink zone from the current sources are zero isopotential lines. These lines correspond to regions of zero voltage demarcated by that portion of the potential crossing the baseline on the CRT (see Fig. 6–3).

An action potential with its local circuit current and associated isopotential lines propagating past an electrode can be considered essentially equivalent to a stationary action potential sequentially sampled with a recording electrode moving through its electric field (see Fig. 6–3). We shall use the latter situation as an example for discussion purposes because it is easier to visualize the ensuing action

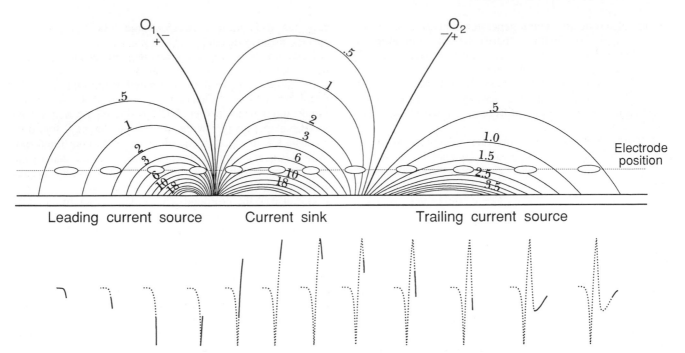

FIGURE 6–3   A propagating nerve or muscle action potential generates a characteristic pattern of voltages associated with the corresponding current flows. Passing an electrode through a hypothetically stationary action potential *(open ovals)* results in the recording of a triphasic extracellular waveform. This basic conceptualization of extracellular waveforms applies equally to nerve and muscle tissue. (From Dumitru D: Electrodiagnostic Medicine. Philadelphia, Hanley & Belfus, 1995.)

potential waveform. Suppose a propagating nerve or muscle action potential is frozen for an instant in time. A characteristic pattern of isopotential voltage lines is described in the region of the body surrounding the nerve or muscle. We can then move a recording electrode through the activated tissue's electric field to simulate a propagating action potential (see Fig. 6–3). The final waveform morphology associated with an action potential propagating along a straight portion of nerve or muscle is a triphasic waveform with a large negative spike flanked by an initial large and subsequent terminal small positive phase. For our discussion purposes, positive is a downward CRT deflection while an upward CRT deflection designates a net negative potential difference between the two recording electrodes. This examples implies that for both nerve and muscle, when an action potential approaches, reaches, and then travels past a recording electrode, the fundamental waveform morphology is a triphasic potential. These same simple principles can be applied to understand the morphologic generation of essentially all potentials likely to be observed during the electrodiagnostic medicine examination.

NERVE AND MUSCLE WAVEFORM MORPHOLOGIES AND CHARACTERISTICS

Nerve Potentials

Sensory Nerve Action Potentials

CLINICAL RECORDINGS. SNAPs can be obtained with either antidromic or orthodromic techniques.[8] The term *antidromic* implies that the induced neural impulse propagates along the nerve in a direction opposite to its physiological direction. Remember that the nerve will conduct an impulse proximally and distally when stimulated by a depolarizing current. On the other hand, stimulating the median sensory fibers on the second digit and recording from the wrist is an example of an orthodromic technique. In orthodromic recordings, the sensory fiber impulses are detected at a location proximal to the stimulus as they travel physiologically from the finger, through the wrist region, on their way to the central nervous system.

SNAP MORPHOLOGY. Antidromic and orthodromic bipolar SNAP waveform recordings are typically biphasic rather than triphasic. The biphasic, negative-positive potential is a result of the bipolar recording technique and not a violation of volume conductor theory. Biphasic SNAP waveforms can best be understood by use of bipolar and referential recording montages for median nerve stimulation at the wrist[12] (Fig. 6–4). The median SNAP is indeed a triphasic waveform and conforms to the principles of volume conduction, but only appears biphasic because of the recording montage used.

It is also possible to predict the optimal interelectrode separation to maximize the biphasic potential's amplitude in the bipolar recording.[15] The critical factor in this instance is the rise time, baseline to negative peak, of the biphasic potential. The recording electrodes must be located at a distance greater than the spatial extent represented by the rise time duration. The rise time of most SNAPs approaches 0.8 ms which represents a longitudinal extent of 40 mm for a conduction velocity of 50 m/sec (50,000 mm/ 1000 ms = D/0.8 ms; D = 40 mm). If the two recording electrodes are separated by a distance of less than 40 mm, some similar information regarding the main peaks of the

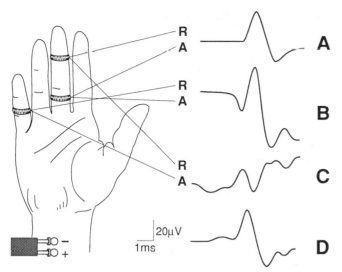

FIGURE 6–4 The median nerve is stimulated at the wrist with an antidromic sensory recording montage. Active (A) and reference (R) electrodes are located on fingers as designated above. *A,* Bipolar recording with the commonly observed biphasic median nerve sensory nerve action potential (SNAP). *B,* The same active electrode location in A is referenced to the fifth digit, resulting in a triphasic SNAP. *C,* An active electrode placed on the fifth digit, but referenced to the third digit, permits the observation of what this electrode records when the median nerve is stimulated. An inverted triphasic potential of small magnitude is detected. It is inverted because of its connection to the inverting amplifier port. *D,* Electronically summating the potential recorded in *B* and *C* yields that recorded with a bipolar montage in *A.* (From Dumitru D: Volume conduction: Theory and application. *In* Dumitru D (ed): Physical Medicine and Rehabilitation State of the Art Reviews: Clinical Electrophysiology. Philadelphia, Hanley & Belfus, 1989.)

two potentials will be recorded by both electrodes and result in mutual cancellation of data, producing a potential with a smaller amplitude. A portion of the nerve will be depolarizing under the reference electrode while still in some degree of depolarization under the active electrode. At interelectrode separations greater than 40 mm where the reference electrode is located more distally on the finger and the active electrode remains unchanged, the biphasic potential's negative peak amplitude will no longer grow, but the terminal positive phase will enlarge slightly and may change its morphology. These findings can be demonstrated by varying the distance between recording electrodes and observing the results (Fig. 6–5). In effect, as the recording distance decreases below 40 mm, the amplitude of the potential declines, and the peak latency shortens.

Activating the median nerve at the wrist will yield the expected biphasic SNAP of a particular duration and amplitude. Relocating the neural stimulator sequentially at more proximal activation sites results in a series of SNAPs with a progressively declining amplitude, and area of the negative phase. This effect occurs because of increasing phase cancellation between the individual SNAPs contained within the peripheral nerve secondary to temporal dispersion manifesting over large distances. The significant reduction in SNAP amplitude with progressive increases in distance between the stimulating and recording electrodes precludes SNAP amplitudes being used as accurate predictors of conduction block or axonal loss from widely separated stimulation sites within the same arm. Corresponding left-right amplitude comparisons for the same stimulus site, however, can be utilized to assess possible axonal loss.

Muscle Potentials

Needle Insertional Activity

NORMAL INSERTIONAL ACTIVITY. Placing a needle (monopolar or standard concentric)-recording electrode into healthy muscle tissue and advancing it in quick but short intervals results in brief bursts of electrical potentials referred to as insertional activity[13] (Fig. 6–6). The observed electrical activity is believed to result from the needle electrode mechanically depolarizing the muscle fibers surrounding its leading edge as it pierces and pushes aside the tissue. Minimal and localized muscle tissue damage may occur from direct needle trauma and is the basis for the synonymous term of "injury potentials." The purpose of including insertional activity analysis as part of the electromyographic examination is that the probing needle may provoke transient or sustained membrane instability prior to this abnormal activity being present with the muscle at rest.

DECREASED INSERTIONAL ACTIVITY. Muscle that has been replaced by fibrous tissue will no longer be capable of electrical activity. Consequently, the needle electrode is incapable of mechanically depolarizing this tissue. The result is that few if any electrical potentials will be detected following needle movement (see Fig. 6–6). This tissue may also have a "gritty" or fibrous feel during needle insertion. One may also detect decreased insertional

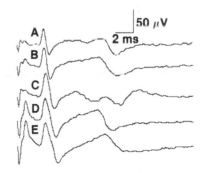

Trace	Interelectrode distance	Latency		Amplitude
		Onset	Peak	
	cm	*ms*		*µV*
A	1.0	2.7	3.0	56
B	2.0	2.7	3.1	72
C	3.0	2.7	3.3	77
D	4.0	2.7	3.3	86
E	5.0	2.7	3.3	86

FIGURE 6–5 The effect of interelectrode separation can be easily demonstrated by evoking an antidromic median sensory nerve action potential (SNAP) and progressively increasing the interelectrode separation between the active and reference electrode. The active electrode remains in the same location while the reference electrode is sequentially displaced more distally on the digit. As can be seen, the SNAP amplitude increases, peak latency increases, and the onset latency remains the same. (From Dumitru D, Walsh NE: Practical instrumentation and common sources of error. Am J Phys Med Rehabil 1988; 67:55–65.)

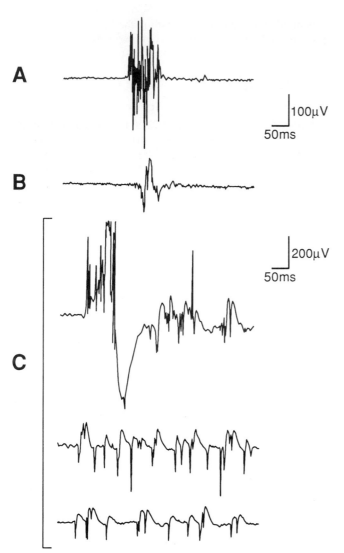

FIGURE 6–6 *A,* Inserting a monopolar needle in healthy muscle tissue results in mechanical depolarization of muscle tissue, which generates a brief burst of electrical activity designated as insertional activity. *B,* Inserting the same needle in fibrotic muscle or subcutaneous fatty tissue results in decreased insertional activity. *C,* Inserting a monopolar needle in denervated muscle tissue produces not only the initial burst of electrical activity, but associated positive sharp waves and fibrillation potentials that abate over several hundred milliseconds. (From Dumitru D: Electrodiagnostic Medicine. Philadelphia, Hanley & Belfus, 1995.)

activity in electrically silent tissue in metabolic or electrolyte abnormalities, as seen in attacks of periodic paralysis.

INCREASED INSERTIONAL ACTIVITY. Practitioners have noted that insertional activity may appear to be prolonged in a number of pathological conditions. This finding has led to the term "increased insertional activity." In disease states where the muscle is no longer connected to its nerve or the muscle membrane is inherently unstable from primary muscle disease, the increased insertional activity completes a temporal continuum from the previously normal insertional activity to the development of sustained membrane instability potentials (see Fig. 6–6).

End-Plate Potentials

MINIATURE END-PLATE POTENTIALS (MEPPs). An active electrode located in the end-plate region can record two distinct potentials. One of the potentials that can be observed is a short-duration (0.5–2.0 ms), small (10–50 mV), irregularly occurring (once every 5 seconds per axon terminal), monophasic negative waveform.[13] These potentials represent the random release of acetylcholine vesicles. Volume conduction theory suggests that for a potential to be monophasic and negative, the current sink would have to start and finish within the active electrode's recording area (Fig. 6–7A).

Clinically, multiple MEPPs are usually observed with an intramuscular recording electrode, and the sound is referred to as end-plate noise or "seashell murmur." Numerous MEPPs are detected despite a firing frequency of 0.2 Hz per end-plate because the recording electrode is relatively large with respect to the end-plate region and detects MEPPs from multiple end-plates firing simultaneously (Fig. 6–7B).

END-PLATE SPIKES. A second potential that can be detected with an active electrode placed in the end-plate region is relatively short in duration (3–4 ms), of moderate amplitude (100–200 mV), irregularly firing, and biphasic with an initial negative deflection.[13] The biphasic potential has an initial negative phase, produced when a current sink originates in the vicinity of the active electrode and then propagates away (Fig. 6–8). Triphasic end-plate spikes may also occur if the active electrode induces an action potential in the terminal axon but the electrode's recording surface is some distance from the end-plate. End-plate spikes and MEPPs are frequently observed together because they arise from the same region (Fig. 6–9).

SINGLE MUSCLE FIBER. The single muscle fiber's extracellular waveform morphology, like nerve tissue, depends on the characteristics of the muscle's intracellular action potential. A muscle's action potential is approximately 4 to 20 times longer than a nerve's, due in particular to the prolonged repolarization process.[13] Aside from the longer duration of local circuit currents compared to neural tissue, the concept of a current sink surrounded by two source currents (source-sink-source) remains unchanged. Because of the local circuit current's longer duration of flow, one may anticipate that the terminal source current will be expanded, thereby diminishing its density and producing a potentially small third or positive phase. A triphasic waveform with a small terminal phase should then be recorded from an extracellular active electrode placed adjacent to a propagating single muscle fiber action potential at some distance from the end-plate region (Fig. 6–10). Single muscle fiber recordings are typically triphasic potentials with a pattern of (large positive-large negative-small positive phase). One may also record biphasic initially positive, or biphasic initially negative single muscle fiber potentials.

Motor Unit Potential Morphology

ANATOMY. One anterior horn cell gives rise to a peripheral axon that splits into multiple terminal axons, each of which innervate a single muscle fiber. The anterior horn cell, its axon, and all the single muscle fibers supplied by that nerve are referred to as a motor unit. When the anterior horn cell fires, or the nerve that arises from it is stimulated, all of the muscle fibers that belong to that motor unit

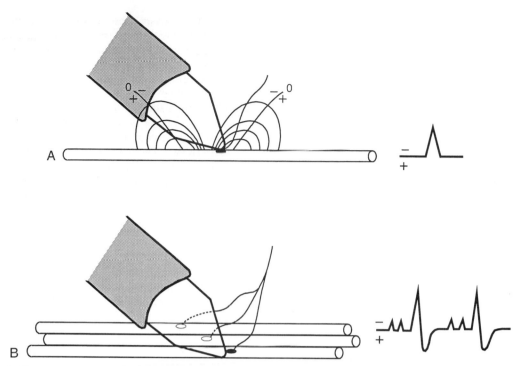

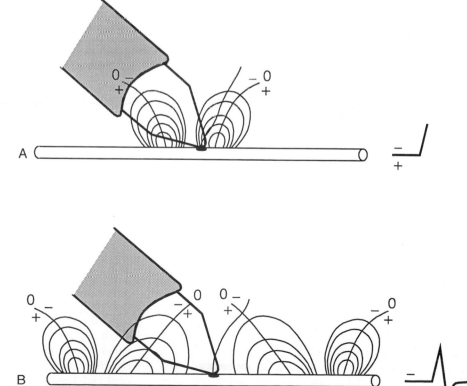

FIGURE 6–7 *A,* Monopolar needle electrode located over a muscle's end-plate records the spontaneous depolarization of a miniature end-plate potential. As the electrode is located over this potential's subthreshold central current sink, and hence does not propagate, a monophasic negative potential is recorded. *B,* The large recording electrode is usually positioned over several end-plates, thus recording multiple miniature end-plate potentials and end-plate spikes. (From Dumitru D: Electrodiagnostic Medicine. Philadelphia, Hanley & Belfus, 1995.)

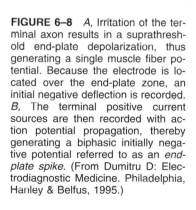

FIGURE 6–8 *A,* Irritation of the terminal axon results in a suprathreshold end-plate depolarization, thus generating a single muscle fiber potential. Because the electrode is located over the end-plate zone, an initial negative deflection is recorded. *B,* The terminal positive current sources are then recorded with action potential propagation, thereby generating a biphasic initially negative potential referred to as an *end-plate spike.* (From Dumitru D: Electrodiagnostic Medicine. Philadelphia, Hanley & Belfus, 1995.)

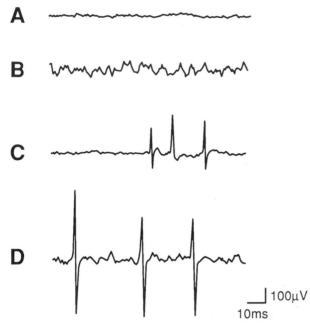

FIGURE 6–9   *A*, Monopolar needle located in a healthy muscle at rest. *B*, Slight needle movement positions the electrode in an end-plate region with the recording of multiple miniature end-plate potentials of a negative spike configuration. *C*, Repositioning the needle electrode to a slightly different region primarily records biphasic initially negative end-plate spikes. *D*, Advancing the needle electrode slightly permits the simultaneous recording of both potentials noted individually in *B* and *C*. (From Dumitru D: Electrodiagnostic Medicine. Philadelphia, Hanley & Belfus, 1995.)

depolarize. The electrical activity from all of these muscle fibers summate to produce a motor unit action potential (MUAP). The anatomical distribution of the terminal axons with respect to the muscle fibers they innervate is particularly relevant to the morphological characteristics of the MUAP.

Let us consider one motor unit belonging to a human biceps muscle[6, 7] (Fig. 6–11*A*). Upon reaching the muscle tissue, the peripheral nerve divides into a large number of terminal axons. Each terminal axon will form an end-plate region with a single muscle fiber. The length of an individual terminal axon from the point it divides to the end-plate is quite variable for each muscle fiber innervated (Fig. 6–11*B*). As a result, the spatial extent of the end-plate region from one motor unit may reach 30 mm longitudinally along the muscle. Additionally, the muscle fibers of a single motor unit are randomly distributed in an oval territory 4 to 6 mm in circumference (see Fig. 6–11*A*). The random distribution implies that the single muscle fibers may be in groups of different numbers or singly arranged within the 4 to 6 mm. Five to 10 or more different motor units may share this area. It is also important to note that the muscle fibers constituting a single motor unit are randomly interspersed with the muscle fibers of the other motor units sharing its oval territory.

AMPLITUDE AND RISE TIME.   The morphology of an MUAP can be described in terms of its *amplitude* (maximum peak-to-peak CRT trace displacement), *rise time* (temporal aspect of a potential's peak), *duration* (departure from and return to baseline), and number of *phases* (baseline crossings plus one) (Fig. 6–12). In the volume conduc-

tor of muscle tissue, the amplitude of potentials declines exponentially with increases in distance from the current generator. This occurs because the surrounding muscle and its supportive tissues impede potentials that change rapidly over a short period of time. The tissue acts as a high-frequency filter. As a result, the peak-to-peak MUAP's amplitude is believed to arise from fewer than 12 and possibly just one or two single muscle fibers located within 0.5 mm of the electrode's recording surface.

DURATION.   The MUAP's duration depends on the (1) shortest and longest lengths of terminal axons from the point they separate from the parent nerve to the end-plate, and (2) conduction velocities of the terminal axons and muscle fibers with respect to the recording electrode (see Figs. 6–11 and 6–12). These factors summate to produce a rather complex situation, but we can simplify matters by considering the sum total of electrical events passing an electrode at one location (see Fig. 6–11*B*). A motor unit with an end-plate expanse of 30 mm will require an action potential traveling at 4.3 m/sec approximately 7 ms to cross this distance.[6, 7] A single muscle fiber potential may have a duration of 3 to 4 ms. The total duration of the MUAP will be the summation of the end-plate time crossing (7 ms) plus the duration of the last few muscle fibers (4 ms) to approximate 11 ms from initial baseline departure to final baseline return.

PHASES.   As previously stated, the single muscle fiber usually has a triphasic appearance when recorded outside of the end-plate zone and away from the tendinous insertion. The voltages from all of the single muscle fibers belonging to one motor unit summate to yield a MUAP that is also usually triphasic: positive-negative-positive. This voltage summation does not always produce a smooth result and small serrations or *turns* can occasionally be seen as part of a MUAP's major phase (see Fig. 6–12). Recall that the number of phases is defined as the number of CRT trace baseline crossings plus one. Normal MUAPs are considered to have four or fewer phases. MUAPs with five or more phases are called *polyphasic potentials.* Recordings of multiple MUAPs from normal muscle tissue can have between 12% (concentric needle) and 35% (monopolar needle) polyphasic potentials depending upon the type of recording electrode used.[13] Slightly different MUAP morphologies can be expected depending upon the exact location of the recording electrode with respect to different single muscle fibers within the motor unit territory.

Pathologic changes can also alter the number of phases a MUAP waveform can have. The motor unit can be affected in two general ways following injury or disease. A pathological condition may affect either the anterior horn cell or peripheral nerve, or the muscle fibers composing the motor unit. If the neural component of a motor unit is compromised severely enough to experience degeneration, all of the muscle fibers innervated by the parent nerve will become denervated. These denervated muscle fibers somehow induce nearby terminal axons of intact nerves to send out neural projections to reinnervate the orphaned muscle fibers. Through peripheral sprouting, the total number of muscle fibers belonging to a specific motor unit may increase dramatically (Fig. 6–13). Neurogenic diseases can

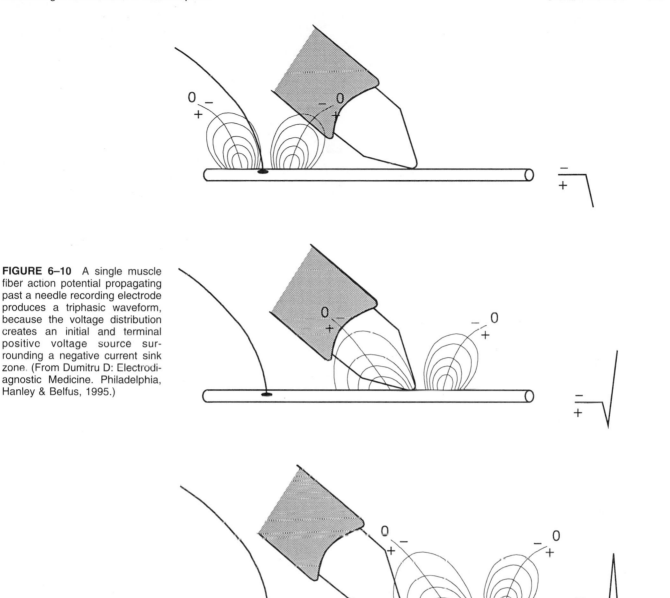

FIGURE 6–10 A single muscle fiber action potential propagating past a needle recording electrode produces a triphasic waveform, because the voltage distribution creates an initial and terminal positive voltage source surrounding a negative current sink zone. (From Dumitru D: Electrodiagnostic Medicine. Philadelphia, Hanley & Belfus, 1995.)

lead over time to larger-amplitude, longer-duration, and highly polyphasic MUAPs.

If the muscle fibers constituting a motor unit undergo a random degeneration, as occurs in some myopathies, the total number of fibers belonging to that motor unit decrease (Fig. 6–14). A decrease in muscle fibers would most likely result in a reduction of the MUAP's maximum amplitude. It is also conceivable that fibers at the extremes of the end-plate region would be involved. The result of these fibers degenerating would cause a shortening of the MUAP duration. Finally, the dropout of single muscle fiber waveforms would produce less voltage with respect to the spatial summation of single fiber potentials. Fewer muscle fibers could lead to "gaps" in the MUAP waveform, causing an increase in the number of phases. A primary myopathic process tends to yield a shorter-duration, highly polyphasic, low-amplitude MUAP.

COMPOUND MUSCLE ACTION POTENTIAL. To elicit a CMAP from a particular muscle, the active electrode is located on the skin's surface directly over the muscle's motor point (end-plate region).[13] The end-plate region typically lies midway between the muscle's origin and insertion. The reference electrode is usually placed on or distal to the tendinous insertion of the muscle so as not to record electrical activity from the activated muscle. Stimulating the peripheral nerve innervating the muscle under investigation results in a relatively large, biphasic waveform with an initial negative deflection (Fig. 6–15).

Occasionally a positive deflection can precede the CMAP's negative phase. Volume conductor theory can explain this observation (Fig. 6–16). The active electrode may not be located directly over the motor point but displaced longitudinally away from it. The region of muscle surrounding the end-plate zone serves as that portion of the volume conductor from which the source currents initially arise to complete the local circuit currents into the

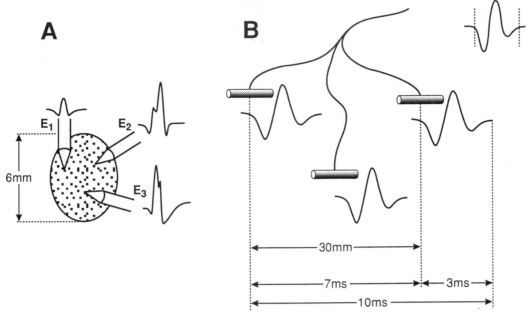

FIGURE 6–11   *A,* The single muscle fibers *(small dots)* comprising a single motor unit in the biceps brachii muscle are depicted. Three needle recording positions are shown, each with a slightly different motor unit action potential (MUAP) morphology for the same motor unit. *B,* The total duration of an MUAP is dependent on the spatial expanse of the end-plate zone, terminal axon conduction velocity, and single muscle fiber conduction velocity. (From Dumitru D, DeLisa JA: Volume conduction. Muscle Nerve 1991; 14:605–624.)

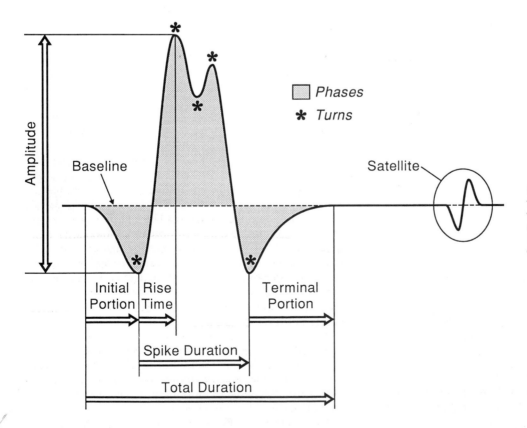

FIGURE 6–12   A motor unit action potential is depicted, with various morphological aspects measured. (From Dumitru D: Electrodiagnostic Medicine. Philadelphia, Hanley & Belfus, 1995.)

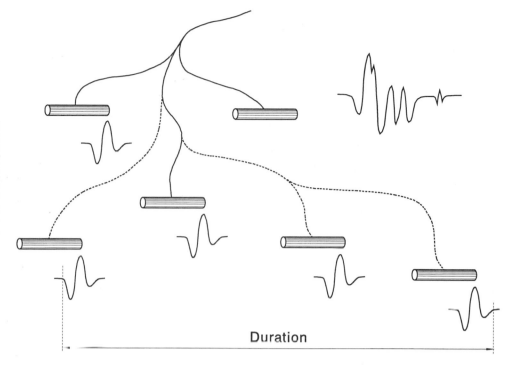

FIGURE 6–13 Several muscle fibers are denervated. Growth of collateral terminal nerve sprouts from an intact motor unit *(dotted lines)* reinnervates denervated muscle fibers. The end result is a large-amplitude long-duration potential with more phases. (From Dumitru D: Electrodiagnostic Medicine. Philadelphia, Hanley & Belfus, 1995.)

current sink. An active electrode located off the motor point will first record some portion of one of the source currents "feeding" the current sink. Recall that the leading portion of the source current will result in a positive deflection of the CRT trace. As propagation ensues in the muscle, the current sink will eventually reach the active electrode, resulting in a negative deflection. Finally, the terminal source current is detected producing a positive

deflection. Instead of the anticipated biphasic potential, a triphasic positive-negative-positive waveform is recorded. Relocating the active electrode over the anticipated motor point region will usually remedy the situation.

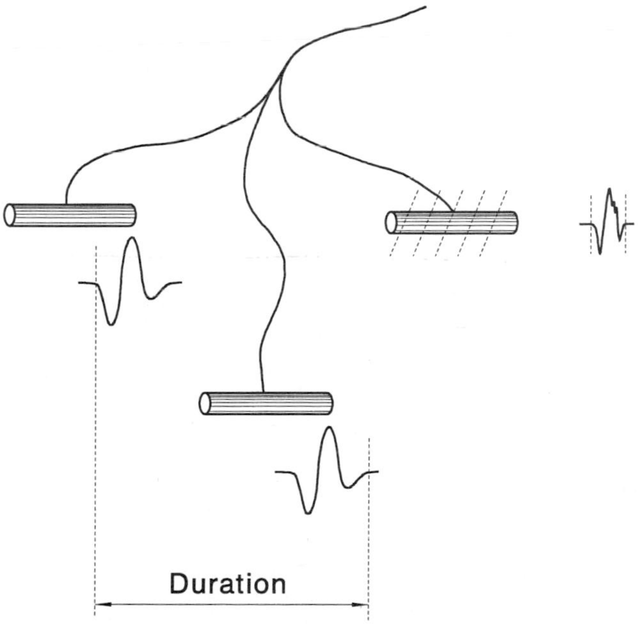

MUSCLE GENERATORS OF ABNORMAL SPONTANEOUS POTENTIALS

FIBRILLATION POTENTIALS. In vitro observations have shown that about 6 days or so after denervation the muscle fiber's resting membrane potential decreases to a less negative level of -60 mV compared to the normal value of -80 mV.[5, 41] Additionally, the resting membrane potential begins to oscillate. Since the threshold level for starting the all-or-none self-sustaining action potential is now closer to the new resting membrane potential, the oscillating membrane potential will eventually reach the threshold level. Once threshold is achieved, a propagating action potential is induced in the muscle fiber which is referred to as a fibrillation potential. The repolarization phase of denervated muscle results in a temporarily more hyperpolarized (-75 mV or more) level than the previous resting membrane potential of -60 mV. Additionally, the muscle's repolarization actually hyperpolarizes the threshold level to that of -60 mV or slightly more negative. As the hyperpolarized membrane level (-75 mV or more) begins to return toward its resting membrane level of -60 mV (the new threshold level), an action potential is again produced. This process repeats regularly on a time interval dependent on the repolarization-to-threshold turnaround time. Fibrillation potentials may be reduced in number following a decrease in temperature, muscle ischemia, or *d*-tubocurarine administration.

The difference between the resting membrane potential and threshold level is less in the former end-plate region

FIGURE 6–14 Loss of single muscle fibers from a motor unit results in the generation of motor unit action potentials with smaller amplitude, shorter durations, and possibly more phases. (From Dumitru D: Electrodiagnostic Medicine. Philadelphia, Hanley & Belfus, 1995.)

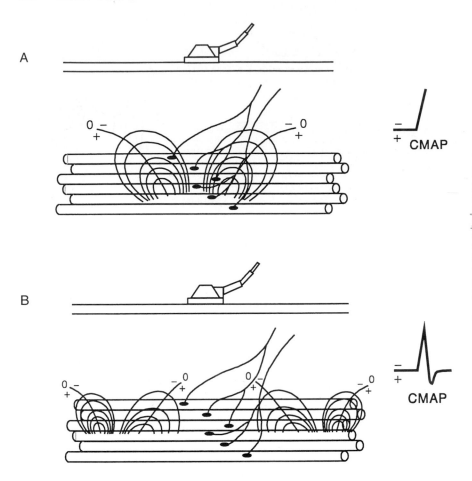

FIGURE 6–15 *A,* Locating an active recording electrode over the motor point of a muscle places this electrode over the central region of the negative current sink generating all of the muscle's action potentials. An initial negative deflection is recorded because of this location, thereby producing the compound muscle action potential's characteristic morphology. *B,* A terminal positive phase is then recorded as the action potential propagates away from the electrode. (From Dumitru D: Electrodiagnostic Medicine. Philadelphia, Hanley & Belfus, 1995.)

than along the muscle fiber. This may explain why fibrillation potentials appear to arise more commonly from the previous end-plate than at other portions of the muscle. Irregularly firing fibrillation potentials occur at times and are less well understood, but are thought to arise from spontaneous depolarizations within the transverse tubule system.

Fibrillation potentials are simply spontaneous depolarizations of a single muscle fiber and demonstrate waveform morphologies similar to those of single muscle fibers that are voluntarily activated (Fig. 6–17). Fibrillation potentials occur not only spontaneously but also can be provoked by electrode movement in pathological tissue. Fibrillation potentials are typically short in duration (less than 5 ms), less than 1 mV in amplitude, and fire at rates between 1 and 50 Hz. They have a typical sound likened to a high-pitched "tick" like "rain on a tin roof" when amplified through a loudspeaker. When the recording electrode is located in the previous end-plate zone of a denervated muscle, fibrillation potentials can be biphasic with an initial positive deflection. A recording electrode outside of the end-plate zone, but far from the tendinous region, will detect fibrillation potentials that are either biphasic (positive-negative) or triphasic (positive-negative-positive).

POSITIVE SHARP WAVES (PSWs). A potential that can be recorded from a single muscle fiber having an unstable muscle membrane potential secondary to denervation or intrinsic muscle disease typically has a large primary sharp positive deflection followed by a small prolonged negative potential. These potentials are called positive sharp waves (see Fig. 6–17). This waveform is believed to have the same clinical significance as a fibrillation potential in that it is a single muscle fiber discharge.[14] Amplified through a loudspeaker, positive sharp waves have a regular firing rate (1–50 Hz) and a dull thud sound. Their durations are from several milliseconds to 100 ms. Although observed to fire spontaneously, PSWs are more often provoked by electrode movement.

A number of other potentials can be observed that have the morphology of a positive sharp wave. As we have already described, a MUAP recorded from the tendinous region can also have an initial positive deflection followed by a negative potential because the current sink cannot pass beyond the recording electrode.[13] It is also possible for the recording electrode to damage a number of muscle fibers in close proximity to the recording surface. This results in a primarily positive potential. An additional possibility is for the cannula of a concentric needle-recording electrode to preferentially be located in the motor unit territory and invert the negative spike (cannula = reference electrode), making it appear positive and simulating a positive sharp wave. These three potentials can be distinguished from a positive sharp wave in that they are MUAPs and subject to voluntary control, whereas a positive sharp wave is not. Asking the subject to contract and relax the muscle under investigation should demonstrate that the potential has a variable firing rate. A positive sharp wave typically fires at a regular rate. If any doubt remains, the electrode

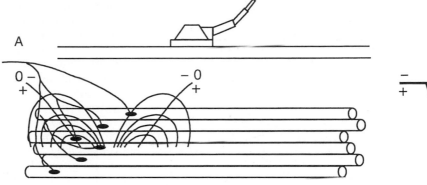

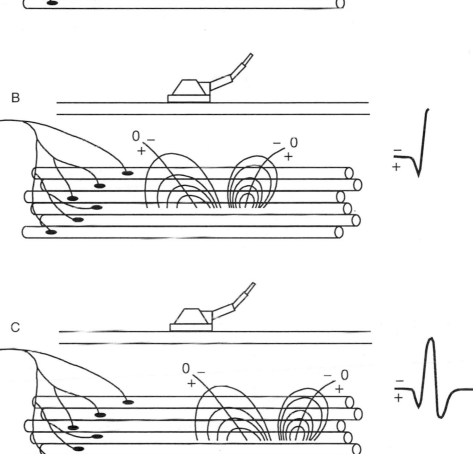

FIGURE 6–16 *A,* Relocating the active electrode in Figure 6–15 off the motor point results in a compound muscle action potential with an initial positive deflection as some of the muscle's action potentials no longer originate under the electrode but propagate toward it. *B,* When the main negative sink reaches the electrode, the potential's main negative spike is detected. *C,* Finally, the terminal positive source currents are recorded generating the potential's terminal positive phase. (From Dumitru D: Electrodiagnostic Medicine. Philadelphia, Hanley & Belfus, 1995.)

should be repositioned until successful recordings are obtained. Transient runs of "positive sharp wave–appearing potentials" may be seen in healthy skeletal muscle, particularly in the paraspinal muscles. The "nonpathologic" positive sharp waves are believed to arise because the needle electrode is oriented in such a manner as to irritate a terminal axon, but extend along the muscle fiber while injuring the tissue and preventing action potential conduction. The induced end-plate spike looks like a positive sharp wave.

COMPLEX REPETITIVE DISCHARGE. A complex repetitive discharge (CRD) is a spontaneously firing group of action potentials (formerly called a bizarre high-frequency discharge, or pseudomyotonic discharge).[13] The morphology of these potentials is that they are continuous runs of simple or complex spike patterns that regularly repeat at

0.3 to 150 Hz. The repetitive pattern of spike potentials has the same appearance with each firing and bears the same relationship to its neighboring spikes (Fig. 6–18). A distinct sound likened to heavy machinery or an idling motorcycle is produced by the firing of CRDs. In addition to the sound and repetitive pattern, a hallmark of these waveforms is that they start and stop abruptly. CRDs may begin spontaneously or be induced by needle movement, muscle percussion, or muscle contraction. Nerve block and curare do not abolish CRDs, suggesting that the origin of these potentials is in muscle tissue.

MYOTONIC DISCHARGES. The phenomenon of delayed muscle relaxation following muscle contraction is referred to as myotonia or action myotonia.[13] The finding of delayed muscle relaxation after reflex activation or induced by striking the muscle belly with a reflex hammer is

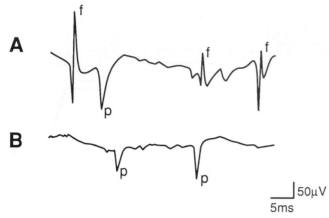

FIGURE 6–17 *A,* Monopolar needle recording of positive sharp waves (p) and fibrillation potentials (f). *B,* Only positive sharp waves are depicted. (From Dumitru D: Electrodiagnostic Medicine. Philadelphia, Hanley & Belfus, 1995.)

called percussion myotonia. Clinical myotonia is usually accentuated by energetic muscle activity following a period of rest. Continued muscle contraction lessens the myotonia and is known as the "warmup." It is believed that cooling the muscle accentuates myotonia, but this finding has only been objectively documented in paramyotonia congenita.

Myotonic discharges may present in one of two waveform types (Fig. 6–19).[38] The myotonic potential induced by needle electrode insertion usually assumes a morphology similar to that of a positive sharp wave. It is believed that the needle movement induces a repetitive firing of the unstable membranes of multiple single muscle fibers. This is because the recording needle is thought to have damaged

that portion of the muscle fiber with which it is in contact. Myotonic potentials may also appear as a series of rapidly firing triphasic single muscle fiber potentials following muscle contraction. Regardless of the waveform type, the hallmark of myotonia is the waxing and waning in both frequency and amplitude. The myotonic discharge has a characteristic sound likened to a dive bomber and is easily recognized. Amplitudes can be several hundred microvolts and firing rates range from 20 to 100 Hz.

Myotonic discharges can occur with or without clinical myotonia. Observation of these potentials requires needle movement or muscle contraction. These potentials persist after nerve block, neuromuscular block, or frank denervation. This suggests that their site of origin is the muscle membrane itself. Although the exact mechanism of myotonic discharge production remains unclear, it is proposed that decreased chloride conductance is responsible at least in part for the findings in myotonia congenita. In addition to the syndromes noted above, myotonic discharges can also be detected at times in acid maltase deficiency and polymyositis.

NEURAL GENERATORS OF ABNORMAL SPONTANEOUS POTENTIALS

FASCICULATION POTENTIALS. The visible spontaneous contraction of a portion of muscle is referred to as a fasciculation. When these contractions are observed with an intramuscular needle-recording electrode they are called fasciculation potentials.[13] A fasciculation potential is the electrically summated voltage of depolarizing muscle fibers belonging to all or part of one motor unit. Occasionally

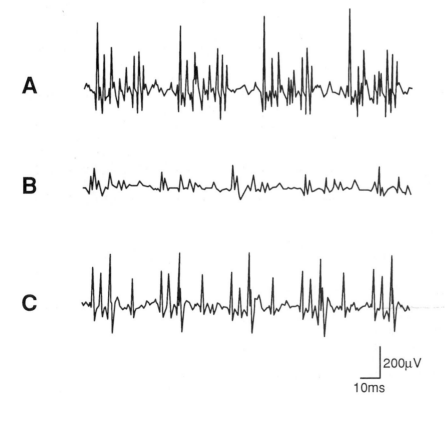

FIGURE 6–18 *A–C,* Several examples of complex repetitive discharges. Note how the same pattern of potentials repeats. The sound of the discharges is like that of heavy machinery, and they start and stop abruptly. (From Dumitru D: Electrodiagnostic Medicine. Philadelphia, Hanley & Belfus, 1995.)

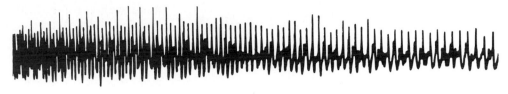

FIGURE 6–19 A run of myotonic potentials demonstrating both the positive sharp waves and negative spike form of the potentials. (From Streib EW: Differential diagnosis of myotonic syndromes. Muscle Nerve 1987; 10:603–615.)

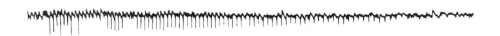

fasciculation potentials may only be documented with needle electromyography because they lie too deep in muscle to be seen.

Fasciculation waveforms can be characterized with respect to polyphasicity, amplitude, and duration (Fig. 6–20).[4] Their discharge rate (1 Hz to many per minute) is irregular. They are not under voluntary control, nor are they influenced by mild contraction of the agonist or antagonist muscles. The site of origin of fasciculation potentials remains unclear, although it appears that the spontaneous discharge may arise from the anterior horn cell, or along the entire peripheral nerve (particularly the terminal portion), and at times within the muscle itself.

Fasciculation potentials occur in normals and in patients with a variety of diseases. Typical diseases in which fasciculation potentials may be found include motor neuron disorders, radiculopathies, entrapment neuropathies, and spondylotic cervical myelopathy. Fasciculation potentials have also been described in metabolic disturbances, including tetany, thyrotoxicosis, and anticholinesterase overdoses. Studies have attempted, unsuccessfully, to distinguish between benign (normal) and pathological fasciculation potentials. There is no reliable way to categorize whether fasciculation potentials indicate a disease state just by considering their inherent characteristics based on routine needle electromyography. Fasciculations with increased jitter or blocking on single fiber electromyography may, however, be considered abnormal. Perhaps the best way to evaluate fasciculation potentials is to analyze the "company they keep." That is, a careful analysis of voluntary motor unit action potential morphology combined with a search for abnormal spontaneous potentials is required prior to concluding that fasciculation potentials are either a normal or an abnormal finding.

MYOKYMIC DISCHARGE. Myokymia is a readily observable vermicular (like a bag of live worms) or rippling movement of the skin. It is usually associated with myokymic discharges.[13] The myokymic discharge consists of bursts of normal-appearing motor units with interburst silent intervals. Typically the firing rate is 0.1 to 10 Hz in a semirhythmic pattern. Two to 10 potentials within a single burst may fire at 20 to 150 Hz.[1] These potentials are not affected by voluntary contraction (Fig. 6–21). The sound associated with these potentials is a type of sputtering often heard with a low-powered motorboat engine. The actual discharge may be distinguished from CRDs in that myokymic discharges do not display a regular pattern of spikes from one burst to the next nor do they typically start and stop abruptly. Myokymic discharges are groups of motor units, whereas CRDs represent groups of single muscle fibers discharging. The groups of motor units within a burst may fire only once or possibly several times. The sputtering bursts of myokymic discharges sound quite different from the continuous drone of a CRD.

Myokymic potentials can be observed in the face (facial myokymia) arising from multiple sclerosis or a brainstem neoplasm. Segmental myokymic discharges can be noted in syringomyelia or radiculopathies. Generalized myokymic discharges have been detected in uremia, thyrotoxicosis, and inflammatory polyradiculoneuropathy. Limb myokymic discharges have also been described associated primarily with radiation plexopathy.

CONTINUOUS MUSCLE FIBER ACTIVITY. A number of relatively rare syndromes producing continuous muscle fiber activity associated with muscle stiffness have been reported.[13] Portions of both the central and peripheral nervous system have been implicated in generating the sustained firing of motor units. One syndrome with continuous

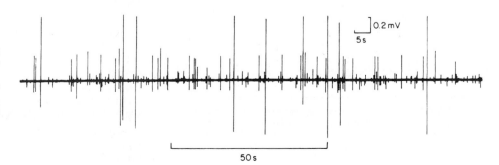

FIGURE 6–20 Multiple fasciculation potentials from a patient with amyotrophic lateral sclerosis are depicted. Note the random firing pattern of individual potentials. (From Brown WF: The Physiological and Technical Basis of Electromyography. Boston, Butterworth, 1984, pp 317–368.)

0.2 mV

5 s

50 s

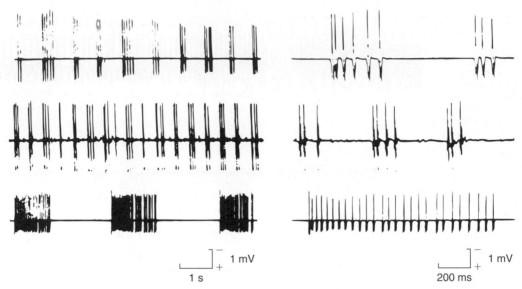

FIGURE 6–21   Multiple examples of myokymic discharges as recorded in patients with radiation plexopathy. Each burst of motor unit activity is relatively regular; however, the motor unit action potential content of each burst is somewhat variable. (From Albers JW, Allen AA, Bastron JD, et al: Limb myokymia. Muscle Nerve 1981; 4:494–504.)

muscle fiber activity is known as "stiff-man syndrome." The motor unit discharges in this condition are believed to have a central origin, as they are abolished or attenuated by peripheral nerve block, neuromuscular block, spinal block, general anesthesia, and sleep. The continuous motor unit firing is diminished by diazepam but not by phenytoin or carbamazepine. The patient can voluntarily control motor unit activity, but when relaxing the overriding involuntary motor unit firing returns. Progressive muscle stiffness involving all muscles (including the chest wall and pharynx) eventually occurs, resulting in contractures and profound impairment. A needle electrode recording reveals normal motor unit potentials producing a sustained interference pattern in both the agonist and antagonist muscles.

A "peripheral" form originating in the peripheral motor axon is referred to as Isaac's syndrome, or neuromyotonia (Fig. 6–22).[11] The continuous motor unit activity is eliminated by neuromuscular block, but not by peripheral nerve

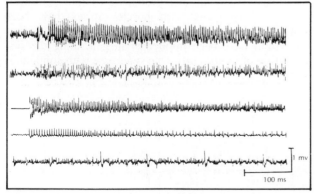

FIGURE 6–22   An example of neuromyotonia as recorded from a patient with Isaac's syndrome. The numbers of motor unit action potentials declines with time as the muscle's metabolic processes become exhausted. (From Daube JA: Needle Examination in Electromyography. Rochester, Minn, AAEM, 1979.)

block, spinal or general anesthesia, or sleep. The motor unit activity usually begins in the lower extremities in the late teens and progresses to all skeletal muscles. Needle recordings demonstrate motor unit discharges with frequencies up to 300 Hz associated with a characteristic "pinging" sound during needle electromyographic analysis. The amplitude of the firing motor unit potentials eventually declines as single fibers become exhausted and fail to fire. Similar neuromyotonic discharges have been described in tetany and anticholinesterase overdose, and in spinal muscular atrophy.

CRAMPS.   A sustained and possibly painful muscle contraction of multiple motor units lasting seconds or minutes may appear in normal persons or specific disease states.[31] In healthy subjects a cramp usually occurs in the calf muscles or other lower extremity muscles following exercise, abnormal positioning, or maintaining a fixed position for a prolonged period of time. Cramps may also be induced by hyponatremia, hypocalcemia, vitamin deficiency, or ischemia. They also occur in early motor neuron disease and peripheral neuropathies. Familial syndromes have been reported that involve fasciculations and cramps; alopecia, diarrhea, and cramps; and simply autosomal dominantly inherited cramps.

A needle-recording electrode placed into a cramping muscle shows multiple motor units firing synchronously between 40 and 60 Hz and occasionally reaching 200 to 300 Hz (Fig. 6–23). A large portion of the muscle is simultaneously involved in a cramp as opposed to the asynchronous excitation of motor units during voluntary activation. Cramps are believed to arise from a peripheral portion of the motor unit. A cramp that results in a taut muscle with electrical silence is the physiological contracture seen in McArdle's disease.

MULTIPLET DISCHARGES.   A clinical syndrome manifested by spontaneous muscle twitching, cramps, and carpopedal spasm is known as tetany.[13] This entity usually results from peripheral or central nervous system irritability

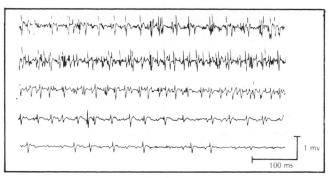

FIGURE 6–23 A characteristic muscle cramp as recorded with an intramuscular needle electrode. There is an initial burst of motor unit activity, which eventually subsides as the cramp dissipates. (From Daube JA: Needle Examination in Electromyography. Rochester, Minn, AAEM, 1979.)

associated with systemic alkalosis, hypocalcemia, hyperkalemia, hypomagnesemia, or local ischemia. Clinically one may induce tetany by tapping the facial nerve (Chvostek's sign), the peroneal nerve at the fibular head (peroneal sign), or inducing limb ischemia (Trousseau's sign).

In the above conditions, characteristic motor unit potentials may be observed. A single motor unit potential may fire rather rapidly with an interdischarge interval of 2 to 20 ms. If the motor unit fires twice it is referred to as a doublet; three times denotes a triplet; and more than three firings is called a multiplet (Fig. 6–24). These potentials can be seen following voluntary contraction or be observed spontaneously from the induction maneuvers noted above (Chvostek's sign or Trousseau's sign) in which MUAPs may fire in long trains or short bursts of 5 to 30 Hz (tetany). A motor unit with an interdischarge interval of 20 to 80 ms is called "paired discharges" but can arise in similar states as previously described.

NERVE INJURY CLASSIFICATION

Peripheral nerve injury is one of the most common pathologic conditions likely to be encountered during an electrodiagnostic medicine classification. It is necessary to be familiar with the various classification systems available to categorize an insult to neural tissue.

Seddon's Classification

The degree to which a nerve is damaged has obvious implications with respect to its present function and potential for recovery. There are, essentially, two general classification systems[32, 35, 39] (Table 6–2). One classification is that of Seddon, and considers neural injury from the perspective of a combination of functional status and histological appearance. In Seddon's scheme, there are three degrees or stages of injury to consider: (1) *neurapraxia*, (2) *axonotmesis*, and (3) *neurotmesis* (see Table 6–2).

NEURAPRAXIA. The term *neurapraxia* is used to designate a mild degree of neural insult which results in blockage of impulse conduction across the affected segment. It is also acceptable to simply designate this type of neural insult as *conduction block*. The most important

aspect of conduction block is its reversibility. The conducting properties of the nerve above and below the lesion site are normal in neurapraxia, and the continuity between the cell body and end-organ is maintained. Wallerian degeneration does not result from a conduction block because the axon is still in continuity. Investigators have mimicked this type of neural lesion by carefully compressing nerves to various degrees such that only a focal demyelination occurs with little or no axonal injury. The end result of a focal demyelinating lesion is action potential slowing or failure across the compressed portion of nerve.

The clinical onset of motor control and sensory functional loss can be either abrupt or gradual. Depending on the degree of injury, it is possible to have partial or complete disruption of either motor or sensory modalities. This variability of motor or sensory loss is believed to be due to the fact that different fibers are more or less susceptible to injury depending on their location within the nerve as well as the focal nature of the lesion. Muscle wasting usually does not occur in conduction block because muscle innervation is maintained, and secondly, recovery is typically rapid enough to avoid disuse atrophy. Fibrillation potentials should not be observed in pure conduction block, since the axon is not disrupted.[42] Keep in mind that many nerve injuries are mixed lesions in which some fibers have conduction block and some have axonal loss. In this case, it is certainly possible to observe fibrillation potentials.

AXONOTMESIS. The second degree of neural insult in Seddon's classification is axonotmesis (see Table 6–2). Axonotmesis is a specific type of nerve injury in which only the axon is physically disrupted, with preservation of the enveloping endoneurial and other supporting connective tissue structures (perineurium and epineurium). Compression of a profound nature or traction on the nerve are typical causes of lesions. Once the axon has been disrupted, the characteristic changes of wallerian degeneration occur. Recovery of function is directly dependent upon the time required for the process of wallerian degeneration and neural regeneration to eventually reach the denervated motor or sensory end-organ. Of course, autonomic function is also lost and must be reestablished. The fact that the endoneurium remains intact is a very important aspect of this type of injury. A preserved endoneurium means that once the remnants of the degenerated nerve have been

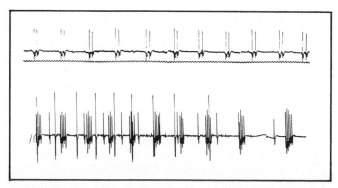

FIGURE 6–24 Doublet *(upper trace)* and multiplet *(lower trace)* motor unit action potentials resulting from voluntary contraction. (From Daube JA: Needle Examination in Electromyography. Rochester, Minn, AAEM, 1979.)

TABLE 6–2   Nerve Injury Classification

Type	Function	Pathological Basis	Prognosis
LUNDBORG Physiological conduction block			
Type a	Focal conduction block	Intraneural ischemia; metabolic (ionic) block; no nerve fiber changes	Excellent; immediately reversible
Type b	Focal conduction block	Intraneural edema; increased endoneurial fluid pressure; metabolic block; little or no fiber changes	Recovery in days or weeks
SEDDON/SUNDERLAND Neurapraxia			
Type 1	Focal conduction block; primarily motor function and proprioception affected; some sensation and sympathetic function may be present	Local myelin injury, primarily larger fibers; axonal continuity; no wallerian degeneration	Recovery in weeks to months
Axonotmesis			
Type 2	Loss of nerve conduction at injury site and distally	Disruption of axonal continuity with wallerian degeneration; endoneurial tubes, perineurium, and epineurium intact	Axonal regeneration required for recovery; good prognosis since original end-organs reached
Type 3	Loss of nerve conduction at injury site and distally	Loss of axonal continuity and endoneurial tubes; perineurium and epineurium preserved	Disruption of endoneurial tubes, hemorrhage, and edema produce scarring; axonal misdirection; poor prognosis; surgery may be required
Type 4	Loss of nerve conduction at injury site and distally	Loss of axonal continuity, endoneurial tubes, and perineurium; epineurium intact	Total disorganization of guiding elements; intraneural scarring and axonal misdirection; poor prognosis; surgery necessary
Neurotmesis			
Type 5	Loss of nerve conduction at injury site and distally	Severance of entire nerve	Surgical modification of nerve ends required; prognosis guarded and dependent on nature of injury and local factors

Modified with permission from Lundborg G: Nerve Injury and Repair. Edinburgh, Churchill Livingstone, 1988.

removed, the regenerating axon simply has to follow its original course directly back to the appropriate end-organ. With this type of injury, there is no misdirection of regenerating axons. A good prognosis can be expected when limited neural damage results only in axonotmesis.

The physical disruption of the axon in axonotmesis results in denervation of the corresponding musculature and complete absence of all sensory modalities. Because of wallerian degeneration, all nerve tissues distal to the site of injury become unexcitable. The time of recovery is dependent mainly upon the distance between the lesion site and the end-organs. Motor recovery occurs proximal-to-distal as the nerve regrows. It is often possible to trace the nerve's recovery clinically based on the advancing Tinel's sign. This results from the sensory fibers being sensitive to percussion at their growing tips. Although the prognosis for recovery in axonotmesis is good, there are occasions when retrograde neuronal degeneration occurs and results in the loss of some cell bodies. In this instance, less than complete recovery can be expected.

NEUROTMESIS. The greatest degree of nerve disruption is designated in Seddon's system as neurotmesis. This is complete disruption of the axon, and all supporting connective tissue structures, including the endoneurium, perineurium, and epineurium, are no longer in continuity. A neurotmetic lesion has a poor prognosis for complete

functional recovery. Surgical reapproximation of the nerve ends will likely be required. Surgery does not guarantee proper endoneurial tube alignment, but at least it improves the chances that axonal growth will occur across the injury site.

Sunderland's Classification

A second popular and somewhat more detailed classification is that proposed and subsequently modified by Sunderland (see Table 6–2).[40] This classification is based on the results of trauma with respect to the axon and its supporting connective tissue structures. Basically, Sunderland's classification is divided into five types of injury, based exclusively on which connective tissue components are disrupted (Fig. 6–25). Type 1 injury corresponds to Seddon's designation of neurapraxia. Seddon's axonotmesis is subdivided by Sunderland into three forms of neural insult (types 2–4). A type 2 injury involves loss of axonal continuity with preservation of all supporting neural structures including the endoneurium (closely corresponds to Seddon's axonotmesis; see Table 6–2). Type 3 and 4 injuries result in progressively more neural disruption. Sunderland's type 5 injury corresponds to Seddon's neurotmesis (complete neural disruption).

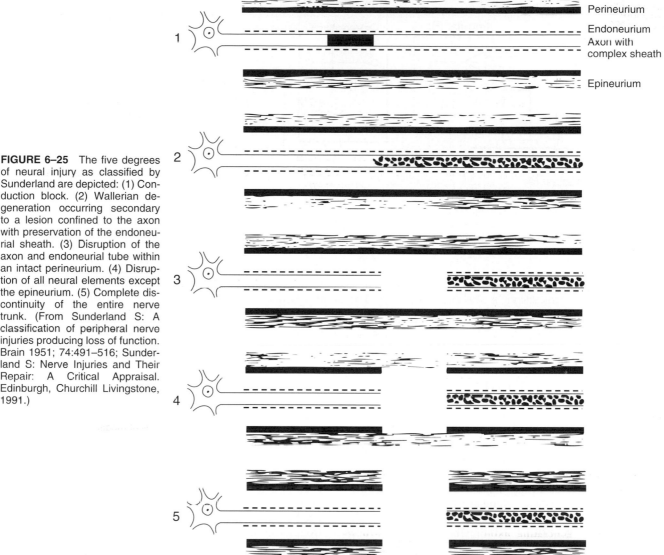

FIGURE 6–25 The five degrees of neural injury as classified by Sunderland are depicted: (1) Conduction block. (2) Wallerian degeneration occurring secondary to a lesion confined to the axon with preservation of the endoneurial sheath. (3) Disruption of the axon and endoneurial tube within an intact perineurium. (4) Disruption of all neural elements except the epineurium. (5) Complete discontinuity of the entire nerve trunk. (From Sunderland S: A classification of peripheral nerve injuries producing loss of function. Brain 1951; 74:491–516; Sunderland S: Nerve Injuries and Their Repair: A Critical Appraisal. Edinburgh, Churchill Livingstone, 1991.)

Perineurium
Endoneurium
Axon with complex sheath
Epineurium

INSTRUMENTATION

An electrodiagnostic instrument is actually comprised of many separate components. The most important of these are the electrodes, amplifier, filters, speaker, analog-to-digital (A/D) converter, CRT, and stimulator[15, 16, 37] (Fig. 6–26).

Electrodes

The two basic types of electrodes are surface and needle. Surface electrodes are manufactured in various sizes and shapes so as to best conform to the body part under investigation. The most commonly applied materials are metals that are good conductors of electricity such as gold, silver, tin, steel, lead, or platinum. A surface electrode with a depression for the electrolyte paste is believed to be superior as it minimizes movement artifact between the patient and electrode and displaces any movement to the skin-electrolyte interface. This prevents the discharge of a potential that can build up between the skin and the electrode's metal surface. The electrode is secured to the patient with tape sufficient to ensure a movement-free placement. Well-secured electrodes minimize movement artifact that could contaminate the desired signal. Commercially available disposable self-adhering electrodes are now available and eliminate the need for tape.

Two basic types of needle-recording electrodes are commonly used: (1) monopolar and (2) concentric (Fig. 6–27). The monopolar needle is a solid stainless steel shaft coated completely with Teflon except for the bare metal tip. It is this bare metal tip which acts at the recording surface. The needle is typically 12 to 75 mm in length and 0.3 to 0.5 mm in diameter with a recording surface of 0.15 to 0.6 mm^2. The recording region of the monopolar needle is a sphere with a radius approximating 2.25 mm. Separate reference and ground electrodes are required. The concentric needle electrode is a hollow stainless steel hypodermic needle with a central platinum or nichrome-silver wire about 0.1 mm in diameter, surrounded by epoxy resin acting as an insulating material from the surrounding cannula. The cannula has a length and diameter similar to that

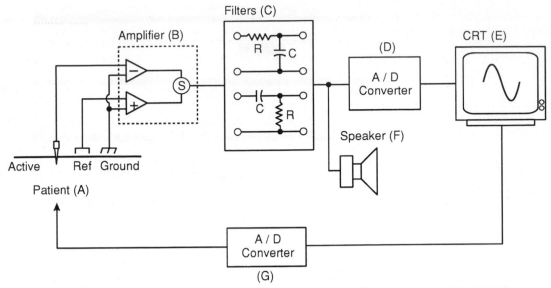

FIGURE 6–26 The subcomponents of the electrophysiological instrument are depicted. Electrodes (A) on or in the patient detect bioelectric changes, which are transmitted to a differential amplifier (B). This signal is filtered (C), undergoes analog-to-digital conversion (D), and is displayed on the cathode ray tube (E) as the sound is being presented through a loudspeaker (F). Time-locked evoked potentials can be generated with the stimulator (G). (From Dumitru D, Walsh NE: Electrophysiologic instrumentation. *In* Dumitru D (ed): Physical Medicine and Rehabilitation State of the Art Reviews: Clinical Electrophysiology. Philadelphia, Hanley & Belfus, 1989, pp 684–699.)

of the monopolar needle. The uptake area of the concentric electrode is a hemisphere with a radius of approximately 1.0 to 2.5 mm and is directional. A separate ground is required, but the cannula serves as the reference electrode.

There has been considerable discussion about the respective merits of these electrodes. Each has its advantages and disadvantages, depending on the clinical circumstances. Monopolar needle electrodes have a wider recording territory and have a distant reference, thereby making the recording "noisier" with respect to distant activity and interference. On the other hand, the Teflon coating reduces patient discomfort. The concentric needle electrode has the active and reference electrodes close together, making them quieter than monopolar needles. Concentric electrodes typically cause more patient discomfort. Concentric needle

electrodes give the following as compared to monopolar needle electrodes: smaller potential amplitudes, possibly fewer phases, comparable durations, and less distant activity. Note that the durations of potentials recorded with monopolar and concentric needle electrodes are the same. The introduction of commercially available disposable monopolar and concentric needle electrodes has eliminated such worries as Teflon peeling back on the monopolar needles and hook formation on the tip of the concentric needle electrodes. The quality of disposable needle electrodes has improved, eliminating the need to use nondisposable needle electrodes. If electrodes are reused, they should be properly sterilized with presoaking in sodium hypochlorite and steam autoclaving.[13]

Single-fiber electrodes are essentially modified concen-

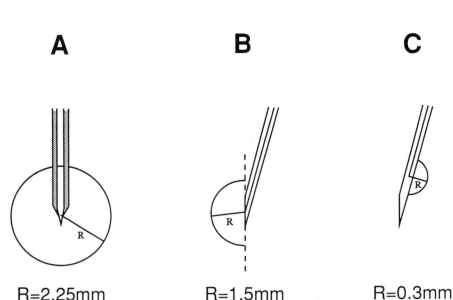

FIGURE 6–27 Various needle electrodes and recording areas are displayed. *A,* A monopolar needle electrode requires a separate reference and ground electrode. *B,* The concentric needle electrode uses the cannula as the reference and a separate ground is required. *C,* The single fiber electrode is essentially a modified concentric needle electrode. (From Dumitru D, Walsh NE: Electrophysiologic instrumentation. *In* Dumitru D (ed): Physical Medicine and Rehabilitation State of the Art Reviews: Clinical Electrophysiology. Philadelphia, Hanley & Belfus, 1989, pp 665–682.)

tric needle electrodes. A small 25-μm recording port is placed opposite the electrode's bevel and several millimeters from the tip. This makes this special electrode capable of recording the electrical activity from a single muscle fiber. The uptake area for this electrode is approximately 300 μm (see Fig. 6–27). Occasionally subdermal electroencephalographic needle electrodes may be used to record somatosensory evoked potentials. The potentials detected with these electrodes are identical to those recorded with surface electrodes.[13] In the case of somatosensory evoked potentials, all reusable electrodes (both surface and needle) must be sterilized. Surface electrodes are exposed to patients' serum if proper techniques are used to abrade the skin so as to reduce the skin's impedance.

Amplifier

The size of biological signals is on the order of microvolts or millivolts and thus must be amplified prior to being analyzed. An amplifier is simply a device with the ability to magnify the detected signal so that it can be displayed on the CRT. Amplification is expressed as gain or sensitivity. Gain is a ratio of the signal's output divided by the input. For example, an output of 1 V for an input of 10 mV implies that the amplifier has a gain factor of 100,000 (output/input = 1 V/0.00001 V = 100,000). Sensitivity is the ratio of the input voltage to the size of deflection on the CRT and is usually measured in centimeters. For example, an amplifier that produces a 1-cm deflection for an input of 10 mV has a sensitivity of 10 mV/cm or 10 mV/division. The sensitivity or gain setting used is important because it can influence the onset latency. Increasing the sensitivity for a given waveform results in the instrument detecting the potential's initial departure from baseline as occurring earlier in time.

One of the most important aspects of the amplifier is input impedance. For our purposes, the terms *impedance* and *resistance* will be considered as equivalent. The resistance of the amplifier must be significantly greater than that of the recording electrodes, so that most of the electrical activity recorded in the body is detected by the amplifier and little, if any, is lost in the electrodes. The electrodes and amplifier can be thought of as resistors in series with the biological signal. As you may recall from simple physics, two resistors in series in an electrical circuit equate to the same current crossing each resistor but with a different voltage dropping across each, forming a so-called voltage divider. Ohm's law can be used to better understand this concept where voltage (V) is equal to resistance (R) times current (I) ($V = I \cdot R$). For biological systems resistance is replaced with impedance (Z) with Ohm's law being $V = IZ$. Recall that for a series circuit the resistances (impedances) are additive in a circuit. Taking all of the factors into account and solving for what the amplifier detects equates to:

$$E_{amp} = \left(\frac{Z_{amp}}{Z_{amp} + Z_{elec}} \right) E_{tot}$$

The potential observed on the CRT (E_{amp}) is proportional to the signal generated in the body (E_{tot}) by a factor of the electrode's impedance divided by the sum of the imped-

ances for the electrode (Z_{elec}) and amplifier ($Z_{amp} \div [Z_{amp} + Z_{elec}]$). This means that for the practitioner to observe what is occurring in the body with little distortion, the amplifier's impedance must be very large compared to that of the electrode. Let us suppose that the signal in the body is 100 mV and the electrode and amplifier have impedances of 100 Ω. Plugging the numbers into the above equation means that the observed signal (E_{amp}) is only half of what it is in the body (50 mV). On the other hand, if the amplifier has an impedance considerably larger than the electrode (e.g., 10,000 Ω), then using this figure in the above equation for the same biological signal and electrode impedance results in the instrument displaying a potential with an amplitude of 99 mV, which is essentially the same as that occurring in the body. As Z_{amp} increases to values considerably larger than Z_{elec}, the value of Z_{amp} divided by the sum of Z_{amp} and Z_{elec} equates to unity with the above equation simplifying to $E_{amp} = E_{tot}$. As a result, if the electrode's impedance is high (dirty, broken, or corroded lead wires), a considerable portion of the signal is lost to the electrode. The resulting reduction in amplitude could cause one to assume that there is loss of nerve or muscle tissue, when indeed there is simply a dysfunctional electrode present.

The standard electromyograph has two amplifiers. The amplifier connected to the active electrode is known as the noninverting amplifier, while the reference electrode is connected to the inverting amplifier. The inverting amplifier magnifies the signal presented to it in the same manner as the noninverting amplifier with the exception of inverting the signal. Both amplified signals (inverted and noninverted) are then electronically summated and like signals are canceled. This is the concept of differential amplification. When the same signal is presented to both amplifiers, theoretically there should be no output from the instrument because there is elimination of the same or common signals. For example, 60-Hz interference recorded by the active and reference electrodes is eliminated as a common mode signal. It is impossible to build two amplifiers with identical properties, so common mode rejection can never be perfect. The ratio of the instrument's output when the same signal is presented to both amplifiers is the common mode rejection ratio. This number should exceed 10,000:1.

Filters

Perhaps the most misunderstood and ignored aspect of the instrument are the filters. The main purpose of filters is to form a window or bandwidth of frequencies contained within the desired waveform, but excluding those frequencies not containing the signal of interest ("noise"). Low- and high-frequency filters are used to prevent those frequencies below and above the respective filter settings from being amplified and subsequently presented for display.

Any biological signal can be conceptualized as a series of sine waves of various frequencies and amplitudes. The combination of "appropriate" sine wave amplitudes and frequencies can result in the formation of essentially any waveform. In this way the biological signal recorded by the instrument consists of multiple subcomponent waveforms with specific frequency and amplitude characteristics. Eliminating any of these subcomponent waveforms results in a distortion of the waveform's appearance. This is exactly what can happen if the high or low frequency is set such that the desired biological waveform has various subcomponent frequencies eliminated. The examples provided below apply equally well to nerve and muscle potentials.

In our example a recorded median SNAP and CMAP are sequentially distorted by altering the low- and high-frequency filter settings. Let us begin with an arbitrary low-frequency filter setting of 1 Hz and a high-frequency filter cutoff of 10,000 Hz. Sequentially elevating the low-frequency filter from 1 Hz to 10 Hz, 100 Hz, and finally to 300 Hz while maintaining a high-frequency filter of 10,000 Hz results in characteristic waveform distortions (Fig. 6–28). The onset latency does not change, the peak latency decreases, amplitude is serially reduced, and the total potential duration decreases. Also, an additional phase is created. The use of higher low-frequency filters removes low frequencies from the SNAP. In other words, the remaining potential now has a predominance of high frequencies contained in it as compared to the original potential. The onset of the potential is a quick departure from baseline and is not influenced by an alteration in the low-frequency content of the waveform. The remainder of the potential, however, is influenced by low-frequency subcomponent waveforms. By taking out the low frequencies, the amplitude is reduced as subcomponent waveforms are removed. The entire waveform is shifted to a earlier time of occurrence because of the high frequencies left in the SNAP. A third phase is created as the potential begins to appear more like a sine wave as the higher frequencies

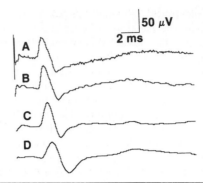

Trace	High frequency filter	Latency		Amplitude
		Onset	Peak	
	Hz	ms		μV
A	10,000	2.7	3.3	76
B	2,000	2.8	3.4	76
C	1,000	2.8	3.8	75
D	500	3.0	4.2	64

FIGURE 6–29 An antidromic median sensory nerve action potential is recorded from the third digit with a constant low-frequency filter of 10 Hz, but different high-frequency filters are employed. Note how the onset and peak latencies are sequentially delayed with decreasing high-frequency filter settings. The potential's amplitude also decreases. (From Dumitru D, Walsh NE: Practical instrumentation and common sources of error. Am J Phys Med Rehabil 1988; 67:55–65.)

begin to emerge. A similar occurrence is noted for the CMAP.

Eliminating high frequencies results in a somewhat different set of alterations. Because we are removing waveforms from the total potential, a reduction in amplitude can be anticipated. The SNAP is thus biased toward a potential with more low frequencies and hence takes longer to occur in time. This results in a delay of both the onset and peak latencies (Fig. 6–29). Lowering the high-frequency filter while maintaining a constant low-frequency filter results in a waveform with a comparatively smaller amplitude, longer onset latency, and longer peak latency. Similar findings can be observed for a CMAP.

There are no universally agreed-upon filter settings for any electrodiagnostic medicine procedure. Arriving at optimal filter settings is highly empirical. The high- and low-frequency filters are lowered and raised respectively until waveform distortions are observed. The filters are then expanded until no waveform changes are noted. The goal is to include the major components of the waveforms while eliminating undesired signals or noise. The most important factor is to reproduce all filter settings originally described by those investigators whose normative data are being used (Table 6–3).

Sound

After the biological signal is filtered it is fed to a loudspeaker. The acoustic analysis of both normal and abnormal potentials is extremely important. It is not uncommon for practitioners to "hear" an abnormality prior to viewing it on the CRT. The instrument must have a relatively good

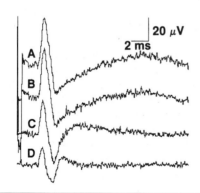

Trace	Low frequency	Latency		Duration negative spike	Amplitude
		Onset	Peak		
	Hz	ms		ms	μv
A	1	2.6	3.3	1.4	65
B	10	2.6	3.3	1.4	65
C	100	2.6	3.1	1.0	54
D	300	2.6	3.0	0.8	30

FIGURE 6–28 An antidromic median sensory nerve action potential is evoked from the third digit while the low-frequency filter is sequentially elevated with a constant high-frequency filter of 10,000 Hz. Note how the onset latency does not change; however, the peak latency decreases, as does the potential's amplitude. A third phase is also produced at the low-frequency filter setting of 300 Hz. (From Dumitru D, Walsh NE: Practical instrumentation and common sources of error. Am J Phys Med Rehabil 1988; 67:55–65.)

TABLE 6–3   Recommended Filter Settings

Procedure	Low Frequency (Hz)	High Frequency (Hz)
NCV (motor)	2–10	10,000
NCV (sensory)	2–10	2000–10,000
EMG (routine)	20–30	10,000
EMG (quantitative)	2–5	10,000
SFEMG	500–1000	10,000–20,000
SEP	1–10	500–3000

Abbreviations: NCV, nerve conduction velocity; EMG, needle electromyography; SFEMG, single fiber electromyography; SEP, somatosensory evoked potential.

From Dumitru D, Walsh NE: Practical instrumentation and common sources of error. Am J Phys Med Rehabil 1988; 67:55–65. Used by permission.

speaker so as to accurately present the sounds associated with the biological signals.

Analog-to-Digital (A/D) Conversion

All of today's commercially available instruments employ the conversion of a real-time analog signal to a digital representation of the recorded waveform. This is accomplished by sampling the potential at a given rate or frequency and assigning a digital representation of the waveform in the computer's memory. Complex signals with many changes over time and high frequencies must be sampled very fast in order to accurately reproduce them. If the sampling frequency is below that of the recorded waveform, considerable distortion can occur. The sampling frequency of the instrument must be at least twice as fast as the highest frequency contained in the waveform and is referred to as the Nyqvist frequency. For example, suppose the rise time, fast subcomponent, of a MUAP is 500 μs. This rise time converts to a frequency of

$$2000 \text{ Hz } (1 \text{ time}/500 \text{ μs} \times \frac{1000 \text{ ms}}{1 \text{ sec}} = 2000 \text{ Hz})$$

The Nyqvist frequency for this potential is 4000 Hz. The sampling frequency of the instrument, therefore, must be at least 4000 Hz. This means that the instrument has to have a sweep speed capable of sampling the potential at the given frequency. For example, suppose our instrument has 1000 points (pts) of resolution across the screen for a sweep speed of 10 ms/division for a total screen of 10 division (100 ms). Our sampling frequency in this case is 10,000 Hz which is more than enough to adequately resolve the waveform (1000 pts/100 ms × 1000 ms/1 sec = 10,000 pts/1 sec or 10,000 Hz). As noted above, the most useful conversion factor is 1000 ms/1 sec as this converts how many times something happens per second into the appropriate number of hertz (= Hz, cycles per second).

Averager

Most modern instruments typically have the capacity for averaging multiple responses. The goal of averaging a number of responses is to improve the size of the signal compared to the background noise, that is, improve the signal-to-noise ratio. Responses can be averaged by taking advantage of the fact that the desired signal can be time-locked to appear in constant time referenced to a delivered electrical stimulus or internal instrument marker. The responses can thus be added while the random occurring noise phase cancels, thus improving the signal compared to the surrounding noise. This can be expressed mathematically as deriving the signal (S) to noise (N) ratio which is directly proportional to the square root of the number of averages (n):

$$S/N = \frac{S \times \sqrt{n}}{N}$$

For example, if a signal has an amplitude of 2 mV while that of the noise is 4 mV, a single stimulus results in a signal-to-noise ratio (S/N) of 1/2 (S/N = [2 mV $\sqrt{1}$] ÷ 4 mV = 1/2). If four averages are performed, S/N becomes 1/1. The S/N improved by the square root of the number of averages. Similarly, averaging 64 times results in an improvement by a factor of 8 ([2 mV × $\sqrt{64}$] ÷ 4 mV = 4/1, and 1/2 × $\sqrt{64}$ = 4/1).

Stimulator

Two different types of stimulators are commercially available: (1) constant current, and (2) constant voltage. For both types of devices, neural tissue is activated under the cathode (negative pole) while the anode (positive pole) completes the stimulating circuit. A constant current stimulator effectively delivers the desired current output for each stimulus irrespective of the resistance between the skin and cathode or anode. This is accomplished by varying the voltage or current driving force as is necessitated by any alterations in the resistance of the skin-stimulator interface. Similarly, a constant voltage stimulator is designed to deliver the same voltage with each stimulus even if the resistance between the skin and stimulator changes. A compensatory increase or decrease in current is provided so as to maintain the same voltage level. In short, a constant current stimulator is effectively a variable voltage stimulator, while a constant voltage stimulator is also a variable current stimulator. Both stimulators are acceptable for most purposes. The constant current stimulator is preferred when the same current must be delivered for each stimulus in clinical situations requiring quantification of current delivery, for example, somatosensory evoked potentials, research, or evaluating side-to-side stimulation thresholds during facial nerve excitability testing.

An important problem associated with stimulators is the stimulus artifact. There is commonly a large potential recorded during the delivery of the stimulus, referred to as the shock or stimulus artifact. At times the magnitude of the potential is large enough to compromise the desired neural or muscular response. In such situations, it is necessary to minimize the shock artifact. An effective method of reducing the shock artifact is to employ fast-recovery amplifiers which act to suppress this artifact by quickly recovering from the overwhelming voltage delivered. These amplifiers are not available on all instruments and so other means must be found to deal with the artifact. The skin surface must be dry and any perspiration, body lotion, makeup, or other surface conductors should be removed.

Wiping a large portion of the body segment under investigation with alcohol usually removes all surface conducting films. A ground electrode is best placed between the stimulus site and the active recording electrode. Wire leads between the patient and stimulator should be separated to avoid any type of capacitive interaction. The stimulator circuit should be isolated from the instrument's ground circuit, which is true of virtually all commercially manufactured instruments. Perhaps the most effective method of reducing stimulus artifact, once all of the above have been addressed, is to rotate the anode about the cathode. This optimizes the stimulator's voltage output as recorded by the active and reference electrode to take advantage of differential amplification and the elimination of the shock artifact as a common mode signal. An attempt is made to have both the active and reference electrodes record similar voltages, thereby minimizing the stimulator's signal from being amplified and displayed along with the signal.

Anodal block is an interesting concept that has been widely discussed, but which has little supporting experimental data. Theoretically the anode hyperpolarizes the neural tissue in its immediate vicinity and should result in an action potential failing to conduct past the anode. In humans, investigations employing bipolar and monopolar anodal current stimulation at the highest current outputs failed to document any type of anodal block. Since the anode is capable of stimulating neural tissue and not blocking it, at this time it appears that anodal block does not occur during the routine electrodiagnostic medicine consultation.

CONCLUSION

Mastering the above information gives the practitioner a firm grasp of the fundamental principles that underpin the electrodiagnostic medicine consultation. Appreciating the formation and generation of an action potential is not a trivial matter. Of equal importance is the manner in which the electrophysiological instrument processes the biological signal of interest. Less than a functional understanding of how the instrument can potentially distort the biological signal predisposes the practitioner to errors in diagnosis.

References

1. Albers JW, Allen AA, Bastron JD, et al: Limb myokymia. Muscle Nerve 1981; 4:494–504.
2. Baer RD, Johnson EW: Motor nerve conduction velocities in normal children. Arch Phys Med Rehabil 1965; 46:698–704.
3. Bolton CF, Carter KM: Human sensory nerve compound action potential amplitude: variation with sex and finger circumference. J Neurol Neurosurg Psychiatry 1980; 43:925–928.
4. Brown WF: The Physiological and Technical Basis of Electromyography. Boston, Butterworth, 1984, pp 317–368.
5. Buchthal F: Fibrillations: clinical electrophysiology. In Culp WJ, Ochoa J (eds): Abnormal Nerves and Muscle Generators. New York, Oxford University Press, 1982, pp 632–662.
6. Buchthal F, Guld C, Rosenfalck P: Volume conduction of the spike of the motor unit potential investigated with a new type of multielectrode. Acta Physiol Scand 1957; 38:331–354.
7. Buchthal F, Guld C, Rosenfalck P: Multielectrode study of the territory of a motor unit. Acta Physiol Scand 1957; 39:83–104.
8. Buchthal F, Rosenfalck A: Evoked action potentials and conduction velocity in human sensory nerves. Brain Res 1966; 3:1–122.
9. Campbell WW, Ward LC, Swift TR: Nerve conduction velocity varies inversely with height. Muscle Nerve 1981; 4:520–523.
10. Cummins KL, Dorfman LJ: Nerve fiber conduction velocity distributions: studies of normal and diabetic human nerves. Ann Neurol 1981; 9:67–74.
11. Daube JA: AAEM minimonograph #11: Needle Examination in Electromyography. Rochester, Minn, American Association of Electrodiagnostic Medicine, 1979.
12. Dumitru D: Volume conduction: theory and application. In Dumitru D (ed): Physical Medicine and Rehabilitation State of the Art Reviews: Clinical Electrophysiology. Philadelphia, Hanley & Belfus, 1989, pp 665–682.
13. Dumitru D: Electrodiagnostic Medicine. Philadelphia, Hanley & Belfus, 1995.
14. Dumitru D, DeLisa JA: Volume conduction. Muscle Nerve 1991; 14:605–624.
15. Dumitru D, Walsh NE: Practical instrumentation and common sources of error. Am J Phys Med Rehabil 1988; 67:55–65.
16. Dumitru D, Walsh NE: Electrophysiologic instrumentation. In Dumitru D (ed): Physical Medicine and Rehabilitation State of the Art Reviews: Clinical Electrophysiology. Philadelphia, Hanley & Belfus, 1989, pp 684–699.
17. Falco FJE, Hennessey WJ, Braddom RL, et al: Standardized nerve conduction studies in the upper limb of the healthy elderly. Am J Phys Med Rehabil 1992; 71:263–271.
18. Falco FJE, Hennessey WJ, Goldberg G, et al: H reflex latency in the healthy elderly. Muscle Nerve 1994; 17:161–167.
19. Halar EM, DeLisa JA: Peroneal nerve conduction velocity: The importance of temperature control. Arch Phys Med Rehabil 1981; 62:439–443.
20. Halar EM, DeLisa JA, Brozovich FV: Nerve conduction velocity: relationship of skin, subcutaneous and intramuscular temperatures. Arch Phys Med Rehabil 1980; 61:199–203.
21. Halar EM, DeLisa JA, Soine TL: Nerve conduction studies in upper extremities: skin temperature corrections. Arch Phys Med Rehabil 1983; 64:412–416.
22. Henrikson JD: Conduction velocity of motor nerves in normal subjects and patients with neuromuscular disorders, thesis. University of Minnesota, Minneapolis, 1956.
23. Hille B: Introduction to physiology of excitable cells. In Patton HD, Fuchs AF, Hille B, et al (eds): Textbook of Physiology, ed 21. Philadelphia, WB Saunders, 1989, pp 1–80.
24. Hodgkin AL, Huxley AF: A quantitative description of membrane current and its application to conduction and excitation in nerve. J Physiol 1952; 117:500–544.
25. Hodgkin AL, Katz B: The effect of temperature on the electrical activity of the giant axon of the squid. J Physiol 1949; 109:240–249.
26. Jewett DL, Rayner MD: Basic Concepts of Neuronal Function. Boston, Little, Brown, 1984.
27. Johnson EW, Olsen KJ: Clinical value of motor nerve conduction velocity determination. JAMA 1960; 172:2030–2035.
28. Katz B: Nerve, Muscle, and Synapse. New York, McGraw-Hill, 1966.
29. Koester J: Resting membrane potential and action potential. In Kandel ER, Schwartz JH (eds): Principles of Neural Science, ed 2. New York, Elsevier, 1985, pp 49–57.
30. Lang AH, Forsstrom J, Bjorkqvist SE, et al: Statistical variation of nerve conduction velocity: an analysis in normal subjects and uraemic patients. J Neurol Sci 1977; 33:229–241.
31. Layzer RB, Rowland LP: Cramps. N Engl J Med 1971; 285:30–31.
32. Lundborg G: Nerve Injury and Repair. Edinburgh, Churchill Livingstone, 1988.
33. Oh SJ: Clinical Electromyography: Nerve Conduction Studies, ed 2. Baltimore, Williams & Wilkins, 1993.
34. Schoepfle GM, Erlanger J: The action of temperature on the excitability, spike height and configuration, and the refractory period observed in the responses of single medullated nerve fibers. Am J Physiol 1941; 134:694–704.
35. Seddon H: Three types of nerve injury. Brain 1943; 66:237–288.
36. Soudmand R, Ward LC, Swift TR: Effect of height on nerve conduction velocity. Neurology 1982; 32:407–410.
37. Stolov W: Instrumentation and measurement in electrodiagnosis. Minimonograph #16. Rochester, Minnesota, American Association of Electrodiagnostic Medicine, 1981.
38. Streib EW: AAEM Minimonograph #27: Differential diagnosis of myotonic syndromes. Muscle Nerve 1987; 10:603–615.

39. Sunderland S: A classification of peripheral nerve injuries producing loss of function. Brain 1951; 74:491–516.
40. Sunderland S: Nerve Injuries and Their Repair: A Critical Appraisal. Edinburgh, Churchill Livingstone, 1991.
41. Thesleff S: Fibrillation in denervated mammalian muscle. *In* Culp WJ, Ochoa J (eds): Abnormal Nerve and Muscle as Impulse Generators. New York, Oxford University Press, 1982, pp 678–694.
42. Trojaborg W: Motor nerve conduction velocities in normal subjects with particular reference to the conduction in proximal and distal segments of median and ulnar nerve. Electroenceph Clin Neurophysiol 1964; 17:314–321.
43. Waxman SG: Action potential propagation and conduction velocity—new perspectives and questions. *In* Trends in Neuroscience, vol 6. New York, Elsevier, 1983, pp 157–161.
44. Waxman SG, Foster RE: Ionic channel distribution and heterogeneity of the axon membrane in myelinated fibers. Brain Res Rev 1980; 2:205–234.

7

Electrodiagnostic Medicine II: Clinical Evaluation and Findings

LAWRENCE R. ROBINSON, M.D.

CLINICAL ASSESSMENT

The electrodiagnostic medical consultation is unique compared with many other types of medical consultations or with laboratory testing. Conceptually, the electrodiagnostic medical consultation should be viewed as a history and physical examination extended by the unique capabilities of electrophysiological testing. The electrophysiological testing may include nerve conduction studies, needle electromyography (EMG), somatosensory evoked potentials (SEPs), single-fiber EMG, and other studies. The consultation starts with a directed history and physical examination and uses electrophysiological testing to help distinguish among the possible differential diagnoses in a more sensitive fashion than is possible with clinical examination alone.

The electrodiagnostic consultation has important distinctions from laboratory tests. It depends greatly on the consultant's history and physical examination and is a dynamic process. Specific methods employed depend on the clinical assessment and the outcomes of some of the initial tests. These may change dynamically throughout the consultation. In contrast, other types of laboratory testing (e.g., serum chemistries or electroencephalography [EEG]) are usually performed in a standard fashion and findings are interpreted after the patient leaves the office or hospital.

As with any other type of testing, the electrodiagnostic medical consultant must try to find electrophysiological abnormalities, preferably multiple ones, that are consistent with the patient's clinical presentation. Diagnoses should not be made solely on electrophysiological "abnormalities" and must always be made in the context of the patient's clinical presentation.

History

A directed history is extremely helpful in generating a list of differential diagnoses and planning the electrophysi-

ological examination. The history should be initially directed toward the presenting chief complaint. A number of components of the history are especially pertinent to the electrodiagnostic medical consultation. The time since onset of symptoms is extremely important, because the electrophysiological findings evolve over time. For instance, a radiculopathy studied 5 days after onset of symptoms would not be expected to show nearly as much electrophysiological evidence of denervation as when studied 21 days after onset of symptoms. Finding out whether symptoms are intermittent or constant is important, as there is a higher likelihood of finding abnormalities on the electrophysiological examination in the case of constant symptoms. Although symptoms are usually reported initially in one or two limbs, one should also ask about other limbs. The patient with hand numbness, for example, could have entrapment neuropathy in the upper limbs. However, if the lower limbs are also involved, then the examiner should do a wider search for a peripheral polyneuropathy. The quality and distribution of symptoms, combined with an intimate knowledge of peripheral nervous system anatomy, are the critical information necessary to narrow the list of differential diagnoses.

Although an extensive search of the past medical history is not always productive for the electrodiagnostic medical consultation, several points should always be raised. The examiner should routinely ask about patient medications. This not only brings up other pertinent diagnoses, but may also uncover possible toxic exposures and the possibility of anticoagulation (which is critical to know before starting a needle examination). A history of systemic disease that might contribute to the chief complaint, such as a history of diabetes mellitus, extensive alcohol intake, or rheumatologic disease, should be sought. Also, it is important to know whether or not the presenting symptoms have occurred in the past, so finding old electrophysiological changes is not confusing.

The examiner should always inquire about the family history of similar or congenital diseases. Some peripheral polyneuropathies and myopathies that are frequently referred for an electrodiagnostic medical consultation are inherited disorders. It occasionally becomes necessary to also examine or test potentially affected family members.

Physical Examination

Whereas the history contributes most significantly to establishing a differential diagnosis, physical examination is useful in providing more objective evidence of peripheral nervous system dysfunction.

In most cases, the four most important examinations are muscle strength, sensation, muscle stretch reflexes, and provocative signs. The strength examination (manual muscle testing) should be directed to all four limbs, to look for widespread abnormalities as well as to assess any underlying poor effort. In most cases the weakness is mild or subtle, although in some cases weakness is severe. Accordingly, muscles should be tested near their "break" points, as opposed to in positions in which resistance cannot be overcome. The examiner must be sure to obtain a maximum mechanical advantage in performing the muscle strength testing by applying force as far as possible from the joint to obtain a maximal lever arm, putting particularly strong muscles at added stretch to put them at a mechanical disadvantage, and using gravity and body weight as an aid to maximally stress antigravity muscles. Simply testing dorsiflexion or plantar flexion at the ankle against manual resistance, for example, is insufficient; one must have the patient walk on the heels and the toes or do 10 toe rises in a row.

Sensory testing should be directed at eliciting subtle deficits in sensation. In distinction to the patient with spinal cord injury, patients with entrapment neuropathies or radiculopathies often have mild or difficult-to-assess sensory losses. Finding out whether the patient can distinguish pinprick from dull touch is usually of insufficient sensitivity, except in cases in which severe deficits are present. Pinprick and light touch sensation in a questionable area should be compared with that of an asymptomatic area (such as the cheek or forehead) or with the same location on the other side if it is not symptomatic. A useful technique is to first touch the asymptomatic area and then the symptomatic area, asking the patient, "If this (asymptomatic) area is 100%, how much is this (the symptomatic area)?" Two-point discrimination has been shown to pick up milder deficits in sensation than simple pinprick testing. Testing vibration is useful if particular involvement of large fibers (e.g., in peripheral polyneuropathy) is expected or if the dorsal column pathways are expected to be spared (e.g., in syringomyelia).

Muscle stretch reflexes are probably the most objective finding in examination of the peripheral nervous system in that they are not as easily influenced by patient cooperation or reporting. In addition to the commonly elicited reflexes in the upper limb (biceps, brachioradialis, and triceps) and lower limb (knee and ankle), other muscle stretch reflexes should be considered. In the lower limbs, the most common

level for radiculopathy is L5. Because the knee jerk largely represents L4 input and the ankle jerk largely S1 input, it is quite easy to miss reflex changes in an L5 radiculopathy unless the medial hamstring or tibialis posterior reflexes are checked routinely. In the upper limb, C7 is the most common level for radiculopathy. Although the triceps reflex is useful in this regard, the pronator teres reflex (elicited by tapping the neutrally positioned forearm into supination and palpating over the pronator teres) can be useful for detecting C6 or C7 changes. Other reflexes, such as Hoffmann's or Babinski's reflexes, are useful to distinguish upper motor neuron from lower motor neuron changes (see Chapter 1 for additional information).

Several useful provocative tests can be employed in the physical examination prior to electrophysiological studies. When considering entrapment neuropathies, Phalen's test is a moderately sensitive and specific test for detecting median nerve compression at the wrist; this is performed by keeping the wrist in sustained flexion for 60 seconds and monitoring for paresthesias. Tinel's sign (which was originally developed for detecting the most distal site of peripheral nerve regeneration) is sensitive but not very specific. It can be elicited over the median nerve at the wrist or ulnar nerve at the elbow in the case of entrapment, but many asymptomatic control subjects also have a positive test over many peripheral nerves. When considering the possibility of cervical radiculopathy, Spurling's sign should be looked for by bringing the neck into extension and lateral flexion toward the side being tested; if one applies pressure to the top of the head and elicits pain extending out to the shoulder or beyond, this is a positive test and may indicate the presence of cervical radiculopathy. In the lower limb, straight leg raising tests or other provocative maneuvers may provide additional useful information about the presence of a lumbosacral radiculopathy.

Depending on the clinical presentation, other parts of the physical examination may be employed. For example, when looking for neuromuscular junction disease or motor neuron disease, a thorough cranial nerve examination should be performed. In suspected myopathies, one should look for muscle tenderness.

Differential Diagnosis

After reviewing the referring physician's request and performing a history and physical examination, one should generate a credible list of differential diagnoses. Even if the consultant does not feel the referring diagnosis is very likely, it is usually wise to perform testing to specifically address it, as the referring physician is expecting a response about this specific diagnosis.

Initial Plan

Based on the list of differential diagnoses, one should plan the electrophysiological examination to look for and distinguish between the possibilities listed. This could start off with either electromyographic (EMG) or nerve conduction studies, depending on the differential diagnoses. The initial goal is to get as much pertinent information as possible in the shortest amount of time (and thus at the lowest cost for the patient). For focal or distal problems where one can stimulate areas proximal and distal to the suspected problem and compound nerve or muscle action potentials distal to the possible lesion (such as in carpal tunnel syndrome or ulnar neuropathy), it is usually best to begin with nerve conduction studies. For predominantly proximal lesions, such as radiculopathies, it is often best to start with needle EMG. For potentially diffuse or multifocal processes, one may want to obtain a rapid estimation of how widespread the problem is. Needle EMG is a more rapid way to obtain this information than nerve conduction studies. There is a great interindividual variation among examiners as to whether it is better to start with nerve conduction studies or EMG. The underlying principle should, however, be to obtain the most useful information with the smallest number of tests, so that the marginal gain of each test is maximized and few or no unnecessary tests are performed.

Although one might come up with an *initial* plan at the beginning of the consultation, this often changes as information is obtained. It is also inappropriate to use a single standardized protocol for all patients. Because the electrodiagnostic medical consultation is a dynamic process, one must be ready to change the testing strategy quickly as new information is obtained and items on the differential diagnosis are either added or deleted.

NEEDLE ELECTROMYOGRAPHY

Preparing the Patient

Preparing the patient for needle EMG is a critical first step in performing this examination. One must explain to the patient what is to be performed and what the experience is like. There are some very good explanatory pamphlets available (such as from the American Association of Electrodiagnostic Medicine), but an additional verbal explanation is usually required to establish an appropriate level of rapport between the examiner and patient. Although the wording used to explain the procedure varies from one examiner to another, it may be useful to avoid words with strong negative connotations. For example: "pin" electrode is preferable to "needle," electrical "pulse" or "stimulus" is preferable to "shock," "uncomfortable" may be better than "painful." It is also helpful to give the patient some measure of control (e.g., "Let me know if I get into an especially uncomfortable area and I will try to move to another location"). It's usually not helpful to show the patient the needle electrode, as most patients erroneously associate needle length with level of discomfort. While it is not standard practice to have the patient sign a consent form for the procedure, it is advisable to inform the patient of any risks that might be involved as well as the potential benefits. If one is performing a high-risk procedure (e.g., intercostal muscle EMG), then informed consent should be obtained.

Patient position is important for patient comfort as well as for ease and accuracy of the examination. The patient should be in a relaxed position, with the muscles to be examined easily accessible. Patients should be gowned and appropriately covered with a blanket or sheet. The room should be reasonably warm, both to prevent distortion of the electrophysiological findings by cooling and to keep the patient comfortable.

Deciding on an Electrode to Use

Assuming that the electrodiagnostic instrument is ready and the patient is prepared and adequately positioned, the next step is to choose an electrode for needle EMG: that is, a monopolar or concentric needle. Each has advantages, with differences predominantly in recording surface area, price, and, possibly, level of discomfort.

The monopolar needle EMG electrode is composed of a single solid-core needle, which is Teflon coated except for an exposed tip. Electrical potentials are usually measured with reference to a nearby surface electrode. The monopolar electrode, compared with the concentric electrode, has a larger recording area, is less expensive, and is felt by many to be less painful. The larger recording area is advantageous with recording potentials that might be distant, such as fibrillations or positive sharp waves. However, the larger recording surface area is a disadvantage in performing quantitative motor unit potential analysis, because extraneous noise from distant potentials is incorporated into the signal. Quantitative EMG reference data has generally been obtained with concentric, rather than monopolar, electrodes, although motor unit action potential durations may not be very different when the two needles are compared. When reusable needle EMG electrodes are used, price can be a factor, as disposable monopolar electrodes are currently about one-fourth the cost of disposable concentric electrodes.

The concentric EMG needle electrode has a more standardized, smaller recording surface area. It does not use a surface reference electrode. The wire running through the center of the insulated shaft is electrically referenced to the exposed outside shaft of the needle. The concentric needle electrode is most useful in performing quantitative motor unit potential analysis, or if, for any reason, a recording is desired from a restricted area near the tip of the needle. Electrodiagnostic consultants should feel comfortable using either type of needle electrode for EMG and should be able to switch between the two types, depending on the clinical circumstances. Disposable needle electrodes have gained widespread acceptance due to fear of spreading infectious disease through reusable needles. The risk of spreading infection through properly sterilized reusable electrodes, however, is probably no greater than that for reusable surgical instruments. A review of proper sterilization techniques can be found in the *Guidelines in Electrodiagnostic Medicine*, published by the American Association of Electrodiagnostic Medicine.

When performing the needle examination, it is advisable to use appropriate safety precautions for exposure to bodily fluids. Both of the examiner's hands should be gloved during the examination, and needles should not be recapped using a two-handed technique. Needle electrodes that facilitate one-handed recapping are available. Another technique is to tape the cap onto the side of the electrodiagnostic instrument and to insert the needle using a one-handed technique. When the examination is finished the needle should be disposed of in an appropriate container without recapping.

Steps of the Needle EMG Examination

For examination of each muscle, the needle EMG examination for each muscle can usually be divided into four distinct steps: (1) insertional activity; (2) spontaneous activity; (3) examination of motor unit potentials; and (4) assessment of recruitment. An excellent summary of the findings on needle EMG examination can be found in a recently published review article.[6]

Insertional Activity

Insertional activity is examined by moving the needle through the muscle briefly and observing the amount and duration of the electrical potentials produced. These potentials are mechanically evoked due to the advancement of the needle. Usually, insertional activity and spontaneous activity should be examined using three to four insertions for each of the four different muscle quadrants. The duration of insertional activity varies from one examiner to another. After a brief, small movement of the needle, insertional activity usually persists for no more than 300 msec. The electrodiagnostic consultant can practice assessing the duration of insertional activity by using a slow sweep speed (such as 100 msec/division).

Insertional activity may be decreased or prolonged in duration. Decreased insertional activity means that the usual degree of injury potentials are not elicited. Decreased insertional activity can result from not being in muscle or from being in a muscle that has fewer viable fibers than normal. Muscles that have become atrophied, been replaced by fat, or become fibrotic have reduced insertional activity. Muscles that have become necrotic due to a compartment syndrome or other causes of ischemia also have reduced insertional activity, and prognosis for recovery of function is poor. Muscles that have become electrically silent, such as during attacks of periodic paralysis, also have reduced insertional activity.

Increased insertional activity is usually considered to be prolonged muscle membrane activity lasting more than 300 msec after the needle movement stops. Prolonged or increased insertional activity, as an isolated finding, is a "soft" finding. No diagnosis can usually be made solely on the basis of this "abnormality." Known as the *syndrome of diffusely abnormal increased insertional activity*, an autosomally dominant inherited syndrome without any clear associated symptomatology,[36] it may be seen in some asymptomatic individuals. Increased insertional activity can also be seen in association with fibrillations or positive sharp waves, in which cases it supports the impression of denervation or primary muscle pathological lesions. Some authors feel that increased insertional activity is an early finding after denervation, before sustained positive sharp waves or fibrillations become apparent.

Spontaneous Activity

Spontaneous activity consists of electrical discharges that are seen without needle movement or voluntary contraction. These are usually looked for after each needle movement when the needle is stationary. Some spontaneous activity, recorded near the end-plate zone (end-plate noise and end-plate spikes), is normal.

End-plate noise (reflecting miniature end-plate potentials, or MEPPs) and end-plate spikes (reflecting nonpropagated end-plate potentials, or EPPs) are normal findings. It is critical to recognize these for several reasons. First, the end-plate zone is a painful area, and staying in this region increases the discomfort of the examination. Second, end-plate spikes, with their short-duration biphasic morphological characteristics, can be mistaken for fibrillation potentials to the inexperienced examiner. In contrast to fibrillation potentials, however, end-plate spikes are almost always initially negative (whereas fibrillations are initially positive) and they discharge in an irregular, sputtering rhythm. Third, if one enters the end-plate zone and proceeds through it (instead of pulling back and going in a different direction, as one should), the end-plate spikes recorded from a distance can assume the morphological characteristics of fibrillation potentials with an initial positivity. It is important to recognize end-plate noise and end-plate spikes and to withdraw the needle from that area of the muscle quickly and proceed to another area.

Fibrillation potentials represent abnormal spontaneous single muscle fiber discharges. They are short in duration (usually less than 5 msec) and biphasic, with an initial positivity in almost all instances. Whereas fibrillation potentials are essentially always abnormal, they are a nonspecific finding. They represent abnormal muscle membrane irritability, which can occur in many disorders. Fibrillation potentials are often seen in denervated muscles. Myopathies may be associated with fibrillation potentials. This is especially common in inflammatory myopathies, but in almost any myopathy, except for, possibly, chronic steroid myopathy or thyroid myopathies, fibrillation potentials may be produced. Direct muscle trauma, intramuscular injections, or intramuscular bleeding has been noted to produce immediate and chronic fibrillations. Neuromuscular junction disorders, particularly presynaptic disorders (e.g., botulism) or occasionally severe postsynaptic defects (e.g., myasthenia gravis), may produce fibrillation potentials. Upper motor neuron lesions, such as stroke and spinal cord injury, have also been shown to produce fibrillation potentials. These are usually seen early after onset of the lesion and can be confusing when trying to diagnose a peripheral nerve lesion superimposed on an upper motor neuron disorder.

Fibrillation potentials, as well as positive sharp waves, are usually graded on a subjective, qualitative scheme. Usually this ranges from 1+ to 4+, with 1+ representing a reproducibly observed fibrillation in an isolated area and 4+ representing sustained fibrillation potentials, often obscuring the baseline, throughout the muscle. Grading schemes vary somewhat from one laboratory to another. It should be remembered, however, that this is an ordinal, nonquantitative, noninterval scale. Thus, a finding of 2+ fibrillation potentials does not necessarily represent twice as much denervation as a 1+, or finding half as much denervation as a 4+ finding. Because each axon supplies many muscle fibers, the loss of only a few axons can produce many fibrillation potentials. It takes relatively little axon loss to produce 4+ fibrillation potentials. In clinical studies comparing functional outcome with the grading of fibrillation potential, there has not been a very good correlation, because density of fibrillations does not reliably estimate the degree of axon loss. The size of the compound muscle action potential (CMAP) elicited distal to the lesion is a better reflection of the viable axon population than is the grading of fibrillation potentials.

Fibrillation potentials decrease in size over time.[17] Large-amplitude fibrillation potentials (greater than 100 μV) are seen within the first year after onset of denervation, and smaller amplitudes (less than 100 μV) are seen later. It has been postulated that this relationship reflects muscle fiber atrophy over time, with smaller-diameter fibers producing smaller-amplitude fibrillations. Consequently, large-amplitude fibrillations in the presence of a neuropathic lesion suggest recent denervation.

Fibrillation potentials after denervation are probably related to acetylcholine hypersensitivity. After denervation, extrajunctional receptors appear on muscle fibers and the muscle fiber membrane comes closer to its firing threshold. The time course for the appearance of fibrillation potentials is similar to that for the development of acetylcholine hypersensitivity. However, some debate exists as to whether this represents the true mechanism.[24] In the case of myopathies, segmental necrosis is thought to account for fibrillation potentials. A myopathic fiber may become necrotic only over a focal portion of its length, leaving a portion of viable muscle fiber (distal to the necrotic area and separated from the motor end-plate by the necrotic area) functionally denervated. Experimental evidence in human and animal models supports this hypothesis.[8, 26] For patients with upper motor neuron lesions, the etiology of fibrillations is less well-delineated. Some authors have proposed that fibrillations are due to transsynaptic degeneration, whereby the lower motor neuron receives less trophic influence from the upper motor neuron.[34]

Positive sharp waves can be thought of in much the same way as fibrillation potentials. They also represent abnormal single-muscle fiber discharges, although they are often evoked by needle movement and may be recorded in a different way (see Chapter 6). Positive sharp waves can be seen in essentially all of the same disorders in which fibrillation potentials are seen. In addition, positive sharp waves may be seen in some cases in which fibrillations are not typically seen.[18] In the autosomally dominantly inherited syndrome of diffusely abnormal insertional activity, positive sharp waves are abundant, but fibrillations are not.[36] Early after denervation, particularly when recording with a monopolar electrode, positive sharp waves are much more predominant than fibrillation potentials; fibrillations become more prominent later. In some cases of muscle trauma, positive sharp waves may be seen in isolation, without associated fibrillations. Positive sharp waves are thought to have the same pathophysiology as fibrillation potentials and can be graded using the same scheme.

Complex repetitive discharges (CRDs), formerly known as bizarre high-frequency discharges, probably represent groups of muscle fibers firing in near synchrony. Single-fiber electromyography has suggested that complex repetitive discharges are produced by a fibrillating muscle fiber that acts as a "pacer" and ephaptically (membrane to membrane, without any neurotransmitter-modulated synapse) discharges adjacent muscle fibers; the phenomenon has been likened to the reentry phenomenon associated with some cardiac arrhythmias. These groups of muscle fibers then discharge in near synchrony with constant interspike intervals. A hallmark of CRDs is that they start and stop abruptly, unlike positive sharp waves or myotonia. CRDs can have any wave shape, with rates varying from 0.3 to 150 Hz. Complex repetitive discharges are a nonspecific finding. They are usually seen in chronic neuropathic or myopathic conditions; however, they are occasionally seen acutely in inflammatory myopathies. When seen in isolation, CRDs are a nonspecific but usually abnormal finding, similar in diagnostic meaning to positive sharp waves and fibrillations. It should be noted that some authors report observing CRDs in the iliopsoas muscle in normal individuals.[16] This author has also noted CRDs in levator scapulae in several individuals without lower motor neuron lesions (personal observation).

Myotonia is a rarely seen discharge that is characteristic for its waxing and waning in both amplitude and frequency. Its sound, when heard on the electrodiagnostic instrument, has been likened to a dive-bomber or to a motorcycle being revved up. Myotonia can be seen in a variety of myotonic disorders, such as myotonic dystrophy, paramyotonia, or congenital myotonia,[31] but it may also be seen rarely in inflammatory myopathies.[6] Acid maltase deficiency has also been reported to produce myotonic discharges, particularly in the paraspinal muscles.

Myotonia may be accentuated by tapping the muscle or by needle movement. In cases of clinically or electrophysiologically mild myotonia, cooling the limb often produces myotonic bursts of increased amplitude that persist longer. In many myotonic conditions the intrinsic hand muscles (e.g., thenar muscles) show the highest incidence of myotonia. Myotonia exists in many mammals, but its pathophysiology is not well understood. There is some evidence that abnormal chloride conductance at the muscle fiber membrane may be involved.[16]

Fasciculation potentials represent spontaneous discharges of all or of part of a single motor unit. As opposed to a fibrillation potential (in which just a single muscle fiber fires), a fasciculation potential involves multiple muscle fibers of the motor unit. Fasciculations produce enough muscle contraction that they can often be seen through the skin on clinical examination. Because a fasciculation potential often involves the discharge of an entire motor unit, a single fasciculation potential cannot be distinguished from a single voluntary motor unit action potential. It is only by their firing patterns that the two can be distinguished. Voluntary motor unit potentials fire in a regular, semirhythmic pattern, typically at rates from 5 to 15 Hz during early recruitment, whereas fasciculation potentials fire in a random pattern that is not under voluntary control. Fasciculation potentials are often generated at the anterior horn cell, as in motor neuron diseases, but they may also be generated ectopically distally along the axon, possibly even in intramuscular axons.

Fasciculation potentials can be seen in a variety of neuromuscular disorders. They can be "benign" fasciculations that occur in otherwise healthy individuals in whom there are no other associated signs, symptoms, or electrophysiological abnormalities. They are often seen in healthy people who are stressed, tired, lack sleep, or who are sensitive to chemicals in the diet (e.g., caffeine). Benign fasciculation potentials tend to fire more rapidly than in patients with motor neuron disease, but the difference in rate of firing is not sufficient to permit unequivocal distinction between the two syndromes. More reliable is the presence or absence of associated electrodiagnostic findings. Motor neuron disease is typically expected to show fibrillation potentials, positive sharp waves, and abnormal motor unit potentials in association with fasciculations. "Benign" fasciculations are seen in individuals who have no other electrophysiological findings. Complex fasciculation (polyphasic, long duration) potentials may be a reason for concern, because these indicate that the motor units that are discharging spontaneously have undergone some axonal sprouting and reinnervation; these are more likely to be seen in a lower motor neuron disorder than in benign fasciculation syndromes. In addition to motor neuron disease and the syndrome of benign fasciculations, fasciculation potentials can be seen in chronic radiculopathies, peripheral polyneuropathies, thyrotoxicosis, and overdosage of anticholinesterase medications.

Myokymia results from groups of motor units firing synchronously in a regular bursting pattern. This can often be seen through the skin surface as a worm-like (or vermicular) movement. When heard over the loudspeaker of the electrodiagnostic instrument, myokymia sounds like marching soldiers. The pathophysiology of myokymia is poorly understood, but it probably arises in the lower motor neuron cell body (in the anterior horn of the spinal cord or the brainstem nucleus) or axon.

Myokymia is a rare finding, but can be seen in a variety of neurological disorders. It can best be classified into two distinct groups: facial myokymia and limb myokymia. Facial myokymia has been reported with multiple sclerosis, brainstem neoplasia (pontine gliomas), facial palsy, and hemifacial spasm. Limb myokymia has been reported in radiation plexopathy/neuropathy and some chronic compression neuropathies as well as in gold polyneuropathy (patients with rheumatologic disorders treated with gold agents). Knowledge of the association with radiation treatment becomes especially important when trying to identify whether a new brachial plexopathy after radiation treatment for malignancy (e.g., breast cancer) represents a recurrence of tumor or radiation plexopathy. Patients with radiation plexopathy usually have myokymia, upper trunk lesions, and paresthesias, whereas those with recurrent tumor typically have painful lower trunk lesions without myokymia but with Horner's syndrome.[20]

Motor Unit Analysis

A great deal of information can be obtained from analysis of voluntarily activated motor unit action potentials (MUAPs). Usually, this information is more specific for neuropathic or myopathic changes than is assessment of spontaneous activity at rest.

Theoretically, in neuropathic conditions in which partial denervation and reinnervation has occurred, one will see changes representative of the underlying process of axonal sprouting (Fig. 7–1). Within days after partial denervation,[24] intramuscular axons that remain unaffected send out sprouts, usually emanating from distal nodes of Ranvier, to reinnervate nearby denervated muscle fibers. These sprouts are initially not well myelinated and conduct slowly. Con-

sequently, in the early phases of reinnervation, motor unit action potentials will have increased polyphasicity and duration. This is the direct result of temporal dispersion in these newly formed sprouts and poor synchronization of muscle fiber discharges. The neuromuscular junctions at the terminals of these new sprouts are not yet mature and are unreliable in terms of always transmitting across the myoneural junction. This results in unstable MUAPs, that is, the morphological characteristics and size vary with repetitive firing. As these sprouts mature, synchronization of muscle fiber discharges improves, and the polyphasicity is somewhat reduced. The final status of reinnervated MUAPs is that they are typically high in amplitude, long in duration, and sometimes polyphasic. The increase in amplitude is a result of the increased density of muscle fibers belonging to the same motor unit within the recording area of the tip of the EMG needle.

Myopathic changes in the MUAP result from loss of individual muscle fibers, impairment to muscle fibers, or temporal dispersion of conduction along muscle fibers. In myopathic conditions, the MUAPs are typically small in amplitude and short in duration; fewer muscle fibers from the same motor unit fire within the recording area of the needle electrode. Polyphasicity is increased, although the reasons behind this are not completely understood. In part, polyphasicity may result from dropout of muscle fibers, causing loss of the normally smooth synchronous discharge of all the muscle fibers firing together. Additionally, the affected muscle fibers may conduct more slowly than usual, increasing temporal dispersion and, consequently, polyphasicity within the MUAP.

Neuromuscular junction (NMJ) diseases tend in many ways to mimic the changes seen with myopathy. Because some of the individual muscle fibers in the motor unit may not fire with the rest of the motor unit, the duration may be shortened and the amplitude reduced. Consequently, NMJ disease should also be considered whenever short-duration, low-amplitude MUAPs are observed. Motor unit variability or instability are also increased in NMJ defects as a result of intermittent blocking of NMJ transmission.

The three most commonly used parameters of MUAPs are amplitude (peak to peak), duration, and number of phases. Amplitude is the easiest parameter to measure, but the amplitude is a reflection of just those muscle fibers that are closest to the tip of the needle. This is due to the high-frequency components of more distant muscle fiber discharges being filtered out during passage through the volume conductor of the body (i.e., the intervening tissue acts like a low-pass filter). An analogy can be made with sound waves transmitted through the air. The most bothersome part of a neighbor's overly loud stereo system is the low-frequency components (e.g., drums) rather than the high-frequency components (e.g., piccolo), which are filtered out in transmission through the air. Likewise, the high-frequency spike component of the MUAP where the amplitude is measured can only be representative of the few muscle fibers very close to the recording surface. Muscle fibers that are distant are recorded with much lower amplitudes and predominantly low-frequency components.

Electromyographers note empirically that amplitude is very dependent on distance and one can record an MUAP as having a small amplitude or large amplitude, depending

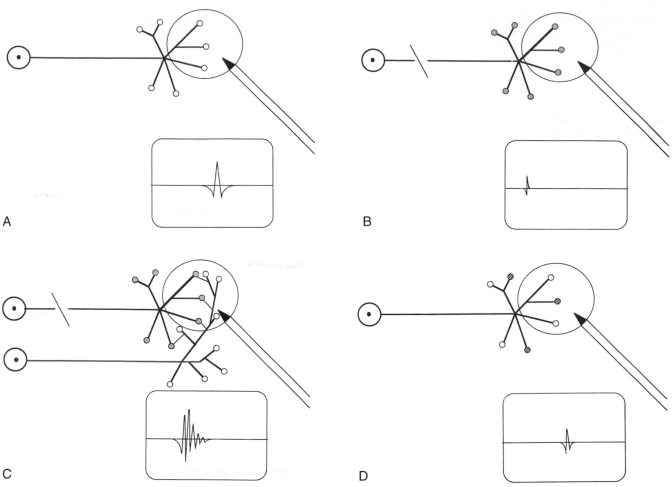

FIGURE 7–1 *A,* The normal motor unit action potential (MUAP). A needle electrode records from muscle fibers within the recording area of the needle. *B,* After denervation, single muscle fibers spontaneously discharge, producing fibrillations (or positive sharp waves). *C,* When reinnervation by axon sprouting has occurred, the newly formed sprouts conduct slowly, producing temporal dispersion (i.e., prolonged motor unit potential duration) and polyphasicity in the MUAP. The higher density of muscle fibers within the recording area of the needle that belong to the enlarging second motor unit result in an increased-amplitude MUAP. *D,* In myopathies, some muscle fibers in the motor unit become necrotic or dysfunctional and no longer contribute to the MUAP, producing shorter durations and smaller amplitudes.

on how much effort is put into focusing the needle close to the discharging muscle fibers. Although amplitude is to some extent a reflection of the density of muscle fibers within the MUAP, it is relatively unreliable as compared with other measures because it depends on how much effort one puts into "focusing" on the potential. Typically the needle is moved to obtain the largest amplitude possible for an MUAP, which usually occurs when the potential sound is sharp rather than dull on the electrodiagnostic instrument. This sharp sound comes from the higher amplitude and rapid rise time of the chief spike of the MUAP.

Duration from onset to end of the motor unit action potential is a better reflection of the number active muscle fibers within the motor unit, i.e., the motor unit territory. Measurement of mean motor unit duration is probably the most reliable routine electrophysiological feature to use in distinguishing between "neuropathic" and "myopathic" conditions. It is less dependent on distance from the motor unit, because duration is being measured from both the initial and terminal low-frequency components of the potential conducted from distant muscle fibers. A problem with duration, however, is the technical difficulty inherent

in its measurement. It is difficult to measure MUAP duration when watching voluntary motor units fly by on a regular sweep speed, except for detecting gross changes. One cannot easily tell where one motor unit starts and another stops when multiple potentials are present, and often baseline noise obscures the start or finish of the motor unit (Fig. 7–2). For an accurate representation of MUAP duration, a trigger and delay line should be used, and to reduce random baseline noise, multiple discharges of a motor unit should be averaged together. It has been shown repeatedly that mean values for at least 20 different MUAPs must be taken to develop reliable measures.

Polyphasicity as an isolated finding is nonspecific and is often overreported and overinterpreted. The phases of a motor unit may be counted as the baseline crossings plus one. When MUAPs have more than five phases, they are termed *polyphasic potentials.* Most normal muscles have at least 10% polyphasic MUAPs, depending on the muscle examined and the type of needle electrode used. Increased polyphasicity can be seen in both neuropathic and myopathic conditions, but it is not specific for either. The electrodiagnostician should be reluctant to make a diagnos-

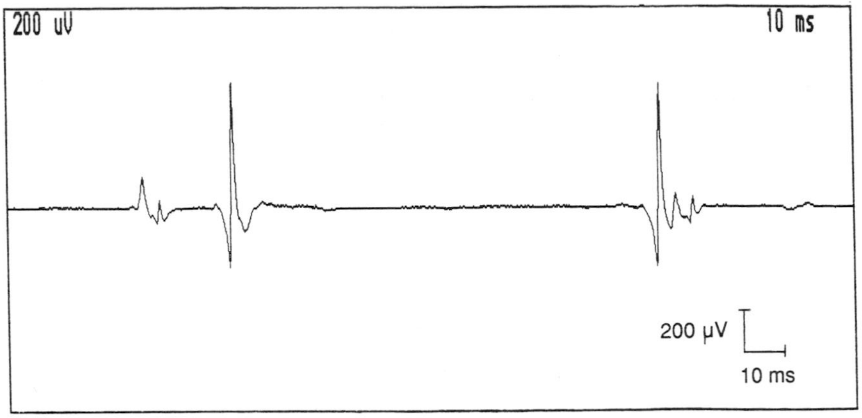

FIGURE 7–2 Two motor unit action potentials (MUAPs) examined during free sweep of the electromyograph. Note that the two potentials superimpose on the right, making it possible to erroneously identify the last potential as a long-duration, polyphasic MUAP.

tic statement only on the basis of an isolated finding of increased polyphasicity.

Motor unit variability or instability is manifested as a change in amplitude or morphological characteristics of MUAPs during repetitive firing. This is usually due to instability or unreliability in neuromuscular junction (NMJ) transmission, either as a result of a primary defect in the NMJ or as a result of recent reinnervation.

Several different methods are available to assess voluntary MUAPs during performance of an EMG. The optimal method may vary and depends on the clinical question being asked, the equipment and software available, the experience of the examiner with various techniques, and the probable subtlety of the findings expected.

The most commonly used method, usually when assessing for possible radiculopathy or entrapment neuropathy, is "semiquantitative." Several MUAPs are examined as they fire during low effort, without a trigger and delay line or any actual quantitative measurement (except possibly for peak-to-peak amplitude of a few of the larger MUAPs). The experienced examiner will notice marked changes in MUAPs, but this method is not sufficient to find more subtle changes. These semiquantitative methods are often acceptable if one is looking for neuropathic conditions in which other indications of neuropathy are typically present (such as positive sharp waves and fibrillations or changes on nerve conduction studies) or if the MUAP changes are marked.

An incremental improvement to this method is the employment of a trigger and delay line and to visually examine several motor units (Fig. 7–3). The trigger feature allows the instrument to store selected MUAPs (exceeding a designated amplitude) for later analysis. If a trigger were used only for storage, a problem would occur with visualizing the entire MUAP, because only the part of the MUAP occurring after the trigger would be displayed. A delay line permits the instrument to "remember" what happened for several milliseconds before the trigger and to display the entire MUAP. Although this still does not provide reliable quantitative information when only a few potentials are analyzed, it does permit closer examination of the motor units and better examination of the duration and morphological characteristics of the potentials.

Traditional quantitative methods were developed in the 1950s by Buchthal and colleagues.[3, 4] These methods involve recording at least 20 different MUAPs and taking

mean values of their measurements. Motor unit potentials are recorded with concentric needle electrodes with wide filter settings (Fig. 7–4). The low-frequency filter is set at 2 Hz, rather than 20 Hz, to include the low-frequency initial and terminal phases of the potential (although this makes the baseline less stable). Display sensitivity is set at a consistent level of 100 μV per division. Since duration measurements are dependent on sensitivity of the display, increasing the sensitivity (such as to 50 μV/division) produces longer durations, and lower sensitivity (such as 200 μV/division) produces shorter durations. During MUAP collection one should not select for only the biggest MUAPs; one should attempt to collect a representative sampling of all MUAPs near the tip of the needle.

Reference values have been studied extensively using these methods; they are available for many different muscles and vary according to age.[28] Mean values are usually given. If a patient's mean value for MUAP duration in a muscle varies by more than 20% from the mean, it is determined to be outside the reference range. The primary role of this type of quantitative analysis is in the evaluation of myopathy.

There are newer, automated techniques that allow extraction of single MUAPs from contractions during which several motor units are firing simultaneously.[9] These allow for collection of more MUAPs in a rapid fashion. Often, five or more motor units can be recorded from a 10-sec epoch during a moderate muscle contraction. However, the MUAPs that are selected with this technique, as well as the subsequent computational methodology employed, may be different from those of Buchthal and colleagues. The normal values to be used with each methodology of MUAP analysis have to be those that are standardized for that technique.

It is traditional to study at least 20 different MUAPs, but methods developed by Stålberg suggest that measurement of the number of outlier potentials with automated sampling may provide similar information using a lower number of analyzed potentials.[30] Those choosing to use this relatively new method should use the same motor unit sampling algorithm as that used by the original authors. The sensitivity of this technique vs. that of more traditional methods is unknown.

Some automated methods for motor unit analysis do not depend on analysis of individual MUAPs. Stålberg and others[29] have studied computerized methods of looking at

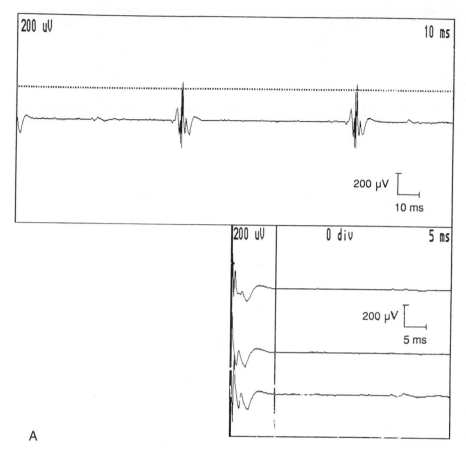

A

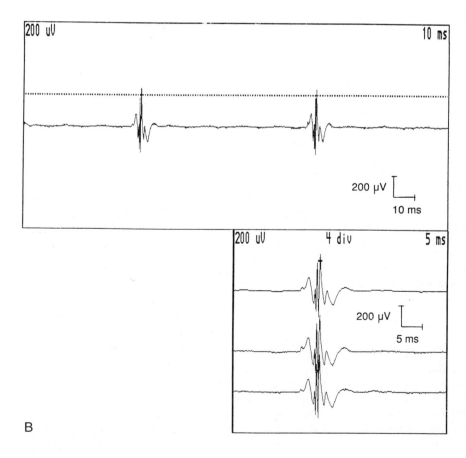

B

FIGURE 7–3 Examination of motor unit action potentials (MUAPs) with a free sweep *(top, A and B)*, trigger only *(bottom, A)*, and trigger and 40-msec delay line *(bottom, B)*. When the trigger is used alone *(A)*, only the part of the MUAP that occurs after the trigger is displayed. However, with both the trigger and the delay line *(B)*, the whole MUAP can be clearly seen for measurement of duration, amplitude, and number of phases.

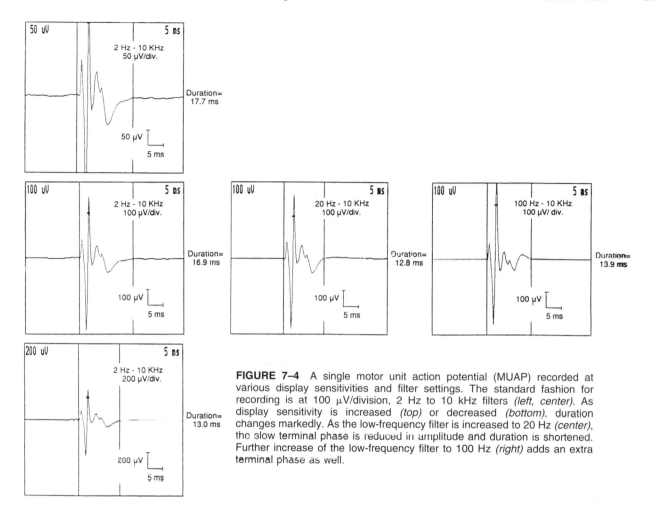

FIGURE 7–4 A single motor unit action potential (MUAP) recorded at various display sensitivities and filter settings. The standard fashion for recording is at 100 μV/division, 2 Hz to 10 kHz filters *(left, center)*. As display sensitivity is increased *(top)* or decreased *(bottom)*, duration changes markedly. As the low-frequency filter is increased to 20 Hz *(center)*, the slow terminal phase is reduced in amplitude and duration is shortened. Further increase of the low-frequency filter to 100 Hz *(right)* adds an extra terminal phase as well.

turns, defined as a change in direction of more than 100 μV, during minimal to moderate contractions (Fig. 7–5). Turns usually represent MUAPs or phases of MUAPs, but they are not resolved as MUAPs by the instrument and could represent noise or other types of discharges. Computationally, the mean amplitude for each turn (theoretically an index of MUAP amplitude) is plotted (on the *y*-axis) against the number of turns measured per second (theoretically an index of the strength of contraction or number of motor units recruited on the *x*-axis). This is done for 20 different 1-sec epochs. If more than 2 of the 20 samples fall outside the reference distribution ("normal cloud"), then the test result is probably abnormal. If the reference data supplied by Stålberg and colleagues are being used, one must of course use the same methods and the same type of needle (concentric) used in the collection of their reference values. Myopathic conditions produce small-amplitude potentials and are below the normal cloud, whereas neuropathic conditions produce large-amplitude potentials above the cloud. This type of analysis might be somewhat better than simple "semiquantitative" analysis of amplitude, depending on the experience of the examiner. In effect, by plotting the amplitude per turn vs. turns per second, one is controlling MUAP amplitude for the strength of voluntary contraction (larger-amplitude MUAPs are recruited with stronger contractions). Interference pat-

tern analysis has been shown to be about as sensitive as conventional needle EMG, but it is probably not much more sensitive. It is probably not as sensitive as using the quantitative analysis methods as applied by Buchthal and colleagues.

Recruitment

Assessment of motor unit recruitment has a number of important purposes.[25] Most importantly, it can assess whether reduced strength is due to a reduction in the lower motor neuron pool vs. poor central effort. Moreover, in myopathies, recruitment analysis allows some qualitative assessment about how much force is being provided by each motor unit.

In distinguishing between reductions in the lower motor neuron pool vs. poor central drive, the primary feature that should be measured is the rate of motor unit firing. This can be measured in several different ways, but the electromyographer should be facile at measuring these quickly. For measuring the firing rate of a motor unit, one could take 1000 msec and divide it by the interpeak interval of two consecutive discharges of a MUAP. For instance, motor unit whose potentials have an interpeak interval of 100 msec would be firing at 10 Hz (1000/100 = 10). If the sweep speed of the instrument is set at 10 msec/division, a

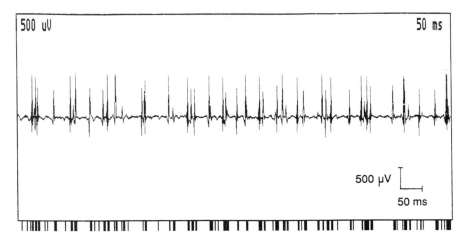

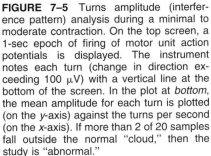

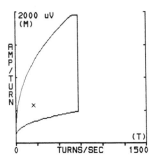

FIGURE 7–5 Turns amplitude (interference pattern) analysis during a minimal to moderate contraction. On the top screen, a 1-sec epoch of firing of motor unit action potentials is displayed. The instrument notes each turn (change in direction exceeding 100 μV) with a vertical line at the bottom of the screen. In the plot at *bottom*, the mean amplitude for each turn is plotted (on the *y*-axis) against the turns per second (on the *x*-axis). If more than 2 of 20 samples fall outside the normal "cloud," then the study is "abnormal."

quick way of estimating this is to count the number of divisions between the two motor units, and divide the number into 100. If there are 10 divisions between the potentials, the rate would be 10 Hz, 9 divisions would be about 11 Hz, 8 divisions would be 12 Hz, etc. A second way to estimate firing rates is to count the number of discharges of a given potential on the screen and multiply this number appropriately to arrive at the number that would be expected in 1 sec (1000 msec). Thus, if an MUAP fires twice during a 100 msec analysis time, the firing rate is about 20 Hz. The second method is less precise, because it does not take into account the possible variable position of the motor units across the screen.

There are several ways to use measurement of firing rates to obtain a quantitative estimate of firing patterns. One method is to measure the firing rate of the first recruited motor unit just before the second MUAP starts to fire. This *recruitment frequency* is faster than normal in diseases that reduce the size of the available motor neuron pool. The upper limit of normal for recruitment frequency varies from one muscle to another. In most limb muscles it is in the range of 12 to 15 Hz, but in the facial muscles it may be as high as 30 Hz. Consequently if one MUAP is firing at 20 Hz in a limb muscle, it is likely that the motor neuron pool is reduced, that is, some axons are not able to fire and others are driven to fire faster to try to provide the requested force.

There are other alternative methods for measuring recruitment. The recruitment ratio compares the number of motor units firing during a minimal to moderate contraction with their frequencies. A rule of thumb is that (for moderate contraction) the rate of motor units firing divided by the number of motor units firing should be less than 5. A number higher than 10 is fairly clear evidence of a loss of motor units. Assessment of the interference pattern looks at how many motor units are firing at maximum voluntary contraction, but it is a more subjective measure. Whichever method is used, motor units' firing rates should be estimated.

After assessing the firing rate, one should classify the recruitment as normal or full, central, reduced or discrete, or early (Fig. 7–6). Normal or full recruitment implies the patient can give a full effort, with many MUAPs firing at normal rates.

Central recruitment implies that reduced numbers of motor units are firing but that they are firing at a normal or slow speed. This is by far the most common "abnormality" in recruitment, but in isolation the finding is completely nondiagnostic. The central pattern of recruitment can be seen in patients with upper motor neuron lesions, pain, or poor voluntary effort.

Reduced and discrete recruitment patterns are pathologically significant and imply reduced numbers of rapidly firing motor units; "reduced" recruitment is less severe than "discrete" recruitment (in which just a few clearly identifiable motor units are firing rapidly, with baseline between them).

Assessment of recruitment is particularly useful in myopathies. In a myopathy each motor unit is "weak," and it takes more of them firing faster to accomplish a task. Consequently, in a myopathy, many MUAPs are activated to provide minimal levels of force. In a severe myopathy, it may be difficult for the patient to fire only a single motor unit as others are recruited quickly at low levels of force.

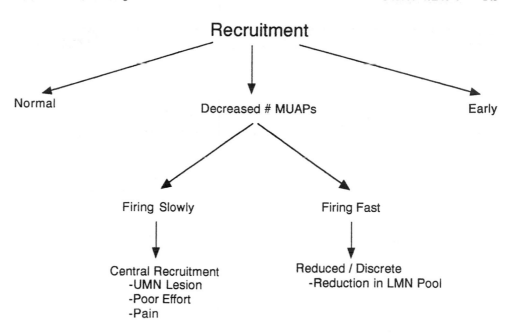

FIGURE 7–6 Assessment of recruitment. By examining firing rates, number of motor units firing, and level of force produced, recruitment should be classified as normal, central (nondiagnostic), reduced or discrete (suggesting reduction in the motor neuron pool), or early (reduced levels of force produced by each motor unit action potential, as seen in myopathy).

False-Positive and False-Negative Findings on Needle EMG

False-positive or false-negative needle EMG findings are common and have many potential causes. False-positive findings are usually related to overreading of "soft" or subtle changes. Most commonly, this includes overreading increased insertional activity, mistaking end-plate potentials for fibrillation potentials, overestimating the percentage of polyphasic motor units or overinterpreting the finding of a few polyphasic potentials, and overreading central or reduced recruitment. False-negative findings are often related to timing. Needle EMG performed too early after the onset of symptoms may produce false-negative results, as it often takes 2 to 3 weeks for obvious findings such as positive sharp waves and fibrillations to develop. False-negative findings may also be produced if subtle MUAP changes are missed in a semiquantitative examination. Obviously, false-negative results could also come from insufficient breadth of the examination (e.g., too few muscles examined or each muscle insufficiently examined) or from not examining areas that are clinically involved.

In general, referring physicians prefer that the electrodiagnostic medical consultant "underread" findings. They tend to be understanding if a patient is subsequently found to have a condition that could not be initially confirmed electrodiagnostically (false-negative findings or type I errors). They are not as forgiving of a specific diagnosis that later is proven not to be present (false-positive findings or type II diagnostic errors).

NERVE CONDUCTION STUDIES

Nerve conduction studies are a very valuable part of the electrodiagnostic consultation. The instrumentation for these is discussed in Chapter 6. Specific case examples of the uses of nerve conduction studies are presented in Chapter 8.

Measurement of Compound or Sensory Nerve Action Potentials

There are usually two measures of nerve action potentials (NAPs): (1) speed of conduction (latency or velocity), and (2) size of the evoked response (amplitude). Traditionally, the speed of conduction for compound nerve action potentials (CNAPs) or sensory nerve action potentials (SNAPs) has been measured using peak latencies; that is, the time between onset of stimulation and the peak of the potential. This is technically the easiest latency measurement to make because it is independent of display sensitivity, and on older instruments it was often the only measurement that could be clearly discerned. The peak latency, however, is not always optimal in that it does not represent the arrival of the fastest-conducting fibers and it is affected by interelectrode separation (overly short active-reference separation produces shortened peak latencies, see Chapter 6). Onset latency, although more difficult to measure (particularly for small potentials or those with noisy baselines), does have the physiological advantage of representing arrival of the fastest-conducting fibers and being less influenced by electrode separation.

Assuming that distance is held constant (e.g., 14 cm), CNAP latency can be used as an index of speed of conduction or it can be used to directly calculate conduction velocity. Conduction velocity for CNAPs (in meters per second) can be derived in two ways. One method is to simply provide a single stimulus and to divide the distance between the stimulation site (cathode) and the active (also sometimes referred to as G1) electrode by the onset latency:

$$CV = \frac{d}{t}$$

where CV = conduction velocity in meters per sec; d = distance between cathode and active electrode in millimeters; and t = onset latency in milliseconds. Onset latency should usually be used for these calculations because it is well understood physiologically and it is thought to represent the fastest fibers.

There is some controversy as to whether one should introduce into the calculation a time for activation of the nerve (activation time). Some authors advocate subtracting a 0.1-msec activation time from the onset latency, although it is not clear whether this number is constant or if it may actually be longer than 0.1 msec.[19] Accounting for activation time, one would alter the equation to:

$$CV = \frac{d}{t - AT}$$

where AT = activation time.

Another method for obtaining conduction velocity involves using two points of stimulation and dividing the distance between the two points by the difference in onset latencies. This method simply looks at the *difference* in latencies, so it cancels out any activation time inherent in both points of stimulation. Because it measures velocity between two points of stimulation rather than one, it is more difficult to measure conduction velocities over distal segments. Whatever method is used for measuring latency or conduction velocity, it should be well standardized and as close as possible to the methods that were used in developing reference (normal) values.

Latency and conduction velocity can be affected by a number of physiological and pathological factors, as discussed in Chapter 6. In healthy control subjects, slower conduction can be a result of cold limbs, aging, or increased height. Pathologically, demyelination produces slowing, as does loss of faster-conducting axons.

Amplitude of the CNAP can be measured from (1) baseline to peak, (2) from initial positive peak to subsequent negative peak if an initial positive peak is present, or (3) from initial negative peak to subsequent positive peak. In the setting of unstable or poorly defined baselines the peak-to-peak measures are often easier to make, although any subsequent motor volume conducted response makes the later positive phase difficult to measure.

Amplitude can also be affected by a number of physiological and pathological factors. Cold increases amplitude of the SNAP when the nerve at the active (G1) electrode is cooled. This is thought to result from a selective effect on Na$^+$ channel inactivation producing longer duration potentials from each axon and a larger summated compound nerve action potential.[7] Whenever a prolonged latency or slowed conduction velocity is encountered in the face of a clearly normal or larger than usual amplitude, a cold limb is the probable cause. *Pathological* causes for slowed velocities or prolonged latencies usually produce small amplitudes. Amplitude is also influenced by the distance between the nerve and the recording electrode, that is, the volume of tissue lying between nerve and electrode. This is because amplitude declines exponentially with distance. Accordingly, subjects with smaller finger circumferences have larger-amplitude SNAPs.[1] Aging produces smaller amplitude SNAPs, probably as a result of loss of large myelinated axons.

In general, the size of the CNAP is roughly proportional to the number of axons depolarizing under the active electrode. Loss of axons reduces the size of the CNAP accordingly. Distal lesions, occurring between the sites of stimulation and recording, drop the amplitude of the CNAP immediately. Proximal lesions (e.g., brachial plexus lesions) that separate the sensory axons from their cell bodies (in the dorsal root ganglion) produce distal axon loss due to axonal degeneration.[24] A reduced-amplitude SNAP can be the result of an axonal lesion anywhere distal to the dorsal root ganglion.

Measurement of Compound Muscle Action Potentials

Principles of stimulation and recording for motor nerve conduction studies are similar to those used for sensory nerve conduction studies with several exceptions. The primary difference is that motor nerve conduction studies involve recording a CMAP over muscle rather than recording directly from nerve. Consequently, the distal latency involves not only conduction along the nerve from the point of stimulation, but also includes neuromuscular junction transmission time (which takes about 1 msec) and conduction along muscle fibers (~3 to 5 m/sec). Although the onset latency from a distal stimulation site can easily be measured, this cannot be converted into a nerve conduction velocity as it can with the SNAP. To obtain conduction velocities, motor nerves are typically stimulated twice, and the distance between the two stimulation sites is divided by the difference in latency. The neuromuscular junction transmission time and the time for muscle fiber conduction are canceled out in this process.

Because each axon supplies many muscle fibers (usually hundreds or more) the compound muscle action potential is usually several hundred times the size of the corresponding nerve action potential. As a consequence, the onset latency of the CMAP is easy to delineate and it, rather than the peak, is usually used for measurement. Amplitudes of the response can be measured either from baseline to peak or from peak to peak, although the former is more common.

Although many of the same factors affect motor nerve conduction studies as affect sensory nerve conduction studies (see preceding discussion), some important differences exist. One difference is that because motor neuron cell bodies reside in the anterior horn of the spinal cord rather than in the dorsal root ganglion, the amplitude of the response is diminished by axon loss at the anterior horn cell or distally (not at the dorsal root ganglion). Another difference is that because the recording is from muscle, neuromuscular junction transmission defects or primary myopathies may reduce the amplitude of the CMAP.

The unusual finding of intact sensory nerve amplitudes with decreased motor amplitudes is encountered occasionally. Conceptually, it is helpful to think about areas in the spinal cord or along the peripheral nervous system that could account for these findings. Motor neuron disease or other intraspinal processes (such as tumor, syrinx, or carcinomatous meningitis) reduce CMAP amplitudes, but because these are pre-ganglionic lesions they do not affect SNAPs. If severe enough, radiculopathies, which almost always occur pre-ganglionically, produce small motor amplitudes but intact sensory responses. More peripherally, selective motor axonopathies produce a similar discrepancy, although these are relatively rare (e.g., heavy metal neuropathies, porphyria, and some of demyelinating neuropathies). Neuromuscular junction defects (usually presynaptic) or primary myopathies may also selectively reduce motor amplitudes, because the CMAP is recorded over muscle and the SNAP over sensory axons.

The CMAP and SNAP amplitudes are useful to estimate the degree of axon loss. The degree of axon loss is roughly proportional to the drop in CMAP or SNAP amplitude elicited with distal stimulation (assuming that enough time for wallerian degeneration has occurred).

Late Responses

There are several "late" responses (i.e., those that occur late after the CMAP or M-wave), that sometimes provide useful information. These include the F-wave, the H-wave, and the A-wave.[11]

The F-wave (so named because it was first recorded in foot muscles) is a late response usually recorded from distal muscles. Physiologically, when a motor nerve is stimulated distally, axons are depolarized in both directions: distally (orthodromically) and proximally (antidromically). Whereas the orthodromic volley activates the muscle distally, the antidromic volley proceeds proximally to the anterior horn cell. It is thought that the F-wave occurs when a small percentage (3% to 5%) of antidromically activated motor cell bodies discharge and produce orthodromic activation of their motor axons. This is noted as a small-amplitude (about 100 to 200 μV) late (about 30 msec in the distal upper limb) potential.

The technique for obtaining F-waves is similar to that for motor nerve conductions with several important differences. First, because the F-wave involves such a small percentage of the motor neuron pool, the sensitivity of the recording instrument needs to be greater (e.g., 200 μV/division vs. a customary 2 to 5 mV/division for conventional motor studies). Second, since the F-wave is a late response, having gone from the distal stimulation site to the spinal cord and back, the sweep speed needs to be slower so that a total of 50 msec (in the upper limbs) or 100 msec (in the lower limbs) can be measured in each sweep. Nerve stimulation for the F-wave is typically at the same point in the limb as for distal motor latencies. However, it is customary practice to turn the stimulating electrode around with the anode facing distally rather than proximally. Although anodal block is probably not a very common phenomenon in clinical nerve conduction studies, the concern for this possibility has made it standard practice to reverse the stimulating electrodes. The small percentage of axons in the motor neuron pool that are activated are not always the same with every stimulation. Consequently, to avoid sampling error, multiple stimulations need to be performed and multiple F-waves measured. Some debate exists as to the number of F-waves that needs to be recorded,[11] but standard practice usually involves 10 to 20 recordings.

Multiple parameters can be measured in the 10 to 20 or more F-waves that are collected. The most widely measured and probably most reliable parameter is the minimal latency, as the shortest latency out of 10 or 20 stimulations.

Some authors[11] advocate using the mean onset latency rather than the minimal latency. Other parameters that can be measured include penetrance (percentage of responses obtained), chronodispersion (the range between the shortest and longest latencies), and number of repeater F-waves (frequency of obtaining the same F-wave over time). Amplitude of the F-wave is probably not very useful, but when it is measured it is usually expressed as a ratio of the corresponding supramaximal CMAP amplitude.

F-wave measurements usually find their greatest applicability in the assessment of multifocal or diffuse processes, especially those affecting proximal areas of the peripheral nervous system. F-waves are particularly helpful in assessing acquired or inherited demyelinating polyneuropathies, which produce multifocal or diffuse slowing of conduction velocity. In Guillain-Barré syndrome (acute inflammatory demyelinating polyradiculoneuropathy), abnormalities in F-wave measures may be the only electrophysiological abnormality early in the disease course. F-waves are also useful in the assessment of syringomyelia, in which prolongation or absence of F-waves can result from impaired turnaround time (central delay) at the anterior horn cell.[22]

Although it would seem appealing to use F-wave measurements for the diagnosis of brachial plexopathy or some entrapment neuropathies, they typically are not of significant help in these applications, nor do they offer information that cannot be obtained by conventional nerve conduction studies. There are two basic reasons for this: First, because the F-wave is produced by only a small percentage of the motor axons, presence of just a few normally conducting fibers mask slowing of other fibers, resulting in a normal F-wave latency. Second, the F-wave volley traverses such a long distance of peripheral nerve that a focal lesion, unless it has severe demyelination, cannot be expected to produce marked abnormalities in F-wave latencies. Another limitation of F-wave measurements is that they usually can be recorded reliably only from distal muscles. As one attempts to record F-waves from proximal muscles, the latency becomes so short that the response is buried within the CMAP.

The H-reflex, unlike the F-wave, does involve synaptic transmission at the spinal cord level. The H-reflex is in many ways analogous to the muscle stretch reflex. However, instead of activating stretch receptors within the muscle mechanically, the large-diameter afferent nerve fibers are activated electrically (many other fibers are probably also activated as well). After the afferent volley reaches the spinal cord, a monosynaptic reflex excites alpha motor neurons and a late response is produced in the muscle. The H-reflex in adults can usually only be elicited in the soleus muscle, although in some subjects it can also be recorded from the flexor carpi radialis. The H-reflex can be seen in many more muscles in children, possibly because the descending inhibitory pathways are not yet fully myelinated.

The H-reflex is recorded using somewhat different techniques than for F-wave recording. For recording from the soleus muscle, stimulation is performed of the tibial nerve in the popliteal fossa; although many authors report using a hand-held stimulator, we have found it preferable to use a disk electrode taped over the middle of the popliteal

supramaximal

fossa with an anode placed anteriorly over the knee, thus driving the current through the knee.[21] Recording is at a standardized site that is half the distance between the popliteal fossa and the medial malleolus.[2] As opposed to the F-wave, the H-reflex is largest in amplitude with stimulation levels that are submaximal for the corresponding M-wave. Usually, the H-reflex should be higher in amplitude than the corresponding M-response. As one increases the intensity of stimulation further, the H-reflex amplitude falls. The reason for this decrease with high levels of stimulation is not clearly known, but it probably involves activation of inhibitory phenomena at the spinal cord level.

Because the H-reflex depends on a reflex at the spinal cord level, some unique concerns are applicable to obtaining these responses. The patient should be relaxed; minimal contractions, particularly the of the ankle dorsiflexors, markedly reduce the amplitude of the response. Some authors, however, utilize a minimal contraction of the ankle plantar flexors to facilitate the response. There also must be ample time between stimuli for the response to recover. Stimulating at rates more than about 0.2 Hz (one every 5 sec) alters the morphological characteristics of the H-reflex (except for the first one). Stimulation usually involves long-duration pulses, optimally between 0.5 and 1.0 msec, to preferentially activate the type Ia afferent fibers.

When performing the H-reflex studies, a late response is sometimes seen after the M-wave, and it may be unclear whether this is an H-reflex or an F-wave. To differentiate the two, the size, the consistency of the response in latency and shape, and the current required to obtain the response should be considered. H-reflexes tend to be large and are usually (but not always) greater in amplitude than the corresponding M-wave seen when the H-reflex is elicited. They tend to be stable with little variability from one stimulation to the next, and they are best elicited at submaximal stimulation intensities and attenuate with higher intensities of stimulation. In contrast, the F-wave is small (usually only about 3% to 5% of the M-wave amplitude), variable in morphological characteristics, and best seen with supramaximal stimulation intensities.

Since the H-reflex latency is dependent on the age of the subject as well as on leg length, reference values have been developed that account for these variables[2] and produce the mean expected latency. It is unusual, however, for a subject to have an H-reflex latency that exceeds the mean and 2 SD generated by this calculation, except in severe neuropathies. More commonly, side-to-side differences exceed the reference range. Side-to-side latency differences exceeding 1.2 msec are probably abnormal.[2] H-reflex amplitude is dependent on the intensity of stimulation as well as on the level of relaxation. This makes it difficult to compare an H-reflex amplitude to absolute reference (normal) values, but it has been found that side-to-side amplitude comparison is also useful.[14] The amplitude on the side with the smaller-amplitude response should not be less than 40% of the amplitude on the side with the larger amplitude response in normal, asymptomatic subjects.

The H-reflex can be abnormal in a variety of peripheral nervous system lesions. Tibial neuropathy, sciatic neuropa-thies, and lumbosacral plexopathies can all create abnormalities in the H-reflex latency, amplitude, and shape. The most useful application of the H-reflex is in the detection of S1 radiculopathy. It has been shown that the H-reflex is more sensitive than needle EMG in the assessment of S1 radiculopathy,[2] probably related to the fact that the H-reflex can detect conduction block and demyelination, whereas needle EMG can detect only motor axon loss.

The A-wave, formerly termed the *axon reflex*, is a rarely seen late response, usually observed in the setting of a peripheral nervous system lesion.[12] In most cases, the A-wave is thought to represent aberrant innervation after peripheral nerve injury such that single axons branch to two different groups of muscle fibers. Consequently, when one stimulates over the regenerated area of nerve, one may be able to stimulate one branch that then depolarizes antidromically and, at the site of branching, activates the other axon branch. This type of A-wave is usually seen only at submaximal stimulation, because supramaximal stimulation activates both branches and causes collision based on the refractory period. The A-wave, when present, is usually abnormal, as it reflects axon branching, although Sunderland has demonstrated axon branching in some normal subjects.[33] The A-wave can be easily missed in routine clinical nerve conduction studies if the sweep speed is too fast to permit the observation of these late responses.

Another proposed etiology for the A-wave is ephaptic transmission. It has been proposed that the A-wave may result from distally activating an axon in a partially demyelinated nerve. When the volley reaches a demyelinated segment, slower-conducting myelinated fibers could ephaptically activate nearby large-diameter faster-conducting fibers (Fig. 7–7). This could be seen even in the case of supramaximal stimulation, in which both branches are activated; the refractory period in the faster fiber may already be over by the time the slow fiber is activated at the site of ephaptic transmission. Ephaptically generated A-waves have been reported in early cases of Guillain-Barré syndrome.[35]

REPETITIVE STIMULATION STUDIES

Physiological Basis

Repetitive stimulation studies are most commonly used to search for abnormalities in neuromuscular junction transmission. To understand repetitive stimulation studies, it is first necessary to review the basic synaptic physiology at the neuromuscular junction (see Chapter 6 and reviews[15, 23]).

When a motor axon is activated, the depolarization proceeds down the axon to the presynaptic terminal. This depolarization produces a large influx of calcium into the presynaptic terminal, which in turn facilitates the release of acetylcholine-containing vesicles. A key point to remember when considering rates of stimulation is how long the calcium stays in the presynaptic terminal: usually about 100 to 200 msec. Given this timing, stimulation rates in excess of 5 to 10 Hz (interstimulus intervals of less than 100 to 200 msec) result in a buildup of calcium intra-axonally and a facilitation of release of acetylcholine to a greater degree than would otherwise occur. However, with stimulation at slow rates (below 5 Hz) calcium egresses from the presynaptic terminal between each stimulation, and no accumulation occurs.

At the time of synaptic transmission, acetylcholine is released to travel across the neuromuscular junction and reaches receptors at the postsynaptic end-plate. Normally, about 3 to 5 times as much acetylcholine is released than is needed to fully activate the postsynaptic membrane. This margin of safety ensures that even though the amount of acetylcholine released during repetitive depolarizations progressively decreases, the muscle fiber is still fully activated.

Stimulation at slow rates (less than 5 Hz) is usually done to detect postsynaptic neuromuscular junction defects. With slow rates of stimulation, a normal successive decrease occurs in the amounts of acetylcholine released. When the safety factor of release is normal, muscle fibers are still fully activated. When the safety margin is less than normal, progressively fewer and fewer muscle fibers are activated during repetitive stimulations at slow rates.

Fast rates of stimulation (e.g., 20 to 50 Hz) are primarily used to detect presynaptic defects in neuromuscular junction transmission. With these rates of stimulation, Ca^{2+} concentrations are progressively increased in the presynaptic terminal and more acetylcholine is released. Presynaptic defects, such as Lambert-Eaton myasthenic syndrome (LEMS) or botulism, produce marked increments (at least two-fold) in amplitude of the CMAP with high rates of stimulation.

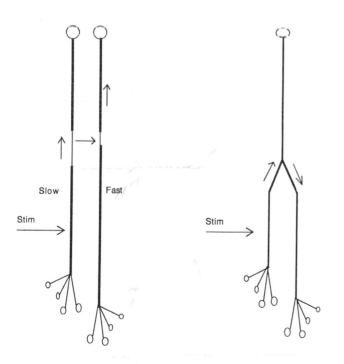

Ephaptic Transmission   Axon Branching

FIGURE 7–7 Axon waves may result from two different mechanisms. When demyelination is present, slowly conducting fibers may ephaptically activate nearby faster conducting fibers. In other cases, in which there is axon branching; selective stimulation of one branch activates the other branch; stimulation of both branches, however, causes collision and the A wave will be absent.

Technical Considerations

A number of important technical variables should be kept in mind when performing repetitive stimulation studies. First, because acetylcholinesterase is sensitive to temperature changes, the limb must be adequately warmed before studies are performed. When the limb is too cold (usually under 34 °C), defects in neuromuscular junction transmission can be hidden. There is no correction factor for an overly cold limb, so the problem must be corrected by warming the limb to 34 °C or greater. Movement artifact is probably the most common technical difficulty in repetitive stimulation studies. This can be reduced by securely taping down all electrodes. Stimulation should be via a block electrode taped to the limb rather than a hand-held electrode whenever possible. When performing stimulation distally, such as in the hand, it is also advisable to use an arm board to stabilize the limb. Submaximal stimulation can be a potential problem. Using stimuli around the maximal level (rather than the supramaximal level) can, result in intermittent submaximal stimuli and "pseudodecrements" with limb movement during stimulation. To avoid the problem, stimulation intensities should be at least 30% above the maximal level.

Although distal muscles are usually the least difficult technically to study, they are also the least sensitive. It is often necessary to perform a progression of studies, starting with the ulnar nerve, which is technically easy to study, then moving proximally to the shoulder (e.g., Erb's point to deltoid or spinal accessory nerve to trapezius), and finally to the facial muscles (nasalis). Facial muscles are the most sensitive for detecting postsynaptic defects of neuromuscular transmission, but they have technical problems due to difficulty with stabilization and movement. If abnormal results are clearly seen in distal muscles, it is often not necessary to move to more proximal studies.

Exercise has a marked effect on repetitive stimulation studies. Immediately after exercise (usually applied as 30 sec of isometric exercise) a brief period of postexercise potentiation occurs, acetylcholine release is facilitated, the margin of safety is improved, and initial deficits may be reduced. Later, 2 to 4 minutes after exercise, a period of postexercise exhaustion occurs, during which release of acetylcholine from the presynaptic terminal is reduced and any defects in neuromuscular transmission become more apparent. Thus, it is useful and customary to perform slow (2 to 3 Hz) repetitive stimulations preexercise, immediately postexercise (during postexercise facilitation), and then at 1-minute intervals for 4 minutes to look for postexercise exhaustion.

Changes in Disease States

Presynaptic disorders of neuromuscular junction transmission are rare. Lambert-Eaton myasthenic syndrome is an autoimmune disorder that is often, but not always, associated with malignancy or autoimmune disease. Botulism results from exposure to the toxin from the bacterium *Clostridium botulinum*. These disorders have in common a reduced release of acetylcholine from the presynaptic terminal. Myasthenia gravis is an example of a postsynaptic neuromuscular junction disorder. In this disorder not only are the postsynaptic receptors blocked by specific antibodies, but the cleft between the presynaptic and postsynaptic terminals is also widened and an increased breakdown of acetylcholine occurs as it crosses the synaptic cleft.

Presynaptic disorders such as LEMS or botulism are characterized by their potentiation with high-frequency stimulation and exercise (Table 7–1). When studied either immediately after exercise or during high-frequency stimulation, the CMAP potential increases at least two-fold, and often several-fold, in affected muscles. Presynaptic disorders also display a decrement with slow rates of stimulation, but this is usually less marked than in postsynaptic disorders.

Postsynaptic disorders such as myasthenia gravis usually have a progressive decrement on slow repetitive stimulation studies, which is exacerbated during postexercise exhaustion. In some cases a decrement may become apparent only during postexercise exhaustion 2 to 4 minutes after exercise. Postsynaptic disorders also manifest postexercise facilitation, but this is far less marked than in presynaptic disorders. Repetitive stimulation studies are moderately sensitive for the diagnosis of myasthenia gravis; most studies would suggest that the sensitivity ranges from 60% to 70%, although single-fiber EMG is probably more than 90% sensitive.

Abnormalities on repetitive stimulation studies are not entirely specific to neuromuscular junction (NMJ) disorders. After reinnervation, newly developed axon sprouts have immature and unstable NMJs, and may produce a decrement during repetitive stimulation at slow rates. Patients with motor neuron disease, peripheral polyneuropathy, or entrapment neuropathies may have decrements unrelated to any specific neuromuscular junction defect. Similar decrements have also been reported in myopathies.

INTERPRETATION

Normal vs. Abnormal

As with any other type of testing, nerve conduction studies and quantitative measurements on EMG are not always conclusively normal or abnormal. Reference values have been derived for most quantitative measurements, but these do not unequivocally differentiate a healthy subject from one with disease.[5] Reference values rather give the

probability of a result's coming from a healthy subject vs. from a patient with disease. If, for instance, one uses the 2 SD level to determine reference values, 97.5% of the subjects will fall on the normal side of that reference value (no diagnoses will be made based on too short a latency, too large an amplitude, or too fast a conduction velocity; hence, a one-sided probability is used). However, 2.5% of the time, someone from the healthy control subject group will have a result outside of the reference values, and be considered "abnormal." Accordingly, a single value outside of the reference range does not indicate disease. It is the finding of multiple "abnormalities" that are consistent with the clinical presentation that help to establish a diagnosis.

The use of 2 SDs to produce reference values at the 97.5 percentile level assumes there is a normal (gaussian) distribution to the data. It has been shown, however, that nerve conduction study data (and probably EMG data) do not follow a gaussian distribution.[27] Consequently, the use of mean and 2 SDs for determining reference values is usually not appropriate and may lead to an increased number of false-positive or false-negative results. Appropriate adjustments to the data can be made to obtain more reliable reference values, but this has usually not been performed in the past.

Given these considerations, when deciding whether or not a study is "normal," one must consider all reference values with some degree of healthy skepticism and avoid making a diagnosis based on a single unusual finding. Diagnoses based on the electrophysiological examination are best made when multiple "abnormalities" are demonstrated in a pattern consistent with the clinical presentation.

Principles of Localization

A number of principles are useful for localizing peripheral nerve lesions based on the electrophysiological examination.

Conventionally, in motor lesions that are primarily axonal or proximal, in which case it is not possible to perform stimulation both proximal and distal to an entrapment site, needle EMG is often used to diagnose and localize abnormalities. One usually examines muscles supplied by multiple peripheral nerves, roots, or areas of the plexus, and a localization is based on the distribution of abnormalities.

TABLE 7–1   Expected Findings on Single and Repetitive Nerve Stimulation*

| | CMAP Amplitude | CMAP After 10 sec Exercise | 2–3 Hz Stimulation | | | 30–50 Hz Stimulation |
			Pre-exercise	*Immediate Postexercise*	*2–4 min Postexercise*	
Normal	Normal	No change	No change	No change	No change	Mild increment (pseudo-facilitation)
Presynaptic defect	Very small	Markedly increased	Decrement, 1st to 4th stimulation	Markedly increased initial CMAP amplitude	Decrement similar to pre-exercise	Marked increment
Postsynaptic defect	Normal	No change	Decrement, 1st to 4th stimulation	Less decrement than pre-exercise	Decrement more than pre-exercise	Mild increment

*Recording the CMAP in normal subjects, patients with presynaptic lesions, and patients with postsynaptic lesions.
Abbreviation: CMAP, compound motor action potential.

Sciatic neuropathy can be distinguished from peroneal neuropathy, for example, if evidence is found of denervation in muscles supplied by both the peroneal and tibial nerves, although more proximal muscles (e.g., gluteal muscles) are normal. Thus, localization is based on finding abnormalities distal to a branch point with normal findings proximally.

Although this approach often results in correct localization, there are many instances in which it leads to choosing an erroneous site. Sunderland[32, 33] has shown that fascicles within peripheral nerves intertwine considerably as they move proximally through the limbs. Fascicles supplying the flexor carpi ulnaris muscle, for example, are not uniquely placed proximally within the ulnar nerve as it joins the medial cord of the brachial plexus. However, fascicles do become organized within peripheral nerves several centimeters prior to branch points. In this example, fascicles destined to supply flexor carpi ulnaris become organized within the ulnar nerve several centimeters prior to supplying the muscle. Consequently, even though ulnar nerve entrapment at the elbow usually occurs proximal to the branch to flexor carpi ulnaris, this muscle is usually spared in ulnar neuropathy at the elbow. The fascicles for this muscle are isolated in a relatively protected area of the nerve at the entrapment site. If localization were based only on EMG using the known branch points, these lesions would be erroneously placed distal to the branch point and in the forearm (Fig. 7-8).

The ulnar nerve is not unique with regard to its specific intraneural topography causing potential problems in localization. Cases have been reported of neuropathy of the common peroneal nerve occurring proximal to the popliteal fossa but resulting in only deep peroneal deficits clinically.[10] Sciatic neuropathies, even when they occur near the hip joint, can result in a clinical picture of predominantly peroneal nerve lesions. The fascicular structure within the peroneal division of the sciatic nerve may make it more predisposed to injury than is the tibial division.[32] Although conventional EMG does make use of known anatomical branch points to arrive at localization, the electromyographer should be aware of the intraneural topography within the nerve and recognize that a partial lesion might be more proximal than predicted by the electrophysiological data.

Nerve conduction studies are best at localizing the site of pathological lesion when demyelination is present. Demyelination causes focal slowing and conduction block. When present, these findings allow precise localization of a focal entrapment. A problem with localizing lesions based on nerve conduction studies arises when there is predominantly axon loss and little demyelination. In such cases, conduction velocity throughout the nerve is mildly slowed due to loss of the faster-conducting fibers, but is not focally or markedly slowed. Although a diffuse reduction is seen in CMAP or SNAP amplitude at all sites of stimulation (due to axon loss and subsequent wallerian degeneration), there is no focal drop in amplitude across the lesion site. Conduction block—in which a drop in amplitude of the CMAP is seen in moving from distal to proximal stimulation—is related only to demyelination and neurapraxia, and is not present in axon loss lesions after wallerian degeneration has occurred (about 7 days after onset).

This difficulty is exemplified when an attempt is made to localize an ulnar neuropathy at the elbow that is predominantly due to axon loss (e.g., post-traumatic lesions). Because there is no focal demyelination across the elbow, all segments of the ulnar nerve tested demonstrate mild slowing and have reduced-amplitude CMAPs. Given the fact that there are only two ulnar-innervated muscles in the forearm and none in the arm, and because of complications introduced by the complex intraneural topography (see preceding discussion), localization by EMG is also difficult.

Localization of proximal lesions such as radiculopathies or plexopathies is usually best done utilizing needle EMG results and SNAPs. Study of motor nerve conduction studies and recording of CMAPs is less useful in localization because it is usually difficult to stimulate proximal to the site of the lesion. CMAP amplitude, however, is useful for assessing the degree of motor axon loss, and, consequently, for making a prognosis.

A common problem in proximal localization is in distinguishing between plexus and root lesions. In most cases, only two findings distinguish between these two possibilities. One is the paraspinal needle EMG, which, if abnormal, speaks strongly for a lesion at or proximal to the posterior primary ramus (such as a root lesion). However, there are patients with root lesions in whom paraspinal muscles are reportedly normal on EMG. The second is the study of the sensory nerve action potential, assuming that there has been enough time for axonal degeneration after injury. This helps to distinguish between preganglionic and postganglionic (dorsal root ganglion) lesions. Plexopathies are usually expected to have small sensory nerve action potentials, and radiculopathies usually have normal potentials. Some

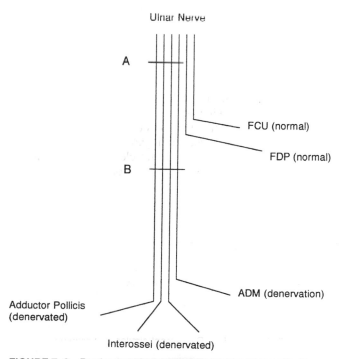

Ulnar Nerve

A

FCU (normal)

FDP (normal)

B

ADM (denervation)

Adductor Pollicis
(denervated)

Interossei (denervated)

FIGURE 7–8 Predominantly axonal ulnar neuropathies with denervation in hand muscles and normal forearm muscles may be difficult to localize. Lesions in the forearm distal to the branches to flexor carpi ulnaris (FCU) and flexor digitorum profundus (FDP) may produce these findings (site *B*). More commonly, the lesion is at a higher location (site *A*), which spares the fascicles supplying the two forearm muscles.

cervical radiculopathies that occur laterally enough to involve the dorsal root ganglion, however, produce small-amplitude SNAPs. Moreover, postganglionic lesions, such as brachial plexopathies, must have marked axon loss if axonal degeneration is to produce reduction of distal SNAPs. Because there is a wide range of "normal" SNAP amplitudes, a drop in amplitude from 60 to 30 μV, for example, might still leave the SNAP within "normal limits."

Deducing the Pathophysiology from the Electrophysiological Results

Whenever possible, it is helpful to provide to the referring physician some indication of the pathophysiology within the peripheral nervous system (e.g., neurapraxia, demyelination, or axon loss) (Fig. 7–9).

Neurapraxia or focal conduction block is seen on nerve conduction studies when a larger-amplitude CMAP or SNAP is elicited with stimulation distal to the site of the lesion, compared to proximally. Purely neurapraxic injuries show no electrophysiological evidence for axon loss (fibrillation potentials or positive sharp waves) or reinnervation.

Demyelination is best demonstrated by slowing of conduction, often with conduction block. Slowing of conduction may take the form of slowed conduction velocities, prolonged distal latencies, increased temporal dispersion, or prolonged late responses. Slowing of conduction does not always mean that demyelination has occurred; axon loss, particularly of the faster-conducting fibers, similarly produces mild slowing of conduction as well.

Axon loss lesions are usually demonstrated by evidence of denervation on needle EMG examination as well as by

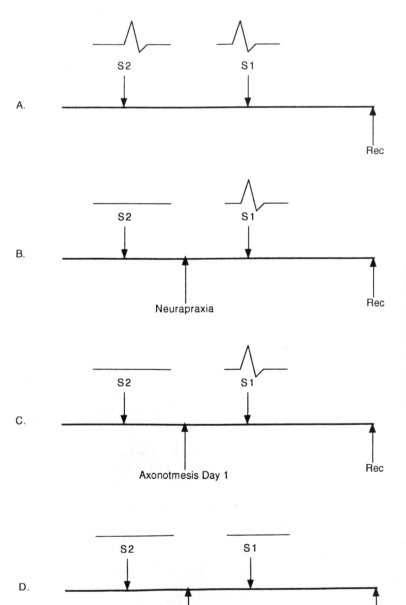

FIGURE 7–9 Normally, stimulation at two different points along a peripheral nerve produces similar-sized responses when recording distally from muscle *(A)*. After a neurapraxic lesion *(B)*, the distal nerve segment remains excitable, but a small-amplitude or absent response is elicited from proximal stimulation until recovery occurs. Similar findings are seen immediately after the occurrence of a lesion producing axonotmesis or neurotmesis *(C)*. After sufficient time for axonal degeneration has elapsed, usually 7 to 10 days *(D)*, the distal segment is inexcitable and no response is produced with distal stimulation.

small-amplitude CMAP and SNAP responses with stimulation and recording distal to the site of the lesion. Although needle EMG is a more sensitive indicator for motor axon loss, measurement of CMAP and SNAP amplitude is a better measure of the *degree* of axon loss and of prognosis.

Timing of Electrophysiologic Changes

The time course of electrodiagnostic changes after onset of a neuropathic lesion should always be kept in mind when planning the electrophysiological examination. Neurapraxia, demyelination, and severe axon loss produce electrophysiological changes immediately if one can perform stimulation both proximal and distal to the lesion. Very proximal lesions, in which it is not possible to access a site both proximal and distal to the lesion, do not immediately produce changes on distal nerve conduction studies or EMG. Distinction between neurapraxia and axonotmesis cannot be made until after wallerian degeneration has occurred.

DAY 1 AFTER AN AXON LOSS LESION. Immediately after onset of an axon loss lesion, some electrophysiological changes may be noted. On needle EMG the only potential abnormality is change in recruitment, with reduced or discrete recruitment if enough axon loss has occurred. Mild lesions do not produce noticeable changes in recruitment. Nerve conduction studies distal to the site of the lesion are unchanged, but stimulation proximal to a lesion with recording distally may produce a small-amplitude response. Otherwise, nerve conduction studies and EMG are usually unremarkable.

DAYS 7 TO 10 Seven days after a complete nerve lesion, wallerian degeneration will have progressed to a point at which stimulation of motor axons elicits no motor responses. Ten days after onset of a complete lesion, SNAPs will be absent as well. Incomplete lesions produce less marked changes, but with similar timing. Seven to 10 days after onset a neurapraxic injury can be distinguished by nerve conduction studies (in which case the distal amplitudes will be normal) from an axonotmetic lesion (in which case the distal amplitudes will be reduced).

DAYS 14 TO 21. Two to 3 weeks after onset of injury the needle EMG starts to show fibrillation potentials and positive sharp waves. Proximal muscles typically demonstrate these abnormalities first and more distal muscles show them later. Radiculopathies, for example, may show paraspinal abnormalities at days 10 to 14 after onset, but distal limb muscle changes may not be apparent until 3 to 4 weeks after onset. In studies of peripheral nerve lesions in animal models, it has been documented that the longer the segment of nerve left attached to a muscle after section, the longer the interval before the appearance of fibrillation potentials. This has raised the question of the existence of some type of "antifibrillation" trophic factor stored in peripheral nerves, with fibrillations occurring only after it is depleted.

Fibrillations and positive sharp waves may be persistent for several months or even many years after a single injury, depending on the extent of reinnervation. Although the presence of positive sharp waves or fibrillations indicates that there has been some denervation, it does not indicate that there is "active" or "ongoing" loss of axons over time. Fibrillation amplitudes are sometimes helpful in determining the chronology of the lesion, because fibrillation potentials larger than 100 µV indicate an onset less than 1 year ago.[17]

REINNERVATION. The timing and type of electrophysiologic changes consequent to reinnervation depend in part on the mechanism of reinnervation. When reinnervation is a result of axonal regrowth from the site of the lesion, as in complete lesions, the appearance of new MUAPs does not occur until motor axons have had sufficient time to grow the distance between the lesion site and the muscle (usually proceeding at 1 mm/day or 1 in./month). When these new axons first reach the muscle, they innervate only a few muscle fibers, producing short-duration, small-amplitude potentials, sometimes referred to as *nascent potentials*. With time, as more muscle fibers join the motor unit, the MUAPs become larger, more polyphasic, and longer in duration.

Motor unit potential changes also develop when reinnervation occurs by axonal sprouting. Polyphasicity and increased duration develop first as newly formed, poorly demyelinated sprouts supply the recently denervated muscle fibers. As the sprouts mature, large-amplitude, long-duration MUAPs develop and persist indefinitely.

Estimating Prognosis

Prognosis of a peripheral nerve lesion is related to the pathophysiological problem that has occurred, the time since onset, and the distance between the lesion and the target muscles. Those lesions that have had extensive axon loss are less likely to have recovery of function. Estimation of the extent of axon loss, however, should not be based solely or predominantly on findings during needle EMG, as it takes very little axon loss to produce profuse fibrillation potentials and positive sharp waves. Rather, the extent of axon loss should be chiefly determined by the distal CMAP amplitude.

Unfortunately, electrophysiological measures cannot assess the integrity of supporting structures around the nerve and cannot distinguish axonotmesis from neurotmesis. Neurotmesis, which has complete or near-complete disruption of supporting structures, carries a much worse prognosis for regeneration than axonotmesis, in which the supporting structures are largely intact. In these cases, careful periodic re-examination of proximal muscles (those expected to reinnervate first) give the best information as to ultimate prognosis for full reinnervation.

Lesions that are predominantly neurapraxic have a much better prognosis, because conduction block in these lesions rarely lasts more a few months. Demyelinating lesions also have a better prognosis than axon loss, but specific prognosis depends on what intervention is taken (e.g., release of entrapment sites).

When axon loss is present, it is important to remember that a critical window of time exists for peripheral nerve regeneration, after which the target muscles cannot be reinnervated any longer; this "window" is usually in the range of 18 to 24 months. Because peripheral nerves regenerate roughly 1 in./month, proximal lesions with a great deal of axon loss have a poor chance of reinnervating distal hand or foot muscles. Brachial plexus injuries, for example, when complete, have very little chance of reinnervating ulnar-innervated hand muscles. As a consequence, most neurosurgical interventions in brachial plexus lesions are directed at reinnervating proximal upper limb muscles. When looking for any electrophysiological evidence of reinnervation, it is important to keep in mind both the distance between the lesion and the muscle being examined and the time since injury, to know whether reinnervation should be expected at the time of the examination.

WRITING THE ELECTRODIAGNOSTIC MEDICAL CONSULTATION REPORT

Guidelines for writing the electrodiagnostic medical consultation report can be found in the American Association for Electrodiagnostic Medicine guidelines for electrodiagnostic laboratories.[13] The report should identify the patient, state the referring problem and indication for the study, and list the findings from the electrophysiological examination. The conclusion should specify whether the study results are normal or abnormal, answer the referring physician's question (e.g., whether or not a specific diagnosis is present), and report any other diagnoses that may have come to light during the clinical or electrophysiological examination. Whenever possible, the pathophysiological basis of the lesion and the prognosis for recovery should be included, if known.

References

1. Bolton CF, Carter KM: Human sensory nerve compound action potential amplitude: Variation with sex and finger circumference. J Neurol Neurosurg Psychiatry 1980; 43:925–928.
2. Braddom RL, Johnson EW: Standardization of H reflex and diagnostic use in S1 radiculopathy. Arch Phys Med Rehabil 1974; 55:161–166.
3. Buchthal F, Guld C, Rosenfalk P: Action potential parameters in normal human muscle and their dependence on physical variables. Acta Physiol Scand 1954; 32:200–218.
4. Buchthal F, Pinelli P, Rosenfalk P: Action potential parameters in normal human muscle and their physiological determinants. Acta Physiol Scand 1954; 32:219–229.
5. Campbell WW, Robinson LR: Issues and opinions: Deriving reference values in electrodiagnostic medicine. Muscle Nerve 1993; 16:424–428.
6. Daube JR: AAEM minimonograph no. 11: Needle examination in clinical electromyography. Muscle Nerve 1991; 14:685–700.
7. Denys EH: AAEM minimonograph no. 14: The influence of temperature in clinical neurophysiology. Muscle Nerve 1991; 14:795–811.
8. Desmedt JE, Borenstein S: Relationship of spontaneous fibrillation potentials to muscle fibre segmentation in human muscular dystrophy. Nature 1975; 258:531–534.
9. Dorfman LJ, McGill KC: AAEE minimonograph no. 29: Automatic quantitative electromyography. Muscle Nerve 1988; 11:804–818.
10. Esselman PC, Tomski MA, Robinson LR, et al: Selective deep peroneal nerve injury associated with arthroscopic knee surgery. Muscle Nerve 1993; 16:1188–1192.
11. Fisher MA: AAEM minimonograph no. 13: H reflexes and F waves: Physiology and clinical applications. Muscle Nerve 1992; 15:1223–1233.
12. Fullerton PM, Gilliat RW: Axon reflexes in human motor nerve fibers. J Neurol Neurosurg Psychiatry 1965; 28:1–11.
13. Guidelines in Electrodiagnostic Medicine. Rochester, Minn, American Association of Electrodiagnostic Medicine, 1994.
14. Jankus WR, Robinson LR, Little JW: Normal limits of side-to-side H-reflex amplitude variability. Arch Phys Med Rehabil 1994; 75:3–7.
15. Keesey JC: AAEM Minimonograph no. 33: Electrodiagnostic approach to defects of neuromuscular transmission. Muscle Nerve 1989; 12:613–626.
16. Kimura J: Electrodiagnosis in Diseases of Nerve and Muscle: Principles and Practice, ed 2. Philadelphia, FA Davis, 1989.
17. Kraft GH: Fibrillation potential amplitude and muscle atrophy following peripheral nerve injury. Muscle Nerve 1990; 13:814–821.
18. Kraft GH: Fibrillation potentials and positive sharp waves: Are they the same? Electroencephalogr Clin Neurophysiol 1991; 81:163–166.
19. Krarup C, Horowitz SH, Dahl K: The influence of the stimulus on normal sural nerve conduction velocity: A study of the latency of activation. Muscle Nerve 1992; 15:813–821.
20. Lederman RJ, Wilbourn AJ: Brachial plexopathy: Recurrent cancer or radiation? Neurology 1984; 34:1331–1335.
21. Little JW, Hayward LF, Halar E: Monopolar recording of H reflexes at various sites. Electromyogr Clin Neurophysiol 1989; 29:213–219.
22. Little JW, Robinson LR: Electrodiagnosis in post-traumatic syringomyelia: Case report and review of the literature. Muscle Nerve 1992; 15:755–760.
23. MacLean IC: Neuromuscular junction. In EW Johnson (ed): Practical Electromyography. Baltimore, Williams & Wilkins, 1980.
24. Miller RG: AAEM minimonograph no. 28: Injury to peripheral motor nerves. Muscle Nerve 1987; 10:698–710.
25. Petejan JH: AAEM minimonograph no. 3: Motor unit recruitment. Muscle Nerve 1991; 14:489–502.
26. Robinson LR: AAEM case report no. 22: Polymyositis. Muscle Nerve 1991; 14:310–315.
27. Robinson LR, Temkin NR, Fujimoto WY, Stolov WC: Effect of statistical methodology on normal limits in nerve conduction studies. Muscle Nerve 1991; 14:1084–1090.
28. Rosenfalk P: Electromyography in normal subjects of different age. Methods Clin Neurophysiol 1991; 2:47–52.
29. Stålberg E, Chu J, Bril V, et al: Automatic analysis of the EMG interference pattern. Electroencephalogr Clin Neurophysiol 1983; 56:672–681.
30. Stålberg E: Outliers, a way to detect abnormality in quantitative EMG. Muscle Nerve 1994; 17:392–399.
31. Streib EW: AAEE minimonograph no. 27: Differential diagnosis of myotonic syndromes. Muscle Nerve 1987; 10:603–615.
32. Sunderland S: The relative susceptibility to injury of the medial and lateral popliteal divisions of the sciatic nerve. Br J Surg 1953; 41:300–302.
33. Sunderland S: Nerves and Nerve Injuries, ed 2. Edinburgh, Churchill-Livingstone, 1968.
34. Taylor RG, Kewalramani LS, Fowler WJ: Electromyographic findings in lower extremities of patients with high spinal cord injury. Arch Phys Med Rehabil 1972; 53:558–562.
35. Wang L, Robinson LR: Axon reflexes resulting from ephaptic transmission in acute demyelinating polyneuropathy. Arch Phys Med Rehabil 1993; 74:1250.
36. Wright KC, Ramsey-Goldman R, Nielsen VK, et al: Syndrome of diffusely abnormal insertional activity: Case report and family study. Arch Phys Med Rehabil 1988; 69:534–536.

Electrodiagnostic Medicine III: Case Studies

KATHRYN A. STOLP-SMITH, M.D.

The ability to perform nerve conduction studies (NCS) and needle electromyography (EMG) in a clinical setting significantly enhances our role as clinicians. Knowledge and skill in clinical neurophysiology allows the clinician a physiological extension and confirmation of the clinical examination. An analytical and sequential thought process, application of medical knowledge of anatomy, physiology, and pathophysiology, and familiarity with electrodiagnostic equipment are necessary to properly perform and interpret NCS and EMG. Clinical neurophysiological studies allow us immediate physiological feedback and confirmation of clinically suspected problems. The decision to perform electrophysiological studies is based on many factors. Confirming a clinical impression, exploring and excluding disorders in a differential diagnosis, highlighting findings that will alter clinical management, and, in some cases, providing objective evidence of a disorder for medicolegal reasons are all ways in which NCS and EMG can facilitate the practice of medicine.

The principal goal of the electrodiagnostic medicine consultation is to reach a diagnostic conclusion efficiently and reliably. Selection of NCS and muscles for EMG should be based not only on the anatomy and suspected pathophysiology but on the patient's ability to tolerate the study, the ease and reliability with which these studies can be performed, and the time allotted by the patient and clinician for the study.

Patient tolerance is to a large extent a function of the examiner's "bedside manner." If the examiner shows patience, good technique, and a thoughtful approach to the study, all procedures are usually well tolerated. As a rule, when no disorder of the neuromuscular system is suspected based on the history and clinical examination, clinical neurophysiological studies are unnecessary. The precise NCS chosen and the muscles examined by EMG are determined by the clinical findings, knowledge of pathophysiology, and factors of patient compliance, positioning, and tolerance. The procedure performed can change depending on the data obtained as each step is completed. A "cookbook" approach to electrodiagnosis is flawed by lack of the necessary customization for each case, and is rarely if ever satisfactory for accurate results or for patient tolerance. Standard techniques may even have to be varied in some situations depending on the type of information sought. Studies performed can be limited by patient compliance, tolerance, coagulopathies, the presence of central vascular catheters, pacemakers, lymphedema, and other factors. Clinical judgment and knowledge of the risk of electrodiagnostic studies apply in all cases. In some cases, other types of studies may prove more useful and appropriate in reaching a diagnosis and determining a management plan.

The following case reports and discussions are meant to highlight these principles. Each patient is unique and the approach differs from patient to patient and from clinician to clinician. The approaches used are examples and not protocols. The purpose of the case reports is to display the logic of performing electrodiagnostic medicine studies and how the sequence of steps is reflected by findings from the preceding step. The cases described are meant to represent problems commonly encountered in the clinical neurophysiological laboratory. Some examples are classic cases, others are focal presentations of generalized problems, and the problem of coexisting disorders is described. Problems of the neuromuscular system are highlighted. Disorders of other organ systems, in particular the musculoskeletal system, are not discussed but often must be considered in the differential diagnosis.

Disorders most readily assessed by NCS and EMG include diseases of the neuron—the anterior horn cell or dorsal root ganglion; the nerve roots; plexus; and the peripheral nerves, including entrapments, discrete proximal conduction block, distal nerve disorders, and neuromuscular junction and muscle disorders. The cases reported here demonstrate how to apply the basic science and techniques described in Chapters 6 and 7 to a clinical situation.

UPPER LIMB PROBLEMS

Many disorders affecting the upper extremity can be diagnosed during the electrodiagnostic medicine consultation. Common problems involving one or both upper limbs include cervical radiculopathy or root avulsion, brachial plexopathy, and radial, ulnar, and median nerve entrapments or compression. Entrapments or compression of other upper limb nerves can be determined, including the spinal accessory, long thoracic, dorsal scapular, suprascapular, axillary, musculocutaneous, thoracodorsal, and pectoral nerves. Cutaneous neuropathies of the lateral and medial antebrachial cutaneous, superficial radial, and dorsal ulnar sensory cutaneous nerves can also be seen. Disorders which may present in but are not limited to the upper limbs include motor neuron disease, multifocal motor neuropathy with conduction block, polyradiculoneuropathies, multiple multifocal mononeuropathies of acquired or hereditary cause, neuromuscular junction disease such as myasthenia gravis, and congenital, acquired, metabolic, or structural disorders of muscle. Clinical symptoms and signs may be acute or chronic, constant or intermittent, focal or generalized, and include numbness, paresthesias, weakness, pain, fatigue, cramps, fasciculations, and position- and posture-related symptoms. Sensory loss, weakness, atrophy, depressed reflexes, fasciculations, myokymia, myotonia, and tremor can result from these disorders.

Neck or Arm Pain (Case 1)

THOUGHT PROCESS. The principal consideration in the differential diagnosis for this case is a right cervical radiculopathy at the C7 level. However, other root level involvement cannot be excluded by the history and examination alone because of overlap of myotomes and dermatomes and individual anatomical variation. An idiopathic or traumatic brachial plexopathy affecting primarily the posterior cord should also be considered. Radial nerve entrapment is a possibility. Median nerve entrapment at the wrist can cause shoulder symptoms, but there is little to suggest this disorder in our current evaluation. The history and physical examination do not support a diagnosis of root avulsion. A central nervous system (CNS) disorder

with spinal cord injury at a cervical level or a discrete lesion rostral to the spinal cord could potentially explain these findings, and although these should not be ignored, they would be unlikely given the time course of the history and the focal findings, and would only rarely produce pain.

Selection of appropriate electrodiagnostic studies is based on the differential diagnosis. Needle EMG is an essential component of the evaluation to specifically define involved myotomes. Sensory nerve conduction studies are important to exclude plexopathy and mononeuropathy. Motor nerve conduction studies denote the severity of axonal loss and assist with myotome definition. F-wave studies, if included, can be useful in highlighting proximal slowing or conduction block in unsuspected areas of involvement. Given the sensory symptoms and findings, tests such as repetitive stimulation to study neuromuscular junction transmission are not indicated. The studies performed in this patient are listed in Table 8–1.

DISCUSSION. As is typical for all but the most severe radiculopathies, the nerve conduction studies are normal.[61] Median and ulnar motor NCS were performed to study nerves commonly entrapped in the upper extremity, which can lead to pain, weakness, and numbness. The compound muscle action potentials from these muscles allow assessment of axonal integrity of the C8 and T1 nerve roots. F-wave studies assess slowing in proximal nerve segments as may be seen in radiculopathy, plexopathy, or multifocal motor neuropathy with conduction block. The median and ulnar antidromic sensory NCS were performed to evaluate the upper and lower trunks of the brachial plexus as well as to exclude common focal entrapments. The specific distribution of numbness by history and physical examination for this patient led to consideration of a radial neuropathy and the radial antidromic sensory NCS was performed. These studies are well tolerated and are technically reliable.

Needle examination should be as focused as possible yet help to appropriately include or exclude disorders noted in the differential diagnosis. Needle examination performed in at least two muscles of the suspected involved myotome increase the chances of finding an abnormality and better define the root level involved. Needle examination of muscles that are clinically involved should always yield some

CASE 1

A 45-year-old male carpenter developed gnawing right-sided neck pain one day following a day of repetitive lifting and stacking lumber. The pain began as a dull ache and gradually became more severe with radiation down the right arm to the dorsum of the hand. Discomfort was exacerbated by turning the head to the right and was associated with transient tingling and numbness along the extensor forearm and dorsum of the hand. He had not found any measures that reduced the pain. Occasionally, the arm felt heavy though not particularly weak. The pain became more severe and 6 weeks after onset he sought a medical evaluation.

Clinical examination showed decreased cervical lordosis and decreased active neck range of motion. Passive range of motion was limited, and Spurling's maneuver significantly increased his neck pain with paresthesias and pain radiating down the arm to the dorsum of the right hand. Shoulder range of motion was normal. Muscle stretch reflexes were normal except for an absent right triceps reflex. Sensory examination revealed decreased pain and touch sensation of the extensor forearm and dorsum of the hand, including the third digit. Manual muscle testing showed mild right triceps weakness.

TABLE 8–1   Case 1: Neck and Arm Pain

NERVE CONDUCTION STUDIES

Nerve Stimulation (Record)	Amplitude (μV)	Conduction Velocity (ms)	Latencies (ms)	
			Distal	*F-Wave*
Motor				
Median (thenar)	6800	52	3.5	29.0
Ulnar (hypothenar)	8300	54	3.0	29.5
Sensory Antidromic				
Radial (hand dorsum)	28	—	3.3	—
Median (index)	42	63	3.0	—
Ulnar (fifth)	20	63	2.8	—

ELECTROMYOGRAPHY*

Muscle	Insertional Activity	Spontaneous Activity		Motor Unit Potentials		
		Fibrillation Potentials	*Fasciculation Potentials*	*Recruitment*	*Duration/ Amplitude*	*Phases/ Turns*
First dorsal interosseous (manus)	Normal	0	0	Normal	Normal	—
Pronator teres	Increased	0	0	Normal	Slightly increased	—
Triceps	Increased	+ +	0	Reduced	Increased	Increased
Biceps	Normal	0	0	Normal	Normal	—
Extensor digitorum communis	Increased	+	0	Reduced	Increased	Increased
Deltoid	Normal	0	0	Normal	Normal	—
Midcervical paraspinal muscles	Increased	+ +	0	Not evaluated	Normal	—

*All needle examinations performed with a concentric needle.

abnormal finding. Severely involved muscles that are fibrotic provide abnormal but limited findings.

EMG can include the first dorsal interosseous of the hand, pronator teres, triceps, biceps brachii, deltoid or infraspinatus, cervical paraspinal muscles, and possibly a finger extensor muscle. Increased insertional activity in the pronator teres resulted in suspicion that a C6 or C7 radiculopathy was present and was evidence against a radial neuropathy. The myotome involved was further defined by the triceps abnormalities. Abnormal findings in the paraspinal muscles taken together with the abnormalities in anterior myotomes limited principally to a single myotome directed us away from the diagnosis of plexopathy and provided good evidence for a radiculopathy. Since the most severe findings were in the triceps with only mild pronator teres abnormalities and a normal biceps, and since there was the presence of both fibrillation potentials and motor unit potential (MUP) changes, the best explanation was an active or chronic and incompletely reinnervated radiculopathy at the right C7 root level.

Arm Numbness and Weakness (Case 2)

THOUGHT PROCESS. The most likely diagnosis for this patient is posttraumatic brachial plexopathy with primarily lower trunk involvement. Elbow flexor weakness with normal strength noted in other upper trunk innervated muscles could indicate more extensive plexus involvement. The most important disorder to exclude in the differential diagnosis is that of root avulsion, since prognosis and further treatment would be significantly altered by this possibility. Given the humerus fracture, multiple mononeuropathies at the level of the fracture could also explain these findings. The history of trauma and the physical

examination findings suggest plexopathy or root avulsion coupled with a musculocutaneous neuropathy.

When considering a less clear-cut brachial plexopathy, other causes must be considered based on the clinical history, course, and portion of the plexus involved. Traction plexopathies typically involve the upper trunk of the brachial plexus.[37] Gunshot wounds more commonly affect the cords.[30] Nontraumatic onset of upper extremity pain with weakness and numbness, occasionally following a viral illness, leads to consideration of an idiopathic plexopathy, or neurologic amyotrophy, as described by Turner and Parsonage.[57] This disorder can also involve the long thoracic nerve and phrenic nerve or cervical roots, resulting in findings which could be attributed to root involvement. Idiopathic brachial plexopathies often present bilaterally,[60, p. 934] and subclinical involvement of the contralateral extremity can be demonstrated using NCS and EMG.[57]

Lower trunk plexopathies that develop insidiously can be due to an apical lung tumor or metastatic breast carcinoma or primary plexus tumors such as neurofibroma or schwannoma.[60, p. 93] Often, differentiating recurrent tumor infiltration from postradiation plexopathy is challenging, but postradiation plexopathy is more likely to demonstrate myokymic discharges on EMG and can occur up to 34 years post radiation therapy.[24, 36] Healthy persons with droopy shoulders can develop symptoms of intermittent lower trunk compromise that can be due to vascular or lower trunk encroachment in the shoulder girdle by a rudimentary cervical rib or fibrous band.[19] Electrophysiological hallmarks of this disorder, known as thoracic outlet syndrome, are a low median compound muscle action potential (CMAP) and markedly reduced or absent ulnar sensory nerve action potential (SNAP) with needle examination abnormalities in lower trunk–innervated muscles.[18]

CASE 2

A 60-year-old farmer developed left upper extremity weakness and numbness after falling from his tractor. His sleeve caught in the tractor doorframe and caused him to dangle freely before falling to the ground. He landed on his shoulder, fracturing the clavicle and humerus. The fractures required surgical fixation and he presented for an evaluation when the surgical wounds were healed.

Clinical examination revealed deformity of the shoulder with limited range of motion. Muscle stretch reflexes were absent in the affected upper limb. Manual muscle testing demonstrated normal strength with shoulder abduction, rotation, and no scapular winging.

Moderate weakness of elbow flexion, forearm pronation, supination, elbow and wrist extension, and severe weakness of wrist flexion, finger extension and flexion, and hand intrinsics were noted. Atrophy of weak muscles, and swelling and clawing of the hand were present. Sensory examination showed reduced pain and touch sensation of the forearm and hand with relative sparing of the thumb, and completely absent sensation of the lateral forearm, medial hand, and fourth and fifth digits. Proximal to the elbow, the medial aspect of the arm demonstrated significant sensory loss.

The NCS and EMG performed in this case are outlined in Table 8–2.

DISCUSSION. One of the electrodiagnostic challenges posed by this case is to completely assess the degree of the lesion without performing excessive NCS and to limit the needle examination. Both median and ulnar motor NCS were performed because (1) both median motor and ulnar motor and sensory nerve fibers course through the lower trunk of the brachial plexus; (2) the median CMAP reflects integrity of primarily C8 axons and the ulnar CMAP represents primarily T1 axons; (3) F waves are readily obtain-

able with both; (4) both NCS are technically reliable; and (5) the ulnar nerve is ideally suited for stimulation at multiple points along its course, including the plexus and root level. Because of the suspected musculocutaneous neuropathy, this nerve and the lateral antebrachial cutaneous nerves were specifically studied.

The abnormalities on these studies alone do not exclude an upper trunk brachial plexopathy. This could be further defined using the needle examination. The normal axillary NCS pointed toward a musculocutaneous neuropathy, though upper trunk plexopathy still could not be completely

---

TABLE 8–2   Case 2: Arm Numbness and Weakness

NERVE CONDUCTION STUDIES

Nerve Stimulation (Record)	Amplitude (μV)	Conduction Velocity (ms)	Latencies (ms) Distal	Latencies (ms) F-Wave
Motor				
Median (thenar)	1500	45	4.0	NR
Ulnar (hypothenar)	NR	NR	NR	—
Musculocutaneous (biceps)	1300	45	4.2	
Axillary (deltoid)	5200	—	—	
Sensory				
Ulnar (fifth)	NR	NR	NR	
Lateral antecubital (forearm)	NR	—		
Median (index)	18	57	3.2	

ELECTROMYOGRAPHY

Muscle	Insertional Activity	Spontaneous Activity Fibrillation Potentials	Spontaneous Activity Fasciculation Potentials	Motor Unit Potentials Recruitment	Motor Unit Potentials Duration/ Amplitude	Motor Unit Potentials Phases/ Turns
Deltoid	Normal	0	0	Normal	Normal	—
Biceps brachii	Increased	+ +	0	Reduced	Increased/low	Increased
Pronator teres	Increased	+	0	Reduced	Increased	Increased
First dorsal interosseous (manus)	Increased	+ + +	0	None activated	—	—
Flexor pollicis longus	Increased	+ +	0	Reduced	Normal	Increased
Triceps	Increased	+	0	Reduced	Increased	Increased
Brachioradialis	Increased	+	0	Reduced	Increased	Increased
Infraspinatus	Normal	0	0	Normal		—
Midcervical paraspinals	Normal	0	0	—		—
Low cervical paraspinals	Increased	+ + +	0	—		—
High thoracic paraspinal muscles	Normal	0	0	—		—

Abbreviation: NR, no response.

excluded. Abnormal sensory NCS indicated a lesion distal to the dorsal root ganglion. In root avulsion without plexopathy, SNAPs should be preserved.[59]

Nerve root stimulation may be indicated to better define the level of involvement in some cases of brachial plexopathy. Nerve root stimulation can be technically difficult and uncomfortable for the patient and generally should not be performed unless the examiner is comfortable with the technique and the technical pitfalls that could affect the results. Root stimulation was not performed in this case.

The needle examination provided evidence of extensive denervation in the upper limb with sparing of upper trunk–innervated muscles except for those innervated by the musculocutaneous nerve. Muscles representing all plexus levels were examined. Relatively normal MUPs with reduced recruitment in the flexor pollicis longus indicated a lack of reinnervation.[29, p. 633] The presence of MUPs in this muscle was evidence against a complete C8 root avulsion. Long-duration, low-amplitude, highly polyphasic MUPs in the biceps are characteristic of nascent MUPs indicating early reinnervation. Low cervical paraspinal fibrillation potentials indicated root involvement and indeed likely avulsion at this level.

The conclusion from these studies was that of a middle and lower trunk brachial plexopathy with probable root avulsion of the C8 or T1 nerve root.

Arm Weakness (Case 3)

THOUGHT PROCESS. The patient's age, history, and examination findings are most characteristic of acquired myasthenia gravis.[20] Lambert-Eaton myasthenic syndrome (LEMS) could also produce these symptoms, but usually displays dysautonomia and less pronounced bulbar symptoms. Weakening, rather than facilitation, of muscle strength and muscle stretch reflexes with repetitive testing were present on clinical examination.[16, 34] The time of weakness onset was most consistent with an acquired disorder of muscle, although a congenital myopathy or dystrophy can present in later years.[6, 58] Myotonic dystrophy or other myotonic disorder of muscle can present in this way, but the examination findings and lack of cramping were not suggestive of this family of disorders.[22] Inflammatory myopathy, motor neuron disease, and motor neuropathy or

inflammatory polyradiculoneuropathy must also be included in the differential diagnosis. Facial weakness is not characteristic of early motor neuron disease or inflammatory myopathy. Motor neuropathy or polyradiculoneuropathy usually present with depressed reflexes[15, 45] and polyradiculoneuropathy is rarely only motor. Multifocal motor neuropathy with conduction block can present with normal or slightly increased reflexes.[35] The NCS and EMG performed in this case are presented in Table 8–3.

DISCUSSION. Myasthenia gravis is the most likely diagnosis given the clinical presentation. It is important to consider disorders of the neuromuscular junction when evaluating a patient for vague or more pronounced complaints of upper limb weakness. Myasthenia gravis can present initially with weakness in the upper extremity.[20] The patient presented here has the more classic presentation with facial and some lower extremity involvement as well.

The key to the electromyographer's approach is to determine whether the neuromuscular junction is involved, whether it is confined to the face or upper or lower limbs, and to prove that motor neuropathy, polyradiculoneuropathy, motor neuropathy, or myopathy is not present. The examiner must also demonstrate the characteristic pattern of decrement on repetitive nerve stimulation in at least two nerves to avoid false-positive results. A decrement greater than 10% is generally used, as technical limitations of repetitive stimulation can produce a small decrement, and a small decrement can be seen in some other disorders. The decremental response must be demonstrated to repair with exercise and to follow a pattern where the greatest incremental percentage of decrement occurs between the first and second CMAP.[41] Decrement is calculated by comparing the amplitude or area of the first CMAP with the fourth or fifth CMAP resulting from a train of four or more stimuli.[50]

The nerves selected were chosen because the (1) ulnar nerve is technically the most reliable for repetitive stimulation (because of distal recording it may not show an abnormality); (2) the accessory nerve is a reliable and well-tolerated proximal NCS and is relatively sensitive (the axillary nerve may be more sensitive but is technically more difficult); (3) facial NCS evaluate facial symptoms and signs; (4) peroneal NCS can demonstrate lower limb

CASE 3

A 42-year-old woman complained of fatigue and upper limb weakness which developed over the past 6 months. She occasionally noted double vision, particularly later in the day, and had difficulty with overhead activities. Although she denied difficulty walking, her legs felt heavy and she described some difficulty climbing stairs. There was no family history of a similar disorder.

Clinical examination revealed a healthy-appearing woman with a transverse smile. Muscle stretch reflexes, gag reflexes, and sensory examination were normal. Manual muscle testing of facial muscles

showed mild orbicularis oculi and oris weakness. With prolonged upward gaze the patient developed ptosis bilaterally. Prolonged phonation and repetitive lingual motions resulted in palatal weakness and dysarthria. Extraocular motions were full and conjugate. Upper extremity strength was normal distally. There was mild weakness of the shoulder rotators and abductors, and repeated contraction of these muscles resulted in moderate weakness. Lower extremity manual muscle testing was normal but repeated squat and rise from the floor became progressively more difficult.

TABLE 8–3   Case 3: Arm Weakness

NERVE CONDUCTION STUDIES

Nerve Stimulation (Record)	Amplitude (μV)	Conduction Velocity (ms)	Latencies (ms)	
			Distal	*F-Wave*
Motor				
Ulnar (hypothenar)*	8800	60	3.0	27.0
Facial (nasalis)*	2800	—	3.0	
Accessory (trapezius)	6000	—	4.2	
Peroneal (EDB)*	4000	46	5.1	55.5
Sensory				
Medial (index)	32	58	3.2	
Medial-plantar (ankle)	10	—	4.4	

Repetitive Stimulation	Ulnar	Facial	Accessory	Peroneal
Rest (% decrement)	10	18	20	3
Exercise duration (sec)	60	15	15	60
Postexercise (% decrement)				
Immediate	0	3	4	3
30 sec	0	6	8	2
1 min	2	10	12	1
2 min	8	18	19	3
3 min	10	22†	27†	3

ELECTROMYOGRAPHY

Muscle	Insertional Activity	Spontaneous Activity		Motor Unit Potentials	
		Fibrillation Potentials	*Fasciculation Potentials*	*Recruitment*	*Duration/Amplitude*
Anterior tibial	Normal	0	0	Normal	
Vastus medialis	Normal	0	0	Normal	
First dorsal interosseous (manus)	Normal	0	0	Normal	
Biceps brachii	Normal	0	0	Normal but slight variation in MUP amplitude	
Upper trapezius	Normal	0	0	Slight short-duration MUP with amplitude varying	
Cervical paraspinals	Normal	0	0	—	

*Repetitive stimulation—2 Hz, % decrement (no increment).
†10-second exercise repeated and repair of decrement reproduced.
Abbreviations: EDB, extensor digitorum brevis; MUP, motor unit potential.

involvement; (5) median antidromic sensory study could be involved early in a polyradiculoneuropathy[2]; and (6) medial plantar NCS can exclude a subtle sensory neuropathy. Ideally, proximal lower limb NCS should be performed, but it is technically difficult and more uncomfortable for the patient. The femoral NCS may show significant findings as one of the first abnormal nerves in LEMS. LEMS usually displays an initial low CMAP at rest, and a more profound decremental response than seen in myasthe-

nia gravis, with a marked incremental response following brief periods of exercise.[26, 42]

The needle examination should include the proximal and distal muscles of the upper and lower limbs to exclude myopathy, motor neuron disease, and define the extent of involvement. Myasthenia gravis is essentially an inflammatory myopathy and can present with EMG findings of occasional fibrillation potentials and short-duration, polyphasic, low-amplitude MUPs leading to confusion with

CASE 4

A 50-year-old dentist presented with weakness of the nondominant left hand and heaviness of the right arm. He denied sensory symptoms and felt this had progressed over the past 6 months. He jogged regularly and noticed that this seemed to be more difficult, although his running distance remained the same. He had no difficulty chewing or swallowing and denied bowel or bladder difficulties. He complained of left-hand muscle loss and occasional cramps and muscle twitches.

Clinical examination showed normal sensory findings, brisk upper and lower extremity muscle stretch reflexes, positive Babinski signs in both feet, and a normal cranial nerve examination. Manual muscle testing demonstrated moderate weakness of the median- and ulnar-innervated left-hand intrinsics and forearm pronators, and mild right ulnar-innervated hand weakness, although the wrist and long finger flexors remained normal. Fasciculations were present in the calves and both upper extremities.

inflammatory myopathy.[53] Repetitive stimulation is necessary to differentiate these disorders. Looking for variation of amplitude with repetitive firing of a single MUP is a sensitive but nonspecific finding of neuromuscular junction involvement.[29, p. 265]

The diagnosis in this case is a postsynaptic disorder of neuromuscular junction transmission characteristic of the type seen in myasthenia gravis.

Arm Weakness (Case 4)

THOUGHT PROCESS. The primary concern in the differential diagnosis is motor neuron disease, specifically amyotrophic lateral sclerosis (ALS). Multifocal motor neuropathy with conduction block could present in this manner and warrants exclusion given the prognostic implications, but is unlikely to present with brisk reflexes.[35] Other causes of motor neuropathy, polyradiculoneuropathy, neuromuscular junction disorders, and myopathies or dystrophies should be considered. Inclusion body myositis[38] could present in this manner, but the brisk reflexes and distribution of weakness would be somewhat unusual. Cervical spondylosis may also present with lower motor neuron findings in the upper limbs and upper motor neuron findings in the lower limbs.[47] The electrophysiological evaluation is noted in Table 8–4.

DISCUSSION. Nerve conduction studies were selected to assess motor nerves for degree of axon integrity and to exclude conduction block. The ulnar nerve was stimulated at the wrist, elbow, upper arm, and supraclavicular fossa to look for proximal conduction block. A search for proximal conduction block was also the purpose of the F-wave studies. Repetitive stimulation can be helpful to determine whether the disorder is more rapidly progressive. A decremental response and motor unit variability indicate immaturity and instability of neuromuscular junctions which occur with rapid denervation and reinnervation.[13]

The diagnosis of ALS is a clinical diagnosis and cannot be made based solely on NCS and EMG data. The findings on these studies are sensitive and often uncover evidence of denervation in clinically unaffected muscles. In early motor neuron disease, MUP morphology often changes without fibrillation or fasciculation potentials being present. Given the prognosis of this disorder, fulfilling Lambert's EMG criteria of fibrillation potentials in at least two muscles innervated by different nerves and root levels in at least three limbs is recommended.[33] When bulbar symptoms are present, findings in cranial muscles, usually the tongue, can substitute for one of the three limbs. This finding is more specific for ALS. Fasciculation potentials in and of themselves are nonspecific and can be present normally and in many other disorders affecting the motor unit (see Chapter 7).[48, 49]

ALS can present with unilateral hand weakness.[11] Occasionally, shoulder girdle weakness is the principal early finding and shoulder girdle neuropathies such as long thoracic, spinal accessory, or suprascapular neuropathies should be considered and excluded if the clinical examination warrants. The NCS and muscles for needle examination should be selected based on the clinical findings.

Inclusion body myositis (IBM) is sometimes confused

TABLE 8–4   Case 4: Arm Weakness

NERVE CONDUCTION STUDIES

Nerve Stimulation (Record)	Amplitude (μV)	Conduction Velocity (ms)	Latencies (ms)	
			Distal	*F-Wave*
Motor				
peroneal (EDB)	4400	42	4.9	52.5
L ulnar* (hypothenar)	**4700**	54	3.0	28.0
L median (thenar)	**4300**	52	3.8	27.5
Sensory				
sural (ankle)	10	45	4.0	27.5
L ulnar (fifth)	25	63	2.8	

ELECTROMYOGRAPHY

Muscle	Insertional Activity	Spontaneous Activity		Motor Unit Potentials		
		Fibrillation Potentials	*Fasciculation Potentials*	*Recruitment*	*Duration/ Amplitude*	*Phases/ Turns*
L anterior tibial	Increased	0	+	Reduced	Increased	—
L vastus medialis	Increased	0		Reduced	Increased	—
L gluteus medius	Increased	+	+	Reduced	Increased	Increased
L medial gastrocnemius	Increased	+	+ +	Reduced	Increased	—
L first dorsal interosseous (manus)	Increased	+ + +	+ +	Reduced	Increased	Increased
L flexor pollicis longus	Increased	+	+	Reduced	Increased	—
L pronator teres	Increased	+ +	+ +	Reduced	Increased	—
L biceps brachii	Increased	+	+	Reduced	Increased	—
R first dorsal interosseous (manus)	Increased	+ +	+ +	Reduced	Increased	—
R triceps	Increased	+	+ +	Reduced	Increased	—
R deltoid	Increased	+	+	Reduced	Increased	—
R cervical paraspinals	Increased	+	+			—
R midthoracic paraspinals	Increased	+ +	+ +			—

*Includes four-point stimulation to Erb's point and 2-Hz repetitive stimulation at rest—15% decrement noted.
Abbreviations: EDB, extensor digitorum brevis; L, left; R, right.

with motor neuron disease. The history of slowly progressive weakness and findings on EMG of diffuse fibrillation and fasciculation potentials may cause confusion. The fasciculation potentials seen in IBM are typically fewer in number than in ALS. IBM can show long-duration, high-amplitude MUPs that distract the electromyographer from the simultaneous presence of short-duration, low-amplitude MUPs. The clinical examination in IBM generally demonstrates more severe involvement of the iliopsoas, quadriceps, biceps brachii, and triceps, and does not show hyperreflexia or other upper motor neuron signs.[38]

The findings in this case are classic for a diffuse disorder of motor neurons and, given the clinical history and examination, a diagnosis of ALS is most appropriate.

Hand Numbness and Weakness (Case 5)

Nerve conduction studies and EMG are very useful in determining the cause of hand numbness and weakness. Often the patient's report of symptoms is definite, yet vague in terms of distribution. Anatomical variation may also lead to confusion in clinical evaluation and diagnosis of hand symptoms. The following cases illustrate the benefit of an electrophysiological evaluation.

THOUGHT PROCESS. The differential diagnosis in this case is complicated by many symptoms that could be attributed to a musculoskeletal etiology. The sensory loss in the entire hand can be characteristic of median neuropathy though not clearly median only. Her symptoms are common for carpal tunnel syndrome[46] but a median neuropathy in the forearm or plexopathy or concomitant ulnar neuropathy should also be considered. She could have a radiculopathy, but the history and examination do not support this diagnosis. Burning pain in the hands could be due to a small fiber neuropathy or other peripheral neuropathy, but this is highly unusual without simultaneous lower extremity symptoms. The results of the electrophysiological evaluation are presented in Table 8–5.

DISCUSSION. Starting the evaluation with a median motor conduction study guides the examiner to select the most appropriate sensory nerve conduction study. Stevens[54] has demonstrated that when comparing median and ulnar motor distal latencies in the same hand, values should be within 1.8 ms of each other. In this case, the distal latencies

obtained in the right hand show a clear median-to-ulnar discrepancy. However, this does not necessarily mean the lesion is at the wrist. Because of the severity of median nerve involvement, we no longer need a sensitive test to assess median nerve function. We need an accurate and reliable method to assess sensory axons remaining in the median nerve. Therefore, a median antidromic sensory study was performed. Findings in the left hand showed no significant discrepancy in motor distal latencies. A very sensitive test which assesses conduction across the carpal tunnel was selected—palmar sensory studies.[25]

The purpose of doing ulnar motor and sensory conduction studies is to exclude ulnar neuropathy, plexopathy, peripheral neuropathy, assist in exclusion of a C8 radiculopathy, and to serve as a means of comparison of conduction at the wrist. When these nerve conduction studies fail to reveal a clinically suspected abnormality, other conduction studies comparing median-to-radial sensory distal latencies at the thumb, ulnar-to-median latencies to the fourth finger, wrist-to-palm latency and amplitude to the middle finger, and antidromic digital nerve studies to the involved digits can be useful.[25]

The needle examination was initiated in the first dorsal interosseous nerve of the hand, as this is relatively well tolerated by the patient and helps exclude ulnar neuropathy or C8 radiculopathy. Examination of the abductor pollicis brevis (APB) is important to measure motor axon integrity and further define the severity of the neuropathy. If this is abnormal, a median neuropathy in the arm or forearm cannot be excluded. Therefore, the pronator teres was also studied. Pronator teres examination also allows assessment for a C6 or C7 radiculopathy which can also present with index and middle finger numbness. To completely study all components of the median nerve, examination of the flexor pollicis longus can be performed to assess anterior interosseous function. Given the clear-cut median neuropathy at the right wrist, and a much milder median neuropathy at the left wrist by NCS, only the left APB was examined. Given the normal findings, further studies were not performed. Other coexisting problems could be present and clinical judgment should be used to determine if further studies are needed. In the case of hand numbness with normal nerve conduction studies and APB needle examina-

CASE 5

A 38-year-old woman working in a meatpacking plant described a 6-month history of forearm, wrist, and hand pain which began in the right hand and more recently occurred in the left. She had burning pain in the palms of both hands and frequently awakened at night with numbness of the entire hand and fingers. The numbness was often relieved by changing positions or shaking her hands. The pain was usually worse by the end of the day after working, where she performed repetitive activities throughout her shift. She also complained of neck pain and headaches. Her symptoms were getting progressively worse.

Clinical examination revealed normal upper limb muscle stretch reflex and motor examination. Sensory examination revealed decreased pain and touch sensation along the palmar surface of the index and middle fingers of the right hand and positive Tinel's and Phalen's signs at the right wrist. A Tinel sign was also present at both elbows, although less pronounced. Neck and shoulder examination, including foraminal compression and thoracic outlet maneuvers, was normal except for soft tissue tenderness and some limited active range of motion of the neck.

TABLE 8–5   Case 5: Hand Numbness and Weakness

NERVE CONDUCTION STUDIES

Nerve Stimulation (Record)	Amplitude (µV)	Conduction Velocity (ms)	Latencies (ms)	
			Distal	F-Wave
Motor				
R median (thenar)	6200	52	**7.8**	32.5
R ulnar (hypothenar)	7400	54	2.8	29.5
L median (thenar)	8000	54	4.0	29.5
L ulnar (hypothenar)	8000	54	3.0	29.5
Sensory				
R median (index)	**NR**			
R ulnar (fifth)	20	65	3.0	
L median (palm)	80	60	**2.5**	
L ulnar (palm)	50	63	1.8	

ELECTROMYOGRAPHY

Muscle	Insertional Activity	Spontaneous Activity		Motor Unit Potentials		
		Fibrillation Potentials	Fasciculation Potentials	Recruitment	Duration/ Amplitude	Phases/ Turns
R first dorsal interosseous (manus)	Normal	0	0	Normal	Normal	—
R abductor pollicis brevis	Increased	+	0	Decreased	Increased	Increased
R pronator teres	Normal	0	0	Normal	Normal	—
R flexor pollicis longus	Normal	0	0	Normal	Normal	—
L abductor pollicis brevis	Normal	0	0	Normal	Normal	—

tion, a more thorough study of the upper limb is indicated to exclude radiculopathy.

The results of this evaluation demonstrate a focal median neuropathy at each wrist, more pronounced on the right, typical of carpal tunnel syndrome.

Hand Numbness and Weakness (Case 6)

THOUGHT PROCESS. The differential diagnosis in this case includes ulnar neuropathy, most likely due to compression at the elbow as a result of positioning during back surgery. Though the nerve is most vulnerable at the elbow, the patient could have compression at other sites along the course of the ulnar nerve. This patient may have had intravenous or intra-arterial catheters placed in the arm at the time of surgery, and depending on the location, could have a more distal ulnar nerve lesion. However, weakness of the wrist flexors indicates a lesion at the elbow or proximal to the elbow. Other considerations include a low cervical radiculopathy or lower trunk or medial cord plexopathy. The electrophysiological examination is described in Table 8–6.

DISCUSSION. The findings are most consistent with a focal ulnar neuropathy with conduction block proximal to the below-elbow stimulation site. To further define the location of the conduction block, "short segment stimulation" was performed as demonstrated in Figure 8–1. Conduction block was found at the level of the medial epicondyle.

The borderline ulnar and median SNAP amplitudes, with slight slowing of conduction velocities and mild changes found in distal muscles of both upper limbs, could represent a peripheral neuropathy. If this finding does not clearly correlate with the clinical history and examination, further studies in the lower extremity are indicated to demonstrate electrophysiologically whether a neuropathy is present. To assess the presence of generalized neuropathy, one may begin NCS in the lower limb at the risk of performing multiple additional studies. This was not necessary in this case. The other possibility explaining these findings is median neuropathy at the wrist, but given a lack of discrepancy in median and ulnar sensory distal latencies, knowing that these were determined over the same distance, and with slowing of conduction velocities, and first dorsal interosseous involvement, it is unlikely that a median neuropathy at the wrist explains these findings.

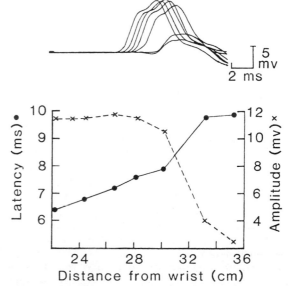

FIGURE 8–1 Ulnar neuropathy at the elbow. Localization with short segment stimulation.

CASE 6

A 60-year-old diabetic man complained of left-hand numbness and weakness in the postoperative period following lumbar spinal fusion. He described neck pain which was worse when sitting and noted paresthesias along the medial aspect of the hand and fifth digit.

Clinical examination revealed focal findings in the left upper extremity with moderate weakness of the dorsal interossei, mild weakness of wrist flexors and lumbricals, and normal thumb opposition and flexion. Pain and touch sensation were diminished in the fifth digit and the medial aspect of the fourth digit and hand. Tinel's sign was not present at the wrist or elbow. Shoulder and neck examinations were remarkable only for some soft tissue tenderness in the posterior cervical musculature.

The needle examination was extended to additional upper extremity muscles to assure that a more proximal process was not influencing the findings, particularly given the history of diabetes. The flexor digitorum profundus was examined because the flexor carpi ulnaris may be spared in ulnar neuropathy at the elbow.[10] The opposite extremity was studied, since the manner of positioning for spine surgery puts both ulnar nerves at risk and because many patients have bilateral ulnar neuropathies at the elbows given anatomical, and in this case, a diabetic predisposition.[39]

The conclusion of these studies is that the patient has an ulnar neuropathy at the level of the left medial epicondyle. Reduced MUP recruitment in the flexor carpi ulnaris and flexor digitorum profundus muscles indicates that this is most likely an acute conduction block lesion which will likely resolve. The severity and distribution of EMG findings in hand muscles is likely due to an underlying peripheral neuropathy.

Hand Numbness and Weakness (Case 7)

THOUGHT PROCESS. The most likely diagnosis in this case is a radial nerve injury due to improper use of axillary crutches, since compression in the axilla by axillary crutches can result in radial nerve injury at this level. However, in this case, the sparing of the triceps and brachioradialis indicates that the radial nerve lesion is distal to the axilla, possibly at the humeral groove where the radial nerve courses laterally and anterior to the humerus.[14] A classic cause of wristdrop is lead neuropathy, which

TABLE 8–6   Case 6: Hand Numbness and Weakness

NERVE CONDUCTION STUDIES

Nerve Stimulation (Record)	Amplitude (μV)	Conduction Velocity (ms)	Latencies (ms)	
			Distal	F-Wave
Motor				
L median (thenar)	5600	55	3.8	29.5
L ulnar (hypothenar)			3.5	32.0
Wrist	8700	45		
Below elbow	8400	**48**		
Elbow	**5800**	**46**		
Upper arm	**5600**	**48**		
Supraclavicular	**5300**	**50**		
R ulnar (hypothenar)				
Wrist	8700		3.5	29.0
Elbow	8400	53		
Sensory				
L ulnar (fifth)	10	52	3.8	
L median (index)	12	52	3.8	

ELECTROMYOGRAPHY

Muscle	Insertional Activity	Spontaneous Activity		Motor Unit Potentials	
		Fibrillation Potentials	Fasciculation Potentials	Recruitment	Duration/Amplitude
R first dorsal interosseous (manus)	Increased	+	0	Reduced	Increased
R abductor pollicis brevis	Increased	+	0	Normal	Mildly increased
R flexor pollicis longus	Normal	0	0	Normal	Normal
R flexor carpi ulnaris	Normal	0	0	Reduced	Normal
R pronator teres	Normal	0	0	Normal	Normal
R triceps	Normal	0	0	Normal	Normal
L first dorsal interosseous (manus)	Increased	+	0	Reduced	Increased
R lower cervical paraspinals	Normal	0	0		

CASE 7

A 27-year-old skier fractured his right tibia, requiring ambulation with axillary crutches. One month after the fracture, he noticed tingling over the dorsum of his left hand. He ignored this and 2 weeks later awoke with a left wristdrop. He was otherwise symptom-free.

Clinical examination showed impaired pain sensation over the dorsum of the hand, thumb, index, and middle fingers. Motor examination revealed moderate weakness of the wrist and finger extensors with normal elbow flexion and extension, pronation, supination, and wrist and finger flexion. Upper extremity reflexes were normal except for a decreased left brachioradialis reflex.

despite being a systemic illness tends to have a predilection for asymmetrical involvement of the radial nerves.[51] Cervical radiculopathy, incomplete posterior cord plexopathy, inflammatory neuropathy, and hereditary tendency to pressure palsies are other considerations. The nerve conduction studies and EMG are presented in Table 8–7.

DISCUSSION. The median antidromic sensory study was performed first. Since the radial SNAP may be technically more difficult to obtain, proving that the upper extremity sensory nerves are generally normal can make radial nerve findings easier to interpret later. In addition, since these findings could be explained by a plexopathy, early demonstration that nonradial sensory nerve fibers are normal contributes to the exclusion of plexopathy and peripheral neuropathy. With focal neurological examination findings, directing studies to the radial nerve is the next most logical step. Generally, in performing radial sensory and motor conduction studies, stimulating at the elbow is sufficient unless one specifically suspects a conduction block. In this case, more proximal stimulation demonstrates a site of conduction block at an anatomically vulnerable site. The ulnar motor conduction study was performed to complete the study of brachial plexus levels and to exclude plexopathy.

The EMG was initiated by deltoid examination since this muscle is innervated by the axillary nerve, the other branch of the posterior cord of the brachial plexus. Normal findings here indicated that a plexopathy involving the posterior cord was unlikely. The biceps was examined to further assess the midcervical roots. Radial innervated muscles were examined, starting with the most proximally innervated, the triceps. The triceps is innervated proximal to the humeral groove and was normal. The brachioradialis was then examined and found to be abnormal. The normal biceps brachii study supports a diagnosis of radial neuropathy rather than a C5 or C6 radiculopathy. The pronator teres was examined to study a median-innervated muscle which could be involved in a C6 or C7 radiculopathy or plexopathy. It was normal. A distal radial-innervated muscle was then examined which showed severe involvement. Finally, the anconeus, saved for last since it is a relatively

TABLE 8–7   Case 7: Hand Numbness and Weakness

NERVE CONDUCTION STUDIES

Nerve Stimulation (Record)	Amplitude (μV)	Conduction Velocity (ms)	Latencies (ms)	
			Distal	F-Wave
Motor				
Radial (extensor indicis proprius)				
Elbow	4000	52	4.2	
Humeral groove*	NR			
Ulnar (hypothenar)	12000	53	3.2	29.0
Sensory				
Median (index)	57	68	3.0	
Radial (dorsum of thenar)	NR			

ELECTROMYOGRAPHY

Muscle	Insertional Activity	Spontaneous Activity		Motor Unit Potentials	
		Fibrillation Potentials	Fasciculation Potentials	Recruitment	Duration/Amplitude
Deltoid	Normal	0	0	Normal	Normal
Biceps brachii	Normal	0	0	Normal	Normal
Triceps	Normal	0	0	Normal	Normal
Brachioradialis	Increased	+	0	Decreased	Increased
Pronator teres	Normal	0	0	Normal	Normal
Extensor indicis proprius	Increased	+ + +	0	Decreased	Increased
Anconeus	Increased	+	0	Decreased	Increased

*Inching shows conduction block between the humeral groove and elbow stimulation sites.
Abbreviation: NR, no response.

difficult muscle to examine, was studied to determine at which level the axonal loss affecting the radial nerve occurred, because it is the next radial muscle innervated after the triceps branches.

The NCS findings indicate a radial neuropathy with conduction block at the humeral groove. The EMG showed evidence of axonal loss sparing the triceps but involving those muscles innervated distal to the radial nerve as it courses through the groove. These findings are also commonly seen in "Saturday night palsy," a compression neuropathy of the radial nerve at the humeral groove.

LOWER LIMB PROBLEMS

As in the upper extremities, disorders that affect the lower extremities may be localized or represent generalized processes. Lumbar and sacral radiculopathies are more often bilateral than are cervical radiculopathies, but lumbar or sacral plexopathies are less often bilateral than are brachial plexopathies. Entrapment neuropathies in the lower limbs and mononeuropathies are also less common than in the upper limbs. Peroneal nerve compression at the fibular head is the most common lower extremity mononeuropathy. Less common lower extremity mononeuropathies include involvement of the femoral, tibial, sciatic, plantar, saphenous, and lateral femoral cutaneous nerves.

Generalized disorders that can begin or present with lower limb weakness or numbness include inflammatory myopathies, most peripheral neuropathies and polyradiculoneuropathies, inclusion body myositis, motor neuron disease, and neuromuscular junction disorders, particularly LEMS. The following cases serve to illustrate more common lower limb problems.

Case 8

THOUGHT PROCESS. The differential diagnosis includes chronic lumbosacral radiculopathy or polyradiculopathy from spinal stenosis or perhaps diabetes. A diabetic peripheral neuropathy could be present, but the examination and history are not suggestive. Peripheral neuropathies of other types should be considered. Other causes of polyradiculopathy such as conus ependymoma, other intraspinal tumors, or infectious disorders including meningeal sarcoidosis, could present in this fashion, but would usually have other features not present in this case. An inflammatory polyradiculopathy or vasculitis could cause these examination findings, but usually also involve the upper extremities and demonstrate a more stuttering course with acute or subacute worsening.[9, 44] These disorders are unlikely to cause neurogenic claudication of which this patient appears to be complaining. A lumbosacral plexopathy could be present but is unlikely to be bilateral, and in diabetes it usually presents with acute and severe pain affecting a single lower extremity.[56, pp. 1228–1229] Cauda equina tumors or perhaps even conus medullaris tumors could present with some of these features, but usually more severe neurological findings and bladder and bowel symptoms would result. Spinal cord arteriovenous malformation is an important consideration. Of course, vascular disease as a cause of leg pain must also be considered. The NCS and EMG are presented in Table 8–8.

DISCUSSION. NCS were performed to assess the degree of axonal loss from the suspected polyradiculopathy and to help exclude peripheral neuropathy, lumbosacral plexopathy, or nonstructural causes of polyradiculopathy. The peroneal motor study recording from the extensor digitorum brevis provided an assessment of the L5 root and sciatic and peroneal nerves. The tibial study provided information about the S1 root and sciatic and tibial nerves. A femoral NCS could have been done, but it is technically more difficult, more uncomfortable for the patient, and does not assist us in excluding problems affecting distal peripheral nerves. The sural sensory conduction study was performed since it is the most reliable lower extremity sensory conduction study, and it helped exclude lumbosacral plexopathy or peripheral neuropathy. Even though the sural SNAP was normal, a mild distal neuropathy could still be present as the sural SNAP is recorded along the nerve trunk at the ankle and not along its most terminal

CASE 8

A 77-year-old woman with a 2-year history of non-insulin-dependent diabetes who was otherwise healthy presented with a 10-year history of low back pain which increased in the past year. She also noted leg pain during the last 6 months. When walking more than one block, she developed aching in the posterior thighs and calves. If she stopped, leaned forward over a fence, or sat on a park bench, the pain resolved over 10 to 15 minutes. She noted less difficulty with leg pain while pushing a grocery cart while shopping. She noted some transient tingling in the legs and was not certain of the distribution or of exacerbating factors. She also experienced occasional stress incontinence but this had not changed in 15 years. Coughing or sneezing did not exacerbate the pain. Sitting was more comfortable than standing but any static position for prolonged periods irritated her back. She denied weight loss, fatigue, or night pain.

Clinical examination showed normal lower extremity pulses and temperature. Spine examination showed limited lumbar range of motion and mild scoliosis with the major curve in the lumbar spine. There was no spine percussion pain. Straight leg raising was negative bilaterally. Muscle stretch reflexes were normal in the upper extremities and knees, but depressed internal hamstring and Achilles reflexes were present bilaterally. Mild calf and foot intrinsic atrophy was present. Sensory examination was remarkable only for decreased vibratory sensation in the toes.

TABLE 8–8   Case 8: Low Back and Leg Pain

NERVE CONDUCTION STUDIES*

Nerve Stimulation (Record)	Amplitude (µV)	Conduction Velocity (ms)	Latencies (ms)	
			Distal	F-Wave
Motor				
Peroneal (EDB)	**1700**	42	5.3	58.0
Tibial (AH)	2300	42	4.9	60.0
Sensory				
Sural (ankle)	8		4.0	

ELECTROMYOGRAPHY

Muscle	Insertional Activity	Spontaneous Activity		Motor Unit Potentials		
		Fibrillation Potentials	Fasciculation Potentials	Recruitment	Duration/Amplitude	Phases/Turns
R anterior tibial	Normal	0	0	Reduced	Increased	—
R medial gastrocnemius	Increased	0	+	Reduced	Increased	—
R peroneus longus	Increased	+	+	Reduced	Increased	Increased
R vastus medialis	Normal	0	0	Reduced	Increased	—
R adductor longus	Normal	0	0	Normal	Normal	—
R tensor fascia lata	Decreased	0	0	Reduced	Increased	—
R gluteus maximus	Normal	0	+	Reduced	Increased	—
R lower lumbar paraspinals	Increased	+	0			—
R high lumbar paraspinals	Increased	+	0			—
R lower thoracic paraspinals	Normal	0	0			—
L peroneal longus	Increased	0	0	Reduced	Increased	—
L medial gastrocnemius	Increased	0	0			—
L vastus medialis	Normal	0	0			
L adductor longus	Normal	0	0	Normal	Normal	

*No conduction block or temporal dispersion noted.
Abbreviations: EDB, extensor digitorum brevis; AH, abductor hallucis.

fibers. A medial-plantar SNAP could be attempted, particularly in a younger person to exclude peripheral neuropathy, although is not likely to be present in normal persons at this age.[40] Further NCS were not performed given the symmetry of the symptoms and signs. However, when findings include generally low CMAPs, LEMS should be considered. If weakness had been the predominant feature of this case, further motor conduction studies and repetitive stimulation would have been performed. An H-reflex can be performed if the needle examination is negative.

The needle examination strategy is to study muscles innervated by the principal nerve roots and nerves to the legs. The anterior tibial provides peroneal and L4–5 root assessment; the medial gastrocnemius, L5–S1 root and tibial nerve. Other L5-innervated muscles, such as the peroneus longus, posterior tibial, or extensor hallucis longus, could be examined. Given abnormalities in the L5–S1 distribution, the next level to assess is L4, so the vastus medialis was studied. With further abnormality here, we have not yet defined the level of the lesion. A severe peripheral neuropathy can explain these findings, so the proximal muscles were examined. The adductor longus provides information about the L2–3 roots and obturator nerve. Assessment of more proximal muscles innervated by L5, the tensor fascia lata, and S1, the gluteus maximus, were also abnormal. Based on the information obtained so far, this appeared likely to be due to a root level disorder, but a plexopathy could not be completely excluded. Of concern in a diabetic patient is that multiple neurological problems can coexist.[56, pp. 1219–1230] To place the level of the disorder at the root, paraspinal muscles were examined. Because of the concern regarding a more widespread diabetic polyradiculopathy, paraspinous muscle examination was extended into the thoracic level to exclude generalized spinal level involvement.[29, pp. 449–450]

The conclusion of the electrophysiological studies is that this patient has multiple chronic lumbosacral radiculopathies, more severe on the right. Given the clinical symptoms and signs, this is most likely structural, related to spinal stenosis. Further studies, including imaging of the lumbar spine, are warranted to exclude an intraspinal lesion, including arteriovenous malformation.[4]

Lower Extremity Weakness (Case 9)

THOUGHT PROCESS. The differential diagnosis includes polyradiculopathy or polyradiculoneuropathy. A primarily motor polyradiculopathy, such as an inflammatory polyradiculopathy, could present in this manner. Motor neuron disease is certainly a consideration, although, without hyperactive reflexes, this is not classic for ALS.[11] A myopathy or late-onset dystrophy or early LEMS could present in this way. Of particular note is the pattern of weakness which is typical in IBM.[38] A disorder of the spinal cord, particularly involving anterior horn cells, could produce this picture. A combination of a motor disorder and a peripheral neuropathy must be considered given the abnormal sensory examination. The electrophysiological findings are presented in Table 8–9.

DISCUSSION. NCS were initiated with the peroneal

[handwritten marginalia: Lambert-Eaton; Inclusion body myositis]

CASE 9

A 60-year-old man with a 50-pack-year history of smoking complained of leg weakness which began approximately 6 months previously. He denied pain, sensory, or bowel or bladder changes, and primarily noted that his legs felt heavy and fatigued. Ascending or descending stairs was more difficult. The right leg seemed worse to him than the left leg. He denied difficulty chewing, swallowing, breathing, or double vision.

Clinical examination revealed normal mental status and cranial nerves. Muscle stretch reflexes were slightly depressed from normal in the lower limbs. Vibratory and touch sensations were mildly diminished distally. Motor examination revealed mild weakness of the triceps and most lower extremity muscle groups. The quadriceps was weaker than any other muscle group and the anterior thighs demonstrated significant atrophy.

motor study to assess distal motor axons (proximal L5 root, peroneal nerve) and because this study lends itself to easy repetitive stimulation testing. The borderline amplitude could represent any of the above disorders or be normal. Repetitive stimulation performed at rest to screen primarily for a presynaptic neuromuscular junction disorder was normal. The absent sural SNAP is likely due to a neuropathy. To further examine the sensory nerves, a median antidromic study was done. Low amplitude and slow conduction velocity correlate with a peripheral neuropathy, but a median neuropathy could also produce these findings. An ulnar SNAP was obtained which demonstrated an abnormality and supported the conclusion that a peripheral neuropathy was likely. An ulnar motor study was conducted to determine the extent of upper limb neuropathy.

On needle examination, the mixture of MUPs of both

increased and decreased amplitude and duration in the anterior tibial muscle could represent a combined myopathy and neuropathy, chronic myopathy, or IBM. The medial gastrocnemius was examined to explore findings in a muscle at a comparable distal anatomical level and similar findings were noted. Because of the question of a coexisting peripheral neuropathy, a foot muscle was studied and was more severely involved with only large MUPs present. This favored a coexisting neuropathy. Proximal lower limb muscles showed that the quadriceps was most severely involved. Moving to the upper limb becomes important, since subclinical findings of neuropathy and myopathy may be present. Here, more subtle changes were noted and again, a mixture of large and small MUPs in some muscles were noted with the most severe involvement in the triceps.

Based on the electrophysiological studies alone, a coex-

TABLE 8–9   Case 9: Lower Extremity Weakness

NERVE CONDUCTION STUDIES

Nerve Stimulation (Record)	Amplitude (μV)	Conduction Velocity (ms)	Latencies (ms)	
			Distal	F-Wave
Motor				
R peroneal (EDB)*	2300	42	4.8	55.0
R tibial (AH)	3600	41	5.2	56.0
R ulnar (hypothenar)	7200	52	3.2	
Sensory				
L sural (ankle)	NR			
R median (index)	10	53	3.4	
R ulnar (fifth)	5		3.0	

ELECTROMYOGRAPHY

Muscle	Insertional Activity	Spontaneous Activity		Motor Unit Potentials		
		Fibrillation Potentials	Fasciculation Potentials	Recruitment	Duration/Amplitude	Phases/ Turns
R anterior tibial	Increased	+	0	Reduced	Increased and decreased	—
R medial gastrocnemius	Increased	+	0	Reduced	Increased and decreased	—
R abductor hallucis	Increased	+ +	0	Reduced	Increased	—
R rectus femoris	Increased	+ + +	+	Reduced	Increased and decreased	Increased
R tensor fascia lata	Increased	+	0		Increased and decreased	—
R first dorsal interosseous (manus)	Normal	0	0	Reduced	Increased	—
R triceps	Increased	+	+	Reduced	Increased and decreased	—
R biceps	Normal	0	+	Normal	Normal	—
R midthoracic paraspinals	Increased	0	+			—

*2-Hz repetitive stimulation at rest and following brief exercise is normal.
Abbreviations: EDB, extensor digitorum brevis; AH, abductor hallucis; NR, no response.

CASE 10

A 20-year-old college student awakened with right leg and ankle weakness and numbness. She had attended a party, where she used alcohol heavily, and had fallen asleep on her bedroom floor. She sought evaluation 3 days after onset of these symptoms.

Clinical examination was normal except for a patch of sensory loss on the dorsum of the right foot and weakness of the ankle dorsiflexors, evertors, and toe extensors.

---

isting myopathy and peripheral neuropathy is the most likely diagnosis. However, taken together with the clinical pattern of weakness and the more severe involvement of the quadriceps and triceps confirmed by needle examination, IBM must be considered. This can be confirmed only on muscle biopsy.

IBM is often associated with some neuropathic findings and fasciculation potentials, which can be confusing. Sensory studies are often not as significantly affected as in the case presented here. A not uncommon mistake is to ignore or not recognize the presence of short-duration, low-amplitude MUPs in the face of others of long duration and high amplitude, resulting in an incorrect conclusion of motor neuron disease. There is no cure for either condition but the prognosis for IBM is more positive than for motor neuron disease.[38]

Foot Numbness and Pain (Case 10)

THOUGHT PROCESS. The diagnosis here is almost certainly a peroneal neuropathy most likely due to compression at the fibular head. Included in the differential diagnosis is a more proximal peroneal or sciatic neuropathy or an L5 radiculopathy. With a radiculopathy, the ankle invertors should also be weak. A lumbosacral plexopathy is unlikely to present with such isolated findings. Hereditary tendency to pressure palsies should also be considered, but in this patient there was no history of prior nerve palsies or family history of nerve problems. Table 8–10 outlines the electrophysiological findings.

DISCUSSION. Starting with the peroneal motor conduction study was the most logical first step, given the high clinical suspicion that a peroneal neuropathy was present. The large discrepancy between the ankle and knee

CMAP amplitudes requires stimulation distal to the site most common for compression. Stimulation at or just below the fibular head showed an amplitude similar to the ankle amplitude, indicating a conduction block proximal to this point of stimulation. Short segment stimulation was performed to specifically localize the lesion. The superficial peroneal nerve was studied to evaluate which divisions of the peroneal nerve were involved, and to help exclude peripheral neuropathy or plexopathy. The tibial NCS was performed strictly to help exclude plexopathy, radiculopathy, or sciatic neuropathy.

The needle examination was performed in muscles that would (1) assess both deep and superficial divisions of the peroneal nerve; (2) explore the tibial division of the sciatic nerve; (3) differentiate an L5 radiculopathy from a peroneal neuropathy; and (4) demonstrate the level of the peroneal neuropathy. The relative acuity of the symptoms did not allow the examiner to define the degree of axonal loss, as the duration of the problem was not sufficient to significantly alter distal axon excitability or cause wallerian degeneration.[79, pp. 64–69] The conduction block signifies at least a neurapraxic lesion at the fibular head. If recovery does not ensue, a repeat study to assess for level of axonal loss and axonotmesis would be useful. The problem was diagnosed as a focal common peroneal neuropathy with conduction block 1 cm proximal to the fibular head.

Generalized Weakness (Case 11)

THOUGHT PROCESS. The most likely diagnosis was thought to be a proximal myopathy or dystrophy. Given the history of an autoimmune thyroid disease, the most likely possibility is another autoimmune disorder such as inflammatory myopathy or myasthenia gravis. The degree

---

CASE 11

A 55-year-old woman presented with a 3-month history of steadily increasing difficulty performing overhead activities such as washing her hair and reaching cupboards. She also noted difficulty arising from low chairs and climbing stairs. She had a history of goiter but was currently euthyroid and otherwise in good health. She denied sensory symptoms, or difficulty with speech or swallowing, although on occasion she felt solids "sticking" in her esophagus. Her weakness did not fluctuate and was not exercise-related. She

denied cramps and had no family history of similar problems.

The clinical examination was remarkable for normal facial strength, muscle stretch reflexes, and sensory examination. Motor examination showed moderate weakness of neck flexors, shoulder girdle, biceps brachii, and triceps muscles, hip girdle, quadriceps, and hamstring muscles. These muscles were not fatigable. Proximal muscle bulk appeared somewhat reduced. Myotonia was not present.

TABLE 8–10   Case 10: Foot Numbness and Pain

NERVE CONDUCTION STUDIES

Nerve Stimulation (Record)	Amplitude (μV)	Conduction Velocity (ms)	Latencies (ms)	
			Distal	F-Wave
Motor				
R peroneal (EDB)				
Ankle	6000		5.2	53.0
Knee	**2500**	**40**		
Fibular head*	5800	51		
R tibial	8800	50	5.2	53.0
Sensory				
R Superficial peroneal (ankle)	20		4.5	

ELECTROMYOGRAPHY

Muscle	Insertional Activity	Spontaneous Activity		Motor Unit Potentials	
		Fibrillation Potentials	Fasciculation Potentials	Recruitment	Duration/Amplitude
Anterior tibial	Normal	0	0	Reduced	Normal
Medial gastrocnemius	Normal	0	0	Normal	Normal
Peroneal longus	Normal	0	0	Reduced	Normal
Posterior tibial	Normal	0	0	Normal	Normal
Biceps femoris, short head	Normal	0	0	Normal	Normal

*Inching demonstrates focal conduction block 1 cm proximal to the fibular head.
Abbreviation: EDB, extensor digitorum brevis.

of limb involvement without facial involvement is more characteristic of polymyositis than of myasthenia gravis (as described in Case 3).

Other considerations in the differential diagnosis include late-onset dystrophy, motor neuron disease, motor neuropathy or polyradiculoneuropathy, thyroid-related myopathy, or a neuromuscular junction defect such as LEMS. The NCS and EMG are presented in Table 8–11.

DISCUSSION. The approach used (1) demonstrated the degree of involvement of both the upper and lower limbs; (2) excluded motor neuropathy or a neuromuscular junction defect; and (3) proved the sensory system was not involved. The peroneal CMAP amplitude was at the lower limits of normal. The sural SNAP was normal. The ulnar motor conduction study was performed because of the ease of performing repetitive stimulation and was normal. Patchy

involvement may be present in myasthenia gravis, so it is necessary to perform repetitive stimulation in an area that is clinically involved. The accessory NCS was chosen because the trapezius was clinically involved, and because of the relative technical ease of performing this study.

The needle examination was performed in proximal and distal muscles of the upper and lower limbs to define the distribution of involvement. It is important in performing a needle examination in inflammatory myopathy to recognize that within a muscle, findings may be fairly localized, with some areas severely involved and other areas that are normal. A careful search in each muscle is important. In subtle cases, the only abnormality found may be in the paraspinous muscles.[1, 55] Paraspinous muscles were not examined in this case owing to the obvious abnormalities in other proximal muscle groups. It is also important to remember that in more

CASE 12

A 33-year-old female assembly line worker presented with forearm pain and hand cramps and noted that fine motor tasks were becoming increasingly more difficult. She denied sensory symptoms or symptoms characteristic of carpal tunnel syndrome. She denied cramps and weakness. She denied a family history of any nerve or muscle problems.

Clinical examination was normal except for weakness of the finger flexors. Obesity impeded the ability to assess for percussion myotonia in the limbs, though tongue myotonia was not present. She did exhibit a delayed relaxation of grip.

Further review determined that the patient had become amenorrheic in her late teens. She also noted increased hand cramping in the cold. She did not have a family history of muscle disease to her knowledge, but did have a family history of diabetes and fertility problems. On examination, the patient had long hair covering the forehead, but on lifting the hair from her forehead, significant frontal balding was noted. The obese face did not display the atrophy that can be characteristic of myotonic dystrophy, but a lid lag was present after tightly closing the eyes.

TABLE 8–11   Case 11: Generalized Weakness

NERVE CONDUCTION STUDIES

Nerve Stimulation (Record)	Amplitude (μV)	Conduction Velocity (ms)	Latencies (ms) Distal	Latencies (ms) F-Wave
Motor				
Peroneal (EDB)	2500	44	5.2	56.0
Ulnar (hypothenar)*	10,500	53	3.2	32.0
Accessory (trapezius)*	3600		4.0	
Sensory				
Sural (ankle)	18		4.0	

ELECTROMYOGRAPHY

Muscle	Insertional Activity	Fibrillation Potentials	Fasciculation Potentials	Recruitment	Duration/Amplitude	Phases/Turns
Anterior tibial	Increased	+	0		Decreased	—
Vastus medialis	Increased	+ +	0	Rapid	Decreased	Increased
Gluteus medius	Increased	+ +	0	Rapid	Decreased	Increased
First dorsal interosseous (manus)	Normal	0	0	Normal	Normal	—
Biceps	Increased	+	0	Rapid	Decreased	Increased

*2-Hz repetitive stimulation at rest and following 1 minute of exercise did not produce a decrement or increment.
Abbreviation: EDB, extensor digitorum brevis.

chronic myopathies, some long-duration, high-amplitude MUPs can be seen, and should not dissuade the examiner from a diagnosis of myopathy.[8] Myasthenia gravis can rarely present with needle examination findings similar to those seen in this case, highlighting the importance of performing repetitive stimulation to assure that this disorder is not overlooked. The most likely diagnosis in this case is a myopathy that results in fiber splitting, vacuolization, and fiber necrosis, as is seen in polymyositis.[7]

Case 12

THOUGHT PROCESS.   This was a puzzling case, given the limited features in a patient who was predisposed to have an overuse syndrome. If finger flexor weakness is not effort-related, a selective distal myopathy or perhaps incomplete nerve entrapment syndrome can produce these findings. The delayed grip relaxation could be a sign of a metabolic disturbance of muscle such as a myotonic disorder or tetany. A peripheral neuropathy could produce these findings, but the lack of sensory features and lower extrem-

ity involvement would be highly atypical. As the electrophysiological studies (Table 8–12) are initiated, the most likely diagnosis is not clear.

DISCUSSION.   NCS were performed on the median and ulnar nerves looking for a nerve entrapment which would explain finger flexor weakness. These studies were normal. The needle examination was somewhat surprising and clearly demonstrated myotonic discharges and myopathic MUP changes affecting the distal muscles most severely. Given these findings, a return to the clinical history and examination was necessary.

These findings are all characteristic of myotonic dystrophy. Myotonic dystrophy is a primarily distal myopathy and may have many associated features which include endocrine, dermatologic, and cardiac complications. Dominantly inherited with incomplete penetrance, some of these features may present in some family members and not others.[22, 23] This case demonstrates that at times the EMG shows unexpected findings, forcing the electrodiagnostician to "go back to the drawing board" by returning to the history and physical examination. This instant feedback on

CASE 13

A 29-year-old man noted tingling of the toes upon awakening one morning. While walking to work, he noted a tendency to catch his toes on sidewalk cracks. By midday, his feet felt numb and walking was generally uncoordinated. Some hand tingling was also noted and by that evening hand clumsiness was present. The patient decided to wait until morning to seek a medical evaluation, and upon awakening the next morning, was unable to get out of bed unassisted and could not walk. He was emergently admitted to a local

hospital and over the next week continued to get weaker and eventually was electively placed on mechanical ventilation. He was in general good health but 3 weeks prior to the onset of these symptoms had experienced a flulike illness.

An EMG was requested 10 days into the course. Clinical examination showed generalized areflexia, sensory loss to all modalities which was worse in the distal upper and lower limbs, and flaccid quadriparesis.

the veracity of one's history and physical examination makes the electrodiagnostician a better clinician over the course of time.

Generalized Numbness (Case 13)

THOUGHT PROCESS. The primary diagnostic consideration in this case was acute inflammatory demyelinating polyradiculoneuropathy (AIDP) or Guillain-Barré syndrome. An idiopathic or inflammatory etiology could be presumed, but other possibilities had to be considered, including arsenic toxicity; axonal neuropathy from a vasculitis; other toxins, including other heavy metals; or porphyria. A dysproteinemia or paraneoplastic syndrome can also present in this manner.[5] The history was strongly in favor of an acquired rather than a hereditary process. The pattern of electrophysiological findings was imperative in guiding the differential diagnosis, because the findings allowed differentiation of axonal from demyelinating and sensory from motor involvement (Table 8–13).

DISCUSSION. This patient was far enough into the course (10 days) to assure that fairly obvious electrophysiological features would be present and identifiable. These findings often lag behind the clinical course. As a rule, starting the NCS and EMG in the lower extremities and then moving to the upper extremities is fairly typical for a peripheral neuropathy assessment. However, if the severity of findings predicted in the legs is so severe that the examiner anticipates lack of evoked action potentials, beginning in the arms is often more feasible. It is also advisable in cases of suspected AIDP to perform studies on multiple motor nerves to define the presence of conduction block and to avoid common sites for conduction block due to compression.[2]

In this case, we were able to obtain reasonable CMAPs from the lower extremities. All studies showed significant temporal dispersion, and focal conduction block was identified in the peroneal nerve just distal to the fibular head. The normal amplitude discrepancy between proximal and distal stimulation of the tibial nerve makes this nerve difficult to assess for conduction block and temporal dispersion unless they are pronounced. The sural SNAP was present and the median SNAP was absent, a finding not uncommon in AIDP. Sensory and motor nerves showed significant slowing. Motor nerves also showed temporal dispersion and conduction block in the upper limbs. Prolonged F-wave latencies were also noted. These were prolonged when correcting for conduction velocity using F-wave estimation, and demonstrated slowing in proximal nerve segments. A musculocutaneous conduction study was performed to demonstrate that proximal slowing was present. Given the severe limb involvement, blink reflexes were recorded and were prolonged, indicating a very proximal peripheral nerve lesion.

The needle examination showed primarily recruitment abnormalities related to conduction block. Given some of the low CMAPs recorded distally over the next few weeks one could expect fibrillation potentials to occur distally and in paraspinal muscles. Studying paraspinal muscles is important to place part of the lesion proximally to confirm the diagnosis of polyradiculoneuropathy. The findings in this case were characteristic of AIDP.

CRANIOFACIAL PROBLEMS

Case 14

Disorders of the head and face present less commonly in the clinical neurophysiological laboratory, but are important to recognize. Disorders that cause facial numbness, pain, twitching, or weakness are the most likely referrals for electrophysiological evaluation. Disorders that result in dysphagia, dysarthria, or vocal cord paralysis can also be

TABLE 8–12   Case 12: Generalized Weakness

NERVE CONDUCTION STUDIES

Nerve Stimulation (Record)	Amplitude (μV)	Conduction Velocity (ms)	Latencies (ms)	
			Distal	*F-Wave*
Motor				
Median (thenar)	6800	56	3.2	31.5
Ulnar (hypothenar)	10,300	55	2.8	31.0
Sensory				
Median (palm-wrist)	160	65	1.8	
Ulnar (palm-wrist)	90	67	1.8	

ELECTROMYOGRAPHY

Muscle	Insertional Activity	Spontaneous Activity		Motor Unit Potentials		
		Fibrillation Potentials	*Fasciculation Potentials*	*Recruitment*	*Duration/ Amplitude*	*Comment*
First dorsal interosseous (manus)	Increased			Difficult to assess	Difficult to assess	Marked myotonic discharges
Pronator teres	Increased	+	0	Rapid	Decreased	Myotonic discharges
Biceps	Increased	0	0	Normal	Normal	Occasional myotonic discharges
Anterior tibial	Increased	+	0	Rapid	Decreased	Myotonic discharges
Gluteus medius	Increased	0	0	Normal	Normal	Occasional myotonic discharges
L cervical paraspinals	Increased	0	0			Myotonic discharges

TABLE 8–13 Case 13: Generalized Numbness

NERVE CONDUCTION STUDIES

Nerve Stimulation (Record)	Amplitude (μV)	Conduction Velocity (ms)	Latencies (ms) Distal	Latencies (ms) F-Wave
Motor				
Peroneal (EDB)	1800	**28**	**6.5**	NR
Tibial (AH)	2700	**32**	**6.5**	77.5
Ulnar (hypothenar)	6600	**44**	**3.8**	51.0
Median (thenar)	4900	**42**	4.4	55.0
Musculocutaneous (biceps)	4500	58	5.2	
Sensory				
Sural (ankle)	**8**			
Median (index)	**NR**			
Ulnar (fifth)	15	52	3.5	
Blink reflex				
R trigeminal (R orbicularis oculi)			$R_1 =$ **18.0** $R_2 =$ 42.5	

ELECTROMYOGRAPHY

Muscle	Insertional Activity	Spontaneous Activity Fibrillation Potentials	Spontaneous Activity Fasciculation Potentials	Motor Unit Potentials Recruitment	Motor Unit Potentials Duration/Amplitude
Anterior tibial	Normal	0	0	None	
Tensor fasciae latae	Normal	0	0	Reduced	Normal
First dorsal interosseous (manus)	Normal	0	0	Reduced	Normal
Biceps	Normal	0	0	Reduced	Normal
L lumbar paraspinals	Normal	0	0		

Abbreviations: EDB, extensor digitorum brevis; AH, abductor hallucis; NR, no response.

evaluated less routinely. The case presented here is of Bell's palsy, since NCS and EMG may be useful in the diagnosis and prognosis of this disorder. Other disorders which lend themselves to evaluation include trigeminal and facial neuropathies from idiopathic, inflammatory, or compressive etiologies such as posterior fossa tumors, most commonly acoustic neuromas. Hemifacial spasm can be well-defined and differentiated from blepharospasm and synkinesis using NCS and EMG, and is usually the result of vascular compression of the facial nerve. As previously discussed, facial weakness can be due to myasthenia gravis or myasthenic syndrome as well as myopathies or dystrophies involving the face. Techniques that can be used for evaluating these problems include facial NCS; EMG of facial, ocular, laryngeal, pharyngeal, and palatal muscles; reflex responses, including the blink reflex, masseter reflex, masseteric inhibitory reflex, and lateral spread response; as well as electrophysiological demonstration of synkinesis.

Visual, brainstem, and trigeminal evoked potentials may also be used in assessing these disorders.

THOUGHT PROCESS. The history, signs, and symptoms are classic for an idiopathic facial neuropathy, or Bell's palsy. Other possibilities include a posterior fossa tumor, multiple sclerosis, brainstem stroke, and less likely, an infectious-related facial neuropathy such as herpes zoster or Lyme disease.[28] Nerve conduction studies to evaluate the facial nerve and exclude other cranial neuropathies were performed (Table 8–14).

DISCUSSION. Bilateral facial nerve conduction studies should be performed first. A low facial amplitude CMAP was recorded over the right orbicularis oculi. Blink reflexes (Fig. 8–2) are also important to define the site of the lesion relative to the facial nucleus. The right efferent limb of this reflex was impaired, that is, the facial nerve. The fact that there was a normal facial nerve distal latency yet prolonged ipsilateral blink reflex latency is important.

CASE 14

A 50-year-old woman awoke one morning and on looking in the mirror noticed a right facial droop which was especially pronounced when she smiled. She did not experience numbness but noted that it was difficult to completely close the right eye. Pursing her lips while eating was also difficult. She decided she had "slept wrong" and did not seek medical attention until 3 days later.

Clinical examination at that time revealed intact extraocular motions and visual fields, facial sensation, hearing, taste, and palatal and tongue motions. The right nasolabial fold was flattened and there was little movement of the right side of the face with smiling. The orbicularis oculi and oris were weak and she could not raise the right eyebrow.

TABLE 8–14   Case 14: Craniofacial Problems

NERVE CONDUCTION STUDIES

Nerve Stimulation (Record)	Amplitude (μV)	Distal Latency (ms)
R facial orbicularis oculi	**1500**	3.4
L facial orbicularis oculi	2900	3.2

Blink Reflex Latency (ms)	R_1	Ipsilateral R_2	Contralateral R_2
L trigeminal	10.7	36.0	**47.0**
R trigeminal	**23.1**	**48.1**	39.1

ELECTROMYOGRAPHY

		Spontaneous Activity		Motor Unit Potentials	
Muscle	Insertional Activity	Fibrillation Potentials	Fasciculation Potentials	Recruitment	Duration/Amplitude
R orbicularis oculi	Normal	0	0	Reduced	Normal
R orbicularis oris	Normal	0	0	Reduced	Normal
R frontalis	Normal	0	0	Reduced	Normal
R mentalis	Normal	0	0	Reduced	Normal
L orbicularis oculi	Normal	0	0	Normal	Normal

These findings suggest a lesion proximal to the stylomastoid foramen. Further studies to evaluate the bony segment and intracranial portion of the nerve are important. Depending on the clinical situation, brainstem auditory evoked potentials, the masseter reflex, and accessory NCS can be performed to show that other cranial nerves are not involved.

Needle examination showed only reduced MUP recruitment given the relatively early course of the problem. Because of future prognostic considerations, needle examination of muscles innervated by multiple branches of the facial nerve was performed to assess the extent of involvement, since routine facial NCS allows us to look only at a single branch.

NCS can be used prognostically in some cases. This is related to whether the lesion is merely demyelinating or includes axon loss. The facial CMAP amplitude measured after adequate time for wallerian degeneration to occur is probably the most useful prognostic measure. A facial CMAP amplitude that is less than 10% of the healthy side denotes delayed recovery for at least 6 to 12 months with significantly limited function. An amplitude of 10% to 30% of the unaffected side heralds mild to moderate dysfunction at 2 to 8 months. Facial CMAP amplitude greater than 30% of normal usually predicts full recovery within 2 months.[41] The electrophysiological findings are consistent with a right facial neuropathy.

PEDIATRIC ELECTROMYOGRAPHY

Case 15

Clinical neurophysiological testing in children is in many respects a specialty unto itself. The basic techniques of NCS and needle EMG are similar but require smaller electrodes and use of shorter distances, depending on the age and size of the patient. The basic physiological principles are similar to those in adults, but the clinician must understand age-related changes in the anatomy and physiology of nerve, neuromuscular junction, and muscle. Patient tolerance is a critical issue and it requires a skilled examiner to glean crucial electrophysiological data in the most efficient manner possible. Each age group displays behavioral characteristics which must be recognized and managed skillfully to achieve the greatest level of cooperation possible for a complete study. Understanding and cooperation of the parents should not be overlooked.

The range of disorders that can exist in children is extensive and normal electrophysiological parameters differ with age. Those in the 12- to 18-year-old age range will generally have amplitudes, conduction velocities, distal latencies, MUP morphology, and neuromuscular junction characteristics that are similar to normal adult values because nerves, muscles, and neuromuscular junctions have matured.[56; pp. 1219–1230] This age does not necessarily guarantee adult levels of cooperation, however.

L. Supraorbital nerve

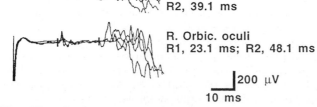

L. Orbic. oculi
R1, 10.7ms; R2, 36 ms

R. Orbic. oculi
R2, 47 ms

R. Supraorbital nerve

L. Orbic. oculi
R2, 39.1 ms

R. Orbic. oculi
R1, 23.1 ms; R2, 48.1 ms

200 μV
10 ms

R. Facial nerve lesion

FIGURE 8–2   Blink reflexes.

Prior to age 12, development of the motor unit is not complete and CMAP amplitudes and MUP morphology differ from those of adults. Myelination begins in utero at 15 weeks' gestation. By age 3 to 5 years, peripheral nerve myelination is complete and conduction velocities and distal latencies approach normal adult values.[17] It is important to recognize that distal latencies are generally shorter than in adults because of shorter distances. Infants and toddlers have conduction velocities that are approximately 50% of normal adult values, but this varies in different nerves and with motor vs. sensory nerves. SNAP amplitudes generally approach adult values by age 7 months.[27]

Results of repetitive stimulation vary with age. Low rates of stimulation should not produce a decrement in normal persons of any age. Premature and full-term infants normally exhibit post-tetanic facilitation and exhaustion to repetitive stimulation at rates of 50 Hz. This is related to a reduced safety factor for neuromuscular transmission resulting from an immature neuromuscular junction and possibly poorly myelinated nerves. At 20 Hz, only premature infants demonstrate these findings. This becomes an issue when studying a floppy infant, especially when coupled with the technical problems of performing these studies in the neonatal intensive care unit.[31]

Disorders having onset at birth generally present with hypotonia, weakness, poor respiration, feeding problems, and often skeletal deformities. Disorders occurring in the neonate include hereditary disorders of nerve, muscle, and the neuromuscular junction most commonly, but acquired disorders such as acute or chronic inflammatory demyelinating polyradiculoneuropathy, infantile botulism, and neonatal myasthenia gravis can also occur.[3] Developmental and dystrophic disorders such as hypomyelinating neuropathy, motor neuron disease and spinal muscular atrophy, myotonic dystrophy, and other congenital myopathies, both metabolic and structural, can present in neonates. Mononeuropathies, although most often traumatic in this age group, can also occur, and the clinician should be alert for evidence of nerve or muscle hypoplasia.

Children aged 1 to 5 years can exhibit problems with delayed developmental milestones or begin to show deterioration in gait, coordination, and ability to keep up with peers. The classic disorder which presents in this age range is Duchenne's muscular dystrophy. Other disorders, both acquired and hereditary, present in this age range, as can essentially any acquired disorder that adults develop.

A complete discussion of the multitude of disorders affecting children is beyond the scope of this chapter. The following case demonstrates a typical situation that may be encountered.

THOUGHT PROCESS.   In a child of this age, the diagnosis usually depends on the clinical and family history, examination, electrophysiological studies, and nerve or muscle biopsy. The electrophysiological studies can be very helpful in the decision to pursue a biopsy and to order various biochemical studies. Because the study may be limited by cooperation, the first consideration is to determine whether the disorder is neuropathic, myopathic, or a neuromuscular junction disorder. The second consideration is to determine the extent and severity of involvement.

In the case of a truly floppy infant, the ability to conduct a complete study is facilitated by the child's inability to resist. However, the examiner must respect the fact that fear by both patient and parents and discomfort remain factors and one should select the minimum number of studies necessary. The NCS and EMG data are listed in Table 8–15.

DISCUSSION.   The first step was to confirm the clinical impression that the disorder involved motor units with sparing of the sensory system. The medial plantar sensory NCS was selected because it is often easily performed in a child and reduces the problems with positioning required to perform a sural nerve study. The normal plantar study probably confirmed that this was primarily a motor disorder, although it did not totally rule out a multifocal neuropathy. A median antidromic sensory study was performed which was also normal. The peroneal motor conduction study is also easily performed in most children and in this case showed only a low CMAP amplitude and was otherwise normal.

Repetitive stimulation could have been performed here but, depending on the child, foot and leg movement may preclude adequate repetitive stimulation recordings at this site. The ulnar motor study was used for repetitive stimulation, as it was technically more feasible. A low ulnar CMAP was noted with normal repetitive stimulation at slow rates. A decrement could indicate immaturity of neuromuscular junctions in reinnervating nerve.[32] The findings of low CMAPs with normal sensory studies indicated a disorder of muscle, motor nerve, or motor neurons that affects both the upper and lower extremities. Normal repetitive stimulation with low-amplitude CMAPs excludes most disorders of neuromuscular junction transmission in this age

---

CASE 15

A 1-month-old infant was referred for an electrophysiological evaluation because of ongoing problems with weakness. The infant was the product of a normal, full-term pregnancy, but had respiratory problems at birth requiring 1 week of intensive care. The mother reported relative lack of fetal movements in utero as compared to her previous pregnancies. Since birth, the infant had fatigued quickly when sucking, often drooling and coughing while swallowing. The mother denied a family history of neuromuscular disorders.

The infant was bright and alert. The infant showed little volitional movement of the extremities and was supine with legs abducted in a froglike position. There was little recoil of the limbs when stretched and released, and no effort to align the head with the torso when pulled from supine to sitting. Muscle bulk was decreased. The infant withdrew the limbs from noxious stimuli, although not vigorously, and had a weak cry.

TABLE 8–15   Case 15: Pediatric Electromyography

NERVE CONDUCTION STUDIES

Nerve Stimulation (Record)	Amplitude (μV)	Conduction Velocity (ms)	Latencies (ms)	
			Distal	*F-Wave*
Motor				
Peroneal (EDB)	**1100**	25	2.0	**NR**
Ulnar (hypothenar)*	**3200**	28	1.6	18.5
Sensory				
Median plantar (ankle)	10		1.8	
Median (index)	22	35	1.4	

ELECTROMYOGRAPHY

Muscle	Insertional Activity	Spontaneous Activity		Motor Unit Potentials		
		Fibrillation Potentials	*Fasciculation Potentials*	*Recruitment*	*Duration/ Amplitude*	*Phases/ Turns*
R anterior tibial	Increased	+ +	0	Reduced	Increased	—
R quadriceps	Increased	+ + +	+	Reduced	Increased	Increased
R first dorsal interosseous (manus)	Increased	+ +	0	Reduced	Increased	Increased
R biceps	Increased	+ +	0	Reduced	Increased	—

*2-Hz repetitive stimulation at rest was normal.
Abbreviations: EDB, extensor digitorum brevis; NR, no response.

group. Other rates of stimulation could be performed at this point, but in this case, the decision was made to return to this only if the needle examination was unrevealing.

The goal of the needle examination was to demonstrate the severity and extent of involvement and to define whether the disorder was primarily one of muscle, motor axons, or neurons. The findings of generalized fibrillation potentials, reduced recruitment, and large MUPs were most consistent with a disorder of motor axons or neurons. Given the clinical history and examination, the findings were typical of those seen in infantile spinal muscular atrophy as described by Werdnig and Hoffmann.[21]

Infantile neuronal degeneration and genetic or acquired neuropathies also demonstrate similar clinical and electrophysiological findings, but generally present with much slower conduction velocities due to dysmyelination or demyelination.[52] Other disorders to consider which could show similar electrophysiological features include some congenital myopathies such as central core disease, although this generally lacks spontaneous activity, or acid maltase deficiency, though generally myotonic discharges would be seen. Poliomyelitis must also be included in the differential diagnosis. Had fibrillation potentials been less prominent, and low-amplitude, short-duration MUPs been the predominant finding, repetitive stimulation at high rates to exclude infantile botulism would have been performed.[12]

OTHER USES OF ELECTRODIAGNOSTIC STUDIES

Routine electrodiagnostic medicine techniques can be applied in evaluating many other types of conditions affecting the peripheral and central nervous systems. Combining information from NCS and EMG with data obtained using other electrodiagnostic techniques may be necessary. Basic techniques of NCS and EMG, evoked potentials, and surface EMG can be useful for diagnosis in many situations.

Surface EMG is useful in the assessment of movement disorders. Patterns of EMG activity can characterize tremor patterns and distinguish organic from functional tremor. This technique assists in determining patterns of muscle activation in dystonia, which significantly enhances choice of muscles for denervation with botulinum toxin or via surgery. A combination of NCS techniques to elicit various types of reflexes and surface EMG recording may be useful in defining disorders causing spasticity and rigidity.

Some patients experience episodic weakness. Routine NCS techniques are applied in exercise testing for periodic paralysis.

Patients with incontinence may benefit from electrodiagnostic assessment to determine the neurologic process responsible for incontinence or to characterize anal sphincter coordination. Pudendal nerve conduction studies and evoked potentials coupled with sphincter EMG to determine appropriate levels of sphincter activation and relaxation with voluntary activation and Valsalva maneuvers can be performed. Anal sphincter EMG is probably most useful for determining if sphincter denervation is present.

Cranial nerves can also be assessed using these techniques. EMG of muscles innervated by cranial nerves, including cranial nerves V, VII, XI, and XII, is easily performed. Less readily accessible muscles include those innervated by cranial nerves IX and X. Fine-wire EMG of palatal muscles is useful in palatal myoclonus and for intraoperative monitoring during posterior fossa or other head and neck surgery. The extraocular muscles can be examined as well. Reflex studies, including the blink reflex, masseter reflex, and masseter inhibitory reflex, can be performed, although the masseter reflexes require a reflex hammer which triggers the oscilloscope. The two-channel recording available on most standard EMG equipment is useful for demonstrating synkinesis and the lateral spread response, the latter characteristic of hemifacial spasm. Trigeminal somatosensory evoked potentials and visual and brainstem auditory evoked potentials are additional techniques which can assist in cranial nerve assessment.

The phrenic nerve can be assessed using NCS of each phrenic nerve in addition to needle EMG of the diaphragm. Intercostal EMG is also possible but caution should be used because of the risk of pneumothorax. These techniques are useful in patients with respiratory symptoms, particularly if diaphragm dysfunction is suspected (as in patients with failure to wean from mechanical ventilation). Excluding more generalized nerve or muscle disease in these patients is critical.

Patients with thoracic pain or paresthesia may have radiculopathy or polyradiculopathy at this level. The most frequent cause of thoracic radiculopathy is diabetes mellitus and is often associated with a neuropathy which can be subclinical. NCS and EMG are useful in defining both problems. Thoracic paraspinal EMG and EMG of abdominal muscles, when appropriate, should be performed.

Various techniques are useful for assessing CNS involvement. High-voltage or high-frequency stimulation of small myelinated fibers can elicit a withdrawal reflex in flexor muscles and assist in characterizing disorders of the CNS and the stiff-man syndrome. Stimulation of a nerve during a muscle contraction in the upper limb results in suppression of activity for 90 to 130 ms (the silent period), which may be altered in some central disorders. In some subjects, a variable C-response occurs during the silent period at 40 to 70 ms. This so-called long loop reflex has also been reported to be abnormal in some central disorders. The H-reflex is useful for assessing proximal conduction, and comparing the amplitude of the maximum H-reflex with the maximum M-wave amplitude provides a ratio that may reflect central excitability, which may be useful in quantification of spasticity. Evoked potential techniques are also used for CNS study.

Intraoperative monitoring during peripheral nerve surgery, spine, and the aforementioned posterior fossa surgeries can be performed using relatively routine NCS, EMG, and evoked potential techniques.

SUMMARY

The practice of electrodiagnostic medicine plays an important role in patient diagnosis and management. Training in neuromuscular disease and electrophysiological techniques is critical for useful diagnostic results from NCS and EMG. The ability to customize each study and alter the course of the study based on results obtained at each step is critical to a well-conducted evaluation. Electrodiagnosis plays a significant role in the practice of physical medicine and rehabilitation.

References

1. Albers JW, Mitz M, Sulaiman AR, Chang GJ: Spontaneous electrical activity and muscle biopsy abnormalities in polymyositis and dermatomyositis. Muscle Nerve 1979; 2:503.
2. Albers JW, Donofrio PD, McGonagle TK: Sequential electrodiagnostic abnormalities in acute inflammatory demyelinating polyradiculoneuropathy. Muscle Nerve 1985; 8:528–539.
3. Al-Quadah AA, Shahar E, Logan WJ, Murphy EG: Neonatal Guillain-Barré syndrome. Pediatr Neurol 1988; 4:255–256.
4. Armon C, Daube JR: Electrophysiologic signs of arteriovenous malformations of the spinal cord. J Neurol Neurosurg Psychiatry 1989; 52:1176–1181.
5. Asbury AK, Arnason BGW, Karp HR, McFarlin DE: Criteria for diagnosis of Guillain-Barré syndrome. Ann Neurol 1978; 3:565.
6. Banker BQ: The congenital myopathies. In Engel AG, Banker BQ (eds): Myology. New York, McGraw-Hill, 1986, pp 1527–1581.
7. Bohan A, Peter JB: Polymyositis and dermatomyositis. N Engl J Med 1975; 292:403–407.
8. Bradley WG. The limb girdle syndromes. In Unken PJ, Broyn GW (eds): Handbook of Clinical Neurology. Diseases of Muscle. Amsterdam. North-Holland, 1979, pp 433–469.
9. Bradley WG: Low back and lower limb pain. In Bradley WG (ed): Neurology in Clinical Practice. Boston, Butterworth-Heinemann, 1991, p 412.
10. Campbell WW, Pridgeon RM, Riaz G, et al: Sparing of the flexor carpi ulnaris in ulnar neuropathy at the elbow. Muscle Nerve 1989; 12:965–967.
11. Caroscio JT, Mulvihill MN, Sterling R, Abrams B: Amyotrophic lateral sclerosis: Its natural history. Neurol Clin 1977; 5:3.
12. Cornblath DR: Disorders of neuromuscular transmission in infants and children. Muscle Nerve 9:606–611, 1986.
13. Daube JR, Mulder DW: Clinical electrophysiologic factors in prognosis in amyotrophic lateral sclerosis. Muscle Nerve 5:S107, 1982.
14. Dawson DM, Hallett M, Millender LH: Entrapment Neuropathies. Boston, Little, Brown, 1990, pp 199–203.
15. Dyck PJ, et al: Chronic inflammatory polyradiculoneuropathy. Mayo Clin Proc 1975; 50:621–627.
16. Eaton LM, Lambert EH: Electromyography and electric stimulation of nerve in diseases of motor units. Observations on myasthenic syndrome associated with malignant tumors. JAMA 1957; 163:1117.
17. Gamble HJ, Breathnach AS: An electron-microscopic study of human foetal peripheral nerves. J Anat 1965; 99:573–584.
18. Gilliatt RW: Thoracic outlet compression syndrome. Br Med J 1976; 1:1274–1275.
19. Gilliatt RW, Willison RG, Dietz V, Williams IR: Peripheral nerve conduction in patients with a cervical rib and band. Ann Neurol 1978; 4:124–129.
20. Groh D, Brunner NG, Namba T: The natural course of myasthenia gravis and effect of therapeutic measures. Ann N Y Acad Sci 1981; 377:652.
21. Harding AE: Inherited neuronal atrophy and degeneration predominantly of lower motor neurons. In Dyck PJ, et al (eds): Peripheral Neuropathy, Philadelphia, WB Saunders, 1993, pp 1053–1054.
22. Harper PS: Myotonic Dystrophy. In Walton HN (ed): Major Problems in Neurology. Philadelphia, WB Saunders, 1979, pp 14–36.
23. Harper PS: The Myotonic Disorders. In Walton JN (ed): Disorders of Voluntary Muscle. New York, Churchill-Livingstone, 1988, pp 569–587.
24. Harper CM, Thomas JE, Cascino TL, Litchy WJ: Distinction between neoplastic and radiation-induced brachial plexopathy with emphasis on the role of EMG. Neurology 1989; 39:502–506.
25. Jablecki CK, Andary MT, So YT, et al: AAEM Quality Assurance Committee: Literature review of the usefulness of nerve conduction studies and electromyography for the evaluation of patients with carpal tunnel syndrome. Muscle Nerve 1993; 16:1392–1414.
26. Jablecki C: Lambert Eaton myasthenia syndrome. Muscle Nerve 1984; 7:250–257.
27. Jones HR: Pediatric Electromyography. In Brown WF, Bolton CF (eds): Clinical Electromyography, ed 2. Boston, Butterworth-Heinemann, 1993, pp 698–704.
28. Karnes WE: Diseases of the seventh cranial nerve. In Dyck PJ, et al (eds): Peripheral Neuropathy, ed 3. Philadelphia, WB Saunders, 1993, pp 826–830.
29. Kimura J (ed): Electrodiagnosis in Diseases of Nerve and Muscle, ed 2. Philadelphia, FA Davis, 1989.
30. Kline D: Civilian gunshot wounds to the brachial plexus. J Neurosurg 1989; 70:166.
31. Koenigsberger MR, Patten B, Lovelace RE: Studies of neuromuscular function in the newborn. A comparison of myoneural function in the fullterm and premature infant. Neuropediatrics 1973; 4:350–361.
32. Kuntz NL, Gomez MR, Daube JR: Prognosis in childhood proximal spinal muscular atrophy. Neurology 1980; 30:378.
33. Lambert EH. Electromyography in amyotrophic lateral sclerosis. In Norris FH, Kurland LT (eds): Motor Neuron Diseases: Research on Amyotrophic Lateral Sclerosis and Related Disorders. New York, Grune & Stratton, 1969, pp 135–153.

34. Lambert EH, Eaton LM, Rooke ED: Defect of neuromuscular transmission associated with malignant neoplasms (abstract). Am J Physiol 1956; 187:612.

35. Lange DJ: Multifocal motor neuropathy with conduction block: is it a distinct clinical entity? Neurology 1992; 42:497–505.

36. Lederman RJ, Wilbourn AJ: Brachial plexopathy: recurrent cancer or radiation? Neurology 1984; 34:1331.

37. Leffert RD: Brachial plexus injuries. N Engl J Med 1974; 291:1059.

38. Lotz BP, et al: Inclusion body myositis: observations in 40 patients. Brain 1989; 112:727–747.

39. Odesate K, Eisen A: An electrophysiological quantitation of the cubital tunnel syndrome. J Can Sci Neurol 1979; 6:403–410.

40. Oh SJ: Clinical Electromyography: Nerve Conduction Studies. Baltimore, University Park Press, 1984, p 231.

41. Olsen PZ: Prediction of recovery in Bell's palsy. Acta Neurol Scand Suppl 1975; 61:90.

42. O'Neill JH, Murray NMF, Newsom-Davis J: The Lambert-Eaton myasthenic syndrome: a review of 50 cases. Brain 1988; 111:577–596.

43. Ozdemir C, Young RR: The results to be expected from electrical testing in the diagnosis of myasthenia gravis. Ann N Y Acad Sci 1976; 274:203.

44. Parry GJ: Diseases of spinal roots. In Dyck PJ, et al (eds): Peripheral Neuropathy, ed 3. Philadelphia, WB Saunders, 1993, pp 899–907.

45. Parry GJ, Clarke S: Multifocal demyelinating neuropathy masquerading as motor neuron disease. Muscle Nerve 1988; 11:103–107.

46. Phalen GS: Reflections on 21 years experience with the carpal tunnel syndrome. JAMA 1970; 212:1365.

47. Preston DC, Kelly JJ: Atypical motor neuron disease. In Dyck PJ, et al (eds): Peripheral Neuropathy, ed 3. Philadelphia, WB Saunders, 1993, p 458.

48. Reed DM, Kurland LT: Muscle fasciculations in a healthy population. Arch Neurol 1963; 9:363–367.

49. Richardson AT: Muscle fasciculation. Arch Phys Med Rehabil 1954; 35:281–286.

50. Rivner MH, Swift TR: Electrical testing in disorders of neuromuscular transmission. In Brown WF (ed): Clinical Electromyography, ed 2. Boston, Butterworth-Heinemann, 1993, pp 630–631.

51. Seto DSY, Freeman JM: Lead neuropathy in childhood. Am J Dis Child 1964; 107:337.

52. Sladley JT: Chronic sensory-motor polyneuropathies in children. American Association of Electrodiagnostic Medicine Course A: Pediatric Electromyography, 1993, pp 7–12.

53. Stalberg E: Clinical electrophysiology in myasthenia gravis. J Neurol Neurosurg Psychiatry 1980; 43:622–633.

54. Stevens JC: AAEE minimonograph #26: The electrodiagnosis of carpal tunnel syndrome. Muscle Nerve 1987; 10:99–113.

55. Streib EW, Wilbourn AJ, Mitsumoto H: Spontaneous electrical muscle fiber activity in polymyositis and dermatomyositis. Muscle Nerve 1979; 2:14–18.

56. Thomas PK, Tomlinson DR: Diabetic and hypoglycemic neuropathy. In Dyck PJ, et al (ed): Peripheral Neuropathy, ed 3. Philadelphia, WB Saunders, 1993.

57. Turner AJW, Parsonage MJ: Neurologic amyotrophy (paralytic brachial neuritis) with special reference to prognosis. Lancet 1957; 1:209.

58. Walton JN, Gardner-Medivin D. Muscular dystrophies. In Walton JN (ed): Disorders of Voluntary Muscle, ed 5. New York, Churchill-Livingstone, 1988, pp 519–569.

59. Warren J, Guttmann L, Figueroa AF Jr, Bloor BM: Electromyographic changes of brachial plexus root avulsions. J Neurosurg 1969; 31:137–140.

60. Wilbourn AJ: Brachial plexus disorders. In Dyck PJ, et al (eds): Peripheral Neuropathy, ed 3. Philadelphia, WB Saunders, 1993.

61. Wilbourn AJ, Aminoff MJ: AAEE minimonograph #32. The electrophysiologic examination in patients with radiculopathy. Muscle Nerve 1988; 11:1099–1114.

9

Employment of Persons With Disabilities

DONNA JO BLAKE, M.D., and DAN D. SCOTT, M.D.

In the United States, disability is a significant public health and social issue. The prevalence of Americans who experience activity limitations secondary to chronic illnesses or impairments has risen while mortality has declined. Approximately 35 million Americans have a mental or physical impairment that interferes with daily activities. Nine million of these Americans have limitations severe enough to prevent them from working, attending school, or maintaining a household. Based on these two measures, disability ranks as the nation's largest public health problem.[5, 16, 20, 23, 38]

The growing numbers of Americans with disabilities present new challenges to the medical, social, and political arenas. The major activity limitations presented by disability include an inability to look after one's own personal care, an inability to work and be financially self-supporting, and an inability to integrate socially and enjoy leisure.[27] These limitations have medical, behavioral, social, and economic implications. In order to help people with disabilities restore functional capacity, avert further deterioration in functioning, and maintain or improve their quality of life, programs in any arena must emphasize rehabilitation and prevention of secondary conditions.[20] These programs must respect disability as multifaceted and foster an interdisciplinary approach.

Within the medical arena, the specialty of physical medicine and rehabilitation has been concerned with the establishment of physiological, psychological, and social equilibrium for persons with disabilities.[15] As stated by Rusk,[23] "A rehabilitation program is designed to take a disabled person from his bed back to his job, fitting him for the best life possible commensurate with his disability and more importantly with his ability." In order to help all persons with disabilities achieve their maximum level of independence, avert further deterioration in functioning, and maintain or improve their quality of life, the physiatrist and the medical rehabilitation team must appreciate the multifaceted character of disability. We must accept the responsibility

to initiate appropriate referrals to other collaborating programs which will support these goals beyond the medical arena. One such program is *vocational rehabilitation*.

In this chapter, we examine the subject of employment of people with disabilities. Specifically, we:

- Discuss the concept of disability
- Review national data on disability and employment
- Consider the economic impact of disability
- Review policies supporting employment of persons with disabilities
- Discuss economic assistance strategies
- Discuss vocational rehabilitation strategies
- Enumerate the incentives and disincentives for returning to work
- Postulate that vocational rehabilitation serves as an actual rehabilitation treatment as well as a disability prevention strategy for people with disabilities

CONCEPT OF DISABILITY

Disability itself is not always precise and quantifiable. The concept of disability is not agreed upon by persons who consider themselves to have a disability, professionals who study disability, or the general public.[16] This lack of agreement on the concept of disability is an obstacle to all studies of disability and to the equitable and effective administration of programs and policies intended for people with disabilities.[8, 9, 16, 20]

There are two major conceptual frameworks in the field of disability: the Nagi framework of "functional limitation" and the International Classification of Impairments, Disabilities, and Handicaps (ICIDH), a trial supplement to the World Health Organization's (WHO) International Classification of Disease. Each of these conceptual frameworks has four basic concepts. In the Nagi framework the four concepts are pathology, impairment, functional limitation, and disability. The four concepts in the ICIDH framework are disease, impairment, disability, and handicap. The first two concepts in each framework are similar, while the second two conceptual categories characterize each framework. Both frameworks, however, recognize that whether a person performs a socially expected activity depends on an interaction between the person and his or her social and physical environment.[4, 16, 19, 20, 39]

The Committee on a National Agenda for the Prevention of Disabilities, in 1991,[20] proposed an alternative conceptual framework of disability drawing on both the Nagi and ICIDH frameworks. This framework also has four basic concepts: pathology, impairment, functional limitation, and disability. *Pathology* refers to interruption or interference of normal bodily processes or structures. *Impairment* is defined as loss or abnormality of mental, emotional, physiological, or anatomical structure or function. *Functional limitation* is the restriction or lack of ability to perform an action or activity in the manner or within the range considered normal. *Disability* is the expression of the physical or mental limitation in a social context. Table 9–1 summarizes these concepts.[20]

The committee's conceptual framework of disability represents a "disabling process." As depicted at the center of Figure 9–1, the disabling process begins with pathology and then progresses toward impairment, functional limitation, and disability.[20] The rate and direction of this process depends on the interaction of risk factors and quality of life with the disabling process. Risk factors include biological, social, and physical environment, and lifestyle and behavioral characteristics. Risk factors influence each stage of the disabling process.[2,20] For example, a lifestyle that includes violence is a risk factor for traumatic brain injury. Traumatic brain injury is a risk factor for work disability. The disabling process also affects and is affected by the quality of life. For example, with a chronic disease like multiple sclerosis in which the impairments may not improve, assistive technology and accommodations in the environment can have a large impact on the individual's quality of life. Quality of life is not the endpoint in this conceptual framework of disability but an integral part of the process. The concept of a disabling process recognizes that disability is not inherent in a person, but is the result of a complexity of factors.

The concept of disability continues to be one about which there are many interpretations and opinions. This lack of agreement about the concept of disability affects epidemiological studies of disability and the development of effective disability treatment and prevention strategies. The model recommended by the Committee on a National Agenda for the Prevention of Disabilities (see Fig. 9–1) provides a standardization of concepts and terminology. Instituting this model will support effective communication, sound research, and appropriate disability treatment and prevention strategies.[20] This is the conceptual framework of disability referred to throughout this chapter.

DATA: IMPAIRMENT AND DISABILITY

Estimates of impairment and disability come from many sources. The National Health Interview Survey (NHIS), in 1990, found at least 120 million persons with impairments. An estimate of the number of people with limitations in life activities according to the NHIS was, in 1989, 34 million, or 14% of the U.S. population.[1] The Survey of Income and Program Participation (SIPP) from the U.S. Bureau of the Census, 1984–1985, estimated that 37 million people, or 21% of the U.S. population, aged 15 years and older had functional limitations.[29] Inability to walk was the most prevalent functional limitation, with 19 million reporting this limitation. The International Center for the Disabled (ICD) surveyed 12,500 households in 1986 and found the prevalence of disability to be 15% (27 million) among Americans aged 16 years and older.[10] While the concept of disability was different for each survey, the results indicate that at least 35 million Americans have disabilities.

Impairments due to chronic disease have become increasingly significant as risk factors of disability.[5, 16] Table 9–2 depicts the 15 conditions with the highest prevalence of functional compromise or disability.[16] The prevalence of disability with these conditions appears due to the prevalence of the condition itself and the chance that the condition will cause a disability. Table 9–3 shows the ranking of persons by percent of specific condition who have functional limitations secondary to that condition.[16] In general, many of the conditions that are significant risk factors for

TABLE 9–1   Concepts of the Disabling Process

Pathology	Impairment	Functional Limitation	Disability
Interruption or interference of normal bodily processes or structures	Loss/abnormality of mental, emotional, physiological, or anatomical structure or function; includes all losses or abnormalities, not just those attributable to active pathologic processes; also includes pain	Restriction or lack of ability to perform an action or activity in the manner or within the range considered normal that results from impairment	Inability or limitation in performing socially defined activities and roles expected of individuals within a social and physical environment
LEVEL OF REFERENCE Cells and tissues	Organs and organ systems	Organism—action or activity performance (consistent with the purpose or function of the organ or organ system)	Society—task performance within the social and cultural context
EXAMPLE Denervated muscle in arm due to trauma	Atrophy of muscle	Cannot pull with arm	Change of job; can no longer swim recreationally

From Pope AM, Tarlov AR (eds): Disability in America: Toward a National Agenda for Prevention. Washington, DC, National Academy Press, 1991. Used by permission.

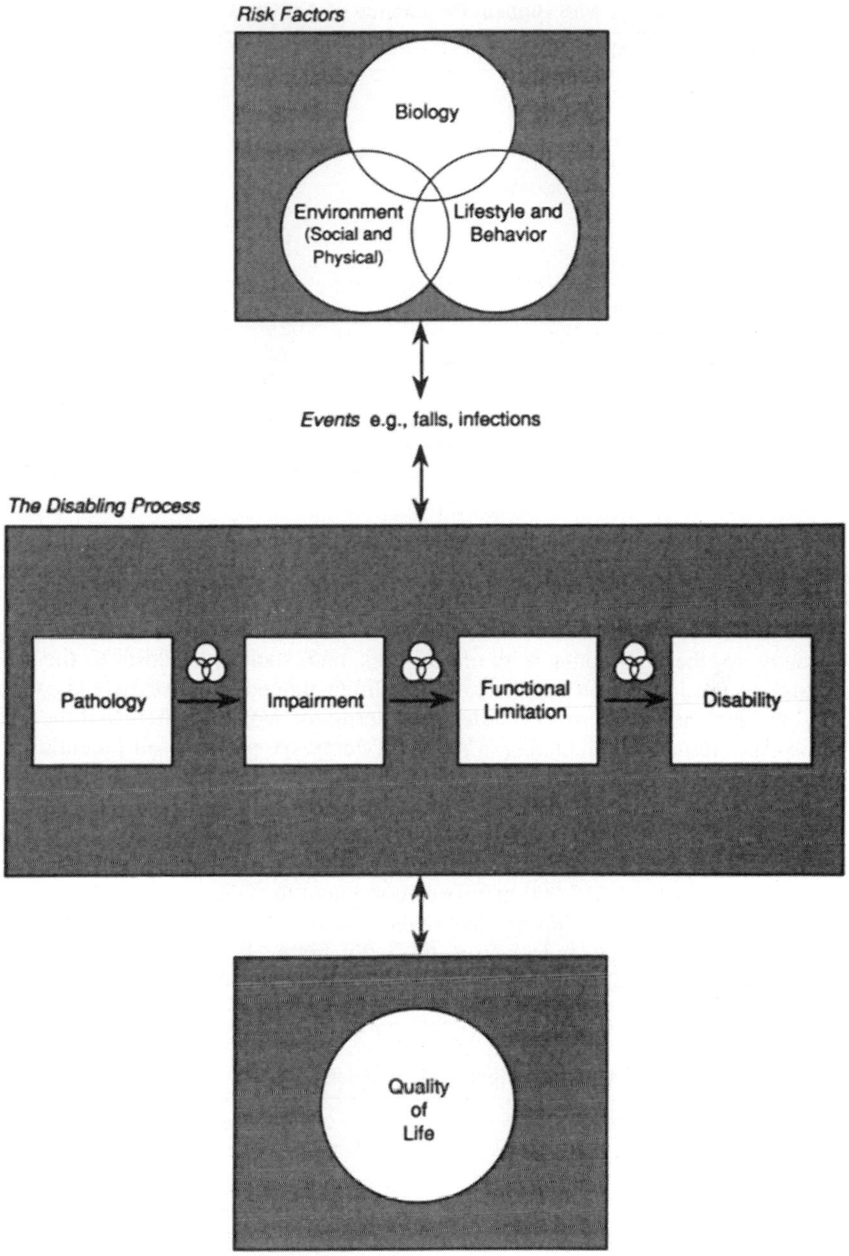

FIGURE 9–1 Interactions of the disabling process, risk factors, and quality of life. (From Pope AM, Tarlov AR (eds): Disability in America: Toward a National Agenda for Prevention. Washington, DC, National Academy Press, 1991.)

disability are low in prevalence. For example, multiple sclerosis has a low overall prevalence but is a significant risk factor for disability. Examination of this ranking shows 7 out of the top 10 disabling conditions to be conditions frequently managed by the physiatrist and the rehabilitation team. These conditions or diseases are, in general, chronic, requiring a lifetime of rehabilitative management in order to have an effect on the disabling process, prevent secondary conditions, and maintain quality of life.

SOCIOECONOMIC EFFECT OF DISABILITY

The disabling process has significant socioeconomic consequences for the individual with disabilities and for soci-

ety. When a person is unable to perform his or her social role as a worker or homemaker because of a physical or mental condition, then that person is said to have a work disability.[4] Work disability results in dependency and loss of productivity for that person. Society, in turn, incurs direct and indirect costs.

The direct expenditures include medical and personal care, architectural modification, assistive technology, institutional care, and income support for the person with a disability. For the individual, these expenses contribute to impoverishment.[3, 33] Society's response to the expenditures related to the disabling process includes disability-related programs such as Social Security Disability Insurance (SSDI), Supplemental Security Income (SSI), Medicare, and Medicaid. Direct expenditures incurred by our economy in 1986 totaled $169.4 billion.[4] These specific disabil-

TABLE 9–2   Conditions With Highest Prevalence of Activity Limitation

Main Cause	%	All Causes	%
Orthopedic impairments	16.0	Orthopedic impairments	21.5
Arthritis	12.3	Arthritis	18.8
Heart disease	22.5	Heart disease	17.1
Visual impairments	4.4	Hypertension	10.8
Intervertebral disc disorders	4.4	Visual impairments	8.9
Asthma	4.3	Diabetes	6.5
Nervous disorders	4.0	Mental disorders	5.6
Mental disorders	3.9	Asthma	5.5
Hypertension	3.8	Intervertebreal disc disorders	5.2
Mental retardation	2.9	Nervous disorders	4.9
Diabetes	2.7	Hearing impairments	4.3
Hearing impairments	2.5	Mental retardation	3.2
Emphysema	2.0	Emphysema	3.1
Cerebrovascular disease	1.9	Cerebrovascular disease	2.9
Osteomyelitis/bone disorders	1.1	Abdominal hernia	1.8

From La Plante MP: The demographics of disability. Milbank Q 1991; 69:55–77.

ity-related programs are discussed in the next section and are outlined in Table 9–4.

In addition to direct expenditures, the disabling process is costly to the individual with disabilities and society because of the loss of productivity. The indirect monetary costs for the individual are considered in terms of losses in job earnings and homemaker services. Twenty-six percent of persons with a work disability in 1978 were at or below the poverty line, while only 8% of nondisabled persons were at the same level.[33] In 1986, the ICD survey found that 50% of all people with disabilities reported household incomes of $15,000 or less as compared to 25% of nondisabled with incomes in that range.[10] The indirect monetary cost to society is loss from the labor force.[3] For example, in 1988, spinal cord injury alone was estimated

to have cost our economy $2.4 billion in lack of productivity.[11]

The disabling process imposes indirect nonmonetary costs to the individual and to society. Fifty-seven percent of persons with disabilities surveyed by Harris[10] in 1986 believed their disability prevented them from reaching their full potential. Work disability, specifically, places the individual in a position of dependency on insurance payments or government benefits for income support and medical care. Dependency affects people's feelings about themselves and their overall satisfaction with life.

Pressure from the customer and the third-party payers for accountability in medical care focuses attention on outcome and cost-effectiveness. Interventions directed at the disabling process should be assessed with the same

TABLE 9–3   Conditions With Highest Risk of Disability

Chronic Condition	No. of Conditions*	% Causing Activity Limitation	Rank	% Causing Major Activity Limitation	Rank	% Causing Need for Help in Basic Life Activities	Rank
Mental retardation	1202	84.1	1	80.0	1	19.9	9
Absence of leg(s)†	289	83.3	2	73.1	2	39.0	2
Lung or bronchial cancer	200	74.8	3	63.5	3	34.5	4
Multiple sclerosis†	171	70.6	4	63.3	4	40.7	1
Cerebral palsy†	274	69.7	5	62.2	5	22.8	8
Blind in both eyes	396	64.5	6	58.8	6	38.1	3
Partial paralysis in extremity†	578	59.6	7	47.2	7	27.5	5
Other orthopedic impairments†	316	58.7	8	42.6	8	14.3‡	12
Complete paralysis in extremity†	617	52.7	9	45.5	9	26.1	6
Rheumatoid arthrilis†	1223	51.0	10	39.4	12	14.9	11
Intervertebral disc disorders†	3987	48.7	11	38.2	14	5.3	—
Paralysis in other sites (complete/partial)†	247	47.8	12	43.7	10	14.1‡	13
Other heart disease disorders§	4708	46.9	13	35.1	15	13.6	14
Cancer of digestive tract	228	45.3	14	40.3	11	15.9‡	15
Emphysema	2074	43.6	15	29.8	—	9.6	15
Absence of arm(s)/hand(s)†	84	43.1	—	39.0	13	4.1‡	—
Cerebrovascular disease†	2599	38.2	—	33.3	—	22.9	7

*In thousands.
†Conditions frequently managed by physiatrists.
‡Figure has low statistical reliability or precision (relative standard error > 39%).
§Heart failure (9.8%), valve disorders (15.3%), congenital disorders (15.0%), other ill-defined heart conditions (59.9%).

TABLE 9–4   Disability-Related Programs

Type of Program	Specific Programs
Cash transfer	Social insurance: Social Security Disability Insurance Private insurance Indemnity compensation Income support: Supplemental Security Income, veterans' pensions, Aid to Families With Dependent Children
Medical care	Medicare Private disability insurance Veterans' programs Workers' compensation Tort settlements Medicaid
Direct services	Rehabilitation and vocational education Veterans' programs Services for persons with specific impairments General funded programs, e.g., food stamps, developmental disabilities, blind, mentally ill Employment assistance programs, i.e., Comprehensive Employment Training Program

From Berkowitz M, Hill MA: Disability and the labor market: an overview. *In* Berkowitz M, Hill MA (eds): Disability and the Labor Market: Economic Problems, Policies, and Programs. New York, ILR Press, 1989, pp 1–28.

scrutiny of outcome and cost-effectiveness. Disability is more than a medical phenomenon, it is a complex socioeconomic process. Assessment of the outcome and cost-effectiveness of an intervention must take into consideration quality of life and indirect monetary costs, as well as direct expenditures.

Vocational rehabilitation is an intervention which can limit work disability. Employment is the expected outcome of vocational rehabilitation, but the impact of this intervention goes beyond simple employment. The positive effects of working are demonstrated when comparing characteristics between working and nonworking persons with disabilities. Those who work are better educated, have more money, are less likely to consider themselves disabled, and, in general, are more satisfied with life.[10]

Comprehensive rehabilitation of persons with disabilities must include strategies like vocational rehabilitation which limit work disability. The outcomes will include increased independence and increased productivity. The cost-effectiveness of comprehensive rehabilitation must be measured in direct and indirect monetary and nonmonetary costs over the lifetime of the individual.[2]

DISABILITY-RELATED PROGRAMS AND POLICIES

Programs

There is a plethora of disability-related programs and policies. Each program and policy has its own definition of disability, and therefore differs in the eligibility and application criteria. The programs can be characterized as ameliorative or corrective.[12] Ameliorative programs provide payment for income support and medical care. Correc-

tive programs facilitate the individual's ability to return to work and to reduce or remove the disability. Whether ameliorative or corrective, all programs affect the disabling process.

Disability-related programs can be categorized into three basic types: (1) cash transfers, (2) medical care programs, and (3) direct service programs. Table 9–4 presents specific programs within these three basic types of programs.[4] Estimates of the expenditures of these disability-related programs provide insight into expenditure trends. In 1970, 61.4% of the disability dollar went for cash transfers, 33% for medical care, and 5.4% for direct services. By 1986, the proportion of the disability dollar for direct services had decreased to 2.1% as the proportion for medical care increased.[4]

The trend toward ameliorative programs capturing more resources is a concern. Studies of the socioeconomic consequences of disability support rehabilitating people with disabilities to allow them to enter the labor market and to decrease dependency and loss of productivity. The physiatrist has an important supportive role in initiating referrals to the corrective programs. These programs are in keeping with the philosophy of rehabilitation, which is to maximize individual functioning and lessen disability.

Public Disability Policies

Public policy in the United States has begun to recognize that many barriers to integration faced by persons with disabilities are the result of discriminatory policy and practices. Furthermore, the view that disability is an interaction between an individual and the environment has become fundamental in shaping public policy toward disability over the last 20 years. Since the late 1960s, Congress has passed a series of laws aimed at enhancing the quality of life for persons with disabilities. These laws have mandated that housing and transportation be accessible, that education for children with disabilities be appropriate, and that employment practices be nondiscriminatory.[6, 7, 35]

Three legislative actions deserve to be highlighted. The Rehabilitation Act of 1973 extended civil rights protection to persons with disabilities. This legislation included antidiscrimination and affirmative action in employment. The Rehabilitation Act Amendments of 1978 broadened the responsibility of the Rehabilitation Services Administration (RSA) to include independent living programs and created the National Council of the Handicapped (the National Council of the Handicapped became the National Council on Disability, January 1989). The capstone of this legislative tradition is the Americans with Disabilities Act of 1989. This legislation established a clear and comprehensive prohibition of discrimination on the basis of disability.[6, 31, 35, 36] Table 9–5 reviews the federal disability laws since 1968.[6, 31]

VOCATIONAL REHABILITATION

The objective of vocational rehabilitation is to allow persons with physical disabilities to engage in gainful employment. Historically formal vocational rehabilitation services were instituted to provide returning World War II

TABLE 9–5 Federal Disability Laws

Year	Public Law No.	Title Of Law	Key Provisions
1968	90–480	Architectural Barriers Act	Requires that buildings built with federal funds or leased by the federal government be made accessible
1970	91–453	Urban Mass Transportation Act	Requires eligible local jurisdictions to plan and design accessible mass transportation facilities and services
1973	98–87	Federal Aid Highway Act	Requires that transportation facilities receiving federal assistance under the act be made accessible; allows highway funds to be used to make pedestrian crosswalks accessible
1973	93–112	Rehabilitation Act	Prohibits discrimination against qualified people with disabilities in programs or receiving services, and benefits that are federally funded; created Architectural and Transportation Barriers Compliance Board
1975	93–391	Department of Transportation Appropriations Act	Prohibits purchase of mass transit equipment or construction of facilities unless they are accessible to elderly and people with disabilities
1975	94–103	Developmental	Establishes protection and advocacy systems for developmentally disabled people; establishes representative councils in each state for developmentally disabled people
1975	94–142	Education for All Handicapped Children Act	Provides for a free appropriate education for handicapped children in the least restrictive setting possible
1975	94–173	National Housing Act Amendments	Provide for the removal of barriers in federally supported housing; establish Office of Independent Living for disabled people in Department of Housing and Urban Development
1978	95–602	Rehabilitation, Comprehensive Services, and Developmental Disability Amendments	Establish independent living as a priority for state vocational rehabilitation programs; provide federal funding for independent living centers
1980	96–265	Social Security Disability Amendments	Remove certain disincentives to work by allowing people with disabilities to deduct independent living expenses in computing income benefits
1990	101–336	Americans with Disabilities Act	Establishes a clear and comprehensive prohibition of discrimination on the basis of disability

Data from DeJong G, Lifchez R: Physical disability and public policy. Sci Am 1983; 248:40–50; and U.S. Equal Employment Opportunity Commission and the U.S. Department of Justice: Americans with Disabilities Act Handbook (EEOC-BK-19). Washington, DC, US Government Printing Office, 1991.

veterans with disabilities assistance in obtaining suitable occupations.[35]

Prior to the 1970s, jobs earmarked for persons with disabilities were provided through government-subsidized sheltered workshops. The Comprehensive Employment Training Act of 1973 (CETA) provided public service jobs for persons with disabilities and for the disadvantaged, along with training programs for this population. At its peak in 1980, CETA and sheltered workshops provided over 1 million jobs to a broadly defined "disabled" population. The CETA program lasted from 1973 to 1982, and the federal government subsequently returned to state-run vocational rehabilitation agencies for provision of these services to persons with disabilities.

The Rehabilitation Act of 1973 authorized federal funding for state rehabilitation agencies to provide a variety of services to qualified persons with disabilities. Table 9–6 lists the services provided. The federal government supplies 80% of the funding for state vocational rehabilitation agencies, while the states must provide the remaining 20%. State agencies administer the programs under the Rehabilitation Services Administration (RSA) in the Department of Education. The intent of the rehabilitation act was to provide services to persons with disabilities with emphasis placed on serving those with more severe disabilities (General Accounting Office [GAO] testimony).[32] State agencies are usually located in the state division of vocational reha-

bilitation. The state division provides direct services, and also refers individuals to private rehabilitation agencies and training programs when indicated.

Traditional Approaches to Vocational Rehabilitation

A variety of approaches to vocational rehabilitation have been developed over the years. The traditional approach will be discussed first. It begins with referral of a person with a disability to a vocational rehabilitation counselor. This referral can be generated by the person with a disability, or by a physician, social worker, or case manager. The initial referral includes medical records, documentation of disabilities and capabilities, and neuropsychological testing (when performed).

TABLE 9–6 Services Provided by Vocational Rehabilitation Specialists

Diagnosis and Evaluation	Adjustment Training
Counseling and guidance	Business or vocational training
Restoration*	Miscellaneous training
Transportation	Placement
College or university training	Referrals
Income maintenance	On-the-job training

*Includes medical treatment, prosthetic devices, or medically necessary services to correct or modify a physical or mental disorder.

The initial interview between the counselor and the client (person with a disability) establishes rapport and provides background information about previous job skills and experiences. The interview also provides information about educational level, motivation, perceived abilities and disabilities, and areas of interest of the individual. If the client was employed prior to his disability, the potential for placement with the former employer exists. The prior employer should be contacted to learn of employment opportunities for the person with a disability. The vocational rehabilitation counselor also assesses the skills the person had premorbidly and the skills needed prior to placement in a suitable position. If no positions are available, vocational testing is performed.

Aptitude Matching vs. Work Sample

Vocational testing is performed to assess the client's level of general intelligence, achievement, aptitudes, interests, and work skills. Formal testing consists of administering a battery of paper-and-pencil standardized tests, examples of which are listed in Table 9–7. This type of approach is known as "aptitude matching." It determines the client's aptitudes or traits in the areas of general intelligence, visuospatial perception, eye-hand coordination, motor coordination, and dexterity. Performance on the tests is compared against a list of essential aptitudes, grouped by occupation, in the *Dictionary of Occupational Titles* (DOT) published by the Department of Labor.[17] When a client's aptitudes match a particular occupation, a job search is undertaken by the counselor.

A work sample approach is often used in conjunction with aptitude batteries. The work sample approach measures general characteristics such as size discrimination, multilevel sorting, eye-hand-foot coordination, and dexterity. The Valpar Component Work Sample Series (VCWSS) is a good example of the work sample approach. The VCWSS uses complex work apparatuses to measure almost exclusively motor responses. There is less focus on general intelligence, aptitude, or academic performance. Work samples can also evaluate the type of "work group" in which the client is most skilled. This simulated work requires performance of a series of tasks, for example, drill press operation, circuit board or bench assembly.[17]

Once the client's skills have been evaluated and his or her interests have been explored, a vocational goal is developed. First, the requirements of the potential position

TABLE 9–7   Tests Administered by Vocational Rehabilitation Counselor or Neuropsychologist

Test	Type
Wechsler Adult Intelligence Scale–Revised (WAIS-R)	Intelligence
General Aptitude Test Battery (GATB)	Aptitude
Differential Aptitude Test (DAT)	Aptitude
Wide Range Achievement Test (WRAT)	Achievement
Strong-Campbell Interest Inventory (SCII)	Interest
Career Assessment Inventory (CAI)	Interest
Minnesota Multiphasic Personality Inventory (MMPI)	Personality
Halstead-Reitan	Cognitive evaluation
Luria-Nebraska	Cognitive evaluation

must be determined. This is accomplished by performing a job analysis of the position, identifying the physical and mental requirements and any necessary job site modifications; for example, adaptive equipment. If training is proposed, it must be accessible and available to the client. Transportation must be arranged and can be paid for by the vocational rehabilitation agency. Tuition, books, and adaptive equipment to allow performance of the position can also be provided by the agency.

Training programs vary in length depending on the potential vocational goal. They can last from a few weeks to several years. Training can be conducted at a trade school, college, or university, or on the job with state vocational rehabilitation agency funding.

On-the-job training requires job development. The counselor or the client explores community business resources to develop suitable positions. Tax incentives for potential employers can help convince industry to offer training. Sliding-scale wages can be arranged to assist in developing positions. For example, the state rehabilitation agency may fund 100% of salary for 3 to 6 months. The employer gradually assumes that responsibility over the next 3 to 6 months as the new employee becomes trained. Many employers want to keep the employees they have trained, but some prefer to act in the capacity of trainers for a series of persons with disabilities. In this case, the counselor still has the task of placing the newly trained people.

Once an individual has completed training and has been placed for 60 days, the state vocational rehabilitation agency considers the case a "success" and closes its file. No follow-up is typically provided.

Sheltered Workshops

One of the problems with the traditional approach of the vocational rehabilitation agency has been its poor record of success, especially for persons with severe disabilities. There were 45% fewer people successfully vocationally rehabilitated in 1988 than in 1974 despite increased financial support and larger numbers of persons with disabilities.[35] A 1987 GAO survey found that of SSDI recipients receiving vocational rehabilitation, less than 1% left the SSDI rolls.[26] The ICD survey reported that although 60% of persons with disabilities knew about vocational rehabilitation services, only 10% took advantage of those services. Of those using the services, more than 50% felt they were not useful in securing gainful employment.[10]

As a result of the poor placement record, alternative strategies have been developed for enabling persons with disabilities to obtain gainful employment. These include sheltered workshops, day programs, transitional and supported employment, projects with industry, independent living center–directed employment, and others. Funding for these programs has come from public nonprofit and private industry, state and federal social service programs, religious entities, corporate and foundation contributions, and individual donations.

A sheltered workshop is a "public non-profit organization certified by the U.S. Department of Labor to pay 'sub-minimum' wages to persons with diminished earning capacity."[13] There are over 5000 workshops, including Goodwill, Inc., and they serve approximately 250,000 persons with disabilities. This form of employment serves persons with severe disabilities, including limited vision, mental illness, mental retardation, and alcoholism. While sheltered workshops provide job experience and income, critics report that sheltered workshops rarely lead to competitive, integrated employment. People with severe disabilities can be competitively employed in the community through the use of some modern strategies, as outlined below.

Day Programs

Day programs have existed since before the 1970s and are meant to provide supervised vocational activity for persons with severe disabilities, usually those with mental retardation or mental illness. These programs are funded by private and corporate sponsors, as well as by state and federal agencies. They are not designed as a transition into competitive employment nor do they allow community integration. They are geared toward providing supervised day activities while caretakers of these persons work or perform their own daily routines. Activities are performed in facilities which serve only persons with disabilities.

Home-Based Programs

Another more traditional method for assisting persons with severe disabilities to obtain employment is the home-based program. Home-based programs can be funded by state vocational rehabilitation, insurance carriers, foundations and societies, or by other agencies. The person with a disability can perform a variety of jobs, including telephone solicitation, typing, or computer-assisted occupations; for example, graphics, accounting, or drafting.

Of these programs—sheltered workshops, day programs, and homebound programs—none emphasizes gainful employment in a nonsheltered integrated setting. It was the failure of these programs to reintegrate their clients into competitive community employment that resulted in the emergence of transitional and supported employment models.

Other Programs for Employment

Projects with Industry (PWI) is a federally sponsored collaborative program established by the Vocational Rehabilitation Act. Employers design and provide training projects for specific job skills in cooperation with rehabilitation agencies. The goal of PWI is competitive employment for the participants.

Job fairs have been somewhat successful in matching vacant positions with capable individuals with disabilities. Businesses in a community spend 1 day interviewing applicants with disabilities who have been prescreened by a participating placement agency. The placement agency may provide further services such as transportation for the potential employee and make recommendations for work accommodations to the potential employer.

Transitional and Supported Employment

Transitional and supported employment are two newer strategies for returning disabled persons to competitive, integrated gainful employment. Transitional employment

consists of providing the job placement, training, and support services necessary to help persons move into independent or supported employment.[28] Independent employment provides at least a minimum wage to the employee and requires no job subsidy or ongoing support. Transitional employment is a short-term provision of services for a period not to exceed 18 months and culminates in an independent or supported employment position.

Supported employment has been utilized as a successful strategy for placing or returning the most severely disabled individuals to competitive, integrated community employment. It requires ongoing support after placement, including counseling for the employee and co-workers, and assistance with transportation, housing, and other non–work-related activities.

It began as an alternative to sheltered workshops or day programs and has grown to have modest federal funding and broad community support. This support comes from groups of persons with disabilities, state vocational rehabilitation agencies, and state departments for the developmentally disabled. This concept became a permanent part of the Rehabilitation Act of 1973 with the passage of the 1986 amendments, and final regulations published in June 1992.[37]

Supported employment is meant to provide ongoing support for persons with severe disabilities. According to Wehman and co-workers,[37] it must meet five critical criteria (Table 9–8). The first is that all interventions, including training, placement, and counseling, be provided at the job site rather than in a therapy room or vocational school. Second, the intervention and services are provided on a permanent or long-term basis as the individual requires them. Third, these programs are intended to serve only those individuals with the most severe disabilities who have been unable to enter the competitive labor market with their disability in the past. Fourth, the work provided is real and meaningful for the employee, and compensation is received equal to that of an able-bodied co-worker for the same duties. Fifth, work must occur in an integrated setting allowing interaction with co-workers without disabilities.[37]

The Department of Education's operational definition of supported employment requires the employee to be paid for working an average of at least 20 hours per week in a position which provides interactions with persons who are not disabled and are not paid caregivers. There must be eight or fewer people with disabilities working together at the job site, and there must be ongoing public funding for providing intervention directly related to sustaining employment. Supportive employment defines the type and

TABLE 9–8   Critical Criteria for Supported Employment

Interventions provided at the job site
Assistance will be long-term or permanent
Programs will serve only severely disabled
Real pay for real work
Work is performed in an integrated setting

From Wehman P, Sherron P, Kregel J, et al: Return to work for persons following severe traumatic brain injury: Supported employment outcomes after five years. Am J Phys Med Rehabil 1993; 72:355–363.

level of support needed by an individual to be employable now, not after a nonintegrated training program.

Four models of supported employment have been developed. The "enclave" model consists of a small group of persons with disabilities working together at an integrated job site. The "mobile work crew" model uses a small group of workers who travel from job to job and offer contractual services under the direction of a supervisor. The "small business or entrepreneurial" model creates a new small business which produces goods or services using both workers with and without disabilities. The most frequently used model is the "job coach with individual placement."[13]

The job coach, or employment specialist, is an employee of the agency providing supported employment services. The coach works with an individual at the job site to provide interpersonal and coping skills as well as job skills. The coach performs job development prior to placement. Once placement occurs, job training and ongoing job retention services are provided. Job coaches may initially be required to complete the duties the worker with a disability has not yet mastered.

Depending on the disability, behavior modification or cognitive training can be required to enable learning of vital skills. These become the responsibility of the job coach. The job coach must be able to evaluate the ecology of the job site, that is, attitudes of co-workers, accessibility of the job site, and the necessity for adaptive equipment. The job coach must then be able to educate co-workers and ensure implementation of appropriate accommodations for the person with a disability.

Job coach intervention time can be very significant (almost 8 hours/day) initially. Wehman and others conducted a 5-year study of supported employment for persons with traumatic brain injury (TBI).[37] They documented an average requirement of 249.1 hours per person of job coach time over 6 months. The job coach's intervention time decreased steadily with time on the job to an average of less than 3 hours per week per person after 30 weeks of employment.

Some persons require continued significant intervention to assist them in meeting difficulties which arise from changes at the job site, that is, new job duties or changes in personnel or goods produced. However, some workers are able to depend on support from employers and co-workers and require little or no direct job coach support. Supportive employment has been highly successful in allowing persons with severe disabilities to participate competitively in the job market and improve their quality of life and economic situation.

Independent Living Centers

The independent living center (ILC) movement has traditionally provided a core of nonvocational services such as housing, independent living skills, advocacy, and peer counseling. Just as supported employment has broadened its scope, so has the ILC movement. Both philosophies provide a combination of nonvocational and vocational services to persons with severe disabilities. ILCs often employ workers with disabilities as peer counselors and program administrators. The small business approach of supported employment has been successfully implemented by ILCs to place their clients in competitive community employment. As these two philosophies continue to merge and provide similar services to persons with severe disabilities, cooperative ventures will be seen between them to allow persons with severe disabilities to fully achieve their maximum level of independence.

Provision of vocational rehabilitation services to persons with disabilities requires a diversity of strategies. The more severe the disability, the more intensive the support and services have to be. Full participation in society is a right of all people. This participation includes being employed in a meaningful job that is both satisfying to the worker and that contributes to society as a whole. The methods for returning persons with disabilities to work vary, but creative strategies have proved significantly more successful than noncreative strategies.

DISINCENTIVES FOR VOCATIONAL REHABILITATION

Public and political opinion has changed in recent years regarding the ability of persons with disabilities to work. Both persons with disabilities and policymakers have demonstrated a desire to returning persons with disabilities to gainful employment. The change of opinion is reflected by statements of past Presidents of the United States. In 1973 Richard M. Nixon was quoted concerning the Rehabilitation Act of 1973, saying it "would cruelly raise the hopes of the handicapped [for gainful employment] in a way that we could never hope to fulfill."[13] Advocacy by groups for the rights of persons with disabilities has achieved significant policy changes as reflected by Ronald Reagan's November 1983 proclamation of the "Decade of Disabled Persons" in which the economic independence of all people with disabilities was to become a "clear national goal."[28] With the passage of the Americans with Disabilities Act (ADA) in July 1990, George Bush proclaimed the "end to the unjustified segregation and exclusion of people with disabilities from the mainstream of American life."[13]

Despite the obvious changes in public and political policies and attitudes, disincentives to entering "the mainstream" abound for persons with disabilities. In order to become eligible for cash and medical benefits through SSI and SSDI, persons with disabilities must prove that they have total and permanent or long-term disability and must meet strict eligibility criteria. In addition, prior to meeting those criteria, the individual and the family must have suffered a series of indignities including exhausting all personal resources and submitting to significant bureaucratic red tape. "Red tape" means completing substantial paperwork, obtaining medical reports verifying disability, and enduring long waiting periods for commencement of benefits. This is usually a long and arduous process. Once the person with a disability finally achieves a modest degree of security, an "opportunity" to give it all up and enter the work force is made available. Naturally the person with a disability is suspicious about the assurance that benefits will be preserved and eligibility will not be taken away because of returning to or entering the job market.

Stereotypes about persons with disabilities being unproductive in society are pervasive. Individuals with disabilities often come to view themselves as totally dependent and unable to work. After all, they are placed in a position to prove their dependency and inability to be productive. The government disability entitlement policies state that if you are unable to work, the government will take care of you. In fact, many government policymakers believe the person with a disability cannot and should not have to work. Some even believe that sending a person with a disability a check is much simpler than implementing the provisions of the ADA.

Employers' attitudes serve as another disincentive. Obstacles to qualified applicants with disabilities who want to participate in the work force include employers' ignorance about the capabilities of a potential employee with a disability, inaccessible work sites, transportation inaccessibility, and discrimination in hiring. The ADA will be instrumental in changing much of this behavior, and removing some of these disincentives. As disabled employees take their places, employers and co-workers will become educated, and attitudes will change.

The physiatrist and other physicians also provide disincentives for persons with disabilities by labeling them as "totally and permanently disabled" or by restricting their activities. Emphasis should be on the capabilities of persons with disabilities and documentation of their functional abilities, both mental and physical.

INCENTIVES FOR VOCATIONAL REHABILITATION

In an effort to overcome disincentives, government policymakers have created incentives for persons with disabilities and for potential employers. These incentives are often voluminous and very specific in wording in order to avoid abuse. An attempt will be made here to briefly discuss various incentive programs.

Incentives for the Individual

Incentive programs are applicable depending on whether the person with a disability receives SSDI or SSI benefits, or both. SSDI work incentives will be discussed first. Table 9–9 presents a summary of the terminology and abbreviations for easy reference. Additional references are given here for those wanting more detailed information.[18, 21, 22, 25, 26, 30]

The initial incentive toward a return to work involves a trial work period (TWP) (see Table 9–9). The TWP lets people test their ability to work or run a business without affecting their benefits. This TWP maintains cash benefits for 9 months (not necessarily consecutive) of trial work earning greater than a specified amount ($200/month currently) in a 60-month period.

Upon completion of the TWP and continued employment at or above the substantial gainful activity (SGA) level (see Table 9–9), benefits continue to be paid for 3 more months and are then terminated.[18, 30] Any earnings from work below the monetary limit of the SGA level described in Table 9–9 are excluded when figuring monthly benefit amounts.

The extended period of eligibility (EPE) is a period of 36 consecutive months during which cash benefits can be reinstated if, during that period, the individual's earnings fall below the SGA level (see Table 9–9). If the individual is unable to maintain earnings at the SGA level, benefits resume automatically, and no waiting periods are required.

Benefits cease at the end of the EPE, but Medicare continues for 3 additional months.[18, 30] The elimination of a second waiting period for both cash benefits and Medicare benefits is also an incentive to perform a trial of work.

Under certain circumstances, the person might be able to participate in a Medicare "buy-in." The client must have completed both the TWP and the EPE (see Table 9–9). In addition, the extended 3 months of Medicare benefits must have passed. Once these conditions are met, Medicare A and B coverage can be purchased for approximately $200 per month. This medical coverage is for those who cannot otherwise obtain health insurance because of preexisting conditions.[18]

Another major incentive program for those receiving SSDI or SSI is for impairment-related work expenses (IRWE) (see Table 9–9). This allows the cost of certain items and services to be deducted from earnings when determining the SGA level. Examples include attendant care, medical devices, equipment, and prostheses.[18]

For those persons with disabilities receiving SSI benefits, a different, but often similar set of incentives apply. These incentives provide SSI recipients with assurances that working will not disadvantage them. Section 1619 of the Social Security Act was made permanent by the Employ-

---

TABLE 9–9 Summary of Incentives for the Individual Receiving Benefits to Enter Work Activities

Social Security Disability Insurance (SSDI)	Disability benefits program based on medical disability and a worker's earnings covered by Social Security (Title II—Social Security Act)
Supplemental Security Income (SSI)	Disability benefits program based on medical disability and the amount of income a person receives (Title XVI—Social Security Act)
Trial work period (TWP)	Allows trial return to work to test work ability without affecting benefits (SSDI)
Substantial gainful activity (SGA)	Performance of significant and productive physical or mental work for pay or profit (over $500/mo for nonblind [SSDI and SSI] and $810/mo for blind recipients [SSDI only])
Extended period of eligibility (EPE)	Allows reinstatement of cash benefits without a waiting period if the worker's earnings fall below SGA level within 36 mo after TWP (SSDI)
Impairment-related work expenses (IRWE)	Allows costs for certain items to be deducted from earnings when figuring SGA level (SSI and SSDI)
Earned income exclusion (EIE)	Allows exclusion of a portion of earned income when figuring an individual's monthly benefit (SSI)
Blind work expenses (BWE)	Allows work-related expenses when figuring benefits (SSI)

ment Opportunities for Disabled Americans Act passed in November 1986. The incentive of Section 1619 allows receipt of SSI cash benefits, even though earned income exceeds the SGA level (see Table 9–9). Cash benefits are calculated using the earned income exclusion discussed below. Medicaid benefits continue as an additional incentive even after wages become high enough to cause cessation of SSI cash benefits if their continuation is needed to allow the recipient to maintain employment.[22, 30]

The earned income exclusion (see Table 9–9) allows most of a recipient's earned income to be excluded, including pay received from a sheltered workshop or day activity center, when figuring the SSI monthly amount.[30] Blind work expenses (see Table 9–9) is an incentive that allows a person who is blind to pay for work expenses, for example, visual aids, guide dogs, or Braille translations. These allowable expenses are then excluded when calculating benefit amounts.

In an effort to prevent work disincentives, benefit caps have been implemented to decrease excessively generous benefits. These caps utilize various formulas to reduce or limit maximum benefits paid by Social Security. These formulas take into account other sources of income, such as workers' compensation benefits, but do not exclude veterans' benefits or disability pensions from government jobs.

Another incentive program, Plans for Achieving Self-Support (PASS), allows an SSI recipient to set aside income and resources necessary to achieve a work goal. The plan must be approved by the Social Security Administration.[21, 30]

Incentives for Industry

Various attempts have been made by government policymakers to offer tax incentives to business and industry. These incentives have mainly been directed at making the workplace accessible. Section 190 of the Internal Revenue Code, enacted in 1976 and revised by the Revenue Reconciliation Act of 1990, allowed $35,000 per year deductible for any expenses incurred in barrier removal, that is, making a business or public transportation accessible. This amount was reduced to a $15,000 per year deductible by the 1990 legislation.[24]

The Revenue Reconciliation Act of 1990 (passed 3 months after the ADA) allows an "access" tax credit with Section 44 of the Internal Revenue Code. It allows credit against income taxes for 50% of eligible expenditures greater than $250, but less than $10,250 (auxiliary services for the disabled employee and aids are covered). This access credit is only allowed for expenses incurred for the purpose of enabling a business to comply with the ADA. It applies only to small businesses, not to large firms.[24]

Tax credits have also been utilized as incentives to encourage hiring of target groups including the "hardcore" unemployed—persons with disabilities and homeless populations. The Targeted Jobs Tax Credit (TJTC), originally enacted in 1978, is meant to encourage employers to hire members of these groups. It provides approximately $1600 per person per year for targeted persons, including those persons receiving SSI benefits and vocational rehabilitation referrals (both groups containing large numbers of persons with disabilities). This credit only provides benefits to an employer for 1 year per employee. Many employers use the credit as a windfall, that is, hiring anyone they want and later checking to see if the new employee falls into a targeted group. This practice is called "retroactive certification."[24]

Unfortunately, the TJTC has not been particularly useful in increasing the number of disabled people hired. In fact, legislative incentives in general have not been very successful in achieving the goal of vocationally rehabilitating persons with disabilities. Approximately 80% of SSI recipients work prior to applying for SSI, and 20% work after they start receiving payments.[25] Scott Muller of the Social Security Administration performed a retrospective analysis of a cohort of over 4000 people who were initially entitled to benefits.[18] Approximately 10% worked during the initial period of entitlement. Of those, 84% were granted a TWP, and of that group, over 70% completed the TWP. Greater than 50% did not leave the rolls as a result of their efforts. Less than 3% had benefits terminated as a result of return to work.[18]

It is clear from the research conducted by the Social Security Administration that legislating incentives are not the complete answer to rehabilitating persons with work disability. Potential employers and persons with disabilities alike must take the initiative.

DISABILITY PREVENTION

With disability ranking as the nation's largest public health problem it seems reasonable to apply the public health model of prevention to disability. The public health model defines three categories of prevention: primary, secondary, and tertiary.

Primary prevention is intended for healthy persons to avoid the onset of a pathologic condition. In persons with disabilities, primary prevention efforts for other health issues need to be in place.

Secondary prevention is aimed at early identification and treatment of a pathologic condition and reduction of risk factors for the disabling process. For persons with disabilities, there are many opportunities for secondary preventive measures in reducing the risk factors. The ameliorative and corrective programs discussed above, including vocational rehabilitation strategies, are aimed at reduction of risk factors for disability and improvement in quality of life. The policies, such as the Americans with Disabilities Act, are also efforts to reduce environmental and social risk factors for disabilities. Interventions in medical rehabilitation focused on risk factors for the disabling process, such as provision of assistive technology, can be considered secondary prevention.

Tertiary prevention focuses on arresting the progression of a pathologic condition and on limiting further impairment within the disabling process. Medical rehabilitation is traditionally considered a tertiary prevention strategy. Indeed, efforts in rehabilitation to prevent secondary conditions or to prevent further impairment are tertiary prevention.[20, 34]

In considering the disabling process and the close interaction with risk factors and quality of life, there are many opportunities for the physiatrist and the medical rehabilitation team to intervene. The physiatrist has a responsibility to be actively involved in therapeutic and public health management of disability.[14]

CONCLUSION

Comprehensive rehabilitation is an intervention directed at the disabling process. The desired outcome is to maximize the physical, mental, social, and economic function of the individual with disabilities. The physiatrist is the team leader of the comprehensive rehabilitation team. It is the responsibility of the physiatrist to take a holistic approach to the person with disabilities. The holistic approach includes collaboration with professionals outside of the traditional medical rehabilitation team, such as those who can facilitate vocational rehabilitation for persons with disabilities.

Vocational rehabilitation strategies are interventions also aimed at the disabling process, risk factors for the disabling process, and the quality of life for the individual. Work disability has significant socioeconomic consequences for the individual and for society. Employment of persons with disabilities supports a better quality of life and limits the progression of the disabling process. Even for people with severe disabilities, vocational rehabilitation strategies have been successful in limiting work disability.

Disability is the largest public health problem in the United States. The demands of this public health issue have captured the attention of public policymakers. This has resulted in implementation of significant federal disability laws. The nation's public policies on disability reflect the policymakers' acceptance of disability as a complex process. Disability is considered to be the result of an interaction between an individual and his or her environment.

The physiatrist is positioned to serve a primary role in the disabling process. As persons with disabilities become a greater segment of our society, the opportunities for physiatrists' involvement are expanded. It is the physiatrists' responsibility to be active in disability prevention, in care and advocacy for persons with disabilities, and in the development of public policy on disability.

References

1. Adams PF, Benson V: Current estimates for the national health interview survey. Vital Health Stat [10] 1989;
2. Anderson TP: Quality of life of the individual with a disability. Arch Phys Med Rehabil 1982; 63:55.
3. Berkowitz M: The socioeconomic consequences of SCI. Paraplegic News 1994; January, pp 18–23.
4. Berkowitz M, Hill MA: Disability and the labor market: an overview. In Berkowitz M, Hill MA (eds): Disability and the Labor Market: Economic Problems, Policies, and Programs. New York, ILR Press, 1989, pp 1–28.
5. Colvez A, Blanchet M: Disability trends in the United States population 1966–76: analysis of reported causes. Am J Public Health 1981; 71:464–471.
6. DeJong G, Lifchez R: Physical disability and public policy. Sci Am 1983; 248:40–50.
7. Funk R: Disability rights: from caste to class in the context of civil rights. In Gartner A, Joe T (eds): Images of the Disabled, Disabling Images. Westport, Conn, Praeger, 1987, pp 7–30.
8. Haber LD: Identifying the disabled: concepts and methods in the measurement of disability. Soc Secur Bull 1988; 51:11–28.
9. Haber LD: Issues in the definition of disability and the use of disability survey data. In Daniel LB, Aitter M, Ingram L (eds): Disability Statistics, An Assessment: Report of a Workshop. Washington, DC, National Academy Press, 1990, pp 1–71.
10. Harris L: The ICD Survey of Disabled Americans: Bringing Disabled Americans into the Mainstream. New York, Louis Harris and Associates, 1986.
11. Harvey C: The business of employment: employment after traumatic SCI. Paraplegic News 1993; October, pp 10–14.
12. Haveman RH, Halberstandt V, Burkhauser RV (eds): Public Policy Toward Disabled Workers: Cross-National Analyses of Economic Impacts. New York, Cornell University Press, 1984.
13. Hearne PG: Employment strategies for people with disabilities: a prescription for change. Milbank Q 1991; 69:111–128.
14. Joe TC: Professionalism: A new challenge for rehabilitation. Arch Phys Med Rehabil 1981; 62:245–250.
15. Kottke FJ: Philosophic considerations of quality of life for the disabled. Arch Phys Med Rehabil 1982; 63:60–63.
16. La Plante MP: The demographics of disability. Milbank Q 1991; 69:55–77.
17. Menchetti BM, Flynn CC: Vocational evaluation. In Rusch FR (ed): Supported Employment. Sycamore, Ill, Sycamore, 1990, pp 111–131.
18. Muller LS: Disability beneficiaries who work and their experience under program work incentives. Soc Secur Bull 1992; 55:2–19.
19. Nagi SZ: Disability concepts revisited: implication to prevention, appendix A. In Pope AM, Tarlov AR (eds): Disability in America: Toward a National Agenda for Prevention. Washington, DC, National Academy Press, 1991, pp 306–327.
20. Pope AM, Tarlov AR (eds): Disability in America: Toward a National Agenda for Prevention. Washington, DC, National Academy Press, 1991.
21. Rigby DE: SSI work incentive participants. Soc Secur Bull 1991; 54:22–29.
22. Rocklin SG, Mattson DR: The employment opportunities for disabled Americans act: legislative history and summary of provisions. Soc Secur Bull 1987; 50:25–35.
23. Rusk HA: The growth and development of rehabilitation medicine. Arch Phys Med Rehabil 1969; 50:463–466.
24. Schaffer DC: Tax incentives. Milbank Q 1991; 69:293–312.
25. Scott CG: Disabled SSI recipients who work. Soc Secur Bull 1992; 55:26–36.
26. Social Security Administration: Report of Disability Advisory Council: Executive Summary. Soc Secur Bull, 1988; 51:13–17.
27. Symington DC: The goals of rehabilitation. Arch Phys Med Rehabil 1984; 65:427–430.
28. Thornton C, Maynard R: The economics of transitional employment and supported employment. In Berkowitz M, Hill MA (eds): Disability and the Labor Market: Economic Problems, Policies, and Programs. New York, ILR Press, 1989, pp 142–170.
29. US Bureau of the Census: Disability, Functional Limitation, and Health Insurance Coverage: 1984–85. Current Population Reports, series P-70, No. 8. Washington, DC, Government Printing Office, 1986.
30. US Department of Health and Human Service. Social Security Administration: Redbook on Work Incentives. Washington, DC, Government Printing Office, 1992.
31. US Equal Employment Opportunity Commission, US Department of Justice: Americans with Disabilities Act Handbook (EEOC-BK-19). Washington, DC, Government Printing Office, 1991.
32. US General Accounting Office: Testimony Before the Subcommittee on Select Education, Committee on Education and Labor, House of Representatives. Vocational Rehabilitation Program: Client Characteristics, Services Received, and Employment Outcomes. Washington, DC, Government Printing Office, November 1991.
33. Vachon RA: Inventing a future for individuals with work disabilities: the challenge of writing national disability policies. In Woods DE, Vandergoot D (eds): The Changing Nature of Work, Society and Disability: The Impact on Rehabilitation Policy. New York, World Rehabilitation Fund, 1987, pp 19–45.
34. Vachon RA: Employment assistance and vocational rehabilitation for people with HIV or AIDS: policy, practice, and prospects. In O'Dell MW (ed): HIV-Related Disability: Assessment and Management. Physical Medicine and Rehabilitation: State of the Art Reviews. Philadelphia, Hanley & Belfus, 1993, pp s203–s224.
35. Vachon RA: Employing the disabled. Issues Sci Technol 1989–1990; winter: 44–50.

36. Verville R: The rehabilitation amendments of 1978: what do they mean for comprehensive rehabilitation? Arch Phys Med Rehabil 1979; 60:141–144.

37. Wehman P, Sherron P, Kregel J, et al: Return to work for persons following severe traumatic brain injury: supported employment outcomes after five years. Am J Phys Med Rehabil 1993; 72:355–363.

38. Wilson RW: Do health indicators indicate health? Am J Public Health 1981; 71:461–463.

39. World Health Organization: International Classification of Impairments, Disabilities and Handicaps: A Manual of Classification Relating to the Consequences of Disease. 1980; Geneva: World Health Organization.

Practical Aspects of Impairment Rating and Disability Determination

ROBERT D. RONDINELLI, M.D., PH.D.

Within the field of physical medicine and rehabilitation, the topics of impairment rating and disability determination have generally been overlooked in terms of availability of formal teaching materials and preceptorships within the major training programs, key reference textbooks or chapters written for and by physiatrists within the current rehabilitation literature, and attention given by the board of examination. Physiatric representation and participation on the physician advisory panel to the American Medical Association's *Guides to the Evaluation of Permanent Impairment* (AMA Guides), which is the standard reference manual for rating compensable injuries under Workers' Compensation within the United States, appears disproportionately low (approximately 5% of physician contributors to a text with approximately 40% of its content devoted to the musculoskeletal system). This is particularly problematic when one considers that impairment, disability, and handicap are the conceptual linchpins of our specialty and the clinical focal point of virtually all rehabilitative problem solving. This chapter is a practical attempt to provide the user with a working vocabulary and conceptual understanding of the processes of impairment rating and disability determination, to highlight their inherent shortcomings and pitfalls at the present time, to provide orientation to the AMA Guides, and to focus on key aspects of the examination and reporting requirements for the physician examiner in cases of compensable injury. It is also an attempt to heighten our awareness of the importance of these topics to our field and to call attention to the need for more formalized didactic treatment and research efforts by physiatrists in these areas.

DEFINITIONS AND TERMINOLOGY

Definitions

The World Health Organization[39] (WHO) definitions are as follows:

Impairment: ". . . any loss or abnormality of psychological, physiological, or anatomic structure or function."

Disability: ". . . any restriction or lack (resulting from an impairment) of ability to perform an activity in the manner or within the range considered normal for a human being."

Handicap: ". . . a disadvantage for a given individual, resulting from an impairment or a disability, that limits or prevents the fulfillment of a role that is normal (depending on age, sex, and social and cultural factors) for that individual."

The fourth edition of the AMA Guides[2] provides the following working definitions for purposes of medical reporting:

Impairment: ". . . the loss, the loss of use, or derangement of any body part, system or function" (p. 315).

Permanent impairment: ". . . impairment that has become static or well stabilized with or without medical treatment, and is not likely to remit despite medical treatment" (p. 315).

Disability: ". . . a decrease in, or the loss or absence of the capacity of an individual to meet personal, social, or occupational demands or to meet statutory or regulatory requirements" (p. 317).

Permanent disability: ". . . occurs when the limiting loss or absence of capacity becomes static or well stabilized and is not likely to change in spite of continuing use of medical or rehabilitative measures" (p. 317).

Handicap: ". . . refers to 'obstacles to accomplishing life's basic activities that can be overcome only by . . . compensation or accommodation'" (p. 2).

Impairment can be considered as a tangible entity, but its relationship to disability and handicap remains a relative one. Disability and handicap should perhaps be viewed in the context of performing specific tasks or functions (Table 10–1). If the impaired individual can perform a required task or function without specific accommodation, no disability or handicap exists. If the impaired individual can successfully perform only in the presence of specific accommodation, and if that accommodation is provided, no disability or handicap exists relating to that task. If the impaired individual can successfully perform only in the presence of specific accommodation, and if that accommodation is not provided, both disability and handicap exist relating to that task. If the impaired individual cannot successfully perform even in the presence of "reasonable accommodation," a disability exists and a handicap might exist, depending on whether the accommodation is limited by "undue hardship" or poses a "direct threat" (see Terminology).

Although disability may arise out of impairment, it is not determined solely (or for that matter, in large part) by the impairment. In fact, similar levels of impairment can give rise to substantially differing disabilities. Handicap can be considered the degree to which social barriers to accommodation exist and, in a sense, bears an inverse relationship to accommodation.

Terminology

The following terminology includes frequently used items central to the process and procedures of impairment evaluating and reporting:

AGGRAVATION: A circumstance or event that (temporarily or permanently) worsens a pre-existing or underlying and susceptible condition.[2]

APPORTIONMENT: A determination of percentage of impairment directly attributable to pre-existing or resulting conditions and directly contributing to the total impairment rating derived.[2]

CAUSALITY: An association between a given cause (an event capable of producing an effect) and effect (a condition that can result from a specific cause) within a reasonable degree of medical probability. Causality requires determination that:

An event took place
The claimant experiencing the event has the condition (impairment)
The event could cause the condition (impairment)
It is medically probable that the event caused the condition (impairment)[2, 29]

DIAGNOSIS-RELATED ESTIMATES (DRE): Estimates of impairment assigned on the basis of a diagnosis rather than findings on physical examination.[2(p.84)] The AMA Guides provides DREs for regional impairments affecting the spine

and extremities. The rating physician must choose between the impairment estimate derived by diagnostic or examination criteria for a specific region; the physician is encouraged to use whichever approach yields the greater estimate.

ERGONOMICS: The science of matching the job to the worker and the product to the user.[32] An effective match optimizes efficiency, safety, comfort, and ease of use.

FUNCTIONAL CAPACITY ASSESSMENT (FCA): A generic assessment of an individual's job-related functional abilities that include strength, flexibility, endurance, and overall capability to perform physical work. The FCA can be useful in case disposition in which no specific job is available to an impaired individual, and general guidelines and restrictions are needed for purposes of job counseling and vocational rehabilitation.[18]

FUNCTIONAL CAPACITY EVALUATION (FCE): A comprehensive assessment of an individual's strength, flexibility, endurance, and job-specific functional abilities. An FCE includes a feasibility assessment of the impaired individual's ability to perform the essential functions of a specific job and could be the most valid predictor of return-to-work potential and restrictions applicable in a given case.[1]

INDEPENDENT MEDICAL EVALUATION (IME): In cases involving Workers' Compensation in which either party disputes maximum medical improvement (MMI; see following text), an administrative law judge may refer to a separate physician examiner for a second opinion regarding MMI and impairment rating.[2, 29] Some regard an IME as any examination done for evaluation purposes by a physician other than the treating physician.

JOB DESCRIPTION: A formal listing of the essential functions that constitute a particular job in terms of their specific physical performance requirements.[18]

JOB SITE EVALUATION (JSE): An on-site analysis of the workplace to determine optimal ergonomic design and to validate specific physical performance requirements of the job. JSE may be useful in concert with FCE to determine applicable return-to-work restrictions and to help ensure employer/employee compliance when necessary.[18]

MAXIMUM MEDICAL IMPROVEMENT (MMI): The point at which medically determined impairment resulting from injury becomes stable and at which no further treatment is reasonably expected to improve the condition. MMI is felt to occur when the following criteria have been satisfied:

The healing period has ended (the AMA Guides recognizes a minimum documented duration of 6 months since injury onset);
The medical condition has fully resolved; or
No further reasonable progress occurs or is expected to occur toward resolution of the medical condition.

TABLE 10–1   Interrelationships Between Impairment, Disability, and Handicap

Impairment Present	Can Perform Essential Functions	Accommodation Necessary to Perform	Accommodation Provided	Disability	Handicap
Yes	Yes	No	No	No	No
Yes	No	Yes	No	Yes	Yes
Yes	No	Yes	Yes	No	No
Yes	No	Yes*	Yes	Yes	Possibly

*May not be able to perform even in presence of accommodation.

MMI does not preclude the deterioration of a condition that is expected to occur with the passage of time; neither does it preclude allowances for ongoing follow-up or maintenance care.[2, 29]

MEDICAL POSSIBILITY: Something could occur due to a particular cause (probability of 50% or less).[2]

MEDICAL PROBABILITY: Something is more likely to occur than not (probability exceeds 50%).[2]

SCHEDULED LOSS: Allocation of a specified value for purposes of indemnification to a regional anatomical or functional unit to which an impairment rating can be assigned. The specified value allowed for a given unit may be expressed in terms of weeks or months of lost wages.[2]

UNSCHEDULED LOSS: Estimated functional loss to the "whole person" for purposes of indemnification and accorded to a physiological system rather than to a regional anatomical or functional unit.[2] The cardiopulmonary, gastrointestinal, and central nervous systems are examples of systems to which an unscheduled loss might apply.

"WADDELL'S SIGNS": Findings on physical examination that are thought to reflect a "nonorganic" basis of physical complaints and collectively serve to invalidate the examination itself.[38]

Five markers are described to include:

1. Tenderness that is provoked by superficial palpation and/or that is non-anatomical in distribution.
2. Pain on simulated provocation by axial loading or sham rotation of the spine.
3. Inconsistency of findings with patient distraction.
4. Regional weakness or sensory loss.
5. Overreaction to the examination

WORK HARDENING: A work-oriented treatment program, delivered in a highly structured environment that simulates the workplace, designed to improve job productivity of an injured or deconditioned worker. Productivity goals may pertain to work tolerance, job proficiency, or job efficiency.[18]

WORK SIMULATION: An individually focused work hardening exercise program that simulates specific components of the workers' job for purposes of making a transition to work-ready status and documenting work-ready status.[18]

HISTORICAL DEVELOPMENT OF IMPAIRMENT RATINGS AND DISABILITY DETERMINATIONS

Workers' Compensation

Workers' compensation is the earliest known disability system,[25] with origins dating at least to Roman times. By the late 1600s, the buccaneers of the West Indies had written "articles" of agreement that stipulated compensable sums to which injured crew members would be entitled for injuries and losses suffered during the course of a particular voyage. For example, 600 pieces-of-eight would be awarded for loss of a right arm, 500 for loss of a left arm, 500 for loss of a right leg, and 100 for loss of an eye.[13]

Von Bismarck first introduced a comprehensive social insurance system in Europe that included provisions for workers' compensation in the 1880's. Contemporary developments in England included the Employers' Liability Act of 1880 followed by the Workers' Compensation Law in 1887. Prior to that time, injured employees were unlikely to receive help from their employer unless they filed suit and could demonstrate that the employer was at fault and the claimant was free from "contributory negligence." Unsuccessful claims went uncompensated, whereas successful litigants might receive large monetary rewards that could jeopardize the financial viability of a company and the jobs available to other constituent workers. A "no-fault" system was adopted to resolve this dilemma whereby eligibility for coverage was automatic if the claim could be shown to have arisen directly during the course of one's employment activity.[25]

In St. Petersburg, Russia, a disability indemnification schedule was developed in 1907 in which regional injuries and resulting physical impairments could be awarded a specified percentage of total "disability" according to the whole person concept.[25]

The United States system of Workers' Compensation was created in 1908 under the Federal Employees Compensation Act. Subsequently, the California Industrial Accident Act of 1914 created a schedule of impairment indemnification according to claimant's age, specific occupation, and physical impairment rating. By 1949, Workers' Compensation was available to all states.[25]

Workers' Compensation is a federally mandated system of health and disability insurance administered at the state level. Its purpose is to provide benefits to disabled workers for any and all claims of injury or illness arising directly out of employment. Under Workers' Compensation, a disability is defined as the ". . . immediate inability, because of work-related injury, to perform gainful activity as defined by one's most recent occupation" or similar suitable occupation for the claimant's level of training and experience.[31] Recipients are eligible for three types of benefits, which include the following:

1. Benefits to an employee's survivor in cases of death.
2. Coverage of expenses of hospitalization and medical and rehabilitative care.
3. Wage-loss compensation.

Wage-loss compensation benefits are of four types[2, 22] and include the following:

1. *Temporary total*—Benefits are typically equal to two thirds of the usual and customary wages up to a maximum allowable cap, which varies by state. For example, temporary benefits are payable monthly from onset of injury until MMI is reached if the claimant is judged medically to be unable to continue working during the specified period of coverage.
2. *Temporary partial*—Benefits paid during the period of onset of injury through MMI if the injured worker is returned to modified duty. Benefits are generally equal to two thirds of the difference between pre-injury vs. modified duty wages up to the temporary total cap for each state.
3. *Permanent partial*—Benefits may be "scheduled" or "unscheduled." Scheduled benefits are awarded in specific amounts associated with specific impairments affecting particular body parts and in accordance with predetermined

disability tables that specify the number of weeks for which benefits must be paid at an average weekly wage rate. Unscheduled benefits typically require the estimation of percentage of impairment to the "whole person," from which proportional compensation against total possible loss can be determined. Benefits are payable at MMI.

4. *Permanent total*—Benefits awarded up to a state-recognized percentage of pre-injury wages if the employee is found to be permanently incapable of returning to work at a level suitable to his or her training and experience. Benefits are payable at MMI.

Other Disability Systems

Social Security

The Social Security Disability Act of 1954, and subsequent establishment of Social Security Disability Income (SSDI) in 1956, provided for a federally administered disability insurance program within the Social Security Administration (SSA) with benefits for individuals who are unable to work because of a disability. The SSA defines disability as the ". . . inability to engage in any substantial gainful activity by reason of any medically determinable physical or mental impairment which can be expected to result in death or has lasted or can be expected to last for a continuous period of not less than 12 months."[31(p. 38)]

SSDI is available to claimants who meet the definition of disability according to the SSA:

- Can demonstrate a recent work history (actively working for at least 5 of the preceding 10 years)
- Have remained unemployed for the previous 6-month period
- Have a current income of less than $300 per month

Entitlement is based on the claimant's contributions from prior earnings to Old Age, Survivors and Disability Insurance (OASDI) or by meeting criteria of a "means test." Benefits include a monthly stipend, Medicare supplemental insurance, and coverage for vocational rehabilitation.[31]

Supplemental Security Income (SSI) provides SSA disability benefits to individuals who meet the SSA definition of disability but lack evidence of a recent work history. Entitlement is based on financial need according to the means test, and benefits include a monthly stipend, Medicaid insurance supplement, and coverage for vocational rehabilitation.[31]

For both SSDI and SSI, a physician must render an impairment rating according to a List of Impairments Schedule (or estimate of equivalent rating) as provided by the SSA.

Department of Veterans' Affairs

The Department of Veteran's Affairs (VA) maintains a federally-administered disability program available to veterans whose disability is recognized as any condition ". . . which is sufficient to render it impossible for the average person to follow a substantially gainful occupation, but only if it is reasonably certain that such disability will continue throughout the life of the disabled."[31(p. 58)] Service-connected entitlement requires determination that the disability be shown to arise during the course of military service, whereas non-service-connected entitlement requires determination that disability is permanent and total (60% or more) and is shown to arise after the course of military service. Benefits awarded to eligible veterans include a monthly stipend, medical care at VA facilities, prosthetic/orthotic devices, durable medical equipment, and home and motor vehicle modifications as appropriate. The rating physician must estimate the nature and severity of impairment according to a VA schedule.

Americans With Disabilities Act

With the passage of the Americans With Disabilities Act (ADA) in 1990, disabled Americans are guaranteed equal rights to employment opportunities, transportation, and public access. The ADA defines disability as ". . . a physical or mental impairment that substantially limits one or more of the major life activities of such individual, a record of such impairment or being regarded as such an impairment."[3] Although it is broad and somewhat imprecise, this definition is narrowed under Title 1 of ADA (Employment) to recognize employment as a major life activity, and views disability within the context of performance of the "essential functions" of an employment position with or without "reasonable accommodation." Reasonable accommodation can include structural modifications at the work site to improve accessibility, availability of modified duty options, and acquisition of adaptive equipment or devices to enable disabled workers to perform the essential functions of their jobs. Accommodations exempted under ADA include those that would impose "undue hardship" on the employer in terms of cost or feasibility of implementation, or those that would pose a "direct threat" to the health and safety of the disabled individual or co-workers.[3]

Impairment Rating Systems

Early Systems

The earliest attempts at impairment rating systems were anatomically based and regional in scope, with emphasis on the musculoskeletal system. This regional approach lent itself well to the concept that a schedule of discrete disability values could be assigned to anatomical units or subunits of the spine and extremities. For example, Smith[36] provided a system for Workers' Compensation to evaluate industrial "disability" according to scheduled losses affecting the extremities (expressed as functional units or "radicals"), eyes, or ears, and according to unscheduled losses affecting other organ systems. Structural criteria (amputation, ankylosis) and joint active range of motion (ROM) formed the basis for rating the extremities. In 1962, the American Academy of Orthopedic Surgeons (AAOS)[1] published a manual devoted entirely to scheduled impairments of the spine and extremities using structural criteria (amputation, ankylosis), ROM, and sensory losses as criteria for rating. Subsequently, Rice[33] described an anatomical system of impairment rating for the spine and extremities whose sole criterion was loss of ROM.

In 1963, McBride[28] introduced additional functional criteria for impairment rating to include strength, coordination, speed of movement, dexterity, and endurance. However he failed to provide a precise methodology to follow when impairment determinations were made according to these additional criteria. Kessler[23] carried the notion of functionally based impairment ratings forward by considering losses due to strength, sensation, and coordination as well as to ROM. Strength was assessed relative to contralateral limb via strain gauge testing or manual muscle testing (MMT), and functional prehension and precision grip testing was also employed. Losses due to coordination and sensation remained poorly defined.

American Medical Association (AMA) Guides

In 1956, the AMA created an ad hoc committee to address medical impairment rating practices, and this resulted in 13 separate publications in the JAMA from 1958 to 1970. These publications were subsequently compiled into the AMA Guides, the first edition of which was published in 1971. By 1981, an advisory panel was formed to update and revise the AMA Guides, and four subsequent revisions appeared[2] from 1984 through 1993. Although traditionally anatomically based, the most recent edition seeks to surmount many pitfalls inherent in that system through the introduction of the "diagnosis-related model" (DRE) as described below.

APPLICATION OF THE AMA GUIDES (MUSCULOSKELETAL SYSTEM)

General Considerations

Qualitative Impairments

Qualitative impairments are anatomically based and belong to discrete, mutually exclusive categories that can only be measured in descriptive terms. Nominal or ordinal scales of measurement may apply to such groupings to yield hierarchical assembly, but the actual magnitude of difference between groupings is non-uniform and lacks true proportionality to assigned numeric value. Examples of qualitative impairments pertaining to the extremities and recognized by the AMA Guides include amputation, joint ankylosis, sensory change (present vs. absent), and cosmetic disfigurement (present vs. absent).

Quantitative Impairments

Quantitative impairments are also anatomically based. They are measured according to continuous scales (interval or ratio) whose units represent fixed values, the ordering of which reflects a uniform and consistent increase in magnitude. The AMA Guides recognizes loss of motion (in degrees) in each cardinal plane of function for a given joint as representing quantitative impairment relative to the normally accepted range of motion for that joint.

Diagnosis-Based Impairments

The most recent edition of the AMA Guides has advanced a diagnosis-related model (DRE) as an alternative approach to impairment rating; it is categorical in nature, less dependent on findings during physical examination,

and, instead, emphasizes the key elements of history of injury and corroborative, objective findings on diagnostic testing. Where applicable, the DRE model has advantages of simplicity and ease of determination, and it is perhaps less biased in terms of the concrete rating guidelines provided.

Shortcomings and Pitfalls

Any person who uses the AMA Guides should recognize the following key shortcomings.

First and foremost, the process whereby functional loss is inferred and extrapolated from anatomically determined impairment might not be valid. More specific and objective determinations concerning normal functioning of an organ system and the impact of impairments on same are needed. The contributors to the AMA Guides have ". . . estimated the extent of impairments on the basis of clinical experience, judgment, and consensus. The estimates of the well qualified persons contributing to . . . [the AMA Guides], most of them physicians . . . [are judged to be] more convincing than those of most others in estimating the severity of people's impairments."[2(p. 3)] Such validation by consensus is, in general, unsupported by rigorously collected, behaviorally based data and lacks a sound scientific foundation at this time. This shortcoming applies to both anatomically based and diagnosis-based impairments.

Second, concerns abound with regard to the validity and reliability of the impairment measures conventionally in use. For example, surface inclinometry is the adopted procedure of choice for determining spinal mobility according to the AMA Guides; however, the degree to which surface inclinometry reflects underlying spinal mobility has been questioned.[27] Furthermore, loss of spinal flexibility may not predict back pain disability, and one study has even suggested an inverse relationship between pain-induced disability and lumbar flexibility.[24] High inter-rater and intra-rater reliability have been reported using the two-inclinometer method to measure lumbar flexion and extension.[21] However, other authors have shown the presence of significant measurement error and unacceptably low reliability estimates for this technique (based on intraclass correlations), even when applied by experienced observers to healthy and fully compliant subjects.[35]

Subjectivity of the patient and examiner and performance effort put forth during any examination and testing can have a negative impact on the validity of impairment measures derived. Whereas true malingering/complaint fabrication can be considered an exceptional occurrence, the examiner can expect to frequently encounter elements of symptom magnification,[26] particularly in compensable injury cases.[36] Such exaggeration and inconsistencies need to be recognized and discounted, hopefully without penalizing the patient who exhibits them. Waddell's signs[38] can aid the examiner in this regard, and meticulous record-keeping of observations on successive visits, when possible, can serve as a further internal check on consistency of findings during examination. Isokinetic ergometers have gained acceptance as an exercise and evaluation tool for assessment of consistency of effort based on coefficients of variability established for healthy subjects. However, a recent review[30] questions the applicability of these coefficients to subjects experiencing back pain or symptom magnification.

Finally, the issue of pain as it pertains to impairment deserves further consideration. The role of pain in disability determinations has been dealt with extensively,[31] and the logistical and conceptual issues surrounding the measurement of pain behavior are beyond our immediate scope, though they are well-documented elsewhere.[14] Simply stated, pain as a phenomenon is entirely subjective and cannot be measured directly. Consequently, pain behavior or complaints should not serve as the only basis for ratable impairment determination in the absence of corroborative objective criteria.[2]

Extremities as Regional Units

The Hand and Upper Extremity

The AMA Guides has adopted a system for evaluating hand and upper extremity impairment, which was originally developed and approved by the International Federation of Societies for Surgery of the Hand in association with the American Society for Surgery of the Hand. This regional unit is divided for purposes of separate evaluation into five regional units: thumb, finger, wrist, elbow and shoulder.

Qualitative impairments are as follows: Total loss of motion or sensation within a regional unit or ankylosis/malposition that precludes functional use of same is equated to total functional loss, as would result from amputation of that unit. Ankylosis of a unit or subunit in optimal functional position is considered the least impairment of that unit. The impairments are assigned numeric values that are presented in tabular form for each regional unit.

Estimates of impairment resulting from peripheral nerve dysfunction involve losses attributable to sensory deficits, pain, or weakness. Sensory loss estimates are equated to 50% of comparable functional loss due to amputation. To be ratable, pain or sensory deficits must be shown to interfere with functional performance of the unit, to follow recognizable neuroanatomical pathways, and to be corroborated by other objective signs of peripheral nerve dysfunction. Similarly, objective and reproducible deficits in strength enable ratable estimates of functional loss attributable to motor weakness if the pattern of weakness is consistent with dysfunction along a peripheral nerve pathway.

Quantitative impairment in terms of restricted ROM for a given member is presented in tabular form as a percentage loss of the normative range for that member. Estimates of ROM are determined goniometrically, using procedures illustrated in the AMA Guides. The AMA Guides specifies that active ROM determination takes precedence over passive ROM whenever possible, and ROM estimates are rounded to the nearest 10 degrees. Although the AMA Guides fails to specify this, the unaffected contralateral extremity (if applicable) may serve as a more valid baseline reference for a given individual's expected ROM than the normative range estimated for that particular joint. Consequently, I recommend using contralateral range loss estimates as the basis for comparison whenever possible.

In some cases, categorical losses due to joint instability, implants, or other connective tissue disorders not covered in the preceding discussion are ratable according to the appropriate tables of the AMA Guides.

The Lower Extremity

The lower extremity is considered in terms of five regional units: hip, knee, ankle, foot, and toes. Qualitative impairments for amputation and ankylosis are recognized, and tabular references for these are provided. Losses due to peripheral nerve dysfunction affecting the lower extremities and attributable to sensory deficits, pain, or weakness are treated in similar fashion to those affecting the upper extremity. In addition, categorical impairment estimates according to limb-length discrepancies, gait "derangements," and muscle atrophy are separately recognized and tabulated. Quantitative impairments due to losses against expected arc of motion can be goniometrically determined and interpreted according to tables provided for each member, and in a manner similar to that for the upper extremity.

Diagnosis-Based Estimates

The AMA Guides separately recognizes diagnosis-based categories of impairment of the lower extremity, including fractures of the regional units, endoprosthetic replacement of the hip or knee, and major skin-grafting procedures. Separate reference tables are provided. The examiner is encouraged to use diagnosis-based ratings as an alternative to (*never* in addition to) anatomically based ratings for each specific impairment and to select whichever option yields the greater impairment in any given case.

Spine as Regional Units

Qualitative Impairments and Diagnosis-Related Estimates (DRE)

The AMA Guides has developed the DRE approach to the assessment of impairments of the spine in an attempt to recognize and differentiate clinical findings due to illness or injury from those that accompany the normal aging process. The DRE or *injury model* recognizes specific diagnostic categories (e.g., vertebral body compression graded according to severity; fracture of vertebral posterior elements or transverse processes; loss of motion segment integrity; cauda equina syndrome; paraplegia) for which diagnosis-based ratings can be derived. The spine is treated as three regional units (cervicothoracic, thoracolumbar, and lumbosacral) for which maximal impairment estimates of 35%, 20%, and 75%, respectively, can be derived. Eight categories of gradation of severity are developed that are applicable to recognized disorders of each regional unit; categorical differentiators for each emphasize objective and reproducible evidence of neurological dysfunction or loss of structural integrity. For example, loss of reflexes or focal atrophy (≥ 2 cm), although recognized, is weighted less than electrodiagnostic findings of acute or chronic nerve root compromise (e.g., multiple positive sharp waves or fibrillation potentials, H-wave absence or delay >3 mm/sec, polyphasic waves). Similarly, cystometrogram findings outweigh those from physical examination. Loss of motion segment integrity is defined according to anteroposterior translations in flexion/extension views of at least 3.5 mm for cervical or at least 5 mm for thoracic or lumbar regions in the sagittal plane. Specific angular displacements identified radiographically between adjacent motion segments in the sagittal plane are also recognized. The DRE system enables the examiner to rate appropriate diagnoses according to region and severity with all ratings rendered according to whole person estimates (see following discussion).

Quantitative Impairments and Inclinometry

The traditional, anatomically based approach to impairment rating of the spine is termed the *range of motion model,* and the AMA Guides currently recommends its use ". . . only if the Injury Model is not applicable, or if more clinical data are needed."[2(p. 112)] Under this model the three regions of the spine are cervical, thoracic, and lumbar, for which maximal ratings for loss of motion of 80%, 40%, and 90%, respectively, are attributed. All impairment ratings are rendered to the whole person (see following discussion) and detailed procedural descriptions are provided for one- and two-inclinometer techniques to determine regional spinal motion in flexion/extension, lateral flexion, and rotation as applicable. Normative tables are provided by region to determine impairment according to degrees of motion loss.

Impairments Due to Specific Spine Disorders

In situations where the range of motion model is being applied, four categories of diagnoses (separate from the DRE model) are recognized, including fractures, intervertebral disk or soft-tissue, spondylolysis/spondylolisthesis (unoperated), and spinal stenosis/segmental instability/spondylolisthesis (operated) for the cervical, thoracic, and lumbar regions, respectively. In contrast to the DRE model, this option enables the examiner to take into account surgical intervention and multiple operative procedures in developing the final impairment rating.

Combining Impairments and Whole Person Ratings

Impairment ratings derived independently for each regional unit or subunit of the spine and extremities are expressed in terms of scheduled values for each unit (exceptions being the unscheduled expressions of whole person ratings derived by the DRE model or other diagnosis-based ratings described earlier). It is possible for the examiner to combine these scheduled and unscheduled ratings to achieve a single cumulative impairment rating to the whole person according to a *combined values chart* provided by the AMA Guides. The chart is designed to ensure that cumulative scheduled ratings of regional subunits do not exceed the total value of the unit itself, and that a cumulative whole person impairment rating does not exceed 100%. In using the combined values chart, all scheduled impairments must first be converted to whole person equivalents using the appropriate conversion charts provided in each section of the AMA Guides. When two whole person ratings from different regional units are combined, the larger value serves to indicate the appropriate row and the smaller value the appropriate column from which to determine the appropriate combined value. The process is repeated until all unit values have been included.

IMPAIRMENT AND DISABILITY REPORT WRITING

Worksheet for History and Physical Examination

A sample worksheet is provided (Fig. 10–1) that is intended to aid the physician examiner and ensure that a consistent, systematic, and complete data base is gathered during the IME. If it is used as a teaching aid for preceptorships in industrial rehabilitation, the preceptor should validate key items of the history and physical examination and ensure that adequate and appropriate documentation takes place. The worksheet also serves as a reference to enable rapid, thorough, and accurate dictation of the IME report.

A number of risk factors for *delayed recovery* syndromes have been described[12, 16] and are important items to address in the IME patient history as follows:

Occupational:
- Time off of work
- Low job satisfaction
- Patient perception of mismatch between physical capacity and job demands
- Lack of modified duty options

Psychosocial:
- Poor English proficiency
- Disabled spouse
- Anger toward system
- Ongoing or prior litigation/compensation
- Disability convictions by patient or physician

Medical:
- Prior history of injury
- History of substance abuse
- Poor cardiovascular fitness

The history serves as an important screening tool to identify patients as high risk and, consequently, should address these items inclusively.

It is well documented that likelihood of return to work following injury decreases precipitously as time off of work following injury increases, regardless of the illness or injury.[15] Specifically, probability decreases to 50% or less at 6 months and to 20% at 1 year postinjury. Strang[37] has shown that 6 or more consecutive months out of work in the presence of amotivation, symptom magnification, and pain unaccompanied by secondary medical conditions presents a chronicity syndrome for which the prognosis for functional recovery is guarded (see Chapter 44). The IME physician must be circumspect about recommending continued therapy in such cases and should judiciously monitor functional progress achieved if therapies are to continue. Justification for discontinuing therapy may be based, in part, on knowledge and documentation of the above.

Symptom magnification[26] refers to embellishment (conscious or otherwise) of the patient's subjective pain and suffering and displays of pain behavior that are out of proportion to what is supported by objective data in a particular case.

Text continued on page 202

WORKSHEET FOR HISTORY AND PHYSICAL EXAMINATION
Date:
Patient Name: ID#
Referred by:
Date of onset of injury/illness:
Employer:
Nature of injury/illness:
Medical/diagnostic/therapeutic treatment rendered:
Present symptoms/complaints:
Pain:
locality   quality
severity (0 - 5 point scale)   duration (constant/intermittent)
aggravating factors   palliating factors
Weakness:
distribution (regional vs focal)
Sensory changes:
numbness/paresthesias   distribution (regional vs focal)
Bladder/Bowel dysfunction
Present treatment strategies:
Medications: type/frequency:
Therapies: exercise/modalities:
type/frequency
Equipment: corset   TENS   other
Review of Systems:
Sleep habits/changes since onset of injury/illness:
Weight gain/loss/appetite changes
Present disability:
Basic mobility/self-care activity
Work related: Duration of time out of work:
modified duty/restrictions (if applicable):
Avocational:
Employment History:
Nature of job
Time on-the-job at onset of injury/illness:
Job satisfaction/performance history
Previous employers/duration of employment
Educational level/English proficiency
Major Life Stressors:
Financial:
Marital/familial:

FIGURE 10–1 Worksheet for history and physical examination.

Past Medical History:
Constitutional illness/symptoms
Use of tobacco   alcohol   caffeine   illicit drugs
Allergies to foods or medications
Peptic ulcer disease/aspirin intolerance
Pregnancies
Past Surgical History:
Family History of Major Illness:
Psychiatric/psychological treatment or medications:
Prior history of injury:
Work related:
Non-Work Related:
Previous compensation/impairment rating:
Present litigation:
Social History:
Marital status:
Active dependents:
Child support?
Other disabled family members?
Patient's goals/expectations:

PHYSICAL EXAM - General:
Height: **Weight:**   **Vital Signs:**
HEENT:
Cardiopulmonary:
Abdominal:
Extremities: Pulses: Erythema/edema/trophic changes:
Affect/cognitive:
Neurological: Tone: Coordination:
Muscle stretch reflexes: upper extremity: lower extremity: sacral:
Sensory: touch: pinprick: proprioception: vibration:
Musculoskeletal: Posture
lordosis/kyphosis: scoliosis: abdominal tone:
guarding/protective/splinting/spasm:
tender points: location/distribution: "jump sign":

Flexibility (Spine:)	**Cervical**	**Thoracic**	**Lumbar**
flexion/extension:			
lateral flexion:			
rotation:			

FIGURE 10–1   *Continued*

Illustration continued on following page

R.O.M. (Extremities)

Upper	L	R	Lower	L	R
Shoulder			Hip		
Elbow			Knee		
Wrist			Ankle		
Hand			Foot		

Muscle Bulk/Symmetry

Upper	L	R	Lower	L	R

Manual Muscle Testing

Upper	L	R	Lower	L	R
Scapulothoracic			Hip flex/ext		
Deltoid			Hip abd/add		
Bicep			Quad		
Tricep			Hamstring		
Wrist flex/ext			Ankle dorsiflex /evert		
Intrinsic			Ankle plantarflex /invert		

Special Tests	Pos	Neg	Functional Gait	Normal	Abnormal
Spurling's:			Heel / toe		
Adsen's:			Tandem		
Tinel's:					
Phalen's:			Trendelenburg/		
Yergason's:			stationary		
Straight leg raise:			dynamic		

Waddell's Signs	Positive	Negative
Superficial/non-anatomic tenderness		
Sham provocation of pain/discomfort		
Inconsistencies		
Regional weakness/sensory loss		
Overreaction		

FIGURE 10–1 *Continued*

Diagnostic Database

Labs:

Radiographic:

Other:

Assessment:

Rehabilitation diagnoses:

Functional prognosis/goals:

Recommendations:

Additional diagnostic/consultative procedures:

Additional therapeutic intervention:

MMI determination (if appropriate):

Final impairment rating:

Case Disposition:

Return-to-work restrictions:

Vocational rehabilitation referral:

Other recommendations:

FIGURE 10–1 *Continued*

PHYSICIAN RESPONSIBILITIES/ REPORTING REQUIREMENTS

IME

In cases involving dispute between claimant and insurer concerning MMI determination or impairment rating derived, a physician examiner unfamiliar with the case can accept a referral from an administrative law judge or other official in order to review the case records, examine the claimant independently, and render a second opinion concerning the findings. In some cases, additional testing and treatment is authorized to be undertaken by the examiner to satisfy an MMI determination at that point.

MMI Determination

The physician examiner is required to complete a physicians initial report, supplemental interim reports, and a maximal medical improvement form at the time of case disposition.[29] Reporting requirements vary by state, but they are generally similar and must include an estimate of when MMI occurred or is expected to occur. The decision of MMI must be rendered before case closure can be achieved. It has been my experience that as long as expectations for further functional improvement continue to be met by demonstrable and ongoing performance gains, the claimant is deemed not to be at MMI. The distinction between functional vs. pain-oriented goal setting must be maintained so that progress toward goal achievement can be measured and monitored objectively. When functional progress is no longer evident or tenable and at least a 6-month healing period has been completed, MMI is felt to have occurred.

The physician examiner is also required to determine the exact date of MMI and to address issues of medical stability from that point forward. Deterioration that might normally be expected with the passage of time (e.g., progression of an osteoarthritic condition) does not preclude MMI determination. The physician must further address issues of future medical management and follow-up that are anticipated to be necessary to maintain MMI for a given condition.

Impairment Rating, Causality, and Apportionment

The physician examiner must determine the nature and degree of physical impairment, if any, according to the guidelines outlined earlier. Impairments can be expressed in terms of functional loss to the unit or to the whole person.

The physician examiner might be asked to render a medical opinion "within reasonable certainty" as to causality of a specific impairment. A direct or "proximate" causal relationship is thought to exist if a medical probability exists that the impairment is a direct result of reported illness or injury.[2] Consequently, examiners must distinguish between medical probability vs. medical possibility in such cases, and to their best ability according to guidelines stated earlier.

In cases involving pre-existing conditions and/or recurrent injury, apportionment is necessary and involves the physician's best estimate of the relative contributions of pre-existing or resulting conditions to the impairment rating that is ultimately derived. McBride[28] has recommended an impartial and objective solution to this problem that requires the development of three contingent "ratings" from which the apportioned percentage can be extracted:

- A total impairment rating is derived irrespective of pre-existing/resulting conditions
- A second rating is derived in which pre-existing conditions are discounted
- A third rating is derived that accounts solely for pre-existing conditions and progression over time without associated or aggravating re-injury

The physician might logically choose to award the greater of the two differences between the first minus the second rating or the first minus the third rating as the amount of total impairment apportioned to the resulting condition. To illustrate, the anatomical model for rating whole person impairment due to disorders of the spine[2(p. 113)] can be applied as follows to determine additional impairment caused by a third operation following a recurrent intervertebral disk injury:

- An overall impairment rating of 13% is first determined (10% for surgically treated disk at one level, 2% additional for second procedure, and 1% for third procedure)
- A second rating of 10% is determined by discounting two prior operations
- A third rating of 12% (10% plus 2%) is determined by discounting the final re-injury and the third operative procedure

In the preceding example, the examiner might render a 13% whole person impairment rating and apportion 3% (the greater difference between 13% minus 10% or 13% minus 12%) for resulting reinjury and a third operation.

Disability Determination/Return-to-Work Restrictions

The AMA Guides recognizes that disability benefits in terms of wage-loss compensation for work-related impairment are independent of the impaired individual's capacity to work and are formulated in terms of expected long-term negative financial impact of a given impairment category.[2] Indemnification schedules exist and vary by individual states with stipulations of the maximum number of weeks of average lost wages payable for loss of use of body parts. Consequently, the impairment rating and other medical information rendered by the physician ultimately assists a legal and administrative panel that is involved in making such determinations in any given case.

During the initial, interim, and MMI phases of reporting, the physician examiner is asked to complete a work status report, an example of which is provided in Figure 10-2.[34] If treatment is ongoing and transitional work is available, the physician can recommend *modified duty* in terms of restrictions on the number of hours of work and permissible activities during the transitional healing period. If modified duty options are unavailable, the physician might be required to render a *temporary total disability* determination until MMI is reached. The probability of returning to work

PATIENT STATUS:

PATIENT NAME: _____ DATE OF INJURY:_____

DIAGNOSIS:_____   STATUS: ☐ Improved ☐ Same ☐ Worse ☐ Resolved

WORK STATUS:

☐ RETURN TO FULL DUTY

☐ RETURN TO LIMITED DUTY   NUMBER OF HOURS/DAY:_____

☐ (OFF) UNABLE TO WORK UNTIL FOLLOW-UP   PROJECTED RETURN TO WORK DATE:_____

RESTRICTIONS:

CHECK THE FREQUENCY AND NUMBER OF HOURS/DAY THE WORKER IS ABLE TO DO THE FOLLOWING ACTIVITIES:

Activity	FREQUENCY		NUMBER OF HOURS/DAY								
	Continuous	Intermittent (with rest)	0	1	2	3	4	5	6	7	8
Sitting											
Standing											
Walking											

	Never	Occasionally (up to 33%)	Frequently (34-66%)	Continuously (67-100%)
Movements:				
Bend/Stoop				
Squat				
Kneel				
Crawl				
Climb				
Pushing/Pulling				
Reach above shoulder level				
Lift:				
Up to 10 lbs				
11 - 25 lbs				
26 - 50 lbs				
> 50 lbs				
Carry:				
Up to 10 lbs				
11 - 25 lbs				
26 - 50 lbs				
> 50 lbs				

RETURN APPOINTMENT:

RETURN APPOINTMENT (DATE):_____   TIME:_____

IS PATIENT AT MMI?   ☐ YES   ☐ NO   IF NOT, PROJECTED MMI DATE:_____

_____   _____
Provider signature/MD   Date of Exam

FIGURE 10–2 Example of typical work status report. (From Rondinelli R: Impairment evaluation and disability assessment. *In* Bonfiglio R (ed): Industrial Rehabilitation Medicine. Philadelphia, Hanley & Belfus, 1995.)

decreases precipitously as time out of work increases,[4] so the physician should make every effort to return the claimant safely to a transitional work setting as soon as possible. In cases in which transitional return to work options are unavailable, work hardening should be considered as a viable alternative to forced inactivity and should be implemented whenever feasible and medically necessary (see Chapter 44). At the point of MMI determination and case closure, the physician must render a final opinion on permanent restrictions applicable from that point forward.

A number of standardized assessment tools are available to assist the physician in determining valid and reliable physical performance expectations for an injured worker:

> *FCE* is a comprehensive assessment of the individual's strength, flexibility, endurance, and safety in performing job-specific activities, and it is perhaps the most valid predictor of appropriate restrictions to activity during various points of recovery and at MMI. In cases in which no specific job exists or is available, FCA provides suitable alternative information of a generic nature. The impaired individual's performance during an FCE or FCA can be assessed with respect to degree of effort, consistency, and reliability during testing.[18] In situations in which lack of consistency or incomplete effort results in questionable validity of performance measured, return-to-work restrictions must remain speculative and subjective.

> A *job description* is frequently available from the employer and can provide a useful list of the essential functions of the job in question for purposes of assessing functional capacities and addressing specific restrictions that can apply.

> *Job site evaluation* can be carried out by a specially trained therapist to validate the essential functions listed in the job description with respect to critical physical demands and relative amounts of time spent performing specific activities of each essential function. In some cases, ergonomic analysis may be useful to quantify physical demands relative to observed physical capacities and to enable specific recommendations for reasonable accommodation in terms of job redesign or workplace modification. Finally, employer and employee willingness to comply with recommended restrictions and accommodation can be addressed.

Physician examiners should avail themselves of these assessment tools in order to ensure that their prognostic inferences and sanctions are founded on valid, empirical, and functionally based data to the fullest extent possible.

LEGAL, ETHICAL, AND OTHER CONSIDERATIONS

Because of the medicolegal nature of many, if not most, Workers' Compensation referrals, the physician examiner can frequently expect to serve as an expert witness and to undergo deposition and courtroom testimony. The physician can be expected to testify with respect to even minute details of a specific case, often months or years after completion of the IME. A systematically collected, thorough, and well-organized data base and record file could significantly reduce the need for additional testimony[6] and can facilitate preparation for testimony and enable rapid retrieval of key items of information by the physician deponent under questioning.

At time of deposition or courtroom testimony, the physician is required to submit evidence attesting to credibility as an expert witness. A curriculum vitae that adequately reflects relevant training and experience and highlights accomplishments pertaining to the area of claimed expertise is helpful. The physician examiner should be prepared to disclose information concerning customary fee schedules, percentage of practice devoted to Workers' Compensation claims and medicolegal testimony,[6] and percentage of referrals generated from plaintiff vs. defendant camps.

Johnston[20] offers the following tips to physicians engaging in medical testimony:

- Always know your file.
- Listen to the question and answer only the question asked.
- Answer yes/no whenever appropriate, and keep answers short and to the point.
- Always elaborate on questions that go to the main issue of the case.
- Always be ready to concede the weak points, but never concede points that are the foundation of your opinion.

In effect, good testimony is provided when an honest and well-prepared physician is willing to give honest answers to hard questions.[20]

The physician examiner must also confront the ethical challenge posed by the patient as a claimant. The traditional paternalistic view of the physician as the zealous advocate of the patient's best interests has given way to a contractual view encompassing patient autonomy, informed consent, and rights to privacy and self-determination. More recently,[9] an *educational model* has been proposed for patients rehabilitated within a team framework; it emphasizes shared responsibility and decision making while recognizing team leadership and authority. Although such a model seeks to preserve patient autonomy it must be ". . . carried out in an environment where financial considerations are playing an increasingly important role in determining access to and discharge from rehabilitation."[9(p. 317)] The examiner who seeks to uphold the changing moral imperatives of the doctor-patient relationship must also be sensitive and responsive to the paradox of compensable injury—that financial compensation can discourage return to work and thereby promote disability.[5] Furthermore, the prolongation of an open claim (through inappropriate and excessive diagnostic and/or therapeutic endeavors, however well intended) may further serve to legitimize disability in the claimant's mind and may also inhibit the likelihood of functional recovery and return to work. Decisions to terminate treatment of compensable injury and reach MMI might not always be mutually agreeable to claimant and examiner, and decisions in such cases are more likely to rest with the final authority of the physician rather than that of the patient. Perhaps the most useful beacon to guide decision making when treating compensable injuries is to promote functional recovery to the fullest extent, to terminate treatment when functional recovery is no longer tenable, and to render impairment ratings and return-to-work decisions that empower the patient to use his or her residual abilities (through accommodation when necessary) as soon as possible and to the fullest extent possible.

The physician examiner is empowered to determine

MMI, impairment rating, if any, and when and to what extent an injured worker can return to work or continue working. Physicians are becoming increasingly accountable for their medical opinions in this arena; this is hardly surprising considering the disproportionately high healthcare costs of occupationally related temporary total and permanent partial disability compensation.[4] Physician impairment rating practices have been shown to vary widely with respect to acceptance of rating criteria, methods of application, and time of rating determination.[7, 11, 17] Lack of uniform standards of application and the resulting inconsistencies have been a source of embarrassing frustration to the physicians themselves,[10] and the process of impairment rating often appears reduced to "educated guesswork."[8] Ideally, rating parameters should meet the standards of objectivity, reliability, and content validity of measurements currently established in the field[19] and should be widely accepted and employed by the rating community. The AMA Guides continues to reflect shortcomings in several of these areas, as discussed earlier in this chapter. These ideals can perhaps be realized if the body of qualified examiners continues to adopt uniform standards for acceptable rating criteria, reference materials, and methods of application, and is prepared to undergo specialized training and certification to promote quality and uniformity of the impairment rating process.[29]

References

1. American Academy of Orthopedic Surgeons: Manual for Orthopedic Surgeons in Evaluating Permanent Physical Impairment. Chicago, American Academy of Orthopedic Surgeons, 1975.
2. American Medical Association: Guides to the Evaluation of Permanent Impairment, ed 4. Chicago, American Medical Association, 1993.
3. Americans With Disabilities Act (ADA): Part 1: Employment. 29CFR Part 1630. Federal Register, July 26, 1991, pp 35726–35756.
4. Andersson GB, Pope MH, Frymoyer JW, et al: Epidemiology and cost. In Pope MH, Andersson GB, Frymoyer JW, et al (eds): Occupational Low Back Pain: Assessment, Treatment, and Prevention. St Louis, Mosby–Year Book, 1991, pp 95–113.
5. Beals RK: Compensation and recovery from injury. West J Med 1984; 140:233–237.
6. Bonfiglio RP, Bonfiglio RL: Medical testimony in Workers' Compensation matters. In Johnson EW (ed): Phys Med Rehabil Clin North Am 1992; 3:665–676.
7. Brand RA, Lehmann TR: Low-back impairment rating practices of orthopaedic surgeons. Spine 1983; 8:75–78.
8. Burd JG: The educated guess: Doctors and permanent partial disability percentage. J Tenn Med Assoc 1980; 73:441.
9. Caplan AL: Informed consent and provider-patient relationships in rehabilitation medicine. Arch Phys Med Rehabil 1988; 69:312–317.
10. Carey TS, Hadler NM: The role of the primary physician in disability determination for Social Security Insurance and Workers' Compensation. Ann Intern Med 1986; 104:706–710.
11. Clark WL, Haldeman S, Johnson P, et al: Back impairment and disability determination: Another attempt at objective, reliable rating. Spine 1988; 13:332–341.
12. Derebery VJ, Tullis WH: Delayed recovery in the patient with a work compensable injury. J Occup Med 1983; 25:829–835.
13. Esquemeling J: The Buccaneers of America, 1684–5. In Stallybrass

14. Fordyce WE: Behavioral Methods for Chronic Pain and Illness. St Louis, CV Mosby, 1976.
15. Frymoyer JW, Andersson GB: Clinical classification. In Pope MH, Andersson GB, Frymoyer JW, et al (eds): Occupational Low Back Pain: Assessment, Treatment, and Prevention. St Louis, Mosby–Year Book, 1991, pp 44–70.
16. Frymoyer JW, Cats-Baril W: Predictors of low back pain disability. Clin Orthop Rel Res 1987; 221:89–98.
17. Greenwood JG: Low-back impairment-rating practices of orthopaedic surgeons and neurosurgeons in West Virginia. Spine 1985; 10:773–776.
18. Isernhagen SJ: Work Injury Management and Prevention. Rockville, Md, Aspen Publishers, 1988.
19. Johnston MV, Keith RA, Hinderer SR: Measurement standards for interdisciplinary medical rehabilitation: Part I. General principles and technical standards. Arch Phys Med Rehabil 1992; 73(suppl):3–12.
20. Johnston W: Importance of communication between physician and attorney. In Johnson EW (ed): Phys Med Rehabil Clin North Am 1992; 3:677–694.
21. Keely J, Mayer T, Cox R, et al: Quantification of lumbar function: Part 5. Reliability of range of motion measures in the sagittal plane and an in vivo torso rotation measurement technique. Spine 1986; 11:31–35.
22. Kemp JD, Pope MH: Workers' Compensation. In Kemp JD, Pope MH (eds): Occupational Low Back Pain: Assessment, Treatment and Prevention. St Louis, Mosby–Year Book, 1991, pp 296–304.
23. Kessler HH: Disability-Determination and Evaluation. Philadelphia, Lea & Febiger, 1970.
24. Lankhorst GJ, Van de Stadt RJ, Van der Korst JK: The natural history of idiopathic low back pain. Scand J Rehabil Med 1985; 17:1–4.
25. Luck J, Florence D: A brief history and comparative analysis of disability systems and impairment rating guides. Orthop Clin North Am 1988; 19:839–844.
26. Matheson LN: Symptom magnification syndrome structured interview: Rationale and procedure. J Occup Rehabil 1991; 1:43–56.
27. Mayer T, Tencer A, Kristoferson S, et al: Use of non-invasive techniques for quantification of spinal range-of-motion in normal subjects and chronic low back dysfunction patients. Spine 1984; 9:588–595.
28. McBride ED: Disability Evaluation and Principles of Treatment of Compensable Injuries, ed 6. Philadelphia, JB Lippincott, 1963.
29. Mueller KL, Goldman B (eds): Division of Workers' Compensation Level II Accreditation Course. Denver, State of Colorado Department of Labor & Employment, Division of Workers' Compensation, 1993.
30. Newton M, Waddell G: Trunk strength testing with iso-machines. Part I: Review of a decade of scientific evidence. Spine 1993; 18:801–811.
31. Osterweis M, Kleinman A, Mechanic D (eds): Pain and Disability: Clinical, Behavioral, and Public Policy Perspectives, Washington, DC, National Academy Press, 1987.
32. Pheasant S: Ergonomics, Work and Health. Gaithersburg, Md, Aspen, 1991, p 4.
33. Rice CO: Calculation of Industrial Disability of the Extremities and the Back, ed 2. Springfield, Ill, Charles C Thomas, 1968.
34. Rondinelli R: Impairment evaluation and disability assessment. In Bonfiglio R (ed): Industrial Rehabilitation Medicine. Philadelphia, Hanley & Belfus, 1995.
35. Rondinelli R, Murphy J, Esler A, et al: Estimation of normal lumbar flexion with surface inclinometry: A comparison of three methods. Am J Phys Med Rehabil 1992; 71:219–224.
36. Smith WC: Principles of Disability Evaluation. Philadelphia, JB Lippincott, 1959.
37. Strang JP: The chronic disability syndrome. In Aronoff GM (ed): Evaluation and Treatment of Chronic Pain. Baltimore, Urban & Schwartzenberg, 1985, pp 603–623.
38. Waddell G, McCulloch J, Kummel E, et al: Nonorganic physical signs in low-back pain. Spine 1980; 5:117–125.
39. World Health Organization: International Classification of Impairments, Disabilities and Handicaps. Geneva, Switzerland, 1980.

W (ed): Broadway Translations. London, G. Routledge & Sons, 1924, p 60.

11

Imaging Studies for the Physiatrist

ANDREW J. COLE, M.D., DAMON C. SACCO, M.D.,
CHARLES P. HO, PH.D., M.D., AND
BETSY A. HOLLAND, M.D.

A thorough rehabilitation plan geared to the clinical presentation of an injury and physiological and psychological patient needs requires the physiatrist to make an accurate diagnosis as soon as possible. The diagnoses must be anatomically specific (e.g., impingement syndrome secondary to subacromial osteophytosis), *not* generic (e.g., "shoulder strain"), so that the rehabilitation plan is structured to adequately and thoroughly address all aspects of the injury. Accurate histories help form initial differential diagnostic impressions that might explain degrees of pain and disability. Well-planned and focused physical examinations are then performed. Working diagnoses, based on a history and physical examination, offer a further refinement of differential diagnoses and determine what additional testing might be required to arrive at a correct final diagnosis.[17]

Radiological imaging studies constitute one subset of additional testing that can help the physiatrist to arrive at a correct diagnosis. The information contained in an imaging study can help the physiatrist to prescribe the most appropriate initial rehabilitation program, alter an ongoing program, or suggest that further rehabilitation might not result in significant clinical gains. In the latter situation, imaging can help the physiatrist to decide whether surgery might be a feasible option for a patient.

A variety of imaging studies are available to help more accurately define pathomorphological changes of different tissues. The physiatrist chooses the single best study or constellation of studies that will yield the most clinically relevant information while simultaneously seeking to minimize cost.

None of the imaging studies discussed in this chapter determines whether a particular structure is the source of a patient's pain. Rather, these studies provide anatomical information that must be correlated with the patient's history, physical examination findings, and response to rehabilitation and medication, as well as the results of any prior studies. This combination of information allows the astute physiatrist to more accurately define the most likely source of pain. Only contrast-enhanced fluoroscopically guided injection procedures that administer local anesthetic can positively identify a source of pain. The anesthetic, placed at the painful locus, should cause significant or complete relief of a patient's pain.

This chapter is intended to help the physiatrist to determine which radiographic studies to order for a wide variety of commonly encountered disorders.

IMAGING OF THE SPINE

Degenerative Disorders of the Spine and Intervertebral Discs

The initial screening examination of the spine should include plain film studies. Computed tomography (CT) and magnetic resonance imaging (MRI) represent complementary and extremely powerful tools in the evaluation of degenerative spinal disorders. In general, MRI excels in evaluation of soft tissue structures such as the intervertebral discs, ligaments, and spinal cord. CT provides excellent osseous detail and is useful in evaluation of spinal fractures, osseous degenerative changes such as osteophytosis, and facet arthropathy. With the advent of thin-section spiral CT scanning of the spine, excellent-quality multiplanar reformatted two-dimensional images and three-dimensional renderings of the spine are now possible (Fig. 11–1).

Both CT and MRI are able to depict the morphology of the disc annulus. However, MRI has the added capability of assessing the degree of disc hydration and evaluating for internal disc disruption (e.g., annular fissures, which are tears through the annulus fibrosus) (Fig. 11–2). CT is

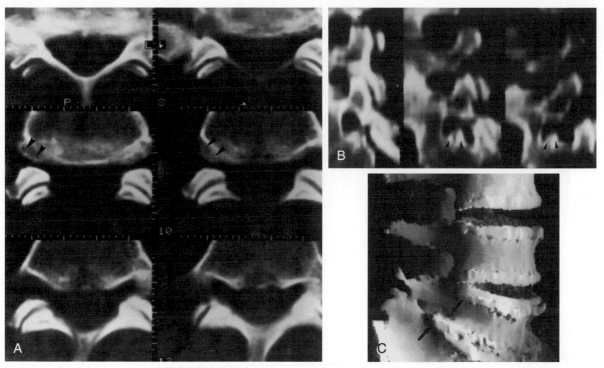

FIGURE 11–1 CT scan of degenerative osseous changes with two- and three-dimensional reformatted images. *A,* Six axial CT images through the level of the L5–S1 disc. Osseous ridging appears off the posterolateral aspects of the adjacent end-plates *(arrowheads). B,* Computerized sagittal reconstructed images from axial images again demonstrate osseous ridging extending into the right neural foramen at the L5–S1 level *(arrowheads). C,* Computerized reformatted three-dimensional image of lumbar spine from axial images (not same case) demonstrates prominent osseous ridging along posterolateral aspect of end-plate adjacent to the L5–S1 disc *(arrows).*

only able to identify an annular fissure after injection of the nucleus pulposus with contrast material as in discography (Fig. 11–3).

Disc pathology is currently described as bulges, protrusions, extrusions, and free fragments. The term *disc bulge* implies that no evidence of an annular fissure exists, and symmetrical bulging of the annulus is identified throughout the circumference of the disc. The term *disc protrusion* implies the presence of an annular fissure with extension of nuclear material into or through the outer annular fibers, but which is limited by the posterior longitudinal ligament.[45] Disc protrusions are associated with an asymmetrical outward extension of the annulus. The term *disc extrusion* implies the presence of an annular fissure with extension of the nuclear material through the annular fibers and also through the posterior longitudinal ligament. The nuclear material remains in continuity with the intervertebral disc and is identified as a focal mass extending from the intervertebral disc space. The term *free fragment* implies extension of disc material through the outer annular fibers with loss of continuity of the nuclear material with the disc space. Disc fragments can migrate either cephalad or caudal to the disc space of origin and can be subligamentous or extend through the posterior longitudinal ligament.[59]

Schmorl's nodes represent prolapse or extension of the intervertebral disc into the adjacent vertebral body end-plates. The most common cause of Schmorl's node formation is compressive loading of the disc with extension of disc material through an end-plate defect. Schmorl's nodes are thought not to be symptomatic; however, they might be indicative of a previous compressive injury and might

possibly accelerate disc degeneration.[24] Schmorl's nodes are readily detected on sagittal MRI images as extension of disc material into the end-plate of an adjacent vertebral body. Schmorl's nodes can be identified on CT as a lucent end-plate defect with a surrounding rim of sclerosis.

Advances in MRI have resulted in improved resolution of the internal disc anatomy. On sagittal T2-weighted images, on which well-hydrated or fluid-containing structures are of increased signal intensity, fissures within the annulus can be identified (see Fig. 11–2). MRI has the added capability of visualizing the outer annular fibers, posterior longitudinal ligament, and dura as separate structures. On T2-weighted images, the outer annular fibers are identified as a rim of decreased signal intensity surrounding the brighter, well-hydrated nucleus pulposus. The posterior longitudinal ligament is identified as a linear area of diminished signal intensity extending along the posterior aspect of the vertebral bodies that merges with the outer annular fibers. The sagittal T2-weighted MRIs through the spine produce the so-called *MR myelogram* effect. On these images, the cerebrospinal fluid (CSF) is of increased signal intensity, with the spinal cord being of intermediate signal intensity. This imaging sequence produces excellent images for evaluation of the cord morphology and also has the ability to demonstrate areas of demyelination or cord edema as focal regions of increased signal intensity within the cord (Fig. 11–4). On T1-weighted sagittal images, the CSF is of diminished signal intensity with the cord being of intermediate signal intensity. These images are also excellent in demonstrating cord morphology but are less sensitive to the presence of a region of demyelination or

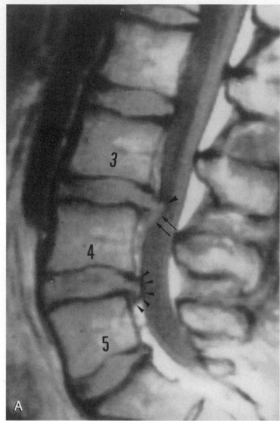

FIGURE 11–2   MRI of disc protrusion, extrusion, and free fragments. *A,* T1-weighted sagittal image of lumbar spine demonstrates disc extrusion with extension of disc material *(arrows)* through torn and elevated posterior longitudinal ligament *(single arrowhead)* at the L3–L4 level. A midline posterior disc protrusion is present at the L4–L5 level; the posterior longitudinal ligament is intact *(arrowheads).* Slight bulging of the annulus at the L5–S1 level is also noted. *B,* T1-weighted *(left)* and T2-weighted *(right)* sagittal images of the lumbar spine reveal a free fragment just caudal to the L5–S1 intervertebral disc space *(arrows).* On the T2-weighted images, loss of continuity of the disc material with the intervertebral disc space is best appreciated. The extruded disc material is identified within the ventral epidural space and is of relatively diminished signal intensity. Note the disc degeneration at the L4–L5 level with degenerative changes involving the inferior end-plate of L4.

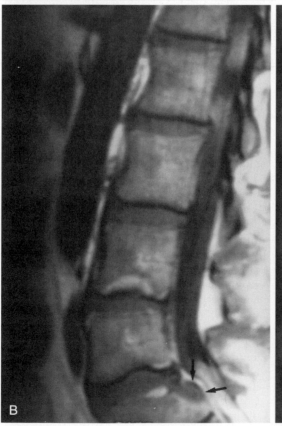

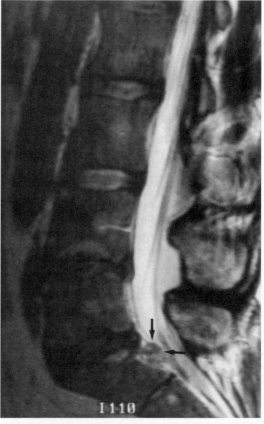

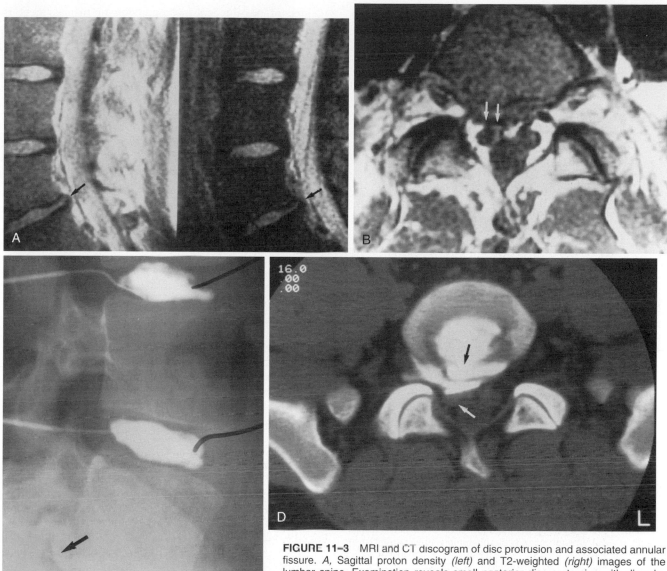

FIGURE 11–3 MRI and CT discogram of disc protrusion and associated annular fissure. *A,* Sagittal proton density *(left)* and T2-weighted *(right)* images of the lumbar spine. Examination reveals small posterior disc protrusion with disc degeneration at the L5–S1 level *(black arrow). B,* Axial T1-weighted MR image through L5–S1 disc demonstrates small right paracentral disc protrusion at the L5–S1 level *(white arrows). C,* Lateral radiograph of lumbar spine obtained following discography in same patient. Note posterior annular fissure at the L5–S1 level. *D,* At CT image through L5–S1 disc of the same patient following discogram. The examination reveals a left paracentral annular fissure *(black arrow)* with contrast noted to extend predominantly along the right posterolateral outer annular fibers. Slight posterior displacement of the right S1 nerve root is seen *(white arrow).* Neither the MRI study nor the CT scan produces any appreciable neural element compression. However, the patient did complain of concordant right lower extremity pain during injection of the L5–S1 disc with contrast.

cord edema. On T1-weighted images, the nucleus pulposus and inner annular fibers are of intermediate signal intensity, with the outer annular fibers and posterior longitudinal ligament remaining low in signal intensity. The fat within the marrow spaces of the vertebral bodies is well demonstrated on the sagittal T1-weighted images, with areas of cancellous bone edema or tumor seen as regions of diminished signal intensity within the normally high–signal-intensity marrow space.

Lumbar disc degeneration and, to a slightly lesser degree, thoracic disc degeneration are seen as diminished signal intensity of the nucleus pulposus on T2-weighted images. This is related to disc desiccation with resultant loss of signal. This finding is less reliable in the cervical spine, where the intervertebral discs are smaller in size and can have a more variable signal intensity.

Axial CT images through the spine can demonstrate disc protrusions, extrusions, and free fragments, but the distinction is more difficult and less reliable than with MRI. The disc material is seen as a soft tissue structure of intermediate density against the lower-density epidural fat. The posterior longitudinal ligament, outer annular fibers, and dura are not identified as individual structures on CT. Additionally, disc hydration cannot be assessed by CT

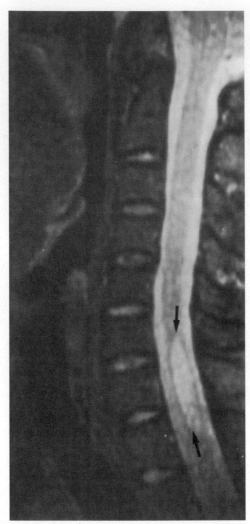

FIGURE 11–4   Sagittal T2-weighted MRI scan of the cervical spine reveals a focal area of increased signal intensity within the lower cervical cord *(black arrows)*. The appearance is consistent with a demyelinating process such as multiple sclerosis.

scanning. However, CT is able to demonstrate other signs of disc degeneration, such as gas within the intervertebral disc (vacuum phenomena) and calcifications within the disc.

For the evaluation of degenerative changes, including atlantoaxial subluxation and basilar invagination at the craniovertebral junction, the procedure of choice is MRI. This is due primarily to its ability to obtain direct sagittal, coronal, and axial images through this region. Although thin-section axial CT images through this area with computerized reformatted sagittal and coronal images can provide some information as to the degree of subluxation or displacement of osseous structures, the cervical cord and brainstem, as well as the posterior fossa structures, are best imaged by MRI. Subtle degenerative changes, including sclerotic and erosive changes involving the osseous structures, are better identified by CT. However, as has been stated, what is perhaps more clinically important is the effect of these changes on the adjacent neural structures. Atlantoaxial subluxation, as with rheumatoid arthritis, can be easily identified by both MRI and CT. However, the

degree of possible cord compression or displacement is best assessed by MRI.

With administration of intrathecal contrast (CT myelography), CT can help evaluate the spinal cord and nerve roots. However, this invasive procedure requires injection of contrast into the subarachnoid space (Fig. 11–5), and it is generally reserved for patients who are unable to undergo an MRI scan. This includes patients who are obese, experience claustrophobia, or have cardiac pacemakers or biostimulating devices in place. Patients with metallic hardware in the region of the spine to be imaged are also referred for a CT myelogram, because metal can create MRI artifacts that render the MRI images uninterpretable.

Spinal Stenosis

Spinal stenosis results in compression or encroachment of the neural elements by osseous or soft tissue structures. This can result in narrowing of the central canal or neural foramen. Most commonly, spinal stenosis is secondary to degenerative changes of the spine with associated osteophytosis and facet degeneration accompanied by hypertrophy or buckling of the ligamenta flava. In the patient presenting with spine pain, it becomes necessary not only to evaluate the presence of stenosis, but also to determine what factors are contributing to the stenotic process.

High-resolution CT is the study of choice for evaluation of stenosis secondary to osseous encroachment on the neural elements. CT is extremely accurate in detecting osteophytosis of the vertebral body end-plates throughout the spine and of the uncovertebral joints of the cervical spine. Hypertrophic and degenerative changes involving the facets are easily identified. Sagittal and coronal reconstructed images are also helpful in evaluating the degree and type of foraminal stenosis. Precise measurements of the anteroposterior (AP) diameter of the central canal also can be obtained (Fig. 11–6).

Although osseous stenosis does not necessarily cause neural element compression, the advantage of MRI over CT in the evaluation of stenosis is its ability to visualize soft tissue structures, including the neural elements. Many patients who present with back pain have degenerative osseous changes throughout the spine that may not cause or contribute to symptoms. MRI is capable of identifying which, if any, neural structures are being compressed. MRI can also identify any compression and edema of the spinal cord. Chronic spinal cord compression can also result in a localized area of cord atrophy (compressive myelomalacia). CT myelography has increased sensitivity in the detection of cord or nerve root compression but is an invasive procedure. An early study comparing MRI to CT myelography showed that MRI provided an amount of information that was equal to, if not more than, that provided by myelography.[58]

The entire neural foramen must be evaluated when foraminal stenosis is being sought. Stenosis can occur anywhere along the length of the foramen from its entrance to its exit zone. The entrance zone represents a sagittal two-dimensional plane just medial to the pedicle where the nerve root enters the foramen. The *mid-zone* is defined as the area caudal to the pedicle, extending from its medial to lateral aspect. The *exit zone* is a two-dimensional area that

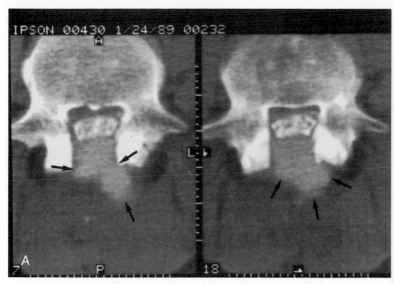
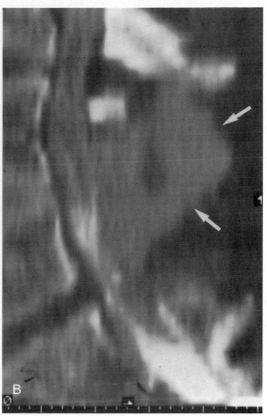

FIGURE 11–5   CT myelography. *A,* Two axial images through the lumbar spine were obtained following injection of contrast into the subarachnoid space (CT myelogram). Mild enhancing fluid collection is seen posterior to the thecal sac *(black arrows).* The appearance is compatible with a postoperative dural leak. *B,* Sagittal reconstructed images of same patient. Enhancing fluid collection is noted again posterior to the thecal sac *(white arrows).* The collection is seen to extend into the region of the laminectomy defect.

FIGURE 11–6   Axial CT images through the cervical spine reveal degenerative changes along the uncovertebral joints with uncinate spurring *(black arrows)* and osseous ridging along the posterior aspect of the vertebral body end-plates *(black arrowheads).* The examination easily demonstrates central canal stenosis as well as foraminal stenosis.

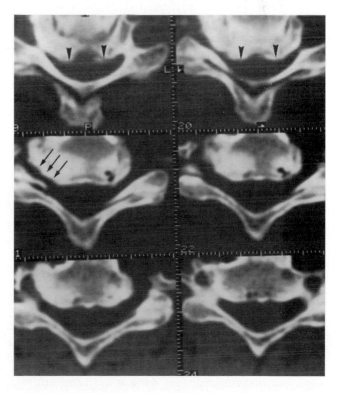

lies just lateral to a sagittal plane through the lateral margin of the pedicle. Although foraminal stenosis typically is related to osteophytosis, foraminal disc protrusions can also cause or contribute to foraminal stenosis. Extracanalicular or *far out* stenosis refers to nerve root impingement that occurs beyond the exit zone of the neural foramen. This type of stenosis is most commonly caused by excessive lateral osteophytosis of the vertebral body end-plates. In addition, far out stenosis can be caused by compression of the L5 nerve root between the L5 transverse process and the sacral ala.

Spondylolysis

The term *isthmic spondylolysis* refers to a fracture or defect within the pars interarticularis. This may or may not be associated with spondylolisthesis. The term *spondylolisthesis* refers to either anterior or posterior subluxation of one vertebral body in relation to another. Spondylolysis of the pars interarticularis is frequently associated with central canal stenosis as well as foraminal stenosis. Hypertrophic changes involving the pars interarticularis and any anterior spondylolisthesis can also contribute to foraminal stenosis. Associated degenerative changes involving the facets and adjacent vertebral body end-plates can also contribute to stenosis.[23]

Plain radiographic oblique views can demonstrate the pars defect as a break in the neck of the "scotty dog." (On oblique images, the transverse process, superior and inferior articular facets, pars interarticularis, and lamina have an appearance that is reminiscent of a silhouette of a scotty dog.) CT with reformatted sagittal images is probably the most sensitive study in detecting small spondylolytic defects and associated fragmentation of the pars interarticularis. These defects can be missed unless thin-section orthogonal images are obtained. However, T1-weighted sagittal images are also sensitive in the detection of spondylolytic defects of the pars interarticularis.[35] MRI, like CT, is also extremely sensitive in evaluating the degree of spondylolisthesis and the presence of associated stenosis with neural element compression (Fig. 11–7). Bone scans are highly sensitive but are relatively nonspecific. Single proton emission computed tomography (SPECT) adds sensitivity and specificity to the planar bone scan. SPECT can help confirm the presence of active pars lesions, such as acute spondylolysis or pars stress reactions.[7, 18]

Epidural Hematomas

With the advent of MRI, epidural hematomas have been seen with increasing frequency. This is due in part to the increased sensitivity of MRI to the presence of blood and blood by-products. Epidural hematomas can be seen after trauma to the spine or in association with a disc protrusion/extrusion (Fig. 11–8). In general, the epidural hematoma on T1-weighted images is of increased signal intensity relative to the intervertebral disc. Its borders are generally not as well defined as those of a disc fragment. And what is perhaps most important, the epidural hematoma typically resolves with time and can eventually disappear on follow-up examinations (see Fig. 11–8). Occasionally, disc extrusions and free fragments are difficult to distinguish from an epidural hematoma. However, with delayed imaging at approximately 3 to 6 months, an epidural hematoma will usually resolve completely, whereas a disc fragment will not resolve completely but will get smaller as a result of desiccation of the extruded disc material.

POSTOPERATIVE SPINE

Postoperative Disc Protrusions

MRI is considered the study of choice for evaluation of recurrent back pain following surgery. The presence of a recurrent disc protrusion can be difficult to assess in the presence of scar tissue. On CT and non–contrast-enhanced MRIs of the spine following surgery, postoperative scar tissue can appear as a diffuse mass of intermediate signal intensity that is indistinguishable from the adjacent disc. Therefore, MRI images of the postoperative spine are generally obtained prior to and after intravenous infusion of gadolinium diethylenetriamine penta-acetic acid (DTPA). Gadolinium DTPA is an MR contrast agent that, on T1-weighted images, results in enhancement or increased signal intensity of structures that are vascular or well profused. Following infusion of gadolinium DTPA, the vascular fibrous tissue and granulation tissue have increased signal intensity whereas the disc material remains low in signal intensity (Fig. 11–9), thus distinguishing a recurrent disc protrusion from postoperative fibrosis. Often, the protruding disc material is encased in or covered by the enhancing fibrous tissue. Postoperative gadolinium DTPA imaging should not be performed earlier than approximately 6 weeks postoperatively, because the presence of seromas, hematomas, and edema can make image interpretation difficult.

Arachnoiditis

The presence of arachnoiditis or arachnoid adhesions is best detected by MRI. Although CT myelography is also sensitive in detecting arachnoiditis, it is an invasive procedure. These studies are sensitive to the presence of arachnoiditis involving the lumbar region and have a limited ability to detect the presence of arachnoiditis throughout the cervical or thoracic spine. The nerve roots of the cauda equina are normally identified as fine linear structures along the posterior and lateral aspects of the thecal sac. They should be seen as distinct individual structures. With arachnoiditis or arachnoid adhesions, clumping and abnormal positioning of the nerve roots of the cauda equina are seen. An additional indication of arachnoiditis is the so-called empty sac sign, in which the nerve roots of the cauda equina are adherent to the dura and are not identified as individual structures within the thecal sac (Fig. 11–10).

Postoperative Complications

During the initial postoperative period, areas of increased signal intensity can be seen on T2-weighted MRI images involving the paravertebral soft tissue structures. These generally remain isointense with muscles on T1-weighted images. On CT, these areas are usually associated with a diffuse soft tissue prominence generally of the same density as the paraspinal muscles. This finding is consistent with

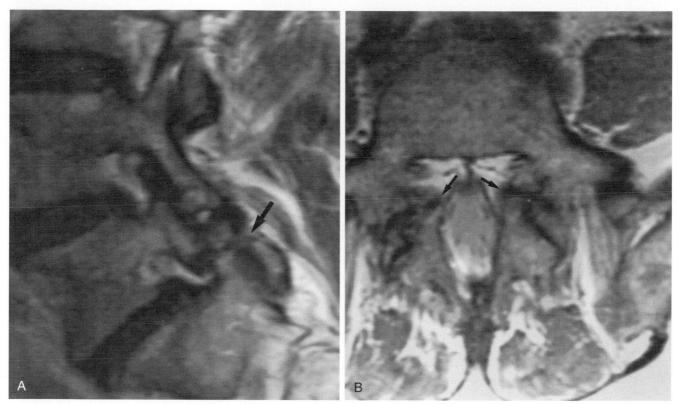

FIGURE 11–7 MRI of spondylolysis. *A,* Sagittal T1-weighted MRI scan of the lumbar spine demonstrates mild (grade I) anterior spondylolisthesis of L5 on S1. A spondylolytic defect through the pars interarticularis of L5 is also noted *(black arrowhead). B,* Proton density axial MR image of the same patient; note diminished signal intensity through the region of the pars interarticularis of L5 *(black arrows).* The appearance is compatible with a spondylolytic defect of the pars interarticularis.

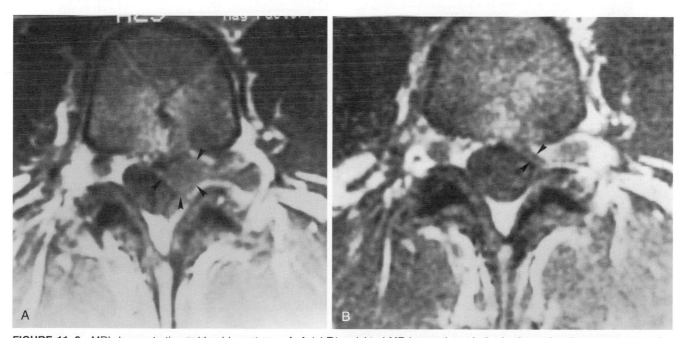

FIGURE 11–8 MRI demonstrating epidural hematoma. *A,* Axial T1-weighted MR image through the lumbar spine demonstrates a rather large epidural mass within the left lateral recess. Patient had complaints of left lower extremity pain. The suspected hematoma is of intermediate signal intensity. As an epidural hematoma was suspected, a follow-up examination was recommended prior to any surgery. *B,* Axial MR image obtained 6 weeks later through approximately the same level as in *A* demonstrates near-complete resolution of the previously identified mass within the left lateral recess. Only a small linear area of residual fibrosis is noted along the left ventrolateral aspect of the thecal sac *(black arrowheads).* The patient no longer had left lower extremity pain at the time of examination.

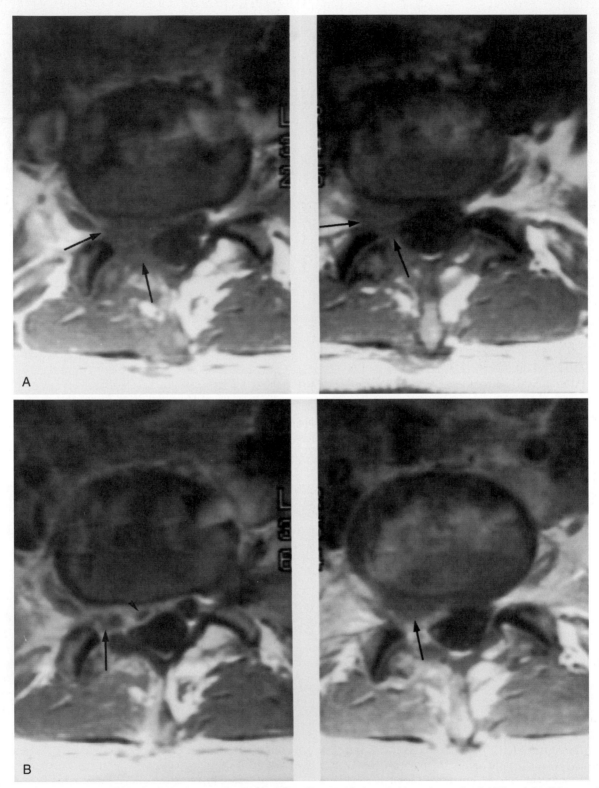

FIGURE 11–9 MRI of postoperative spine to evaluate for recurrent disc herniation. *A,* Nonenhanced axial T1-weighted images through the lumbar spine following surgery demonstrate a rather large irregular mass of intermediate signal intensity extending along the right lateral aspect of the thecal sac. The appearance is compatible with postoperative fibrosis and scarring. However, without gadolinium, it would be difficult to rule out a recurrent/residual disc herniation. *B,* T1-weighted axial images through the same lumbar level following infusion of gadolinium DTPA demonstrate enhancement of the fibrosis and granulation tissue. However, the herniated disc material *(black arrows and arrowheads)* does not enhance. The appearance is consistent with a recurrent/residual postoperative disc herniation.

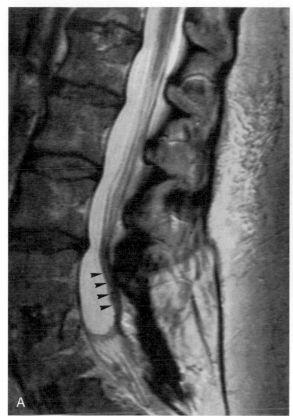
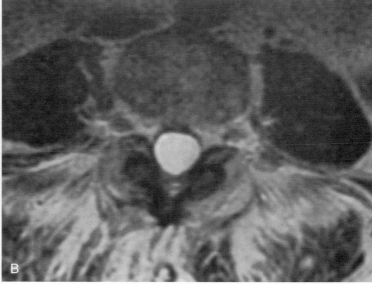

FIGURE 11–10 MRI of arachnoiditis. *A,* Sagittal T2-weighted MR scan of the lumbar spine. Note postoperative changes involving the lower lumbar spine with findings consistent with anterior interbody fusion and a posterior laminectomy defect. The nerve roots of the cauda equina are clumped and appear to be displaced along the posterior aspect of the thecal sac *(black arrowhead).* A more normal appearance of the cauda equina is noted above the level of surgery. The appearance is consistent with arachnoiditis with arachnoid adhesions. *B,* T2-weighted axial MR scan of the same patient demonstrates an apparently empty thecal sac. The nerve roots of the cauda equina are adherent to the dural sac, giving the impression of an empty thecal sac.

postoperative edema, which typically resolves with time, and should not be confused with areas of increased signal intensity within the paraspinal structures on T1-weighted images. As previously discussed, areas of subacute hemorrhage are associated with increased signal intensity on T1-weighted MR images. This finding is helpful in distinguishing postoperative hematoma from a seroma or pseudomeningocele (Fig. 11–11). On CT, a paraspinal hematoma may be isodense or slightly increased in density compared with the adjacent paraspinal muscles, making the distinction between hematoma and seroma on CT alone difficult.

Postoperative pseudomeningoceles are related to leakage of CSF from a hole or a tear within the dura.[88] Pseudomeningoceles are generally well defined and located directly posterior to the thecal sac. On MRI images, the signal intensity of a pseudomeningocele is similar to that of CSF, which is low in signal intensity on T1-weighted images and high in signal intensity on T2-weighted images. MRI recognizes the distinction between the hematoma and a pseudomeningocele. The distinction among a pseudomeningocele, a seroma, and a wound abscess can be difficult with MRI alone, as all of these collections would have similar signal intensities. The site of the communication with the subarachnoid space can be difficult to image. The accurate diagnosis of a pseudomeningocele by CT generally requires injection of contrast medium into the subarachnoid space (CT myelography) with subsequent

scanning through the region of the suspected pseudomeningocele. The contrast material leaks into the collection, indicating a communication with the subarachnoid space.

Evaluation of Hardware

Because of artifacts created by ferromagnetic material within the magnetic field, MR imaging is not used in the evaluation of metallic hardware. Generally, plain film studies are adequate for evaluating a broken or fractured pedicle screw or plate. CT scanning of metallic hardware is also limited by the presence of beam-hardening artifacts. However, by using appropriate window and level settings (image contrast settings), the position and appearance of metallic hardware can be assessed. Misplaced pedicle screws that extend into the neural foramen can be detected by CT as well as by plain film studies.

Plain film studies that include lateral flexion and extension views can reveal a fragmented or incomplete fusion mass. Additionally, the presence of motion at a fused level on flexion and extension views is indicative of a failed fusion. Osseous fusions, either anterior or posterior, can be evaluated by MRI, CT, and plain film studies. However, CT scanning with reformatted sagittal and coronal images is more sensitive in the detection of subtle fractures or of small areas of incomplete osseous union. On CT, an anterior fusion is seen to be solid when a complete osseous

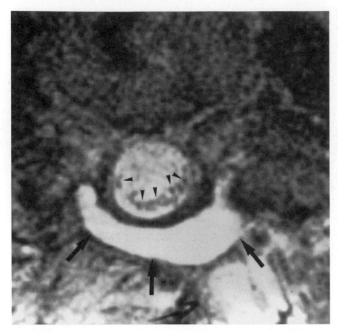

FIGURE 11–11 T2-weighted axial MR image through the lumbar spine. Note relatively normal appearance of the nerve roots of the cauda equina within the thecal sac *(black arrowheads)*. A fluid collection in the area of the laminectomy defect is noted to extend posterior to the thecal sac *(black arrows)*. The differential diagnosis would include a dural leak, postoperative seroma or hematoma, or abscess. A dural leak could be evaluated by a CT myelogram (see Fig. 11–5).

fusion mass is identified to extend from one vertebral body to another. The presence of gas (vacuum phenomenon) or soft tissue density extending across the fusion mass is indicative of a failed fusion. Posterolateral fusion masses are also best evaluated on reformatted sagittal and coronal CT images. These are seen as solid osseous fusion masses extending along the posterolateral elements. Fragmentation or lucent defects within the fusion mass are indicative of a failed or incomplete fusion (Fig. 11–12).

Trauma

Plain film studies remain the screening study of choice in the evaluation of acute spine trauma. If the initial plain film studies are abnormal and further evaluation is required, or if the plain films do not demonstrate traumatic changes but neurological findings persist, CT is generally performed through the region of interest. In the evaluation of spine trauma, both CT and MRI provide complementary data. However, CT is superior in the demonstration of fracture lines, particularly those that involve the posterior elements. CT, with its excellent bone detail, is better at determining the extent and location of spine fractures. Position of osseous fragments can also be determined by CT. Both two-dimensional and three-dimensional reformatted images are also helpful in defining the extent and position of spine fractures.

Although CT excels in the evaluation of the osseous structures, it is limited in the evaluation of the soft tissue structures of the spine. MRI, because of its excellent soft tissue resolution, is able to directly image the spine in any plane. Direct visualization of the spinal cord enhances the identification of any injury to the cord. Areas of cord contusion or compression are easily identified. Direct visualization of ligamentous tears is also possible. With MR imaging, the presence of a cord contusion can be distinguished from traumatic cord compression from either bone or epidural hematoma. In the past, compression of the cord could only be determined by administration of intrathecal contrast, with or without CT. This distinction is not trivial, as rapid surgical decompression of a compressive lesion can result in improvement or resolution of neurological deficits.[51]

In acute trauma, MRI is capable of distinguishing between cord edema and cord hemorrhage. On T2-weighted images, cord edema is identified as areas of increased signal intensity within the cord. Acute intramedullary hemorrhage can be seen as an area of diminished signal intensity on T2-weighted images with increased signal intensity on T1-weighted images. The presence of an intramedullary hematoma is generally considered to carry a worse prognosis than simple cord edema[11] (Fig. 11–13).

The late sequela of spinal cord trauma is best evaluated by MRI. MRI is the study of choice for the evaluation of post-traumatic syrinx. The syrinx is identified as a linear area of diminished signal intensity within the cord on T1-weighted images. The craniocaudal extension of a syrinx is well delineated by MR imaging. Post-traumatic cysts of the cord are also easily identified. These lesions are easily distinguished from myelomalacia, which is seen as an area of focal cord atrophy.

Discitis

MRI has a high level of sensitivity and specificity for diagnosing discitis.[62] Disc space infections have a typical appearance on both T1- and T2-weighted images. On T1-weighted images, a loss of signal intensity involving the intervertebral disc and the marrow within the adjacent vertebral bodies is noted. A lack of definition or disruption of the typical low signal intensity of the vertebral body end-plates is seen. Narrowing of the intervertebral disc space can also occur. On T2-weighted images, increased signal intensity involving the disc is noted, with loss of the normal internal disc anatomy. Increased signal intensity is also identified within the marrow of the adjacent vertebral bodies (Fig. 11–14).

The signal changes identified within the marrow spaces of the adjacent vertebral bodies are most likely related to associated marrow edema. One could argue that these MRI findings could be seen with an infiltrating neoplasm, but tumors generally do not extend across the vertebral body end-plates.

MRI can also accurately detect the presence of an associated epidural or paravertebral abscess. The abscess can be contiguous with the disc space infection. With the ability of MRI to provide multiplanar imaging, the precise location and extent of the abscess can be determined noninvasively. Involvement or compression of the adjacent neural structures can also be determined.

Spinal Tumors

For the evaluation of intramedullary lesions of the spinal cord, MRI is the study of choice. Although both CT mye-

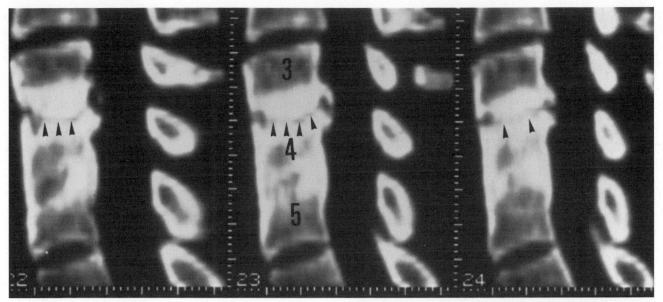

FIGURE 11–12   CT scan of cervical spine demonstrates a failed fusion at the C3–C4 level *(black arrowheads)*. Note lucent defect along caudal aspect of attempted interbody fusion. Posterior osteophytic spurring off the adjacent end-plates is also present. A solid interbody fusion is identified at the C4–C5 level.

lography and MRI are able to depict the morphological characteristics of the spinal cord, MRI has the added capability of determining the presence of intramedullary pathological lesions by evaluating for the presence of abnormal signal intensity within the cord. The presence of blood, tumor, and cystic structures within the cord can alter the normal signal intensity of the cord on both T1- and T2-weighted examinations. For example, a small cord tumor might result in no alteration of the cord morphology and hence go undetected on a CT myelographic study. However, the same small cord tumor could result in an alteration of the normal homogeneous signal intensity of the cord and would be detected on MRI. Similarly, cystic lesions involving the cord, such as a syrinx, can go undetected on a routine CT scan of the spine. MRI, however, is extremely sensitive and specific to the presence of a cystic lesion within the cord and is thus more likely to detect it.

A further improvement in the detection and delineation of intramedullary and extramedullary lesions uses intravenous gadolinium DTPA. Gadolinium DTPA is able to detect areas of blood-brain barrier breakdown, which results in enhancement of cord tumors on T1-weighted examinations. This can be helpful in distinguishing between an area of cord edema or demyelination and a cord tumor.[73]

IMAGING OF THE EXTREMITIES

Imaging of the Shoulder

The shoulder is subject to a wide variety of derangements, and patients with shoulder pathological lesions often present with poorly defined or nonspecific pain. The patient presenting with shoulder pain can be screened with conventional radiographs for gross osseous lesions, including osseous degenerative change of the glenohumeral and acromioclavicular joints, fractures or dislocations, erosions, or

unsuspected tumor. In many instances, however, the sources of shoulder pain involve soft tissue derangements for which plain radiographs might be unrevealing. Other imaging modalities might then be needed.

Fractures/Dislocations

In acute bony trauma, plain radiographs can be used to assess fracture size, displacement/distraction, or rotation of major fragments. Frontal films in internal and external rotation of the humerus are invaluable for this assessment. Gross dislocation or associated impaction fractures of the humeral head, such as Hill-Sachs lesions[100] of the posterolateral humeral head and osseous Bankart fractures of the anterior inferior glenoid rim, may be evaluated with these internal and external humeral head rotation views. The less frequent reverse Hill-Sachs and reverse Bankart/trough fractures can also be evaluated. When more precise delineation of fracture fragment size and orientation is needed, or when subtle avulsion fragments might be present, CT scan resolution and tomographic capability provide greater osseous detail. In the event of equivocal fractures or other bone lesions, scintigraphy/bone scan can be helpful in confirming the presence of osseous pathological lesions and can be sensitive and cost-effective (although often nonspecific). MRI is also sensitive for subtle/occult fractures or bone contusions and can be more specific.

Rotator Cuff Derangement and Impingement Syndrome

When rotator cuff derangement is suspected, conventional radiographs are often of limited use. Radiographs can reveal gross osseous changes, such as prominent hypertrophic degenerative change of the acromioclavicular joint with inferior osteophyte formation, subacromial spur or enthesophyte formation, and close apposition of the high-riding humeral head with the inferior margin of the acro-

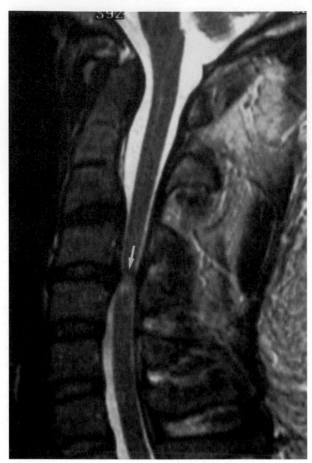

FIGURE 11–13 Sagittal T2-weighted MRI image through the cervical spine demonstrates a focal area of increased signal intensity within the cervical cord following a hyperextension injury. The appearance is compatible with a small area of cord edema secondary to contusion *(white arrowhead)*. There is evidence of central canal stenosis at this level as well, which is in part related to a posterior disc protrusion. Incidental note is made of developmental fusion of the C2 and C3 cervical vertebral bodies.

mion. Gross narrowing of the subacromial space to less than about 5 to 7 mm on plain radiographs supports the clinical diagnosis of impingement syndrome[30, 66] and possible associated rotator cuff derangement. Unfortunately, these radiographic findings can occur late in the evolution of impingement syndrome and rotator cuff pathological changes. These radiographic findings are indirect, as they fail to demonstrate or visualize the rotator cuff itself. Also, the other components of the coracoacromial arch that can contribute to clinical impingement are not well delineated on plain radiographs. For example, the shape of the acromial undersurface[5, 65] has been implicated in the natural history of rotator cuff tears and also possibly in clinical impingement. Yet conventional radiographs, including scapular Y views or outlet views, have not been found to be a reliable indicator of acromial shape. MRI, by its multiplanar tomographic capability, accurately evaluates acromial shape as well as tilt/orientation. The shape and orientation of the coracoid process is difficult to determine by conventional radiographs. Yet when it is prominent, broad, and elongated, the coracoid can come into close apposition to the lesser tuberosity and encroach on and

pinch the subscapularis tendon with forward flexion and horizontal adduction of the humerus. This less common form of more anterior or coracoid impingement syndrome can require CT scan or MRI for adequate delineation of the coracoid process morphology. (In addition, coracoid fractures may be extremely difficult to detect on radiographs; CT scan might be needed to find the fracture and to assess fracture fragment orientation and displacement.)

Soft tissue structures can also contribute to clinical impingement of the rotator cuff. The coracoacromial ligament, when thickened and scarred, can narrow the coracoacromial arch and cuff outlet and encroach on the rotator cuff. However, this and other soft tissue structures, such as extrinsic masses (which can also contribute to narrowing of the coracoacromial space and cuff outlet), cannot be assessed by plain radiographs, CT scan, or bone scan. Ultrasound can be used for more superficial soft tissue structures but can be inadequate for deeper soft tissue components. MRI might be needed for full evaluation of all soft tissue structures or masses that might encroach on the rotator cuff and contribute to clinical impingement.

In the case of rotator cuff tears, the plain film findings of the high-riding humeral head are not seen until late in

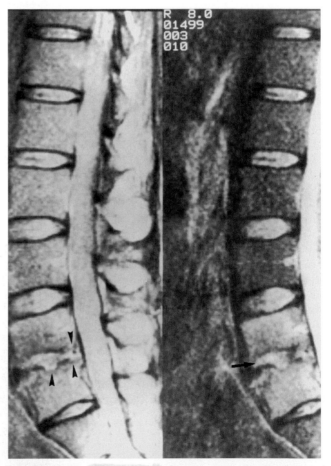

FIGURE 11–14 MRI of discitis. Sagittal proton density *(left)* and T2-weighted *(right)* images of the lumbar spine demonstrate increased signal intensity *(black arrow)* of the narrowed L4–L5 disc. There is irregularity involving the adjacent end-plates *(black arrowheads)*. On the T2-weighted images, increased signal intensity is present throughout the marrow spaces of the adjacent L4 and L5 lumbar vertebral bodies.

the process (Fig. 11–15). At this point, tears can be massive, with retraction and atrophy of the cuff. The muscle bellies can be atrophic and infiltrated with fat. Such tears might not be repairable, and the prognosis could be poor.

More direct imaging and visualization of the cuff is needed for earlier detection and clinical intervention in the natural history of rotator cuff derangement. Arthrography is accurate for detection of full-thickness cuff tears. Partial-thickness tears of the articular margin of the cuff can also be detected by glenohumeral joint space arthrography, but sensitivity can be less. Partial tears of the superior/bursal margin of the cuff cannot be seen by glenohumeral joint injection, and require a separate subacromial/subdeltoid bursal injection of contrast. Assessment of the precise size of rotator cuff tears in both medial/lateral and anterior/posterior dimensions can be helpful for operative planning. Such assessment by arthrography is difficult and can be inadequate.

Ultrasound has been used in assessment of rotator cuff tears. In experienced hands sonography can be accurate for evaluation of lateral tears close to the greater and lesser tuberosities. More medial tears under the acromion can be more difficult to evaluate because of penetration limits or artifact formation due to the intervening sound-reflecting osseous structures.

MRI is becoming the gold standard advanced imaging procedure for direct visualization and full evaluation of the rotator cuff[15, 16, 25, 40, 42, 48, 92] when more detailed anatomical information beyond that contained in initial screening radiographs is needed. As previously noted, all of the components of the coracoacromial arch, as well as other structures that might encroach on the rotator cuff and contribute to clinical impingement, can be assessed. The cuff itself can be assessed for morphological and signal changes in more acute tendinitis or tendon or muscle strain or contusion. More chronic tendinosis with atrophy and degeneration can be delineated. Full-thickness or partial-thickness tears (including both superior/bursal and inferior/articular margin partial tears) can be accurately determined (Fig. 11–16).

Cuff tear size and location can also be accurately evaluated to aid in preoperative planning. The relatively late findings of muscle atrophy and fatty infiltration, difficult to detect by other imaging modalities, can also be determined by MRI and can have prognostic significance.

Instability

Clinical instability is another major category of shoulder pain and dysfunction. Acute traumatic dislocations or more chronic recurrent dislocations can present with the humeral head still displaced, which might be apparent clinically. Plain radiographs serve to confirm the degree and direction of dislocation. Once the dislocation is reduced, plain radiographs can reveal gross associated Hill-Sachs or bony Bankart fractures. More subtle impaction fractures or bony fragments might require CT scan for adequate visualization. Soft tissue injury, such as labral tears or detachments,[85] or capsular tears or stripping are more difficult to image, as plain radiographs can be unrevealing. Conventional arthrography in more acute injuries can show gross extravasation of contrast through large capsular or labral defects. In more chronic instances, CT arthrography, with its tomographic capability and high resolution, might be needed for detection of labral tears or attenuation (Fig. 11–17). Sonography has not been shown to be useful, because it is limited by depth of penetration as well as by intervening osseous structures. MRI is very promising as an accurate and sensitive means of visualizing the labral and capsular surfaces and substance[67] for degeneration, fraying, and tears. MRI is particularly useful in the assessment of more acute disorders when large joint effusions might be present. These effusions help to outline the labral and capsular surfaces and, in essence, serve as a native intra-articular contrast agent (Fig. 11–18). In the assessment of more chronic disorders, MRI arthrography with intra-articular injection of saline or diluted gadolinium/saline solutions can be used to delineate more subtle labral tears.

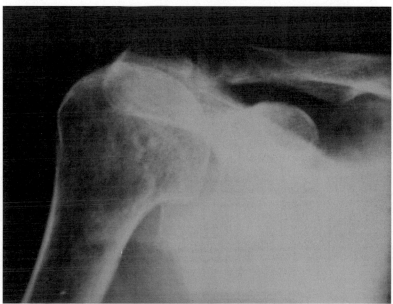

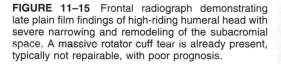
FIGURE 11–15 Frontal radiograph demonstrating late plain film findings of high-riding humeral head with severe narrowing and remodeling of the subacromial space. A massive rotator cuff tear is already present, typically not repairable, with poor prognosis.

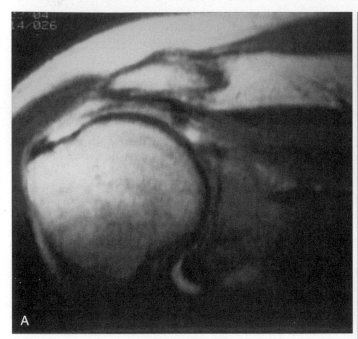

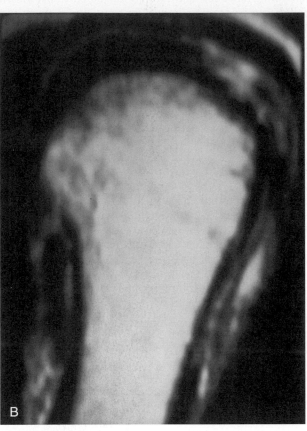

FIGURE 11–16 MRI accurately assesses location and size of full-thickness tear of supraspinatus portion of rotator cuff. *A,* Coronal T2-weighted image demonstrates medial/lateral size of tear with bright/high signal fluid in tear. *B,* Sagittal T2-weighted image reveals anterior/posterior size of tear.

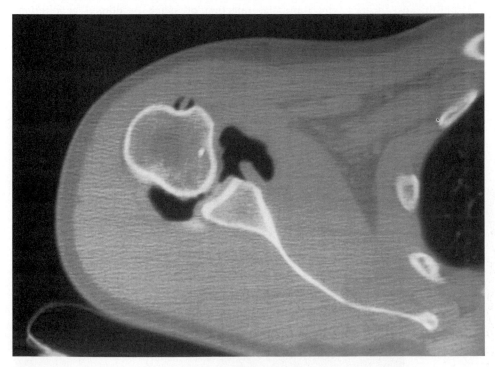

FIGURE 11–17 CT arthrography demonstrates chronic tear of anterior labrum with injected air and contrast outlining the labral and capsular margins.

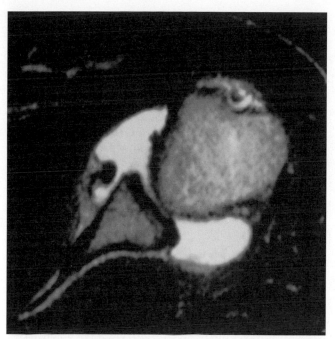

FIGURE 11–18 Axial T2-weighted MRI image reveals acute anterior labrum detachment/Bankhart lesion. Large effusion typically seen with acute injuries is helpful as native intra-articular "contrast" to outline the capsulolabral complex.

The more difficult problem of shoulder laxity/instability, typically seen in younger individuals, remains a difficult clinical and imaging diagnosis. No imaging modality has been shown to reliably or sensitively make this diagnosis—particularly because there can be no gross anatomical or morphological abnormalities. Preliminary dynamic motion or kinematic pseudomotion studies with MRI have been used to analyze motion of the humeral head relative to the glenoid fossa. This imaging study holds great promise to help in the diagnosis of instability, particularly subtle instability.

Other Causes of Shoulder Pain

Patients can also present with less common causes of shoulder pain that can be difficult to diagnose clinically. Screening radiographs can reveal an unexpected osseous lesion, such as a mass or tumor. Although not sensitive, these plain radiographs might be most specific in differentiating among possible bone tumors. CT scan can be helpful for subtle cortical erosion or periostitis as well as for subtle matrix calcification or ossification. Bone scan, although not specific, is quite sensitive for subtle bone tumors as well as for screening for bony metastases. In general, soft tissue tumors or the extent of soft tissue involvement by osseous masses is not well evaluated by these imaging modalities, which have poor soft tissue contrast. Ultrasound can occasionally be helpful in assessing relatively superficial cystic vs. solid soft tissue involvement. MRI, with its exquisite soft tissue contrast and multiplanar imaging capability, can be helpful (although it is often nonspecific) in evaluating soft tissue masses. The extent and anatomical relationships of soft tissue lesions as well as the presence and extent of adjacent osseous cortical or marrow involvement are

accurately and sensitively demonstrated by MRI, particularly with the newer fat-signal suppression MRI sequences.

Many of the other less common causes of shoulder pain involve soft tissue derangements that are not well detected or evaluated by plain radiographs, bone scan, or CT scan. Biceps tendon tears can occasionally be seen by arthrography or CT arthrography. The more superficial/lateral tears might also be seen by ultrasound. Tendinitis or tendinosis/degeneration, as well as tendon dislocation,[14] can be better demonstrated by MRI. Extra-articular soft tissue lesions, such as para-articular ganglion cysts (likely associated with labral or capsular tears/defects), may entrap the suprascapular nerve within the suprascapular notch or spinoglenoid notch,[29] producing nonspecific deep shoulder pain that can be associated with atrophy and weakness of the supraspinatus and infraspinatus muscles. Such cysts are difficult to detect by physical examination because of their location and are not reliably demonstrated by most imaging modalities because they are located deep in the soft tissue. Again, MRI is the optimal imaging modality for accurate evaluation of ganglion cysts or other soft tissue lesions along the course of the suprascapular nerve.

Imaging of the Elbow

Traumatic Injuries

The traumatized elbow can be evaluated by conventional radiographs for gross fractures and joint effusions. Fracture orientation, possible intra-articular extension, and fracture fragment displacement or angulation can be assessed. However, complex comminuted fractures with supracondylar and intra-articular involvement can be difficult to fully appreciate because of the projectional nature of radiographs. CT is helpful for more precise delineation of fracture fragment size and orientation. CT can also identify "loose bodies" within the joint (Fig. 11–19). Subtle fractures, such as radial head fractures, can be more difficult to demonstrate on plain radiographs. In this situation, specialized radial head views might be required. When findings on radiographs are equivocal or clinical suspicion is high, bone scan can be a more cost-effective and sensitive, although less specific, modality for identifying abnormal

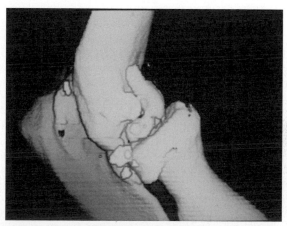

FIGURE 11–19 Three-dimensional reformation with surface rendering/shading of CT scan of elbow, demonstrating position and orientation of multiple large osseous bodies.

osseous lesions. CT scan and MRI can be more specific and provide excellent anatomical resolution.

Trauma to the skeletally immature elbow presents special challenges. Physeal injuries can be occult and not seen on either plain radiographs and CT. MRI might be needed for accurate evaluation of possible injury to the cartilaginous growth plates. Gross osteochondral lesions or osteochondritis dissecans of the elbow, at the capitellum, can also be demonstrated by screening plain radiographs. More subtle lesions can require CT scan to evaluate irregularity or disruption of the cortical margins. MRI can be a powerful tool for evaluating these lesions. Extension of joint fluid into the bed of the lesion typically indicates full-thickness disruption of the overlying articular cartilage and instability of the osteochondral fragment. In equivocal settings, MRI arthrography or CT arthrography with injection of intra-articular contrast might be needed. The injection of large amounts of the appropriate contrast under some pressure could be required for optimal visualization of the cartilage surface and of disruption extending into the bed of the osteochondral lesion.

In less severe osteochondral injuries, MRI is likely more revealing for incomplete lesions with osseous contusion, rather than osteochondral fragmentation, which might not be seen on CT scan or plain radiographs. Bone scan can demonstrate the presence of such lesions, but lacks specificity.

Epicondylitis and Instability

Acute traumatic and chronic overuse injuries can involve primarily the soft tissues supporting the elbow. Frequently, the common flexor and extensor tendons and the corresponding medial and lateral collateral ligaments at their attachments at the medial and lateral epicondyles, respectively, can be injured.[19, 63, 64, 69, 71, 89, 94] The resulting inflammation, pain, and tenderness in the region of the medial and lateral epicondyles is termed *epicondylitis*. Unfortunately, this is a somewhat nonspecific term, as assessment and differentiation of degree of tendon vs. ligament injury can be difficult by physical examination. Radiographs, CT scan, or bone scan might offer little for such soft tissue injuries. Ultrasound may be used to demonstrate changes in morphology and echo texture of the tendons and underlying ligaments. However, sonography can be highly dependent on the experience and interest of the sonographer, likely more so than with other imaging modalities. MRI, however, provides exquisite soft tissue definition. Tendinitis, tendinosis/degeneration, partial tears, or complete tears/detachments of the common flexor or common extensor tendons at the medial and lateral epicondyles, respectively, can be fully assessed (Fig. 11–20). The components of the medial and lateral collateral ligament complexes can be evaluated for partial or full tears, as well as for more chronic degeneration and scarring. In more acute disorders, extravasation of joint fluid through capsular defects can also be demonstrated. Historically, arthrography could be used in acute settings for demonstration of such capsular defects and associated ligament injuries. However, the sensitivity of arthrography diminishes rapidly with chronicity and scarring, whereas MRI can visualize

the ligaments more directly, even in more chronic conditions.

Other regional soft tissue injuries of the elbow, such as of the distal biceps tendon[9] or the triceps tendon,[87] can benefit from MRI evaluation to determine the precise level and extent of injury. For example, MRI can help distinguish tendinitis from tendinosis/degeneration and partial from complete tears. Such information can be of significant benefit when initiating or modifying a rehabilitation program or developing a surgical plan. Again, other imaging modalities might have little to offer for such soft tissue derangements.

Neuropathies

Injuries to the ulnar, median, or radial nerves can be clinically suspected on physical examination. The level or nature of the injury might require additional studies, including imaging to determine whether any structural abnormalities are present. Radiographs or CT scan can reveal gross osseous or soft tissue lesions and can be valuable for detection of calcification or ossification within gross mass lesions. However, these studies provide limited soft tissue detail and can miss more subtle structural causes of neuropathy. Bone scan and sonography might have little to offer in this setting. Because of its exquisite contrast and resolution, MRI is able to visualize the courses of the ulnar, median, and radial nerves. Extrinsic masses encroaching on the nerves can be demonstrated and the precise anatomical relationships of such masses to the neurovascular structures characterized. Such masses can also be excluded by MRI, and other nerve lesions can also be delineated. Ulnar nerve contusions along the relatively shallow and exposed ulnar groove behind the medial epicondyle can be demonstrated. The presence of the anomalous anconeus epitrochlearis muscle or a thickened cubital tunnel retinaculum predisposing to static or dynamic compression of the ulnar nerve as in cubital tunnel syndrome[57, 72] can be noted. Similarly, extrinsic mass encroachment vs. dynamic compression of the median nerve in pronator teres muscle syndrome can also be demonstrated (Fig. 11–21). Nerve entrapment syndromes or neuropathies such as carpal tunnel syndrome[60] can be evaluated by MRI for intrinsic vs. extrinsic causes when other imaging techniques are of limited use. Nerve edema/inflammation or hemorrhage can be identified. Acute denervation signal changes and chronic atrophy and fatty infiltration of the affected muscle bellies can also be detected and characterized.

Imaging of the Wrist and Hand

Traumatic Injuries

Conventional radiographs serve to demonstrate gross fractures of the wrist and hand, as well as possible unexpected patterns of erosions, osteopenia, or osteophyte formation or osseous "whiskering," which is seen in the rheumatoid or seronegative rheumatoid variant arthritides and osteoarthrosis. Unexpected tumors can also be demonstrated, with plain radiographs being perhaps the most specific of the imaging modalities. Subtle fractures might require specialized radiographs such as scaphoid views. Bone scanning can demonstrate subtle fractures, but gener-

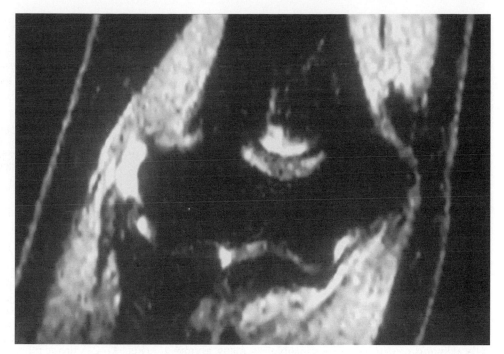

FIGURE 11–20 Coronal fat-suppression short time inversion recovery (STIR) image reveals location, extent, and high signal edema/hemorrhage in partial tear of common extensor tendon at lateral epicondyle.

ally does so with little specificity. When needed, CT scan can be invaluable for demonstration of subtle fractures or more precise characterization of fracture fragment size and orientation. Small avulsion fractures of the triquetrum or hook of the hamate can be difficult to demonstrate by plain radiographs but can be seen on CT scan (Fig. 11–22).

Plain radiographs and CT scan can also reveal the relatively late findings of sclerosis and possible fragmentation of osteonecrosis or osteochondroses, such as Kienböck disease of the lunate. Post-traumatic osteonecrosis and possible osseous nonunion of the scaphoid can also be revealed. Bone scan can be helpful in earlier or more equivocal cases, but again, with relative lack of specificity. MRI can be both sensitive and specific for earlier or radiographically equivocal or occult findings suggestive of marrow edema, contusion, or osteonecrosis[76] (Fig. 11–23).

Triangular Fibrocartilage and Intrinsic Ligament Injuries

In many acute traumatic and chronic degenerative or overuse settings, injuries of the wrist and hand can involve primarily the soft tissues. A common source of pain involves tears of the triangular fibrocartilage complex or the scapholunate or lunotriquetral ligaments of the wrist. Wrist arthrography can demonstrate such tears by leakage of injected contrast. Single radiocarpal joint space injection can demonstrate most tears, but three compartment injections have been reported to be more sensitive, as tears can be partial or might allow only a unidirectional flow of contrast via a ball valve mechanism. MRI has also been touted as a noninvasive means of demonstrating such triangular fibrocartilage or ligament tears. Although wrist arthrography remains the gold standard, improved hardware, software, and coil design should permit higher reso-

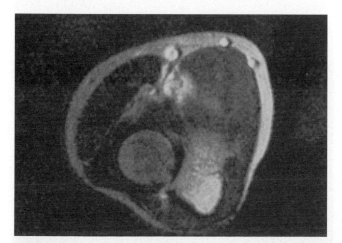

FIGURE 11–21 Axial T2-weighted image demonstrates edema/inflammation of median nerve (but absence of extrinsic masses) presumably from dynamic compression in pronator teres muscle syndrome.

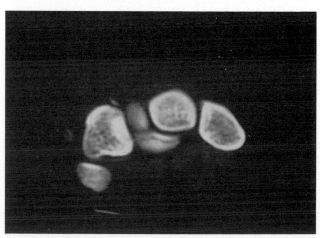

FIGURE 11–22 Occult fracture of triquetrum revealed by CT scan when conventional radiographs were unrevealing.

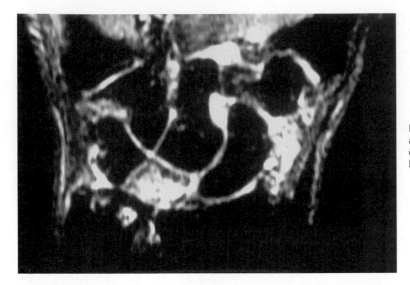

FIGURE 11–23 Coronal fat suppression STIR MR image demonstrates prominent high signal cancellous edema of lunate (which may be an early change of Kienböck disease or osteonecrosis).

lution and more accurate MRI examinations of the wrist.[6, 49, 97] However, the clinical significance of these radiographically demonstrated tears is questionable, as many asymptomatic patients, particularly older individuals, can have such tears on a degenerative basis. Operative management of such tears is limited, and conservative treatment might be chosen regardless of the presence or absence of such tears.

Other Soft Tissue Lesions

Imaging study results can directly influence the choice of treatment prescribed. For example, because the prognosis of tendon tear repair typically favors earlier rather than later intervention, early assessment of the degree and extent of tendon tears is especially important. Tenography can demonstrate complete or partial tears but might be less revealing of intrasubstance tears or degeneration. It is also an invasive and sometimes difficult examination to perform. Ultrasound can be beneficial when properly directed and localized and when performed by an experienced and interested sonographer. MRI can be more widely applicable, with its high soft tissue contrast and resolution demonstrating both morphology and signal changes of the tendons and of tenosynovitis involving the tendon sheath.

Extrinsic ligament injury, such as ulnar collateral ligament injury of the thumb (as seen in gamekeeper's or skier's thumb), can also benefit from imaging to demonstrate the level and extent of ligament tears and possible displacement of the ligament remnants. This injury can require operative repair (e.g., a Stener lesion of the thumb).[68] Stress radiography is an indirect means of demonstrating complete ligament tears, but it offers little information about partial tears or displacement of complete tears. Arthrography can be helpful in acute settings, but it might be of little value in more chronic cases. Arthrography is also invasive and might be painful in the acutely traumatized joint. Again, MRI holds great promise as a noninvasive comprehensive examination of the collateral ligaments and joint capsules.

Soft tissue masses of the wrist and hand can also be demonstrated and their anatomical relationships character-

ized by MRI. With some exceptions MRI is very sensitive, though it might be relatively nonspecific. Ganglion cysts (Fig. 11–24) are a relatively common lesion of the wrist and hand; they have characteristic fluid intensity, well-defined lobulations, and, at times, an appearance of septation, often with a neck extending toward a joint space or tendon sheath. Sonography can also be beneficial in differentiating cystic from solid lesions. Other imaging modalities generally have little to offer in evaluation of such soft tissue processes.

Imaging of the Hip

Traumatic Injuries

Screening frontal and lateral radiographs serve to detect and assess gross fractures of the femoral head and neck for fracture orientation, displacement, and varus/valgus angulation. Nonreduced fracture dislocations are assessed for displacement of the femur and associated gross fractures of

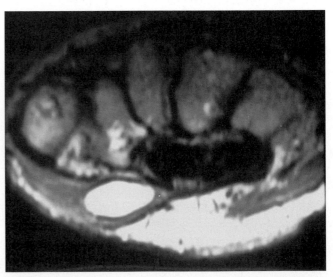

FIGURE 11–24 Axial T2-weighted MRI image reveals characteristic well-defined high signal mass (fluid) of ganglion cyst extending into thenar muscles of hand.

the femoral head and acetabulum. When needed, CT scan accurately determines the degree of rotation of fractures of the femoral head and neck. CT scan also can demonstrate more subtle impaction fractures of the femoral head. Subtle avulsion fragments of the femoral head or acetabulum that can become trapped in the hip joint on reduction of fracture dislocations can also be accurately detected. This helps guide surgical planning for removal of the fragment. CT scan is also valuable for demonstrating bony and soft tissue injuries about the remainder of the pelvis that are often associated with hip trauma.[41]

When plain radiographs are unrevealing and clinical suspicion is high, conventional tomography can, at times, be helpful for detecting subtle fractures. Bone scan is a sensitive modality for detecting radiographically occult fractures and osseous contusions, but it can be relatively nonspecific. MRI is likely of equal sensitivity and is more specific for both fractures and contusions.[21] MRI is also the modality of choice for assessment of associated soft tissue injuries, because it is more sensitive and accurate than CT scan (although less capable of detecting and localizing small avulsion fragments). Muscle strains or contusions,[1, 28, 34, 43] hemorrhage/hematomas, joint effusions/synovitis, or bursitis can all be accurately evaluated by MRI when other imaging modalities might have little to offer.

Stress reactions or stress fractures[52, 86] can present a diagnostic dilemma. Radiographs or CT scan can be relatively specific in later stages, when relatively well-defined bandlike sclerosis or frank fracture lines develop and extend across the femoral neck, but can be unrevealing in early stages. Bone scanning, again, can be sensitive in early stages, but might lack specificity until such time as linear bandlike activity can be detected. MRI is both sensitive and more specific, ranging from the early, poorly defined edematous or inflammatory change along the endosteal or periosteal margin of the cortical bone in stress reactions to the better-defined bandlike or linear abnormal cancellous and cortical signal change in later, more discrete or complete stress fractures.

At times, trauma can be incidental to underlying processes such as rheumatoid arthritis or rheumatoid variants. In such settings, plain radiographs detecting typical erosions and osteopenia can be the most specific of the imaging modalities. CT scan may be helpful for more subtle erosions, but it adds little specificity. MRI is able to demonstrate the synovitis and pannus formation as well as more subtle erosions, but it might add little specificity.

When relatively minor trauma produces pathological fractures, the unexpected underlying lesion might be documented with the most specificity by plain radiographs. CT scan can add greater detail in assessment of osseous margins and degree of cortical disruption of the underlying lesion. MRI is the most accurate test to assess any associated soft tissue mass and the extent of marrow involvement. Bone scan has relatively little to offer in evaluating the underlying lesion, but it is very helpful for screening for the presence of other osseous lesions in metastatic disease.

Avascular Necrosis

Unfortunately, avascular/ischemic necrosis of the femoral head, whether primary or post-traumatic, might show little or no conventional radiographic or CT findings until late in its course, when gross sclerosis or subcortical fracture lines or frank irregularity/collapse of the weightbearing surface of the femoral head can be detected. Bone scan is a sensitive modality and can be specific when a characteristic scintigraphic appearance is found in the appropriate clinical setting of underlying risk factors. MRI[33, 61] is more specific than and at least as sensitive as scintigraphy in detecting early changes of osteonecrosis, with typical findings of poorly defined marrow edema. In later stages, very characteristic and specific geographic lesions, centered on the anterosuperior weight-bearing portion of the femoral head, may be detected well in advance of the late stages of overlying cortical irregularity and collapse of the head (Fig. 11–25).

Imaging of the Knee

In trauma or other sources of knee pain, plain radiographs are a good screen for gross fractures or dislocations. Osteophytosis, sclerosis, and loss of joint space in osteoarthrosis can be detected. Gross erosions and joint effusions in rheumatoid arthritis or rheumatoid variants can be characterized. The unexpected primary or metastatic bone tumor is also evaluated (Fig. 11–26) with greatest specificity by radiography, although not necessarily with great sensitivity. CT scan can complement radiography by providing more accurate evaluation of the degree of cortical erosion or disruption in traumatic or pathological fractures and, in the case of tumor, evaluation of possible matrix calcification.

In many instances, however, knee pain in both acute trauma and more chronic or repetitive microtrauma can primarily involve internal derangement of the soft tissues about the knee, for which radiography, CT scan, or scintigraphy have little to offer. MRI is now the gold standard for comprehensive evaluation of internal derangement of the knee.[8, 27, 95] Arthrography still has a limited role for

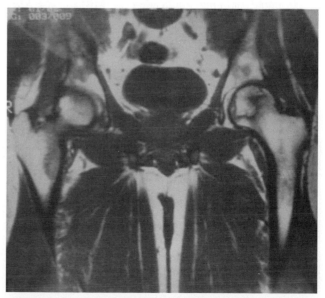

FIGURE 11–25 Coronal T1-weighted MRI image of characteristic geographic lesion of avascular necrosis of hips, including unsuspected asymptomatic lesion of contralateral hip.

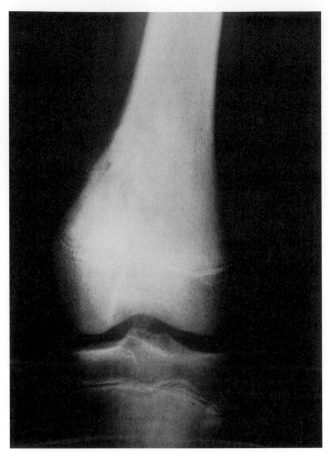

FIGURE 11–26   Radiograph demonstrates sclerotic bone-forming tumor (osteosarcoma) of distal femur.

patients with severe claustrophobia or contraindications to MRI.

Meniscal Tears

The initial defining application of MRI in the knee was evaluation of meniscal pathological conditions (Fig. 11–27). Tears can be imaged directly for location, configu-

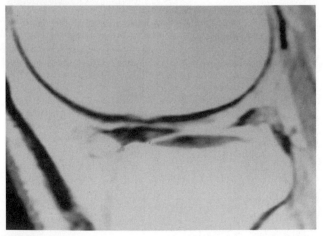

FIGURE 11–27   Sagittal T1-weighted MRI image reveals bucket-handle tear of low signal meniscus posterior horn displaced anteriorly to the adjacent anterior horn.

ration, size, and displacement of tears, all of which can have implications for the course of management. Potentially unstable tears, such as bucket handle or flap tears, should be reported accurately, as such tears can be at risk of extending or displacing to produce locking or meniscal fragments, and can require operative intervention. Accurate reporting of tears in the periphery of the meniscus is important, as residual vascularity can be present, and such tears are more likely to heal rather than be resected.

Arthrography is still a useful means of evaluating the menisci, although MRI in experienced hands can be more accurate. Accurate positioning and manipulation of the knee in arthrography for demonstration of all parts of the meniscus is vital. Such manipulation can be strenuous for both examiner and patient, and can be difficult or impossible in the acutely traumatized knee.

Ligament Tears

Arthrography is limited in its ability to evaluate the supporting soft tissues about the knee, such as ligaments. MRI has been proved a highly reliable and accurate imaging modality for demonstration and evaluation of the precise location and extent of partial to complete tears of the cruciate and collateral ligaments.[93] The accuracy of such information has important implications for operative planning for repair vs. reconstruction of such ligaments, and can be an important supplement to the clinical examination. Physical examination can reveal anterior cruciate ligament (ACL) instability, for example, but fail to reveal the precise location of the tear or the quality of the remaining ACL substance. Physical examination can be difficult and equivocal in the acutely traumatized knee with prominent edema/swelling or patient guarding. MRI can reliably localize proximal tears, which are more likely to be repaired successfully. Tears in the mid-substance (Fig. 11–28), with poor vascularity, are less likely to heal or be repaired successfully and may warrant reconstruction. In distal avulsions of the ACL, indistinguishable on clinical examination from frank ligament substance tears, the size and degree of elevation of the avulsed bone fragment and the degree of damage of the ligament substance can be evaluated. This is helpful for operative planning for reattachment of the bone fragment and ligament (vs. reconstruction when extensive ligament substance damage is also revealed).

Capsular and Retinacular Injury

Arthrography can demonstrate acute capsular or retinacular tears by extravasation of contrast, but can be unrevealing in late settings in which scarring and granulation tissue can be present to block the leakage of contrast. MRI can demonstrate capsular sprains and tears in acute settings, with high-signal intrasubstance and surrounding hemorrhage and edema. More chronic injuries can also be revealed, with low-signal irregularity and thickening and scarring. Lateral and posterior capsule tears, not uncommonly associated with ACL injuries, can also be revealed accurately. The plain film finding of the small Segund avulsion fracture fragment of the distal lateral capsule attachment at the tibia can also be detected by MRI. The posterolateral corner complex, consisting of posterolateral

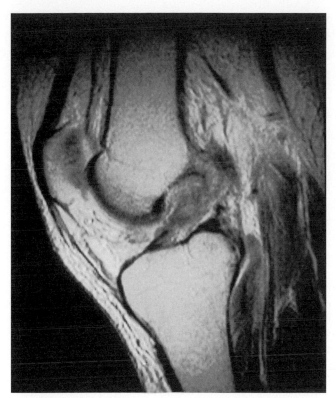

FIGURE 11–28 Sagittal T2-weighted MRI image shows complete mid-substance tear of anterior cruciate ligament that is unlikely to heal or be repaired successfully and likely will require reconstruction.

capsule, arcuate ligament, and popliteus and lateral gastrocnemius muscles, is an important ancillary support of the knee and is also not uncommonly injured with ACL tears. This complex can also be well evaluated by MRI when other imaging modalities might have little to offer. In acute settings, prominent thickening with hemorrhage/edema is seen. Assessment is more difficult in more chronic settings, but irregular low-signal thickening and scarring can be detected.

Tendon and Muscle Injuries

The muscles and tendons of the knee are frequently injured. Plain film radiography, CT, scintigraphy, and arthrography generally are not helpful in identifying such injuries. MRI accurately demonstrates alterations from the normal smooth morphology and low signal of tendons and low to intermediate signal of muscles.[28] Thickening and increased signal can be detected in tendinitis or tendinosis and in muscle strains or contusions. Frank tendon or muscle tears can also be evaluated accurately for precise location and extent, with important implications for planning management and operative intervention.

Chondral Lesions

Gross osteochondral lesions can be detected by plain radiographs, with CT scan being helpful for more precise evaluation of location and size of such lesions. More subtle osteochondral lesions or purely chondral lesions generally are difficult to evaluate by such modalities. CT arthrogra-

phy adds sensitivity and accuracy but is limited by the general confinement of CT imaging to the axial plane. MRI has been proved an accurate means of evaluating the chondral surfaces (particularly in acute chondral lesions, in which sharply marginated defects may be seen) and chondral substance.[101] In acute settings, large joint effusions are likely to outline the sharp edges of such lesions (Fig. 11–29). In more chronic settings, chondral thinning might be more diffuse, with gradually tapered edges, and minimal joint fluid might be present. Examination is then more difficult and generally less accurate. Intra-articular injection of contrast in MRI arthrography[50] can improve visualization and accuracy and is particularly helpful in more chronic settings.

Imaging of the Ankle and Foot

In ankle trauma, plain film radiography is helpful in screening for gross fractures or dislocations. Gross soft tissue swelling or talar tilt or subluxation can imply associated ligamentous injury. CT scan adds additional information on fracture size and orientation (Fig. 11–30), and is particularly sensitive for small avulsion fragments. Such information can be extremely important. For example, subtle avulsion fragments about the tarsometatarsal joint can be the only findings in Lisfranc's injury or fracture dislocation. Bone scanning, again, is sensitive but nonspecific. This can be a problem, particularly about the ankle and foot, where typical degenerative changes on bone scan might be difficult to differentiate from traumatic findings or contusions or subtle fractures. MRI is both sensitive and more specific for osseous injury ranging from fractures to contusions.

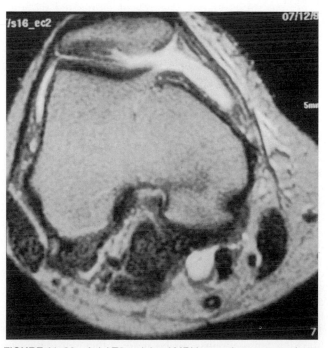

FIGURE 11–29 Axial T2-weighted MRI image demonstrates large, sharply marginated, acute chondral defect over patella that is well-delineated by high-signal acute joint effusion.

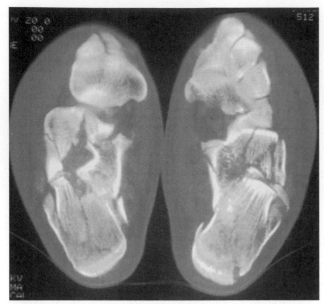

FIGURE 11–30 CT scan best demonstrates fracture fragment size and position in bilateral comminuted fractures of calcaneus.

Ligament Injuries

Plain film radiographs can reveal gross soft tissue swelling indicating acute ligament injuries. Stress views can be inspected for talar tilt or drawer findings for ligament tears. Such tests can be difficult and limited in the acute setting because of patient pain and extensive hemorrhage and edema. Stress views can also be equivocal in more chronic settings in which scarring or fibrosis is often present. Arthrography can be useful in acute capsule and ligament tears by demonstrating leakage of contrast, but is generally unrevealing in more chronic settings in which scarring is present. Scintigraphy can reveal associated osseous injuries, but is of little value in assessment of the ligaments themselves. MRI[70] is able to directly delineate the components of the medial and lateral collateral ligament complexes for precise location and extent of injuries or tears in both acute and chronic settings.

Tendon Injuries

Tenography has been used for evaluation of both traumatic and inflammatory or fibrotic tendon and tendon sheath processes.[77] Tendon tears, tenosynovitis, or fibrosing tenosynovitis have been successfully demonstrated. Tenography is limited in application, as it is an invasive procedure that is dependent on the experience and interest of the examiner. Also, more chronic intrasubstance tendon changes, such as tendinosis, can be difficult to assess, as the tendons are not directly imaged in tenography.

MRI is able to identify directly intrasubstance tendon changes as well as the precise location and extent of frank tears (Fig. 11–31) of the Achilles and other tendons of the ankle and foot.[75, 78] Tenosynovitis is revealed by prominent fluid within the tendon sheaths, with somewhat irregular and indistinct margins. The findings in more chronic fibrosing tenosynovitis can be more difficult to delineate by MRI, with lower sensitivity and accuracy than those of tenography.

Stress Fractures, Osteochondral Lesions, and Other Osseous Lesions

As previously mentioned in discussions of the knee and hip, late or gross stress fractures, osteonecrosis,[82] and osteochondral lesions[2, 20] can be detected by plain film radiography and more accurately evaluated by CT scan. Bone scanning is sensitive, although relatively nonspecific, but can be appropriate in the proper clinical setting. MRI is sensitive, more specific, and useful in evaluating the overlying articular cartilage in osteochondral lesions of the talar dome or tibial plafond. Such information has important implications for potential instability of osteochondral fragments, which can dictate earlier operative intervention. CT arthrography and MRI arthrography can accurately detect intra-articular fragments.

Tarsal coalitions can have characteristic findings on plain film radiographs, such as prominent talar beaking and remodeling of the talar dome and tibial plafond. Osseous coalitions can be seen on plain film radiographs, including oblique views. Talocalcaneal sustentacular coalitions can be difficult to discern by plain radiographs, but they are well demonstrated by CT scan in the direct-angled coronal plane. Less common coalitions and fibrous or cartilaginous coalitions can be difficult to delineate confidently with radiographs or CT scan, and can benefit from the multiplanar capability and contrast resolution of MRI.

Tarsal Tunnel Syndrome, Plantar Fasciitis, Sinus Tarsi Syndrome, and Other Soft Tissue Lesions

Compromise of the tibial nerve in tarsal tunnel syndrome can be detected by nerve conduction studies. The cause of the neuropathy might be more of a diagnostic dilemma. MRI can be beneficial for resolving the more diffuse processes, such as vasculitis and diabetic neuropathy, from structural lesions that reduce the volume of the tarsal tunnel or directly encroach on the tibial nerve.[80] Talocalcaneal sustentacular coalition (which may also be found by CT

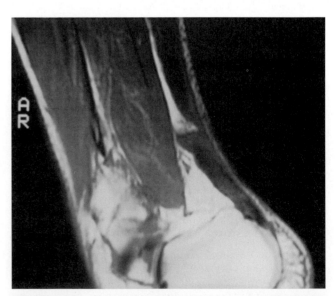

FIGURE 11–31 Sagittal T2-weighted MRI image best shows location and extent of near-complete partial tear of Achilles tendon.

scan) or soft tissue mass lesions, such as ganglion cysts or lipomas, may be identified when other imaging modalities are generally unrevealing.

At times, tarsal tunnel syndrome can also be mimicked by other lesions, such as plantar fasciitis. MRI can aid in differentiating as well as in evaluating the other lesions, whereas other imaging can be negative. Plantar fasciitis can show more acute focal thickening or disruption of the fascia with high signal hemorrhage and edema, or more chronic diffuse thickening and scarring by MRI.

The sinus tarsi and talocalcaneal interosseous ligament can also be accurately evaluated for ligament sprain/tear with surrounding edema or hemorrhage in sinus tarsi syndrome.

Other soft tissue lesions of the ankle and foot are best imaged by MRI (although CT scan may be beneficial in demonstrating of subtle calcifications or associated osseous erosions). Soft tissue masses can be localized and evaluated for anatomical relationships when needed for preoperative planning, although MRI lacks specificity for tissue characterization. Some lesions can have a relatively specific appearance, such as lipomas and other fatty tumors. The appearance of cystic lesions, such as ganglion or synovial cysts, can be highly suggestive. However, in general, many soft tissue masses, including neuromas, neurofibromas, or sarcomas, can have similar or overlapping MRI appearance. A relatively characteristic location and appearance of Morton's interdigital neuroma or fibroma is of relatively well-defined intermediate signal masses along the plantar aspect of the interdigital spaces, typically in the third interspace.

IMAGING OF THE BRAIN

Cerebral Infarction (Ischemic)

Cerebral ischemia and infarction result in transitory or permanent neurological dysfunction. The most common etiology is atherosclerosis with focal ischemia due to arterial stenosis or secondary embolic phenomenon. Diffuse cerebral ischemia can occur in generalized hypoxemia associated with states of hypoperfusion, such as cardiac arrest or shock. In the acute phase, the radiological evaluation is useful in confirming the presence of an infarction, the assessment of its size and location, and the exclusion of associated hemorrhage. In the later stages, imaging is useful in demonstrating the location and extent of the infarcted region and the exclusion of other clinically "silent" infarctions.

The CT findings within the first 24 hours of onset of infarction vary, depending on the size of the ischemic injury. Findings range from a normal scan with no change in parenchymal density to a scan with ill-defined areas of diminished density, sulcal effacement, loss of gray-white differentiation, and mass effect[96] (Fig. 11–32). The low density demonstrated in the acute phases is the result of cytotoxic edema associated with cell death. The cytotoxic edema and its secondary mass effect are greatest at approximately 5 days and subside within 3 weeks. As the cytotoxic edema resolves, a period can occur in which the infarcted area is isodense with normal brain.[4] The infarction

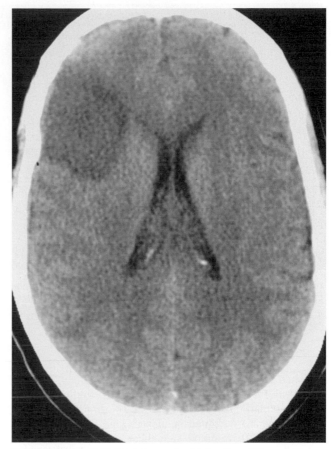

FIGURE 11–32   CT of acute cerebral infarction. CT scan demonstrates a wedge-shaped area of low density in the right frontoparietal region with effacement of adjacent gyri.

results in transient damage to the blood-brain barrier. Consequently, contrast enhancement of the area can be demonstrated at 3 to 5 days, resolving by 8 weeks.[83] As cell death and the resorption of dead neurons progresses, the infarction becomes progressively lower in density, with enlargement of adjacent cerebrospinal fluid spaces.

The MRI findings in acute infarction include regions of subtle increased signal intensity on proton density sequences, usually within gray matter only. In the subacute stage, the signal intensity becomes more intense with the development of white matter abnormalities and gyral effacement as a result of edema (Fig. 11–33). The signal intensity changes in the acute and subacute stage are due to increased intracellular water associated with cell death. MRI is more sensitive than CT in the demonstration of acute infarctions. MRI is positive in 80% of cases; CT in 60%.[13] In the chronic stage, the infarction demonstrates even greater signal intensity on proton density and T2-weighted sequences, and its margins are more clearly demarcated as a result of the increased water content of encephalomalacic brain.

Lacunar infarctions, due to small-vessel occlusive disease, generally occur in the basal ganglia, brainstem, internal capsule, and periventricular white matter. In the acute stages, a CT scan is usually normal because of the small size of the infarctions. In the later stages, the CT can demonstrate multiple, usually bilateral, small areas of di-

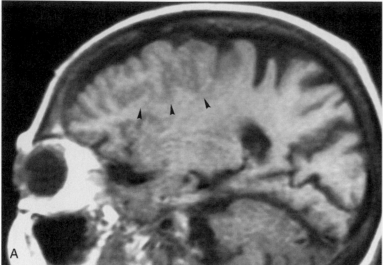

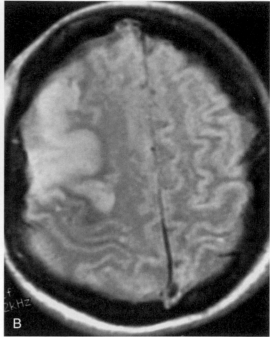

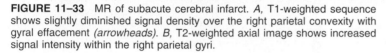

FIGURE 11–33   MR of subacute cerebral infarct. *A,* T1-weighted sequence shows slightly diminished signal density over the right parietal convexity with gyral effacement *(arrowheads). B,* T2-weighted axial image shows increased signal intensity within the right parietal gyri.

minished density. MRI is more sensitive than CT in the detection of lacunar infarctions.[12] The MRI findings include multiple small and confluent foci of diminished signal intensity on T1-weighted sequences and increased signal intensity on T2-weighted sequences in the basal ganglia and periventricular white matter. Because of the high sensitivity of MRI, such signal-intensity changes are commonly seen in patients as an age-related phenomenon.

Generalized cerebral hypoxia can result in deep gray matter infarctions, infarctions in the watershed zones between cerebral artery territories, or diffuse cerebral edema. CT findings include low density in the basal ganglia, somewhat wedge-shaped areas of diminished density in the watershed zones, or diffuse cerebral low density with loss of gray-white differentiation and sulcal effacement.

Nontraumatic Intracranial Hemorrhage

Parenchymal Hemorrhage

In the acute stage (1 to 3 days), a parenchymal hematoma consists of intact red blood cells containing oxyhemoglobin, which is rapidly desaturated to deoxyhemoglobin. The intracellular deoxyhemoglobin is subsequently oxidized to methemoglobin. At 4 to 5 days (the subacute stage), lysis of the red blood cells occurs with release of free methemoglobin. Reactive and inflammatory changes occur along the peripheral aspect of the hematoma. Macrophages appear and rapidly become hemosiderin laden. Subsequently, vascular proliferation and reactive astrocytosis result in capsule formation.[90]

The CT finding in an acute hematoma is a hyperdense mass. It can demonstrate adjacent low-density edema and mass effect (Fig. 11–34). Initially, the hematoma is of high density because of the high protein content of intact red blood cells. As the red blood cells lyse, the hematoma gradually diminishes in density. In the later stage, a well-demarcated area of marked low density or encephalomala-

cia is seen. Contrast enhancement of the hematoma, particularly along the periphery, can be seen in the first 6 weeks, initially as a result of perivascular inflammation and subsequently as a result of vascular proliferation.[102]

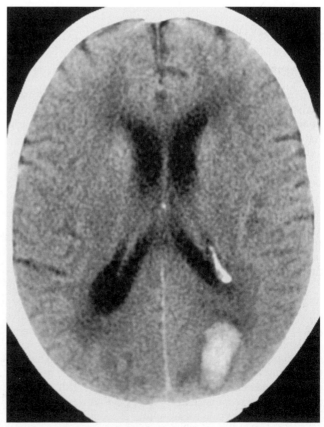

FIGURE 11–34   CT of acute hemorrhagic infarct. High-density right occipital hemorrhage with surrounding low-density edema.

The MRI findings of parenchymal hemorrhage are complex because the field strength of the magnet and the chemical constituents of the hematoma affect the signal intensity characteristics (Fig. 11–35). The presence, in varying proportions, of oxyhemoglobin, deoxyhemoglobin, intracellular methemoglobin, and free methemoglobin can change the appearance of the hematoma. Simplistically, in the first 24 hours, the hematoma can be of high signal intensity on T2-weighted sequences due to secondary edema. In the first 1 to 3 days, the hematoma is of diminished signal intensity on T2-weighted sequences because of the presence of deoxyhemoglobin. After 3 days, the hematoma demonstrates a high–signal-intensity component on T1-weighted images and a low–signal-intensity component on T2-weighted images due to intracellular methemoglobin. As the red blood cells lyse, releasing free methemoglobin, the hematoma shows high–signal-intensity components on T2-weighted sequences. As the hematoma further matures, a low–signal-intensity rim of hemosiderin (which persists indefinitely) is seen on T2-weighted sequences.[90]

Subarachnoid and Intraventricular Hemorrhage

Subarachnoid and intraventricular hemorrhage can occur as a result of an aneurysm, an arteriovenous malformation, the extension of an intracerebral hemorrhage, trauma, or hypertension.

CT is the imaging modality of choice for the evaluation of subarachnoid and intraventricular hemorrhage in the acute stage. In subarachnoid hemorrhage, noncontrast CT demonstrates increased density in the basilar cisterns, sulci, and fissures because of the high attenuation of clotted blood (Fig. 11–36). In intraventricular hemorrhage, CT demonstrates high-density blood layers posteriorly in the ventricles. As the blood is resorbed, CT is less sensitive in its detection. Consequently, in the first 24 hours, CT detects 95% of subarachnoid hemorrhage; at 7 days, it detects slightly more than 50%.[53, 54]

In the acute stage, MRI is relatively insensitive to the detection of subarachnoid and intraventricular hemorrhages.[3] The conspicuousness of an acute hemorrhage is dependent on the presence of deoxyhemoglobin. Because of the relatively high partial pressure of oxygen within cerebrospinal fluid, conversion of oxyhemoglobin to deoxyhemoglobin in subarachnoid and intraventricular blood is delayed, rendering the hemorrhage relatively isointense to cerebrospinal fluid.[90] Additionally, cerebrospinal fluid pulsation artifacts can further diminish the sensitivity of MRI. However, in the subacute stage, T1-weighted MR images demonstrate linear hyperintensity in the subarachnoid space or high–signal-intensity blood layering posteriorly in the ventricles. In the chronic phase, peripheral low signal intensity can be demonstrated on T2-weighted sequences as a result of hemosiderin deposition.[90]

Hemorrhagic Infarction

A hemorrhagic infarction can occur after an embolic infarction with subsequent lysis of the embolus and reper-

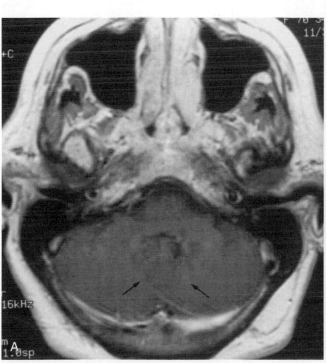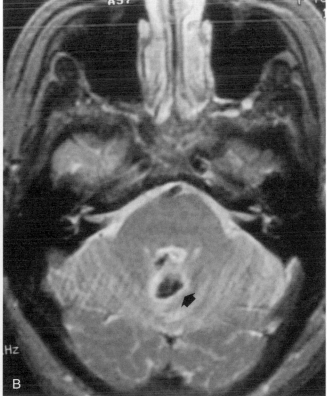

FIGURE 11–35 MR of acute hemorrhagic Infarct. *A,* T1-weighted image shows mass effect on posterior aspect of the fourth ventricle *(arrows). B,* T2-weighted image shows acute hematoma of decreased signal intensity as a result of the presence of deoxyhemoglobin with linear high–signal-intensity rim of edema *(arrow).*

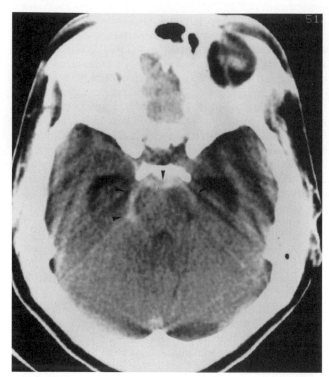

FIGURE 11–36 Subarachnoid hemorrhage. CT scan demonstrates high-density subarachnoid hemorrhage surrounding the pons *(arrowheads)*. Dilatation of the temporal tips as a result of communicating hydrocephalus is also demonstrated.

fusion, or after a thrombotic infarction with reperfusion of an infarcted area by collateral vessels. The acute CT and MRI findings are of a parenchymal hemorrhage of variable size with associated mass effect (see Fig. 11–34). Contrast enhancement can occur subacutely, persisting for as long as 4 to 6 weeks; it can render differentiation from a hemorrhagic neoplasm difficult in the early stage.

Hypertensive Hemorrhage

Hypertensive hemorrhage occurs as a result of bleeding from small arteries secondary to degenerative changes in the vessel wall media and of rupture of microaneurysms. The CT and MRI findings are primarily those of intraparenchymal hemorrhage. The hemorrhage usually occurs in the basal ganglia, and less commonly, in the cerebral white matter, brainstem, cerebellum, and thalamus. The hemorrhage can extend into the subarachnoid and intraventricular spaces.

Aneurysm

Aneurysm rupture is the most common cause of spontaneous intracranial hemorrhage. The most common locations of aneurysms are at the anterior communicating artery, posterior communicating artery, middle cerebral artery trifurcation, supraclinoid carotid, and distal basilar artery. Because the most common radiographic finding is subarachnoid hemorrhage, CT is far more sensitive than MRI in the acute stages (see Fig. 11–36). Parenchymal and intraventricular hemorrhage can also occur. Complications of subarachnoid hemorrhage include hydrocephalus and

infarction. Hydrocephalus associated with subarachnoid hemorrhage can be either communicating (due to obstruction of pacchionian granulations by the high protein content of hemorrhagic cerebrospinal fluid) or obstructive (due to outlet obstruction by blood clots). Vasospasm, which occurs in approximately 40% of patients after subarachnoid hemorrhage, can result in cerebral infarction.[98]

Head Trauma

The role of radiological imaging in head trauma in the acute stages is the assessment of the presence of extra-axial hematomas, parenchymal hematoma or contusion, or diffuse brain swelling. CT is the imaging modality of choice in the acute stages, because CT is as sensitive as MRI in the detection of acute parenchymal hemorrhage and more sensitive than MRI in the detection of subarachnoid hemorrhage, intraventricular hemorrhage, and skull fractures. Additionally, acutely injured patients are frequently unable to cooperate, and CT scans are less sensitive than MRI to degradation by patient motion. Furthermore, the patient can be monitored more easily during CT scanning. It should be noted, however, that after the acute phase, MRI is more sensitive than CT in detecting nonhemorrhagic white matter injuries and small hematomas.

Extra-axial Hematoma

A subdural hematoma (SDH) occurs when trauma results in disruption of veins or superficial cerebral arteries bridg-

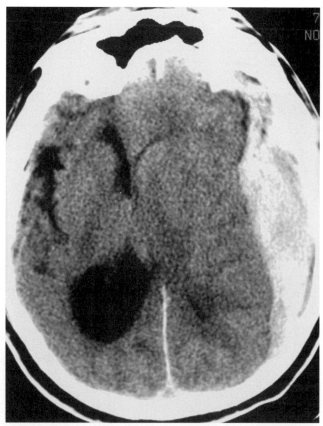

FIGURE 11–37 Subdural hematoma. CT scan demonstrates a large crescentic high-density subdural hematoma with shift of the midline structures to the right (parafalcine herniation), flattening of the left lateral ventricle, and dilatation of the right lateral ventricle.

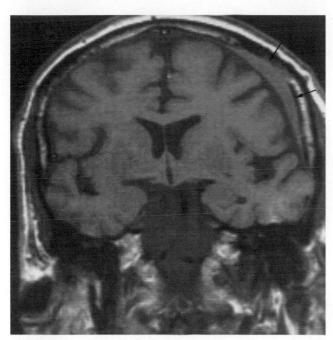

FIGURE 11–38 MR of subdural hematoma. Coronal T1-weighted scan shows a small, acute subdural hematoma over the left convexity *(arrows)*.

ing the potential subdural space between the dura and arachnoid. CT findings in acute SDH include a high-density crescentic collection along the inner aspect of the calvarium, most commonly over the cerebral convexities (Fig. 11–37). Associated abnormalities are due to secondary mass effect, including effacement of cortical sulci, flattening and medial displacement of the adjacent lateral ventricle, and shift of midline structures to the contralateral side. At 2 to 3 weeks, as the red blood cells lyse, the SDH can be isodense with brain. At more than 3 weeks, the SDH is considered chronic. Chronic SDHs usually occur in elderly patients. The chronic SDH is of low density and may have a well-defined capsule.

Epidural hematomas (EDHs) occur when trauma results in disruption of meningeal arteries and veins coursing between the dura and the inner table of the calvarium. EDHs usually occur in younger patients. The CT findings in an acute EDH include a biconvex, hyperdense peripheral collection with secondary mass effect. Associated fractures are commonly present.

MRI is more sensitive than CT in the detection of extra-axial hematomas.[32] Because MRI is capable of direct multiplanar imaging, hematomas in the sagittal or coronal planes (i.e., subfrontal, subtemporal, tentorial hematomas) are better demonstrated by MRI (Fig. 11–38). Small hematomas adjacent to the high-density calvarium or hematomas isodense with brain, which are difficult to detect with CT, are also readily apparent by MRI.[32, 37] However, MRI is usually appropriate only in patients with subacute or chronic extra-axial fluid collections.

Parenchymal Contusion and Hematoma

Intracerebral contusions occur from the traumatic impact of the brain against the calvarium or from angular accelera-

tion. The CT findings of a contusion include an ill-defined parenchymal area of diminished density, most frequently involving the frontal and temporal lobes. The density of the contusion can be heterogeneous if petechial hemorrhage is superimposed on the concussive edema. Associated mass effect can be seen. The early findings in a traumatic parenchymal hematoma include a hyperdense mass with peripheral edema and mass effect (Fig. 11–39). The hematoma diminishes in density over time. In the late phase, residual low density is usually seen as a result of encephalomalacia. The MRI appearance of intracerebral contusions and hematomas depends on the age of the lesion and the various constituents of edema and hemorrhage, as previously discussed.[39, 90]

Diffuse Brain Injury

Shearing injury or diffuse axonal injury results from differential movement of adjacent cerebral tissues at high angular acceleration. Axonal disruption and swelling ensue. Such injuries are most common in the lobar white matter at the gray-white junction, the corpus callosum, and the brainstem. Even when the injury is severe, the CT findings are relatively mild, ranging from a normal scan to a scan demonstrating small, multifocal hemorrhages.[56] MRI, which is more sensitive than CT in the detection of shear injury, demonstrates multifocal lesions of variable signal intensity depending on the content of edema and hemorrhage.[39, 46, 84]

Diseases of White Matter

Myelin is a component of the cell wall membrane of oligodendroglia in the central nervous system. Diseases of myelin can be due to demyelinating or dysmyelinating processes. Demyelinating diseases are those in which myelin is formed normally but is subsequently destroyed. Primary demyelinating processes include multiple sclerosis and diffuse sclerosis. Secondary demyelination can be the result of infection, vascular insults, or toxins. Dysmyelinating diseases are those in which normal myelin either is not formed or is not maintained once it is formed, usually as the result of a single enzymatic deficiency. The dysmyelinating disorders can affect gray and white matter or white matter only. Included in this group are metachromatic leukodystrophy, Krabbe's disease, and adrenoleukodystrophy.

Multiple sclerosis is the most common demyelinating disorder. MRI is more sensitive than CT in the detection of characteristic lesions. CT is positive in 25% to 50% of patients with definite multiple sclerosis; MRI is positive in 50% to 100%.[38, 81] The radiographic findings in multiple sclerosis include lesions of low density by CT or high signal intensity on T2-weighted MRI, a few millimeters to a few centimeters in diameter. The lesions are commonly located in the cerebral hemispheres and are frequently periventricular in distribution. Plaques can also be demonstrated in the internal capsule, brainstem, and cerebellar white matter. In general, acute and chronic multiple sclerosis plaques cannot be distinguished without intravenous contrast material (Fig. 11–40). Acute multiple sclerosis plaques are enhanced due to transient breakdown in the blood-brain barrier. Serial scans can show progression and regression in activity. Contrast-enhanced MRI is more sen-

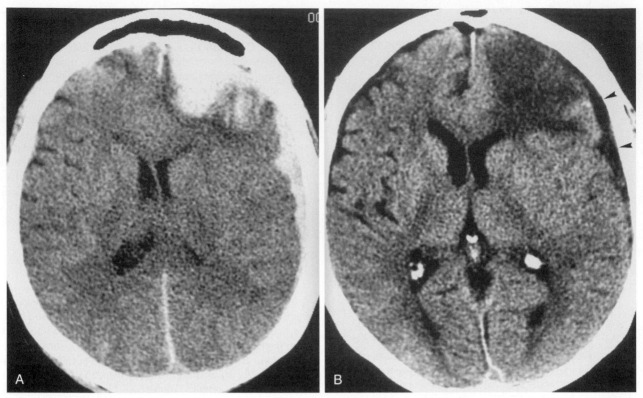

FIGURE 11–39 Hemorrhagic contusion. *A,* In the acute stage, CT scan demonstrates a large, high-density left frontal hematoma with mild generalized cerebral edema. Also seen is a small left subdural hematoma *(arrow). B,* Four weeks later, CT scan shows resorption of the hematoma with residual left frontal edema. Note interval increases in size of the ventricles with the resolution of cerebral edema. A small subdural hygroma is seen *(arrowheads).*

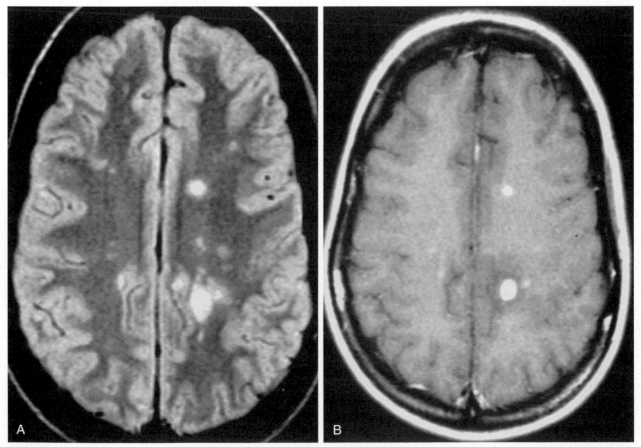

FIGURE 11–40 Multiple sclerosis. *A,* T2-weighted MR demonstrates multiple punctate foci of high signal intensity adjacent to the lateral ventricles and in the centrum semiovale. *B,* T1-weighted postintravenous contrast MR shows contrast enhancement of foci of active demyelination.

sitive than contrast-enhanced CT in the detection of active multiple sclerosis.[79] In advanced disease, cerebral atrophy can be seen.

Aging and Dementing Disorders

The brain undergoes significant atrophic changes in the normal course of aging.[91] Imaging studies using both CT and MRI have demonstrated quantitative enlargement of the ventricles and cortical sulci. Commonly, periventricular low-density foci can be demonstrated by CT and, even more commonly, high–signal-intensity periventricular and subcortical foci of increased signal intensity may be seen on T2-weighted MRI images. These lesions have been ascribed variously to demyelination associated with arteriolar hyalinosis, white matter gliosis, or small vessel infarctions.

Alzheimer's Disease

The radiographic findings in Alzheimer's disease include cerebral atrophy with ventricular and sulcal enlargement.[31, 44] Abnormalities of the mesial temporal lobe/hippocampal region can be seen with enlargement of the temporal horns of the lateral ventricles and sylvian fissures and increased signal intensity in the hippocampal and sylvian cortex on T2-weighted images.[26, 47] Periventricular and subcortical white matter lesions are also more common in patients with Alzheimer's disease than in nondemented elderly persons.[10, 26] However, the extent of white matter abnormalities does not correlate with the severity of dementia, and extensive white matter changes can be seen in nondemented elderly persons.[10]

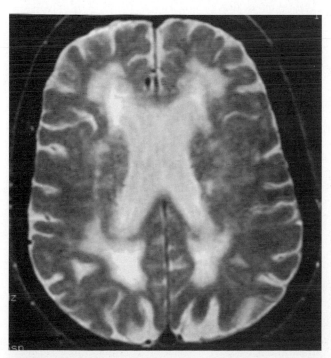

FIGURE 11–41 Multi-infarct dementia. T2-weighted MR shows confluent areas of increased signal intensity in periventricular white matter as a result of extensive small-vessel infarctions.

Multi-infarct Dementia

Multi-infarct dementia can occur in patients with multiple infarctions, particularly if cortical gray matter is involved.[55] The CT and MR findings are nonspecific, including multiple periventricular and subcortical white matter infarctions and lacunar infarctions (Fig. 11–41). The lacunar infarctions can involve the basal ganglia, thalamus, and brainstem.

CONCLUSION

Radiological imaging procedures play a significant role in helping to further define pathomorphological tissue changes. The information contained in these studies can assist the physiatrist in making a complete, correct, and anatomically specific diagnosis. The physiatrist can then use this information to plan further rehabilitation, order subsequent tests, and determine whether surgical care is required.

Although current imaging technology is a powerful tool, the physiatrist is trained to treat a patient's entire injury and disease complex—not just the findings of imaging studies.

Acknowledgments

Andrew Cole, M.D., would like to thank Bradley L. Hundley and Associates for their editorial assistance and Joyce Heiser and Carolyn A. Cole, M.S., M.F.A., for their invaluable and timely assistance in the preparation of this manuscript.

References

1. Agre JC: Hamstring injuries: Proposed aetiological factors, prevention, and treatment. Sports Med 1985; 2:21–23
2. Anderson IF, Crichton KJ, Grattan-Smith T, et al: Osteochondral fractures of the dome of the talus. J Bone Joint Surg Am 1989; 71:1143–1152.
3. Barkovich AJ, Atlas SW: Magnetic resonance imaging of intracranial hemorrhage. Radiol Clin North Am 1988; 26:801–820.
4. Becker H, Desch H, Hacker H, et al: CT fogging effect with ischemic cerebral infarcts. Neuroradiology 1979; 18:185–192.
5. Bigliani LU, Morrison DS, April EW: The morphology of the acromion and its relationship to rotator cuff tears. Orthop Trans 1986; 10:216.
6. Binkowitz LA, Ehman RL, Cahill DR, et al: Magnetic resonance imaging of the wrist: Normal cross section imaging and selected abnormal cases. Radiographics 1988; 8:1171–1202.
7. Bodner RJ, Heyman S, Drummond DS, et al: The use of single photon emission computed tomography (SPECT) in the diagnosis of low-back pain in young patients. Spine 1988; 13:1155.
8. Boeree NR, Watkinson AF, Ackroyd CE, et al: Magnetic resonance imaging of meniscal and cruciate injuries of the knee. J Bone Joint Surg Br 1991; 73:452–457.
9. Bourne MH, Morrey BF: Partial rupture of the distal biceps tendon. Clin Orthop 1991; 271:143–148.
10. Bowen BC, Barker WW, Lowenstein DA, et al: MR signal abnormalities in memory disorder and dementia. Am J Neuroradiol 1990; 11:283–290.
11. Brodkey JS, Miller CF, Halmody RM: The syndrome of acute cervical spinal cord injury revisited. Surg Neurol 1980; 14:251–257.
12. Brown JJ, Hesselink JR, Rothrock JR: MR and CT scan of lacunar infarcts. Am J Neuroradiol 1988; 9:477–482.
13. Bryan RN, Levy LM. Whitlow WD, et al: Acute Stroke: Magnetic Resonance Imaging and Diagnosis. Presented at the American Society of Euroradiology Annual Meeting. Los Angeles, 1990, p 23.
14. Cervilla V, Schweitzer ME, Ho C, et al: Medial dislocation of the biceps brachii tendon: Appearance at MR imaging. Radiology 1991; 180:523.

15. Chandnani V, Ho C, Gerharter J, et al: MR findings in asymptomatic shoulders: A blind analysis using symptomatic shoulders as controls. Clin Imaging 1992; 16:25–30.

16. Clark JM, Harryman DT II: Tendons, ligaments, and capsule of the rotator cuff. J Bone Joint Surg Am 1992; 74:713–725.

17. Cole A, Herring S: The role of the physiatrist in the management of musculoskeletal pain. In Tollison CD (ed): Handbook of Pain Management, ed 2. Baltimore, Williams & Wilkins, 1994, pp 85–95.

18. Collier BD, Johnson RP, Carrera GF, et al: Painful spondylolysis or spondylolisthesis studies by single photon emission computerized tomography. Radiology 1985; 154:207.

19. Conway JE, Jobe FW, Glousman RE, et al: Medial instability of the elbow in throwing athletes: Treatment by repair or reconstruction of the ulnar collateral ligament. J Bone Joint Surg Am 1992; 74:67–83.

20. DeSmet AA, Fisher DR, Burnstein MI, et al: Value of MR imaging in staging osteochondral lesions of the talus (osteochondritis dissecans): Results in 14 patients. Am J Radiol 1990; 154:555–558.

21. Deutsch AL, Mink JH, Waxman AD: Occult fractures of the proximal femur: MR imaging. Radiology 1989; 170:113–116.

22. Dines DM, Warren RF, Inglis AE, et al: The coracoid impingement syndrome. J Bone Joint Surg Br 1990; 72:314–316.

23. Edelson TG, Nathan H: Nerve root compression in spondylolysis and spondylolisthesis. J Bone Joint Surg Am 1986; 68:596–599.

24. Fan HF, Hubirdeau RM, DuBow HI: Lumbar intervertebral disc degeneration: The influence of geometrical features on the pattern of disc degeneration: A post mortem study. J Bone Joint Surg Am 1972; 54:492–510.

25. Farley TE, Neumann CH, Steinbach LS, et al: Full-thickness tears of the rotator cuff of the shoulder: Diagnosis with MR imaging. Am J Radiol 1992; 158:347–351.

26. Fazekas F, Chawluck JB, Alavi A, et al: MR signal abnormalities at 1.5 T in Alzheimer's dementia and normal aging. Am J Neuroradiol 1987; 8:421–426.

27. Fischer SP, Fox JM, Del Pizzo W, et al: Accuracy of diagnoses from magnetic resonance imaging of the knee: A multi-center analysis of 1014 patients. J Bone Joint Surg Am 1991; 73:2–10.

28. Fleckenstein JL, Weatherall PT, Parkey RW, et al: Sports-related muscle injuries: Evaluation with MR imaging. Radiology 1989; 172:793–798.

29. Fritz RC, Helms CA, Steinbach LS, et al: Suprascapular nerve entrapment: Evaluation with MR imaging. Radiology 1992; 182:437–444.

30. Fu FJ, Harner CD, Klein AH: Shoulder impingement syndrome: A critical review. Clin Orthop 1991; 269:162–173.

31. Gado M, Hughes CP, Danziger W, et al: Aging, dementia and brain atrophy: A longitudinal computed tomographic study. Am J Neuroradiol 1983; 4:699–702.

32. Gentry LR, Godersky JC, Thompson B, Dunn VD: Prospective comparative study of intermediate-field MR and CT in the evaluation of closed head trauma. Am J Neuroradiol 1988; 9:91–100.

33. Glickstein MF, Burk DL, Schiebler ML, et al: Avascular necrosis versus other diseases of the hip: Sensitivity of MRI. Radiology 1988; 169:213–216.

34. Greco A, McNamara MT, Escher MB, et al: Spin-echo and STIR MR imaging of sports-related muscle injuries at 1.5 T. J Comp Assist Tomogr 1991; 15:994–999.

35. Grenier N, Kressel HT, Schieber ML, et al: Isthmic spondylosis of the lumbar spine: MR imaging at 1.5T. Radiology 1989; 170:489–493.

36. Grossman RI, Kemp SS, Yu IC, et al: The importance of oxygenation in the appearance of acute subarachnoid hemorrhage on high-field magnetic resonance imaging. Acta Radiol 1986; 369(suppl):56–58.

37. Han JS, Kaufman B, Alfidi R, et al: Head trauma evaluated by magnetic resonance and computed tomography: A comparison. Radiology 1984; 150:71–77.

38. Haughton WM, Ho KC, Williams AL, et al: CT detection of demyelinated plaques in multiple sclerosis. Am J Radiol 1979; 132:213–215.

39. Hesselink JR, Dowd CF, Healy ME, et al: MR imaging of brain contusions: A comparative study with CT. Am J Neuroradiol 1988; 9:269–278.

40. Ho CP: Applied MRI anatomy of the shoulder. J Orthop Sports Phys Ther 1993; 18:351–359.

41. Ho C, Sartoris D: Modern assessment of hip fractures. Postgrad Radiol 1990; 10:87–97.

42. Iannotti JP, Zlatkin MB, Esterhai JL, et al: Magnetic resonance imaging of the shoulder. J Bone Joint Surg Am 1991; 73:17–29.

43. Ishikawa K, Kai K, Mizuta H: Avulsion of the hamstring muscles from the ischial tuberosity: A report of two cases. Clin Orthop 1988; 232:153–155.

44. Johnson KA, David KR, Buonanno FS, et al: Comparison of magnetic resonance and roentgen ray computed tomography in dementia. Arch Neurol 1987; 44:1075–1080.

45. Kamblin P, Nixon JE, Caait A, et al: Annular protrusion: Pathophysiology and roentgenographic appearance. Spine 1988; 13:671–675.

46. Kelly AB, Zimmerman RD, Snow RB, et al: Head trauma: Comparison of MR and CT—experience in 100 patients. Am J Neuroradiol 1988; 9:699–708.

47. Kido DK, Caine ED, LeMay, et al: Temporal lobe atrophy in patients with Alzheimer disease: a CT study. Am J Neuroradiol 1989; 10:551–555.

48. Kjellin I, Ho CP, Cervilla V, et al: Alterations in the supraspinatus tendon at MR imaging: Correlation with histopathologic findings in cadavers. Radiology 1991; 181:837–841.

49. Koenig H, Lucas D, Meissner R: The wrist: A preliminary report on high-resolution MR imaging. Radiology 1986; 160:463–467.

50. Kramer J, Stiglbauer R, Engel A, et al: MR contrast arthrography (MRA) in osteochondrosis dissecans. J Comp Assist Tomogr 1992; 16:254–260.

51. Kulkarni M, McArdle CB, Kopanick D, et al: Acute spinal cord injury: MR imaging at 1.5T. Radiology 1987; 164:837–843.

52. Lee JK, Yao L: Stress fractures: MR imaging. Radiology 1988; 169:217–220.

53. Lilliequist B, Lindquist M, Valdimarsson E: Computed tomography and subarachnoid hemorrhage. Neuroradiology 1977; 14:21–26.

54. Lim ST, Sage DJ: Detection of subarachnoid blood clot and other thin flat structures by computed tomography. Radiology 1977; 123:79–84.

55. Liston EH, La Rue A: Clinical differentiation of primary degenerative and multi-infarct dementia: A critical review of the evidence: Part II: Pathological studies. Biol Psychiatry 1983; 18:1467–1484.

56. Lobato RD, Sarabia R, Rivas JJ, et al: Normal computerized tomography scans in severe head injury: Prognostic and clinical management implications. J Neurosurg 1986; 65:784–789.

57. McPherson SA, Meals RA: Cubital tunnel syndrome. Orthop Clin North Am 1992; 23:111–123.

58. Masaryk TJ, Modic MT, Geisinger MA, et al: Cervical myelopathy: A comparison of MR and myelography. J Comput Assist Tomogr 1986; 10:184–194.

59. Masaryk TJ, Ross JS, Modic MT, et al: High resolution MR imaging of sequestered lumbar intervertebral disks. Am J Radiol 1988; 150:1155–1162.

60. Middleton WD, Kneeland JB, Kellman GM, et al: MR imaging of the carpal tunnel: Normal anatomy and preliminary findings in the carpal tunnel syndrome. Am J Radiol 1987; 147:307–316.

61. Mitchell DG, Rao VM, Dalinka MK, et al: Femoral head avascular necrosis: Correlation of MR imaging, radiographic staging, radionuclide imaging, and clinical findings. Radiology 1987; 162:709–715.

62. Modic MT, Felglin DH, Piraino DW, et al: Vertebral osteomyelitis: Assessment using MR. Radiology 1985; 157:157–166.

63. Morrey BF, An KN: Articular and ligamentous contributions to the stability of the elbow joint. Am J Sports Med 1983; 11:315–319.

64. Morrey BF, An KN: Functional anatomy of the ligaments of the elbow. Clin Orthop 1985; 201:84–90.

65. Morrison DS, Bigliani LU: The Clinical Significance of Variations in Acromial Morphology. Presented at the Third Open Meeting of the American Shoulder and Elbow Surgeons, San Francisco, 1987.

66. Neer CS: Impingement lesions. Clin Orthop 1983; 173:70–77.

67. Neumann CH, Petersen SA, Jahnke AH: MR imaging of the labral-capsular complex: Normal variations. Am J Radiol 1991; 157:1015–1021.

68. Newland CC: Gamekeeper's thumb. Ortho Clin North Am 1992; 23:41–48.

69. Nirschl RP, Petrone FA: Tennis elbow: The surgical treatment of lateral epicondylitis. J Bone Joint Surg Am 1979; 61:832–839.

70. Noto AM, Cheung Y, Rosenberg ZS, et al: MR imaging of the ankle: Normal variants. Radiology 1989; 170:121–124.

71. O'Driscoll SW, Bell DF, Morrey BF: Posterolateral rotatory instability of the elbow. J Bone Joint Surg Am 1991; 73:440–446.

72. O'Driscoll SW, Horii E, Carmichael SW, et al: The cubital tunnel and ulnar neuropathy. J Bone Joint Surg Am 1991; 73:613–617.

73. Parizel PM, Beleriaux D, Rodesch A, et al: Gadolinium DTPA–enhanced MR imaging of spinal tumors. Am J Radiol 1989; 252:1087–1096.
74. Pech P, Haughton VM: Lumbar intervertebral disk: Correlative MR and anatomic study. Radiology 1985; 150:699–701.
75. Quinn SF, Murray WT, Clark RA, et al: Achilles tendon: MR imaging at 1.5 T. Radiology 1987; 164:767–770.
76. Reinus WR, Conway WF, Totty W, et al: Carpal avascular necrosis: MR imaging. Radiology 1986; 16:689–693.
77. Resnick D, Niwayama G: Diagnosis of Bone and Joint Disorders, ed 2. Philadelphia, WB Saunders, 1988, p 414.
78. Rosenberg ZS, Cheung Y, Jahss MH, et al: Rupture of posterior tibial tendon: CT and MR imaging with surgical correlation. Radiology 1988; 169:229–235.
79. Runge VM, Price AC, Kirschner HS, et al: The evaluation of multiple sclerosis by magnetic resonance imaging. Radiographics 1986; 6:203–212.
80. Sammarco JG, Stephens MM: Tarsal tunnel syndrome caused by the flexor digitorum accessorius longus. J Bone Joint Surg Am 1990; 72:453–454.
81. Sheldon JJ, Siddharthan R, Tobias J, et al: MR imaging of multiple sclerosis: Comparison with clinical CT examination in 74 patients. Am J Neuroradiol 1985; 6:683–690.
82. Sierra A, Potchen J, Moore J, et al: High-field magnetic resonance imaging of aseptic necrosis of the talus. J Bone Joint Surg Am 1986; 68:927–928.
83. Skiver EB, Olsen TS: Contrast enhancement of cerebral infarcts: Incidence and clinical value in different states of cerebral infarction. Neuroradiology 1982; 23:259–265.
84. Snow RB, Zimmerman RD, Gandy SE, et al: Comparison of magnetic resonance imaging and computed tomography in the evaluation of head trauma. Neurosurgery 1986; 18:45–52.
85. Snyder SJ, Karzel RP, Del Pizzo W, et al: SLAP lesions of the shoulder. Arthroscopy 1990; 6:274–279.
86. Stafford SA, Rosenthal DI, Gebhardt MC, et al: MRI in stress fracture. Am J Radiol 1986; 147:553–556.
87. Tarsney FF: Rupture and avulsion of the triceps. Clin Orthop 1972; 83:177–183.
88. Teplick JG, Pryster RG, Teplick S, et al: CT identification of post laminectomy pseudomeningocele. Am J Neuroradiol 1981; 4:179–182.
89. Thorson EP, Szabo RM: Tendinitis of the wrist and elbow. Occup Med 1989; 4:419–431.
90. Thulborn KR, Atlas SW: Intercranial hemorrhage. In Atlas SW (ed): Magnetic Resonance Imaging of the Brain and Spine. New York, Raven Press, 1991, pp 175–222.
91. Tomlinson BE, Blessed G, Roth M: Observations on the brains of nondemented old people. J Neurol Sci 1968; 7:343–356.
92. Traughber PD, Goodwin TE: Shoulder MRI: Arthroscopic correlation with emphasis on partial tears. J Comput Assist Tomogr 1992; 16:129–133.
93. Vahey TN, Broome DR, Kayes KJ, et al: Acute and chronic tears of the anterior cruciate ligament: Differential features at MR imaging. Radiology 1991; 181:251–253.
94. Vangsness CT, Jobe FW: Surgical treatment of medial epicondylitis. J Bone Joint Surg Am 1991; 73:409–411.
95. Vellet AD, Marks PH, Fowler PJ, et al: Occult posttraumatic osteochondral lesions of the knee: Prevalence, classification, and short-term sequelae evaluated with MR imaging. Radiology 1991; 178:271–276.
96. Wall SD, Brant-Zawadzki M, Jeffrey RB, et al: High frequency CT findings within 24 hours after cerebral infarction. Am J Neuroradiol 1981; 2:553–557.
97. Weiss KL, Beltran J, Lubbers LM: High-field MR surface coil imaging of the hand and wrist: Part II. Pathologic correlations and clinical relevance. Radiology 1986; 160:147–151.
98. Wier BKA: The effect of vasospasm on morbidity and mortality after subarachnoid hemorrhage from ruptured aneurysms. In Williams RH (ed): Cerebral Arterial Spasm. Baltimore, Williams & Wilkins, 1980, pp 385–393.
99. Wiltse LL, Guyer RD, Spencer CW, et al: ALAR transverse process impingement of the L5 spinal nerve: The far out syndrome. Spine 1984; 9:31–41.
100. Workman TL, Burkhard TK, Resnick D, et al: Hill-Sachs lesion: Comparison of detection with MR imaging, radiography, and arthroscopy. Radiology 1992; 185:847–852.
101. Yulish BS, Montanez J, Goodfellow DB, et al: Chondromalacia patellae: Assessment with MR imaging. Radiology 1987; 164:763–766.
102. Zimmerman RD, Leeds NE, Naidich TP: Ring blush with intracerebral hematomas. Radiology 1977; 14:21–26.

12

Quality and Outcome Measures for Medical Rehabilitation

CARL V. GRANGER, M.D.,
MARGARET KELLY-HAYES, Ed.D., R.N., C.R.R.N.,
MARK JOHNSTON, Ph.D.,
ANNE DEUTSCH, M.S., R.N., C.R.R.N.,
SUSAN BRAUN, M.L.S., O.T.R., AND
ROGER C. FIEDLER, Ph.D.

THE CHALLENGE OF REVIEWING AND ASSURING QUALITY

Reviewing and assuring quality of healthcare delivery are daunting issues, not just for physical medicine and rehabilitation but for all of healthcare. The Peer Review Organization (PRO) was created as a national program in the early 1980s to review delivery of care and to assure quality of care for Medicare recipients. Audet and Scott[4] point out that we still lack evidence of the PRO's effect on quality of care. They indicate that the Health Care Financing Administration (HCFA) is committed to reform. At the time of this writing, HCFA proposes to change to the use of a Uniform Clinical Data Set (UCDS) as a national data base for Medicare's quality review program. Five years in the making, the UCDS can accommodate 1800 clinical variables per patient, although it is expected that approximately 200 to 600 elements will actually be used. The elements cover (1) patient identification, (2) history and physical examination, (3) laboratory results, (4) diagnostic test results, (5) endoscopic procedures, (6) surgical interventions, (7) therapeutic interventions, (8) in-hospital medications, (9) recovery phase, and (10) discharge planning and discharge status.

Audet and Scott conclude that although the UCDS can potentially improve the accuracy and reliability of data abstraction and the validity of reviews, it remains to be seen whether this will be the case. They suggest that while the UCDS has a unique but limited role in national surveillance of practice patterns, detailed assessments of quality are more appropriately done at local or institutional levels.[4]

Almost two decades ago medical rehabilitation adopted a facility-based model of program evaluation with certain common elements. In doing so, the case-by-case review, which was the hallmark of the PRO system, was bypassed. The case-by-case review system is now viewed by HCFA as being punitive. HCFA plans to replace it with a model similar to program evaluation that emphasizes education and continuous quality improvement. Since an important purpose of medical rehabilitation is to improve the functional status of patients, reliable and valid methods of functional assessment are necessary.

DEFINITION OF FUNCTIONAL ASSESSMENT

Functional assessment is a method for describing an individual's abilities and limitations. The essence of it is the measurement of an individual's use of the variety of skills included in performing tasks necessary to daily living, leisure activities, vocational pursuits, social interactions, and other required behaviors. For a comprehensive functional assessment, selected diagnostic descriptors, performance (skill or task) descriptors, and social role descriptors are used to assemble the information desired. The technique includes coding the component skills and tasks according to categories of activities required to support quality of daily living. The data help formulate judgments as to how well these essential skills are used, and to gauge the degree to which tasks are accomplished and social role expectations are met.

Figure 12–1 proposes that an individual's fulfillment and quality of daily living are a result of balancing functional opportunities (*left*) and functional requirements or demands (*right*). We have chosen the term "quality of daily living" in preference to the more common term "quality of life" because it is less expansive, more subject to empirical investigation, and is analogous to another commonly used term, "activities of daily living (ADL)." Functional opportunities are expressed as an individual's choices, options, and expectations. Functional requirements are expressed in physical, cognitive, and emotional terms. In order to achieve fulfillment and to maximize the quality of daily living, there must be a balance between improved opportunities through individual health and functioning (*on the left*) and the reduction or removal of life's barriers causing constraints (*on the right*).

A clinician who is proficient in using functional assessment can obtain a performance-oriented data base that can be analyzed in conjunction with diagnostic descriptors of pathological conditions and impairment states. This integration of medical status with status in performance of tasks and fulfillment of social roles, together with knowledge of the individual's level of social supports, allows for the construction of a set of data that profiles the whole person. Given this profile, problems and areas of need can be identified more accurately and reviewed in an orderly manner. Following analysis, interventions and long-range coordination strategies (e.g., case management and critical pathways) can be developed that maximize personal independence and subjective well-being.

It is possible to compare the changes in status over periods of time for an individual or a group of individuals by assessing function at appropriate intervals. In this manner, outcomes of professional interventions of healthcare, rehabilitation, education, or psychological and social counseling may be described and monitored. Outcomes that are measurable are manageable.

The objectives of a functional assessment instrument that Donaldson and her co-workers summarized in 1973[9] still hold today. They are (1) objective description of functional status at a given point in time, (2) serial repetition allowing detection of changed functional status, (3) data collected through observation relevant to and useful in monitoring the treatment program, (4) enhancement of communication among treatment team members and between referral agen-

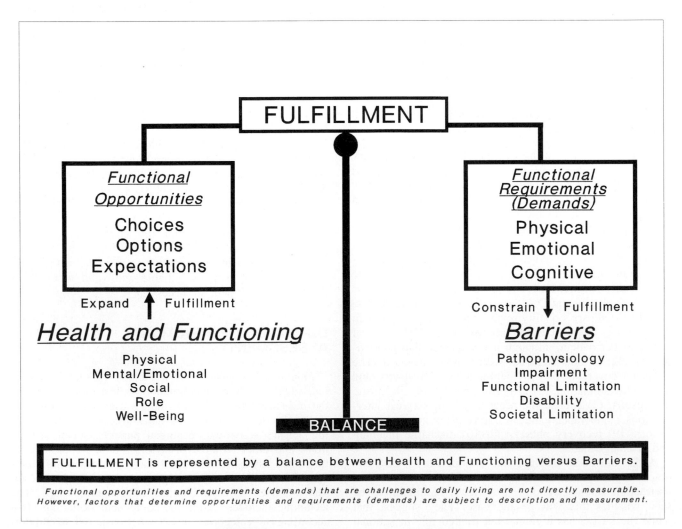

FIGURE 12–1 Challenges to quality of daily living.

cies, and (5) comparable clinical observations compatible with research questions.

The conceptual underpinnings for functional assessment are provided by disablement models proposed by Nagi,[47] Wood for the World Health Organization (WHO),[59] and the National Center for Medical Rehabilitation Research (NCMRR).[48] Although constructed slightly differently, the continuum from organ biology to the whole person and the social context is constant in each. The model of the NCMRR is the most recent and is intended to facilitate research efforts that probe how persons with a disability might interact with the rehabilitation process to achieve optimal accommodation with the environment. The terms specific to the NCMRR model are listed in Table 12–1.

Social norms are defined in the WHO document[59] within six key roles or dimensions of experiences in which competence is expected of the individual for survival: orientation, physical independence, mobility, occupation, social integration, and economic self-sufficiency. To satisfy these social roles, the individual employs a variety of functional skills that result in complex behaviors and in performance of tasks.

According to the WHO formulation, certain fundamental accomplishments or behaviors related to the existence and survival of people as social beings are expected in virtually every culture. The individual is expected to:

1. Receive signals from surroundings (such as seeing, listening, smelling, or touching), to assimilate these signals, and to express a response to what is assimilated.

2. Maintain a customarily effective independent existence with regard to the more immediate physical needs of the body, including eating, personal hygiene, and various other ADL.

3. Move around effectively in the environment.

4. Occupy time in a fashion appropriate to his or her gender, age, and culture, including following an occupation such as tilling the soil, laboring for others, running a

household, bringing up children, and carrying out activities such as play or recreation.

5. Participate in and maintain social relationships with others.

6. Sustain socioeconomic activity and independence by virtue of labor or exploitation of material possessions, such as natural resources, livestock, or crops. This economic self-sufficiency customarily includes obligations to sustain others, such as members of the family.

MEASUREMENT STANDARDS AND PRINCIPLES OF SCALING

There have been many attempts to improve the quality of measurement in rehabilitation over the last 30 years.[14, 27, 36–38, 46] Experts have repeatedly warned that functional assessment scales and procedures now in common use have distinct failings. The empirical properties of scales—including basic validity, reliability, scaling characteristics, and standardization—have been insufficiently developed. In this chapter, functional assessment instruments or tools are referred to as scales. The term "measure" is reserved for those scales that have been constructed or converted so that they have equal interval characteristics, in order that "adding one more always adds the same amount."[60] Sometimes, the domains of functional assessment scaling have been stated in global, indistinct terms, such as "quality of life" or "function," without specification of the exact meaning of these terms. Rehabilitation facilities have commonly relied on locally developed scales and documentation procedures that lack formal study or development. Even simple clinical terms such as "mild," "moderate," and "severe," when applied without specific or objective reference, are used inconsistently.[57] All of the disciplines involved in medical rehabilitation face similar technical problems in the assessment of human function and performance.

Researchers and other leaders in rehabilitation had been communicating about problems in functional assessment for many years. Attempts to write specific measurement standards applicable to rehabilitation did not coalesce until the end of the 1980s, when the American Congress of Rehabilitation Medicine formed the Task Force on Measurement and Evaluation. This interdisciplinary task force included members of the Congress and the American Academy of Physical Medicine and Rehabilitation. Disciplines represented in the task force included physiatry, psychology, physical therapy, occupational therapy, rehabilitation nursing, rehabilitation counseling, and others. After several years of work, "Measurement Standards for Interdisciplinary Medical Rehabilitation" was published in a special issue of the *Archives of Physical Medicine and Rehabilitation* in December 1992.[29]

The interdisciplinary standards document presents guidelines for development and use of assessment procedures for measurement for the several disciplines involved in medical rehabilitation. Its purpose is to facilitate improved assessment in all of the disciplines. The interdisciplinary standards were designed to serve as a resource in courses and to guide the development, choice, use, and interpretation of assessments, both in research and clinical practice.[28]

TABLE 12–1 Disablement Model Definitions

Term	Definition
Pathophysiology	Any interruption of, or interference with, normal physiological and developmental processes or structures
Impairment	Any loss or abnormality at the organ or organ system level of the body
Functional limitation	Any restriction or lack of ability to perform an action in the manner or within a range consistent with the purpose of an organ or organ system
Disability	Any limitation in performing tasks, activities, and roles to levels expected within physical and social contexts
Societal limitation	Any restriction attributable to social policy or barriers (structural or attitudinal) that limits fulfillment of roles or denies access to services and opportunities associated with full participation in society

Modified with permission from National Institutes of Health, National Institute of Child Health and Development: Research Plan for the National Center for Medical Rehabilitation Research. US Department of Health and Human Services, Public Health Service (NIH) publication no. 93-3509. Rockville, Md, National Institutes of Health, March 1993.

A remarkable degree of consensus was reached and now there are standards that distinguish quality assessment scales from merely hopeful ones.

The relationship between pathophysiological processes and wider life issues is crucial to medical rehabilitation, both in research and in practice. Interdisciplinary measurement standards are intended to apply to the assessment of impairment (specific anatomical, physiological, and psychological functional limitations) as well as to assessment of broader domains such as disability, societal limitations, and quality of daily living.

Similar measurement standards have been developed for psychology[2] and for physical therapy.[56] The interdisciplinary standards were designed to be consistent with the specific standards of these disciplines. Physical therapy standards are more stipulative than the interdisciplinary standards. The psychology standards are similar to the rehabilitation standards in that both are phrased primarily at the level of scientific principles; the two differ in the examples used to give content to the principles.

The documents addressing measurement standards differ fundamentally from systems that infer the impact on the "whole person" based on expert evaluation of severity of impairment alone. Some examples can be seen in the American Medical Association's Evaluation of Permanent Impairment, which is well-established and periodically revised.[3] On the other hand, WHO's constructs of impairment, disability, and handicap have defined concepts that incorporate the whole person in a way that is understandable and scientifically defensible.[59] Current scientific understanding requires empirical testing of the reliability and validity of *disablement* and health-related scales.[1, 26, 28, 29, 39, 50, 60]

Validity and Related Guidelines

"Validity is the paramount criterion for choice and use of a measure. Validity is commonly regarded as the extent to which a test measures what it is intended to measure."[29] Validation involves linking a concept with specific operations involved in the assessment procedure and accumulating evidence that supports the logical inferences from the measurement procedure.

Scales of human function or performance may be quite broad or robust across diagnoses,[25, 42, 45] but they still cannot be assumed to have universal or unlimited validity. Validity is delimited by a particular construct, setting, and population or problem. Validity always relates to a specified use. Measurement standards are based on scientific validity principles. The initial standard (1.1) in the 1992 document states that a measure should have evidence of validity that is appropriate to its intended use.[29] Content validity, predictive validity, and construct validity are three types of validity that have stood the test of time.

Content validity is the extent to which a test contains items critical or appropriate to a domain. The content of a functional assessment domain must be examined to choose a scale that has items that are appropriate to the clinical problem. For example, an item addressing indoor mobility is appropriate to include in a basic functional assessment tool that measures independence in ADL. However, it is not an item that is sufficient to measure the abilities of

persons who need speed and endurance in moving about in the community. A knowledge of pathophysiology is also helpful in analyzing functional assessment scales logically. Careful analysis of the sensibility of scales is essential in medical application.[12] Even though content validity is often established by a panel of experts representing experience and authority, only empirical evidence will resolve the many disputes about the validity and uses of functional assessment scales.

Predictive or criterion-referenced validity is the extent to which a scale is related to some outcome or external criterion. A truly useful assessment procedure should predict something outside of itself in the future. This is an acid test of the information provided by functional assessment scales. For example, a Barthel Index or Functional Independence Measure (FIM) rating can help to predict the likelihood of a patient's returning to the community vs. going to a nursing home after discharge from a stroke rehabilitation program.[49] Occasionally, concurrent validity—the ability to predict something that occurs at the same point in time—is of interest. For instance, one may be interested in patient performance at home, but it is impractical to leave the outpatient clinic to observe actual home performance. The outpatient clinic assessment should then be shown to correlate with home performance.

Construct validity is the extent to which a scale behaves as it should according to a theory. It involves study of the interactions of theoretically important constructs. A well-developed theory typically states that a construct should converge toward certain empirical criteria (convergent validity) on the one hand, but, on the other hand, the construct should be distinguishable by diverging from different criteria (divergent validity). Therefore, for a given scale there should be an accumulation of evidence of convergent and divergent relationships.[1, 26, 29] Construct validation involves study of the interactions of parameters that are theoretically important. For instance, one expects certain disease processes to affect related aspects of function, while unrelated aspects of function are not affected. This is an example of the dynamic logic by which rehabilitation is developing as a science. Tools that measure a physical quantity can often be validated against a single "gold standard" criterion. An inexpensive way to measure efficiency of ambulation can, for instance, be validated against an expensive and cumbersome laboratory measure of oxygen uptake. However, scales of complex concepts such as disability and societal limitation cannot be fully validated against a single ideal criterion. More complex construct validation analyses are required.

Guidelines for Reliability and Scaling

Functional assessment tools must have more than external validity characteristics such as predictive validity. They must also have internal validity characteristics such as reliability and internal homogeneity of the dimensional structure. Rehabilitation measurement standards require that adequate scales have numeric estimates of reliability (Standard 2.1).[29]

Reliability is usually defined as freedom from random error.[1, 39] It may be thought of as the extent to which the data contain relevant information with a high signal-to-noise ratio vs. irrelevant static and confusion. Reliability is a necessary but not sufficient condition for validity. Although assessment tools of narrow physical quantities or impairments can attain high reliability coefficients, one cannot assume that such tools are more reliable or valid than assessment tools of the wider and more complex behaviors, which often reveal much more about daily life and the priority needs of persons with disabilities.

Empirical testing of reliability begins with computation of the degree of agreement when a test is administered more than once under similar circumstances.[26] Agreement, however, is not precisely the same as reliability. Agreement means that the results of testing are similar despite variances in raters, time, or subjects tested. Percent of agreement is affected by population base rates, number of categories in the rating scale, and other factors that are not relevant to the balance between information and error in the measurement procedure. Several texts discuss the statistics that are used to estimate underlying reliability from surface-level agreement data.[11, 26, 39]

There are several ways of estimating reliability. Interrater reliability is crucial for rating scales which can be applied differently by various observers. Ratings of physical independence in basic ADL have shown high reliability coefficients in the range of .89 to .95.[45] (The coefficients are Pearson correlations, which are acceptable summaries of reliability only if there are no significant differences in rater means or variabilities, i.e., a normal distribution of the values.) Test-retest reliability is a critical form of reliability when results of the measurement procedure fluctuate over short periods of time, such that the ability to measure gain in basic status or ability is unlikely. When more than one form of a test is used, then parallel form reliability is needed.

A great deal hinges on the internal structure of tests involving multiple items. Internal consistency or unidimensionality is essential to a scale formed by adding up ratings from a series of items. If one adds up item ratings that are unrelated, the resulting sum is likely to fail to predict anything, even if some constituent items are in fact highly related to the criterion. Statistics such as split-half correlations and Cronbach's alpha have been used to estimate internal consistency.[1, 11, 26, 50] Factor analysis and Rasch analysis are used to identify latent factors or dimensions, that is, items that fit together.[1, 49]

The degree of ability or disability can be gauged by relating a person's performance to that of a wider age-gender-severity–adjusted comparison group. Explicit norms enhance the value of a test. Whenever possible, the characteristics of the comparison group used for evaluating patient performance should be explicitly stated (Standard 3.1).[29]

Guidelines for Clinical Application of Scales

Although measurement standards are based in science and apply most directly to researchers and developers of scales, they also have important implications for clinical practice. Simply stated, the idea is that scientific findings, when they exist and are relevant, should be applied to clinical assessment procedures. The first standard for use

of measures is that "Users of measures should read the technical manual or relevant available documentation . . ." (Standard 6.1).[29] Users need to understand the scientific basis for the inferences they make from their clinical assessments (Standard 6.2) and the boundaries of this knowledge (Standards 6.3–6.6).

Scales used in rehabilitation often need to be altered to fit unusual impairments or problems, and these modifications ought to be made within bounds understood by the user (Standards 6.22–6.25). Additionally, it must be kept in mind that persons being assessed have rights that must be respected (Standards 7.1–7.4).

Guidelines for Program Evaluation, Quality Improvement, and Group Applications

Formal measures are frequently applied at a group or systems level, rather than at the level of individual patients. Group applications include program evaluation, quality improvement, ongoing utilization review, and policymaking by government and managed-care organizations. Evidence of validity and reliability should be provided for measures used in all group applications, and the measures used should be shown to be relevant to the client populations involved (Standard 8.1).

The most respected scientific methodologies are based and validated on group rather than on single-subject studies. Usually individual outcomes are aggregated into some form of an average. When individual function varies greatly from the average, however, knowledge of the average may tell little about the individual. Standard 8.2 provides a caution, stating that comparisons of an individual with a group average need explicit justification.

Outcomes are affected by many factors other than the effectiveness of treatment. One can rarely infer effective treatment from outcomes alone. Rather, the effectiveness of rehabilitative interventions is based on a pattern of input, process, and outcome measures compared to some measured or assumed comparison.[31] One must adjust for case severity. Although severity adjustment is important everywhere in outcomes research, nowhere is it more critical than in rehabilitation, which specializes in treatment of persons with severe, permanent impairment. Standard 8.3 warns against evaluation of service providers on the basis of outcome scores alone in the absence of any other data.

The movement to improve and standardize measurement in rehabilitation should result in a smaller number of better-developed scales and measures. Quality and outcome monitoring will be facilitated by large sample sizes and valid comparisons.

STEPS IN INSTRUMENT DEVELOPMENT

A sound functional assessment instrument is required if useful data are to be generated.[15] Although functional assessment instruments have been developed in a variety of ways, most have followed a definable series of steps. Details in the sequence of steps may vary, but an ideal series is as follows:

1. DEVELOP CONCEPTUAL DEFINITIONS. The chief

aim is to define the entity to be measured. A well-defined construct allows the items to relate to a testable hypothesis for validation. A comprehensive review of the literature is needed to reveal work of a like nature done on similar or different populations. Extensive theorizing is necessary to clarify the meaning of a term such as "disability." For example, use of an instrument to collect empirical data about disability has served to support continued use of such instruments. The kinds of patients, problems, and behaviors, and the settings for using an instrument should be defined early. In particular, the developer should envision future uses of the instrument in actual practice.

2. DEVELOP A RESEARCH PLAN. Conceptual foundations lead to operational definitions and a research plan. The appropriate type and number of subjects must be identified. The appropriate type and range of behaviors to be included needs specification. Methods of selection of assessors, of determination of competence of assessors, timelines, and budgets should be established.

A decision should be made as to whether the scale will measure one or several parameters. Later on, the use of factor analysis, Rasch analysis, and internal consistency reliability estimates, such as Cronbach's alpha, will help to confirm if the instrument has one or more dimensions. A scaling technique, either categorical (choices between either one or another quality) or ordinal (choices along gradations) must be chosen. Categorical choices can elicit false-positive or false-negative information, which might be more tolerable for screening purposes than for seeking more definitive interpretations. Ordinal scaling is typically used in functional assessment scales. Here items should be selected on the basis of a continuum from easy to difficult in order that the "floor" and "ceiling" of the test are not too close together. Patients of varying abilities can be tested using the same scale. Later on, testing with empirical data allows a determination of the psychometric properties of the instrument.

Measurement standards for interdisciplinary medical rehabilitation state that both reliability and validity data are required for a professional scale, but do not impose an arbitrary order in which such data must be obtained.[29] In some circumstances it is advantageous to conduct a small study of predictive (criterion) validity before extensive testing of internal scaling characteristics. If such testing shows promise for offering predictive relationships, then one has evidence for a scale that is likely to be useful and further efforts to develop robustness can be justified.

3. CREATE A PILOT INSTRUMENT. Item generation is a creative process, calling on experience, imagination, and modification of items from previous instruments. Experienced individuals or a committee of experts can be invaluable in developing good items. Feedback is essential to the process. The response format must be determined. For example, using a yes/no answer format for numerous detailed items that vary in difficulty may be more desirable than requiring graded, multipoint judgments for a fewer number of items. What degree of rigidity will be allowed when using a checklist as opposed to a more liberal degree of response? Directions for collecting accurate responses should be clearly and concisely written.

4. COLLECT AND TEST PILOT DATA. As few as 10 to 20 cases can be used to obtain pilot data, but the process may need to be repeated several times in order to develop an easily understood and administered scale. This experience uncovers problems and limitations which should lead to improvements and solutions. The pilot data must be evaluated for feasibility (degree of user-friendliness), sensibility (face validity), and content validity of the scale. Are the data consistent with current knowledge and experience regarding disease, function, and clinical processes? Are there problems with accuracy and completeness? Misunderstandings must be identified and plans made for clarification. Feedback from data collectors, other professionals, and study participants is important. A final draft version of the scale must be prepared for formal testing.

5. FORMALIZE TEST RELIABILITY AND INTERNAL SCALE VALIDITY CHARACTERISTICS. Testing internal validity—reliability and scaling properties—is essential to the development of a useful measure. It is especially important when error or bias in assessment is a concern, as with some subjective rating scales. The form of reliability to be tested depends on the most likely problem with the scale. For instance, low inter-rater reliability is a common problem with more complex scales. Stability of responses from week to week is a matter of concern with satisfaction and mood scales.

Studying dimensionality (e.g., via factor analysis followed by Rasch analysis) is essential to understanding the scale and knowing whether one actually has a measure or not.[60] This is accomplished with a computer model that applies latent trait analysis. Usually data from a single point in time are used. Since most functional assessment scales are used to assess change in patients over time, the assessment items need to be tested at two points in time to detect whether the scale is sensitive to change. Hopefully, the dimensionality of the items does not change on pre- and post-testing, because if it does, that phenomenon should be understood.

6. TEST CRITERION–ORIENTED VALIDITY. Study of the criterion validity of a scale is required to determine whether the scale is actually valid for its purpose.[29] Reliability is a necessary, but not sufficient, condition for a valid scale. Internal scaling studies may similarly establish that a set of items constitutes an equal-interval measure, but cannot show that this measure is useful or valid for any particular application or inference. External validity can be established only by demonstrating relationships to external criteria.

In order for scales to be useful, they must predict something outside of themselves. The functional independence measure (FIM), for instance, predicts the approximate help in minutes per day that a person with a certain level of disability needs.[18, 19] It is a valid measure of physical assistance or substituted effort from one person to another. Improved FIM ratings indicate decreased support time and it follows that they have a relationship to the cost-effectiveness of the treatment program. Prediction of a criterion in the future is a vastly more convincing test of validity than showing that a scale relates to some other item applied at the same point in time.

The choice of criterion depends on what one intends to measure (the construct) and how it is to be used. A scale that strives to show improvement of cognitive abilities might address problems in instrumental ADL or some element of stress as reported by family members. A scale that is relevant to vocational assessment should predict success in work or school.

Sensitivity to change is usually proof that a scale is applicable to a clinical rehabilitation setting or population. For instance, the FIM has been shown to be quite sensitive to change in inpatient rehabilitation, even with patients who have traumatic brain injuries.[24] On the other hand, the Galveston Orientation and Amnesia Test (GOAT) was not found to be sensitive to change, as the majority of patients were no longer in severe post-traumatic amnesia on admission to rehabilitation.[40]

The need for sensitivity to change is not absolute. An overly sensitive measure focusing on a small element of function (e.g., leg acceleration in degrees per second per second) may be unstable from day to day or from task to task and may poorly reflect the social value of the intervention. Similarly, manual muscle tests may show change but their objectivity and connection to social value have been questioned.[26]

7. COMPLETE AND SUMMARIZE STUDIES. Data on the internal and external validity of the scale should be written for publication and peer review. Conclusions can be drawn regarding the internal validity and generalizability (external validity) of the instrument. The results of the formal testing may suggest further changes or improvements.

8. FORMALIZE THE INSTRUMENT AND WRITE A MANUAL. The publication of manuals is one of the key steps needed to improve functional assessment in rehabilitation and medical care. A chief purpose of the manual is to serve as a self-guided training resource. Users may still need guidance in interpretation of the items on a scale or the results obtained by administration of the scale. A manual should summarize key evidence of the characteristics, reliability, and validity of a scale. It should also state key limitations. Policies regarding distribution, support services, and costs need to be established.

9. CONTINUE DEVELOPMENT. Scale development is an ongoing process. Over time, as a successful scale is used repeatedly in practice and in research, one learns more about its strengths and limitations. Construct validation, in particular, involves testing whether a scale, shown to be valid in basic developmental studies as discussed above, behaves as expected according to the initial conceptualization. It involves study of the interactions of theoretically important constructs. One learns, for example, how disease processes affect function, and how therapeutic interventions affect the course of recovery. This is the whole dynamic enterprise of development of rehabilitation as a science.

CHARACTERISTICS OF EXISTING FUNCTIONAL ASSESSMENT INSTRUMENTS

Functional assessment methods have been influenced by changes in the concept of rehabilitation and technological developments. With the expanded scope of rehabilitation, there has been an increase in the number of domains routinely assessed as part of the rehabilitation process. It is currently common practice in rehabilitation services to utilize a large number of assessment instruments to document impairments, the ability to complete basic and more complex daily living skills, and perceptions of quality of daily living. The combination of these instruments provides the evaluation of the critical components that make up independent or interdependent active life. Although the assessment instruments can either be generic to rehabilitation patients or disease-specific, most documentation of functional abilities is determined using generic tools.

Comprehensive functional assessment is an essential clinical management component. It goes beyond disease categories and physical impairments to address the resultant disability which rehabilitation efforts target. The rationale or goal of treatment intervention guides the choice of instruments employed. Information from assessment instruments can be utilized for descriptive, evaluative, or predictive purposes. The use of functional assessment for descriptive purposes is a common screening method in rehabilitation and chronic illness, documenting the type and severity of disabilities at a given point in time. Assessment instruments are also used to set therapeutic goals and to monitor the clinical course of the disease, while measuring clinical changes over time. The predictive use of assessment instruments provides objective criteria to plan the treatment and evaluate the goals that have been set. Regardless of the instrument chosen, they should be practical, simple to administer, and yield meaningful results that can direct the rehabilitation process. The guiding principles in choosing a functional assessment scale are: that the scale be a valid measure of the function being tested, that previous studies document validity and adequate reliability, and that the measurement be sensitive enough to document clinically important change.[33]

The ability to distinguish between the concepts of functional capacity and functional performance is an important consideration for test administration. Methodological differences in obtaining the assessment measures and the type of populations being assessed are two sources of discrepancies. Often measures do not clearly differentiate between the presence of a functional impairment that makes an activity impossible to carry out and the actual performance of an activity. As a simple example, a low score in locomotion could mean either that the subject had severe paralysis of limbs or else lacked the will or ability to use limbs that were otherwise intact. Performance ADL was shown to have an integral cognitive component in the Framingham study of noninstitutionalized persons who have had strokes, and in patients after traumatic brain injury.[34, 37] This factor is a major consideration in rehabilitation. In addition, Nagi[47] has documented that disability, unlike functional limitation, has a major social component. Since disability reflects performance within a sociocultural context, one could expect that daily performance would be strongly influenced by social as well as physical factors. The goals and rationale for choosing a specific functional assessment instrument need to take these considerations into account. One needs to be aware that performance-based functional assessment takes the social and physical contexts into account.

The functional assessment scale employed should be able to measure disability, monitor progress, enhance communications, measure the effectiveness of treatment, and document the benefits of rehabilitation interventions. Since assessment instruments are used repeatedly during the course of rehabilitation, the results should be reliable and valid measures for the disabilities being treated.

EXISTING ADULT FUNCTIONAL ASSESSMENT SCALES

Activities of Daily Living (ADL) Scales

Activities of daily living refer to those basic skills that a person must possess in order to care for oneself independently. Instruments that assess ADL usually assess abilities in self-care (eating, bathing, grooming, dressing, etc.), transfers, continence, and, in most cases, locomotion. ADL scales are usually hierarchical in arrangement. They include easier activities such as eating, and more difficult tasks such as climbing stairs. The Functional Independence Measure and the Patient Evaluation and Conference System (PECS) are examples of recently developed scales that include the domains of functional communication and social cognition. Information is collected by observing actual performance rather than capacity as demonstrated in an artificial setting such as during therapy. There are a number of valid and reliable scales that document ADL. Most are administered by trained clinicians, although there are some that are based on subjective judgment. The utility of these instruments is that they provide a minimum number of items set for describing physical functioning and can be used to track a clinical course of treatment.

Table 12–2 displays a description of selected ADL scales that are currently in use in rehabilitation and that meet adequate validity and reliability standards.

Instrumental Activities of Daily Living (IADL) Scales

The ability to accomplish activities related to maintaining one's living environment is tested using IADL scales. These tasks can include using a telephone, shopping, preparing meals, and managing money. Developing and restoring these skills are often part of a rehabilitation program but are difficult to evaluate until the individual returns home. IADL scales may be rated by either an interviewer or by the individual, depending on the disability and circumstances. These scales may not be sensitive to change as not all activities are pertinent to everyone. Also, they do not take safety into account as a feature of performance.

Table 12–3 describes three IADL scales utilized in rehabilitation services.

Quality of Life Scales

Quality of life scales denote a wide range of capabilities, symptoms, and psychosocial characteristics that describe functional ability and satisfaction with life. Components of quality of life include social roles and interactions, functional performance, intellectual functioning, perceptions, and subjective health. Indicators can include standards of living and general satisfaction with life. Although there is controversy over the measurement of quality of life, it is a powerful indicator of successful rehabilitation. The relevance of these types of scales to populations with permanent disability has not yet been established. Rather than being criterion-referenced, these scales generally ask the subject to compare himself or herself with a prior healthy state.

Although several measures have been developed, only a few have been well validated. Two that meet these criteria are described in Table 12–3 (descriptions are found in Table 12–4).

PROGRAM EVALUATION AND CONTINUOUS QUALITY IMPROVEMENT

Definition

The Commission on Accreditation of Rehabilitation Facilities (CARF) defines *program evaluation* as a systematic procedure for measuring the outcomes of care.[8] The directives for achieving quality healthcare through program evaluation from CARF, the Joint Commission on Accreditation of Healthcare Organizations (JCAHO), state health departments, and other agencies have been a major stimulus for documentation of outcomes in medical rehabilitation.

Quality assessment and quality improvement are "ongoing activities designed to objectively and systematically evaluate the quality of patient care and services, pursue opportunities to improve patient care and services and resolve identified problems."[32] In 1992, Gonnella[16] described program evaluation as a branch of quality assessment and improvement. Other branches include utilization review, risk management, infection control, and documentation.

Program evaluation is one way to measure the effectiveness and efficiency of rehabilitation services. Structure, process, outcome, or a combination of these factors can be addressed in the evaluation. Structural evaluation data include information about certification of professional healthcare providers. Process evaluation data include information about the provision of treatment in terms of number and type. Outcome evaluation data include information about the level of functional independence achieved or the level of patient satisfaction. Good patient outcomes are the culmination of the combined effects of structure and process. For practical purposes, then, program evaluation in medical rehabilitation has come to mean a comparison of the measurement of the functional performance of patients, as well as related variables, at the beginning of rehabilitation and after care has been completed.

Elements of Program Evaluation

The elements of program evaluation include a description of the purpose of the program (mission statement), program structure, program goals, program objectives, methods of applying measures, and utilization of outcome data in various reports and communications.[8]

The program mission statement is a broad summary of the rehabilitation program, the patients served, and the treatments provided. The program structure describes the

TABLE 12–2   Selected Measures of Activities of Daily Living (ADL)

Scale	Description and Type of Scale	Reliability, Validity, and Sensitivity	Time and Administration	Comments
Barthel Index (BI)[43]	Ordinal scale with total scores ranging from 0 (totally dependent)–100 (independent); 10 weighted items: feeding, bathing, grooming, dressing, bladder control, bowel control, toileting, chair/bed transfer, mobility, and stair climbing	Well-documented reliability and validity; not sensitive to minor changes at higher levels of ADL functioning	Clinician observation: < 40 min; appropriate for screening, formal assessment, monitoring, maintenance	Widely accepted scale for disability; strong reliability and validity
Index of Independence in ADL[35]	Dichotomous rating in hierarchical order of dependency: bathing, dressing, toileting, transfer, continence, and feeding; cases ranked from A (independent in all 6 items) to G (dependent in all 6 items)	Documented reliability and validity; limited range of activities assessed; not as sensitive to change as BI or other instruments	Clinician observation: < 20 min; appropriate for screening, formal assessment, monitoring, maintenance	Widely accepted scale, especially in geriatrics; assesses some basic skills but not walking and climbing stairs
Kenny Self-Care Evaluation[54]	Ordinal scale with 17 specific activities under 6 major categories: bed activities, transfers, locomotion, personal hygiene, dressing, and feeding; measured on 5-point scale, 0 = dependence–4 = independence; range of total scores: 0–24	Documented reliability and validity; reasonable sensitivity	Clinician observation or judgment: > 30 min; appropriate for formal assessment, monitoring, maintenance	Range of inclusive categories, geared to rehabilitation assessment; ratings can be subjective
Functional Independence Measure (FIM)[22]	Ordinal scale with 18 items, 7-level scale with scores running from 18–126; areas of evaluation include self-care, sphincter control, transfers, locomotion, communication, and social cognition	Well-documented reliability and validity; able to detect minor changes with 7 levels; physical and cognitive components able to detect increments of change; can be converted into two Rasch-derived measures	Clinician observation: < 20 min; appropriate for screening, formal assessment, monitoring, maintenance, and program evaluation	Widely accepted in medical rehabilitation, including international; proven measure of ADL and social cognition; standardized interobserver reliability by credentialing of clinicians; extensive training materials
Level of Rehabilitation Scale (LORS) and LORS American Data System (LADS) (LORS/LADS)[5]	Five interval subscales assessing ADL, mobility, communications, cognitive ability and memory, measured on 5-point scale from 0 = unable to perform activity–4 = able to perform	Documented reliability and validity; specific to physical and cognitive measures in medical rehabilitation setting	Clinical observation: 10 min per subscale, > 60 min total; appropriate for screening, monitoring, maintenance, and program evaluation	Measures broad functional outcome categories; provides separate scores for subscales; does not measure bladder or bowel incontinence
Patient Evaluation and Conference System (PECS)[51]	Ordinal scale with 115 items in a 6-step scale ranging from total dependence to total independence; major headings include medicine, nursing, physical mobility, ADL, communication, medications, device utilization, pay, neuropsychology, social issues, therapeutic recreation, procedures, nutrition, pain, pulmonary	Documented reliability and validity; broad range of categories relating to medical rehabilitation services	Discipline-specific evaluations: < 60 min for most disciplines; appropriate for formal assessment, monitoring, maintenance, and program evaluation	Extensive number of items evaluated; focuses on long-term needs and program evaluation; an ADL subscale has been Rasch-analyzed

organizational framework. This includes the type of facility, admission criteria, patients served, and services provided.[8] The program goals are derived from the mission statement and are written for each rehabilitation program (e.g., the stroke program). The goal statements are expressed in achievable terms.

Program objectives follow the program goals and are stated in terms that are measurable according to expected results. Achievement of objectives should relate to effectiveness and efficiency of the program and to satisfaction of the individuals served. Effectiveness objectives address the extent to which outcomes are attained. Efficiency objectives indicate the quantity of resources used to attain program goals.

TABLE 12–3   Selected Measures of Instrumental Activities of Daily Living (IADL)

Scale	Description and Type of Scale	Reliability, Validity, and Sensitivity	Time and Administration	Comments
Functional Health Status[53]	Guttman scale containing 25 questions indicating ascending dependency; questions include out-of-home activities such as going to the movies, walking half a mile, and doing heavy work	Documented reliability and validity	Interviewer: < 30 min; appropriate for maintenance in community setting	Simple scale design with general functioning questions; limited utility with disabled population; difficult to validate in an institutional setting
Older Americans Resources and Services Multidimensional Functional Assessment Questionnaire (OARS MFAQ)[10]	Multidimensional assessment tool containing 105 questions in 5 domains: social resources, economic resources, mental health, physical health, and ADL	Documented reliability and validity	Interviewer: > 10 min; appropriate for maintenance in the community	Measures broad base of information necessary for independent living; complex domains assessed
Philadelphia Geriatric Center Instrumental Activities of Daily Living[41]	Guttman scale includes questions on use of telephone, walking, shopping, food preparation, housekeeping, laundry, public transportation, and medicine	Documented reliability and validity	Time: < 30 min	Strength: measures broad base of information necessary for independent living

For example, program objectives of a stroke program might be to (1) optimize self-care skills, (2) optimize sphincter management, (3) optimize transfer skills, (4) optimize locomotion skills, (5) optimize communication skills, (6) optimize social cognition skills, (7) return patients to the community, (8) optimize vocational independence, (9) ensure appropriate length of stay, and (10) optimize the average cost per unit of improvement (gain in function).

Functional assessment scales are used to determine whether these objectives have been achieved. They may reflect improvement from admission to discharge or else represent criterion levels to be matched or exceeded. Typically, this information is derived from using a functional assessment instrument that compares admission and discharge levels of independence. On the other hand, criterion measures indicate improvement to a predetermined level. An example of criterion measures might be a facility's objective to achieve a certain percentage of community discharges. From past performance, a facility might choose a level of 72% as minimally acceptable, with a goal of 80%, and an optimal level of 88%. A facility with less severely affected or younger patients might choose a percentage that is closer to 100% as optimal. Some facilities choose a criterion based on a regional or national average. To handle more than one objective, CARF recommends using relative weighting (either by assigning weights or ranking the objectives in order of importance).[8]

Additional data to be collected and analyzed for the program evaluation reports include demographic data and descriptors of the problems or barriers to individual success. Typically, demographic data include (1) average age and age distribution, (2) gender distribution, (3) average time from onset of impairment to admission to rehabilitation, (4) frequency of program interruptions, (5) vocational status prior to impairment, and (6) payment sources.

Having collected and aggregated the outcome data, feed-

TABLE 12–4   Selected Measures of Quality of Life

Scale	Description and Type of Scale	Reliability, Validity, and Sensitivity	Time and Administration	Comments
MOS 36-Item Short Form Survey (SF-36)[58]	Assesses 8 health domains including physical and social activities, mental health, general health perceptions, vitality, and discomfort	Documented reliability and validity	Interviewer in person or phone: < 30 min; appropriate for maintenance in community setting	Items well-standardized; widely used in community; utility for following persons with disability not known
Sickness Impact Profile (SIP)[6]	Subscales evaluate the following areas: ambulation, self-care, emotions, communications, alertness, habits, home and recreation, vocation, and social interactions	Adequate reliability and validity	Interviewer in person or phone: < 30 min; appropriate for maintenance in community setting	Comprehensive evaluation; behavioral rather than subjective health items; focus on community life; utility for following persons with disability not known

back reports must be compiled to summarize the findings. The data are then used for management reports, quality improvement and research, and communications to the community and third-party payers.

Rationale and Usefulness

Forer,[13] in 1992, succinctly described the benefits of program evaluation:

1. Ensure that a program is functioning within predetermined standards.
2. Provide guidance for alignment of program goals and objectives with patient needs.
3. Facilitate collecting outcome data systematically for research purposes.
4. Make information available for evaluation of cost-effectiveness.
5. Plan for the future with the help of informed decision making.
6. Support marketing efforts with objective data.
7. Promote understanding and acceptance of the rehabilitation program by the community.

Program evaluation reports form the basis for monitoring the rehabilitation program. For example, they can be used to identify patients whose outcomes did not meet previously established goals and expectations. Identification of these patients can lead the quality improvement committee to suggest revision of existing programs, treatments, or interventions. By following certain indicators over time, administrators and clinicians may monitor the impact of those revisions and make further adjustments. It is important to establish a baseline of values with which results may be compared before and after a change of program is implemented.

Using outcome data to understand and improve the results of patient care is the most significant reason for doing program evaluation. Outcome data can identify those patients who fail to attain maximal benefits from the program as well as those patients who exceed expectations. Patients who may have had adjustment problems, medical complications, or who have deteriorated in functional status may be identified and the program improved to serve them better.[13]

Outcome data from several facilities can be pooled to support research studies. For example, Granger et al.[20] and Johnston et al.[30] studied characteristics that predict outcomes for stroke patients in rehabilitation. The existence of a large and current data pool, such as the Uniform Data System for Medical Rehabilitation, allows investigators to study the interactions of many different factors in order to identify characteristics of patients with selected outcomes such as functional status, placement at discharge, and estimated length of stay.[55]

Outcome data can also be used to address a facility's operational issues such as the effectiveness and efficiency with which care is provided in relation to outcomes. The average cost per patient, the average length of stay, and the average cost per unit of improvement are important parameters for managing a facility. In these days of rapid changes in the manner of providing and paying for healthcare, planning for future program needs is another critical use of outcome data. Data should be used to monitor for changes in the following[13]:

1. Distribution of patient characteristics such as age and gender
2. Diagnostic mix
3. Case severity
4. Number of patients treated
5. Length of stay
6. Charges or costs per patient
7. Frequency of program interruptions
8. Discharge patterns
9. Intensity, modalities, and types of clinicians involved in treatment

UNIFORM DATA SYSTEM FOR MEDICAL REHABILITATION

In 1983, a national task force was established to develop a uniform data system for medical rehabilitation that would document the outcomes and costs of medical rehabilitation. The task force recognized the need for the creation of a tool that could be used uniformly to measure the functional status of the person with long-term needs.[22] The work of the task force, supported by a grant from the National Institute of Handicapped Research (NIHR), resulted in the development of the Functional Independence Measure (FIM) (see Table 12–2) and the creation of the Uniform Data System for Medical Rehabilitation (UDSMR). This data set is now used on a regular basis in approximately 55% of the medical rehabilitation facilities across the United States.

The UDSMR includes admission, discharge, and follow-up FIM ratings (Fig. 12–2), as well as demographic, diagnostic, financial, and length-of-stay variables. Since its inception in 1987, complete data have been collected on almost 600,000 medical rehabilitation patients with a variety of diagnoses. The collection and analysis of comparable data from clinical sites across the country represented the next step in the development of an appropriate functional assessment scale for patients with disability. The opportunity to accumulate the data across sites and over time within a single data base allows for a wide variety of comparisons to be made, including within-site, across-site, regional, national, and even international comparisons. These same data sets also may be compared over time to examine for trends. Further uses of data bases with comparable data include development of predictive models to test for improvements that may be occurring in healthcare and rehabilitative practices.

What are the advantages of a data base, what can it be used for, and how can it be applied to rehabilitation of patients over the long run? Data bases store information for subsequent analyses by both clinicians and research experts. Ongoing data bases allow data to accumulate over time and across sites, which is particularly advantageous for studying patterns of care over time. One key advantage of accumulated data is that sample size is increased by pooling data across sites and over time to make comparisons. Statistical research often depends on the availability of large sample sizes to reach substantive conclusions about healthcare outcomes.

LEVELS	
7 Complete Independence (Timely, Safely) 6 Modified Independence (Device)	NO HELPER

Modified Dependence
  5 Supervision
  4 Minimal Assist (Subject = 75% +)
  3 Moderate Assist (Subject = 50% +)
 	
Complete Dependence
  2 Maximal Assist (Subject = 25% +)
  1 Total Assist (Subject = 0% +)
	HELPER

	ADMIT	DISCHG	FOL-UP
Self-Care A. Eating B. Grooming C. Bathing D. Dressing - Upper Body E. Dressing - Lower Body F. Toileting			
Sphincter Control G. Bladder Management H. Bowel Management			
Transfers I. Bed, Chair, Wheelchair J. Toilet K. Tub, Shower			
Locomotion L. Walk/Wheelchair M. Stairs	Walk Wheelchair Both	Walk Wheelchair Both	Walk Wheelchair Both
Motor Subtotal Score			
Communication N. Comprehension O. Expression	Auditory Visual Both Vocal Non-vocal Both	Auditory Visual Both Vocal Non-vocal Both	Auditory Visual Both Vocal Non-vocal Both
Social Cognition P. Social Interaction Q. Problem Solving R. Memory			
Cognitive Subtotal Score			
Total FIM			

NOTE: Leave no blanks; enter 1 if patient not testable due to risk

FIGURE 12–2 Functional independence measure (adult FIM). (From Uniform Data System for Medical Rehabilitation: Guide for the Uniform Data Set for Medical Rehabilitation (Adult FIM), version 4.0. Buffalo, NY, State University of New York, 1993.)

Another key advantage resulting from the use of ongoing data bases such as the UDSMR is that clinical sites can contribute to the pool of data accumulated nationally, while at the same time keeping their own data in a readily accessible form for in-house data analysis and research efforts. This allows for improvements at both the local and national level, and allows for comparisons of the trends at each clinical site with regional and national trends. These comparisons can be immediately made over the last quarter or can be examined in trend form over a number of years. Obviously, the sooner a data base is initiated, the longer the time periods available for comparisons.

The UDSMR data base provides quarterly summary data on such variables as FIM items; subscale, domain, and total scores; demographics; charges; length of stay; and program evaluation models for each subscribing clinical site. The data are contained in reports that allow for direct comparisons of the clinical site with regional and national data. Since the data set is uniform across clinical sites, these comparisons provide critical evaluation and planning data for any one site at any single point in time and across time from admission to discharge to follow-up.

The data base can also be used as a tracking device by examining trends across reporting periods. Comparisons within sites allow clinicians and administrators to determine patterns of care within their facilities, while tracking across reports of regional and national data allows the same staff to be aware of changes in either regional or national medical rehabilitation policies and procedures. Of course, owing to the unique reporting by type of impairment across all diagnoses, the facilities can use the data to focus, with considerable detail, on their individual patient groups, and make comparisons within impairment types with regional and national trends. The unique uniformity of data allows direct comparisons with confidence in the FIM item, subscale, domain, and total scores across the population of UDSMR data.

Perhaps most important, large ongoing data bases such as the UDSMR can provide national data of sufficient sample size that key indicators at admission can be incorporated into statistical models to predict more precisely the course of medical rehabilitation and the outcomes at discharge and follow-up. This predictive power of the FIM has been developed into models of Function Related Groups (FIM-FRG) through the work of Stineman and colleagues.[55] The appearance of FIM-FRGs signals the next step in putting the national data base to work for improving rehabilitative care. Not only does the data base provide site-specific, regional, and national data, and data trends across reporting periods, comparisons within sites allow clinicians and administrators to determine patterns of care and trends over time. The data base currently provides the data for prediction models with enough data left over for cross-validation studies of these predictive models to verify their accuracy and report their confidence.

In 1987, the FIM was adapted for use in pediatrics by a multidisciplinary team of physicians, nurses, and therapists.[23] The resulting scale, known as the Functional Independence Measure for Children (WeeFIM), is a measure of functional abilities and the need for assistance that is associated with levels of disability in children 6 months to 7 years of age. It can also be used with children well beyond the age of 7 when delays in functional performance are evident.

The WeeFIM utilizes the same items and rating scale as the FIM. The 18 items are organized into six subscales of self-care, sphincter control, transfers, locomotion, communication, and social cognition. Each item is scored on a seven-level ordinal scale ranging from complete independence to total assistance.

Pilot studies involving 111 children without documented disabilities were conducted in 1987–1988 in a hospital-based ambulatory care clinic, two daycare centers, and a nursery school. The results revealed a strong association between WeeFIM scores and age. Items on the WeeFIM appeared to progress in a developmental sequence. Less complex tasks, such as ambulation and eating, were performed independently at younger ages, while more complex tasks, such as dressing and problem-solving, were completed at older ages.

In 1991, the first phase of a normalization study was completed when 417 nondisabled children were assessed by 10 pediatric nurses trained in the use of the WeeFIM. The data were obtained by interviewing parents and primary caregivers at 11 pediatric primary care sites in Buffalo and its suburbs. Rasch analysis of the data led to the development of WeeFIM norms for the Motor and Cognitive Subscales, the Total WeeFIM, and for each of the individual items. The subscale and Total WeeFIM norms are included in the WeeFIM manual as look-up tables. Individual age-related norms are automatically calculated in the UDSMR software program entitled FIMware.

In 1991, McCabe[44] concluded that the relationship between growth in functional independence and age in months, in nondisabled children, is logarithmic. She also determined that test-retest and inter-rater reliabilities were satisfactory, and that functional independence growth curves distinguish between nondisabled and disabled children.

Although comparative follow-up assessments are available through UDSMR, increasing attention needs to be given to the follow-up of patients to study the impact of medical rehabilitation after discharge. Examination of both the short- and long-term impacts of medical rehabilitation on its patients becomes even more valuable when considering linkages of data bases. When connections can be made between the UDSMR and other national data sets, as has been done with the ongoing study that is enhancing evaluation of the trauma system by incorporating the rehabilitation component,[21] then increasingly more detailed studies become available. The development of UDSMR data bases for skilled nursing facilities, outpatients, and children[23] allows for a broad perspective on patients from birth through old age. The advantages of uniformity and matching measuring tools (FIM and WeeFIM) allow for a unique opportunity to develop secondary prevention models by linking WeeFIM data bases to adult data bases to study lifetime outcomes.

The measurement of functional changes over time has received considerable attention in the statistical literature[7, 52] owing to the complicated nature of repeated measures statistics. The application of good measurement principles to the FIM and WeeFIM has resulted in tools that investigators can have confidence in using over time with little measurement error. The UDSMR can be used with considerable statistical power and measurement confidence to provide unique insights into long-term care of patients in medical rehabilitation. The advantages of uniformity and large numbers of patients allow for a broad range of clinical research to be applicable across the life span, from childhood to old age. This unique uniformity of measurement across time will provide an important key to understanding and meeting the needs of a diverse population with disabilities.

SUMMARY

Reviewing and assuring quality of healthcare delivery are daunting issues for all providers of healthcare. Almost two decades ago, medical rehabilitation adopted a model of program evaluation that is facility-based with certain common elements. Since an important purpose of medical rehabilitation is to improve the functional status of patients, reliable and valid methods of functional assessment are necessary.

Functional assessment is a method for describing a person's abilities and limitations. The essence of functional assessment is the measurement of a person's use of the variety of skills included in performing tasks necessary to daily living, leisure activities, vocational pursuits, social interactions, and other required behaviors. The data are used to help formulate judgments as to how well these essential skills are being used, and to gauge the degree to which tasks are accomplished and social role expectations are being met. Performance-based functional assessments take the social and physical contexts of the person into account.

It is possible to compare changes in status over periods of time for an individual or a group of individuals by assessing function at appropriate intervals. In this manner, outcomes of professional interventions of healthcare, rehabilitation, education, or psychological and social counseling may be described and monitored. Once outcomes become measurable they become manageable. However, care must be exercised in applying standards derived from group studies to the management of an individual. Factors that are unique to a particular case must be taken into account.

There have been many attempts to improve the quality of measurement in rehabilitation over the last 30 years. Validity is the paramount criterion for choice and use of a measure. Reliability is usually defined as freedom from random error and is necessary but not sufficient. The acid test of the utility of a functional assessment tool is that it predicts something into the future that is outside of itself.

Development of a sound functional assessment instrument involves having a good idea that is conceptually clear and feasible, operationalizing the idea in the form of a stable instrument with logical procedures, tedious testing, and, finally, dissemination, with opportunities to follow the consequences of use of the instrument.

The design of an effective program evaluation system involves many ingredients. Program evaluation data must be presented in a clear, concise, and timely manner. The information must be relevant and understandable to those reviewing the information. Some form of the information should be shared with managers, clinical staff, and others. Presentation may take a variety of formats including statistics, graphs, matrices, and narrative descriptions. This information should be used by providers to solve problems and improve the quality of care delivered to patients. The results of program evaluation could prove useful for evaluating alternative treatment modalities within a rehabilitation facility but will become crucial for evaluating outcomes among different types of rehabilitation settings.

In 1985, Granger[17] predicted that by the year 2000

. . . all healthcare workers will be using standardized terminology to describe the problems consequent to chronic disease and we will be employing systematic computerized methods for tracking individuals' functional abilities and their unmet needs over time. Medical rehabilitation programs will be mandated into the healthcare plans of individuals disabled by accident or disease. However, authorization for payment by third parties will entail requirements for (a) an organized system of care with a comprehensive plan of management, (b) a functional prognosis in terms of probabilities for therapeutic gains in terms of quality of life, (c) efficient delivery of services, and (d) documentation of outcomes through periodic assessments of functional status in order to determine the most favorable benefit/cost ratios.[17]

As standardized functional assessment measures are developed that closely approximate the clinical situation, they will be used to predict the outcomes of care and they will be a part of the cost/benefit analysis that will be integral to decision making in the health and rehabilitative care systems. Functional assessment will allow comparison of the effectiveness and efficiency of alternative therapeutic interventions and settings. Finally, predictable relationships will emerge between the "dose" of rehabilitative services and the "response" of the patient.

References

1. Allen MJ, Yen WM: Introduction to Measurement Theory. Monterey, Calif., Brooks/Cole, 1979.
2. American Educational Research Association, American Psychological Association, National Council on Measurement in Education: Standards for Educational and Psychological Testing. Washington, DC, American Psychological Association, 1985.
3. American Medical Association: Guide to the Evaluation of Permanent Impairment, ed 3, revised. Milwaukee, American Medical Association, 1990.
4. Audet AM, Scott HD: The Uniform Clinical Data Set: an evaluation of the proposed national database for Medicare's quality review program. Ann Intern Med 1993; 119:1209–1213.
5. Carey RG, Posavac EJ: Program evaluation of a physical medicine and rehabilitation unit: a new approach. Arch Phys Med Rehabil 1978; 59:330–337.
6. Carter WB, Bobbitt RA, Bergner M, Gilson BS: Validation of an interval scaling: The Sickness Impact Profile. Health Serv Res 1976; 11:515–528.
7. Collins LM, Horn JL (eds): Best Methods for the Analysis of Change. Washington, DC, American Psychological Association, 1991.
8. Commission on Accreditation of Rehabilitation Facilities (CARF): Program Evaluation: A Guide to Utilization. Tuscon, CARF, 1982.
9. Donaldson SW, Wagner CC, Gresham GE: A unified ADL form. Arch Phys Med Rehabil 1973; 54:175–179.
10. Duke University Center for the Study of Aging and Human Development: Multidimensional Functional Assessment: The OARS Methodology. Durham, Duke, 1978.
11. Dunn G: Design and Analysis of Reliability Studies. New York, Oxford University Press, 1989.
12. Feinstein AR: Clinimetrics. New Haven, Yale University Press, 1987.

13. Forer S: How to make program evaluation work for you. NeuroRehabil. 1992; 2:52–71.

14. Frey WD: Functional assessment in the '80s: a conceptual enigma, a technical challenge. *In* Halpern AS, Fuhrer MJ (eds): Functional Assessment in Rehabilitation. Baltimore, Paul H. Brookes, 1984, pp 11–43.

15. Gable RK: Instrument Development in the Affective Domain. Boston, Kluwer-Nijhoff, 1986.

16. Gonnella C: Program evaluation. *In* Fletcher GF, Banja JD, Jann BB, Wolf SL (eds): Rehabilitation Medicine: Contemporary Clinical Perspectives. Philadelphia, Lea & Febiger, 1992, pp 243–268.

17. Granger CV: Medical rehabilitation: Predicting needs and measuring outcomes for quality of life. *In* Gaitz CM, Niederehe G, Wilson NL (eds): Aging 2000: Our Health Care Destiny. Vol 2: Psychosocial and Policy Issues. New York, Springer-Verlag, 1985, p 255.

18. Granger CV, Cotter AC, Hamilton BB, Fiedler RC: Functional assessment scales: a study of persons after stroke. Arch Phys Med Rehabil 1993; 74:133–138.

19. Granger CV, Cotter AC, Hamilton BB, et al: Functional assessment scales: a study of persons with multiple sclerosis. Arch Phys Med Rehabil 1990; 71:870–875.

20. Granger CV, Hamilton BB, Fiedler RC: Discharge outcome after stroke rehabilitation. Stroke 1992; 23:978–982.

21. Grant #R49-CCR 304550-03, Centers for Disease Control and Prevention. Enhancing Trauma System Evaluation: Incorporating the Rehabilitation Component (Wayne Copes, PI, ongoing).

22. Guide for the Uniform Data Set for Medical Rehabilitation (Adult FIM), Version 4.0. Buffalo, State University of New York at Buffalo, 1993.

23. Guide for the Uniform Data Set for Medical Rehabilitation for Children (WeeFIM). Version 4.0—Inpatient/Outpatient. Buffalo, State University of New York at Buffalo, 1993.

24. Hall KM, Hamilton BB, Gordon WA, Zasler ND: Characteristics and comparisons of functional assessment indices: Disability Rating Scale, Functional Independence Measure, and Functional Assessment Measure. J Head Trauma Rehabil 1993; 8:60–74.

25. Heinemann AW, Linacre JM, Wright BD, et al: Relationships between impairment and physical disability as measured by the Functional Independence Measure. Arch Phys Med Rehabil 1993; 74:566–573.

26. Hinderer SR, Hinderer KA: Objective measurement in rehabilitation: Theory and application. *In* DeLisa J, Gans BM, Currie DM (eds): Rehabilitation Medicine: Principles and Practices, ed 2. Philadelphia, JB Lippincott, 1993.

27. Johnston MV, Findley TW, deLuca J, Katz R: Research in physical medicine and rehabilitation. XII. Measurement tools with application to brain injury. Am J Phys Med Rehabil 1991; 70:40–56.

28. Johnston MV, Keith RA: Measurement standards for medical rehabilitation and clinical applications. Phys Med Rehabil Clin North Am 1993; 4:425–449.

29. Johnston MV, Keith RA, Hinderer S: Measurement standards for interdisciplinary medical rehabilitation. Arch Phys Med Rehabil 1992; 73(suppl):S3–S23.

30. Johnston MV, Kirshblum S, Zorowitz R, Shiflett SC: Prediction of outcomes following rehabilitation of stroke patients. NeuroRehabil 1992; 2:72–97.

31. Johnston MV, Wilkerson DL, Maney M: Evaluation of the quality and outcomes of medical rehabilitation programs. In DeLisa J, Gans BM, Currie DM (eds): Rehabilitation Medicine: Principles and Practices. Philadelphia, JB Lippincott, 1993.

32. Joint Commission on Accreditation of Healthcare Organizations (JCAHO): 1993 Accreditation Manual for Hospitals. Oakbrook Terrace, Ill, JCAHO, 1992.

33. Kane RA, Kane RL: Assessing the Elderly: A Practical Guide to Measurement. Lexington, Mass, Lexington Books, 1981.

34. Kaplan CP, Corrigan JD: The relationship between cognition and functional independence in adults with traumatic brain injury. Arch Phys Med Rehabil 1994; 75:643–647.

35. Katz S, Lord AB, Moskowitz RW, et al: Studies of illness in the aged: the index of ADL: A standardized measure of biological and psychological function. JAMA 1963; 185:914–919.

36. Keith RA: Functional assessment measures in medical rehabilitation: current status. Arch Phys Med Rehabil 1984; 65:74–78.

37. Kelly-Hayes M, Jette A, Wolf PA, et al: Functional limitations and disability among elders in the Framingham Study. Am J Public Health 1992; 82:841–845.

38. Kelman HR, Willner A: Problems in measurement and evaluation of rehabilitation. Arch Phys Med Rehabil 1962; 63:172–181.

39. Kraemer HC: Evaluating Medical Tests: Qualitative and Objective Guidelines. Newbury Park, Calif, Sage, 1992.

40. Kreutzer JS, Gordon WA, Rosenthal M, Marwitz J: Neuropsychological characteristics of patients with brain injury: preliminary findings from a multicenter investigation. J Head Trauma Rehabil 1993; 8:47–59.

41. Lawton MP: Assessing the competence of older people. *In* Kent E, Kastenbaum R, Sherwood S (eds): Research Planning and Action for the Elderly. New York, Behavioral Publications, 1972.

42. Linacre JM, Heinemann AW, Wright BD, et al: The structure and stability of the Functional Independence Measure. Arch Phys Med Rehabil 1994; 75:127–132.

43. Mahoney FI, Barthel D: Functional evaluation: The Barthel Index. Md Med J 1965; 14:61–65.

44. McCabe MA: Evaluating the validity and reliability of the Pediatric Functional Independence Measure, dissertation, Rush University, Chicago, 1991, UMI order no. PUZ9125959.

45. McDowell I, Newell C: Measuring Health: A Guide to Rating Scales and Questionnaires. New York, Oxford University Press, 1987.

46. Merbitz C, Morris J, Grip JC: Ordinal scales and foundations of misinference. Arch Phys Med Rehabil 1989; 70:308–312.

47. Nagi S: Disability concepts revisited. *In* Sussman MB (ed): Sociology and Rehabilitation. Washington, DC, American Sociological Association, 1965, pp 100–113.

48. National Institutes of Health, National Institute of Child Health and Human Development. Research Plan for the National Center for Medical Rehabilitation Research. US Department of Health and Human Services, Public Health Service (NIH) publication no. 93-3509. Rockville, Md, National Institutes of Health, March 1993.

49. Norusis MJ (ed). SPSS Guide to Data Analysis for SPSS-X. Chicago, SPSS, 1988.

50. Nunnally J: Psychometric Theory. New York, McGraw-Hill, 1978.

51. Patient Evaluation and Conference System (PECS). Available from Marianjoy Rehabilitation Hospital and Clinics, PO Box 795, Wheaton, IL 60189.

52. Rogosa DR, Willett JB: Understanding correlates of change by modelling individual differences in growth. Psychometrica 1985; 50:203–228.

53. Rosow I, Breslau N: A Guttman health scale for the aged. J Gerontol 1966; 21:556–559.

54. Schoening HA, Iversen IA: Numerical scoring of self-care status: a study of the Kenny self-care evaluation. Arch Phys Med Rehabil 1968; 49:221–229.

55. Stineman MG, Escarce JJ, Goin JE, et al: A case mix classification system for medical rehabilitation. Med Care 1994; 32:366–379.

56. Task Force on Standards for Measurement in Physical Therapy: Standards for tests and measurements in physical therapy practice. Phys Ther 1991; 71:589–622.

57. Wanlass RL, Reutter SL, Kline AE: Communication among rehabilitation staff: "mild," "moderate," or "severe" deficits? Arch Phys Med Rehabil 1992; 73:477–481.

58. Ware JE, Sherbourne CD: The MOS 36-item short form survey (SF-36): conceptual framework and item selection. Med Care 1992; 30:473–483.

59. World Health Organization: International Classification of Impairments, Disabilities, and Handicaps. Geneva, World Health Organization, 1980.

60. Wright BD, Masters GN: Rating scale analysis. Chicago, Mesa, 1982.

Research in Physical Medicine and Rehabilitation

RICHARD T. KATZ, M.D.,
DENISE I. CAMPAGNOLO, M.D.,
GARY GOLDBERG, M.D.,
JERRY C. PARKER, PH.D.,
ZACHARY M. PINE, M.D., AND
JOHN WHYTE, M.D., PH.D.

As recently delineated in the supplement on research published by the *American Journal of Physical Medicine and Rehabilitation*,[1] there are several key reasons why physiatrists and others in rehabilitation research must concentrate on research. Recently there has been an unprecedented growth of specialists in physical medicine and rehabilitation and in rehabilitation-related fields. These investigators require a solid research base on which to practice.

For physical medicine and rehabilitation to thrive as a specialty, it must maintain a strong presence in medical schools, where academic physiatrists are carrying out research and education in contact with peers in other specialties. Physiatric research must demonstrate that the treatments we offer are clinically and cost-effective, so they will be eligible for payment in an age of unrelenting fiscal restraint.

There is a long-standing need to increase the number of physiatrists engaged in research. A recent survey of physiatrists showed virtual unanimity for this sentiment.[8] Only 2% of physiatrists were spending more than one fourth of their time in research. The most common impediments were lack of funding and insufficient equipment.

Finally, research is critical for improving the day-to-day practice of medicine. The skills of clinical research are core knowledge for the improvement of clinical care, and should be part of the repertoire of every physician, starting with residency. Leaders in our field have argued strongly that a foundation of basic research skills should be included as part of residency training, and incorporated into "lifelong learning" of every physiatrist.[7]

This chapter serves as a primer to the broad knowledge base listed in Table 13–1. The chapter is divided into five sections: (1) introduction to rudimentary statistics, (2) reading the medical literature, (3) designing a research study, (4) grant writing and funding, and (5) ethical issues.

INTRODUCTION TO RUDIMENTARY STATISTICS

There is a clear rationale why every physiatrist should have a working knowledge of statistics. As technology progresses, medicine is becoming increasingly quantitative.

TABLE 13–1   Basic Research Skills

Defining a research question and formulating testable hypotheses	Ethical issues
	Project management
	Use of descriptive statistics
Critical review of the scientific literature in a selected area	Use of analytic statistics
	Use of statistical consultants
Specifying subjects and sampling techniques	Organizing a pilot study—pretest, quality control
Precision and accuracy of measurements	
Development and use of questionnaires	Technical skills in equipment, procedures, and questionnaires
Using secondary data	Scientific writing
Cohort study design	Oral presentation
Cross-sectional and case-control design	Grant preparation
	Computer use—word processing, data base, statistics
Evaluation of diagnosis tests	
Observational studies and inferences of causality	Library reference search
Experimental sample size	

From Findley TW, DeLisa JA: Research in physical medicine and rehabilitation: XI. Research training: Setting the stage for lifelong learning. Am J Phys Med Rehabil 1991; 70(suppl):S165–S168.

Medical research is reliant on statistical methodology, and statistics pervade the medical literature. The myriad of statistical methods may seem at first to be overwhelming, but studies have shown that the vast majority of studies in leading journals depend on a relatively small number of statistical concepts.[6]

Descriptive statistics refers to the organization, presentation, and summarization of data. One type of descriptive statistics of interest to medicine is vital statistics, such as birth rates, mortality rates, and life expectancy. Another important concept is that of statistical inference, by which an investigator draws conclusions about a certain *target population* (e.g., all persons with spinal cord injury, SCI) by studying a *sample population* of that group (e.g., SCI patients drawn from model SCI centers). Obviously there may be differences between the sample and target populations, which is generally referred to as *bias*. One method of minimizing sample bias is to obtain a *random sample*, where each member of the sample population has an equal and independent chance of being selected.

Data Collection

Data can be collected in several different ways:

1. *A nominal scale* (also called enumeration or attribute data) is where the data fit into a certain category or classification. For example, after a cerebrovascular accident patients may have no weakness, right hemiplegia, left hemiplegia, or bilateral hemiplegia.

2. *An ordinal scale* is one where there is a predetermined order among the response classifications. For example, a patient who undergoes a total joint replacement may be independent, need minimal assist, moderate assist, maximal assist, or be fully dependent for ambulation on the seventh postoperative day. In an ordered classification one need not assume equal distances between categories (see below).

3. *A full ranking scale* orders the members of a group from high to low. For example, if there are 12 attendings in a physiatry group, an administrative analysis is done to see which physicians are seeing the most outpatients. The physicians can be ranked from 1 through 12 according to their average monthly outpatient visits over the last 4 months.

4. *An interval scale* is one in which the distances between any two numbers are of equal size. For example, an increase in pinch strength from 5 to 10 lb is equal to one of 10 to 15 lb. Pinch strength is also an example of a *ratio scale*, because a pinch strength of 20 lb is exactly double the force of 10 lb.

Data may be numerically *discrete* (e.g., the number of irregular heart beats per minute after acute quadriplegia) or *continuous* (e.g., the creatine kinase level in a patient with polymyositis).

The way in which we collect data is very important, but not without pitfalls. Functional assessment scales are commonly 7-point ordinal scales. Ordinal scales suffer from "nonlinearity," that is, the distance from class to class is not known—an improvement from "3" to "4" may not be equivalent to improvement from "4" to "5".[17] This has prompted a great deal of discussion in the rehabili-

tation literature where outcome measurement is extremely important. One solution has been to use a strategy called *Rasch analysis* where ordinal can be transformed into interval data.[24]

When choosing a certain measure in data collection, one should have some idea as to its *validity*.[12] Validity refers to the *appropriateness*, meaningfulness, and usefulness of the specific inferences made from the test score. For example, the validity of IQ (intelligence quotient) scores has frequently been challenged as a predictor of school performance and achievement. *Reliability* refers to the *reproducibility* of those data. Suppose, for example, an electromyographer were to perform a nerve conduction study on a patient and record the results on the visual display. If the examiner manually moves the cursor to the takeoff of the compound muscle action potential on two occasions, how close will the results of the first placement be in comparison with those of the second (*intrarater reliability*)? If two electromyographers move the cursor to the takeoff of the same tracing, how close will the results be between examiners (*interrater reliability*)? If one electromyographer stimulates the patient on two occasions and measures the takeoff, how stable will the results be (*test-retest reliability*)?

Probability

Basic concepts of probability are an important element of statistical knowledge. Probability involves a random process—a repetitive process or operation that in any one trial may result in any one of a number of possible outcomes. These outcomes are determined by chance and are impossible to predict. For example, when a coin is tossed (assuming that it cannot land on its side) it will randomly land on heads or tails. The probability of a certain outcome (e.g., heads) occurring can be determined as a ratio of that outcome divided by all possible outcomes (1/2). This is true only if the two outcomes are mutually exclusive, that is, one outcome precludes the other (if the outcome is heads, the outcome cannot also be tails). If the probability of a spinal cord injury patient surviving 1 year is 0.9, there is a 1 in 10 or 10% chance that person will not survive 1 year.

One of the most important concepts of probability is that of *independent events*. Events are independent if the occurrence of one does not affect the probability of occurrence of the other. For example, it is extremely common for spinal cord–injured patients to also suffer a minor traumatic brain injury (TBI), so the likelihood of these occurring in one person means that they are *not* independent events. However the possibility of suffering SCI and having had septic sore throat as a child are almost certainly unrelated, and can thus be considered independent events. Given two independent events A and B, the probability of *both* occurring is the product of the probability of A times the probability of B (*multiplicative law of probability*). Thus if the probability of developing septic sore throat as a child is 0.4, and that of developing spinal cord injury is 0.01, the probability of one person being inflicted with both conditions in a lifetime would be the product $(0.4)(0.01) = 0.004$.

One has to be careful using the multiplicative law of probability. Examine two examples:

If the possibility of surviving a cataract removal is 0.9 (or 90%), and the chance of surviving a tonsillectomy is 0.7 (or 70%), then (assuming the two procedures are independent events) a patient would have a $(0.7)(0.9) = 0.63$ or 63% chance of surviving both procedures.

However, examine a different example:

The probability of contracting a urinary tract infection (UTI) after catheterization is 0.1 (10%). The probability of contracting a UTI after two separate catheterizations is *not* $(0.1)(0.1) = .01$ (1%). The correct way of applying the multiplicative law (again assuming that these are independent events) is to recognize that the probability of *not* contracting a UTI is 0.9 (90%), and the probability of *not* contracting a UTI after two separate catheterizations would be $(0.9)(0.9) = 0.81$ (or 81%). The probability of contracting a UTI after two separate catheterizations would then be $1 - 0.81 = 0.19$ (or 19%).

Another possibility that often arises in probability analysis is in a situation in which one or another of a group of mutually exclusive events may occur. The *additive law of probability* states that the probability of A *or* B occurring is the sum of the probability of A and the probability of B. For example, if we were to examine the relative frequency of 100% of confirmed lumbar radiculopathies in a series of patients, we might find that 1% occurred at L2, 2% at L3, 5% at L4, 42% at L5, and 50% at S1. The additive law of probability allows us to state that the probability of suffering a radiculopathy at L5 *or* S1 is $0.42 + 0.50 = 0.92$ (or 92%).

Displaying Data

Numerically discrete or numerically continuous data can be summarized in a *frequency distribution*. Table 13–2 shows uric acid levels for men with their first attack of gouty arthritis. After creating such a frequency distribution, the data can be charted on a bar-type graph (*histogram*) or *frequency polygon*, as in Figure 13–1A and B.

Summarizing Data

Once data have been plotted, there are several useful measurements to help summarize the data. The mean, median, and mode are the most useful measures of central tendency or location. The *mean* or *arithmetic mean* (μ) is simply the total of the scores of the observations divided by the number of observations ($\Sigma x/n$, where Σ = summation sign, x = variable measured, and n = number of x values). The *median* is the observation "in the middle."

TABLE 13–2   Example of Frequency Distribution

Uric Acid Level (mg/dL)	No. of Men (N = 100)
8.0–8.4	10
8.5–8.9	17
9.0–9.4	23
9.5–9.9	22
10.0–10.4	20
10.5–10.9	8

TABLE 13–3   Example of Data Needed to Calculate Variance and Standard Deviation

Trial	x (lb)	x^2
1	3	9
2	4	16
3	7	49
4	8	64
5	3	9
	$\Sigma x = 25$	$\Sigma x^2 = 147$

The *mode* is the most popular value. For example, pinch strength is measured five times with measured values of 3, 4, 7, 8, and 3 lb. The mean would be 5 (25 divided by 5), the median 4 (middlemost number), and the mode 3 (most commonly observed value). The mean is most often used in statistics but can be seriously affected by extreme values or *outliers*. The median is unaffected by outliers but is less amenable to statistical treatment.

The second important parameter in summarizing data is the spread or *variation*. The *range* of the data refers to the difference between the highest and lowest values (e.g., the pinch strengths ranged from 3 to 8 lb with a range of 5 lb). Two other useful indices are the *variance* (σ^2) and its square root, the *standard deviation* (σ). The mathematical formulas for these are

$$\sigma^2 = \frac{\Sigma x^2 - (\Sigma x)^2/n}{n - 1} \quad \text{and} \quad \sigma = \sqrt{\frac{\Sigma x^2 - (\Sigma x)^2/n}{n - 1}}$$

The reader is referred to standard texts for their derivation, and for further details of "sample" vs. "population" standard deviations. An example of data needed to calculate variances and standard deviations of pinch strengths is shown in Table 13–3. It is easy to plug these numbers into our equations and determine the variance (σ^2) = 5.5, and the standard deviation (σ) = 2.34. The standard deviation is the most commonly used measure of variation in the medical literature.

Normal Distribution

The concept of a gaussian or *normal distribution* is very important to statistical inference. The normal distribution is a symmetrical bell-shaped curve that can be characterized by its mean (μ) and standard deviation (σ). The normal distribution is very important empirically because many medical measurements in a given population approximate this curve (e.g., blood pressure, height, weight). While the exact formulation of the normal distribution is beyond the scope of this discussion, there are several characteristics worth mentioning. In Figure 13–2A, normal curves A and B have identical means but differing standard deviations. Curves A and C have identical standard deviations but different means. Many statistical tests are derived with the assumption that the variables being tested have a normal distribution. These tests are sometimes referred to as *parametric* tests.

In normal curves as well as other curves that are relatively bell-shaped, the $\mu \pm 1\sigma$ represents approximately 68% of observations that are charted (Fig. 13–2B). The

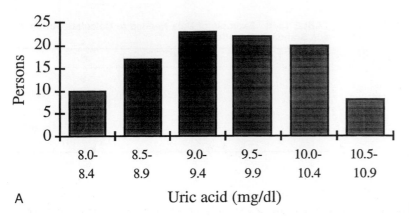

A

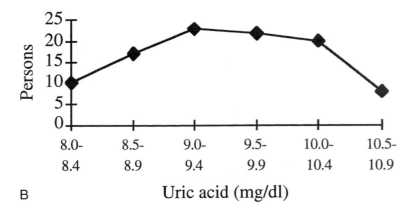

B

FIGURE 13–1 *A,* Histogram (or bar graph) demonstrating uric acid levels in 100 men with their first attack of gouty arthritis. *B,* Frequency polygram or line chart using the same data.

mean $\mu \pm 2\sigma$ represents approximately 95%, and the $\mu \pm 3\sigma$ represents 99% of all observations. For example, if a sampling of body weights in 100 spinal cord–injured women was found to be in a normal distribution with $\mu = 120$ lb and $\sigma = 10$ lb, approximately 68% of all subjects would range in weight from 110 to 130 lb, 95% from 100 to 140 lb, and 99% from 90 to 150 lb. These relationships do *not* hold true for curves that are asymmetrical (have a large degree of *skewness*). Such distributions are not well described by the mean and standard deviation. Remember that the term "normal" refers to a *mathematical model, and has no biological or clinical connotation.*

Normal Limits

In distributions that are normal, the mean ± 2 standard deviations are frequently defined as the *upper and lower limits of normal.* In this context normal refers to *clinical normalcy.* Since $\mu \pm 2\sigma$ encompasses 95% of the subjects studied, this would represent the population between the 2.5 and 97.5 percentiles. Again, these concepts hold true *only if the population studied falls into a normal distribution.* Cholesterol values and motor nerve conduction velocities are examples of values that are *not* in a bell-shaped or normal distribution.

Normal distributions may often be of use in studying differences between two populations. For example, suppose a new blood test (serum factor H) was being assessed for the detection of heterotopic bone (Fig. 13–3). Suppose that the normal distribution of serum factor H values obtained from 100 patients is represented by curve HO($-$), and the

normal distribution of serum factor H values from those with heterotopic ossification is HO($+$). Note that the curves overlap. Our goal for this new diagnostic test is to find an upper limit of normal for serum factor H. Clearly, anywhere we draw an arbitrary vertical line to signify the upper limit of normal serum factor H values is going to involve certain compromises. Our goal is to find a line where all patients without heterotopic bone are going to fall to the left of the line (*true-negatives*) and all with heterotopic bone are going to fall to the right (*true-positives*). As the HO($-$) and HO($+$) curves overlap, this is not possible. A small number of persons who do not have heterotopic bone are going to fall to the right of our upper limit discretionary value (*false-positives*), and some with heterotopic bone will fall to the left of the line (*false-negatives*).

With an ideal laboratory test the cutoff point distinguishes entirely between true-negatives and true-positives. However, more often tests suffer from some degree of false-positives and false-negatives. The *sensitivity* of this test is the ratio of true-positives divided by the sum of true-positives and false-negatives. The *specificity* of the test is a ratio of true-negatives divided by the sum of true-negatives and false-positives. Suppose for our sample above we created the illustration shown in Table 13–4. The sensitivity of the test is represented by 80 divided by (80 + 20) = 80%. The specificity is 90 divided by (90 + 10) = 90%. Note that if we move our vertical line or cutoff to the right, we would increase our identification of true-negatives, and decrease the number of false-positives (spec-

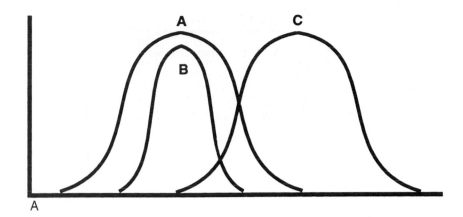

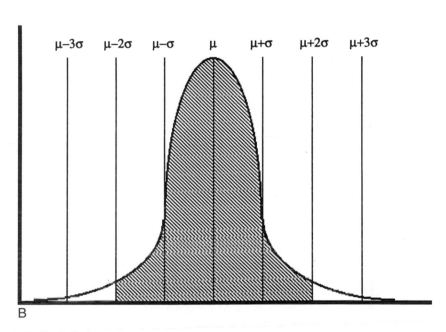

FIGURE 13–2 Three normal curves. Curves *A* and *B* have identical means (μ) but differing standard deviations (σ). Curves *A* and *C* have identical σ but different μ. *B*, Normal curve with vertical lines denoting the mean, μ, and standard deviations (σ) above/below the mean. The *cross-hatched area* represents 95% of the area under the curve.

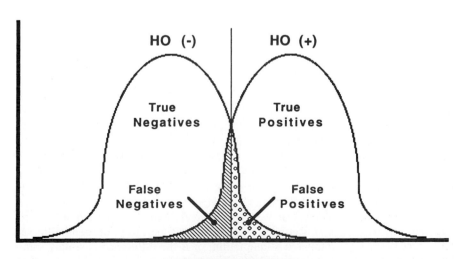

FIGURE 13–3 The distribution of serum factor H level is recorded for patients with [HO(+)] and without [HO(−)] heterotopic bone. The *vertical line* is arbitrarily placed to represent the upper limit of normal. As the two curves overlap, the upper limit of normal determines the relative number of true negatives, true positives, false negatives, and false positives.

TABLE 13–4　Sample of Table Needed to Calculate Sensitivity and Specificity

Result of Serum Factor H Test	Persons With HO	Persons Without HO
Positive	80	10
Negative	20	90

ificity will improve, sensitivity will decrease). If we move it to the left, the opposite happens.

Sources of Variation

There are many sources of variation in a defined group of data. One type is true *biological variation* which represents the actual differences that exist in different subjects. For example, if an investigator was studying weight fluctuation after SCI, actual weight loss in a group of patients might be found to vary from 0 to 20 lb in the first 3 weeks postinjury.

Other types of variation may occur, however. *Temporal variation* is the natural variation that occurs over time. For example, owing to physiological fluid changes, women may gain weight due to retained fluid during the menstrual cycle, and this may "confound" the observation of weight loss after SCI. Variation may result from *measurement error* on the part of the observer (e.g., one who reads the scale incorrectly) or the measurement instrument (e.g., a faulty scale).

Sampling variation is yet another important type of variation, and can occur when we are studying large populations. Suppose we wished to study the level of a blood factor, serum factor K, in the American public. We could attempt to sample each and every one of the 250+ million Americans. Obviously this is impossible, but let us assume we could do it, and it was represented by a normal distribution with $\mu = 100$ and $\sigma = 10$. This would represent the *true* mean and standard deviation of factor K in the American public. The reality of the situation is that we are *not* able to study all Americans and have to select a random sample of Americans and sample their blood. We obtain samples from 100,000 Americans on five separate occasions and find the data shown in Table 13–5. None of the samples precisely represent the true mean and standard deviation, but they come quite close. The *central limit theorem* states that the *distribution* of these sample means (98.6, 100.1, 97.3, 103.1, and 100.2) will fall in a normal distribution around our true mean (100). This means that we can construct a normal curve (Fig. 13–4) not out of the actual data, *but of the mean values for each of our samples.* This curve has its own mean (which hopefully is very close

TABLE 13–5　Example of Data From Five Samples of a Large Population

Sample	$\mu \pm \sigma$
1	98.6 ± 10.3
2	100.1 ± 9.9
3	97.3 ± 9.8
4	103.1 ± 8.9
5	100.2 ± 11.0

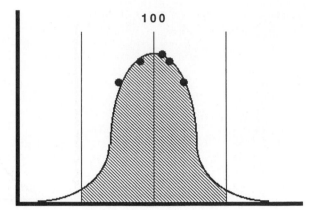

FIGURE 13–4　A normal curve of sample means derived from samples of serum factor K in the American population. The sample means are close to, but not exactly identical to, the true mean = 100. The central limit theorem states that the distribution of the sample means fall in a normal distribution about the true mean.

to the true mean of 100) and standard deviation (called the *standard error*).

The construction of such a normal curve of sample means allows us to define *confidence intervals*. From the previous discussion of normal distributions, we know that 95% of all observations fall within 2 standard deviations of the mean. Using the concept of the central limit theorem, we know that if we find the mean and standard deviation of our *curve of sample means*, we can then state that there is a 95% chance that the *true* mean of serum factor K in the American public (100) would fall within the mean plus or minus twice the standard error of our curve. This is the concept of defining a 95% confidence interval, and the values at each end of that interval are the *confidence limits*. It is a way of quantitating how "confident" we are that the true mean (of 100) falls within our sample estimate. From this discussion it is obvious that confidence limits provide a probability of specifying how successfully we have sampled the true mean value (in this case of serum factor K). Sample means based on a large sample have a better chance of truly estimating our mean value than smaller samples. A sample with a large number of observations typically has a *narrower* confidence interval.

Comparing Groups

Often in medicine we are asked to see if a new drug or treatment is superior to an older method, and we must design studies to assess the superiority of one of two (or more) methods. Suppose we had a new antibiotic, genticillin, to treat UTIs, and wished to compare it to a second antibiotic, ampicillin. If genticillin cured 8 out of 10 patients, and ampicillin, 1 out of 10, we would strongly suspect genticillin to be the superior drug. However if genticillin cured 6 out of 10 and ampicillin, 5 out of 10, we would be less convinced of that superiority. Our question is, Can we use statistical methods to determine if there is a statistically significant superiority of genticillin as compared to ampicillin, or if the difference is simply sampling variation (as discussed above)?

One way of doing this is to construct a *null hypothesis* (abbreviated H_0 that there is *no* difference between our two treatments. If through statistical methods we can show there is an extremely low probability that the null hypothesis is correct (i.e., that there is no difference between genticillin and ampicillin), it follows that there is an extremely high probability that the converse is true (i.e., that there is a significant treatment difference between genticillin and ampicillin). This concept of *rejecting the null hypothesis* is the statistical hallmark of determining differences between various types of treatment.

COMPARING PERCENTAGES. The *chi-squared test* is one such tool for determining statistical differences between two percentages (as compared to actual *measurement* data; see below). Suppose we were to compare our two antibiotics (Table 13–6): The question is whether the success rate for genticillin (8/10) is superior to that for ampicillin (1/10). For any 2 × 10 table (two treatments—genticillin, ampicillin; two potential outcomes—success, failure), the chi-squared value (χ^2) may be computed by the following formula*:

$$\chi^2 = \frac{(|ad - bc| - n/2)^2 n}{(a + c)(b + d)(a + b)(c + d)}$$

The larger the treatment difference between the two drugs, the larger the χ^2 value will be. It can be determined from statistical tables of χ^2 values that only 5% of values will exceed 3.84 (for our sample size). If we compute from our example that the $\chi^2 = 7.27$, there is less than a 5% chance that there is no treatment difference between genticillin and ampicillin. (In our example there is actually less than a 1% chance that there is no treatment difference between genticillin and ampicillin.) It is more reasonable then to *reject* our null hypothesis (no treatment difference) and accept the converse—that there *is* a treatment difference between genticillin and ampicillin. To put it another way, there is less than a 1 in 100 chance that the treatment difference between genticillin and ampicillin is due to sampling variation, and greater than a 99 in 100 chance that it is due to a difference in drug efficacy. Using χ^2 values of 5% (or .05) or 1% (or .01) as a criterion for accepting or rejecting the null hypothesis is the basis of determining statistically significant differences between groups. *This is commonly expressed as being statistically significant at the .05 (P < .05) or .01 (P < .01) level.*

COMPARING MEASUREMENTS. There are many statistical significance tests for testing a null hypothesis when measurements are involved. The most commonly used method is the *Student's t-test*. There are different *t*-tests for *paired measurements* and *unpaired measurements*.

---

*The chi-squared formula presented here uses the Yates correction. Readers are referred to statistical texts for details concerning use of the Yates correction.

TABLE 13–6   Example of 2 × 2 Table to Compare the Results of Two Alternative Treatments

Antibiotic	Successes	Failures	Total
Genticillin	a	b	a + b
Ampicillin	c	d	c + d
Total	a + c	b + d	n

where a = 8, b = 2, c = 1, d = 9 and n = a + b + c + d = 20

TABLE 13–7   Example of a Data Table for a Paired Measurement Study

Patient No.	Calcitonin (A)	Placebo (B)	Difference (A − B)
1	1.5	2.0	− 0.5
2	3.0	2.0	1.0
3	1.0	0.4	0.6
4	2.5	2.0	0.5
5	1.2	1.0	0.2
	ΣA/n = 1.84	ΣB/n = 1.48	Σ[A − B]/n = 0.36

Paired measurements involve an experimental design in which each subject in group A has a correlate in group B. These are discussed further below in the section on study design, but examples of paired measurements are twin studies (one of each pair of identical twins in each treatment group) and crossover design (where a patient may take either the active drug or placebo during phase 1, and then the opposite during phase 2). Suppose we examined the effect of calcitonin in treating immobilization hypercalcemia after SCI in five patients. Calcitonin and placebo treatment were each administered for 1 week in each patient; the order of treatment was randomized and both the patient and investigator were blinded to the identity of the drug. The reduction in serum calcium during calcitonin administration is shown in Table 13–7. If the null hypothesis states there is no difference between the active drug (calcitonin) and placebo in lowering serum calcium, we would expect the *mean difference* in calcium reduction to be zero. That is, if there are five paired comparisons, perhaps calcitonin would be better in two, placebo in two, and the same result in one. However, the arithmetic *mean* of those five (Σ(A − B)/n) would be zero. In our example the mean difference is 1.8/5 = 0.36.

The *paired t-test* helps us evaluate the question, Is our mean difference in calcium reduction readily explainable by random chance, or due to a statistically significant treatment effect? The derivation of the *t*-test is beyond the scope of this discussion (see references for further information), but suffice it to say that the *t* test uses a distribution curve which is shaped much like a gaussian distribution, and whose mean value is zero. Note that we can denote critical values which mark off the extreme 5% (2.5% in each tail) in the distribution with a sample size of n. The *t*-test will then tell us whether our calculated mean difference (0.36) is different enough from the mean difference of the perfect null hypothesis (zero) to justify rejecting the null hypothesis. If the disparity between our calculated mean difference and the "ideal" mean difference of the null hypothesis is significant at the 5% or .05 level, there is a less than a 1 in 20 chance that this difference can be explained on the basis of random chance alone. Thus we would usually reject the null hypothesis. (In our case the difference is not statistically significant.) Unlike chi-squared values, *t*-values can be (+) or (−).

The *unpaired Student's t-test* allows us to compare treatment effects on two groups when the individual members are not paired. Suppose we compare five patients taking calcitonin with five taking placebo (for convenience, we use the same data as for the previous example). The null hypothesis—that there is no difference between calcitonin and placebo—would argue that the average reduction in calcium in the treatment group would be equal to the reduction in the placebo group. Once again, the *t*-test could examine whether there is a statistically significant difference between the calcitonin group (mean reduction, 1.84) and the placebo group (mean reduction, 1.48). The *t*-test values are calculated using tables or a statistical computer program, and are dependent on the numbers of subjects in the group.

To be used appropriately, the *t*-test requires that the observations in both the treatment and control groups be normally distributed and that the variances be approximately the same. If this is not believed to be the case, other statistical tests are available.

Another feature to examine is the one-tailed vs. the two-tailed *t*-test. Suppose, for our example, we assume that the calcitonin will lower the hypercalcemia more than placebo, and we are trying to prove that to be the case. We can use a *one-tailed* t-*test* to prove the decline in calcium with calcitonin is greater. However, we may be making a critical error! Perhaps calcitonin has some sort of paradoxical effect and raises the calcium level. A *two-tailed* t-*test* lets us test the hypothesis that calcitonin is significantly more *or* less effective than placebo in lowering calcium levels. The one-tailed test only examines the statistical significance of calcitonin being *more* effective. The two-tailed *t*-test is the more conservative approach, and if there is any doubt about which *t*-test to use, it should be the two-tailed.

Tests of comparison such as a *t*-test must be used judiciously. Suppose, as an investigator, we were to collect a huge data set and then arbitrarily perform multiple *t*-tests looking for significant differences between measurements. As the number of *t*-tests increases, so does the likelihood that a "significant" difference may be found purely by random chance (when in actuality no significant difference really exists). When performing multiple simultaneous comparisons within a data set, special corrections must be used.

ANALYSIS OF VARIANCE. Yet another way of comparing differences is *analysis of variance (ANOVA)*. ANOVA allows us to compare more than two groups at once, or more than one intervention at once. It is now the most frequently encountered statistical test in the rehabilitation literature. For example, suppose we were to measure the effect of four diets on post-SCI immobilization hypercalcemia. The four diets might be high calcium, low calcium, high sodium, and low sodium. Our null hypothesis would be that there would be *no difference in calcium levels in patients randomized to each of the four treatment groups*. A simple *one-way ANOVA* would be the statistical tool to compare each of the groups to one another, and determine whether there is a significant likelihood that a *single* intervention (in this example, a type of diet) is effective in altering immobilization hypercalcemia.

In a simple one-way ANOVA, we compute a mean and variance for each dietary treatment group (high calcium, low calcium, high sodium, and low sodium). We then compare the means and the variance between the dietary treatment groups using the *F-statistic*. The F-statistic is a ratio of the variance *between the means* of each of the treatment groups, and the variance within each of the treatment groups. The F-statistic lets us answer the question, Is the difference between the means among the four treatment groups due to chance, or is it most likely due to a treatment effect? Similarly, we could investigate the role of two different treatments (e.g., diet and diuretics) simultaneously using a *two-way ANOVA*. More than two dependent variables can be assessed using a *multivariate* ANOVA, or *MANOVA*.

NONPARAMETRIC STATISTICS. There are occasions when a body of data does not conform with the assumptions underlying traditional parametric statistical methods. Such a body of data does not fit in a normal distribution, because the data may be greatly skewed in one direction, or may have a large number of outliers. Such a body of data can be statistically analyzed using *nonparametric tests*. The *Wilcoxon rank sum test* is an example of such a nonparametric method, and is the nonparametric equivalent of the unpaired *t*-test. It essentially compares the ranking in one group with the ranking in another. For example, examine 20 physicians sitting for a board examination, 10 from program A and 10 from program B. Our question might be, Do physicians in group A perform superiorly? In the rank sum test we would rank the scores from 1st place to 20th place, and attempt to prove that the group A physicians have significantly higher *rankings* than do the physicians in group B. An alternative version of the Wilcoxon rank sum test is the *Mann-Whitney test*. The *Wilcoxon signed rank test* is the nonparametric equivalent of the paired *t*-test. Yet another nonparametric technique is *Spearman's rank correlation*.

Nonparametric statistics are simpler to calculate for small groups, they make fewer assumptions of the data (remember *t*-tests are used when one assumes there is approximately a normal distribution in the data), and they can be used when only rankings or ordinal data are available. For example, if you knew from the test data that program A had taken places 1, 3, 4, 5, 6, 7, 11, 12, 13, 14, you could demonstrate that this is significantly superior to program B's placements of 2, 8, 9, 10, 15, 16, 17, 18, 19, 20. In summary, nonparametric statistics may be viewed as valuable alternatives to *t*-tests.

TYPE I AND TYPE II ERROR. In this section we have postulated a null hypothesis (e.g., calcitonin and placebo have no difference in therapeutic efficacy) which we attempt to show with a statistical tool (e.g., the *t*-test) to be an extremely unlikely possibility. As previously mentioned, we often choose that value of probability to be less than 1 in 20 (abbreviated $P < .05$) or less than 1 in 100 ($P < .01$). If we find our null hypothesis to be suitably unlikely, we feel comfortable rejecting our null hypothesis, and accepting that the converse is most likely true (e.g., calcitonin is effective in lowering post-SCI hypercalcemia). It is obvious that occasionally we may *reject a null hypothesis that is actually true*! At the .05 level of significance we have a 5% probability of rejecting a null hypothesis that is correct (e.g., accepting the therapeutic difference between calcitonin and placebo when in reality there is none). This first error of erroneously rejecting a true null hypothesis is called *type I error* or α *error*. Conversely, we can make a *type II error* or β *error* by erroneously failing to reject a null hypothesis that is, in fact, false (e.g., concluding there is no difference between calcitonin and placebo when indeed there is).

Type I and type II errors are inherent in every study, and we attempt to minimize them by increasing the number of observations or subjects (N) in the experimental design. Also, the more powerful the treatment effect (e.g., the more dramatic the difference in efficacy between calcitonin and placebo), the less important type I and type II errors turn out to be. Beginning researchers often wonder how large an N must be used in any particular study. One can design a study with an appropriate N by determining the level of type II error that is acceptable, and estimating the difference in efficacy one can expect from the two treatment choices. This is called the *power* of a study, and can be easily calculated for a variety of statistics. Lack of statistical power has been shown to be an important pitfall in the analysis of stroke rehabilitation clinical trials, where small numbers of subjects limit the researcher's ability to detect small or medium treatment effects.[16]

CLINICAL (PRACTICAL) VS. STATISTICAL SIGNIFICANCE. Statistics can offer us a way of assessing the probable "truth" of a null hypothesis, but it cannot substitute for clinical judgment in assessing the practical value of that observation. Suppose we were to study the effect of a hypothetical new drug, cognexin, in improving cognition after traumatic brain injury. We study a huge number of patients (perhaps 100,000) and find that those given cognexin have a 2-point greater score on the Wechsler Memory Scale at 1 year, and this is statistically significant at the .05 level. Nonetheless, as clinicians, we can state that we are not sure that any practical significance is to be found in this study unless other benefits are found from taking the drug. In this case we have discovered a statistically significant difference between the groups, which our common sense correctly tells us is of no clinical significance.

Linear Regression and Correlation

Sometimes, while surveying certain groups, we may note certain factors or characteristics that seem to be "related." For example, if we study the incidence of diabetes mellitus and obesity, there appears to be a positive relationship between these two conditions. If we were to plot 8 AM blood glucose on the y-axis as a function of pounds in excess of ideal body weight for 40 subjects, we might find a relationship such that shown in Figure 13–5A.

Eyeballing the *scattergram* would confirm our suspicion that the incidence of hyperglycemia increases with the degree of obesity. We can estimate a line which most closely fits this data according to the formula $y = ax + b$, which is the simple algebraic formula for a line where a = slope and b = y intercept. The formula for this line that most closely fits our data is called a *simple linear regression*, and can be estimated statistically in several ways, one of which is called the *method of least squares*. The straight line that is selected is that which minimizes the sums of the squares of the vertical deviations between the points and the line (Fig. 13–5B).

Depending on the scattergram, certain linear regressions will fit the data very neatly, while others will fit poorly. The strength of a linear regression between x and y is expressed as the r-*value*, also called the *Pearson correlation coefficient*. Formulas for the calculation of r may be found in a statistics book, but the important thing to remember is that $-1 \le r \le 1$. An $r = 1$ implies a perfect correlation between two variables (e.g., the number of birthday parties one might have had and one's age). An $r = -1$ implies a perfect inverse correlation. For example, if one has 10 pieces of candy, how many pieces of candy are left after eating each piece? After eating one there would be nine left, after eating two there would be eight left, etc. An $r = 0$ implies absolutely no correlation between the x and y variable.

Another statistic useful in the study of linear relationships is the *coefficient of determination* or r^2. The r^2 value provides a more useful measure of the predictability of y as a function of x than does the correlation coefficient alone. It follows that if $-1 \le r \le 1$, then $0 \le r^2 \le 1$.

We can use computer programs to calculate 95% confidence limits for a linear regression (95% confidence limits are commonly used), just as we can develop 95% confidence limits for our sample mean as discussed above. The 95% confidence interval for a linear regression implies that there is less than 1 chance in 20 ($P < .05$) that the true algebraic formula for the linear regression ($y = ax + b$) *does not* fit within the curved lines denoting the confidence limits. We can also build more complex linear equations or models using more than one x variable. For example, if we measure nerve conduction velocity and collect a set of data about our subjects (e.g., age, sex, height, shoe size, arm span), we could perform a series of linear regressions to show how y (nerve conduction velocity) correlates with a series of x variables (age, sex, height, shoe size). We can perform such analyses one x at a time—*stepwise linear regression*, or for all of the x variables at once—*multiple linear regression*.

Linear regression models assume that a linear fit is the best fit for the data, but this may not be the case. For example, relationships between x and y may be better fit using quadratic or logarithmic instead of linear solutions. Secondly, as a general rule, *causal inferences* cannot be drawn without *experimentation*. That is, just because a strong correlation is found between x and y does not imply that x is the cause of y or vice versa. To test causal relationships generally requires an experimental paradigm.

Vital Statistics

Vital statistics comprise another important area of descriptive statistics. *Mortality rates* may be estimated by the *crude annual death rate*, which is the ratio of total deaths for a given year divided by the population at risk in that year (usually measured at the midyear point). It is often helpful to stratify death rates by age group—*age-specific death rate*—because of the varying constitution of certain populations. Another special example of death rates is *cause-specific death rate*. An example of this would be the number of deaths from motor vehicle accidents each year for the total population.

Morbidity rates are a ratio of the number of cases of a certain disease divided by the number of persons at risk for the disease. Morbidity rates can be reported as incidence and prevalence. The *incidence* is the number of new cases occurring during a given time period divided by the number at risk for the disease at that time. The *prevalence*

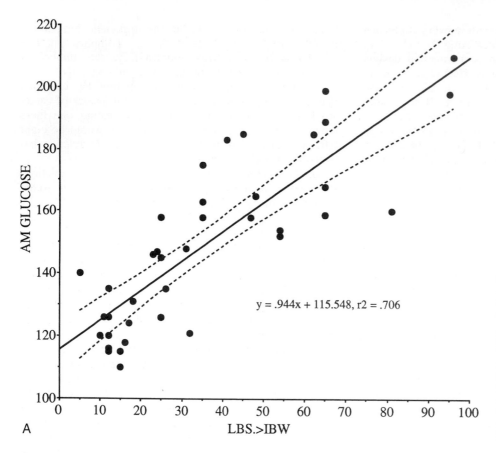

A

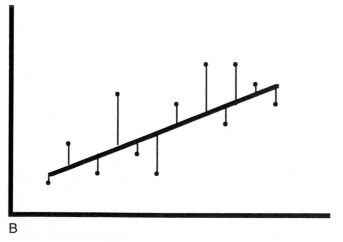

B

y = .944x + 115.548, r2 = .706

FIGURE 13–5 *A,* A scattergram plotting morning (AM) glucose values as a function of pounds above ideal body weight (IBW). The *solid line* is the regression line and is represented by the linear formula displayed on the figure. The *dotted curvilinear boundaries* represent the 95% confidence intervals for the regression line. *B,* A depiction of the method of least squares. The *straight line* used for the regression line is that which minimizes the sums of the squares of the vertical deviations between the points and the line.

of a disease represents the number of cases that exist at a specific point in time divided by the number at risk for the disease. For example, in Table 13–8 two new patients suffered from the disease during the month of March, an incidence of 20%, with a prevalence of 50%.

Experimental Design

Scientific studies may be divided into *experimental* and *observational* (nonexperimental) studies. In an experimental study the investigator has control over the major variables, for example, a drug or treatment. In nonexperimental studies researchers look for associations between variables, often in a search for causal relationships. As previously

mentioned, once a possible causal relationship is suspected, it may then be tested in an experimental design.

Clinical trials are experiments in which the subject is a human being. The prototype of clinical trials is the controlled clinical trial where the treatment group or groups are compared with a similar group of *controls*. Controlled trials have many advantages over uncontrolled observations, since controlled trials allow causal inferences to be drawn, and bias can be minimized through proper *randomization* (assignment of subjects into treatment and control groups purely by chance) and design methods. Randomized controlled trials can offer a persuasive argument that differences in treatment effect are not due to inherent differences between treatment and control groups, and are not due to

TABLE 13–8 Occurrence of a Disease by Month in 10 Patients

Patient	Jan	Feb	Mar	Apr	May	June	July	Aug	Sept	Oct	Nov	Dec
1	xxxxxx	xxxxxx	xxxxxx									
2									xxxxxx	xxxxxx	xxxxxx	
3												
4		xxxxxx	xxxxxx	xxxxxx	xxxxxx	xxxxxx						
5												
6			xxxxxx	xxxxxx								
7	xxxxxx	xxxxxx	xxxxxx	xxxxxx	xxxxxx							
8												
9			xxxxxx									
10												

differences in the handling of the groups during the course of an investigation (both of which might bias the study results).

Randomization is best carried out by using a random number list. An example of failure to adequately randomize treatment and control groups would be to compare treatment A on one hospital ward vs. treatment B on another. Are the same socioeconomic-diagnostic groups of patients admitted to both wards? Similarly, the assignment of alternate cases to the study or control group might be biased; did the referring physicians prefer one treatment method over the other and "load" one treatment group? With paired samples, randomization can be carried out using a *crossover design* in which the patients serve as their own controls. When drugs A and B are compared, one half of the subjects are randomized to receive the drugs ordered A–B, and the other B–A.

Another method of randomization that is sometimes useful is *stratification*, also known as *randomized complete block design*. For example, if one were to design a study to assess the effect of the drug GM-1 in minimizing neurotrauma in SCI, we might want to stratify our treatment and control groups by level of injury or completeness of injury, or both. Subjects would then be randomly assigned within each of these strata. Stratification is especially important with small samples where straight randomization may still lead to unbalanced groups.

Matched controls are sometimes used as substitutes for true randomization. This appears to be attractive at first, but should be used with caution. For example, we can place a subject with five "attributes" in one treatment group, and a second subject with the same attributes in the control group. Unfortunately, we cannot always be sufficiently informed that we can identify all of the important attributes. For example, suppose we identify two groups whose attributes are: (1) round shape, (2) found in a tree, (3) edible, (4) 3 to 5 in. in diameter, and (5) approximately 0.5 lb in weight. Although we might create a matched control group, we could still be comparing apples with oranges![4]

One type of control that is often used in drug trials is a *placebo* control. In this type of study a chemically inert "sugar" pill is formulated to look identical to the active drug to control for the *placebo effect*—the positive psychological benefit derived from receiving a pill from a caregiver. In a *single blind clinical trial* the *subjects but not the investigators* are blinded to the treatment identity for each subject. In a *double blind clinical trial, both* the investigators and the subjects are blinded.

SINGLE-SUBJECT DESIGN. The randomized controlled study is often less suitable in the rehabilitation setting, because there are typically a large number of variables that would require substantial subject populations for randomization. One solution is to use a patient as his or her own control throughout the study, a strategy called *single-subject design* (SSD). These are also called *idiographic* or *within-subject designs*. Figure 13–6 shows an example of such a design. The effect of 75 mg/day of amitryptiline vs. placebo is being assessed in a TBI patient for the control of agitation. A single patient is observed for several days to establish a baseline (days 0–5). A drug is started on day 5, and both patient and investigator might be blinded as to whether it is amitriptyline or placebo. The drug is stopped on day 10 and a 5-day "washout" ensues.

FIGURE 13–6 A data summary for a single subject design or idiographic study. The *x*-axis represents a 30-day time period. The *y*-axis is a 10-point scale summarizing the patient's agitation for that day (Agitation Rating Scale). After a 5-day observation period, placebo administration is started on day 5. Placebo administration is stopped on day 10 and a 5-day "washout" ensues. Amitriptyline administration is started on day 15. This is followed by a subsequent washout at day 20 and a second baseline observation period from days 25 through 30.

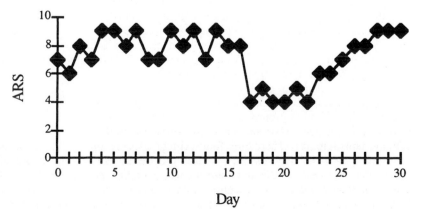

The second drug (in this case, amitriptyline) is started on day 15. This might similarly be followed by a subsequent washout at day 20 and a second baseline observation period from day 26 through 30. There are obviously many variations of baseline periods (A) and intervention periods (B) which could be constructed; some examples are AB, ABA, ABAB.

The obvious advantage of SSD is that efficacy can be demonstrated without the benefit of large numbers of patients, or in settings where a control group is difficult to define. One disadvantage is that the investigator must then prove that the results are generalizable to larger groups. Another disadvantage is that statistical methods for manipulating SSD are available but less well-accepted and less robust than for traditional statistics. Nonetheless, SSDs are especially attractive in the rehabilitation research setting.[15, 19]

META-ANALYSIS. There have been a burgeoning number of *meta-analysis* studies in the medical literature recently.[3] Meta-analysis combines the data from smaller studies into a larger sample size, which can then be statistically evaluated in a more robust fashion than can be done with smaller samples. For example, suppose there are five studies of stroke outcome, each with a sample size between 20 and 40. Perhaps there was no clinical benefit from speech therapy, and the investigator hypothesized that this was because the sample size (N) was too small to demonstrate a statistically significant effect (this would be a type II error). However, by grouping several studies together and reanalyzing the data, we might have a large enough N to gain the statistical power to demonstrate that the effect is statistically significant. Meta-analysis may be undermined when the original smaller studies vary in quality, when incongruous data are inappropriately lumped together, or when negative studies fail to be published (*publication bias*).

EPIDEMIOLOGICAL STUDIES. Epidemiology is the study of the distribution of disease in a population and of those factors that influence that distribution. Epidemiologists often have the difficult task of making educated inferences about disease causation, *even though they are making these inferences without the benefit of an experimental method.*

Case control studies are an example of *retrospective* studies where the numbers of persons in a certain population suffering from a certain disease are compared with another group not suffering from that disease. Both groups are then assessed for their exposure to a certain variable or variables—factors suspected of being causally related to that disease. For example, suppose we want to assess the contribution of excess alcohol consumption as a risk for TBI. We could perform a retrospective analysis of 1000 persons with TBI and 1000 normal controls to assess whether the incidence of excessive alcohol intake is higher or lower in the TBI group. We could then compare the treatment and control groups to determine if the *relative risk* of suffering a TBI is higher in persons with higher alcohol consumption. There are four critical aspects of performing retrospective studies: (1) How did the investigator select the study (TBI) and control cases? (2) Are the study cases and control cases comparable (e.g., are they from similar demographic backgrounds)? (3) How did the

investigator define the factor under study (e.g., excess alcohol consumption)? (4) How accurate were the histories of exposure (e.g., to alcohol) in the study (TBI) and control groups.

Cohort studies are an example of *prospective* studies. Instead of "looking backward," as in a retrospective study, we "look forward." We assess certain risk factors (e.g., risk factors for cardiovascular disease) in a certain population, and then follow this group of patients over time. We can then assess in long-term follow-up the relative risk of each of the potential risk factors (e.g., smoking, hypertension, obesity) in the development of a certain disorder (e.g., angina, myocardial infarction, stroke). The Framingham studies of cardiovascular disease are perhaps the most famous examples of this type of study. Prospective studies are less susceptible to bias than retrospective studies, but often require very large populations in order to have an adequate sample size. One of the most difficult features of epidemiological studies is minimizing or eliminating bias in the control or comparison group (see Reading the Medical Literature below).

READING THE MEDICAL LITERATURE

When reading research papers using experimental design in the medical literature, the physiatrist must examine each research paper critically with the following principles in mind. These principles are similarly applicable for investigators preparing their own research paper.[2] (See also Additional References.)

- *There should be a clear statement of the objectives* (e.g., it is the hypothesis of this study to determine whether calcitonin is superior to placebo in the control of post-SCI immobilization hypercalcemia). This should include a brief review of the current medical literature demonstrating a synthesis of present medical knowledge.

- *If treatment and control groups are used, they should be clearly stated* (e.g., 100 male and 100 female spinal cord–injured persons between 10 and 50 years of age with no history of previous metabolic disorders). The demographic and socioeconomic features of the experimental subjects, as well as *inclusion* and *exclusion criteria*, should be clearly identified.

- *If treatment and control groups are used, there should be random allocation of subjects* (e.g., the 200 subjects were randomized using a random number generator into treatment and control groups). The authors should demonstrate that there were no inherent differences between the treatment and control groups, and that they were similarly handled throughout the investigation. In criticizing a paper in a medical journal, it is not necessary to prove that there was bias in randomization of the treatment and control groups. It is enough to provide a cohesive argument that there *may* have been substantial bias in the way the treatment and control groups were compared.

- *There should be a rationale for choice of the particular experimental design* (e.g., a double blind crossover study in which each patient serves as his or her own control). The methodology, including the variables studied and the method of quantitating these variables, should be sufficiently explained so that the work can be replicated by others. The type and range of values that can be obtained from each measurement instrument should be explained. This is especially important in rehabilitation research where outcomes may be measured in quality of life or other idiosyncratic ways.[11, 12, 14]

- *The resulting data should be clearly and objectively presented, and the methods of statistical analysis explained.* The methods of data collection, the strength and weakness of the data, figures, tables, and photographs should all be presented in a manner which facilitates understanding by the reader.

- *The conclusion should explain why the null hypothesis was accepted or rejected* (e.g., the data clearly demonstrated that daily subcutaneous calcitonin was effective in the control of immobilization hypercalcemia in persons suffering from acute SCI). There should be a justification of the worthiness of the analysis, and a statment of conclusions justified by the data. The results should be discussed in light of previous research, and the implications of the work explained.

DESIGNING A RESEARCH STUDY

The following outline may be helpful in providing an overview of the design and completion of a research study. This material is covered in more detail in "Physiatric Research: Hands-on Approach," a supplement to the *American Journal of Physical Medicine and Rehabilitation* (see Additional References).

- *Formulate a research question.* Pose a question in a fashion that can be answered. Identify methods of answering the question. Determine that the necessary data can be collected. Assure that the planned analysis will answer your question. Ask yourself where the results of the study might be published and who will benefit from the answer? Table 13–9 summarizes one author's "ten commandments" for picking a research project.

- *Review of the literature.* Place your question in the context of existing scientific literature by performing a literature search. It may be useful to locate two to four highly relevant articles as a starting point, then do a computerized literature search. A *MEDLINE* search can be performed on CD-ROM in the medical library, or through an on-line computerized search service such as *Grateful Med* or *BRS Colleague*. Ask other experts in the field for pertinent literature. Computer searches may miss important articles that do not share "keywords" used in the search strategy. Integrate your literature review into a "conceptual review," where the merits and value of various studies are weighed (see Reading the Medical Literature above)

- *Preliminary (pilot) study.* Consider performing a pilot study, perhaps a retrospective chart review. Decide on your research variables, sample size, and how you will collect your data.

TABLE 13–9 Ten Commandments for Picking a Research Project

I.	**Anticipate the results before doing the first study** If you are not prepared to follow up with successful results of the study, it is probably not worth beginning
II.	**Pick an area on the basis of the interest of the outcome** Pick an area which is of interest to more than a handful of people
III.	**Look for an underoccupied niche that has potential** Even well-studied areas have very important aspects that remain understudied
IV.	**Go to talks and read papers *outside* your area of interest** This offers new ideas and suggests new avenues
V.	**Build on a theme** Try to publish more than one paper in the same area
VI.	**Find a balance between low-risk and high-risk projects, but always include a high-risk, high-interest project in your portfolio** This offers the opportunity to make a "seminal" observation and move in front of the field
VII.	**Be prepared to pursue a project to any depth necessary** Be prepared to learn the new skills or technologies that may be required to complete your study
VIII.	**Differentiate yourself from your mentor** Although a strong mentor is crucial in early development as a researcher, define your project in an area that is complementary but not directly competitive with your mentor
IX.	**Do not assume that outstanding, or even good, clinical research is easier than outstanding basic research** It is often more difficult to design well-controlled and informative clinical studies, and they may take longer
X.	**Focus, focus, focus** Few people are able to make an impact in three or four different areas

Adapted with permission from Kahn CR: Picking a research problem: the critical decision. N Engl J Med 1994; 330:1530–1533.

- *Selection of project design.* Determine the number of subjects needed, and ensure that an adequate substrate of patients is available to the investigation. Determine selection (inclusion and exclusion) criteria for subjects and controls. If randomization is part of the study design, how will the treatment group and controls be randomized? Select the appropriate measurement scales and method of statistical analysis. Plan to assure like treatment of treatment and control groups. Consultation with a statistician should be considered before proceeding with the project.

- *Data entry and early exploratory data analysis.* Identify appropriate computer software and develop data entry format for the computer. Design data entry forms. Ensure that the program has adequate statistical capabilities. Perform a preliminary data analysis to verify data accuracy.

- *Research budgeting.* Identify what funding resources are available, whether from extramural or intramural sources (see below). Develop a budget.

- *Regular meetings and ongoing project analysis.* Meet periodically with the entire research team to discuss progress, problems, and ongoing needs.

- *Synthesis of data and results.* Place aside an appropriate block of time to pore over your data, critically evaluate it, and synthesize results. Relate the significance of these results to present medical knowledge.

- *Dissemination of results.* Prepare an abstract of the results for submission to a professional conference.

Gather the suggestions and criticisms from your peers when presenting at the conference. Prepare the final manuscript, and submit the paper to a peer-reviewed journal of suitable readership.

GRANT WRITING AND FUNDING

The grant writer must approach grantsmanship as a business. Granting agencies are in the business of providing funding and support for projects that both meet their needs and fulfill their mission. The grant applicant is in the business of pursuing his or her goals, and at the same time fulfilling the needs of the granting agency. A successful grant applicant must not only possess the research skills needed to complete the task but must also be able to convince the granting agency that the research idea is worth funding.

There are several key components to good grantsmanship: (1) understanding the mission of the potential funding agency, (2) understanding the grant review process, and (3) having the ability to write for the grant reviewer. We will examine each of these factors more closely with the perspective of identifying common deficiencies in grant writing.

Understanding the Mission

The potential researcher should stay informed and up-to-date as to the needs of the funding agencies from which he or she intends to seek support. For example, the mission of the National Institutes of Health (NIH) is to improve the health of the people in the United States; funding good science is simply a means to this end. The potential grantee must demonstrate ingenuity and flexibility to take advantage of current NIH priorities. Researchers can be placed on the mailing list for the *NIH Guide for Grants and Contracts*, and should stay current with revisions of the

NIH grant application form (PHS-398). It is extremely important for a first-time grant applicant to visit the office for grants and contracts (sponsored programs) at his or her university or institution. The people and resources in this office can make the grant-writing process smoother, and often have substantial experience to share.

The grant writer should be aware of the political overtones of grantsmanship. The major funding agencies are composed of federal employees within the executive branch of the federal government. There are times when political priorities and pressures may have a bearing on what types of research are funded. For example, women's health issues (i.e., cardiovascular disease in women, breast cancer) and acquired immunodeficiency syndrome (AIDS) are two areas in which national funding agencies have responded to strong political movements with increased funding support.

It is helpful to understand the structural hierarchy of the federal government agencies that fund rehabilitation research (Fig. 13–7). The NIH is an agency of the Public Health Service (PHS), which is within the U.S. Department of Health and Human Services. In 1990, legislation was signed which created the National Center for Medical Rehabilitation Research (NCMRR) within the National Institute of Child Health and Human Development (NICHHD) at the NIH.[9] The National Institute on Disability and Rehabilitation Research (NIDRR) is an agency of the office of Special Education and Rehabilitation Services of the U.S. Department of Education. NIDRR was founded in 1978 as an outgrowth of the Rehabilitation Research and Demonstration Program administered by the Rehabilitation Services Administration.[22] The mission of NIDRR is to generate, disseminate, and promote new knowledge that will substantially improve the capacities of people with disabilities to perform work and other activities in the community.[9] Their annual research priorities are published in the *Federal Register*.

There are two general methods of obtaining funding

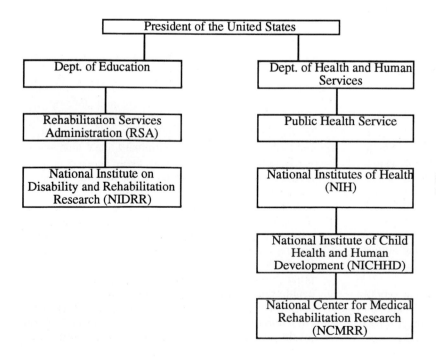

FIGURE 13–7 Federal agencies that primarily fund rehabilitation research.

from these federal agencies. One can apply for *center-directed research* in which the agency issues a request for grant applications or contract proposals (RFA or RFP respectively) and the investigator submits an application fitting the needs of this request. The other main type of application is an *investigator-initiated research* award (referred to by NIH as an R-01). This is the most common mechanism for funding research at the NIH.

Understanding the Grant Review Process

The NIH grant review process is typical of the steps used in a variety of federal granting agencies. A grant proposal is written and initiated by a principal investigator, and then submitted to the NIH Division of Research Grants (DRG). The DRG is an advisory group responsible for setting up study sections to review grant proposals. The NIH has a two-tiered review process: the first level is the scientific merit review by the study section, also called the initial review group. The second level is the priority and relevance review by the advisory council. When a grant proposal is received by the DRG, it is assigned a number which includes an abbreviation for the particular institute from which funding is sought (Table 13–10).

The DRG has approximately 12 referral officers who assign applications to the appropriate study section. Each study section has a scientific review administrator and approximately 14 to 20 basic and clinical scientist members, one of whom serves as a chairperson. The administrator of the study section, usually a scientist, is responsible for the administrative and technical review of the applications, and preparation of a summary statement with final recommendations.

Each grant application is assigned two to three primary reviewers. These persons present a written report to the study session which encapsulates the scientific and technical merits of the proposal. Members serve as the primary reviewer on several proposals, but additionally may serve as a secondary reviewer for scores of applications. It is extremely important to write grants in a "reader-friendly"

fashion. After the reports are read by the reviewers and their merits are evaluated, a vote is taken. Possible outcomes include (1) "not recommended for further consideration"; (2) deferred for additional information; and (3) assignment of a "priority score."

Occasionally, a site visit is arranged when the application involves a complex coordination of individuals, or inspection of the proposed site of research is needed to make a recommendation for funding. Approximately 2 weeks after the study session meets, the priority scores are tabulated, percentile ranks are calculated, and the results are forwarded to the applicant. Summary statements generally require 6 to 8 weeks to reach the principal investigator. Only the top 70% of grant applications assigned a priority score go on to the next stage of the review process. These are sent on to the advisory council meeting of the assigned institute (center, division) to be considered for funding by a panel which includes both scientists and nonscientists. Generally, the order of priority scores is respected and funds are appropriated from top to bottom until exhausted.

The grant review process at NIDRR is somewhat different.[22] The NIDRR peer review process is based on policies contained in the Education Department Grant Administration Regulations (EDGAR), and detailed in the *Federal Register*. A short-term ad hoc review panel is established for each announced competition. Once applications are received in the application control center, they are inspected for completion and appropriateness by designated program staff. Selected reviewers read and score all assigned applications before the scheduled panel meeting in Washington, D.C. During this formal panel meeting discussion takes place and the applications are ranked for approval or disapproval. The panel manager checks all scores and evaluation materials. The panel's recommendations, as well as those of the program staff, are reviewed by the NIDRR director and other departmental officials in a prefunding conference. The final selections are then forwarded to the Department of Education's Grants and Contracts Services for negotiation and award.

Writing for the Grant Reviewer

Writing with the grant reviewer in mind is a necessary part of successful grantsmanship. Preparation of a grant application is a scholarly endeavor that combines scientific skills with clear, disciplined writing style.[5] Grant reviewers have a very difficult and time-consuming job. It is essential to make the reviewer's job as easy as possible. The following suggestions seem timely for the potential grantee:

- Follow the instructions on the grant application precisely. Inability to follow directions makes a negative first impression.
- Keep to the page limits and use the specific font and line spacing called for to make a neat and pleasing document. Carelessness in writing or presentation may suggest to the reviewer a potential carelessness in research.
- Begin to write the grant proposal early. Use an outline for each section of the proposal so that the logic of the discussion flows from section to section. It is much easier to detect logical errors when the manuscript is in skeletal form than when it is fully fleshed out

TABLE 13–10 Abbreviations and Two-Letter Designations of the NIH Institutes and Their Funding Components

NEI (EY)	National Eye Institute
NIA (AG)	National Institute on Aging
NIDR (DE)	National Institute of Dental Research
NHLBI (HL)	National Heart, Lung, and Blood Institute
NCI (CA)	National Cancer Institute
NIGMS (GM)	National Institute of General Medical Sciences
NIEHS (ES)	National Institute of Environmental Health Sciences
NIAID (AI)	National Institute of Allergy and Infectious Diseases
NINDS (NS)	National Institute of Neurological Disorders and Stroke
NIDDK (DK)	National Institute of Diabetes, Digestive, and Kidney Diseases
NICHD (HD)	National Institute of Child Health and Human Development
NIAMS (AR)	National Institute of Arthritis, Musculoskeletal, and Skin Diseases
NIDCD (DC)	National Institute of Deafness and Other Communication Disorders

with prose. It may help to prepare figures, tables, and photographs before writing the actual text of the proposal.

- Writing should be clear and concise, providing the reviewer with the maximum amount of information in the least number of words. Avoid redundancy and ambiguity, while being consistent with terminology and abbreviations. Many persons reading the grant application will not be physicians, so it is wise to avoid medical jargon. Ask more senior colleagues from the basic and clinical science communities to read and critique your proposal—a "mock review" by a knowledgeable scientist in the field may be very helpful.

- It has been estimated that approximately 90% of applications submitted to the NIDRR are rejected for technical deficiencies each year.[22] Five types of errors account for 76.8% of all the deficiencies noted in these applications: (1) poor conceptualization of problem or approach, (2) inadequate control of variables, (3) research design errors, (4) methodological errors, and (5) inappropriate statistical analysis.

Funding Sources

It is always difficult to decide where to apply for funding support. The university office of grants and contracts and the dean's office are good starting points to find out what intramural funding is available. Small seed grants may be available to younger faculty and fellows to serve as startup funds for new research initiatives. Private foundations may serve as the source for startup funds when a new investigator works in a facility that is not part of a larger academic arena. Funding priorities in such organizations are often made by executive process rather than by peer review, and final decisions are ratified by a board of directors. The *Foundation Directory*[18] is the standard reference work for information about private and community grant-making foundations in the United States, and is available at most libraries.

Extramural funding is commonly solicited from the federal government through health research agencies such as NIH and NIDRR. The private sector is also often interested in promoting research when it is related to the development of potential new drugs, products, services, or specific interests. Unfortunately, there is no central source of information for such funding sources and the potential grantee needs to seek these out on an individual basis. Funding is also available through the Small Business Innovation Research program of the Department of Health and Human Resources, and the National Science Foundation has partial listings of small businesses with research interests. An extensive list of resources is available in texts.[20]

ETHICAL ISSUES

The final section of this chapter deals with perhaps the most important aspect of clinical research. There are three general ethical principles which serve as guidelines for clinical research: (1) *respect for persons* (subjects), (2) *beneficence*, and (3) *justice*.

RESPECT FOR PERSONS.   Patients who are enrolled in a clinical trial must be *volunteers* and must be free to withdraw from the study at any time. *Informed consent* must be obtained before a human being may become part of a clinical experiment. In the case of persons who lack full autonomy because of brain injury, dehabilitated state, or immaturity, consent *by proxy* must be given by the legal guardian or his or her appointee. All information collected must be strictly confidential.

BENEFICENCE.   Investigators are obligated to design protocols that will produce valid and generalizable knowledge. Recognizing that *inherent risk* cannot be eliminated for volunteers in a clinical trial, the standard should be that the researcher has taken steps to preclude all *unnecessary* risks to the participants. For example, before a surgical technique or drug is tried in a clinical trial, it is usually assessed first in animal studies. Also, the benefits of the study to the patient, mankind, or science should clearly *outweigh* the risks to the subjects participating in the trial.

Federal law requires approval by an *institutional review board (IRB)* of any research project involving human subjects. It is the IRB's responsibility to review the entire research proposal, including the consent form, and weigh the potential benefits and risks to patients who are participating in the study. Experimental devices or drugs additionally may require approval from the Food and Drug Administration.

JUSTICE.   The benefits and burdens of research should be distributed fairly among all members of society. Disadvantaged, disabled, or minorities should not be asked to bear a disproportionate share. Scientific discoveries often have great societal impact. Nowhere is this more visible than in the work done with AIDS patients. Science and technology are integral parts of society and so investigators are often thrust into the public arena. They need to provide a successful interface so that the scientific value and merit of their work are not distorted in the public eye.

The question sometimes arises whether it is ethical to have a control group, or what type of control to use. This question is apropos in a rehabilitation research setting. Some examples are illustrative:

> While it is relatively easy to argue that the effect of a new antidepressant should be compared with an older antidepressant or a placebo, or both, should speech therapy be compared to placebo speech therapy, or to the absence of speech therapy?
>
> Studies are presently underway investigating the use of a ganglioside, GM-1, as a method of minimizing SCI. Since there is no present evidence that GM-1 is effective, a clinical trial is necessary to accept or reject the null hypothesis that GM-1 is *not* effective. Yet a prominent football player was able to obtain the drug outside of the experimental protocol.
>
> How far can one go with placebos and dummy treatments? Should we perform sham back surgery as a control in comparison to a new surgical technique?

CONFLICTING AND PROPRIETARY INTERESTS. Most journals and symposia require that the authors or lecturers disclose whether they have any financial or other type of interest that might bias the results. For example, a researcher who receives all of his or her research funding from a drug company might have difficulty reporting the uselessness of that company's product. Sometimes drug companies reserve the right to prohibit a clinical trial from being published if the results are adverse to their financial interests.[23]

In other scenarios investigators may be constrained to share data or other research tools because of proprietary interests. A new drug, reagent, or procedure may have significant financial potential, and a scientist or institution may reserve certain legal rights as to its future use. For example, a Wisconsin opthalmologist was the innovator of using botulinus toxin for the treatment of strabismus. The rights to this treatment have since been acquired by a drug company because of its marketability, not only to opthalmologists but for disorders such as torticollis, spasticity, and other movement disorders.

COMMUNAL REVIEW OF SCIENTIFIC RESULTS. The hallmark of scientific progress is the ability to communicate. Researchers communicate with others in their fields through informal dialogue and presentations at conferences, but most important, through the submission of their work to peer-reviewed journals. This critical examination provides the only reliable method of self-correcting the march of scientific progress. Information transmitted first through the mass media (e.g., trials of high-dose steroids in the treatment of acute SCI) may grossly prejudice the evaluation of these results, and how the public perceives them. Many journals will not accept scientific papers without an agreement that they must be published before being presented to the lay press.

ERROR AND FRAUD. Error caused by the inherent limits of scientific theory can only be ascertained by the advancement of science. Despite the utilization of scientific method, mistakes will inevitably occur. These errors should not be tolerated when they are the result of negligence. There is a clear distinction between preventable error and outright fraud. *Fraud* may be defined as a conscious effort to publish inaccurate or misleading results. It is the most grave violation of the ethos of science.

ALLOCATION OF CREDIT IN COLLABORATIVE RESEARCH. When scientific papers are published, credit is given in the list of authors, in an acknowledgment at the end of the text, and in the reference citations. As the lists of authors in multidisciplinary or multicenter studies continue to increase, the issue of authorship ranking has arisen. In some fields the senior author is listed first, while in other fields the leader's name is last. Generally, these issues are handled most productively by discussing them early in the development of a research project, and by ranking authors based on their contributions to the generation of the study idea, solicitation of funding, data collection and analysis, and finally the synthesis of results and writing of the manuscript(s).[10, 21] Unfortunately, "authors" of scientific papers may be added for political reasons, and the ranking of non-first authors often is not based on their contribution to the research effort.[20] The most blatant misappropriation of credit in research is *plagiarism*, intentionally seeking credit for another scientist's intellectual property.

CONCLUSIONS

This chapter was constructed to serve as a steppingstone for young physiatrists. Although vast treatises on statistical techniques cannot be summarized in a book chapter, we hope we have concisely stated the majority of introductory concepts required to review a research paper or begin a research project. Similarly, a textbook chapter cannot substitute for formal training in research, or for experience in soliciting grants from public or private sources. A career as a basic scientist requires apprenticeship with one or more mentors who can instill the rigor of the scientific method into bright young minds. Many worthy research projects in the physical medicine and rehabilitation literature have been completed with little or no funding. Nonetheless, a successful research career within a university often requires physicians who are able to obtain or collaborate in funded research studies. Herein lies the future of physical medicine and rehabilitation as a viable specialty.

References

1. Braddom RL: Why is physiatric research important? Am J Phys Med Rehabil 1991; 70(suppl):S2–S3.
2. Braddom CL: Framework for writing and/or evaluating research papers. Am J Phys Med Rehabil 1991; 70(suppl):S169–S171.
3. Bulpitt CJ: Medical statistics: Meta-analysis. Lancet 1988; 2:93–94.
4. Deyo RA: Practice variations, treatment fads, rising disability. Spine 1993; 18:2153–2162.
5. Eaves GN: Preview of research grant applications at the National Institutes of Health. Fed Proc 1972; 31:2–9.
6. Emerson JD, Colditz GA: Use of statistical analysis in the *New England Journal of Medicine*. N Engl J Med 1983; 309:709–713.
7. Findley TW, DeLisa JA: Research in physical medicine and rehabilitation: XI. Research training: Setting the stage for lifelong learning. Am J Phys Med Rehabil 1991; 70(suppl):S107–S113.
8. Grabois M, Fuhrer MJ: Physiatrists' views on research. Am J Phys Med Rehabil 1991; 70(suppl):S165–S168.
9. Gray DB, Graves WH, Cole TM: Federal funding of medical rehabilitation research: NCMRR and NIDRR. Phys Med Rehabil State of the Art Rev 1993; 70:381–392.
10. Huth EJ: Guidelines on authorship of medical papers. Ann Intern Med 1986; 104:269–274.
11. Johnston MV, Findley TW, DeLuca J, Katz RT: Research in physical medicine and rehabilitation. XII. Measurement tools with application to brain injury. Am J Phys Med Rehabil 1991; 70(suppl):S114–130.
12. Johnston MV, Keith RA, Hinderer SR: Measurement standards for interdisciplinary medical rehabilitation. Arch Phys Med Rehabil 1992; 73(suppl):S1–S23.
13. Kahn CR: Picking a research problem: The critical decision. N Engl J Med 1994; 330:1530–1533.
14. Keller RB, Rudicel SA, Liang MH: Outcomes research in orthopaedics. J Bone Joint Surg [Am] 1993; 75:1562–1574.
15. Larson EB, Ellsworth AJ, Oas J: Randomized clinical trials in single patients during a two-year period. JAMA 1993; 270:2708–2712.
16. Matyas TA, Ottenbacher KJ: Confounds of insensitivity and blind luck: Statistical conclusion validity in stroke rehabilitation clinical trials. Arch Phys Med Rehabil 1993; 74:559–565.
17. Merbitz C, Morris J, Grip JC: Ordinal scales and foundations of inference. Arch Phys Med Rehabil 1989; 70:308–312.
18. Olson S, Feczko MM (eds): Foundation Directory, ed 13. New York, Foundation Center, 1991.
19. Ottenbacher KJ: Clinically relevant designs for rehabilitation research: The idiographic model. Am J Phys Med Rehabil 1991; 70(suppl):S144–S150.
20. Reif-Lehrer L: Writing a Successful Grant Application, ed 2. Boston, Jones & Bartlett, 1989.
21. Shapiro DW, Wenger NS, Shapiro MF: Contributions of authors to multiauthored biomedical research papers. JAMA 1994; 271:438–442.
22. Thomas JP, Lawrence TS: Common deficiencies of NIDRR research applications. Am J Phys Med Rehabil 1991; 70(suppl):S161–164.
23. Witt MD, Gostin LO: Conflict of interest dilemmas in biomedical research. JAMA 1994; 271:547–551.
24. Wright BD, Linacre JM: Observations are always ordinals; measure-

ments, however, must be interval. Arch Phys Med Rehabil 1989; 70:857–867.

Additional References

Monographs for Further Reading

Bailar JC III, Mosteller F: Medical Uses of Statistics, ed 2. Boston, New England Journal of Medicine Books, 1992.

Colton T: Statistics in Medicine. Boston, Little, Brown, 1974.

Committee on the Conduct of Science, National Academy of Sciences: On Being a Scientist. Washington, DC, National Academy Press, 1989.

Duncan RC, Knapp RG, Miller MC: Introductory Biostatistics for the Health Sciences, ed 2. New York, John Wiley & Sons, 1983.

Edwards AL: Multiple Regression and the Analysis of Variance and Covariance, ed 2. New York, WH Freeman, 1985.

Hulley SB, Cummings SR: Designing Clinical Research: An Epidemiologic Approach. Baltimore, Williams & Wilkins, 1988.

Krauth J: Distribution-Free Statistics. An Application-Oriented Approach. Amsterdam, Elsevier, 1988.

Leaverton PE: A Review of Biostatistics: Program for Self-Instruction, ed 2. Boston, Little, Brown, 1978.

Sokal RR, Rohlf FJ: Biometry. The Principles and Practices of Statistics in Biological Research, 2nd ed. New York, WH Freeman and Company, 1981.

Journal Series on Research and Critical Reading of the Medical Literature

Cook DJ, Guyatt GH, Oxman AD, Sackett DL, and Evidence-Based Medicine Working Group: User's guides to the medical literature. JAMA 1993; 271:59–63, 389–391, 703–707, 1615–1619; 1994; 270: 2093–2095, 2598–2601 [Series in progress].

O'Brien PC, Shampo MA: Statistics for clinicians. Mayo Clin Proc 1981; 56:45–49, 126–128, 196–197, 274–276, 324–326, 393–394, 452–454, 513–515, 573–575, 639–640, 709–711, 753–756.

O'Brien PC, Shampo MA: Statistics series. Mayo Clin Proc 1988; 63:813–820, 918–920, 1043–1045, 1140–1143, 1245–1249.

Physiatric research: hands-on approach. American Journal of Physical Medicine and Rehabilitation 1991; 70(suppl):S1–S171.

Sackett DL, Haynes RB, Tugwell PX, Trout KS: How to read clinical journals. Can Med Assoc J 1981; 124:555–558, 703–710, 869–872, 985–990, 1156–1162.

Victoria CG, Grisso JA, Carpenter LM, et al: Facts, figures and fallacies. Lancet 1993; 2:97–99, 157–160, 221–223, 286–288, 345–348, 418–421, 479–481, 530–532.

Treatment Techniques and Special Equipment

Upper Limb Amputee Rehabilitation and Prosthetic Restoration

ALBERTO ESQUENAZI, M.D.

INCIDENCE AND DEMOGRAPHICS

Based on the most recent information available from the National Center for Health Statistics, approximately 1,230,000 amputees are living in the United States (all levels of amputation) with an annual incidence of approximately 50,000 new amputations.[28] The ratio of upper limb to lower limb amputation estimated from this information is 1:4.9. The most frequent causes of upper limb amputation are trauma and cancer, followed by vascular complications of disease. The most common major upper limb amputation is that at the transradial level, which accounts for 57% of all arm amputations. Transhumeral amputation accounts for 23% of all amputations. The right arm is more frequently involved in work-related injuries. Sixty percent of arm amputees are between the ages of 21 and 64 years, and 10% are younger than 21 years.[11, 18]

Congenital upper limb deficiency has an incidence of approximately 4.1 per 10,000 live births.[28] The congenital limb deficiencies are best classified according to the International Organization of Standards and the International Society of Prosthetics and Orthotics classifications as modified from Frantz-O'Reilly. The limb deficiencies can be transverse or longitudinal. The term *terminal* is used to describe the fact that the limb has developed normally to a particular level, beyond which no skeletal element exists. In intercalary limb deficiency, a reduction or absence of one or more elements occurs within the long axis of the limb, and in this case normal skeletal elements may be found distal to the affected segments.[19] The most common congenital limb deficiency is the left terminal transverse radial limb deficiency (Table 14–1).

LIMB SALVAGE VS. AMPUTATION SURGERY

Severe hand injuries frequently challenge the skills of the surgeon to the point of having to consider amputation. The absolute surgical indication for amputation in trauma is ischemia in a limb with unreconstructible vascular injury. As reconstruction techniques have improved, more attempts at limb salvage have been made, although amputation is often ultimately required after multiple surgical procedures. Such surgical procedures also represent a substantial investment of time, money, and emotional energy. Massively crushed or burned muscle[10] and ischemic tissue release myoglobin and cell toxins, which can lead to renal failure, adult respiratory distress syndrome, and death. In addition, the risk of infection, contractures, and nerve injuries that interfere with function need to be considered. Recent studies show the value of early amputation not only in saving lives, but also in preventing the emotional, marital, and financial disasters and narcotic analgesic addictions that can follow desperate attempts at limb salvage.

In establishing guidelines for immediate or early amputation of mangled limbs the surgeon must bear in mind that for the upper limb, salvage should be based on providing an extremity that has sufficient sensation to provide protective feedback, has a durable soft tissue cover, and can be used to interact with the environment. An upper limb with limited motion, multiple scars, or lack of sensation functions poorly because of the constant risk of tissue injury. This type of limb often functions worse than a modern prosthetic replacement. Recently, grading scales for mangled lower limbs have been developed and should serve as guidelines

TABLE 14–1   International Terminology for the Classification of Congenital Limb Deficiencies

International Organization of Standards and the International Society of Prosthetics and Orthotics Classifications
Terminal: The limb has developed normally to a particular level, beyond which no skeletal elements exist. **Intercalary:** There is a reduction or absence of one or more elements within the long axis of the limb, and normal skeletal elements may be present distal to affected segment.

to help the surgeon assess the gravity of the injury and the subsequent risk of salvage.[13]

Amputation should never be viewed as surgical failure but rather as the means to return the patient to a more functional status. The value of approaching amputation with a positive and reconstructive approach cannot be overemphasized. The decision to amputate is an emotional process for all involved, and the rehabilitation team should stand ready to respond and assist early in the process.

The selection of the surgical level of amputation is probably one of the most important decisions that must be made for the amputee. The viability of soft tissue and the amount of skin coverage with adequate sensation usually determine the most distal possible functional level for amputation. After surgery, the patient with an upper limb amputation should ideally be able to use a prosthesis (either body or externally powered) during most of the day. Bony prominences, skin scars, soft tissue traction, shear, and perspiration can complicate prosthesis use. For these reasons the residual limb must be surgically constructed with care to optimize the intimacy of fit, maintain muscle balance, and allow assumption of stresses necessary to meet the limb's new function. New surgical techniques that permit myocutaneous transfers, skin expansion methods, and bony lengthening procedures are available to optimize the residual limb shape, size, and function.[15] This optimization should preferably be done at the time of the amputation, but it can be done in a second stage. Using a staged approach delays prosthetic fitting and can decrease the success of prosthetic restoration. Early prosthetic fitting after arm amputation (1 to 3 months) is imperative if successful prosthetic restoration is to be expected.[25] Once healing has occurred, prevention of scar tissue adhesion formation is critical.

Levels of Amputation

Finger amputation can occur at the distal interphalangeal, proximal interphalangeal, and metacarpophalangeal levels (Fig. 14–1). Transcarpal amputation and wrist amputation are seen less frequently because of their limited functional outcome. Multiple finger amputations, including thumb and partial hand amputations and those through the wrist, need to be considered carefully in view of the possible functional and cosmetic implications of prosthesis fitting and restoration. Inappropriate choice of amputation site can result in a prosthesis with disproportional length or width. It can also preclude the use of externally powered devices.

The transradial amputation is preferred in most cases; it

can be performed at three levels (resulting in long, medium, and short residual limbs). The long forearm residual limb is preferred when optimal body-powered prosthetic restoration is the goal. It is the ideal level for the patient who is expected to perform physically demanding work. The medium forearm residual limb is preferred when optimal externally powered prosthetic restoration is the goal. This length typically permits good function and cosmesis. The short transradial amputation level can complicate suspension and limit elbow flexion strength and elbow range of motion. These three amputation levels require the same type of rehabilitation interventions and make use of similar prosthetic components. The suspension system for each one of them can be different. Transradial amputation is the most common level and allows the highest level of functional recovery in the majority of cases.

The elbow disarticulation has some surgical and prosthetic advantages and disadvantages. The surgical technique permits reduction in surgery time and blood loss, provides improved prosthetic self-suspension while permitting the use of a less encumbering socket, and reduces the rotation of the socket on the residual limb, as compared with the transhumeral level of amputation.[37] Major disadvantages are the marginal cosmetic appearance caused by the necessary external elbow mechanism, as well as the current limitations in technology that impede the use of externally powered elbow mechanisms at this level of amputation. These drawbacks often outweigh the advantages

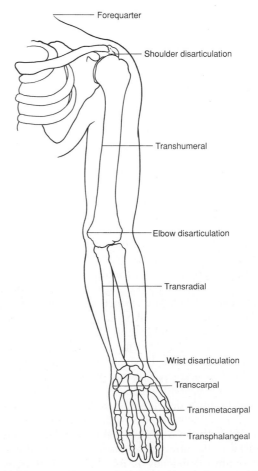

FIGURE 14–1   New terminology and levels for amputation.

in the long run. In the patient for whom bilateral transhumeral amputation is the alternative, the elbow disarticulation is a more desirable level when feasible, despite the possible cosmetic problems.

The transhumeral amputation can be performed at three levels (long, medium, and short residual limbs). The long arm residual limb (7 to 10 cm from the distal humeral condyle) is preferred for optimal prosthetic restoration. These three amputation levels require the same type of rehabilitation interventions and, in most cases, require similar prosthetic components, which can be externally powered, body powered, passive, or have a combination of these.

The shoulder disarticulation and forequarter amputations fortunately are seen less frequently than amputations at other levels. In most cases they are made necessary as part of the surgical intervention to remove a malignant lesion. Patients with these levels of amputation are the most difficult to fit with a functional prosthesis, due to the number of joints to be replaced and the problems related to maintaining secure suspension of the prosthesis.

In regard to surgical techniques, soft tissue handling is especially critical to wound healing and functional outcome in amputation surgery. When tissues are excessively traumatized, the risk of wound failure and infection are high. Flaps should be kept thick, and unnecessary dissection between the skin, subcutaneous, fascial, and muscle planes should be avoided. All bone edges should be rounded, and prominences should be beveled for optimal force transmission during prosthetic use. Split-thickness skin grafts are generally discouraged except as a means to save essential residual limb length and with the understanding that future surgical revision might be necessary. Skin grafts do best with adequate soft tissue support and are most durable when not adherent to bone. Muscle loses its contractile function when the skeletal attachments are divided during amputation. Stabilizing the distal insertion of muscle can improve residual limb function and comfort. *Myodesis* is the direct suturing of muscle or tendon to bone. This technique is most effective in stabilizing muscles that are needed to counteract strong antagonistic muscular forces. *Myoplasty* involves suturing of muscles to periosteum. Myoplasty does not provide as secure a distal stabilization of the muscle as does myodesis. Care must be taken to prevent having a mobile sling of muscle over the distal end of the bone, which can result in formation of a painful bursa that could interfere with prosthetic fitting and use.

All transected nerves form a neuroma. Nerves should be transacted cleanly, allowing the cut end to retract into the soft tissues away from the scar and prosthetic pressure points. The integrity of the peripheral nervous system should be assessed as early as feasible after traumatic amputation, because traction injuries frequently result in temporary or permanent nerve injury that have direct implications on arm function as well as on rehabilitation and prosthetic restoration programs.

The Amputee Rehabilitation Program

The amputee rehabilitation program should ideally be designed to cover the wide spectrum of care from pre-

amputation to reintegration into the community. The proposed stages are outlined in Table 14–2.[26]

Preamputation Counseling

During this stage it is essential to develop direct communication involving the patient, the family, and the surgeon regarding the need for amputation and the expected surgical outcome. Communication with the physiatrist, therapists, and other members of the treatment team should be facilitated. At this point, it is appropriate for the clinician to have introductory discussions about phantom limb sensation, prosthetic devices, prosthesis fitting and training, and the timing of these events. When possible, a demonstration of a prosthesis by a trained volunteer with a similar level of amputation and discussion of realistic expected functional outcomes should be arranged. Family involvement throughout this process should be encouraged. For all levels of amputation a "prehabilitation" program should include strengthening exercises to the trunk and remaining upper limb musculature and range of motion exercises for the involved glenohumeral, scapulothoracic, and elbow joints (if present).

Amputation Surgery

Partial hand amputations should be carefully planned to ensure adequate residual sensation and movement. There is little point in salvaging a partial hand if no metacarpals are present to provide pinch. Prosthetic restoration of the thumb should be attempted before any pollicization procedures or toe transfers are attempted. Many patients find that a thumb prosthesis provides adequate functional restoration, and they choose to forego further surgical reconstruction.[26] In addition, toe transfers can result in the partial loss of the normal foot function during walking.

Selecting a transhumeral level amputation over a transradial amputation presents a number of important dilemmas in rehabilitation. The lack of an anatomical elbow joint requires increased effort and cost for prosthetic restoration and results in greater impairment. The selection of the level of amputation should take into consideration the amount of space necessary for the appropriate prosthetic components with adequate cosmesis. The amputation has to be a minimum of 5 cm proximal to the distal radius to accommodate an externally powered terminal device. Transhumeral amputations should be performed 7 to 10 cm proximal to the distal humeral condyles to accommodate most of the prosthetic elbows. Longer residual limbs affect the

TABLE 14–2   **Stages of Amputee Rehabilitation**

Stages of Upper Limb Amputee Rehabilitation Program
1. Pre-amputation counseling
2. Amputation surgery
3. Acute post-amputation period
4. Preprosthesis training
5. Preparatory prosthesis fitting
6. Prosthesis fitting and training
7. Reintegration to the community
8. Long-term follow-up

location of the artificial elbow joint center of rotation, which can compromise cosmesis.

Transradial and Transhumeral Amputations

In the traumatic transradial and transhumeral amputation, it is not uncommon to find a more proximal fracture, a dislocation, or, occasionally, a peripheral nerve injury that can temporarily or permanently interfere with optimal prosthesis fitting and arm motion. Early diagnosis of these problems is needed to ensure inclusion of the necessary appropriate prosthetic modifications and alterations to the rehabilitation program.

Shoulder Disarticulation and Forequarter Amputation

Shoulder disarticulation is performed in severe trauma cases and in tumor surgery. Prosthetic replacement in these cases is more successful in those who are healthy, young, and male. In the majority of cases, the loss of the anatomical shoulder necessitates the use of an external prosthetic shoulder joint. This joint requires control mechanisms in addition to the body-powered or externally powered control mechanisms needed for the elbow, wrist, and hand.

Forequarter amputation is rarely performed, but it can be required in some cases of severe trauma or malignant lesion involving the shoulder. Functional prosthetic use is uncommon after this procedure, as suspension is difficult to maintain. Special considerations should be made for providing a shoulder cap to allow the patient to wear clothing more easily and to improve cosmesis. The use of an ultralight passive prosthesis is usually well accepted by the patient.

Acute Post-amputation Period

Pain control, maintenance of range of motion and strength, and promotion of wound healing (Table 14–3) are the goals of this stage, which begins with the surgical closure of the wound and culminates with wound healing. Pain control and residual limb maturation should be pursued aggressively. Immediate application of postoperative plaster of Paris rigid dressing (IPORD) or soft elastic bandage and subsequent pneumatic compression are indicated for edema control. An increasingly popular method of wound protection, swelling control, early shaping and soft tissue shrinking, and return to function is the immediate postoperative prosthesis, as reported by Malone and others.[24] Soft compressive dressings or Unna bandages are used in many centers.[9] The dressing should be extended to the proximal joint to better control swelling and to improve

the joint suspension. Proper postoperative positioning and rehabilitation are essential to prevent elbow flexion and shoulder adduction contractures when wounds are present over or close to the joints. This is most important if the wounds are caused by burn injuries.

Acute Pain Management

Pain control can be best achieved initially with a patient-controlled analgesia (PCA) system, followed by the use of scheduled parenteral and oral analgesia. A skin desensitization program that includes gentle tapping, massage, soft tissue and scar mobilization, and lubrication is recommended for the patient with a soft or elastic dressing.

When the patient's condition is medically stable, early mobilization, general endurance, and strengthening exercise are started. Special attention is paid to the shoulder and scapulae and to the prevention of joint contractures. It is also important to carefully observe the remaining limbs, especially their strength and function, with attention to switching hand dominance if necessary. At this time, emotional counseling for the patient and the family should begin, with special focus on the significant other and children. Psychosocial evaluation of the patient and family should be initiated to assess and manage depression and/or anxiety. It is important during this phase to promote patient participation in the decision-making process to encourage independence and a sense of control.

Postoperative Care

Postoperative edema is common following amputation. If soft dressings are used they should be combined with elastic wrapping to control edema, especially if the patient is a candidate for a prosthesis. The ideal shape of the upper extremity residual limb is cylindrical, not conical. The major complication from elastic wrapping is applying the bandage too tightly at the proximal end in an attempt to improve bandage suspension. This causes congestion, worsens edema, and results in a dumb-bell shaped residual limb. The recommended elastic dressing involves the use of a figure-of-8 wrapping technique that extends over the proximal joint and that is reapplied every 4 to 6 hours.

The use of an IPORD to control postoperative edema, promote healing, protect the limb from trauma, decrease postoperative pain, desensitize the limb, and allow early mobilization and rehabilitation is the preferred treatment approach (Table 14–4). In some centers, the rigid dressing is applied and managed by a team of specialists that includes the surgeon, the physiatrist, and the prosthetist. In other facilities where the team approach to amputee

---

TABLE 14–3   Frequently Utilized Wound Dressing Systems

Postoperative Wound Dressings
Immediate postoperative rigid dressing
Immediate postoperative prosthesis
Elastic bandage dressing
Unna bandage
Soft dressing

TABLE 14–4   Indications for IPORD (Immediate Postoperative Rigid Dressing)

IPORD Functions
Pain control
Promote wound healing
Protection from trauma
Edema control
Desensitization
Prevent contractures

management has not been implemented, the dressing can be applied by a trained clinician. The dressing is made out of plaster of Paris bandages that extend beyond the proximal joint for suspension. An IPORD should be replaced at 1-week intervals. By the time the second dressing is replaced, the prosthesis can be casted and a few days later it can be fitted. If the patient has a fever for which no other apparent cause can be determined, the IPORD should be removed and the wound inspected. The IPORD should be reapplied if the wound shows no signs of infection.

Phantom Limb, Phantom Pain, and Painful Residual Limb

Phantom limb sensation is the feeling that all or a part of the amputated limb is still present. This sensation is felt by nearly all "acquired" amputees, but is not always bothersome.[27] Phantom sensation usually diminishes over time, and telescoping (the sensation that the phantom hand has moved proximally) commonly occurs. Phantom sensation is not necessarily painful. As many as 70% of amputees perceive phantom pain in the first few months after amputation. However, such pain usually disappears or decreases sufficiently so that it does not interfere with prosthesis fitting and day-to-day activities.[5] A smaller percentage of patients experience long-term pain, whereas others have recurrent pain later in life. When pain persists for more than 6 months, the prognosis for spontaneous improvement is poor, and it can be extremely difficult to treat successfully. Perceived pain intensity is closely related to anxiety level, depression, prosthesis fitting problems, and other personal factors.[36]

The traditional explanation for phantom sensation and pain is that the remaining nerves in the amputated limb continue to generate impulses that flow through the spinal cord and the thalamus to the somatosensory areas of the cerebral cortex. Another theory suggests that the phantom arises from excessive, spontaneous firing of spinal cord neurons that have lost their normal sensory input from the missing body part. Another suggests that the phantom sensation is caused by changes in the flow of signals through the somatosensory circuit in the brain.[27]

Appropriate management of phantom limb begins by preventing prolonged periods of pain before the amputation, because preamputation pain often ends in postoperative phantom pain. Treatment includes prosthetic socket revisions, desensitization techniques, transcutaneous nerve stimulation, neuropharmacological intervention, and the voluntary control of the phantom limb (mental imaging). For severe cases, nerve blocks, steroid injections, and epidural blocks can be useful. Nonsurgical interventions are far more successful than surgical ones.[17] Clearly, the etiology of the phantom limb phenomenon is more complex than any of the theories here presented would suggest, and treatment can be complex. An important issue to discuss with the patient is normal phantom sensation, phantom pain, and the relationship between phantom pain and tension, anxiety, stress, and pain perception.

Joint Contractures

Joint contractures can occur between the time of amputation and prosthesis fitting. Efforts should be directed at preventing contractures with aggressive rehabilitation efforts, beginning soon after surgery. If burns or severe trauma with proximal fractures are the cause of amputation, special attention should be given to the prevention of frozen shoulder and contractures induced by scar tissue formation. In the case of peripheral nerve or brachial plexus injury, appropriate positioning, splinting, and passive and assisted range of motion should be implemented to preserve joint mobility.

Preprosthetic Rehabilitation

It is not unusual for patients with amputations to be provided with artificial limbs without much attention being paid to prosthetic training or other special needs. With the advent of specialized treatment teams, regional centers, and new prosthetic devices, the outlook for the upper limb amputee has improved. A preprosthesis rehabilitation program must be initiated as soon as possible.[8] Pain control and residual limb maturation should be promoted during this phase. An IPORD or soft elastic bandages are indicated for edema control. This is also a time for the patient to initiate emotional adaptation to a body image without the artificial limb, and to learn basic skills without a prosthesis, which is essential for the times when the device is not worn. Soft tissue desensitization, early mobilization, improving general endurance, strengthening, avoidance of joint contractures, and emotional counseling are the key goals of this phase.

Often, limb loss is interpreted in our society as punishment for a misdeed. An amputation typically causes patients to initiate a process of introspection and reassessment of goals. This process can result in an individual taking a more mature approach toward life goals and actively pursuing plans. Occasionally, however, a patient can become so emotionally disturbed by the limb loss that the result can be a chronic failure to cope. This can have a very negative effect on the rehabilitation outcome.[6]

The use of the first prosthesis should be implemented as soon as possible in this stage. The early fitting of the prosthetic device is intended to promote prosthesis use. As reported by Malone and others[24, 25] there is a direct relationship between the time of fitting and long-term prosthetic use. There is a 3- to 6-months window of opportunity for the unilateral upper limb amputee. If a prosthesis is fitted during this period, there is a much greater rate of acceptance of the artificial arm.

The first prosthesis is intended to promote residual limb maturation and desensitization, to build up wearing tolerance, and to allow the patient to become a functional user. Commonly, this is done with a body-powered or a switch-controlled externally powered prosthesis. Suction suspension or myoelectric control is not practical at this stage because of limb volume fluctuation that results in the loss of the necessary intimate contact of the socket and electrodes with the soft tissues. When no significant volume fluctuation is noted in the residual limb over a period of 2 months, consideration should be given to proceeding with fitting of the first permanent prosthesis. Serial circumferential measurements of the limb at pre-established locations is the simplest method of determining residual limb size stability. Volumetric measurements in a water displacement chamber or with a computer-aided design system are more precise, although more time-consuming, techniques.

Prosthesis Fitting and Training

Prosthesis prescription options for the amputee have changed greatly since the mid-1980s. Selecting the most appropriate componentry for prosthetic restoration of the upper limb is an extremely challenging task in view of the variety and complexity of available prosthetic components (prosthetic terminal devices, wrists, elbows, and shoulders), socket fabrication techniques, suspension systems, and sources of power and control. This task should be accomplished by an expert team of professionals in close communication with the patient. Members of the team ideally should include the surgeon, a physiatrist who devotes time in practice to amputee rehabilitation and prosthetics, a certified prosthetist, an occupational therapist, a physical therapist, a recreational therapist, a psychologist, a social worker, and the patient and family. Other specialists can be added to the team as needed. The team members can best service the needs of the patient if they have significant experience in the specialized rehabilitation techniques for the upper limb amputee and prosthetic fabrication and training. This typically occurs most commonly in large, specialized regional rehabilitation centers.

Terminal Devices

The functional capacity of the upper limb is determined by the development of multiple integrated spheres of action by the shoulder complex, elbow, wrist, and hand. Given the normal proportions of limb segments, this capacity is limited in relation to the surrounding space. The functional activities of the hand are extensive, but they can be grouped into non-prehensile and prehensile activities. The former include touching, feeling, pressing down with the fingers, tapping, vibrating the cord of a musical instrument, and lifting or pushing with the hand. Prehensile activities are grouped into precision and power grips. Three-jaw chuck involves grip with the thumb and index and middle fingers. A lateral or key grip involves contact of the pulp of the thumb with the lateral aspect of the corresponding finger. These two patterns provide precision prehension. Power grip predominantly involves the ulnar aspect of the hand, with less involvement of the ring and little fingers. The hook power grip involves flexion of both interphalangeal joints and minimal participation of the metacarpophalangeal (MCP) joint. This grip pattern is used in carrying a briefcase. The spherical grip is very much like the power grip but with minimal flexion of the fingers, which are abducted and rotated; the thumb is used to stabilize the object and to provide counterpressure.

Most patients who suffer an upper limb amputation and undergo prosthetic restoration require a terminal device for their prosthesis. The human hand is a very complex anatomical and physiological structure whose functions cannot be replaced by the current level of prosthetic technology. A variety of prosthetic terminal devices are available and include passive, body-powered, and externally powered hooks and hands (Fig. 14–2). They all lack sensory feedback and have limited mobility and dexterity. Prosthetic hands provide a three-jaw chuck pinch and

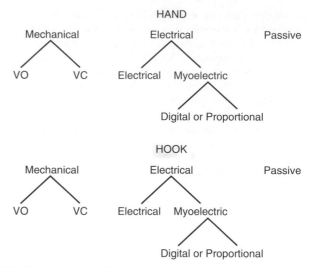

FIGURE 14–2 Classification of terminal devices. Abbreviations: VO, voluntary opening; VC, voluntary closing.

hooks provide the equivalent of lateral or tip pinch. Body-powered terminal devices can be voluntary-opening (most common and practical) or voluntary-closing (most physiological). The voluntary-opening device is maintained in the closed position by rubber bands or tension springs. The patient can open the device by "pulling" with the cable on the harness system in preparation to grasp. To grasp, the patient releases the opened terminal device on an object; the rubber bands or spring provide the prehensile force. The maximum prehensile force possible is predetermined by the number of springs or rubber bands. To control the amount of prehensile force, the patient must generate an opening force all the time. Voluntary-closing terminal devices, require that the patient close the device by "pulling" with the cable on the harness system to grasp an object. To release, the patient releases the pull on the harness, and a spring in the terminal device opens it. The maximum prehensile force possible is determined by the strength of the individual. One major disadvantage of this system is that prolonged prehension requires constant pull on the harness. The human hand normally does not reach out to grasp an object in the closed position, but rather uses the semi-open position to facilitate the interaction with the environment.

Externally powered devices can have digital (on/off) or proportional (stronger signal = faster action) control systems.

Prosthetic Wrists

The type of prosthetic wrist (Table 14–5) most commonly used allows passive pronation and supination. Spring-assisted rotation is available for the bilateral amputee. Quick-disconnect wrists are also available. The friction control permits for ease of positioning, but it can rotate when lifting heavy objects. This is particularly problematic when the wearer is carrying a plate or tray. Quick-disconnect wrists permit rapid interchange of different terminal devices. In addition, when it is locked, the quick-disconnect wrist provides a secure control for wrist rotation. An externally powered, switch, or myoelectric control wrist prono-

TABLE 14–5   Types of Prosthetic Wrists

MECHANICAL
   Pronosupination
      Friction
      Quick-disconnect
      Spring-assisted
   Flexion
      Spring-assisted internal or external
ELECTRIC
   Pronosupination
      Myoelectric
      Switch control

supination system exists, but it is prescribed infrequently. A mechanical spring-assisted wrist flexion unit is indispensable for the bilateral upper limb amputee. This device permits the patient to reach the body's midline for grooming, feeding, hygiene activities, and buttoning of clothing.

Prosthetic Elbows

The prosthetic elbows available in the treatment of transhumeral amputation have either external or internal joints. These joints can be passive, body-powered, or externally powered (Figs. 14–3 and 14–4). These devices are controlled via mechanical cables, electric switches, or myoelectric signals (Table 14–6). The externally powered systems have digital or proportional control mechanisms. The mechanical elbows have a locking mechanism that is manually applied using the contralateral hand, the chin, or the ipsilateral shoulder via a cable system. Electric elbows have an electromechanical brake or a switch-controlled lock mechanism to maintain the selected position. The rotation function of the arm (internal/external rotation) is provided through the use of a turntable. This device is useful to provide reach to the body midline. Electric elbows have limited active flexion force. The flexion force across a mechanical elbow is dependent on the wearer's strength, the comfort of the socket fit, and the ability to efficiently transfer the power from the residual limb to the prosthesis.

For elbow disarticulation, the external elbow joint is indicated in an attempt to maintain the optimal length of the arm. This joint is larger and protrudes in the medial aspect. Limited flexion strength and increased maintenance are some of the problems with this type of joint.

Prosthetic Sockets

Socket configuration and materials have improved greatly since the mid-1980s. The key functions of a pros-

TABLE 14–6   Classification of Prosthetic Elbows

BODY-POWERED ELBOW
   External, with or without spring-assisted flexion
   Internal, with or without spring-assisted flexion
   Internal, with rotating turntable

EXTERNAL-POWERED ELBOW
   Digital switch control
   Proportional switch control
   Digital myoelectric control
   Proportional myoelectric control

PASSIVE ELBOW
   Manual lock

TABLE 14–7   The Key Functions of the Prosthetic Socket

Comfortable residual limb–prosthesis interface
Efficient energy transference to the prosthesis
Secure suspension of the prosthesis
Adequate cosmesis

thetic socket include comfortable total contact interface with the residual limb, efficient energy transfer from the residual limb to the prosthetic device, secure suspension, and cosmetic appearance (Table 14–7). A patient often fails to accept the prosthesis if the socket does not provide most of these characteristics.

Sockets used in the past were carved of wood. These sockets had the disadvantage of being open-ended, which promoted distal residual limb swelling with potential development of chronic edema and trophic skin changes. With the development of high-temperature rigid plastic materials such as polyester resin, sockets with decreased weight and increased durability could be molded to have total contact. More recently, acrylic lamination, the use of carbon graphite, and the introduction of flexible thermoplastics have permitted the design of sockets with windows that are lined with flexible materials and are more comfortable, lighter, and durable. Most upper limb prosthetic sockets have two layers. The first one is closely contoured to the residual limb, whereas the external layer is used to give the necessary length and shape to the socket. It is to this external layer that the necessary prosthetic components (e.g., elbow, wrist) are attached.

Sockets are custom made by obtaining a negative impression of the residual limb by plaster of Paris wrap. This is then converted to a positive mold that can be modified by the prosthetist to appropriately distribute pressure throughout the entire surface of the residual limb. Routinely, a transparent plastic socket is first manufactured to permit direct visualization of the soft tissues. The transparent socket can be modified to ensure comfortable total contact. Eventually a final socket is fabricated. The concepts of computer-assisted design (CAD) and computer-assisted manufacturing (CAM) have been adapted to prosthesis fabrication. Direct surface video imaging of the residual limb, ultrasound and/or magnetic resonance imaging, and direct digitization from a plaster of Paris mold are being used in some centers as sources of digital data to be manipulated in a computer environment. From that point, a computer-controlled carver can create a positive mold of wax or plaster from which a socket can be manufactured from vacuum-formed thermoplastics.[2]

New flexible plastic materials have made sockets lighter and more comfortable.[11] The use of these new materials in prosthetics has resulted in the development of improved socket construction techniques.[16, 21, 30] The inner socket provides total contact with the residual limb and is the interface that provides suction suspension if desired. The outer socket or frame is made of a more rigid material, thermoplastic or resin, and provides the structural integrity of the socket. When double sockets are used, windows can be cut out in the exterior frame to allow muscles to expand during contraction and to improve comfort and sensory feedback. The elasticity of the thermoplastic material re-

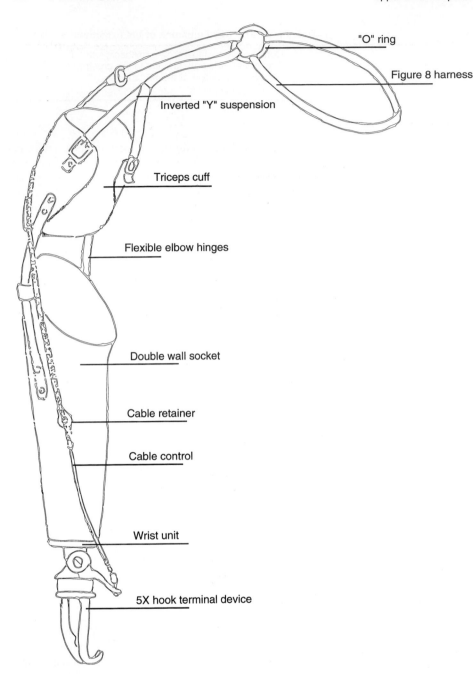

"O" ring

Figure 8 harness

Inverted "Y" suspension

Triceps cuff

Flexible elbow hinges

Double wall socket

Cable retainer

Cable control

Wrist unit

5X hook terminal device

FIGURE 14–3 Transhumeral level body-powered prosthetic components.

sults in a more comfortable fit. Although more costly and time-consuming to fabricate initially, the frame socket design has the added advantage of allowing replacement of the inner socket to accommodate small residual limb changes without changing the external frame to which the other prosthetic components are attached. It is a fairly simple process to pull out the old liner and slip in a new one. The inner socket is usually held in place by Velcro or another removable fastener. The frame socket design is particularly appealing for externally powered prostheses and self-suspended ones (wrist and elbow disarticulation and Muenster sockets). One disadvantage of these materials is their poor temperature insulation characteristics, which make them uncomfortable during cold weather. This can be partially corrected by using clothing layers to cover the arm.

Suspension Systems

The suspension and control system of a body-powered prosthesis needs to provide two distinct important functions to make the prosthetic device work. One of these is suspension, which is the means of securing the prosthetic device to the body. The other is to permit control of the prosthesis, including the terminal device. The more secure the suspension system the more prosthetic control and comfort can be expected by the patient. The upper limb amputee has traditionally been provided with suspension systems that are uncomfortable and that limit mobility. They consist mostly of straps with metal and plastic attachments. The traditional suspension mechanisms (Table 14–8) for the upper limb sockets include a strap that suspends the prosthesis over the shoulder (figure-of-8 harness). The

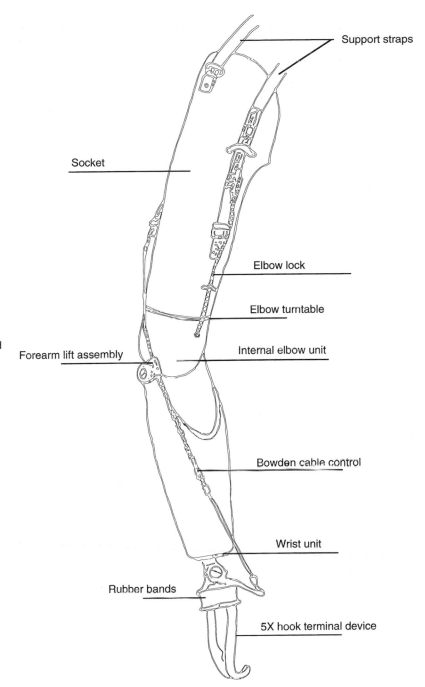

Support straps

Socket

Elbow lock

Elbow turntable

Forearm lift assembly

Internal elbow unit

Bowden cable control

Wrist unit

Rubber bands

5X hook terminal device

FIGURE 14–4 Transradial level body-powered prosthetic components.

harness is used as a control mechanism to transmit body power to the terminal device and elbow. For the more proximal level amputation, a chest strap or shoulder saddle can be used to further improve suspension. Patients with wrist or elbow disarticulation or transradial amputations can use bony prominences for suspension. The Muenster[14] or condylar suspension is perhaps the best of these. When this type of suspension is used, a figure-of-9 harness can be used for control purposes only.

The transradial Muenster socket design was developed in Germany in the early 1950s[14] and was later modified at Northwestern University. This socket configuration provides excellent suspension by encasing the elbow condyles. The main disadvantage is the limitation in elbow range of

motion for terminal extension and flexion. This can prevent its use as the preferred type of suspension for the patient with bilateral transradial amputations. This type of suspension works extremely well with externally powered, myoelectric control prostheses, as the patient can be completely free of straps.

In most cases, a sock is used as an interface between the residual limb and the socket. Using different numbers of sock layers can adjust for the physiological volume changes that occur from day to day. Socks also protect the skin and improve hygiene. The only exceptions are suction sockets, for which direct skin-to-socket contact is required, and socks cannot be used.

Hypobaric and semi-suction suspension is best thought

TABLE 14–8 Prosthetic Suspension Systems

Harness	Semisuction
Figure-of-8	Hypobaric
Chest strap	Semisuction
Shoulder saddle	Suction
Self-suspension	Full suction
Condylar	Silicone sock
Muenster	
Northwestern	

of as a transition between nonsuction and full-suction suspension. This suspension system utilizes socks that have a special silicone band in them, and the socket is provided with a one-way valve that permits the expulsion of air during donning. The band creates a seal between the socket and the skin of the residual limb and permits the development of suction that can be used for suspension. The advantage of this suspension system is that changes in residual limb volume that typically occur early in the rehabilitation process can be accommodated simply by altering the number of plies (thicknesses) of socks used.

Control Mechanisms

When a body harness is used as a control mechanism for a body-powered prosthesis, the patient needs to be able to produce movements that generate the power requirements to activate the terminal device or elbow. These movements include scapular abduction; chest expansion; shoulder depression, extension, and abduction and humeral flexion; and elbow flexion and extension (Fig. 14–5). These movements can be difficult to perform if the residual limb is short, painful, or has limited motion, or if the prosthetic socket does not fit well. A poorly adjusted harness decreases the power transmission of the movements.[7]

Electric switch control mechanisms can be activated with residual limb movements that depress a switch inside the socket. For other cases, a chest strap, waist belt, or figure-of-9 harness can be used. Servo controls that sense tension have been introduced to clinical use.

Myoelectric controls use the electrical activity generated during a muscle contraction to control the flow of energy from a battery to a motor in the prosthetic device. The control signals come from muscle sites in the amputated limb that still have normal innervation and voluntary con-

trol.[31] Ideally, muscles in the more distal portion of the residual limb should be used. Antagonistic muscles are best for this function (i.e., wrist or elbow flexor/extensor). This ensures that the control is easy to use, physiological, consistent, and precise. At times, more proximal muscles or muscles in the trunk or other limb can be used. Systems that use single-channel control mechanisms use two electrode sites; one to trigger hand closure or elbow flexion and the other to trigger hand opening or elbow extension. Multi-channel systems permit the use of one muscle to control two different functions. This requires that the patient be able to produce a slow, gentle muscle contraction for one function and a strong, faster one for the other function. Myoelectronic prosthetic components, such as the Utha arm, use an "electronic switch" to alternate between the hand and the elbow function. Some systems also include proportional controls, which respond to the speed and strength of the muscle contraction by correspondingly producing a faster or slower movement of the hand or elbow. A very snug fit of the socket is required to avoid shift of the muscles in reference to the electrodes for proper function. Hybrid systems combine two or more of the available control mechanisms, either electric or body-powered.

Suction Suspension

For the transhumeral amputee, suction suspension (negative pressure) without the use of straps is the preferred type of suspension. For this system to work well, and to be able to don the prosthesis independently, the patient should have good contralateral upper limb strength, endurance, and coordination. The socket is made small enough and provided with a one-way valve that permits the expulsion of air during donning. The amputee dons the socket using a pull sock or ace bandage or with a wet fit (using a lubricant liquid or powder). The intimate fit between the socket and the skin of the residual limb, especially distally, results in a tight seal between the socket and skin. Doffing requires breaking the vacuum seal. To maintain proper suspension over time, the residual limb must be mature and volume stable.[9]

The silicone suction sock is also useful for prosthetic suspension. It requires less effort to don and functions well with a less intimate fit. The silicone is moistened with alcohol or powder for lubrication and rolled over the skin. Then it is covered with at least one sock to allow sliding of the residual limb with the silicone sock into the socket. A distal pin or strap is then used to attach the prosthesis to the silicone sock and, in turn, to the patient. Silicone socks can also be used without the suspension system.

Shoulder Disarticulation and Forequarter Amputation

There has been little change in the basic socket design for shoulder disarticulation or forequarter amputation since it was designed. The main changes have been modification of the socket trim lines and suspension and use of lighter materials to construct the socket. As in sockets for other levels of amputation, thermoplastic and silicone materials are being used to provide lighter, more secure, and more comfortable sockets at these proximal levels of amputation.

- Scapular abduction = Terminal device activation

- Chest expansion = Terminal device activation

- Humeral flexion = Terminal device activation

- Shoulder depression, extension, and abduction = Elbow lock activation

---

FIGURE 14–5 Body control motions typically used for prosthesis activation.

Most of the advances in prosthetic design for these levels have occurred with externally powered components, which are described elsewhere in this chapter. A shoulder joint with a manual lock that provides improvement in the arm control and position is now available.

Cosmetic Covers

Cosmetic covers can be manufactured for a single digit, for the hand, or to extend to the elbow. They should be considered an integral part of the prosthesis, because for many patients the cover is the factor that determines success or failure of prosthetic restoration. Custom-made silicone cosmetic covers can provide excellent cosmetic results, but they can be very expensive and difficult to maintain, and they deteriorate over time. Intrinsic coloration is a newer technique that provides a more realistic look. The colors are integrated at the time of fabrication instead of painting the cover after it has been applied to the arm.

Activity-Specific Devices

To optimally perform at work, sports, or recreational activities, it may be necessary to provide the patient with a specially designed terminal device. Many devices are commercially available that are designed for participation in sports (e.g., golf, fishing, skiing). Many more have been designed by the users for activities such as construction, cooking, archery, and photography.

Prosthetic Prescription

The prosthetic prescription should be carefully prepared to satisfy the needs and desires of the patient. A team approach to prescription writing should be used. The prescription should clearly spell out the components, control system, suspension, materials, and any special features that might be required. The prescription should serve to clearly communicate with the prosthetist and the insurance company. A clear, well-thought-out, organized prescription should achieve this.

Prosthetic Training

Training is integral to the rehabilitation process. A new amputee or an experienced one who receives a prosthetic device that has different components should participate in such training. In most cases, this program should be a coordinated effort among the occupational, physical, and recreational therapists and the prosthetist, with frequent physiatric input (kinesiotherapists are also used at some centers). Each of the team members uses different techniques to teach what needs to be learned by the amputee. Before initiating a program of upper limb prosthetic training, one must realistically orient the patient to what the prosthesis can and cannot do.[1] The patient should learn prosthetic management, including the basic principles behind the function, care, and maintenance of each of the components in the prosthesis. The patient should practice independently putting on and taking off the prosthesis. Skin care and inspection techniques are also reviewed. For the body-powered devices, dismounting the harness for washing and replacing it should be practiced. Written in-

struction can be useful for explaining the care and maintenance of the batteries used in externally powered devices. A review and practice of the use of the prosthesis for bimanual activities, such as grooming, dressing, feeding, driving, sports, work, and recreation activities, should always be included in the training process.

Special Considerations for the Bilateral Upper Limb Amputee

For the bilateral upper limb amputee, training should promote the development of a dominant prosthesis and skills for independent donning. Alternative techniques for putting on the prosthesis are frequently required. This might include using the bed for setup and suspending the prosthetic devices from special wall hooks or frames. The prosthesis should have a wrist flexion device that permits access to the body midline.

For bathing activities, the patient with bilateral upper limb amputations ideally should have a modified shower with wall brushes and liquid soap dispensers. In some cases, simplified shower prostheses (devices that are waterproof), are a medical necessity, because they allow the patient to perform this activity independently.

Brachial Plexus and Other Nerve Injuries

Brachial plexus injuries can be the result of many different causes, which can be divided into two main categories: closed injuries and open penetrating trauma (see Chapter 47). The majority of cases are caused by closed injuries. Traction on the upper plexus and the C5 and C6 roots occurs when the head and neck are stretched away from the shoulder. When the arm is stretched overhead, traction to the lower plexus and C8 and T1 roots occurs most frequently. The injuries can be pre-ganglionic (indicating injury or avulsion of the nerve root proximal to the spinal ganglion) with resulting severe or even complete motor and sensory loss. This can also be accompanied by Horner's syndrome. Postganglionic injuries occur distal to the spinal ganglion and tend to have a more favorable prognosis (Table 14–9).

Reintegration to the Community

Reintegration to the community is best done as a gradual process over a few weeks or months. This process can be initiated early in the rehabilitation program with the supervision of the team members during organized trips for shopping, recreation, and part-time work or school. When possible, the use of "day hospital" rehabilitation

TABLE 14–9   Types and Common Causes of Brachial Plexus Injuries

Brachial Plexus Injuries	
Closed Injuries	*Penetrating Injuries*
Traction	Gunshot
Compression	Fracture
Combined	Knife
Radiation	

programs, in which the patient participates in rehabilitation for 6 hours/day, 5 days/week (with return to home every evening and weekend) is a good system to foster community reintegration.

The patient can return to work when safety concerns are met.[20] Initially, modified or restricted work should be provided, but the patient should not be discouraged from returning to the premorbid work level if it is safe to do so. The use of a partial "day hospital" rehabilitation program in which the patient participates in rehabilitation for 3 hours/day, 5 days/week or 6 hours/day, 2 to 3 days/week also encourages and allows time for the return to part-time work in the community. The availability of psychological counseling and/or assistance from the team members during each of these steps is important for the smooth transition of patients and their families to independent functioning.

Functional Outcomes

Realistic goals for the majority of unilateral transradial or transhumeral amputees include independence in all activities of daily living, most household activities, driving, and work (Table 14–10). Some restrictions should be imposed in relationship to handling delicate, heavy, or voluminous objects. The typical patient with a transradial amputation can be expected to lift 20 to 30 lb, unless the residual limb is very short or sensitive. The typical patient with a transhumeral amputation can be expected to lift 10 to 15 lb, unless the residual limb is very short or sensitive. This is also affected by the type of elbow used.

For the bilateral transhumeral amputee, realistic goals include independence in most activities of daily living after assisted donning, some household activities, driving with a spin ring, and most types of sedentary work. Restrictions should be imposed in relationship to handling delicate, heavy (15 lb, unless the residual limb is very short or sensitive), or voluminous objects.

If work is to take place where magnetic fields or large electrical currents are present, myoelectric prostheses may not work well unless special shielding materials are used during fabrication, to prevent interference.

Long-Term Follow-up

The patient who has successfully completed a rehabilitation program should be seen for follow-up by a minimum of two of the team members at least every 3 months for the first 18 months. These visits might need to be more frequent and include other members of the team if the patient is having difficulties with prosthesis fitting, the residual limb, specific activities, or psychosocial adjustment. After this critical period, the patient should be seen at least every 6

TABLE 14–10   Typical Functional Outcomes for Upper Limb Amputation With Prosthesis

Unilateral transradial or transhumeral
Independent ADLs, household activities, driving, and work, with some limitations
Bilateral amputation
After assisted donning of prosthesis, independent ADLs, household activities, driving, and work, with many limitations

months to ensure adequate prosthetic fit and function and to assess the need for maintenance and the overall medical condition and functional level of the patient. When the patient's condition is stable it may be necessary to replace a prosthesis or parts of it every 18 months to 3 years for body-powered devices and every 2 to 4 years for myoelectric prostheses.

Neuromas

Neuroma is the formation of scar tissue around the distal end of the severed nerve. As previously mentioned, every time a nerve is cut it forms a neuroma. Good surgical technique results in the neuroma being buried under large soft tissue masses that serve to protect it from irritation. At times, because of limited soft tissue coverage or very large neuroma formation with compression of the nerve, adhesion of the tissues, or complications from the surgical technique, a neuroma may become symptomatic. This results in pain that can be perceived at the site of the neuroma and that radiates distally to the end of the residual limb (or, at times, into the phantom limb). A painful neuroma is palpable most of the time, and pressure over it reproduces the symptoms. Desensitization techniques, prosthetic modifications, and, at times, use of flexible materials with windowed frame construction to decrease pressure over the neuroma may help. Injection of the neuroma with a mixture of long-and short-acting local anesthetics and a corticosteroid should reduce the scar tissue pressure on the nerve and produce symptomatic improvement. When correctly performed, this technique reproduces the presenting symptoms with increasing severity as the needle is advanced. The injection can be repeated three times at 6- to 8-week intervals. Surgical removal of the neuroma with careful retraction of the nerve prior to cutting it should be reserved for those cases in which all other interventions have failed and in which the tissues allow repositioning of the neuroma to a less-exposed location.

Support Groups

Support groups are a source of information, peer counseling, and motivation for many patients. These groups ideally should constitute one more component of the comprehensive rehabilitation approach to the patient with an amputation. Patients who have recently sustained an amputation benefit from the exposure to members who are experienced amputees; at the same time, the veteran amputee enjoys serving as a resource. This forum can also be used effectively as a resource for the family of the patient with an amputation.

Dermatological Problems

The skin of a patient who wears a prosthesis is subject to much abuse. Most prosthetic sockets prevent appropriate air circulation, thereby trapping perspiration moisture. This can result in a variety of problems such as hyperhidrosis, folliculitis, allergic dermatitis, and even skin breakdown where adherent scars are present. Poor hygiene is frequently the cause of some of these problems, and for this reason the patient should be trained in the proper washing technique for the residual limb, socks, and the socket and its interfaces. A daily routine of washing the skin and the internal wall of the socket with a mild soap might suffice. It can be necessary at times to use concentrated antiperspirants, bacteriostatic or bactericidal soaps, and, in some cases, antibiotics. Topical antibiotics or steroids should not generally be used if the prosthesis has silicone components as part of the socket materials that are in direct contact with the skin. Contact dermatitis frequently occurs because of this.[23]

PEDIATRIC LIMB DEFICIENCY AND AMPUTATION REHABILITATION

The pediatric patient can have an acquired or congenital limb deficiency. The child with a congenital limb deficiency has no sense of loss and does not have to go through the psychological adjustment process. The prosthesis is perceived as an aid rather than as a replacement. If the device cannot serve in this role it will be discarded. These children try to engage in the same types of activities as other children. Their only limitations are usually those imposed by adults. In contrast, the child with an acquired limb deficiency goes through the natural readjustment process of limb loss. How well they are able to adjust has a direct impact on their acceptance of an artificial limb.[36] Some special considerations should be made for the pediatric patient with upper limb deficiency or amputation.[12] Three specific points to consider in this population are (1) normal growth and development, which will necessitate frequent prosthetic adjustments or replacements; (2) bony overgrowth; and (3) the more rigorous use that the device will be subjected to. It can be expected that a prosthesis (socket only, or all of it) will need to be replaced yearly in the first 5 years of life, every 18 months from 5 to 12 years of age, and every 2 years until age 21 years.[3] To address growth problems, multilayered sockets (onion sockets) for body-powered devices can be used. These allow removal of one layer at a time to accommodate growth. This results in gradual enlargement of the socket to coincide with periods of growth. The socket made in this fashion increases the life span of the prosthesis from 6 months to as much as 18 months. Length adjustment is also important, although it is not as critical as with lower limb prostheses. This can be adjusted by adding material at the wrist or elbow sites when necessary. Harnesses and cables need to be adjusted for length and replaced more frequently.[4] For bony overgrowth, surgery with bony capping may be necessary.[22] For myoelectric devices, two problems are noted: (1) the limitation imposed by weight and size of the components[29] and (2) the necessary frequent alterations to the socket to maintain optimal electrode contact as the residual limb size changes. Frequently required socket replacements can make myoelectric devices less practical for this population due to their cost. Terminal devices and elbows might need to be replaced frequently. Prosthetic component banks are available in some countries, which make myoelectric prosthetic component replacement less expensive.

Parental counseling and support are integral components in the rehabilitation of the pediatric amputee. The prosthetic fitting for the pediatric patient with upper limb deficiency or the pediatric amputee should be initiated at 3 to 9 months of age. This should coincide with sitting and the initiation of bimanual activities. The use of a passive mitten, hand, or inactive hook or California Amputee Pediatric Project (CAPP) terminal device and a preflexed fixed elbow are indicated at this stage. The terminal device can be activated at ages 18 to 24 months and the elbow at ages 36 to 48 months.[32] Myoelectric devices have been used at these young ages with good results.[34] For very proximal upper limb deficiency the use of the feet should be encouraged.

SUMMARY

The rehabilitation process for the patient with an upper limb amputation is a complex one, and it is best accomplished by the patient who is able to work in a close cooperative relationship with a comprehensive, multidisciplinary, specialized treatment team. The team members should be ready and able to assist the patient throughout the rehabilitation program, from preamputation to community reintegration. The availability of psychological counseling and/or assistance from the team members during each one of these steps is very important for the smooth transition of the patient back into the community.

References

1. Atkins D: Adult upper-limb prosthetic training. *In* Atkins DJ, Meier RH (eds): Comprehensive Management of the Upper-Limb Amputee. New York, Springer-Verlag, 1989, pp 39–59.
2. CAD-CAM special issue. Prosthet Orthot 1989; 1:116–190.
3. Challenor Y: Limb deficiencies in children *In* Molnar G (ed): Pediatric Rehabilitation. Baltimore, Williams & Wilkins, 1992, pp 400–424.
4. Curran B, Hambrey R: The prosthetic treatment of upper limb deficiency. Prosthet Orthot Int 1991; 15:82–87.
5. Davis RW: Phantom sensation, phantom pain and stump pain Arch Phys Med Rehabil 1993; 74:79–91.
6. Dise-Lewis J: Psychological adaptation to limb loss. *In* Atkins JD, Meier RH III (eds): Comprehensive Management of the Upper-Limb Amputee. New York, Springer-Verlag, 1989, pp 165–172.
7. Dobner DL: A prosthetic harness adaptation. Arch Phys Med Rehabil 1990; 71:436–438.
8. Edelstein JE: Preprosthetic management of patients with lower or upper limb amputation. Phys Med Rehabil Clin North Am 1991; 2:285–297.
9. Esquenazi A: Geriatric amputee rehabilitation. Clin Geriatr Med 1993; 9:731–743.
10. Fletchall S, Hickerson WL: Early upper-extremity prosthetic fit in patients with burns. J Burn Care Rehabil 1991; 12:234–236.
11. Glatly HW: A statistical study of 12,000 new amputees. South Med J 1964; 57:1373–1378.
12. Gover AM, McIvor J: Upper limb deficiencies in infants and young. Infant Young Child 1992; 5:58–72.
13. Gregory RT, Gould RJ, Peclet M, et al: The mangled extremity syndrome (MES): A severity grading system for multisystem injury of the extremity. J Trauma 1985; 25:1147–1150.
14. Hepp O: Prothesen der oberen Extremitat. *In* Hohmann G, Hoackenbrock K, Lindemann L (eds): Handbuck der Orthopadie, vol 1. Stuttgart, Georg Thieme Verlag, 1957.
15. Illizarov GA: Possibilities offered by our method for lengthening various segments in upper and lower limbs. Basic Life Sci 1988; 48:323.
16. Jendrzejczyk D: Flexible socket systems. Clin Prosthet Orthot 1985; 9:27–31.
17. Kamen LB, Chapis GJ: Phantom limb sensation and phantom pain. PM&R State Art Rev 1994; 8:73–88.
18. Kay HW, Newman JD: Relative incidence of new amputations: Statistical comparisons of 6,000 new amputees. Orthot Prosthet 1975; 29:3–16.

19. Kay H, Working Group, ISPO: A proposed international terminology for the classification of congenital limb deficiencies. Orthot Prosthet 1974; 28:33–48.

20. Kejlaa GH: The social and economic outcome after upper limb amputation. Prosthet Orthot Int 1992; 16:25–31.

21. Kristinsson O: Flexible above-knee socket made from low density polyethylene suspended by a weight-transmitting frame. Orthot Prosthet 1983; 37:25–27.

22. Lambert C: Amputation surgery in the child. Orthop Clin North Am 1972;3:473–482.

23. Levy WS: Skin Problems of the amputee. *In* Bowker JH, Michael JW (eds): Atlas of Limb Prosthetics, ed 2. St Louis, Mosby–Year Book, 1992, pp 681–688.

24. Malone JM, Childers SJ, Underwood J, et al: Immediate postsurgical management of upper extremity amputation: Conventional, electric and myoelectric prosthesis. Orthot Prosthet 1981; 35:1.

25. Malone JM, Fleming LL, Roberson J, et al: Immediate, early and late postsurgical management of upper limb amputation. J Rehabil Res Dev 1984; 21:33.

26. Meier RH: Upper limb amputee rehabilitation. PM&R State Art Rev 1994; 8:165–185.

27. Melzack R: Phantom limbs. Sci Am, April 1992, pp 120–126.

28. National Center for Health Statistics: Washington, DC, Current Estimates from the National Health Interview Survey, US Department of Health and Human Services, 1990.

29. Patton J, Shida-Tokeshi J, Setoguchi Y: Prosthetic components for children. Phys Med Rehabil 1991; 5:2.

30. Pritham CH, Fillauer C, Fillauer K: Experience with the Scandinavian flexible socket. Orthot Prosthet 1985; 39:17–32.

31. Scott RN: Biomedical engineering in upper-extremity prosthetics. *In* Atkins DJ, Meier RH (eds): Comprehensive Management of the Upper-Limb Amputee. New York, Springer-Verlag, 1989, pp 173–189.

32. Setoguchi Y, LeBlanc M: Upper limb strength of young limb deficient children as a factor in using body powered terminal devices—a pilot study. J Assoc Child Prosthet Orthot Clin 1992; 27:89–96.

33. Setoguchi Y, Rosenfelder R (eds): The Limb Deficient Child. Springfield, Ill, Charles C Thomas, 1982.

34. Sherman AR, Sherman JC, Gall GN: A survey of current phantom limb pain treatment in the United States. Pain 1980; 8:85–99.

35. Sorbye R: Myoelectric prosthetic fitting in young children. Clin Orthop 1980; 148:34–40.

36. Varni JW, Setoguchi Y: Effects of parental adjustment on the adaptation of children with congenital or acquired limb deficiencies. J Dev Behav Pediatr 1993; 14:13–20.

37. Wilson AB Jr: Limb Prosthetics, ed 6. New York, Demos, 1989, pp 69–90.

Lower Limb Prostheses

ROBERT D. McANELLY, M.D., AND
VIRGIL W. FAULKNER, C.P.O.

The types of amputation by level are partial foot, Syme, transtibial (below-knee), knee disarticulation (through-knee), transcondylar/supracondylar, transfemoral (above-knee), hip disarticulation, transpelvic (hemipelvectomy), and translumbar (hemicorporectomy). The 1977 National Health Survey found 358,000 persons with major amputations living in the United States, yielding a rate of 1.7 major amputations per 1000 persons.[103] Of the major amputations, 91,000 were upper extremity, 92,000 were transfemoral, 113,000 were transtibial, 22,000 were partial foot, 36,000 were bilateral lower extremity, and 4000 were combined lower and upper extremity amputations. An estimated 205,000 persons used an artificial leg or foot.[104] The subsequent 1990 National Health Survey unfortunately failed to differentiate finger amputations from major extremity amputations.[101] Nonfederal hospitals in the year 1989, however, discharged patients with 30,000 transfemoral amputations, 24,000 transtibial amputations, and 11,000 partial foot amputations.[102]

Kaye and Newman surveyed 5830 new amputees for the causes of amputation.[47] They found that vascular disease and infection accounted for 70% of all amputations; trauma, 22%; tumor, 5%; and congenital deformity, 3%. The largest number of amputations for disease occurred in the 61- to 70-year age group; for trauma, the 21- to 30-year age group; and for tumor, the 11- to 20-year age group. Male amputees outnumbered female amputees in the disease group 2.1:1; in trauma, 7.2:1; in tumor, 1.3:1; and in congenital deformity, 1.5:1. The ratio of lower- to upper-limb amputations was 11:1. The distribution of lower-limb amputations by level was Syme, 3%; transtibial, 59%; knee disarticulation, 1%; transfemoral, 35%; and hip disarticulation, 2%.

The oldest discovered prosthesis was made of bronze and iron with a wooden core, and was dated about 300 BC from a tomb in Capua, Italy.[87] Prosthesis development accelerated in the United States after World War II because of a 1945 research program founded jointly by the National Academy of Sciences, the Veterans Administration, the Department of Health, Education, and Welfare, and the Armed Services. In 1970, the American Academy of Orthotists and Prosthetists formed as a professional association to improve quality and education. The International Society of Prosthetics and Orthotics (ISPO), formed in 1972, sponsors conferences on prosthetics and publishes the journal *Prosthetics and Orthotics International*.

Vascular diseases requiring amputation include diabetes mellitus, arteriosclerosis, and Buerger's disease. Diabetics not only experience vascular compromise, but also suffer motor, sensory, and autonomic neuropathy, all of which lead to ulceration.[6] Antibiotic drugs have greatly improved the control of infection in vascular cases, allowing amputation to be performed at a lower level. (For further information, see Chapter 56.)

In malignancy cases, it was common in the past to amputate well proximal to the neoplastic lesion. Advances in chemotherapy and radiation therapy with better tumor staging now make it possible, in many cases, to perform segmental limb resection with wide local excision of the tumor. Segmental limb resection in the region of the knee can allow options such as total knee arthroplasty or van Ness tibial rotationplasty (Fig. 15–1), in which the anatomical ankle joint is rotated 180 degrees to become a functional knee joint. Post-tumor amputees who have received doxorubicin (Adriamycin) require cardiac screening prior to prosthesis fitting.[54] Amputees on chemotherapy have residual limb volume fluctuation, and it is important to coordinate prosthetic and chemotherapy programs. Transfemoral socket fit and gait training should be done when the patient is feeling well, usually prior to chemotherapy.[14] For the transtibial amputee, after alignment and initial gait training, chemotherapy if indicated, can begin on the same day.[14] Almost every post-tumor amputee deserves a prosthesis trial, regardless of prognosis.[44, 49] The permanent prosthesis should not be prescribed until 6 weeks after termination of chemotherapy (with resolution of transient edema). (For further information, see Chapter 57.)

All combinations of congenital limb deficiency occur, including missing intermediate parts. For example, the thigh or upper arm may be missing, whereas the other parts

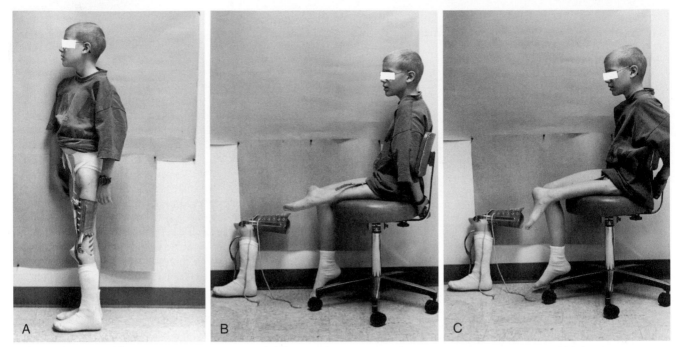

FIGURE 15–1 *A–C,* van Ness rotationplasty after tumor resection. (Courtesy of R. P. Williams, M.D.)

of the limb may be present but malformed. If a malformed part is nonfunctional, then surgical options may have to be considered for amputation or reconstruction.

Trauma to a limb often involves vascular or nerve injury, burn injury, cold injury, and nonhealing fracture. These may render the limb permanently less functional than an artificial limb. In such cases, early amputation, rather than attempts at limb salvage, is often the best option.

In trauma cases in which a limb has been reimplanted, the limb is often less functional than the amputated limb with a prosthesis would have been. Surgical reimplantation requires meticulous internal bone fixation, vascular anastomosis, tendon repair of muscles, and nerve repair. Postreplantation therapy includes limb elevation to prevent swelling once the arterial supply is intact, avoidance of constricting dressings, and prevention of infection. Gentle passive range of motion exercises typically begin on day 4. Splints can be used to help prevent deformity or to improve function. Skin observation is necessary for the even temporarily anesthetic limb.

PREOPERATIVE MANAGEMENT

Psychological Aspects

Preoperative counseling by the rehabilitation team and peer counseling by other amputees facilitates recovery. Preoperative therapy includes range of motion exercise, strengthening, and ambulation with an assistive device. Keep in mind that a new amputee typically experiences depression, especially if he or she is unaware of the prosthetic options for future function and ambulation.

Surgical Decisions and Level of Amputation

The rule of amputation is to save as much of the limb as possible, consistent with satisfactory healing and function.

"Dry" gangrene is ischemia and presents as mummification, showing few signs of infection. In "wet" gangrene infection is always present, as is the potential for life-threatening sepsis.

In cases of trauma, surgeons choose the amputation option after consideration of the difficulties of fracture fixation and vessel and nerve repair, especially if months or years of the patient's undergoing multiple muscle and skin flaps would be required. Surgeons too often view amputation of a traumatized lower limb as a defeat instead of seeing it as one therapeutic alternative.[39] Limb salvage has increased morbidity with multiple operations and high cost that may be financially and psychosocially ruinous. It is often better to choose early amputation and prosthetic fitting over limb salvage of questionable functional benefit.[5, 6, 33, 35, 36, 38, 56, 57] If the posterior tibial artery is severed and the leg is perfused only by the anterior tibial artery, then necrosis of the posterior musculature can occur. It is usually best to treat posterior tibial nerve disruption coupled with severe foot and ankle trauma with amputation. If bony loss with associated muscle damage involves more than 6 cm of bone length, then amputation should usually be performed.

In cases of severe peripheral vascular disease, placing a distal bypass to patent tibial arteries at the ankle may salvage the foot, with requirement of perhaps only a minor digital amputation. The main deliberation is usually to decide between a partial foot, transtibial, or transfemoral amputation. Diabetic patients without significant large vessel disease may be able to heal a partial foot amputation despite not qualifying for a vascular bypass.

It is difficult to accurately select the optimum level of amputation based on clinical assessment of tissue viability. Criteria such as poor skin edge bleeding during surgery and absence of pulses do not always correlate with failure to heal.[11] Many noninvasive vascular studies are available to determine level of amputation.[67, 77] Adequate nutrition and immunocompetence, as measured by albumin and total lymphocyte counts, also contribute to healing.

Preamputation arteriography in peripheral vascular disease is done chiefly to guide possible arterial reconstruction, as it is of limited value for amputation level selection, because distal vessels are commonly not detected.[3] Despite angiography's limited prognostic value,[76] occlusion of both the deep and superficial femoral vessels indicates a poor prognosis for healing in transtibial amputation.[84]

Doppler-determined ankle blood pressure measurements are of little value in assessing partial-foot amputation viability,[41, 70, 109] probably due to arteriovenous shunting that results in artificially elevated ankle blood pressures. Thigh blood pressure measurements above 70 mm Hg and possibly between 50 and 70 mm Hg, however, are predictive of success in transtibial amputation surgery.[88]

Intradermally injected radioisotope traces (^{133}Xe, ^{131}I, or ^{125}I-iodoantipyrine) provides a direct measure of skin blood flow, though it is not easily performed. Skin blood flow greater than 2.5 mL/100 g/min is correlated with healing at multiple amputation levels.[67, 71] Skin blood flow technique may be the most accurate measurement to assess skin viability, particularly around the knee joint,[65] but it is not as reliable in assessing regional blood flow.[64] Absolute skin perfusion pressure is also valuable,[34, 42, 100] and healing occurs in 90% of patients with skin perfusion calf pressure over 30 mm Hg, and in 67% with skin perfusion pressure from 20 to 30 mm Hg.[43]

Transcutaneous oxygen pressure (TcPO$_2$) is easy to measure but difficult to interpret. TcPO$_2$ levels greater than 35 mm Hg at the calf predict that a transtibial amputation will heal, but values below this are not predictive.[11, 12, 23, 82, 110] Adding 100% oxygen inhalation to the test improves test reliability dramatically, with successful healing predicted with a rate of change of 9 mm Hg/min on switching to 100% oxygen from room air, or with a rise in TcPO$_2$ of at least 10 mm Hg after 10 minutes of 100% oxygen inhalation compared with room air values.[37, 66]

Infrared thermography, intravenous fluorescein dye, and laser Doppler are less commonly utilized vascular studies. Infrared thermography is less valuable because much of the heat derives from deeper structures,[113] but it is a good indicator of skin flap viability.[65] Fluorescein dye can be injected intravenously to provide quantitative fluorometry criteria for skin flap viability,[68, 96] but this is rarely used because interpretation is difficult. Laser Doppler studies also provide some information about the microcirculation in a noninvasive mode.[40]

Preoperative noninvasive vascular studies are crucial in preserving limb length, so that the level selected is at the edge of tissue viability. If limb infection is present, then the limb blood flow should be evaluated to assess whether healing will occur.

Proper surgical technique requires suturing of cut muscles to each other and to the periosteum at the end of the cut bone (myoplasty) or to the bone itself (myodesis). In the most functional residual limbs, the muscles and their fascia are sutured directly to the bone through drill holes. In myoplasty, the muscles are joined to each other with minimal tension, which takes less operating time. The surgeon should taper the muscle mass to reduce distal bulk.

Prognosis

After the immediate period for deaths directly related to surgery, Roon and co-workers found the expected 5-year survival rate after lower extremity amputation to be 45% compared with 85% for the age-adjusted normal population.[84] They also reported that the 5-year survival for nondiabetic amputees was almost normal at 75%, whereas the 5-year survival for diabetic amputees was only 39%. Others report a mortality rate of 30%, 50%, and 70%, after 5, 10, and 15 years, respectively, in those with critical limb ischemia.[4, 15, 21, 48, 78] The mortality is chiefly due to the comorbidity of cardiovascular and cerebrovascular disease. Risk factors include smoking, diabetes, and hypertension.[22] Of the survivors, critical limb ischemia will develop in the remaining limb in 18% to 28% within 2 years of amputation.[62] Diabetics not only experience vascular compromise, but also suffer sensory neuropathy leading to ulceration.[7] Follow-up care of the contralateral dysvascular limb includes nail and callus trimming, counseling regarding skin care of the feet, use of only electric razors to shave the legs, tight control of diabetes, and referral for the oxford extra-depth shoe fitted with a wide toe box, a blucher-type throat and a molded insert. (See Chapter 56 for further information.)

In the 1960s, 5-year survival for osteogenic sarcoma was less than 20%, but 3-year survival has improved to 60% to 85%,[24, 55] with similar survival improvements for other bone and soft tissue sarcomas.[52] There are similar overall survival results for patients who undergo amputation vs. those who undergo segmental limb resection,[55, 63, 97, 111] although en bloc resection may be contraindicated for large tumors and minimal response to preoperative chemotherapy.[31] Limb salvage options for tumor include (1) autologous tissue transfers, (2) intercalary amputation ("internal amputation") and reconstruction (such as the van Ness procedure), (3) intercalary bone allografts (cadaveric) and osteoarticular allografts, (4) custom and modular endoprostheses (also called *megaprostheses*), and (5) composite allograft endoprostheses (standard joint replacement prostheses by use of an intercalary allograft).[49]

POSTOPERATIVE MANAGEMENT

The history should include reason for and date of amputation, dates of revisions, prior ambulatory status, self-care status, cardiopulmonary status, neurological status, psychiatric status, peripheral vascular status, diabetic control, previous surgical procedures, residual limb pain, phantom sensation, and pain. The physical examination should include an evaluation of vision and mental status, peripheral vascular status, surgical incision and drainage, skin lesions, residual limb skin mobility, edema and pitting, induration, tenderness, skin redundancy, graft and graft donor sites, passive range of motion, joint stability, sensation, and strength in all extremities.

The ideal transtibial residual limb is cylindrical, whereas the ideal transfemoral residual limb is conical. Records should be kept of several circumferential measurements of the residual limb at specific distances from the greater trochanter for a transfemoral amputee, or from the medial knee joint line for a transtibial amputee. The residual limb soft tissue status and bony length should also be assessed.

Wound Healing

Wound healing is maximized by evaluating and optimizing nutrition, anemia, diabetic control, and antibiotic use. Whirlpool treatment with debridement is helpful for an infected wound but not for an uninfected wound, because whirlpool causes residual limb edema. An open incision or wound should be covered with a Telfa pad under the shrinkage device or prosthesis. The Telfa should not be placed between a wound and a prosthetic socket if the wound is over a bony prominence, but rather a thinly cut 2 × 2-in. sterile gauze sponge should be used. Blisters on the residual limb should never be punctured. The wound should be inspected regularly for odor, drainage, warmth, redness, and dehiscence.

Delayed wound healing can be due to inappropriate level selection, skin or muscle closure under tension, excessive use of sutures, early removal of sutures, inadequate nutritional status, immunocompromise, tobacco use, or infection. Infections require adequate surgical drainage and appropriate antibiotics. For diabetic patients, if baseline transcutaneous oxygen pressure ($TcPO_2$) is less than 40 mm Hg on room air, but exceeds 40 mm Hg with 100% O_2 at 1 atm for 20 minutes, the use of postoperative hyperbaric oxygen therapy should be considered. For non-diabetic patients, the critical value is 30 mm Hg.[80] A chronically draining sinus may be the result of a superficial suture abscess, a bone spur, or localized osteomyelitis. The opening should be probed to determine its depth, and plain films and bone scans should be obtained to determine bony involvement.

Residual Limb Management

A postoperative plaster of Paris or fiberglass rigid dressing prevents edema, protects from trauma, and decreases postoperative pain. Postoperative edema occurs within a few minutes, so immediate replacement of the dressing is necessary. Once they are removed for inspection or suture removal, rigid dressings must be replaced within minutes to prevent recurrence of edema.

The removable rigid dressing (RRD) for the transtibial amputee consists of a plaster of Paris or fiberglass cast suspended by a stockinet and supracondylar cuff, and is adjusted by adding or removing socks to maintain compression.[115, 116] The RRD provides good edema control with the advantage of allowing daily inspection.

When a rigid dressing is not being used, one may wrap cotton-elastic bandages around the residual limb if the patient is physically and mentally able to learn this technique (Figs. 15–2 and 15–3). Elastic bandages are typically the least effective shrinkage device, because many patients fail to master the wrapping technique, which requires reapplication many times a day. Poorly applied elastic bandages also can cause circumferential constriction with distal edema. Double-length 4-in. bandages should be used for the transtibial limb and double-length 6-in. bandages for the transfemoral limb.

Elastic shrinker socks are easy to apply and provide uniform compression, but are more expensive than elastic

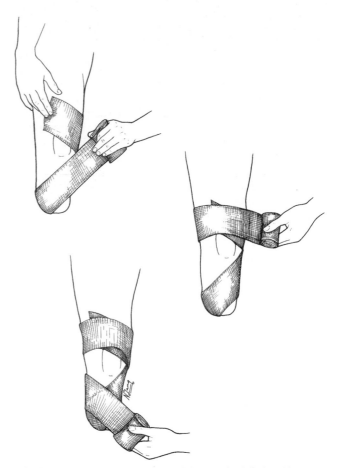

FIGURE 15–2 Wrapping a transtibial residual limb with elastic bandage in a figure-of-8 pattern to reduce edema. (Courtesy of the University of Texas Health Science Center at San Antonio.)

bandages (Fig. 15–4). They should fit snugly, and should reach the groin in the transfemoral amputee. They may also cause skin damage with constriction if not properly fitted and maintained.

The amputee should wear a shrinkage device 24 hours/day except for bathing or for ventilating an open sore for short periods during the day. A shrinkage device for the non–prosthesis candidate helps control pain and edema and facilitates healing. The shrinkage device can be discontinued after fitting the definitive prosthesis if the amputee wears the prosthesis regularly. It can be used at night if overnight edema occurs.

A contracture is easy to prevent but difficult to correct. The amputee must not lie on an overly soft mattress, use a pillow under the back or thigh, or have the head of the bed elevated. Standing with a transfemoral residual limb resting on a crutch should be avoided. All of these practices lead to hip flexion contractures. The amputee must not place a pillow between the legs, because this creates a hip abduction contracture. A transtibial amputee must not lie with the residual limb hanging over the edge of the bed, with a pillow placed under the knee, or with the knees flexed, and must not sit in a wheelchair with the knee flexed, because these positions lead to knee flexion contractures. The transtibial amputee should sit with the knee extended on a board under the wheelchair cushion, with a towel wrapped over the board. Crutch walking with or without a prosthesis

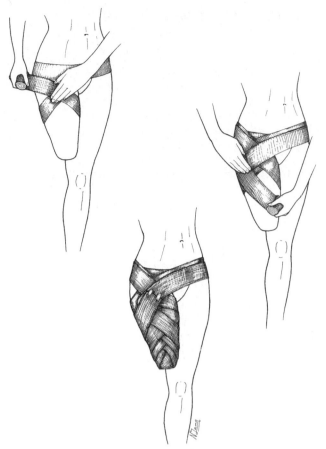

FIGURE 15–3 Wrapping a transfemoral residual limb with elastic bandage in a figure-of-8 pattern to reduce edema. (Courtesy of the University of Texas Health Science Center at San Antonio.)

promotes good range of motion and, when feasible, is preferred over wheelchair mobility. Amputees should lie prone for 15 minutes three times a day to help prevent hip flexion contractures. The amputee who cannot lie prone should lie supine and actively extend the residual limb while flexing the contralateral leg.

After suture removal, the residual limb should be cleansed daily with bland soap and tepid water; one can add an antiseptic cleanser. The limb should be patted completely dry before application of any shrinkage device. Gentle massage decreases sensitivity to pressure, and deep friction massage perpendicular to the scar prevents scar adhesions. Be sure that the residual limb scar has mobility in all directions, because adherent scars can cause pain. One may use a thin layer of emollient to decrease the friction from massage, but discourage the use of thick creams. For very dry skin, a thin emollient can be applied in the evening for absorption overnight. Shaving of the residual limb should be discouraged.

Preprosthetic Training

Preprosthetic training includes active range of motion exercises, positioning, muscle strengthening, skin care, wheelchair mobility, transfers, ambulation with assistive devices, self-care, and patient and family education. Goals should be realistic but individualized to challenge each

amputee to his or her maximum potential based on functional considerations of age and health.

Immediate Postoperative and Early Prosthetic Training

In 1963, Weiss reported success in fitting amputees with prostheses immediately after surgery and beginning ambulation training the next day.[112, 117] The immediate postoperative weightbearing required by this technique has lost popularity due to concerns over wound healing, but it is still commonly used for pediatric and clean post-traumatic amputees. The usual technique is to apply a rigid plaster of Paris or fiberglass dressing postoperatively to prevent edema and to promote healing. A pylon and foot are attached to the rigid dressing for immediate postoperative weightbearing. It should be noted that patients should never be fully weightbearing on this type of socket. At 10 to 14 days after surgery, a preparatory prosthesis is provided if the wound has closed. If the wound has not closed, a new rigid dressing should be applied for 10 additional days. Others recommend waiting at least 21 days postoperatively for the temporary prosthesis.

The amputee must learn to adjust the number of plies of prosthetic socks, to use a nylon sheath against the skin to prevent friction, and to don and doff the prosthesis and inserts. The amputee dons the nylon sheath before the prosthetic socks. The socks must have no wrinkles, and seams should not be over bony areas or scars. The amputee must wash socks and sheaths daily, wipe the socket and

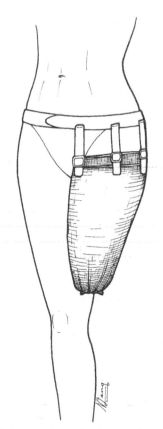

FIGURE 15–4 Elastic shrinker for the transfemoral residual limb. (Courtesy of the University of Texas Health Science Center at San Antonio.)

insert daily with a damp cloth, and air non-gel inserts overnight. Gel inserts left out of the socket overnight may deform.

Gait Training

Training for an efficient, cosmetically acceptable gait begins with the parallel bars and includes training in sit-to-stand transfers, balance, knee control, lateral weight shifting, and forward progression. Balancing techniques are taught first, with progression to limited weightbearing. The amputee should use open hands to avoid pulling up on the bars.

Advanced gait training progresses through gait aids (e.g., walker, crutches, canes) to ramps, curbs, stairs, clearing obstacles, and, if indicated, falling safety and floor-to-standing transfers. In stair climbing and ramp walking, the amputee ascends by leading with the sound foot, and descends by leading with the prosthesis. If skin pressure problems occur, the prosthesis wearing time should be temporarily decreased and the problem identified and corrected. Patients fitted immediately postoperatively should ideally be wearing the prosthesis at least 3 hours/day before discharge.

THE PROSTHESIS

Preparatory/Temporary Prosthesis

When there is uncertainty about a patient's potential success at using a prosthesis, a preparatory prosthesis should still be provided as a trial. All limb prostheses consist of a suspension device, a socket, rigid components, and a terminal device (foot), and it may include artificial joints. Most amputees also require a prosthetic sheath and socks over the residual limb. The prosthesis-patient interface is the "fit," and the geometry of the components is the alignment.

The preparatory or temporary prosthesis is usually uncosmetic, but is used during the period of residual limb shrinkage. The amputee uses the preparatory prosthesis until maximal shrinkage has been attained, usually 3 to 6 months postsurgery. Outpatient follow-up is done best with a prosthetic clinic team, including a physician, prosthetist, therapist, and social worker. When the patient is wearing 10- to 15-ply socks due to residual limb shrinkage, the amputee should be given a new socket, because this many plies cause a tendency to piston.

Definitive/Permanent Prosthesis

The definitive or permanent prosthesis is cosmetically finished. Its fit, alignment, and components are chosen based on the amputee's experience with the preparatory prosthesis. A test or check socket is usually made to test fit just prior to fabricating the definitive socket. If the definitive prosthesis is fitted too early, the limb continues to shrink and the prosthesis becomes too large, necessitating replacement. Weight loss or gain of 5 lb can alter the fit. Diuretics, hemodialysis, chemotherapy, and alcohol consumption can also cause fluctuations in residual limb size. The definitive prosthesis typically requires replacement about every 3 years.[61]

PARTIAL FOOT AMPUTATIONS

Surgical Procedures

Amputation of a single small toe results in little loss of function. The amputation of any single ray still permits good function. The exception to this is the first ray, where as much metatarsal length as possible should be preserved to allow for an effective medial arch. Rather than resect two or more rays, a transmetatarsal amputation may give a more functional result.

In transmetatarsal amputation, the surgeon sections the metatarsals transversely, usually just proximal to the metatarsal heads, and bevels them inferiorly. Tendons are allowed to retract. The longer sensate plantar flap is sewn to the shorter dorsal flap.

The Lisfranc amputation is a tarsometatarsal disarticulation. The Chopart amputation is a disarticulation at the midtarsal joint through the talonavicular and calcaneocuboid joints (Fig. 15–5). In both of these procedures, the remaining foot often develops a significant equinovarus deformity resulting in excessive anterior weightbearing with breakdown. Adequate extensor tendon implantation with Achilles tendon lengthening has been advocated to prevent this deformity. Such patients frequently require a postoperative rigid dressing for several weeks to try to prevent the equinus deformity.

The Boyd amputation consists of excision of all tarsals except the calcaneus. After removal of a portion of the sustentaculum tali, the calcaneus is internally fixated into the ankle mortise. Weightbearing is then allowed on the distal heel pad without the concern for heel pad migration seen in the Syme amputation. The Boyd amputation is rarely performed in the adult due to residual limb length problems, but is commonly performed in the pediatric congenital amputee.

Prosthetic and Orthotic Prescription

For patients with toe amputation, wool, sponge rubber, or foam should be inserted in the shoe to function as a spacer and to prevent toe deformity. For an amputated great toe, a long steel spring shank, a metatarsal pad, and a rocker sole improve function. The transmetatarsal

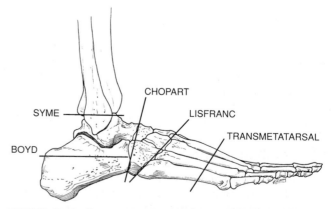

FIGURE 15–5 Syme and partial foot amputations: Boyd, Chopart, Lisfranc, and transmetatarsal. (Courtesy of the University of Texas Health Science Center at San Antonio.)

amputation requires a custom molded insole and toe filler. The stiff insole should prevent shoe hyperextension proximal to the natural toe break. A thin, lightweight carbon fiber shank can be incorporated directly in the insert. The slipper-type prosthesis contains flexible and semi-flexible materials, and provides a plantar lever arm and cosmesis.

For the Lisfranc or Chopart amputee, modified shoe or molded plastic socket, or a combination of the two, should be provided. Modern slipper-type prostheses terminate at the ankle joint, whereas the older devices, such as the prosthetic boot and ankle-foot orthosis (AFO), may extend up the ankle and inhibit subtalar and tibiotalar motion. The ground reaction force AFO with anterior and posterior plastic shells gives maximal control with minimal ankle motion and some limited proximal weightbearing, and is indicated for the muscularly imbalanced, active, or pressure-sensitive amputee.[2]

The Boyd amputation is fitted as a Syme amputation—described next—and it requires a contralateral shoe lift in adults because of leg length discrepancy.

SYME AMPUTATION

Surgical Procedures

Syme amputation is an ankle disarticulation for destructive and infective lesions of the foot that cannot be treated with a transmetatarsal amputation. The original Syme procedure is the best for this level. Taking great care in separating the heel flap from the calcaneus preserves it for end-bearing. The surgeon disarticulates the tarsal bones, removes the malleolar projections, and removes a thin slice of tibia connecting the malleoli. The heel flap is attached firmly to the cut end of the tibia, usually permitting full weightbearing on the distal residual limb. One difficulty with Syme amputation is that the heel pad may migrate posteriorly or mediolaterally if it is not adequately anchored to the cut end of the tibia. One may manage this by careful, total-contact prosthetic fitting or by surgical repositioning of the heel pad. Syme amputation prostheses are uncosmetic, because of the inability to match the shape of the contralateral leg. This amputation level compromises cosmesis in favor of function, and may not be suitable for some persons.

Prosthetic Prescription

The Syme prosthesis usually has a removable medial window that allows the patient to push the residual limb into the socket (Fig. 15–6). The window, when replaced, provides suspension over the malleoli. The prosthesis gives excellent function. The Syme amputation also allows the amputee to walk on the residual limb alone for household distances. The prosthetic heel should be soft to accommodate lack of ankle motion. Feet for the Syme amputee include all of the solid ankle cushion heel (SACH)–type feet as well as some energy-storing feet, and are similar to the feet of the same name described under Transtibial Amputation, but have a lower profile.

Gait speed is typically decreased 32% and oxygen consumption increased 13% per distance walked in the vascu-

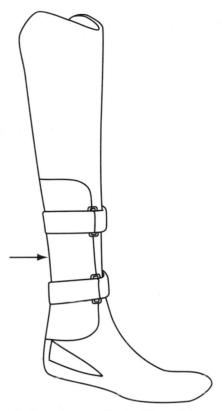

FIGURE 15–6 Syme-type prosthesis with medial opening socket. (From Cestaro JM: The Illustrated Guide to Orthotics and Prosthetics. Alexandria, Va, National Office of Orthotics and Prosthetics, 1992, p 234.)

lar Syme amputee with a prosthesis, compared with normal subjects without vascular disease.[108]

TRANSTIBIAL (BELOW-KNEE) AMPUTATION

Surgical Procedures

Transtibial amputation is usually performed at the junction of the upper and middle third of the tibia (Fig. 15–7). Some advocate a longer residual limb to provide a longer lever arm and more efficient gait, but this is harder to fit. The surgeon should cut the fibula only slightly shorter than the tibia to provide a cylindrical residual limb. A long posterior flap meets a shorter anterior flap to allow the gastrocnemius-soleus muscles to form the distal soft tissue. The wound should be closed by myodesis or myoplasty. Myodesis fixes the posterior muscle to the tibia and prevents retraction, with better function than myoplasty.[8]

Nearly full use of the knee allows the transtibial amputee to have a more efficient gait. In debilitated elderly persons with no walking or transfer potential, knee disarticulation is preferable to transtibial amputation to prevent knee flexion contracture and distal residual limb breakdown.[73] Unlike Syme amputation, the end of the transtibial residual limb cannot bear total body weight. Transtibial residual limbs as short as 2½ in. can be successfully fitted with a prosthesis. Ertl recommended a distal tibiofibular synostosis to prevent

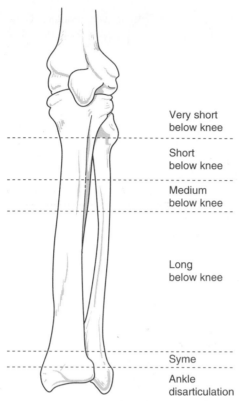

FIGURE 15–7 Categories of transtibial residual limb based on length. (From Epps CH: Surgery of the Musculoskeletal System, 2. New York, Churchill Livingstone, 1990, p 5124.)

fibular hypermobility and to improve weightbearing in the traumatic amputee.[19]

Prosthetic Prescription

Foot-Ankle Assemblies

Prosthetic feet are classified into five types: (1) the SACH foot, (2) the single-axis foot, (3) the multi-axis foot, (4) the solid ankle flexible keel foot, and (5) the energy-storing foot.[72] The SACH foot has a cushioned heel that compresses during heel-strike, simulating plantar flexion, and a rigid anterior keel to roll over during late stance (Fig. 15–8). It is light, durable, and inexpensive, and is most often prescribed for juvenile and geriatric amputees.

The single-axis foot has a single mechanical axis for plantar flexion and dorsiflexion motion limited by anterior and posterior bumpers, allowing quicker foot flat, which results in a more stable knee (Fig. 15–9). The single-axis foot is heavier and less durable than the SACH foot, and finds use most often in transfemoral prostheses, but seldom in transtibial prostheses.

Multi-axis feet, such as the Greissinger, Endolite Multiflex, and stationary attachment flexible endoskeleton (SAFE) II allow dorsiflexion, plantar flexion, inversion, eversion, and transverse rotation (Fig. 15–10). Multi-axis feet are good for walking on uneven ground or for an excessively scarred and sensitive residual limb, because of better shock absorption. They are heavier, less durable, and more costly than SACH feet.

Feet such as the Kingsley stored-energy (STEN) and

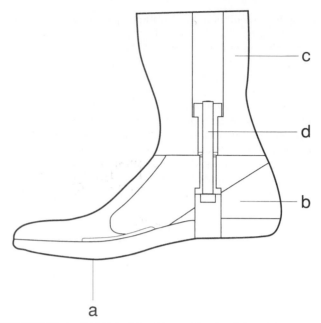

FIGURE 15–8 SACH (solid ankle cushion heel) foot. The plastic cover (a) is over a wooden core. The heel wedge (b) is elastic. The foot is attached to the wooden ankle block (c) by a bolt (d). (Courtesy of Otto Bock Orthopadische Industrie GmbH and Co.)

Otto Bock 1D10 Dynamic foot are similar to the SACH foot but have a flexible anterior keel (Fig. 15–11). Solid ankle flexible keel feet are lighter than multi-axis feet, and provide limited inversion, eversion, and transverse rotation. They offer shock absorption in late stance and benefit the moderately active or obese amputee.

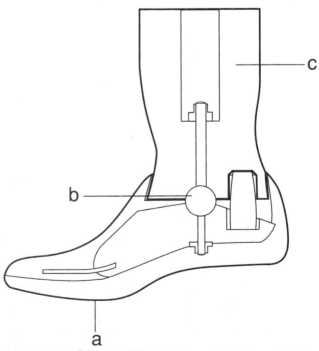

FIGURE 15–9 Single-axis foot allowing plantar and dorsiflexion. The foam cover (a) is over a wooden core. The single-axis joint (b) connects the foot to the ankle block (c). A rubber bumper limits plantar flexion, and a rigid stop limits dorsiflexion. (Courtesy of Otto Bock Orthopadische Industrie GmbH and Co.)

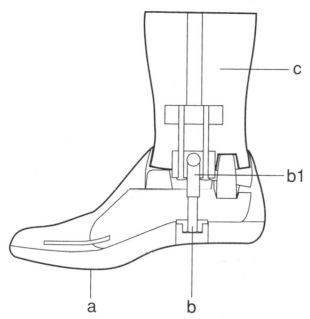

FIGURE 15–10 Multi-axis Greissinger foot. The foam cover *(a)* is over a wooden core. The Greissinger foot joint *(b)* connects the foot to the ankle block *(c)*. Movement in all directions is permitted by the U-joint *(b1)*. Rubber bumpers limit plantar flexion and dorsiflexion. (Courtesy of Otto Bock Orthopadische Industrie GmbH and Co.)

Energy-storing feet (dynamic response feet) store and release energy as the limb is weighted and unweighted, giving a "springy" feeling (Fig. 15–12).[114] Examples include the Seattle foot, Seattle Light, Carbon Copy II, Carbon Copy II Light, Carbon Copy III, Quantum Foot, Flex Walk, Flex Foot (Fig. 15–13), and Springlite. Energy-storing feet result in a higher self-selected walking speed and

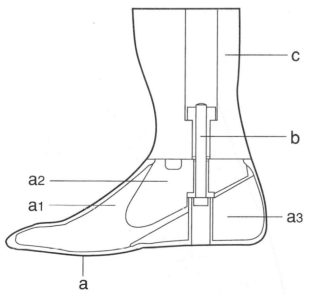

FIGURE 15–11 The Otto Bock 1D10 Dynamic foot is an example of a foot with a flexible keel. The foot *(a)* consists of a plastic inner foot *(a1)* with a wooden core *(a2)*, and is coated by an exterior plastic material. The heel wedge *(a3)* is elastic. The foot is attached to the ankle block by a steel and titanium bolt *(b)*. (Courtesy of Otto Bock Orthopadische Industrie GmbH and Co.)

are indicated for the more active amputee. They may be slightly more energy efficient than SACH feet at normal speeds, with increased relative efficiency at higher speeds, though not all studies concur.[13, 75]

Shanks: Exoskeletal ("Crustacean") vs. Endoskeletal (Modular)

The two basic designs for the shank are (1) the exoskeletal ("crustacean") and (2) the endoskeletal (modular). The exoskeletal "crustacean" system has a hard outer plastic shell. It is very durable, but does not allow alignment changes in the finished prosthesis. The endoskeletal system has a pylon covered by contoured, soft foam. The endoskeletal system is generally lighter and more cosmetic, and can be more easily accessed for adjustment and component change-out.

Sockets

Patellar Tendon–Bearing Socket

The conventional total contact patellar tendon–bearing (PTB) socket is characterized by a bar in the anterior wall designed to apply pressure to the patellar tendon. The trimline extends anteriorly to the midpatella level, may extend mediolaterally to the femoral condyles, and extends posteriorly to below the level of the PTB bar. Pressure-sensitive areas include the tibial crest, tubercle and condyles, the fibular head, the distal tibia and fibula, and the hamstring tendons. Pressure tolerant areas include the patellar tendon, the pretibial muscles, the gastrocnemius-soleus muscles, the popliteal fossa, the lateral flat aspect of the fibula, and the medial tibial flare (Fig. 15–14). Despite the name *patellar tendon–bearing*, pressure should be equally distributed over the pressure-tolerant areas and relieved over the pressure-sensitive areas. The PTB socket is a total-contact socket, because the distal part of the residual limb is in contact with the socket with minimal end-weightbearing. This socket may incorporate a soft, foamed distal pad to protect the distal residual limb as it settles and to increase comfort. Suspension of the PTB socket can be by a supracondylar cuff strap, a cuff strap with a waist belt, a suspension sleeve, or a silicone suction suspension system.

Soft and Hard Sockets

A plastic socket without an insert is a *hard socket,* and when fitted with an insert it is a *soft socket*. An insert provides extra protection for the residual limb, but reduces the intimate contact between limb and prosthesis. It is often fabricated from polyethylene foam, though a silicone gel insert protects the sensitive residual limb better. Inserts should be prescribed when peripheral vascular disease, extensive scarring, or reduced subcutaneous tissue is present.

Flexible Socket

Flexible sockets provide a softer, thermoplastic material for weight transmission. The flexible socket sits in a rigid frame and is described in greater detail in the section

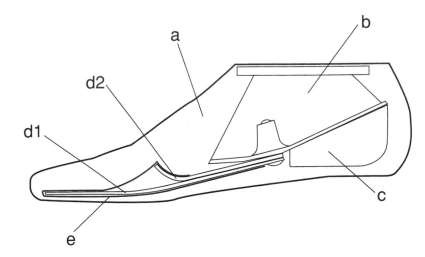

FIGURE 15–12 The Carbon Copy II is an example of an energy-storing foot. The flexible foam urethane foot *(a)* is over a rigid composite keel *(b)*. The heel wedge *(c)* is elastic. Primary *(d1)* and secondary *(d2)* deflection plates store and release energy as the fore-foot is weighted and unweighted. A Kevlar sock *(e)* prevents the plates from punching through the ure-thane. (Courtesy of Ohio Willow Wood Co.)

Transfemoral Amputation. Note that the term *flexible* refers to the socket material and not to the socket shape.

Suspension

Flexible Attachment

The supracondylar cuff is a simple cuff or strap fitted just above the femoral condyles that suspends the prosthesis during swing phase (Fig. 15–15). It may have a Velcro or buckle closure. A waist belt and elastic strap can be added for extra security.

Neoprene or rubber suspension sleeves provide excellent suspension, fitting snugly over the proximal prosthesis and several inches up onto the thigh (Fig. 15–16). Sleeves should not be used for very short residual limbs or for amputees who need added knee stability with proximal trim lines. Perspiration and hygiene problems may occur, especially in hot, humid climates, and kneeling shortens the life of the sleeve.

The silicone suction suspension system (3S, ICEROSS, ALPS) is a thin-walled, highly compliant, closed-end insert or liner of silicone (Fig. 15–17).[28] The amputee rolls the silicone liner onto the bare residual limb, and then can attach it to the socket by a shuttle lock system. The ampu-

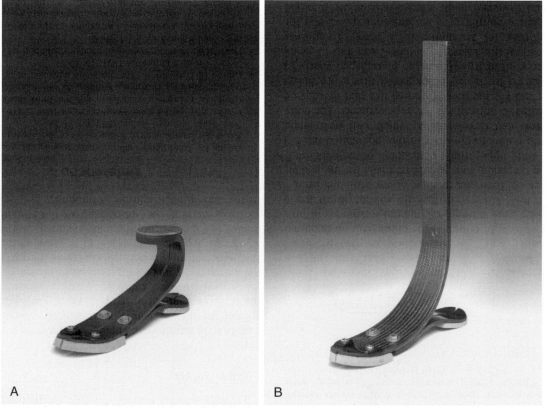

A   B

FIGURE 15–13 Flex-Walk II *(A)* and Flex-Foot Modular III *(B)* energy-storing feet store and release energy by way of graphite composite springs. There is also a cosmetic foam cover. (Courtesy of Flex-Foot, Inc.)

PRESSURE-TOLERANT AREAS   PRESSURE-SENSITIVE AREAS

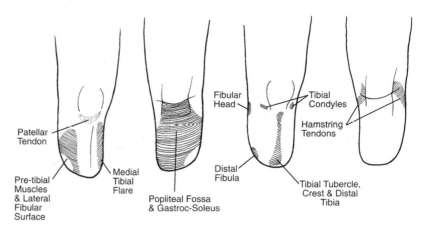

FIGURE 15–14 Pressure-tolerant and pressure-sensitive areas of the PTB socket. (Courtesy of the University of Texas Health Science Center at San Antonio.)

tee pushes the residual limb into the prosthesis until a click (or clicks) is heard. The amputee pushes a button to doff the socket. The liner provides friction suspension and absorbs moderate impact and shear forces on the residual limb. The silicone suction suspension system is more expensive than most suspension systems, but it provides excellent suspension for the athlete and excellent skin protection for the scarred residual limb.

Suction suspension is very difficult to achieve in the transtibial amputee due to the presence of many bony channels, but has been achieved by using a flexible socket.

Brim Contour

SUPRACONDYLAR. The patellar tendon–bearing socket with supracondylar wedge (PTB-SC) extends its mediolateral trimlines above the femoral condyles for suspension (Fig. 15–18). A wedge is either built into the liner or is

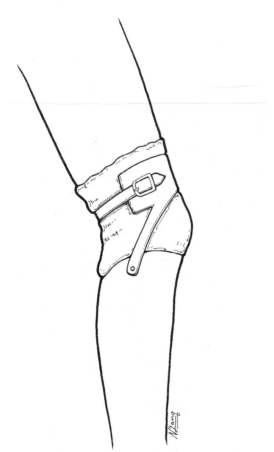

FIGURE 15–15 Supracondylar cuff for the transtibial amputee. (Courtesy of the University of Texas Health Science Center at San Antonio.)

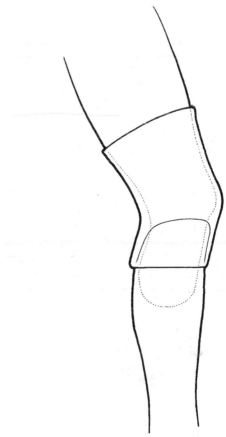

FIGURE 15–16 Elastic sleeve suspension for the transtibial amputee. (Courtesy of the University of Texas Health Science Center at San Antonio.)

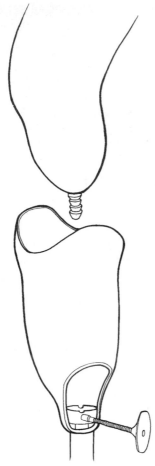

FIGURE 15–17 The 3S is an example of a silicone suction suspension system for the transtibial amputee. It attaches to the socket by a shuttle lock system. Silicone suction suspension systems are also available for the transfemoral amputee. (Courtesy of Durr-Fillauer Orthopedic Inc.)

completely separate, and is positioned above and over the medial femoral condyle. The PTB-SC provides extra mediolateral support and is helpful for short residual limbs and in overweight amputees.

SUPRACONDYLAR/SUPRAPATELLAR. The patellar tendon–bearing socket with supracondylar/suprapatellar trimline (PTB-SC/SP) is a PTB-SC socket with suprapatellar trimlines (see Fig. 15–18). The alternative name, from France, is *prothèse tibiale supracondylien* (PTS). The suprapatellar trimline helps suspend the prosthesis and increases socket wall support of the expected stance phase varus moment; it is helpful for short residual limbs and for controlling genu recurvatum.

Thigh Corset

The patellar tendon–bearing socket with joints and corset (PTB w/J&C) adds a femoral corset to decrease residual limb weightbearing by 40% to 60%. It gives less knee control and worsens gait and is therefore the socket suspension of last resort (see Fig. 15–18). It provides control of significantly lax collateral ligaments and protects the knee from varus stresses during stance. It also provides additional mediolateral support for the patient with a short

residual limb. The PTB w/J&C relieves weight on a residual limb with poor pressure tolerance, and it is often used for amputees involved in heavy manual labor.

Bent Knee or Kneeling Prosthesis and Bypass Prosthesis

The bypass prosthesis receives all pressure from the thigh, ischium and gluteus, and bypasses the tibia. If the bypass is due to severe knee flexion contracture, then it is called a *bent knee* or *kneeling prosthesis*. Protruding external knee hinges are necessary. The biomechanics are the same as for the transfemoral prosthesis, with poorer cosmesis.

Transtibial Prosthetic Care

The amputee must be taught to adjust the prosthetic socks so that the patellar tendon bar is over the midpoint of the patellar tendon. The insert should be donned before the prosthesis is donned. Inserting a clay ball the size of a pea, wrapped in plastic, at the bottom of the socket during weightbearing is a way to test fit. If the ball is partly but not totally flattened, then distal contact is adequate.

Gait Deviations: Static and Dynamic Analysis

Fit and Alignment

The weightbearing surface is increased by aligning the PTB socket to hold the knee in 5 to 10 degrees of flexion. During mid-stance there should be a slight varus moment at the knee, pushing the knee laterally. The socket applies a counterposing force to the medial femoral condyle and the lateral fibular shaft. The foot is set medial to the socket center. Moving the foot medially increases the varus moment. Moving the foot laterally decreases the moment but may create a valgus moment, resulting in pressure over sensitive areas. Sagittal plane forces within the socket progress from anteroproximal and posterodistal in early stance, to anterodistal and posteroproximal in late stance.

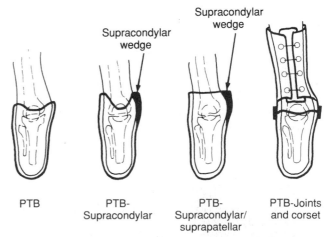

FIGURE 15–18 Examples of the variations of the PTB socket design. (From Karacoloff LA, Hammersley CS, Schneider FJ: Lower Extremity Amputation. Gaithersburg, Md, Aspen Publishers, 1986, p 27.)

Pistoning should be checked by marking the posterior brim of the socket against the sock while the amputee is standing. Pistoning of more than ¼ in. indicates inadequate suspension or loose socket. If suspension is by elastic sleeve, then a portion of the proximal sleeve should be in direct contact with the amputee's skin.

Gait Analysis

Table 15–1 lists gait problems, causes, and solutions in the transtibial amputee.

Energy Expenditure

The average measured gait velocity of the vascular transtibial amputee is decreased 44%, with oxygen consumption increased 33% per distance walked. The gait velocity of the traumatic transtibial amputee is decreased only 11%, with oxygen consumption increased 7% per distance walked, as compared with normal subjects without vascular disease.[108] Longer residual limbs have lower oxygen requirements than short residual limbs, ranging from 10% to 40% increased oxygen requirement per distance walked.[30]

KNEE DISARTICULATION (THROUGH-KNEE AMPUTATION)

Surgical Procedures

Knee disarticulation is removal of the tibia and fibula at the knee. As in the Syme procedure, knee disarticulation provides the capacity for partial end-weightbearing. Knee disarticulation is used for trauma and for infection. A transtibial amputation should be done if 2½ in. of tibia can be saved, because of the value of a functional knee, and so this level is rarely indicated for the dysvascular patient. The knee disarticulation level keeps the thigh musculature intact with more control and with a longer lever arm than at the transfemoral level. Medial and lateral skin flaps are best if the blood supply is marginal. The patellar tendon is sewn to the cruciate ligaments. Over time, some muscle atrophy develops, making the distal surfaces more bony.

Prosthetic Prescription

The socket is usually a modified quadrilateral socket with some ischial weightbearing, and a soft socket liner with supracondylar buildups to provide suspension. Proximal socket trim lines prevent socket rotation on the limb, though ischial weightbearing is not an absolute requirement, if the femoral condyles provide suspension. The problem in prosthetic fitting of a knee disarticulation is that the prosthetic knee's center of rotation needs to go through the distal residual limb. Fitting a knee unit distal to the residual limb has caused problems in the past, but the four-bar polycentric knee has helped to solve the problem (Fig. 15–19). The polycentric knee, unlike the single-axis knee, has an instantaneous center of rotation that changes, and is proximal and posterior to the knee unit itself. This allows greater knee stability, a more symmetrical gait and equal knee length when sitting. Fluid control can be added for the active amputee.

TABLE 15 1   Gait Analysis of the Transtibial Amputee

Problem	Cause	Solution
Delayed, abrupt, and limited knee flexion after heel-strike	Heel wedge is too soft; foot is too far anterior	Stiffen heel wedge; move foot posterior
Extended knee throughout stance phase	Too much plantar flexion	Dorsiflex foot
Toe stays off floor after heel-strike	Heel wedge too stiff; foot too anterior, too much dorsiflexion	Soften heel wedge; move foot posterior; plantar flex foot
"Hill-climbing" sensation toward end of stance phase	Foot too anterior; too much plantar flexion	Move foot posterior; dorsiflex foot
High pressure against patella throughout most of stance phase; heel is off floor when patient stands	Foot too plantar flexed	Dorsiflex foot
Knee too forcefully and rapidly flexed after heel strike; high pressure against anterodistal tibia at heel-strike and/or prolonged discomfort at this point	Heel wedge too stiff; foot too far posterior; foot too dorsiflexed	Soften heel; move foot anterior; plantar flex foot
Hips level, but prosthesis seems short	Foot too far posterior; foot too dorsiflexed	Move foot anterior; plantar flex foot
Drop-off at end of stance phase	Foot too far posterior	Move foot anterior
Toe off of floor as patient stands or knee flexed too much	Foot too dorsiflexed	Plantar flex foot
Valgus moment at knee (knock-kneed) during stance phase; excessive pressure on distomedial limb and proximolateral surface of knee	Foot too outset	Inset foot
Excessive varus moment at knee (bow-legged) during stance phase (a varus moment at the knee should occur in stance phase but should never be excessive); the distolateral residual limb is painful	Mediolateral dimension of socket too large; foot too inset	Fit of socket should be checked; outset foot

Courtesy of Northwestern University Prosthetic-Orthotic Center, Chicago.

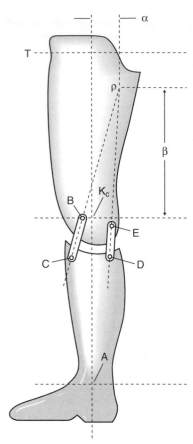

FIGURE 15–19 Four-bar polycentric knee with superiorly and posteriorly displaced instantaneous center of rotation. (From Greene MP: Four bar linkage knee analysis. Orthot Prosthet 1983; 37:17.)

Waters and colleagues found the average measured gait velocity for the traumatic through-knee amputee to be decreased 24%, with oxygen consumption increased 53% per distance walked, compared with normal subjects without vascular disease.[108]

TRANSCONDYLAR/SUPRACONDYLAR AMPUTATION

Surgical Procedures and Prosthetic Prescription

The Gritti-Stokes procedure provides partial but not total end-weightbearing, and eliminates the bulbous prosthetic profile seen in knee disarticulation. The amputation is done through the femoral condyles, and the patella is attached directly over the cut end of the femur. Gritti-Stokes amputation is a very difficult procedure and is now seldom used.[87]

In the transcondylar and supracondylar amputation, a conventional single-axis knee unit almost fits distal to the residual limb, though the prosthetic thigh is still slightly longer than the normal thigh. Suspension is also more difficult than in knee disarticulation.

TRANSFEMORAL (ABOVE-KNEE) AMPUTATION

Surgical Procedures

Transfemoral amputation is usually performed with equal anterior and posterior length flaps. This amputation does not tolerate total end-weightbearing. The surgeon typically transects the quadriceps just proximal to the patella, transects the adductor magnus from the adductor tubercle, and transects the smaller muscles 1 to 2 in. longer than the bone cut. If severed muscles are not sutured, they retract. An abduction contracture is likely to develop if most of the adductor muscles have been severed and have not been reattached. Flexion-abduction contracture can be minimized by reattaching the adductor magnus to the lateral aspect of the femur.[32]

With myoplasty or myodesis, hamstrings are able to assist in hip extension and thereby stabilize the prosthetic knee. Myoplasty produces a smoother, more rounded cylindrical residual limb, though best results appear to be with myodesis or bony attachment. Muscle strength is proportional to its cross-section and its length, and shortened muscle in a shortened residual limb is weaker (Fig. 15–20).

Prosthetic Prescription

The residual limb should be at least 8.5 to 13.6 cm in length, measured from the groin, to fit a transfemoral prosthesis; but no absolute measurement is prescriptive, because success is dependent on soft tissue volume.[87]

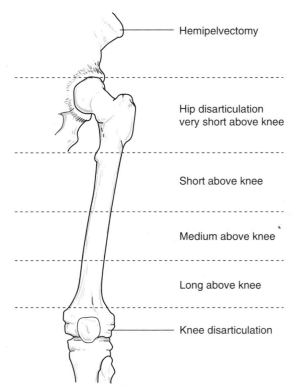

FIGURE 15–20 Categories of transfemoral residual limb based on length. (From Epps CH: Surgery of the Musculoskeletal System, 2. New York, Churchill Livingstone, 1990, p 5124.)

Foot-Ankle Assemblies

Compared with a transtibial amputee, a transfemoral amputee needs softer plantar flexion to enhance knee stability. The single-axis foot therefore offers more knee stability than the SACH foot, but is also heavier. If a SACH foot is used, then a softer heel is necessary. Energy-storing feet should also be considered. An ankle unit torque-absorber may be used to reduce transverse friction forces for the short residual limb.

Shanks

The choice between an endoskeletal (modular) and an exoskeletal ("crustacean") shank is similar to that for the transtibial amputee. The hard shell of the exoskeletal system is more durable, whereas the endoskeletal system is lighter, more cosmetic, and allows easier prosthetic adjustment. The endoskeletal shank has gradually gained popularity over the exoskeletal shank, and lightweight or ultralight prostheses are generally prescribed for geriatric amputees.

Knee Units

Knee units are either single axis or polycentric. They are also either mechanical or fluid-controlled. All knee units, except for the hydraulic stance control units such as the Mauch S-N-S, attempt to keep the knee flexion-extension fixed at one angle (without relative motion) throughout the stance phase.

Mechanical Knee Units

Conventional constant friction single-axis knees are light, durable, and inexpensive. Single-axis knees rely on alignment for stability, and work best at one speed. Exces-

sive heel rise in early swing phase, as well as terminal swing impact in late swing phase, may occur at faster cadences. These problems can be corrected by manually adjusting the constant friction unit, which can only be set for one optimum cadence. The amputee must prevent knee buckling by activating the hip extensors. The debilitated amputee or amputee with a short residual limb cannot adequately contract the hip extensors, and requires a knee that is set posterior to the trochanter-knee-ankle (TKA) line (Fig. 15–21). This alignment has the disadvantage of causing difficulty in flexion of the knee for swing phase, which causes increased energy expenditure compared to other knee units.

A manual locking knee provides maximum stability for the debilitated or elderly amputee, but this is accompanied by the worst gait efficiency and increased energy consumption. The knee can be manually unlocked for sitting. This knee is typically reserved for those with weakness, and for those who are likely to sustain severe injuries if they fall.

The weight-activated stance control knee (*limited slip* or, formerly, *SAFETY knee*) may provide stable stance for up to 20 degrees of knee flexion by producing friction when weight increases during stance (Fig. 15–22). This knee design is for amputees with weak hip extensors or for geriatric amputees. The stance control is not automatic, and the amputee must be able to initiate and maintain control of the knee.

The four-bar polycentric knee, previously mentioned in the section on knee disarticulation (see Fig. 15–22), works well for patients with very long residual limbs as well as for those with poor stability due to short residual limbs, poor balance, or weak hip extensors. Fluid control can be added, and some polycentric knees can be manually locked.

Extension aids are sometimes used with single-axis knees and polycentric knees, and are usually located within

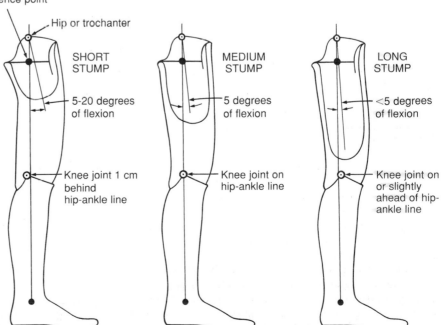

FIGURE 15–21 Trochanter-knee-ankle (TKA) alignment for the short, medium, and long transfemoral residual limb. (From Radcliffe CW: Biomechanics of above-knee prostheses. *In* Murdoch G (ed): Prosthetic and Orthotic Practice. London, Edward Arnold, 1970, p 191.)

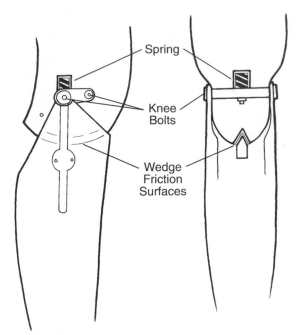

FIGURE 15–22 One type of weight-activated stance control knee (limited slip or, formerly, SAFETY knee).

the shank. The extension aid is usually a compressible spring with screw adjustments that give constant resistance to knee flexion until flexion reaches 90 degrees, then it assists flexion. Extension aids improve knee stability at the expense of gait efficiency.

Hydraulic- and Pneumatic-Control (Fluid-Control) Knee Units

Both hydraulic- and pneumatic-control (fluid-control) knee units are cadence-responsive through cadence-dependent resistance. Pneumatic units are air-filled and are lighter in weight, but they cannot support the heavier or more athletic amputee as well as the hydraulic units can. Fluid-control knees are helpful for the active amputee who varies cadence and who can tolerate the extra weight and expense. Most fluid-control knees control the knee velocity during swing phase only, although hydraulic stance control knees (such as the Mauch S-N-S hydraulic knee) (Fig. 15–23) give gradually yielding resistance to knee flexion during late stance phase as well. The Endolite pneumatic intelligent prosthesis has a computer-controlled valve that adjusts knee swing phase speed based on cadence. The Hydracadence knee is unique in that it also hydraulically controls ankle dorsiflexion and plantar flexion.

Sockets

An adjustable hinged socket for the temporary prosthesis is an option that allows adjustment for edema reduction. The quadrilateral socket is the usual choice. The choice for socket shape in the definitive prosthesis is between the traditional quadrilateral socket and the newer ischial containment socket. Both the quadrilateral and ischial containment sockets are total-contact sockets with ischiogluteal weightbearing.

Socket Shape

QUADRILATERAL SOCKET. The traditional quadrilateral socket has a flat, horizontal posterior shelf on which the ischial tuberosity and gluteal muscles rest. There is an inward bulge over the femoral triangle, and a channel for the rectus femoris. The femoral triangle bulge keeps the ischial tuberosity on the posterior shelf. Medially, there is an anterior channel for the adductor longus tendon. If an "adductor roll" of soft tissue is present over the medial brim, then the medial wall needs higher extension or the roll needs to be pulled inside the socket. The quadrilateral socket has a wide mediolateral and a narrow anteroposterior dimension at the proximal socket edge.

ISCHIAL CONTAINMENT SOCKET. The ischial containment socket (Narrow M-L socket) was developed as the normal shape normal alignment (NSNA) socket by Long and as the contoured adducted trochanteric-controlled alignment method (CAT-CAM) by Sabolich (Fig. 15–24).[59, 60, 86] The posterior wall is ¾ to 1¼ in. proximal to the ischial level and is contoured to support the ischium and gluteal muscles. Compared with the quadrilateral socket, the ischial containment socket gives mediolateral control, or "bony lock," at the minor expense of increased anteroposterior movement, and has a narrow mediolateral dimension and wide anteroposterior dimension at the level of the ischial ramus. It does not, however, alter femoral adduction angle within the socket as compared to the quadrilateral socket.[29] The ischial containment socket gives more en-

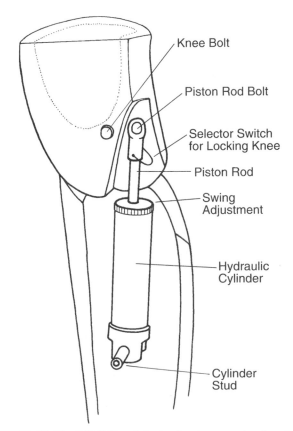

FIGURE 15–23 S-N-S Mauch hydraulic stance and swing-phase control knee unit. (Courtesy of the University of Texas Health Science Center at San Antonio.)

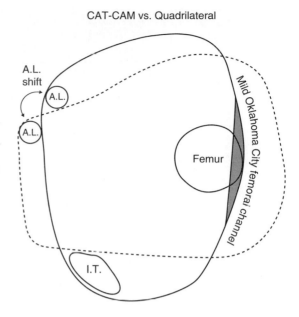

CAT-CAM vs. Quadrilateral

FIGURE 15–24 Comparison of CAT-CAM and quadrilateral sockets in a transverse view. The CAT-CAM is a type of ischial containment socket. In the CAT-CAM socket, the femur and ischial tuberosity are fixed, whereas the adductor longus tendon shifts a small amount compared with the quadrilateral socket. Note the Oklahoma City channel about the femur. (From Sabolich J: Contoured adducted trochanteric-controlled alignment method (CAT-CAM): Introduction and basic principles. Clin Prosthet Orthot 1985; 9:17.)

ergy-efficient ambulation at high speeds[29] for the active amputee, and is helpful for the short residual limb or weak gluteus medius.

BYPASS PROSTHESIS. For transfemoral amputees with a non-weightbearing lesion in the femur or insufficient pressure tolerance of the residual limb, a complete bypass of weightbearing allows fitting of a hip disarticulation–type prosthesis.

Socket Materials: Laminated vs. Flexible

The choice in materials is between the traditional rigid plastic-laminate socket and a flexible thermoplastic socket. The flexible socket originated with the ISNY (Icelandic–Swedish–New York) transfemoral socket consisting of two separate structures: a thin, pliable, vacuum-formed thermoplastic socket to interface with tissues, and a rigid, outer supporting frame for weight transmission (Fig. 15–25).[46, 52] The soft, flexible socket is often translucent or transparent and is more comfortable. It gives better total contact, enables one to better sense external objects through the socket, and feels cooler, with better heat dissipation. Flexible sockets can be more rapidly fabricated and modified, but they are also more expensive. They are especially beneficial for the patient with scarring of the residual limb, and because of better adherence, they provide better suction suspension. The frames usually do not permit a hip joint and pelvic band to be attached.

Suspension

Suspension systems for the transfemoral amputee include suction or partial suction, total elastic suspension (TES) belt, Silesian band, hip joint with pelvic band and waist belt, silicone suction suspension system, and hypobaric silicone suction system (Fig. 15–26).

Suction

The amputee usually dons a total suction prosthesis while standing. It requires that a pull sock or elastic ban-

dage cover the residual limb. The sock or bandage is passed through the valve hole and is used to pull the limb into the socket. Alternatively, a wet fit can be used. The wet fit procedure uses a gel that turns into a liquid or powder after the prosthesis is donned. A one-way valve placed in the valve hole seals the socket by allowing air to escape but not to enter. Total suction is the best suspension biomechanically, but it requires minimal volume fluctuation of the residual limb, good hand strength and dexterity, good balance, and good skin tissue integrity.

Any socket that has a suction valve but that requires the user to wear prosthetic socks is called "partial suction" but provides only minimal suspension (except for the hypobaric silicone system described later), and so auxiliary suspension is needed.

The hypobaric silicone suction system consists of a prosthetic sock impregnated with a proximal ring of silicone to provide an air seal for suction suspension. The amputee dons it while either sitting or standing. Once the residual limb is all the way in the socket, the amputee replaces the air valve. The hypobaric system allows suction in a looser-fitting socket.

The silicone suction suspension system, previously described for transtibial suspension, is a roll-on silicone sock attached to the distal socket, and is only occasionally used for transfemoral amputees.

No Suction

The TES belt is a neoprene belt attached to the prosthesis and pulled around the waist, providing a relatively cosmetic auxiliary suspension. The Silesian belt is a soft belt that encircles the pelvis and is attached proximally to the posterolateral aspect of the socket wall, and to the proximal anterior wall at the midline. The hip joint with pelvic band and waist belt gives excellent mediolateral stability for the frail amputee or for the amputee with a short residual limb, but it is bulky, heavy, constricting, and cumbersome. Placement of these suspension mechanisms over bypass

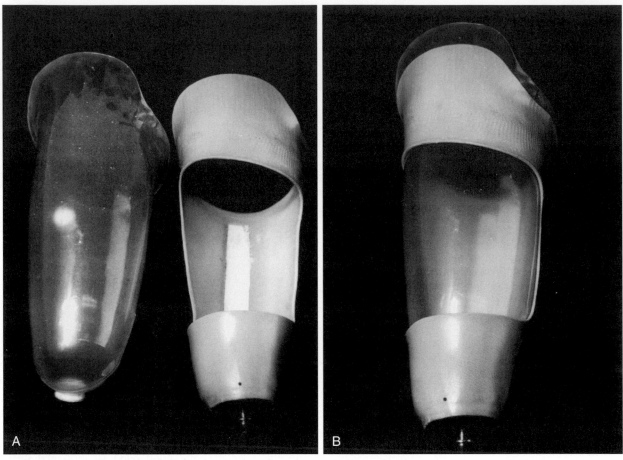

FIGURE 15–25   *A* and *B,* Flexible socket in a rigid frame for the transfemoral amputee. (Copyright Robert D. McAnelly, M.D.)

graft surgery sites and use in pregnant women are contraindicated.

Gait Deviations: Static and Dynamic Analysis

Fit and Alignment

For the quadrilateral socket, the ischium should rest on the posterior shelf, with firm but not excessive pressure between the tuberosity and socket. Insufficient pressure indicates the use of too many plies of socks or a palpable adductor roll, whereas excessive pressure indicates insufficient ply. The adductor longus tendon should be rotated to lie in the anteromedial corner.

For the ischial containment socket, the pubic ramus should be identified where it exits the medial wall. As the patient unweights the residual limb, he or she should check to see that the ischial tuberosity rests inside the ischial pocket or flare.

If a valve is present, the valve should be removed to see that the residual limb is in contact with the bottom of the socket. If there is no valve, the clay ball procedure, as described previously for the transtibial amputee, should be performed. The pelvis may be ¼ in. lower on the prosthesis side to allow toe clearance during swing phase.

To allow the amputee to walk with an erect trunk and with a normal stride length, the initial socket flexion is set at 5 degrees of socket flexion plus the amputee's angle of hip flexion contracture. This puts the hamstrings on stretch, giving the amputee greater stance control. Sagittal plane forces within the socket progress from anteroproximal and posterodistal in early stance, to anterodistal and posteroproximal in late stance.

The TKA line is a line drawn in the sagittal plane through the greater trochanter and mid-ankle (see Fig. 15–21). If the knee joint is on this line, then the knee is in *intermediate alignment.* If it is anterior to this line, then it is said to be in *voluntary alignment,* because the amputee must actively extend the hip during stance to prevent knee buckling. If the knee is posterior to this line, then the knee is in maximum stability, and is said to be in *involuntary alignment.*

In the coronal plane, the center of rotation of the transfemoral amputee within the socket is about the ischium. A varus moment about the hip joint occurs naturally and must be stabilized by the lateral socket wall. Lack of intimate contact between the lateral femur and the socket wall makes the hip abductors inefficient and weak. The farther the foot is inset, or the heavier the amputee, the greater the varus moment. In the transverse plane, foot toe-out should match that of the sound limb.

Gait Analysis

Table 15–2 lists gait problems and causes in the transfemoral amputee.

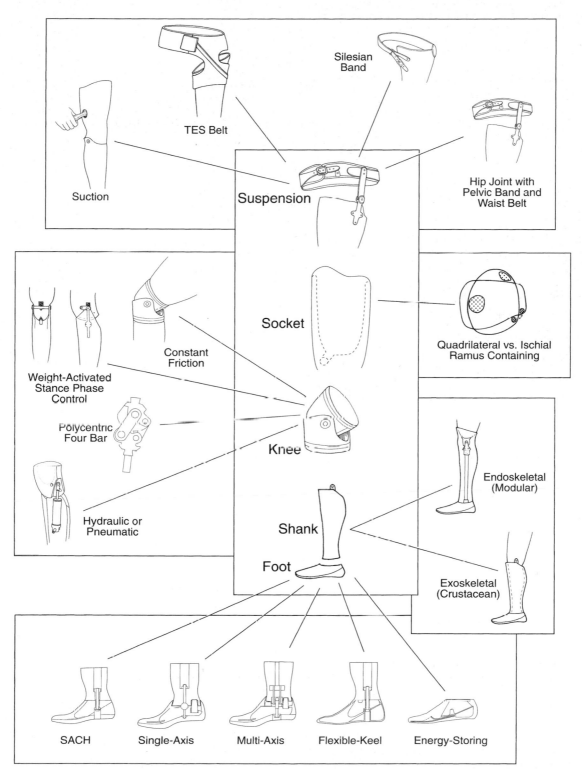

FIGURE 15–26 Prosthetic options for the transfemoral amputee. (Courtesy of the University of Texas Health Science Center at San Antonio.)

TABLE 15–2 Gait Analysis of the Transfemoral Amputee

Problem and Characteristics	Prosthetic Causes	Amputee Causes
Lateral bending of trunk: excessive bending occurs laterally from midline, generally to prosthetic side	• Prosthesis may be too short • Improperly shaped lateral wall may fail to provide adequate support for femur • High medial wall may cause amputee to lean away to minimize discomfort • Prosthesis aligned in abduction may cause wide-based gait, resulting in this defect	• Amputee may not have adequate balance • Amputee may have abduction contracture • Residual limb may be oversensitive and painful • Very short residual limb may fail to provide a sufficient lever arm for pelvis • Defect may be due to habit pattern
Abducted gait: very wide-based gait with prosthesis held away from midline at all times	• Prosthesis may be too long • Too much adduction may have been built into prosthesis • High medial wall may cause amputee to hold prosthesis away to avoid ramus pressure • Improperly shaped lateral wall can fail to provide adequate support for femur • Pelvic band may be positioned too far away from patient's body	• Patient may have abduction contracture • Defect may be due to habit pattern
Circumducted gait: prosthesis swings laterally in wide area during swing phase	• Prosthesis may be too long • Prosthesis may have too much alignment stability or friction in knee, making it difficult to bend knee in swing-through	• Amputee may have abduction contracture of residual limb • Patient may lack confidence for flexing prosthetic knee because of muscle weakness or fear of stubbing toe • Defect may be due to habit pattern
Vaulting: rising on toe of sound foot permits amputee to swing prosthesis through with little knee flexion	• Prosthesis may be too long • Socket suspension may be inadequate • Excessive stability in alignment or some limitation of knee flexion, such as knee lock or strong extension aid, may cause this deficit	• Vaulting is fairly frequent habit pattern • Fear of stubbing toe may cause this defect • Residual limb discomfort may be a factor
Uneven heel rise: prosthetic heel rises quite markedly and rapidly when knee is flexed at beginning of swing phase	• Knee joint may have insufficient friction • Extension aid may be inadequate	• Amputee may be using more power than necessary to force knee into flexion
Terminal swing impact: rapid forward movement of shin piece allows knee to reach maximum extension with too much force before heel-strike	• Knee friction is insufficient • Knee extension aid may be too strong	• Amputee may try to assure himself or herself that knee is in full extension by deliberately and forcibly extending the residual limb
Instability of the prosthetic knee creating a danger of falling	• Knee joint may be too far ahead of trochanter-knee-ankle (TKA) line • Insufficient initial flexion may have been built into socket • Plantar flexion resistance may be too great, causing knee to buckle at heel-strike • Failure to limit dorsiflexion can lead to incomplete knee control	• Amputee may have hip extensor weakness • Severe hip flexion contracture may cause instability
Medial or lateral whips: whips best observed when patient walks away from observer; a medial whip is present when heel travels medially on initial flexion at beginning of swing phase; a lateral whip exists when heel moves laterally	• Lateral whips may result from excessive internal rotation of prosthetic knee • Medial whips may result from excessive external rotation of knee • Socket may fit too tightly, thus reflecting residual limb rotation • Excessive valgus or "knock" in prosthetic knee may contribute to this defect • Badly aligned toe break in a conventional foot may cause twisting on toe-off	None
Drop-off at end of stance phase; downward movement of trunk as body moves forward over prosthesis	• Limitation of dorsiflexion of prosthetic foot is inadequate • Heel of SACH-type foot may be too short, or toe break of a conventional foot may be too far posterior • Socket may have been placed too far anterior in relation to foot	None

TABLE 15–2 Gait Analysis of the Transfemoral Amputee *Continued*

Problem and Characteristics	Prosthetic Causes	Amputee Causes
Extensive trunk extension: amputee creates an active lumbar lordosis during stance phase	• Improperly shaped posterior wall may cause forward rotation of pelvis to avoid full weightbearing on ischium • Insufficient initial flexion may have been built into socket	• Amputee may have hip flexor tightness • Amputee may have weak hip extensors and may be substituting with lumbar erector spinae muscle; abdominal muscles may be weak • Defect may be due to habit pattern • Amputee may be moving shoulders backward in an effort to obtain better balance • Weak abdominal muscles may contribute to this defect

Courtesy of Northwestern University Prosthetic-Orthotic Center, Chicago.

Energy Expenditure

The average measured gait velocity for the vascular transfemoral amputee is decreased by 55%, with oxygen consumption increased by 87%. The average measured gait velocity for the traumatic transfemoral amputee is decreased by 35% with oxygen consumption increased by 33%, as compared with those of normal subjects without vascular disease.[108] Individual energy expenditure per distance walked increases with a shorter residual limb or with age. The energy expended walking with a prosthesis is usually less than walking with crutches and without a prosthesis.[108] As a rule of thumb, if a patient can ambulate without the prosthesis and with crutches, he or she has strength and endurance to ambulate with a prosthesis. Geriatric amputees are best fitted with lightweight "modular" prostheses using titanium or carbon fiber components. Stress testing is indicated for the patient with serious cardiac compromise to see if the energy level needed for ambulation can be tolerated.[16]

HIP DISARTICULATION AND TRANSPELVIC AMPUTATION (HEMIPELVECTOMY)

Surgical Procedures

A true hip disarticulation involves removal of the entire femur, but in practice the proximal femur is usually left to provide prosthetic stabilization and to avoid an uncosmetic cavity. Transpelvic amputation is the surgical removal of the lower limb and part or all of the ileum. These surgical procedures are usually done for malignant tumor, major trauma, or uncontrolled infection.

Boyd first described the basic operation for hip disarticulation.[9] The standard racquet incision is anterior, just inferior to the inguinal ligament, and extends to the ischial tuberosity. Soft tissue padding is provided by suturing the gluteus maximus to the remnants of the adductor muscles.

Transpelvic amputation uses more variable surgical technique, but the incision usually follows the inguinal ligament and continues along the iliac crest. The transpelvic amputation is closed by suturing the gluteal flap to the abdominal muscles. Postoperative treatment is by soft compression or by a plaster of Paris or fiberglass rigid dressing to reduce edema.

Prosthetic Prescription

The hip disarticulation amputee bears weight in the socket through the ischial tuberosity and gluteal muscles, whereas the transpelvic amputee bears weight on the soft tissue and lower rib cage. The hip disarticulation socket usually has good contact just above the iliac crest inside the socket rim, though reduced trim line socket designs are available for young, active amputees (Fig. 15–27). Velcro socket closures secure the socket to the torso to prevent pistoning.

The transpelvic socket requires careful contouring, with gluteal bearing on the contralateral side (Fig. 15–28). The proximal border of the socket may be trimmed below the

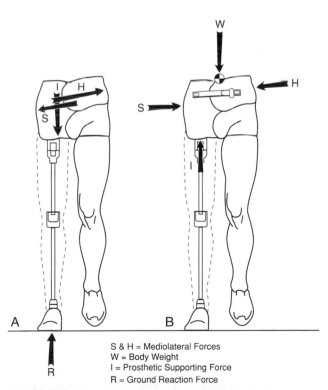

S & H = Mediolateral Forces
W = Body Weight
I = Prosthetic Supporting Force
R = Ground Reaction Force

FIGURE 15–27 Mediolateral forces in the hip-disarticulation prosthesis during stance. *A,* Forces acting on the prosthesis. *B,* Forces acting on the amputee. (From Radcliffe CW: The biomechanics of the Canadian-type hip-disarticulation prosthesis. Artificial Limbs 1957; 4:34.)

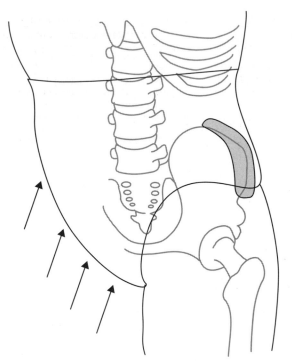

FIGURE 15–28 Transpelvic (hemipelvectomy) socket pressures. (From Lower Limb Prosthetics, New York, New York University, 1975, p 246.)

traditional second rib margin if distal contours provide precise fit.

The older Canadian-type exoskeletal hip disarticulation prosthesis has been replaced by the lightweight and ultralight endoskeletal prosthesis. Hip joint mechanisms for the hip disarticulation and transpelvic amputee are similar. The free hip joint has a posterior bumper extension stop and an anterior flexion stop, but allows no abduction or rotation. The hip joint is made to be stable by placing it anteriorly. A hip extension assist and lockable or four-bar polycentric hip joint are options.

Most of the knee units used with the transfemoral prosthesis can also be used with the hip disarticulation or transpelvic prosthesis, as can most prosthetic feet.[71] The active amputee may need a hydraulic knee, but otherwise the four-bar polycentric knee is an excellent choice. Adding a transverse rotation unit above the knee allows rotation of the distal prosthesis to assist in donning and doffing shoes and to allow cross-legged sitting. A torque-absorber may be added to prevent transverse shear forces at the socket-limb interface.

Successful gait training depends on successfully mastering a posterior pelvic tilt to advance the prosthesis, and then mastering prosthetic swing-through and weight-shift (Fig. 15–29). *Vaulting,* or intentionally rising up on the toes of the sound foot during prosthetic swing to clear the prosthesis, should be avoided.

The average measured gait velocity for the surgical hip disarticulation amputee is decreased by 41%, with oxygen consumption increased by 60% per distance walked. The average measured gait velocity for the surgical transpelvic amputee is decreased by 50%, with oxygen consumption increased by 93% per distance walked, as compared with

normal subjects without vascular disease.[108] Due to the high energy requirements of hip disarticulation and transpelvic amputation ambulation, motivation and cardiopulmonary status are extremely important for prosthetic use. Most young men abandon these prostheses in favor of crutch-walking, whereas 50% of women retain their prosthesis for cosmesis.

TRANSLUMBAR AMPUTATION (HEMICORPORECTOMY)

Surgical Procedures

Translumbar amputation is usually performed for pelvic malignancy, intractable decubitus ulcers, infection, or trauma. It is unique for the resultant loss of the rectum and bladder as well as of most of the body mass. A segment of distal sigmoid colon can be used to create a continent urinary diversion.[107] A colostomy is also formed. The amputation is usually closed by approximating the anterior abdominal wall fascia to the lumbodorsal fascia. The need for considerable advanced psychological preparation for this procedure is obvious.

Prosthetic Prescription

Prosthetic training begins with a sitting device to increase sitting tolerance. The socket must accommodate and allow free access to the ostomy stomas. The amputee should learn stoma care and transfers in and out of the socket. Regular weight reliefs within the socket prevent skin breakdown. Attaching legs to the socket for limited ambulation impairs transfers, and so a second socket is needed if ambulation training is attempted. Successful ambulation is difficult, but cases of household and limited

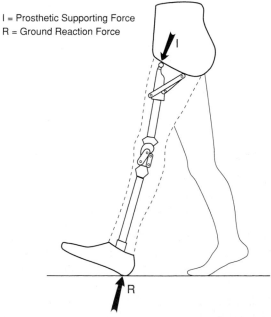

I = Prosthetic Supporting Force
R = Ground Reaction Force

FIGURE 15–29 Hip disarticulation prosthesis at heel-strike. The ground reaction force R creates no flexion moments at the knee or hip, allowing the amputee to remain stable. (From Murdoch G (ed): Prosthetic and Orthotic Practice. London, Edward Arnold, 1970, p 287.)

community ambulation are reported.[20] Prosthetic components should be lightweight and adjustable, and are similar to hip disarticulation components.

BILATERAL TRANSTIBIAL, TRANSFEMORAL, OR TRANSTIBIAL AND TRANSFEMORAL AMPUTATION

Prosthetic Prescription

For the bilateral amputee as for the unilateral amputee, as much of the limb should be saved as will satisfactorily heal and be functional. For the bilateral hip disarticulation amputee, a molded jacket or bucket socket may be necessary to maintain sitting. If the bilateral hip disarticulation is from pressure ulcers related to spinal cord injury, then the socket should be open-ended to relieve pressure over insensate areas and should distribute weight over the chest wall without compromising respiration. A walking prosthesis is rarely indicated for the bilateral hip disarticulation amputee owing to excessive energy costs.

Bilateral transfemoral amputees are sometimes limited functional ambulators, but those in the geriatric population rarely ambulate. Lightweight or ultralight componentry should be used. The Mauch S-N-S knee and four-bar polycentric knee provide more stability than does the weight-activated stance control knee. Most dysvascular bilateral transfemoral amputees lack the cardiopulmonary reserve to ambulate. "Stubbies" are short, basic transfemoral prostheses without knee joints and with rocker bottom feet. They require less energy to ambulate than standard transfemoral prostheses, but stubbies leave the amputee at an uncosmetic and less functional height and result in energy-inefficient gait. Wheelchairs for bilateral transfemoral amputees and other proximal amputees require anti-tip devices and/or offset rear axles to maintain rolling stability.

Healthy bilateral transtibial amputees rarely require assistive devices, although the dysvascular amputee may require a cane. Bilateral transtibial amputees are generally better ambulators than unilateral transfemoral amputees, though limited data in the literature make direct metabolic comparisons difficult.[106, 108]

The combination transfemoral-transtibial amputee obviously has less function than a bilateral transtibial amputee or a unilateral transfemoral amputee, but has more function than a bilateral transfemoral amputee. The transfemoral-transtibial amputee usually ambulates with at least the help of a cane. Ambulation with this combination is usually done only by younger or post-traumatic amputees.

Hemiparesis on either side may prevent prosthetic ambulation in the unilateral amputee, depending on the predictive factors of severity of hemiparesis, level of amputation, and bowel and bladder continence.[1, 76, 105] In the unilateral amputee, amputation of the contralateral arm limits use of assistive devices, and so limits ambulation.

PROBLEMS OF AMPUTEES AND THEIR TREATMENT

Skin Problems

Skin lesions of the residual limb can expand rapidly, so early intervention is required, particularly for diabetic patients. Daily residual limb and socket washing are mandatory. In adults, split-thickness skin grafts cannot tolerate pressure, particularly over bony prominences, and require socket modifications. Painful bursae are common and are best managed by socket modifications, but surgical excision of a troublesome bony prominence might be necessary.

Choke Syndrome

Lack of total contact with proximal restriction results in distal edema called *choke syndrome*. The distal, strangulated residual limb becomes darkened with hemosiderin. Treatment might involve adding a distal pad, improving suspension, or changing sockets.

Verrucous hyperplasia is a wart-like skin overgrowth, usually of the distal residual limb, resulting from inadequate external compression and edema; it can be reversed with total contact within the socket.

Skin Infection

Folliculitis is a hair-root infection resulting from poor hygiene, sweating, poor socket fit, or pistoning. It is important to clean the area with antiseptic cleanser, to keep it dry, and to consider administration of oral antibiotics. Treat boils and abscesses with limited prosthetic use. Epidermoid cysts occur when sebaceous glands are plugged by keratin, and usually do not appear until months or years after a prosthesis is worn. They grow up to 5 cm in diameter and may break to discharge purulent fluid. They should be treated with topical or oral antibiotics, and in some cases with incision and drainage.

Tinea corporis and tinea cruris mainly result from sweating; they may be confirmed through culture or microscopy and are treated by topical or oral fungicides as well as by good residual limb and socket hygiene.

Excessive residual limb sweating can be controlled with cornstarch or unscented talc, but astringents and rubbing alcohol should be avoided. Antiperspirants or iontophoresis with copper sulfate or formalin might also be helpful.

Contact Dermatitis

Allergic contact dermatitis may arise from topical medications or from agents used in prosthetic manufacture. Eczema may appear acutely with small blisters, and later with scaling and erythema. Topical corticosteroids should be applied, and the offending agent should be identified and removed.

Bone Problems

Symptomatic bone spurs may arise from bone from which the periosteum was incorrectly stripped during surgery or that was stripped during trauma. Bone pain may also result from a hypermobile fibula that is left longer than the tibia. If a balanced myodesis was not performed in the transfemoral amputation, the femur may extrude through the muscle and present subcutaneously. If prosthetic adjustments, such as a flexible socket, are inadequate for the extruded femur, then surgical intervention might be needed. If the amputee has severe hip joint arthritis, then total hip arthroplasty is an option. If the sound limb and the prosthetic limb are of unequal length, then a functional scoliosis occurs on standing, and requires shortening or lengthening of the prosthesis.

Pain

Incisional pain should subside with healing, although shear forces on an adherent scar can be painful. Deep massage helps prevent scar adhesions. Intermittent claudication pain in parts of the residual limb may be experienced by the amputee. After tumor amputation, local recurrence of tumor might also be an explanation for a painful residual limb. Remember that not all residual limb pain is the result of poorly fitting prosthesis.

Neuromas

Every severed nerve develops a pressure-sensitive neuroma. The surgeon should sever nerves proximally to avoid socket pressure. Palpating directly over the neuroma typically elicits lancinating pain. The treatment for neuromas is socket adjustment. Direct injection of local anesthetic, with or without steroids, is helpful and aids in making the diagnosis. Neurolysis with phenol may be tried after multiple anesthetic injections have failed. If conservative measures fail, surgery to move the neuroma to a deeper or more proximal site should be considered.

Phantom Pain and Phantom Sensation

The amputee usually has the sensation of the amputated part, or "phantom sensation," but this usually diminishes with time. Occasionally, new amputees have such a dramatic phantom sensation that they transfer out of bed in a darkened room at night and fall when the phantom limb fails to support them. A night light may prevent such a fall.

Phantom pain may accompany the phantom sensation, localizing in the phantom limb rather than in the residual limb. This pain has been described as cramping, aching, burning, and, occasionally, lancinating, and it is felt to be caused by neuron deafferentation hyperexcitability. The longer a person has pain in a limb before it is amputated, the more likely he or she is to have phantom pain. Phantom pain usually diminishes with time, and chronic phantom pain is rare. Occasionally, medical intervention is required, though tricyclic antidepressants, mexiletine, anticonvulsants, capsaicin, propranolol, and chlorpromazine are of limited benefit.[17] Because the etiology is not precisely known, phantom pain is difficult to treat.[45, 58, 91–95] Vigorous desensitization techniques of the residual limb are usually of great benefit, and if the patient can move the perceived phantom limb, then "isometric exercise" of the phantom ankle in all planes might benefit.[73] Psychological support with relaxation therapy and biofeedback may be indicated in severe cases, although phantom pain is not considered a psychosomatic complaint. Ambulation on a temporary prosthesis can alleviate phantom pain. Transcutaneous electrical stimulation over the tibial nerve in the popliteal fossa and lumbar paravertebral sympathetic block at the L2 level should be considered if the phantom pain is burning and of a character similar to that of reflex sympathetic dystrophy.[79] Intravenous regional guanethidine or reserpine blocks have been tried with little success.

Contractures

Maintaining the residual limb in extension is necessary to prevent flexion contractures. For severe knee flexion contractures beyond 25 degrees in an amputation without vascular disease, hamstring lengthening with posterior knee capsule release or a bent-knee prosthesis should be considered. Less severe contractures can be treated with stretching, with or without simultaneous ultrasound. When a contracture is less than 10 degrees, the patient should be encouraged to walk as much as is tolerated, as this might further reduce the contracture. More than 15 degrees of hip flexion contracture in the transfemoral amputee requires marked compensatory lumbar lordosis. Hip flexion contractures up to 25 degrees can be accommodated in the short transfemoral amputee with resulting loss of hip extensor power, but contractures are more difficult to accommodate for longer residual limbs. Hip flexion contractures result in knee instability and poor cosmesis, and often require that the prosthesis have a lockable knee. Contractures in children may lead to scoliosis.

Psychosocial Adjustments

Amputees may develop a sense of inferiority, inadequacy, or repulsiveness. They should learn to discuss problems openly. Their sexual identity and body image are altered, and phantom pain may occur with orgasm. Some amputees need psychological counseling. Attention to cosmesis, such as the cosmetic "New Skin" prosthetic skin covering, may facilitate psychological adjustment.[98] The clinician should also remember never to refer to the residual limb as a "stump."

Activities of Daily Living and Vocational Adjustments

To dress, the patient dons underwear first. Trousers are then put on the prosthesis before the prosthesis itself is donned. Shoe heel height cannot be changed unless foot wedges are used or unless an adjustable foot or second foot is available for the prosthesis. Driving a car may require moving the gas or brake pedal for the unilateral amputee, or installing hand controls for the bilateral amputee. Velcro closures are often needed for patients with poor hand dexterity.

The team must be aware of how much lifting, bending, climbing, and carrying of heavy objects is necessary in the patient's job, both for prosthetic training and for prosthetic prescription. Fine balance while standing may also be a job requirement to be addressed. Cosmesis may also be a significant part of the requirement. Retraining manual laborers for more sedentary work is often necessary (see Chapter 9).

Recreational Activities

The capacity for sports activities requires a careful evaluation of the amputee by the physician and prosthetist. The transfemoral amputee with a mechanical knee must run with a hop-skip pattern, but with a hydraulic knee the person may run with a more normal motion. Recreational opportunities for the amputee are endless. The main U.S. organization for amputee sports is National Handicapped

Sports (NHS), whereas the National Wheelchair Athletic Association offers wheelchair competition. The International Sports Organization for the Disabled (ISOD) organizes international competitions. The Paralympics began as an official competitive event sponsored by the International Olympics Committee in 1988.

PEDIATRIC AMPUTEE

Kaye and Newman's national survey of 5830 new amputees found that 3% of new amputees were in the first decade of life, and 7% were in the second decade.[47] In the first decade, 68% of new amputations were from congenital deformity, 27% from trauma, 3% from tumor, and 2% from disease. In the second decade, 63% of new amputations were from trauma, 22% from tumor, 9% from disease, and 6% from late surgery for congenital deformity.

Differences Between Adult and Pediatric Amputees

Major pediatric amputee concerns include skill development, growth, and psychosocial issues. Just as for adults, all possible functional residual limb length should be preserved. A contraindication to lower extremity amputation is severe upper extremity deformities that make lower extremity prehension necessary.

Pediatric bony overgrowth refers to pressure-related periosteal appositional growth, not epiphyseal growth. Bony overgrowth is a problem of the skeletally immature, particularly after mid-shaft amputation of the fibula or tibia. It occurs frequently enough in acquired amputations to require residual limb revision about 10% of the time, and it also can occur in congenital amputation. Bony overgrowth may cause the skin to become thin and shiny and be accompanied by pain, making prosthetic fitting difficult. The bone can even break through the skin. This overgrowth might require excision or reamputation, and capping or transplanting an amputated epiphysis over the bone end can limit the problem of recurrence.[81] To preserve the epiphysis, amputations should be done through a joint rather than through a bone. Unlike those in adults, the residual condyles in children tend to atrophy, resulting in a more cosmetic fitting prosthesis.

Leg length discrepancy from epiphyseal growth asymmetries can be substantial in the pediatric amputee. The epiphyseal plates about the knee give the greatest contribution to growth, with the distal femoral plate contributing 70% to femoral growth lengthening and the proximal tibial plate contributing 56% of tibial growth lengthening. Some residual limbs, such as a short transtibial limb, can be improved by skeletal lengthening. This procedure often requires a muscle flap for adequate skin coverage.

Unlike the case in adults, pediatric split-thickness skin grafts provide good residual limb coverage, even on end-bearing surfaces, and surgical incisions tolerate more tension. Symptomatic neuromas are rarely a problem in children, and socket modifications can usually relieve neuroma pain. Phantom limb pain is less frequent and of shorter duration in children. Knee and hip flexion contractures in children can largely be ignored and the affected limb fitted for conventional alignment, as those contractures usually stretch out with walking and growth.

Classification of Congenital Deformity

The new International Standard, ISO 8548–1:1989, "Method of Describing Limb Deficiencies at Birth," is a classification system to describe every level and type of congenital deficiency in simple terms.[18] This system categorizes congenital deformities as transverse and longitudinal (Figs. 15–30 and 15–31). A transverse deficiency has no distal skeletal elements, whereas otherwise it is a longitudinal deficiency. The transverse level is named after the segment beyond which no bony elements exist. Digital buds do not count. Longitudinal level names the bones affected, and whether the bones are partly or totally affected.

Congenital limb deformities may be genetic or environmental. Embryologically, the limbs appear at about day 26 and are completely formed during the first 8 weeks of gestation. An estimated 1 of every 2000 human births have limb malformations,[25] primarily from unknown etiologies.[89]

Krebs and Fishman surveyed 679 new amputees referred to specialized pediatric amputee clinics, where they found that 48% of the patients were age 0 to 3 years and 11% were 4 to 6 years.[51] In these specialized clinics, congenital limb deficiencies outnumbered acquired amputations 1.6:1. They reported 41% were unilateral upper limb amputees, 40% were unilateral lower limb amputees, and 19% were multiple limb amputees. Boys outnumbered girls 2.1:1 for acquired amputations and 1.5:1 for both congenital unilateral lower limb and multiple limb deficiencies. Girls outnumbered boys 1.1:1 for congenital unilateral upper limb deficiencies. Because previous attempts at surveying congenital anomalies by scientific classification had failed due to the sheer number of different anomalies, Krebs and Fishman instead asked in their survey for the prosthetic fitting of congenital amputees. They reported that 2% of congenital unilateral lower extremity amputees were fitted as hip disarticulation, 21% as transfemoral, 6% as knee disarticulation, 37% as transtibial, 26% as Syme, and 8% as partial foot amputations.

Corrective Surgery: Surgical Possibilities

The goal of surgery is to improve the function of the child. Reasons for corrective surgery include bony overgrowth, better prosthetic fit, leg-length discrepancy, severe contracture, unstable joints, feet in a non-weightbearing position, limb malrotation, severe neurological anesthesia, polydactyly, and cosmesis.[90] Surgery may be indicated to change a congenital anomaly to an amputation. The family may offer valuable insight into the potential effects of surgery. Surgery for congenital deformity should be planned, if possible, so that all surgical procedures can be carried out in one stage. Surgery for limb lengthening should be preceded by calculating the mature predicted discrepancy. Surgery done as early as 1 year of age provides early fitting and adaptation. Joint disarticulation is preferred over the long shaft of bones to preserve normal bone growth, to prevent bony overgrowth, and for distal end-bearing. The Ilizarov device increases length, epiphysi-

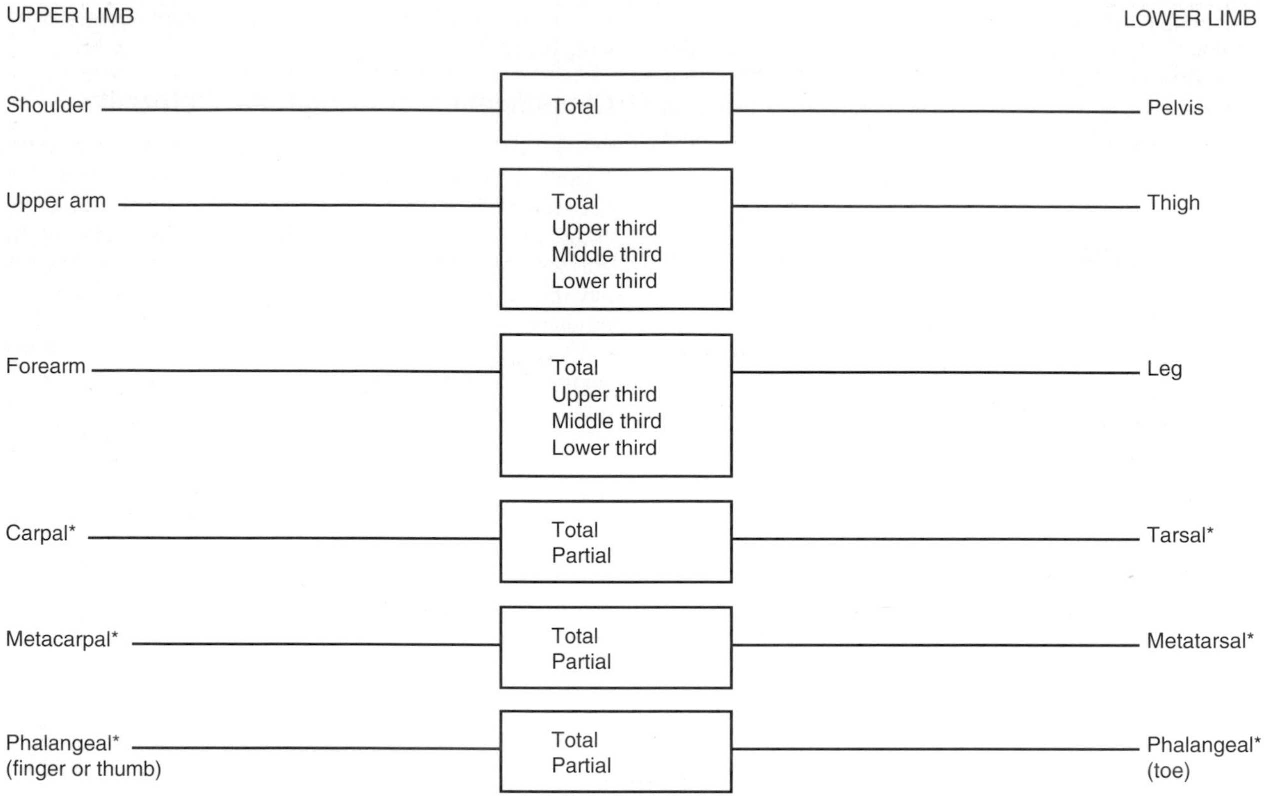

UPPER LIMB

LOWER LIMB

Shoulder	Total	Pelvis
Upper arm	Total Upper third Middle third Lower third	Thigh
Forearm	Total Upper third Middle third Lower third	Leg
Carpal*	Total Partial	Tarsal*
Metacarpal*	Total Partial	Metatarsal*
Phalangeal* (finger or thumb)	Total Partial	Phalangeal* (toe)

FIGURE 15–30 Designation of levels of congenital transverse deficiencies of the upper and lower limbs. Note that skeletal elements marked with an *asterisk* are used as adjectives in describing transverse deficiencies (e.g., tarsal transverse deficiency, total). A total absence of the shoulder or hemipelvis (and all distal elements) is a transverse deficiency. If only a portion of the shoulder or hemipelvis is absent, the deficiency is of the longitudinal type. (From Day HJB: The ISO/ISPO classification. *In* Bowker JH, Michael JW (eds): Atlas of Limb Prosthetics: Surgical, Prosthetic, and Rehabilitation Principles, ed 2. St Louis, Mosby–Year Book, 1992, p 744.)

odesis stunts bone growth, osteotomy corrects malalignment, and joint fusion improves stability. Acetabuloplasties, shelf procedures, and femoral osteotomies can be used to stabilize the hip.

Prostheses

Several specialists are necessary to fully meet the needs of the pediatric amputee, including physicians, prosthetists, therapists, and social workers.

Timing of Prosthetic Fitting

Children generally do not need a lower limb prosthesis until they are ready to stand. Most children sit at about 6 months, crawl on all fours at about 8 to 9 months, and walk at about 1 year. Children are ready for a lower extremity prosthesis between 9 and 12 months for standing. Some, however, fit pediatric transfemoral amputees at 6 months of age to promote a symmetrical sitting posture. A child with a high-level amputation is often fitted with a locked knee joint once he or she appears to be ready to ambulate. At age 3 years, the child can usually handle a constant friction knee joint with an extension strap. Children tolerate immediate postoperative fitting well, owing to good vascularity and sensation. Crutches may be tried at about 4½ years of age.

Pediatric Prosthetic Components

Flexible thermoplastic transfemoral sockets within a rigid frame allow for some growth. Children are active and have prominent fat, and often require auxiliary suspension such as waist belts, bilateral shoulder suspension, elastic sleeves, or the silicone suction suspension system. Suction is more difficult to achieve due to growth. Alignment must be age-specific, because toddlers ambulate with legs externally rotated, abducted, and flexed. The prosthesis must adjust to the child's rapidly changing needs and challenges, such as to the prosthetically destructive teenager. Most prefer the greater durability of exoskeletal construction, unless the patient feels that cosmesis is a high priority. The ideal prosthesis for a young child should be lightweight and easily modified with growth.

Many common adult components, such as feet and mechanical knee joints are also available in pediatric sizes. A good first nonlocking knee unit around age 3 years is a constant friction hinge using an elastic extension aid to help prevent buckling. The active child and teenager is likely to want a hydraulic knee for activities, and will test prosthetic durability to the maximum. Hip disarticulation in children is accompanied by similar problems as in the adult.

Growth Considerations

Children require a new lower limb prosthesis at least annually up to age 5 years, biannually until age 12 years,

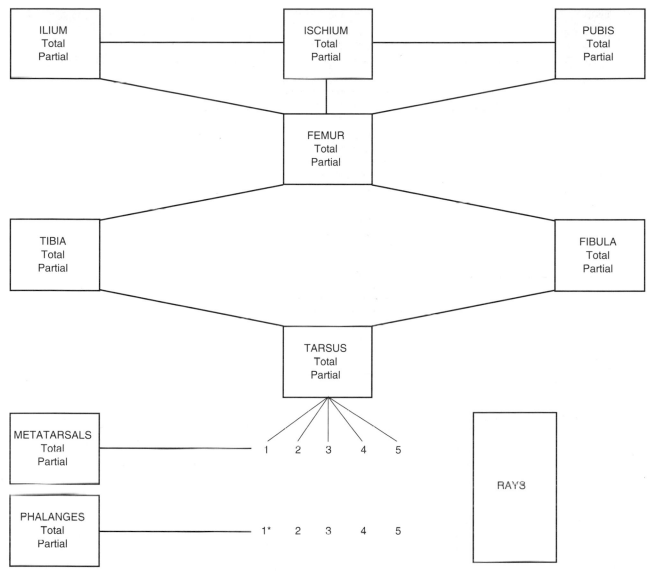

FIGURE 15–31 Description of congenital longitudinal deficiencies of the lower limb. The *asterisk* indicates the great toe, or hallux. (From Day HJB: The ISO/ISPO classification. *In* Bowker JH, Michael JW (eds): Atlas of Limb Prosthetics: Surgical, Prosthetic, and Rehabilitation Principles, ed 2. St Louis, Mosby–Year Book, 1992, p 746.)

and every 3 or 4 years until age 21 years.[53] Pediatric prostheses must be altered or replaced depending on the growth rate (or when the prosthesis has become more than 1 cm shorter than the sound limb). Pediatric limbs grow faster longitudinally than circumferentially. Growth may be accommodated by removing distal end pads or liners, extending an endoskeletal pylon, or adding wedges between the foot and exoskeletal shank. Scoliosis on standing that is not present on sitting might indicate unequal leg length.

Common Longitudinal Deficiencies

Fibular Longitudinal Deficiency, Total/Partial (Formerly Fibular Hemimelia)

Fibular longitudinal deficiency is the most common congenital deficiency, and is bilateral in 25% of cases (Fig. 15–32). It consists of complete or partial absence of the fibula. The clinical picture is that of a shortened tibia with an anteromedial bow, foot equinovalgus deformity,

occasionally a shortened femur, and leg length discrepancy. There may be a ball and socket ankle joint, fusion of tarsal bones, absent lateral rays, ankle instability, genu valgum, and abnormal distal tibial epiphysis. Anatomically, there is often a cartilaginous or a fibrous rudimentary fibula. The muscles originating on the fibula, such as the peroneals and flexor hallucis longus, may be deficient. Care is needed not to confuse this deformity with delayed ossification of the fibula.

The leg length inequality can be severe. The amount of inequality is roughly correlated with the percent of the fibular aplasia. There can also be some correlation with the severity of foot deformity, particularly the number of absent lateral rays. Conservative treatment is indicated if the final shortening is not expected to be greater than 7.5 cm.[99] Most of the treatment is to correct the limb length inequality with considerations of a shoe lift, bracing, contralateral epiphysiodesis (to stunt growth), ipsilateral limb lengthening, or Syme or Boyd amputation. The bow tends to

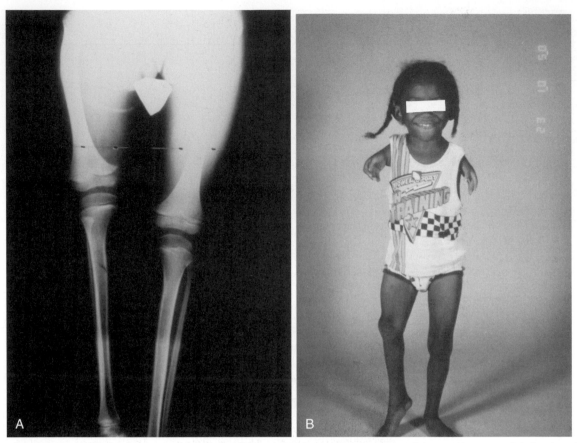

FIGURE 15–32 *A* and *B,* A patient with a longitudinal fibular deficiency and upper limb deficiency. (Courtesy of J. Sanders, M.D.)

straighten with growth after Syme or Boyd amputation. If the foot is retained intact, then the surgeon can correct the bow with a tibial osteotomy. The Gruca procedure reinforces an unstable ankle with an osteotomy through the distal tibia and epiphysis, but may worsen leg length discrepancy. In most unilateral cases, the Gruca procedure is an interim procedure that does not compromise the result of subsequent Syme or Boyd amputation, but it may be considered definitive in cases of bilateral deformity.[99]

Proximal Femoral Focal Deficiency or Femoral Longitudinal Deficiency, Partial

Proximal femoral focal deficiency (PFFD) is characterized by partial deficiency of the proximal femur and involves the hip joint (Fig. 15–33). It comprises a spectrum of deformities ranging from mild hypoplasia to complete absence of the proximal femur, classified as Aitken class A (mild) through D (severe).[10] The femur is typically short and held in flexion, abduction, and external rotation. Partial fibular absence and foot deformity are often present, with possible tibial shortening, hip and knee flexion contractures, and an unstable knee joint.[50] The incidence is about 1 in 50,000 births. About 10% to 15% are bilateral. Embryologically, this deformity is a failure of the proximal femoral growth plate and the chondrocytes to migrate proximally. Treatment depends on whether PFFD is unilateral or bilateral, if a hip joint is present, the amount of coxa vara, the presence of pseudarthrosis, and the estimated ultimate leg length inequality.[85]

Bilateral deformities should usually not be treated by amputation unless there is great likelihood the patient can walk with prostheses after bilateral amputations. For bilateral PFFD, the child with symmetrical shortening often is able to ambulate without a prosthesis. If the upper limbs are either absent or severely deformed, then both feet must be saved for self-care activities.

Options for PFFD include special prostheses to lengthen the leg, surgical limb lengthening, surgical correction of the coxa vara and the pseudarthrosis, hip stabilization with an iliofemoral fusion, Syme or Boyd amputation, knee disarticulation and prosthetic fitting, and knee fusion with a van Ness rotationplasty. The length of the shortened femur grows as a constant proportion to the length of the contralateral normal femur. If the predicted foot position at maturity is below the level of the opposite knee and the ankle is normal, then a knee arthrodesis and van Ness tibial rotationplasty (see Fig. 15–1) allow fitting as a transfemoral amputee. One may try fitting a child with an unstable hip joint with an ischial containment socket to prevent the femur from pistoning.

Tibial Longitudinal Deficiency, Total/Partial (Formerly Tibial Hemimelia)

Tibial longitudinal deficiency occurs in approximately 1 in 1 million births and is characterized by complete or partial absence of the tibia (Fig. 15–34). Clinically, the foot is in severe varus, the leg is shortened, and there may be instability of the knee, ankle, or both. It may occur with

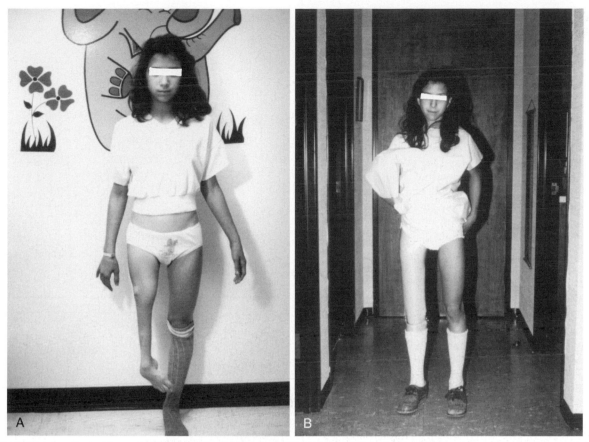

FIGURE 15–33 A patient with proximal femoral focal deficiency (PFFD) before *(A)* and after *(B)* Syme amputation with knee fusion. The patient was fitted as a knee disarticulation amputee. (Courtesy of K. Wilkins, M.D.)

FIGURE 15–34 Sisters with the familial form of tibial longitudinal deficiency. The older sister has a short transtibial amputation; the younger sister, whose deformity was less severe, later had a Syme amputation. (Courtesy of K. Wilkins, M.D.)

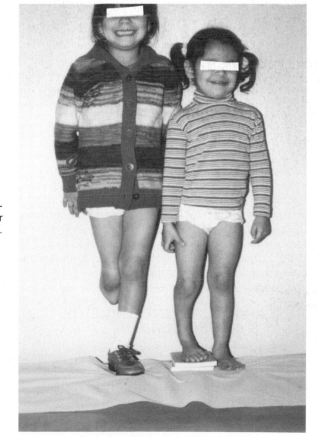

PFFD and coxa valga. Associated upper extremity deformities include supernumerary digits, partial adactyly (floating thumb), and central aphalangia of the hands ("lobster-claw" hands). Longitudinal tibial deficiency may be part of an inherited autosomal dominant syndrome, and 30% of cases are bilateral. Treatment depends on the anatomical abnormalities.

Treatment depends on the presence of any proximal tibia, the presence of a quadriceps mechanism, whether the foot and ankle are salvageable, and what the anticipated leg length discrepancy will be. The foot and ankle are usually not salvageable, and therefore require a Syme or Boyd amputation. If a proximal tibia and quadriceps mechanism are present, then the patient can function as a transtibial amputee by fusing the fibula to the remaining tibia. With no proximal tibia and no quadriceps mechanism, a knee disarticulation provides a functional amputation.

Training and Treatment Goals

Most children require minimal training, because they adapt quickly and easily to new devices. Play is a primary motivation, and so games with the prosthesis may keep the child's attention and increase proficiency.

Toddlers should be encouraged, but not forced, to wear a prosthesis, because they will wear a prosthesis if it truly helps them. Remember the milestones of the normal child: heel-to-toe gait at age 2 years, standing on one foot with help at 20 months, and standing on one foot momentarily at 3 years.

Children should be encouraged to participate in as many activities as possible. Transtibial or more distal pediatric amputees may excel at athletics. They can develop valgus knee deformities and patellar instability, which rarely need surgical treatment.

When prostheses are contraindicated in severely handicapped multiple amputees, alternative mobility should be provided at approximately 16 months of age. The alternative may be a caster cart, swivel-rocker, or electrically powered cart.[26]

Psychosocial Issues

Peer counselors make a significant difference in acceptance of the prosthesis. Congenitally limb-deficient children accept their deficiency more readily than does the acquired amputee. Children deal with limb loss better if they are adequately prepared. Adolescents, of course, place a high priority on cosmesis. The child should be encouraged by the parents to engage in as much normal physical activity as possible. Although most limb deficiencies occur sporadically, cases of tibial deficiency with a known heritable defect require genetic counseling.

RESEARCH AND DEVELOPMENT: WHAT'S ON THE HORIZON

Computer-aided design/computer aided manufacturing (CAD-CAM) of prostheses has been in the making for 20 years (Fig. 15–35).[27, 69] The first step in CAD-CAM is for

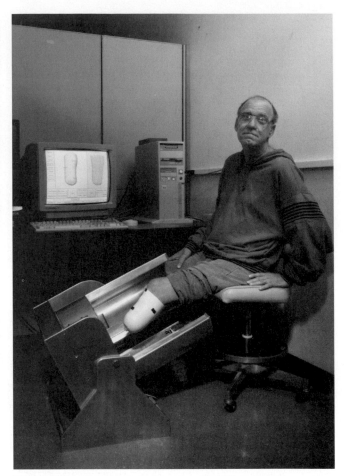

FIGURE 15–35 San Antonio computer-aided design/computer-aided manufacture (CAD-CAM) video laser imager and SOCKETS software. (Copyright Robert D. McAnelly, M.D.)

the computer to gather information about the residual limb. The second step is for the computer to manipulate this information to generate specifications for fabricating a socket. In the third step, a model is produced on an automated carver for immediate socket manufacture. A fourth step is modification of a socket design, if needed, after checking it on the residual limb. The biggest advantage in CAD-CAM is the data bank of information about each patient's previous limbs and fittings, which constantly updates and improves the technique. Current shortcomings of CAD-CAM include the continued dependence on input from the prosthetist (with the associated expense and possibility of human error), software and hardware that is currently limited to transtibial or transfemoral sockets, and the inability of most CAD-CAM data input sensors to detect the location of bones and the density of deep tissues. When these problems are overcome, the amputee will reap the rewards of continued improvement in the understanding of the socket-residual limb interface, and the payer will reap the rewards of a time-, labor-, and cost-saving process.

The editors dedicate this chapter to the memory of Lawrence W. Friedmann, M.D., who throughout his career, until his death in 1995, championed improvements in prosthetic care for his patients and ours.

References

1. Altner PC, Rockley P, Kirby K: Hemiplegia and lower extremity amputation: Double disability. Arch Phys Med Rehabil 1987; 68:378.
2. Ayyappa E: Prosthetic Desk Reference, rev ed 5. Long Beach, Calif, West VA Regional Medical Education Center, 1995.
3. Beard J, Scott DJA, Evans JM, et al: Pulse-generated runoff: A new method of determining calf vessel patency. Br J Surg 1988; 75:361.
4. Bodily KC, Burgess EM: Contralateral limb and patient survival after leg amputation. Am J Surg 1983; 146:280.
5. Bondurant FJ, Cotler HB, Buckle R, et al: The medical and economic impact of severely injured lower extremities. J Trauma 1988; 28:1270–1272.
6. Border J, Allgower M, Hanse ST, et al: Blunt Multiple Trauma: Comprehensive Pathophysiology and Care. New York, Marcel Dekker, 1990.
7. Boulton AJM, Kubrusly DB, Bowker JH, et al: Impaired vibratory perception and diabetic foot ulceration. Diabetic Med 1986; 3:335–337.
8. Bowker JH, Keagy RD, Pooneker PD: Musculoskeletal complications in amputees: Their prevention and management. In Bowker JH, Michael JW (eds): Atlas of Limb Prosthetics: Surgical, Prosthetic, and Rehabilitation Principles. ed 2. St Louis, Mosby–Year Book, 1992.
9. Boyd HB: Anatomic disarticulation of the hip. Surg Gynecol Obstet 1947, 84:364.
10. Bryant DD, Epps CH: Proximal femoral focal deficiency: Evaluation and management. Orthopedics 1991; 14:775.
11. Burgess EM, Matsen FA, Wyss CR, et al: Segmental transcutaneous measurements of pO_2 in patients requiring below-the-knee amputation for peripheral vascular insufficiency. J Bone Joint Surg Am 1982; 64:378.
12. Cina C, Katsamouris A, Megerman J, et al: Utility of transcutaneous oxygen tension measurements in peripheral arterial occlusive disease. J Vasc Surg 1984; 1:362.
13. Colborne GR, Naurmann S, Longmuir PE, et al: Analysis of mechanical and metabolic factors in the gait of congenital below knee amputees. Am J Phys Med Rehabil 1992; 71:272.
14. Cole WG, Klein RW, ValLith M, Jarvis R: Prosthetic program after above-knee amputation in children with sarcomata. J Bone Joint Surg Br 1982; 64:586–589.
15. Couch NP, David JK, Tilney NL, et al: Natural history of the leg amputee. Am J Surg 1977; 133:469.
16. Currie DM, Gilbert DML: Aerobic capacity with two leg work vs. one leg plus both arms work in peripheral vascular disease. Arch Phys Med Rehabil 1992; 73:1081–1084.
17. Davis RW: Phantom sensation, phantom pain, and stump pain. Arch Phys Med Rehabil 1993; 74:79–89.
18. Day HJB: The ISO/ISPO classification of congenital limb deficiency. Prosthet Orthot Int 1991; 15:67–69.
19. Deffer PA: More on the Ertl osteoplasty. Amputee Clin 1970; 2:7–8.
20. DeLateur BJ, Lehman JF, Winterscheid LC: Rehabilitation of the patient after hemicorporectomy. Arch Phys Med Rehabil 1989; 50:14.
21. Dormandy J: Natural history of intermittent claudication. Hosp Update, April 1991, pp 313–315.
22. Dormandy J, Mahir M, Ascady G, et al: Fate of the patient with chronic leg ischemia. J Cardiovasc Surg 1989; 30:50.
23. Dowd GSE, Linge K, Bentley G, et al: Measurement of transcutaneous oxygen pressure in normal and ischaemic skin. J Bone Joint Surg Br 1983; 65:79.
24. Eilber FR, Eckhardt J, Morton DL: Advances in the treatment of sarcomas of the extremity: Current status of limb salvage. Cancer 1984; 54:2695.
25. Evans DGR, Thakker Y, Donnai D: Heredity and dysmorphic syndromes in congenital limb deficiencies. Prosthet Orthot Int 1990; 15:70–77.
26. Faulkner V, Walsh N, Currie D: Early mobility aid for non-walking children. Clin Prosthet Orthot 1987; 11:106–108.
27. Faulkner V, Walsh NE, Gall NG: A computerized ultrasound shape-sensing mechanism. Orthot Prosthet 1988; 41:57–65.
28. Fillauer CE, Pritham CH, Fillauer KD: Evolution and development of the silicone suction socket (3S) for below-knee prostheses. J Prosthet Orthot 1989; 1:92–103.
29. Gailey RS, Lawrence D, Burditt C, et al: The CAT-CAM socket and quadrilateral socket: A comparison of energy cost during ambulation. Prosthet Orthot Int 1993; 17:95–100.
30. Gonzalez EG, Corcoran PJ, Reyes RL: Energy expenditure in below

31. Goorin A, Abelson H, Frei E: Osteosarcoma—15 years later. N Engl J Med 1985; 313:1637.
32. Gottschalk FA, Kourosh S, Stills M: Does socket configuration influence the position of the femur in above-knee amputation? J Prosthet Orthot 1989; 2:94–102.
33. Gregory RT, Gould RJ, Peclet M, et al: The mangled extremity syndrome (M.E.S.): A severity grading system for multi-system injury of the extremity. J Trauma 1985; 25:1147–1150.
34. Hammersgaard E, Baadsgaard K: Healing of below knee amputations in relation to perfusion pressure of skin. Acta Orthop Scand 1977; 48:335.
35. Hansen ST: Overview of the severely traumatized lower limb. Clin Orthop 1989; 243:17–19.
36. Hansen ST: The type IIIC tibial fracture. J Bone Joint Surg Am 1987; 69:799–780.
37. Harward TRS, Volny J, Golbranson F, et al: Oxygen inhalation-induced transcutaneous pO_2 changes as a predictor of amputation level. J Vasc Surg 1985; 2:220.
38. Helfet DL, Howey T, Sanders R, et al: Limb salvage versus amputation: Preliminary results of the mangled extremity severity score. Clin Orthop 1990; 256:80–86.
39. Hicks JH: Amputation in fractures of the tibia. J Bone Joint Surg Br 1964; 46:388–392.
40. Holloway GA, Burgess EM: Preliminary experience with laser Doppler velocimetry for the determination of amputation levels. Prosthet Orthot Int 1983; 7:63.
41. Holstein P: Distal blood pressure as guidance in choice of amputation level. Scand J Clin Lab Invest 1973; 31:245.
42. Holstein P, Lund P, Larsen B, et al: Skin perfusion pressure measured as the external pressure required to stop isotope washout. Scand J Clin Lab Invest 1977; 37:649.
43. Holstein P, Sager P, Lassen NA: Wound healing in below-knee amputations in relation to skin perfusion pressure. Acta Orthop Scand 1979; 50:49.
44. Jain AS, Stewart CPU: Tumor related lower limb amputation: A 23 year experience. Prosthet Orthot Int 1989; 13:82–85.
45. Jensen TS, Krebs B, Nielsen J, Rasmussen P: Immediate and long term phantom limb pain in amputees—incidence, clinical characteristics, and relationship to pre-amputation limb pain. Pain 1985; 21:267–278.
46. Kawamura I, Kawamura J: Some biomechanical evaluations of the ISNY flexible above-knee system with quadrilateral socket. Orthot Prosthet 1986; 40:17–23.
47. Kaye HW, Newman JD: Relative incidences of new amputations: Statistical comparisons of 6,000 new amputees. Orthot Prosthet 1975; 29:3–16.
48. Kihn RB, Warren R, Beebe GW: The "geriatric" amputee. Ann Surg 1972; 176:305.
49. King JC, Williams RP, McAnelly RD, Leonard EI: Rehabilitation of tumor amputees and limb salvage patients. In Garden FH, Grabois M (eds): Physical Medicine and Rehabilitation: State of the Art Reviews, vol. 8, No. 2, Cancer Rehabilitation. Philadelphia, Hanley & Belfus, 1994.
50. Krajbich I: Proximal femoral focal deficiency. In Kalamachi A (ed): Congenital Lower Limb Deficiencies. New York, Springer-Verlag, 1989.
51. Krebs DE, Fishman S: Characteristics of the child amputee population. J Pediatr Orthop 1984; 4:89–95.
52. Kristinsson O: Flexible above-knee socket made from low-density polyethylene suspended by a weight-transmitting frame. Orthot Prosthet 1983; 37:25–27.
53. Lambert C: Amputation surgery in the child. Orthop Clin North Am 1972; 3:473–482.
54. Lane JM, Kroll MA, Rossbach PG: New advances and concepts in amputee management after treatment for bone and soft-tissue sarcomas. Clin Orthop 1990; 256:22–28.
55. Lane RH, Harsh B, Boland P, et al: Osteogenic sarcoma. Clin Orthop 1986; 204:93.
56. Lange RH: Limb reconstruction versus amputation decision making in massive lower extremity trauma. Clin Orthop 1989; 243:92–99.
57. Lange RH, Bach AW, Hansen ST, et al: Open tibial fractures with associated vascular injuries: Prognosis for limb salvage. J Trauma 1985, 25:203–208.
58. Loeser JD: Pain after amputation: Phantom limb and stump pain. In

(Continued from previous column)
knee amputees: Correlation with stump length. Arch Phys Med Rehabil 1974; 55:111–119.

Bonica JJ (ed): The Management of Pain, ed 2. Philadelphia, Lea & Febiger, 1990, p 244.

59. Long IA: Allowing normal adduction of the femur in above-knee amputations. Orthot Prosthet 1975; 29:53.

60. Long IA: Normal shape normal alignment (NSNA) above-knee prosthesis. Clin Prosthet Orthot 1985; 9:9.

61. Lowry R: Durability of lower extremity prostheses. Arch Phys Med Rehabil 1966; 47:742–743.

62. Malone JM: Complications of lower extremity amputation. In Moore WS, Malone JM (eds): Lower Extremity Amputation. Philadelphia, WB Saunders, 1989, pp 208–214.

63. Marcove R, Rosen G: En bloc resection for osteogenic sarcoma. Cancer 1980; 3040.

64. McCollum PT, Spence VA, Walker WF, et al: Amputation for peripheral vascular disease: The case for level selection. Br J Surg 1988; 75:1193.

65. McCollum PT, Spence VA, Walker WF, et al: Circumferential skin blood flow measurements in the ischaemic lower limb. Br J Surg 1985; 72:310.

66. McCollum PT, Spence VA, Walker WF, et al: Oxygen induced changes in the skin as measured by transcutaneous oxymetry. Br J Surg 1986; 73:882.

67. McCollum PT, Walker WF: Major limb amputation for end-stage peripheral vascular disease: Level selection and alternative options. In Bowker JH, Michael JW (eds): Atlas of Limb Prosthetics, ed 2. St Louis, Mosby–Year Book, 1992, pp 29–30.

68. McFarland DC, Lawrence PF: Skin fluorescence: A method to predict amputation site healing. J Surg Res 1982; 32:410.

69. Medhat MA, McAnelly RD: What's new in lower extremity amputation and prosthetics: IV. CAD-CAM. Surg Rounds Orthop, July 1990, pp 37–39.

70. Mehta K, Hobson RW, Jamil Z, et al: Fallibility of Doppler ankle pressure in predicting healing of transmetatarsal amputation. J Surg Res 1980; 28:466.

71. Michael J: Component selection criteria: Lower limb disarticulations. Clin Prosthet Orthot 1988; 12:99–108.

72. Michael J: Energy storing feet: A clinical comparison. Clin Prosthet Orthot 1987; 11:154–168.

73. Mooney V, Wagner FW, Waddell J, et al: The below-the-knee amputation for vascular disease. J Bone Joint Surg Am 1976; 58:365.

74. Moore WS, Henry RE, Malone JM, et al: Prospective use of xenon[133] clearance for amputation level selection. Arch Surg 1981; 116:86–88.

75. Nielson DH, Schurr DG, Golden JC, et al: Comparison of energy cost and gait efficiency during ambulation in below-knee amputees using different prosthetic feet: A preliminary report. J Prosthet Orthot 1989; 1:24–31.

76. O'Connell PG, Gnatz S: Hemiplegia and amputation: Rehabilitation in the dual disability. Arch Phys Med Rehabil 1989; 70:451.

77. Oishi CS, Fronek A, Golbranson FL: The role of non-invasive vascular studies in determining levels of amputation. J Bone Joint Surg Am 1988; 70:1520.

78. Otteman MG, Stahlgrew LH: Evaluation of factors which influence mortality and morbidity following major lower extremity amputation for atherosclerosis. Surg Gynecol Obstet 1965; 120:1217.

79. Personal oral communication, N. Gall, M.D., 1995.

80. Personal oral communication, R. Heimbach, M.D., 1995.

81. Pfeil J, Marquardt E, Holtz T, et al: The stump capping procedure to prevent or treat terminal osseous overgrowth. Prosthet Orthot Int. 1991; 15:96–99.

82. Ratcliff DA, Clyne CAC, Chant ADB, et al: Prediction of amputation wound healing: The role of transcutaneous pO_2 assessment. Br J Surg 1984; 71:219.

83. Robbs JV, Ray R: Clinical predictors of below knee stump healing following amputation for ischaemia. S Afr J Surg 1982; 20:305.

84. Roon AJ, Moore WS, Goldstone J, et al: Below-knee amputation: A modern approach. Am J Surg 1977; 134:153.

85. Rossi TV, Kruger L: Proximal femoral focal deficiency and its treatment. Orthot Prosthet 1975; 29:37–57.

86. Sabolich J: Contoured adducted trochanteric-controlled alignment method (CAT-CAM): Introduction and basic principles. Clin Prosthet Orthot 1985; 9:15.

87. Sanders GT: Lower Limb Amputations: A Guide to Rehabilitation. Philadelphia, FA Davis, 1986.

88. Schwartz JA, Schuler JJ, O'Connor BJA, et al: Predictive value of distal perfusion pressure in the healing of amputation of the digits and forefoot. Surg Gynecol Obstet 1982; 154:865.

89. Scott CI: Genetic and familial aspects of limb defects with emphasis on the lower extremities. In Kalamachi A (ed): Congenital Lower Limb Deficiencies. New York, Springer-Verlag, 1989.

90. Setoguchi Y, Rosenfelder R: The Limb-Deficient Child. Springfield, Ill, Charles C Thomas, 1982.

91. Sherman RA: Phantom limb pain mechanism–based management. Clin Podiatr Med Surg 1994; 11:85–106.

92. Sherman RA, Sherman CJ, Gall NG: A survey of current phantom limb treatment in the United States. Pain 1980; 8:85–99.

93. Sherman RA, Sherman CJ: A comparison of phantom sensations among amputees whose amputations were of civilian and military origins. Pain 1985; 21:91–97.

94. Sherman RA, Sherman CJ: Prevalence and characteristics of chronic phantom limb pain among American veterans. Am J Phys Med Rehabil 1983; 62:227–238.

95. Sherman R, Sherman CJ, Parker L: Chronic phantom and stump pain among American veterans: Result of a survey. Pain 1984; 18:83–95.

96. Silverman DG, Roberts A, Reilly CA, et al: Fluorometric quantification of low-dose fluorescein delivery to predict amputation site healing. Surgery 1987; 101:335.

97. Simon MA: Limb salvage for osteosarcoma in the 1980s. Clin Orthop 1991; 270:264–270.

98. Staats TB: Advanced prosthetic techniques for below knee amputations. Orthopedics 1985; 8:249–258.

99. Thomas IH, Williams PF: The Gruca operation for congenital absence of the fibula. J Bone Joint Surg Br 1987; 69:587.

100. Thyregod HC, Holstein P, Steen Jensen J, et al: The healing of through-knee amputations in relation to skin perfusion pressure. Prosthet Orthot Int 1983; 7:61.

101. US Department of Health and Human Services: Current Estimates from the National Health Interview Survey, 1990, series 10, 181. Washington, DC, Vital and Health Statistics, 1991, p 94.

102. US Department of Health and Human Services: Detailed Diagnoses and Procedures: National Hospital Discharge Survey, 1989, series 13, 108. Washington, DC, Vital and Health Statistics, 1989, p 119.

103. US Department of Health and Human Services: Prevalence of Selected Impairments: United States—1977, series 10, 134. Washington, DC, Vital and Health Statistics, 1981, pp 14–17, 28–29.

104. US Department of Health and Human Services: Use of Special Aids: United States—1977, series 10, 135. Washington, DC, Vital and Health Statistics, 1980, pp 12–13, 15–16, 23–25.

105. Varghese G, Hinterbuchner C, Mondall P, et al: Rehabilitation outcome of patients with dual disability of hemiplegia and amputation. 1978; 59:121.

106. Volpicelli L, Chambers R, Wagner F: Ambulation levels of bilateral lower extremity amputees. J Bone Joint Surg Am 1983; 65:599.

107. Wagman LD, Terz JJ: Hemipelvectomy and translumbar amputation. In Moore WS, Malone JM (eds): Lower Extremity Amputation. Philadelphia, WB Saunders, 1989, pp 157–176.

108. Waters RL, Perry J, Chambers R: Energy expenditure of amputee gait. In Moore WS, Malone JM (eds): Lower Extremity Amputation. Philadelphia, WB Saunders, 1989, pp 250–260.

109. Welch GH, Leiberman DP, Pollock JG, et al: Failure of Doppler ankle pressure to predict healing of conservative forefoot amputations. Br J Surg 1985; 72:888.

110. White RA, Nolan L, Harley D, et al: Noninvasive evaluation of peripheral vascular disease using transcutaneous oxygen tension. Am J Surg 1982; 144:68.

111. Williard WC, Hajdu SI, Casper ES, et al: Comparison of amputation with limb-sparing operations for adult soft tissue sarcoma of the extremity. Am Surg 1992; 215:269–275.

112. Wilson AB: Limb Prosthetics, ed 6. New York, Demos Publications, 1989.

113. Wilson SB, Spence VA: Dynamic thermographic imaging method for quantifying dermal perfusion: Potential and limitations. Med Biol Eng Comput 1989; 27:496.

114. Wing DC, Hittenberger DA: Energy-storing prosthetic feet. Arch Phys Med Rehabil 1989; 70:330–335.

115. Wu Y, Keagy RD, Krick HJ, et al: An innovative removable rigid dressing technique for below-knee amputation. J Bone Joint Surg Am 1979; 61:724–729.

116. Wu Y, Krick H: Removable rigid dressing for below-knee amputees. Clin Prosthet Orthot 1987; 11:33–44.

117. Zettl JH: Immediate postoperative prostheses and temporary prosthetics. In Moore WS, Malone JM (eds): Lower Extremity Amputation. Philadelphia, WB Saunders, 1989, pp 177–207.

CHAPTER

16

Upper Limb Orthoses

KATIE D. IRANI, M.B.B.S.

An orthosis, as defined by the International Standards Organization of the International Society for Prosthetics and Orthotics, is an externally applied device used to modify structural and functional characteristics of the neuro-musculoskeletal system.[12] Orthoses are used with the primary goal of restoration of function.

There has been a remarkable expansion recently in the types of orthotic materials available, especially the low-temperature thermoplastics. There has also been a marked increase in the number of different commercially available upper extremity orthoses. This has made it easier to modify and custom-fit many of the commonly used orthoses. It has also been one of the factors in the increased use of orthoses, especially for trauma, sports, work-related musculoskeletal problems, and arthritis.

It is likely that with the aging of our population there will be even greater use of orthoses in the future.

FUNCTIONS OF ORTHOSES

The goal of using an orthosis is to improve function, either immediately or as part of a treatment program that will lead to improved function in the future.[8]

TO IMMOBILIZE OR SUPPORT. Orthoses can be used to rest or immobilize a joint or body part to allow healing, to prevent or correct deformity, or to maintain a joint in a more functional position. The position of an orthosis can also help prevent deformity by maintaining ligaments and muscles and other soft tissues at an appropriate length.

TO APPLY TRACTION. Traction can be used to increase range of motion (ROM) of a joint or stretch a tight or contracted muscle. This orthosis permits the full available ROM and attempts to increase ROM or length with some added tension. This is not typically a comfortable orthosis and the patient's tolerance has to be increased gradually with increases in wearing time. The tension can be adjusted every few days if more ROM is needed.

TO ASSIST WEAK OR PARTIAL SEGMENTS. In some cases an orthosis can assist a weak or partial body segment. The orthosis should not override the weakened muscle, but should assist in providing an enhanced function when there is reasonable expectation of recovery. If the weakness is permanent, an orthosis providing a strong overriding force to achieve the function might be necessary.

TO SUBSTITUTE FOR ABSENT MOTOR FUNCTION. When there is very weak or paralyzed muscle function in one direction and usable strength in the opposite direction, a dynamic orthosis is often used. The patient moves the joint in one direction, and when relaxed, the orthotic device moves the segment in the opposite direction. An example of this is a dynamic finger extension splint in radial nerve injury.

TO PERMIT CONTROLLED DIRECTIONAL MOVEMENT. This type of orthosis is used to allow movement in one plane, while restricting motion in other planes. An example of this is an orthosis that allows flexion and extension, but prevents abduction and adduction of meta-carpophalangeal (MP) joints after implant surgery.

TO ALLOW ATTACHMENT OF ASSISTIVE DEVICES. This orthosis functions as a base to which different assistive devices can be attached (e.g., a universal cuff) (Fig. 16–1).

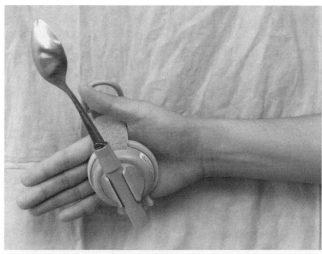

FIGURE 16–1 Universal cuff orthosis with swivel attachment pocket.

321

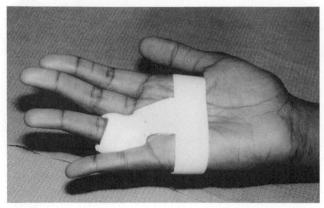

FIGURE 16–2   Orthosis with a single-finger MP stop to isolate PIP flexion. It allows strengthening of the flexor digitorum sublimis.

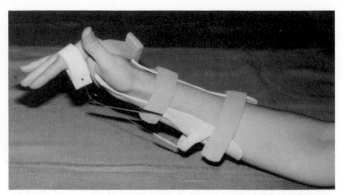

FIGURE 16–4   Wrist-hand orthosis of low-profile design with dynamic MP flexion of the index finger.

TO BLOCK A SEGMENT.   This orthosis is used to prohibit movement in a joint so that adjacent joints can be exercised. This is used primarily in the hand as, for example, when an MP joint is blocked to prevent flexion so that the proximal interphalangeal (PIP) joint can be exercised (Fig. 16–2).

TYPES OF SPLINTS

There are two basic types of orthoses used: static and dynamic. Some orthoses use both principles.

Static means that the orthosis is rigid and gives support without allowing movement (Fig. 16–3). These are commonly used to rest a part after trauma, surgery, and for acutely inflamed joints and tendons. These are typically conforming orthoses which accommodate to the available static position. When mild traction is needed, the static orthosis can be made to be nonconforming to stretch a contracture of a joint or stretch a muscle.[10]

Dynamic orthoses allow a certain degree of movement. Often the terms *functional orthoses* and *dynamic orthoses* are incorrectly used synonymously. Functional orthoses are those that improve function whether or not they allow motion or have moving parts.[8] Many times dynamic orthoses are used primarily to stretch a contracture and do not provide any functional skill (Fig. 16–4). A functional orthosis often utilizes rubber bands, springs, movable joints, cables, or batteries to give added function. These are used commonly in patients with permanent residual dysfunction after injury, in slowly recovering conditions, or with chronic disease.[1]

Many functional orthoses are complex, need proper fit and design, and are more difficult to make than the simple dynamic orthoses.

CONSIDERATIONS IN PRESCRIPTION OF ORTHOSES

SENSATION.   An orthotic device does not provide sensation. In fact, it often covers skin areas and decreases sensory feedback. This is of particular importance in the volar aspect of the hand.

GRAVITY.   Gravity plays an important role in upper limb orthoses, especially in those joints with the heaviest movement masses like the shoulder and the elbow. Gravity and the weight of the upper extremity act to distract joints.

COMFORT.   The orthosis should be comfortable. Pressure should be distributed over the largest area possible.[3, 6]

SIMPLICITY.   The design should be simple for easy donning and doffing.

DURABILITY.   The orthosis should be durable and easy to maintain.

UTILITY.   The orthosis must be useful and serve a real purpose. A well-functioning opposite extremity is a major deterrent to the use of an orthosis as most activities of daily living (ADL) can be performed with the "good" hand. The critical question is what the patient can do with the orthosis vs. what can be done without it (in relation to what the patient wishes to perform). Patients typically discontinue the use of an orthosis that does not add significantly to their function.

TOLERANCE.   Consider the extent of the patient's tol-

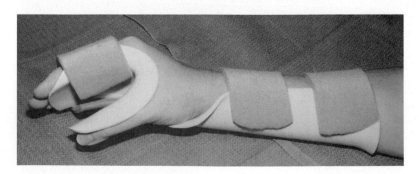

FIGURE 16–3   Static wrist-hand orthosis.

erance. The more complicated the "gadget," the less likely it is to be accepted for permanent use.

COSMESIS. Cosmesis is important, especially in hand orthoses. A functional but unsightly orthosis is often rejected if the patient values appearance over function.

Unless these above criteria are addressed, the best-made orthosis is doomed to be ineffective, since the patient is likely to reject it. An orthosis is most likely to be accepted and used consistently by the patient if it reduces pain or provides improvement in a desired function.

THE UPPER LIMB: KINESIOLOGIC CONSIDERATIONS

The functional activity of the hand and its placement in an infinite number of positions is a combined, integrated activity of the entire upper limb. The role of the shoulder is limb orientation in space. The shoulder positions the upper limb in different positions so that the hand, for example, can reach in front to wash or high enough to access the top shelf of a cabinet. The elbow acts like a caliper to regulate the distance between the hand and the body. At least 45 to 50 degrees of elbow flexion is needed for the hand to reach the mouth if there is normal wrist movement. The forearm and wrist govern the orientation of the hand. The hand has innumerable combinations of motion and the greatest amount of motion occurs at the MP joint of the thumb. The motor component of the hand and wrist form a single functional unit to provide a precision force that is volitional and proportional to the task performed.

Release is almost as important as grasp. For example, in radial nerve palsy, one can grasp an object but will have difficulty in releasing and placing it precisely.

Extension stability of the wrist is important for optimal function of the hand. Most activities of the hand are carried out with the wrist in neutral to 10 degrees of extension, while strong grasp activities need 20 to 30 degrees of wrist extension.

Contouring and opposition are integral parts of hand function. There are two basic types of hand grips—power and precision. In power grip the wrist is held in dorsiflexion with the fingers wrapped around an object held in the palm. In a precision grip, the thumb is held against the tips of the index and middle fingers. Functional hand splinting is typically aimed at improving pinch. There are three types of pinch: (1) palmar pad pinch, (2) palmar tip pinch, and (3) lateral pinch. It is usually best to splint toward palmar pad pinch. This allows the best compromise between very fine precision tip pinch without force (e.g., picking up a needle), and a strong lateral pinch without precision (holding a pen). There is no practical orthosis that can substitute for, or improve, thumb adduction.

The wrist joint is the "key" to the hand. The prehensile force of the hand is greatest when the wrist is in 20 to 30 degrees of extension. If the wrist is allowed to fall into flexion, the MP joints hyperextend, the PIP and DIP (distal interphalangeal) joints flex, the metacarpal arch flattens, and the thumb falls into adduction. Obtaining wrist stability by muscle power or splinting is imperative if optimal hand function is to be achieved.

The MP joint is the key joint for finger function. When MPs are hyperextended, the interphalangeal joints flex, owing to the tension of the flexors and the delicate muscle balance between the finger extensors and flexors. For example, this is seen in the "intrinsic minus hand" having a combined median and ulnar nerve injury. Contracture of the MP joint in extension occurs typically as the collateral ligament of the MP joint is relaxed in extension and taut in flexion. The MP joints are typically maintained in about 45 degrees of flexion in a completely paralyzed hand.

SHOULDER AND ARM ORTHOSES

The most common orthosis for the shoulder is a sling, and many varieties of slings are available. Some slings tend to hold the shoulder in adduction and internal rotation with the elbow flexed. Since they simply support the upper extremity, shoulder and elbow joint stiffness can result. When treating shoulder subluxation with a sling, there should be enough pull on the arm cuff or push-up at the elbow to hold the humeral head against the glenoid cavity of the scapula. A subluxated shoulder can also be treated with a humeral cuff and chest straps (Fig. 16–5).

An airplane splint is a static shoulder orthosis. It consists of a body piece that is connected by a static part to an arm support trough which holds the shoulder in the desired degree of abduction and flexion. It is often used after burns of the axilla and after shoulder surgery.

With trapezius muscle loss the shoulder tends to droop downward and forward. A simple figure-of-8 orthosis with anterior inferior padding can hold the shoulder back, decrease muscle pull and pain in the neck, and improve posture.

Shoulder dynamic orthoses are rarely indicated. Many have been tried in the past but they are bulky, complex, cumbersome, and provide limited additional function. They are typically not accepted by patients. The only dynamic shoulder orthoses used are as part of the mobile arm

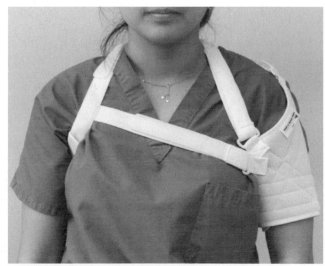

FIGURE 16–5 Sling with humeral cuff and chest straps that can be used for supporting a subluxed shoulder. This orthosis does not support the elbow or hand.

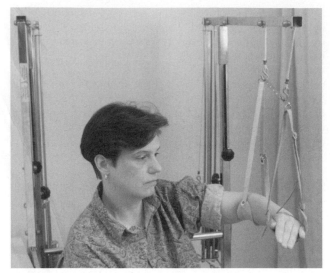

FIGURE 16–6 Overhead sling with two straps for supporting the upper limb. This can be mounted to a wheelchair.

orthotic systems, or balanced forearm orthoses (BFOs). With severe weakness of the upper limb, overhead slings, friction feeders, or BFOs can be used. Overhead sling suspension is used to support very weak proximal muscles and reduce the effect of gravity (Fig. 16–6). This is often used as a training apparatus prior to use of a BFO.

A balanced forearm orthosis can be attached to a wheelchair. It consists of a forearm trough which is attached by a hinge joint to a ball-bearing swivel mechanism and a mount.[1] It supports the weight of the forearm and arm against gravity. With only minimal muscle force requirement at the shoulder girdle and trunk, the patient can move the arm horizontally and flex the elbow to bring the hand to the mouth. This orthosis is primarily used for patients with severe upper limb weakness, as in high quadriplegia or other severe neuromuscular conditions. The orthosis must be precisely adjusted for effective use, and the patient must be trained in its use. The patient must also have sufficient range of motion of the shoulder and elbow, as well as adequate trunk stability while sitting. The BFO also adds width to the wheelchair.

In ambulatory patients with severe proximal shoulder girdle and elbow weakness (as occurs with the central cord syndrome), a simple orthosis consisting of a figure-of-8 shoulder harness and forearm cuffs can be made. The forearm cuffs are connected to the harness by flexible rubber tubing. Clamps on the cuffs allow for variable arm positioning.[9]

The humeral orthosis is a static bivalve orthosis that encircles the arm, and is typically fitted in a healing fracture of the midhumerus. It can be fabricated proximally over the shoulder joint to limit motion of the shoulder if desired.

ELBOW ORTHOSES

Most static elbow orthoses are used to increase elbow range of motion in flexion or extension. A simple volar or dorsal conforming splint can be used, or one can use a three-point orthosis with cuffs and bars. Joints, dials, and turnbuckles can be used to gradually change the elbow joint angle and increase the force applied. A functional dynamic orthosis can be fitted for the patient with weak elbow flexion. It consists of a forearm cuff and an arm cuff which are connected to a pivot joint by springs or rubber tubing. If the elbow flexors are less than antigravity, an elbow assist can be used with an elbow-locking mechanism. This holds the elbow in a functional position to allow the hand to carry a load. A Bowden cable housing system can be utilized as in an above-elbow prosthesis.[1]

An orthosis to assist or substitute for elbow extension is not usually necessary as gravity is adequate to achieve extension in most patients. A static elbow wrist orthosis is used to stabilize the elbow and prevent supination and pronation of the forearm. This is used to give rest to the elbow region in inflammatory conditions, as well as after surgeries around the elbow and proximal forearm.[13]

WRIST ORTHOSES

The most frequently used upper limb orthosis is a wrist support. Most of those on the market can be fitted to a patient who requires only simple support in the case of a painful wrist. The wrist can be splinted with either a dorsal or volar splint (Fig. 16–7). Volar splints support while dorsal splints suspend the part. Volar splints obstruct the palm in gripping objects and decrease the available surface for palmar sensation and interfere with grasp. Most of the attachments for the hand and fingers are on the dorsal side, except for those that assist finger flexion. Palmar wrist support should not extend beyond the distal palmar crease (which corresponds to the MP joints).[2] This allows free movement of these joints. The wrist splint should be about two-thirds the length of the forearm proximally for good leverage. It also helps in distributing the pressure over a larger surface area. A radial- or ulnar-based orthosis is used in different conditions around the radial or ulnar aspect of the wrist (Fig. 16–8).

A dynamic wrist orthosis is used to support the wrist and control flexion and extension. It prevents ulnar and radial deviation. It is used after wrist arthroplasty, synovectomy, and fractures. It is also used to increase range of motion of the wrist.[6, 10]

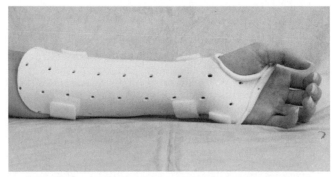

FIGURE 16–7 Static volar wrist orthosis with thumb cutout.

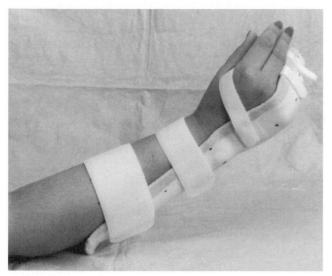

FIGURE 16–8 Static ulnar "gutter" splint made of thermoplastic material and Velcro straps.

HAND ORTHOSES

Many different kinds of hand orthoses can be made and a number of innovative, individualized forms are currently utilized, especially by hand therapists. A few components are used in all designs, including the basic hand component, web spacer, thumb flexor and extensor, finger MP, PIP, and DIP flexor and extensor orthoses.

Since most ADL can be performed by one normal hand, a hand orthosis is often rejected by the patient. Hand orthoses are frequently utilized in the early stages after an injury or surgery. Once the pain is resolved and healing has occurred, patients will use an orthosis only if it allows them to do activities which otherwise could not be done.

Static hand orthoses can be used to hold the hand in a particular position or immobilize a digit or a single joint.

Short opponens hand orthoses are made of either metal or plastic. The Bennett types of metal hand orthoses have a dorsal part that extends over the fifth metacarpal to the hand and over the lateral aspect of the thumb to act as an opponens bar.[1] It also has a web spacer that extends below the thumb and the index finger. The Rancho type also has an opponens bar, a C bar, and a volar strap across the hand. The Engen type is made of thermoplastic material and comes in various sizes. These preformed thermoplastic shells fit in the palm of the hand over the palmar arch, extend to the base of the thumb, and are held by a dorsal strap. Many different attachments can be added to the basic hand unit.

A static wrist-hand orthosis is used to rest an injured hand, prevent contracture, or stretch a contracture. Since there is a fine balance between finger flexors and extensors, the positions of the finger joints depend on the position of the more proximal joints. If the PIP joint is held in flexion, a secondary hyperextension of the DIP joint can occur (e.g., in the rheumatoid hand with a boutonnière deformity). Splinting for tightness of flexors or extensors requires splinting both of the wrist and the fingers. If only the wrist is splinted (in extension), it can accentuate flexion

of the fingers, especially in the presence of flexor tightness. Single joints with joint or capsular tightness can be splinted. A simple gutter splint or a trough can be fitted for PIP or DIP joints. A boutonnière or swan-neck deformity of the PIP joint can be stabilized by a three-point orthosis made of rings attached together on the dorsum or palm of the hand (Fig. 16–9).

Dynamic wrist hand orthoses (WHOs) are complex and challenging to fit. Each has to be evaluated for the multiple and various combination of movements encountered. Every deformity does not require orthotic correction, and overzealous splinting can interfere with hand function. The goals of splinting have to be carefully evaluated. Dynamic splints are used to substitute for absent or weak finger extensors or to provide traction of finger joints in flexion or extension. A basic wrist-hand orthosis is used to which dynamic outriggers are attached.

A wrist-extension, finger-flexion reciprocal orthosis is used in C6 quadriplegia, as in any patient who can extend the wrist but cannot flex the fingers. It is a dynamic, functional, wrist-hand orthosis that in the older literature was called the "flexor hinge splint." It utilizes the wrist extension force which is translated into finger flexion at the MP joints of the index and middle fingers (Figs. 16–10 and 16–11). It consists of a basic hand orthosis with wrist and MP joints. The index and middle fingers are held together in slight flexion at the PIP and DIP joints. A telescopic rod connects the forearm piece to the fingers and can be adjusted according to the size of the object to be held. When the wrist is extended the fingers go into flexion to provide a pulp pinch. When the wrist goes into flexion, the fingers open and release the object. This orthosis uses the principle of a parallelogram.

A similar orthosis with a ratchet is used to set the wrist passively to give the desired pinch. This is used chiefly in C5 quadriplegic patients who do not have active wrist extension.

An MP flexion orthosis is commonly used to stretch out MP extension contractures (Fig. 16–12). It is not usually used for loss of one of the flexors at the MP joint, as there are four flexors of the MP joint (the interossei, lumbricals, and flexor digitorum superficialis and profundus). A basic palmar wrist-hand orthosis is used with a volar projection to which finger loops and rubber bands are attached. The loops are placed over the proximal phalanges and the pull

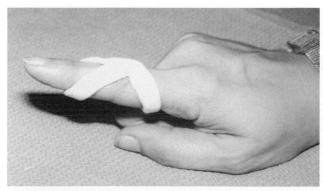

FIGURE 16–9 Static three-point PIP orthosis to prevent hyperflexion (e.g., boutonnière deformity). It allows MP and DIP movement. Rotated 180 degrees it prevents PIP hyperextension (e.g., swanneck deformity).

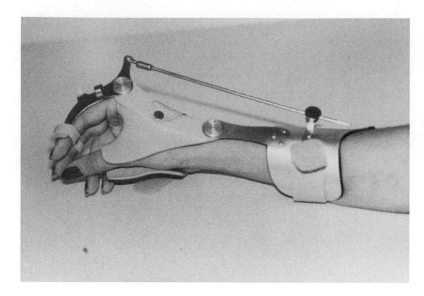

FIGURE 16–10 Wrist extensor, finger flexor orthosis with adjustable rod. Note that the wrist is in extension and the fingers are in a three-point pinch position. This is also called a "flexor hinge splint." Its function is to use available wrist extension strength to power finger flexion and pinch.

FIGURE 16–11 Wrist extensor, finger flexor orthosis with adjustable rod. Note that the wrist is in flexion and the fingers are in an open position, to release an object (see also Fig. 16–10).

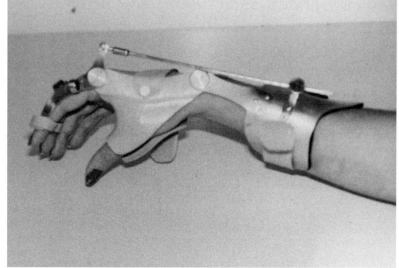

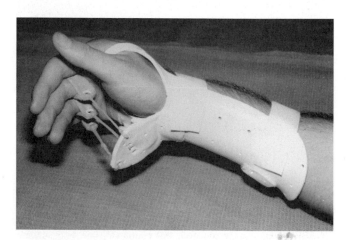

FIGURE 16–12 Dynamic MP flexion orthosis. Note that each finger is pulled into a slightly different degree of flexion.

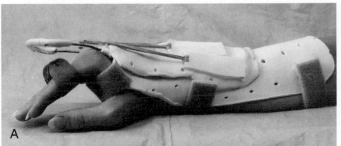
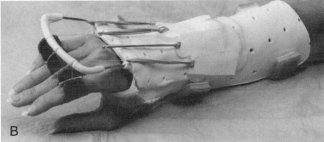

FIGURE 16–13   Dynamic MP extension splint, low-profile design. *A*, Lateral view. *B*, Dorsal view.

is kept perpendicular to the proximal phalanx. The greater the extension contracture, the larger the volar projection required to achieve a perpendicular force. This kind of splint allows individual control of MP joints with varying pull.

A low-profile MP flexion splint can be fabricated by adding a triangular-shaped metal wire, the base of which lies at the level of the base of the thumb. The finger loop is attached to a nylon wire which is pulled over this metal bar and is attached proximally to a short rubber band that is anchored to the volar surface. Tension adjustment can be done for individual joints.

Ready-made MP flexor orthoses, commonly called "knuckle benders," are commercially available. These consist of two metal plates that fit over the dorsum of the hand and over the proximal phalanges. The two plates are connected by metal wires to a rigid palmar bar. Rubber bands are attached at the ends of the plates. This orthosis does not allow tension adjustment of individual fingers. Most of the traction force affects the most contracted or lagging finger. The other fingers do not get much or even any traction until the lagging finger improves. This splint is useful when a custom-made splint is not available.

An MP extension orthosis is used as a functional splint in patients with absent or weak finger extensors, and also as a traction splint for flexion contracture of the MP joint. The same principle as in the MP flexor orthosis is used, but on the dorsal side (Fig. 16–13A and B). A dorsal wrist-hand orthosis with dorsal outrigger is used to which finger loops and rubber bands are attached. The finger loop is placed on the proximal phalanx and the pull should be perpendicular. A low-profile splint can be fabricated, and many outrigger designs are available. These use thermoplastic materials in combination with rubber bands, nylon thread, and metal wire.

An MP extension block, called a "lumbrical bar," is used dorsally over the proximal phalanges to block the MP joint from hyperextending. This is useful in conditions having MP hyperextension such as an intrinsic minus hand.

An IP joint extension (Fig. 16–14) or flexion orthosis (Fig. 16–15) is used to stretch a contracted joint. The orthosis must block the MP joint to prevent movement and allow traction force to act solely on the IP joint. Dynamic traction is achieved with a finger loop and rubber band over the middle phalanx. These are dynamic, nonfunctional, traction splints. Elastic bands and cuffs can be used as static IP flexion splints. A number of commercial splints for IP joints are available and can be tried if there is only single-joint involvement.

DIP joint flexion in patients with DIP extension contractures is best achieved by cuffs and bands. A static DIP extension splint is commercially available and is commonly used after injury of the extensor tendon (as in mallet finger) (Fig. 16–16).

ORTHOSES USED FOR HAND INJURIES

Flexor Tendon Injuries

Tendon injuries occur commonly in the hand. Flexor tendon injuries are far more serious than extensor tendon

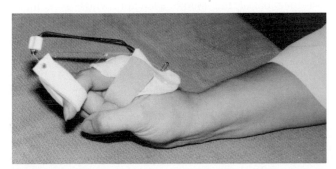

FIGURE 16–14   Dynamic PIP extension orthosis with low-profile construction design.

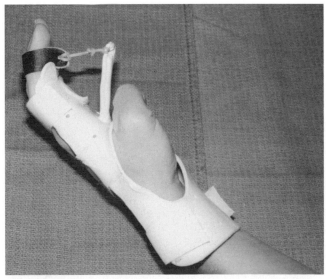

FIGURE 16–15   Dynamic PIP flexion orthosis. Note the perpendicular pull of the rubber bands and the long volar outrigger.

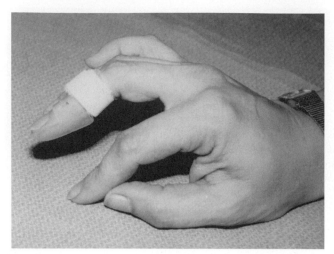

FIGURE 16–16 Commercially available static volar DIP extension orthosis. Note that it allows PIP movement.

injuries because of the specific anatomical nature of the flexor tendons and the tendon sheaths in the fingers. Emphasis is placed on preventing loss of tendon excursion caused by adhesions, which can limit finger function.

Rehabilitation is directed toward early guarded passive motion to allow tendon glide inside the sheath. This must be done without imposing any tension on the repair site and without stretching the repaired tendon.[14] Splinting is an integral part of the rehabilitation of flexor tendon injuries. A postoperative orthosis is applied from the forearm to the involved fingers. The wrist joint is flexed about 40 degrees, the MP joint, about 45 degrees, the PIP joint, 90 degrees, and the DIP joint, to full flexion. A finger hook is attached via a nylon string and rubber band to the base of the forearm (Fig. 16–17). The rubber band acts as a passive flexor and full active extension is limited by the dorsal block. After 3 to 4 weeks, the passive pull is discontinued and the dorsal block is adjusted to allow a gradual increase in wrist and finger extension. Later, to strengthen the flexor digitorum sublimis and profundus individually, a volar MP block and PIP block orthosis is used.

Extensor Tendon Injuries

The same principles are used with extensor tendon injury. A dorsal WHO with the wrist in 20 degrees of

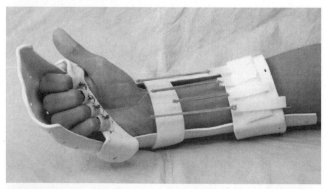

FIGURE 16–17 Dynamic orthosis used after flexor tendon repair. It allows active extension and passive flexion of the repaired tendons. The patient can resist the rubber bands to gain extension of the PIP joints without excessive tension at the tendon repair site(s).

extension, dorsal outrigger, and rubber bands are used to allow controlled passive extension and partial active flexion.[4]

ORTHOSES USED FOR NERVE INJURIES

Injury to any of the three nerves supplying the hand results in loss of function. Careful assessment of what functions are missing is essential. First, determine if there is a natural substitute for what is missing. Then determine whether an orthotic device could substitute for the lost function and improve overall hand function. Keep in mind the vocational and avocational demands put on the hand. The purposes of orthotic use in the care of the hand with a nerve injury are to (1) prevent deformity from occurring in an imbalanced hand, (2) restore full passive range of motion in the affected areas and achieve full active range of motion and strength in the nonaffected surrounding areas, (3) add mechanical assistance by positioning the hand so that it can be used more effectively, and (4) substitute for lost muscle power.

Radial Nerve Injury

The most obvious deformity with a radial nerve injury is a wristdrop and drop finger. If the wrist is held in a neutral or slightly extended position, the patient can make a strong full fist but is unable to open the hand and release the object. A dorsal wrist support with dynamic extension force at the MP joints gives a very functional hand (Fig. 16–18A and B).

In case of posterior interosseus nerve injury or in radial nerve injury following recovery of the wrist extensors, a dynamic MP extensor dorsal hand orthosis without a wrist support is appropriate (Fig. 16–19).

Ulnar Nerve Injury

The classic deformity is "clawing" of the fourth and fifth digits, often called the "benediction hand" or "static papal sign." The goal of the orthosis is to prevent hyperextension of the MP joints of the fourth and fifth two digits to allow proper wrapping of the fingers around an object (Fig. 16–20A and B). A dorsal MP block (lumbrical bar) to the fourth and fifth digits with a soft strap on the palmar aspect is usually quite effective.

There is no orthotic device that can substitute for the lost function of the thumb adductor, which is a major deficit in ulnar neuropathy.

Median Nerve Injury

The deformity seen with a distal median nerve injury is often called an "ape hand." This is because of the flat appearance of the hand with wasting of the thenar eminence and loss of palmar abduction and opposition of the thumb. The splinting principle is to put the thumb in an abducted, opposed position. A C bar or a thumb post static orthosis or a dynamic thumb orthosis can be utilized. Since lateral pinch is preserved, many patients prefer not to use an orthosis except during specific fine-pinch activities.

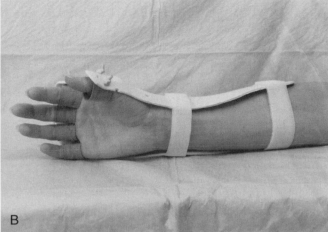

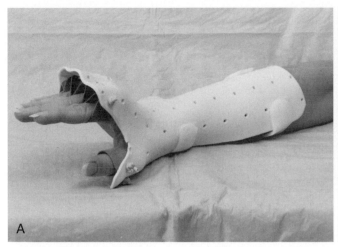

FIGURE 16–18 *A,* "Radial nerve glove" orthosis used in cases of radial nerve injury with weakness or paralysis (side view of the fingers extended passively by the rubber sheaths). *B,* Palmar view of the same orthosis.

With proximal median nerve injury, there is also loss of DIP flexion of the index and middle fingers. The index finger remains extended when the patient makes a fist. This is often called the "active papal sign" because it is noted only on active flexion and not in a relaxed hand. (The "passive papal sign" occurs in ulnar nerve injury.) Simply taping the index and middle fingers together (buddy splint) can also be helpful.

A median and ulnar nerve injury together gives a "clawhand" or an intrinsic minus hand. The hand intrinsics are not functioning and the finger extensors work unopposed at the MP joints. This gives hyperextension at the MP joints and secondary flexion at the interphalangeal joints. A hand orthosis with an MP block (lumbrical bar) over all the digits can improve grasp.

Combinations of different nerve injuries can cause complicated and variable deformities. The patient's acceptance of an orthosis is poor unless the orthosis gives a definite improvement in function. Just holding a deformity in a

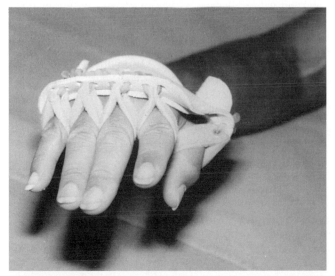

FIGURE 16–19 Dorsal hand orthosis that is used in posterior interosseous nerve injury. It provides dynamic extension of the MP joints.

better position is not a sufficient reason for most patients to continue wearing the splint.

ORTHOSES USED FOR INFLAMMATION OF JOINTS AND TENDONS

A static wrist support orthosis can be used in acute inflammation of the wrist. A WHO is useful in inflammation of the hand.

TENDINITIS. Inflammation of any of the extensor tendons and associated synovium can occur in the six dorsal compartments of the wrist. De Quervain's disease is stenosing tenosynovitis of the tendons of the abductor pollicis longus and extensor pollicis brevis in the first dorsal compartment. Pain is typically present over the radial styloid, and the Finkelstein sign is positive. A thumb spica WHO orthosis can be used with the wrist held in neutral position, and with the thumb radially abducted. The IP joint is left free (Fig. 16–21).

Tendinitis of the other extensor tendons and the intersection syndrome are treated with simple static wrist orthoses to rest the inflamed structures.

TRIGGER FINGER. Digital stenosing tenosynovitis of the flexor tendon causes clicking, locking, or snapping, usually at the proximal end of the flexor sheath, where maximal flexor force occurs with a full fist. This is most commonly found in the middle and ring fingers. A volar static hand orthosis can be used to immobilize the MP joint in a neutral position and allow full interphalangeal flexion. This gives rest, relieves the flexor force, and reduces friction between the tendon and the pulley system by altering the flexor biomechanics and encouraging differential tendon gliding between the flexor digitorum sublimis and profundus muscles.[5]

ORTHOSES USED FOR CARPAL TUNNEL SYNDROME

A static wrist orthosis with the wrist in 0 to 15 degrees of extension often provides dramatic relief from carpal

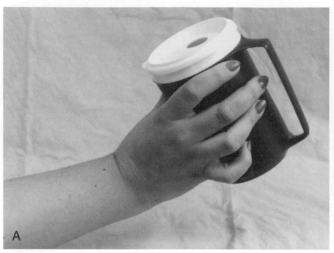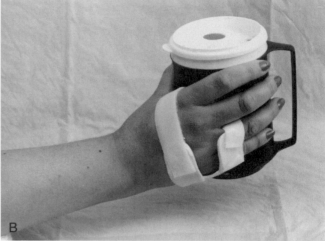

FIGURE 16–20   *A,* Patient with ulnar nerve injury and resulting clawing of the fourth and fifth digits, attempting to grasp a cup. *B,* Same patient with an orthosis providing MP "block," which provides for a stronger grip.

tunnel syndrome symptoms. The splint can be worn during the day or at night, or day and night, depending on the clinical situation.

ORTHOSES USED FOR BURNS

During the early postburn period the aim is to hold the hand in a neutral position and prevent stiffening of the MP joints in an extended position. This is the position of comfort since the collateral ligaments of the MP joints are relaxed in extension. A static volar WHO is used with the wrist 15 degrees in extension, the MP joints in 65 degrees of flexion, and the PIP and DIP joints in neutral position. With finger extensor tendon burns, the finger is held in an extended position and the tendon is kept moist to allow primary healing of the extensor tendon. Later, if contractures develop, the use of paraffin heating and stretching and serial splinting with a stretch-out orthosis is recommended.

Burns around the elbow joint are initially treated by a volar conforming splint. Dynamic elbow splinting can be used later if a contracture is present.

Axillary burns are treated with an airplane splint, with the shoulder held in abduction and in 20 degrees of forward flexion. There is danger of a stretch injury of the brachial

plexus with full abduction of the shoulder (see also Chapter 58).

ORTHOSES USED IN RHEUMATOID ARTHRITIS

During the acute inflammatory stage of rheumatoid arthritis (RA), a support orthosis is given to immobilize the affected part. In the chronic stage, orthoses might be of little help in improving function even if severe deformities are present. Use of antideformity splinting is controversial. With one or a few joints involved as in boutonnière or swan-neck deformities, a simple three-point orthosis can be helpful in enhancing pinch (see Fig. 16–9). With severe deformity of the thumb in MP hyperflexion and IP extension, often described as a "duck-bill" deformity, a thumb post is used to hold the thumb in an opposed, abducted position. This gives a stronger, less painful cylindrical grip. This is especially useful if the patient is weightbearing on the hand with the use of a cane or walker. With a painless MP ulnar deviation deformity, an ulnar deviation orthosis with ulnar block or loop over the individual finger can be used to give a more effective grip (Fig. 16–22).

After implant surgery of the MP joints, a dorsal WHO with a dynamic extension orthosis is used to control movements, allowing flexion and extension but preventing abduction and adduction (see also Chapter 35).

ORTHOSES USED FOR STROKE AND BRAIN INJURY

A shoulder sling is often used for stroke patients having a flail extremity with a subluxated shoulder joint. Any of the commercially available slings can be used, with special attention to the position of the humeral head against the glenoid cavity. The sling is used when the patient is ambulatory (see Fig. 16–5). When sitting, the upper limb can be supported with pillows, lapboard, or wheelchair arm support. Use of a sling is discouraged when lying down and sitting.

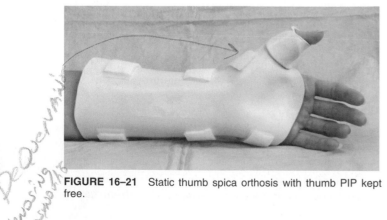

FIGURE 16–21   Static thumb spica orthosis with thumb PIP kept free.

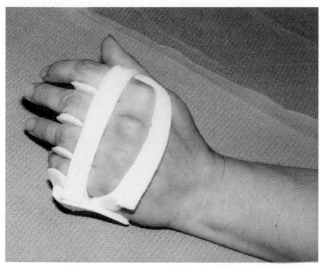

FIGURE 16–22 Dorsal hand orthosis with ulnar aspect MP block and individual finger stops, which helps prevent ulnar deviation at the MP joints.

A spastic upper extremity in traumatic brain injury is difficult to treat orthotically. A simple static WHO or an antispastic orthosis may be used. Inhibitive casting followed by static splinting is also often used.

ORTHOSES USED IN SPINAL CORD INJURY

A number of different types of orthoses are used in spinal cord injury depending on the level of injury and the condition of the functioning muscles and joints. The following is a list of different orthoses used with different levels of injury. (See also Chapter 55.)

C1–C4

- Mouthsticks. Their best success is achieved with C3 and C4 quadriplegic patients. They can cause dental and temporomandibular joint problems.

C4–C5

- BFO or mobile arm support. Some deltoid and biceps function is required to use this effectively.

C5

- Overhead slings (see Fig. 16–6).
- Electrically powered wrist extension, flexor-hinge reciprocal orthosis.
- Long opponens orthosis (ADL orthosis) for positioning of the wrist and hand. It is used with an attachment holder.
- Dorsal wrist support with a pocket that swivels.
- Ratchet WHO. The wrist angle is set passively, which allows the desired pinch.
- Long Wanchik.

C6

- Wrist extension, finger-flexion reciprocal orthosis. It requires at least 3+ strength of the wrist extensors.

DIP range of motion is essential. It is difficult to don if the DIP joints are tight (see Figs. 16–10 and 16–11).
- Short opponens orthosis.
- Short Wanchik.
- Universal cuff.
- Futuro wrist brace without the metal piece.

C7

- Short Wanchik.
- Short opponens orthosis.
- Universal cuff.
- Clip-on U cuff.

C8–T1

- Built-up utensils.

C5 and C6 quadriplegic patients most commonly can do basic ADL like feeding and grooming with the use of the above-mentioned orthoses. Writing and keyboard activities are also achieved. Patients who tend to use them the most are homemakers, students, and the employed. Sometimes, the orthosis is only used to do a single activity on the job.[7]

ORTHOSES USED IN SPORTS AND PERFORMING ARTS

Protective orthoses and taping are used to prevent injuries, especially when hand contact is crucial for performance, as in gymnastics, baseball, golf, and racquet sports. These activities create a considerable, repetitive stress on the wrist and hand joints. Wrist taping is often used in these sports. A glove with proper padding can be used. MP taping is done by gymnasts, as these joints are repetitively stressed in their routines. The ultimate decision on the kind of material used for a sports orthosis depends upon how flexible or rigid the system needs to be. Immobilization of an injured part requires a rigid support, while flexible taping material is used for prophylactic support of joints.[11]

Thumb injuries are quite common in sports. Mild injuries can be treated by taping. Severe injuries of the thumb require immobilization in a thumb spica splint. (See also Chapter 43.)

SUMMARY

An orthosis will be well accepted by the patient if it relieves pain or improves function. The patient, therapist, and physician must determine the specific deficits posed by the condition and the goals of the use of an orthosis. Active participation of the patient in the orthotic treatment enhances compliance and produces more efficacious outcomes.

References

1. Bender LF: Upper extremity orthotics. *In* Kottke FJ, Stillwell GK, Lehmann JF (eds): Krusen's Handbook of Physical Medicine and Rehabilitation, ed 3. Philadelphia, WB Saunders, 1982.
2. Bennett RL, Stephens HR: Assistive and adaptive devices for upper extremities. Phys Ther Rev 1955; 35:626–640.

3. Brand PW: The forces of dynamic splinting: Ten questions before applying a dynamic splint to the hand. *In* Hunter JM, Schneider LH, Mackin EJ, et al (eds): Rehabilitation of the Hand: Surgery and Therapy, ed 3. St Louis, Mosby–Year Book, 1990, pp 1095.

4. Browne E Jr, Ribik C: Early dynamic splinting for extensor tendon injuries. J Hand Surg 1989; 14:72–76.

5. Evans R, Hunter J, Burkhalter W: Conservative management of the trigger finger: A new approach. J Hand Ther Jan–March 1988, pp 59–68.

6. Fess EE, Gettle KS, Strickland JW: Hand Splinting: Principles and Methods. St Louis, Mosby–Year Book, 1981.

7. Garber S, Gregario T: Upper extremity assistive devices: Assessment of use by spinal cord injured patients with quadriplegia. Am J Occup Ther 1990; 44:126–131.

8. Irani KD: Wrist and hand orthoses. *In* Redford JB (ed): Physical Medicine and Rehabilitation State of the Art Reviews, vol 1. 1987, pp 137.

9. Kohlmeyer K, Weber C, Yarkony G: A new orthosis for central cord syndrome and brachial plexus injuries. Arch Phys Med Rehabil 1990; 71:1006–1009.

10. Long C, Schutt A: Upper limb orthotics. *In* Redford JB (ed): Orthotics Etcetera, ed 3. Baltimore, Williams & Wilkins, 1986.

11. Press J, Weisner S: Prevention: Conditioning and orthotics; hand injuries in sports and performing arts. Hand Clin 1990; 6:383–392.

12. Redford JB: General principles. *In* Redford JB (ed): Physical Medicine and Rehabilitation State of the Art Reviews, vol 1. 1987.

13. Schutt A: Upper extremity and hand orthotics. Phys Med Rehabil Clin North Am 1992; 3:223–240.

14. Strickland J: Flexor tendon injuries, part 2. Orthop Rev 1986; 15:49–69.

17

Lower Limb Orthoses

**WILLIAM J. HENNESSEY, M.D., AND
ERNEST W. JOHNSON, M.D.**

An orthosis is defined as a device that is attached or applied to the external surface of the body to improve function, restrict or enforce motion, or support a body segment.[27] Lower limb orthoses are indicated to assist gait, reduce pain, decrease weightbearing, control movement, and minimize worsening of a deformity. Lower limb orthoses are able to help ambulatory patients walk more safely. Ambulation aids may be used in combination with lower limb orthoses to help patients ambulate more safely. Ambulation aids represent extensions of the upper limb and are technically upper limb orthoses; however, they are discussed in this chapter due to their importance in gait.

PRINCIPLES OF LOWER LIMB ORTHOSES

Orthoses should be used for specific management of selected disorders. They should be used only as indicated and for as long as necessary. Joint movement should be allowed wherever it is possible and appropriate. Orthoses should be functional throughout all phases of gait. Placement of orthotic joints should approximate that of anatomical joints. Compromise occurs at the ankle joint because an oblique axis is present (unlike the transverse orthotic ankle joint), with the lateral malleolus located posterior and inferior to the medial malleolus. The orthotic ankle joint should be centered over the tip of the medial malleolus. Placement of the orthotic knee joint is also compromised because the knee has two axes on which it rotates, in comparison to the single axis offered by most orthotic knee joints. The orthotic knee joint should be located at the prominence of the medial femoral condyle.[38] The hip joint should be located in a position that allows the patient to sit upright with the hip joints positioned at 90 degrees. Patient compliance is enhanced if the orthosis is comfortable, cosmetically acceptable, and functional. A summary of these principles is presented in Table 17–1.

Most orthoses utilize a three-point system to ensure proper positioning of the limb within the orthosis. For example, a knee that has a tendency to be "back-bent" can be treated with a knee orthosis that applies force posterior to the knee, but that also applies forces anteriorly along the leg distally and the thigh proximally. This ensures adequate control of the knee by exerting these forces proximal to, distal to, and at the knee joint.

TERMINOLOGY

Orthoses have frequently been incorrectly referred to as "orthotics." *Orthotic* is the adjective of the noun *orthosis*. An orthosis may be referred to as an *orthotic device*. An orthosis is made in an *orthotic laboratory*.

Terminology pertinent to the anatomy of the lower limb is also frequently used incorrectly. The term *lower extremity* specifically refers to the foot. The term *leg* should be used to refer to the portion of the lower limb between the knee and ankle joints. The thigh is located between the hip and knee joints. *Lower limb* refers to the thigh, leg, and foot.

Pathological abnormalities regarding angulation have also been referred to incorrectly as *varus* and *valgus* deformities at the knee and hip. Correct use of the Latin-derived terminology for these deformities requires use of the suffix "*-us*" at the ankle, "*-um*" at the knee, and "*-a*" at the hip. Varus and valgus deformities of the foot are

TABLE 17–1 Principles of Lower Limb Orthoses

1. Use only as indicated and for as long as necessary
2. Allow joint movement wherever possible and appropriate
3. Orthoses should be functional throughout all phases of gait
4. Orthotic ankle joint should be centered over tip of medial malleolus
5. Orthotic knee joint should be centered over prominence of medial femoral condyle
6. Orthotic hip joint should be in a position that allows patient to sit upright at 90 degrees
7. Patient compliance will be enhanced if orthosis is comfortable, cosmetic, and functional

described for both the hindfoot and the forefoot (e.g., hindfoot valgus or forefoot varus). Bow-leggedness is correctly referred to as *genu varum*. Deformity at the hip is referred to as *coxa valga* and *coxa vara*.

Lower limb orthoses are frequently referred to by their acronyms. Standard orthotic nomenclature uses the first letter of each joint that the orthosis crosses from proximal to distal. It then lists the first letter of the limb to which it is affixed (e.g., "f" for foot). Lastly, the letter "o" is used to signify it is an orthosis. Thus, an AFO refers to an ankle-foot orthosis, KAFO refers to a knee-ankle-foot orthosis, and HKAFO refers to a hip-knee-ankle-foot orthosis.

The orthotic literature uses variable medical terminology, which can make it difficult to understand the literature unless one knows which of these terms are used interchangeably. The calcaneus is frequently referred to as the *os calcis*. A plantar flexion deformity is referred to as an *equinus deformity*. Torsion and rotation have been incorrectly used as interchangeable terms. *Torsion* refers to twisting of a portion of a limb. *Rotation* of a limb only occurs at a joint. *Pronation* has been referred to as in-rolling, whereas *supination* has been referred to as out-rolling. An orthosis is not put on and taken off but rather is donned and doffed. *Checkout* refers to an examination of the patient after the orthosis is fitted.

MATERIALS FOR LOWER LIMB ORTHOSES

Plastic materials have become, by far, the most commonly used materials in the orthotic industry. Thermosetting and thermoplastic are the two common types of plastics used by orthotists. Thermosetting plastics are designed to be set after heating. They are not meant to be reheated for further molding. They will not return to their original consistency if reheated, but they will soften. Thermoplastics, such as polypropylene, are used more commonly than thermosetting plastics. Polypropylene is the most common type of plastic used, and it is frequently used in combination with other plastics to make orthoses. Thermoplastics soften when heated for molding purposes. They can be remolded when necessary by warming them. Plastic orthoses designed for long-term use are typically made of high-temperature thermoplastics.[26] The plastic orthoses are often lined internally with a thin layer of padding.

Combination plastic/metal orthoses are being used more frequently to reduce the weight of the orthosis but still provide the added strength of metal components where necessary, such as at the joints. Aluminum alloy is the most common type of metal used. Stainless steel may be needed for durability in very heavy individuals and for joint components.

Carbon graphite is also used in orthotic fabrication. It offers strength and low weight as desirable features. Graphite compounds have a very narrow temperature window at which they can be shaped and set without compromising strength. This is why the knee joints are usually made of stainless steel in order to ensure strength, while the uprights may be made of carbon graphite. Graphite currently costs significantly more than its metal counterparts, but its cost

is expected to decrease over time with increasing usage. Carbon graphite inserts are frequently incorporated into plastic AFOs at the ankle to increase rigidity and thereby minimize plantar and dorsiflexion.

SHOES

The purpose of wearing shoes is to protect the feet. The normal foot does not require support from shoes. The sole should be pliable so as not to interfere with the normal biomechanics of the foot. The ability to apply an index fingertip between the tip of the great toe and the toe box is a practical method of ensuring that a shoe is of adequate length.[42] The presence of calluses indicates areas of friction from poorly fitting (loose) shoes. The presence of corns indicates areas of friction over bony prominences, most often from tight-fitting shoes. Leather shoes are good choices for all types of activity. They are durable, allow ventilation, and mold to the feet with time. A good pair of shoes may eliminate the need for foot orthoses and should be considered before orthotic prescription.

Shoe Parts

The shoe can be divided into lower and upper parts. The lower part can be divided into the sole, shank, ball, toe spring, and heel (Fig. 17–1). The sole is often made of leather for dress shoes and of rubber for athletic shoes. Leather soles are best for modification and attachment of orthoses. They provide a firm surface against which the leverage of bars and wedges can be exerted. The shank is the narrowest portion of the sole between the heel and ball. It can be reinforced with metal for attachment of metal ankle-foot orthoses (AFOs). The ball is the widest part of the sole located in the region of the metatarsal heads. It can be modified internally or externally to help alleviate forefoot pain. The toe spring is the space between the outer sole and the floor. It helps produce a rocker effect during toe-off. The heel helps to prevent the shoe from "wearing out" and shifts weight to the forefoot. The use of high heels can contribute to forefoot pain, and it can make the subtalar joint less stable and make the wearer more predisposed to injury. Heels are not present on athletic and children's shoes because they interfere with natural gait.

The upper shoe can be divided into the quarter, heel counter, vamp, toe box, tongue, and throat (see Fig. 17–1). The quarter is the posterior portion of the upper and is often reinforced with a heel counter. A high quarter is referred to as a "high top" and is used by athletes for greater sensory feedback. It does not offer significant mediolateral stability. The heel counter provides posterior stability to the shoe. It reinforces the quarters of the shoe and helps support the calcaneus. The vamp is the anterior portion of the upper and is often reinforced with a toe box. The toe box is a reinforcement of the vamp that can serve to help protect the toes from trauma. The tongue may be part of the vamp or may be a separate piece attached to the vamp. The throat is the entrance of the shoe. It is located at the base of the tongue. The farther anteriorly it is located, the more room is present for internal modification or insertion of an orthosis. Special shoes, known as

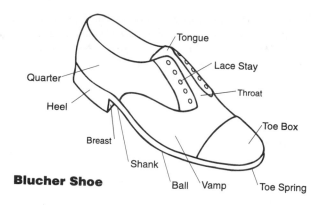

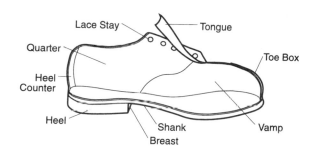

Blucher Shoe

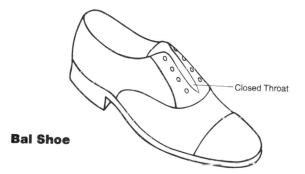

Bal Shoe

FIGURE 17–1 Shoe types and components. The open throat of the blucher shoe accommodates an orthosis better than the bal shoe.

extra depth shoes, also allow more room inside the shoe for orthotic intervention.

There are two types of dress shoes commonly worn, the blucher and the bal (see Fig. 17–1). The tongue is part of the vamp in the blucher shoe. The quarters overlap the vamp. This type of dress shoe should be recommended to most patients who require an orthosis because there is more room to don and doff the shoe and orthosis. Another popular shoe style, the bal, has its quarters meet at the throat. The vamp is stitched over them at the throat, thereby limiting the ability of the shoe to open and accommodate an orthosis.

A shoe with a welt should also be recommended to patients. A welt is a narrow strip of leather used to unite the upper part of the shoe, the inner sole, and the outer sole of a shoe by means of stitching.[44] The welt design allows the orthotist to disassemble the shoe for modifications more easily than with other types of shoes. The presence of a welt can be easily noted by the horizontal

stitching just above the sole. It is also present in most athletic shoes, at least along the anterior half of the shoe, to provide reinforcement for activities requiring frequent "cutbacks."

FOOT ORTHOSES

Foot orthoses (FOs) range from arch supports, found at a local pharmacy or athletic store, to customized orthoses, fabricated by an orthotist. The effectiveness of an orthosis depends on the proper diagnosis of the foot condition, the appropriate selection of orthotic material, and proper molding. FOs affect the ground reactive forces acting on the joints of the lower limb. They also have an effect on rotational components of gait. A foot imprint is a simple, useful way of demonstrating abnormal pressure point areas to be targeted by orthotic intervention (Fig. 17–2).

Mild conditions may be treated with over-the-counter orthoses. More severe problems require customized orthoses, which are available in three types. A soft type is most commonly used in over-the-counter orthoses. Orthotists usually provide semi-rigid orthoses that provide more support than the soft type but still absorb shock. A rigid orthosis is indicated only for a problem that requires aggressive bracing to control the deformity.

To make a custom foot orthosis, the subtalar joint should be placed in a neutral position prior to casting. This position minimizes abnormalities related to foot and ankle rotation, such as hyperpronation, and is also the position in which the foot functions best.[29] The foot is then covered

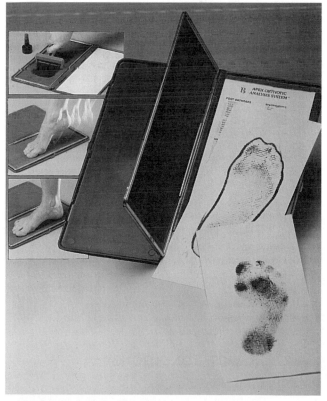

FIGURE 17–2 Foot imprint system. (Courtesy of Apex Foot Health Industries, South Hackensack, NJ.)

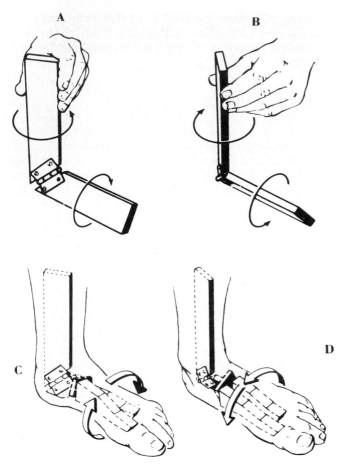

FIGURE 17–3 Analogy of subtalar axes to an oblique hinge. *A* and *C,* Outward rotation of the upper stick (tibia) results in inward rotation of the lower stick (calcaneus). This results in elevation of the medial border of the foot and depression of the lateral border. *B* and *D,* Inward rotation of the upper stick (tibia) results in outward rotation of the lower stick (calcaneus). This results in depression of the medial side of the foot with elevation of the lateral side. (Modified from Mann RA: Biomechanics of the foot. *In* American Academy of Orthopaedic Surgeons (eds): Atlas of Orthotics. St Louis, Mosby–Year Book, 1985, p 118.)

with a parting agent, such as a stockinette or a clear plastic wrap, and wrapped in either plaster of Paris strips or fiberglass tape and allowed to harden. Fiberglass casting is also used for difficult orthotic cases in which the fiberglass casting itself can be used as a temporary orthosis to demonstrate if the mold properly controls the deformity. This negative mold is then removed to allow a positive mold to be made from it. The positive mold may be modified to increase the effectiveness of the orthosis. The custom orthosis is obtained by heating and form-fitting (often by use of a vacuum) the plastic to the positive mold.

It should be noted that research has not determined the length of time that an orthosis remains effective. The orthosis should be examined at each follow-up to determine when a new one is necessary.

COMMON FOOT CONDITIONS

Pes Planus ("Flatfoot")

Symptomatic relief of pain is obtained by controlling excess pronation of the foot. Pronation of the foot may be

defined as a rotation of the foot in the longitudinal axis resulting in a lowering of the medial aspect of the foot. Pronation is also referred to as *inrolling*. Pronation and abduction of the foot occur at the subtalar joint. Foot pronation is a component of eversion. Eversion involves pronation and abduction (at the subtalar joint) and dorsiflexion (at the ankle joint). The key to controlling excess pronation is controlling the calcaneus to keep the subtalar joint in a neutral position.

Pes planus may be due to abnormalities such as excessive internal torsion of the tibia (which results in pronation of the foot) or malalignment of the calcaneus. It is the interaction between the tibia and the foot at the subtalar joint that allows pathology outside the foot to cause inrolling of the foot (Fig. 17–3).

The reduction of pronation is accomplished by maintaining the calcaneus and the subtalar joint in correct alignment. The subtalar joint must be in a neutral position during the custom molding process. The subtalar joint neutral position prevents occurrence of rotational deformities associated with excessive pronation or supination (see parts *C* and *D* of Fig. 17–3). Elevation of the anteromedial calcaneus exerts an upward thrust against the sustentaculum tali to help prevent inrolling.[5] The orthosis should extend beyond the metatarsal heads to provide better leverage for control of the deformity. A custom-made foot orthosis designed to prevent hyperpronation is also referred to as a *UCBL* (or *UCB*) *orthosis,* which stands for University of California Biomechanics Laboratory, where original work regarding this type of orthosis was performed in the 1940s.

Some cases of pes planus are due to ligamentous laxity within the foot. For these cases, a medial longitudinal arch support can be helpful for alleviating pain. Initial use of an arch that is too high can cause discomfort. The height of the arch can be increased as necessary as the foot develops a tolerance for the inlay. A Thomas heel extension (Fig. 17–4) may also offer medial support, particularly for heavier individuals.

Pes Cavus ("High-Arched" Foot)

A typical complication of pes cavus is excess pressure along the heel and metatarsal head areas, which could lead

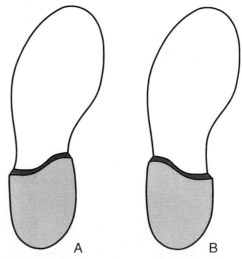

FIGURE 17–4 *A,* Thomas heel. *B,* Reverse Thomas heel.

to pain. This can be prevented by making the height of the longitudinal support just high enough to fill in the space between the shank of the shoe and the arch of the foot to distribute weight more effectively (Fig. 17–5). Weight should also be evenly distributed over the metatarsal heads. The lift is extended just to the metatarsal head area to help distribute and alleviate pressure over the metatarsal weightbearing area. Because the tendency to pronate as in pes planus is lacking, the high point of the arch is located at the talonavicular joint. If the tibia is externally rotated (see Fig. 17–3), it can give the appearance of an elevated arch as the foot supinates and the lateral aspect of the foot assumes additional weightbearing responsibility. In these cases, a foot orthosis is custom molded with the subtalar joint in a neutral position to prevent excess supination from occurring.

Forefoot Pain (Metatarsalgia)

Relief of pain in the forefoot is accomplished by distributing the weightbearing forces proximal to the metatarsal heads. This can be done by either internal or external modification. A metatarsal pad (also referred to as a *cookie*) should rest inside the shoe just posterior to the second, third, and fourth metatarsal heads. It should also be just posterior to the lateral aspect of the first metatarsal head and medial to the fifth metatarsal head (Fig. 17–6). A metatarsal bar (Fig. 17–7) is recommended for cases in which the foot is too sensitive to tolerate a pad inside the shoe. The metatarsal bar is typically ¼ in. thick and tapers distally. The distal edge must be proximal to the metatarsal heads. It is often applied to a leather or neoprene sole. The metatarsal bar may also be used for forefoot pain associated with pes cavus.

Prevention of forefoot pain should also be emphasized to patients. Patients should avoid shoes with high heels and/or pointed toes, which place excess stress on the metatarsal heads.[3]

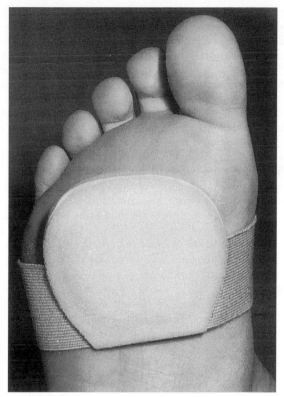

FIGURE 17–6 Metatarsal pad for forefoot pain. (Courtesy of Apex Foot Health Industries, South Hackensack, NJ.)

Heel Pain

The painful area may be alleviated by using an orthosis to help distribute weight. Rubber heel pads may be applied inside the shoe to offer relief in cases associated with minor discomfort. A calcaneal bar is recommended for cases in which the foot is too sensitive to tolerate a pad inside the shoe. The calcaneal bar is placed distal to the painful area to prevent the calcaneus from assuming a full weightbearing status.

A common cause of heel pain along the anteromedial calcaneus is plantar fasciitis. Pain occurs at the attachment site of the fascia along the medial aspect of the heel. Point tenderness, which is located over the anteromedial calcaneus, is common in people whose feet hyperpronate,

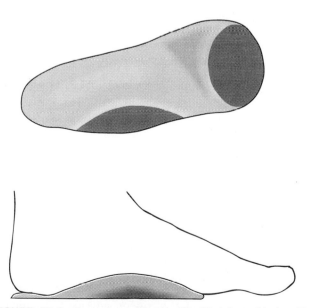

FIGURE 17–5 Pes cavus orthosis. (Modified from Diveley RL: Foot Appliances and Shoe Alterations: Orthopaedic Appliances Atlas. Ann Arbor, Mich, Edward Brothers, 1952, p 464.)

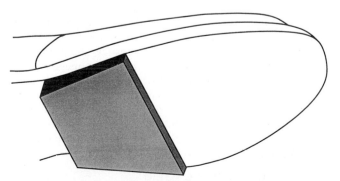

FIGURE 17–7 Metatarsal bar. (Modified from Pfeffinger LL: Foot orthoses. *In* American Academy of Orthopaedic Surgeons (eds): Atlas of Orthotics. St Louis, Mosby–Year Book, 1985, p 350.)

thereby placing excess stress on the medial longitudinal arch.[8] A custom made orthosis with the subtalar joint in a neutral position (such as that described for pes planus) helps prevent excessive inrolling from occurring and reduces the stress placed along the proximal arch. A custom made orthosis is indicated for cases in which conservative treatment has failed.

Plantar fasciitis is also common in patients with high arches. For these patients, the medial longitudinal arch undergoes marked stress during weightbearing. This may be treated with either an elevated arch support or a heel well, which helps distribute pressure along the medial longitudinal arch.

Heel spurs are frequently mistaken to be the source of heel pain. Heel spurs related to plantar fasciitis are the result of mechanical stress acting through the plantar fascia onto its origin at the calcaneus and are not the source of the pain.[28] Inferior heel spurs are related to advancing age and are not painful in nature.

Heel lifts help some causes of Achilles tendon pain by decreasing the amount of stretch placed on the Achilles tendon (by keeping the ankle joint plantar flexed). A heel lift may be used to treat Achilles enthesitis, an inflammatory reaction at the insertion of the tendon into the periosteum of the calcaneus. A heel lift may also be helpful for treating plantar flexion spasticity/contracture by increasing the total heel height to help ensure that the patient has a heel-strike prior to toe touch during gait.

Toe Pain

The goal of orthotic intervention in toe pain is to decrease pain via immobilization. This is done by extending the steel shank forward to reduce mobility of the distal joints. A metatarsal bar may also be used for partial immobilization.[9] Common conditions associated with toe pain include hallux rigidus, gout, and arthritis.

Leg Length Discrepancy

A symptomatic leg length discrepancy must first be evaluated with proper measurement. True leg length is measured from the distal tip of the anterior superior iliac spine to the distal tip of the medial malleolus. Apparent leg length is measured from a midline point such as the pubic symphysis or umbilicus to the distal tip of each malleolus. This finding may be abnormal in cases in which the true leg length is normal but in which pelvic obliquity is present secondary to conditions such as scoliosis, pelvic fracture, or muscle imbalance.

Leg length discrepancies less than ½ in. do not need correction. The total discrepancy is never corrected. At most, 75% of the leg length discrepancy should be corrected. The first ½ in. discrepancy can be managed with a heel pad. Additional correction requires the heel to be built up externally. The sole should also be built up proportionally when the heel is built up externally, to provide a comfortable, stable gait. A taller sole should have a rocker bottom to help normalize the gait pattern at toe-off (see Fig. 7–14).

Osteoarthritis of the Knee

Although osteoarthritis of the knee is not a foot condition, it is mentioned here because pain related to it may be alleviated with foot orthoses. Foot orthoses alter the ground reaction forces affecting the more proximal joints, such as the knee, and this must be considered when prescribing a foot orthosis. Lateral heel wedges can be used for conservative treatment of osteoarthritis when medial compartment narrowing results in genu varum. The heel wedges used are ¼ in. thick along the lateral border and taper medially. Relief was obtained with heel wedges in 74 of 121 knees from 85 patients in one study.[10] Relief of pain was noted to be most frequently obtained in mild osteoarthritis, but pain relief was also documented in some cases with complete obliteration of the medial joint space. Wedge use widened the gait pattern.

Pediatric Shoes

Children's shoes should have a simple design. To facilitate gait, a heel should not be present. Soft soles are recommended to permit the natural development of feet. Tennis shoes are adequate for most children. A high quarter or three quarter shoe will stay on a child's foot better than a low-cut shoe and is recommended during the first few years of life.

It is a common misconception that all flat feet need to be treated in children. Flat feet are usual in infants, common in children, and occur occasionally in adults.[35] Flat feet improve over time, due in part to the loss of subcutaneous fat and the reduction of laxity of the joints that occur with growth[35] and the maturation of gait pattern. Intensive treatment with corrective shoes or inserts for a 3-year period did not alter the natural history of flat feet in 129 children who were 1 to 6 years of age.[41] Frequent shoe size change is necessary in the first few years of life.[42]

ANKLE-FOOT ORTHOSES

Ankle-foot orthoses (AFOs) are the most commonly prescribed lower limb orthoses. They were formerly known as *short-leg braces*. Metal or plastic AFOs can be used to effectively control ankle motion. Metal AFOs are relatively contraindicated in children because the weight of the brace may cause external tibial rotation. Plastic AFOs are now more common in all age groups.

AFOs should provide mediolateral stability as a safety feature.[11] Although much emphasis with AFOs is placed on controlling the amount of dorsiflexion and plantar flexion, movements at the subtalar joint also have a significant influence on the biomechanics of gait. Supination and adduction occur at the subtalar joint, which results in the foot's being in a varus position. Pronation and abduction occur at the subtalar joint, resulting in the foot's being in a valgus position. Rotation at the subtalar joint is also accompanied by rotation of the tibia (see Fig. 17–3).

AFOs can also stabilize the knee during gait.[17] They are prescribed for conditions affecting knee stability, such as weak quadriceps or genu recurvatum. An AFO should be considered for conditions affecting the knee, particularly when a problem exists concurrently at the ankle or subtalar joints. A proper AFO prescription considers the biomechanical influence of the orthosis at the foot, ankle, and knee in all planes of movement.

Metal AFOs

Metal AFOs are used infrequently. They are discussed here for the following three reasons: (1) Much of the research regarding the biomechanics of AFOs on gait was performed with metal AFOs. These principles also apply to plastic orthoses. (2) Metal components (especially joints) are frequently used in combination with plastic orthoses. (3) Some older patients wish to continue to use the metal orthoses to which they have become accustomed.

The metal AFO consists of a proximal calf band, two uprights, ankle joints, and an attachment to the shoe to anchor the AFO (Fig. 17–8). The posterior metal portion of the calf band should be 1½ to 3 in. wide to distribute pressure.[7] The calf band should be 1 in. below the fibular neck to prevent a compressive common peroneal palsy. A leather strap with Velcro is used to close the calf band and provides ease of closure for patients with only one functional upper limb.

Ankle joint motion is controlled with the insertion of pins or springs into channels (Figs. 17–9 and 17–10). The pins are adjusted with a screwdriver to set the desired amount of plantar flexion and dorsiflexion. The spring is also adjusted with a screwdriver to provide the proper

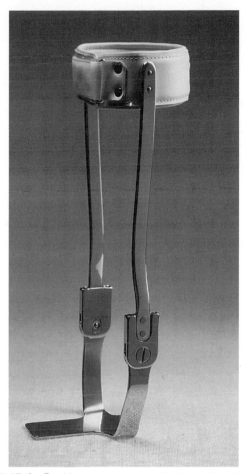

FIGURE 17–9 Double action metal ankle joint with solid stirrup. (Courtesy of Becker Orthopedic Co., Troy, Mich.)

amount of tension necessary to aid motion at the ankle joint (used to assist dorsiflexion). Longer channels help prevent the spring mechanism from "bottoming out" and provide more precise control of ankle motion.

A solid stirrup is a U-shaped metal piece permanently attached to the shoe. Its two ends are bent upward to articulate with the medial and lateral ankle joints (see Fig. 17–9). The proximal stirrup attachment sites are shaped to enforce the desired movements at the ankle joint (Fig. 17–11). The sole plate may be extended beyond the metatarsal head area for conditions requiring a longer lever arm for better control of plantar flexion (such as plantar spasticity).

A split stirrup may be used instead of a solid stirrup (Fig. 17–12). The split stirrup has a sole plate with two flat channels for insertion of the uprights. The two uprights are now called calipers, as they can open and close distally to allow donning and doffing of the AFO. A split stirrup allows removal of the uprights from the shoes so that the AFO can be worn with other shoes (see Fig. 17–7). Other pairs of shoes must also have the sole plate with channels for calipers incorporated into the heel area. The split stirrup is not as stable as the solid stirrup.

Ankle Stops and Assists

The ankle joint may be positioned so that it is in a neutral, dorsiflexed, or plantar flexed position depending

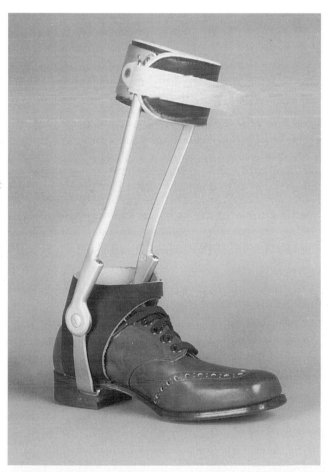

FIGURE 17–8 Metal double upright dorsiflexion assist AFO on left shoe with medial T strap for control of valgus deformity. The metal dorsiflexion assist ankle joint is also referred to as a *Klenzak ankle joint.* Note the split stirrup in the heel that allows the wearing of the orthosis with other shoes.

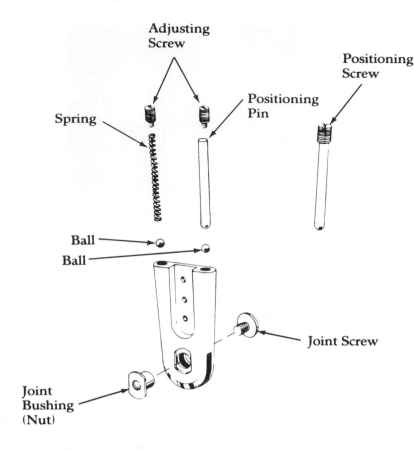

FIGURE 17–10 Schematic drawing of metal ankle joint components. This type of ankle joint has also been referred to as a *double action ankle joint*, a *double Klenzak ankle joint*, and a *BiCAAL* (bichannel adjustable ankle locking) joint. (Courtesy of USMC, Pasadena.)

on the gait disturbance. It can be set to permit a partial range of motion or to eliminate a certain motion. An understanding of the effect on the placement of pins and screws into the two channels of an ankle joint (see Fig. 17–10) facilitates the proper orthotic prescription for the patient. This section reviews the common uses of the posterior stop, the anterior stop, and the posterior dorsiflexion assist. A spring in the anterior channel has not been demonstrated to be of clinical value.

Plantar Stop (Posterior Stop)

The plantar stop is most commonly set at 90 degrees. A pin is inserted into the posterior channel of an ankle joint,

such as that in Figure 17–9, to limit plantar flexion. It is used to control plantar spasticity and to help incrementally stretch plantar contractures. An AFO with a plantar stop at 90 degrees produces a flexion moment at the knee during heel-strike. Because the dorsiflexors cannot eccentrically activate to permit the foot to make contact with the ground, the ground reactive force remains posterior to the knee after heel-strike, which creates a flexion moment at the knee (and possibly an unstable gait). The proximal portion of the AFO also has an effect on knee stability. The posterior portion of the proximal AFO exerts a forward push on the proximal leg to increase the knee flexion moment after heel-strike (Fig. 17–13). The opposite occurs

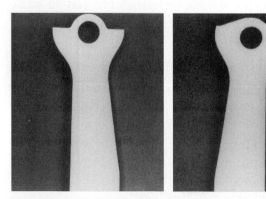

Stirrup for Double Action   **Stirrup for Toe Lift**

FIGURE 17–11 Dorsiflexion assist and double action stirrups, used with the ankle joints shown in Figures 17–9 and 17–8, respectively. (Courtesy of USMC, Pasadena.)

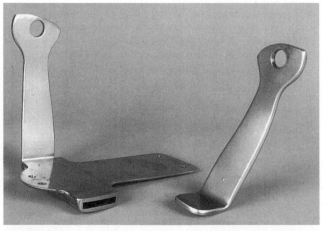

FIGURE 17–12 Split stirrup. Note how the stirrup extends anteriorly to attach at the shank area of a shoe for stability.

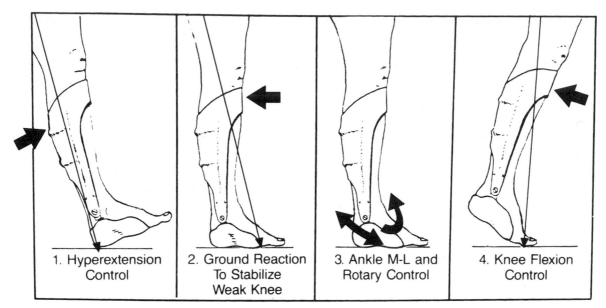

| 1. Hyperextension Control | 2. Ground Reaction To Stabilize Weak Knee | 3. Ankle M-L and Rotary Control | 4. Knee Flexion Control |

FIGURE 17–13 Ground reaction AFO dynamic illustration. Note the effect of the proximal portion of the AFO on the knee throughout gait. (Courtesy of Oregon Orthotic System, Albany, Ore.)

at toe-off, with an extension moment created at the knee (see Fig. 17–13). This concept has been used to develop what has been referred to as a *plastic ground reaction AFO* with a solid proximal anterior tibial closing, which provides a greater influence on the knee. This is discussed in more detail later.

The greater the plantar flexion resistance, the greater the flexion moment at the knee at heel-strike, and the greater the need for active hip extensors to prevent the body from collapsing forward on a buckling knee.

A solid ankle cushioned heel (SACH heel) wedge (Fig. 17–14) can be used to reduce the flexion moment at the knee. The SACH heel serves as a shock absorber at heel-strike and thereby is able to partially substitute for the dorsiflexors that cannot be activated when the ankle plantar stops of an AFO are set at 90 degrees. The SACH heel also helps move the ground reactive force more anteriorly. If the ground reactive force is anterior to the knee, then the knee enters extension and becomes more stable during

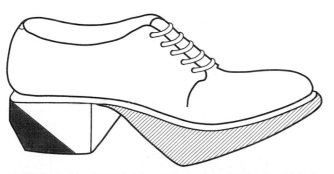

FIGURE 17–14 SACH heel and rocker bottom. Note that the elevated heel requires an elevated sole with rocker bottom to facilitate gait. The heel must also slant inward to prevent an excessive flexion moment at the knee at heel-strike. (Modified from Pfeffinger LL: Foot orthoses. *In* American Academy of Orthopaedic Surgeons (eds): Atlas of Orthotics. St Louis, Mosby–Year Book, 1985 p 350.)

the stance phase of gait. The SACH heel can be used with an AFO to minimize the amount of plantar flexion spasticity present after heel-strike. The term *SACH* is a misnomer borrowed from the prosthetic literature. The "SA" (*solid ankle*) refers to the type of prosthetic ankle joint. The SACH heel wedge should be appropriately referred to as a cushioned heel.

The posterior stop should be set at the minimal amount of plantar flexion required to clear the foot during swing-through.[12] This minimizes the bending moment at the knee after heel-strike and provides a more stable gait than when the ankle plantar stops are set in any amount of dorsiflexion.

A balanced decision must be made between providing resistance to plantar flexion to clear the foot during the swing phase of gait, and increasing the amount of instability at the knee during the stance phase of gait. No AFO is effective in reducing the amount of knee flexion to normal levels during the stance phase of gait due to restriction of range of motion at the ankle.[14]

Dorsiflexion Stop (Anterior Stop)

An anterior stop is used to substitute for the function of the gastrocnemius-soleus complex. It is used in conditions with weak calf muscles or weak quadriceps (due to its effect on the knee). Weak calf musculature causes the ankle to enter dorsiflexion. The anterior stop set at 5 degrees of dorsiflexion best substitutes for gastrocnemius-soleus function.[12, 14]

The anterior stop assists with push-off and assists the knee joint into extension. It must be used in combination with a stirrup with a sole extension to the metatarsal heads to simulate the action of the calf muscles. The dorsiflexion stop simulates the gastrocnemius-soleus function by causing the heel to rise during the latter part of stance, when it would otherwise remain flat on the ground. The shoe pivots over the metatarsal heads, creating an extension moment at the knee that helps stabilize the knee from mid-stance to toe-off.

The earlier the dorsiflexion stop occurs during the stance phase, the greater the extension moment at the knee. This is useful in clinical situations in which quadriceps weakness is also present. If the extension moment at the knee is too great for too long, then genu recurvatum ("back knee") may occur. A balance must be obtained in the amount of extension at the knee that is necessary to stabilize the knee in extension and the amount that is necessary to prevent genu recurvatum. If too much dorsiflexion is permitted by the anterior stop, too much knee flexion will be present during gait from mid-stance to toe-off.

Dorsiflexion Assist (Posterior Spring)

The posterior spring serves two purposes. It substitutes for concentric contraction of dorsiflexors to prevent flaccid footdrop after toe-off. It also substitutes (inadequately) for the eccentric activation of the dorsiflexors after heel-strike. The metal dorsiflexion assist ankle joint is also known as a Klenzak ankle joint (see Fig. 17–8).

The posterior spring prevents rapid plantar flexion at heel-strike during its compression in the posterior channel. The posterior spring is again compressed during plantar flexion during late stance prior to toe-off. The posterior spring assists with toe clearance during the swing phase of gait by providing a downward thrust posterior to the ankle joint at toe-off, which results in dorsiflexion anterior to the ankle joint. The longer the channel, the greater the ability to control dorsiflexion.

A summary of some of the common indications for the various channel components is found in Table 17–2.

Metal AFO Varus/Valgus Control

Varus and valgus deformities are associated with rotation at the subtalar joint. A T strap is attached along the side of the shoe distal to the subtalar joint to help minimize the deformity (see Fig. 17–8). T straps are also used to help prevent worsening of the deformity. Last, they help distribute pressure properly along the foot during weightbearing.

T straps are referred to as either *medial* or *lateral*. A medial T strap is sewn to the medial aspect of the shoe and the belt is cinched around the lateral upright of the AFO (see Fig. 17–8). A medial T strap is used to control a valgus deformity. The belt is secured with a buckle around the lateral upright. This translates a force directing the subtalar joint inward, which counteracts the pronation and abduction tendency that would result in excess valgus.

The opposite is true for a varus deformity, with the T strap being laterally located. A pressure sore can develop over the malleolus if the T strap is buckled too tightly.

The T strap inadequately substitutes for the foot pronators, supinators, abductors, and adductors because it does not have an attachment on the plantar surface of the foot to create the mechanical advantage offered by the plantar-attached muscles and tendons.

Plastic AFOs

Plastic AFOs are the most commonly used AFOs because of their cost, cosmetic acceptability, light weight, ability to be interchangeable with shoes, ability to control varus and valgus deformities, better foot support with the customized foot portion, and ability to accomplish what is offered by the metal AFO. Energy consumption is equal in patients using a plastic solid AFO and in those using a metal double-stop AFO.[2] Although the weight of the plastic orthosis is less than that of its metal counterpart, the weight of the orthosis is not as important as the influence of the ground reactive force created by the presence of the orthosis. The same orthotic principles apply to orthoses made of plastic or metal. The effect of the plastic AFO on knee stability should be recognized. The plastic AFO prescribed for toe clearance should be just rigid enough to provide resistance for toe clearance. Excessive resistance to plantar flexion can make the knee unstable (create a flexion moment) after heel-strike.[15]

Plastic AFOs can be prefabricated or custom made. The reasons for prescribing a custom molded orthosis include long-term need, conformed molding for comfort or for insensate feet, placement of the orthosis in a fixed amount of plantar flexion or dorsiflexion, better control of rotational deformities, and further reduction of weightbearing for a tibial fracture. The custom made process is similar to that previously described in this chapter for foot orthoses, with the positive mold serving as the model for the orthosis.

A few practical pieces of advice should be offered to the patient regarding the use of a plastic AFO. If changing shoes, it is best to have another pair with a similar heel height to prevent alteration of the biomechanical effects at the foot, ankle, and knee. Tennis shoes are most accommodating for donning and doffing of the AFO. However, if dress shoes are to be worn, patients should also be told that their shoe size may need to be a half size greater and the next width larger to accommodate the orthosis. A blucher style dress shoe will also help accommodate the orthosis (see Fig. 17–1).

TABLE 17–2 Clinical Indications for Various Metal Ankle Channel Components

Channel	Rod or Spring	Function	Clinical Indications
Posterior	Rod	Limits plantar flexion	Plantar spasticity, toe drag, pain with ankle motion
Posterior	Spring	Assists dorsiflexion	Flaccid footdrop, knee hyperextension
Anterior*	Rod	Limits dorsiflexion	Weak plantar flexors, weak knee extensors, pain with ankle motion
Anterior	Spring	Assists plantar flexion	None

*Used in combination with an extended sole plate to metatarsal head area to help substitute for weak plantar flexors.

Plastic AFO Components

The foot component of the AFO should extend beyond the metatarsal heads. The foot plate can be extended beyond the toes to reduce the spasticity aggravated by toe flexion. The shape and molding of the foot portion will have an influence on the biomechanics of more proximal joints.

The ankle and subtalar joints can be made more stable under four circumstances: (1) the trim line extends more anteriorly at the ankle level (a trim line is the anterior border of the plastic AFO); (2) the plastic material is thicker; (3) carbon inserts are placed along the medial and lateral aspects of the ankle joint (Fig. 17–15); and (4) corrugations are made within the posterior leaf of the AFO. The strength of the AFO must be matched with the patient's weight and activity.

Plastic AFOs can also be hinged at the ankle (Figs. 17–16 and 17–17). These allow full or partial ankle motion, which can permit a more natural gait. They should be considered when complete restriction of ankle motion is not required. Newer designs allow for a quick and precise exchange of cams that alter the limit of plantar flexion and dorsiflexion, without the necessity of having to adjust the height of pins (see Fig. 17–16). Newer designs also have a single midline posterior spring mechanism (see Fig. 17–

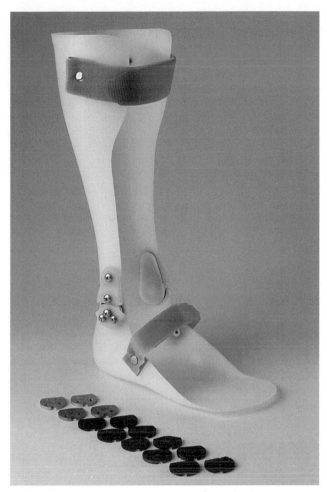

FIGURE 17–16 Natural Select articulated AFO. The color-coded cams each allow a set amount of plantar and dorsiflexion and are interchangeable with use of a screwdriver. (Courtesy of USMC, Pasadena.)

17). The midline spring functions like the more traditional medial and lateral dual posterior spring assist mechanism (see Fig. 17–7). This makes the AFO narrower in the mediolateral direction and slightly longer in the anteroposterior direction, which better conforms to the fit of most pants. Free ankle motion is also offered via plastic joints (see Fig. 17–17).

The leg component should encompass three quarters of the leg and should be padded internally.[7] The proximal extent should end 1 in. below the fibular neck to prevent a compressive common peroneal nerve palsy.

The Solid Plastic AFO

The solid plastic AFO is the most commonly prescribed plastic AFO (see Fig. 17–15). It can be made to serve several purposes. The term *solid* refers to an AFO that is made of a single piece of plastic. It does not have ankle joints. A solid AFO can still be flexible enough to allow some ankle motion.

Prefabricated solid AFOs set at 90 degrees are commonly used for footdrop. Less obvious, but equally important, is the ability of the solid AFO to treat conditions affecting the knee. The AFO may be fixed in a few degrees

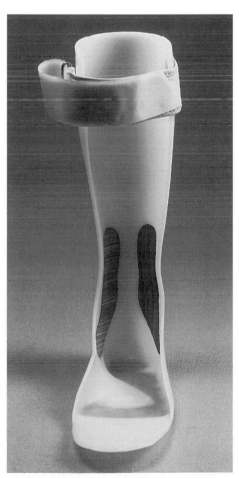

FIGURE 17–15 Plastic solid AFO with carbon inserts for ankle joint and subtalar joint stability. (Courtesy of Becker Orthopedic Co., Troy, Mich.)

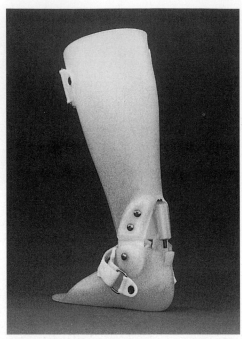

FIGURE 17–17 Elite midline dorsiflexion assist articulated AFO. Note the use of a plastic ankle joint to further decrease weight. (Courtesy of Precision O & P Components, Tempe, Ariz.)

of plantar flexion to provide stability at the knee during the stance phase of gait. Genu recurvatum may also be treated with a solid AFO. The more rigid the AFO, the greater the flexion moment at the knee at heel-strike, which helps reverse the extension moment at the knee associated with genu recurvatum. The flexion moment at the knee also becomes greater during mid-stance if the ankle is placed in a few degrees of dorsiflexion.

Plastic AFO Varus/Valgus Control

The goal of orthotic intervention is to alter the ground reactive forces with custom molding to help maintain proper alignment of the lower limb by "building up" selected portions of the AFO. A three-point system is used to provide the counterforces necessary to oppose the forces of the deformity (Fig. 17–18).[22] Some orthotists believe that an orthosis should be firm ("not conforming") to control a deformity. Pressure points should be present in expected areas at follow-up visits if the orthosis is serving its purpose. A custom ground reaction orthosis provides appropriate foot support that influences the rotation of more proximal joints (Fig. 17–19). The anterior tibial shell closing helps to stabilize the knee during gait (see Fig. 17–11).

An equinovarus deformity is controlled by applying forces medially at the metatarsal head area and the calcaneus. The next force is applied more proximally along the lateral aspect of the fibula. This helps to prevent inversion at the subtalar and ankle joints. A more proximal medial tibial force is applied to provide stabilization of the leg portion of the plastic AFO by providing an opposing force to the fibular area (see Fig. 17–18). A three-point system also exists at the foot level to help prevent supination of the foot related to the equinovarus deformity (see Fig. 17–18). A three-point system is again applied to control the plantar flexion deformity associated with equinovarus (see Fig. 17–18).

The reverse of the previously described three-point system to control varus can be used to control valgus at the foot. Movements in all joints should be considered when prescribing an orthosis.

Patellar Tendon–Bearing AFOs

A patellar tendon–bearing (PTB) AFO uses the patellar tendon and the tibial condyles to partially relieve weight-

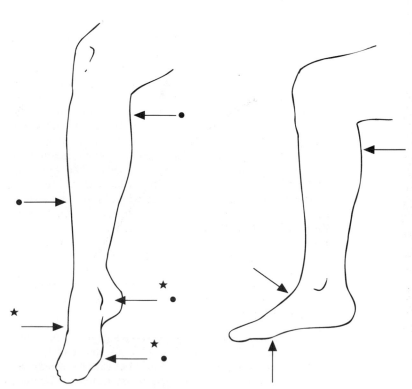

FIGURE 17–18 Three-point system control of equinovarus deformity. *Left*, Control of varus rotational component at the foot (*) and subtalar joint (●). *Right*, Control of equinus deformity. (Modified from Marx HW: Lower limb orthotic designs for the spastic hemiplegic patient. Orthot Prosthet 1974; 28:14.)

bearing stress on skeletal structures distally, with more weightbearing distributed along the medial tibial condyle. PTB is a misnomer for this orthosis because only about 10% of the weight is distributed along the patellar tendon and the medial tibial condyle. Most of the weightbearing is distributed throughout the soft tissues of the leg that are compressed by an appropriately fitted orthosis. Compression of the soft tissues of the leg is also responsible for maintaining alignment and length of the tibia after a fracture.[32, 33]

PTB AFOs are prescribed for diabetic ulcerations of the foot, tibial fractures, and relief of a weightbearing surface in painful heel conditions, such as calcaneal fractures, postoperative ankle fusions, and avascular necrosis of the foot or ankle. The orthoses are made of plastic due to its light weight and durability. They are bivalved and fit snugly with the use of Velcro straps or buckles similar to those seen on ski boots (Fig. 17–20).

Custom made PTB AFOs are indicated when maximum weightbearing reduction is necessary to ensure proper healing (such as in a debrided diabetic heel ulcer) and to decrease pain. It must first be determined that the painful condition is associated with weightbearing rather than with range of motion. If pain occurs with range of motion, then the pain-producing range of motion should be eliminated.

The solid plastic orthosis makes contact with the ground before the reactive force is absorbed significantly by the

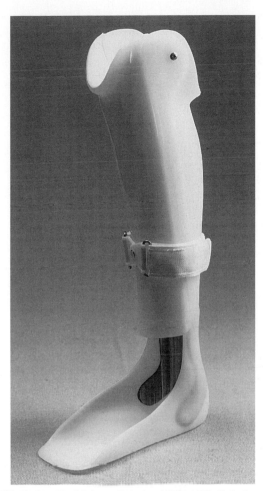

FIGURE 17–20   Prefabricated bivalved PTB AFO. Note the carbon inserts that help eliminate ankle motion and therefore help eliminate active push-off. (Courtesy of Becker Orthopedic Co., Troy, Mich.)

foot; then it distributes the force more proximally along the leg. A custom made PTB AFO (compared with a prefabricated PTB AFO) more effectively distributes pressure over a greater surface contact area for maximal weightbearing reduction. Additional weightbearing reduction is obtained by eliminating ankle movement (i.e., by the use of carbon graphite inserts as in Figs. 17–15 or 17–20) and by using a rocker bottom (see Fig. 17–14), which eliminates active push-off.[20] A rocker bottom is incorporated into the plastic orthosis.

Checkout

The patient must be examined after fitting and use of the orthosis. The orthotic ankle joint should coincide with the tip of the medial malleolus. The patient is to be checked for ability to easily don and doff the orthosis. While the orthosis is off, the skin should be observed for areas of breakdown. If the AFO was prescribed to control spasticity, the orthotic evaluation should be thorough to determine its effectiveness in a dynamic setting, because spasticity may worsen with ambulation.

KNEE-ANKLE-FOOT ORTHOSES

Knee-ankle-foot orthoses (KAFOs) were formerly referred to as *long-leg braces*. The components are the same

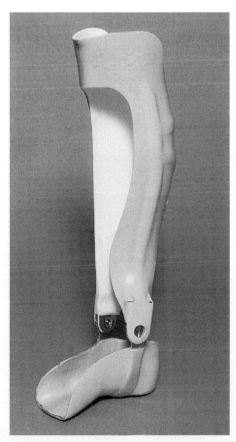

FIGURE 17–19   OOS rotational control AFO. Note the corrugations that add strength to the orthosis. Also note the metal ankle joint that is similar to those in Figures 17–9 and 17–10. (Courtesy of Oregon Orthotic System, Albany, Ore.)

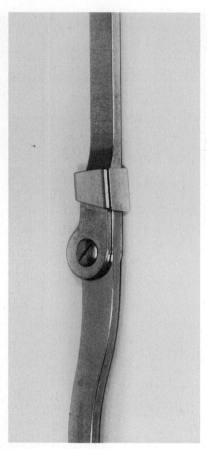

FIGURE 17–21 Straight set knee with drop lock. (Courtesy of USMC, Pasadena.)

as those of an AFO, but they also include a knee joint, thigh uprights, and a proximal thigh band. Various knee joints and knee locks are available for a variety of conditions. KAFOs are used for patients with severe knee extensor weakness, structural knee instability, and knee flexion spasticity. The purpose of the KAFO is to provide stability at the knee, ankle, and subtalar joints during ambulation. They are most commonly prescribed bilaterally for patients with spinal cord injuries and unilaterally for patients with polio.

KAFOs may be prescribed for functional ambulation and/or exercise. The benefits of exercise to the patient requiring bilateral KAFOs include the prevention of lower limb contractures, cardiovascular fitness, maintenance of upper body strength for activities of daily living, delay of osteoporosis development, and decrease in medical complications, such as deep venous thromboses.

The use of KAFOs often complements the use of a wheelchair for ambulation. The proprioceptive level is a reliable indicator of which spinal cord–injured patients will achieve ambulation.[39] It is helpful to have sensation and proprioception of the lower limbs in order to ambulate safely with KAFOs. The level of the spinal injury is also important in predicting the ability to ambulate. Adult spinal cord–injured patients with lesions at or above T12 generally are not functional ambulators due to the metabolic cost involved.[23] Children have a higher center of gravity and thus can have a functional gait with a higher spinal cord lesion.

Muscle function is a predictor of the quality of ambulation. Good trunk control and upper body strength are needed to ambulate with KAFOs because they are used in combination with ambulation aids, such as walkers and quad canes.

Some paraplegic patients are able to avoid the need for KAFOs for ambulation (i.e., those with lower lumbar lesions with some knee extensor strength). Ambulation in these patients can often be accomplished with the use of bilateral plastic ground reaction AFOs (see Figs. 17–13 and 17–19) with the ankles fixed in 10 to 15 degrees of plantar flexion. The plantar flexion provides an extension moment at the knee during gait for stability with ambulation. The proximal anterior tibial shell closing provides further stability at the knee from mid-stance to toe-off (see Fig. 17–13, part 4). A walker or two quad canes are used for additional support and balance.

Knee Joints

There are three basic types of knee joints. The straight set knee joint provides rotation about a single axis (see Fig. 17–21). It allows free flexion but prevents hyperextension. It is often used in combination with a drop lock, which keeps the knee in extension throughout all phases of gait for further stability (see Fig. 17–21).

The polycentric knee joint uses a double axis system to simulate the flexion/extension movements of the femur and tibia at the knee joint (Fig. 17–22). Although this concept is theoretically sound, it has not been proven to be advantageous over the straight set knee joint and is used less commonly. It also adds bulk to the orthosis. It is most frequently used in sport knee orthoses.

The third type of knee joint is the posterior offset knee joint (Fig. 17–23). It is prescribed for patients with weak knee extensors and good hip extensor strength. It allows free flexion and extension of the knee during the swing phase of gait and helps keep the ground reactive force in

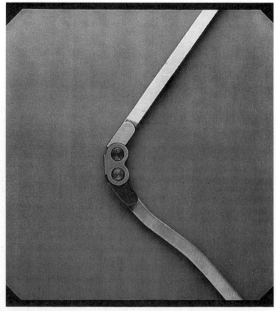

FIGURE 17–22 Polycentric knee joint. (Courtesy of Becker Orthopedic Co., Troy, Mich.)

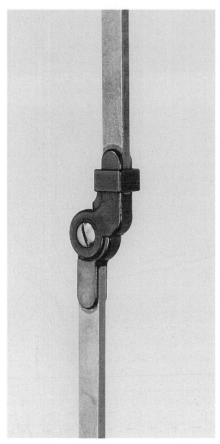

FIGURE 17–23 Offset knee joint with drop lock. (Courtesy of USMC, Pasadena.)

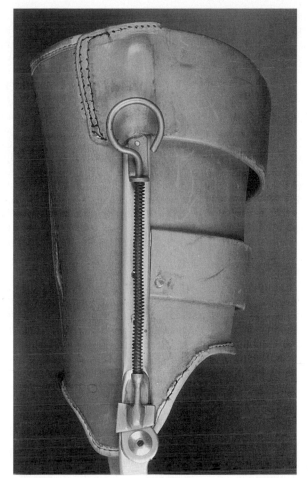

FIGURE 17–25 Drop lock with spring-loaded pull rod.

front of the knee axis for stability during stance. The center of gravity is normally posterior to the knee at heel-strike, creating a flexion moment at the knee that requires knee extensor muscle contraction to counteract the force. The offset knee joint component of the KAFO helps place the ground reactive force anterior to the orthotic knee joint, creating an extension moment at the knee during stance to compensate for the weak knee extensors. The offset knee joint has a hyperextension stop to help prevent genu recurvatum.

Occasionally, the offset knee joint is not an adequate provider of stability at the knee. The ankle component of the KAFO can then be set in 10 to 15 degrees of plantar flexion to further help create an extension moment at the knee for stability (Fig. 17–24).

Knee Locks

Knee locks are used to provide complete stability at the knee in cases in which quadriceps weakness is severe or when no strength is present, as in some spinal cord injuries. There are three common types of knee locks.

The drop lock (ring lock) is used most commonly in both the medial and the lateral uprights of the KAFO (see Fig. 17–21). Its advantage is simplicity of design without bulk. However, it can require fine coordination skills to lock the knee in complete extension. The drop lock may then "settle" after ambulation and can be difficult to pull up to unlock the knee. A spring-loaded pull rod may be used to assist with drop lock management (Fig. 17–25),

FIGURE 17–24 Plastic-metal KAFO. The 10 degrees of plantar flexion and the posterior offset knee joint initially provided stability at the knee for the patient. A drop lock had to be added due to advancing knee extensor weakness.

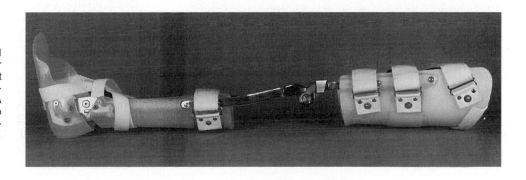

but it also adds bulk to the orthosis. The drop lock is pushed into place by the spring and is released by pulling on the rod. A drop lock can be used unilaterally along the lateral upright in instances in which the patient is of relatively low weight and has a low activity level.

The bail lock (Swiss, French, Schweitzer, or pawl lock) provides an easy method of simultaneously unlocking the medial and lateral knee joints of a KAFO (Figs. 17–26 and 17–27). Lifting up the bail posteriorly releases the knee joint to permit flexion to allow the patient to sit down (see Fig. 17–27). The patient can also catch the bail on the edge of a chair to release the lock mechanism to permit sitting. The locking mechanism is often spring-loaded to assist locking the knee into extension (see Fig. 17–27). The bail is often padded with rubber to protect the clothing from being torn or soiled. The KAFO with a bail lock can be worn over or under clothes, depending on the size of the bail lock and the size of the clothing.

The dial lock (formerly known as a *turnbuckle*) is used to stabilize the knee in varying amounts of flexion (Fig. 17–28). It can be adjusted every 6 degrees. Its uses include helping to prevent worsening of a flexion contracture and assisting with the gradual reduction of a flexion contracture.

Thigh Component of KAFO

The thigh band needs to be wide enough to adequately distribute the pressure of the ground reactive force trans-

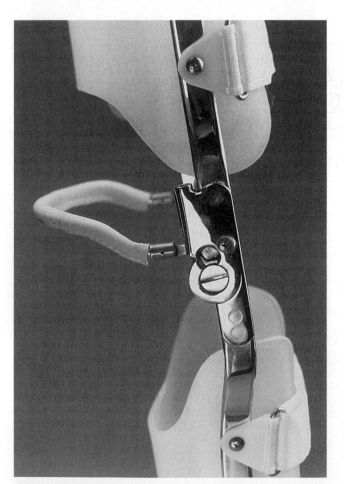

FIGURE 17–26 Spring-loaded bail lock. (Courtesy of Becker Orthopedic Co., Troy, Mich.)

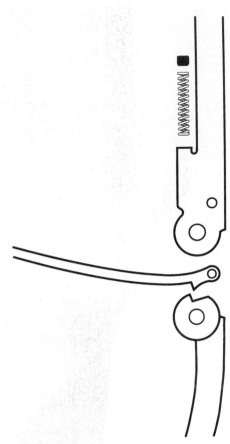

FIGURE 17–27 Spring-loaded bail lock mechanism. Lifting the bail permits free flexion for sitting and the spring mechanism helps lock the knee joint into extension.

mitted through the knee axis. If properly fitted, a partial plastic thigh shell can provide a greater contact area and decrease high-pressure areas (see Fig. 17–24). Plastic/metal combination KAFOs also decrease the weight of the KAFO, which may add to patient comfort and usage. A low thigh band is used for prevention of genu recurvatum.

Scott Craig Orthosis (Fig. 17–29)

This orthosis was designed to provide the paraplegic patient who has a complete neurological level at L1 or higher with a more functional and comfortable gait.[34] It was also designed to reduce unnecessary hardware by making a KAFO of lighter weight, which also facilitated donning and doffing.

The orthotic design consists of an ankle joint with anterior and posterior pin stops, a sole plate extending to the metatarsal heads, a crossbar added to the metatarsal head area for mediolateral stabilization, and an offset knee joint with a bail lock.[34] A rigid anterior tibial band is positioned directly below the tibial tubercle and a rigid, proximal thigh band is positioned posteriorly and closed anteriorly by a soft strap secured with Velcro. These two bands must be shallow enough to hold the knee in extension. A three-point system helps keep the knee in extension with pressure applied at the proximal thigh posteriorly, at the proximal tibia anteriorly, and at the calcaneus posteriorly.[16] The ankle joint functions with a dorsiflexion stop used to simulate

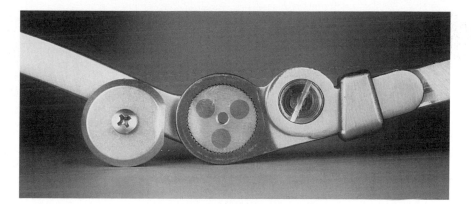

FIGURE 17–28 The dial lock may be adjusted every 6 degrees for precise control of knee flexion.

the triceps surae function (as previously described) and with a posterior stop set at 90 degrees to prevent toe drag.

A group headed by Lehmann analyzed the Scott Craig orthosis and found that it was the most easily donned and doffed of the KAFOs tested.[18] This orthosis in its original design is still frequently prescribed for paraplegic patients.

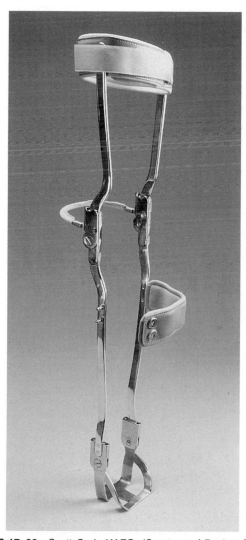

FIGURE 17–29 Scott Craig KAFO. (Courtesy of Becker Orthopedic Co., Troy, Mich.)

KNEE ORTHOSES

Swedish Knee Cage

The Swedish knee cage (Fig. 17–30) is a knee orthosis (KO) that is used to control minor to moderate genu recurvatum due to ligamentous or capsular laxity. It is available in nonarticulated and articulated forms. The nonarticulated version does not allow any knee flexion or extension and therefore is no longer the recommended version of the Swedish knee cage for genu recurvatum. The articulated version allows full knee flexion and prevents hyperextension. The articulated version is recommended for the treatment of genu recurvatum. It uses a three-point system with two bands placed anterior to the knee axis (one above and one below the knee) and a third band placed posterior to the knee joint in the popliteal area (see Fig. 17–30). It also has an additional thigh band with longer uprights to obtain better leverage at the knee joint. Severe genu recurvatum may need to be controlled with longer lever arms, such as those offered by a KAFO.

Genu recurvatum can also be controlled with a solid plastic AFO that resists plantar flexion. This may be used in cases where pathological conditions also affect the ankle or subtalar joints. The more rigid the AFO, the greater the flexion moment at the knee during heel-strike (which counters the extension moment of the recurvatum). An additional flexion moment at the knee may be obtained by fixing the AFO in a few degrees of dorsiflexion.

Sport Knee Orthoses

An abundance of widely marketed sport orthoses are available; however, definitive research regarding their role in athletics is lacking. This can lead to much confusion regarding their prescription unless the knee orthosis is reviewed systematically. Sport knee orthoses can be divided into prophylactic, rehabilitative, and functional categories.[25]

Prophylactic knee bracing attempts to prevent or reduce the severity of knee injuries. No evidence supports the use or cost benefit of these orthoses. Studies have indicated that the use of these orthoses has actually increased the number of athletes with knee injuries.[31, 36] It is theorized that knee-braced players may put themselves in compromising positions due to overconfidence in the orthosis, and this may contribute directly to the increasing injury rates

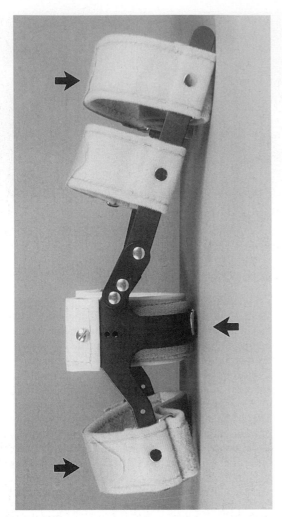

FIGURE 17–30 The articulated Swedish knee cage, which uses a three-point system to control genu recurvatum.

observed. The use of prophylactic knee bracing has also been associated with increased energy consumption, which may impair athletic performance.[8]

Rehabilitative knee bracing is used to allow protected motion within defined limits.[25] It is useful for postoperative and conservative management of knee injuries.

Functional knee bracing is designed to assist or provide stability to the unstable knee. Functional knee bracing does not replace the need for rehabilitation of the knee. Functional braces are used most commonly to stabilize a laterally subluxing patella or an anterior cruciate ligament–deficient knee (Fig. 17–31). Their use has only been shown to be effective at loads much lower than those placed on the knee during athletic participation. In summary, functional knee bracing may play a role in pathological laxity by possibly decreasing the frequency of episodes of instability.[25]

PEDIATRIC ORTHOSES

Caster Cart

Disabled children should experience and identify early with motion in order to encourage a natural progression of

ambulatory skills. Without familiarity with motion, disabled children will not have a desire to ambulate once placed in a parapodium or reciprocating gait orthosis (discussed below).

The caster cart (Fig. 17–32) is used for children with a developmental delay in ambulatory skills, and it serves as an initial mobility aid. It is most often prescribed for children with spina bifida. Most children are upright and cruising by age 10 months.[9] Children with paraplegia should be fitted for a caster cart once they have obtained enough upper limb strength and trunk balance to propel themselves. If balance is a problem for the child, a deep seat bucket may be prescribed to help provide balance so that the child can use the upper limbs for propulsion (see Fig. 17–32).

The caster wheel at the back of the cart facilitates multidirectional movement. Initially, the child can be pushed around in the cart and a handle can be attached posteriorly so that the cart serves functionally as a stroller.

Standing Frame

The use of a standing frame (Fig. 17–33) follows successful use of a caster cart. The age range for initial use is roughly 8 to 15 months. Patients may continue to use their caster carts during this period. Children who are pulling

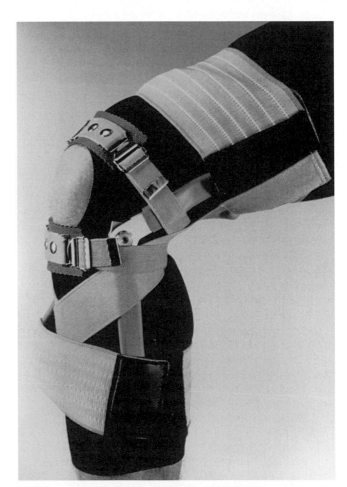

FIGURE 17–31 Lenox Hill Spectralite knee orthosis, which is commonly prescribed for anterior cruciate–deficient knees and for patellas with a tendency to lateral subluxation. (Courtesy of Lenox Hill Brace Co., Bethesda, Md.)

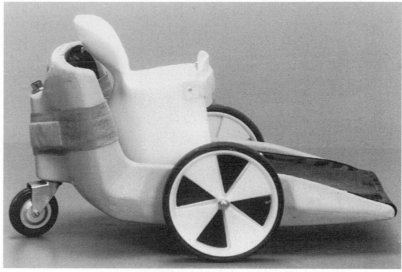

FIGURE 17–32 Caster cart. This is an initial mobility aid for the disabled child. The child uses it as a "pre-wheelchair device." The deep seat bucket stabilizes the seated ataxic child while permitting free use of the upper limbs for ambulation. (Courtesy of The Hugh MacMillan Rehabilitation Center, Toronto.)

themselves up along furniture, which is the first sign that they are interested in standing and moving, are typically ready for use of a standing frame.[9]

The standing frame helps balance the body in space and allows free use of the upper limbs for participation in activities. Children with thoracic level lesions need AFOs to provide good ankle and foot support in the standing frame or parapodium (see following discussion). Initial gait training can occur with the use of the standing frame via a swing-through gait with the assistance of parallel bars.

Parapodium

The parapodium (Fig. 17–34) has also been referred to in the past as a *swivel orthosis*. Children must first demonstrate adequate use of a standing frame and have a desire to ambulate prior to the prescription of a parapodium. A child's standing frame can be evaluated for wear and tear to determine if it has been used sufficiently for the child to advance to a parapodium. A frequently used standing frame (or any orthosis) looks dirty and scratched up and has lint in the Velcro straps. It is important to note this, because parents frequently set expectations that are too high for the disabled child. A child who has not used a standing frame will likely be unable and unwilling to ambulate with a parapodium.

A parapodium is appropriate to prescribe for children who are unlikely to become functional walkers due to the severity of their impairment. It often complements wheelchair use.[20] It is most commonly prescribed for children between ages 2½ and 5 years.

A parapodium allows crutchless gait. Ambulation occurs by the child pivoting the hips and using "body English" to swivel one side of the oval-based stand forward; the child then repeats the same event for the other side. Its design is similar to that of the standing frame, but it has hip and knee joints. The hip and knee joints remain locked in extension to permit ambulation in the upright position, but they can be unlocked (simultaneously in some models) to permit sitting. The difficulties experienced with the use of this orthosis include those encountered in donning and doffing and rising from a seated to a standing position.

Reciprocating Gait Orthosis

The reciprocating gait orthosis (RGO) (Fig. 17–35) was formerly known as a *hip-guided orthosis* (HGO). It may also be referred to as a *bilateral hip-knee-ankle-foot orthosis* (HKAFO). The purpose of the RGO is to provide

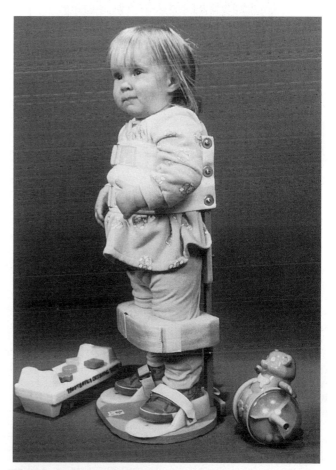

FIGURE 17–33 A standing frame being used by a spina bifida toddler with a T12 neurosegmental level lesion. (Courtesy of The Hugh MacMillan Rehabilitation Center, Toronto.)

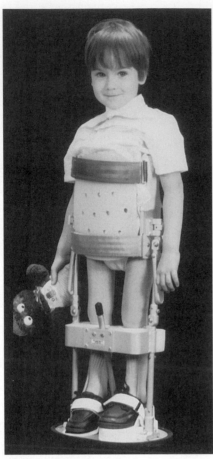

FIGURE 17–34 Parapodium. Note the lift on the left leg to compensate for a leg length discrepancy and the wide abdominal support pad to assist in upright posture. (Courtesy of The Hugh MacMillan Rehabilitation Center, Toronto.)

contralateral hip extension with ipsilateral hip flexion. The RGO is appropriate for children who have used the standing frame, have developed good trunk control and coordination, can safely stand, and are mentally prepared for ambulation. Good upper limb strength, trunk balance, and active hip flexion have been shown to be important positive variables for ambulation.[6] Obesity, advanced age, lack of patient or family motivation, scoliosis, spasticity,[6] and contractures have been found to be significant negative factors in the long-term use of the RGO.

Spinal cord injury level is not a very reliable predictor of ambulation capability for children. As children with spinal cord injuries grow taller, they may experience more difficulty walking as their center of gravity becomes lower.

The RGO is prescribed most commonly for children ranging from 3 to 6 years of age. The concept of the RGO was developed during work with a patient who had active hip flexion and no hip extension. Gait is initiated with unilateral hip flexion and can be assisted by swaying the trunk when hip flexion is inadequate. This type of gait pattern may also be considered to be a form of physical therapy because hip extension occurs passively with each step, which helps to reduce flexion contractures. Cables were initially used to provide the necessary hip motion, but newer mechanical methods of reciprocal gait employ a

"teeter-totter" concept (see Fig. 17–35). This type of RGO has been reported to be more energy-efficient than an RGO with cables.[43]

Crutches are used with the RGO to provide a control mechanism, taking advantage of the forward momentum to produce small propulsive forces when needed.[21] This is a disadvantage of this orthosis (compared with the parapodium), because the upper limbs are not free for other activities. The patient with an RGO is able to negotiate a greater variety of surfaces than would be possible with the parapodium.[30]

The hip joints of the RGO have hip flexion and abduction capabilities on release of the locking mechanisms (Fig. 17–36). It is recommended that one hip joint have abduction capability to permit catheterization and to allow sitting in a hip-flexed and abducted position.

Twister

A twister (Fig. 17–37) may be prescribed for lack of control of internal or external rotation or torsion of the lower limb. Its use is not to be regarded as corrective but rather as supportive. It is most commonly used in a patient with excessive internal rotation, to prevent tripping over the feet. Older models are made with cables placed outside

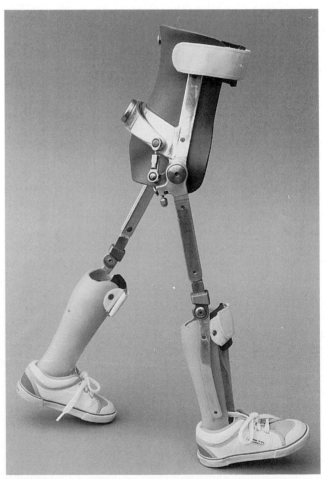

FIGURE 17–35 Isocentric reciprocating gait orthosis (RGO): dynamic view. (Courtesy of Center for Orthotic Design, Redwood City, Calif.)

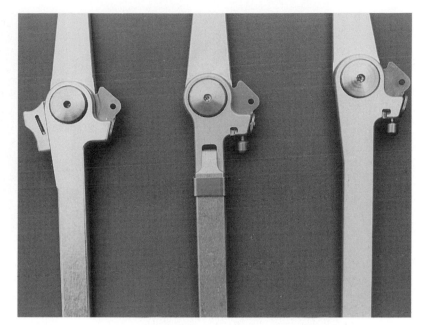

FIGURE 17–36 Unique hip joints for use with the Isocentric RGO. *Left*, "Pre-selected" with easy-to-lock and -unlock lever. *Middle*, "Abduction hinge" hip joint for easy catheterization without removal of the brace. *Right*, Conventional hip joint as used on cable braces. (Courtesy of Center for Orthotic Design, Redwood City, Calif.)

the clothing. Newer models are made of canvas straps that can lie underneath the clothing. Twisters can be worn as long as necessary during maturation. Internal tibial-femoral torsion often decreases spontaneously with growth.[1, 40] Tibial osteotomies can be performed for severe cases of tibial torsion.

AMBULATION AIDS

The purpose of using ambulation aids (Figs. 17–38 and 17–39) is to increase the area of support for patients who have difficulty maintaining the center of gravity safely over their own support area. A variety of aids are available

for the individual needs of the patient (see Fig. 17–38). Ambulation aids improve balance, redistribute and extend the weightbearing area, reduce lower limb pain, provide small propulsive forces, and provide sensory feedback. They should be considered to be an extension of the upper limb. Therefore, good upper limb strength and coordination are needed. An exercise program for the upper limbs is useful and may complement ambulation with the aid to increase endurance and stability. A supervised period of training is recommended after prescription of an aid.

The type of aid needed depends on how much balance and weightbearing assistance is needed. The body weight transmission for a unilateral cane opposite the affected side is 20% to 25%.[4] It is 40% to 50% with the use of a forearm

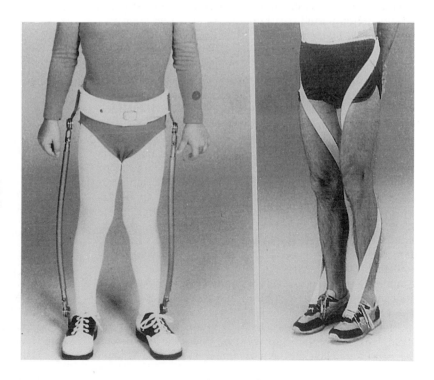

FIGURE 17–37 *Left*, Traditional cable twister. (Courtesy of Hanger Orthopedic, Columbus, Ohio.) *Right*, Canvas twister. (Courtesy of JA Preston Corp., Jackson, Mich.)

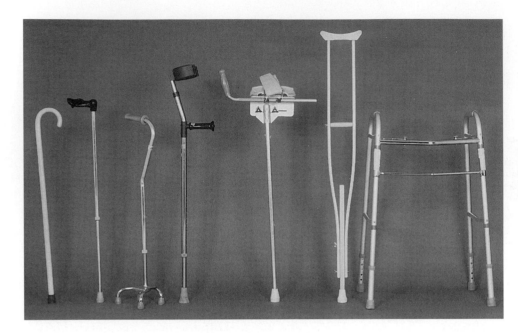

FIGURE 17–38 Ambulation aids. From *left* to *right*, C cane, functional grip cane, quad cane, Lofstrand forearm orthosis, platform forearm orthosis, crutch, and walker.

or arm cane.[4] Body weight transmission with bilateral crutches is estimated at up to 80%.[4]

Canes

PRESCRIPTION

1. Measure the tip of the cane to the level of the greater trochanter with the patient in an upright position.[37]

The elbow should be flexed approximately 20 degrees, which is a desirable elbow position for all ambulation aids. Canes are made of wood or aluminum, with the aluminum alloy cane having adjustable notches so that "one cane fits all."

There are three common types of canes. The C cane is most commonly used (see Fig. 17–38). It is also known as a *crook top cane* or a *J cane*. A functional grip cane offers the patient a grip that may be more comfortable than that of the C cane (see Fig. 17–38). A quad cane provides an increased area of support compared with other canes (see Fig. 17–38). Quad canes also come in narrow- and wide-based forms for different degrees of support. The lateral two legs are directed away from the body.

A cane is used on the side opposite the supporting lower limb. It is advanced with the opposite lower limb. It is usually held on the patient's unaffected side. This can be done to lessen the force exerted on a hip with a pathological condition. The load is increased by four times the body weight on the stance side during gait, owing to the gravitational forces and the gluteus medius-minimus force exerted across the weightbearing hip.[4] The cane helps to decrease the force generated across the affected hip joint by decreasing the work of the gluteus medius-minimus complex. This occurs when the upper limb exerts force on the cane to help minimize pelvic drop on the side opposite the weightbearing lower limb.

Patients should be instructed how to ascend and descend stairs. The mnemonic "up with the good and down with the bad" serves as an easy reminder. The patient should

always have the "good" lower limb assume the first full weightbearing step.

Walker

PRESCRIPTION

1. Place the front of the walker (which should partially surround him or her) 12 in. in front of the patient.
2. The proper height is determined with the patient standing upright with the shoulders relaxed and the elbows flexed 20 degrees.[37]

A walker provides maximum support for the patient but also necessitates a slow gait. It is useful for hemiplegic and ataxic patients. Wheels can be added to the walker's front legs to facilitate movement of the walker for patients who lack coordination in the upper limbs. Patients using wheeled models must be supervised initially to ensure safety. Some walkers also have a U-shaped front extension with extra supports to provide stability for stair climbing. A patient needs to be motivated and have good strength and coordination to use this model walker.

Visual Impairment Cane

PRESCRIPTION

1. Flex the shoulder until the upper limb is parallel to the floor.
2. The distance from the hand to the floor is the proper length.

This cane should be lightweight, flexible, and easily collapsible. The distal portion of the cane is red.

Crutches

PRESCRIPTION

1. Crutch length. The distance is measured from the anterior axillary fold to a point 6 in. lateral to the fifth toe while the patient stands with the shoulders relaxed.
2. Handpiece. This is measured with the elbow flexed

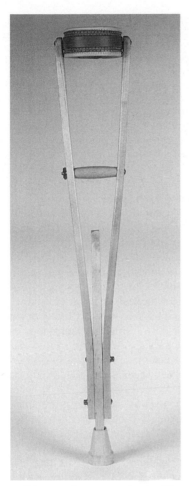

FIGURE 17–39 Wooden forearm orthosis (Kenny stick). The leather band encloses the proximal forearm.

30 degrees, the wrist in maximal extension, and the fingers forming a fist. This is measured after the total crutch height is determined with the crutch 3 in. lateral to the foot.

A crutch is defined as a device that provides support from the axilla to the floor. The term *axillary crutch* is redundant. Although there are different types of crutches and canes, they may all be referred to as *orthoses* because they are applied to the external surface of the body to improve function.

The patient should be able to raise the body 1 to 2 in. by complete elbow extension. Despite the popularity of placing padding on the axillary area of the crutch, this should not be done. It needs to be emphasized to the patient that crutches are not designed to be rests for body support. This point must be made to patients to reduce the incidence of compressive radial neuropathies.

Nonaxillary Crutches

Nonaxillary crutches should be named more appropriately *forearm* or *arm canes*. They may also be referred to as *forearm* or *arm orthoses*. The Lofstrand forearm orthosis, Kenny sticks, the Everett (or Warm Springs) orthosis, the Canadian crutch, and the platform forearm orthosis are discussed in the following text (see Figs. 17–38 and 17–39).

FOREARM ORTHOSES

Lofstrand Forearm Orthosis

PRESCRIPTION

1. The handpiece is measured as previously described for crutches, with the elbow in 20 degrees of flexion and the patient standing upright.

The proximal portion of the orthosis is also angled at 20 degrees to provide for a comfortable, stable fit. The Lofstrand forearm orthosis is often made of tubular aluminum. It provides less support than crutches for ambulation but is sufficient for many patients. These orthoses are most often used bilaterally. The open end of the cuff is placed on the lateral aspect of the forearm to permit elbow flexion and grasping without dropping the orthoses.

Wooden Forearm Orthosis (Kenny Stick)

Another forearm orthosis option is the Kenny stick (see Fig. 17–39). It was named after Sister Kenny, who sawed off the top half of wooden crutches and placed a leather band around the proximal portion of the forearm. It was designed for polio patients who had satisfactory proximal upper limb musculature but who may have been weak distally and unable to effectively hold and control the orthosis. Its advantage over the Lofstrand orthosis is the presence of a closed leather band, which ensures that the patient (more so than with the Lofstrand forearm orthosis) will not drop the ambulation aid.

Platform Forearm Orthosis

PRESCRIPTION

1. Have the patient stand upright with the shoulders relaxed and the elbows flexed 90 degrees. The distance from the ground to the forearm rest is the proper length.

This orthosis is helpful for patients with painful wrist and hand conditions as well as those with elbow contractures. Velcro straps are applied around the forearm, especially for patients with weak hand grips.

Triceps Weakness Orthoses (Arm Orthoses)

These orthoses, also known as *triceps weakness crutches*, were originally developed for poliomyelitis patients. The metal version is known as a *Warm Springs* or *Everett crutch*. The wooden version is known as a *Canadian crutch*. These crutches resemble "axillary" crutches in style but end proximally with a cuff at the mid-arm level. These ambulation aids help prevent flexion (buckling) of the elbow during gait.

Crutch Tips and Hand Grips

The purpose of using crutch tips is to absorb shock and prevent slippage. Crutches are only as safe as the quality of their tips. Special crutch tips are available for rainy and icy conditions (Fig. 17–40). At each routine checkup, the physician must make sure that they are not worn out. Hand grips are used to reduce pressure on the hands and are also safety features, because they help prevent slippage.

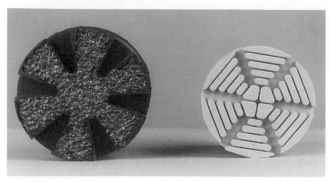

FIGURE 17–40   *Left*, Snow Boot crutch tip for use in snowy and icy conditions. *Right*, Rain Guard crutch tip for use in wet conditions. (Courtesy of Hi-Trac Industries, Holley, Mich.)

Crutch Gaits

Strength, balance, coordination, and walking surfaces all have an effect on deciding which crutch gait should be used under which circumstance. Each patient should be comfortable with more than one type of crutch gait. There are two-point, three-point, and four-point crutch gaits. The swing-through, swing-to, and drag-to gaits are also discussed. Although these have traditionally been referred to as crutch gaits, their use applies to the other ambulation aids as well.

The four-point crutch gait follows the sequence left crutch → right foot → right crutch → left foot → repeat. Its advantage is stability: three points are always in contact with the ground. It is useful for ataxic patients and for those with marked lower limb weakness. It is more difficult to learn than the other gait patterns and provides a relatively slow form of ambulation.

The three-point crutch gait follows the sequence both crutches and the weaker lower limb → "good" lower limb → repeat. Its advantage is the elimination of all weightbearing on the affected lower limb. It is commonly used by patients with lower limb fractures or amputations. It is also known as the non-weightbearing gait. The patient must have good balance to perform this gait.

The alternate two-point crutch gait follows the sequence left crutch and right foot → right crutch and left foot → repeat. This gait pattern provides stability and is useful for ataxic patients and those with decreased lower limb weightbearing capabilities. It is faster than the four-point gait pattern and provides some weightbearing relief to both lower limbs.

Gait may also be classified as swing-through, swing-to, and drag-to. The swing-through pattern sequence is both crutches → advancement of both lower limbs past the crutches. It is very energy-consuming and its use requires functional abdominal muscles. The swing-through gait is the fastest gait (even faster than able-bodied walking). The swing-to gait sequence is both crutches → advancement of both lower limbs almost to the crutch level. There are alternate and simultaneous forms of drag-to gait. The alternate sequence is left crutch → right crutch → drag to crutch level. The simultaneous sequence is both crutches → drag to crutch level. These are useful as initial gait patterns for paraplegic patients, who may advance to an-other gait pattern. They provide stability during gait but are slow and laborious methods of ambulation.

PRESCRIPTION AND COST

A medical diagnosis with delineation of the impairment and any resulting disability must be made before an orthotic prescription is written. The orthotic goals should be documented for the orthotist. An AFO prescription should include the type of ankle (rigid, flexible, or jointed) and the position of the ankle (neutral, dorsiflexed, or plantar flexed). If the ankle is jointed, the range of motion should be specified. In the case of a compressive peroneal nerve palsy, for example, the disability would be a flaccid foot-drop. The ankle should be flexible and held in a neutral position with a plastic AFO. The goals include toe clearance during swing-through and prevention of foot slap during early stance.

The ability to provide a patient a cost-effective service is becoming increasingly important. Physicians should know the costs of the tests they order. Likewise, physicians should know and be able to tell patients how much medical equipment will cost. Table 17–3 provides estimated costs for the various orthoses discussed in this chapter.

Most private insurance companies reimburse 80% of the cost of the orthosis. Medicare pays approximately 75% of the cost of orthoses listed in Table 17–3, whereas Medicaid reimbursement varies by state (but it reimburses consistently less than Medicare). Medicare usually allows orthoses to be replaced as needed. Medicaid has state-by-state laws that differ on the rate of reimbursement as well as on the frequency of replacement. Adjustments in orthoses that are necessary for growing children are usually covered by most payers.

SUMMARY

An appropriate lower limb orthotic prescription requires a thorough biomechanical analysis of gait and knowledge

TABLE 17–3   Orthotic Cost*

Orthosis	Price ($)
Over-the-counter shoe insert for pes planus/pes cavus	10–30
Custom made orthosis for pes planus (UCBL)	280
Over-the-counter foot pads ("cookies")	5
Prefabricated plastic AFO	180
Custom plastic solid AFO	440
Custom hinged plastic AFO	700
Metal AFO	420
Custom PTB AFO	900
Metal/plastic KAFO (per side)	1600
Scott Craig KAFO (per side)	2300
Swedish knee cage	280
Sport knee orthosis	150–1000
Standing frame	800
Parapodium	1400
Reciprocating gait orthosis	3000
Twister (canvas/cables)	350/500
Straight cane	20
Quad cane	45
Walker	75
Wooden crutches (pair)	35
Lofstrand forearm orthoses (pair)	50
Special crutch tips (pair)	10

*Costs listed are estimates obtained from several midwestern orthotic companies in the United States in 1995.

of the available orthotic components available to treat specific conditions. The prescribing physician must maintain a close working relationship with the certified orthotist to make certain that the patient is receiving the best orthotic options available.

Patient complaints about orthoses usually are related to cosmesis, comfort, clothing soil or damage, weight, and difficulty with donning and doffing. All practitioners should work toward the goal of achieving the ideal orthosis for the patient that will enhance comfort, cosmesis, and function, which will in turn enhance compliance. The ideal orthosis would be weightless, invisible, maintenance-free, comfortable, and strong; it would cost nothing and would normalize the gait pattern, with reduction of energy consumption to within normal limits.

Acknowledgments

Bradd L. Rosenquist, C.P.O., Columbus Orthopaedic Prosthetic and Orthotic Center, Inc.; Mike Russell, C.P.O., and colleagues, Hanger Orthopedics; Rosalind Batley, M.D.; and Kurt Kuhlman, D.O.; reviewed this chapter. Steve Brady, medical illustrator, and Jenny Torbett, photographer, made contributions to several figures in this chapter. Pearl Liss, Apex Foot Health Industries, Inc.; R. Douglas Turner, Becker Orthopedic; Wally Motloch, C.O., Center for Orthotic Design, Inc.; Robert Evans, High-Trac Industries; Greg Belbin, C.O., The Hugh MacMillan Rehabilitation Center; Carol Hiemstra-Paez, Hanger Orthopedic Group, Inc.; Deanna Fish, C.P.O., O.O.S., Inc.; Stacey Whiteside, C.O., Precision O & P Components, Inc.; and Wayne Janke, USMC; provided photographs of their products for this chapter.

Product Suppliers

Apex Foot Health Industries, Inc.
170 Wesley Street
South Hackensack, NJ 07606
(800) 526-2739

Center for Orthotic Design, Inc.
1629 Main Street
Redwood City, CA 94063
(800) 346-4746

The Hugh MacMillan Rehabilitation Center
350 Rumsey Road
Toronto, Canada M4G1R8
(416) 425-6220

JA Preston Corporation
P.O. Box 89
Jackson, MI 49204
(800) 866-7522

Precision O & P Components, Inc.
P. O. Box 24566
Tempe, AZ 85285
(602) 897-9007

Becker Orthopedic
635 Executive Drive
Troy, MI 48083-4576
(800) 521-2192

High-Trac Industries
502 North Saginaw Street
Holley, MI 48422
(810) 634-4044

Lenox Brace Company
11-20 43rd Road

Long Island City, NY 11101
(800) 222-8837

Oregon Orthotic System, Inc.
2280 3 Lakes Road
Albany, OR 97321
(800) 866-7522

United States Manufacturing Company
180 North San Gabriel Boulevard
Pasadena, CA 91117
(800) 228-5448

References

1. Bleck EE: Developmental orthopaedics. III: Toddlers. Dev Med Child Neurol 1982; 24:533–555.
2. Corcoran PJ, Jebsen RH, Brengelmann GL, et al: Effects of plastic and metal leg braces on speed and energy cost of hemiparetic ambulation. Arch Phys Med Rehabil 1970; 51:69–77.
3. D'Ambrosia RD: Conservative management of metatarsal and heel pain in the adult foot. Orthopedics 1987; 10:137–142.
4. Deathe AB, Hayes KC, Winter DA: The biomechanics of canes, crutches, and walkers. Crit Rev Phys Rehabil Med 1993; 5:15–29.
5. Diveley RL: Foot appliances and alterations. In American Academy of Orthopaedic Surgeons (eds): Orthopaedic Appliances Atlas, vol 1. Ann Arbor, JW Edwards, 1952, pp 463–464.
6. Guidera KJ, Smith S, Raney E, et al: Use of the reciprocating gait orthosis in myelodysplasia. J Pediatr Orthop 1993; 13:341–348.
7. Halar E, Cardenas D: Ankle-foot orthoses: Clinical implications. Phys Med Rehabil State Art Rev 1987; 1:45–66.
8. Houston ME, Goemans PH: Leg muscle performance of athletes with and without knee support braces. Arch Phys Med Rehabil 1982; 63:431–432.
9. Johnson EW, Spiegel MH: Ambulation problems in very young children. JAMA 1961; 175:858–863.
10. Keating EM, Faris PM, Ritter MA, et al: Use of lateral heel and sole wedges in the treatment of medial osteoarthritis of the knee. Orthop Rev 1993; 22:921–924.
11. Lehmann JF: The biomechanics of ankle foot orthoses: Prescription and design. Arch Phys Med Rehabil 1979; 60:200–207.
12. Lehmann JF, Condon SM, de Lateur BJ, et al: Ankle-foot orthoses: Effect on gait abnormalities in tibial nerve paralysis. Arch Phys Med Rehabil 1985; 66:212–218.
13. Lehmann JF, Condon SM, de Lateur BJ, et al: Gait abnormalities in peroneal nerve paralysis and their correlation by orthoses: A biomechanical study. Arch Phys Med Rehabil 1986; 67:380–386.
14. Lehmann JF, de Lateur BJ, Warren CG, et al: Biomechanical evaluation of braces for paraplegics. Arch Phys Med Rehabil 1969; 50:179–188.
15. Lehmann JF, Esselman P, Ko MJ, et al: Plastic ankle foot orthoses: Evaluation of function. Arch Phys Med Rehabil 1983; 64:402–407.
16. Lehmann JF, Warren CG: Restraining forces in various designs of knee ankle orthoses: Their placement and effect on anatomical knee joint. Arch Phys Med Rehabil 1976; 57:430–437.
17. Lehmann JF, Warren CG, de Lateur BJ: A biomechanical evaluation of knee stability in below knee braces. Arch Phys Med Rehabil 1970; 51:687–695.
18. Lehmann JF, Warren CG, Hertling D, et al: Craig Scott orthosis: A biomechanical and functional evaluation. Arch Phys Med Rehabil 1976; 57:438–442.
19. Lehmann JF, Warren CG, Pemberton DR, et al: Load bearing function of patellar tendon bearing braces of various designs. Arch Phys Med Rehabil 1971; 52:367–370.
20. Liptak GS, Shurtleff DB, Bloss JW, et al: Mobility aids for children with high-level myelomeningocele: Parapodium versus wheelchair. Dev Med Child Neurol 1992; 34:787–796.
21. Major RE, Stallard J, Rose GK: The dynamics of walking using the hip guidance orthosis (HGO) with crutches. Prosthet Orthot Int 1981; 5:19–22.
22. Marx HW: Lower limb orthotic designs for the spastic hemiplegic patient. Orthot Prosthet 1974; 28:14–20.
23. Merritt JL: Knee-ankle-foot orthotics: Long leg braces and their

practical applications. Phys Med Rehabil State Art Rev 1987; 1:67–82.

24. Milgram JE, Jacobson MA: Footgear: Therapeutic modifications of sole and heel. Orthop Rev 1978; 7:57–61.

25. Millet C, Drez D Jr: Knee braces. Orthopedics 1987; 10:1777–1780.

26. Ragnarsson KT: Lower extremity orthotics, shoes, and gait aids. *In* DeLisa JA (eds): Rehabilitation Medicine: Principles and Practice. Philadelphia, JB Lippincott, 1993, p 493.

27. Redford JB: Orthoses. *In* Basmajian JV, Kirby RL (eds): Medical Rehabilitation. Baltimore, Williams & Wilkins, 1984, p 101.

28. Reid DC: Heel pain and problems of the hindfoot. *In* Reid DC (ed): Sports Injury Assessment and Rehabilitation, ed 1. New York, Churchill Livingstone, 1992, pp 196–212.

29. Riegler HF: Orthotic devices for the foot. Orthop Rev 1987; 16:293–303.

30. Rose GK, Stallard J, Sankarankutty M: Clinical evaluation of spina bifida patients using hip guidance orthoses. Dev Med Child Neurol 1981; 23:30–40.

31. Rovere GD, Haupt HA, Yates CS: Prophylactic knee bracing in college football. Am J Sports Med 1987; 15:111–116.

32. Sarmiento A: A functional below the knee brace for tibial fractures: A report of its use in 135 cases. J Bone Joint Surg Am 1970; 52:295–311.

33. Sarmiento A, Gersten LM, Sobol JA, et al: Tibial shaft fractures treated with functional braces: Experience with 780 fractures. J Bone Joint Surg Br 1989; 71:602–609.

34. Scott BA: Engineering principles and fabrication techniques for Scott-Craig: Long leg brace for paraplegics. Orthop Prosthet 1974; 28:14–19.

35. Staheli LT, Chew DE, Corbett M: The longitudinal arch. J Bone Joint Surg Am 1987; 69:426–428.

36. Teitz CC, Hermanson B, Kronmal RA, et al: Evaluation of the use of braces to prevent injury to the knee in collegiate football players. J Bone Joint Surg Am 1987; 69:2–9.

37. Varghese G: Crutches, canes, and walkers. *In* Redford JB (ed): Orthotics Etcetera, ed 2. Baltimore, Williams & Wilkins, 1980, pp 453–463.

38. Von Werssowetz OF: Basic principles of lower extremity bracing. Orthot Prosthet Appl J 1962; 323–350.

39. Waters RL, Miller L: A physiologic rationale for orthotic prescription in paraplegia. Clin Prosthet Orthot 1987; 11:66–73.

40. Weiner DS, Weiner SD: The natural history of internal tibial torsion. Orthop 1979; 2:584–589.

41. Wenger DR, Mauldin D, Morgan D, et al: Foot growth rate in children age 1 to 6 years. Foot Ankle 1983; 3:207–210.

42. Wenger DR, Mauldin D, Speck G, et al: Corrective shoes and inserts as treatment for flexible flatfoot in infants and children. J Bone Joint Surg Am 1989; 71:800–810.

43. Winchester PK, Carollo JJ, Parekh RN, et al: A comparison of paraplegic gait performance using two types of reciprocating gait orthoses. Prosthet Orthot Int 1993; 17:101–106.

44. Zamosky I, Redford JB: Shoes and their modifications. *In* Redford JB (ed): Orthotics Etcetera, ed 2. Baltimore, Williams & Wilkins, 1980, pp 388–452.

Spinal Orthoses in Rehabilitation

**STEVEN V. FISHER, M.D., AND
ROBERT B. WINTER, M.D.**

CLINICAL USE OF SPINAL ORTHOSES

STEVEN V. FISHER, M.D.

Splints are described dating back to ancient Egypt (2700 BC). The Egyptians attempted to protect a damaged body part from further outside injury instead of attempting to hold bone fragments rigidly to allow healing or to prevent further damage from movement of the body parts.[41] In the Middle Ages, the skill of fabrication of armor led to talents in brace making.[50] Ambroise Paré is considered a pioneer in the modern art of brace making. His inventions included metal corsets. Lorenz Heister is credited with developing the first spinal brace in the 15th century with the construction of some of the basic components of today's cervical orthoses with a halolike structure for the head with an axillary sling, shoulder straps, and a waist or pelvic belt for thoracic stabilization. There have not been any significant changes in the basic concept and mechanisms of bracing since that time.[47] In the 19th century, Hugh Owen Thomas, an orthopedic physician, developed a cervical orthosis which has been modified but still bears his name. New materials and research have contributed to more effective bracing. New materials, coupled with the tremendous explosion in spinal surgery, have brought about a significant change in the actual orthoses used for the spine.[47] Relatively few external appliances merit application for the treatment of most spinal deformities. Many devices have been fabricated, however, and are often, unfortunately, known by eponyms based on the inventor's name, the locality where they were designed, or by their description.[50]

The primary objectives for the application of an orthosis include (1) controlling the position of the spine by the use of external forces; (2) applying corrective forces to abnormal curvatures; (3) aiding in spinal stability when soft tissues cannot sufficiently perform their role as stabilizer; and (4) restricting spinal segment movement after acute trauma or after a surgical procedure to protect against further injury.[4, 22] In the case of traumatic spinal injury the most important objective is the protection of the spinal cord and nerve roots. To put this in other terms, the goal of an orthosis is to control the position of the spine by the application of an external force for protection, immobilization, support, or correction of a deformity.[50]

These objectives are gained through the biomechanical effects of trunk and head support, motion control, and spinal realignment.[50] When dealing with the cervical spine an additional biomechanical effect is partial weight transfer of the head to the trunk when the patient is upright.[20, 50]

The negative effects of spinal orthoses include axial muscle atrophy secondary to reduced muscle activity needed to maintain spinal posture. The control of motion by the orthosis also promotes contractures of the immobilized part. Psychological dependency on an orthosis can occur and thereby increase physical dependence on the orthosis. Psychosocial and economic elements may also play a negative role in a patient's continued use of an orthosis.

CERVICAL ORTHOSES

Proper prescription of a cervical orthosis requires knowledge of the general principles of bracing, biomechanics of the cervical spine (see Chapter 36), and an understanding of the indications and limitations of specific cervical orthoses. All spinal orthoses utilize the principle of a three-point pressure system. The corrective component of force is ideally located midway between the opposing forces. As in a first-class lever system, any corrective force applied depends on its point and force of application and the distance from the axis of rotation. The effectiveness of a cervical orthosis is determined by its ability to resist not only gross but also intersegmental motion. As discussed later, it is the control of intersegmental motion that is difficult, especially in the cervical spine because of its extreme flexibility at multiple levels.

The occipito-atlanto-axial complex (C1 and C2) is a very distinct anatomical and functional unit. The occiput-C1 articulation is capable of very significant flexion and extension with minor degrees of lateral bending and very little axial rotation. The atlantoaxial joint (C1–C2) is more complex and also more frequently involved in pathological processes. The primary motion is rotation with a much smaller component being flexion-extension. The rotation at this joint accounts for nearly 50% of the rotation of the entire cervical spine in the adult. The combined movement of the occipito-atlanto-axial complex allows total flexion of approximately 23 degrees and a total axial rotation of 47 degrees. Lateral bending at this complex is approximately 8 degrees of motion. In the lower cervical spine, C3 through C7, each unit functions similarly. The vertebral bodies are wider anteriorly than posteriorly and the facet joints are aligned at an angle to the body that causes lordosis and allows flexion-extension, lateral bending, and axial rotation movement. The greatest flexion-extension takes place at C5 to C6, followed closely by C6 to C7. Lateral bending and axial rotation is greatest in the upper part of the cervical spine (C2–C3 and C3–C4) and decreases in the lower cervical spine.[20, 47, 48]

The biomechanical consequences of the spinal orthosis therefore are dependent on the points of application, direction, and magnitude of the force applied by the device, the tightness with which it is worn, and the amount of force the patient exerts against it. The patient's body habitus also plays a significant role in the effectiveness of the orthosis. Spinal trauma at times produces unpredictable instability and a given orthosis must be "tested" to assure effectiveness of the device. In order for a clinician to judge the effectiveness of an orthosis on a particular patient, radiographs in different positions with the patient wearing the orthosis are required.

The objective of the clinician in applying a cervical orthosis is to control the position of the spine by the use of external force. The cervical spine, however, is the most mobile part of the entire spine and has multiple planes of motion. Also, there is only a small body surface area available for adequate contact of the orthosis. The amount of external force applied over the small surface area of the chin and occiput needs to be limited to prevent local ischemic pressure problems. Anatomically, adequate contact of the orthosis on the bony structures of the skull and thorax is difficult. The occiput is rounded and the chin can easily be lifted away from the mandibular support by extending the upper cervical spine. Additionally, the shoulders and clavicle are mobile. Any strong force which acts

on the head or over the clavicles is unpleasant for the patient. The chin becomes tender rather easily with undue pressure, especially in a male who needs to shave, and there may be complications such as skin breakdown and local pain.

Cervical orthoses may be categorized in several different ways. Some authors have arranged the cervical appliances into four basic designs: (1) cervical collars; (2) poster appliances; (3) cervicothoracic orthoses; and (4) halo devices. Probably the most widely used orthoses are the (1) soft and hard collar; (2) Philadelphia orthosis; (3) SOMI (*s*ternal-*o*ccipital-*m*andibular *i*mmobilizer) orthosis; (4) poster orthosis (two or four); (5) Yale type of cervicothoracic orthosis; (6) thermoplastic Minerva body jacket (TMBJ); and (7) halo jacket or vest. These cervical orthoses will be discussed and compared with one another. Figures illustrate each general category.

There are several basic types of cervical collars. The first is a soft cervical collar (Fig. 18–1) which is made of foam rubber covered by a stockinet cover. It is well tolerated by most patients. It does not restrict cervical motion in any plane (Table 18–1). It is of low cost and is easy to fabricate. It provides warmth and psychological comfort but no support. It probably only serves as a reminder to hold the neck relatively still.

The second type of collar is a hard collar made of a rigid polyethylene. It can have an optional occipital and mandibular support. The hard collar without the mandibular and cervical support does not significantly immobilize the cervical spine. With the two supports it gives more restriction in flexion and extension, but it is not truly effective. It does not limit lateral bending or rotation. It does not

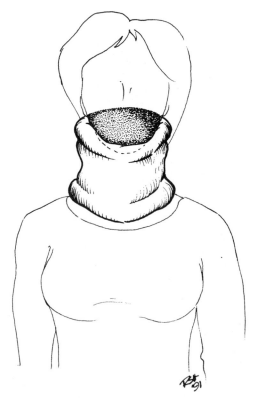

FIGURE 18–1 Soft collar.

TABLE 18–1 Normal Cervical Motion From Occiput to First Thoracic Vertebra and the Effects of Cervical Orthoses

	Mean of Normal Motion (%)		
	Flexion/Extension	*Lateral Bending*	*Rotation*
Normal*	100.0	100.0	100.0
Soft collar*	74.2	92.3	82.6
Philadelphia collar*	28.9	66.4	43.7
SOMI brace*	27.7	65.6	33.6
Four-poster brace*	20.6	45.9	27.1
Yale cervicothoracic brace	12.8	50.5	18.2
Halo device*	4.0	4.0	1.0
Halo device†	11.7	8.4	2.4
Minerva body jacket‡	14.0	15.5	0

*Data from Johnson RM, Hart DL, Simmons EF, et al: Cervical orthoses: a study comparing their effectiveness in restricting cervical motion in normal subjects. J Bone Joint Surg [Am] 1977; 59:332.

†Data from Lysell E: Motion in the cervical spine, thesis. Acta Orthop Scand Suppl 1969; 123.

‡Data from Maiman D, Millington P, Novak S, et al: The effects of the thermoplastic Minerva body jacket on cervical spine motion. Neurosurgery 1989; 25:363–368.

contact onto the thorax. It can press on the clavicles, creating areas of high pressure with subsequent discomfort.

The Philadelphia ("collar") orthosis (Fig. 18–2) is made of plastazote reinforced with anterior and posterior plastic struts. The front and rear halves fasten with Velcro closures. The orthosis has a molded mandibular and occipital support. The anterior and posterior caudal aspects of the brace extend onto the upper thorax. The Philadelphia orthosis does restrict cervical spine motion, particularly in flexion and extension (see Table 18–1). This is probably due to the better fit at the occiput and chin as well as

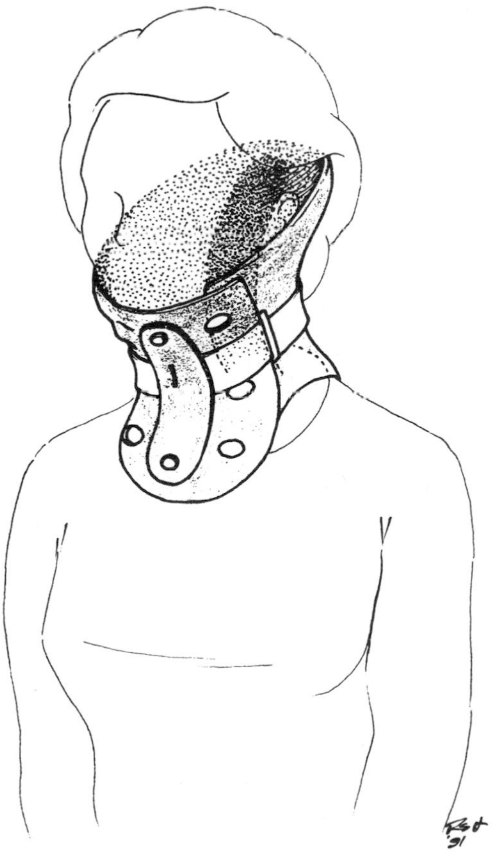

FIGURE 18–2 Philadelphia collar.

the improved contact on the upper thorax. However, the Philadelphia orthosis is relatively ineffective in controlling rotation and lateral bending (see Table 18–1). Depending on the prominence of the clavicles of the individual wearer, the Philadelphia orthosis may be quite uncomfortable.

Another brace in this category is a Jobst Vertebrace constructed from a high-density polyethylene sheet with its periphery cushioned with soft, closed-cell polyethylene foam. It provides full contact along its costal end to the sternum and it closely cups the mandible. A radiological study of 10 normal volunteers showed that this orthosis functioned as well as, or better than, the Yale (see below for description; also see Fig. 18–5) and Philadelphia orthoses. The authors believed it was a good orthotic choice for use in emergency transport situations.[12]

The four-poster brace (Fig. 18–3) represents the first true cervical thoracic orthosis discussed here. It has a molded mandibular and occipital support with adjustable struts attaching to anterior and posterior padded thoracic plates. The mandibular and occipital supports can be held together with straps running below the ears. The anterior and posterior thoracic pads are connected by leather shoulder straps. There are no straps under the axilla. The Guilford brace (Fig. 18–4) is a two-poster brace with a front and back strut connecting the anterior and posterior thoracic plates to the chin and occipital piece. The strapping runs over the shoulder as well as under the axilla. These orthoses are relatively effective in limiting range of motion in flexion and extension (see Table 18–1).

Another true cervical thoracic brace is the Yale orthosis (Fig. 18–5). This cervicothoracic orthosis was originally a modified Philadelphia collar with molded plastazote reinforced with plastic struts. It extends down onto the anterior and posterior thorax with strapping beneath the axilla. The occipital piece can extend higher on the skull than the original Philadelphia orthosis. The increased contact on the body surface at the occiput as well as onto the thorax improves the stability which this brace offers (see Table 18–1).

McGuire et al[25] used fresh cadavers destabilized at C4 to C5 by sectioning the facet capsules, interspinous ligaments, spinal cord, posterior longitudinal ligament, and intervertebral disc. They used a constant flexion force and studied

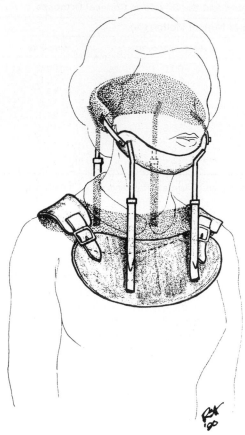

FIGURE 18-3   Four-poster collar.

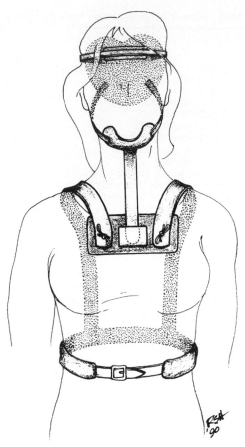

FIGURE 18-4   Two-poster orthosis (Guilford).

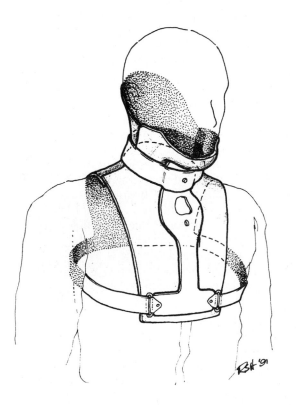

FIGURE 18-5   Yale cervicothoracic orthosis.

movement radiographically. They found that the Philadelphia Collar Halo System was superior to the Philadelphia Collar, and two other collars (Necloc and Stifneck). They concluded that the increased length and chest pieces counteract the deformity forces, thereby best preventing flexion. Both the Yale and the Philadelphia Collar Halo System orthoses improve stability because of their thoracic extensions.

The SOMI orthosis (Fig. 18–6) is also a cervicothoracic orthosis. It has a rigid anterior plastic chest piece and shoulder straps. The occipital piece is attached with two posters which run anteriorly. The mandibular piece has a single poster which also attaches anteriorly. These posts are made of rigid aluminum. The strapping crosses under the arms to the base of the chest piece. The SOMI brace is well tolerated. This brace can be applied without moving the patient from the supine position, and this is an advantage in the spinal cord–injured patient in skeletal tong traction. It is supplied with an optional headpiece that snaps onto the occipital rest and passes around the forehead which can be used to allow removal of the mandibular support while eating. It is relatively effective in restricting flexion-extension (see Table 18–1).

There have been several studies in the last 15 years documenting the effectiveness of cervical orthoses. The most widely referenced study was performed by Johnson and associates[12] (Table 18–1). Normal subjects were fitted with a soft collar, Philadelphia collar, SOMI brace, four-poster brace, cervicothoracic brace, and a halo with plastic body vest. Flexion-extension and lateral bending were measured radiographically and rotation was measured using

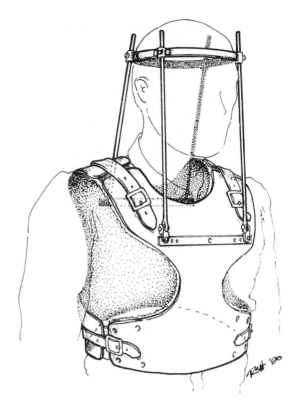

FIGURE 18–7   Halo device/vest.

overhead photography. Fisher et al[9] studied normal subjects radiographically using the polyethylene hard collar, plastazote Philadelphia orthosis, a four-poster, and a SOMI orthosis. This study measured only flexion and extension. Although there were some differences in the range of motion at specific cervical levels, the results of the two separate studies generally agree and trends can be recognized. It is known that no cervical orthosis totally immobilizes the cervical spine. There is a recognized "snaking" of the cervical spine with some segments moving into flexion and others into extension, especially when forced flexion and extension is attempted against the orthosis. The differences noted in these studies at specific cervical levels are probably due to the variable degree of snaking of the spine with forced movements against the orthosis.

Soft collars allow 75% to 100% of normal unrestricted flexion and extension motion, while plastic collars allow 25% to 30%. Four-posters, two-posters, and the SOMI allow 10% to 28%. The Yale orthosis and the TMBJ, discussed later, provide more restriction in this plane (see Table 18–1).

In the United States the halo brace (Fig. 18–7) has become the most frequently used method of treating cervical fractures or dislocations. It was first described by Perry and Nickel[36] in 1959 and reviewed by them again in 1968.[37]

There are basically two types of halo orthotic devices currently used to control neck motion. They are the halo cast and halo vest. The halo component is the same on each type and consists of a rigid metal or graphite ring attached to the skull with four fixation pins, two anteriorly, usually in the frontal region, and two posteriorly in the parieto-occipital area. The ring is bolted to four posters which run down onto either a rigid polyethylene vest or

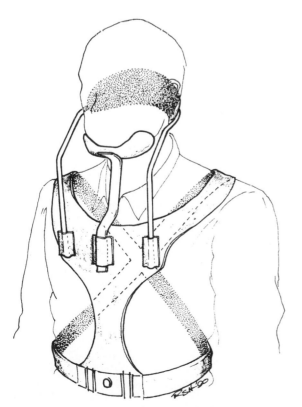

FIGURE 18–6   Sterno-occipital mandibular immobilization orthosis (SOMI).

onto a plaster cast, both of which extend to about the umbilicus. If further intimate contact on the thorax is needed, a body cast is fabricated distally with contact onto the pelvis.

Johnson et al[12] and Lysell[23] studied the restriction of motion provided by the halo. Their results are summarized in Table 18–1. Koch and Nickel[15] first studied forces within the halo vest device coupled with range-of-motion measurements. There was a strikingly wide variety of values in different patients and a wide range of values for each individual in different positions. The variability was partially related to the fit of the vest. The forces could be either compressive or distractive. They also found that the absolute motion in the halo vest had been underestimated in previous studies using normal subjects and that an average of 31% of normal spine motion was observed in their patient population.

Walker and co-workers[45] found the same magnitude of vertical forces noted by Koch and Nickel,[15] but noted that these forces would be applied infrequently over a typical day. The vest was again thought to be the weak link in terms of movement and distortion. The forces on the pins in the skull are primarily shear forces acting in multiple directions which explains why pinholes enlarge in a craterlike fashion.

Lind and others[18] found the same snakelike motion described by Johnson et al[12] and great individual variability as noted above. Using a different measurement technique, they found maximal cervical motion in a halo apparatus of 70% of the normal motion was greatest in the upper cervical spine area. Rehabilitation exercises did not cause any greater movement to the spine than did daily motion and activity.

Wolf and Jones[51] studied seven patients in a halo cast and 14 in a plastic body jacket. There was no significant difference found in the amount of motion in flexion-extension and lateral bending as determined radiographically. Patient acceptance and comfort was greater in the plastic jackets. The frequency of pin loosening was twice as high in the heavier halo cast.

Wang and associates[46] studied the influence of vest length on the stability of the cervical spine. A half-vest to the level of the nipples was compared with a short extended vest to the 12th rib and a full vest extended to the iliac crests in 12 normal subjects. There was no rotation of the cervical spine regardless of vest length. There was a variable amount of flexion and extension of the upper cervical spine regardless of vest length. More motion was seen in the lower cervical spine than in the upper. The authors concluded that a lesion of the upper cervical spine could be treated with a half-vest which improves comfort and ease of patient care. However, they recommended a full vest.[46]

With the overestimation of restriction in motion and the variability noted, it is not surprising that the literature on treatment of cervical fractures is unclear on the indications for halo alone, or for surgical intervention coupled with halo immobilization. Sears and Faz[40] studied 173 acute cervical injuries. They found that those patients with facet joint dislocation formed a distinct subgroup in which only 44% achieved stability with halo alone, but even half of these had a poor anatomical result. Of the patients without facet joint dislocation, 70% achieved stability and 75% had good results anatomically.

Clark and White[5] studied patients with fractures of the dens, which is another area of management controversy. Their results support the surgical approach of type II (fractures of the junction of the dens and central body of the axis) with either angulation or displacement. Unstable type III (fractures which go deep into the body of the axis) are also believed to require surgery.

When one realizes that the halo device does not immobilize as well as was first thought and that most motion occurs in the upper cervical spine, it is not surprising that upper cervical spine injuries require frequent surgical intervention as well as halo immobilization.

Glaser and others[11] reviewed 245 cases treated with halo vests and they concluded that halo vests protect cervical fracture patients from neurological injury, but do not absolutely immobilize or even prevent deformity. After 3 months of halo immobilization, surgery might be required in cases of ligamentous and osseous injuries to achieve stability.

The United Kingdom has been very cautious in adopting the halo device but a relatively recent publication suggests acceptance of this device vs. the more traditional skull caliper–bed immobilization treatment.[34]

The Minerva molded type of orthosis is not new (Fig. 18–8). It did not contact the head or thorax any better than the more traditional Philadelphia or four-poster. The newer design of the TMBJ shown in Figure 18–9 runs down the thorax to a level similar to that of the halo vest and provides significant contact on the head with its circumferential forehead adaptation. It is obviously much lighter in weight than its forerunner, the plastic Minerva jacket. It offers an advantage over the halo device in not being

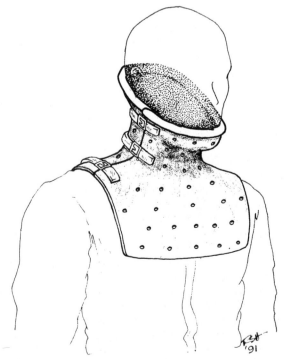

FIGURE 18–8 Custom-molded cuirass orthosis (original Minerva design).

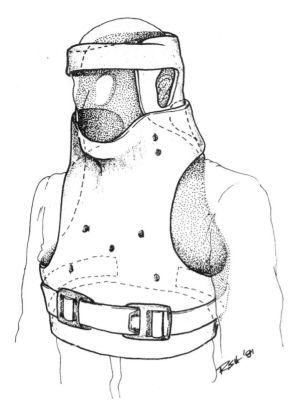

FIGURE 18–9 Thermoplastic Minerva body jacket (TMBJ).

invasive with the inherent pin problems of infection and slippage.

Millington and colleagues[27] introduced the TMBJ in 1987 and later Maiman et al[24] studied 21 normal subjects in terms of the effectiveness of this device. That study is summarized in Table 18–1. The authors doubted the accuracy of their rotation measurements secondary to inadequate stabilization of the trunk. They believed, however, that flexion-extension compared favorably with the halo device studies of other researchers. The authors caution that this study was on normal subjects and this has to be considered when applying their findings to patients.

Benzel and co-workers[2] compared the TMBJ and halo devices in 10 ambulatory patients with an unstable cervical spine. The patients initially underwent 6 to 8 weeks of immobilization with a halo device followed by the TMBJ. Prior to removal of the halo flexion-extension, radiographs were taken. Two to 3 weeks later similar films were taken in the TMBJ. The average spine movement in the TMBJ was less than in the halo. The authors believed the difference was attributable to the snaking of the cervical spine noted in the halo device.

Pringle, in a review article,[38] stated that both the Minerva and the halo vest are far superior to other cervical thoracic orthoses and are the treatment of choice in the ambulant management of the unstable cervical spine. Additionally, there is literature that supports the use of the Minerva vest in preference to the halo vest in preschool-age children. This is due to the Minerva vest providing necessary stabilization and yet being lightweight, with maximal comfort, and allowing early mobilization of the patient for rehabilitation.[10]

It seems that the TMBJ can be an alternative to the halo in selected patients. Further clinical studies certainly are required, but the TMBJ seems to be a promising addition to cervical orthotic management.

There is very little published on the management of upper thoracic fractures. The typical thoracic orthoses such as the Jewett hyperextension device or the chairback brace with sternal pad provide immobilization up to the level of T6 at the maximum and are therefore of no value in the upper thoracic spine. The ribs act as support struts in the thorax, but many times there are associated rib fractures which reduce the desired stability. If neurological compromise is a risk in a given upper thoracic fracture with instability, a halo device is needed. Surgical stabilization can also be required.[6] Other orthoses can be utilized for attempted posture control if the spinal cord is not in jeopardy of compromise. Upper thoracic fractures require either a halo cast to the pelvis or a Milwaukee-type orthosis (cervicothoracolumbosacral orthosis, CTLSO) if surgery is not selected.[49]

THORACOLUMBOSACRAL ORTHOSES

Lumbosacral (LSO) and thoracolumbosacral (TLSO) orthoses are prescribed more frequently than cervical orthoses. There are more variations of design for each type and therefore there are more eponyms. This discussion focuses on the most commonly prescribed and the representative types of design and material.

As with cervical orthoses, proper prescription of a thoracolumbar orthosis (TLO) requires knowledge of the general principles of bracing, biomechanics of the thoracic and lumbar spine, and an understanding of the indications and limitations of specific thoracic and lumbar orthoses. It is outside the scope of this chapter to deal in detail with these subjects, but a few general considerations are necessary.

The sacrum can be considered the "foundation" of the spinal column. The sacrum is attached to the ilium to very rigidly form the pelvis, which rotates freely on the femoral heads. In the upright standing posture, flexion of the pelvis on the femur causes a compensatory extension of the lumbar spine (increased lumbar lordosis with an increase in the lumbosacral angle). Likewise, if there is an increase in lumbosacral lordosis, there can be an increased thoracic flexion or kyphosis.

As in the cervical spine, the range of motion of each spinal segment is directly related to the anatomy of the region. In the thoracic spinal column, the facets are primarily oriented in the horizontal plane. Each vertebra is bilaterally attached to a rib, with the upper 10 ribs attaching directly to the sternum, and the spinous processes are overlapping. These factors severely limit thoracic spine mobility in flexion and extension. The rib cage plays a great role in enhancing the stiffness of the thoracic spine. It has been demonstrated that the spine is 27%, 45%, 31%, and 132% stiffer in flexion, lateral bending, axial rotation, and extension, respectively, owing to the rib cage.[1] Rotation and lateral bending is the predominant movement possible: about 6 degrees of lateral bending at each segment, and 8 to 9 degrees of axial rotation. There is an average of 4 degrees of flexion and extension in the upper portion and

6 degrees in the middle segments of the thoracic spine. The transitional segments from thoracic to lumbar spine (T10–T12) have much greater flexion and extension (average, 12 degrees). There is also increased lateral bending (average, 8 degrees), and less rotation (2 degrees). This is in part because the ribs do not articulate with the sternum in the last segments and the facet joints are in transition from the alignment in the thoracic spine to that of the lumbar spine.

The lumbar spine has five large vertebrae, large intervertebral discs, and nearly sagittally placed articular processes with posteriorly directed spinous processes. Because of the anatomical alignment of the facets, there is between 12 degrees of flexion and 17 degrees of extension, 3 to 6 degrees of lateral bending, and only 1 to 2 degrees of axial rotation at any given level. The greatest flexion and extension, and the least lateral bending and axial rotation occur at L5 to S1.[47]

The objectives of TCLOs are similar to those of the cervical region: to control the position of the spine by the use of external forces, to apply corrective forces to abnormal curvatures, to aid in spinal stability when soft tissues cannot sufficiently perform their role as stabilizer, and to restrict spinal segment movement. In the case of trauma the most important objective is the protection of the spinal cord, cauda equina, and nerve roots.

The work of Norton and Brown[33] was the first and remains one of the most important dealing with the effectiveness of back braces. There is very significant variability in the effectiveness of back braces. This relates to an individual's lumbar flexion pattern. Orthotic devices that are well fixed to the chest but inadequately so to the pelvis leave the lumbosacral segments unsupported. Braces such as the chairback brace, which has shorter supports, tend to pull away from the pelvis less, thereby giving more support to the lumbosacral (LS) area.[33] No brace can totally immobilize, but can limit, interspinous motion. If an orthosis is to be effective, it must supply sufficient pressure over bony prominences to remind the wearer to change position or maintain posture.[21] All braces employ a three-point pressure system. The more contact the brace has with the wearer, the more evenly the pressure is distributed and the better the control achieved. The total contact custom-molded thermoplastic orthosis is an example of an orthosis in which the three-point pressure principle is diffused by the total contact against the patient.

Morris and associates[29] demonstrated that increasing the abdominal pressure by using an orthosis decreases the net force applied to the spine when lifting a weight from the floor. However, when extra loading of the spine occurs, the amount of compression necessary is not well tolerated. They believed that since the spinal column is attached to the sides of the abdominal and thoracic cavities, the action of the trunk muscles converts the thoracic and abdominal chambers into nearly rigid containers. These containers transmit part of the forces (generated in loading the spine when lifting), thereby relieving the load directly on the spine.[28]

Nachemson and co-workers,[32] however, noted that no LSO significantly raised intragastric pressure. Intra-abdominal pressure increases only with closure of the glottis during muscular activity. The LS support, when tightened within patient tolerance, decreases the intradiscal pressure at the lumbar spine by approximately 30%.[30] Nachemson et al demonstrated that wearing an LSO reduces disc pressure values during about two thirds of a set of exercises and increases pressure during the remaining third.[32]

Morris and associates[29] found that the chairback brace and the LS corset decreased or had no effect on the electrical activity of back muscles. Nachemson et al[32] also found no consistent trends when studying four normal volunteers performing six tasks while using an orthosis. The erector spinal myoelectrical activity was at times increased and at other times reduced by a like amount.[32]

Lantz and Shultz[17] also found inconsistent changes in the myoelectrical activity with normal volunteers and some of the increased activity was thought to be due to antagonistic muscle activity. It was considered, but not verified experimentally, that low back pain patients wearing an orthosis daily "relax into the brace" and perhaps reduce antagonistic muscle activity.[17] Segmental motion can be increased at each end of the immobilized spine as the spine moves, possibly exacerbating a condition the orthosis is attempting to treat.[20]

The studies mentioned earlier of TLOs were in large part carried out on normal volunteers. The authors did not take into consideration important complicating factors such as pain, decreased muscular strength, insensate skin, altered biomechanics secondary to trauma and instability, or surgical changes.[43] Since there is significant variability of fit and effectiveness, radiographic analysis of spinal motion is

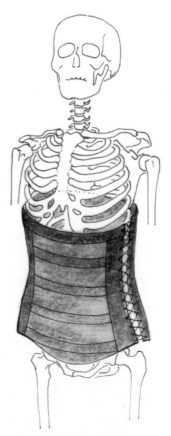

FIGURE 18–10 Chairback lumbosacral orthosis with side lacing attachment to an abdominal apron.

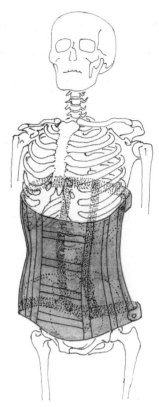

FIGURE 18–11 Chairback lumbosacral orthosis with paraspinal uprights in addition to the midaxillary line supports.

necessary for a given patient to determine the effectiveness of the device in limiting unwanted motion.

These appliances can be classified as corsets, rigid braces, hyperextension braces, hyperflexion braces, and jackets. All spinal orthoses with the exception of hyperextension braces give abdominal support. The ability of these devices to restrict motion has not been measured in as great detail as with the cervical orthoses. The evaluation of effectiveness is therefore more subjective.

The most commonly prescribed LS support is the LS corset.[35] In general, a corset is made of canvas with rigid backstays often made of steel. There is adjustable side or back lacing. A corset is a stock item and can usually be fitted by a corsetier without difficulty. The corset can be LS or TLS. The stays can be either rigid or semirigid. Fidler and Plasmans[7] and Lantz and Schultz[16] found that a corset significantly reduced spinal motion by as much as two thirds. The stays actually give only a little amount of support, but they supply painful stimuli if the patient leans against them, especially the lateral ones. The corset gives minimal actual support and its effectiveness might be more related to the discomfort it can produce for patients[33] because it reminds them to maintain adequate posture.

LUMBOSACRAL ORTHOSES. The chairback brace is the most popular of the rigid braces. It consists of an anterior corset or apron front with midaxillary metal uprights (Fig. 18–10) or of two paraspinal uprights and two uprights in the midaxillary line (Fig. 18–11). It is designed to control flexion-extension and lateral motion.

Another LSO commonly prescribed is the William's back brace, which is used primarily to control extension

and lordosis, and to give some lateral control (Fig. 18–12). It is a specialized orthosis in that it allows free flexion but limits extension and uses a lever action and abdominal support to reduce lumbar lordosis.

THORACOLUMBOSACRAL ORTHOSES. There are two major types of TLSOs. The more common is the Taylor orthosis, which is constructed to restrict flexion and extension (Fig. 18–13). This type of orthosis is relatively ineffective for limiting lumbar spine motion.[33] The Taylor orthosis limits thoracic motion only if the axillary straps are tightened to the point of discomfort. When the patient loosens the straps because of discomfort, the orthosis unfortunately becomes ineffective. This orthosis appears to be a poor choice for TLS immobilization. The chairback brace with cowhorn or sternal pad attachments (Fig. 18–14), which transmit pressure through the sternum and ribs directly to the spine, provides better LS and thoracic immobilization than a brace by which force is transmitted through the pectoral girdle (which is attached to the spinal axis only by muscles and the sternoclavicular joints).

Molded jackets are made either of plaster of Paris or a thermoplastic material to conform to the contours of the body (Fig. 18–15). If made properly, they become a nearly total contact type of orthotic device. The pressure distribution is more uniform and more support is provided. Fidler and Plasmans[7] and Lantz and Schultz[16] verified that the molded TLSO restricts spinal movement better than a corset or chairback brace. A spica attachment to the molded TLSO not unexpectedly was best at restricting movement, presumably by partially immobilizing the pelvis. These jackets are used frequently for patients with spinal fractures or low back fusions to allow early mobilization and rehabil-

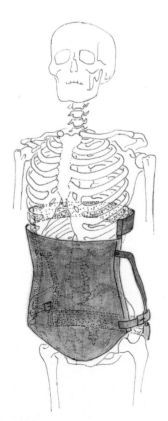

FIGURE 18–12 William's hyperextension lumbosacral orthosis.

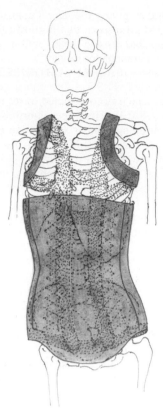

FIGURE 18–13 The Taylor thoracolumbosacral brace.

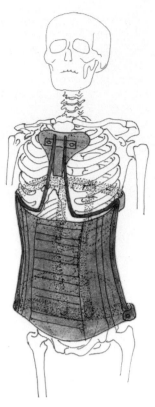

FIGURE 18–14 Chairback brace with sternal pad transmitting bony support to the lower thoracic spine.

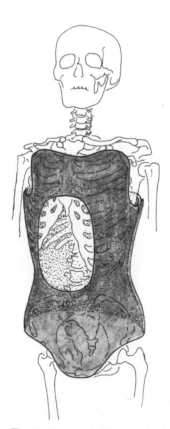

FIGURE 18–15 The custom-molded thermoplastic jacket-type thoracic lumbosacral orthosis.

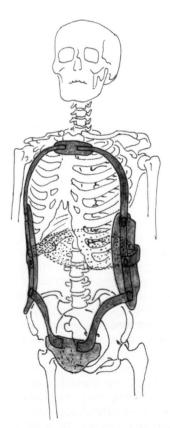

FIGURE 18–16 Jewett hyperextension orthosis restricts spinal flexion by anterior pressure over the sternum and pubic symphysis, and posterior pressure across the lower thoracic/upper lumbar region.

itation. They also may be of value when there are metastases in vertebrae, to provide support and control pain. Donning and doffing the molded jacket are more difficult than with other orthoses.

The hyperextension orthosis differs from other devices because it does not have an abdominal apron and does not give abdominal support. It functions to give a hyperextension moment (Fig. 18–16). This hyperextension brace applies three-point pressure over the sternum and the pubis anteriorly and over the upper lumbar spine posteriorly. This hyperextension orthosis is used to permit the upright position, while preventing flexion after a compression frac-

ture of a vertebral body. It is not recommended in the management of compression fractures in osteoporotic elderly patients because it can place excessive hyperextension forces on lower lumbar vertebrae, which can induce posterior element fractures or exacerbate a degenerative arthritis condition.

It should be stressed that orthoses only partially limit rather than immobilize the spine. Spinal orthoses should be considered to be temporary devices. At the same time that the orthotic device is prescribed, a rehabilitation treatment plan should be outlined to attempt to rid the patient of the need for the device in the future.

SPINAL ORTHOSES FOR SPINAL DEFORMITY

ROBERT WINTER, M.D.

The purpose of this section is to describe the orthoses used for the management of spinal deformities, as well as to indicate the goals, indications, contraindications, and problems. Thirty years ago, bracing was purely empirical. There has been adequate clinical research from around the world since the 1960s to now make the orthotic management of spinal deformities a well-established, proven technique.

HISTORY

Bracing for spinal deformity has gone through many historical stages. Prior to the first spinal fusion for scoliosis by Hibbs in 1915, bracing was the only treatment method available and highly sophisticated orthoses were available, especially in Germany. As surgery became better refined and increasingly safe, there was an understandable diminution in enthusiasm for bracing. Surgery, however, still had significant risks and was a very unpleasant experience for the patient, especially the many months in bed in a heavy plaster cast.

A major milestone took place in the late 1940s when Blount and Schmidt, in Milwaukee, collaborated on a new brace design. It was first used for postsurgical correction and stabilization, and then secondarily was modified for nonoperative treatment.

As evidence slowly accumulated that braces could not only halt the progression of curvatures but sometimes even create lasting improvement, there was a tremendous surge

of enthusiasm for brace management. This was actually an overzealous swing of the pendulum away from surgery toward bracing.

By the late 1970s, considerable pessimism began to be heard which reached its maximum in the late 1980s and early 1990s. This was so pronounced that many orthopedic surgeons were saying that braces were "of no use at all" and that "bracing really did not affect the natural history of scoliosis." However, thanks to diligent work over many years in several centers, it has been amply demonstrated that orthotic management can have a very positive effect on many spinal deformities.

Methods proved to be of no value in the treatment of scoliosis include exercise, spinal manipulation, electrical stimulation, biofeedback, acupuncture, holistic medicine, vitamins, and religious prayer.

BIOMECHANICS

There is an unfortunate tendency in scoliosis management to make drawings of lateral curvatures and then to apply arrows showing the direction of forces and some numbers to indicate the magnitude of those forces. Scoliosis is always a three-dimensional problem. Rotation of vertebrae is an integral component of all structural scolioses. The frontal plane radiograph, anteroposterior (AP) or posteroanterior (PA), as well as lateral films, must be studied. Most important, the physical examination of the patient reveals the rotational aspects far better than radiographs.

Another common mistake is to think only in terms of *passive* forces. Many orthoses, especially the Milwaukee brace (CTLSO), are designed to stimulate *active* corrective forces on the part of the patient.

A third common mistake is to look only at spinal radiographs rather than to realize all of the organs involved in the human torso. For example, an orthosis might produce a nice-looking radiograph but cause a marked reduction in vital capacity. Berg and Aaro[3] showed decreased renal function, and Kennedy et al[13, 14] showed decreased pulmonary function with use of the Boston brace.

Biomechanics are quite dynamic. For example, in a well-fitted Milwaukee brace for a right thoracic idiopathic scoliosis, there is a constant force only in the pelvic section. It is a circumferential force, but mild enough that there are no pressure sores on the skin and the patient has no discomfort related to pressure. The design is such that the patient's neck "floats" within the neck ring, that is, there are usually zero forces anywhere on the neck. The main corrective force pad, that is, the right thoracic pad, is broad, thus distributing the force over a wide area of skin. The patient can, at any time, shift the thorax to the left so that there are zero forces under the pad.

This ability to "get away from the pad" guarantees that there will not be any skin sores, and the patient is actively using trunk muscles only in a way that corrects the curvature. This is one example of the "active" component of the brace.

The second active component is the neck ring. If the patient slumps in the brace, the throat will come down onto the throat mold, which produces an uncomfortable feeling. The patient will instinctively elongate the spine again, using trunk muscles in a way that is curve-correcting.

In a well-fitting Milwaukee brace, trunk muscles are constantly being used, but always in a positive mode relative to the curve. These muscles are quiet only at night. It is incorrect to state that such a brace produces "severe muscle atrophy," which is a common statement made by people unfamiliar with the true nature of corrective spinal bracing. Such "muscle atrophy" has never been shown.

These concepts of dynamic muscle activity can be carried over into underarm orthoses (TLSOs) if they are carefully designed using the same concepts. The great virtue of the Milwaukee brace is its open design, and its lack of circumferential torso constriction. The torso is allowed to shift to the left (in a typical right thoracic curve pattern) since there is no "wall" of plastic on the left to block the shift.

Thus a TLSO can be designed which incorporates a "space" into which the torso can shift. The counterforce opposing the right thoracic pad must therefore be a high axillary padded margin of the TLSO above the "space" area. Because this high axillary contact point can be an irritant if the patient sags down, the patient will tend to elongate and lean the upper thorax to the right, thus adding to the effectiveness of the right thoracic pad.

Lumbar pads, whether in a TLSO or a Milwaukee brace, tend to be much more passive than thoracic pads. Both the TLSO and the Milwaukee brace should, however, be

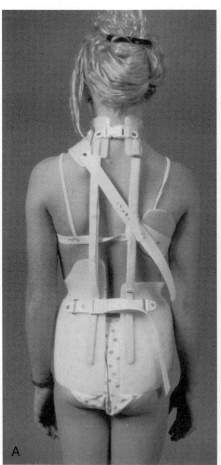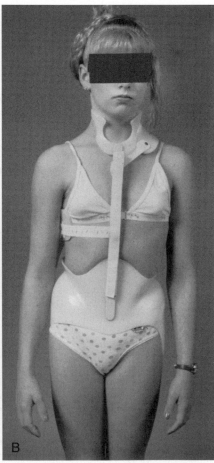

A   B

FIGURE 18–17 *A,* Posterior view of a modern Milwaukee brace showing the pelvic section, a lumbar pad, a right thoracic pad, a left trapezius pad, and the new style plastic neck-ring. *B,* Frontal view of the same patient, again showing the pelvic section, the anterior upright, the trapezius pad, and the modern plastic neck-ring, which avoids all dental problems and is much more aesthetically acceptable to the patient.

designed to provide a "space" into which the patient can actively shift the spinal segments.

The above-mentioned dynamic concepts apply, of course, only to those patients with active muscle power and a good sense of muscle control. Patients with neuromuscular problems are quite different and the orthoses used in these patients are purely passive.

TYPES OF ORTHOSES FOR SPINAL DEFORMITIES

Milwaukee Brace

The Milwaukee brace (TLSO) was the first to have statistically proven positive results in spinal deformity, and is thus a "gold standard" against which other orthoses can be compared. It consists of a well-molded pelvic section, originally made of leather, but now almost universally made of some type of plastic; two posterior uprights; a single anterior upright; and a neck ring. These components are always made in straight alignment, that is, the pelvic section is level, the uprights are all perfectly vertical, and the neck ring is centered over midpelvis.

Curve correction is achieved by one or more pads which are attached to the basic frame. In an ideal sense, the deformed spine is brought to the perfect vertical alignment. A patient with a leg-length difference should have a shoe lift such that the pelvis is leveled.

The two most common corrective pads for scoliosis are the thoracic pad and the lumbar pad. Other pads less often used are the oval pad, the trapezius pad, and the shoulder ring. The axillary sling is not a corrective pad, but rather a device the patient pushes against in order to center the neck within the neck ring. For kyphosis, two thoracic kyphosis pads are used, one on each posterior upright (Fig. 18–17A and B).

The Thoracolumbosacral Orthosis

The TLSO reaches only to the axillary level and is thus incapable of exerting any corrective action on the upper thoracic spine. It is typically used for scolioses having their apex at T9 or lower, and for kyphoses having their apex at the thoracolumbar junction.

Many different styles exist, often named for the city or institution in which they were developed, for example, Gillette, Lyon, Cuxhaven, Boston, Dupont, Minnesota Spine Center, etc. The names are not as important as the design concepts. Any orthosis worth its salt *must* have a positive effect on the curve to be treated, and *must* not be harmful.

There are corrective types designed primarily for adolescents with idiopathic scoliosis and passive TLSOs made with the patient held in a corrected alignment (Fig. 18–18A and B). These latter types are most commonly used for neuromuscular deformities. The mold is usually taken on some type of traction table.

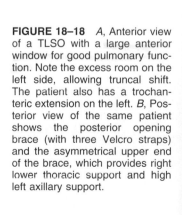

FIGURE 18–18 *A*, Anterior view of a TLSO with a large anterior window for good pulmonary function. Note the excess room on the left side, allowing truncal shift. The patient also has a trochanteric extension on the left. *B*, Posterior view of the same patient shows the posterior opening brace (with three Velcro straps) and the asymmetrical upper end of the brace, which provides right lower thoracic support and high left axillary support.

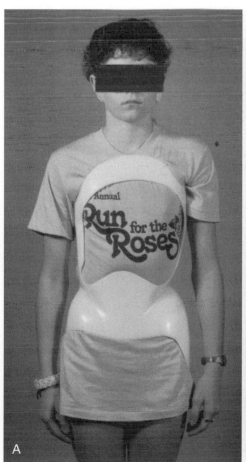

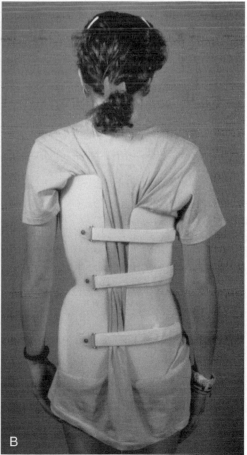

The Lumbosacral Orthosis

The LSO is a specific design *only* for lumbar scolioses. It is firmly locked to the pelvis, has a strong force pad against the apex of the lumbar curve, and *no* thoracic extension on the opposite side. The correction is done by the patient's own active righting reflexes and muscle power. It is intended only for idiopathic scoliosis patients (Fig. 18–19A and B).

BRACING FOR INFANTILE IDIOPATHIC SCOLIOSIS

By definition, idiopathic *infantile* scoliosis is an idiopathic curvature occurring in a child under 3 years of age. There must be no anomalous vertebrae, and magnetic resonance imaging (MRI) or myelogram must demonstrate the absence of a syrinx, tumor, or any other neurological abnormality.

Since 80% to 85% of infants with this type of scoliosis have spontaneous resolution of their curvature, it is important to avoid bracing a mild curve that will disappear on its own. Similarly, it is important to aggressively treat those children with progressive curves. One useful sign of a bad prognosis curve is the measurement of the angle between the proximal portion of the rib at the apex of the curve and the superior margin of the corresponding vertebra. If the angle on the convexity is greater than the angle on the concavity by 20 degrees or more, a bad prognosis exists (Mehta's rib–vertebral angle difference [RVAD]).

Curves progressing past 30 degrees should also be treated. Although Mehta prefers serial plaster casts, the author favors the use of the classic Milwaukee brace. It requires a skilled orthotist to create such a brace for children age 6 months or older.

The brace is worn on a full-time schedule (23½ hours/day), removed only for the daily bath. Normal developmental activities are encouraged. These children readily adapt to the brace and soon largely forget that life existed without it.

Many of these children will have a cure of their problem with a vigorous brace program. The spine gradually becomes straight in the brace as it is held straight for many months, and then gradually the brace is removed (the "weaning" process). The spine remains straight from then onward.

Another outcome of treatment is successful curve control, but this is not a cure. The spine does well as long as the brace is on, but deforms with attempts at weaning. This necessitates long-term bracing until the pubertal growth spurt. At this point the curve usually gets worse despite the brace, and surgical fusion is necessary.

The third possible outcome is brace failure with the curve simply not responding to the brace from the beginning. For such patients serial Risser corrective scoliosis casts should be used, then another brace trial. When all such nonoperative attempts fail, surgery should be performed.

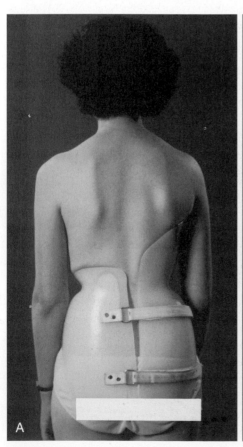
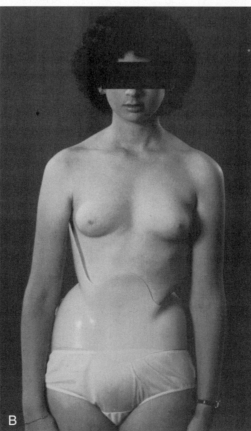

FIGURE 18–19 *A*, Posterior view of a lumbosacral orthosis fitted for a left lumbar curve. Note the pad in the region of the left lumbar prominence, the pelvic section, and the counterpoint on the right thoracic area. *B*, Anterior view of the same brace showing the total lack of any constriction of the thorax.

BRACING FOR JUVENILE IDIOPATHIC SCOLIOSIS

Juvenile idiopathic scoliosis is far more common in North America than infantile idiopathic scoliosis, and more likely to affect females than males. Curves developing after age 3 years, but before puberty onset, are in this category.

Unlike infantile idiopathic scoliosis, the juvenile type almost never spontaneously resolves, and owing to the many years of growth during which progression can take place, extremely severe curves can develop.[8, 44] In North America, this is the type of idiopathic scoliosis most likely to cause adult cor pulmonale and early death. Because of the very poor prognosis of this scoliosis, and the great desire to avoid fusion at a young age, bracing becomes an extremely important method of management.

Thoracic curves predominate, although a compensatory lumbar curve can become quite significant. Because of the thoracic curve, and because the rib cage is soft and pliable, it is critical to use a Milwaukee brace rather than any type of TLSO. The two most common errors made by physicians are failure to start bracing soon enough and failure to use the correct brace.

Brace treatment should begin when the curve reaches approximately 25 degrees. It is not necessary to brace curves less than 20 degrees, and curves as high as 60 degrees can still respond to a brace. This is a much higher value than for successful bracing of adolescent idiopathic scoliosis where the upper limit is 40 to 45 degrees (discussed immediately below).

The outcomes in juvenile idiopathic scoliosis are similar to those of infantile idiopathic scoliosis: totally successful brace management without ever having to consider surgery; successful bracing until the pubertal growth spurt, then surgery; or complete failure of bracing, with surgery needed before the onset of puberty.

Brace wearing always begins with a full-time (23 hours/day) schedule with subsequent adjustments according to the curve's response. It is not unusual for a child to require 5 to 8 years of full-time brace wearing. This may seem unduly harsh; however, children this age do not have psychological problems wearing the brace, and the alternative outcome of curve progression with early death from cor pulmonale is unacceptable (Figs. 18–20A, B, and C, and 18–21A–D).

BRACING FOR ADOLESCENT IDIOPATHIC SCOLIOSIS

This is the most common diagnosis for which scoliosis bracing is used. Thousands of braces are prescribed yearly in North America for its treatment. The indications for bracing are a *growing* child with a curve of between 25 and 45 degrees. Below 25 degrees there are too many curves that are nonprogressive to justify treatment, and above 45 degrees bracing is ineffective. The highest-risk child for progression is the premenstrual girl with a thoracic curve of 25 to 35 degrees. In this patient population brace treatment should be most aggressive. A lumbar curve in a boy who is nearly complete in his growth is so unlikely to progress that bracing is not indicated.

These adolescent scolioses are associated with a variety of highly standardized curve patterns: single thoracic (almost always to the right), single lumbar (almost always to the left); single thoracolumbar (apex at the thoracolumbar junction); double thoracic (high left thoracic T1–T5 and low right thoracic T5–T12); and double major right thoracic and left lumbar.

As stated earlier, curves with an apex at T9 or lower can be managed with a TLSO, but curves with an apex higher than that require a Milwaukee brace. The high left curve T1 to T5 of the double thoracic pattern requires a trapezius pad mounted on a Milwaukee brace. Single lumbar curves do best with the dynamic LSO; low thoracic and thoracolumbar curves, with the TLSO; and higher thoracic curves, with the Milwaukee brace.

Bracing should begin in most cases with a 22-hours-per-day schedule and then after a year some modification can sometimes be done. Some children require the full 22-hour schedule until growth has stopped. Miller et al[26] showed a distinct advantage of bracing over natural history in 1983.

Nighttime-only bracing has been advocated by some, but there is no scientific evidence of its effectiveness. In fact, there is a large body of evidence showing poor results with nighttime and half-time bracing. Currently there is a fad for nighttime bracing with the Charleston Bending Brace. There is no documentation of success with this brace.

There is *excellent* documented scientific evidence of the effectiveness of quality brace treatment vs. the natural history. The first of these two works is the classic paper by Lonstein and Winter[19] on the effectiveness of the Milwaukee brace on adolescent idiopathic scoliosis in 1020 patients. They clearly demonstrated ($P = .0001$) that even in the highest-risk group, the premenarcheal female with a right thoracic curve of 20 to 39 degrees, bracing was highly effective in preventing curve progression. They also simultaneously demonstrated that treatment by electrical stimulators (popular in the 1970s and early 1980s) gave results no different from the natural history of the disease.

In 1993, Nachemson and Peterson[31] presented to the Scoliosis Research Society, the sponsoring society, the results of a prospective, controlled, international, multicenter clinical comparison of natural history, electrical stimulation, and bracing for adolescent idiopathic girls with a curve of 25 to 35 degrees. They again demonstrated that bracing can affect the natural history of this condition ($P = .0001$)[31] (Fig. 18–22A, B, and C).

BRACING FOR SCHEUERMANN'S DISEASE

Second only to adolescent idiopathic scoliosis, Scheuermann's disease is the most frequent diagnosis for which bracing is prescribed. There are two locations of the condition, the classic midthoracic with apex at T7, T8, and T9, and the less common thoracolumbar apex. The latter is more likely to present with pain, the former with deformity.

Scheuermann's disease is a developmental disorder of the discs and vertebral end-plates occurring in adolescents. The cause is unknown, but there is a strong genetic tendency. Males and females are affected equally.

The indications for bracing are a growing child with an

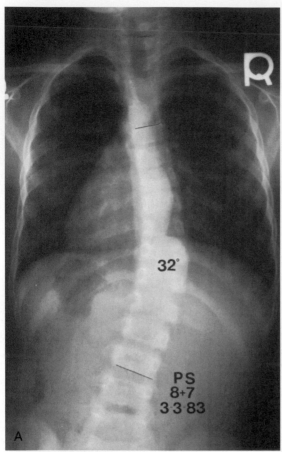

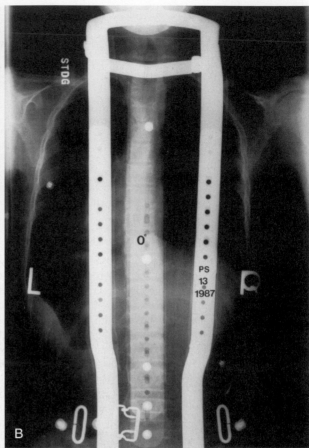

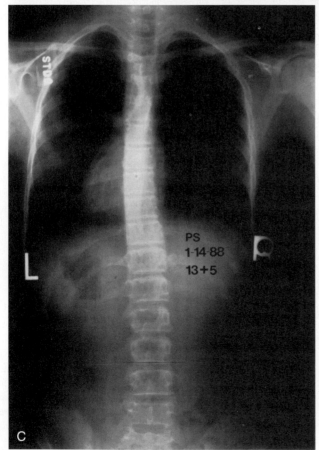

FIGURE 18–20 This 8-year, 7-month-old girl presented with progressive 32 degree low thoracic juvenile idiopathic scoliosis. *B,* After 5 years in a brace, her spine was corrected to a totally straight alignment. *C,* After removal of the brace, the spine remained straight.

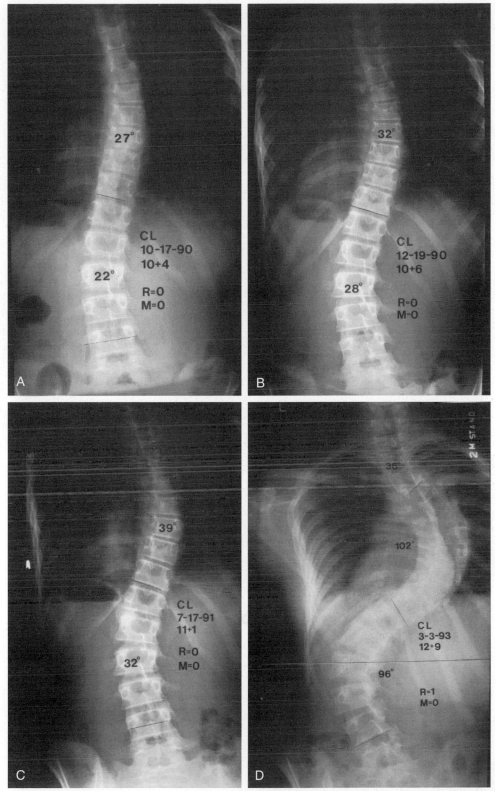

FIGURE 18–21   *A,* When first seen at the age of 10 years, 4 months, this girl had a 27 degree right thoracic and 22 degree left lumbar curve. Her menses had not begun and the Risser sign was zero. Despite her young age, it was elected not to brace her at this time. *B,* Just 2 months after she was seen for a check up, the curves had increased to 32 degrees thoracic and 28 degrees lumbar. Despite this obvious increase, it was unfortunately decided not to institute bracing. *C,* A radiograph taken 7 months later showed an increase of the thoracic curve to 39 degrees and the lumbar to 32 degrees. The Risser sign was still zero and menses had not begun; the patient was without signs of secondary development. At this point, a Charleston nighttime bending brace was prescribed, to be worn at night only. *D,* When seen by the author 1 year and 8 months later, the patient's curves had increased to 102 degrees thoracic and 96 degrees lumbar. This case represents a situation in which bracing was started too late, the wrong brace was prescribed, and bracing persisted for too long, resulting in a severe curve with major pulmonary function deficit. (From Winter RB: The pendulum has swung too far. Orthop Clin North Am 1994; 25:202–203).

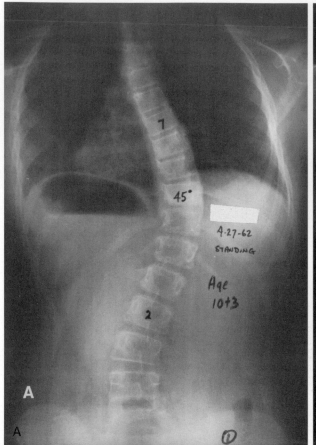

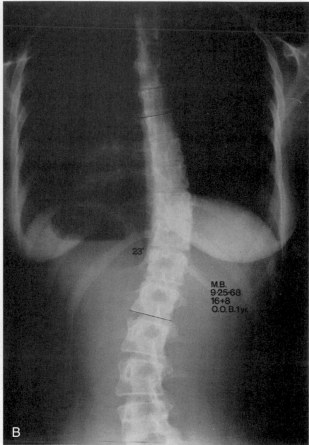

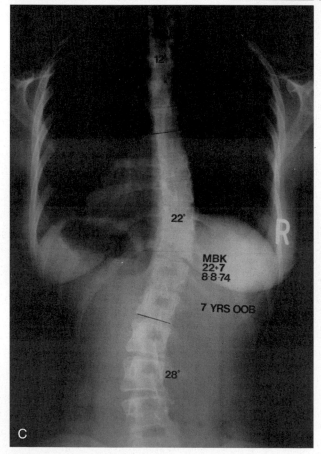

FIGURE 18–22   *A*, This 10-year-old girl presented to Gillette Children's Hospital in 1962 with a 45 degree right thoracic curve. She was immediately placed in a Milwaukee brace, which she wore until she was 15½ years old. *B*, This radiograph of the same patient was taken at age of 16 years 8 months, at which time she had been out of the brace 1 year, and shows her curve to be 23 degrees. *C*, This radiograph of the same patient was taken at age 22 years, 7 years after removal of the brace; it shows maintenance of full correction with curves of 22 degrees thoracic and 28 degrees lumbar.

increasing deformity, pain, or both. The upper limit of normal thoracic kyphosis is 50 degrees. For midthoracic disease a brace candidate is one in whom there is a deformity with radiological evidence of disc space narrowing, end-plate irregularity, vertebral body wedging, and lack of normal extension flexibility.

For lesions at the thoracolumbar junction, the degree of kyphosis is not relevant, since any kyphosis at this level is pathological. The old definition of "three consecutive vertebrae wedged 5 degrees or more" is no longer considered valid, since this represents end-stage disease.

For the classic midthoracic disease, the only brace of proven value is the Milwaukee brace. All underarm braces (TLSOs) have failed for deformity at this level, but are the braces of choice for lesions at the thoracolumbar junction.

The duration of bracing depends greatly on the time of onset of the problem, since bracing to the end of growth is usually necessary.[39] Short-duration programs, (i.e., 18 months) have failed. The intensity and duration of bracing are also related to the severity of the disease process, since there is a wide spectrum within the diagnosis (Figs. 18–23A and B and 18–24A, B, and C).

BRACING FOR NEUROMUSCULAR SCOLIOSIS

Neuromuscular spine deformities include a very large number of different diagnoses, not all having the same natural history and not all having the same response to bracing. Flaccid deformities are different than spastic, and children with absent skin sensation present a different problem for bracing than those with intact sensation.

The original experience with neuromuscular curves was largely with poliomyelitis, a flaccid paralysis with intact skin sensation. Given an early curve diagnosis, a responsive curve pattern, a good orthosis, and a good wearing schedule, most of these children responded well to a brace until the pubertal growth spurt, at which time the curve would "get out of control" and surgery was necessary. This pattern of adequate curve control until the pubertal growth spurt with subsequent surgery has proved to be quite consistent in the neuromuscular diagnoses. Rarely, if ever, is bracing done to prevent surgery entirely.

Good brace results are seen in cerebral palsy, myelomeningocele, traumatic paraplegia, and spinal muscular atrophy. Bracing has *not* proved to be of value in Duchenne's muscular dystrophy, Friedreich's ataxia, or syringomyelia.

Virtually all bracing in neuromuscular diseases is achieved with TLSOs. These can be back-opening, front-opening, or bivalved. The mold is customarily obtained in the corrected alignment on a Risser frame or Cotrel table.

BRACING FOR CONGENITAL SPINE DEFORMITY

Bracing is totally useless for congenital kyphosis or congenital lordosis, but does have limited value in some congenital scolioses.

The curvatures most likely to benefit from bracing are the long curve (10 vertebrae or more) which demonstrates considerable flexibility (at least 50% on a supine bending radiograph as compared to an upright radiograph). Much like the neuromuscular scolioses, bracing in congenital scoliosis is done as a method of "buying time," that is,

FIGURE 18–23 *A*, This patient is wearing a Milwaukee brace for a typical midthoracic kyphosis of Scheuermann's disease. Note the plastic pelvic section, the single strap, the two kyphosis pads (one mounted on each upright), and the modern plastic neck-ring. *B*, A frontal view of the same patient shows the pelvic section, the single, narrow upright, and the modern plastic neck-ring.

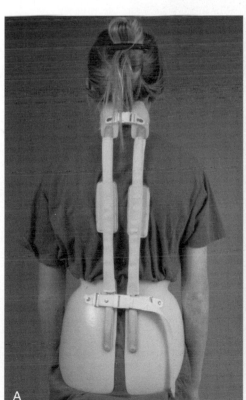

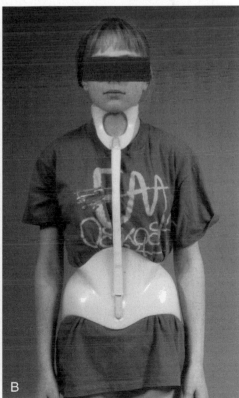

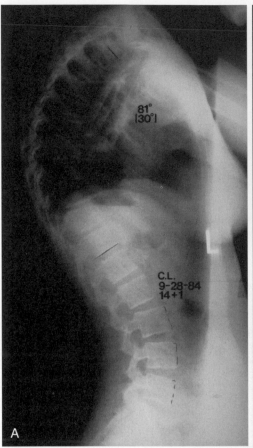

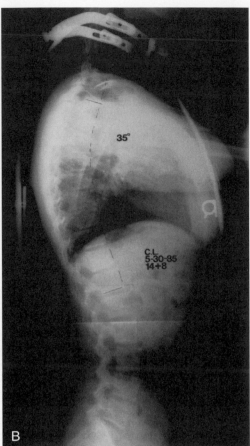

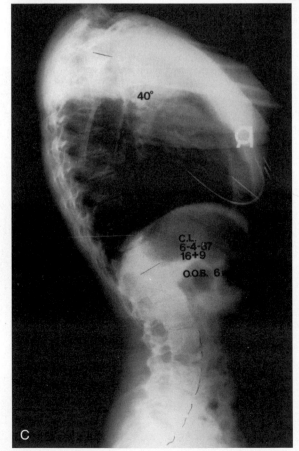

FIGURE 18–24   *A*, This girl presented at age 14 years with progressive thoracic kyphosis due to Scheuermann's disease. The curve measured 81 degrees on the standing lateral film but the spine was significantly flexible, hyperextending to 30 degrees. *B*, She was immediately placed in a Milwaukee brace. Due to her flexibility, we were able to correct her to within the normal range of thoracic kyphosis, 35 degrees. She wore the brace 22 hours a day for 2 years, and 12 hours a day for a third year. *C*, On brace removal only mild setting of the curve occurred, measuring 40 degrees at 6 months after brace removal. Further follow-up 6 years later showed that the curve remained at 40 degrees.

controlling the curve until the adolescent growth spurt, at which time fusion is done. Bracing is also used to control compensatory curves after fusion of the primary congenital scoliosis.

BRACING FOR OTHER SCOLIOSES

The previous material has covered the more common diagnoses, but there still remain a large number of children with various problems in which curvatures exist and bracing can be considered. In general terms any child with a progressive curvature at an age when fusion is undesirable or when there is hope that surgery can be prevented is a candidate for bracing. The exceptions are those conditions previously mentioned where bracing is useless: Duchenne's muscular dystrophy, congenital kyphosis, and congenital lordosis. Additionally, bracing is known to be useless in dystrophic neurofibromatosis and Marfan's syndrome. Inadequate medical care occurs when attempts are made to treat these problems with a brace when abundant scientific evidence exists to the contrary. These patients typically require surgical fusion. In progressive problems involving loss of respiratory function (as in Duchenne's muscular dystrophy), the fusion should be done early while there is adequate vital capacity. Waiting until the patient has a low pulmonary function greatly increases the surgical morbidity and mortality.

References

1. Andriacchi TP, Schultz AB, Belytschko TB, Galante JO: A model for studies of mechanical interactions between the human spine and rib cage. J Biomech, 1974; 7:487.
2. Benzel EC, Hadden TA, Saulsberry CM: A comparison of the Minerva and halo jackets for stabilization of the cervical spine, J Neurosurg 1989; 70:411–414.
3. Berg U, Aaro S: Long term effect of Boston brace treatment on renal function in patients with idiopathic scoliosis. Clin Orthop 1983; 180:169–172.
4. Berger N, Lusskin R: Orthotic components and systems. In American Academy of Orthopaedic Surgeons (eds): Atlas of Orthotics: Biomechanical Principles and Applications. St Louis, Mosby–Year Book, 1975.
5. Clark CR, White AA III: Fractures of the dens. J Bone Joint Surg [Am] 1985; 67:1340–1348.
6. Denis F: Personal communication, Minnesota Spine Center, Minneapolis, May 1991.
7. Fidler MW, Plasmans CMT: The effects of four types of supports on the segmental mobility of the lumbosacral spine. J Bone Joint Surg [Am] 1983; 65:943–947.
8. Figueredo UM, James JIP: Juvenile idiopathic scoliosis. J Bone Joint Surg [Br] 1981; 63:61–72.
9. Fisher SV, Bowar JF, Awad EA, Gullickson G: Cervical orthoses effect on cervical spine motion: roentgenography and goniometric method of study. Arch Phys Med Rehabil 1977; 58:109–115.
10. Gaskill SJ, Marlin AE: Custom fitted thermoplastic Minerva jacket in the treatment of cervical spine instability in preschool age children. Pediatr Neurosurg 1990; 91:35–39.
11. Glaser JA, Whitehill R, Stamp WG, Jane JA: Complications associated with the halo-vest, a review of 245 cases. J Neurosurg 1986; 65:762–769.
12. Johnson RM, Hart PL, Owen JR, et al: The Yale cervical orthosis, a study comparing their effectiveness in restricting cervical motion in normal subjects. J Bone Joint Surg [Am] 1977; 59:332–339.
13. Kennedy JD, Robertson CF, Hudson I, Phelan P: Effect of bracing on respiratory mechanics in mild idiopathic scoliosis. Thorax 1989; 44:548–553.
14. Kennedy JD, Robertson CF, Olinsky A, et al: Pulmonary restrictive effect of bracing in mild idiopathic scoliosis. Thorax 1987; 42:959–961.
15. Koch RA, Nickel UL: The halo vest, an evaluation of motion and forces across the neck. Spine 1978; 3:103–107.
16. Lantz SA, Schultz AB: Lumbar spine orthosis wearing. Restriction of gross body motion. Spine 1986; 11:834–837.
17. Lantz SA, Schultz AB: Lumbar spine orthosis wearing. II. Effect on trunk muscle myoelectric activity. Spine 1986; 11:838–842.
18. Lind B, Shlbom H, Nordwall A: Forces and motions across the neck in patients treated with the halo vest. Spine 1988; 13:162–167.
19. Lonstein JE, Winter RB: Milwaukee brace treatment of adolescent idiopathic scoliosis: a review of 1020 patients. J Bone Joint Surg Am 1994; 76:1207–1221.
20. Lucas BD: Spinal bracing. In Licht S (ed): Orthotics, Etcetera. New Haven, Conn, E. Licht, 1966, pp 275–305.
21. Lumsden RM, Morris JM: An in vitro study of axial rotation and immobilization at the lumbosacral joint. J Bone Joint Surg [Am] 1968; 50:1591–1602.
22. Lusskin R, Berger N: Prescription Principles. In American Academy of Orthopaedic Surgeons: Atlas of Orthotics: Biomechanical Principles and Applications. St Louis, Mosby–Year Book, 1975.
23. Lysell E: Motion of the cervical spine, thesis. Acta Orthop Scand Suppl 1969; 123.
24. Maiman D, Millington P, Novak S, et al: The effects of the thermoplastic Minerva body jacket on cervical spine motion. Neurosurgery 1989; 25:363–368.
25. McGuire RA, Degnan G, Amundson GM: Evaluation of current extrication orthoses in immobilization of the unstable cervical spine. Spine 1990; 15:1064–1067.
26. Miller JAA, Nachemson A, Schultz AB: Effectiveness of braces in mild idiopathic scoliosis. Presented to the Scoliosis Research Society, New Orleans, 1983.
27. Millington P, Ellingsen J, Hauswirth B, Fabian P: Thermoplastic Minerva body jacket—a practical alternative to current methods of cervical spine stabilization. Phys Ther 1987; 67:223–225.
28. Morris JM: Low back bracing. Clin Orthop 1974; 102:126–132.
29. Morris JM, Lucas DB, Bresler B: Role of the trunk in stability of the spine. J Bone Joint Surg [Am] 1961; 43:327–351.
30. Nachemson A, Morris JM: In vivo measurement of intradiskal pressure: discometry, a method for the determination of pressure in the lower lumbar discs. J Bone Joint Surg [Am] 1964; 46:1077–1092.
31. Nachemson A, Peterson K: A prospective, controlled, international multicenter study of the non-operative treatment of adolescent idiopathic scoliosis. Presented to the Scoliosis Research Society, Dublin, 1993.
32. Nachemson A, Schultz A, Andersson G: Mechanical effectiveness studies of lumbar spine orthoses. Scand J Rehabil Med Suppl 1983; 9:139–149.
33. Norton PL, Brown T: The immobilization efficiency of back braces, their effect on the posture and motion of the lumbosacral spine. J Bone Joint Surg [Am] 1957; 39:111–139.
34. Parry H, DeLargy M, Burt A: Early mobilization of patients with cervical cord injury using the halo brace device. Paraplegia 1988; 26:226–232.
35. Perry J: The use of external support in the treatment of low back pain. J Bone Joint Surg [Am] 1970; 52:1440–1442.
36. Perry J, Nickel VL: Total cervical spine fusion for neck paralysis. J Bone Joint Surg [Am] 1959; 41:37–60.
37. Perry J, Nickel VL, Garrett A, Heppenstall M: The halo—a spinal skeletal traction fixation device. J Bone Joint Surg [Am] 1968; 50:1400–1409.
38. Pringle RG: Review article: halo versus Minerva—which orthosis? Paraplegia 1990; 28:281–283.
39. Sachs B, Bradford DS, Winter RB, et al: Scheuermann's kyphosis: long-term results of Milwaukee brace treatment. J Bone Joint Surg [Am] 1987; 69:50–57.
40. Sears W, Fazi M: Prediction of stability of cervical spine fracture managed in the halo vest and indications for surgical intervention. J Neurosurg 1990; 72:426–432.
41. Smith GE, Cantab MA: The most ancient splints. BMJ 1908; 1:732–734.
42. Solot JA, Winzelberg GG: Clinical and radiologic evaluation of vertebrae R extrication collar. J Emerg Med 1990; 8:79–83.
43. Stillo JV, Stein AB, Ragnarsson KT: Low back orthoses. In Lehman JF (ed): Orthotics. Phys Med Rehabil Clin North Am 1992; 3:57–94.

44. Tolo VT, Gillespie R: The characteristics of juvenile idiopathic scoliosis and results of its management. J Bone Joint Surg [Br] 1978; 60:181–188.

45. Walker PS, Lamser D, Hussey RW, et al: Forces in the halo vest. Spine 1984; 9:773–777.

46. Wang GJ, Moskal JT, Albert T, et al: The effect of halo-vest length on stability of the cervical spine. J Bone Joint Surg [Am] 1988; 70:357–361.

47. White, AA III, Panjabi, MM: Clinical Biomechanics of the Spine. Philadelphia, JB Lippincott, 1990.

48. White AA III, Panjabi MM, Brand RA: A system for defining position and motion of the human body parts. Med Biol Eng 1975; 13:261.

49. Winter RB: Personal communication, Minnesota Spine Center, Minneapolis, April 1994.

50. Wolf JW, Johnson RM: Cervical orthoses. *In* The Cervical Spine Research Society (eds): The Cervical Spine. Philadelphia, JB Lippincott, 1983, pp 54–61.

51. Wolf JW, Jones HC: Comparison of cervical immobilization in halo-cast and halo-plastic jackets. Orthop Trans 1981; 5:118.

Prescription of Wheelchairs and Seating Systems

RALPH BUSCHBACHER, M.D.,
JUDY ADKINS, O.T.R., BRIAN LAY, AND
RANDALL L. BRADDOM, M.D., M.S.

Having the optimal wheelchair and seating system is critical to the habilitation or rehabilitation and ongoing well-being of patients with mobility impairment and many other types of disorders. Because a wheelchair is often used during all waking hours and during all activities, having the right one can make the difference between independence and dependence. A patient of one author once confided that "having the wrong wheelchair is worse than having the wrong spouse." Due to the myriad number of brands and types that are now available, the wheelchair user has never had more choices. For the same reason, it has never been more difficult for the practitioner to prescribe a wheelchair.

Although the types, brands, and choices of components are numerous, constantly changing, and can seem overwhelming to the practitioner, the basic principles of prescribing wheelchairs have not changed. This chapter discusses the types of wheelchairs and seating systems that are available and the principles of prescription.

PURPOSES OF WHEELCHAIRS AND SEATING SYSTEMS

Britell[1] cites the five following major goals of wheelchair prescription (Table 19–1):

MAXIMIZATION OF EFFICIENT INDEPENDENT MOBIL-

TABLE 19–1 Purposes of Wheelchair and Seating Prescription

1. Maximization of efficient independent mobility
2. Prevention/minimization of deformity or injury
3. Maximization of independent functioning
4. Projection of a healthy, vital, attractive "body image"
5. Minimization of short-term and long-term equipment cost

ITY. The wheelchair should provide mobility in the environment with as little energy consumption as possible and with minimal assistance from others.

PREVENTION/MINIMIZATION OF DEFORMITY OR INJURY. The wheelchair and seating system should help to prevent pressure ulcers, contractures, joint deformities, and other injuries.

MAXIMIZATION OF INDEPENDENT FUNCTIONING. The wheelchair should allow the user to meet the environment in the most functional manner. As use of the head and upper extremities is essential for function, the wheelchair should maximize stable positioning and limit abnormal tone or dysfunctional movements.

PROJECTION OF A HEALTHY, VITAL, ATTRACTIVE BODY IMAGE. Because able-bodied individuals often view the wheelchair user and the wheelchair as a unit, the wheelchair and seating system should have as esthetically appealing an appearance as possible.

MINIMIZATION OF SHORT-TERM AND LONG-TERM EQUIPMENT COST. With the current emphasis on containing healthcare costs, the practitioner should prescribe wheelchairs that are the most cost-effective, not necessarily the least expensive. The overall expense of a wheelchair includes not only the purchase price, but also maintenance and repair.[1]

Practitioners have to be assertive in explaining to third-party payers how it is "penny wise and pound foolish" to prescribe an inappropriate, stripped-down, or nondurable wheelchair because of its lower purchase cost. Teenagers and young adults in particular can test the physical limits of a wheelchair. Prescribing a nondurable wheelchair will likely result in such patients frequently having a "broken" chair, which adds considerable repair costs. However, patients getting a wheelchair for the first time often pressure the practitioner to prescribe every available option. Patients rapidly learn that a wheelchair that has too many options is not always better, as it is heavier, more prone to break down, often more difficult to propel, and more difficult to place in vehicles.

HISTORY OF WHEELCHAIRS

Perry[10] has provided a summary of the likely history of wheelchairs. The development of the wheelchair first required the invention of the chair (documented as early as 2900 BC) and the wheel/axle (documented as early as 3500 BC). The wheelbarrow was the most-used vehicle for mobility-impaired persons in the Middle Ages and the Renaissance (it was probably invented in China in the third century AD and used in Europe by the 12th century AD). Putting wheels on chairs probably occurred in the 15th century AD, with the addition of a hand-crank mechanism in the 17th century, to permit propulsion by the user.

By the 18th century, a manually powered wheelchair with two large front wheels and a small rear wheel was developed. The 19th century saw the introduction of smaller and lighter wheelchairs made of wood, with bicycle-type wheels that had hand rims. During the American Civil War, the wheelchair was typically a manually powered nonfolding wooden type, with large front wheels and two small rear wheels (Fig. 19–1). The first folding wheelchair is believed to have been developed in the United States by the father of a mobility-impaired daughter, in collaboration with the superintendent of a wheelchair manufacturing company, who also had a mobility-impaired daughter. The wheelchair was made of steel, and, when folded, it was 20 in. wide.[10]

The next major advance in wheelchair design occurred in 1933 when Herbert A. Everest (a person with paraplegia), and Harry C. Jennings (a mechanical engineer), invented the modern folding metal wheelchair.[10] Although the wheelchair has been developed over thousands of years, modern advances in materials and design are causing improvements to occur at a dizzying and accelerating pace.

COMMONLY USED WHEELCHAIR TYPES

The types of wheelchairs now available can be variously categorized in the following ways: adult/pediatric, heavy/moderate/lightweight/ultralight, manually propelled/powered, folding/nonfolding/standup frame, reclining/nonreclining, tilting/nontilting, and metal/composite. Table 19–2 lists the major types of wheelchairs on the market that are prescribed commonly. These wheelchairs are described in more detail later in the chapter.

MANUAL WHEELCHAIR COMPONENTS

Frames

The most common type of wheelchair frame in use is the folding type (Table 19–3). Rigid wheelchairs are more energy-efficient because they have less internal wasted motion during movement; however, they are not as easy to transport as a folding frame type. The rigid chair (Fig. 19–2) can have quick-release wheels and a folddown back to make it more compact and transportable, but it is still more cumbersome than the folding type. Folding chairs (Fig. 19–3) utilize a cross-linkage (X-shaped) bar frame assembly. The chair is folded by lifting the center of the seat, which to some extent limits the seating support and cushions that can be fitted to the chair. Because the folding chair has more parts, it is typically heavier than the rigid type, and usually weighs around 27 lb.

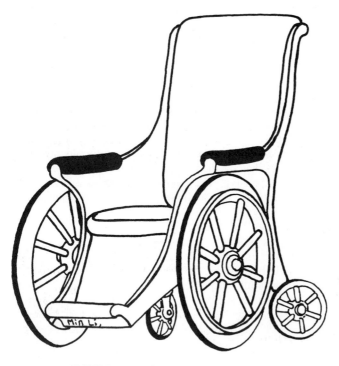

FIGURE 19–1   Civil war era wheelchair.

TABLE 19–2   Basic Types of Wheelchairs and Their Characteristics

Wheelchair Type	Characteristics
Rigid frame	Nonfolding; commonly used in institutions; used in sports chairs
X-frame	Common folding wheelchair
User-propelled	User propels chair
Assistant-propelled	Assistant pushes chair, usually large wheels are placed forward (or has 4 small wheels); commonly used in institutions
Motorized	Various types of battery-powered scooters or chairs available
Standard weight	Usual configuration
Ultra–lightweight	For especially active individuals
Sports chairs	For specific events
Adult chairs	Usual configuration
Pediatric chairs	Various sizes available
Standing frame	Allows user to gain height; motorized and nonmotorized units available
Nonreclining	Usual configuration
Reclining	Useful in patient with hypotension and for pressure relief, though some units increase shear force on sacrum
Nontilting	Usual configuration
Tilting	Useful in high-tone patients, for pressure relief, for pulmonary posture changes

TABLE 19–3   Types of Frames and Their Common Uses, Advantages, and Disadvantages

	Uses	Common Advantages	Disadvantages
Rigid	Institutions	More stable, energy efficient	Difficult to transport
Folding	Community mobility	Compact transport	Heavier, more energy use

In the past, most wheelchairs were made of steel and wood. They were strong, inexpensive, and easy to construct, but were too heavy for ordinary use. The wooden and steel wheelchair is still used by many hospitals and other institutions for internal patient transport, primarily because the wheelchair is very durable and tends to be stolen much less frequently than the more modern styles.

Most wheelchairs are now constructed of aluminum. This makes the chair durable enough for ordinary use and lighter than the steel chair, and it can be purchased at a reasonable cost. Even lighter chairs, made of titanium, are available. They are very durable, but are also very expensive. The lightest chairs are made of composite materials, although these are currently prohibitively expensive and are not very durable. In underdeveloped nations, ease of construction and the ready availability of replacement parts are of greatest importance. Wheelchairs in these countries are often constructed of various bicycle parts.

Wheels and Tires

Two basic types of wheels are available: "mag" wheels and spoked wheels (Table 19–4). The most commonly used is the mag wheel. The mag wheel was first made out of magnesium, which is how it got its name. It was also first used in bicycles. Now most mag wheels are actually made out of plastic. Although these wheels are typically heavier than their spoked counterparts, they require virtually no maintenance. Spoked wheels are lighter, but the spokes tend to loosen and must be retightened periodically. Mag wheels are very durable and, unlike spoked wheels, are unlikely to bend with heavy use.

Three types of tires can be fitted to the wheels (Table 19–5): hard rubber, pneumatic, and pneumatic with flat-free inserts. Hard rubber tires are very durable and have a low rolling resistance, especially on flat, smooth surfaces. On rough terrain they create a harsh ride. They are also relatively heavy.

Pneumatic tires utilize an outer tire casing with an innertube. They are lightweight and give the best ride on most surfaces, though on flat, smooth surfaces they have a higher rolling resistance than hard rubber tires. Unfortunately they can have "flats." To solve this problem, the flat-free insert has been developed, which is basically a piece of soft rubber or latex gel that takes the place of the

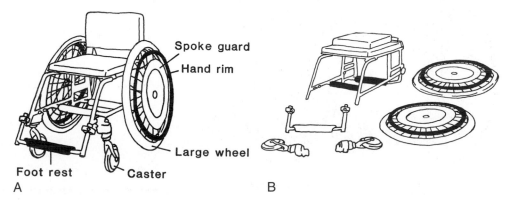

FIGURE 19–2 Rigid chair. *A*, Assembled. *B*, Disassembled with casters, wheels, and footrest removed and seatback folded.

Spoke guard
Hand rim
Large wheel
Foot rest   Caster
A   B

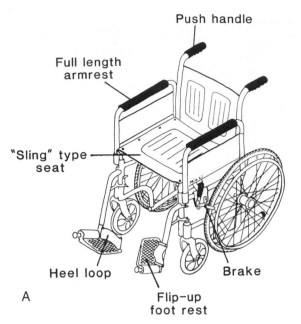

Push handle

Full length
armrest

"Sling" type
seat

Heel loop

Brake

Flip-up
foot rest

A

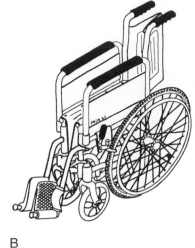

B

FIGURE 19–3 Folding chair. *A*,
Open. *B*, Folded.

innertube. It provides nearly as good a ride as the pneumatic tire, without the risk of flats. Because it is heavier than the innertube, it also carries added weight, however.

Wheels and tires come in several size options, the most common being 24 in. in diameter; 22 and 20 in. wheels are also commonly used to vary the height of the chair.

Wheel placement is an important consideration in chair construction. Many chairs allow for adjustment of the wheel up and down as well as forward and backward (Fig. 19–4). Up and down adjustments are used to vary the height of the chair. This can improve positioning and, in the case of chairs for patients with hemiplegia, allow a user to reach the floor with the "good" foot. Forward and back wheel adjustments alter the stability of the chair. The further forward the wheel is placed, the more easily the chair will tip backward. This can be desirable for a patient with paraplega who does "wheelies" to negotiate curbs. It is undesirable in the bilateral lower extremity amputee, as the lack of forward-placed (leg) weight makes it even easier to tip the chair backward. The wheels also need to be placed posteriorly for some types of reclining or poste-

rior-tilting wheelchairs. Unfortunately, the further posterior the rear wheels are placed, the greater the rolling resistance and the greater the turning radius. The tradeoff of stability vs. rolling ease must be factored into the wheel-placement decision.

Camber is the angle the wheel makes from the vertical axis. A wheelchair demonstrating increased camber is shown in Figure 19–2A. The further the bottom of the wheel is moved outward, the greater its camber and stability. Increasing the camber makes it easier to manually propel the chair and is especially useful in sports chairs. A greater camber also improves the user's ability to propel the wheelchair at higher speeds and tightens the turning radius. The tradeoff is a wider chair and greater wear and tear (mainly on the tires, but also on doorways and furniture).

Handrims

Handrims are placed slightly lateral to the wheel and are smaller in diameter than the wheel (Table 19–6). The larger

TABLE 19–4   Types of Wheels and Their Common Uses, Advantages, and Disadvantages

		Common Uses	Advantages	Disadvantages
Mag		Community mobility	Durable, low maintenance	Heavier
Spokes		Community, institutions, sports	Lighter	Greater maintenance, less durable

TABLE 19–5   Types of Tires and Their Common Uses, Advantages, and Disadvantages

		Common Uses	Advantages	Disadvantages
Hard rubber		Institutions	Low rolling resistance	Harsh ride on rough terrain, heavy
Pneumatic		Community mobility	Best all-around ride, lightweight	Tendency to develop flats
Pneumatic with flat free inserts		Community mobility	Good ride with no flats	Moderately heavy

the handrim's diameter, the easier it is to propel the chair, but the greater the number of arm strokes required to cover a given distance. Larger handrim diameters are the most practical for general use, but wheelchair athletes often opt for smaller-diameter rims to maximize the distance covered with each stroke.

Handrims can be varied in thickness, and different coatings can be used to foster optimal grip. The thicker the rim the easier it is to grip, but weight and width are added to the chair. Some patients with very poor grip, such as those with quadriplegia, benefit from the attachment of knobby projections to the rim.

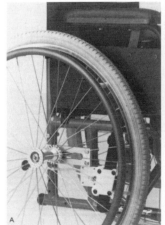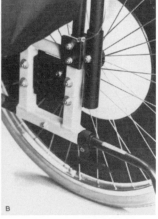

FIGURE 19–4   Wheel adjustment devices. *A,* Axle lies in a plate with a groove for forward/backward adjustment. The plate can be moved up or down. *B,* Plate with multiple holes. Axle can be fitted into any of the holes. (From Britell CW: Wheelchair prescription. *In* Kottke FJ, Lehmann JF (eds): Krusen's Handbook of Physical Medicine and Rehabilitation, ed 4. Philadelphia, WB Saunders, 1990, pp 548–563.)

Casters

Casters are the small wheels typically found on the front of the chair (Table 19–7). They come in different diameters, widths, and materials. In general, the smaller casters are suited for rapid maneuverability; these are often used on sport chairs. Narrow, hard casters are good on smooth, level surfaces, but perform poorly on rough terrain or on outside surfaces. They also tend to shimmy (wobble) when moving longitudinally along a grade, as is often the case on slightly tilted sidewalks. Larger and wider casters are easier to use on rough terrain, although on smooth, level surfaces they increase rolling resistance. For most purposes an 8 in. diameter caster of relatively wide configuration is optimal.

Seats and Backs

The seats and backs that are standard on most wheelchairs are referred to as *sling upholstery* or *hammock* style (see Fig. 19–3A). They consist of a piece of material that is suspended between the frame posts of the chair and are lightweight and easy to fold. The most common material used for such slings is vinyl, which is inexpensive, durable, and easy to clean, and comes in a number of colors. Vinyl tends to become quite warm with use and promotes perspiration. Because of this problem, materials such as Dacron and nylon are often used instead as they are lighter in weight and more breathable. They are not as easy to clean however, and tend to accumulate dirt and stains.

Since sling-type chairs provide little support, a solid seat is often placed on top of them. This solid support can be removed when the chair is folded. Other styles utilize a solid folding seat; however, this adds weight to the chair and cannot easily be modified.

TABLE 19–6   Types of Handrims and Their Common Uses, Advantages, and Disadvantages

		Common Uses	Advantages	Disadvantages
Large diameter		Community, institutions	Easy to propel	Less distance per stroke
Small diameter		Active individual, sports	Greater distance per stroke	More force required
Thick		Poor hand grip	Easier to grip	More weight and width
Knobby		Poor hand grip	Easier to push	More weight and width

Seat Cushions

A number of more specialized seating surfaces are available (Table 19–8). They include air cell cushions, which can help prevent local pressure-induced skin breakdown. The pressure in each cell can be individually adjusted to provide proper pressure distribution.

Another seat cushion that provides improved pressure distribution is the gel-filled type, which can be fitted with modular components to optimize the configuration. Custom molded seats and seat backs can also provide optimal pressure distribution while helping to control posture. Wheelchairs can also be customized with lateral supports and headrests (Fig. 19–5A and B). Pelvic and leg position can be maintained with abductor wedges and a proper cushion.

Seat backs vary in height, depending on the level of control and mobility that is desired. The higher the back, the more support, and the less freedom of mobility. If the back is too low, it leads to a slumped "sacral seating" posture with a tendency toward development of thoracic kyphosis. If the back is too high, it pushes the scapulae forward. Most wheelchair users require seat backs that come to mid-back or to a level a few inches below the inferior poles of the scapulae. Quadriplegic persons require higher back heights, and paraplegic persons sometimes do

TABLE 19–7   Types of Casters and Their Common Uses, Advantages, and Disadvantages

		Common Uses	Advantages	Disadvantages
Large		Community, institutions	Rough terrain	Increased rolling resistance
Small		Sports	Maneuverability	Poor outdoor performance

TABLE 19–8   Types of Cushions and Their Common Uses, Advantages, and Disadvantages

		Common Uses	Advantages	Disadvantages
Foam		General use	Good stability, low cost	Pressure relief not optimal
Coated, contoured foam		General use	Excellent stability, cleanability, durability	Heat build-up, expensive
Gel filled		General use	Good pressure relief, cleanability, heat dissipation	Expensive
Contoured foam with gel insert		When improved pressure distribution needed	Good pressure relief, stability, cleanability, durability	Expensive, heat build-up
Air-filled villous		Optimal pressure relief needed	Excellent pressure relief, cleanability, heat dissipation	Expensive, suboptimal seating stability

From Britell CW: Wheelchair prescription. *In* Kottke FJ, Lehmann JF (eds): Krusen's Handbook of Physical Medicine and Rehabilitation, ed 4. Philadelphia, WB Saunders, 1990, pp 548–563.

well with a lower height. Seat backs are usually fitted with push handles to allow an aide to maneuver the chair.

Reclining Backs

Persons prone to development of pressure ulcers or orthostatic hypotension often benefit from the reclining or semireclining posture. Semireclining and reclining chairs are available (Fig. 19–5A) and come with a variety of release mechanisms, including cable releases and hydraulic units that help hold the weight of the patient. Not all chairs recline equally, and this must be considered when ordering a chair. Reclining chairs also add weight, width, and bulk, and can make transport more difficult. Simple reclining chairs may create shear stress over the back and sacrum

during position changes. In the person at risk for pressure ulcers, special nonshear recliners are indicated. They allow the seat or back to slide during movement, instead of having only a simple hinge.

Tilt-in-Space Seats

An alternative to the reclining seat back is the tilt or tilt-in-space chair (Fig. 19–5B), which utilizes a system whereby the entire seat and back are tilted posteriorly as a single unit. Such systems generally utilize a hydraulic cylinder to aid in movement. The advantage of tilt systems is that they do not create shear stress during movement. Like reclining units, they also help with pressure release and orthostasis and are sometimes used for patients in need

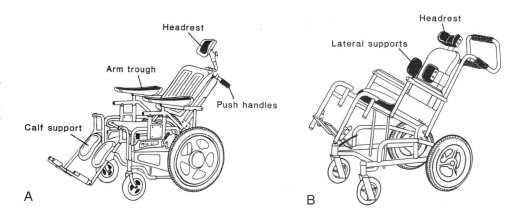

FIGURE 19–5   *A,* Reclining chair with modular supports added. Unit shows headrest and arm troughs. *B,* Tilt chair with modular headrest and lateral trunk supports.

of help with pulmonary secretions. They may offer an advantage over the reclining units in patients with tone or spasticity problems in whom reclining can trigger spasticity. Tilt models tend to be unstable if used for large persons. They also require a higher seating position and do not allow the patient's body to straighten toward the supine position.

Footrests/Legrests

Fixed and Swingaway Footrests

Footrests and legrests help provide balance and positioning and afford protection to the wheelchair user. Swingaway footrests (Fig. 19–6A) are used most commonly. They allow the footrest to be moved out of the way, which makes transfers easier, as the user can position the chair closer to chairs, beds, or toilets. Removable footrests can also improve the portability of the wheelchair.

Fixed, or nonremovable, footrests are available as well. They generally make the chair lighter and more rigid but interfere with transfers and portability.

Elevating Footrests

Elevating footrests (Fig. 19–6B) are available for situations in which the knee cannot or should not be flexed. They can also be used to help minimize dependent edema. Elevating legrests are of two types: one is level with the seating surface, called the *low pivot-point* style; the other projects higher than the seat, called the *goose neck* style. The goose neck is less desirable as it can interfere with transfers and provides a point of pressure contact with the leg. Elevating footrests usually come with calf supports to hold the lower leg, and for this reason they are often referred to as "legrests."

Other Footrests

Specialized footrests are available for many clinical situations. In a chair for paraplegics, the footrest is generally a single bar that connects the two sides of the chair (see Fig. 19–2A). This improves structural rigidity but eliminates the folding option. When more leg and foot control is necessary, the footrest can be ordered with special loops or pads. Heel loops (see Fig. 19–3A) are often used instead of the legrest portion of the unit, as they reduce weight.

Most footrests can also be flipped up to aid in transfers (see Fig. 19–3A).

Armrests/Laptrays

Armrests are added to wheelchairs for a number of reasons (Fig. 19–7). They help provide balance and stability by allowing the user to rest the elbows. They also help provide a point of pushoff for weight shifting and pressure release. Many types and styles of armrests are available. The choice of armrest style can affect the patient's independence level, function, and the ability to use certain seating systems.

Fixed Armrests

The main advantages to fixed armrests are that they are inexpensive and cannot be lost. Their chief disadvantages are that they can make fitting of a seating system more difficult and can also hinder transfers.

Removable Armrests

Removable armrests make transfers easier. They can generally be adjusted in height or replaced to accommodate growth. Their disadvantage is that they increase the width and weight of the chair.

Wraparound Armrests

The wraparound armrest design reduces the width of the wheelchair. This is accomplished by attaching the armrest behind the seatback rather than next to the seat. These armrests can generally be moved or detached for transfers.

Desk Length Armrests

Both fixed and detachable armrests are available in full or desk lengths. Full-length armrests extend from the seatback to the front of the chair. They provide more area for resting the arm or for pushing the body forward in a transfer. However, full-length armrests interfere with the ability to maneuver the chair close to tables and desks. Desk-length armrests extend forward only partially, and allow the user to slide the knees under a desk. Because elbow and shoulder positioning is important, adjustable height armrests are available to accommodate individuals of different sizes.

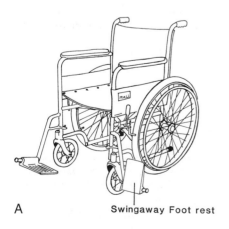

A — Swingaway Foot rest

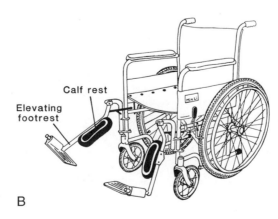

B

Calf rest
Elevating footrest

FIGURE 19–6 Footrests/legrests. *A,* Standard swingaway. *B,* Elevating.

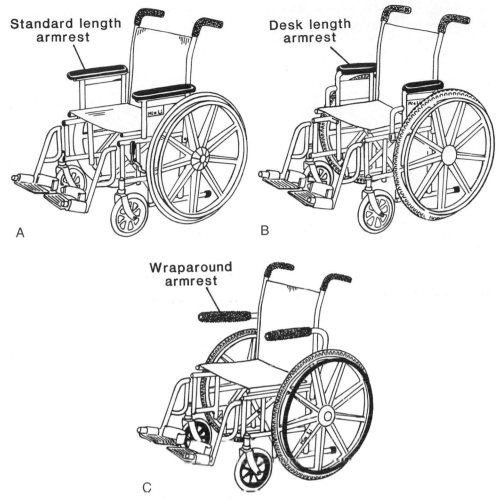

FIGURE 19–7   Armrests. *A,* Standard. *B,* Desk length. *C,* Wraparound.

Other Armrests

In addition to the styles described previously, there are swingaway or flip-up armrests. Young persons with paraplegia often prefer chairs with no armrests at all. Persons who need more control of their limbs often require trough-style armrests (see Fig. 19–5*A*) to hold the forearms in place. In power chairs, one armrest generally has an attached joystick control unit. Hemiplegic individuals often do well with a laptray instead of regular armrests. The tray provides a larger surface on which to rest the arm and may help prevent the pain of shoulder subluxation. It can also be used to hold a communication board or a daily schedule. If a laptray is to be used, proper armrests that can accommodate such a tray are needed.

Brakes/Grade Aids

All wheelchairs are available with wheel locks, commonly known as *brakes* (Fig. 19–8). This mechanism is a very important safety feature. Wheel locks are devices that put pressure on the larger wheels or tires to lock them into position. They are installed to prevent unintended rolling of the chair, either on a grade or during transfers. They are not, however, foolproof, and they should not be used as a substitute for good wheelchair technique.

Wheel locks attach to the sideframe of the chair and are available in either a "push-to-lock" or a "pull-to-lock" mechanism. They are also available in a low mounting style, which places them out of the way so they do not interfere with transfers. Persons who do not have the cognitive ability to decide when to lock and unlock the chairs can have the brakes placed in the rear of the chair where the brakes can be activated only by an attendant or caregiver. Persons with hemiplegia who are not able to activate or release the brake on one side often benefit from an extended handle so that their "good" arm can reach both brakes. In cases in which greater stability is required, the casters can be locked as well.

Wheel locks are available in both a lever style and a toggle style. The lever can be set in different notches to provide varying degrees of holding power. This can be an advantage on a steep grade, but its use requires greater control and strength. Toggle style brakes are used more commonly. The "power" of the lock is preset, but can be adjusted.

Grade aids, or "hill holders," are devices that prevent the chair from rolling backward but do not interfere with forward motion. They are useful for persons with poor strength or endurance on inclines, where the chair might roll backward between forward thrusts (Fig. 19–9).

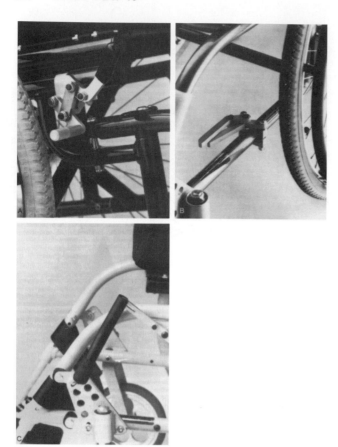

FIGURE 19-8   Several designs of wheelchair brakes. (From Britell CW: Wheelchair prescription. *In* Kottke FJ, Lehmann JF (eds): Krusen's Handbook of Physical Medicine and Rehabilitation, ed 4. Philadelphia, WB Saunders, 1990, pp 548–563.)

Anti-tippers

Patients at risk of falling backward in the chair often benefit from the addition of anti-tippers (Fig. 19–10). These devices can be fixed or removable, and they are capable of

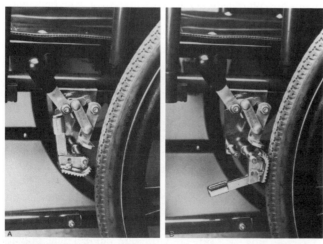

FIGURE 19-9   Grade aid connected to a wheel lock (upper mechanism). *A,* Disengaged. *B,* Engaged. (From Britell CW: Wheelchair prescription. *In* Kottke FJ, Lehmann JF (eds): Krusen's Handbook of Physical Medicine and Rehabilitation, ed 4. Philadelphia, WB Saunders, 1990, pp 548–563.)

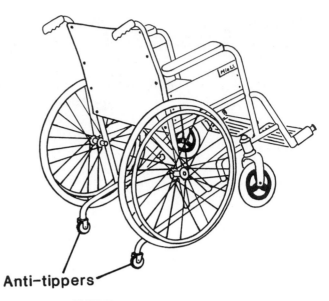

Anti-tippers

FIGURE 19-10   Anti-tipper device.

being turned. Turning the anti-tipper to the "up" position can help during such maneuvers as negotiating curbs, when the device might interfere. Anti-tippers are useful for above-knee amputees, who have a more posterior center of gravity. They are generally not used for paraplegic patients who practice "wheelies" to help in climbing curbs. In rare cases, forward facing anti-tippers are necessary.

One-Arm Drive

Patients who have the ability to propel a wheelchair with one arm only are sometimes given one-arm drive chairs (Fig. 19–11). On these chairs, both propelling rims are on one side. When both are turned, the chair moves straight ahead. Turning one or the other steers the chair. One-arm drive chairs are wider and heavier than standard chairs, and they often require a longer wheel base. They are rarely used successfully, as propelling them requires a fairly high degree of strength and coordination. A practical alternative in most hemiplegic patients is to use one hand rim and one foot to properly guide the chair. A motorized chair is also sometimes a more practical solution than the one-arm drive wheelchair.

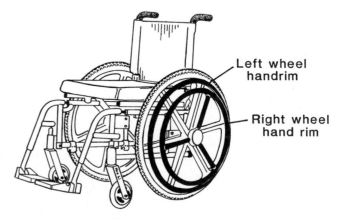

Left wheel handrim

Right wheel hand rim

FIGURE 19-11   One-arm drive chair.

Hemichair

Hemiplegic patients are often able to utilize the "good" leg to help propel the chair, but the seat height in a regular chair is too high for their legs to reach the floor effectively. Hemichairs are made lower to the ground and allow the user to propel the chair with the "good" arm and ipsilateral leg.

Stand-up Chairs

The stand-up design allows the patient to stand within the frame of the chair (Fig. 19–12). Patients can benefit from being able to stand for a number of reasons, including having access to more jobs and experiencing an improved psychological outlook. Standing chairs also provide weight-bearing benefits on bone and improved pressure release. They are available in both motorized and manual versions, but have drawbacks of increased weight, width, cost, and complexity.

MOTORIZED WHEELCHAIRS AND SCOOTERS

Individuals who do not have the strength or dexterity to efficiently propel a manual wheelchair usually need a motorized wheelchair. Such chairs can provide a high degree of independence, and with modern reclining and tilting models, even severely impaired persons can perform pressure release maneuvers.

Although manual wheelchairs permit much needed exercise, many users are better served in the long run with a motorized model. Although they may be able to operate a manual chair for short distances, they might not have the endurance for long distance travel. Manual wheelchair use can also hasten the deterioration of the shoulders, so that in the long term the patient may lose function for such critical activities as transfers and activities of daily living.[9, 11] This is becoming an ever more prevalent problem in active paraplegic patients, who typically have a high incidence of shoulder problems and compressive neuropathies.

Three types of motorized wheelchairs are available: (1) direct drive, (2) belt driven, and (3) add-on units; scooters constitute a separate category.

Direct-Drive Motorized Wheelchairs

Direct-drive wheelchairs (Fig. 19–13A) are commonly referred to as *power base chairs*. They have a rigid main frame that contains the drive components and provides the base for the required seating system. Direct-drive chairs commonly have four small balloon tires, but some newer models offer larger wheels in the rear. They are durable and suited for rough terrain.

Belt-Driven Motorized Wheelchairs

Belt-driven wheelchairs (see Fig. 19–13B) usually have large rear tires and small front casters. They are more stable than direct-drive units and are generally capable of reaching greater speeds, but they tend to be less durable. Belt-driven chairs are more versatile than direct-drive versions, because the frames are better suited to modification and the addition of different components.

Add-on Power Packs

For individuals requiring a motorized chair that is easily transported, a few add-on power packs are available (see Fig. 19–13C) that convert a manual chair to a motorized chair. These units give the user an advantage in transportability, but they are not as durable as standard electrically powered wheelchairs. They are mainly helpful for individuals who use a manual chair most of the time, but who occasionally need power assistance for long distance travel or rough terrain. They can be mounted on folding or rigid frames and are less expensive than conventional power chairs. They are also not as durable, have less power and smaller batteries, and are less adaptable than standard power chairs.

Motorized Scooters

Three- and four-wheeled scooters (see Fig. 19–13D) are a good choice of powered mobility for individuals who

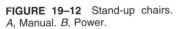

FIGURE 19–12 Stand-up chairs. *A,* Manual. *B,* Power.

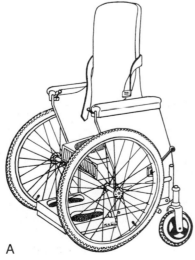

A

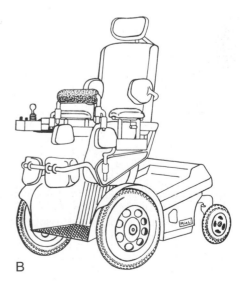

B

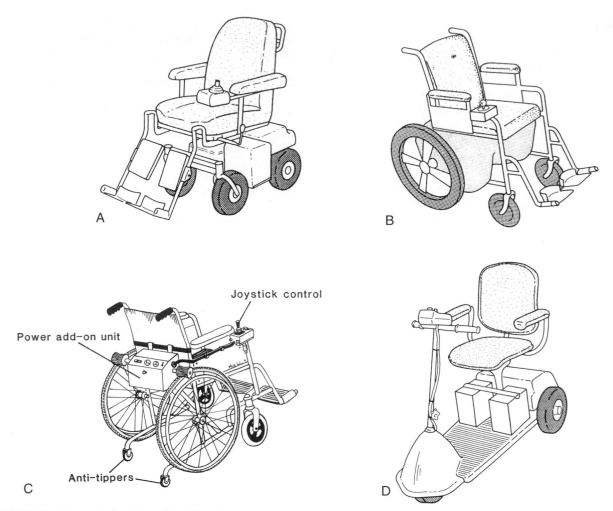

FIGURE 19–13   Power chairs: direct-drive *(A)*, belt-drive *(B)*, add-on power unit *(C)*, and three-wheeled scooter *(D)*. (*A, B,* and *D* (from Britell CW: Wheelchair prescription. *In* Kottke FJ, Lehmann JF (eds): Krusen's Handbook of Physical Medicine and Rehabilitation, ed 4. Philadelphia, WB Saunders, 1990, pp 548–563.)

have the upper body dexterity and strength to manually steer the unit. They are not available with as much "custom fitting" as other wheelchairs and generally do not have as good a seating position. They are more difficult to transfer into and out of than most other motorized chairs. They are optimally used by the person who can ambulate, transfer, and perform most activities of daily living, but who lacks the endurance to ambulate for long distances or to use a manual wheelchair. They are also useful in persons who must avoid overuse of their limbs. They are well suited to many patients with rheumatoid arthritis or severe cardiac or degenerative joint disease, and to some patients with multiple sclerosis or motor neuron or neuromuscular junction disease.

Three-wheeled scooters are available with both front- and rear-wheel drive. Front-wheel drive is less powerful and limits the user to smooth, flat terrain. Front-wheel drive units can be built with smaller dimensions and are best suited to indoor or light use.

Four-wheeled scooters are available in both rear- and four-wheel drive models. These units are more stable than three-wheeled models, but they are not as compact and are harder to transport. Despite their greater stability than that

of three-wheeled scooters, caution is still advised. All scooters have a tendency to be top-heavy and can tip easily, especially when operating at high speed.

Control Systems for Motorized Chairs

Control systems for motorized wheelchairs can be classified as either proportional (graded response) or nonproportional (on/off). Proportional systems are used most commonly. They require the ability to incrementally control the push or pull of a joystick (see Fig. 19–13*C*) by the hand, head, or foot. Pushing the joystick further increases the speed of the wheelchair or the angle of a turn. Proportionally operated power chairs are generally fitted with what is known as a *high brake bias*. When there is no input to propel the chair, it brakes automatically.

Nonproportional systems are used when an individual cannot operate a joystick. They basically have an "on-or-off" type of control. As little as one switch can be used, along with a scanning system. Several switches are usually used, each for a different command or direction. Switches can be placed at any point of the body at which the person can generate enough movement to activate them. Switch sensitivity can be controlled, and in patients with severe spasticity (for safety reasons), the unit can be programmed to ignore excessively rapid movements. Air-controlled "sip-and-puff" drive controls are nonproportional controls used for individuals with high-level quadriplegia who have the capacity to control their breathing. They are sometimes used even in conjunction with ventilator use.

Voice-controlled wheelchairs are only experimental at this time, but practical voice-controlled units will probably be available in the future.

SPORT WHEELCHAIRS

Sport wheelchairs have a rigid frame and are usually made of lightweight material, such as titanium. They are usually not the primary chair of the user. These chairs are generally expensive, cannot easily be modified, and are of limited use outside their intended sport. Basketball chairs have thin indoor-type wheels with little tread and small casters. Camber is large, and depending on the type of impairment (usually level of paraplegia), these chairs allow fairly unrestricted upper body mobility.

Racing chairs (Fig. 19–14) are highly specialized. They compress the athlete's body into a compact shape, have a large camber, and have small-diameter handrims to help get maximum distance from each arm stroke. Due to body position, wheelchair racers tend to have problems with skin irritation and breakdown. Incidentally, because wheelchairs propel the body mass with little or no vertical or side-to-side displacement of the center of gravity, they are more efficient than running, and in long-distance events, such as marathons, the wheelchair athletes routinely have shorter finishing times than the runners.

Wheelchair exercise provides both physical and psychological benefits to the participant, and if it is properly structured, such exercise can provide training comparable to standard aerobic exercise.[2]

ENERGY CONSIDERATIONS IN WHEELCHAIR USE

As described in previous sections, certain wheelchair modifications and styles affect rolling resistance and energy consumption. The most important of these is probably tire

and caster width. Narrower tires have less rolling resistance and are ideal for use on hard, flat surfaces, such as within institutions. They require much more force to propel through uneven surfaces (such as gravel) and are not suited for outdoor use. The same holds true for small casters, which are mainly used for maneuverability in sports such as basketball. Weight obviously is another consideration in calculating energy consumption, and for sports applications, very lightweight chairs are available. In one study,[6] sports chairs were found to require 17% less energy to propel than standard chairs.

The energy consumption of wheelchair use is lowest on a flat, hard surface. Carpeting, rough terrain, and even small inclines or slopes greatly increase the energy cost of mobility.[4, 5, 15] This increase can be prohibitive in elderly or debilitated patients. Powered mobility may be a more realistic option in these patient populations.

To optimize energy consumption, careful selection of all components of the wheelchair is important.[8] Alternative wheelchair propulsion designs have been investigated. Although some of these have been shown to be more energy efficient than those currently in use,[7, 12, 14] none have yet gained wide popularity.

GENERAL CONSIDERATIONS IN WHEELCHAIR SELECTION

When prescribing wheelchairs for adults it is important to note whether the mobility impairment is of adult onset or has existed since birth or childhood. Developmentally disabled adults present with problems of abnormal muscle tone, deformity, and contractures. Some require custom molded seating to correct or accommodate these abnormalities.

Adults with traumatic paraplegia are typically best fitted with high-strength lightweight wheelchairs. High-level quadriplegic persons usually need powered mobility with sophisticated control systems such as chin controls or sip-and-puff systems. Adults with multiple sclerosis often do well with powered scooters, and adults with stroke typically use a hemi-height manual wheelchair, which they propel with the "good" arm and leg.

Traumatic brain injury patients often initially require a complex wheelchair system, but frequently progress to needing a less sophisticated system or no wheelchair over the course of time.

The most important prescribing considerations in all cases include the diagnosis, clinical picture, living situation, family involvement, funding, and previous experience of the patient/caregiver with wheelchairs. Tables 19–9 and 19–10 list some of the indications for choosing either a manual or power chair. Table 19–11 lists some of the issues important in prescribing a power chair, whereas Table 19–12 lists some of the disadvantages of powered chairs.

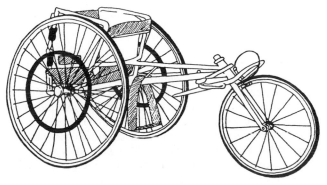

FIGURE 19–14 Racing chair.

TABLE 19–9 Indications for Manual Mobility

1. Physical limitation not compatible with ambulation
2. Need for increased independence at work or school
3. Poor endurance/distance walking

TABLE 19–10   Indications for Powered Mobility

1. Physical limitations not compatible with manual wheelchair mobility
2. Need for increased independence level at school and work
3. To improve self esteem
4. To increase efficiency of mobility
5. To spare the upper limb joints from premature deterioration

TABLE 19–12   Potential Disadvantages of Powered Mobility

1. Relatively high cost
2. Weight
3. Transportation difficulty
4. Maintenance
5. Technological dependence
6. Limited environmental accessibility
7. Lack of physical exercise

PEDIATRIC CONSIDERATIONS IN WHEELCHAIR PRESCRIPTION

Pediatric patients present with all of the challenges in wheelchair selection seen in adults, but with specific additional concerns. These include accommodating the patient's growth, fostering development of self-esteem, and enabling proper interaction with peers and the environment. Children have different needs based on their developmental level and age. They need physical contact and handling (as do adults), and the equipment they use should not limit that physical contact. For example, wheelchair laptrays used in classrooms can sometimes cause peers to keep their distance, and they do not permit the same interaction as occurs at a desk or a table or in a circle on the floor.

Cosmetic Concerns

Children are very conscious of their appearance and like brightly colored equipment. Most adults are more concerned about the reliable operation of equipment, with appearance being a somewhat secondary concern. Children, however, have very definite ideas about the appearance and color of their equipment. They frequently reject the traditional chrome frame wheelchair "look." Manufacturers have responded to this concern with brightly colored choices. Some vendors monogram the name of the child at no extra charge.

Growth Concerns

Manufacturers offer both manual and power-drive wheelchairs with "growth potential," and decisions should be made on the basis of whether the child can self-propel the chair or will be able to in the future. Some chairs can be expanded in width and depth with modular and expanding frames. Growth of the legs can be accommodated with longer footrest hangers. Prescribers of wheelchairs for children should be familiar with which products "grow," how they grow, and their growth ranges. In general, one should strive to obtain a chair that meets the child's needs for a 5-year period. However, prescribing a chair that is initially

TABLE 19–11   Evaluation Factors for Powered Mobility

1. Physical ability
2. Intelligence level
3. Age
4. Judgment
5. Perception
6. Transportability of device
7. Reimbursement
8. Follow-up availability/maintenance
9. Family acceptance

too large can be counterproductive, as it decreases the child's independence and makes propelling the chair more difficult.

Family Concerns

Dealing with children requires carefully listening to the parents or primary caregivers regarding function, appearance, and utility of the end product. It is often psychologically difficult for a parent with a very young child to use a device that looks like a wheelchair. The parents are usually still hopeful that the child will learn to sit, have head control, and walk. Although they realize the need for good positioning and proper body alignment to help prevent contractures and added deformity, they often want the seating components fitted into a device that looks more like a stroller. They might also want the capacity to use the seating system as a car seat. Some manufacturers make FDA-approved car seats that interface with a mobility base for transport, which may or may not be the best choice for the child. Most parents want to be intimately involved in the wheelchair decision-making process.

Ventilators and Wheelchairs

Growing numbers of children are ventilator dependent. For these children not only must one choose the best seating system to support function, growth, and positioning needs, but the system must also "house" and transport the ventilator and other support equipment. If respiratory status improves, one should be able to modify the system for increased independence and function.

Progressive Disorders

Functional independence is always a goal in working with children, but for children who have degenerative or progressive disorders, future loss of control has to be considered. Sometimes it is not possible to predict how quickly changes will be required, but the system of choice should be adaptable to those changes when they occur.

Power Chairs

Power chairs should be considered for children who have adequate intelligence and judgment but lack the necessary muscle control to propel a manual wheelchair. Varying opinions exist about how early a child has the judgment and control to use a power chair. Many 3-year-olds can safely use power chairs, and power has even been successfully used with some 2-year-olds. It is obviously important that the wheelchair should not be allowed to pose a safety threat to the child or others.

Powered mobility should be considered in children with

a number of diagnoses, including cerebral palsy, muscular dystrophy, hemiplegia, severe arthrogryposis, traumatic quadriplegia, or bronchopulmonary dysplasia. Children with severe juvenile arthritis or cardiac dysfunction often need powered mobility for more freedom of movement. A scooter often meets their needs, as a special seating system is typically not needed. However, most children who require powered mobility also require a special seating system for support and control. The optimal type of system is determined by considering the diagnosis, degree of deformity, functional ability, and overall clinical picture.

TRANSPORTING THE WHEELCHAIR

Manual Wheelchairs

Manual wheelchairs are easily transported in motor vehicles. Most manual wheelchairs have folding frames and can be lifted into a trunk or back seat. The lifting weight can be lessened by removing the footrests, the armrests, and, on some models, the rear wheels. Trunk lifts are also available for those who lack the strength to put the chair in the trunk by themselves.

Although rigid frame wheelchairs do not fold, they are usually fitted with quick-release axles for easy removal of the rear wheels. Their backs can also be folded down. If necessary, the push handles can be made to turn down, and casters can be made with quick-release mechanisms.

Transporting tilt wheelchairs is very similar to transporting rigid frame wheelchairs. Tilt wheelchairs can be made with a seating system that snaps out, armrests and backs that fold down, and rear wheels that can be removed. This generally leaves a manageable size for storage in the trunk or on the back seat of a car.

Power Wheelchairs

Power wheelchairs present complex transport problems. Although some can be disassembled, this is not practical or recommended on a daily basis. Transport of power wheelchairs generally is best done with a van, van lift, and an approved tie-down system. A ramp system can be used instead of a lift, but for safety reasons, the wheelchair has to be pushed or driven up the ramp by someone other than the user. The width of the van door and roof clearance are critical measurements to consider when a power wheelchair is purchased. Roof clearance can be increased with an extra top on the vehicle, but because the resultant seating and transfer position is usually too high, the van must often be modified by lowering the floor. Some vans, such as the Volkswagen Eurovan, do not require modification in most cases.

Adolescents and adults who operate their own vans generally remove the driver's seat so that they can substitute their wheelchair. They use a lift and tie-down so that they can drive while seated in the restrained wheelchair. The tie-down system in these cases is usually an automatic system that can be operated by a driver-controlled button. This system promotes maximum independence for individuals who can drive.

Power Add-on Units

Power add-on systems do not decrease portability, because the unit is easily removed. These systems have worked well with many patients and have become popular when used with high-strength lightweight wheelchairs.

Scooters

Scooters can usually be disassembled for relatively easy transport in a car. They are often too heavy for the user to lift, so trunk lifts are often prescribed. However, lifts of any variety are rarely funded by third-party payers, making them difficult for many patients to procure. Vocational rehabilitation programs can sometimes help in the purchasing of a lift, especially if it is necessary to provide work access.

TRANSPORTING THE WHEELCHAIR USER

Adults or children who use wheelchairs and seating systems can usually be transferred to the car seat (or child safety seat) and wear a regular seatbelt. Sometimes, large children or adults with cognitive problems must be restrained with a vest in combination with the auto seatbelt. Persons who must be transported in their wheelchairs require vans with an FDA-approved tie-down system. Although manufacturers do not recommend that individuals be in their wheelchairs for transport, it is often the most acceptable or the only practical method.

Airline Travel

For air travel, the wheelchair user is advised to call ahead to let the airline know that specific accommodations might be necessary. Most major carriers have aids to assist the traveler in this regard. When power chairs are to be transported they must have approved batteries, because airlines will not allow some batteries to be transported on board.

Bus Travel

When traveling by bus, the same general considerations apply as for air travel. The user should call ahead to learn about any specific requirements. Most municipal bus systems now offer wheelchair-accessible facilities. Cities also often provide alternative transport with a van, if necessary, although this usually has to be arranged in advance.

For school bus transportation, the parents should contact their local school district for any specific recommendations or requirements. In some states, safety standards recommend using forward-facing four-point tie-downs. Weight restrictions might apply as well. Upper extremity supports, such as lap trays, might be prohibited due to their potential for causing injury in the case of an accident. The child should be safely secured in the seating system, and the wheelchair and seat should be secured to the bus. Special accommodations might be necessary for ventilator-dependent children.

SIZING THE WHEELCHAIR

Determining the size of the mobility base and seating system components requires careful measurement of the patient. The measurements that should be taken are depicted in Figure 19–15. The thickness of cushions and padding should be taken into consideration and added to the chair's dimensions.

MAINTENANCE AND SAFETY CONSIDERATIONS

Wheelchairs have many moving parts that must regularly be lubricated, cleaned, and maintained. The user (or caregiver) must make sure that the chair is in proper working order, to maximize both durability and safety. Wheelchairs should not be immersed in water, as some parts can rust. They should periodically have their bearings replaced. Power chairs should be taken out of gear when not in use.

SEATING SYSTEMS

A proper seating system is important for the patient, both in and out of the wheelchair. Proper seating is necessary in the young child who does not yet need a wheelchair for mobility (Fig. 19–16). In the elderly, seating is important for general care and to prevent deformity. This section addresses the seating prescription, both as a subset of the wheelchair selection process and as an independent need.

Goals of Seating Systems

Selection of a seating system is a complex process that requires input from the patient, family, primary caregiver, physician, therapists, vendor, and educator. The team ap-

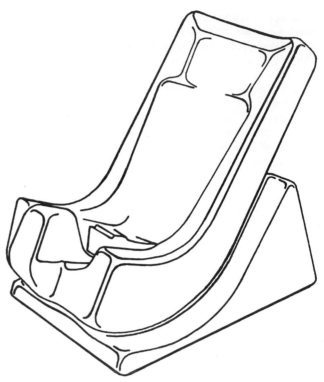

FIGURE 19–16 Tumbleform pediatric seating device.

proach can help to ensure a more positive outcome. Goals of seating include the following.

Control Abnormal Tone and Reflexes

Proper support can help normalize tone and inhibit abnormal reflexes. Abnormal tone and reflexes produce abnormal movement patterns and poor posture, which in turn contribute to the development of muscle contractures and skeletal deformities. Maintaining proper alignment can help to prevent these deformities.

Correct or Accommodate Deformities

The seating position should help correct or prevent deformities, such as hip adduction contractures and ankle plantar flexion contractures. When a deformity cannot be prevented or corrected, it has to be accommodated to prevent its worsening or the development of new compensatory deformities.

Above all, the seating system should not cause new deformity. One of the problems with the commonly used "hammock" or "sling" wheelchair seat is that it can promote poor posture (Fig. 19–17), and it should be avoided in patients at risk for such deformity.

Enhance Function and Improve Control

Function is enhanced by optimum posture and position. For example, proper support to the head and neck can improve swallowing and decrease the risk of aspiration during eating. Proper alignment and support can also free the upper extremities for self-care activities or for self-propulsion.

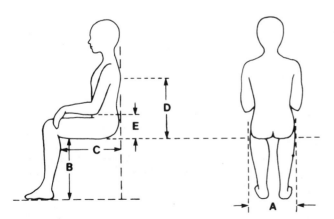

FIGURE 19–15 Standard measurements required for wheelchair dimensions. Seat width: 1 in. wider than the width of the widest part of the buttocks (A). Seat height: 2 in. higher than the distance from the bottom of the heel to the popliteal area (B). Seat depth: 1 to 2 in. longer than the distance from the popliteal area to the back of the buttocks (C). Back height: 2 in. less (may vary) than the distance from the bottom of the scapulae to the sitting surface (D). Armrest height: Distance from bottom of buttocks to elbow (E). (From Britell CW: Wheelchair prescription. *In* Kottke FJ, Lehmann JF (eds): Krusen's Handbook of Physical Medicine and Rehabilitation, ed 4. Philadelphia, WB Saunders, 1990, pp 548–563.)

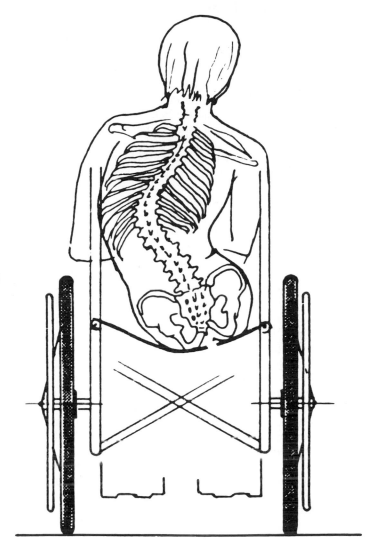

FIGURE 19–17 Sling effect of standard chairs, which can promote deformity. (From Letts RM (ed): Principles of Seating Prescription. Boca Raton, Fla, CRC Press, 1991.)

Improve Comfort and Improve Sitting Tolerance

A seating system should provide the necessary support with the least possible restriction of movement. Proper support should provide a secure, stable base and enhance the patient's sitting tolerance.

Provide Pressure Relief and Skin Protection

The able-bodied child or adult shifts position frequently to redistribute pressure and prevent skin breakdown. Individuals with a lack of sensation or with physical and/or cognitive limitations are not always capable of such weight shifts, nor do they always understand the need for them. A seating system that equalizes pressure distribution, prevents shear force, and provides proper support decreases the incidence of pressure ulcers.

Facilitate Management and Care

Seating cannot improve function or control in some patients with very severe neurological impairments. A proper seating system can, however allow them to be placed in an upright position to improve respiration, digestion, and urinary function. It also allows them to be transported more easily and helps others to do their care and hygiene.

Principles of Seating

Types of Systems

Sitting should provide the necessary support to the body while fostering a comfortable, symmetrical midline posture. Proper sitting position is generally considered to be with the head in midline, trunk erect, hips flexed to 90 degrees, knees at 90 to 100 degrees, and feet in neutral position, with the spine stable and the pelvis level. Seating systems are traditionally grouped into three categories: (1) planar systems (see Fig. 19–5B for an example), (2) contoured systems (see Fig. 19-16 for an example), and (3) custom molded systems.

Planar, also known as *linear, seating systems*, are constructed of a support covered with upholstery to provide a relatively flat surface. Possible planar components include seats, seatbacks, lateral/head/sternal supports, abductor supports, laptrays, footrests, and cushions. The planar components are generally inexpensive and can readily be modified, repaired, or replaced.

Contoured seating systems are used when patients require a more customized shape to accommodate their bodies. They can be simple or complex. Simple contours can be constructed by using varying densities of foam in the seat cushions to accommodate the body (see Table 19–8). More commonly, however, a more complex design is required. Preformed bases can be obtained with curves to better fit the body. These are then covered with foam or gel to which special add-on pads can be applied, such as lateral supports and thigh abductors. Contoured systems are useful for patients who require mild to moderate support and who are free of severe deformity.

If more support is necessary, or if the patient's deformity is such that standard seating systems will not fit, a custom molded seat is needed. Custom molded systems tend to be used with patients who have more severe deformities and a history of skin breakdown. They are not usually advisable for use in very young children due to their cost and the inability to change the system to accommodate growth. Most of these systems cannot be modified and require replacement if they do not fit properly.

The covering of the seating system is important. Some patients are allergic to and do not tolerate materials such as latex or neoprene. Incontinence is a problem for some patients, and the material used must be either easily cleaned or impervious to urine. Some coverings can cause increased shear pressure in transfers, which presents a problem in the patient at risk for pressure ulcers.

Assessing patients for wheelchairs typically requires removal of their clothing. Clothing can hide gastrostomy tubes, bony deformities, and pressure ulcers. Patients or families often fail to mention these factors, and they are essential for making a good seating choice.

Prescribing Seating Systems

The availability of numerous wheelchair bases combined with multiple seating options requires that the seating team thoroughly assess the patient to successfully prescribe the best system. Prescription of the system is further compounded by funding limitations and family resources. Modern technology can enhance the user's potential for independence, but it is not always affordable or practical based on funding restrictions and the environment in which such equipment is to be operated. Clinical assessment should include the following items (also summarized in Table 19–13).

Tone/Spasticity

Patients presenting with tone or spasticity problems often require special seating considerations, such as rolled seats

(thinner over the ischial tuberosities to properly position the pelvis), anti-thrust seats, abduction devices, and special back-to-seat angles. They also require parts that are reinforced or made of stronger and more durable materials. Patients with low tone often require lumbar supports to promote spinal extension, tilt mechanisms to improve head and trunk control, or custom headrests. Patients with athetosis may require stabilization of an upper and lower extremity to effectively use the remaining upper extremity functionally. Other patients have fluctuating tone, and the seating system should support this flexibility. Tone can also change over time as the patient's medical condition changes.

Contracture

Contractures create a number of problems for the patient and for the clinician prescribing or recommending equipment. Knee flexion contractures can affect caster size and type of footrest that can be used. Hip extension contractures require a more open hip angle and might necessitate a reclining back feature. Assessment of contractures should include whether the patient has a fixed deformity or abnormal posturing.

Pathological Reflexes

The presence of abnormal or pathological reflexes, such as an asymmetrical tonic neck reflex (ATNR) directly affects posture and control. Many cognitively aware patients can utilize these reflexes to enhance function, whereas others are hindered by them. The type of headrest used can position the head to allow the patient to effectively "break through" these abnormal reflexes for added postural control.

Impaired Sensation/Body Awareness

Sensation has a direct impact on positioning, and sensory deficits can impair balance as well as predispose to pressure ulceration. A proper sense of body awareness is important. Patients with perceptual problems, such as hemineglect, often injure themselves in their wheelchairs. They might drag a foot on the floor without realizing that it has fallen from the footrest. Sometimes they injure a hand or arm as it dangles and gets caught in the wheel. Special seating and wheelchair restrictions are needed to prevent these problems.

Skin Integrity

Tissue integrity should also be assessed. Children and adults with no history of breakdown usually tolerate regular planar seating systems. Clients with current ulcers or a history of previous pressure ulcers require more creative seating and the use of foam, air-cell, or pressure pads.

Other Seating Considerations

A number of other items should be noted, as they can necessitate special seating or wheelchair arrangements. These items include the status of vision and hearing, need for orthoses, presence of deformities, and behavior problems. Table 19–14 lists some of the more common prob-

TABLE 19–13 Items to Consider in the Clinical Assessment for Wheelchair or Seating Systems

1. Muscle tone	6. Visual impairments
2. Contractures	7. Hearing impairments
3. Abnormal reflexes	8. External orthotics
4. Sensory deficits	9. Bony deformities
5. Tissue integrity	10. Behavioral problems

TABLE 19–14   Troubleshooting in Postural Seating and Wheelchair Prescription

	Problem	Possible Causes	Possible Solutions
Pelvis	Posterior tilt (sacral sitting or sliding out of chair)	Hypotonia	Decrease seat length
		Tonic labyrinth prone (TLP) reflex (producing flexed posture)	Reduce seat wedge/roll height
		Limited active hip flexion (causing compensatory loss of low lumbar curve)	Lumbar or sacral pad
			Change position of head in space and thereby influence TLP
		Tight hamstrings with seat too long or with too high a wedge in seat, footrests preventing knee flexion	Raise height of tray
			Adjust position of footrests to allow more knee flexion
		Improper positioning in seat	Reposition pelvis (flex pelvis)
		Lap belt located too high	Lower lap belt attachment point
	Lateral tilt (weight on one buttock)	Asymmetrical muscle tone	Solid base to seat
		Scoliosis with pelvic obliquity	Midline orientation by using lateral pelvic blocks
		Dislocated or subluxated hip	
		"Hammock" of wheelchair seat	Three-point pressure support of trunk and pelvis
			Contour seat to facilitate equal weight distribution
Trunk	Scoliosis	Postural	Midline pelvic orientation
		Position of pelvis not midline	Three-point support
		Hypotonia-hypertonia asymmetrical muscle tone (asymmetrical tonic neck reflex, asymmetrical distribution of tone, hemiplegia, etc.)	Midline trunk or chest harnesses
			Recessed back or midline orientation
			Tray to help with midline orientation
			Reduce abnormal tone
			Hip angle
		Environmental or functional demands	Neck collar
		Structural	Change orientation of functional work
		Persistent asymmetrical posture (fixed deformity)	Recline back to reduce effects of gravity
	Kyphosis	Postural	Surgery or orthotic management
		Posterior pelvic tilt	See previous solutions, pelvic tilt
		Structural	Add chest panel or bandolier harnesses
		Fixed deformity	Lumbosacral pad
			Surgery or orthotic management
Shoulder girdle	Retraction	Thoracolumbar scoliosis	Reduce extensor tone
		Extensor thrust	Roll or wedge seat
		Asymmetrical tonic neck reflex	Decrease hip angle
		Instability of upper trunk	Neck collar
			Alter head position in space (gravity)
			Protract shoulders
			Tray extensions or rounded seatback with wings
			Lower tray
			Stabilize upper trunk with straps
	Protraction	TLP	Lumbosacral pad
		Kyphosis	Raise tray height
			Chest panel
			Change attitude of body in space (gravity)
Head and neck	Hyperextension	Extensor hypertonicity	Neck collar positioned just below occipital region
		Poor flexor control	
		Headrest or neck collar positioned too low	Reduce total extensor hypertonicity at pelvis (see above)
		Improper neck or head support (i.e., headrest placed on occipital)	Position neckrest slightly anterior
			Alter position of head in space (gravity)
		Thoracolumbar scoliosis	
	Protraction	Hypotonia	Lower neckrest and align in neutral position
		Neckrest too high or too far forward	
		TLP	Raise and/or tilt tray
		Tray work too low	Low lumbosacral pad
		Kyphosis	Alter position of head in space (gravity)
	Rotation	Atonic neck reflex	Inhibit atonic neck reflex
			Midline orientation of pelvis and trunk
			Protraction of shoulders
		Sensory deficit	Thoughtful positioning for function
		Visual	Reduce general hypertonicity
		Auditory	
		Unstable spine	
		Generalized domination of primitive pathosis	
	Side flexion	Hypertonicity	Reposition of neck or headrest
		Hydrocephalus	Larger neck or headrest
		Severe retardation	More stable chest support
		Sensory deficits	Recline body in space (gravity)

Table continued on following page

TABLE 19–14 Troubleshooting in Postural Seating and Wheelchair Prescription *Continued*

	Problem	Possible Causes	Possible Solutions
Hips	Extension-adduction Internal rotation	Thoracolumbar scoliosis Positive supporting reaction Extensor thrust Dislocated hip Seat too short Seat belt too long or poorly positioned	Roll seat, with roll one finger width behind knee Increase hip flexion by Higher roll Wedge Flexing seatback anterior of vertical Pommel (as a last resort); keep it short enough so it is nowhere near groin area Platform shoes to reduce positive supporting reaction (PSR) Seat belt at 45 degrees to thigh Alter attitude of body in space to affect tonic labyrinth supine reaction (gravity) Have removable footrests for initial fittings Caution: watch pelvis as you increase hip flexion if hamstrings are tight
	Flexion-abduction	Hypotonia Adductor releases	Adduction blocks with good foot position (footpads or straps)
Knees	Flexion	Primitive patterns Flexion contractures	Inhibit flexor tone by adjusting (roll or wedge) Position feet in neutral (if tight hamstrings, watch effect on pelvis) Surgery
	Extension	Extension patterns (usually dynamic response to abnormal tone)	Inhibit extensor tone with roll or wedge Decrease hip angle Neutral strapping of feet Shorten seat
Feet	Plantar flexion	Extension pattern Positive supporting reaction Heel cord contractures Footrest too low	Check footrest height and place foot in slight dorsiflexion to inhibit PSR Surgery Inhibit tone with roll/wedge Platform shoes
	Inversion-eversion	Same as above	Footrest height Platform shoes Footpads or straps Ankle-foot orthosis

From Letts RM (ed): Principles of Seating Prescription. Boca Raton, Fla. 1991.

lems in seating along with their causes and possible solutions.

CONCLUSION

The wheelchair and seating options currently available are numerous and increasing rapidly. It is nearly impossible for one person to keep abreast of all the latest developments, but by adhering to the basic principles outlined in this chapter and by listening to the patient and family, it is possible to achieve better outcomes than ever before. This is most efficient and effective with the use of a wheelchair team approach that includes the patient, family, physician, therapist, and vendor, all working toward the common goal of prescribing the best wheelchair and seating system available for each patient.

References

1. Brittell CW: Wheelchair prescription. *In* Kottke FJ, Lehmann JF (eds): Krusen's Handbook of Physical Medicine and Rehabilitation. Philadelphia, WB Saunders, 1990, pp 548–563.
2. Cardus D, McTaggart WG, Ribas-Cardus F, et al: Energy requirements of gamefield exercises designed for wheelchair-bound persons. Arch Phys Med Rehabil 1989; 70:124–127.
3. DuBow LL, Witt PL, Kadaba MP, et al: Oxygen consumption of elderly persons with bilateral below knee amputations: Ambulation vs wheelchair propulsion. Arch Phys Med Rehabil 1983; 64:255–259.
4. Glaser RM, Barr SA, Lauback CC, et al: Relative stresses of wheelchair activity. Hum Factors 1980; 22:177–181.
5. Glaser RM, Sawka MN, Wilde SW, et al: Energy cost and cardiopulmonary responses for wheelchair locomotion and walking on tile and on carpet. Paraplegia 1981; 19:220–226.
6. Hilbers PA, White TP: Effects of wheelchair design on metabolic and heart rate responses during propulsion by persons with paraplegia. Phys Ther 1987; 67:1355–1358.
7. Linden AL, Holland GJ, Loy SF, et al: A physiological comparison of forward vs reverse wheelchair ergometry. Med Sci Sports Exerc 1993; 25:1265–1268.
8. McLaurin CA, Brubaker CE: Biomechanics and the wheelchair. Prosthet Orthot Int 1991; 15:24–37.
9. Nichols PJR, Norman PA, Ennis JR: Wheelchair user's shoulder. Scand J Rehab Med 1979; 11:29–32.
10. Perry RAF: The history of wheelchairs. *In* Letts RM (ed): Principles of Seating the Disabled. Boca Raton, Fla, CRC Press, 1991, pp 331–337.
11. Rodgers MM, Gayle GW, Figoni SF, et al: Biomechanics of wheelchair propulsion during fatigue. Arch Phys Med Rehabil 1994; 75:85–93.
12. Sawka MN, Glaser RM, Wilde SW, et al: Metabolic and circulatory responses to wheelchair and arm crank exercise. J Appl Physiol 1980; 49:784–788.
13. Smith PA, Glaser RM, Petrofsky JS, et al: Arm crank vs handrim wheelchair propulsion: Metabolic and cardiopulmonary responses. Arch Phys Med Rehabil 1983; 64:249–254.
14. Van Der Woude LHV, DeGroot G, Hollander AP, et al: Wheelchair ergonomics and physiological testing of prototypes. Ergonomics 1986; 29:1561–1573.
15. Waters RL, Lunsford BR: Energy cost of paraplegic locomotion. J Bone Joint Surg Am 1985; 67:1245–1250.

Therapeutic Exercise

BARBARA J. DE LATEUR, M.D., M.S.

THEORETICAL CONSIDERATIONS

It is common knowledge that strength is somehow related to the ability to lift objects in a gravitational field. It is intuitive that this strength is greater with larger muscles and is also related to the technique of lifting. Scientific research and research-based practice, however, require greater precision of definition.

One- and Ten-Repetition Maxima

A useful definition is the one-repetition maximum (1 RM), that is, the largest weight that can be lifted once and only once through the full range of motion of a given joint. The 1 RM lends itself to use in highly technical isokinetic equipment, an example of which would be the peak torque developed at any point in the range of a given joint at a given contraction velocity. It could also be given as an angle-specific torque, for example, the torque developed by the quadriceps at 60 degrees/sec at an angle of 60 degrees of flexion. Another useful definition is the 10 RM, that is, the highest weight that can be lifted through the full range of motion 10 times only. The 10 RM is useful where only a set of weights is available but not an isokinetic apparatus or other dynamometer.

Determinants of Strength

Absolute Muscle Strength

It has been known from antiquity that larger muscles are stronger. It has been known since the late 19th century that strength or the ability to develop force is related to the cross-sectional area of the muscle. This has been further refined to relate muscle strength to the physiological cross-sectional area, which is the cross section at the bulkiest part of the muscle for long parallel muscles such as the sartorius (Fig. 20–1). For pennate muscles, multiple cross sections must be taken at right angles to the fibers until all fibers have been included (Fig. 20–2). Because many more (necessarily shorter) muscle fibers can be packed into a pennate muscle of the same volume as a parallel muscle, such muscles are said to be adapted to force rather than

speed. While figures vary in the literature, a generally accepted value for the absolute muscle strength is 3.6 kg/cm^2 of physiological cross-sectional area.[1, 47] This should be listed technically as 3.6 kp/cm^2, noting that a kilopond (kp) is the force exerted by the mass of 1 kg in earth's gravitational field. This is generally implied rather than stated, and the convention is simply to give the force in kilograms.

Neural or Learning Factors in Strength

Gordon and co-workers[30] showed, in rats, that high-force or high-intensity performance could be enhanced without substantial overall increase in muscle bulk. This work has

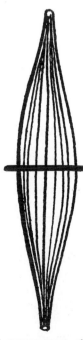

FIGURE 20–1 Parallel arrangement of muscle fibers. "Physiological" cross section is equal to cross-section of muscle belly. (From Brunnstrom S: Clinical Kinesiology, ed 2. Philadelphia, FA Davis, 1966.)

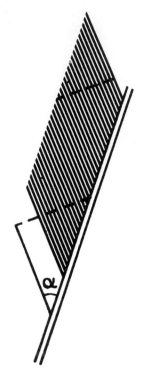

FIGURE 20–2 In pennate muscle, the physiological cross-section is determined by multiple sections at right angles to the fibers until all are included (From Brunnstrom S: Clinical Kinesiology, ed 2. Philadelphia, FA Davis, 1966.)

been confirmed in humans by Moritani and deVries[39] and by Milner-Brown et al.[38] Moritani and deVries make use of the fact that if one assesses integrated surface electromyographic activity (IEMG) over the same spot of the same muscle with the same angle of the joint, and keeps the contraction purely isometric, there will be a linear relationship between force and integrated electromyographic (EMG) activity. Figure 20–3(A–C) shows theoretically possible outcomes of training. In Figure 20–3A there is, as a result of training, an increase in the amount of EMG activity that can be produced at maximal effort. There is no change in the amount of force achieved for any given amount of effort. The line is simply extended upward. Figure 20–3B shows another theoretically possible outcome in which the amount of force generated for any given amount of EMG activity is greater. This *electrical efficiency*, as Moritani and deVries term it, presumably reflects hypertrophy. Figure 20–3C shows how one can determine the relative contributions of increased EMG activity reflecting neural or learning factors, and increased efficiency, reflecting hypertrophy.

Figure 20–4A shows data from trained and untrained arms of a female subject over the course of 8 weeks of training. Note that the IEMG-force relationships between the baseline (week 0) and at the end of 2 weeks of training virtually superimpose, but the line of week 2 extends beyond that of week 0. This suggests that there was no hypertrophy in the first 2 weeks of training, but something happened with learning or the ability to recruit or rapidly fire motor units or a combination of these. By week 4 the IEMG-force line has moved to the right, indicating that hypertrophy had taken place, and for any given level of

effort (IEMG), greater force results. The same happens for subsequent weeks. There is little or no further upward extension of the line beyond week 4 in this subject.

CROSS-TRAINING. The question of whether strengthening one limb results in strength increases in the opposite, untrained limb is of practical as well as theoretical interest. Current use of the term *cross-training* means the extent to which training in one sport benefits performance in another sport. In the older literature, cross-training meant the extent to which training one limb benefited the opposite limb. This might be of concern, for example, where the untrained side is in a cast. The series of measurements shown in Figure 20–4B show that there is a learning effect, but no hypertrophy. This is reasonable since it is, after all, the same brain that is being utilized and trained, but one would not expect hypertrophy when muscles are not subjected to tension-producing activity.

Endurance, Fatigue, and the Relationship of Endurance to Intensity of Activity

Endurance is the ability to continue a prescribed task in the desired manner. Virtually all definitions of endurance are variations on this theme. In contrast, *fatigue* can be defined in more than one way. For example, fatigue could be defined as the number of seconds in an attempted sustained contraction (or the number of contractions in a dynamic task) until that point where the peak force or torque reaches a specified percentage of the initial force or torque, for example, the time at which 60% of the initial value is reached. This definition is useful in assessing the response to training or to various therapeutic interventions. A broader definition of fatigue, useful to coaches and others concerned with athletic competition, is any decrement in performance resulting from previous performance.[42]

Figure 20–5 shows the results of a subject attempting to sustain a maximal isometric contraction for 5 sec. Note from the figure that it takes (for this muscle group) approximately 1 sec to reach the peak force and that this true peak can be held for only 1 sec despite sustained effort. The decrement in force over the next 4 sec reflects fatigue in the broadest sense. Thus defined, fatigue need not imply total exhaustion. The latter would be a very narrow definition and also a rare occurrence. In the figure, fatigue is also reflected in the fact that following 10 min of 1-sec-on, 1-sec-off contractions at only 5% of maximal effort, a lower peak force is generated upon attempted maximal contraction. It should be observed that the general configuration of the curve remains the same as the pre-exercise attempted maximal curve.

Absolute Endurance vs. Relative Endurance

Absolute endurance is the time that a subject can sustain a given workload; or, the number of seconds a given force can be held; or, the number of repetitions of a given load. Examples would be the number of seconds that a given bicycle ergometer can be pedaled by a subject at 100 W; the number of seconds a force of 50 N can be held; or the number of times a subject can lift a loaded barbell weighing

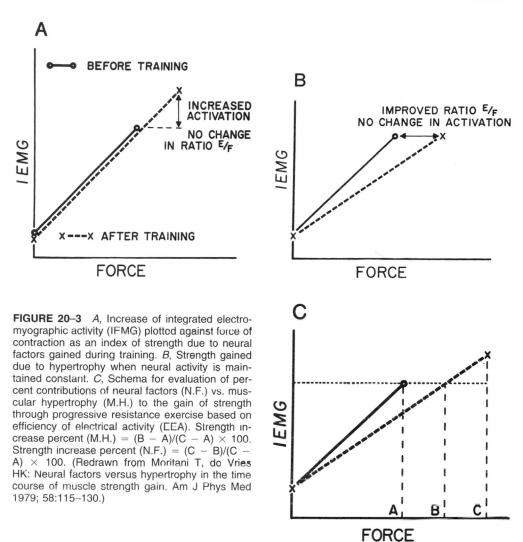

FIGURE 20–3 *A*, Increase of integrated electromyographic activity (IFMG) plotted against force of contraction as an index of strength due to neural factors gained during training. *B*, Strength gained due to hypertrophy when neural activity is maintained constant. *C*, Schema for evaluation of percent contributions of neural factors (N.F.) vs. muscular hypertrophy (M.H.) to the gain of strength through progressive resistance exercise based on efficiency of electrical activity (EEA). Strength increase percent (M.H.) = (B − A)/(C − A) × 100. Strength increase percent (N.F.) = (C − B)/(C − A) × 100. (Redrawn from Moritani T, de Vries HK: Neural factors versus hypertrophy in the time course of muscle strength gain. Am J Phys Med 1979; 58:115–130.)

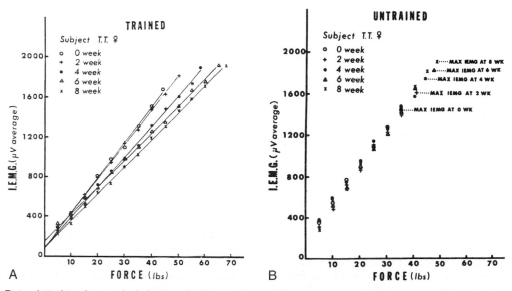

FIGURE 20–4 Data plotted to show typical changes in the trained arm *(A)* as compared with the untrained arm *(B)*. Both arms gained in strength, but only the trained arm showed significant changes in the E/F ratio (hypertrophy). (From Moritani T, de Vries HK: Neural factors versus hypertrophy in the time course of muscle strength gain. Am J Phys Med 1979; 58:115–130.)

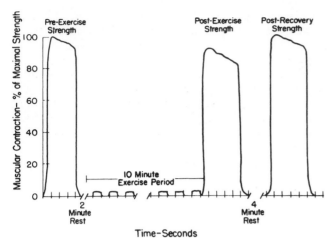

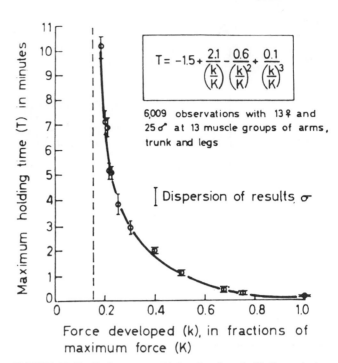

FIGURE 20–5 Maximal tension can be maintained during a voluntary maximal contraction of hand grip for less than 1 sec before evidence of fatigue appears as the available supply of ATP is exhausted. Fatigue (unavailability of ATP) increases in proportion to the intensity of activity but can be demonstrated following 10 minutes of intermittent contractions at 5 percent of maximal. (From Mundale MO: The relationship of intermittent isometric exercise to fatigue of hand grip. Arch Phys Med Rehabil 1970; 51:532–539.)

$$T = -1.5 + \frac{2.1}{\left(\frac{k}{K}\right)} - \frac{0.6}{\left(\frac{k}{K}\right)^2} + \frac{0.1}{\left(\frac{k}{K}\right)^3}$$

6,009 observations with 13♀ and 25♂ at 13 muscle groups of arms, trunk and legs

⌶ Dispersion of results, σ

FIGURE 20–7 Endurance and intensity of work. Static work: tension at fractions of maximum strength. (From Simonson E: Recovery and Fatigue. Springfield, Ill, Charles C Thomas, 1971, pp 440–458.)

10 lb with the right biceps. Note that these activities all have units, such as watts, newtons, pounds, etc.

Figure 20–6A and B and Figure 20–7 show the relationship of endurance to intensity of activity. In Figure 20–6A and B, absolute units are recorded on the abscissa. In Figure 20–7 the abscissa reflects relative force from 20% to 100% of the maximal voluntary contraction (MVC). In relative endurance, strength and endurance are not related because no matter how strong or weak one is, 100% is still 100% and the true maximal isometric contraction can be held only for 1 sec, as seen in Figure 20–5. On the other hand, if one looks at absolute endurance, for example, how long one can hold a given weight, strength and endurance are very much related. If the MVC of my right biceps is 20 lb and I go on a strength-training program and double the strength of my MVC to 40 lb, then I will be able to hold the force of 20 lb for more than 1 min. My new MVC of 40 lb, which is now 100% of the MVC, can be held for only 1 sec. This distinction between absolute muscle endurance and relative muscle endurance should resolve much of the apparent conflict in the literature about the relationships of strength and endurance.

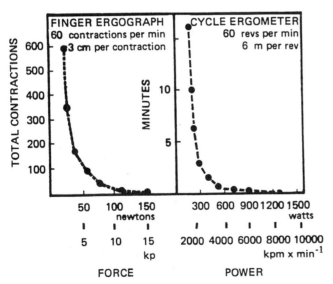

FIGURE 20–6 A, Relationship of endurance (as total contractions) of repeated flexion of third digit to effective force of contraction. B, Relationship of endurance (as minutes to fatigue) of cycle ergometer exercise to external power production. In both panels, the intercept with the abscissa represents the exercise intensity for which the maneuver could be performed only once (and, therefore, the strength of the concentric movement). In both panels, endurance could be presented as either total contractions or minutes to fatigue and, as the contraction rate and velocity are designated, either abscissa could be designated as force (per individual repetition) or power (work per unit time). (From Knuttgen HG: Development of muscular strength and endurance, In Knuttgen HG (ed): Neuromuscular Mechanisms for Therapeutic and Conditioning Exercises. Baltimore, University Park Press, 1976, pp 97–118.)

Length-Tension Relationships

Figure 20–8 shows the classic force-velocity relationships, also known as a Blix diagram. Attention is directed to curve C. In this relationship the tendon of insertion of the relaxed muscle of the anesthetized animal is removed from the insertion and connected to a tension-measuring device. At very short lengths no tension registers in the muscle-tendon relationship. That length at which tension just begins to exceed zero is known as the "resting length." As the muscle is drawn out (stretched) further and further, tension increases exponentially. If the muscle then is returned to a much shorter length (in the figure to 88% of the resting length), and a tetanizing volley of electrical stimuli is given to the motor nerve, tension is developed in the muscle. This is known as the "active" tension. At all

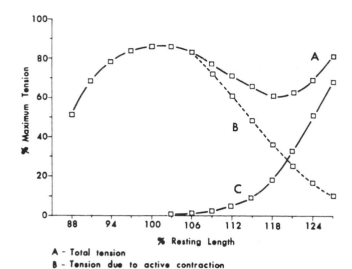

FIGURE 20-8 Length-tension diagram for passive stretch of an unsimulated muscle is shown in lower curve *C*. Curve *A*, showing total isometric tension when the muscle was stimulated at various lengths from maximal stretch through moderate shortening, represents the summation of active contraction plus passive tension due to the stretch. Active tension due solely to muscular contraction is obtained by subtracting passive tension *(C)* from total tension *(A)* and is represented by curve *B*. Normal resting length is 100, represented by curve *B*. Normal resting length is 100 percent. (Redrawn from Schottelius BA, Senay LC: Effect of stimulation-length sequence on shape of length-tension diagram. Am J Physiol 1956; 186:127–130.)

points below 100% of the resting length, the active and total tension are the same. At a point beyond 100% of the resting length, the active tension (*B*) is obtained by subtracting the passive tension (*C*) from the total tension (*A*). It can be seen that the tension (total) that can be developed in the muscle is greatest at this theoretical resting length, and it is inferred that the active tension drops off markedly at greater than 100% of the resting length. It is difficult to determine this theoretical resting length in living subjects and the term "resting length" can be misleading, since the muscle can be at rest (relaxed) at many lengths. As a practical matter, the resting length, sometimes called the neutral length, of the intact subject could be considered to be about midpoint of the joint range or slightly longer.

Leverage Effect

Leverage curves that were determined by looking at the angle of application of the tendon of insertion at various joint angles are shown in Figure 20–9. Any muscle force can be broken down into two forces normal (perpendicular) to each other: a rotatory force and a stabilizing force. The rotatory force is equal to the product of the total muscle force times the sine of the angle of application. Since the sine of 90 degrees is 1, the full muscle force is converted to rotatory force only if the angle of insertion is 90 degrees. Leverage is a function of the site of application of the tendon of insertion, that is, the perpendicular distance of the site of application from the joint.

Before isokinetic devices were available, these torque-angle curves had to be measured isometrically. Examples

are shown in Figures 20–10, 20–11, and 20–12. Leverage is determined by this site of application as well as the angle of application. If the leverage so defined were the only determinant of torque, it would be inferred from Figure 20–9 that the brachioradialis was the strongest of the elbow flexors. However, the force or tension developed by the muscle is, as we have seen, a function of the physiological cross-sectional area of the muscle. The torque developed (the effectiveness of the muscle for producing rotation about the joint) is the net result of muscle size (physiological cross-sectional area) and leverage.

Torque-Velocity Relationships

Modern isokinetic devices allow easy measurement of torque as it varies throughout the range of motion. They also permit the measurement of such torque-angle curves at varying velocities of contraction. Consequently, there are whole families of torque-angle-velocity curves. The point of maximum torque even shifts with the velocity of contraction. It is as though, at higher velocities, especially when the muscle is working against gravity (as when the seated subject uses the quadriceps to extend the knee), the

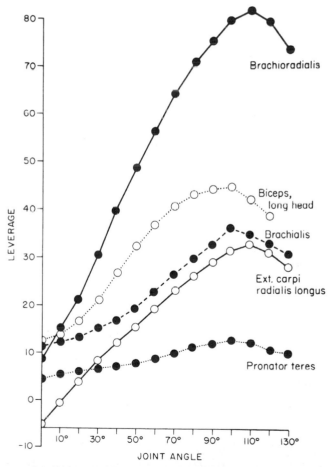

FIGURE 20-9 Leverage curves of elbow flexors; 0 degrees: elbow extended. Leverage is effective lever arm length: I*f* × sine α where I*f* is the distance from joint axis to site of application of tendon of insertion and α is the angle of insertion of the tendon at that joint angle. (From Brunnstrom S: Clinical Kinesiology, ed 2. Philadelphia, FA Davis, 1966.)

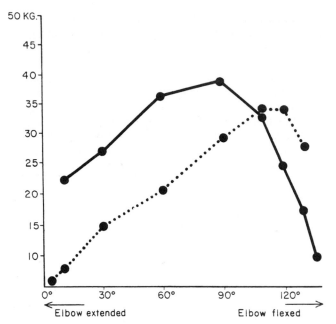

FIGURE 20–10 Torque curves for flexion and extension of right elbow, from determinations of four male subjects. *Solid curve*, elbow flexion curve; *dotted curve*, elbow extension. (From Brunnstrom S: Clinical Kinesiology, ed 2. Philadelphia, FA Davis, 1966.)

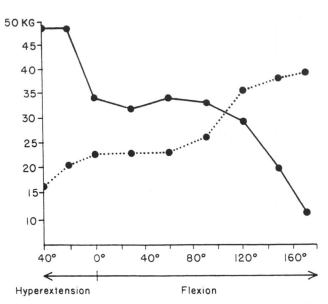

FIGURE 20–12 Torque curves for flexion and extension of right shoulder, derived from determinations on four male subjects. *Solid curve*, flexion; *dotted curve*, extension. (From Brunnstrom S: Clinical Kinesiology, ed 2. Philadelphia, FA Davis, 1966.)

muscle has to "catch up" with the resistance lever of the isokinetic device. Examples are shown in Figures 20–13, 20–14, and 20–15. Figure 20–16 shows the torque-angle curve for the quadriceps and hamstrings of a seated subject at 3 rpm (18 degrees/sec), 10 rpm (60 degrees/sec), and 30 rpm (180 degrees/sec). The displacement or position angle in degrees is shown in the lower set of curves. With these synchronized curves one can see the point of maximal torque for the quadriceps and the hamstrings. Of greater importance, however, is the fact that in spite of full effort the subject can produce less torque at 10 rpm than at 3 rpm, and less torque at 30 rpm than at 10 rpm. This illustrates the well-known torque-velocity relationships which are plotted out in Figure 20–17. This plot shows

that one can develop less torque with a fast shortening (concentric) contraction than with a slow shortening contraction; less torque with a slow shortening than with an isometric contraction; less torque with an isometric than with a slow lengthening (eccentric) contraction; and less torque with a slow lengthening than with a rapid lengthening contraction. This relationship has important implications for therapeutic exercise for development of strength and for hypertrophy (see discussion of the overload principle, below).

Muscle Fiber and Motor Unit Types

In the human there appear to be two muscle fiber types, generally designated type I (slow oxidative or SO) and type II (fast-twitch or FT). There is at least one subdivision

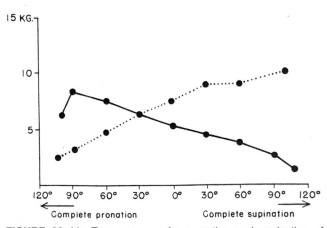

FIGURE 20–11 Torque curves for pronation and supination of right elbow, derived from determinations on four male subjects. Elbow at 90 degrees of flexion. *Solid curve*, supination; *dotted curve*, pronation; 0, thumb upward. (From Brunnstrom S: Clinical Kinesiology, ed 2. Philadelphia, FA Davis, 1966.)

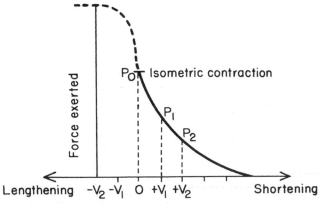

FIGURE 20–13 Force velocity curve of human muscle. *Solid line*, data obtained from elbow flexors of human subjects. At the time this curve was drawn, the *dotted line* was made by extrapolation. This portion of the curve has subsequently been confirmed experimentally (see Fig. 20–5). (From Brunnstrom S: Clinical Kinesiology, ed 2. Philadelphia, FA Davis, 1966.)

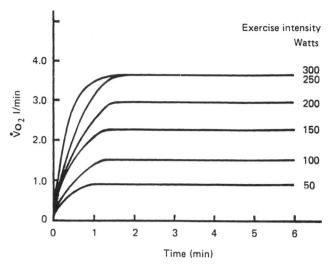

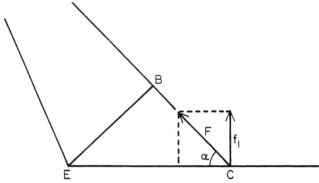

FIGURE 20–15 Two methods of computing torque. Torque equals f1 × EC or F × EB. (From Brunnstrom S: Clinical Kinesiology, ed 2. Philadelphia, FA Davis, 1966.)

FIGURE 20–14 Relationship of oxygen uptake to various exercise intensities utilizing several muscle groups in reciprocal concentric contractions. There is no additional increase in oxygen uptake with further increase in exercise intensity (external work) once maximal oxygen uptake is reached. (From Soule RG: Physiological response to physical exercise. In Knuttgen HG (ed): Neuromuscular Mechanisms for Therapeutic and Conditioning Exercise. Baltimore, University Park Press, 1976, pp. 79–96.)

of fibers into fast glycolytic (FG) and fast oxidative-glycolytic (FOG). The categorization into types I and II is made on the basis of the twitch characteristics, that is, fast or slow, illustrated in Figure 20–18. The characteristics of the muscle fibers are determined by the type of motor unit, as illustrated in Table 20–1. These characteristics include such things as their metabolic processes and sources of fuel, along with the enzymatic activity, speed of contraction, and rate of fatigue. Descriptions of differences in muscle color and muscle fiber diameter relate more consistently or at least more obviously to animals rather than to humans in whom the differences are more subtle. The distinction between light and dark meat in the Thanksgiving turkey is well known. The FOG motor unit including the muscle fiber can be thought of as a sort of hybrid which is defined as type II by its FT characteristics, but it retains some of the fatigue resistance associated with the oxidative phosphorylation seen in the type I or SO motor unit types.

Twitch characteristics of muscle are not easily determined in the intact subject and one generally uses histochemical markers to determine whether units in a given micrograph are type I or type II. Figure 20–19 shows, in the illustration on the left, the designation of type I (light-staining fibers) vs. type II (dark-staining fibers). Serial sections can then be stained for other enzymatic features (see illustration on the right in Fig. 20–19) which shows that the type I fibers have greater NADH diaphorase. The fuel utilized by the various motor units has important implications for therapeutic exercise, particularly fat reduction (see Exercise for Fat Reduction, below).

The Motor Unit Size Principle

Henneman[33] first enunciated the size principle, which has been supported by subsequent investigators. The smaller motor units have fewer muscle fibers, smaller motor unit action potentials, somewhat smaller cross-sectional areas, and have a lower threshold of recruitment. In needle EMG, as motor units are recruited in succession, the smaller motor units come in first and the larger motor units later. Some later motor units appear smaller because of their distance from the exploring electrode. With needle adjustment to focus on the motor unit, it becomes much larger. Another way of stating this is that one is able to recruit smaller units without the larger, but one cannot

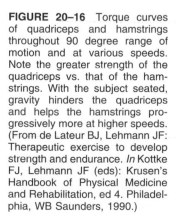

FIGURE 20–16 Torque curves of quadriceps and hamstrings throughout 90 degree range of motion and at various speeds. Note the greater strength of the quadriceps vs. that of the hamstrings. With the subject seated, gravity hinders the quadriceps and helps the hamstrings progressively more at higher speeds. (From de Lateur BJ, Lehmann JF: Therapeutic exercise to develop strength and endurance. In Kottke FJ, Lehmann JF (eds): Krusen's Handbook of Physical Medicine and Rehabilitation, ed 4. Philadelphia, WB Saunders, 1990.)

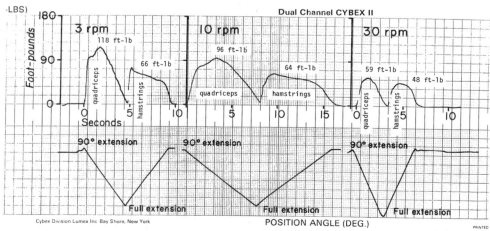

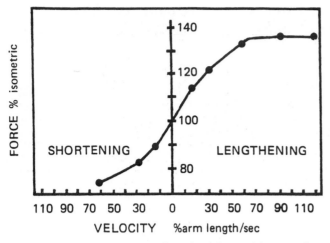

FIGURE 20–17 Relationship of maximal force of human elbow flexor muscles to velocity of contraction. Velocity on abscissa is designated as a percentage of arm length per second. (From Knuttgen HG: Development of muscular strength and endurance. *In* Knuttgen HG (ed): Neuromuscular Mechanisms for Therapeutic and Conditioning Exercises. Baltimore, University Park Press, 1976, pp. 97–118.)

recruit larger units without the smaller. Some variation of this can be seen among motor units of similar size.

Metabolic Aspects of Exercise

The work of Gollnick et al.[28] has shown that the point of recruitment of the larger type II fibers depends on the type of exercise. With sustained isometric contractions, type II motor units are brought in at 20% of the MVC. However, if the isometric effort is sustained long enough, type II fibers can be brought in at thresholds somewhat below 20% of MVC. With aerobic exercise, as on a bicycle ergometer, the reliance is on type I motor units below 100% of the maximal aerobic capacity ($\dot{V}O_2$max). Beyond this aerobic capacity, both type I and type II are relied upon, and the subject will rapidly go into an oxygen debt secondary to anaerobic metabolism. However, the threshold

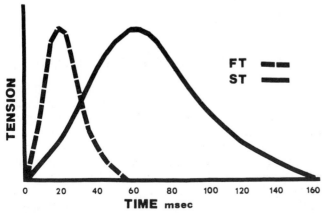

FIGURE 20–18 Twitch characteristics (contraction relaxation curves) of slow twitch (type I) and fast twitch (type II) muscles. (From Ianuzzo CD: The cellular composition of human skeletal muscle. *In* Knuttgen HG (ed): Neuromuscular Mechanisms for Therapeutic and Conditioning Exercise. Baltimore, University Park Press, 1976, pp. 31–53.)

TABLE 20–1 A Characterization of Skeletal Muscle Fibers Based Upon Their Metabolic and Mechanical Properties

	Muscle Fiber Characteristics		
	Slow Oxidative (SO)	Fast Glycolytic (FG)	Fast Oxidative-Glycolytic (FOG)
Major source of ATP	Oxidative phosphorylation	Glycolysis	Oxidative phosphorylation
Mitochondria	Numerous	Few	Numerous
Myoglobin content	High	Low	High
Capillarity	Dense	Sparse	Dense
Muscle color	Red	White	Red
Glycogen content	Low	High	Intermediate
Glycolytic enzyme activity	Low	High	Intermediate
Myosin ATPase activity	Low	High	High
Speed of contraction	Slow	Fast	Fast
Rate of fatigue	Slow	Fast	Intermediate
Muscle fiber diameter	Small	Large	Intermediate

Abbreviations: ATP, adenosine triphosphate; ATPase, adenosine triphosphatase.
From Kidd G, Brodie P: The motor unit: A review. Physiotherapy 1980; 66:146–152.

for bringing in anaerobic pathways is generally about 70%, although it may be higher in endurance-trained (aerobic-trained) athletes.

Application of Principles to Therapeutic Exercise for Strength, Local Muscle Endurance, and Hypertrophy

STRENGTH. Improvement of muscle performance, including performance on tests of strength, can be enhanced in various ways. These include increases in the amount of weight lifted (progressive resistance exercise, or PRE), increases in the number of repetitions or sets, or both; and increases in the contraction velocity (while keeping the resistance and number of repetitions the same).

PROGRESSIVE RESISTANCE EXERCISE. This type of exercise was described and popularized by T. L. De-Lorme, who at the time was a captain in the U.S. Army. It requires the determination, usually once a week, of the 10 RM. For each session, carried out 3 to 5 days per week, the subject performs 10 repetitions at each of a series of fractions of the 10 RM. In the early stages this was 10 repetitions each at 10%, 20%, 30%, . . . all the way up to 100% of the 10 RM.[19, 20] Because of the enormous amount of time necessary to train multiple muscles with this technique, a number of modifications of this program were devised and the final form was 10 repetitions each at 50%, 75%, and 100% of the 10 RM. This program has much to recommend it, including the fact that there is a built-in warmup at a lower intensity and the likelihood of fatigue limiting the number of contractions in the final set at 100%. Nevertheless, some workers were concerned about the inability to carry out the full prescribed 10 RM at 100% and thus the "Oxford technique"[48] was developed. It begins with 10 repetitions at 100% and progresses down in weight to 10 repetitions at 75% and 50% of the 10 RM. The work of Esselman and others[23] showed that as many as 40 extra repetitions at a lower resistance had virtually no effect upon the results of 12 weeks of training. This strongly suggests that the DeLorme technique is more effective than the Oxford technique, although the critical study in this

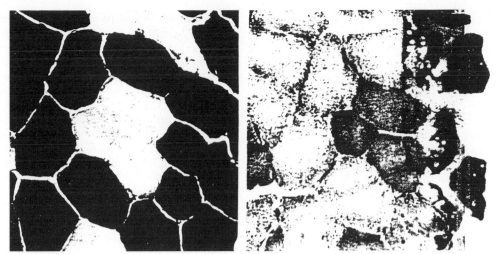

FIGURE 20–19 Histochemical micrograph illustrating the fast twitch (FT) and slow twitch (ST) muscle fibers in human skeletal muscle. The micrograph on the left has been stained for myofibrillar ATPase. The light and dark stained cells are ST and FT fibers, respectively. The micrograph at the right is from a serial section of the muscle and has been stained for DPNH-diaphorase, which indicates the aerobic potential of the fibers. These micrographs illustrate that in human skeletal muscle ST fibers have a relatively high aerobic capacity, whereas FT fibers have a low capacity. (From Ianuzzo CD: The cellular composition of human skeletal muscle. In Knuttgen HG (ed): Neuromuscular Mechanisms for Therapeutic Conditioning Exercise. Baltimore, University Park Press, 1976, pp. 31–53.)

regard has apparently not been done. The reader is advised to determine what type of exercise training is actually performed when progressive resistive exercise is requested.

INCREASING THE NUMBER OF REPETITIONS. There is essentially 100% transfer-of-training when there is a comparison of relatively high weights with few repetitions compared with relatively low weights with more repetitions, as long as the exercise is carried out to the point of fatigue.[17] However, two points should be noted. The first is that far more repetitions have to be carried out with lower weights than with the higher to reach the point of fatigue. It is likely that the subject will stop low-weight exercise for reasons other than true muscle fatigue. The amount of mechanical work done will be much greater with the lower weight. Mechanical work is far less relevant to muscle training than is the stimulus of muscle failure, that is, a short-lasting inability to carry out the task. There may be some circumstances in which the subject should avoid the risk of training that might occur with the higher weights. In general, however, use of higher weights to failure is both more effective and more efficient than lower weights to failure. One can also do multiple sets, going to fatigue with each set, with the higher weights. This might be necessary once a plateau is reached in training.

PROGRESSIVE RATE TRAINING OF HELLEBRANDT. Hellebrandt[32] showed that muscle performance can be improved by selecting a relatively high weight and using a metronome to control the contraction velocity. A fixed number of repetitions can be used, such as 10 or, at most, 20. The metronome is set initially at the lowest rate and the weight is lifted on "tick" and lowered on "tock." Each day the metronome rate is set one notch higher. Almost imperceptibly the contraction velocity is thereby increased and the entire torque-velocity curve is shifted upward. This technique has the additional advantage that the exercise time required is shorter every day. It is also unnecessary to keep redetermining the 10 RM. With these advantages it is somewhat surprising that this technique is rarely used, but that is apparently the case.

A variation on this type of training could theoretically be carried out by using an isokinetic device with the initial velocity limit set very low. One might therefore start out at an 18 degrees/sec velocity limit and gradually increase this to as much as 360 degrees/sec, or the upper limit of the machine.

OTHER APPROACHES. A simple but highly effective technique[16] is to find a relatively high weight, one that can be lifted three to five times prior to failure (temporary inability to lift the weight further) and record the number of repetitions. The exercise should be carried to the point of muscle fatigue or failure each session. One records or graphs the number of repetitions to fatigue each day. When the subject can perform some 15 to 20 repetitions, the weight is increased approximately 10% and the process is repeated. A variation on this process, useful when strength begins to reach a plateau, is to carry out multiple sets during a session, with each set going to fatigue.

CLINICAL AND SPORTS APPLICATIONS

The practice of sports medicine is characterized by a number of maxims, and perhaps one of the most important and useful of these is the following: "Get in shape to play. Do not play to get in shape." This should also be applied to clinical rehabilitation practice. Following this one maxim would likely do more to prevent injury than virtually any other practice. By doing so, one builds up a reserve in the mechanical, metabolic, and neuromuscular aspects of performance, and this reserve goes a long way toward preventing overuse injuries, strains, sprains, and so forth.

Are Athletes Born or Made?

Marked differences between athletes participating in different types of sports can be detected by the casual observer or the devotee of sport and in greater detail by the scientist in the human performance laboratory. The weightlifter is heavy and extremely strong. The distance runner is slight of build with very little body fat and relatively low strength but has the ability to continue running, literally for hours. Definite but more subtle changes are observed between the sprinter and the distance runner. Differences in local metabolic capacity of the muscle as well as fiber type differences have been determined by large-needle biopsy.[3] Gollnick et al.[27] sampled the upper and lower extremity muscles of athletes participating in various sports. A total of 74 trained and untrained men were studied. The quantitative chemical studies that were carried out included succinate dehydrogenase (SDH) and phosphofructokinase (PFK), representing, respectively, the oxidative and glycolytic capabilities of the muscle sample as a whole, without distinction between fiber types. Histochemical studies included myosin adenosine triphosphatase (ATPase) for fiber-typing, as well as NADH diaphorase and alpha-glycerophosphate dehydrogenase for estimating (semiquantitatively only) relative (type I vs. type II) oxidative and glycolytic capabilities. The distribution of glycogen was estimated (in serial sections) from the periodic acid–Schiff

(PAS) reaction. Standard photographs were made so that planimetry could be used for fiber areas. In addition, each subject's $\dot{V}O_2$max was determined while he was either running on a treadmill or pedaling a bicycle. Whereas only minor differences existed for PFK (glycolytic capacity), remarkable differences were found in local muscle oxidative capacity (SDH) and in $\dot{V}O_2$max. The SDH and $\dot{V}O_2$max of the weightlifters were no greater than those of the untrained men; in fact, they were slightly less. The endurance-trained athletes had much higher $\dot{V}O_2$max and local muscle SDH activity than the untrained men or the weightlifters.

Of particular interest is the selective effect upon the muscles used predominantly in the sport. For instance, in the group of bicyclists the SDH activity of the vastus lateralis (11.0 ± 1.0 μmol/g/min) was much greater than that of the deltoid (6.1 ± 0.2), whereas in canoeists, the SDH activity of the deltoid (7.9 ± 0.6) was much higher than that of the vastus lateralis (5.8 ± 0.9). Table 20–2 show the fiber sizes, populations, and contributions to muscle area of several individual subjects. Note that in the untrained men, the weightlifters, and the sprinter, the slow-twitch (ST) fibers (type I) occupied a relatively small

TABLE 20–2 Relationship of Exercise Training of Upper and Lower Extremity Muscles to Fiber Diameters, Total Cross-Sectional Areas, and Percentage of Slow Twitch and Fast Twitch Muscle Fibers*

Subject	Sample Site	Group	Fiber Diameter (μm) ST	Fiber Diameter (μm) FT	Area (μm²) ST	Area (μm²) FT	ST Fibers (%)	Area of ST Fibers (%)
PG	L	Untrained	75.2 ± 2.9 (47.1–96.1)	85.8 ± 2.0 (69.3–101.7)	4567.5 ± 343.2 (1740–7250)	5843.0 ± 273.9 (3770–8120)	34.0	28.7
CS	L	Untrained	80.3 ± 3.3 (54.4–112.2)	93.2 ± 2.2 (71.9–110.4)	5234.5 ± 440.3 (2320–9860)	6902.0 ± 329.9 (4060–9570)	30.0	24.5
MKS	L	Untrained	63.4 ± 2.4 (47.1–79.4)	67.7 ± 2.4 (47.1–86.0)	3057.5 ± 273.6 (1740–4930)	3683.0 ± 250.0 (1740–800)	34.0	30.0
GK	A	Untrained	63.6 ± 2.0 (38.0–76.0)	67.3 ± 1.7 (53.8–79.2)	3234.0 ± 181.2 (1135–4540)	3594.0 ± 177.8 (2270–4918)	48.3	45.7
	L		72.2 ± 3.5 (43.9–98.2)	75.0 ± 1.4 (65.9–87.8)	4275.0 ± 382.1 (1513–7566)	4445.0 ± 169.1 (3405–6053)	48.6	47.6
NP	L	Sprinter	79.5 ± 2.6 (54.4–98.0)	89.4 ± 2.1 (74.4–101.7)	5060.5 ± 314.0 (2320–7540)	6336.5 ± 284.2 (4350–8120)	26.0	21.9
DM	L	Distance runner	67.1 ± 1.7 (54.4–83.3)	58.0 ± 1.3 (47.1–69.3)	3581.1 ± 186.2 (2320–5510)	2668.0 ± 1220 (1740–3770)	75.0	80.1
DS	L	Distance runner	85.1 ± 3.5 (57.7–105.3)	105.2 ± 2.5 (81.5–124.6]	5858.0 ± 445.8 (2610–8700)	8776.1 ± 403.2 (5220–12,179)	70.0	60.9
DF	L	Middle-distance runner	95.5 ± 3.2 (74.4–121.6)	87.9 ± 3.4 (47.1–115.3)	7307.8 ± 499.6 (4350–11,599)	6235.0 ± 448.2 (1740–10,439)	55.0	58.9
RP	L	Middle-distance runner	59.2 ± 2.7 (27.2–79.2)	71.6 ± 2.5 (50.9–98.0)	2856.5 ± 231.8 (580–4830)	4118.0 ± 295.9 (2030–540)	47.0	38.1
BA	L	Former weightlifter	107.1 ± 3.8 (83.8–135.9)	108.9 ± 3.4 (92.2–160.8)	9199.1 ± 656.7 (5510–14,499)	9482.9 ± 666.9 (6670–20,299)	24.0	23.5
MH	L	Weightlifter	85.6 ± 4.9 (47.1–113.7)	110.8 ± 3.0 (86.0–135.9)	6035.6 ± 629.4 (1740–10,149)	9758.1 ± 516.6 (5800–14,499)	25.3	23.5
	A		83.5 ± 2.4 (60.8–98.0)	105.0 ± 3.3 (74.4–135.9)	5553.5 ± 303.8 (2900–7540)	8917.2 ± 543.1 (4350–14,499)	48.4	36.9
JR	A	Bicyclist	83.1 ± 1.4 (71.9–96.1)	96.2 ± 1.9 (76.9–108.7)	5467.0 ± 187.9 (4060–7250)	7337.0 ± 273.7 (4640–9280)	52.1	48.6
	L		104.6 ± 2.3 (86.0–127.5)	112.2 ± 2.2 (98.0–137.2)	8651.5 ± 763.9 (5800–12,759)	9946.6 ± 401.5 (7540–14,789)	51.3	44.0
BL	A	Canoeist	101.9 ± 2.6 (86.3–129.5)	102.9 ± 2.3 (88.6–118.2)	8244.0 ± 570.3 (5850–13,162)	8391.0 ± 361.9 (5484–10,968)	57.9	74.6
	L		90.5 ± 2.7 (68.2–107.9)	80.3 ± 1.5 (68.2–91.6)	6544.0 ± 387.5 (3656–9140)	5100.0 ± 190.1 (3656–6581)	69.9	57.5
SH	A	Swimmer	88.0 ± 1.7 (71.6–101.2)	91.0 ± 2.4 (77.8–105.7)	6124.0 ± 233.9 (4022–8043)	6552.0 ± 263.2 (4753–8774)	85.3	84.4
	L		79.0 ± 2.0 (61.9–91.6)	93.6 ± 1.9 (74.8–105.7)	4954.0 ± 237.6 (2925–6581)	6928.0 ± 266.9 (4387–8774)	79.7	73.7

*Values are means ± SE. Values in parentheses are highest and lowest observations.
Abbreviations: ST, slow twitch; FT, fast twitch; L, leg; A, arm.
Modified from Gollnick PD, Armstrong RB, Sanbert CW IV, et al. Enzyme activity and fiber composition in skeletal muscle of untrained and trained men. J Appl Physiol 1972; 33:312–319.

percentage of the muscle fiber area (21.9%–30%), whereas in the endurance-trained athletes the ST fibers occupied as much as 84% of the area.

This study examined the athletes as they were and did not constitute a before-and-after experiment. It might be argued that very early in their athletic careers these athletes found that they were able to compete much more effectively in one type of sport than in another and therefore, because of positive reinforcement, selected the sport at which they were successful. However, there is some suggestion that the changes seen in their muscles were at least to some extent the result of training, because one would anticipate genetically a more or less constant ratio of ST to FT fibers in the upper and lower extremities. This is not to say that the same ratio of ST to FT in the deltoid and in the vastus lateralis would be expected. However, if the ST/FT ratio is X in the deltoid and Y in the vastus lateralis in one subject, and if the ST/FT ratio in the deltoid is A and the ST/FT in the vastus is B in another subject, then, if differential usage (training) has no effect, one might expect X/Y to equal A/B. However, those athletes who used the upper or the lower extremity more in a specific sport had enhancement of the metabolic capability and a larger percent area of ST fibers in the muscles used.

Gollnick et al.[26] also carried out a 5-month training program with biopsy studies before and after training. The training program was 1 hour/day for 4 days a week at a load requiring 75% to 90% of maximal aerobic power. The subsequent biopsies showed an increase in the ratio of the areas of ST to FT fibers from 0.82 to 1.11 ($P < .01$). Oxidative capacity increased in both fiber types; anaerobic capacity increased only in the FT fibers. This study indicates the possibility of great enhancement of local muscle metabolic capability, particularly oxidative capacity, with endurance training, and strongly supports the notion of some degree of specificity of training. In studies with human subjects, fiber number does not appear to increase. However, in an animal study, Gonyea et al.[29] were able to excise and tease apart the fibers of an entire muscle using nitric acid digestion, and they found a small but significant increase in fiber number in response to unilateral exercise. The fact that they found significance means either that a rare thing had happened (the animals had been born with more fibers on one side than on the other) or that there was an actual increase in fiber number in response to exercise.

Regarding the question of whether athletes are born or made, it appears that the genotype sets the rather wide limits, with the actual performance capability determined by the extent and type of training.

Studies on the Specificity of Training

The exercise literature as well as clinical experience strongly supports the notion that the poorer the initial condition of the subject (provided that no specific neuromuscular disorder is present), the greater the percentage response to training and the greater the generalizability of the training. Conversely, the more elite the athlete or performer, the greater the requirement for specific training (see also Coordination, below). With very deconditioned subjects, aerobic training leads to increases in strength, and

strength training leads to improved aerobic performance as well as enhanced local muscle endurance.[10, 14, 46]

High Weights vs. Low Weights: "The DeLorme Axiom"

One study illustrates the transferability of training on relatively high weights to performance under low-weight conditions (and vice versa) utilizing a study design known as double-shift transfer-of-training design.[17] This type of design, long utilized by investigators in the realm of motor skills learning, requires the best performance a subject can produce during each training session. In this way each session yields a score and no other assessment is required. This type of design was utilized during World War II to see, for example, the extent to which training in flight simulators transferred to performance in airplanes (which were in relatively short supply). A similar design was used to determine whether gunnery training should be performed on small targets, which were thought to make the shooters sharp, or on large targets, which were reinforcing because of the higher time spent on target. Such transfer-of-training designs are ideally suited to test the DeLorme axiom, which states: "High weight (intensity), low repetition programs build strength; low weight (low intensity) high repetition exercises build endurance."[19] Each of these types of exercise is wholly distinct and wholly incapable of producing the results obtained by the other. In the extreme, this axiom must be true. However, there is a large middle ground in which this axiom is untrue, that is, in which there is a high degree of transferability of relatively low to relatively high weight conditions as long as the subject goes to the point of fatigue. It should be noted that 50 lb lifted 10 times will have a different training effect from 10 lb lifted 50 times, even though the mechanical work performed by the muscle is the same. What counts is the relative intensity or tax on the muscle (see discussion of intensity-endurance relationships, above).

In a study, "A Test of the DeLorme Axiom," the authors randomly assigned a relatively homogeneous group of young, sedentary males to four training groups: two groups who trained on 55-lb weights and two groups who trained on the relatively low weight of 26 lb[17] (26 lb was selected as the low weight because much below this level, even these sedentary subjects would have been able to repeat the exercise indefinitely without muscle failure). Paced by a metronome, seated subjects raised the weighted limb to full extension of the knee on the count of 1, held it through the count of 6, lowered the weight on 7, and repeated the process at the next beat. In order to encourage maximal performance, subjects were paid per repetition and received more pay per high-weight repetition. At the end of the series of training sessions, one low-weight group switched to the high-weight condition, and one high-weight group switched to the low-weight condition, and all groups continued performing their best for several more (test) sessions. Figure 20–20 shows that there was a 100% transfer from one condition to another. It could be said that the strength-trained group gained as much endurance as the endurance-trained group, and the endurance-trained group gained as much strength as the strength-trained group. Although one training condition was as *effective* as the

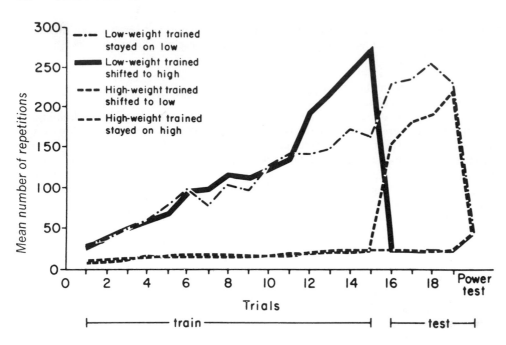

FIGURE 20–20 Mean scores for each of the four groups for each of 15 training trials and each of 4 test trials. The mean score for each of the four groups on the power test is also shown. (From de Lateur BJ, Lehmann JF, Fordyce WE: A test of the DeLorme axiom. Arch Phys Med Rehabil 1968; 49:245–248.)

other, the high-intensity (and therefore, necessarily, low-repetition) group took far less time and was therefore much more efficient.

Isometric vs. Isotonic

A double-shift, transfer-of-training design is also well suited to sort out the controversy between the proponents of isometric and those of isotonic exercise. During the height of this controversy, one could find studies that purported to show the superiority of isometric over isotonic and other studies that purported to show the reverse. It was stated that "one 6-sec maximal isometric contraction was worth more than hours and hours in a weight room." The issue of test bias or training-to-task was generally not considered. In a 1972 study, the authors randomly assigned healthy sedentary young adult males to one of four groups, two of which trained on a 50-lb isometric task and two of which trained on a 50-lb isotonic task.[18] The weight was kept the same to avoid confounding by low-vs.-high weights. For those training on the isometric condition, the experimenters lifted the weighted limb to the point of full extension of the knee and by the count of 3 the subject had to hold the weight himself. The extended limb lifted a light bar which triggered the stopclock, and the subject was paid per second held. This constituted the training task and yielded the score for each day. For those training on the isotonic task, the knee was fully extended and lowered to the count of a metronome. When the bar was lifted, however briefly, the repetition was counted and the subject was paid per repetition. There was no "hold" for the isotonic group. Each task was kept pure (no lift for the isometric group and no hold for the isotonic group). At the end of the series of training sessions, two of the four groups shifted to the opposite condition and all groups continued to perform their best for several more sessions.

The result, shown in Figure 20–21, was very interesting in that subjects always did better on the task on which they had trained. Figures 20–22 and 20–23 break out the results

as though they had been performed as two single-shift, transfer-of-training studies. If one saw only Figure 20–22, one would conclude that isometric was superior. If one saw only Figure 20–23, one would conclude that isotonic was superior. This clearly illustrates the effect of training-to-task. From these results it can be concluded that for qualitatively identical tasks, as in the DeLorme axiom study, there are comparable results, as long as subjects go to the point of fatigue in training (remember that it will take much longer to go to true muscle fatigue for lower weights). For qualitatively different tasks (or for extreme quantitative differences), the best training for a task is that task itself. This is a good illustration of Aristotle's maxim, "Men become builders by building, lyre players by playing the lyre, and virtuous by doing virtuous acts."

Isokinetic Programs: Strength, and Hypertrophy; Specificity of Velocity of Training

Isokinetic programs require special isokinetic equipment. The type of training and testing involved is not reflected in everyday, nontechnical experience. This is in contrast to isotonic and isometric exercise, which reflects the ordinary activity of lifting or holding objects against gravity. Training to task and learning to perform on the isokinetic devices are heavily involved in isokinetic programs. Consequently, it is theoretically possible, and such seems to be the case,[13, 23] that isokinetic performance can be greatly enhanced without significant hypertrophy. This is especially true if there is no eccentric component. Early isokinetic devices involved purely concentric exercise since performance of knee extension was carried out by the quadriceps (concentric), and knee flexion by the hamstrings (also concentric). In contrast, raising and lowering a weight has both a concentric and an eccentric component. More recent equipment, such as the Kin-Com, Lido (Loredan), and Biodex, allow either a mixed mode or a purely concentric mode. Although studies are conflicting,[36, 37] the preponder-

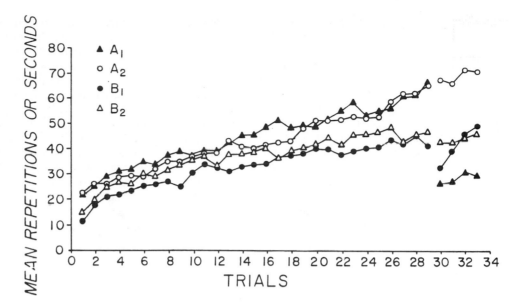

FIGURE 20–21 Results of the isotonic-isometric comparison. Groups A1 and A2 were isotonically trained. Groups B1 and B2 were isometrically trained. Group A1 shifted to the isometric task on day 30. Group B1 shifted to the isotonic task on day 30. (From de Lateur BJ, Lehmann J, Stonebridge J, Warren CG: Isotonic vs. isometric exercises: A double-shift, transfer-of-training study. Arch Phys Med Rehabil 1972; 53:212–217.)

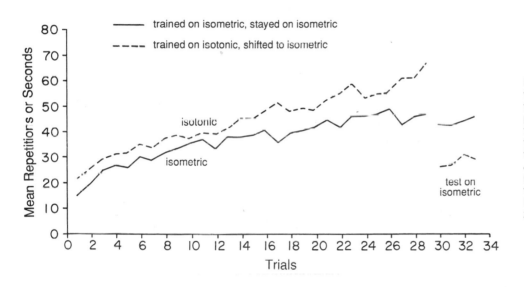

FIGURE 20–22 Results of isotonic-isometric comparison. Group trained on isometric *(solid line)* performed better on isometric than did the group trained on isotonic *(dashed line).* (From de Lateur BJ, Lehmann J, Stonebridge J, Warren CG: Isotonic vs. isometric exercises: A double-shift, transfer-of-training study. Arch Phys Med Rehabil 1972; 53:212–217.)

FIGURE 20–23 Results of isotonic-isometric comparison. Group trained on isotonic *(solid line)* performed better on isotonic than did the group trained on isometric *(dashed line).* (From de Lateur BJ, Lehmann J, Stonebridge J, Warren CG: Isotonic vs. isometric exercises: A double-shift, transfer-of-training study. Arch Phys Med Rehabil 1972; 53:212–217.)

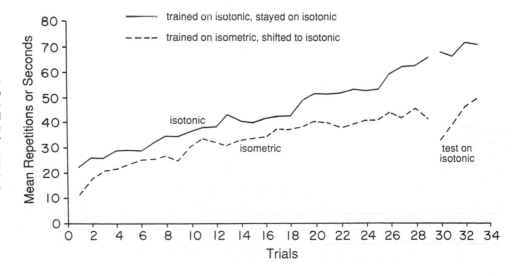

ance of evidence suggests that if hypertrophy is desired, there should be at least a component of eccentric exercise in the training.

SPECIFICITY OF VELOCITY OF TRAINING. If the best training for a task is that task itself, and if the task requires exerting force at high velocities, it would seem advantageous to train at high contraction velocities. The intrinsic shape of the torque-velocity curve (see Figs. 20–13, 20–14, and 20–15) implies that, regardless of effort, training at high contraction velocities will be less forceful, although the force exerted will gradually, with training, become higher. Esselman et al.[23] randomly assigned healthy sedentary young men to training at 6 rpm (18 degrees/sec) and 18 rpm (108 degrees/sec). Because effort is all-important on isokinetic performance, subjects were paid a small amount per foot-pound of torque for every training or testing contraction. Torque-velocity curves were carried out at baseline and after 12 weeks of training. Subjects who trained at the slower contraction velocity limit (and therefore more forcefully) gained more than those who trained at a faster velocity limit, not only at the velocity at which they trained but throughout the entire torque-velocity curve, even at velocities far greater than those at which either group trained. Is this a violation of the specificity principle? Probably not, since what one was attempting to increase was the ability to produce torque (force). It therefore appears that the more important variable in developing strength (forceful contractions) is the tension (force) produced in the muscle during training. To the extent that a skill is involved, however, such as throwing a baseball, it is extremely important to practice on the task itself.

Coordination

The maxim "Practice makes perfect" would be more accurate if restated, "*Perfect* practice makes perfect." Inaccurate practice leads to inaccurate performance and the wrong notes or skills are learned as readily as the correct ones. Some extremely complex tasks involving more than one limb should be broken down into simpler tasks and

performed slowly enough that the practice is essentially error-free. The simpler tasks should then be brought up to a faster speed following which combined practice is undertaken at a slow speed. This is gradually increased until the combined performance can be carried out at a much faster speed than will be required in recital or concert (in the case of musical performance). This would be appropriate in the case of pipe organ performance for the training of the lower limbs for a pedal task, since the hands have their task separated from the pedals. Care must be taken, however, not to develop some techniques which work at slow speeds or separation of the limbs that would not be sustainable in faster or combined tasks. Accurate repetitions must be carried out until an engram is generated. A useful definition of an *engram* is a precise automatic performance implying a preprogrammed pattern.[35]

The number of repetitions required to generate an engram varies with the complexity of the task, but is probably much higher than ordinarily thought. Figure 20–24 shows the gradually increasing performance of human cigar makers compared with the cigar-making machine.[15] Only with millions of repetitions does the human subject approach the machine's time as a limit. Specificity of training or practice is extremely important with highly coordinated tasks. This is the experience of musicians who go from one woodwind instrument to another or from one type of keyboard to another, such as piano vs. harpsichord, mechanical action pipe organs vs. electropneumatic pipe organs. It is very clear that with this level of required skill, the best training for a given task is that task itself.

APPLICATIONS TO AGING

STRENGTH TRAINING. Evidence is accumulating that older people respond favorably to strength training.[4–8, 14, 24, 25, 40, 41] There were some data from the inferential technique of Moritani and deVries[40] that the improved performance on strength tasks of older subjects was due entirely to

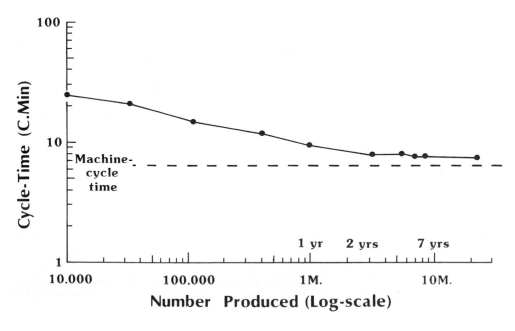

FIGURE 20–24 Practice and speed in cigar-making. Each point is the average cycle-time over 1 week's production for one operator. The ordinate is the total production by the operator since beginning work. (From Crossman ERFW: A theory of the acquisition of speed skill. Ergonomics 1959; 2:163–166.)

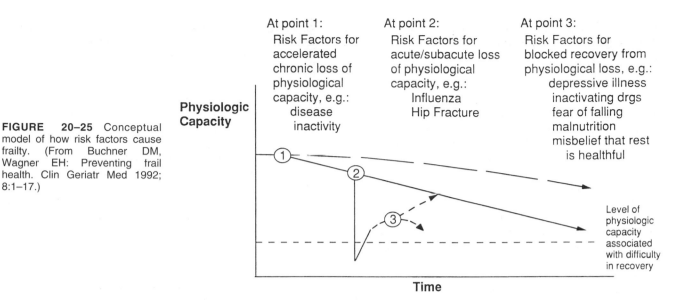

FIGURE 20–25 Conceptual model of how risk factors cause frailty. (From Buchner DM, Wagner EH: Preventing frail health. Clin Geriatr Med 1992; 8:1–17.)

learning or neural factors, not to hypertrophy. However, the direct imaging used by Frontera et al.[25] showed that the muscles of older people can in fact improve their performance by hypertrophy as well as by learning.

PREVENTION OF FRAILTY. Buchner and Wagner[9] defined *frailty* as "the state of reduced physiologic reserve associated with increased susceptibility to disability." This is a more inclusive concept and more useful than the popular notion of frailty as "thin and weak." Although those who are thin and weak are most often frail, there are many obese people who are frail in that they have a poor strength index or strength-to-weight ratio. In either case, because of the loss of reserves, some disruption of their equilibrium by injuries or intercurrent illness might well lead to disability.

CONCEPTUAL MODEL OF FRAILTY. Figure 20–25 illustrates this conceptual model. When subjects drop below a certain level they have difficulty getting back to the minimal strength or aerobic capacity required to carry out their ordinary functions or activities of daily living (ADL). Likewise, the strength index, or power/weight ratio, is much more important than the absolute strength in the matter of self-perceived impairment. Figure 20–26 shows that there is a threshold of relative strength below which subjects are likely to see themselves as impaired and that this threshold is lower in older subjects (the "old" old) than in the younger geriatric subjects.[8] Strengthening muscles beyond this threshold does not yield any less perceived impairment, but would lead to a greater reserve so that they do not as easily slip beyond that threshold. There are two basic ways to improve the strength index. One is by strength training and the other is by weight reduction, especially fat reduction in the obese.

EXERCISE FOR FAT REDUCTION. Evidence is accumulating[2] that the size of the fat cells is regulated in the same way that many things in the body—such as oxygen tension, carbon dioxide tension, calcium levels, blood sugar, temperature—are regulated, and that this "lipostat"[34] is high in some persons and low in others, with all gradations in between. Efforts in fat reduction by severe caloric restriction have only a temporary result because the body

interprets this restriction as a famine, and mechanisms to defend the fat cell size over the long term are brought into play. The first line of defense is hunger. If this does not succeed in restoring the caloric intake, the next line of defense is energy conservation by decreased production of heat and a strong disinclination to exercise. People who attempt to control their weight without exercise generally have poor long-term results and tend to put on as much or more weight than they took off. In addition, when weight is lost by caloric restriction without exercise, there is some loss of muscle mass as well as fat. When the weight is put back on without exercise, it is mostly fat that is restored. The subject can wind up being more obese, in terms of percentage of body fat, than at the start of the program.

Muscles are the furnaces in which fat is burned. Progressive loss of muscle makes it more and more difficult to burn off even an ordinary intake of calories. The only way to successfully live below a high set-point, that is, to reduce body fat in the face of a high set-point, is by prolonged aerobic exercise.

Gwinup[31] recruited moderately obese subjects who were

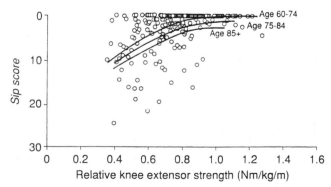

FIGURE 20–26 Relative knee extensor strength vs. SIP physical dimension score. Data from 434 adults aged 60 years or older with only every other point plotted. SIP scale is oriented so that higher scores, which reflect poorer function, are at the bottom. Curves derived from polynomial regression. (From Buchner DM, de Lateur BJ: The importance of skeletal muscle strength to physical function in older adults. Ann Behav Med 1991; 13:91–98.)

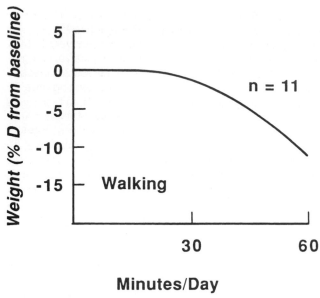

FIGURE 20–27 The relationship between percent change from baseline weight and time spent walking each day. (From Gwinup G: Weight loss without dietary restriction: Efficacy of different forms of aerobic exercise. Am J Sports Med 1987; 15:275–279.)

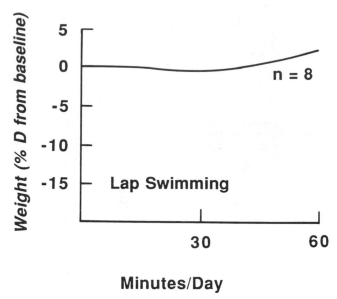

FIGURE 20–29 The relationship between percent change from baseline weight and time spent lap swimming each day. (From Gwinup G: Weight loss without dietary restriction: Efficacy of different forms of aerobic exercise. Am J Sports Med 1987; 15:275–279.)

all long-term failures at repeated dieting, and randomly assigned them to one of three groups: (1) walking or jogging, (2) stationary bicycling, and (3) lap swimming. They were exercised 7 days a week for 6 months. They were told to pay as little attention to dietary intake as they could, and no records were kept of their intake. Figures 20–27 through 20–29 show the results. The threshold for change in body weight was 30 min of exercise per day. Much more marked changes were observed with 60 min/day. The stationary cyclists and walkers lost 10% to 12% of their body weight, all fat. The swimmers, who exercised

60 min/day, showed no change in their body fat, but put on approximately 10% body weight, which was all muscle. This no doubt related to their initial condition of fitness (or lack thereof). The exact numbers varied depending upon greater or lesser extent of initial physical fitness. The figures do not imply that swimming cannot be useful as an adjunct to moderate caloric restriction, and in fact swimming may be the only type of exercise tolerable to those with certain disorders such as arthritis. They do imply that swimming alone is not a useful means of fat reduction.

REACTION TIME. Cross-sectional studies clearly indicate[11, 12, 21, 22] that fitter is faster. Spirduso has shown for such things as simple reaction time or movement time that, although young active subjects are fastest and old sedentary subjects are slowest, old active subjects may be as fast as or slightly faster than young sedentary subjects.[43–45] This does not, however, establish cause and effect. Perhaps the quickness of some subjects makes their motor activity more pleasurable and reinforcing, and actually promotes their participation in activity, rather than the activity promoting the quickness. More research needs to be done to determine whether putting older subjects on a progressive activity or exercise program will, in fact, improve their reaction time and general quickness. This is important to determine, since quick reaction time can be important in the prevention of falls.

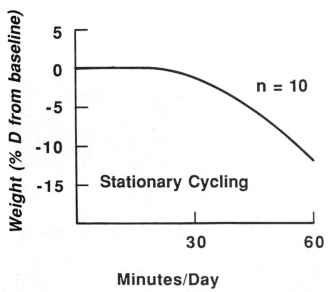

FIGURE 20–28 The relationship between percent change from baseline weight and the time spent each day in stationary cycling. (From Gwinup G: Weight loss without dietary restriction: Efficacy of different forms of aerobic exercise. Am J Sports Med 1987; 15:275–279.)

EQUIPMENT CONSIDERATIONS

Equipment ranges from simple resistance devices to complex electronic and compression devices available for both resistance and metabolic exercise.

SIMPLE RESISTANCE TRAINING DEVICES. These fall into two basic categories: elastic resistance and free weights. *Elastic resistance* devices, whether they involve tension or compression, have resistance that varies with and other information considered of interest. Some form of feedback is of great importance, both for its cue value and for its reinforcement or reward value. One need only look at the response to the daily report of the stock market to see the effect of information feedback about performance.

Relatively simple mechanical devices can be very useful in strengthening some muscles that are ordinarily awkward to subject to resistance training or to give relatively uniform stress and training throughout the range of motion. An example of the former would be the Elgin table, as shown in Figures 20–30 and 20–31. In Figure 20–30 the subject is strengthening his hip extensors in the supine position. The weight-and-pulley system allows exercise throughout at least 60 degrees' range with gradations from a very mild gravity-assisted exercise to severe progressive loading. These muscles, the hip extensors, cannot be satisfactorily trained with the subject in the prone (face downward) position, since the excursion of the muscles and of the joint has been used up in the extended position and the subject winds up forcibly hyperextending the lumbar spine. Likewise, the adductors are difficult to strengthen without special equipment. Figure 20–31 shows the Elgin table being used for adductor strengthening. This allows excursion for at least 45 degrees and perhaps as much as 70 degrees, again with a resistance ranging from a gravity-assisted exercise (the weight does not fully counterbalance the weight of the limb) to a heavy resistance.

Another simple device is the N-K table shown in Figures 20–32 and 20–33. This has at least two advantages, namely, relative safety and ease of attaching weights. A third advantage is the ability to change the point in the range at which the muscle begins to exert substantial force. In Figure 20–32, the force arm and weight arm are parallel and not much force is required in the early part of the range. In Figure 20–33, the relative positions of the force and weight arm have been changed such that a substantial force is required even before the 90-degree flexed position is reached.

Recent years have seen the development of accommodating resistance devices that not only allow concentric but

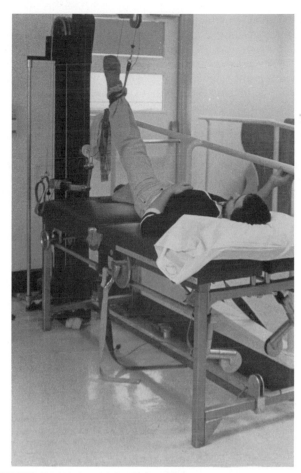

FIGURE 20–30 Use of the Elgin table to strengthen hip extensors in the supine position. (From de Lateur BJ, Lehman JF: Therapeutic exercise to develop strength and endurance. In Kottke FJ, Lehmann JF (eds): Krusen's Handbook of Physical Medicine and Rehabilitation, ed 4. Philadelphia, WB Saunders, 1990.)

displacement. Surgical tubing is a commonly used example of an elastic resistance device. It is available in bulk, and can be cut to the length needed. It has the advantage of portability, ease of use, low cost, and adaptability to a rather wide range of muscles. Such a device can even be used in the weightless environment of space. A disadvantage is the lack of feedback regarding what is done in precise terms or of the progress being made. With *free weights*, there is a similar advantage of simplicity and versatility for upper extremity use. For the lower limb, adaptations must be made such as the quadriceps boot or DeLorme boot, which is a short bar with circular weights and collar attachments with a metal plate and straps for attaching to the foot. The disadvantage is that numerous weights must be used to adapt to muscles of different strength or to the increasing strength of a given muscle. This greatly restricts the portability of such a device. Feedback of progress can be given by counting repetitions or recording the change in the amount of weight lifted.

COMPLEX RESISTANCE TRAINING DEVICES. The last decade has seen the development of a number of complex devices with computerized feedback systems attached. Such devices can be programmed to compare left and right sides, the quadriceps-to-hamstrings strength ratio,

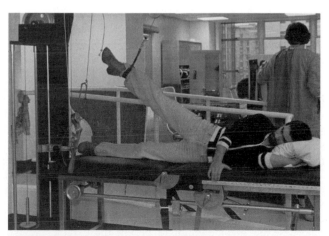

FIGURE 20–31 Use of the Elgin table for adductor strengthening. (From de Lateur BJ, Lehman JF: Therapeutic exercise to develop strength and endurance. In Kottke FJ, Lehmann JF (eds): Krusen's Handbook of Physical Medicine and Rehabilitation, ed 4. Philadelphia, WB Saunders, 1990.)

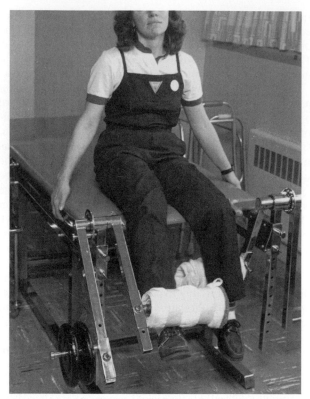

FIGURE 20–32 Little force is required using the N-K table, with the force arm and weight arm parallel. (From de Lateur BJ, Lehman JF: Therapeutic exercise to develop strength and endurance. *In* Kottke FJ, Lehmann JF (eds): Krusen's Handbook of Physical Medicine and Rehabilitation, ed 4. Philadelphia, WB Saunders, 1990.)

also allow eccentric exercise. With accommodating resistance devices, exemplified by the Cybex, Lido, KinCom, and Biodex, the operator presets a maximum contraction velocity. Accommodating resistance is developed when the subject attempts to accelerate the resistance arm beyond the preset limit. Passive devices such as the original Cybex and Cybex II permit only concentric training. For example, with training of the muscles about the knee, extension of the knee is produced by concentric contraction of the quadriceps, and flexion is produced by concentric contraction of the hamstrings. Robotic devices allow eccentric training as well. For example, the subject attempts to accelerate the (robotically moving) resistance arm as it moves toward extension of the knee, and to decelerate (eccentrically) the resistance arm as it moves toward flexion of the knee. This allows development of different levels of force with concentric and eccentric exercise. The latter appears to be very important for hypertrophy as well as for maximum strength training. In the early phases of strength training, however, it would be safer to use an all-concentric mode.

Newer devices involving electronic programming and compressors permit the partial counterbalancing of the subject's weight to permit upper body chin-and-dip exercise for subjects whose upper body strength would not otherwise be great enough to permit these rather severe exercises. Such a device is the Gravitron made by Stairmaster. The subject steps on the platform, turns on the device, and enters his or her accurate body weight, including the weight of the training clothes and shoes. The subject then

selects a level of intensity from 1 to 17. With the lowest level, the machine counterbalances all but a small fraction of the weight. As the subject's strength increases, he or she can increase either the amount of training weight (by decreasing the amount of the body weight counterbalanced), the number of repetitions, or both, with each chin-and-dip routine. It will be valuable when such devices as these are adapted for persons who use wheelchairs.

EQUIPMENT FOR METABOLIC EXERCISE. A wide range of equipment is available for metabolic exercise. Some devices are equipped with computers that estimate the number of calories expended based on body weight or typical efficiencies. Arm ergometers range from simple mechanical devices such as the Monark to the more complex electromechanical devices with attached computer software which not only give caloric readouts but also allow competition with built-in pacers. Depending upon the initial state of training of the subject and the intensity of the activity, strength may be increased as well as aerobic capacity.[10] Similarly, for the lower body, one may use a simple bicycle-type attachment to a chair, or one may go to the much more complex devices made by Cybex, Lifecycle, or other devices such as the Wind Trainer. These devices may be upright or recumbent. A device which allows simultaneous or separate use of the upper and lower limbs is the Schwinn Airdyne. The lower limbs move in a

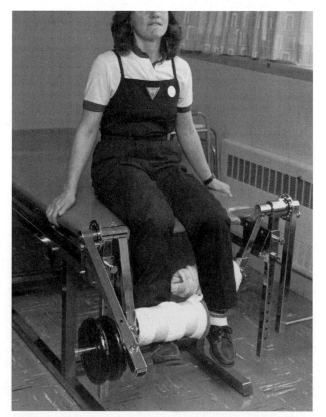

FIGURE 20–33 A substantial force is required even before the 90-degree flexed position is reached, simply by changing the positions of the force and weight arms on the N-K table. (From de Lateur BJ, Lehman JF: Therapeutic exercise to develop strength and endurance. *In* Kottke FJ, Lehmann JF (eds): Krusen's Handbook of Physical Medicine and Rehabilitation, ed 4. Philadelphia, WB Saunders, 1990.)

circular fashion as with any bicycle, and the upper limbs move in a forward-and-back motion as they move long levers. Resistance is provided by calibrated pedals. As with any wind resistance, the resistance is in proportion to the square of the speed. This type of device allows a very smooth aerobic employment of large numbers of muscles in a reciprocal fashion. As such, it is virtually ideal for burning fat (see Exercise for Fat Reduction).

Treadmills allow weightbearing aerobic activity at precise speeds and grades. The subject can clip an infrared-based pulse meter to the earlobe and monitor the pulse. Speed and grade are varied to bring the heart rate into the desired range.

References

1. Arkin AM: Absolute muscle power: The internal kinesiology of muscle, thesis. Department of Orthopedic Surgery, State University of Iowa, 1939.
2. Bennett W, Gurin J: The Dieter's Dilemma. New York, Basic Books, 1982.
3. Bergstöm J: Muscle electrolytes in man. Scand J Clin Lab Invest 1962; Suppl 14 (68):11–13.
4. Buchner DM, Cress ME, de Lateur BJ, et al: Variability in the effect of strength training on skeletal muscle strength in older adults. Facts Res Gerontol 1993; 7:143–153.
5. Buchner DM, Cress ME, de Lateur BJ, et al: The effect of strength and endurance training on gait, balance, fall risk and health services use in community living older adults. JAMA, in review.
6. Buchner DM, Cress ME, Wagner EH, et al: The role of exercise in fall prevention: Developing targeting criteria for exercise programs. In Vellas B, Troupet M, Rubenstein L, et al (eds): Falls, Balance and Gait Disorders in the Elderly. Amsterdam, Elsevier, 1992.
7. Buchner DM, Cress ME, Wagner EH, et al: The Seattle FICSIT/MoveIt Study: The effect of exercise on gait and balance in older adults. J Am Geriatr Soc 1993; 41:321–325.
8. Buchner DM, de Lateur BJ: The importance of skeletal muscle strength to physical function in older adults. Ann Behav Med 1991; 13:91–98.
9. Buchner DM, Wagner EH: Preventing frail health. Health Promotion Dis Prev 1992; 8:17.
10. Clarke DH, Stull GA: Endurance training as a determinant of strength and fatigability. Res Q 41:19–26, 1970.
11. Clarkson PM, Kroll W: Practice effects on fractionated response time related to age and activity level. J Motor Behav 1978; 10:275–286.
12. Clarkson-Smith L, Hartley AA: Relationships between physical exercise and cognitive abilities in older adults. Psychol Aging 1989; 4:183–189.
13. Côté C, Simoneau J-A, Lagassé P, et al: Isokinetic strength training protocols: Do they induce skeletal muscle fiber hypertrophy? Arch Phys Med Rehabil 1988; 69:281–285.
14. Cress ME, Esselman PC, de Lateur BJ, et al: Lower limb strength predicts VO2max in frail elderly. Med Sci Sports Exerc 1992; 24 (suppl 5):S15.
15. Crossman ERFW: A theory of the acquisition of speed-skill. Ergonomics 1959; 2:153–166.
16. de Lateur BJ, Lehmann JF: Therapeutic exercise to develop strength and endurance. In Kottke FJ, Lehmann JF (eds): Krusen's Handbook of Physical Medicine and Rehabilitation, ed 4. Philadelphia, WB Saunders, 1990, p 512.
17. de Lateur BJ, Lehmann JF, Fordyce WE: A test of the DeLorme axiom. Arch Phys Med Rehabil 1968; 49:245–248.
18. de Lateur BJ, Lehmann JF, Stonebridge JB, et al: Isotonic versus isometric exercise: A double-shift, transfer-of-training study. Arch Phys Med Rehabil 1972; 53:212–217.
19. DeLorme TL: Restoration of muscle power by heavy-resistance exercises. J Bone Joint Surg Am 1945; 27:645–667.
20. DeLorme TL, Watkins AL: Progressive Resistance Exercise. East Norwalk, Ct, Appleton-Century-Crofts, 1951.
21. Dustman RE, Emmerson RY, Ruhling RO, et al: Age and fitness effects on EEG, ERPs, visual sensitivity, and cognition. Neurobiol Aging 1990; 11:193–200.
22. Engle VF: The relationship of movement and time to older adults' functional health. Res Nurs Health 1986; 9:123–129.
23. Esselman PC, de Lateur BJ, Alquist AD, et al: Torque development in isokinetic training. Arch Phys Med Rehabil 1991; 72:723–728, 970 [erratum].
24. Fiatarone MA, O'Neill EF, Ryan ND, et al: Exercise training and nutritional supplementation for physical frailty in very elderly people. N Engl J Med 1994; 330:1819–1820.
25. Frontera WR, Meredith CN, O'Reilly KP, et al: Strength conditioning in older men: Skeletal muscle hypertrophy and improved function. J Appl Physiol 1988; 64:1038–1044.
26. Gollnick PD, Armstrong RB, Saltin B, et al: Effect of training on enzyme activity and fiber composition of human skeletal muscle. J Appl Physiol 1973; 34:107–111.
27. Gollnick PD, Armstrong RB, Saubert CW IV, et al: Enzyme activity and fiber composition in skeletal muscle of untrained and trained men. J Appl Physiol 1972; 33:312–319.
28. Gollnick PD, Karlsson J, Piehl K, et al: Selective glycogen depletion in skeletal muscle fibres of man following sustained contractions. J Physiol 1974; 241:59–67.
29. Gonyea WJ, Sale DG, Gonyea FB, et al: Exercise induced increased in muscle fiber number. Eur J Appl Physiol 1986; 55:137–141.
30. Gordon EE, Kowalski K, Fritts M: Protein changes in quadriceps muscle of rat with repetitive exercises. Arch Phys Med Rehabil 1967; 48:296–303.
31. Gwinup G: Weight loss without dietary restriction: Efficacy of different forms of aerobic exercise. Am J Sports Med 1987; 15:275–279.
32. Hellebrandt FA, Houtz SJ: Methods of muscle training: The influence of pacing. Phys Ther Rev 1958; 38:319–322.
33. Henneman E: Peripheral mechanisms involved in the control of muscle. In Mountcastle VB (ed): Medical Physiology, ed 13. St Louis, Mosby–Year Book, 1974.
34. Kennedy GC: The role of depot fat in the hypothalamic control of food intake in the rat. Proc R Soc Lond Biol 1953; 14:579–592.
35. Kottke FJ, Halpern D, Easton JKM, et al: The training of coordination. Arch Phys Med Rehabil 1978; 59:567–572.
36. Lacerte M: Effects of concentric versus combined concentric-eccentric isokinetic training programs on peak torque and hypertrophy of human quadriceps femoris muscle, thesis. University of Washington, Seattle, 1989.
37. Lacerte M, de Lateur BJ, Alquist AD, et al: Effects of concentric versus combined concentric-eccentric isokinetic training programs on peak torque of human quadriceps femoris muscle. Arch Phys Med Rehabil 1992; 73:1059–1062.
38. Milner-Brown HS, Stein RB, Lee RG: Synchronization of human motor units: Possible role of exercise and supraspinal reflexes. EEG Clin Neurophysiol 1975; 38:245–254.
39. Moritani T, DeVries HA: Neural factors versus hypertrophy in the time course of muscle strength gain. Am J Phys Med 1979; 58:115–130.
40. Moritani T, deVries HA: Potential for gross muscle hypertrophy in older men. J Gerontol 1980; 35:672–682.
41. Morris-Chatta R, Buchner DM, de Lateur BJ, et al: Isokinetic testing of ankle strength in older adults: Assessment of inter-rater reliability and of stability of strength over six months. Arch Phys Med Rehabil 1994; 75:1213–1216.
42. Mundale MO: The relationship of intermittent isometric exercise to fatigue of hand grip. Arch Phys Med Rehabil 1970; 51:532–539.
43. Spirduso WW: Reaction and movement time as a function of age and physical activity level. J Gerontol 1975; 30:435–440.
44. Spirduso WW: Physical fitness, aging and psychomotor speed: A review. J Gerontol 1980; 35:850–865.
45. Spirduso WW, Clifford P: Replication of age and physical activity effects on reaction and movement time. J Gerontol 1978; 33:26–30.
46. Stull GA, Clarke DH: High-resistance, low-repetition training as a determiner of strength and fatigability. Res Q 1970; 41:189–193.
47. Von Recklinghausen H: Gliedermechanik und Lähmungsprothesen. Berlin, Springer-Verlag, 1920.
48. Zinovieff AN: Heavy-resistance exercises: The "Oxford" technique. Br J Phys Med 1951; 14:129–132.

Manipulation, Traction, and Massage

**JAMES W. ATCHISON, D.O.,
SCOTT T. STOLL, D.O., PH.D., AND
WOLFGANG G. GILLIAR, D.O.**

In recent years, spinal care for back and neck disorders has moved toward an "aggressive conservative approach." Comprehensive treatment programs, often consisting of multidisciplinary teams, utilize many treatment modalities and activities. Within this conservative (nonsurgical) setting, both the traditional physical therapeutic interventions (heat, cold, exercise, traction, and massage) and "alternative" interventions (manipulation) have seen a growth in interest and research of indications, efficacy, dosage, and frequency. Also emerging within our present medical system is the trend of identifying cost-effective treatment options. The physiatrist needs to be well versed in the medical indications and contraindications for all conservative treatment options.

The physiatrist is not only well trained in the "functional approach" to a patient, but has the added advantage of working closely in a team concept with many of the health professionals who provide the therapeutic interventions discussed in this chapter. The physiatrist is ideally suited to provide efficient and cost-effective musculoskeletal care utilizing each of the conservative "tools" (heat and cold modalities, exercise, manipulation, traction, or massage) when indicated.

MANIPULATION

Definition and Goal of Manipulation

The International Federation of Manual Medicine defines *manipulation* as "the use of the hands in the patient management process using instructions and maneuvers to maintain maximal, painless movement of the musculoskeletal system in postural balance."[116] The goal of manipulation or manual medicine is to help maintain optimal body mechanics and to improve motion in restricted areas in order to enhance maximal, pain-free movement in postural balance and optimize function.[29, 43, 100] This is accomplished by treatments that attempt to both restore the mechanical function of a joint and normalize altered reflex patterns,[73, 77, 100] as evidenced by optimal range of motion, body symmetry, and tissue texture. The indications for and success of manual medicine techniques are determined by structural evaluation before and after treatment.[44, 73, 100]

Manual medicine involves manipulation of both spinal and peripheral joints, although lately most attention has been focused on spinal manipulation. The indications for the use of manual medicine are in part based on the theories of how manual medicine works, and include (1) restoration of normality and symmetry at either the disc or facet level[24, 52, 61]; (2) mechanically restoring optimal muscular and myofascial range and ease of motion to restore function[76]; (3) therapy-induced mechanical afferent signal transmission to the cord, which diminishes pain awareness through a gate theory effect[73, 76, 77]; (4) endorphin release, which increases the pain threshold and reduces pain severity[43, 61, 77]; and (5) placebo effect.[32] Selection of a particular manipulative modality is based on the disorder encountered and the theoretical mechanism of action of each treatment model.

The effectiveness and risks of manual medicine have been and continue to be controversial. As with most other forms of conservative treatment of spinal and other musculoskeletal pain syndromes, good randomized, controlled studies to determine long-term benefit have not been done. Studies have been limited by the variability of the clinical source and length of the pain, the variety of manual medicine techniques utilized, the difficulty of blinding treatments, and the lack of widely accepted or validated outcome measures.* There have been several recent reviews[75,]

---

*References 3, 4, 31, 39, 46, 55, 86, 92, 123.

[106, 118, 120] of manual medicine studies indicating effectiveness in certain subpopulations, especially in persons with low back pain of 2 to 4 weeks' duration.[46, 86] Manual medicine continues to be widely practiced and is in high demand by patients,[30] as evidenced by the estimated 12 million Americans[109] undergoing a total of 90 to 120 million manipulations per year.[50]

History

Manual medicine has regained popularity over the past 30 to 40 years, but it dates back to the time of Hippocrates (460?–377? BC), Galen (AD 131?–202?), and Ambroise Paré (AD 1510–1590).[49, 51] Many other physicians (e.g., Sydenham, Hahnemann, Boerhaave, Shultes) deviated from the traditional disease-oriented form of medicine during the 16th and 17th centuries,[51] but manual medicine fell out of favor until the 19th century. The pioneers of manual medicine at that time included the "bonesetters" of England (Richard Hutton, Wharton Hood, Sir Herbert Baker),[9, 51] Andrew Taylor Still, the founder of osteopathic medicine in 1874,[44] and Daniel David Palmer, the founder of chiropractic in 1895.[44, 51]

Still's philosophy stressed wellness and wholeness of the body and included (1) the unity of the body—all systems depend upon and influence all other systems; (2) the body's natural ability for self-healing; (3) the somatic component of disease; (4) the interrelationship of structure and function; and (5) the use of manipulative therapy.[44, 51] His use of manual medicine was based not only on restoration and maintenance of the structural-functional relationship within the musculoskeletal system but also on the neural-hormonal relationship with all other systems.

"Traditional" medical professionals have also recently become interested in manual medicine. James Mennell[94] and his son John McM. Mennell,[95] as well as Edgar and James Cyriax,[24] espoused the use of joint manipulation within the British medical community. James Cyriax, a British orthopedic surgeon, published several works beginning in the 1940s related to manipulation, which incorporated massage, traction, and injections[24] in the treatment programs. His books are still used today as reference texts for injections, but his use of manual medicine has not been as widely accepted. Travell's[130] use of manual techniques for examination purposes has been well accepted.

This section on manual medicine is intended as a brief introduction to these techniques. These techniques are widely used throughout the world, but clearly need considerable controlled research to establish efficacy and a physiological mechanism of action.

Nomenclature

In general, the benefits, risks, and effectiveness of manual medicine have remained controversial. One of the difficult concepts in learning and teaching manual medicine is to understand exactly what it is that is being manipulated. One of the things that has changed over the years is the nomenclature for the musculoskeletal abnormality or "manipulable lesion." At present, it is labeled "somatic dysfunction," while previous terms include "osteopathic

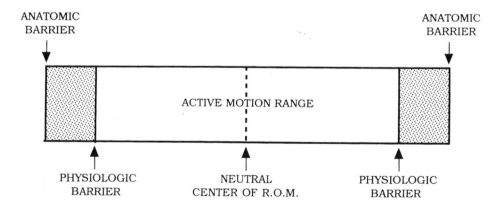

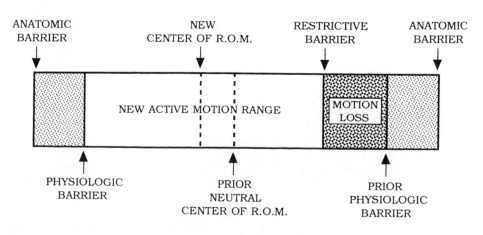

FIGURE 21–1 The barrier concept for normal joint motion *(top)* and with somatic dysfunction *(bottom)*. All joints have an optimal range of motion with a physiological and an anatomical barrier at each end. A restrictive barrier causes motion loss and establishes a new center to the active range of motion. This shift in neutral positioning aids in the diagnosis of somatic dysfunction. (From Kimberly PE: Formulating a prescription for osteopathic manipulative treatment. J Am Osteopath Assoc 1980; 79:508.)

lesion," "subluxation," "joint blockage," "loss of joint play," and "joint dysfunction."[76, 77, 100]

Somatic dysfunction is defined as impaired or altered function of related components of the somatic (body framework) system; skeletal, arthrodial, and myofascial structures; and related vascular, lymphatic, and neural elements.[62] Somatic dysfunction is manifested as *t*enderness, structural *a*symmetry, altered *r*ange of motion, and *t*issue texture changes (TART). There may be decreased mobility at any point along the physiological range of motion of any joint[5, 44, 73] (Fig. 21–1). Joint play[44, 49] is usually decreased and there is muscle contraction or tissue texture changes associated with the restricted joint. Early findings can include vasodilation, edema, pain, and tenderness, while chronically, fibrosis, paresthesia, itching, and persistent tenderness are more often present. These findings are generally asymmetrical, and there may be other reflex effects on the function of tissues that are innervated from the same spinal segmental level as the somatic dysfunction.[43, 73, 76, 77]

In the past, "manipulation" has traditionally been equated with high-velocity, thrusting techniques. There are actually a broad range of manipulative techniques. They have historically ranged from the "barbaric" stretching techniques of Hippocrates,[51] to Cyriax's combinations,[24] to the Mitchells' use of muscle forces[97, 98] (Figs. 21–2, 21–3, and 21–4) and Jones's passive positioning techniques.[7, 64] In the European literature the term *mobilization* means only thrusting procedures, but in the American literature manipulation encompasses mobilization techniques that utilize thrusting (high-velocity, low-amplitude, or impulse) forces (Figs. 21–5 to 21–10) as well as many other nonthrusting procedures (Table 21–1).

Indications and Goals of Treatment

Manual medicine techniques are potentially useful for treatment of any musculoskeletal problem demonstrating a loss of functional range of motion, change in tissue texture, or asymmetry of structural or segmental motion testing. This can include specific conditions such as acute and chronic cervical pain,[2, 88, 90] thoracic pain,[32, 87, 88, 90] rib strain,[44, 88] functional and mechanical low back pain,[4, 32, 55, 87, 90, 92] chronic low back pain,[4, 55, 64, 87, 92] bulging intervertebral disc,[23, 24, 88, 104] facet syndrome,[64] piriformis syndrome,[64] sciatica,[87] headaches,[32, 87, 88, 124, 132] and sacroiliac syndromes.[32, 49, 64, 90] However, classifying patients into clinical profiles of acute, subacute, and chronic pain to determine appropriateness for manipulation, as was recommended by the Rand Corporation study[22, 119] may be most appropriate. While there is no indication for manipulation when there is no evidence of somatic dysfunction,[73, 100] the effects of manipulation could extend beyond the somatic system through somatovisceral reflexes.

The assessment for somatic dysfunction starts with a history and physical examination that includes a careful neuromusculoskeletal examination. This is followed by a detailed structural evaluation which incorporates observation, palpation, and segmental motion testing. The structural examination requires sophisticated palpatory skills to assess for tenderness, body asymmetry, altered range of motion, and tissue texture changes (Greenman's "ten-step screen"; Table 21–2). Since it is possible to find some evidence of somatic dysfunction in asymptomatic persons[27] and multiple areas in acutely ill patients,[43] the practitioner must determine the clinical significance of each area of dysfunction and decide which areas require treatment.[73]

During the structural evaluation, the practitioner tries to determine the relationship of the physiological and anatomical barriers of the patient, while assessing for potential pathological barriers[5, 44, 73, 100] (see Fig. 21–1). The physiological barrier is at the end of normal, active range of motion. The anatomical barrier is at the end of passive motion, and if exceeded, leads to fracture, dislocation, or ligamentous damage. There is a normal feel of increasing resistance as the physiological and anatomical barriers are approached. A pathological barrier limits the usual range of motion or alters the ability of the tissues to perform throughout the usual range of motion, and is evidence of dysfunction.[43, 73]

Tissue texture changes are assessed by observation and palpation of the tissues from the most superficial tissues

Text continued on page 428

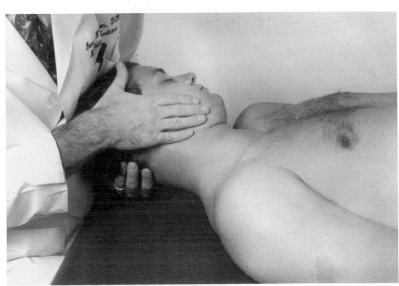

FIGURE 21–2 Hand placement for muscle energy treatment for the cervical spine with left rotation restriction. The right hand is resisting the patient's attempt to rotate the head to the right (midline). The more cephalad the dysfunction, the more the cervical spine is concomitantly flexed.

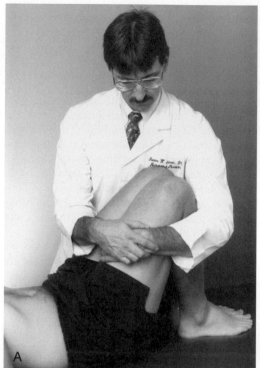

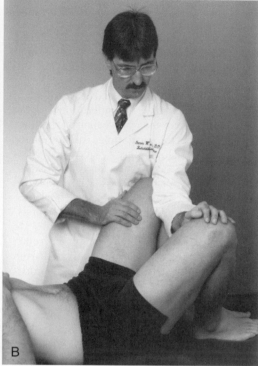

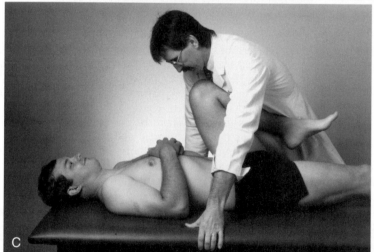

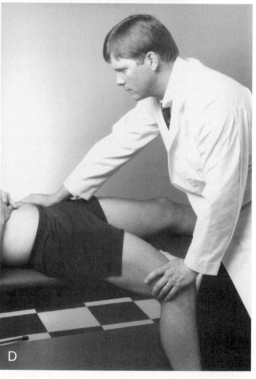

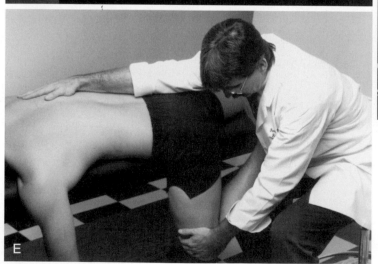

FIGURE 21–3 Muscle energy treatment for the sacroiliac joint may include: *(A)* supine, resisted abduction (both hips); *(B)* supine, resisted adduction (both hips); *(C)* supine, resisted extension (left hip); *(D)* supine, resisted flexion (right hip); and *(E)* prone, resisted flexion (left hip). These maneuvers are used in varying combinations depending on the patient's structural examination findings.

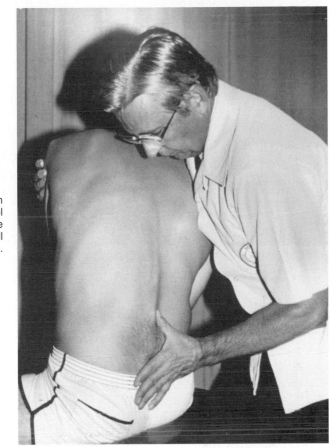

FIGURE 21–4 Muscle energy treatment for the lumbar spine with patient in a seated position. The left hand is stabilizing below the level of the dysfunction, while the thumb monitors segmental motion. The patient is being positioned from above toward the barrier and then will be resisted by the examiner's right arm (not visible in front of patient). (Courtesy of Dr. P. E. Greenman.)

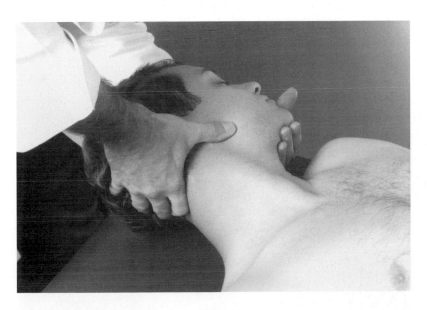

FIGURE 21–5 High-velocity, low-amplitude treatment for cervical spine dysfunction. The thrust is provided by the thumb and the metacarpophalangeal area of the index finger *(right)* through the transverse process being contacted to induce rotation and side-bending. With high cervical dysfunction the opposite *(left)* hand provides distraction prior to the thrust.

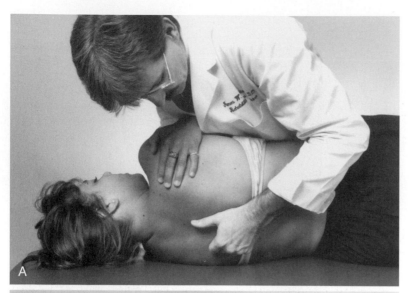

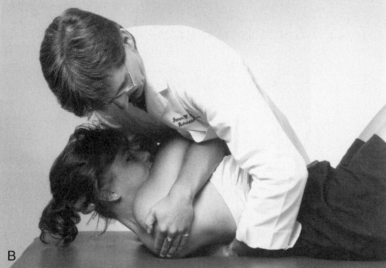

FIGURE 21–6 High-velocity, low-amplitude treatment (crossed-arm technique) for the thoracic spine in a supine position. *A,* The hand is placed with the thenar eminence contacting the transverse process of the dysfunctional vertebrae. *B,* The force is then directed to the hand by thrusting through the patient's ipsilateral (right) arm.

FIGURE 21–7 High-velocity, low-amplitude treatment (crossed-hands technique) for the thoracic spine with the patient in a prone position. The right thenar and left hypothenar areas are in contact with both transverse processes of the same vertebrae. The thrust will be directed through the body (inducing extension), with caudal movement of the right hand to induce side-bending and greater compressive force by the left hand to induce rotation.

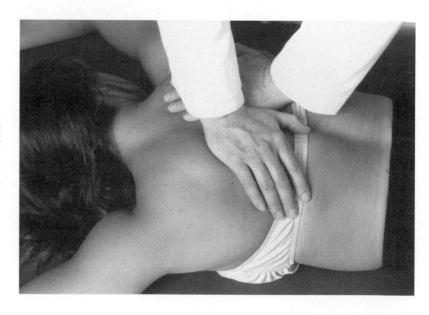

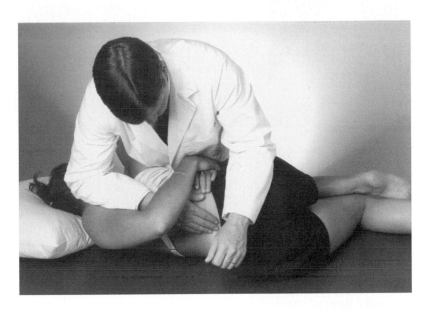

FIGURE 21–8 High-velocity, low-amplitude treatment for the lumbar spine with rotatory thrusting. The patient is positioned below the level of dysfunction in flexion, left rotation, and right side-bending, and above the level in extension, right rotation, and left side-bending. The practitioner thrusts by dropping his shoulders and forcing the patient's shoulder toward the table and the hip toward himself.

FIGURE 21–9 High-velocity, low-amplitude treatment for elevated first rib on the left. *A*, With the patient in a seated position, the right arm over the practitioner's leg allows increased left side-bending. Combined with left cervical rotation, the thrust is directed caudally and toward the midline. *B*, With the patient in a supine position, the head is rotated right to allow the right hand thrust to induce distraction, while the left hand thrusts caudally and toward the midline.

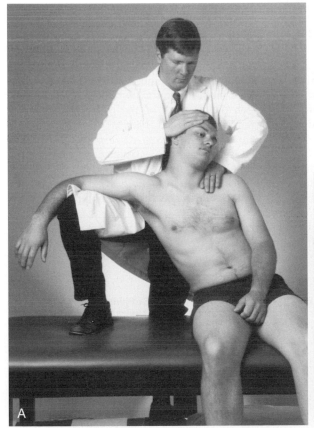

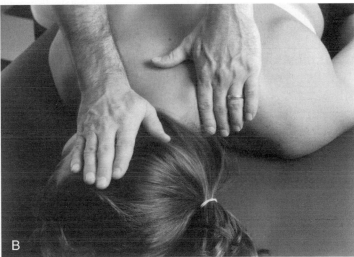

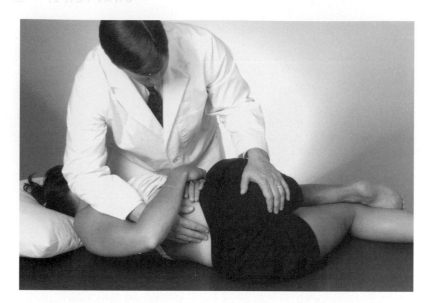

FIGURE 21–10 High-velocity, low-amplitude treatment for the sacroiliac joint. The positioning is similar to that for treatment of the lumbar spine; however, the direction of thrust with the bottom hand is more cephalad.

down to bony prominences. Muscle, tendon, and fascia may show signs of vasodilation, edema, flaccidity, contraction, contracture, or fibrosis individually or in various combinations. These changes lead to changes in skin temperature (hot or cold), moisture (sweating), and bogginess, ropiness, thickening, or firmness of muscles.[5, 44, 100] The examiner's hands must be skilled at assessing the various tissue levels and monitoring their response to treatment.

Musculoskeletal asymmetry can appear as structural or functional asymmetry or both. The examiner should observe for asymmetrical joint range of motion, tenderness, or strength, as well as asymmetrical posture, positioning, or muscle tone. Asymmetry directs the practitioner to an area or segment of somatic dysfunction. Range of motion is assessed grossly and segmentally by palpation and observation. The evaluation is designed to determine multilevel vs. segmental abnormalities and whether the primary dysfunction is hypomobility or hypermobility. A complete structural evaluation of all areas of the body (see Table 21–2) is necessary to differentiate primary and secondary areas of dysfunction. Once a diagnosis is established, the appropriate treatment technique(s) can be applied[5, 44, 73, 100, 105] (Fig. 21–11).

Classification of Manual Medicine Techniques

There are many different types of manual medicine treatments. They can be classified as soft tissue procedures,

articulatory procedures, and specific joint mobilization[44, 45, 73, 100] (see Table 21–1). All techniques can be classified by basic models of interaction with the body, while specific joint mobilization interventions can also be differentiated by the direction and type of treatment force.

The direction of treatment force is related to the barrier concept (see Fig. 21–1). *Direct methods*[43, 44, 73, 100] involve moving the patient toward the pathological barrier or in the direction of increasing resistance. Once the barrier has been engaged, a force is applied to move through the pathological barrier toward the normal physiological or anatomical barrier (see Fig. 21–2). *Indirect methods*[43, 44, 73, 100] involve movement of the patient or segment in the direction of least resistance, away from the pathological barrier. This allows the body's inherent and muscle energy forces to enhance mobility and allow changes in the relationship between the position of the pathological barrier and the normal physiological barrier. Often, *combined methods*[43, 44] are used. *Physiological response methods*,[43, 44, 61, 73, 100] such as respiratory assistance or exaggerated movements, may also be involved with both direct and indirect techniques. These are activities performed by the patient which increase the effect of the simultaneous practitioner-directed techniques.

The type of activating treatment force involved may be extrinsic or intrinsic. *Extrinsic forces*[5, 43, 73] are applied from the outside of the body and may be provided by gravity,

---

TABLE 21–1   Manual Medicine Techniques

Thrusting
    Mobilization with impulse/high-velocity, low-amplitude
Nonthrusting
    Mobilization without impulse/articulatory technique
    Muscle energy
    Counterstrain
    Functional technique
    Myofascial release
    Soft tissue
    Craniosacral

TABLE 21–2   Ten-Step Screening Examination

1. Gait analysis
2. Dynamic trunk mobility—lateral flexion
3. Standing flexion test
4. Seated flexion test
5. Upper extremity functional range of motion
6. Trunk rotation in a seated position
7. Trunk side-bending in a seated position
8. Passive movement of the head
9. Thoracic cage motion with respiratory function
10. Lower extremity range of motion

From Greenman PE: Principles of Manual Medicine. Baltimore, Williams & Wilkins, 1989, pp 20–27.

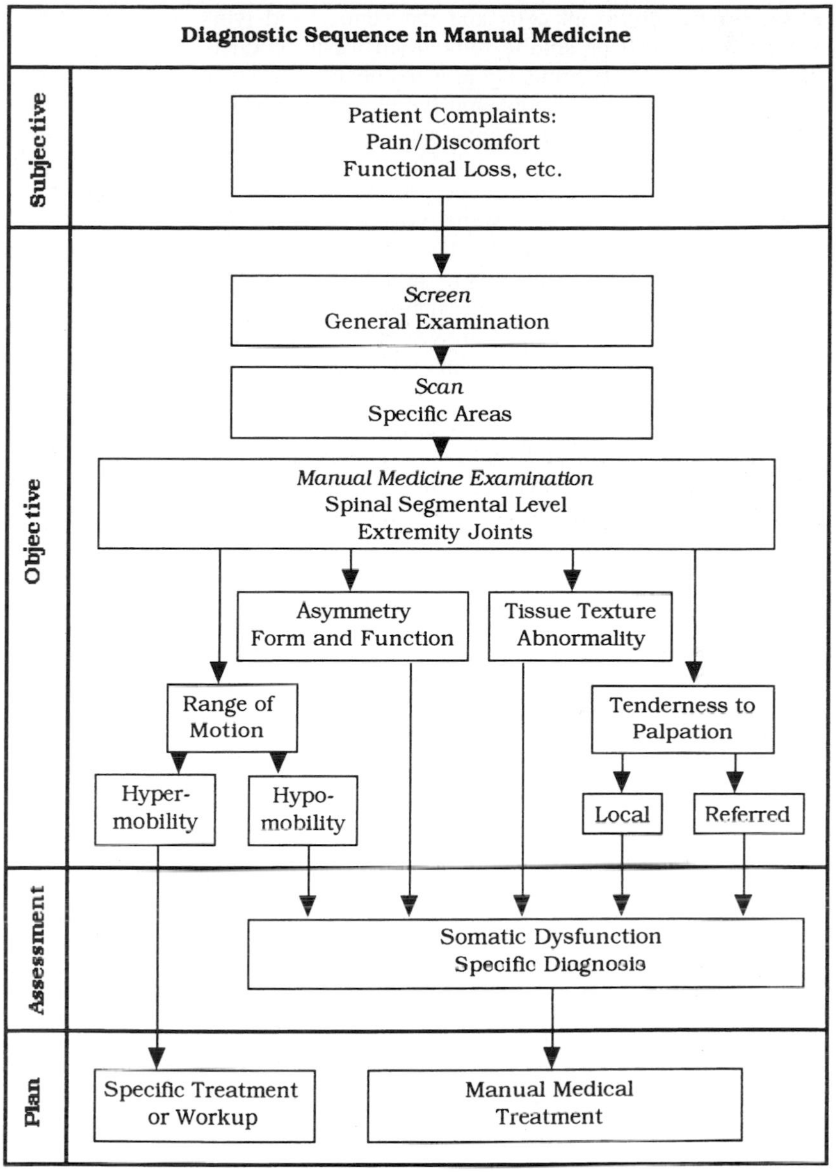

Diagnostic Sequence in Manual Medicine

Subjective

Patient Complaints:
Pain/Discomfort
Functional Loss, etc.

Objective

Screen
General Examination

Scan
Specific Areas

Manual Medicine Examination
Spinal Segmental Level
Extremity Joints

Asymmetry
Form and Function

Tissue Texture
Abnormality

Range of
Motion

Tenderness to
Palpation

Hyper-
mobility

Hypo-
mobility

Local

Referred

Assessment

Somatic Dysfunction
Specific Diagnosis

Plan

Specific Treatment
or Workup

Manual Medical
Treatment

FIGURE 21–11 The diagnostic sequence in manual medicine. The general and/or specific examinations reveal objective changes that help to establish the diagnosis of a specific somatic dysfunction and plan the appropriate treatment. (Modified from Neumann H-D: Introduction to Manual Medicine. Berlin, Springer-Verlag, 1989, p 14.)

straps, pads, or by another person. The practitioner may use a thrusting, springing, or guiding technique.[44] *Intrinsic forces*[43, 73] occur within a person's body and include muscle forces, respiratory forces, and inherent forces, such as fluctuating body fluid pressures.[44]

Manual medicine techniques can be classified by the force (intrinsic or extrinsic), the approach to the barrier (direct or indirect), or the patient contribution (active or passive).[43, 73, 100] The effects of these types of treatments can be conceptualized by five basic theoretical models: (1) postural-structural, (2) neurological, (3) respiratory-circulatory, (4) bioenergy, and (5) psychosocial.[43, 44, 61] Each of the various treatment techniques involves combinations of the models to explain the benefits and effects of the procedure.

The *biomechanical model* (postural-structural) looks at the human body as a linkage of bone, muscle, ligament, and fascia to form joints and allow function. Proper function requires symmetry of joints and other soft tissues as well as symmetrical strength. The therapeutic goal in this model is to restore balanced posture and efficient use of

the musculoskeletal system.[43] This can be accomplished with thrusting, soft tissue, articulatory, muscle energy, or traction techniques, and is especially useful around the pelvis.[44]

The *neurological* model is based on segmental facilitation,[76] proprioceptive function, and axonal transport within the central and peripheral nervous system.[61] An increase in afferent messages due to poor posture, visceral dysfunction, or trauma can lead to altered responses in the somatic or autonomic nervous system. Evidence of resulting increased autonomic efferent responses (sudomotor, pilomotor, or vasomotor) in this model is also used diagnostically to help determine areas of somatic dysfunction. The goal of manipulative treatment is to reduce mechanical stress on the musculoskeletal system, which reduces the altered afferent input.[43, 61] All manual medicine techniques have some effect in this model whether by changes in nociceptive input or by pain inhibition.

The *respiratory-circulatory* model[96] is based on the premise that the arterial system must be able to bring necessary nutrients to all cells and the venous and lymphatic systems must be able to remove all waste products from the tissues. The treatment goal is to enhance muscular function which controls venous and lymphatic circulation, as well as to stabilize the sympathetic nervous system responses that control arterial blood flow.[61] Directed circulatory-respiratory treatments focus on improving diaphragm, rib cage, and thoracic spine movement, especially in the area of the thoracic inlet. The normal body movements with respiration (inhalation straightens vertebral curves, externally rotates limbs; exhalation increases vertebral curves, internally rotates limbs)[44, 100] are also used indirectly with many treatment techniques to enhance their effectiveness.

The *behavioral-psychosocial* model considers the interaction between behavior and the disease process in regard to patients' reactions to environmental and psychological stressors. The body's response to these stressors can manifest itself in musculoskeletal symptoms leading to somatic dysfunction.[11, 122] Manual medicine treatment in this model is aimed at reducing hyperactivity of the sympathetic nervous system.[61] This model is closely related to the concept of "placebo effect," because it is difficult to measure objectively.

The *bioenergy* model[43, 61] is based on attempting to maintain a balance between the external environment and a person's inherent physiological reserves. Increased energy demands can result from trauma, infection, joint restriction, soft tissue dysfunction, or poor posture. This reduces the body's capacity to function at its normal level and its ability to respond or compensate to new stressors. Treatment techniques to reduce energy demands can be directed at muscles,[44, 97] fascia,[9, 134] joints,[5, 24, 44, 94, 95] or fluids (blood,[79] lymph,[140] cerebrospinal [CSF][124, 132]). The restoration of the body's inherent fluid forces by "mobilizing" the brain, meninges, and CSF is the postulated hallmark of craniosacral manipulation.[124, 132]

Specific Types of Manual Medicine Techniques

Mobilization with impulse is more commonly known as the thrust maneuver[52] or the high-velocity, low-amplitude (HVLA) form of manual medicine. This is a direct form of treatment, and is commonly prescribed for cervical[5, 8, 24, 35, 44, 60, 75, 109] (see Fig. 21–5), thoracic[24, 35, 44] (see Figs. 21–6 and 21–7), lumbar* (see Fig. 21–8), rib[5, 35, 44, 87] (see Fig. 21–9), sacroiliac[5, 24, 32, 35, 44, 87] (see Fig. 21–10), and extremity[5, 24, 44, 87] dysfunctions. These are the techniques most commonly associated with the term *manipulation*. They are frequently performed because they are the quickest mode of releasing a dysfunctional segment or region. There is often a resulting "crack" or "pop" that occurs when a restricted joint is released.[93, 115] The noise itself has no effect on the treatment outcome. The reintroduction of movement into the restricted or dysfunctional area is the treatment benefit.[52]

The preparation of the patient for HVLA is as important as the thrust itself.[44, 52, 100] While the positioning by itself may be therapeutic, it also allows the treatment to be

directed to the barrier of the restricted segment, while protecting the other spinal segments[32] (see Figs. 21–5 to 21–10). The more precise the localization by positioning, the less thrusting force necessary for treatment. High thrusting forces should be avoided to prevent possible soft tissue or joint injury. After localizing and engaging the barrier, there is a momentary waiting period to allow the patient to relax the muscles in the area. During this time, the practitioner monitors the patient's respiratory cycle, and delivers the treatment thrust at the point of deepest exhalation. This allows maximal relaxation of the surrounding muscles. The thrust (or impulse) is directed perpendicular or parallel to the tangential plane of the facet joint surface[52, 100] depending on the structural findings. The force of the thrust varies with the location of the treatment, with the cervical area requiring the least and the thoracic area the greatest force.[53] The greater the forces required to position and stabilize the patient in the prethrust position, the greater the thrusting force required.[53] The duration of the thrust is very short, less than 0.5 sec.[129] Immediate relief of pain symptoms may not occur, but an improvement in the range of motion of the treated joint should occur.

The patient has to be relaxed to get maximal effectiveness. Tightening of the muscles, or "guarding," can limit the amount of movement resulting from the thrust and increase the amount of thrusting force required. Treatment should always be provided in a pain-free direction, enhancing relaxation and avoiding guarding. Somatic dysfunction rarely restricts movement along all planes simultaneously.[100] If a patient cannot be positioned without exacerbating pain in any of the three planes (flexion-extension, side-bending, rotation), this is an indication that the pain or restriction is likely to be from a source other than somatic dysfunction[49] (i.e., an inflammatory or destructive process; Table 21–3).

Many other manual medicine techniques have been commonly used by practitioners. These treatment techniques involve use of soft tissue release,[9, 44, 45, 87, 134] as well as

TABLE 21–3　Contraindications to High-Velocity Manipulation Techniques

Unstable fractures
Severe osteoporosis
Multiple myeloma
Osteomyelitis
Primary bone tumors
Paget's disease
Any progressive neurological deficit
Spinal cord tumors
Cauda equina compression
Central cervical intervertebral disc herniation
Hypermobile joints
Rheumatoid arthritis
Inflammatory phase of ankylosing spondylitis
Psoriatic arthritis
Reiter's syndrome
Anticoagulant therapy
Congenital bleeding disorder
Acquired bleeding disorder
Inadequate physical and spinal examination
Poor manipulative skills

From Haldeman S: Spinal manipulative therapy in the management of low back pain. *In* Finneson BE (ed): Low Back Pain. Philadelphia, JB Lippincott, 1980, p 250.

---

*References 4, 5, 24, 31, 35, 39, 44, 46, 55, 75, 86, 92, 109, 120, 123.

positioning,[6, 7, 12, 64] active muscle firing patterns,[5, 40, 44, 97, 98] and low-velocity oscillations.[18, 89, 90, 92, 103, 104, 123] These techniques are more time-consuming than HVLA techniques, but generally have fewer contraindications and require less training to be able to perform them safely. These techniques can be used as first-line treatments or in combination with thrusting techniques to enhance treatment.

The *articulatory technique*,[44, 100] or mobilization without impulse, is a direct segmental technique in which a combination of leverage, patient ventilatory movement, and a fulcrum is used to achieve mobilization of the dysfunctional segment. This is most often done by repeatedly applying a low-velocity, high-amplitude force to directly engage and then move away from the barrier.[89, 90, 103] By repeatedly "tapping" on the barrier, the technique is designed to gently move the pathological barrier toward the physiological barrier (see Fig. 21–1) improving the range of motion. This is the graded oscillation form of the technique, but less commonly a progressive or sustained loading technique is used.[105] These procedures are an extension of the diagnostic evaluation for range of motion, and can be combined with soft tissue or thrust techniques.[44]

The *muscle energy (ME) technique*[40, 97] was introduced by F. L. Mitchell Sr.[98] and involves voluntary contraction of muscles (isometric, concentric, or eccentric) by the patient against resistance supplied by the practitioner (see Figs. 21–3 through 21–5). This is an active manual medicine treatment that can be applied to most muscle groups in the body as either a direct or indirect technique.[97] The goal is to increase the mobility of hypomobile segments, increase functional range of motion, allow the return of symmetrical motion to affected segments, strengthen weakened muscles, and lengthen contracted or spastic muscles.[40, 44] ME is also believed to have an effect on the nervous system.[40, 44, 77, 107] It is a relatively safe technique, with few contraindications, since the patient controls the degree of force applied to the dysfunctional area.

ME involves re-lengthening shortened or hypertonic muscles, which allows the attached bones to return to their normal neutral position and resume a normal range of motion. This is most often performed as an isometric contraction while movement is limited at the distal attachment. The muscle contraction provides a force to move the proximal segment, and following relaxation of the muscle a longer resting length may be acquired. By using an isometric contraction, the segment to be treated can be localized and stabilized, and pain is limited since only segmental movement is occurring. The isotonic form of ME uses either concentric or eccentric contractions and the law of reciprocal innervation and inhibition.[44]

Most practitioners perform the direct form of ME manipulation. The patient is passively moved to the pathological barrier or restriction, and then actively contracts the muscles in an attempt to move away from the barrier while the practitioner resists the movement. The patient tries to maintain a mild-to-moderate degree of sustained contraction for 3 to 7 sec. With instruction by the practitioner the patient chooses the degree of active contraction, avoiding contracting hard enough to induce pain. The practitioner provides only static resistance, and does not try to induce movement during the contraction.

Following the contraction the patient completely relaxes

the muscles, which usually takes 1 to 2 sec. The patient should not be moved during this time. Then the practitioner passively moves the patient to the new barrier. This step-by-step procedure is repeated three to five times, in an attempt to increase muscle length and advance motion past the pathological barrier toward the physiological barrier following each contraction. Physical therapists refer to this technique as "contract-relax."[126]

ME techniques can be used effectively for a somatic dysfunction in nearly any area of the body. The cervical spine[5, 44, 97] (see Fig. 21–2) and sacroiliac and pelvic regions[5, 44, 97] (see Fig. 21–3) respond readily to ME. These areas are more easily treated by novice practitioners and can be learned by patients as part of a home exercise program. Lumbar[5, 44, 97] (see Fig. 21–4) and thoracic spine dysfunctions,[5, 44, 97] rib lesions,[5, 44, 97] and muscle imbalances[5] in the limbs are more difficult to treat with ME and require more practitioner expertise.

Strain and counterstrain (CS) is a manual medicine technique that attempts to passively place a spinal segment or other joint into its position of greatest comfort or ease. This is an indirect, functional technique[6, 44] developed by Jones[64] that tries to relieve painful dysfunction through a reduction in inappropriate afferent proprioceptor activity.[40, 77, 107] The goal of the positioning treatment is to increase functional pain-free range of motion, re-lengthen contracted or hypertonic muscles, allow return of symmetrical segmental motion, and reduce pain.[64] The technique is very well tolerated by patients and has widespread application. It requires no active muscle movement or thrusting and relies on patient interaction to determine the position of maximal relief.[7]

Treatment with CS is based on the hypothesis that somatic dysfunction from an injury does not result from strain of the muscle itself but from the reaction of the body to the strain, that is, the "counterstrain." The body responds to the strain or overstretch by trying to suddenly and forcibly return the joint or spinal segment to neutral. The overstretched muscle's proprioceptors report strain even before returning to neutral owing to the rapid change in the length and velocity.[76] It is postulated that this outpouring of sensory feedback from the annulospiral nerve endings in the muscle spindle maintains continual reflex firing of the gamma motor neuron,[107] maintaining a hypertonic muscle.[40, 77] Treatment of this type of dysfunction aims to return the muscle-joint complex to its original condition prior to the onset of reflex muscle hypertonicity. This allows a reduction in firing of the primary proprioceptive nerve endings, and then a slow re-lengthening of the muscle to its original neutral position so that the muscle spindle can reset itself.

Structural evaluation is required prior to using CS treatment to determine the areas of dysfunction and specify the localization of Jones's "tender points."[7, 12, 64] These are palpably tense and tender areas located deep in the tissue, and may involve muscle, fascia, tendon, or ligament. The tender points may be widely distributed throughout the body, and are not located only in the area of dysfunction. According to Jones the tender points follow a reflex pattern, and their location is reproducible for each specific spinal level of somatic dysfunction. They are different from the "myofascial trigger points" described by Travell.[130] For each tender point there is a position that will relieve the pain, and while the treatment positions for each point have also been predetermined, certain basic principles allow the treatment to be individualized for each patient.

Following localization of a tender point, the practitioner uses one hand on the point as a "monitoring hand" while the other hand moves the patient into various positions trying to shorten and relax the muscle. The monitoring hand discerns tissue relaxation vs. tightening, and verbal interaction with the patient is used to localize the exact position that provides the greatest relief of pain. In general, the nearer the tender point is to the midline, the more flexion or extension is needed for relaxation. The more lateral to the midline, the more side-bending (abduction-adduction) will be needed. Internal or external rotation of the closest appendage may give further relief of pain.

Once the position of relief (ease) is determined, it should be maintained for 90 to 120 sec. During this time, the monitoring hand may continue to provide palpatory pressure on the tender point. This is somewhat controversial, as some practitioners feel this may be associated with a form of acupressure. Continual "fine-tuning" may occur during the 120 sec of positioning, and often as the tender point releases the monitoring hand will feel a pulsatile sensation.

It is essential to return the patient to the neutral position very slowly in order to let the muscle spindles reset themselves.[40, 77] Often it is best to move in only one plane at a time (rotation, then side-bending, etc.). The patient must remain relaxed and should not assist by firing any of the involved muscles. After returning to neutral, the patient should be re-evaluated structurally, as there may be other tender points that still require release, or other forms of manual medicine that may be indicated.

CS has widespread indications for symptomatic relief, and often allows a patient to begin an active back treatment program earlier than would otherwise be possible. The structural evaluation performed with the use of CS includes searching for tender points in the chest, anterior abdomen, and anterior pelvis. Identification and treatment of these anterior tender points, which are associated with thoracic, lumbar, and sacral dysfunction, may contribute to the therapeutic armamentarium of many practitioners.[64]

There are few contraindications associated with this passive, indirect technique, and it can be safely performed by the novice practitioner or incorporated into a home treatment program. A limiting factor to CS treatment is the time required to release each tender point. Since each point requires 1½ to 2 min to treat, a patient with diffuse or multiple tender points may benefit just as readily from other techniques. The other limiting factor with CS treatment is the varying length of time during which the treatment may provide symptomatic relief. These techniques must therefore be prescribed appropriately since some patients become "addicted" to this form of passive release and do not assume enough active responsibility for their own recovery.

Other *functional techniques*[6, 44] also involve the evaluation and treatment of the quality of motion instead of the range of motion. A palpating hand is placed over the dysfunctional segment to "listen" while motion is introduced into the area actively by the patient or passively by the practitioner. The "listening hand" is trying to determine which direction allows easy and free movement (ease) and which direction is difficult (bind). Motion is introduced in every direction in a sequential pattern while monitoring for ease in each direction. Functional techniques are theoretically a part of the neurological model and can be used in both acute and chronic problems because they are not painful and depend on a release of soft tissue rather than a structural change.[44]

Myofascial release[9, 44, 134] involves treatment of the neuromuscular-somatic unit as a whole, and combines soft tissue, ME, and craniosacral principles. It involves the release of somatic dysfunction or related imbalances, whether affecting a discrete region, a vertebral segment level, an entire limb, or the whole body. This can be accomplished by using intrinsic and extrinsic forces with direct or indirect methods. Direct treatment engages the restrictive barrier and pushes against it with a constant force until tissue release occurs. With the indirect technique, dysfunctional tissues are guided along the path of least resistance until free movement is achieved. Each of the techniques uses a combination of manual traction and twisting maneuvers to achieve tension on the soft tissues which will effect biomechanical and reflex changes.[44, 134]

The goal of treatment with myofascial release is to restore myofascial continuity, integrity, and symmetry. This will enhance mobility and strength as well as muscular coordination. Initial treatment is directed at the short, tight muscle groups. The stretch should always follow the long axis of the fascia, and then a twisting force may be added to localize the traction. Palpation throughout the treatment process is important to monitor tissue response, while following the concept that tightness creates and weakness permits asymmetry.[44] The palpating hand focuses on the patient's ability to relax and respond to movement of the tissues. This includes skeletal and soft tissue conformation; neurological status, including pain-related factors; thermoregulatory states; shifting locomotor demands; physical conditioning; and body positioning.[134] The treatment process is a dynamic process which cannot be predetermined by the practitioner, but must be continually adjusted according to the response of the patient's tissues. General principles have been established by Ward[134] and others, but experience and expert palpatory skills are essential to treatment success. This form of manual medicine is becoming widely used by physical therapists in both acute and chronic musculoskeletal pain syndromes, but further research is needed to determine long-term outcome benefits and cost-effectiveness.

Craniosacral therapy[44, 124, 132, 134] is a manual medicine technique for diagnosis and treatment of the body by way of the primary respiratory mechanism. It was pioneered by Sutherland,[124] who perceived that the cranial bones undergo subtle cyclical motion about the cranial sutures at a rate of 8 to 12 Hz. This motion is felt most easily at the cranium and the sacrum, but is palpable everywhere in the body. Sutherland termed this inherent motion the *primary respiratory mechanism* and claimed that it comprised five body components: (1) the articular mechanism of the cranial bones, (2) involuntary motion of the sacrum between the ilia, (3) fluctuation of the CSF, (4) reciprocal tension of the dural membranes, and (5) inherent motion of the central nervous system.

Craniosacral therapy consists of assessing the amplitude, rate, symmetry, and quality of the primary respiratory mechanism. Gentle pressure applied to the body in rhythm with the palpated inherent motion can be used to passively move toward optimal mobility.[124, 132] There has been growing interest by various practitioners as to the applicability and appropriateness of craniosacral therapy in patients following head trauma and with postconcussive syndrome. While there has been basic anatomical and physiological research done on the movement of the cranial sutures and CSF dynamics,[1, 102] craniosacral therapy to date has more hypothetical than hard scientific support.

Soft tissue techniques can involve lateral stretching (Fig. 21–12), linear stretching (Fig. 21–13), deep pressure (Fig. 21–14), or traction (Fig. 21–15), or any combination of these, directed at separating the origin and insertion of a muscle.[44] It incorporates procedures similar to traditional massage, but may also include acupressure, Travell's trigger point release,[130] diaphragmatic release,[44] mesenteric release,[44] and lymphatic drainage techniques.[44, 79, 140] Soft tissue techniques can be used for generalized treatment programs in patients with chronic illnesses such as multiple sclerosis, hemiplegia, or any immobility syndrome. They are also used preceding other forms of more active treatment programs or manipulation.

The *lymphatic pump*[44] is a soft tissue technique that utilizes muscle forces and intrathoracic pressure changes to enhance lymphatic flow. Intermittent compression of the thoracic cage in a rhythmic fashion enhances the return of lymph through the thoracic inlet, which relieves vascular engorgement to allow resumption of normal tissue motion. Other lymphatic techniques can be similarly performed with repetitive movements of the arms or legs. These techniques are often performed distal to proximal, similar to centripetal massage techniques[24, 56, 57, 138] used to relieve edema in the extremities.

Contraindications and Risks

Manual medicine techniques should be used only in patients having a somatic dysfunction. Each type of treatment technique has its own set of contraindications. Mobilization with impulse (HVLA) has the greatest number of contraindications[49] (see Table 21–3). Once the contraindica-

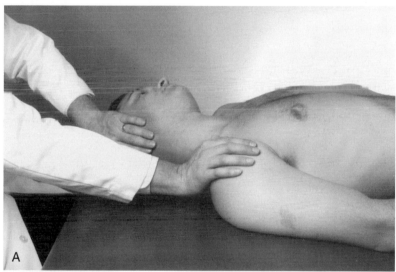

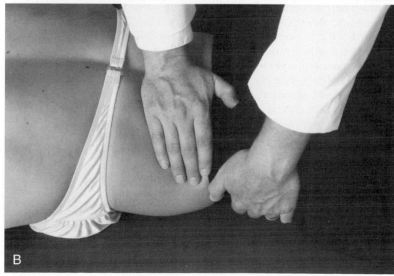

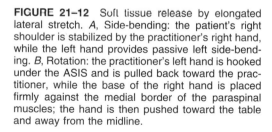

FIGURE 21–12 Soft tissue release by elongated lateral stretch. *A,* Side-bending: the patient's right shoulder is stabilized by the practitioner's right hand, while the left hand provides passive left side-bending. *B,* Rotation: the practitioner's left hand is hooked under the ASIS and is pulled back toward the practitioner, while the base of the right hand is placed firmly against the medial border of the paraspinal muscles; the hand is then pushed toward the table and away from the midline.

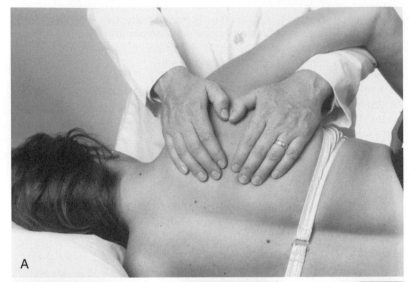

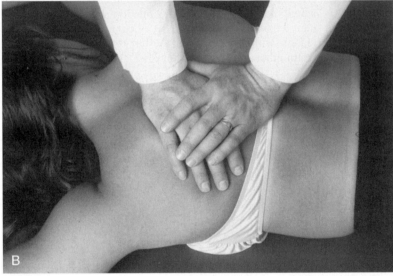

FIGURE 21–13   Linear soft tissue release by scapular mobilization. *A,* Side-lying: the practitioner's finger pads are hooked under the medial border of the scapula and lifted upward. *B,* Prone: the thenar eminences of both hands are placed in contact with the medial border of the scapula and a gentle force is directed toward the table and laterally.

tions and specific treatment procedures have been appropriately established for a particular clinical situation, the incidence of "complications" decreases.[28]

Absolute contraindications to HVLA treatment include malignancy, osteoporosis, and other metabolic bone diseases; fracture; aseptic necrosis; primary joint disease (rheumatoid arthritis, infectious arthritis); genetic disorders with hypermobility (Down syndrome, Ehler-Danlos syndrome, Marfan syndrome); aneurysm; congenital or acquired bleeding disorder; anticoagulant therapy; myelopathy; and cauda equina syndrome.[49, 129] Spondylolisthesis and acute herniated nucleus pulposus with radiculopathy may contraindicate thrusting techniques, but this is not absolute.[49] Soft tissue, ME, CS, and myofascial release techniques have few contraindications, since they have a much lower inherent risk to the patient than HVLA thrusting techniques.

There are a few general precautions to be followed for all manual medicine techniques for safety and effectiveness. Neck positioning is important, especially in elderly patients. Prolonged neck extension should be avoided because of potential vertebral artery abnormalities, and also

the likelihood of irritating arthritic facet joints or compromising cervical nerve roots. Prolonged, extreme neck rotation may be dangerous in patients with carotid artery disease. All levels of the spine should be carefully positioned in persons with significant osteoporosis, as marked or prolonged flexion may lead to compression fractures (see Chapter 40). Extension should be limited in patients with lumbar stenosis (see Chapter 39). With all techniques the patient must be kept relaxed and breathing freely to avoid excessive changes in blood pressure, as well as increased abdominal or spinal canal pressure.

There are potential side effects that can occur even when manual medicine treatment is successful, including increased autonomic effects (hypotension, menses, perspiration, etc.) and a transient increase in discomfort.[48] Other side effects are mostly related to inadequate skill of the practitioner, improper diagnosis, or the use of an inappropriate technique for a particular dysfunction.[48] Catastrophic outcomes have been reported such as stroke,[78, 110, 121] quadriplegia,[109] cauda equina syndrome,[109] cardiac arrest,[41] and even death,[20] mostly the result of manipulation of the cervical spine with improper technique or misdiagnosis, or

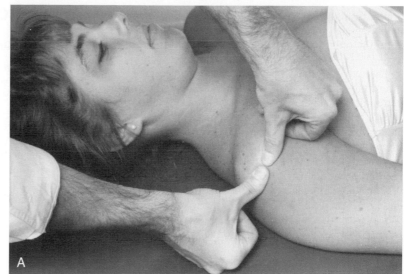

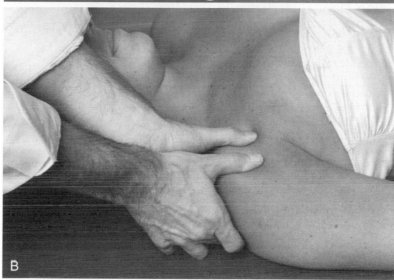

FIGURE 21–14 Soft tissue release by deep friction massage. *A*, Supraspinatus tendon: the thumb pads are placed between the acromion and the humeral head, with deep pressure used to roll the fingers back and forth without losing contact with the skin. *B*, Biceps tendon: the entire thumb is placed on either side of the tendon as it progresses cephalad. Deep pressure is applied by rhythmically bringing the thumbs together without losing contact with the skin.

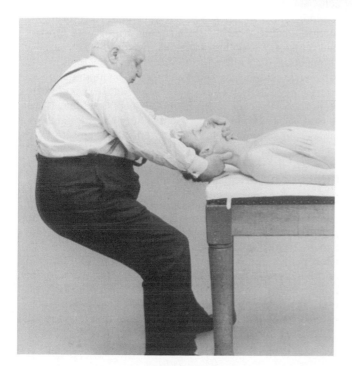

FIGURE 21–15 Manual cervical traction. The force is applied in a straight line, pulling predominantly with the left hand. The right hand is used as a fulcrum to keep the cervical spine in neutral or in slight flexion. (From Cyriax JH, Cyriax PJ: Cyriax's Illustrated Manual of Orthopedic Medicine, ed 2. Oxford, Butterworth-Heinemann, 1993, p 174.)

both.[22] While these cases provide the basis for most arguments against the use of manual medicine, their frequency is rare at only one such case per 1 to 1.5 million manipulations.[109]

There have been reports of manual medicine causing progressive neurological changes in a radicular pattern,[109] vertebral osteomyelitis,[84] compression fractures,[47] and worsening of herniated discs.[59, 111] Since these disorders have a highly variable course, it is very difficult to determine for certain whether the conditions in these cases worsened owing to the manipulation or as a result of the natural course of the disease process. Although some practitioners advocate manipulative procedures in the presence of a disc herniation, the general guideline is to not use thrusting techniques (unless in the hands of a highly trained practitioner). Nonthrusting techniques are typically preferred in these cases.

Using Manual Medicine in Practice

The philosophies of the use of manual medicine and the practice of physical medicine and rehabilitation (PM&R) are consistent in their goals to increase function. In manual medicine this increase in function is gauged by increased motion and body symmetry.

The structural examination to determine dysfunction required for manual medicine is a hands-on approach that can easily be incorporated into the routine physiatric physical examination. Greenman[44] (see Fig. 21–4) has proposed a ten-step examination to screen for structural abnormalities, many of which are already done in a routine physiatric examination. The ten-step screen is outlined in Table 21–2.

Surface landmarks are also helpful in the static examination of posture. These include asymmetry of the shoulders, scoliosis, asymmetry at the lumbosacral junction, joint dysfunction in the legs, and leg length differences.[100] Segmental dysfunction influences the overall motion, loading, and the forces of the rest of the spine and the lower extremities.

The practitioner's goal is to determine whether or not there is a treatable dysfunction. If so, the treatment can be easily incorporated into the office visit immediately following the examination or a patient may be referred to a practitioner trained in manual medicine. Some general guidelines for the duration and frequency of manipulative treatment have been proposed, but these have only addressed HVLA or thrusting techniques.[22, 119] Treatment plans for all types of manual medicine must be developed on an individual basis in relation to the patient's structural diagnosis, the type and location of the somatic dysfunction, the type of manual medicine techniques being performed, and the patient's response to treatment. With each patient visit, the practitioner must re-evaluate these parameters to determine the need for continued manipulative treatment. The indiscriminate use of manual medicine for weeks or months without the proper indications is inappropriate.

As with most types of treatment for musculoskeletal pain, manual medicine assumes but one part of a comprehensive treatment program. Some forms of manual medicine are more easily incorporated into a home program, such as ME and CS. These treatments should be associated with, and can be included in, an active exercise program.[5, 72, 125]

TRACTION

Definition and Goals

Traction is the technique in which a pulling force is used to stretch soft tissues and to separate joint surfaces or bone fragments.[54] The goal of spinal traction is to obtain pain relief and functional improvement. Traction involves applying a force of sufficient magnitude and duration in the proper direction, while simultaneously resisting movement of the body by an equal and opposing force. With proper positioning of the patient and the correct angle of pull, traction may be localized to a specific spinal area. The force is generally applied through a mechanical pulley system with weights, and stabilization by either a chin strap for the cervical spine (Figs. 21–16 and 21–17) or a pelvic belt for the lumbar spine[112] (Figs. 21–18 and 21–19). The various techniques may be performed in the standing, sitting, or lying position (see Figs. 21–16 to 21–19; Fig. 21–20).

History

Traction was originally and more extensively utilized in the treatment of fractures and dislocations. Hippocrates recommended the use of traction with spinal disorders such as scoliosis and excessive kyphosis.[55, 58] The early use of traction was limited by soft tissue or skin interfacing with the traction apparatus, so that any pull on the bone had to be transferred through the soft tissue. This type of traction is effective for conditions such as burn contractures,[81] but it remains a limitation today for most forms of spinal traction. Skeletal traction with the use of hooks (Malgaigne), pins (Steinmann), and wires (Kirschner) has improved traction techniques in the limbs,[54] but is not useful for spinal traction except with surgical stabilization or halo bracing.

Cyriax,[23, 24] in the 1950s, popularized the use of traction for lumbar disc lesions. Since then, Judovich,[66, 68, 69] Colachis and Strohm,[13, 14] and others* have extensively studied the indications for, methods, and effects of traction in both the neck and low back. No consensus with regard to maximal clinical benefit has emerged. Traction can be used in conjunction with other forms of conservative treatment of low back and neck pain to improve symptomatic outcome,[18, 23, 58] but evidence of long-term benefit remains scanty. Most recent changes in the techniques have been related to positioning,[112, 137] the development of stabilizing tables,[36, 128] motorized delivery systems,[112, 137] and inversion techniques.[34]

Indications and Goals of Treatment

It is generally held that any condition involving irritation or compression of nerve roots, whether related to trauma, a degenerative process, or compression from the disc, can benefit from a trial of traction. It is most often used for neck pain secondary to cervical nerve root compression or radiculopathy[66, 87, 99] and low back pain from lumbar radiculopathy.[23, 36, 58] Some practitioners also prescribe traction for patients with nonspecific low back pain, acute cervical or lumbar strain, and other soft tissue abnormali-

---

*References 21, 33, 34, 38, 58, 83, 128, 137, 139.

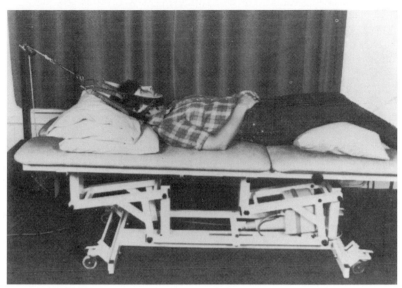

FIGURE 21–16 Mechanical cervical traction. Patient in a supine position with the neck slightly flexed. (Note spring balance in series to monitor the amount of force applied.) (From Grieve GP: Mobilisation of the Spine, ed 5. New York, Churchill Livingstone, 1991, pp 270–271.)

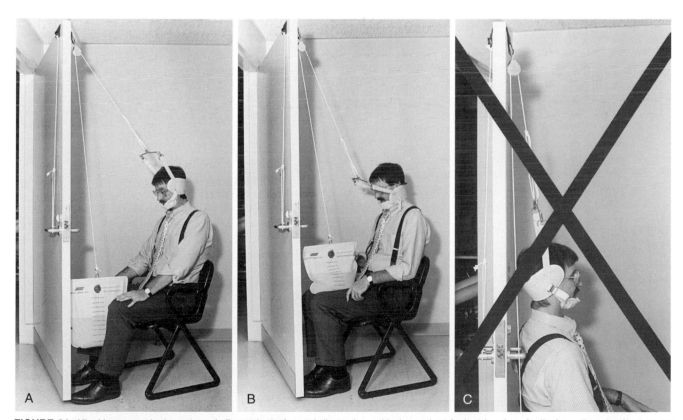

FIGURE 21–17 Home cervical traction. *A,* Properly performed distraction, with the patient facing the door (pulley) to allow the force to be applied through a slightly flexed cervical spine. *B,* To perform intermittent traction, the position of the patient is maintained while the weight (water bag) is placed to allow the rope to be relaxed. *C,* Improper positioning with the neck in extension is not appropriate and may lead to further cervical injury. Make sure the door is not accidentally moved by anyone during the treatment.

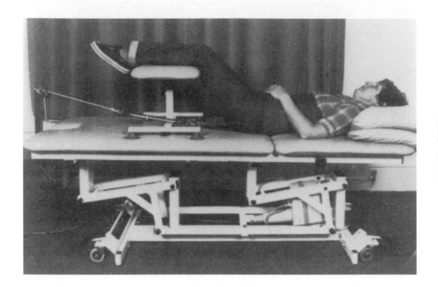

FIGURE 21–18 Motorized lumbar traction with patient in a supine position with hips and knees flexed. The distractive force is directed through the pelvic belt, while the upper belt stabilizes the patient. (From Grieve GP: Mobilisation of the Spine, ed 5. New York, Churchill Livingstone, 1991, p 261.)

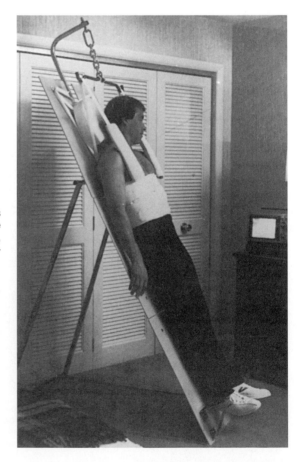

FIGURE 21–19 Gravitational lumbar traction. The patient's weight provides the force of distraction, while the thoracolumbar belt must be able to stabilize the upper body. In this position, the lumbar spine is in neutral or slight extension, which may assist or hinder the treatment process. (From Grieve GP: Mobilisation of the Spine, ed 5. New York, Churchill Livingstone, 1991, p 264.)

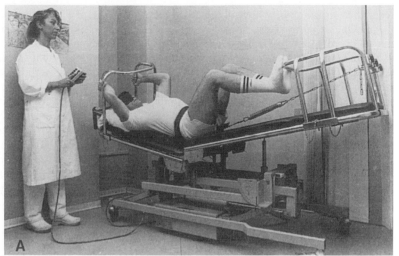

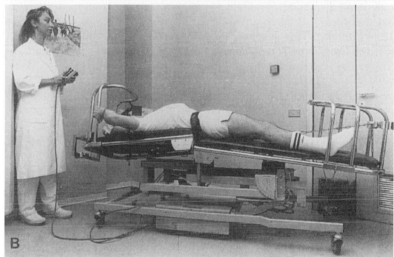

FIGURE 21–20 Autotraction treatment for low-back pain. Patient pulls with the upper limbs while lying on a specially designed traction table. The treatment starts with the patient in the least painful position *(A)*; then traction is provided by the patient through the arm-bar *(B)*. (From Tesio L, Merlo A: Autotraction versus passive traction: An open controlled study in lumbar disc herniation. Arch Phys Med Rehabil 1993; 74:873.)

ties.[19, 33, 45, 87] Some practitioners assert that the main benefit of traction is the associated immobilization.[19, 112]

Although specific clinical indications for traction are controversial, the anatomical basis for the use of traction is well established. Traction has been shown to (1) enlarge intervertebral foramina,[14–17, 137] (2) separate apophyseal joints,[14–17, 137] (3) stretch muscles and ligaments,[17] (4) tighten the posterior longitudinal ligament to exert a centripetal force on the adjacent annulus fibrosus,[54] and (5) enlarge the intervertebral space[14, 17] (possibly producing a suction effect on the disc[63]). Traction is theoretically indicated for any condition that could benefit from these anatomical changes (Table 21–4). The magnitude, duration, position, and direction of pull vary with the treatment goals.

Types of Traction

Spinal traction is used in the cervical (see Figs. 21–16 and 21–17) and lumbar (see Figs. 21–18, 21–19, and 21–20) regions for the conditions listed above. The effects of traction in the thoracic area and sacrum or pelvis are minimal, and use in these areas is limited to stabilization for fractures, dislocations, or correction of congenital deformity or scoliosis. Different methods of delivering

traction to a patient include manual[24, 44, 45, 87] (see Fig. 21–15), mechanized[54, 112] (see Fig. 21–16), motorized or hydraulic[112, 137] (see Fig. 21–18), special tables[36, 54, 112, 128] (see Figs. 21–18, 21–19, and 21–20), and inversion[34] methods. The pull may be continuous, sustained, intermittent, or intermittently pulsed, and can vary based on the magnitude, duration, and direction of pull.[54]

All types of treatment must overcome the body's surface

TABLE 21–4 Theoretical and Observed Changes with Axial Spine Traction

Diminution of disc protrusion
Reduction of cervical disc space pressure
Enlargement of intervertebral foramen
Opening up of the intervertebral disc space
Separation of intervertebral joints
Stretching a tight or painful capsule
Release of entrapped synovial membrane
Freeing of adherent nerve roots
Production of central vacuum to reduce herniated disc
Production of posterior longitudinal ligament tension to reduce
  herniated disc
Relaxation of muscle spasm

From White AA, Panjabi MM: Clinical Biomechanics of the Spine, ed 2. Philadelphia, JB Lippincott, 1990, p 432.

resistance to traction, which is equal to about one half of the weight of the body segment,[67, 68] plus the resistance of the involved soft tissues. This resistance is also a function of the patient's position, and changes depending on whether the patient is supine, inclined or tilted, or sitting. Gravity may be used to either assist or resist the pulling force. The force required is obviously greater for lumbar traction than for cervical traction, but in either type the force necessary for vertebral separation may be more than a patient can safely tolerate.

Continuous traction uses a low force over a long period of time, such as 20 to 40 hours.[54] This is hard for many patients to tolerate, and any change in the patient's position may change the direction of the pull. It is often used in spinal traction for the low back, mostly to assure that a person remains at bed rest, or for orthopedic uses other than for the spine.

Sustained traction uses forces greater than continuous, but less than with intermittent. The pull is maintained for 20 to 60 min.[54] This is still difficult to tolerate if too much force is used. This is a more practical technique timewise for therapy departments. Split traction tables or autotraction tables are typically used. Sustained traction treatments may be given at varying frequencies although it is common practice to treat inpatients daily and outpatients three times per week.

Intermittent traction techniques allow for the use of greater forces, but for a shorter period of time. The force is gradually increased and decreased during each treatment cycle, and can be administered by pulley or motorized system. The duration can be adjusted, and may be on a timed, rhythmic schedule or may be controlled manually by the patient. For a preprogrammed treatment protocol, the time sequences may vary from as little as 7 to 10 sec with a tractive force and 5 sec rest, up to 30 to 60 sec of tractive force followed by 10 to 15 sec rest.[15, 17] The on-off cycle is repeated for 15 to 25 min.[16, 17] The patient-controlled protocol is based more on tolerance, and so the amount of time with a tractive force and resting is variable for each sequence depending on that person's tolerance. Intermittent traction is used in the cervical region to allow the use of progressively higher forces (up to 50 lb) which increases vertebral separation.[15, 66, 82]

Cervical traction can be administered by a manual force[24, 45] (see Fig. 21–15) (often with manipulation) or with the use of a head or chin sling by a mechanized or motorized force (see Fig. 21–16). The sling (the Sayre sling[54, 87] is the most common) should fit so that it does not compress any vascular structures or the ears, and is designed to provide more pull on the occipital region than on the mandible. Colachis and Strohm[14] have demonstrated that posterior vertebral separation is related to the angle of the pull, with maximum separation occurring at 24 degrees of flexion. Clinically, the best relief reportedly occurs between 20 and 30 degrees of cervical flexion.[20, 21] The most common reason clinically for cervical traction to fail or to exacerbate symptoms is applying the force in extension rather than flexion (see Fig. 21–17). There is no effective way to deliver cervical traction with an inversion system.

The optimal force for cervical traction varies depending on the method of delivery. At least 10 lb of force is necessary to counter the effects of gravity on the head,[63] while 25 lb of force is necessary to provide straightening of the cervical lordotic curve and the earliest separation of posterior vertebral segments.[66] Several studies have shown that larger forces definitely cause more separation,[15, 66] but higher forces cannot always be tolerated by patients. When tolerated, the longer a constant force can be applied, the greater the separation.[15] The maximum separation occurs anteriorly at C4 to C5 after 25 min and posteriorly at C6 to C7 after 20 min.[16] The distraction effect is short-lived, since 20 min after traction there is no evidence of posterior separation.[16]

Cervical traction in the inclined position[54] uses the effect of gravity on the body to pull against a stable chin strap. In the supine position,[137] the weight of the head is reduced, but there is increased frictional resistance between the head and the table. This position does give the patient better control of the neck, and allows for better relaxation, but in many cases, if the angle of pull is to remain at 24 degrees of flexion, the patient may have difficulty staying flat on the table. This can cause the patient to actively fire the neck muscles, causing pain and limiting the effect of the traction.

Many clinicians prescribe traction in the seated position because it is easier to position the patient for the correct angle of pull and the patient's body weight counters the force of the pull. In this position, however, the neck is more uncontrollable than in the supine position, and some patients have difficulty relaxing the muscles in this position. The pulley systems and motorized instruments can be used in either the sitting or supine position (see Fig. 21–16). Each patient should be assessed for the position of best individual tolerance.

Once it has been established that a patient is benefiting from cervical traction, it can be performed at home as long as the correct angle for pull is maintained (see Fig. 21–17). The patient should always be facing toward the door to which the pulley is attached; this keeps the cervical spine in flexion. Patients using traction at home should never be alone, as someone else may need to assist them if any untoward effects arise. The optimal frequency of treatments has not yet been established for any of the methods of delivery.

Lumbar traction that provides vertebral separation requires significantly larger forces than cervical traction to overcome the body's resistance.[33, 68, 83] Pelvic belts (see Fig. 21–18) or the use of gravity by tilting[117] (see Fig. 21–19) or inversion[34] is necessary to deliver sufficient tractive force to the lumbar spine. Owing to the large amount of weight necessary to overcome the body's resistance in this area, either a thoracic or chest belt or corset is necessary to hold the upper body in place during distraction of the lower body. These chest harnesses are often uncomfortable and may limit breathing and venous return,[54] affecting a patient's cardiovascular status.

Lumbar traction can be delivered by continuous, sustained, intermittent, or pulsed intermittent methods. Several studies have shown that the larger the force, the greater the vertebral separation, but these high forces (300–400 lb) have to be delivered intermittently for patients to tolerate them.[83] The use of sustained delivery methods with less weight (40,[19] 50,[17] 80,[19] 100,[17] and 132[139] lb) become more effective when surface resistance is reduced by increasing lumbar flexion,[17, 67] using a Scott traction frame,[82] or a standing technique.[83] Split-traction and autotraction tables also reduce the body's surface resistance so that less force is required to provide the same degree of vertebral separation.

Split-traction tables[54, 58, 68] allow the mobile half of a treatment table with the lower body on it to separate from the stationary portion of the table. This stabilizes the upper body and allows vertebral separation with less force at the level where the table is separating. This reduces the force necessary to overcome surface resistance, and treatment can be provided with as little as 80 to 150 lb,[54, 68] rather than 300 to 400 lb.[33, 83] Optimal treatment frequency and duration have not yet been established.

The autotraction table (see Fig. 21–20) allows both sections of the table to move, which induces rotational and side-bending forces into the spine. The patient is assisted by a therapist to assume the most pain-free position, similar to the beginning of a neutral spine exercise program.[113, 114] The patient then provides and controls the amount of tractive force by pulling on an overhead bar for 3 to 6 sec, and can also push or pull with the feet on a bar at the foot of the bed which alternates compressive and distracting forces. The patient rests about 60 sec between each tractive sequence, and repeats the treatment for 30 to 60 min. This is a more active form of traction treatment and has been shown to provide more symptomatic benefit than passive traction.[128] Optimal frequency or length of treatment has not been established, but the studies showing symptomatic benefit have provided treatment every 2 to 3 days for 6 to 10 treatments.[128]

There has been no definitive study of lumbar traction to determine optimal magnitude, duration, frequency, or angle of pull for clinical use. It has been shown that pain relief is quicker with the lumbar spine in flexion,[54] and Colachis and Strohm[17] found that with the hips flexed to 70 degrees an angle of pull of 18 degrees provided the greatest vertebral separation. The duration of beneficial treatment varies with the amount of force used, but there is no evidence of residual effect following removal of the tractive force,[37, 38, 39, 83] even in studies showing a strong clinical benefit. A home treatment table has been proposed,[131] but has not been as widely accepted as home cervical traction. Also, because of the large forces necessary for lumbar vertebral separation, manual traction is not an option.

Contraindications and Risks

Absolute contraindications to traction (Table 21–5) include malignancy[54, 80]; infectious diseases such as tuberculosis, osteomyelitis, or discitis; osteoporosis; rheumatoid arthritis; cord compression; pregnancy; and hypertension or cardiovascular disease. In the cervical region, midline disc herniation[23, 66] is also a contraindication since traction could pull the cord into contact with the disc. Traction should be used with caution in all elderly patients, and not used in those with evidence of significant carotid or vertebral artery disease. Most clinicians recommend that no one have a trial of traction unless radiographs have been obtained to rule out instability, infection, and so forth. Lumbar traction should be performed with caution in persons with abdominal problems, such as peptic ulcer and hiatal or other hernias; aortic aneurysm; or hemorrhoids.[54] Patients

TABLE 21–5   Contraindications to Traction

General
   Osteomyelitis or discitis
   Primary bone tumor or spinal cord tumor
   Unstable fracture
   Severe osteoporosis
   Hypertension
   Cardiovascular disease
   Inadequate expertise
Cervical
   Central intervertebral disc herniation
   Hypermobile joints
   Rheumatoid arthritis
   Carotid or vertebral artery disease
Lumbar
   Pregnancy
   Cauda equina compression

with neurogenic bladder[5] related to nerve root entrapment should not receive lumbar traction.

Traction should be discontinued in those who experience nausea, dizziness, exacerbation of temporomandibular joint dysfunction, or increased pain in the soft tissues of the neck. In the lumbar region, pain may be worsened by the traction itself, at the contact points of the pelvic belt, or at the upper body–belt or corset interface. Frazer[33] reports an "untoward sequelae" rate of only 6 per 25,000 with lumbar traction. Traction still has detractors such as Weinberger,[135] who argues that traction is "irrational, counterproductive, non-physiologic and traumatic." Weinberger states that traction perpetuates new and aggravates already existing skeletal abnormalities. The use of inversion traction[34] involves more risk than standard traction, as it may increase systolic and diastolic blood pressure, decrease heart rate, cause persistent blurred vision, persistent headaches, and periorbital or pharyngeal petechiae. Also, since the center of gravity in adults is at the level of S2, there is a greater weight pulling on the lumbar discs if the patient is hanging upright.

Using Traction in Practice

In clinical practice, traction is used most often for patients who present with signs and symptoms of cervical radiculopathy. It may be used as both a diagnostic and treatment tool, since patients with nerve root compression often receive benefit, while patients with soft tissue or myofascial pain often have an exacerbation of symptoms. The limiting factor for successful cervical traction treatment is often the amount of weight that can be tolerated by the patient. Manual traction during the examination may give an initial indication whether a patient can tolerate cervical traction. Another benefit of cervical traction is that it can potentially be used at home, but initial instruction should always be done under the supervision of a physician or physical therapist.

The use of lumbar traction has become more restricted in recent years.[25] This is due to patient intolerance and the difficulty of stabilizing a patient and delivering the amount of force necessary for traction to be effective. Regulations limiting hospital admissions for low back pain have further decreased its use. In addition, aggressive conservative low back programs for either soft tissue or radicular symptoms have not found it necessary to include the use of lumbar traction. However, it must be considered in some patients as an adjunctive modality so as to enhance their ability to perform an active treatment program. It has been combined empirically with other modalities, such as heat, cold, and massage, but no study has yet been done that proves these combinations improve effectiveness.

MASSAGE

Definition

Graham, in 1884, defined *massage* as "a group of procedures which are usually done with the hands, such as friction, kneading, rolling and percussion of the external tissues of the body in a variety of ways, either with a curative, palliative or hygienic object in view."[42] Massage and manipulation have common ancient roots. In modern times these modalities have become separated, but they continue to share considerable overlap in terminology, philosophy, and technique.

History

Massage has been celebrated in the writings of poets, philosophers, historians, and physicians from ancient to modern times. From its beginnings, massage has waxed and waned as a respected form of health promotion and healing. The philosophy, technical practice, and goals of massage have evolved through the millennia and continue to change today. There is considerable debate as to the etymology of the word *massage*.[70] Most likely it is from the Arabic *massa*, to touch; the Greek *massein*, to knead; or possibly the Sanskrit *makch*, to strike, press, or condense.[42, 70]

The most ancient references to the use of massage come from Babylonia, China, and India, followed later by Greek and Roman literature. Around 900 BC, Babylonian-Assyrian medical writings prescribed massage to expel demons[70] and to aid in healing. In China, documented use of massage dates back to text written on kung fu in 2700 BC.[70] The Nei Ching, written around 1000 BC,[133] and Taoism, originated by Lao-tzu in the 6th century BC,[70] also embraced massage. The Ayur-Veda is the oldest medical writing known in India (1500–1200 BC) and it also makes reference to the use of massage.[70]

References to massage are common in ancient Greek and Roman literature. Hippocrates (460?–377? BC) referred to massage in the treatment of many conditions, stating "the physician must be experienced in many things, but assuredly also in rubbing; for things that have the same name have not the same effects. For rubbing can bind a joint which is too loose and loosen a joint that is too hard."[138] Plato (427?–347? BC) and Socrates (470?–399? BC) refer to the benefits of anointing with oils and rubbing as an "assuager of pain."[42] The Greek physician Asclepiades, considered by some the father of physical medicine, wrote extensively about the three most important treatments he recommended: hydrotherapy, exercise, and massage.[70] Galen, another Greek physician who settled in Rome, wrote extensively about exercise and massage.[70]

In the Middle Ages, under the moral guidance of the Roman Christian authorities, disdain for nudity and preoccupation with bodily health pushed massage out of common favor. Ancient literature on massage and other medical topics was preserved predominantly by Arabic countries during the intellectual suppression of the Middle Ages. The French rediscovered and translated this information for its eventual dissemination throughout Europe. With the Renaissance in the late 15th century came a recounting of ancient recommendations for the use of massage.[65] A series of physicians in the 16th, 17th, and 18th centuries used, promoted, and wrote about massage in the successful treatment of disease.[70]

The most common terminology employed today can be traced to Per Henrik Ling (1776–1839) who was a Swedish teacher of physical education. Ling adopted the French terms for various massage strokes translated from ancient writings. He classified and systematized a series of movements of the soft tissues and then the joints. He used terms such as *rolling*, *slapping*, *pinching*, *shaking*, and *vibration*, and he promoted the use of the French terms *effleurage*, *pétrissage*, *friction massage*, and *tapotement*. Ling emphasized strictly defined massage techniques, employed rationally on a foundation of mechanical and anatomical principles. A royal institute for the practice, promotion, and teaching of what came to be known as Swedish massage was established in Stockholm in 1813 under Ling's direction.[70] Ling's students later opened similar institutes in the capitals of Europe. In 1916 an institute was established in New York.[70]

Other major contributors to the field of massage included Lucas-Championnière (1843–1913), who advocated the use of early mobilization and massage in fractures.[85] Cornelius of Germany first developed the concept of massage treatment of reflex zones, later termed *reflex massage*.[70] Elisabeth Dicke's *Bindegewebsmassage* (connective tissue massage) further promoted the concept of reflex zone therapy.[9, 26, 70]

In the 20th century, many systems of massage have evolved and are currently popular. Massage currently does not enjoy the prominence and prestige that it did during the Roman Empire or in the 1800s. The recent decline may be attributable to several modern trends, including the great emphasis on medications in the medical profession today. Medical schools rarely include massage training in their curriculum. There is also greater interest in the use of therapeutic tools that use advanced technologies rather than the hands. Nevertheless, in recent years, increasing numbers of people are again seeking the benefits of manipulation and massage therapy.[30, 109] If history repeats itself, physicians may once again frequently recommend massage for the health of their patients.

Indications and Goals of Treatment

There are mechanical, reflex, neurological, and psychological effects of massage.[9, 24, 138] Any massage will elicit a combination of these effects. The magnitude and exact characteristics of each of these effects depend on the technique employed and the manner in which it is applied. The goals of treatment can include sedation, reducing adhesions (see Figs. 21–13 and 21–14), mobilizing fluids, muscular relaxation (see Fig. 21–12), and vascular changes. Massage can be useful with any physical diagnosis in which mobilization of tissues, relief of muscle hypertonicity, relief of discomfort, or reduction of swelling would be beneficial to the patient.

The mechanical effects of massage are most evident, easily understood, quantified, and studied. They are based on mobilizing individual muscle fibers and constricting the blood vessels to mechanically squeeze blood and lymph centrally. Deep continuous stroking from distal to proximal of an extremity compresses the low-pressure vasculature and augments venous return.[10, 108, 136] As blood is expressed from the periphery into the central venous system, arterial blood flow is augmented and more freely flows into the vacated tissue capillary beds.[10, 136] Edema is alleviated by massage-induced increase in tissue hydrostatic pressure. Vascular stasis is a risk factor for thrombosis, edema, ischemia, and their consequent morbidities. Massage can be used effectively to help alleviate vascular stasis via the mechanisms described above.

Massage clearly has temporary effects on cutaneous blood flow. This can be readily observed by the hyperemic redness of the skin after vigorous cutaneous stimulation or the increased prominence of superficial veins which results from rubbing the skin over them. The specific mechanisms responsible for changes in cutaneous blood flow are multiple and not well delineated. Mechanical stimulation of mast cells in the skin causes release of histamine. Local histamine release causes the triple response of redness, flare, and wheal formation at the site of cutaneous stimulation. Autonomic neurological reflex changes are also probably involved.

The lymphatic system returns fluids and macromolecules from the interstitium to the vascular system. Stroking techniques performed slowly with deep, constant pressure can mobilize lymphatic flow.[138] There is smooth muscle in the walls of venous and lymphatic vessels to assist in moving fluid centrally. However, the cyclical contraction and relaxation of skeletal muscle through which these vessels travel is a major contributor to the flow of fluid. Many conditions, from pain to paralysis to debilitation, prevent sufficient muscle contractions to mobilize fluid. Massage can be used as a substitute for muscular contractions to augment venous and lymphatic flow in patients who are immobile.[138] Retrograde massage is frequently used to control edema seen in hemiparesis after stroke, in reflex sympathetic dystrophy, or in lymphedema after axillary node dissection.

Deep massage also has mechanical effects on fascia and connective tissue.[9, 138] The fascia surrounds, infiltrates, and supports the musculoskeletal system as well as most of the visceral organs. Restrictions, microadhesions, and scarring in the fascial system lead to diminished musculoskeletal mobility, contracture, and consequent stasis. Fascia is believed to have colloidal properties which enable it to be molded and stretched by sustained pressure. Deep friction massage can, for example, be used to treat shoulder hypomobility secondary to myofascial and tendinous restrictions. Deep friction massage may result in an immediate increase in shoulder mobility and decrease in pain by easing fascial restrictions.

In the past, massage was believed to increase muscle strength,[71, 91] but this is no longer considered valid. Massage has been shown to facilitate the recovery of muscle ability to perform exercise after being fatigued by work or electrical stimulation.[10] Massage has also been shown to improve myofascial flexibility.[101, 138] Massage can aid in developing strength by enabling more exercise with decreased probability of injury. Massage does not stimulate the metabolism of fat, as was once promoted by health spas.

Musculoskeletal hypomobility, intra- and extravascular fluid stasis, and subsequent pain are hypothesized to form a self-perpetuating, positive feedback loop. Pain and splinting of a joint occur after musculoskeletal injury. Decreased movement in the injured muscles around the joint may cause fluid stasis which allows for the buildup of metabolic byproducts. The increasing local concentration of these metabolites is thought to cause irritation and pain, which in turn cause more involuntary splinting. Once initiated, this process can perpetuate itself indefinitely. By mechanically deforming and lengthening connective tissue, massage may alleviate the hypomobility. Massage may also augment the dispersion of the metabolites by its direct effects on venous and lymphatic flow. Pain is relieved as muscle splinting is diminished and noxious metabolites are mobilized. Once the self-perpetuating cycle of hypomobility, stasis, and pain is broken, the body's own restorative mechanisms can complete the healing process.

Further mechanical effects of massage include mobilizing bronchial secretions by a cupping technique (tapotement) to the thorax commonly used in conjunction with postural drainage for airway congestion.[138] The "lymphatic pump"[44] is a vibration type of pétrissage applied to the rib cage in coordination with the breath. The lymphatic pump is designed to draw lymphatic fluid into the chest by causing rapidly alternating positive and negative pressure in the chest.

Neural reflex reactions to massage have also been proposed to explain some of the its widespread effects. Afferent nerves carry information from the somatic system to the spinal cord. This information includes pain sensation and proprioception as well as feedback from the muscle spindle and autonomic afferents. When a given part of the somatic system is dysfunctional, there is a sustained increase in afferent neural input into the spinal column at that given spinal segmental level. This continuous barrage of increased segmental afferent information is hypothesized to have an impact on other neural elements at that same spinal segmental level, creating a "facilitated spinal segment."[76, 77, 107]

A "facilitated spinal segmental level" is one that has a decreased threshold for depolarization of all neurons in that segment because of excessive afferent neural input. At the facilitated spinal segment, any given stimulus for efferent neuronal depolarization causes an exaggerated efferent outflow. This hypothesis implies that all somatic and visceral tissues can be negatively affected if they are innervated by the nerves from a spinal segment that receives afferent information from an area of somatic dysfunction. If this is true, then it follows that alleviation of somatic dysfunction via massage can result in optimized function of somatic and visceral systems that are innervated by the same spinal segment. Neural reflex changes in somatic systems by massage or manipulation are called "somatosomatic" reflex effects. Neural reflex changes in visceral systems by massage are called "somatovisceral" reflex effects.

Many massage strokes are designed not to mobilize fluids, release myofascial restrictions, or initiate reflex neurological effects. These strokes are above all comfortable and relaxing and have their greatest impact on the psychological health of the patient. A positive impact on the psychological state of a patient appears to have widespread benefits. The emerging field of psychoneuroimmunology documents clearly the favorable impact of a positive mental attitude on the immune system.[11, 122] Alternately, pain, depression, and anxiety exert a negative effect on the body's immune system. The uplifting and relaxing experience of an expertly given, painless massage may have much more than psychological benefit, benefits that need to be documented in future studies.

Massage functions via a variety of mechanisms to be of benefit in a wide variety of conditions. Patients with low back pain, neck pain, fibromyalgia, arthritis, bursitis, tendinitis, fasciitis, and even neuromas may benefit from massage techniques. Other conditions associated with multiple sclerosis, cerebral palsy, hemiplegia, and quadriplegia, such as spasticity, reflex sympathetic dystrophy, edema, and contracture may also be significantly improved. Specific techniques for respiratory problems can help persons with chest paralysis. Limited use with varicose ulcers, localized draining infections, and following skin grafting have been reported. Light massage with a lubricant can be useful on a recent skin graft. Deeper massage techniques may be beneficial later on after skin grafting to prevent or model scar tissue. Massage can also release deep scar adhesions and contracture following amputations to improve fitting of prostheses and decrease some of the complications of prosthetic wear.

Types of Massage

The most commonly accepted types of hand movements used in therapeutic massage are from the Swedish system. The four basic stroke types are called (1) effleurage, (2) pétrissage, (3) friction, and (4) tapotement.[57, 138] These manipulations are described below.

Effleurage, or stroking massage,[24, 56, 138] involves lightly running the hand over the skin. This may be performed with either superficial or deep pressure and provides different effects depending on the depth of treatment. Deep stroking involves mechanical effects and should be performed with continuous contact of the hands from distal to proximal on the extremities, the back, or the neck. Once the proximal extent is reached, the hands can be drawn back to the distal position applying light contact or no contact at all. Effleurage is especially effective in assisting return of venous or lymphatic drainage, such as following joint sprains, peripheral muscle strains, or bruising, and vascular congestion related to surgery, peripheral vascular disease, or reflex sympathetic dystrophy.

Superficial stroking may be performed in any direction and involves mostly reflex and psychological effects to enhance relaxation, especially with muscle hypertonicity or spasticity. One or two hands can be used with varying degrees of rate or pressure depending on the desired effect, slow for relaxation or rapid for stimulation. Stroking may also include a rapid hand-over-hand series of short strokes progressing from proximal to distal along a portion of the body.

Pétrissage, or compression massage,[24, 44, 56, 138] includes *kneading*, *picking up*, *wringing*, *rolling*, and *shaking*. The common characteristic is the compression of the body's soft tissues between two hands or between the hand and the underlying skeletal tissue (see Fig. 21–12). The techniques are designed to mobilize fluid and tissue deposits, as well as to break up tissue and muscle adhesions (see Fig. 21–13). *Kneading* indicates circular movements of one hand superimposed on the other, a single hand, the knuckles, the finger pads, or the thumb compressing superficial soft tissues against deeper ones. *Picking up* includes four basic steps: (1) compression of soft tissue against underlying structures, (2) grasping of the soft tissue, (3) release of the soft tissue, and (4) moving the hands to a new position. *Wringing* is performed like picking up, except once the tissue is grasped using two hands side by side, one hand pulls while the other pushes. This generates a shear force in the tissue planes. *Rolling* is the motion of gathering skin alone or muscle and skin between the fingers and thumb and allowing the tissue to "roll" between these digits before releasing and taking another nearby grasp. In *shaking*, once the soft tissue is firmly grasped between thumb and fingers the hands are shaken vigorously side to side as they move down the length of the muscle.

Friction massage[24, 44, 56, 138] is performed by applying circular or transverse motions through the fingers, thumb, or the heel of the palm of the hand to a small area of tissue (see Fig. 21–14). Treatment progresses from superficial to deep by increasing the pressure through the hand to the level of the tissue problem (i.e., muscle, tendon, ligament, or myofascial junction). When applied correctly, no motion should occur between the fingertips and the skin, the movement should occur deeper in the tissues. Deep friction may be uncomfortable and even cause mild bruising, but it is especially effective for soft tissue problems such as tendinitis or fasciitis (i.e., lateral epicondylitis, supraspinatus tendinitis, subacromial bursitis, and plantar fasciitis) and trigger points as described by Travell.[130]

Tapotement, or percussion massage,[24, 56, 138] produces stimulation by rhythmic, alternating movements of the hands on the soft tissue of the patient. *Clapping, hacking, vibrations, beating, pounding*, and *tapping* are all types of tapotement massage. *Clapping*, or cupping, is the technique wherein the open palms are cupped and repetitively strike the surface of the body. Often a sheet or towel is placed between the striking hands and the skin. The cupped hand produces a dull noise and affects deeper tissues. A flat hand makes a sharper, high-pitched noise and stimulates predominantly the skin. *Hacking* consists of repetitively striking the body with the medial border of the hands with the plane of the open hand perpendicular to the surface of the body. The hands alternate as they strike the body at a rate of 2 to 6 Hz, providing superficial stimulation. *Vibrations* should be distinguished from shakings. Vibrations require a rapid up-and-down motion of pressure and release within the soft tissue without losing contact with the skin. Shaking is a side-to-side rapid oscillating motion and is not a form of tapotement. *Beating* and *pounding* are rarely used techniques wherein the loosely clenched fists are used to repetitively strike the body in an alternating manner.

Beating strikes the body palm down and *pounding* strikes the body with the medial border of the fist. *Tapping* uses the finger pads to percuss. The second through fourth fingers of each hand in rapid succession rise and fall in turn in small, sensitive areas such as the face.

Tapotement can have a wide range of effects depending on how it is applied. Deep clapping to the thorax is believed to be of physical benefit in patients with respiratory problems by loosening impacted secretions. Superficial tapotement, such as tapping on the face, is thought to be of more psychological than physical benefit.

There are many different styles of massage other than the commonly employed Swedish forms described above. Alternative techniques include acupressure, shiatsu, reflexology, Rolfing, and *Bindegewebsmassage*.[9, 127]

Acupressure[127] is a technique of applying constant, circular friction pressure to specific points for treatment purposes. It uses the principles and points of acupuncture defined more than 3000 years ago in China. Acupuncture specialists contend that there are hundreds of points energetically aligned within 12 energy meridians which interconnect and course longitudinally throughout the human body. Disease is believed to result from imbalances in the body's energy systems, and therefore the goal of treatment is to balance the flow of energy through the meridians to allow the body to regain homeostasis and heal itself. In traditional acupuncture these points are stimulated by fine needles which are heated or carry electrical impulses. In acupressure, these points are stimulated by a circular friction massage.

Shiatsu massage[127] was developed in Japan as early as 200 BC and also is based on the Chinese system of acupuncture meridians. In shiatsu massage, heavy pressure is applied perpendicularly to the body over a given meridian with the palm of the hand or heel of the foot. It is believed that the use of the upper body musculature to apply the necessary force requires the practitioner to be too tense to adequately sense patient responses and appropriately guide therapy. The mental attitude of the practitioner is believed to be critical to successful balancing of the energy meridians.

Reflexology[127] also has its roots in Chinese acupuncture. The philosophical tenet of reflexology is that there is a homuncular representation of the entire human body mapped out on the sole of the foot and the palm of the hand. By palpating the entire surface of the palm or sole one can readily find areas of point tenderness. These areas of tenderness correspond to organs or tissues in the body which are dysfunctional. Once these areas are identified, they are treated by circular deep friction massage. Massage became the favored manner of treatment in the palms of the hands and soles of the feet because acupuncture needles proved to be intolerable. Reflexology massage must be firm and is often uncomfortable, but the practitioner must take care not to induce extreme discomfort. A 20-minute session to diagnose and treat both hands or feet on a regular basis is believed to have a favorable impact on any dysfunctional area of the body.

Rolfing[9] (structural integration) is a method of restructuring and realigning the deep fascial planes in the body through a variety of deep friction massage techniques. Ida Rolf developed and promoted this type of deep fascial massage. The goal is to balance and align the human body in the gravitational field. The Rolfing treatment consists of a series of deep friction massages described as being notoriously uncomfortable but effective. Rolfing theory adheres to the concept of mind-body integration and tries to favorably influence the psychological state as it corrects physical problems.

Bindegewebsmassage[9, 26, 127] (connective tissue massage) was originated by the German physiotherapist Elisabeth Dicke in the 1920s and was later promoted by Maria Ebner. *Bindegewebsmassage* is a rigidly structured massage system that employs a light, lubricant-free, cutaneous massage. *Bindegewebsmassage* always begins on the low back and sacrum and progresses to the affected area. It is hypothesized to treat musculoskeletal as well as visceral disorders. Effects may result from direct connective tissue deformation and from somatovisceral reflexes. The gentle nature of this massage is very comforting and may aid in relaxing the patient such that deeper fascial work may be employed if necessary.

Contraindications and Risks

There are numerous contraindications to massage. Massage should not be performed over an area of malignancy, cellulitis, or lymphangitis.[74] The effects of massage on mobilizing vascular and lymphatic fluid may only serve to disseminate tumor cells or spread infection.

Areas of recent trauma or bleeding can rebleed if massage is applied too soon after injury or surgery. Massage is commonly used to increase elasticity and mobility in scar tissue, but caution should be taken not to disrupt the incision by beginning massage before healing is complete. When performing massage after joint replacement, make sure the therapist is familiar with the allowable range of motion of the replaced joint. Massage should not be performed over any open area where the therapist can be exposed to bloodborne pathogens.

Massage should not be applied over an area of known deep venous thrombosis or over a known atherosclerotic plaque. Deep massage may dislodge venous or arterial thrombi, which can potentially cause pulmonary, cerebral, or peripheral embolic infarcts.

Massage should be done only when the reason for the massage, the cause of the condition being treated, and the goals of therapy are known. For example, if massage is prescribed as a treatment for edema, the cause of the edema should be known (renal failure, heart failure, reflex sympathetic dystrophy, deep venous insufficiency, lymphatic obstruction, immobility, infection, postoperative, etc.).

Using Massage in Practice

The ability to perform structural diagnosis is not essential for prescribing massage techniques but can be beneficial in determining the type of treatment that is indicated. There are many similarities between massage techniques and manual medicine techniques, such as myofascial release, the lymphatic pump, and other soft tissue release techniques. Knowledge of the indications and contraindications for each treatment approach is essential for safe and effective treatment. There is a risk of psychological patient dependence with these physical modalities just as there is with medications or manipulation.

Massage can be very effective within the context of a comprehensive rehabilitation plan. Since massage is a passive modality, any massage technique must be supplemented with an active treatment program at the proper time. During the initial stages after a fracture or dislocation, tissue mobilization and soft tissue stretching without joint or bone movement is beneficial, but eventually the patient needs to begin an active movement program to resume normal function. Other diagnoses for which massage is commonly prescribed, such as lumbar sprain or strain, cervical sprain or strain, fibrositis or fibromyalgia, supraspinatus tendinitis, and lateral epicondylitis, should have some form of active range-of-motion program started at the time of initial treatment, and should eventually be progressed into a strengthening program when appropriate. There are no studies to date that indicate the optimal treatment frequency or duration, or that document the benefits of any of the massage techniques.

The basic principles of massage treatment are (1) the patient must be comfortable, relaxed, and not too cold; (2) the therapist must be comfortable and able to complete the technique without shifting position; (3) the therapist should have clean hands, short nails, and no areas of broken skin; (4) the use of lubricants may facilitate ease of technique; and (5) the skill of the practitioner is related more to his or her ability to distribute even pressures throughout the hands rather than to strength alone.

The art of massage is a time-consuming process to master. Practice and natural ability to "feel" with the hands are essential. Some techniques may be difficult, and many practitioners argue against instructing patients or families in home programs. However, in a patient who has demonstrated therapeutic response and benefit, it can become part of a complete home program.

References

1. Adams T, Heisey RS, Smith MC, et al: Parietal bone mobility in the anesthetized cat. J Am Osteopath Assoc 1992; 92:599–622.
2. Beal MC, Vorro J, Johnston WL: Chronic cervical dysfunction: Correlation of myoelectric findings with clinical progress. J Am Osteopath Assoc 1989; 89:891–900.
3. Blomberg S, Hallin G, Grann K, et al: Manual therapy with steroid injections—a new approach to treatment of low back pain. Spine 1994; 19:569–577.
4. Blomberg S, Svardsudd K, Mildenberger F: A controlled, multicentre trial of manual therapy in low-back pain. Scand J Prim Health Care 1992; 10:170–178.
5. Bourdillon JF, Day EA, Bookout MR: Spinal Manipulation. Oxford, England, Butterworth-Heinemann, 1992.
6. Bowles CH: Functional technique: A modern perspective. J Am Osteopath Assoc 1981; 80:326–331.
7. Brandt B Jr, Jones LH: Some methods of applying counterstrain. J Am Osteopath Assoc 1976; 75:786–789.
8. Brodin H: Cervical pain and mobilization. Med Phys 1983; 6:67–72.
9. Cantu RL, Grodin AJ: Myofascial Manipulation: Theory and Clinical Application. Gaithersburg, Md, Aspen, 1992.
10. Carrier EB: Studies on physiology of capillaries: Reaction of human skin capillaries to drugs and other stimuli. Am J Physiol 1922; 61:528–547.
11. Chrousos GP, Gold PW: The concepts of stress and stress system disorders. JAMA 1992; 267:1244–1252.
12. Cislo S, Ramirez MA, Schwartz HR: Low back pain: Treatment of forward and backward sacral torsions using counterstrain. J Am Osteopath Assoc 1991; 91:255–259.
13. Colachis SC Jr, Strohm BR: Radiographic studies of cervical spine motion in normal subjects: Flexion and hyperextension. Arch Phys Med Rehabil 1965; 46:753–760.
14. Colachis SC Jr, Strohm BR: A study of tractive forces and angle of pull on vertebral interspaces in the cervical spine. Arch Phys Med Rehabil 1965; 46:820–830.
15. Colachis SC Jr, Strohm BR: Cervical traction: Relationship of traction time to varied tractive force with constant angle of pull. Arch Phys Med Rehabil 1965; 46:815–819.
16. Colachis SC Jr, Strohm BR: Effect of duration of intermittent cervical traction on vertebral separation. Arch Phys Med Rehabil 1966; 47:353–359.
17. Colachis SC Jr, Strohm BR: Effects of intermittent traction on separation of lumbar vertebrae. Arch Phys Med Rehabil 1990; 50:251–258.
18. Coxhead CE, Meade TW, Inskip H, et al: Multicentre trial of physiotherapy in the management of sciatic symptoms. Lancet 1981; 1:1065–1068.
19. Crisp EJ, Cyriax J, Christie BGB: Discussion on the treatment of backache by traction. Proc R Soc Med (Section of Physical Medicine) 1955; 48:805–814.
20. Crue BL: The importance of flexion in cervical traction for radiculitis. U S Air Force Med J 1957; 8:374–380.
21. Crue BL, Todd EM: The importance of flexion in cervical halter traction. Bull Los Angeles Neurol Soc 1965; 30:95–98.
22. Curtis P, Bove G: Family physicians, chiropractors, and back pain. J Fam Pract 1992; 35:551–555.
23. Cyriax J: Conservative treatment of lumbar disc lesions. Physiotherapy 1964; 50:300–303.
24. Cyriax J, Russell G: Textbook of Orthopaedic Medicine, Vol 2: Treatment by Manipulation, Massage and Injection. London, Bailliere Tindall, 1980.
25. Deyo RA, Tsui-Wu Y: Descriptive epidemiology of low-back pain and its related medical care in the United States. Spine 1987; 12:264–268.
26. Dicke E, Schliack H, Wolff A: Bindegewebsmassage. Stuttgart, Thieme, 1975.
27. Dreyfuss P, Dreyer S, Griffin J, et al: Positive sacroiliac screening tests in asymptomatic individuals. Spine 1994; 19:1138–1143.
28. Dvorak J, Dvorak V, Schneider W: Manual Medicine. Berlin, Springer-Verlag, 1984.
29. Dvorak J, Dvorak V: Manual Medicine: Diagnostics. Stuttgart, Thieme, 1990.
30. Eisenberg DM, Kessler RC, Foster C, et al: Unconventional medicine in the United States: Prevalence, costs, and patterns of use. N Engl J Med 1993; 328:246–252.
31. Fisk JW: A controlled trial of manipulation in a selected group of patients with low-back pain favouring one side. N Z Med J 1979; 10:288–291.
32. Fisk JW: Medical Treatment of Neck and Back Pain. Springfield, Ill, Thomas, 1987.
33. Frazer EH: The use of traction in backache. Med J Aust 1954; 41:694–697.
34. Gianakopoulos G, Waylonis GW, Grant PA, et al: Inversion devices: Their role in producing lumbar distraction. Arch Phys Med Rehabil 1985; 66:100–102.
35. Gibbons RW: The evolution of chiropractic: Medical and social protest in America. In Haldeman S (ed): Modern Developments in the Principles and Practice of Chiropractic. New York, Appleton-Century-Crofts, 1980, pp 3–24.
36. Gillstrom P, Ehrnberg A: Long-term results of autotraction in the treatment of lumbago and sciatica. Arch Orthop Trauma Surg 1985; 104:294–298.
37. Gillstrom P, Ericson K, Hindmarsh T: Autotraction in lumbar disc herniation. Arch Orthop Trauma Surg 1985; 104:207–210.
38. Gillstrom P, Ericson K, Hindmarsh T: Computed tomography examination of the influence of autotraction on herniation of the lumbar disc. Arch Orthop Trauma Surg 1985; 104:289–293.
39. Godfrey CM, Morgan PP, Schatzker J: A randomized trial of manipulation for low-back pain in a medical setting. Spine 1984; 9:301–304.
40. Goodridge JP: Muscle energy technique: Definition, explanation, methods of procedure. J Am Osteopath Assoc 1981; 81:249–254.
41. Gorman RF: Cardiac arrest after cervical spine mobilization. Med J Aust 1978; 2:169–170.

42. Graham D: Practical Treatise on Massage. New York, Wm. Wood, 1884.

43. Greenman PE: Models and mechanisms of osteopathic manipulative medicine. Osteopathic Med News 1987; 4:1–20.

44. Greenman PE: Principles of Manual Medicine. Baltimore, Williams & Wilkins, 1989.

45. Grieve GP: Mobilisation of the Spine. New York, Churchill Livingstone, 1991.

46. Hadler NM, Curtis P, Gillings DB, et al: A benefit of spinal manipulation as adjunctive therapy for low-back pain: A stratified controlled trial. Spine 1987; 12:702–706.

47. Haldeman S, Rubinstein SM: Compression fractures in patients undergoing spinal manipulative therapy. J Manipulative Physiol Ther 1992; 15:450–454.

48. Haldeman S, Rubinstein SM: The precipitation or aggravation of musculoskeletal pain in patients receiving spinal manipulative therapy. J Manipulative Physiol Ther 1993; 16:47–50.

49. Haldeman S: Spinal manipulative therapy in the management of low back pain. In Finneson BE (ed): Low Back Pain. Philadelphia, JB Lippincott, 1980, pp 245–275.

50. Haldeman S: Spinal manipulative therapy: A status report. Clin Orthop 1983; 179:62–70.

51. Harris JD: History and development of manipulation and mobilization. In Basmajian JV (ed): Manipulation, Traction and Massage. Baltimore, Williams & Wilkins, 1985, pp 3–21.

52. Heilig D: The thrust technique. J Am Osteopath Assoc 81:244–248, 1981.

53. Herzog W, Conway PJ, Kawchuk GN, et al: Forces exerted during spinal manipulative therapy. Spine 1993; 18:1206–1212.

54. Hinterbuchner C: Traction. In Basmajian JV (ed): Manipulation, Traction and Massage. Baltimore, Williams & Wilkins, 1985, pp 172–201.

55. Hoehler FK, Tobis JS, Buerger AA: Spinal manipulation for low back pain. JAMA 1981; 245:1835–1838.

56. Hofkosh JM: Classical massage. In Basmajian JV (ed): Manipulation, Traction and Massage. Baltimore, Williams & Wilkins, 1985, pp 263–269.

57. Hollis M: Massage for Therapists. Oxford, England, Blackwell, 1987.

58. Hood LB, Chrisman D: Intermittent pelvic traction in the treatment of the ruptured intervertebral disk. Phys Ther 1968; 48:21–30.

59. Hooper J: Low back pain and manipulation: Paraparesis after treatment of low back pain by physical methods. Med J Aust 1973; 1:549–551.

60. Howe DH, Newcombe RG, Wade MT: Manipulation of the cervical spine—a pilot study. J R Coll Gen Pract 1983; 33:574–579.

61. Hruby RJ: Pathophysiologic models and the selection of osteopathic manipulative techniques. J Osteopath Med 1992; 6:25–30.

62. International Classification of Diseases, ed 9. Clinical Modification, ed 3. US Department of Health and Human Services Publication No. (PHS) 89-1260, vol 1, 1989, p 637.

63. Jackson R: The Cervical Syndrome. Springfield, Ill, Thomas, 1958.

64. Jones LH: Strain and Counterstrain. Newark, Ohio, The American Academy of Osteopathy, 1992.

65. Joseph LH: Gymnastics from the Middle Ages to the eighteenth century. Ciba Found Symp, 1949.

66. Judovich BD: Herniated cervical disc: A new form of traction therapy. Am J Surg 1952; 84:646–656.

67. Judovich BD: Lumbar traction therapy and dissipated force factors. Lancet 1954; 74:411.

68. Judovich BD: Lumbar traction therapy—elimination of physical factors that prevent lumbar stretch. JAMA 1955; 159:549–550.

69. Judovich BD, Nobel GR: Traction therapy: A study of resistance forces. Am J Surg 1957; 93:108.

70. Kanemetz HL: History of massage. In Basmajian JV (ed): Manipulation, Traction and Massage. Baltimore, Williams & Wilkins, 1985, pp 211–255.

71. Kellogg JH: The Art of Massage. Battle Creek, Mich, Modern Medical, 1919.

72. Khalil TM, Asfour SS, Martinez LM, et al: Stretching in the rehabilitation of low-back pain patients. Spine 1992; 17:311–317.

73. Kimberly PE: Formulating a prescription for osteopathic manipulative treatment. J Am Osteopath Assoc 1980; 79:506–513.

74. Knapp ME: Massage. In Kottke FJ, Lehmann JF (eds): Krusen's Handbook of Physical Medicine and Rehabilitation. Philadelphia, WB Saunders, 1990, pp 433–435.

75. Koes BW, Bowler LM, Kripschild PG: Spinal manipulation and mobilisation for back and neck pain: An indexed review. Br Med J 1991; 303:1298–1303.

76. Korr IM: Proprioceptors and somatic dysfunction. J Am Osteopath Assoc 1975; 74:638–650.

77. Korr IM: Somatic dysfunction, osteopathic manipulative treatment, and the nervous system: A few facts, some theories, many questions. J Am Osteopath Assoc 1986; 86:109–114.

78. Krueger BR, Okazaki H: Vertebral-basilar distribution infarction following chiropractic cervical manipulation. Mayo Clin Proc 1980; 55:322–332.

79. Kurz W, Litmanovitch YI, Romanoff H, et al: Effect of manual lymph drainage massage on blood components and urinary neurohormones in chronic lymphedema. Angiology 1981; 32:119–127.

80. LaBan MM, Meerschaert JR: Quadriplegia following cervical traction in patients with occult epidural prostatic metastasis. Arch Phys Med Rehabil 1975; 56:455.

81. Larson DL, Evans EB: Skeletal suspension and traction in the treatment of burns. Ann Surg 1968; 168:981.

82. Lawson GA, Godfrey CM: A report on studies of spinal-traction. Med Serv J Can 1958; 14:762.

83. Lehmann JF, Brunner GD: A device for the application of heavy lumbar traction: Its mechanical effects. Arch Phys Med Rehabil 1958; 39:696–700.

84. Lewis M, Grundy D: Vertebral osteomyelitis following manipulation of spondylitic necks—a possible risk. Paraplegia 1992; 30:788–790.

85. Lucas-Championnière J: Traitement des fractures par le massage et la mobilisation. Paris, 1895.

86. MacDonald RS, Bell CMY: An open controlled assessment of osteopathic manipulation in nonspecific low back pain. Spine 1990; 15:364–370.

87. Maigne R: Orthopedic Medicine: A New Approach to Vertebral Manipulations. Springfield, Ill, Thomas, 1972.

88. Maigne R: Manipulation of the spine. In Basmajian JV (ed): Manipulation, Traction and Massage. Baltimore, Williams & Wilkins, 1985, pp 71–134.

89. Maitland GD: Peripheral Manipulation. London, Butterworth-Heinemann, 1991.

90. Maitland GD: Vertebral Manipulation. London, Butterworths, 1986.

91. McMillan M: Massage and Therapeutic Exercise. Philadelphia, WB Saunders, 1925.

92. Meade TW, Dyer S, Browne W, et al: Low back pain of mechanical origin: Randomised comparison of chiropractic and hospital outpatient treatment. Br Med J 1990; 300:1431–1437.

93. Meal GM, Scott RA: Analysis of the joint crack by simultaneous recording of sound and tension. J Manipulative Physiol Ther 1986; 9:189–195.

94. Mennell J: The Science and Art of Joint Manipulation, vol. 2. The Spinal Column. London, J & A Churchill, 1952.

95. Mennell J McM: Joint Pain: Diagnosis and Treatment Using Manipulative Techniques. London, J & A Churchill, 1964.

96. Mitchell FL Jr: The respiratory-circulatory model: Concepts and applications. In Greenman PE (ed): Concepts and Mechanisms of Neuromuscular Functions. Berlin, Springer-Verlag, 1984.

97. Mitchell FL Jr, Moran PS, Pruzzo NA: An Evaluation and Treatment Manual of Osteopathic Muscle Energy Procedures. Valley Park, Mo, Mitchell, Moran, and Pruzzo, 1979.

98. Mitchell FL Sr: Structural pelvic function. AAO Yearbook 71–89, 1958.

99. Nayak NN: Cervical traction: Prescription patterns (abstract). Arch Phys Med Rehabil 1993; 74:1268.

100. Neumann H: Introduction to Manual Medicine. Heidelberg, Springer-Verlag, 1989.

101. Nordschow M: Influence of manual massage on muscle relaxation: Effect on trunk flexion. J Am Phys Ther Assoc 1962; 42:653.

102. Norton JM: A tissue pressure model for palpatory perception of the cranial rhythmic impulse. J Am Osteopath Assoc 1991; 91:975–994.

103. Nwuga VCB: Manipulation of the Spine. Baltimore, Williams & Wilkins, 1976.

104. Nwuga VCB: Relative therapeutic efficacy of vertebral manipulation and conventional treatment in back pain management. Am J Phys Med Rehabil 1982; 6:273–278.

105. Nyberg R: Manipulation: definition, types, application. In Basmajian JV, Nyberg R (eds): Rational Manual Therapies. Baltimore, Williams & Wilkins, 1993, pp 21–47.

106. Ottenbacher K, DiFabio RP: Efficacy of spinal manipulation/mobilization therapy: A meta-analysis. Spine 1985; 10:833–837.

107. Patterson MM: Louisa Burns Memorial Lecture 1980: The spinal cord—Active processor not passive transmitter. J Am Osteopath Assoc 1980; 80:210–215.

108. Pemberton R: The physiologic influence of massage and the clinical application of heat and massage in internal medicine. *In* Principles and Practices of Physical Medicine, vol I. Hagerstown, Md, WF Prior, 1932.

109. Powell FC, Hanigan WC, Olivero WC: A risk/benefit analysis of spinal manipulation therapy for relief of lumbar or cervical pain. Neurosurgery 1992; 33:73–78.

110. Raskind R, North CM: Vertebral artery injuries following chiropractic cervical spine manipulation—case reports. Angiology 1990; 41:445–452.

111. Richard J: Disk rupture with cauda equina syndrome after chiropractic adjustment. N Y State J Med 1967; 67:2496–2498.

112. Rogoff JB: Motorized intermittent traction. *In* Basmajian JV (ed): Manipulation, Traction and Massage. Baltimore, Williams & Wilkins, 1985, pp 201–207.

113. Saal JA: Rehabilitation of sports-related lumbar spine injuries. Phys Med Rehabil 1987; 1:613–637.

114. Saal JA, Saal JS: Nonoperative treatment of herniated lumbar intervertebral disc with radiculopathy: An outcome study. Spine 1989; 14:431–437.

115. Sandoz R: The significance of the manipulative crack and of other articular noises. Ann Swiss Chiropractic Assoc 1969; 4:47–68.

116. Scientific Advisory Committee, International Federation of Manual Medicine: Workshop. Fischingen, Switzerland, 1983.

117. Sheffield FJ: Adaptation of tilt table for lumbar traction. Arch Phys Med Rehabil 1964; 45:469.

118. Shekelle PG: Spine update: Spinal manipulation. Spine 1994; 19:858–861.

119. Shekelle PG, Adams AH, Chassin MR, et al: The appropriateness of spinal manipulation for low-back pain: Indications and ratings by a multidisciplinary panel. Santa Monica, Calif, Rand, 1991.

120. Shekelle PG, Adams AH, Chassin MR, et al: Spinal manipulation for low-back pain. Ann Intern Med 1992; 117:590–598.

121. Sherman DG, Hart RG, Easton JD: Abrupt change in head position and cerebral infarction. Stroke 1981; 12:2–6.

122. Shors TJ, Weiss C, Thompson RF: Stress induced facilitation of classical conditioning. Science 1992; 257:537–539.

123. Sims-Williams H, Jayson MIV, Young SMS, et al: Controlled trial of mobilisation and manipulation for low back pain: Hospital patients. Br Med J 1979; 2:1318–1320.

124. Sutherland Cranial Teaching Foundation of the Cranial Academy: Osteopathy in the Cranial Field. Kirksville, Mo, Journal Printing, 1976.

125. Sweeney T: Neck school: Cervicothoracic stabilization training. Occup Med 1992; 7:43–54.

126. Tanigawa MC: Comparison of the hold-relax procedure and passive mobilization on increasing muscle length. Phys Ther 1972; 52:725–735.

127. Tappan F: Healing Massage Techniques: Holistic, Classic, and Emerging Methods. Norwalk, Ct, Appleton & Lange, 1988.

128. Tesio L, Merlo A: Autotraction versus passive traction: An open controlled study in lumbar disc herniation. Arch Phys Med Rehabil 1993; 74:871–876.

129. Tobis JS, Hoehler F: Musculoskeletal Manipulation: Evaluation of the Scientific Evidence. Springfield, Ill, Thomas, 1986.

130. Travell J: Myofascial Pain and Dysfunction. Baltimore, Williams & Wilkins, 1983.

131. Turner D: New apparatus: A spinal traction treatment table. Br J Phys Med 1957; 20:259.

132. Upledger JE, Vredevoogd JD: Craniosacral Therapy. Seattle, Eastland Press, 1983.

133. Veith I: The Yellow Emperor's Classic of Internal Medicine. Baltimore, Williams & Wilkins, 1949.

134. Ward RC: Myofascial release concepts. *In* Basmajian JV, Nyberg R (eds): Rational Manual Therapies. Baltimore, Williams & Wilkins, 1993, pp 223–241.

135. Weinberger LM: Trauma or treatment? The role of intermittent traction in the treatment of cervical soft tissue injuries. J Trauma 1976; 16:377–382.

136. Wolfson H: Studies on effect of physical therapeutic procedures on function and structure. JAMA 1931; 96:2020–2021.

137. Wong AMK, Leong CP, Chen C: The traction angle and cervical intervertebral separation. Spine 1992; 17:136–138.

138. Wood EC, Becker PD: Beard's Massage. Philadelphia, WB Saunders, 1981.

139. Worden RE, Humphrey TL: Effect of spinal traction on the length of the body. Arch Phys Med Rehabil 1964; 45:318–320.

140. Zanolla R, Monzeglio C, Balzarini A, et al: Evaluation of the results of three different methods of postmastectomy lymphedema treatment. J Surg Oncol 1984; 26:210–213.

Physical Agent Modalities

**DAVID C. WEBER, M.D.,
AND ALLEN W. BROWN, M.D.**

Modalities are physical agents that are utilized to produce a therapeutic response in tissue. They include heat, cold, water, sound, electricity, and electromagnetic waves (including infrared, visible, or ultraviolet [UV] light; shortwaves; and microwaves) (Fig. 22–1). This chapter focuses on these physical agent modalities, except for the therapeutic use of electrical stimulation (which is covered in Chapter 23). These modalities are generally considered adjunctive treatments, rather than primary curative interventions. This chapter reviews the physiological effects, common uses, techniques of application, and precautions for the therapeutic use of modalities.

MODALITY PRESCRIPTION

The elements of a prescription for heat or cold are listed in Table 22–1. The condition for which the modality is

being used should be clearly indicated. The location to be treated influences modality selection in that large areas can preclude the use of modalities such as ultrasound (US) or ice massage. The surface to be treated can also influence selection. If using US over an irregular surface, degassed water may be preferred over a gel coupling agent. If using superficial heat over an irregular surface, hot packs or heating pads may result in focal heating over prominences, so radiant heat may be preferred. Intensity should be indicated where appropriate (e.g., US power output, hydrotherapy, Fluidotherapy, paraffin bath temperature, etc.). Most modalities allow only qualitative dosimetry as currently used in physical medicine, and therefore rely on patient perception of thermal intensity for safety. Duration for most modalities is 20 to 30 min, except for US which is typically 5 to 10 min per site. Frequency is based on the severity of the condition being treated and on clinical

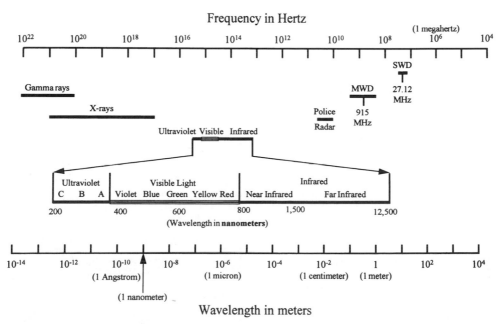

FIGURE 22–1 Electromagnetic spectrum.

TABLE 22–1   Elements of a Prescription for Heat or Cold

Indication/diagnosis	Intensity
Modality	Duration
Location	Frequency

judgment. Although information about duration and intensity of treatment is noted in this chapter, it is intended only as a guideline, and should be modified by clinical experience and the clinical condition.

Modality selection is influenced by multiple factors (Table 22–2). In selecting a modality, one must realize that there are few well-designed clinical trials demonstrating the efficacy of *specific* modalities in *specific* conditions. However, there are numerous studies that review the physiological effects of modalities. Having a firm understanding of the physiological effects of a particular modality allows one to make an educated selection. One must understand the heating or cooling capabilities of the various modalities to ensure that one has selected the proper modality for the target tissue. Body habitus influences modality selection in that subcutaneous adipose affects the depth of penetration of many modalities. Co-morbid conditions should also be considered. For example, both cold and heat may have adverse effects in the patient with significant arterial insufficiency. Cold can have harmful effects via the production of arterial vasoconstriction, and heat can cause complications via the production of increased metabolic activity, which may exceed the potential increase in blood supply and produce ischemia. Age is also a factor in modality selection. In the pediatric population, US should generally be avoided near open epiphyses.[85] In the elderly population, there may be co-morbidities that will affect modality choice. Gender may also play a role in modality use, since fetal malformations have been reported following US near a gravid uterus.[60]

HEAT

Forms of heat can be broadly classified by depth of penetration and form of heat transfer (Table 22–3). Depth of penetration is arbitrarily divided into superficial and deep. Superficial heat includes hot packs, heating pads, paraffin baths, Fluidotherapy, whirlpool baths, and radiant heat. Deep heating agents (or diathermies) include US, shortwave, and microwave. Mechanisms of heat transfer include conduction, convection, radiation, evaporation, and conversion (Fig. 22–2). *Conduction* is the transfer of ther-

TABLE 22–2   Factors to Consider in Modality Selection

Target tissue
Depth of heating or cooling desired
Intensity of heating or cooling desired
Body habitus (i.e., amount of subcutaneous adipose)
Co-morbid conditions (e.g., cancer, vascular disease, neuropathy, etc.)
Specific patient features (e.g., metal implants, pacemaker, cold allergy, etc.)
Age (e.g., open epiphyses)
Sex (e.g., pregnant female)

TABLE 22–3   Classification of Various Types of Heating

	Depth	Main Mechanism of Energy Transfer
Hot packs/heating pads	Superficial	Conduction
Paraffin baths	Superficial	Conduction
Fluidotherapy	Superficial	Convection
Whirlpool baths	Superficial	Convection
Radiant heat	Superficial	Radiation
Ultrasound	Deep	Conversion
Shortwave diathermy	Deep	Conversion
Microwave	Deep	Conversion

mal energy between two bodies in direct contact. *Convection* uses movement of a medium (e.g., water, air, blood, etc.) to transport thermal energy, although the actual transfer of thermal energy is ultimately by conduction. *Radiation* refers to the thermal radiation emitted from any body whose surface temperature is above absolute zero (-273.15 °C or -459.67 °F). *Evaporation* involves the transformation of a liquid to a gas, a process that requires thermal energy. Evaporation is actually a process of heat dissipation, and plays a role in cooling modalities such as vapocoolant sprays. For each gram of water that evaporates from the body surface, approximately 0.6 calorie (kilocalorie) of heat is lost.[34] *Conversion* refers to the transformation of energy (e.g., sound, electromagnetic, etc.) to heat. Likewise, the human body converts protein, carbohydrates, and fats to thermal energy via numerous metabolic processes. This section reviews the physiological effects (Table 22–4), general uses (Table 22–5), and general precautions (Table 22–6) for the therapeutic use of heat, followed by a discussion of agents currently used in physical medicine.

Physiological Effects of Heat

Hemodynamic

Localized heating produces a variety of hemodynamic effects. A two- to threefold increase in forearm blood flow has been demonstrated following hydrotherapy at 44 to 45 °C (111.2–113 °F) or shortwave diathermy.[1] This vasodilation results in increased ingress of nutrients, leukocytes, and antibodies, and increased egress of metabolic byproducts and tissue debris, and may facilitate resolution of inflammatory conditions.[33, 78] Unfortunately, vasodilation

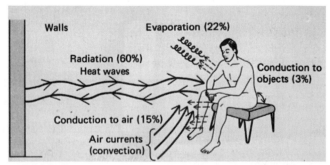

FIGURE 22–2 Mechanisms of heat transfer. (From Guyton AC: Body temperature, temperature regulation, and fever. *In* Guyton AC (ed): Textbook of Medical Physiology, ed 8. Philadelphia, WB Saunders, 1991, pp 797–808.)

TABLE 22–4   Physiological Effects of Heat

Hemodynamic
    Increased blood flow
    Decreased chronic inflammation
    Increased acute inflammation
    Increased edema
    Increased bleeding
Neuromuscular
    ?Increased group Ia fiber firing rates (muscle spindle)
    ?Decreased group II fiber firing rates (muscle spindle)
    ?Increased group Ib fiber firing rates (Golgi tendon organ)
    Increased nerve conduction velocity
Joint and connective tissue
    Increased tendon extensibility
    Increased collagenase activity
    Decreased joint stiffness
Miscellaneous
    Decreased pain
    General relaxation

with heating may also contribute to increased bleeding and increased edema formation, and can exacerbate acute inflammatory conditions.[78] There are a number of experimental animal models of acute and chronic inflammation which support the general clinical impression that acute inflammatory conditions tend to react unfavorably to heat, whereas chronic inflammatory conditions tend to benefit from heat.[78]

Neuromuscular

Animal experiments of localized heating have demonstrated increased firing rates in all group Ia fibers (muscle spindle) and many group Ib (Golgi tendon organ) fibers, while the majority of group II fibers (muscle spindle) had decreased firing rates.[63] It should be noted that all experiments of muscle spindle and Golgi tendon organ firing rates are significantly influenced by the length and tension at which they are performed. This factor likely accounts for many of the differences among investigators.[24, 63] In contrast, the effects of temperature change on nerve conduction velocity are much more consistent. Heating produces modest increases in conduction velocity, whereas cooling is capable of producing dramatic decreases in conduction velocity. Abramson et al.[1] noted increases in conduction velocity of up to 7.5 m/sec following hydrotherapy at 44 to 45 °C (111.2–113 °F) or shortwave diathermy, whereas cooling produced conduction velocity decreases of up to 35.8 m/sec. The effects of temperature in clinical neurophysiology are succinctly summarized elsewhere.[18]

Joint and Connective Tissue

In vitro experiments demonstrate the importance of combined heating and stretching to maximize tendon extensibil-

TABLE 22–5   General Uses of Heat in Physical Medicine

Musculoskeletal conditions (tendinitis, tenosynovitis, bursitis, capsulitis, etc.)
Pain (neck, low back, myofascial, neuromas, postherpetic neuralgia, etc.)
Arthritis
Contracture
Muscle relaxation
Chronic inflammation

TABLE 22–6   General Precautions for the Use of Heat

Acute trauma, inflammation
Impaired circulation
Bleeding diatheses
Edema
Large scars
Impaired sensation
Malignancy
Cognitive or communication deficits that preclude reporting of pain

ity. Lehmann et al.[51] measured tendon extensibility under a variety of temperature and loading conditions. Tendon extensibility was greater at 45 °C (113 °F) than at 25 °C (77 °F). Furthermore, simultaneous use of heating and stretching produced significantly increased tendon extensibility when compared to the isolated use of either agent. Sustaining stretching during the cooldown period also facilitated tendon elongation. Other investigators[95] have demonstrated metacarpophalangeal joint stiffness to decrease by as much as 20% at 45 °C (113 °F) compared to 33 °C (91.4 °F). Temperature also affects enzymatic activity. In vitro experiments have shown a fourfold increase in collagenase activity with a temperature increase from 33 to 36 °C (91.4–96.8 °F).[35]

Miscellaneous Effects of Heat

It is generally accepted that heat produces an analgesic effect. A variety of mechanisms for the analgesic effect of heat have been postulated.[25, 44] These include (1) cutaneous counterirritant effect, (2) vasodilation resulting in decreased ischemic pain, (3) vasodilation resulting in washout of pain mediators, (4) endorphin-mediated response, (5) alteration of nerve conduction, and (6) alteration of cell membrane permeability. Elevation of pain threshold has been demonstrated following therapeutic application of US, microwave, and infrared radiation.[45] Many patients also find heat to have a general relaxation effect, although the specific mechanisms are not well defined.

General Uses of Heat in Physical Medicine

The general uses of heat are summarized in Table 22–5. These uses are based on the physiological effects previously described. Heat is used in a variety of musculoskeletal conditions because of its potential to produce analgesia, muscle relaxation, and facilitate resolution of inflammation. Increased soft tissue extensibility and decreased joint stiffness make heat useful in contractures and a variety of arthritides.

General Precautions for the Use of Heat

The general precautions for the use of heat are listed in Table 22–6. As noted earlier, heat can exacerbate acute inflammation, and should generally be avoided in the acute management stage.[78] In the patient with impaired circulation, increased metabolic activity with heating may exceed the capacity of arterial supply, so heat should be used with caution in this patient population. Vasodilation from heat can result in increased bleeding in persons with bleeding diatheses. Likewise, it may produce increased edema. Since scars can be relatively avascular and have reduced ability for heat dissipation, they can be selectively heated. Heat should generally be avoided in areas of impaired sensation because of obvious potential for thermal injury due to the lack of precise dosimetry in modality use. This same reason justifies caution in using heat in patients with impaired cognition or communication which precludes reporting of pain. Lehmann[44] cautions against the use of heat over malignancies because of the potential for increased rate of tumor growth or hyperemia increasing hematogenous spread. However, this should be distinguished from the use of specific local hyperthermia in the adjunctive treatment of malignancies.[72] It also does not preclude the use of heat for adjunctive analgesia in the terminally ill cancer patient.

SUPERFICIAL HEAT

Superficial heating agents achieve their maximum tissue temperatures in skin and subcutaneous fat. Deeper tissue heating is limited by vasodilation (which dissipates heat), and the insulating properties of fat. Superficial heating agents can heat via conduction (hot packs, heating pads, and paraffin baths), radiation (heat lamps), or convection (Fluidotherapy and whirlpool baths). Superficial heat is used in osteoarthritis, rheumatoid arthritis, neck pain, low back pain, muscle pain syndromes, and a variety of musculoskeletal conditions.[44]

Hot Packs

Commercially available hot packs, such as Hydrocollator packs, typically contain silicon dioxide encased in a canvas pack. They come in a variety of sizes and styles for use over different areas. Hot packs are immersed in tanks at 74.5 °C (166 °F) and applied over several layers of insulating towels.[54] After several minutes, the skin should be inspected briefly to ensure that the heating is not excessive. Total treatment time is usually 30 min. A 30-min application of a Hydrocollator pack to the posterior thigh produced approximately 3.3 and 1.3 °C tissue temperature elevations at 1- and 2-cm depths respectively.[54] Other investigators observed a 1.1 °C temperature rise 4 cm deep in the brachioradialis muscle following 30-min application of a Hydrocollator pack.[2] A 1.2 °C increase in intra-articular temperature (knee) has also been demonstrated following hot pack application.[93] General heat precautions should be observed. The patient should not lie on the pack, as this can squeeze water from the pack, wetting the insulating towels, which increases their thermal conductivity, potentially leading to burns. Likewise, the focal pressure from lying on a hot pack can produce increased heating over bony prominences. Hot packs are one of the more common causes of burns in physical therapy owing to the sedative effects of heat and because the patient is typically not directly supervised when this modality is used.

Heating Pads

Two main types of heating pads are available, electric heating pads and those that circulate a heated fluid such as water. Electric heating pads usually control heat output by regulating current flow. Circulating fluid heating pads usually control heat output thermostatically. Peak temperatures of nearly 52 °C (125 °F) were achieved with an electric heating pad set on the *lowest* setting.[19] Periodic temperature oscillations of up to 5 °C were also noted.[19] General heat precautions should be observed with heating pads. There is an obvious potential for electric shock, particularly when used in conjunction with moist toweling. Many commercially available heating pads are designed to be used in conjunction with moist toweling, but caution should be taken to inspect them regularly to ensure that all insulating materials are intact. The patient should not lie on a heating pad, as this can result in focal temperature increases, leading to burns. This is of particular concern in the slender or cachectic patient with minimal subcutaneous adipose over bony prominences. Figure 22–3 shows a typical heating pad burn. The patient was an elderly woman who had not received adequate instruction in home use of her modalities, and had been repeatedly lying supine on an electric heating pad. Repeated and prolonged skin exposure to heat may result in erythema ab igne, a skin condition characterized by reticular pigmentation, and telangiectasia, which has been noted following the use of a variety of superficial heating modalities.[20]

Radiant Heat

Radiant energy, including infrared radiation (IR), is emitted from any substance with a temperature above absolute zero. IR is the portion of the electromagnetic spectrum adjacent to the long-wavelength, low-frequency (red) end of the visible spectrum. Luminous IR heat lamps emit radiation in the near-infrared spectrum (wavelength, 770–1500 nm) and nonluminous IR heat lamps emit radiation in the far-infrared spectrum (wavelength 1500–12,500

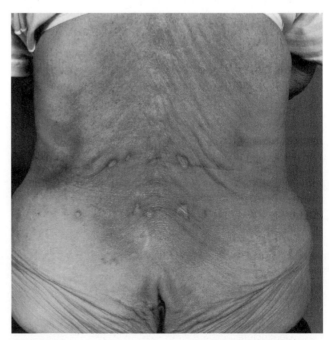

FIGURE 22–3 Typical heating pad burn. Note the focal hypopigmentation from burns at areas of increased pressure. Also note the more diffuse hyperpigmentation changes (erythema ab igne).

nm).[44] IR produces heating by inducing molecular vibration.[20] A 1.3 °C temperature rise has been noted at a depth of 2 cm following heat lamp application.[54]

The main determinants of intensity of radiant heating are distance and angle of delivery. The inverse square law states that the intensity of radiation varies inversely with the square of the distance from the source (Fig. 22–4). This means that doubling the distance from a heat lamp reduces the heating intensity by a factor of 4. Conversely, decreasing the distance from the heat lamp by half would increase the intensity fourfold. Typical distances are 30 to 60 cm from the patient's body, depending on heat lamp wattage.[44] Angle of delivery also affects the intensity of thermal radiation. Maximal radiation is applied when the source of radiation is perpendicular to the surface. As the angle away from perpendicular increases, the intensity of radiation decreases in proportion to the cosine of the angle.

Radiant heat is often preferable in patients who cannot tolerate the weight of hot packs. Caveats for the use of radiant heat include (1) general heat precautions, (2) light sensitivity, (3) skin drying, and (4) dermal photoaging.[20, 44] Some laboratory data suggest a potential for IR acting synergistically with UV radiation in cutaneous photocarcinogenesis, but the clinical significance of this, if any, remains to be determined.[20]

Fluidotherapy

Fluidotherapy is a superficial, dry heating modality that uses convective heating with forced hot air and a bed of finely divided solid particles.[9] This solid-gas system reportedly behaves like a heterogeneous fluid of low viscosity, a phenomenon labeled fluidization.[8] Reputed advantages include the massaging action of the highly turbulent solid-gas mixture, and the freedom to perform range of motion exercises.[8] Peak hand muscle and joint capsule temperatures of nearly 42 °C (107.6 °F) and peak foot

muscle and joint capsule temperatures of approximately 39.5 °C (103.1 °F) have been achieved following 20 min of Fluidotherapy at 47.8 °C (118 °F).[9] Both the temperature and the amount of agitation can be controlled. The typical temperature range is 46.1 to 48.9 °C (115–120 °F). Decreased degrees of agitation can be utilized for sensitive areas. General heat precautions should be observed and infected wounds should probably be avoided because of the risk of cross-contamination.

Paraffin Baths

A paraffin bath is a superficial heating agent that uses conduction as the primary form of heat transfer. Paraffin wax and mineral oil are mixed in a ratio of 6:1 or 7:1.[44] Treatment temperatures are 52.2 to 54.4 °C (126–130 °F). These are tolerated because of the low heat conductivity of the paraffin mixture.[44] A thermometer should be used to ensure proper temperature. A thin film of unmelted paraffin on the tank walls generally indicates a safe temperature. Methods of application include dipping, immersion, and brushing. After removing all jewelry, thoroughly wash and dry the area to be treated. The dipping method involves 7 to 12 dips followed by wrapping in plastic and towels or insulated mitts to retain heat.[2] The immersion method involves several dips to form a thin glove of paraffin, followed by immersion for 30 min.[2] The brushing method involves brushing on several coats of paraffin, followed by covering with towels. The brushing method is more cumbersome and infrequently used in the adult population. However, children may find paraffin brushing to be fun, thereby improving their treatment compliance. Paraffin brushing can also be useful for areas difficult to immerse. For home treatment, patients can use a double boiler, although commercial paraffin tanks are reasonably inexpensive and probably safer. The equipment safety precautions should be carefully reviewed. General heat precautions apply to paraffin use. Open wounds and infected areas should be avoided.

The immersion method produces the greatest quantity and duration of temperature increase, with peak forearm subcutaneous tissue temperatures of 5.5 °C over baseline and brachioradialis temperatures of 2.4 °C over baseline.[2] The dip method produces a 4.4 °C peak forearm subcutaneous tissue temperature rise and a 1.0 °C brachioradialis temperature rise, but these temperature rises decrease significantly by 15 to 20 min post-dipping.[2] In a study of scleroderma patients, paraffin baths in conjunction with friction massage and active range-of-motion exercise resulted in statistically significant improvement in skin compliance and overall hand function.[3] In a study of rheumatoid arthritis patients, statistically significant improvements in range of motion and grip function were noted following paraffin treatment in conjunction with active range-of-motion exercises, whereas paraffin baths alone had no statistically significant effect.[17] This again emphasizes the importance of using exercise in combination with the modality.

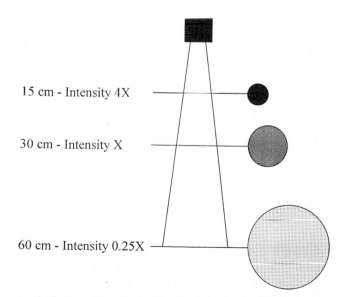

FIGURE 22–4 Example of inverse square law with the intensity arbitrarily defined as x at a distance of 30 cm. With a change in distance from the heat source, the area of heating changes and, therefore, the heat intensity per unit of area changes.

15 cm - Intensity 4X

30 cm - Intensity X

60 cm - Intensity 0.25X

DEEP HEAT

Diathermy is derived from *dia* (through) and *therme* (heat), and refers to several forms of deep heating, namely shortwave, microwave, and US. Since the target tissue in physical medicine is generally muscle, tendon, ligament, or bone (rather than skin or subcutaneous fat), the goal of early investigators was to discover a mode of heating that minimized skin and subcutaneous tissue heating, but maximized heating of deeper tissues.[33] The challenge of diathermy developers was to discover a modality that could penetrate the skin and subcutaneous fat to produce a maximum temperature rise in underlying soft tissues. Conversely, the modality should not produce excessive temperatures in more superficial tissues (subcutaneous fat, being relatively avascular compared to muscle, is unable to adequately dissipate heat via vasodilation). The therapeutic target temperature is generally considered to be 40 to 45 °C (104–113 °F).[33] Lower temperatures may not produce adequate vasodilation and increased metabolism, whereas higher temperatures may result in tissue damage. Since the thermal pain threshold is approximately 45 °C (113 °F), pain perception may be used to monitor intensity of heating.[33] One gradually increases modality intensity to the earliest pain perception, then slightly decreases intensity. However, there is a fine line between the therapeutic temperature range and potential thermal injury.

Ultrasound

Ultrasound is defined as acoustic vibration with frequencies above the audible range (i.e., greater than 20,000 Hz). Medical uses of US can be diagnostic or therapeutic. Diagnostic US is used for a variety of obstetric, urological, cardiovascular, and other imaging studies, and is outside the scope of this chapter. Therapeutic US involves the use of high-frequency acoustic energy to produce thermal and nonthermal effects in tissue. Ultrasonic signals are typically generated using the reverse piezoelectric effect. Certain quartz crystals and synthetic ceramics have piezoelectric characteristics, such that when they vibrate they produce an electric current.[87] Conversely, by passing an electric current across such crystals, vibration at a specific frequency is produced.

As ultrasonic waves travel through tissue, they lose a proportion of their energy, a process called attenuation.[96] *Attenuation* in tissue is produced by several mechanisms: absorption, beam divergence, and deflection.[96] *Absorption* is the major cause of US attenuation.[96] Ultrasonic energy is absorbed by the tissue, and is ultimately converted into heat.[96] For most tissues, attenuation increases as frequency increases, so a 1.0-MHz signal would penetrate deeper than a 3.0-MHz signal because of its lower attenuation by the tissue.[96] *Beam divergence* is the amount that the beam spreads out from the transducer. Beam divergence decreases as frequency increases, so a higher frequency signal has a more focused beam.

Deflection includes the processes of *reflection, refraction*, and *scattering*.[96] The *angle* of the reflected wave is equal to the angle of the incident wave (Fig. 22–5). The *magnitude* of the reflected wave depends on the difference in acoustic impedance between the tissues on each side of the reflecting surface.[96] Acoustic impedance is a measure of the resistance to the transmission of a sound wave and is the product of the velocity of sound and density of

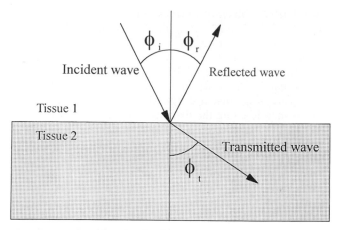

FIGURE 22–5 Example of reflection and refraction at a tissue interface. ϕ_i = Angle of incident wave; ϕ_r = angle of reflected wave; and ϕ_t = angle of transmitted wave.

the medium.[87, 96] The magnitude of the reflected wave is proportional to the following formula[87]:

$$A_2 - A_1/A_2 + A_1$$

where A_2 is the acoustic impedance of tissue 2 and A_1 is the acoustic impedance of tissue 1. Therefore, the greater the mismatch of acoustic impedance of the two tissues, the greater the magnitude of the reflected wave. Since the impedance mismatch between skin and air is extremely high, essentially all of the acoustic signal is reflected if a coupling agent is not used (see below).[96] *Refraction* is a deviation of beam direction as it is transmitted between two media (see Fig. 22–5). The angle of the transmitted (refracted) wave is determined by the velocity of sound in the two media, and is given by Snell's law[96]:

$$\frac{\text{sine 1}}{\text{sine 2}} = \frac{\text{velocity 1}}{\text{velocity 2}}$$

where sine 1 is the sine of the incident wave, and sine 2 is the sine of the transmitted wave, and velocity 1 is the velocity of sound in the first tissue, and velocity 2 is the velocity of sound in the second tissue. *Scattering* is the last mechanism of beam deflection. It occurs when surface irregularities scatter the signal. Scattering is minimized when surface irregularities are small with respect to the wavelength.

Parameters for therapeutic US are noted in Table 22–7. Frequency is generally in the range of millions of cycles per second (or MHz). In the United States, the most commonly used frequencies are in the range of 0.8 to 1.1 MHz, although frequencies around 3.0 MHz are also fairly common. Power is total energy per unit time, whereas intensity is power per unit area. Intensity may be expressed in terms of peak or average intensity, and spatial or temporal intensity, and is indicated in units of watts per square centimeter. These different measures of intensity are defined in Table 22–7. The World Health Organization and the International Electrical Commission both recommend limiting spatial average intensity to 3 W/cm².[38] Most clinically used intensities of therapeutic US are in the 0.5 to

TABLE 22–7   Ultrasound Parameters

Frequency—millions of cycles per second (MHz)
Power—total energy per unit time (W)
Effective radiating area—the area of the transducer which actually radiates ultrasonic waves (cm²)
Intensity—may be expressed in terms of peak or average and spatial or temporal (W/cm²)
    Spatial average intensity—total power output divided by effective radiating area
    Spatial peak intensity—maximal intensity anywhere within the beam
    Temporal average intensity—average intensity of "on" and "off" periods of a pulsed signal
    Temporal peak intensity—maximal intensity of "on" period of a pulsed signal
Duration—generally 5–10 min per site
Additional parameters for pulsed ultrasound
    Pulse duration—time of actual ultrasound pulse ("time on")
    Pulse repetition period—time interval from one pulse to the next ("time on" and "time off")
    Pulse repetition frequency—number of pulses per second
    Duty factor—fraction of total time during which ultrasound is emitted (calculated by dividing pulse duration by pulse repetition period)

2.0 W/cm² range. Temperatures of up to 46 °C (114.8 °F) in deep tissues (e.g., bone-muscle interface) are easily achieved with US.[47–49] If very deep heating (e.g., hip joint) is the goal, US appears to be superior to microwave or shortwave diathermy.[53]

Ultrasound delivery may be continuous or pulsed. Pulsed delivery involves the emission of brief bursts or pulses of US, interspersed with periods of silence (Fig. 22–6). For pulsed US delivery, additional parameters should be indicated.[87] These include pulse duration, pulse repetition period, pulse repetition frequency, and duty factor, and are defined in Table 22–7. In most US units, selecting a duty factor automatically determines the other parameters. Duty factor commonly ranges from 10% to 50%. For example, a 2-ms pulse duration might be interspersed with 8 ms of silence. The pulse repetition period would be 10 ms, the pulse repetition frequency would be 100 Hz, and the duty factor would be 20%. Pulsed delivery, especially at low duty factors, results in less heating than continuous-wave US, and thereby presumably emphasizes nonthermal effects.

The physiological effects of US can be divided into thermal and nonthermal effects. Thermal effects are produced when acoustic energy is absorbed, producing molecular vibration, which results in heat production.[13] Nonthermal effects include cavitation, media motion (acoustic streaming, microstreaming), and standing waves. *Cavitation* is the production of gas bubbles in a sound field.[13] These bubbles can expand and contract with alternating compressions and rarefactions of a sound wave.[13] Stable cavitation refers to bubbles that oscillate in size within the sound field.[22] Unstable cavitation refers to bubbles that continue to grow in size and then collapse. The high temperatures and pressures generated by this can produce platelet aggregation, localized tissue damage, and cell death.[22] Both forms of cavitation are capable of mechanical distortion, movement of material, and alteration of cellular function, but their clinical significance is not yet clearly defined.[13, 65]

Media motion includes acoustic streaming and microstreaming. Acoustic *streaming* is defined as unidirectional movement in an ultrasonic pressure field, and results from an ultrasonic wave traveling through a compressible medium.[22] Acoustic *microstreaming* is produced by stable cavitation. As the stable cavitation bubbles oscillate in size, the surrounding fluid is set in motion, with nearby particles being attracted to the oscillating bubble.[22] In addition to movement of material, acoustic streaming and microstreaming can result in cell membrane damage and accelerate metabolic processes.[22]

Standing waves are produced by the superimposition of incident and reflected sound waves and can result in focal heating at tissue interfaces of different densities.[22] Stasis of red blood cells at one-half wavelength intervals in a sound field has also been demonstrated in the laboratory.[23] Although numerous subcellular, cellular, and tissue nonthermal US effects have been reported, their clinical significance remains to be elucidated.[13, 15, 22, 23, 65] Certain measures can minimize the nonthermal effects of US. Higher frequency, lower intensity, and pulsed delivery mode minimizes acoustic cavitation.[15] Stroking technique of application minimizes standing wave formation.[22]

As noted previously, the amount of US reflected at an interface between two media depends on the difference in acoustic impedance, so the ideal coupling medium is one with an acoustic impedance similar to tissue. Three factors have an impact on the effectiveness of a coupling medium (1) absorption by the medium, which attenuates the ultrasound power; (2) impedance match between the coupling media and the transmitter sound head, which determines the amount of power reflected into the US source; and (3) impedance match between the coupling medium and the body tissue, which determines the amount of power reflected into the medium.[4] Degassed water is a commonly used coupling medium and is used to prevent bubble formation on the skin surface. Allowing tap water to stand overnight should allow for adequate gas evaporation. In tests of acoustic transmissivity, mineral oil and several commercially available coupling gels had similar transmissivities to the reference standard of distilled degassed water.[90] However, the hydrocortisone phonophoresis coupling agents tested had a significantly lower transmissivity, presumably related to microscopic air bubbles introduced to the media. Variation in transducer pressure produced dramatic differences in transmissivity, which outweighed the differences between the various coupling media. These investigators concluded that coupling media can be chosen primarily on the basis of cost and convenience, without compromising function.[90] Encased silicon gel shows promise for use as a coupling agent over irregular body surfaces, sensitive skin areas, and open wounds, if the issue of impedance mismatch with the sound head can be rectified.[4]

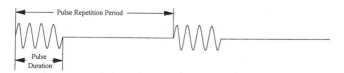

FIGURE 22–6   Example of pulsed ultrasound signal.

In addition to accommodating for impedance mismatches, coupling media also lubricate to permit smooth movement of the transducer over the skin.

The most common technique of US application is the stroking technique. It allows a more even energy distribution over the site being treated. The applicator is moved slowly over an area of approximately 25 cm^2 (4 in.^{2}) in a circular or longitudinal manner.[44] The applicator size (usually 5–10 cm^2) limits the size of the area that can be treated, so multiple fields of treatment may be needed for larger areas (i.e., shoulder and hip anterior, lateral, and posterior ports). The stationary technique generally should be avoided because of the potential for standing waves and the production of hot spots.[69] Intensity is indicated by specifying the particular watts per square centimeter or by titrating to just below pain threshold. In surveys of performance of ultrasonic therapy equipment, variations in frequency and power output were common.[38, 83] Although the frequency of commercially available US applicators was typically within 5% of manufacturer's specifications, the overwhelming majority (85%) of applicators tested had power output variations of over 20%.[83] Therefore, US applicators should be recalibrated regularly.

Over 35 clinical uses of US have been described, but many of these are not well supported by experimental evidence.[85] Falconer et al.[25] recently reviewed and summarized the literature addressing the effectiveness of US in a variety of musculoskeletal conditions including periarticular inflammatory conditions (bursitis, capsulitis, epicondylitis, tendinitis), other "chronic inflammatory conditions" (rheumatoid arthritis, ankylosing spondylitis, nonspecific musculoskeletal pain, low back pain, frozen shoulder), and osteoarthritis. Study differences precluded meta-analysis, so a quantitative synthesis was performed instead. The overall quality of many of the studies was questionable. Only 5 of 35 studies were blinded and placebo-controlled. As one would expect, uncontrolled or unblinded studies were more likely to produce positive outcomes. The authors concluded that pain and range of motion appear to improve following US treatment in acute periarticular inflammatory conditions and osteoarthritis, but not in chronic periarticular inflammatory conditions.[25] Pain relief was theorized to be related to alterations in nerve conduction, washout of pain mediators by increased blood flow, or alterations in cell membrane permeability that result in decreased inflammation.[25] The authors emphasized a significant placebo effect and experimenter expectancy bias and noted that well-designed clinical trials (e.g., randomized, controlled, blinded studies) are necessary to resolve the issue of ultrasound efficacy.[25]

Ultrasound precautions are summarized in Table 22–8.[60, 69, 85] Concern about the use of heat near malignancies was discussed previously. Deep heating over an open epiphysis could result in either increased growth (from hyperemia) or decreased growth (from thermal injury). Avoiding US near pacemakers is reasonable because of potential thermal or mechanical injury to the pacemaker. Ultrasound over laminectomy sites could theoretically result in spinal cord heating. There are also case reports of increased radicular pain with US.[29] There are even case reports of patient abuse of US.[56] The concern with US use over arthroplasties and other metallic implants is the potential for focal heat-

TABLE 22–8 Ultrasound Precautions

General heat precautions
Near brain, eyes, reproductive organs
Gravid or menstruating uterus
Near pacemaker
Near spine, laminectomy sites
Malignancy
Skeletal immaturity
Arthroplasties?
Methyl methacrylate or high-density polyethylene?

ing. Gersten[28] reported that temperature rises near metal were actually lower than temperature rises near bone, so metal per se should not be a contraindication to US. However, Lehmann[44] cautions against the use of US near methyl methacrylate or high-density polyethylene because of their high coefficient of absorption. The effect of US on bony ingrowth arthroplasties is not yet well defined. Since the effects of US on arthroplasties are not yet completely delineated, the most prudent course would be to avoid US over these areas whenever possible.

Shortwave Diathermy

Shortwave diathermy (SWD) is a modality that produces deep heating via conversion of electromagnetic energy to thermal energy. Oscillation of high-frequency electrical and magnetic fields produces movement of ions, rotation of polar molecules, and distortion of nonpolar molecules, with resultant heat generation.[30, 40] The Federal Communications Commission (FCC) limits industrial, scientific, and medical (ISM) use to 13.56 MHz (22-m wavelength), 27.12 MHz (11-m wavelength), and 40.68 MHz (7.5-m wavelength).[42] The 27.12-MHz frequency is most commonly used. The heating pattern produced depends on the type of shortwave unit and on the water content and electrical properties of the tissue. Tissues can be grossly divided into those with high water content (muscle, skin, blood, etc.) and those with low water content (bone, fat, etc.).[40]

Shortwave diathermy units can be inductive or capacitive. Inductive applicators use induction coils which apply a magnetic field to induce circular electrical fields in the tissue.[33] They achieve higher temperatures in water-rich tissues with higher conductivity.[42] These applicators may have a cable or drum configuration.[42] Cables are semiflexible induction coils which can be formed to the contour of the area to be treated. Drum applicators consist of induction coils enclosed in a rigid housing or drum. For a capacitive applicator, the patient is placed between two metal condenser plates (Fig. 22–7). The plates and the patient's intervening tissue act as a capacitor (an object which stores electrical charge), and heat is generated by rapid oscillations in the electric field from one plate to the other.[30] Capacitive applicators may achieve higher temperatures in water-poor tissues such as subcutaneous adipose.[33, 42]

Currently available shortwave applicators do not allow precise dosimetry, so initial pain perception is used to monitor intensity. Terry cloth towels are used for spacing and to absorb sweat, which is highly conductive and could result in potentially severe focal heating.[44] Typical treatment time is 20 to 30 min. Specific applicator configuration can greatly affect the distribution of heating.[42, 52] In a

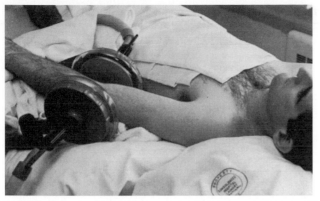

FIGURE 22–7 Example of shortwave diathermy application with capacitive applicator (condenser plates). (From Kothe FJ, Lehmann JF (eds): Krusen's Handbook of Physical Medicine and Rehabilitation, ed 4. Philadelphia, WB Saunders, 1990, p 293.)

review of several different induction applicators, the ratio of muscle heating vs. fat heating ranged from 0.39 to 2.67 for the various applicators tested.[52]

Lehmann et al.[46] evaluated the effect of subcutaneous fat thickness and technique of SWD application. In comparing distance from the applicator, 2 cm of air space between patient and applicator produced a more desirable heating pattern than did 3 mm of terry cloth between patient and applicator. Depth of subcutaneous fat also had a significant effect on temperature distribution. Muscle temperature rise in subjects with less than 1 cm of subcutaneous fat compared to those with more than 2 cm of subcutaneous fat, were 9.5 °C and 5.6 °C, respectively.[46] SWD has been purported to be useful in a variety of musculoskeletal conditions.[30] The precautions are listed in Table 22–9. Metal can result in focal heating and should be strictly avoided. All jewelry should be removed, and the treatment table ideally should not contain metal. Likewise, electromagnetic energy can seriously interfere with pacemaker function, so a pacemaker is an absolute contraindication. Contact lenses are a concern because of the potential for focal heating.[79] The other precautions listed are self-explanatory.

Microwave Diathermy

Microwave diathermy is another form of electromagnetic energy which uses conversion as its primary form of heat production. Thermal energy is produced by increased kinetic energy of molecules within the microwave field.[71] FCC-approved frequencies for therapeutic microwave are 915 MHz (wavelength, 33 cm) and 2456 MHz (wavelength, 12 cm).[44] The lower frequency has the advantage of in-creased depth of penetration, but disadvantages of greater beam dispersion and the requirement of larger applicators.[71]

Temperature distribution in a particular tissue is affected largely by its water content. The fraction of power absorbed in a particular tissue depends on several factors including the frequency of the electromagnetic wave, the dielectric constant, and the electrical conductivity of the tissue.[71] In general, tissues with high water content absorb greater amounts of energy, and are selectively heated.[44] If muscle heating is a primary objective, 915-MHz applicators are preferable to 2456-MHz applicators.[50] Nonthermal effects of microwave diathermy have been documented, but Lehmann points out that there is no evidence that these are of any therapeutic significance.[44] Average temperatures of approximately 41 °C (105.8 °F) at a depth of 1 to 3 cm have been demonstrated.[16] Microwave, although once quite popular, has been largely replaced by other modalities such as US and hot packs.[84] However, a recent study did demonstrate some potential benefit in rheumatoid arthritis. In this study, treatment with 915-MHz microwave to the rheumatoid knee resulted in statistically significant improvements in pain score index and walking speed.[92]

General heat precautions should be observed with microwave. Metal implants, pacemakers, sites of skeletal immaturity, reproductive organs and brain, and fluid-filled cavities (eye, bullae, effusions, etc.) should be avoided.[41, 44]

CRYOTHERAPY

All forms of cryotherapy (therapeutic use of cold) are considered superficial cooling agents, usually transferring thermal energy by conduction. Exceptions include convective cooling in the whirlpool, and evaporative cooling with vapocoolant sprays (Table 22–10). This section reviews the physiological effects (Table 22–11), general uses (Table 22–12), and general precautions (Table 22–13) for cryotherapy, followed by a discussion of the agents currently used in physical medicine.

Physiological Effects of Cold

Hemodynamic

Application of cold to the skin results in immediate cutaneous vasoconstriction through sympathetically mediated reflex mechanisms and by directly stimulating smooth muscle contraction.[34, 73] Lewis[57] observed phasic oscillations of temperature in the fingers after initial vasoconstriction during cold water immersion. The initial vasoconstriction is thought to be due to a cold-induced increase in the affinity of the postjunctional α-adrenergic receptors for

TABLE 22–9   Shortwave Precautions

General heat precautions
Metal (jewelry, pacemakers, intrauterine devices, surgical implants, etc.)
Contact lenses
Gravid or menstruating uterus
Skeletal immaturity

TABLE 22–10   Classification of Various Types of Cooling

	Depth	Main Form of Energy Transfer
Cold packs	Superficial	Conduction
Ice massage	Superficial	Conduction
Cold water immersion	Superficial	Conduction
Cryotherapy-compression units	Superficial	Conduction
Vapocoolant spray	Superficial	Evaporation
Whirlpool baths	Superficial	Convection

TABLE 22–11 Physiological Effects of Cold

Hemodynamic
    Immediate cutaneous vasoconstriction
    Delayed reactive vasodilation
    Decreased acute inflammation
Neuromuscular
    Slowing of conduction velocity
    Conduction block and axonal degeneration with prolonged
      exposure
    Decreased group Ia fiber firing rates (muscle spindle)
    Decreased group II fiber firing rates (muscle spindle)
    Decreased group Ib fiber firing rates (Golgi tendon organ)
    Decreased muscle stretch reflex amplitudes
    Increased maximal isometric strength
    Decreased muscle fatigue
    Temporarily reduced spasticity
Joint and connective tissue
    Increased joint stiffness
    Decreased tendon extensibility
    Decreased collagenase activity
Miscellaneous
    Decreased pain
    General relaxation

existing norepinephrine in vascular smooth muscle.[80] Reactive vasodilation occurs as further cooling interrupts norepinephrine release. Vasodilation warms the tissues, again releasing norepinephrine to sensitized receptors, and the cycle repeats. This "hunting" of temperature is believed to be a mechanism by which peripheral exposed parts of the body are protected from cold injury. Others have demonstrated vasodilation after cooling of the hand and forearm, without the phasic oscillations observed by Lewis.[12, 26] The effects of localized cooling on heart rate and blood pressure are variable, and have been summarized elsewhere.[61] Cryotherapy has also been shown to moderate inflammation, more effectively in the acute phase than in the chronic phase.[78]

Neuromuscular

The initial response of peripheral nerve to cold application is a marked slowing of conduction velocity.[1, 18] With more prolonged exposure there is conduction block, cessation of axoplasmic transport, and eventual axonal degeneration.[68] Decreased muscle spindle (both group Ia and II fibers) and Golgi tendon organ (group Ib fibers) firing rates have been demonstrated after local cooling in animals.[24] The clinical neuromuscular effects of cooling include a decrease in gastrocnemius muscle stretch reflex amplitude,[6, 43] an increase in maximal isometric strength,[11, 59] and slowing in the rate of muscle fatigue.[11] Cold has also been shown to temporarily reduce spasticity in patients with hemiplegia and multiple sclerosis, improving exercise tolerance and

TABLE 22–12 General Uses of Cryotherapy in Physical Medicine

Musculoskeletal conditions (sprains, strains, tendinitis,
    tenosynovitis, bursitis, capsulitis, etc.)
Myofascial pain
Following certain orthopedic surgeries
Component of spasticity management
Emergent treatment of minor burns

TABLE 22–13 General Precautions for the Use of Cold

Cold intolerance
Cryotherapy-induced neurapraxia/axonotmesis
Arterial insufficiency
Impaired sensation
Cognitive or communication deficits that preclude reporting
    of pain
Cryopathies
    Cryoglobulinemia
    Paroxysmal cold hemoglobinuria
    Cold hypersensitivity
    Raynaud's disease/phenomenon

enhancing function.[37, 64] Other investigators also demonstrated generally reduced spasticity following cryotherapy, but cautioned that some subjects had significantly increased spasticity after cold application.[75]

Joint and Connective Tissue

Topical cold application to the knee in dogs induced significant (approximately 4 °C) and sustained depression of intra-articular temperature without significant effect on core temperature.[7] Synovial collagenase activity also decreases with temperature. In vitro experiments demonstrate negligible synovial collagenase activity after cooling to 30 °C (86 °F), suggesting that therapy that decreases intra-articular temperature in inflammatory arthropathies may slow the rate of collagenolysis.[35] However, potentially negative effects such as decreased tendon extensibility and increased joint stiffness have also been demonstrated following cooling.[51, 95]

Miscellaneous Effects of Cold

The analgesic effect of cold may be related to reflex muscle relaxation, cutaneous counterirritation, or its effects on nerve conduction.[61] As with heat, some patients note cold to produce a general relaxation, although the mechanisms are not well defined.

General Uses of Cryotherapy in Physical Medicine

The general uses for therapeutic cold are summarized in Table 22–12. Cryotherapy is most commonly used acutely after musculoskeletal injury to minimize formation of edema, and for symptomatic relief in painful soft tissue and articular inflammatory states.[31, 39, 61, 62, 88] It has also been used for controlling pain and swelling after some orthopedic procedures,[14, 36] and as a component of spasticity management.[37, 64] Cryotherapy in the form of immediate ice water immersion is advocated as emergent primary treatment for minor burns.[82]

General Precautions for the Use of Cold

The general precautions for the use of cold are outlined in Table 22–13. The most common relative contraindication to the use of cold is simple cold intolerance. A patient who does not tolerate cold application will tend to increase muscle guarding and co-contraction, which is directly counterproductive to the therapeutic goals. Simple cold intolerance should be distinguished from true cold hypersensitivity discussed below. Caution should also be used when applying cold over the course of superficial nerves as peroneal and ulnar palsies have been reported following cryotherapy.[21] Application of cold over areas of compromised arterial vascularity can theoretically produce further ischemia from local vasoconstriction and should be avoided. Likewise, because of the potential for cold injury, cryotherapy should be used with caution in areas of impaired sensation, or in patients who have cognitive or communication deficits which preclude reporting of pain.

The cryopathies are also contraindications to the use of cold.[76] Cryoglobulinemia is a condition which results in the precipitation of immune complexes at low temperatures. Paroxysmal cold hemoglobinuria is a rare disorder resulting from an antibody directed against a red blood cell surface antigen, with hemolysis precipitated by cold exposure. Cold hypersensitivity is a mast cell–mediated process producing urticaria and angioedema on exposure to cold. Raynaud's *disease* is an idiopathic condition characterized by arteriolar spasm precipitated by cold exposure or stress. Raynaud's *phenomenon* is secondary to other rheumatologic conditions (such as rheumatoid arthritis, scleroderma, systemic lupus erythematosus, etc.) and is classically manifested by digital pallor, followed by cyanosis and eventual reactive hyperemia.

Cryotherapy Agents

Cold Packs

Cold packs include Hydrocollator packs, endothermic chemical gel packs, and ice packs. Hydrocollator packs are cooled in a freezer to −12 °C (10 °F) and applied over a moist towel.[43] Endothermic chemical gel packs have separate compartments with compounds such as ammonium nitrate and water that, when mixed, undergo a heat-absorbing reaction. They are portable, pliable, and easily used in the field. Although many endothermic chemical gel packs are designed for one-time use, some have the advantage that they can be refrozen and reused as a simple cryogel pack. Ice packs are easily used at home and can be applied by elastic bandage or tape. The duration of application is typically 20 to 30 min. With application of a cooled Hydrocollator pack, the skin is cooled immediately, subcutaneous tissues are cooled within minutes, and muscle at a depth of 2 cm is cooled by approximately 5 °C after 20 min.[43] Precautions for cold packs are as listed in Table 22–13.

Ice Massage

Ice massage is the direct application of ice to the skin using gentle stroking motions. It combines the therapeutic effects of cooling with the mechanical effects of massage. Water is frozen in a paper cup, with the ice being exposed by tearing the top rim of paper off as the ice melts (Fig. 22–8). Alternatively, a wooden tongue depressor can be placed in the water, to be used as a handle after the water is frozen. Ice massage is generally used for localized symptoms and applied for 5 to 10 min per site, depending on the amount of subcutaneous adipose tissue.[58] Typically, there is a phasic response to ice massage, beginning with

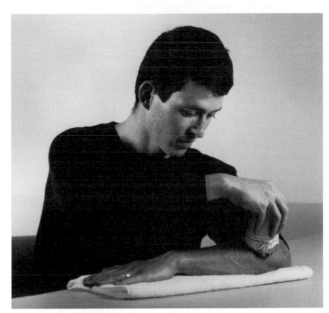

FIGURE 22–8 Example of ice massage.

an initial perception of coolness, followed by a burning or aching, then hypesthesia and analgesia.[31] Intramuscular temperatures at a depth of 2 cm after 5 min of ice massage have been reported to be reduced by 4.1 °C in the posterior thigh[91] to as much as 15.9 °C in the biceps brachii muscle.[58] In his initial description of ice massage, Grant[31] reported a "satisfactory treatment result" in over 80% of a series of over 7000 patients with a variety of painful musculoskeletal conditions treated with ice massage and mobilization exercises, although no statistical analysis was reported. Precautions for ice massage are as listed under general cold precautions.

Cold Water Immersion

Immersion in cold water is best suited for circumferential cooling of the limbs, usually at temperatures of 4 to 10 °C (39.2–50 °F). It is often uncomfortable and poorly tolerated, though reportedly effective with localized burns, as skin temperature rapidly approaches water temperature.[82] Gastrocnemius muscle temperature decreases to approximately 6 °C below baseline after 30 min of cold water immersion.[64, 74] Precautions for cold water immersion are listed in Table 22–13.

Cryotherapy-Compression Units

Cryotherapy-compression units consist of a cuff or boot through which cold water is circulated and can be pneumatically compressed statically or in a serial, distal-to-proximal pumping action (see Fig. 43–10). They are designed to combine the beneficial effects of cryotherapy with the advantages of pneumatic compression. They are used primarily after acute musculoskeletal injury with soft tissue swelling and after some surgical procedures.[77] Typical temperatures of 45 °F (7.2 °C) and pressures up to 60 mm Hg are used.

Vapocoolant Spray

Vapocoolant spray-and-stretch methods are used by some practitioners to treat myofascial and musculoskeletal pain syndromes. The technique consists of a series of unidirectional applications of Fluori-Methane spray, which has replaced the highly flammable ethyl chloride spray in clinical usage.[88] Treatment begins in the "trigger area" (area of deep myofascial hypersensitivity) and extends over the "reference zone" (area of referred pain) while passively stretching the muscle.[88] The spray and stretch is performed parallel to the muscle fibers, at an approximate rate of 4 in./sec. Waiting briefly between applications helps prevent skin freezing. The therapeutic effect of spray and stretch is postulated to result from a counterirritant phenomenon.[88] Precautions include general cold precautions and avoidance of cutaneous freezing.

HYDROTHERAPY

Hydrotherapy is defined as the external application of hot or cold water, in any form, for the treatment of disease.[27] The main forms of hydrotherapy are whirlpool baths, the Hubbard tank, the shower cart, and contrast baths. Their primary uses are in arthritis and a variety of musculoskeletal conditions, and in the cleansing and debridement of burns and other dermal injuries.

Whirlpool Baths and Hubbard Tanks

Whirlpool baths and Hubbard tanks control water temperature and agitate it by aeration, dispersing thermal energy by convection (although as noted previously, the actual transfer of heat to or from the body is by conduction). Whirlpool baths come in a variety of sizes and are typically used for treatment of a limb or localized lesion. Because only a portion of the body is immersed, greater extremes of temperature can be tolerated without significant core body temperature change.[27, 74] As more body surface area is immersed and the extremes of temperature increase, there is increasing potential for alteration of core body temperature. Hubbard tanks are larger tanks generally used for whole-body immersion, so neutral temperatures (34–36 °C or 93–97 °F) should be used to prevent core temperature fluctuations.

An immersed body experiences a vertical antigravity force equal to that of the volume of the displaced water, decreasing stress on bones and joints.[27] This property, along with the therapeutic effects of the water temperature, make hydrotherapy appropriate for adjunctive treatment of degenerative arthritis, acute musculoskeletal injuries, burns, and skin ulceration and infection.[27] Antiseptic conditions can be used for hydrotherapy of burns or infected areas, but truly sterile conditions are not easily achieved. Sodium hypochlorite is the most commonly used antibacterial solution used in burn programs.[86] Likewise, for Hubbard tank treatment of large wounds, salt may be added to minimize fluid shifts. Isotonic saline is 0.9% sodium chloride (0.9 g $NaCl$/100 mL H_2O), so 900 g (approximately 2 lbs) of salt should be added per 100 L (approximately 25 gallons) of water.

Shower Cart

Hydrotherapy has several features that are desirable for treatment of burns or other wounds. It loosens adherent dressings to facilitate removal, allows for removal of antimicrobial cream prior to reapplication, and softens eschar to facilitate debridement.[89] However, there is a risk of autocontamination and cross-contamination with conventional whirlpool baths or Hubbard tanks.[89] The shower cart was developed in response to this risk.[89] It allows for gentle spray or shower hydrotherapy during mechanical debridement of large surface area burns and other wounds under relatively sterile conditions.[89] Typical units have overhead retractable shower heads (Fig. 22–9), with independently adjustable water temperature and pressure. A shower cart also uses significantly less water, less space, and requires less maintenance than a Hubbard tank.

Contrast Baths

Contrast baths consist of alternating immersion of the distal limbs in hot (42–45 °C or 108–113 °F), then cold (8.5–12.5 °C or 47–55 °F) water.[94] The effect is believed to be related to the cyclic vasoconstriction and vasodilation produced by the temperature extremes. Thirty-minute treatment sessions are typical, beginning with a 10-min immersion in hot, followed by alternating immersions of 1 min cold and 4 min hot, ending the session with cold immersion to theoretically limit swelling. The technique may be beneficial in the treatment of rheumatological disease, neuropathic pain, or other chronic pain syndromes such as reflex sympathetic dystrophy.

OTHER MODALITIES

Ultraviolet

Ultraviolet radiation is that part of the electromagnetic spectrum adjacent to the short-wavelength, high-frequency

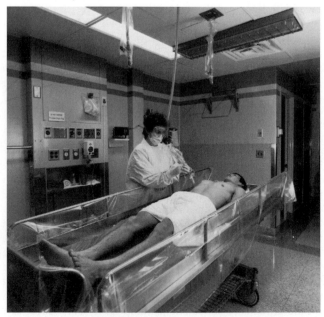

FIGURE 22–9 Shower cart.

(violet) end of the visible light spectrum. Historically, UV radiation has been used in physical medicine for the treatment of skin ulcers, but now its therapeutic use is almost exclusively dermatological.[66] Most current treatments with UV radiation utilize either UVA (wavelength, 320–400 nm) or UVB (wavelength, 290–320 nm) radiation.[66] The minimal erythema dose (MED) may be used to titrate intensity, and is determined by exposing small areas of skin to different durations of UV radiation. The MED is that duration of exposure which produces erythema. Although originally used mainly in the treatment of psoriasis, there are now over 30 dermatological disorders for which UV radiation may be efficacious.[66] Potential adverse effects include premature aging of the skin, non-melanoma skin cancer, and cataracts.[66]

Iontophoresis

Iontophoresis is the migration of charged particles across biological membranes under an imposed electrical field.[55] Proposed advantages include the theoretical ability to direct the active substance to a specific location, and the avoidance of gastrointestinal intolerance of oral medications when delivered iontophoretically.[10] Ionic medications (local anesthetics, corticosteroids, analgesics, antibiotics) or plain tap water have been used with this technique. The ionic solution to be iontophoresed is placed on the electrode of the same polarity, and then the negative, positive, and ground electrodes are applied to the skin. A direct current, typically between 10 and 30 mA, is applied to drive the solution away from the electrode and into the surrounding tissues.[81] The quantity of solution transported appears to be dependent on the local current density, duration of treatment, and the solution concentration.[70] Shrivastava and Singh[81] reported 100% efficacy following treatment of palmar-plantar hyperhydrosis with tap water iontophoresis. Chantraine et al.,[10] in an uncontrolled study of a heterogeneous population of 188 patients with a variety of musculoskeletal conditions, reported 56% "good results" as defined by remission of pain and decreased inflammation using corticosteroid iontophoresis. The authors were unable to demonstrate transcutaneous passage of the corticosteroid in experimental or animal models, so the clinical effects achieved may have been related to the application of the electrical current or to a placebo effect. Iontophoresis is generally well tolerated, and few complications have been reported.[81]

Phonophoresis

Phonophoresis involves the use of US (see Ultrasound, above) to theoretically facilitate transdermal migration of topically administered medications. Although this phenomenon has been demonstrated in animal models, whether this occurs in humans is controversial.[67] Corticosteroids are the most frequently used phonophoresis agents. The therapeutic effects of US and corticosteroids are thought to be synergistic.[67] The actual mechanism of transdermal migration has not been well defined, but may involve increased cell permeability from the thermal effects of US.[67] Standard ultrasonic coupling gel is mixed with 1% or 10% hydrocortisone solution or with 1% lidocaine to produce the phonophoresis coupling agent.[67] Typical pho-

nophoresis treatment parameters are similar to those of standard US–pulsed mode, 1-MHz transducer frequency, stroking technique, at 1.0 to 1.5 W/cm^2, for approximately 5 min per site.[67] Proposed indications for phonophoresis include osteoarthritis, bursitis, capsulitis, tendinitis, strains, fasciitis, epicondylitis, tenosynovitis, contracture, scar tissue, neuromas, and adhesions.[32, 67] Griffin et al.[32] evaluated the efficacy of standard US compared to ultrasonically driven hydrocortisone in 102 patients with a variety of musculoskeletal conditions. They found that 68% of the 10% hydrocortisone phonophoresis group improved, compared with 28% of the "placebo" group which received only US. Precautions for and contraindications to phonophoresis are listed in Table 22–8.

Low-Energy Laser

Laser is the acronym for *l*ight *a*mplification by *s*timulated *e*mission of *r*adiation. It consists of a coherent (inphase), collimated (restricted in area) beam of photons of identical frequency. Low-energy lasers typically deliver less than 90 mW, and should be distinguished from higherpower (10 to 100+ W) lasers utilized in surgery, dermatology, and ophthalmology. Low-energy lasers deliver minimal energies (between 1 and 4 J) and can be considered a form of intense, focal light therapy.[5] They have been shown to affect many subcellular and cellular processes, although the mechanisms have not been well defined.[5] It is important to note, however, that low-energy laser does not produce significant tissue temperature changes, so any potential physiological effects appear to be nonthermal. The equipment, experimental designs, and techniques noted in the low-energy laser literature are highly variable, and Basford[5] advises close attention to treatment parameters when reviewing and comparing these studies. Low-energy laser is not currently approved by the Food and Drug Administration for any therapeutic indication. Protective goggles should be worn by both the patient and treating therapist to protect against potential retinal injury.

CONCLUSION

This chapter has reviewed the physiological effects, common uses, techniques of application, and precautions for the therapeutic use of modalities. It is important to remember that these modalities are adjunctive treatments, to be used in conjunction with appropriate therapeutic exercise and medications. Because of the potential for deleterious effects, their use should generally be preceded by appropriate professional evaluation. Having a firm understanding of the physiological basis of modality selection is crucial to their proper use.

References

1. Abramson DI, Chu LSW, Tuck S, et al: Effect of tissue temperatures and blood flow on motor nerve conduction velocity. JAMA 1966; 198:1082–1088.
2. Abramson DI, Tuck S, Chu SW, et al: Effect of paraffin bath and hot fomentations on local tissue temperatures. Arch Phys Med Rehabil 1964; 45:87–94.
3. Askew LJ, Beckett VL, An K, et al: Objective evaluation of hand

function in scleroderma patients to assess effectiveness of physical therapy. Br J Rheumatol 1983; 22:224–232.

4. Balmaseda MT, Fatehi MT, Koozekanani SH, et al: Ultrasound therapy: A comparative study of different coupling media. Arch Phys Med Rehabil 1986; 67:147–150.

5. Basford JR: The clinical and experimental status of low energy laser therapy. Crit Rev Phys Rehabil Med 1989; 1:1–9.

6. Bell KR, Lehmann JF: Effect of cooling on H- and T-reflexes in normal subjects. Arch Phys Med Rehabil 1987; 68:490–493.

7. Bocobo C, Fast A, Kingery W, et al: The effect of ice on intra-articular temperature in the knee of the dog. Am J Phys Med 1991; 70:181–185.

8. Borell RM, Henley EJ, Ho P, et al: Fluidotherapy: Evaluation of a new heat modality. Arch Phys Med Rehabil 1977; 58:69–71.

9. Borell RM, Parker R, Henley EJ, et al: Comparison of in vivo temperatures produced by hydrotherapy, paraffin wax treatment, and Fluidotherapy. Phys Ther 1980; 60:1273–1276.

10. Chantraine A, Ludy JP, Berger D: Is cortisone iontophoresis possible? Arch Phys Med Rehabil 1986; 67:38–40.

11. Clarke DH, Stelmach GE: Muscular fatigue and recovery curve parameters at various temperatures. Res Q 1966; 37:468–479.

12. Clarke RS, Hellon RF, Lind AR: Vascular reactions of the human forearm to cold. Clin Sci 1958; 17:165–179.

13. Coakley WT: Biophysical effects of ultrasound at therapeutic intensities. Physiotherapy 1978; 64:166–169.

14. Cohn BT, Draeger RI, Jackson DW: The effects of cold therapy in the postoperative management of pain in patients undergoing anterior cruciate ligament reconstruction. Am J Sports Med 1989; 17:344–349.

15. Daniels S, Blondel D, Crum LA, et al: Ultrasonically induced gas bubble production in agar based gels: Part I, experimental investigation. Ultrasound Med Biol 1987; 13:527–539.

16. DeLateur BJ, Lehmann JF, Stonebridge JB, et al: Muscle heating in human subjects with 915 MHz microwave contact applicator. Arch Phys Med Rehabil 1970; 51:147–151.

17. Dellhag B, Wollersjo I, Bjelle A: Effect of active hand exercise and wax bath treatments in rheumatoid arthritis patients. Arthritis Care Res 1992; 5:87–92.

18. Denys EH: AAEM Minimonograph No. 14: The influence of temperature in clinical neurophysiology. Muscle Nerve 1991; 14:795–811.

19. Diller KR: Analysis of burns caused by long-term exposure to a heating pad. J Burn Care Rehabil 1991; 12:214–217.

20. Dover JS, Phillips TJ, Arndt KA: Cutaneous effects and therapeutic uses of heat with emphasis on infrared radiation. J Am Acad Dermatol 1989; 20:278–286.

21. Drez D, Faust DC, Evans JP: Cryotherapy and nerve palsy. Am J Sports Med 1981; 9:256–257.

22. Dyson M: Non-thermal cellular effects of ultrasound. Br J Cancer 1982; 45(suppl):165–171.

23. Dyson M, Woodward B, Pond JB: Flow of red blood cells stopped by ultrasound. Nature 1971; 232:572–573.

24. Eldred E, Lindsley DF, Buchwald JS: The effect of cooling on mammalian muscle spindles. Exp Neurol 1960; 2:144–157.

25. Falconer J, Hayes KW, Chang RW: Therapeutic ultrasound in the treatment of musculoskeletal conditions. Arthritis Care Res 1990; 3:85–91.

26. Folkow B, Fox RH, Krog J, et al: Studies on the reactions of the cutaneous vessels to cold exposure. Acta Physiol Scand 1963; 58:342–354.

27. Franchimont P, Juchmes J, Lecomte J: Hydrotherapy—mechanisms and indications. Pharmacol Ther 1983; 20:79–93.

28. Gersten JW: Effect of metallic objects on temperature rises produced in tissue by ultrasound. Am J Phys Med 1958; 37:75–82.

29. Gnatz SM: Increased radicular pain due to therapeutic ultrasound applied to the back. Arch Phys Med Rehabil 1989; 70:493–494.

30. Goats GC: Continuous shortwave (radiofrequency) diathermy. Br J Sports Med 1989; 23:123–127.

31. Grant AE: Massage with ice (cryokinetics) in the treatment of painful conditions of the musculoskeletal system. Arch Phys Med Rehabil 1964; 45:233–238.

32. Griffin JE, Echternach JL, Price RE, et al: Patients treated with ultrasonic driven hydrocortisone and with ultrasound alone. Phys Ther 1967; 47:594–601.

33. Guy AW, Lehmann JF, Stonebridge JB: Therapeutic applications of electromagnetic power. Proc IEEE 1974; 62:55–75.

34. Guyton AC: Body temperature, temperature regulation, and fever. In

35. Harris ED, McCroskery PA: The influence of temperature and fibril stability on degradation of cartilage collagen by rheumatoid synovial collagenase. N Engl J Med 1974; 290:1–6.

36. Hecht PJ, Bachmann S, Booth RE, et al: Effects of thermal therapy on rehabilitation after total knee arthroplasty. Clin Orthop 1983; 178:198–201.

37. Hedenberg L: Functional improvement of the spastic hemiplegic arm after cooling. Scand J Rehabil Med 1970; 2:154–158.

38. Hekkenberg RT, Oosterbaan WA, vanBeekum WT: Evaluation of ultrasound therapy devices. Physiotherapy 1986; 72:390–394.

39. Hocutt JE, Jaffe R, Rylander CR, et al: Cryotherapy in ankle sprains. Am J Sports Med 1982; 10:316–319.

40. Johnson CC, Guy AW: Nonionizing electromagnetic wave effects in biological materials and systems. Proc IEEE 1972; 60:692–718.

41. Jones SL: Electromagnetic field interference and cardiac pacemakers. Phys Ther 1976; 56:1013–1018.

42. Kantor G: Evaluation and survey of microwave and radiofrequency applicators. J Microwave Power 1981; 16:135–150.

43. Knutsson E, Mattsson E: Effects of local cooling on monosynaptic reflexes in man. Scand J Rehabil Med 1969; 1:126–132.

44. Lehmann JF: Therapeutic Heat and Cold, ed 4. Baltimore, Williams & Wilkins, 1990.

45. Lehmann JF, Brunner GD, Stow RW: Pain threshold measurements after therapeutic application of ultrasound, microwaves and infrared. Arch Phys Med Rehabil 1958; 39:560–565.

46. Lehmann JF, DeLateur BJ, Stonebridge JB: Selective muscle heating by shortwave diathermy with a helical coil. Arch Phys Med Rehabil 1969; 50:117–123.

47. Lehmann JF, DeLateur BJ, Warren CG, et al: Heating produced by ultrasound in bone and soft tissue. Arch Phys Med Rehabil 1967; 48:397–401.

48. Lehmann JF, DeLateur BJ, Warren CG, et al: Therapeutic temperature distribution produced by ultrasound as modified by dosage and volume of tissue exposed. Arch Phys Med Rehabil 1967; 48:662–666.

49. Lehmann JF, DeLateur BJ, Warren CG, et al: Heating of joint structures by ultrasound. Arch Phys Med Rehabil 1968; 49:28–30.

50. Lehmann JF, Johnston VC, McMillan JA, et al: Comparison of deep heating by microwaves at frequencies 2456 and 900 megacycles. Arch Phys Med Rehabil 1965; 46:307–314.

51. Lehmann JF, Masock AJ, Warren CG, et al: Effect of therapeutic temperatures on tendon extensibility. Arch Phys Med Rehabil 1970; 51:481–487.

52. Lehmann JF, McDougall JA, Guy AW, et al: Heating patterns produced by shortwave diathermy applicators in tissue substitute models. Arch Phys Med Rehabil 1983; 64:575–577.

53. Lehmann JF, McMillan JA, Brunner GD, et al: Comparative study of the efficiency of short-wave, microwave and ultrasonic diathermy in heating the hip joint. Arch Phys Med Rehabil 1959; 40:510–512.

54. Lehmann JF, Silverman DR, Baum BA, et al: Temperature distributions in the human thigh, produced by infrared, hot pack and microwave applications. Arch Phys Med Rehabil 1966; 47:291–299.

55. Lekas MD: Iontophoresis treatment. Otolaryngol Head Neck Surg 1979; 87:292–298.

56. Levenson JL, Weissberg MP: Ultrasound abuse: Case report. Arch Phys Med Rehabil 1983; 64:90–91.

57. Lewis T: Observations upon the reactions of the vessels of the human skin to cold. Heart 1930; 15:177–208.

58. Lowdon BJ, Moore RJ: Determinants and nature of intramuscular temperature changes during cold therapy. Am J Phys Med 1975; 54:223–233.

59. McGown HL: Effects of cold application on maximal isometric contraction. Phys Ther 1967; 47:185–192.

60. McLeod DR, Fowlow SB: Multiple malformations and exposure to therapeutic ultrasound during organogenesis. Am J Med Genet 1989; 34:317–319.

61. Meeusen R, Lievens P: The use of cryotherapy in sports injuries. Sports Med 1986; 3:398–414.

62. Melzack R, Jeans ME, Stratford JG, et al: Ice massage and transcutaneous electrical stimulation: Comparison of treatment for low-back pain. Pain 1980; 9:209–217.

63. Mense S: Effects of temperature on the discharge of muscle spindles and tendon organs. Pflugers Arch 1978; 374:159–166.

64. Miglietta O: Action of cold on spasticity. Am J Phys Med 1973; 52:198–205.

Guyton AC (ed): Textbook of Medical Physiology, ed 8. Philadelphia, WB Saunders, 1991, pp 797–808.

65. Miller DL: A review of the ultrasonic bioeffects of microsonation, gas-body activation, and related cavitation-like phenomena. Ultrasound Med Biol 1987; 13:413–470.

66. Morison WL: Phototherapy and photochemotherapy. Adv Dermatol 1992; 7:255–271.

67. Newman JT, Nellermoe MD, Carnett JL: Hydrocortisone phonophoresis. J Am Podiatr Med Assoc 1992; 82:432–435.

68. Nukada H, Pollock M, Allpress S: Experimental cold injury to peripheral nerve. Brain 1981; 104:779–811.

69. Oakley EM: Dangers and contraindications of therapeutic ultrasound. Physiotherapy 1978; 64:173–174.

70. O'Malley EP, Oester YT: Influence of some physical chemical factors on iontophoresis using radio-isotopes. Arch Phys Med Rehabil 1955; 36:310–316.

71. Paliwal BR, Shrivastava PN: Microwave hyperthermia: Principles and quality assurance. Radiol Clin North Am 1989; 27:489–497.

72. Perez CA, Emami B: Clinical trials with local (external and interstitial) irradiation and hyperthermia—current and future perspectives. Radiol Clin North Am 1989;27:525–542.

73. Perkins JF, Li M, Nicholas CH, et al: Cooling as a stimulus to smooth muscles. Am J Physiol 1950; 163:14–26.

74. Petajan JH, Watts N: Effects of cooling on the triceps surae reflex. Am J Phys Med 1962; 41:240–251.

75. Price R, Lehmann JF, Boswell-Bessette S, et al: Influence of cryotherapy on spasticity at the human ankle. Arch Phys Med Rehabil 1993; 74:300–304.

76. Ritzmann SE, Levin WC: Cryopathies: A review. Arch Intern Med 1961; 107:186–204.

77. Scheffler N, Sheitel P, Lipton M: Use of Cryo/Cuff for the control of postoperative pain and edema. J Foot Surg 1992; 31:141–146.

78. Schmidt KL, Ott VR, Rocher G, et al: Heat, cold and inflammation (a review). Z Rheumatol 1979; 38:391–404.

79. Scott BO: Effects of contact lenses on short-wave field distribution. Br J Ophthalmol 1956; 40:696–697.

80. Shepherd JT, Rusch NJ, Vanhoutte PM: Effect of cold on the blood vessel wall. Gen Pharmacol 1983; 14:61–64.

81. Shrivastava SN, Singh G: Tap water iontophoresis in palmo-plantar hyperhidrosis. Br J Dermatol 1977; 96:189–195.

82. Shulman AG: Ice water as primary treatment of burns. JAMA 1960; 173:96–99.

83. Stewart HF, Harris GR, Herman BA, et al: Survey of use and performance of ultrasonic therapy equipment in Pinellas County, Florida. Phys Ther 1974; 54:707–714.

84. Stuchly MA, Repacholi MH, Lecuyer DW, et al: Exposure to the operator and patient during short wave diathermy treatments. Health Phys 1982; 42:341–366.

85. Ter Haar G, Dyson M, Oakley EM: The use of ultrasound by physiotherapists in Britain, 1985. Ultrasound Med Biol 1987; 13:659–663.

86. Thomson PD, Bowden ML, McDonald K, et al: A survey of burn hydrotherapy in the United States. J Burn Care Rehabil 1990; 11:151–155.

87. Thornton KL: Principles of ultrasound. J Reprod Med 1992; 37:27–32.

88. Travell J: Ethyl chloride spray for painful muscle spasm. Arch Phys Med 1952; 33:291–298.

89. Walk EE, Himel HN, Batra EK, et al: Aquatic access for the disabled. J Burn Care Rehabil 1992; 13:356–363.

90. Warren CG, Koblanski JN, Sigelmann RA: Ultrasound coupling media: their relative transmissivity. Arch Phys Med Rehabil 1976; 57:218–222.

91. Waylonis GW: The physiologic effects of ice massage. Arch Phys Med Rehabil 1967; 48:37–42.

92. Weinberger A, Fadilah R, Lev A, et al: Treatment of articular effusions with local deep microwave hyperthermia. Clin Rheumatol 1989; 8:461–466.

93. Weinberger A, Fadilah R, Lev A, et al: Intra-articular temperature measurements after superficial heating. Scand J Rehabil Med 1989; 21:55–57.

94. Woodmansey A, Collins DH, Ernst MM: Vascular reactions to the contrast bath in health and in rheumatoid arthritis. Lancet 1938; 2:1350–1353.

95. Wright V, Johns RJ: Quantitative and qualitative analysis of joint stiffness in normal subjects and in patients with connective tissue diseases. Ann Rheum Dis 1961; 20:36–45.

96. Ziskin MC: Fundamental physics of ultrasound and its propagation in tissue. Radiographics 1993; 13:705–709.

23

Electrical Stimulation

**W. JERRY MYSIW, M.D., AND
REBECCA D. JACKSON, M.D.**

The history of electrical stimulation as an adjunct to traditional medicine has its roots in Greek philosophy. Although early applications with a variety of electricity-generating devices were advocated for use in treatment of many different medical conditions, its initial association with "quackery" limited its general acceptance. Despite this, gradual acceptance has grown as the systematic collection and analysis of scientific and clinical data have helped to define its beneficial impact. Current clinical applications of electrical stimulation therapy have crossed the lines of many specialities, including rehabilitation medicine, neurology, urology, gynecology, orthopedics, dermatology, and pain management.

The publication that laid the framework regarding magnetism and electricity was "DeMagnete" written by William Gilbert in the 16th century. The first studies suggesting the use of electricity for therapeutic purposes date back to Krueger in 1744,[134] but the field began to rapidly expand following Galvani's discovery of the effect of interrupted direct current on muscle contraction, from experiments that showed that placement of a metal connector between the spinal cord and muscle could produce a twitch. Subsequently, Matteucci demonstrated that injured biological tissues were capable of producing electrical current. On the basis of these studies, the application of electrical stimulation to clinical medicine began to flourish.

Throughout the 1800s, electrical stimulation was applied as a treatment for a variety of complaints. Although there was a great debate as to the ideal form of electrical stimulation therapy, with strong proponents for galvanism, faradism, and franklinism (static electricity),[73] many of the claims for general electrical therapy were never substantiated. Electrical stimulation eventually fell out of favor and hindered the progress in determining the scientific basis for some of the benefits that were ascribed to it.

In the early 1900s, Faraday described alternating current generation. This new technology was quickly applied to the treatment of neurological complaints by Duchenne. In 1920, the demonstration of the role of acetylcholine in nerve impulse transmission changed the direction of the field of neurology and rehabilitation medicine and intensified the emphasis on chemical rather than electrical phenomena in neuromuscular physiology.

Despite the interest in neurochemical changes, the field of electrical stimulation has continued to develop and data that have been gathered since the mid-1940s support the efficacy of electrical stimulation as a valuable therapeutic modality. In 1947, Lund expanded the potential role of electrical stimulation in the book, "Bioelectric Fields and Growth," which demonstrated that electrical potentials can control the growth of a biological system. In 1957, Fukada and Yasuda demonstrated that mechanical deformation of bones could induce electrical potentials in regions under compression (negative potentials) and tension (positive potentials).[74] The recognition of endogenous electrical current in both bone and skin was the groundwork for later applications of electrical stimulation in the healing of soft and hard tissue damage.

The first significant application of electrical stimulation to improve muscle function dates back to 1950, with the invention of the cardiac pacemaker.[168] Effective application of functional electrical stimulation (FES) in a rehabilitation system is generally credited to Liberson, who applied electrical stimulation to the peroneal nerve to produce ankle dorsiflexion in hemiplegic patients during the swing phase of gait.[145] This was followed by reports of the use of electrical stimulation of the quadriceps to aid in static standing following spinal cord injury.[118] Together, these are the first reports of functional neuromuscular stimulation utilizing electrical stimulation to serve as a neuro-orthosis or external control of motor function.

Since the 1960s, advances have come rapidly. The gate theory of pain by Melzak and Wall in 1965[159] provided the rationale for the development of such stimulation techniques as transcutaneous electrical nerve stimulation and the use of implanted dorsal column and conus medullaris root stimulators for neurogenic bladder control. Most recently, electrical stimulation has returned to its functional roots in cardiology and has been applied to the development of latissimus dorsi cardiomyoplasty assist devices for treatment of cardiomyopathy.

Over the past several decades, improvements in electronic technology and increased understanding of neuromuscular physiology have worked together to improve the use of electrical stimulation for functional and therapeutic purposes. Today, there is a substantial body of experimental data supporting its application for use and treatment in a variety of medical conditions, based on its unique properties in modifying certain biological and chemical aspects of in vivo biological tissues and increasing the contractile properties of muscle.

PHYSIOLOGICAL EFFECTS OF NEUROMUSCULAR ELECTRICAL STIMULATION

Normal Muscle Physiology

Normal muscle contraction is initiated by propagation of depolarization from the alpha motor neuron to the muscle fiber. At the neuromuscular junction, there is release and diffusion of the neurotransmitter acetylcholine, with depolarization conducted via the acetylcholine receptors to the sarcolemma, an excitable membrane. The action potential is conducted within the muscle fiber via the transverse tubular system (T system), which runs transversely through the myofilament to the sarcoplasmic reticulum (SR) membrane system. Activation of the SR results in a release of calcium, causing force generation. During the actual process of contraction, an interaction between actin and myosin filaments results in a ratchet like rotation of the myosin head at the cross-linkers, sliding the myosin along the actin. This process requires energy in the form of adenosine triphosphate (ATP) that is obtained via aerobic or anaerobic metabolic pathways.[1]

The motor unit involved in contraction consists of an alpha motor neuron, its axon, the myoneural junction, and the muscle fibers that it innervates. The alpha motor neurons differ in size and function with the small motor neurons (which have the lowest activation frequency) innervating slow muscle fibers and the large neurons innervating fast fibers. Muscle fibers within the motor unit can be classified into four main categories[158] based on specific functional, metabolic, and histochemical features of the individual muscle fiber types (Table 23–1). Within each motor unit, all muscle fibers are histologically identical,[32] although within a muscle, all fiber types can be present in varying amounts, resulting in unique contractile characteristics.

During normal muscle contraction, a motor unit with a low axonal conduction velocity (or activation frequency) is recruited before a unit with a higher conduction velocity.[97, 98] This size principle suggests that the axonal conduction of a motor unit is related to the muscle fiber parameters such that a unit with a low conduction velocity has a slow-twitch force, long contraction time, and higher resistance to fatigue. This theory explains the orderly progression of fiber activation with the onset of isometric voluntary contraction. Weak, slowly conducting, fatigue-resistant motor units containing type I fibers are recruited first to allow for slow increases in firing rate and increasing tension in the muscle.[162, 163] This is followed sequentially by the recruitment of the high conduction velocity type IIb fibers, which can increase gain.[165]

When the motor unit is stimulated by artificial rather than voluntary action, this orderly progression of fiber activation does not always occur.[128] With functional neuromuscular stimulation, the order of recruitment can be reversed because activation of the motor unit is dependent on the excitation current threshold, which varies inversely with the diameter of the nerve fiber.[233] This results in initial stimulation of the type II fibers followed by activation of the slow type I fibers with continued stimulation.

Response of Muscle Fibers to Electrical Stimulation

Following chronic, continuous, low-frequency (10 Hz) electrical stimulation of normal, fast-twitch skeletal muscles, a stereotypical series of events occurs, resulting in transformation of the muscle fiber from a fast-twitch type IIb fiber to a composition with slow-twitch type I characteristics (Table 23–2). Although the majority of the data have been derived from studies in animal (mammalian) models with several different low-frequency, continuous stimulation regimens, the consistency of changes reported supports its generalization to many animals and humans.

Within 2 to 4 days of the onset of stimulation, initial changes are noted in the SR. First, there is a decrease in the rate and capacity of ionized calcium uptake, which is associated with a decrease in the activity of the calcium-dependent adenosine triphosphatase (ATPase) and its phosphorylated intermediate.[96, 152, 208, 221] There is an associated decrease in calsequestrin, the major calcium-binding protein in the SR,[95] an increase in specific membrane proteins that are typical of the slow-twitch type I SR[253] and a rearrangement of the membrane phospholipid matrix.[224] The transformation of the SR is associated with a decline in parvalbumin, the calcium-binding cytosolic protein, which almost completely disappears within 3 weeks of stimulation.[127] These histochemical changes result in both a decrease in calcium sequestration in the SR and a reduction in calcium-buffering capacity, which functionally affects contractile properties by increasing the time-to-peak velocity within the first week.[95, 199] The isotonic twitch characteristics, a function of myosin heavy and light chains and

TABLE 23–1   Properties of Muscle Fiber Types

	I	IIa	IIb
Morphology			
Name	Red	Intermediate	White
Capillary density	↑	Intermediate	↓↓
Histochemical			
Myosin ATPase	↓	↑	↑
Mitochondria	↑	↑	↓
Glycogen	Low	Intermediate	High
Myosin HC	HC$_s$	HCfa	HCfb
Myosin LC	LC$_{1a, 1b, 2}$	Lcf$_{1, 2, 3}$	Lcf$_{1, 2, 3}$
Metabolism			
Type	Oxidative Aerobic	Oxidative/glycolytic Mixed	Glycolytic Anaerobic
Contractile properties			
Twitch	Slow	Fast	Fast
Fatigability	Slow	Intermediate	Rapid

TABLE 23–2 Chronic Low-Frequency Stimulation of Fast-Twitch Muscle: Sequence of Events in Transformation

	Acute (0–3 wk)	Subacute (4–8 wk)
Contractile	↑ resistance to fatigue ↑ time-to-peak twitch ↑ time-to-half relaxation ↑ tetanus-to-twitch	↓ maximal velocity of shortening
Ultrastructural	Swelling SR ↑ T system ↓ particle in SR bilayer ↑ mitochondrial fraction ↑ Z band width	Broad Z band Declining mitochondria
Histochemical	↑ Type IIA - ↓ type IIB HC	↓ Type IIA → type I HC ↓ LC$_2$ → ↑ LC$_{2s}$ ↓ LC$_3$ then ↓ LC$_1$ ↓ NCH$_3$-histidine
Metabolic	↑ oxidative enzyme mRNA Δ α, β-tropomysin ↓ Ca-transport + Ca-active ATPase ↓ glycolytic enzymes mRNA	↑ oxidative enzyme activity ↓ glycolytic activity
Morphological	↑ capillary density ↑ blood flow	↓ muscle fiber area ↓ muscle fiber wet weight

other contractile proteins, are unaltered during this early stage of transformation.[2]

Ultrastructurally, there is an early decrease in T-tubuli, terminal cisternae, and SR,[64] as well as a decrease in calcium-transporting membranes. In addition, there is a decrease in high-density intramembranous particles of the SR. These are thought to be oligomers of calcium-pumping ATPase, and their decline is associated with a reduction in the rate and capacity of calcium uptake in the SR.[62]

Although the most rapid-transformation responses to electrical stimulation are centered on the SR, continued low-frequency stimulation must eventually affect the myosin contractile proteins to result in the ultimate transformation to a slow fiber type. Calcium-activated myosin ATPase activity begins to decline by 3 weeks, eventually reaching the low levels typical of slow type I muscle fibers. Concomitantly, there is an increase in the alkali lability of the myosin ATPase corresponding with changes in myosin light chain (LC) patterns.[235] Changes in LC patterns occur at both the level of transcription and translation during the transformation from fast to slow fiber type. In an orderly sequence, the fast DTNB-LC chain (LC–f2) is replaced by its slow counterpart (LC-S2), followed by declines in LC-f3, then LC-f1, with replacement by the corresponding slow LC.[26, 230] The changes in the DTNB-LC occur simultaneously with the initial changes in myosin heavy chain (MHC). MHC messenger RNA (mRNA) expressed in each muscle fiber encodes a unique myosin cross-bridge for type I, IIa, and IIb fibers, which is responsible for the characteristic intrinsic velocity of contraction and economy of force of each muscle fiber type. Within 4 days of the onset of electrical stimulation, there is a decline in the mRNA of the MHC characteristic type IIb fibers (MHC-fb), with eventual suppression of these mRNA levels by 90% after 21 days (Fig. 23–1).[29] This is followed by a decline in MHC-fb protein within 12 days.[94] The decreas-

ing MHC-fb is initially replaced by an MHC reflecting the type IIa fiber (MCH-fa), and only after prolonged stimulation is the phenotypic transformation completed with replacement of MHC-fa by MHC-s.[26] However, if electrical stimulation is combined with stretch, there is a synergistic effect of mechanical and electrical forces leading to a rapid (4-day) stimulation of MHC-s mRNA (Fig. 23–2).[83] This asynchronous transformation from fast to slow type within the different myosin subunits can lead to the coexistence of both slow and fast isoforms of myosin within a single muscle fiber (type IIc fibers).[152, 197, 219]

By 3 weeks after the onset of stimulation, alpha and beta tropomyosin changes from fast to slow type,[218] and Z lines become evident with a corresponding development of the M-band structure. Conversion of fiber type is completed within 8 weeks of chronic, low-frequency stimulation.[195] This new type I muscle fiber composition is functionally associated with both an increase in resistance to fatigue and a decrease in the maximum velocity of shortening.

The changes in ultrastructural and contractile properties from a fast- to a slow-twitch muscle fiber are also associ-

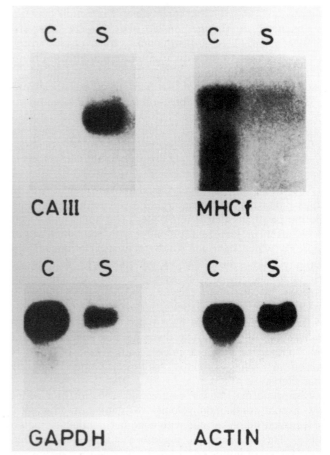

FIGURE 23–1 Northern blot analysis of changes in messenger RNA expression of four different muscle genes in response to 21 days of electrical stimulation of the tibialis anterior muscle. There is a stimulation of carbonic anhydrase III (CAIII) expression and suppression of both glyceraldehyde-3-phosphate dehydrogenase (GAPDH) and the fast myosin heavy chain (MHCf) with electrical stimulation–induced fast-to-slow transition. (From Brownson C, Isenberg H, Brown W, et al: Changes in skeletal muscle gene transcription induced by chronic stimulation. Muscle Nerve 1988; 11:1183–1189.)

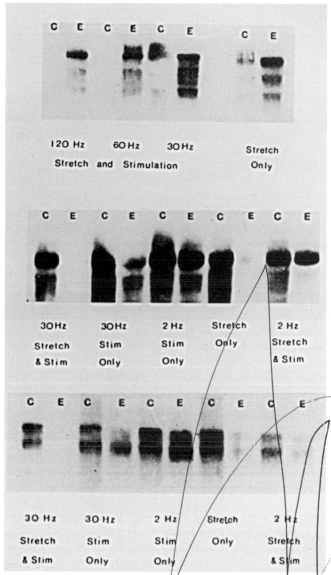

FIGURE 23–2 Northern blot analysis of RNA from normal (C) and electrically stimulated and stretched (E) rabbit tibialis anterior muscle after 4 days. There is activation of slow myosin heavy chain (panel A) with repression of both fast type IIb myosin heavy chain (panel B) and myosin heavy chain genes detected with a myosin light chain 1 and 3 probe (panel C). Note that the two bands in panel C represent the two light chains encoded by the same gene. (From Goldspink G, Scutt A, Martindale J, et al: Stretch and force generation induce rapid hypertrophy and isoform gene switching in adult skeletal muscle. Biochem Trans 1991; 19:368–373.)

ated with important changes in metabolic activity from use of an anaerobic, glycolytic pathway in the type IIb fiber to the aerobic, Krebs cycle–associated pathway of type I fibers. With the onset of continuous, low-frequency electrical stimulation, there is an enhancement of the enzymes responsible for phosphorylation and oxidation of glucose. There is a rapid rise of GLUT-4, a facilitative glucose transporter isoform present in tissues (such as skeletal muscle) that are responsive to insulin stimulation, within 10 days of initiating electrical stimulation.[67] In contrast, activity of citrate synthase (an enzyme in the Krebs cycle) increases more slowly after the onset of electrical stimula-

tion with rises in protein levels over 30 to 40 days and a plateauing of the peak effect by day 60 to 90, reflecting the metabolic change to an aerobic oxidative enzyme system. The mRNA for carbonic anhydrase II, an enzyme that facilitates carbon dioxide(CO_2) movement in muscle, is also rapidly stimulated with electrical stimulation to reach the levels seen in type I fibers over 10 to 20 days (see Fig. 23–1).[29] Finally, there is a pronounced increase in many other enzymes involved in terminal substrate oxidation and fatty acid and ketone body oxidation.[31, 107, 127, 196, 198, 211] These metabolic changes are also associated with pronounced increases in capillary density[27, 109, 211] and oxygen consumption, which in combination may be responsible for the development of increased resistance to fatigue.[108]

In addition to the increase in oxidative capacity, there is a suppression of enzymes involved in anaerobic glycogenolysis. There are progressive declines in the level of phosphorylase kinase (PK),[140] a regulator of glycogen metabolism that promotes glycogenolysis by phosphorylating and activating phosphorylase enzyme. These changes might reflect the very early changes in metabolic activity in the SR in response to electrical stimulation as this enzyme is allosterically activated by calcium through its delta subunit, calmodulin, thus providing a potential link between electrically stimulated calcium changes and glycogenolysis. There are also dramatic changes in mRNA levels of glyceraldehyde-3-phosphate dehydrogenase (GAPDH), a glycolytic enzyme abundant in fast-twitch fibers (see Fig. 23–2).[29] There are steady declines in GAPDH mRNA to the levels seen in slow-twitch fibers after 21 days of electrical stimulation, suggesting that part of the regulation of fast-to slow-twitch fiber transformation is occurring at the level of gene transcription. When comparing temporal data of GAPDH enzyme activity to those of its mRNA, it appears that the declines in mRNA concentration precede the observed protein changes[127, 194]; this is similar to a pattern of events described for aldolase,[255] an enzyme adjacent to GAPDH in the glycolytic pathway. These data suggest that there is a relative delay in the turnover of the glycolytic proteins, which potentially delay the rate of change observed in metabolic activity in response to electrical stimulation.

Several studies have helped to confirm the applicability of some aspects of these data derived from animal models to the effects of electrical stimulation on human muscle in vivo. After 21 days of electrical stimulation (50 Hz, alternating current) in normal muscle, there is a significant increase in total capillary length per tissue volume, a decrease in intercapillary distance, and a decrease in Krogh cylinders, leading to an improvement in capillary supply to muscle;[87] these findings are similar to those changes noted in animal models. Using intermittent electrical stimulation (square wave, 20 to 30 Hz, 0.003-sec pulse, 33% duty cycle) with surface electrodes for 30 minutes twice a day for 90 days in individuals with chronic spinal cord injury, electrical stimulation of the lower extremity has resulted in an increase in the number of type IIa muscle fibers (Fig. 23–3).[84] Munsat and associates have shown a more dramatic change in fiber type in response to electrical stimulation, with an increase in type I muscle fibers from 4% to 48% after FES of the quadriceps in patients with disuse atrophy.[169] Studies using electrical stimulation of the triceps

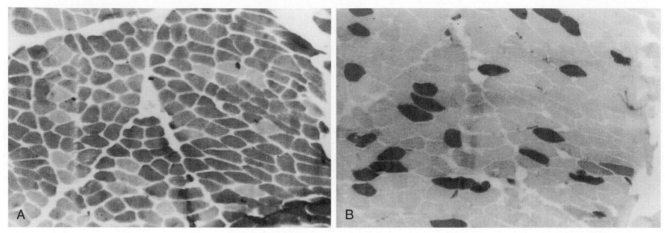

FIGURE 23–3   Biopsy of vastus lateralis of the quadriceps femoris muscle from a subject with a spinal cord injury before *(A)* and after *(B)* undergoing functional electrical stimulation for 90 days. The muscle biopsy was stained with a dye for ATPase myofibrillar activity. Note the increase in type IIa fibers after electrical stimulation. (From Greve JMD, Muszkat R, Schmidt B, et al: Functional electrical stimulation (FES): Muscle histochemical analysis. Paraplegia 1993; 31:764–770.)

surae muscle for 20 days at medium (50 Hz) and high (2500 Hz) frequencies have also shown an increase in fiber size, mitochondrial fraction, and DNA fiber content.[35, 36] Finally, similar changes have also been noted in normal muscle from subjects with scoliosis in whom chronic, low-intensity electrical stimulation resulted in increases in type I and IIC muscle fiber percentages after 6 months of continuous stimulation. In addition to changes in muscle fiber types, an increase was also noted in citrate synthase activity, suggesting a move toward an oxidative metabolism[87] and a more fatigue-resistant muscle.

After discontinuation of electrical stimulation, the muscle fiber type begins to transform to its prestimulation characteristics in a time-course that reflects a "first in–last out" relationship. Within 6 weeks, the former fast-twitch muscle fiber regains its previous contractile behavior with a change in maximum velocity of contraction. This is associated with changes in N-methyl-histidine content, myosin ATPase, and LC. Changes in oxidative and glycolytic enzymes lag behind the contractile protein changes, with a return to an anaerobic metabolic pathway by 12 weeks. Capillary density changes are one of the last features to be modified and may be present for up to several months.[220] If electrical stimulation therapy is discontinued, a series of changes occurs in the muscle fiber that depend on the length of discontinuation of therapy. This may affect the muscle response to resumption of electrical stimulation (detraining effect).

The importance of stimulation frequency on fiber transformation has also been a subject of intense investigation.[221] Application of low-frequency (10 Hz) stimulation for 8 hours/day results in a delay in acquisition of the transformation from fast- to slow-twitch muscle fiber composition in comparison with a continuous (24 hours/day), low-frequency (10 Hz) stimulation protocol.[196] Despite this delay, similar changes in contractile properties eventually occur with both stimulation regimens. If an equal number of stimuli are given per minute as a short burst of high-frequency (40 Hz) stimuli, vs. continuous low-frequency (10 Hz) stimulation, similar histochemical changes reflecting a transition from fast- to slow-twitch muscle fiber

type are noted in both groups.[110] Increases in succinate dehydrogenase activity are also seen in response to each of these stimulation patterns, although the increase in succinate dehydrogenase occurs at a slower rate when the stimulation frequency is 40 Hz.[200] Using even higher frequencies (2.5 sec trains at 60 Hz every 10 sec) with a number of stimuli equivalent to continuous low-frequency (10 Hz) stimulation over a 5-week period, nearly identical changes are seen in ATPase, fiber type, calcium uptake, and contractile properties in each regimen.[234]

The impact of a change in frequency, however, is dramatically different if there is an increase in *both* frequency and number of stimuli. Using the denervated rat soleus model, intermittent high-frequency (100 Hz) electrical stimulation resulted in conversion of the muscle from a slow- to fast-twitch fiber type.[147, 148] In contrast, continuous low-frequency (10 Hz) stimulation of this muscle maintained the slow-twitch characteristics of the denervated soleus muscle.[148] Thus, the selection of both the specific frequency and the number of stimuli per minute with electrical stimulation can dramatically affect the phenotypic expression of the muscle fiber in response to treatment. This switch from slow- to fast-twitch fiber type, at this point, is unique to denervated muscle and has never been reported in innervated muscle.

To exclude the influence of the release of local neurotropic factor(s) on the transformation of muscle fiber type in response to electrical stimulation, investigations have focused on the response of denervated muscle to electrical stimulation. Using a 1-sec train of low-frequency (10 Hz) pulses every 2 sec, electrical stimulation started within 24 hours of denervation results in a decrease in atrophy and maintenance of oxidative enzyme levels at or above normal levels in 95% of samples.[173] More surprisingly, however, were findings that the late-onset initiation of electrical stimulation (28 days postdenervation) using an intermediate frequency (25 Hz) stimulus with a long bi-directional impulse duration (20 msec) markedly retards atrophy and induces a hybrid fiber type with mitochrondrial changes suggestive of a type I fiber and type IIb myofibrillar ATPase expression.[164] These studies and other histological and biochemical data suggest that denervated muscles exhibit some properties of plasticity independent of neurological input.

WAVEFORMS

Therapeutic electricity is characterized according to its waveform, amplitude, duration, and frequency. Three basic types of waveforms exist: direct current, alternating current, and pulsed current. Direct current involves the unidirectional flow of a charge with no change in waveform characteristics over time. This type of uninterrupted direct current waveform is not applicable to FES systems. *Alternating current* refers to an uninterrupted bidirectional flow of charged particles that can be symmetrical or asymmetrical (Fig. 23–4).[136, 170] The pulsed waveforms are the most common waveforms applied for therapeutic purposes.[136] Pulsed waves can be further classified as *monophasic* or *biphasic*. The biphasic waveforms can be symmetrical or asymmetrical with respect to the baseline. The reference to symmetry applies to any combination of parameters, such as current intensity, duration, rise time, or decay of the waveform.[170]

Pulsed or alternating currents can be varied, or modulated, with respect to amplitude, duration, or frequency.[136, 170] These modulations can be sequential, intermittent, or variable. *Ramping* refers to a form of modulation in which either the pulse amplitude or the duration is increased (ramp up) or decreased (ramp down) over time. A *burst* refers to a type of modulation in which a finite series of pulses, or an envelope of alternating current, is delivered at a specific frequency (carrier frequency) over a specified time interval (burst duration). The interval be-

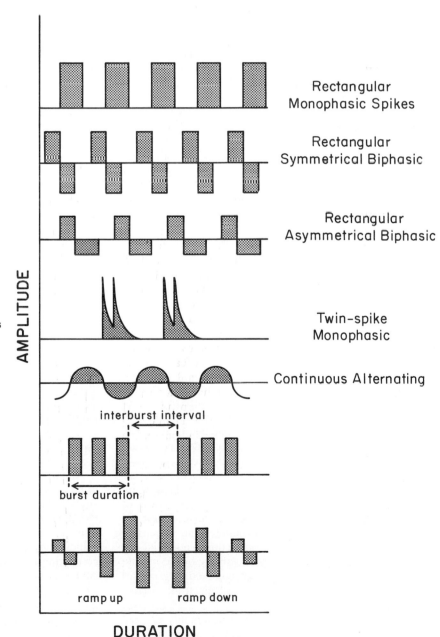

FIGURE 23–4 Diagrammatic representations of waveforms and modulations.

tween bursts is referred to as the *interburst interval* (see Fig. 23–4). The *duty cycle* is defined as the ratio between burst duration and the total cycle time, where the total cycle time equals the duration of the burst duration plus the interburst interval. The duty cycle is often expressed as a percentage; therefore, a duty cycle ratio of 1:4 corresponds to a duty cycle of 20%.

A number of studies have been done to explore the impact of different waveforms and stimulation parameters on patient comfort, force of contraction, strengthening effect, and fatigue. The majority of these studies have been done in normal muscle, and these data are presumably transferable to upper motor neuron and myopathic conditions.

Both burst-modulated alternating current and asymmetrical biphasic pulsed current appear to induce the most forceful contractions.[132, 249] No consensus exists as to which waveform provides the greatest patient comfort; various studies have advocated the burst-modulated alternating current, asymmetrical biphasic pulsed current, symmetrical biphasic pulsed current, and twin spiked monophasic pulsed currents.[9, 87, 259]

The relationship between current amplitude (milliamperes [mA]) and the force of muscle contraction is linear.[136] A stimulus duration in excess of 200 μsec is likely to produce a more forceful muscle contraction; however, waveforms with durations in excess of 60 μsec are also associated with greater pain.[21, 105] Stimulation frequencies of 60 to 100 Hz are necessary to produce the most forceful muscle contraction, but stimulation at these rates rapidly results in muscle fatigue.[17] Muscle fatigue is significantly diminished by utilizing stimulation rates of approximately 20 Hz, but this results in approximately a 35% drop in the force generated at higher stimulation frequencies.[116] In summary, data demonstrate that waveform amplitude, duration, and frequency can all be manipulated to control the force of muscle contraction.

ELECTRODES

The development of neuromuscular stimulation electrodes remains problematic. A number of different types of electrodes are available including surface, epimysial, intramuscular, juxtaneural, nerve cuff, epineural, intraneural/intrafascicular, and intraspinal.[240] The choice of an electrode type is based on the goal of the electrical stimulation program and its ease of use for the patient. In addition, selection criteria for the choice of an electrode type should include general biocompatibility of the electrode and leads, electrochemistry at the electrode-tissue interface, the possibility of actively or passively induced tissue damage by the electrodes or leads, electrode invasiveness, ease of surgical placement, ease of electrode retrieval and/or replacement, electrode reliability and failure rate, selectivity of the desired elicited muscle contractions, potential for side effects, repeatability and reproducibility of the muscle responses over time, dependence of contractile responses on muscle length and joint angle, and electrode system economics.[240]

Surface electrodes remain the most commonly utilized electrode type for most FES therapeutic and functional interventions. The force of muscle contractions induced with surface electrodes is influenced by electrode size and alignment. Longitudinal placement of electrodes produces as much as a 64% increase in the maximal tolerable torque when compared with a transverse placement.[136] Larger surface electrodes result in a more forceful muscle contraction and cause less discomfort as compared with smaller surface electrodes.[136]

Electrical stimulation protocols that require multiple surface electrodes are often impractical if long-term FES utilization is anticipated. In an effort to improve the practicality of surface stimulation, a number of electrode garments have been developed (Fig. 23–5). These garments are particularly useful for FES cycle ergometry and standing and gait protocols in that they decrease preparation time for FES, increase patient independence, and provide more consistent electrode placement.

The lack of precision achieved with surface stimulation is at least in part overcome with implanted electrode systems. Epimysial, intramuscular, and nerve cuff electrodes are the most common examples of implanted electrodes presently utilized. A number of material science issues need to be resolved in designing neuromuscular stimulation electrodes that minimize tissue injury while maintaining electrode reliability. Failure rates of percutaneously inserted intramuscular electrodes have apparently been reduced from an early failure rate of 20% to a subsequent failure rate of approximately 1% per year.[250]

Cuff electrodes, which are placed around peripheral nerves that innervate several muscles, offer the opportunity to activate numerous muscles through a single electrode, thereby diminishing the extent of required hardware. Snug-fitting cuff electrodes are available that can improve selectivity by stimulating portions of a peripheral nerve.[188] Endoscopic implantation techniques are being developed for cuff electrodes that overcome the lack of precision of surface and percutaneous electrodes while avoiding the need for surgical exposure of target nerves.[180] In addition, stimulation techniques such as decreasing the duration of stimulation, stimulating at lower rates (20 Hz vs. 50 Hz), and using an intermittent duty cycle are being developed that minimize neural damage from cuff electrodes.[1]

THERAPEUTIC NEUROMUSCULAR ELECTRICAL STIMULATION FOR MUSCLE STRENGTHENING

Stimulation of Normal Muscle

Although electrical stimulation therapy has been shown to be effective in improving muscle force,[34] no data to date suggest that the use of neuromuscular electrical stimulation (NMES) in a normal healthy human results in substantial improvements in muscle strengths as compared with that achieved by voluntary isometric exercise. Multiple studies comparing the efficacy of NMES with isometric voluntary contraction of the quadriceps have shown that gains in isometric muscle strength occur with both exercise regimens; however, no significant difference in strength is seen when comparing the NMES to the voluntary exercise groups.[52, 53, 89, 132, 135, 139] When a combination of neuromus-

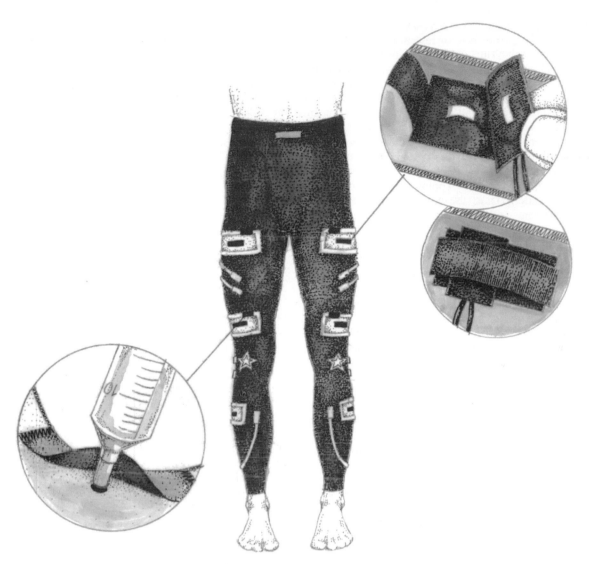

FIGURE 23-5 Example of a custom made electrode garment manufactured by Bioflex, Inc. Electrodes are made of stretch materials and conductive gel is inserted into the pocket on the side of the electrode. Velcro connectors are arranged to allow connection of all anteriorly and posteriorly placed electrodes to stimulators while the patient is seated.

cular stimulation and voluntary exercise are compared to either program alone, no significant augmentation of quadriceps strength is seen after combined training. The lack of additional benefit from NMES in combination with voluntary contraction for strengthening probably reflects the fact that with maximal voluntary contraction, nearly 100% of the recruitable motor units are activated. Thus, the additional stimulation provided by NMES is unable to recruit additional motor units to result in further increments in force.

Despite the fact that NMES and voluntary exercise result in comparable increases in isometric strength, these two training regimens differ. With voluntary training, type I fibers are activated first, followed by the progressive recruitment of type II fibers with increasing force. In contrast, the NMES protocols lead to an activation of type II fibers to a greater extent than type I fibers. As maximal force depends on type II fiber activation, selected augmentation of the type II muscle fibers by NMES might lead to greater increases in the overall strength of the muscle at

submaximal training intensity. This hypothesis has been supported by data showing that voluntary exercise groups train at higher muscle contraction intensity (78% to 119% of initial maximal voluntary isometric contraction [MVIT]) in comparison to that of NMES groups (33% to 68% MVIT) to achieve an equivalent degree of strengthening.[53] These higher workloads have been shown in one study of isometric strength training in the elderly male to result in increases in heart rate during the training sessions. Subjects randomized to NMES, in contrast, had similar gains in strength without a change in cardiovascular work.[38] Thus, NMES strengthening might offer specific advantages in training over voluntary contraction in certain populations of individuals who have cardiovascular disease or other limitations that preclude training at higher workloads.

Studies of the adductor pollicis of the nondominant hand with neuromuscular electrical stimulation or voluntary isometric contraction have shown the importance of understanding the unique contractile properties of the specific muscle involved in the training regimen. Both NMES and voluntary training resulted in increases in muscle force, although the observed increase in response to NMES was significantly smaller. With voluntary training, a greater increase was seen in tetanic force of contraction, speed of contraction and speed of relaxation in comparison to NMES. Training with NMES, however, had no effect on mechanical twitch tension and resulted in no reduction in fatigue. Finally, voluntary training resulted in faster kinetics of contraction, whereas no improvements were noted with NMES. The authors concluded that in small muscles, such as the adductor pollicis,[59] all or nearly all motor units were recruited during voluntary contractions but not during electrical stimulation. Thus, the number of trained motor units was different with the two training regimens. In this specific muscle group, voluntary contraction using activation of synaptic ionic current with excitation contraction coupling was more efficient in stimulating the smaller motor neurons with the higher input resistance that were present in the hand. In contrast, electrical stimulation affected changes in peripheral processes beyond the membrane ionic mechanisms of the muscle excitation contraction coupling, thus recruiting larger cells with lower external input, which reflected a smaller population of the motor units within the hand muscle. Based on these data, it is clearly important to understand the motor unit composition of the muscle to determine the most appropriate therapeutic intervention and response.

NMES might also have a therapeutic application for augmenting strengthening at skeletal regions in which attainment of maximal volitional contraction is difficult to achieve. NMES at both high (2,000 Hz) and moderate (50 Hz) frequencies has been shown to increase maximal isometric force of the triceps surae.[34] NMES with voluntary contraction can also result in significantly higher gains in abdominal strength and endurance when compared with NMES or voluntary exercise alone.[6] Finally, biphasic NMES of the back muscles has been shown to improve isokinetic strength to a degree that is equal to voluntary exercise, with the added benefit of enhanced endurance.[117]

Not only has NMES been shown to increase muscle strength, but it has also been shown to improve functional performance. NMES applied to the quadriceps femoris muscle bilaterally has been shown to improve performance on force measurements from a squat machine, the 25-yard dash time, and vertical jump.[258] Another benefit of NMES in normal muscle is in the prevention of muscle atrophy associated with prolonged immobilization. Individuals undergoing knee immobilization following ligament reconstruction surgery experience significant muscle atrophy as demonstrated by decreases in strength, endurance, muscle mass, and oxidative capacity.[136] Early intervention with NMES of the quadriceps femoris (Fig. 23–6) results in improved preservation of quadriceps muscle strength, muscle mass,[166] and succinate dehydrogenase activity[136] as well as higher isokinetic peak torque values.[93, 254] Using NMES protocols (30 Hz, 300 msec) for isometric quadriceps contraction for a 10 min session four times per day, three times per week, together with voluntary quadriceps contraction vs. exercise alone, the combination of NMES plus voluntary exercise resulted in a significant reduction in muscle wasting, a reduction in the loss of isometric torque, and a preservation of oxidative enzyme activity as defined

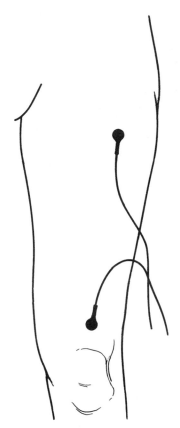

FIGURE 23–6 Electrode placement for isometric quadriceps femoris strengthening. The active electrode is placed proximally and the indifferent electrode is placed both laterally and distally to stimulate the vastus lateralis muscle. The lateral position is utilized to avoid stimulation of the rectus femoris, which if stimulated would cause knee extension and hip flexion.

by the levels of citrate synthase and triphosphate dehydrogenase (TPDH) during the period of immobilization (Table 23–3).[254]

The benefit of NMES appears to be limited to the period of immobilization. In one prospective study of NMES after knee immobilization, although losses of thigh girth and maximal voluntary contraction during immobilization were significantly smaller with the use of NMES, by 12 weeks postsurgery (6 weeks after discontinuation of immobilization), no significant differences were seen in maximal voluntary isokinetic torque or thigh girth between patients randomized to the nonexercise control or NMES group.[57] This suggests that NMES could be of greatest benefit in treatment of elite athletes or other individuals who desire

TABLE 23–3 Effects of Neuromuscular Electrical Stimulation on the Quadriceps Femoris During Immobilization (% Change)

	Isometric Torque	Cross-sectional Area	Citrate Synthesis Activity	TPDH Activity
Electrical stimulation	−39.2	−22.9	−5.8*	−10.1*
Control	−57.8	−25.9	−29.4	−16.8

*$P < 0.05$, electrical stimulation vs. control.

a rapid return to maximal performance levels, but that it might be of little or no benefit in individuals who can afford the delay in return to peak physical activity until after the period of immobilization and reconditioning is complete.

NMES (30 Hz per 18% duty cycle for 1 hour/day), using surface electrodes on the quadriceps femoris, prevents the development of disuse muscle atrophy in individuals immobilized with a long-leg cast for a tibial fracture. This preservation of muscle mass was associated with a maintenance of muscle protein synthesis and rate of muscle protein synthesis per unit of muscle RNA (Fig. 23–7).[79] NMES of the calf muscles (7 Hz for 30 min twice a day) in patients hospitalized in the intensive care unit for postoperative ventilatory failure or cerebral infarctions, decreased urinary 3-methylhistidine and creatinine excretion, reflecting a slowing of negative nitrogen balance and improved preservation of muscle mass, in contrast to nonstimulated controls.[20] These studies taken together suggest a potential role for NMES in preserving muscle mass in individuals undergoing prolonged periods of immobilization for a variety of reasons.

One final application of NMES in normal muscle is to help to evaluate the etiology of weakness in a patient. Under conditions of normal volitional central control, a decrease occurs in electrical stimulation–induced contraction response with increasing voluntary muscle contraction at different levels (Fig. 23–8A).[215] Thus, if a subject is volitionally attempting to maximally contract muscle, leading to an optimal pattern of recruitment of all the motor units, direct electrical stimulation of the muscle will not lead to a further increment in muscle force. If, however, the subject is not maximally trying (or other forces contribute to a drop in volitional muscle force), electrical stimulation will lead to an increase in muscle force. This is best seen as a striking difference in the ratio of the electrically induced torque increment (EITI) in the fourth to first stimulation in response to increases in voluntary contraction in normal controls vs. malingerers (Fig. 23–8B). The decrease in the fourth to first EITI ratio in normal subjects at 75% and 100% voluntary contraction reflects the effect of the development of peripheral fatigue at near-maximal contractions, which subsequently results in a reduced responsiveness of the motor unit to electrical stimulation.[53]

Stimulation of Myopathic Muscle

There remains considerable controversy regarding the benefit of electrical stimulation in preservation of motor function in individuals with neuromuscular disease. Previous studies have suggested that aggressive physical exercise may result in overwork weakness and a loss of physical function.[113, 246] Using dystrophic animal models, low-frequency electrical stimulation has been shown to improve muscle function, delay degeneration of muscle fibers, and increase the quantity of oxidative enzymes.[54, 151, 212, 248] In the genetically dystrophic chicken, NMES applied early after hatching delayed the onset of righting disability, gradually increased muscle mass, increased dystrophic protein by 29%, and increased circulating creatine phosphokinase (CPK) levels. Surprisingly, however, electrical stimulation in this model resulted in a discernible shift toward a glycolytic metabolism, which is the opposite of the effect seen with NMES in normal muscle.[106]

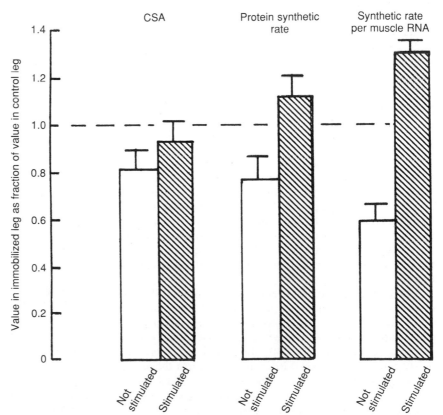

FIGURE 23–7 Effect of 6 weeks of electrical stimulation of the cast-immobilized quadriceps femoris muscle on muscle protein synthesis and quadriceps cross-sectional area in comparison to the same parameters in immobilized controls. (From Gibson JNA, Smith K, Rennie MJ: Prevention of disuse muscle atrophy by means of electrical stimulation: Maintenance of protein synthesis. Lancet 1988; 2(8614):767–769.)

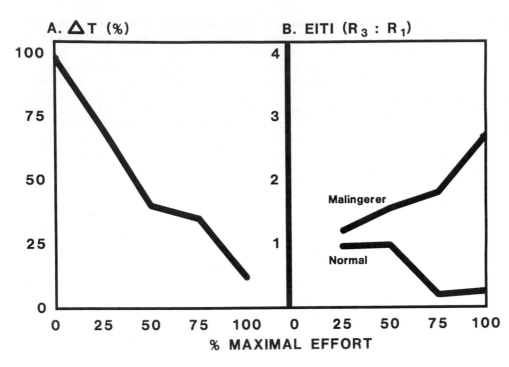

A. ΔT (%)

B. EITI (R$_3$: R$_1$)

Malingerer

Normal

% MAXIMAL EFFORT

FIGURE 23–8 Effect of central and peripheral factors in fatigue elicted by electrical stimulation with voluntary contraction of the quadriceps femoris. *Panel A* reflects the dependence of the amplitude of electrically stimulated torque increments (T) on the percent of maximal voluntary contraction (% MVC). *Panel B* shows the utility of measuring the ratio of the electrically induced torque increments (EITI) in the third to the first trial (R3:R1), to detect malingerers. The amplitude of force at 100% maximal voluntary force drops on successive trials in normal control subjects due to fatigue, but the target torque is dramatically different in the malingerer. (Data from Latash ML, Yee MJ, Orpett C, et al: Combining electrical muscle stimulation with voluntary contraction for studying muscle fatigue. Arch Phys Med Rehabil 1994; 75:29–35.)

When low-frequency electrical stimulation is applied to dystrophic muscle in children with muscular dystrophy, improvements occur in maximal voluntary contraction of the stimulated muscle[161, 225, 226, 260] and in torque, with no increase in fatigue.[260] If, however, electrical stimulation is initiated after significant strength has already been lost, there appears to be no benefit from electrical stimulation treatment. After discontinuation of NMES, strength gains are lost rapidly.[161] Thus, if NMES is to be used for strengthening in neuromuscular disease, the physician should be aware that it is only of benefit in individuals who have retained more than 15% of normal strength and that the benefit is likely to be short-lived, resulting in only a delay of the inevitable outcome.

Stimulation of Denervated Muscle

As previously described in animal models, denervated muscle appears to have some plasticity, as NMES has been shown to facilitate the transformation from fast- to slow-twitch (or slow- to fast-twitch) fiber. This result has been associated with improved maintenance of muscle fiber area[81, 182] and muscle girth[88, 176] for a short interval until re-innervation sets in. NMES, however, has no benefit in maintaining certain isometric contractile properties that are associated with prolongation of the action potential, including the twitch to peak time and twitch half-relaxation time.[45]

The data are mixed on the effect of initiating NMES late after denervation injury. If the electrical stimulation is initiated immediately at the time of injury, the acceleration of the half-life of the slow-degrading acetylcholine receptor can be prevented.[7] If started after the acetylcholine receptor has begun to destabilize, NMES cannot reverse the switch to a faster-degrading receptor nor can it slow the degradation of the rapid acetylcholine receptor. These data suggest that maximal maintenance of normal motor unit character-

istics in a short-term stimulation program depends on very early initiation of stimulation.

In contrast, NMES using an unusually long duration (20 msec), bi-directional, rectangular impulse at a frequency of 25 Hz, begun 28 days after denervation, has been shown to preserve muscle fiber diameter and to induce a hybrid fiber type, with properties of both slow- and fast-twitch muscle.[164] The authors postulate that the relatively dramatic results of this late application of NMES might be due in part to the long impulse duration used in the stimulation protocol. This is consistent with data from a previous study comparing 8 Hz/1 msec with 1 Hz/7 msec stimulation regimens in the denervated rabbit fast-twitch muscle, that found that only the lower-frequency stimulation pattern reduced atrophy.[175] Thus, the consensus of several studies on the dose-response of tetanic stimulation in prevention of muscle atrophy is that stimulation durations ranging from 5 to 45 msec are beneficial, with no utility of shorter-duration impulses.[251] However, although application of NMES for muscle that was denervated 4 to 10 months previously can cause some improvement in muscle tension, the resultant upper end of tension noted in the studies was only 10% of normal values.[3]

Although these data confirm some efficacy in animals, in man, low-frequency NMES started within 7 weeks of injury and continued for more than 35 weeks resulted in no benefit over the long term as measured by clinical muscle force testing, dynamometry, muscle mass measurement (by CT or ultrasound), or maximal amplitude or frequency of denervation activity.[19] In contrast, galvanic stimulation (30 stimulations three times per day) has been reported to maintain hand muscle bulk.[112] The discrepancies among these studies, other data in the literature, and the animal models could reflect differences in stimulation parameters and muscle characteristics. Parameters that have been shown to be most effective for NMES in denervation are high voltage and short duration or long duration and low voltage, both of which can be clinically impractical due to discomfort.[99]

Ultimately, the decision to use therapeutic intervention should depend on evidence of an improved outcome. There are no data to support that NMES of denervated muscles speeds the process of reinnervation.[229] This lack of efficacy, in combination with studies showing that NMES using implanted microelectrodes results in a suppression of peripheral sprouting compared with nonstimulated controls, suggests that no convincing data show that the application of NMES for treatment of denervated muscle is advantageous.

Stimulation of Decentralized Muscle

Electrical stimulation of muscle following central nervous system or spinal cord injury can result in reversal of the muscular atrophy seen in association with the relative immobilization associated with these disorders. Although applications of NMES after cerebral vascular accident have, in general, been limited to use of NMES as an orthotic assist rather than as a therapeutic adjunct to strengthening, it has been used successfully in the small superficial muscles of the hand and wrist to improve strength and decrease atrophy.[183] Recommendations for electrical stimulation in the hand muscles suggest that strength is maintained at greater than 80% of initial value over an 8-month period, using a 1:5 duty cycle with decreases in dorsiflexion force output as duty cycle is equalized to 50%. Thus, modification of electrical stimulation parameters to meet the fatigability of the muscles undergoing training is necessary, especially in situations in which spasticity and severe weakness may limit therapeutic gain.

Much more attention has been paid to the use of NMES as a modality for rehabilitation of paralyzed muscles following spinal cord injury (SCI). Following SCI, a decrease occurs in type I fibers, myofibrillar ATPase, and succinate dehydrogenase activity, and the capillary-to-fiber ratio is reduced in comparison to that of normal control muscles. In addition, a loss of muscle bulk, a reduction in force, and increased fatigability have been noted. Electrical stimulation (20 Hz/15% duty cycle) of a tibialis anterior in individuals with chronic SCI resulted in an increase in the proportion of type I fibers from 14% ± 8% to 25% ± 10% (although the final level was well below that of control muscles), but had no effect on the distribution of fiber sizes or mean fiber area.[157] In addition, NMES enhanced the oxidative capacity of the muscle as defined by an increase in the activity of succinate dehydrogenase. These results are similar to those seen with the application of low-frequency electrical stimulation to normal muscle. Muscle strength and contractile properties also showed a positive response to NMES. Daily NMES increased endurance of the muscle to levels found in able-bodied control subjects, with a slowing of the time course of contraction and half-relaxation.[239] These data suggest substantial increases in fatigue resistance from characteristics of a fast-twitch, fatigable muscle (type IIb) to a fast-twitch fatigue-resistant type (type IIa). Despite these improvements in fatigue, an absence was noted of any marked change in muscle force with a stimulation pattern. This might reflect unique muscle properties of the tibialis anterior muscle, as other studies of NMES in SCI have shown that increases in force are maintained with stimulation.

Although NMES-induced muscle contraction has been shown to increase certain contractile and histochemical properties of decentralized muscle, actual increases in muscle strength and endurance are most dramatically seen when NMES is combined with resistance training or functional activities. Since the mid-1980s, isometric quadriceps strengthening using NMES to move the knees through a 45-degree arc with increasing resistance has resulted in increases in quadriceps endurance and mass. The development of a functional electrical stimulation hybrid cycle ergometry system (FES-CE) (Fig. 23–9) has resulted in further therapeutic benefits. The system uses a rectangular, monophasic waveform of 30 Hz, 0 to 130 mA at 375 msec duration to sequentially stimulate the quadriceps, hamstrings, and gluteal muscles to produce a smooth pedaling motion of a Monark lower extremity cycle ergometer. This closed-loop system is set to maintain a cycling rate of 35 to 50 rpm, with automatic shutoff if the impedence is greater than 16,000 Ω, if the voltage exceeds 220, or if the pedaling rate is less than 35 rpm (suggesting fatigue). Using FES cycle ergometry, several investigators have shown increases in thigh circumference,[189, 190, 206] muscle strength and endurance,[203] quadriceps muscle area (by CT scan),[184] and quadriceps muscle protein synthesis rates (from 0.071% to 0.0985%/hour) with no change in whole body protein turnover.[184] Changes in contractile properties include a decrease in the initial slope of quadriceps twitch, which is assumed to be compatible with a disproportionate increase in the function of slow-twitch fibers.[203]

Not only can FES result in changes in localized muscle mass, but it can affect overall body composition. Following SCI, lean body mass decreases and fat mass increases.

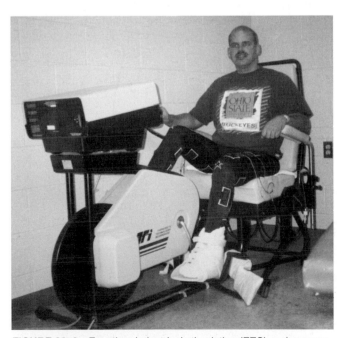

FIGURE 23–9   Functional electrical stimulation (FES) cycle ergometer by Therapeutic Technologies, Inc. Cycling is produced with sequential stimulation of the quadriceps femoris, hamstring, and gluteal muscles, using surface electrodes.

Data from our laboratory have shown, however, that individuals with chronic SCI who were randomized to an FES-CE protocol showed gains in total body lean body mass (LBM) of 7.9% with a decrease in percent body fat of 12.1%. These gains in lean body mass are primarily attributed to gains in the lower extremity LBM, which increases 9.7% over baseline. FES-CE is also a promising intervention to prevent the losses in lean body mass associated with acute SCI.

Finally, the use of NMES to stimulate muscle contraction and maintain muscle mass might be applicable to the prevention of pressure sores. NMES (50 Hz/33% duty cycle) resulted in an increase in blood flow under the ischial tuberosity. During electrical stimulation, in untrained SCI subjects, this change was not statistically significant. Because significant benefits were noted in able-bodied subjects, the authors postulated that fatigue might have contributed to a reduction in the increment of blood flow in the SCI subjects, and that training might improve the hemodynamic benefit. In addition, NMES (50 Hz) of the gluteus maximus (Fig. 23–10) in able-bodied subjects can produce appreciable changes in seating interface pressure distribution and result in substantial shape changes of the buttocks at stimulation levels producing only a small fraction of maximum voluntary contraction.[144] The buttock shape obtained during stimulation more nearly resembles the shape of the suspended buttocks, implying a reduction in tissue distortion. If similar results could be obtained in an SCI population, NMES could have a potential application as a form of "pressure release" to decrease the incidence of pressure sores.

ELECTRICAL STIMULATION FOR PREVENTION OF COMPLICATIONS OF DISUSE

Following a neurological insult, a person is predisposed to a number of complications that arise long-term due to

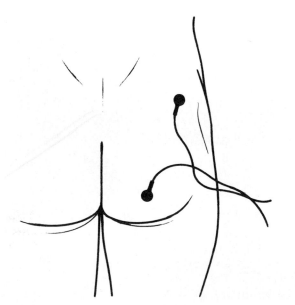

FIGURE 23–10 Hip extension is produced with placement of the active electrode on the gluteus maximus below the posterior superior iliac crest, and the indifferent electrode is placed inferiorly on the muscle.

the resultant decrease in physical activity. Nowhere is the magnitude of this greater than in SCI. With the loss of voluntary bipedal locomotion, individuals with SCI are at greater risk for cardiovascular disease, osteoporosis, pressure ulcers, and thromboembolic disease. In addition, changes in self-image can have a major influence on well-being. In an attempt to reduce these disuse-associated medical conditions, physicians have turned to NMES techniques.

Cardiovascular Deconditioning

During the past few decades, with improvement in bladder and skin management, cardiovascular disease has become the primary cause of death in individuals with SCI. A body of evidence shows that SCI is associated with a decrease in cardiopulmonary performance. Within the first 3 months of SCI, a significant decline occurs in aerobic capacity, with declines in maximal oxygen consumption of more than 40%.[65] After discharge from rehabilitation, the workload of a paraplegic individual performing independent activities of daily living (ADL) is only 24% of the maximal work capacity, which is insufficient to maintain cardiovascular fitness.[102] This cardiovascular deconditioning is even more pronounced in quadraplegic persons, for whom data show a decrease in maximum heart rate, stroke volume, and cardiac output[186] and development of left ventricular atrophy.[172] Studies of maximal oxygen consumption (VO_2) in persons with chronic SCI reveal an inverse relationship to the level of SCI.[103]

Cardiovascular deconditioning, however, is not an inevitable consequence of SCI. Wheelchair athletes have been shown to have significantly higher VO_2, cardiac output, and stroke volume than sedentary SCI individuals.[179, 261] In addition, their lipid levels are nearly the same as those of abled-bodied individuals, with the exception of a lower HDL_3 level.[23] Arm crank ergometry (AE) has been proposed as a means to improve cardiovascular training, but it is inefficient, because recruitment of small muscle mass during exercise results in a VO_2 level that is 15% to 35% lower than that that can be obtained with lower extremity exercises.[50, 66, 205] For quadriplegic individuals, AE may be impractical due to upper limb weakness; attention has therefore turned toward the use of therapeutic NMES as an intervention to improve cardiovascular fitness. Chronic use of AE might also accelerate the deterioration of the shoulder joints seen in chronic SCI.

A consensus has existed since the initial studies in the late 1980s, that short-term training with FES-CE can produce an increase in both endurance and maximal oxygen consumption when stress testing is performed with the lower limb cycle ergometer.[172, 201] In addition, in quadriplegic persons, FES-CE can result in an improvement in left ventricular mass.[172] This lower limb training, however, has not been shown to translate to a cardiovascular improvement when exercise testing is done via AE stress testing.[103] This is consistent with data in abled-bodied individuals that indicate a training effect is specific to the muscle groups that are trained.[42]

During an acute bout of FES-CE, a relative increase occurs in VO_2, pulmonary ventilation, heart rate, and stroke volume, with greater increases noted in paraplegic vs.

quadriplegic persons. The increase in VO_2 is thought to be due to augmented blood flow to the exercised muscles. Work by Petrofsky and Stacy[193] has shown that the respiratory efficiency of FES cycling is only 3.6% (thus, 3.6% of the energy of cycling is converted to energy to move the pedals), which is substantially lower than the value of 20% to 30% for lower limb cycle ergometry in abled-bodied individuals. Despite the low respiratory efficiency, however, prolonged training with FES-CE does result in increases in blood pressure, heart rate, cardiac output, and VO_2 maximum that are linear with the metabolic demand on the muscle.

In an attempt to increase the efficiency of cardiovascular training, studies have combined AE with lower extremity FES. Training with these hybrid systems has shown improved increments in oxygen consumption, minute ventilation, cardiac output, and stroke volume in comparison with AE or FES-CE alone. New approaches include the combination of FES quadriceps extension against 20 lb of resistance with AE at 50 rpm,[63] FES-CE with voluntary AE,[133] or FES-rowing.[137]

In summary, advances in functional electrical stimulation have resulted in the development of several systems that can increase muscle mass, reduce venous pooling, increase stroke volume and cardiac output, and improve cardiorespiratory fitness. Additional long-term data analyzing the efficacy of various FES techniques and treatment protocols are necessary to determine whether the short-term improvements in cardiorespiratory fitness can be maintained over long periods of time and whether they will have a substantial influence on cardiovascular morbidity and mortality.

Osteoporosis

One prominent metabolic consequence of SCI is an acute disruption of normal calcium balance, which contributes to a rapidly evolving osteopenia that is a permanent consequence of the injury. The severe osteopenia results in an increased risk of fractures, and as many as 9% of all SCI patients present with one or more fractures within the first 10 years after injury.[207] Cross-sectional studies of regional bone mass changes have documented that bone mass loss is not uniform below the level of neurological injury, but that the magnitude of loss is determined, at least in part, by the degree of reduction in biomechanical loading.[16] One of the mechanisms thought to contribute to this profound bone loss is the loss of muscle contraction and mechanical loading in the SCI patient. Based on Wolff's law, which states that the form and structure of bone is organized to optimally resist perceived loads from functional demands, attention has been focused on the use of therapeutic NMES as a means of reducing immobilization, increasing biomechanical strain, and potentially improving bone mass at localized skeletal regions.

Initial studies by Leeds and associates[142] and Pacy and colleagues[184] showed no benefit of FES-CE on bone mass at the proximal femur or lumbar spine in individuals with SCI of long duration. More recent data from our laboratory suggest FES-CE can produce small increments in bone mass in patients with chronic SCI, but these benefits are localized to the two skeletal regions (proximal tibia and distal femur) receiving the greatest mechanical strain with

the exercise regimen.[18] In addition, as seen in able-bodied individuals, these increments in bone mass are dependent on achieving a sufficient workload, with gains limited to individuals who were able to cycle at workloads of 18 W or greater. Additional studies by the authors' laboratory suggest that FES-CE could be of greater benefit for the prevention of neurogenic osteopenia. This is consistent with all other forms of osteoporosis for which there are no known strategies to date for reversing significant osteopenia. Early intervention with FES-CE following acute SCI have been reported to significantly slow rates of bone loss and to decrease hypercalciuria.[171] Longer-duration studies with continued use of FES-CE will help to define whether NMES is a practical and an effective means of preventing osteopenia and of reducing the incidence of fractures.

Deep Venous Thrombosis

Another complication associated with the relative immobilization seen after a neurological insult is an increase in the risk of thromboembolic disease. Following a cerebrovascular accident, there is a 23% to 75% incidence of deep venous thrombosis (DVT) and a 10% incidence of pulmonary emboli during the first 6 months. The role of reduced muscle activity is suggested by data that show that the DVT is most commonly localized to the paretic limb (5- to 10-fold increase). The incidence of DVT is even greater following SCI, with an incidence reported between 47% and 100% within the first year post-SCI. Thromboembolic disease accounts for 37.5% of acute deaths in this population. Because certain individuals have contraindications to subcutaneous heparin prophylaxis (e.g., blood in CNS), there has been some exploration of the use of NMES to reduce the incidence of thromboembolic disease. NMES (10 Hz, 50 μsec pulse/33% duty cycle) of the tibialis anterior and gastrocnemius-soleus muscle groups for 23 hours/day over a 28-day period in combination with low-dose heparin in patients with acute SCI showed a significant decrease in the incidence of DVT in comparison with a group receiving low-dose heparin alone.[160] This might be due, in part, to the effects of NMES in increasing plasma fibrinolytic activity.[119] Despite these promising results in SCI patients, studies in other patient populations have failed to confirm a significant efficacy, and in sensate individuals, NMES was associated with pain and local skin irritation.

Psychological Effects

A number of psychosocial problems have been reported in patients following SCI, including mood disorders and diminished social and vocational functioning. It has been proposed that exercise might result in some psychological benefits, such as improved self-esteem. Utilizing FES-CE, 62% of paraplegic and 56% of quadriplegic patients reported improved self-image with participation.[232] Other benefits included increased self-esteem,[92, 232] well-being,[8] and independence[92] and diminished depression.[4] Not all changes, however, are positive, with some subjects also reporting decreased motivation and increased anger and tension. Expectations played an important role in resultant negativity, with individuals with unrealistic expectations (e.g., anticipation of improved neurological function) showing the fewest psychological benefits.[22] The positive feelings noted with FES-CE can have a physiological explanation, as regular exercise with FES-CE has been shown to significantly increase beta-endorphin levels.[245]

THERAPEUTIC FUNCTIONAL ELECTRICAL STIMULATION

Urinary Incontinence

Urinary incontinence is a significant public health problem that carries an economic burden estimated at $10 billion per year.[40] Although Kegel introduced exercises for the management of urinary incontinence in the late 1940s and early 1950s, the primary method of intervention has remained surgical intervention.[30] The conservative management of urinary incontinence is, however, considered to be the wave of the future.[30]

Caldwell was the first to report positive results after implantation of an electrical stimulation system for the correction of urinary incontinence in 1963.[115] A subsequent study treated women with both stress and motor-urge incontinence with intravaginal electrodes. After 12 weeks of stimulation, 20 minutes daily, a markedly diminished leakage of urine was noted in 35% of women with stress incontinence and in 65% of women with motor-urge urinary incontinence.[115] Another study combined pelvic floor exercises with intravaginal maximal electrical stimulation. After 6 weeks of stimulation for 15 minutes daily, 89% of women with stress urge incontinence, 73% with motor instability, and 70% with mixed incontinence demonstrated improvement. Long-term follow-up demonstrated that 80% of women maintained the improvement.[40]

The mechanism for this therapeutic response is believed to be secondary to the fact that incontinence might represent a denervation injury; that is, the observed improvements could be due to the muscle strengthening properties of electrical stimulation.[30] The validity of this hypothesis is questioned in view of the fact that many humans do not tolerate stimulation intensities sufficiently high to directly stimulate motor nerves. Therefore, it is suggested that pelvic floor afferents with reflex connections to the muscle are stimulated.[71]

The stimulation systems for the management of bladder incontinence include electrodes implanted into pelvic floor muscles, intra-anal electrodes, and intravaginal electrodes. The intravaginal electrodes appear to be the most commonly utilized technique. Stimulation programs typically utilize biphasic pulsed waveforms; less than 10 Hz stimulation is optimal for bladder inhibition, whereas stimulation rates approaching 50 Hz are recommended for optimal urethral closure. Mixed stress and urge incontinence protocols utilize stimulation rates of 20 Hz.[71] Pulse duration and amplitude are adjusted to the maximal tolerable level.

In summary, data clearly suggest that the electrical stimulation of pelvic floor muscles is an important adjunct to the conservative management of stress and motor-urge urinary incontinence. It has been suggested that this technique is primarily suited as an adjunct to therapy for individuals who are not able to voluntarily stop urine flow and who cannot actively contract the pelvic floor muscles.[30]

Electrical stimulation has also been utilized extensively for the restoration of bladder function after SCI. Toward this goal, implanted electrodes have been applied to the bladder wall, pelvic splanchnic nerves, conus medullaris, mixed sacral nerves, and sacral anterior roots. The greatest attention is being directed toward stimulation of the sacral anterior roots. This procedure is, however, complicated by the reflex activation of sphincters. A number of techniques have been explored to reduce the subsequent outflow obstruction such as pudendal neurectomy, external sphincterotomy, and developing stimulation parameters that sufficiently maintain the peak contraction of the sphincter and bladder out of phase to produce micturition between bursts.[49]

More recently, posterior root rhizotomy has been advocated in conjunction with sacral anterior root stimulation as a means of abolishing uninhibited reflex bladder contractions, thereby increasing bladder capacity, restoring bladder compliance to normal, and abolishing reflex contraction of the sphincter. The disadvantages of the posterior root rhizotomy include the loss of reflex erection and reflex ejaculation. The combination of these techniques is useful in that they decrease residual urine volume, improve bladder compliance, improve urinary incontinence, and decrease reflux and hydronephrosis. Additional benefits of these two interventions are restoration of full erections sufficient for coitus in 60% of patients and production of defecation with the stimulator alone in 50% of patients.[49]

Ejaculatory Failure

Ejaculatory failure is noted in approximately 95% of SCI survivors. Semen retrieval, however, is possible with subcutaneous physostigmine, vas aspiration, vibratory stimulation, and electrostimulation by rectal probe.[110] Ejaculation via rectal probe stimulation is apparently accomplished with either sinusoidal or pulsed waveforms utilizing a variety of stimulation parameters.[187, 228] Ejaculation via electrostimulation appears to be well tolerated and safe, and it significantly enhances the fertility of SCI survivors.

Management of Spasticity

Electrical stimulation has been used therapeutically for the management of spasticity since Duchenne's first use of it in 1871. Since then, electrical stimulation for the management of spasticity has been administered by epidural, implanted peroneal, subcutaneous, and surface stimulation. Most of the available information regarding the efficacy of this modality is based on observations noted during the application of electrical stimulation for functional purposes. Few studies have attempted to systematically evaluate the therapeutic efficacy of this modality in spasticity. One study did, however, attempt to quantify the short-term effects of surface electrical stimulation in a group of 12 SCI survivors. The stimulation protocol involved an intensity of 100 mA, a duration of 0.5 msec, a stimulation frequency of 20 Hz, a compensated monophasic waveform, and a duty cycle ratio of 1:1. Just after 20 minutes of stimulation a significant improvement was seen in the pendulum drop test, but this improvement did not persist past 24 hours.[216]

The same group evaluated the impact of an 8-week

electrical stimulation protocol in which subjects received 20 minutes of electrical stimulation two times per day, 6 days/week. This protocol demonstrated a tendency toward increasing spasticity with long-term surface electrical stimulation.[217]

These results are not consistent with observations noted in hemiplegic individuals. One study, for example, followed up a group of hemiplegic patients receiving surface stimulation and via an implanted peroneal stimulator for 12 months. The stimulation parameters were described as a pulse width of 0.5 msec and a stimulation frequency of 30 to 33 Hz. This group noted a significant decrease in passive resistance and tonic reflex activity. These changes were thought to result in improved voluntary control in agonist and antagonist muscle groups.[236] A second study applied electrical stimulation to wrist extensors of hemiplegic individuals with flexor spasticity. Their stimulation program involved training individuals for three 30-min periods per day, 7 days/week, with stimulation parameters described as square wave pulses at 33 Hz, a pulse width of 200 μsec, and a pulse amplitude of 100 mA. The stimulation cycle was described as 7 seconds on, followed by a 10-sec rest interval. This group also demonstrated a decrease in flexor spasticity, a decrease in the contractures noted in persons with chronic hemiplegia, and a prevention of flexion contractures noted in "subacute" hemiplegic individuals.[10]

In summary, these data clearly indicate that electrical stimulation results in a short-term decrease in spasticity that may persist for several hours after a treatment session. There also appears to be evidence to suggest that long-term treatment decreases spasticity in hemiplegic individuals. However, the data are less clear regarding the impact of long-term stimulation on SCI survivors. More information is required to determine if the type and completeness of the lesion affects the observed responses from long-term functional electrical stimulation intervention.

Hemiplegic Upper Limb

The most common application of electrical stimulation in the hemiplegic upper limb is in the treatment and prevention of shoulder subluxation. Electrical stimulation is felt to be a superior option in that this type of intervention does not restrict the use of the limb as physical supports do. One study demonstrated that electrical stimulation could reduce existing subluxation. The study protocol involved stimulating the supraspinatus and posterior deltoid muscles (Fig. 23–11) with an asymmetrical biphasic waveform over a 6-week period.[11] The results indicated that electrical stimulation was superior to slings and wheelchair arm supports in reducing subluxation, but this apparently had no impact on reduction of shoulder pain. A subsequent controlled study evaluated the efficacy of electrical stimulation in a group of recent hemiplegic stroke patients. The goal was to evaluate the efficacy of electrical stimulation in the prevention of glenohumeral joint stretching and subsequent subluxation and to facilitate recovery of the flaccid shoulder. The protocol also involved placing the active electrode over the posterior deltoid and the passive electrode over the supraspinatus muscles. Stimulation frequency was set at 33 Hz and intensity was adjusted to elicit

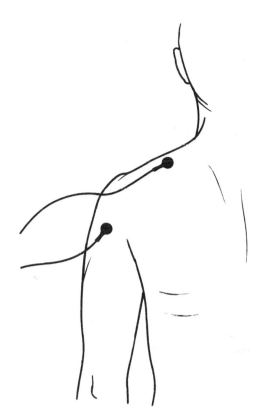

FIGURE 23–11 Use of electrical stimulation for treatment of shoulder subluxation involves placement of electrodes over the supraspinatus and posterior deltoid muscles.

the desired response. The duty cycle varied throughout the duration of the study. Patients were treated 1.5 to 6.0 hours/day over a 6-week period. The results suggested that FES resulted in improvement in arm muscle tone and function as well as in decreased shoulder subluxation, and the data suggested that electrical stimulation facilitated a more rapid recovery of arm function.[68]

It has also been demonstrated that electrical stimulation can improve functional use of a chronically hemiplegic upper limb (more than 6 months after cerebrovascular accident) by combining electrical stimulation techniques with voluntary effort. One particular study assigned subjects into four groups who received electromyographically (EMG) induced electrical stimulation of wrist extensors, low-intensity electrical stimulation of wrist extensors combined with voluntary contractions, proprioceptive neuromuscular facilitation exercises, or no treatment. The EMG-initiated electrical stimulation protocol involved utilizing low-level voluntary EMG activity in target muscles to trigger electrical stimulation of forearm wrist extensor muscles to produce a joint movement. The stimulation protocol involved a 0.2-msec biphasic square wave pulse as 30 to 90 Hz and a constant current of 20 to 60 μV. The group with low-intensity electrical stimulation of wrist extensors with combined voluntary contractions received 30 min of stimulation to the wrist extensors with a 0.3 msec square wave pulse at 30 to 90 Hz. The stimulation intensity was adjusted to increase voluntary range of wrist extension. The subjects were told to perform voluntary wrist extension exercises during the stimulations. The results of this study are compelling in that the electrical stimulation appeared to improve the function of chronically hemiparetic upper limbs. Specifically, subjects who received the EMG-induced electrical stimulation of wrist extensors demonstrated the greatest improvement. In addition, these gains were retained for 9 months.[129]

Phrenic Nerve Stimulation

Modern phrenic nerve stimulation dates to 1948.[177] Since that time, the technique has proved itself a valuable adjunct in the care of the patient with chronic ventilatory insufficiency who has normal phrenic nerve, diaphragm, and lungs. Specifically, this technique is useful in persons with high-level quadriplegia accompanied by respiratory paralysis and central hypoventilation syndromes.[177] It has been estimated that, nationally, 100 SCI survivors would annually meet the criteria for use of a phrenic nerve pacer.[177] The goal of this technique is to circumvent the need for mechanical ventilation. One series demonstrated that 40% of all quadriplegic patients who received the device were supported full-time by the phrenic nerve pacers.

Initial protocols involved pacing a single phrenic nerve with high-frequency stimulation (25 to 30 Hz) at a respiratory rate of 12 to 17 per minute. Problems with this approach included loss of efficiency secondary to paradoxical motion of the contralateral unpaced side and myopathic changes noted in animal diaphragms subjected to the same stimulation program.[82] In 1981, protocols evolved that utilized uninterrupted simultaneous pacing of both hemidiaphragms using low-frequency stimulation (7 to 8 Hz) and a respiratory rate of 5 to 9 per minute. This approach improved minute volumes and resulted in better air mixing.[82] In addition, it is speculated that the low-frequency stimulation converts the normal mixture of fast-twitch and slow-twitch fibers to a preponderance of fatigue-resistant type I fibers.[82] This speculation is in part supported by the fact that endurance and respiratory function improve slowly after initiation of phrenic nerve pacing.

THERAPEUTIC FUNCTIONAL ELECTRICAL STIMULATION AS AN ORTHOTIC DEVICE

Scoliosis

The importance of bracing in the prevention of scoliosis curve progression was documented in the 1970s and 1980s (see Chapter 18). During the same period, studies were initiated that examined the efficacy of FES in the management of scoliosis. The technique involved placement of electrodes along the convex portion of the curve above and below the apex. Stimulation parameters typically approximate a stimulation rate of 35 Hz, a pulse width of 200 μsec, and a pulse amplitude of 0 to 100 mA. In addition, the stimulation was modulated to deliver 5 seconds of stimulation followed by 25 seconds of rest. The advantage of this technique is that the electrical stimulation was performed only for 8 to 10 hours per night.[72]

Although the technique was typically well tolerated with few complications, the efficacy of the technique remains unclear. Some studies have documented that electrostimula-

tion was equal in efficacy to a Milwaukee brace in the treatment of adolescents with mild curves (20 to 40 degrees).[72] However, other studies documented failure rates with electrostimulation that approximated the rates of progression noted in studies examining the natural history of this disorder.[61] Moreover, patients whose curves progressed with electrostimulation then underwent bracing, with a subsequent halting of the progression of the scoliosis.[61, 72]

Therefore, the data examining the efficacy of electrical stimulation in the management of idiopathic scoliosis are inconclusive. Although some data indicate that electrostimulation is as effective as a Milwaukee brace in halting the progression of the disease, other data would imply that electrical stimulation does not alter the natural course of the disorder.[61, 72] Therefore the role for electrical stimulation in the management of idiopathic scoliosis is at best limited to use in a patient who is unable to tolerate appropriate bracing.

Hemiplegic Gait

Electrical stimulation has been utilized as a neural orthosis since 1961.[145] Since that time, NMES has been an important adjunct in the rehabilitation of patients with hemiplegia. Primarily this has involved utilizing NMES to improve the gait pattern of hemiplegics by increasing the torque output of the ankle dorsiflexors and reciprocally decreasing spastic reflexes in the plantar flexors.[58] Additionally, NMES can be applied to gluteal muscles (Fig. 23–12) and/or to the quadriceps muscles in an effort to enhance the stance phase of gait. Finally, NMES can be utilized to facilitate the swing phase of gait in hemiplegia with stimulation of the sole, dorsum of the foot, or lower posterior thigh in an effort to induce the flexion reflex.[58] The greatest role for NEMS in hemiplegic gait appears to be early during the acute rehabilitation phase of recovery.

FUNCTIONAL NEUROMUSCULAR STIMULATION: CLINICAL APPLICATIONS

Standing and Gait

Since the 1970s, FES for gait restoration after SCI has progressed from feasibility studies to the development of a commercially available, FDA-approved ambulation system.[130, 231] Despite the considerable progress, a number of barriers remain that continue to render this a cumbersome clinical application of technology. In addition to requiring a user-friendly system, the ideal FES gait system should be safe (in that it does not cause additional injury, such as degenerative joint changes), reliable, sufficiently functional to provide community ambulation, and both inexpensive and cosmetically acceptable.[15] Many of these goals have not been realized.

The typical components of the FES system include a power source plus cables, a control mechanism, display and ground, stimulator with cables, and electrodes.[202] Additionally, FES systems require a feedback mechanism. In open-loop systems, the feedback is controlled by the patient or therapist in response to observations. More sophisticated, closed-loop systems automatically incorporate feed-

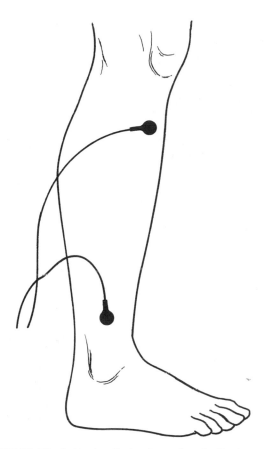

FIGURE 23–12 Ankle dorsiflexion is produced with placement of the active electrode proximally over the anterior tibialis and peroneal muscle groups and placement of the indifferent electrode distally over the tendons of the peroneal muscle.

back into the FES system. This permits the FES system to adjust to changes in muscle spasticity and fatigue. In addition, closed-loop systems likely improve endurance by controlling the stimulation intensity to the minimum necessary to accomplish a given functional task. Finally, closed-loop systems require less concentration on the part of the ambulator. Types of FES feedback systems include input from (1) external sensors, (2) EMG of muscle, (3) sensory nerve, or (4) motor areas of the brain.[156] The most common and practical sensors are externally mounted devices that feed back information regarding limb position and movement.

The number of channels in FES ambulation systems varies according to the sophistication of the system. Two-channel systems typically stimulate the knee extensors while four-channel systems typically activate knee extensors and hip flexors.[100, 231] FES ambulation systems employing more than eight channels often require implanted electrodes to provide more precise stimulation and to avoid the stimulation of adjacent muscles. Finally, the FES ambulation systems available today range from totally external devices (Fig. 23–13) to more experimental systems that are virtually completely implanted.

A survivor of a thoracic-level SCI presently has three options for pursuing the ability to walk. These include utilizing a mechanical orthosis (reciprocal gait orthosis, long-leg brace, etc.), an FES gait system, or a hybrid

system that utilizes a mechanical orthosis with the assistance of FES. Ambulation with a mechanical orthosis alone is impractical, at least in part, because the energy consumption is three to nine times that found in normal controls.[44] However, FES gait systems also consume considerable energy, as it has been estimated that these patients utilize 59% to 75% of their maximum aerobic power.[155] It appears that the energy consumption of some FES systems rival, if not exceed, that required for walking with a mechanical orthosis.

FES ambulation systems are also somewhat impractical because they permit only a limited range of activity. The typical standing time for these systems ranges from minutes to hours.[130] The speed of ambulation is slow, typically in the range of 0.1 to 0.4 m/sec.[130] Finally, the walking distance with these devices is limited to approximately 20 m, although distances of more than 1000 m have been reported.[130, 154]

The fatigue associated with FES ambulation is attributed to several factors. First, considerable energy is expended in stimulating the muscles necessary to maintain a standing position.[155] In addition, the rapid onset of FES-induced muscle fatigue is in part caused by the preferential recruitment of rapidly fatiguing, type II muscle fibers.[154] In an effort to minimize this fatigue, several stimulation techniques have been developed. First, stimulation intensities are limited to the minimum necessary to achieve a desired functional response. Second, stimulation rates are kept within the physiological ranges of 15 to 50 Hz.[155] Specifically, lower stimulation rates are desirable, presumably due to a greater likelihood of stimulating slow-twitch fatigue-resistant muscle fibers.[39] The third approach to diminish muscle fatigue involves an electrode distribution that permits the stimulation of portions of muscles or muscle groups; that is, muscle fatigue is diminished by sequentially activating portions of an individual muscle or muscle group, thereby producing the minimum necessary force to accomplish a functional task.[101, 188]

Because the technology does not yet exist for FES to produce functional community ambulation, most FES systems are hybrid systems that concomitantly utilize FES with a mechanical orthosis. This combination of devices offers several advantages. First, the mechanical orthosis permits standing without considerable energy expenditure.[130] Hybrid systems also appear to utilize less energy than either mechanical orthoses or FES ambulation systems. One study specifically compared the energy consumption during ambulation with a reciprocating gait orthosis (RGO), RGO and FES, FES alone, long-leg braces, and a hip-guided orthosis. The order of energy expenditure (from lowest to highest) was (1) RGO with FES to the thigh muscles, (2) hip-guided orthosis, (3) long-leg brace, and (4) FES systems. The addition of FES to the RGO decreased energy consumption by approximately 16%.[100] Finally, hybrid systems increase the speed of ambulation.[167, 174] The addition of FES to an RGO increases the optimum speed of ambulation from 1.2 km/hour with the RGO to 2.4 km/hour with the hybrid system.[174]

Advances in FES gait systems have extended to the commercial availability of an FDA-approved ambulation system.[231] However, the technology is still not capable of resolving or compensating for issues such as FES-induced

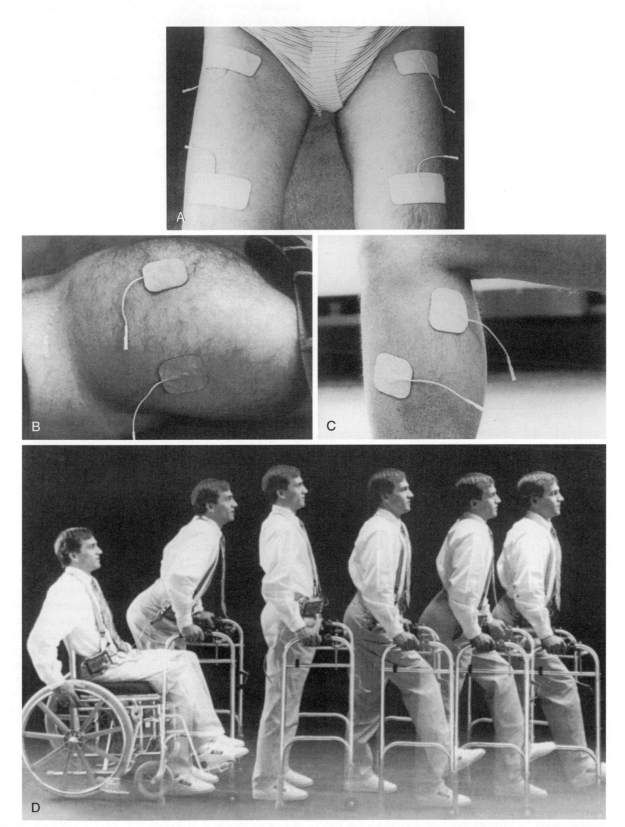

FIGURE 23–13 Parastep system developed by Sigmedics, Inc. These systems use surface electrodes. Both four- and six-channel systems exist that assist spinal cord injury individuals to stand and ambulate with use of a walker. Electrodes are placed over the quadriceps *(panel A)*, peroneal nerve behind the fibula head and tibialis anterior *(panel C)*, and gluteus medius and maximus *(panel B; six-channel system only)* to allow for standing and walking *(panel D)*.

muscle fatigue, excessive energy expenditure associated with FES ambulation, reduced FES-induced joint torques, autonomic hyper-reflexia, osteoporosis, modified reflex activity, and spasticity.[154] Because FES ambulation systems to date are unable to achieve many of the criteria for a truly functional system, the patients who might benefit from existing FES ambulation systems are relatively few. One study estimated that approximately 10% of patients admitted to an SCI service are candidates for an FES gait restoration program. Only half of those, or 5% of survivors in the cohort, eventually learned to walk, but fewer than 3% of those patients ultimately utilized the FES ambulation system functionally within their home.

Restoration of Upper Limb Function

Traditionally, the option for survivors of a high cervical SCI with loss of hand function has included functional restoration via orthotic devices or surgical procedures, such as arthrodesis and tendon transfers. The goal of FES in this population is to provide palmar and lateral prehension grasp and to develop a means to easily change from one type of grasp to the other.[185]

To accomplish this goal, intramuscular or epimysial electrodes have been utilized to stimulate the flexor digitorum superficialis and profundus, flexor pollicis longus, abductor pollicis, flexor pollicis brevis, abductor pollicis brevis, extensor digitorum, and extensor pollicis longus.[185] The stimulation parameters typically involve amplitudes of approximately 20 mA and pulse widths of approximately 200 μsec. Variations in stimulation frequency between 15 and 50 Hz permit smooth transitions in force of muscle contraction.[185]

A position transducer in the contralateral shoulder is utilized to operate the system. Shoulder protraction and retraction are utilized to produce a proportional signal for hand opening and closing. Shoulder elevation and depression movements are then utilized to either maintain or release a set level of stimulation.[120]

Functional ADL skills achieved through this technology have included handling eating utensils, cups, writing instruments, books, and the telephone. More complex tasks, such as pouring, washing, brushing teeth, and handling computer diskettes have also been demonstrated.[185] Many ADL tasks require shoulder and elbow stabilization for their performance, and new stimulation techniques are being developed for synthesizing multi-joint arm movements to ensure stability.[124] Operative procedures such as arthrodesis, tenodesis, and tendon transfers are also available to minimize joint movement and to improve upper limb stability for FES utilization.[185]

A prerequisite for increasing hand functioning in the future is the development of a sensory feedback system for joint position, contact, force, slippage, pressure, and temperature.[120] To date, a single-element subcutaneous electrode in the C5 dermatone has been utilized.[120] A more intriguing feedback mechanism currently under development is an implanted cuff electrode that permits recording from peripheral sensory nerves.[214]

Another upper limb FES modification currently under development involves improvement in the present shoulder transducer control method. The present method is problematic because shoulder movements are often coupled with the desired functional movement of the arm and hand. New techniques to lock or unlock stimulation commands are being developed.[91] In addition, new techniques to control upper limb neuroprostheses are being developed. For example, command input from bilateral sternocleidomastoid muscle electrodes are being explored as a possible technique for the control of bilateral upper limb neuroprostheses.[227]

The results from the upper limb neuroprostheses have been favorable. However, the applicability is limited to patients who have primarily C6-spared SCIs. In addition, problems with peripheral nerve injuries involving the upper limb further limit the utility of this technique.

ELECTRICAL STIMULATION FOR THE TREATMENT OF SOFT AND HARD TISSUE INJURY

Wound Healing

A body of scientific evidence has been accumulating to suggest that electrical stimulation can be used to promote the healing of wounds. Investigators have previously demonstrated that the surface of human skin is electronegative with respect to the inner layers. Wounded skin demonstrates the existence of a natural bioelectric current, with the ionic body fluids allowing for transmission of electricity between outer and inner layers. When electrical stimulation is applied to a wound, a number of biological processes in the wound are modified that might lead to enhanced healing. Electrical stimulation increases the number and function of fibroblasts[51, 76] and collagen, protein, and DNA synthesis,[13] and causes changes in expression of cellular receptors for transforming growth factor beta[70] and enhancing calcium uptake and neurite growth and extension. The fibroblasts and epithelial cells move along the path of the voltage gradient (the galvanotaxic effect)[48, 256] toward the cathode. Electrical stimulation has also been shown to increase the relative number of neutrophilic granulocytes while suppressing the number of mast cells.[252] This suppression of mast cells has been postulated to result in improved wound healing with a decrease in fibrotic scarring and, thus, better cosmetic results. It appears that electrical stimulation can augment the endogenous chemical factors that initiate the inflammatory stage of healing.

Electrical stimulation can also improve blood flow.[111] The improved vascularity has been associated with decreased lipid peroxidation and prevention of damage to oxygen-derived free radicals. Evidence also indicates that electrical stimulation has bacteriostatic and bactericidal properties.[111] Duration of exposure and voltage shows a linear relationship between inhibition of growth of several common wound pathogens when negative polarity is used.[123]

Several studies published since the mid-1960s[247] have demonstrated the effectiveness of electrical stimulation to promote the healing of dermal ulcers (Table 23–4). The initial studies were nonrandomized, prospective trials to determine the safety and efficacy of electrical stimulation on chronic dermal ulcers. Using electrical stimulation for treatment of pressure ulcers or ischemic ulcers in a variety of patient populations showed a significant increase in ulcer

TABLE 23–4 Effect of Electrical Stimulation on Wound Healing

| | Non-randomized Trials | | | |
| | Unilateral Ulcer | | Bilateral Ulcers (% Healed) | |
Type of Ulcer	NO. PARTICIPATING	% HEALING	ELECTRICAL STIMULATION	CONTROL
Chronic[257]	75	13.4	27	5
Ischemic	150	20.0	28.3	8.3
Ischemic[75]	106	28.4	30	14.7
Elderly[244]	223	89.7	—	—

| | | Randomized Trials | | | | | |
| | | Electrical Stimulation | | | Control | | |
Type	No.	%Δ ULCER SIZE	% HEALED	TIME TO HEAL (DAYS)	%Δ ULCER SIZE	% HEALED	TIME TO HEAL (DAYS)
Pressure	8	—	100	50.1	+13.8	—	74
Pressure[126]	16	−38*	100	50	+28.9	—	52
Mixed[245]	17	—	88.9	51.2	—	37.5	77
Pressure[85]	17	−80			−52		
Diabetic[150]	64	−61	42	84	−41	15	84

*Improvement in ulcer size after cross-over of ulcers from sham treatment to electrical stimulation.

healing. When patients entered into the study were noted to have more than one ulcer, several trials utilized those patients to randomize one ulcer to treatment with electrical stimulation and the other to a non–electrical stimulation control group. In these substudies, significant improvements were noted in the rate of ulcer size reduction and number of healed ulcers in the ulcers receiving electrical stimulation in comparison to control ulcers. Recognizing the need for randomized trials, several studies have subsequently been published comparing electrical stimulation to sham-treated ulcers. In general, these studies have shown increased rates and percentages of healing with electrical stimulation in comparison to control populations (see Table 23–4) with no significant complications. Recent studies have focused on use of pulsed galvanic electrical stimulation with demonstration of similar benefits.[78] In summary, the data suggest that electrical stimulation can augment wound healing, and the efficacy appears to be generalizable to ischemic ulcers and pressure ulcers as well as to other types of deep wounds.

The most effective stimulation pattern is pulsed electrical stimulation, because it allows for higher current density without tissue irritation or burning. Recent studies have used alternating polarities beginning with a negative polarity, which is thought to have antibacterial effects and is associated with increased vascular support; when no further improvements in wound healing are noted (*plateauing*), polarity is changed. The absolute charge density needed to cause successful wound healing is on the order of 0.1 to 2.0 coulombs/cm[2, 210] and duration of treatment sessions can vary from 1 to 24 hours/day. Although no specific device has been approved by the FDA for the treatment of wound healing, this might become an important application of electrical stimulation in rehabilitation medicine in the future.

Fracture Healing

It has been known for years that mechanical deformation of bone induces electrical signals that arise from the deformation of crystals that have an asymmetrical lattice (*piezo-*

electric), or that are generated when stress is applied at the interface between the surface of bone and the surrounding ion-containing fluid (*electrokinetic*). In addition, electronegativity was also noted in metabolically active bone, with the greatest electric potential found in growth plates and healing fractures. These observations led to exploration of electrical stimulation for the treatment of fractures. It is now known that electrical stimulation leads to increases in proteoglycan synthesis in bone matrix, matrix calcification, and proliferation of osteoblasts.[25]

The clinical application of electrical stimulation to bone has primarily focused on its use as a therapeutic modality in the treatment of non-union. Many reports have been published since around 1980 on the use of electrical stimulation for the treatment of non-union of a wide variety of fractures. The majority of trials are nonrandomized prospective trials of individuals who have already undergone lengthy periods of fracture immobilization, bone grafting, and/or internal fixation without success. The consensus of these studies is that electrical stimulation, added to meticulous fracture care, improved fracture healing rates,[12, 14, 15, 18, 46, 56, 237] with the highest success rate occurring in tibial lesions (82%). Overall, the most effective use of electrical stimulation for fracture repair is in the lower extremity. Recent studies suggest that applications of pulse magnetic fields may help delay revision hip surgery in patients with loosened cement hip prostheses.[121]

Three primary electrical stimulation approaches are currently utilized for the treatment of non-union: surgical implantation of direct current, noninvasive inductance, and noninvasive capacitance. Contraindications to electrical stimulation include synovial pseudoarthroses, fracture cracks wider than 1 cm, dead bone, avascularity, and severe osteoporosis.[47] Active infections or the presence of metallic hardware is not a contraindication.[24]

TRANSCUTANEOUS ELECTRICAL NERVE STIMULATION

Shortly after the description of the gate control theory of pain in 1965, transcutaneous electrical nerve stimulation

(TENS) developed into an important intervention for the management of pain.[159] TENS remains the most common and important form of electroanalgesia. Despite the widespread utilization and acceptance of TENS, basic issues such as optimal stimulation parameters, electrode placement, and frequency of stimulation remain unresolved.

Several mechanisms have been proposed to explain the palliative properties of TENS. The possibility that a placebo effect contributes significantly to the reported responses has never been completely ruled out due to study design problems and difficulties in developing a creditable placebo. The gate control theory of pain is also frequently postulated as the mechanism for TENS-induced analgesia. According to this theory, TENS preferentially activates peripheral A-beta fibers, thereby modulating pain-carrying A-delta and C-fibers at the level of the dorsal horn.[159] Updates in the gate theory continue to provide a physiological rationale for TENS in that direct noxious stimulation can inhibit pain produced by another noxious stimulus. According to this theory, counterirritation activates neurons in the rostral ventral medulla, which in turn inhibits the activity of dorsal horn nociceptive neurons.[33]

Another intriguing hypothesis explaining the pain-mediating properties of TENS implicates the release of endogenous opioids at CNS sites.[90] In 1979, Cheng and Pomeranz were the first to demonstrate in an animal model that the pain-mediating effect of electroacupuncture may be secondary to endogenous opioids.[41] Specifically, they demonstrated that antinociception produced at 4 Hz stimulation was blocked by an opioid antagonist, naloxone, but antinociception induced at 200 Hz stimulation was not blocked by a similar dose of naloxone. Hence, it was initially theorized that the effect of low-frequency TENS was mediated by the endogenous opioid system, whereas the effect of high-frequency TENS was mediated by other mechanisms, such as gate control. Later studies, however, demonstrated that high-frequency stimulation–induced antinociception was also reversed with naloxone, but that higher doses were required.[41]

More recent studies have confirmed these observations in a human model. Specifically, low-frequency TENS has been shown to result in marked increases in metenkephalin and beta-endorphin.[33, 43] However, high-frequency (100 Hz) TENS has been shown to produce significant increases in dynorphin A.[90] As in the animal model, the antinociceptive effect of low-frequency stimulation is readily reversed by naloxone, and it is therefore postulated that these effects are mediated by naloxone-sensitive mu-receptors. However, the analgesia induced by high-frequency stimulation requires higher doses of naloxone for reversal, thereby implicating naloxone-resistant dynorphin-binding kappa-receptors.[90] Thus, both high- and low-frequency TENS stimulation appears to stimulate the endogenous opioid system, but the type of response is dependent on stimulation frequency.

Other neurotransmitter systems have been implicated in mediating the analgesic effect of TENS. Specifically, CNS changes have been noted in serotonergic and substance P systems secondary to TENS stimulation.[5] However, these other neurotransmitter systems have received comparatively little attention in the literature, and thus their relative importance remains to be determined.

TABLE 23–5   Transcutaneous Electrical Nerve Stimulators

Type	Frequency	Width (msec)	Amplitude
Conventional	50–100	<200	Low
Acupuncture	1–10	200–300	High
Hyperstimulation	50–150	100–200	High
Burst	50–100* 1–10†	75–100	High
Modulated	Variable	<200	Variable

*Carrier frequency.
†Burst frequency.

Several types of TENS units have been developed that offer various stimulation parameters (Table 23–5). The most common type is the so-called *conventional TENS*. This type of unit offers high-frequency, low-intensity stimulation in the 50 to 100 Hz range, a pulse width of up to 200 μsec, and an amplitude capability between 0 and 100 mA that is adjusted to produce the minimum sensation. This type of unit typically decreases pain within 10 to 15 minutes of treatment, and the persistence of pain relief after cessation of treatment is similarly brief. The duration of treatment is typically 30 minutes to many hours. The *acupuncture-like TENS* units offer low-frequency, high-intensity stimulation parameters with stimulation rates of 0 to 10 Hz, a pulse width of 0 to 200 μsec, and an amplitude of sufficient milliamperes to produce discomfort and/or visible muscle contractions. The onset of pain relief from these units can be delayed several hours, but pain relief may persist several hours after treatment cessation, the treatment sessions are typically *30 to 60 minutes in duration. A third category of TENS units is the brief, intense TENS or hyperstimulation TENS.* This unit produces high-frequency, high-intensity stimulation parameters that presumably provide counterirritation, thereby activating C-fibers.[213] Duration of treatment sessions is rarely tolerated for more than 15 to 30 minutes. The *pulse trains TENS* or *burst mode* units provide high-frequency stimulation bursts at low-frequency intervals. As noted with the acupuncture-like TENS, onset of pain relief is delayed by several hours, and the relief can persist for hours after termination of treatment. Again, treatment sessions range between 30 and 60 minutes. The final category of TENS units is the *modulated TENS*, which offers impulses that vary in frequency and intensity in an attempt to avoid neurohabituation.[213]

These different stimulator types have been advocated for specific conditions. For example, the conventional TENS units are advocated for neuropathic pain, whereas the acupuncture-like TENS units are advocated more for acute musculoskeletal conditions. However, the data comparing the different stimulator types as to therapeutic efficacy and patient comfort are too few to draw significant conclusions.[114, 242] Interestingly, it has been observed that the overall efficacy of TENS in diminishing pain has not improved with the addition of new units that provided stimulation parameters other than those found in the original *conventional TENS* units.[178]

Proposed indications for TENS are numerous. Primarily, TENS units are advocated for the relief of pain secondary to neuropathic conditions and for all types of musculoskeletal pain.[149] Unfortunately it remains difficult to assess the efficacy of TENS for these conditions. Estimates of efficacy after 1 year of TENS treatment range between 10% and 50%.[149] Although the efficacy of TENS undoubtedly varies per diagnostic category, it is generally believed that a 30% long-term response rate is achieved in a heterogeneous population.[149] The accuracy of that estimate is easily questionable, as even controlled studies evaluating the efficacy of TENS for the management of chronic low back pain have yielded contradictory results.[55, 153]

TENS has also been advocated as being effective in a wide variety of other conditions. This has included management of pain secondary to CNS injury,[141] relief of spasticity,[143] relief of anginal pain,[223] improvement of blood flow and reduction of edema in skin flaps,[125] improvement of pain management during wound care in burn survivors, use during surgical procedures[122] (as an adjunct to pain control), and to increase the frequency and strength of uterine contractions.[60] TENS has also been advocated for labor pain relief; however, randomized studies have failed to confirm its efficacy despite the reported increase in patient satisfaction.[241]

The potential complications or contraindications to TENS are similar to those of other electrical stimulators. Typically it is advised that high-voltage units should not be used over the carotid sinus and they should not be used in patients who are either pregnant or utilize a cardiac pacemaker.[80] Few studies mention complications such as rashes or burns related to the electrodes. The primary concern regarding TENS safety has involved its utilization in conjunction with permanent cardiac pacemakers. One series of 51 patients with 20 different models of permanent cardiac pacemakers demonstrated that the TENS units had no effect on pacemaker function.[209] However, the authors did caution against using TENS electrodes parallel to the pacemaker electrode vector until studies verify the safety of that positioning.

TENS remains an important tool for the rehabilitation physician in the management of multiple acute and chronic pain conditions. However, the exact role of TENS in the management of these conditions remains unclear. Studies have not yet resolved basic issues, such as where electrodes should be applied, how long a unit should be utilized, or the most appropriate waveform and stimulation parameters. Future studies must report this information clearly if they are to be reproducible. Other issues that must be resolved before TENS is more widely accepted and respected as an important palliative modality include designing studies in which TENS is evaluated in a homogeneous population, in which the efficacy of TENS is compared with that of other modalities, in which the efficacy of TENS is evaluated early in a patient's clinical course (rather than used as a treatment of last resort), and in which the most efficacious stimulation parameters are determined for specific conditions.

CONCLUSION

Electrical stimulation is a historic physiatric modality, but an explosion of new interest in this area has occurred since the mid-1970s. In addition to rehabilitation medicine, a renewed interest in electrical stimulation has been demonstrated in various fields such as physiology, molecular biology, engineering, neurosurgery, neurology, orthopedics, urology, and plastic surgery. The result has been a significant improvement in the technology available for functional applications. In addition, a far greater understanding has developed of the physiological basis for the improvements noted with therapeutic applications of electrical stimulation.

Electrical stimulation appears to have growing importance as a modality in rehabilitation medicine. Continued research is, however, needed to ensure that this technology is maximally utilized. Toward this end, continued advancements in technology, a better understanding of optimal stimulation parameters, and a better understanding of the physiological changes induced by this technology are required.

References

1. Agnew WF, McCreery BB, Yuen TGH, Bullara LA: Histologic and physiologic evaluation of electrically stimulated peripheral nerve: Considerations for the selection of parameters. Ann Biomed Eng 1993; 17:39–60.
2. Al-Almond WS, Buller AJ, Pope R: Longterm stimulation of cat fast-twitch skeletal muscle. Nature 1973; 244:225–227.
3. Al-Amood WS, Lewis DN, Schmalbruch H: Effects of chronic electrical stimulation on contractile properties of long-term denervated rat skeletal muscle. J Physiol 1991; 441:243–256.
4. Alexander CJ, Sipski ML: Electrical stimulation bicycle ergometry with spinal cord injured patients: Potential medical and physiological benefits. Sci Psycho Soc Process 1990; 3:18–20.
5. Almay BG, Johansson F, von Knorring L, et al: Long-term high frequency transcutaneous electrical nerve stimulation (hi-TENS) in chronic pain: Clinical response and effects on CSF-endorphins, monoamine metabolites, substance P-like immunoreactivity (SPLI) and pain measures. J Psychosom Res 1985; 29:247–257.
6. Alon G, McCombe SA, Koutsantonis S, et al: Comparison of the effects of electrical stimulation and exercise on abdominal musculature. J Orthop Sports Phys Ther 1987; 8:567–573.
7. Andreose JS, Xu R, Lomo T, et al: Degradation of two AchR populations at rat neuromuscular junctions: Regulation in vivo by electrical stimulation. J Neurosci 1993; 13:3433–3438.
8. Baker RC, Heinemann AW, Yarkony GM, Jeager R: Functional neuromuscular stimulation for standing and ambulation: Six month evaluation of psychological effects. Proceedings of the RESNA 12th Annual Conference. New Orleans, 1989, pp 401–402.
9. Baker LL, Bowman BR, McNeal DR: Effects of waveform on comfort during neuromuscular electrical stimulation. Clin Orthop Rel Res 1988; 233:75–85.
10. Baker LL, Yeh C, Wilson D, Waters RL: Electrical stimulation of wrist and fingers for hemiplegic patients. Phys Ther 1979; 59:1495–1499.
11. Baker LL, Parker K: Neuromuscular electrical stimulation of the muscles surrounding the shoulder. Phys Ther 1986; 66:1930–1937.
12. Bassett CA, Mitchell SN, Gaston SR: Pulsing electromagnetic field treatment in ununited fractures and failed arthrodeses. JAMA 1982; 247:623–628.
13. Bassett CA, Hermann I: The effect of electrostatic fields on macromolecular synthesis by fibroblast in vitro. J Cell Biol 1968; 39:9A.
14. Bassett CA, Mitchell SN, Schink MM: Treatment of therapeutically resistant non-unions with bone grafts and pulsing electromagnetic fields. J Bone Joint Surg Am 1982; 64:1214–1220.
15. Bess GM, Waugh TR, Melone CP: Treatment of non-union with electrical stimulation. Orthop Rev 1985; 14:392–402.
16. Biering-Sorensen F, Bohr H, Schaadt O: Bone mineral content of the lumbar spine and lower extremities years after spinal cord lesion. Paraplegia 1988; 26:293–301.
17. Binder-MacLeod SA, Guerin T: Preservation of force output through progressive reduction of stimulation frequency in human quadriceps femoris muscle. Phys Ther 1990; 70:619–625.
18. Bloomfield SA, Jackson RD, Mysiw WJ, et al: Can functional

electrical stimulation cycle ergometry reverse disuse osteopenia in chronic spinal cord injury. Am Soc Bone Mineral Res 1990.

19. Boonstra AM, van Weerden TW, Eisma WH, et al: The effect of low-frequency electrical stimulation on denervation atrophy in man. Scand J Rehabil Med 1987; 19:127–134.

20. Bouletreau P, Patricot MC, Saudin F, et al: Effects of intermittent electrical stimulation on muscle metabolism in intensive care patients. J Parenteral Enteral Nutr 1987; 11:552–555.

21. Bowman BR, Baker LL: Effects of waveform parameters on comfort during transcutaneous neuromuscular electrical stimulation. Ann Biomed Eng 1985; 13:59–74.

22. Bradley MB: The effect of participating in a functional electrical stimulation exercise program on affect in people with spinal cord injuries. Arch Phys Med Rehabil 1994; 75:676–679.

23. Brenes G, Dearwater S, Shapera R, et al: High density lipoprotein cholesterol concentration in physically active and sedentary spinal cord injured patients. Arch Phys Med Rehabil 1986; 67:445–450.

24. Brighton CT, Pollack SR: Treatment of recalcitrant non-union with a capacitively coupled electrical field: A preliminary report. J Bone Joint Surg Am 1985; 67:577–585.

25. Brighton CT, McCluskey WP: Cellular response and mechanism of action of electrically-induced osteogenesis. Bone Mineral Res 1986; 4:213–254.

26. Brown MC, Holland RL: A central role for denervated tissues in causing nerve sprouting. Nature 1979; 282:724–726.

27. Brown MD, Cotter MA, Hudlicka O, Vrbova G: The effects of different patterns of muscle activity on capillary density, mechanical properties and structure of slow and fast rabbit muscles. Pfluegers Arch 1976; 361:241–250.

28. Brown WE, Salmons S, Whalen RG: The sequential replacement of myosin subunit isoforms during muscle type transformation induced by longterm electrical stimulation. J Biol Chem 1983; 258:14686–14692.

29. Brownson C, Isenberg H, Brown W, et al: Changes in skeletal muscle gene transcription induced by chronic stimulation. Muscle Nerve 1988; 11:1183–1189.

30. Brubaker L, Kotarinos R: Kegel or cut? Variations on his theme (review). J Reprod Med 1993; 38:672–678.

31. Buchegger A, Nemeth PM, Pette D, Reichmann H: Effects of chronic stimulation on the metabolic heterogeneity of the fibre population in rabbit tibialis anterior muscle. J Physiol 1984; 350:109–119.

32. Burke RE, Levine DN, Tsairis P, Zajac FE: Physiological types and histochemical profiles of motor units of the cat gastrocnemius. J Physiol 1973; 234:723–748.

33. Bushnell MC, Marchand F, Tremblay N, Duncan GH: Electrical stimulation of peripheral and central pathways for the relief of musculoskeletal pain. Can J Physiol Pharmacol 1991; 69:697–703.

34. Cabric M, Appell HJ: Effect of electrical stimulation of high and low frequency on maximum isometric force and some morphological characteristics in man. Int J Sports Med 1987; 8:256–260.

35. Cabric M, Appell HJ, Resic A: Effects of electrical stimulation of different frequencies on the myonuclei and fiber size in human muscle. Int J Sports Med 1987; 8:323–326.

36. Cabric M, Appell HJ, Resic A: Fine structural changes in electrostimulated human skeletal muscle: Evidence for predominant effects on fast muscle fibers. Eur J Appl Physiol 1988; 57:1–5.

37. Cabric M, Appell HJ, Resic A: Stereological analysis of capillaries in electrostimulated human muscles. Int J Sports Med 1987; 8:327–330.

38. Caggiano E, Emrey T, Shirley S, Craik RL: Effects of electrical stimulation or voluntary contraction for strengthening quadriceps femoris muscles in an aged male population. J Orthop Sports Phys Ther 1994; 20:22–28.

39. Campbell J: Efficacy of volitional versus electrically evoked knee extension exercise. In Proceedings of the RESNA 10th Annual Conference. San Jose, Calif, June 19-23, 1987, pp 648–650.

40. Caputo RM, Benson JT, McClellan E: Intravaginal maximal electrical stimulation in the treatment of urinary incontinence. J Reprod Med 1993; 38:667–671.

41. Cheng RSF, Pomeranz B: Electroacupuncture analgesia could be mediated by at least two pain relieving mechanisms: Endorphin and non-endorphin systems. Life Sci 1979; 25:1957–1962.

42. Clausen JP: Circulatory adjustments to dynamic exercise and effect of physical training in normal subjects and in patients with coronary artery disease. Prog Cardiovasc Dis 1976; 18:459–495.

43. Clement-Jones V, McLoughlin L, Tomlin S, et al: Increased beta-endorphin but not met-enkephalin levels in human cerebrospinal fluid after acupuncture for recurrent pain. Lancet 1980; 2:946–948.

44. Clinkingbeard JR, Gersten JW, Hoehn D: Energy cost of ambulation in traumatic paraplegia. Am J Phys Med 1964; 43:157–165.

45. Cole BG, Gardiner PF: Does electrical stimulation of denervated muscle, continued after reinnervation, influence recovery of contractile function? Exp Neurol 1984; 85:52–62.

46. Connolly JE: Electrical treatment of non-unions: Its use and abuse in 100 consecutive fractures. Orthop Clin North Am 1984; 15:89–106.

47. Connolly JF: Selection, evaluation and indications for electrical stimulation of ununited fractures. Clin Orthop Rel Res 1981; 161:39–53.

48. Cooper MS, Schliwa M: Electrical and ionic controls of tissue cell locomotion in DC electric fields. J Neurosci Res 1985; 13:223–244.

49. Cresey GH: Electrical stimulation of sacral roots for micturition after spinal cord injury. Urol Clin North Am 1993; 20:505–515.

50. Crowell LL, Squires WG, Raven PB: Benefits of aerobic exercise for paraplegics: A brief review. Med Sci Sports Exerc 1982; 18:501–508.

51. Cruz NI, Bayron FE, Suarez AJ: Accelerated healing of full thickness burns by the use of high-voltage pulsed galvanic stimulation in the pig. Ann Plast Surg 1989; 23:49–55.

52. Currier DP, Lehman J, Lightfoot P: Electrical stimulation in exercise of the quadriceps femoris muscle. Phys Ther 1979; 59:1508–1512.

53. Currier DP, Mann R: Muscular strength development by electrical stimulation in normal individuals. Phys Ther 1983; 63:915–921.

54. Dangain J, Vrbova G: Effect of chronic electrical stimulation at low frequency on the passive membrane properties of muscle fiber from dystrophic mice. Exp Neurol 1983; 79:630–640.

55. Deyo RA, Walsh ME, Martin BC, et al: A controlled trial of transcutaneous electrical nerve stimulation (TENS) and exercise for chronic low back pain. N Engl J Med 1990; 322:1627–1634.

56. DeHaas WG, Watson J, Morrison DM: Non-invasive treatment of ununited fractures of the tibia using electrical stimulation. J Bone Joint Surg Br 1980; 62:465–470.

57. Delitto A, Rose SJ, McKowen JM, et al: Electrical stimulation versus voluntary exercise in strengthening thigh musculature after anterior cruciate ligament surgery. Phys Ther 1988; 68:660–663.

58. DeVahl J: NMES and rehabilitation. In Gersh M (ed): Electrotherapy in Rehabilitation. Philadelphia, FA Davis, 1992, pp 244–245.

59. Duchateau J, Hainaut K: Training effects of sub-maximal electrostimulation in a human muscle. Med Sci Sports Exerc 1988; 20:99–104.

60. Dunn PA, Rogers D, Halford K: Transcutaneous electrical nerve stimulation at acupuncture points in the induction of uterine contractions. Obstet Gynecol 1989; 73:286–290.

61. Durham JW, Moskowitz A, Whitney J: Surface electrical stimulation versus brace in treatment of idiopathic scoliosis. Spine 1990; 15:888–892.

62. Edstrom L, Grimby L: Effect of exercise on the motor unit. Muscle Nerve 1986; 9:104–126.

63. Edwards BG, Marsolais EB: Metabolic responses to arm ergometry and functional neuromuscular stimulation. J Rehabil Res Dev 1990; 27:107–113.

64. Eisenberg BR, Salmons S: The reorganization of subcellular structure in muscle undergoing fast-to-slow type transformation: A stereological study. Cell Tissue Res 1981; 220:449–471.

65. Ellenberg M, MacRitchie M, Franklin B, et al: Aerobic capacity in early paraplegia: Implications for rehabilitation. Paraplegia 1989; 27:261–268.

66. Emes CG: Fitness and the physically disabled. A review. Can J Appl Sport Sci 1981; 6:176–178.

67. Etgen GJ Jr, Farrar RP, Ivy JL: Effect of chronic electrical stimulation on GLUT-4 protein content in fast-twitch muscle. Am J Physiol 1993; 264:r816–819.

68. Faghri PD, Rodgers MN, Glaser RM, et al: The effects of functional electrical stimulation on shoulder subluxation, arm function recovery, and shoulder pain in hemiplegic stroke patients. Arch Phys Med Rehabil 1994; 75:73–79.

69. Fakhri O, Amin M: The effect of low-voltage electric therapy on the healing of resistant skin burns. J Burn Care Rehabil 1987; 8:15–18.

70. Falanga V, Bourguignon GJ, Bourguignon LY: Electrical stimulation increases the expression of fibroblast receptors for transforming growth factor-beta. J Invest Dermatol 1987; 88:488.

71. Fall M, Lindstrom S: Electrical stimulation: A physiologic approach to the treatment of urinary incontinence. Urol Clin North Am 1991; 18:393–407.

72. Fisher DA, Rapp GF, Emkes M: Idiopathic scoliosis: Transcutaneous muscle stimulation versus the Milwaukee brace. Spine 1987; 12:987–991.

73. Flanagin A: JAMA 100 years ago: A plea for static electricity (editorial). JAMA 1992; 267:1068.

74. Fukada E, Yasuda I: On the piezoelectric effect of bone. Physiol Soc Jpn 1957; 12:1158–1162.

75. Gault WR, Gatens PF: Use of low intensity direct current in management of ischemic skin ulcers. Phys Ther 1976; 56:265–269.

76. Gentzkow GD, Miller KH: Electrical stimulation for dermal wound healing. Clin Podiatr Med Surg 1991; 8:827–841.

77. Gentzkow GD: Electrical stimulation to heal dermal wounds. J Dermatol Surg Oncol 1993; 19:753–758.

78. Gentzkow GD, Pollick SV, Kloth LC, Stubbs HA: Improved healing of pressure ulcers using dermapulse, a new electrical stimulation device. Wound 1991; 3:158–170.

79. Gibson JN, Smith K, Rennie MJ: Prevention of disuse muscle atrophy by means of electrical stimulation: Maintenance of protein synthesis. Lancet 1988; 2(8614):767–769.

80. Gieck JH, Saliba EN: Application of modalities in overuse syndromes. Clin Sports Med 1987; 6:423–486.

81. Girlanda PR, Dattola R, Vita G, et al: Effect of electrotherapy on denervated muscles in rabbits: An electrophysiological and morphological study. Exp Neurol 1982; 77:483–491.

82. Glenn WW, Hogan JF, Loke JS, et al: Ventilatory support by pacing of the conditioned diaphragm in quadriplegia. N Engl J Med 1984; 310:1150–1155.

83. Goldspink G, Scutt A, Loughna PT, et al: Gene expression in skeletal muscle in response stretch and force generation. Am J Physiol 1992; 262:r356–363.

84. Greve JMD, Muszkat PT, Schmidt B, et al: Functional electrical stimulation (FES): Muscle histochemical analysis. Paraplegia 1993; 31:764–770.

85. Griffin JW, Tooms RE, Mendius RA, et al: Efficacy of high voltage pulsed current for healing of pressure ulcers in patients with spinal cord injury. Phys Ther 1991; 71:433–442.

86. Grimby G, Nordwall A, Hulten B, Henriksson KG: Changes in histochemical profile of muscle after long-term electrical stimulation in patients with idiopathic scoliosis. Scand J Rehab Med 1985; 17:191–196.

87. Grimby G, Wigerstad-Lossing I: Comparison of high- and low-frequency muscle stimulators. Arch Phys Med Rehabil 1989; 70:835–838.

88. Gutmann E, Gutmann L: Effects of electrotherapy on denervated and reinnervated muscles in rabbit. Lancet 1942; 1:169–170.

89. Halbach JW, Straus D: Comparison of electro-myostimulation to isokinetic power of the knee extensor mechanism. J Orthop Sports Phys Ther 1980; 2:20–24.

90. Han JS, Chen XY, Sun SL, et al: The effect of low- and high-frequency TENS on Met-enkephalin-Arg-Phe and dynorphin A immunoreactivity in human lumbar CSF. Pain 1991; 47:295–298.

91. Hart RL, Kilgore KL: A lock detection algorithm for shoulder control of a hand grasp neuroprosthesis. In Neural Prostheses: Motor Systems IV. Engineering Foundation Conferences. New York, July 23-28, 1994.

92. Harvey JR, Bradley MB: Staff perceptions of the psychological benefits of FES training: A grounded therapy approach. SCI Psychosoc Process 1992; 5:8.

93. Haug J, Wood LT: Efficacy of neuromusclar stimulation of the quadriceps femoris during continuous passive motion following total knee arthroplasty. Arch Phys Med Rehabil 1988; 69:423–424.

94. Heilig A, Pette D: Changes induced in the enzyme activity pattern by electrical stimulation of fast twitch muscle. In Pette D (ed): Plasticity of Muscle. Berlin, Walter de Gruyter, 1980, pp 409–420.

95. Heilmann C, Pette D: Molecular transformations in sarcoplasmic reticulum of fast-twitch muscle by electro-stimulation. Eur J Biochem 1979; 93:437–446.

96. Heilmann C, Muller W, Pette D: Correlation between ultrastructural and functional changes in sarcoplasmic reticulum during chronic stimulation of fast muscle. J Membr Biol 1981; 59:143–149.

97. Henneman E, Somjen G, Carpenter DO: Functional significance of cell size in spinal motoneurons. J Neurophysiol 1965; 28:560–580.

98. Henneman E, Somjen G, Carpenter DO: Excitability and inhibitability of motoneurons of different sizes. J Neurophysiol 1965; 28:599–620.

99. Herbison GJ, Jaweed MM, Ditunno JF Jr: Exercise therapies in peripheral neuropathies. Arch Phys Med Rehabil 1983; 64:201–205.

100. Hirokawa S, Grimm M, Le T, et al: Energy consumption in paraplegic ambulation using the reciprocating gait orthosis and electric stimulation of the thigh muscles. Arch Phys Med Rehabil 1990; 71:687–694.

101. Hjeltnes N, Lannem A: Functional neuromuscular stimulation in four patients with complete paraplegia. Paraplegia 1990; 28:235–243.

102. Hjeltnes N, Vokac Z: Circulatory strain in everyday life of paraplegics. Scand J Rehabil Med 1979; 11:67–73.

103. Hoffman MD: Cardiorespiratory fitness and training in quadriplegics and paraplegics. Sports Med 1986; 3:312–330.

104. Hooker SP, Figoni SF, Glaser RM, et al: Physiologic responses to prolonged electrically stimulated leg-cycle exercise in the spinal cord injured. Arch Phys Med Rehabil 1990; 71:863–869.

105. Howson DC: Peripheral neural excitability: Implications for transcutaneous electrical nerve stimulation. Phys Ther 1978; 58:1467–1473.

106. Hudecki MS, Caffiero AT, Gregorio CC, Pollina CM: Effects of percutaneous electrical stimulation on functional ability, plasma creatine kinase, and pectoralis musculature of normal and genetically dystrophic chickens. Exp Neurol 1985; 90:53–72.

107. Hudlicka O, Aitman T, Heilig A, et al: Effects of different patterns of long-term stimulation on blood flow, fuel uptake and enzyme activities in rabbit fast skeletal muscles. Pfluegers Arch 1984; 402:306–311.

108. Hudlicka O, Brown M, Cotter M, et al: The effect of long-term stimulation of fast-muscles on their blood flow, metabolism and ability to withstand fatigue. Pfluegers Arch 1977; 369:141–149.

109. Hudlicka O, Dodd L, Renkin EM, Gray SD: Early changes in fibre profile and capillary density in long-term stimulated muscles. Am J Physiol 1982; 243:h528–535.

110. Hudlicka O, Tyler KR, Srihari T, et al: The effect of different patterns of long-term stimulation on contractile properties and myosin light chains in rabbit fast muscles. Pfluegers Arch 1982; 393:164–170.

111. Im MJ, Lee WP, Hoopes JE: Effect of electrical stimulation on survival of skin flaps in pigs. Phys Ther 1990; 70:37–40.

112. Jackson S: Role of galvanism in treatment of denervated voluntary muscle in man. Brain 1945; 68:300–330.

113. Johnson EW, Braddom R: Over-work weakness in fascioscapulohumeral muscular dystrophy. Arch Phys Med Rehabil 1971; 52:333–336.

114. Johnson MI, Ashton CH, Thompson JW: The consistency of pulsed frequencies and pulse patterns of transcutaneous nerve stimulation (TENS) used by chronic pain patients. Pain 1991; 44:231–234.

115. Jonasson I, Larsson B, Pschera H, Nylund L: Short-term maximal electrical stimulation–a conservative treatment of urinary incontinence. Gynecol Obstet Invest 1990; 30:120–123.

116. Jones DA, Bigland-Ritchie B, Edwards RH: Excitation frequency and muscle fatigue: Mechanical responses during voluntary and stimulated contractions. Exp Neurol 1979; 64:401–413.

117. Kahanovitz N, Nordin M, Verderame R, et al: Normal trunk muscle strength and endurance in women and the effect of exercises and electrical stimulation. 2: Comparative analysis of electrical stimulation and exercises to increase trunk muscle strength and endurance. Spine 1987; 12:112–118.

118. Kantrowitz A: Electronic Physiologic Aids. Brooklyn, NY, Maimonides Hospital, 1960, pp 4–5.

119. Katz RT, Green D, Sullivan T, Yarkony G: Functional electrical stimulation to enhance systemic fibrinolytic activity in spinal cord injury patients. Arch Phys Med Rehabil 1987; 68:423–426.

120. Keith MW, Peckham CH, Thrope GB, et al: Functional neuromuscular stimulation neuroprostheses for the tetraplegic hand. Clin Orthop Rel Res 1988; 233:25–33.

121. Kennedy WF, Roberts CG, Zuege RC, Dicus WT: Use of pulsed electromagnetic fields in treatment of loosened cemented hip prosthesis: A double-blind trial. Clin Orthop Rel Res 1993; 286:198–205.

122. Kho HG, Eijk RJ, Kapteijns WMMJ, van Egmond J: Acupuncture and transcutaneous stimulation analgesia in comparison with moderate dose fentanyl anaesthesia in major surgery: Clinical efficacy and influence on recovery and morbidity. Anaesthesia 1991; 46:129–135.

123. Kincaid CB, Lavoie KH: Inhibition of bacterial growth in vitro following stimulation with high voltage, monophasic, pulsed current. Phys Ther 1989; 69:651–655.

124. Kirsch RF: A technique for synthesizing multi-joint arm movement using functional neuromuscular stimulation based on end point limb mechanics. In Neural Prostheses: Motor Systems IV. Engineering Foundation Conferences, New York, July 23-28, 1994.

125. Kjartansson J, Lundeberg T: Effects of electrical nerve stimulation (ENS) in ischemic tissue. Scand J Plast Reconstr Hand Surg 1990; 24:129–134.

126. Kloth LC, Feedar JA: Acceleration of wound healing with high voltage, monophasic, pulsed current. Phys Ther 1988; 68:503–508.

127. Klug G, Wiehrer W, Reichmann H, et al: Relationships between early alterations in parvalbumins, sarcoplasmic reticulum and metabolic enzymes in chronically stimulated fast twitch muscle. Pfluegers Arch 1983; 399:280–284.

128. Knaflitz M, Merletti R, Deluca CJ: Inference of motor unit recruitment order in voluntary and electrically elicited contraction. J Appl Physiol 1990; 68:1657–1667.

129. Kraft GH, Fitts SS, Hammond MC: Techniques to improve function of the arm and hand in chronic hemiplegia. Arch Phys Med Rehabil 1992; 73:220–227.

130. Kralj AR, Bajd P, Munih M, Turk R: FES gait restoration and balance control in spinal cord injured patients. Prog Brain Res 1993; 97:387–396.

131. Kralj A, Bajd T, Turk R: Enhancement of gait restoration in spinal injured patients by functional electrical stimulation. Clin Orthop Rel Res 1988; 233:34–43.

132. Kramer JF, Semple JE: Comparison of selected strengthening techniques for normal quadriceps. Physiol Ther Can 1983; 35:300–304.

133. Krauss JC, Robergs RA, Depaepe JL, et al: Effects of electrical stimulation and upper body training after spinal cord injury. Med Sci Sports Exerc 1993; 25:1054–1061.

134. Krusen FH: Physical medicine: The employment of physical agents for diagnosis and therapy. In Krusen FH (ed): History of Physical Therapy. Philadelphia, WB Saunders, 1941, pp 9–41.

135. Kubiak RJ, Whitman KM, Johnston RM: Changes in quadriceps femoris muscle strength using isometric exercise versus electrical stimulation. J Orthop Sports Phys Ther 1987; 8:537–541.

136. Lake DA: Neuromuscular electrical stimulation: An overview and its application in the treatment of sports injuries. Sports Med 1992; 13:320–336.

137. Laskin JJ, Ashley EA, Olenik LM, et al: Electrical stimulation-assisted rowing exercise in spinal cord injured people: A pilot study. Paraplegia 1993; 31:534–541.

138. Latash ML, Yee MJ, Orpett C, et al: Combining electrical muscle stimulation with voluntary contraction for studying muscle fatigue. Arch Phys Med Rehabil 1994; 75:29–35.

139. Laughman RK, Youdas JW, Garrett TR, Chao EY: Strength changes in the normal quadriceps femoris muscle as a result of electrical stimulation. Phys Ther 1983; 63:494–499.

140. Lawrence JC Jr, Krsek JA, Salsgiver WJ, et al: Phosphorylase kinase isozymes in normal and electrically stimulated skeletal muscles. Am J Physiol 1986; 250:c84–89.

141. Leandri M, Parodi CI, Corrieri N, Rigardo F: Comparison of TENS treatments in hemiplegic shoulder pain. Scand J Rehab Med 1990; 22:69–71.

142. Leeds EM, Klose KJ, Ganez W, et al: Bone mineral density after bicycle ergometry training. Arch Phys Med Rehabil 1990; 71:207–209.

143. Levin MF, Hui-Chan CWY: Relief of hemiparetic spasticity by TENS is associated with improvement in reflex and voluntary motor functions. Electroencephalogr Clin Neurophysiol 1992; 85:131–142.

144. Levine SP, Kett RL, Cederna PS, Books SV: Electric muscle stimulation for pressure sore prevention: Tissue shape variation. Arch Phys Med Rehabil 1990; 67:108–116.

145. Liberson WT, Holmquest HJ, Scot D, et al: Functional electrotherapy: Stimulation of the peroneal nerve synchronized with the swing phase of gait of hemiplegic patients. Arch Phys Med Rehabil 1961; 42:101–105.

146. Lewis SM, Clelland JA, Knowles CJ, et al: Effects of auricular acupuncture like transcutaneous electrical nerve stimulation on pain levels following wound care in patients with burns: A pilot study. J Burn Care Rehabil 1990; 11:322–329.

147. Lomo T, Westgaard RH, Dahl HA: Contractile properties of muscle:

148. Lomo T, Westgaard RH, Engebretsen L: Different stimulation patterns affect contractile properties of denervated rat saveus muscles. In Pette D (ed): Plasticity of Muscle. Berlin, Walter de Gruyter, 1980, pp 297–309.

149. Long DM: Fifteen years of transcutaneous electrical stimulation for pain control. Stereotact Funct Neurosurg 1991; 56:2–19.

150. Lundeberg TCM, Eriksson SV, Malm M: Electrical nerve stimulation improves healing of diabetic ulcers. Ann Plast Surg 1992; 29:328–331.

151. Luthert P, Vrbovà G, Ward KM: Effects of slow frequency electrical stimulation on muscles of dystrophic mice. J Neurol Neurosurg Psychiatry 1980; 43:803–809.

152. Mabuchi K, Szvctko D, Pinter K, Sreter FA: Type IIB to IIA fiber transformation in intermittently stimulated rabbit muscles. Am J Physiol 1982; 242:c373–381.

153. Marchand S, Charest J, Li J, et al: Is TENS purely a placebo effect? A controlled study on chronic low back pain. Pain 1993; 54:99–106.

154. Marsolais EB: FES ambulatory assist. In Neural Prosthesis: Motor Systems IV. Engineering Foundation Conferences. New York, July 23-28, 1994.

155. Marsolais EB, Edwards BG: Energy costs of walking and standing with functional neuromuscular stimulation and long leg braces. Arch Phys Med Rehabil 1988; 69:243–249

156. Marsolais EB, Kobetic R, Barnicle K, Jacobs J: FNS application for restoring function in stroke and head injury patients. J Clin Eng 1990; 15:489–496.

157. Martin TP, Stein RB, Hoeppner PH, Reid DC: Influence of electrical stimulation or the morphological and metabolic properties of paralyzed muscle. J Appl 1992; 72:1401–1406.

158. McDonagh JC, Binder MD, Reinking RM, Stuart DG: Tetrapartite classification of motor units of cat tibialis posterior. J Neurophysiol 1980; 44:696–712.

159. Melzack R, Wall PD: Pain mechanism: A new theory. Science 1965; 150:171–179.

160. Merli GJ, Herbison GJ, Ditunno JF, et al: Deep vein thrombosis: Prophylaxis in acute spinal cord injured patients. Arch Phys Med Rehabil 1988; 69:661–664.

161. Milner-Brown HS, Miller RG: Muscle strengthening through electrical stimulation combined with low-resistance weights in patients with neuromuscular disorders. Arch Phys Med Rehabil 1988; 69:20–24.

162. Milner-Brown HS, Stein RB, Yemm R: The orderly recruitment of human motor units during voluntary isometric contraction. J Physiol 1973; 230:359–370.

163. Milner-Brown HS, Stein RB, Yemm R: The contractile properties of human motor units during voluntary isometric contractions. J Physiol 1973; 228:285–306.

164. Mokrusch T, Engelhardt A, Eichorn KF, et al: Effects of long-impulse electrical stimulation on atrophy and fibre type composition of chronically denervated fast rabbit muscle. J Neurol 1990; 237:29–34.

165. Monster AW, Chan H: Isometric force production by motor units of extensor digitorum communis muscle in man. J Neurophysiol 1977; 40:1432–1443.

166. Morrissey MC, Brewster CE, Shields CL Jr, Brown M: The effects of electrical stimulation on the quadriceps during postoperative knee immobilization. Am J Sports Med 1985; 13:40–45.

167. Mortiemer JT: Extra neural neuromuscular stimulating electrodes. In Neuroprosthesis: Motor Systems IV. Engineering Foundation Conferences. New York, July 23-28, 1994.

168. Mullett K: State-of-the-art in neurostimulation. PACE 1987; 10:162–175.

169. Munsat TL, McNeal D, Waters R: Effects of nerve stimulation on human muscle. Arch Neurol 1976; 33:608–617.

170. Myklebust BM, Kloth L: Electrodiagnostic and electrotherapeutic instrumentation: Characteristics of recording and stimulation systems and principles of safety. In Gersh MR (ed): Electrotherapy in Rehabilitation. Philadelphia, FA Davis, 1992, pp 51–100.

171. Mysiw WJ, Jackson RD: Hypercalciuria permitted by functional electrical stimulation (abstract). Arch Phys Med Rehabil 1990; 71:795.

172. Nash MS, Bilsker S, Marcillo AE, et al: Reversal of adaptive left ventricular atrophy following electrically-stimulated exercise training in human tetraplegics. Paraplegia 1991; 29:590–599.

Control by pattern of muscle activity in the rat. Proc R Soc Lond Biol 1974; 187:99–103.

173. Nemeth PM: Electrical stimulation of denervated muscle prevents decreases in oxidative enzymes. Muscle Nerve 1982; 5:134–139.

174. Nene AV, Patrick JH: Energy cost of paraplegic locomotion using the ParaWalker electrical stimulation "hybrid" orthosis. Arch Phys Med Rehabil 1990; 71:116–120.

175. Nix W: Effect of electrical stimulation on denervated muscle. In Nix WA, Vrbova G (eds): Electrical Stimulation and Neuro-disorders. Berlin, Springer, 1986, pp 115–124.

176. Nix WA: The effect of low-frequency electrical stimulation on the denervated extensor digitorum longus muscle of the rabbit. Acta Neurol Scand 1982; 66:521–528.

177. Nochomovitz ML, Peterson BK, Stellato TA: Electrical activation of the diaphragm. Clin Chest Med 1988; 9:349–358.

178. Noland MF: Selected problems in the use of transcutaneous nerve stimulation for pain control—an appraisal with proposed solutions. A special communication. Phys Ther 1988; 68:1694–1698.

179. Okuma H, Ogata H, Hatada K: Transition of physical fitness in wheelchair marathon competitors over several years. Paraplegia 1989; 27:237–243.

180. Osman SG, Marsolais EB: Endoscopic implantation of cuff electrodes on the hamstring branches of the sciatic nerve in paralyzed subjects. In Neuroprothesis: Motor Systems IV. Engineering Foundation Conferences. New York, July 23-28, 1994.

181. Osterman AL, Bora FW Jr: Electrical stimulation applied to bone and nerve injuries in the upper extremity. Orthop Clin North Am 1986; 17:353–364.

182. Pachter B, Eberstein A, Goodgold J: Electrical stimulation effect on denervated skeletal myofibers in rats: A light and electron microscopic study. Arch Phys Med Rehabil 1982; 63:427–430.

183. Packman-Braun R: Relationship between functional electrical stimulation duty cycle and fatigue in wrist extensor muscles of patients with hemiparesis. Phys Ther 1988; 68:51–56.

184. Pacy PJ, Hesp R, Halliday DA, et al: Muscle and bone in paraplegic patients, and the effect of functional electrical stimulation. Clin Sci 1988; 75:481–487.

185. Peckham PH, Keith MW, Freehafer AA: Restoration of functional control by electrical stimulation in the upper extremity of the quadriplegic patient. J Bone Joint Surg Am 1988; 70:144–148.

186. Pentland B: Quadriplegia and cardiorespiratory fitness. Lancet 1993; 341:413–414.

187. Perkash I, Martin DE, Warner H, Speck V: Electroejaculation in spinal cord injury patients: Simplified new equipment and technqiue. J Urol 1990; 143:305–307.

188. Petrofsky JS: Sequential motor unit stimulation through peripheral motor nerves in the cat. Med Biol Eng Comput 1979; 17:87–93.

189. Petrofsky JS, Phillips CA: The use of functional electrical stimulation for rehabilitation of spinal cord injured patients. Cent Nerv Syst Trauma 1984; 1:57–74.

190. Petrofsky JS, Phillips CA, Heaton HH, Glaser RM: Bicycle ergometer for paralyzed muscle. J Clin Eng 1984; 9:13–19.

191. Petrofsky JS, Smith JB: Physiologic costs of computer-controlled walking in persons with paraplegia using a reciprocating gait orthosis. Arch Phys Med Rehabil 1991; 72:890–896.

192. Petrofsky JS, Phillips CA, Stafford DE: Closed loop control for restoration of movement in paralyzed muscle. Orthopedics 1984; 7:1289–1302.

193. Petrofsky JS, Stacy R: The effect of training on endurance and the cardiovascular responses of individuals with paraplegia during dynamic exercise induced by functional electrical stimulation. Eur J Appl Physiol 1992; 64:487–492.

194. Pette D: Activity-induced fast to slow-transition in mammalian muscle. Med Sci Sports Exerc 1984; 16:517–528.

195. Pette D, Müller W, Leisner E, Vrbova G: Time dependent effects on contractile properties, fibre population, myosin light chains and enzymes of energy metabolism in intermittently and continuously stimulated fast twitch muscle of the rabbit. Pfluegers Arch 1976; 364:103–112.

196. Pette D, Ramirez BU, Müller W, et al: Influence of intermittent long-term stimulation on contractile, histochemical and metabolic properties of fibre populations in fast and slow rabbit muscles. Pfluegers Arch 1975; 361:1–7.

197. Pette D, Schnez U: Coexistence of fast and slow type myosin light chains in single muscle fibres during transformation as induced by long-term stimulation. FEBS Lett 1977; 83:128–130.

198. Pette D, Smith ME, Staudte HW, Vrbova G: Effects of long-term electrical stimulation on some contractile and metabolic characteristics of fast rabbit muscles. Pfluegers Arch 1973; 338:257–272.

199. Pette D, Staudte HW, Vrbova G: Physiological and biochemical changes induced by long-term stimulation of fast muscle. Naturwissenschaften 1972; 59:469–470.

200. Pette D, Tyler KR: Response of succinate dehydrogenase activity in fibres of rabbit tibialis anterior muscle to chronic nerve stimulation. J Physiol 1983; 338:1–9.

201. Phillips CA, Petrosky JS, Hendershot DM, Stafford D: Functional electrical exercise: Comprehensive approach for physical conditioning of spinal cord injured patients. Orthopedics 1984; 7:1112–1123.

202. Polando G, Schiner A, Marsolais EB: Reliability of lower extremity FES systems: Analysis of a current laboratory system. In Neuroprosthesis: Motor Systems IV. Engineering Foundation Conferences. New York, July 23-28, 1994.

203. Pollack SF, Axen K, Spielholtz N, et al: Aerobic training effects of electrically-induced lower extremity exercises in spinal cord injured people. Arch Phys Med Rehabil 1989; 70:214–219.

204. Popovic DB: Finite state model of locomotion for functional electrical stimulation systems. Prog Brain Res 1993; 97:397–407.

205. Ragnarsson KT: Physiologic effects of functional electrical stimulation-induced exercises in spinal cord injured individuals. Clin Orthop Rel Res 1988; 233:53–63.

206. Ragnarsson KT, Pollack SF, O'Daniel W, et al: Clinical evaluation of computerized functional electrical stimulation after spinal cord injury: A multicenter pilot study. Arch Phys Med Rehabil 1988; 69:672–677.

207. Ragnarsson KT, Sell G: Lower extremity fractures after spinal cord injury: A retrospective study. Arch Phys Med Rehabil 1981; 62:418–423.

208. Ramirez BU, Pette D: Effect of long-term electrical stimulation on sarcoplasmic reticulium of fast rabbit muscle. FEBS Lett 1974; 49:188–198.

209. Rasmussen MJ, Hayes DL, Vlietstra RE, Thorsteinsson G: Can transcutaneous electrical nerve stimulation be safely used in patients with permanent cardiac pacemakers? Mayo Clin Proc 1988; 63:443–445.

210. Reich JD, Tarjan PP: Electrical stimulation of skin. Int J Derm 1990; 29:395–400.

211. Reichmann H, Hoppeler H, Mathieu-Costello O, et al: Biochemical and ultrastructural changes of skeletal muscle mitochondria after chronic electrical stimulation in rabbits. Pfluegers Arch 1985; 404:1–9.

212. Reichmann H, Pette D, Vrbova G: Effects of low frequency electrical stimulation on enzyme and isozyme patterns of dystrophic mouse muscle. FEBS Lett 1981; 128:55–58.

213. Rieb L, Pomeranz B: Alterations in electrical pain thresholds by use of acupuncture-like transcutaneous electrical nerve stimulation in pain free subject. Phys Ther 1992; 72:658–667.

214. Riso RR, Gorman PH: Viability of the cutaneous innervation of the fingers in C5 and C6 level quadriplegic subjects studied using evoked sensory nerve action potentials. In Neuroprosthesis: Motor Systems IV. Engineering Foundation Conferences. New York, July 23-28, 1994.

215. Robinson LR, Mustovic EH, Lieber PS, et al: A technique for quantifying and determining the site of isometric muscle fatigue in the clinical setting. Arch Phys Med Rehabil 1990; 71:901–904.

216. Robinson CJ, Kett NA, Bolam JM: Spasticity in spinal cord injured patients: 1. Short-term effects of surface electrical stimulation. Arch Phys Med Rehabil 1988; 69:598–604.

217. Robinson CJ, Kett NA, Bolam JM: Spasticity in spinal cord injured patients: 2. Initial measures and long-term effects of basic electrical stimulation. Arch Phys Med Rehabil 1988; 69:862–888.

218. Roy RK, Mabuchi K, Sarkar S, et al: Changes in tropomyosin subunit pattern in chronic electrically stimulated rabbit fast muscles. Biochem Biophys Res Commun 1979; 89:181–187.

219. Rubinstein N, Mabuchi K, Pepe F, et al: Use of type-specific antimyosins to demonstrate the transformation of individual fibers in chronically stimulated rabbit fast muscles. J Cell Biol 1978; 79:252–261.

220. Salmons S, Henriksson J: The adaptive response of skeletal muscle to increased use. Muscle Nerve 1981; 4:94–105.

221. Salmons S, Sreter FA: Significance of impulse activity in the transformation of skeletal muscle type. Nature 1976; 263:30–34.

222. Salmons S, Vrbova G: The influence of activity on some contractile characteristics of mammalian fast and slow muscles. J Physiol 1969; 210:535-549.

223. Sanderson JE: Electrical neurostimulators for pain relief and angina. Br Heart J 1990; 63:141–143.

224. Sarzala MG, Szymanska G, Wiehrer W, Pette D: Effects of chronic stimulation at low frequency on the lipid phase of sarcoplasmic reticulum in rabbit fast-twitch muscle. Eur J Biochem 1982; 123:241–245.

225. Scott OM, Hyde SA, Vrbova G, Dubowitz V: Therapeutic possibilities of chronic long-frequency electrical stimulation in children with Duchenne muscular dystrophy. J Neurol Sci 1990; 95:171–182.

226. Scott OM, Vrbova G, Hyde SA, Dubowitz V: Responses of muscles of patients with Duchenne muscular dystrophy to chronic electrical stimulation. J Neurol Neurosurg Psychiatry 1986; 49:1427–1434.

227. Scott PRD: Mild electric control of upper extremity neuroprostheses utilizing dual sternocleidomastoid muscles. *In* Neuroprosthesis: Motor Systems IV. Engineering Foundation Conferences. New York, July 23-28, 1994.

228. Seager SW, Halstead LS: Fertility options and success after spinal cord injury. Urol Clin North Am 1993; 20:543–548.

229. Sebrille A, Boudoux-Jahan M: Effects of electrical stimulation in previous nerve injury on motor function recovery in rats. Brain Res 1980; 193:560–565.

230. Seedorf K, Seedorf U, Pette D: Coordinate expression of alkali and DTNB myosin light chains during transformation of rabbit fast muscle by chronic stimulation. FEBS Lett 1983; 158:321–324.

231. Sigmedics: Parastep Update. Northfield, Ill, Sigmedics, 1994.

232. Sipski ML, Delisa JA, Schweer S: Functional electrical stimulation bicycle ergometry: Patient perceptions. Am J Phys Med Rehabil 1989; 68:147–149.

233. Solomonow M: External control of the neuromuscular system. IEEE Trans Biomed Eng 1984; 31:752–763.

234. Sreter FA, Pinter K, Jolesz F, Mabuchi K: Fast to slow transformation of fast muscles in response to long-term phasic stimulation. Exp Neurol 1982; 75:95–102.

235. Sréter FA, Gergely J, Salmon S, Romanul FCA: Synthesis by fast muscle of myosin light chain characteristic of slow muscle in response to longterm stimulation. Nature 1973; 241:17–19.

236. Stefanovska A, Gros N, Vodovnik L, et al: Chronic electrical stimulation for the modification of spasticity in hemiplegic patients. Scand J Rehab Med 1988; 17(Suppl):115–121.

237. Stein GA, Anzel SH: A review of delayed unions of open tibia fractures treated with external fixation and pulsing electromagnetic fields. Orthopedics 1984; 7:428–436.

238. Stein RB: Methods for using feedback to control functional electrical stimulation. *In* Neuroprosthesis: Motor Systems IV. Engineering Foundation Conferences. New York, July 23-28, 1994.

239. Stein RB, Gordon T, Jefferson J, et al: Optimal stimulation of paralyzed muscle after human spinal cord injury. J Appl Physiol 1992; 72:1393–1400.

240. Sweeney JD: Selection criteria for neuromuscular stimulation electrodes. *In* Neuroprosthesis: Motor Systems IV. Engineering Foundation Conferences. New York, July 23-28, 1994.

241. Thomas I, Tyle V, Webster J, Neilson A: An evaluation of transcutaneous electrical nerve stimulation for pain relief in labour. Aust NZ J Obstet Gynecol 1988; 28:182–189.

242. Tulgar M, McGlone F, Bowsher D, Miles JB: Comparative effectiveness of different stimulation modes in relieving pain: II. A double blind controlled long-term clinical trial. Pain 1991; 47:157–162.

243. Twist DJ, Culpepper-Morgan JA, Ragnarsson KT, et al: Neuroendocrine changes during functional electrical stimulation. Am J Phys Med Rehabil 1992; 71:156–163.

244. Unger PG: A randomized clinical trial of the effect of HVPC on wound healing. Phys Ther 1991; 71:S118.

245. Unger PG, Rainastry S: A controlled study of the effect of high voltage pulse current (HVPC) on wound healing. Phys Ther 1991; 71:S119.

246. Vignos PJ, Watkins MP: The effect of exercise in muscular dystrophy. JAMA 1966; 197:843–848.

247. Vodovnik L, Karba R: Treatment of chronic wounds by means of electrical and electromagnetic fields: I. Literature review. Med Biol Eng Comput 1992; 30:257–266.

248. Vrbova G, Ward K: Observations on the effects of low frequency electrical stimulation on fast muscles of dystrophic mice. J Neurol Neurosurg Psychiatry 1981; 44:1002–1006.

249. Walsfley RP, Letts G, Booyf J: A comparison of torque generated by knee extension with a maximal voluntary muscle contraction: Vis-a-vis electrical stimulation. J Orthop Sports Phys Ther 1984; 6:10–17.

250. Weber RJ: Functional neuromuscular stimulation. *In* DeLisa JA, Gans BM (eds): Rehabilitation Medicine: Principles and Practice. Philadelphia, JB Lippincott, 1993, pp 463–476.

251. Wehrmacher WH, Thomson JD, Hines HM: Effects of electrical stimulation on denervated skeletal muscle. Arch Phys Med Rehabil 1945; 26:261–266.

252. Weiss DS, Eaglstein WH, Falanga V: Pulsed electrical stimulation decreases scar thickness at split thickness graft donor sites (abstract). J Invest Dermatol 1989; 92:3.

253. Wiehrer W, Pette D: The ratio between intrinsic 115 kDa and 30 kDa peptides as a marker of fibre type–specific sarcoplasmic reticulum in mammalian muscles. FEBS Lett 1983; 158:317–320.

254. Wigerstad-Lossing I, Grimby G, Jonsson T, et al: Effects of electrical stimulation combined with voluntary contractions after knee ligament surgery. Med Sci Sports Exerc 1988; 20:93–98.

255. Williams RS, Salmons S, Newsholme EA, et al: Regulation of nuclear and mitochondrial gene expression by contractile activity in skeletal muscle. J Biol Chem 1986; 261:376–380.

256. Winter GD: Movement of epidermal cells over the wound surface. Adv Biol Skin 1964; 5:113.

257. Wolcott LE, Wheeler PC, Hardwicke HM, Rowley BA: Accelerated healing of skin ulcers by electrotherapy: Preliminary clinical results. South Med J 1969; 62:795–801.

258. Wolf SL, Ariel GB, Saar D, et al: The effect of muscle stimulation during resistive training on performance parameters. Am J Sports Med 1986; 14:18–23.

259. Wong RA: High voltage versus low voltage electrical stimulation: Force of induced muscle contraction and perceived discomfort in healthy subjects. Phys Ther 1986; 66:1209–1214.

260. Zupan A, Gregoric M, Valencic V, Vandot S: Effects of electrical stimulation on muscles of children with Duchenne and Becker muscular dystrophy. Neuropediatrics 1993; 24:189–192.

261. Zwiren LD, Bar-Or O: Responses to exercise of paraplegics who differ in conditioning level. Med Sci Sports 1975; 7:94–98.

24

Computer Assistive Devices and Environmental Controls

**JAN C. GALVIN, B.A., AND
KEVIN M. CAVES, B.S.M.E.**

Computers have changed the way Americans think, work, and play. They have become a part of our everyday life as components in microwave ovens, ATM machines, remote control units, and children's games, and they are often present in our workstations. Even such a mundane item as an iron now might contain a computer microchip that tells it when to switch off.

For persons with disabilities, computers have opened up tremendous opportunities for independence, community integration, education, and employment. Children with disabilities are using computers in the classroom from preschool to postsecondary school, to play, communicate, and learn. Adults with disabilities are using computers in the workplace to access and disseminate information, design buildings, and teach. Older Americans use computerized environmental control systems in the home for both safety and security, to switch lights on and off, to open and close doors, and to call for help if needed.

A vast array of computer-related equipment is available to assist individuals with disabilities. Ten years ago an individual with quadriplegia and a law degree could not hope to work independently, let alone live independently. Now, through the use of an adapted computer, such an individual can research documents from every law library in the United States, write briefs, and, if the courtroom is wheelchair-accessible, vigorously defend his or her client. After winning the case, the lawyer can go home in an adapted van to a barrier-free, automated environment. An attendant might still be required to assist with bathing, grooming, and eating, but the individual is able to be a productive member of society through the assistance of computers and computer adaptations.

How can you find out what types of computer-related equipment are available? How can you determine the consumer's needs? How do you know if the different components interface with each other? Finally, who pays for computer-related technology? This chapter focuses on the different types of adapted computer technologies available and how to evaluate a patient's need for such equipment, and identifies the primary disability groups most likely to benefit from access to adapted computer technologies.

BACKGROUND

Computers are part of our everyday life. Even if you don't actually use a personal computer, the world surrounding you is full of computer chips. The telephone answering machine and the fax machine both use microchips. Televisions and VCRs also utilize computer technology. The computer revolution has led to medical imaging technology such as magnetic resonance imaging (MRI) and the use of miniature cameras for microsurgery. Computer-aided design has led to improved prosthetic devices, and virtual reality allows a surgeon to simulate an operation before entering the operating room.

It is difficult to imagine life without computers; however, the advent of personal computers took place in 1975 (the IBM PC was introduced in 1981 and the Apple Macintosh in 1984), and mainframe computers started a technology revolution in 1963. Mainframe computers can be the size of a room and cost millions of dollars. Notebook computers can weigh less than 4 lb and cost as little as $1000. As with the industrial revolution of the 19th century, computers are revolutionizing the way we think, act, learn, and earn a living. Although the continuing growth and sophistication of computers is enhancing opportunities for individuals with disabilities, the "downside" is that this revolution is also affecting the way industry does business: robots are being used in place of people on the production line, and jobs are being computerized so that fewer human workers are needed.

COMPUTERS AT SCHOOL, WORK, HOME, AND LEISURE

The growth in computer technology and the changing nature of commerce and industry has and will continue to provide opportunities for individuals with disabilities to be more independent at home, at work, and at play. A few examples of how adapted computers are being used are presented in the following text.

For an individual who is blind, a speech synthesizer allows the computer to speak aloud, a Braille printer translates printed text into Braille, and an optical scanner reads the printed word and speaks it aloud or transmits the text to storage for future retrieval. An individual who is visually impaired might use a magnification system that enlarges the text on the computer screen, making it easier to read.

The lawyer who is a quadriplegic uses a personal computer with a voice-recognition system to control programs including those for the word processor, data bases, spreadsheets, telecommunications, and other applications. Its extensive vocabulary and ability to learn new words enables the lawyer to speak to the computer as a sighted person would type words. Verbal commands are also recognized, such as "delete," "print," and "merge." The workstation consists of a raised-height desk so that the employee in a wheelchair can roll right up to the desk.

For deaf persons, the computer revolution and the upsurge in communications can be frustrating. They may have no problem accessing a regular computer, but they need audible communications to be made visual so they can see the spoken word. A person who is deaf can use a telephone device for the deaf (TDD), a relay service, or a fax machine to communicate.

Modems linked to personal computers allow a wider range of communication alternatives, such as electronic mail. Computer-aided transcription can provide instantaneous hard copy printouts of meetings. Software is available that teaches American sign language. Captioning translates the spoken word into text, making television programming and videotapes more accessible. Visual alarm systems provide a means to monitor the environment.

Assistive technology and adaptive computer technologies are not just used in special education classrooms, but also in the regular classroom. From preschool to college, the computer can be both a teaching tool and a way for individuals with disabilities to learn, communicate, and express themselves in a broad variety of ways. Technology is a tool that can be used to make the learning environment more accessible and enhance individual productivity. Computerized technology can facilitate access and interaction with teachers and peers. People can use it to manipulate their environment by controlling tape recorders and electrical appliances. Computers are helping students to prepare for future vocational settings, and children access computer-related technologies for play, recreation, and leisure. Adaptive controllers for video games allow the child to have fun on an equal footing with able-bodied peers.

Since 1992, a sizable increase has been seen in the number of devices and in software packages available to help children with reading, writing, and computational skills. Computers in school allow students to work at their own pace and to receive immediate feedback. Computers can help to motivate students and to compensate for their disabilities.

Trifiletti and co-workers[6] analyzed the effects of math drills and tutoring on the proficiency of a group of students with disabilities. They found that 40 min of computerized tutoring and math drills was more than twice as effective as an equivalent amount of teacher-delivered math instruction. Jones and colleagues[3] found that computer-based instruction in reading enabled students to increase their reading speed by 26%, vs. a 4% increase for students given teacher-based instruction.

For the home, software packages are available for entertainment, to track monthly budgets, to access information services, and to shop from home. Closed captioning and descriptive video programming have overcome the barriers to enjoying television for those with sensory impairments. Outside of the home, talking computerized credit card readers and paper money identifiers are available for individuals who are visually impaired.

TRENDS IN PREVALENCE OF ASSISTIVE TECHNOLOGY DEVICES

According to findings from the 1990 National Health Interview Survey (NHIS) on Assistive Devices, which was co-sponsored by the National Center for Health Statistics (NCHS) and the National Institute on Disability and Rehabilitation Research (NIDRR), more than 13.1 million Americans (about 5.3% of the population) were using assistive technology devices to accommodate physical impairments.[4] It is also estimated that 37.3 million noninstitutionalized persons aged 15 years and older living in the United States have a chronic health disability that limits their ability to participate fully in life. More than 70 chronic conditions are listed in the NHIS report, and each of these has the potential to cause one or more functional limitations that could be ameliorated by the use of appropriate assistive technology. In addition, a significant number of individuals are surviving catastrophic trauma and living with severe functional losses. More children are being born with learning disabilities resulting from in utero drug addiction or lack of prenatal care. These individuals can potentially benefit from the use of adaptive computer technologies.

The potential of technology to help individuals with disabilities to achieve maximum independent functioning is well recognized in rehabilitation. Several pieces of legislation, notably The Rehabilitation Act of 1973 (as amended), the Americans with Disabilities Act of 1990, the Individuals with Disabilities Education Act of 1990, and the Technology Related Assistance for Individuals with Disabilities Act of 1988, have placed significant emphasis on the use of assistive technology as part of the continuum of services. It is important to remember, however, that as technology is used to increase opportunities for individuals with disabilities to become productive members of society, the needs of the whole person must be taken into account to ensure maximum benefit from the technology. Equally, all professionals in assistive technology service delivery must be technology-literate so that appropriate referrals and selections can be made.[7, 8]

EVALUATING FOR APPROPRIATE PERSON/DEVICE MATCH

To gather the information necessary to identify the appropriate technology for a given person, an evaluation is performed. The purpose of the evaluation is to ensure that the equipment will meet the user's needs. The evaluation can involve persons from several different backgrounds with different areas of expertise. Evaluations are often performed by a team of individuals, including occupational, physical, and speech language therapists, engineers, assistive technologists, rehabilitation counselors, nurses, and physicians. This technology team should include the person for whom the evaluation is being performed, who should be considered an equal partner in the process.

There are as many different styles of evaluation as there are rehabilitation professionals. However, an evaluation should provide enough information to allow the team to identify the appropriate technology. An outline for a typical evaluation is in the following text.

Identify Consumer Goals and Tasks

The first portion of the assessment is used to gather information about the goals of the individual and the need for equipment. This may be the most important step of the process. The needs assessment is used to identify why the individual is seeking technology, in order to be able to identify the most appropriate technology.

Different people use equipment in different ways and for different purposes, and the needs assessment provides the technology team with information about what the user wants to be able to do and about the "type" of user the person will be. For example, a computer programming student's computer technology requirements will likely be greater than those of the home computer user, and therefore the level of control and access may be more complex. It is also important to conduct a task analysis of activities (i.e., to look at the components of the activity and determine what actions are required to do it).

Get Comprehensive Information

Get information about the person, the environment, and the devices. Assess the consumer's functional abilities and personal preferences and environmental barriers and resources; ascertain product availability (Table 24–1).

The information-gathering step is often ongoing, until the final decision is actually made. In most cases, evaluation of functional capabilities rests with the physicians and clinical professionals involved.

A comprehensive evaluation of the consumer's environment is also essential. Clinicians conducting functional evaluations need to consider environmental issues, as does the counselor. The counselor may have special expertise in the work and community settings. Consumers returning to previously held jobs have the best understanding of the work environment and are a crucial source of information.

Establish Criteria for a Successful Choice

Based on the consumer's goals, abilities, and preferences, identify specific, objective criteria by which to judge

TABLE 24–1   User's Functional Abilities

User's Functional Abilities	
Disability	Type, severity, age at onset, prognosis
Motor	Strength, endurance, range of motion, fine and gross motor coordination, positioning to use device, type of control that can be operated
Cognitive	Intelligence, judgment, attention span, problem-solving, memory
Communication	Voice quality, pronunciation, speed
Sensory	Vision, hearing, tactile perception
User's Personal Characteristics	
Psychosocial	Interests/activities, personal values, adjustment to disability, coping style, motivation/desire, attitude toward devices, concept of independence
Family and social support	Family, friends, co-workers, neighbors, etc.
Environment	
Environmental compatibility	Usable in home, work, play, community; architectural barriers, getting into and out of rooms, access to lighting, kitchen, phones, bath
Resources available	Space, electronics, wiring compatible
Impact on others in environment	Family, housemates, co-workers
Service delivery system	Training provided, follow-up provided, user support services available, installation, timely delivery

From Galvin J, Barnicle K, Perr A: Evaluating and Choosing Assistive Technology. Proceedings of the Technology and People with Disabilities Conference. Northridge, Calif, California State University, 1992.

potential solutions. To make the best match, you must consider multiple issues: the tasks to be accomplished, the consumer's functional abilities and personal characteristics, the environment, and the device. The interaction of these issues must then be considered, because they all affect the use of the device. The major areas of concern are summarized in Table 24–2.

Make a Final Selection

Apply the criteria to possible solutions to narrow down the options. Determine which of these solutions best meets

TABLE 24–2   Device Selection Evaluation Criteria

Performance	Effectiveness, reliability, durability, safety, comfort
Ease of use	Easy to set up, learn to use, operate, maintain, repair
Aesthetics	Attractive, quiet, well-designed
Cost	Purchase, maintenance, repairs
Convenience	Easy to store, transport, etc.
Flexibility	Compatible with other devices, expandable

From Galvin J, Barnicle K, Perr A: Evaluating and Choosing Assistive Technology. Proceedings of the Technology and People with Disabilities Conference. Northridge, Calif, California State University, 1992.

the criteria. Equipment trials utilizing loaner or rental equipment are extremely useful, especially in the area of augmentative and alternative communication (AAC). In lieu of equipment trials, recommendations are made and equipment is procured, set up, and configured. Training and appropriate follow-up are integral parts of the evaluation process, to ensure the success of the technology solution.

Although these steps are presented as a linear process, the operation is really iterative (cyclical). Information gathered at each step might necessitate adjustment of decisions made in earlier steps. Additionally, a device selected for one activity might have an effect on another activity. For example, in a work setting, hand-held typing sticks may be the best method for typing. However, if the user must also answer the phone, the typing stick might interfere and make overall activity more difficult. All of the benefits and drawbacks must be weighed within the larger context.

When evaluating for computer-related technologies it is important to ensure that the technologies interface with each other: that is, the hardware, the software, and the user interact for the desired result. It is also important to be aware of other related factors, such as an employer's using only a specific type of computer. Cognitive factors, as well as sensory and motor skills, must also be taken into account. Tables 24-3 and 24-4 illustrate some of the factors affecting computer use.

It is important to realize that any piece of equipment works best when used as designed. When an assistive technology intervention is necessary, the simpler the intervention the better. When looking at computer adaptations, the same rule applies. First, try the device as designed. If this is not workable, try to identify the simplest appropriate intervention and only use more complicated interventions as needed. Avoid the temptation to use the "high-tech" solution when a "low-tech" solution may be best.

COMPUTER ADAPTATIONS

Computer workstations consist of hardware (the actual computer, monitor, and printer) and software (programs such as DOS, WordPerfect, or Lotus). For an individual with a disability, all of these can be used with some adaptations and/or peripheral devices to allow alternative input to the computer and alternative output, enabling the user to receive information from the computer. Computer adaptations range from free to inexpensive software packages, costing less than $100, to hardware adaptations or peripheral devices costing more than $10,000. It is possible to get information in and out of a computer in a number of ways, and many different types of computers are available, from personal computers to minicomputers and mainframe computers. Some use graphical interfaces (such as the Macintosh or Microsoft Windows user interfaces). All of these factors contribute to the decision to use a given solution over another. This section focuses on personal computer solutions and adaptations for input and output (Table 24-5).

Positioning

One of the first areas to evaluate is positioning of the individual and the computer equipment. Ergonomically de-

TABLE 24–3 Cognitive Factors That Affect Assistive Technology Interventions

Cognitive Factors	Impact on Use of Technology
Attention deficits	Failure to follow screen prompts and directions
	Inability to consistently perform multi-step procedures
	Inability to filter information on busy screens
	Difficulty with large amounts of computer speech
Sensory deficits	Inability to separate command menus from other screen data
	Inability to track user information on rapidly changing screens
	Slow visual-motor dexterity
	Difficulty understanding computer speech
Memory deficits	Unable to complete multi-step operations or device commands
	Unable to follow set-up directions
	Unable to locate and recall disk files
	Difficulty recalling knowledge of computer symbols and commands
Abstract reasoning and thinking deficits	Unable to analyze equipment procedures and generalize operations
	Unable to understand scanning methods
	Unable to build abstract symbol sets to infer selections or choices
	Unable to reproduce a sequence of operational tasks
Problem-solving deficits	Unable to operate device because of a hardware or software procedure problem
	Unable to use software or hardware rules to back out of an operation
	Unable to use device prompts or cues to accomplish task
	Unable to sequence steps to complete computer commands

From Church G, Glennen S: The Handbook of Assistive Technology. San Diego, Singular Publishing, 1992.

signed office chairs, footrests, arm supports, and wristrests can help positioning so that equipment is more easily accessed. When used properly, this type of equipment can help to prevent computer-related disabilities, such as repetitive stress syndromes. Devices such as keyboard trays, copy holders, monitor arms, and printer stands can all help to make access easier. Many of these devices are available from computer and stationery stores.

Keyboard Accommodations

The traditional device for computer input is the keyboard. The QWERTY keyboard (named for the letter arrangement of the top left hand row of keys) is the standard computer keyboard and has over 100 keys. The QWERTY keyboard was actually designed to limit typing speed, to prevent jamming on original manual typewriters.

It is preferable to access equipment in the standard way in which it was designed to be accessed, but traditional input devices and methods can be difficult or impossible for persons with disabilities to use. The QWERTY keyboard works very well for people with ten working fingers, but can severely slow down a person who types using a

TABLE 24–4 Motor Factors That Affect Assistive Technology Interventions

Motor Factors	Impact on Use of Technology
Voluntary motor deficits	Inability to make deliberate switch and keyboard selections
	Limited control of trunk and extremities during movement
	Eye twitching resulting in overshooting the mark when reaching for objects
	Limited ability to produce speech communication
Fixed-posture and positioning deficits	Limited hand positioning and stabilization for access to assistive and peripheral devices
Recurring purposeless motion	Accidental triggering of switches and keys
	Limited fine motor control in isolating symbol, key, and button selections
Motor paralysis	Changes in muscle tone interfere with motor movements
	Spastic movements result in poor control and accidental selections
	Limited movement of arm, face, and leg
	Inhibits movement of arm, face, and leg
Low muscle tone	Loss of balanced muscle control in extremity for selection and stability
Rigidity	Inhibits arm and leg movements and good positioning
Spasticity	Limits full range of motion
	Reduces accurate and consistent motor movements for switch, key, and button selection
Tremors	Inhibits the precision of fine and gross motor precision selection tasks

From Church G, Glennen S: The Handbook of Assistive Technology. San Diego, Singular Publishing, 1992.

single hand, or even a single finger. Fortunately, a number of strategies and devices have been developed to accommodate persons with disabilities.

Free software packages are available that modify the way the keyboard responds (e.g., delaying the automatic repeat, or permitting one-finger typists to press the shift key sequentially rather than simultaneously when capitalizing). Programs are available that allow the keyboard layout to be changed from QWERTY to one that is designed to facilitate typing by one-hand typists.

TABLE 24–5 Common Adapted Computer Input and Output Hardware and Software

Alternative computer keyboard	Braille input devices
Braille translation	Braille printers/embossers
Computer keyboard enhancers	CD-ROM
Digitizers	Environmental control unit (ECU)
Expanded keyboards	Facsimile machines
Graphical user interface (GUI)	Keyguards
Keyboard emulators	Large-print software
Magnified CRT displays	Morse code input
Mouse/trackball input	Optical character recognition (OCR)
Refreshable Braille displays	Screen reader software
Signaling systems	Speech synthesizers
Speech recognition	Speech amplification
Telephone amplifiers	Telephone device for the deaf (TDD)
Touch screens	Word prediction software

Many different keyboards are available for individuals who cannot use the standard keyboard. Keyboards come in a variety of sizes and shapes, key type, and layout. Mini-keyboards are available for individuals whose range or strength is limited; expanded keyboards for individuals who lack fine motor control; membrane keyboards (similar to those found on microwave ovens and ATM machines) that enable the typist to slide the hand across other keys without selecting unwanted keystrokes; and keyboards with different layouts that facilitate typing for one-hand or one-finger typists. Keyboards that take advantage of an individual's present keyboarding skills, such as a Braille keyboard, are also available. When access cannot be accomplished through a keyboard, an alternate form of access may be successful (Fig. 24–1).

Alternate Access

Alternative access methods range from using switches to select characters from scanning arrays, to inputting dots and dashes in Morse code, to using voice input. Although these alternate methods can provide access, they are more complex to set up and to learn to use, because they usually require additional hardware and software.

Switches have been designed to capture virtually any movement that a person can make and to translate that movement into a signal to the computer. Switches can be activated by the head, hands, or feet or even by eye movements. Switches can be used to provide input to a computer in one of two ways. The first involves scanning, in which the person uses a switch to make selections from an array of characters. Scanning can allow a severely physically disabled person, who is only able to access a single switch, to use a computer. Switches can also be used to send coded input to the computer. For example, switches are used to send Morse code, which the computer translates into letters and numbers.

Cutting-edge technology, such as optical character recognition (OCR), voice input systems, and handwriting recognition can be used to provide input to computers. With OCR, the computer is programmed to recognize printed material and to convert the printed text to information that the computer can understand. OCR involves using a scanner to "take a picture" of the printed page and then using software that recognizes the picture as letters and numbers. OCR is often limited to certain typefaces and font sizes. Computer systems that can be trained to recognize an individual's handwriting are becoming more common.

Voice input systems allow persons to dictate to the computer. The computer is "trained" to recognize a sound and to provide a word or computer action in response. These high-end systems can be trained to understand tens of thousands of words. It is important to realize that a computer is not nearly as good at "recognition" as the human brain is. Computers can only match to a pattern, and they typically have difficulties if the pattern is varied (e.g., if a word is spoken more softly). People are able to understand spoken and written information even if a substantial portion is missing by "filling in the blanks" using such cues as content or emotion. Again, technological solutions such as voice output are more complex, and can require more training, set-up, and support time.

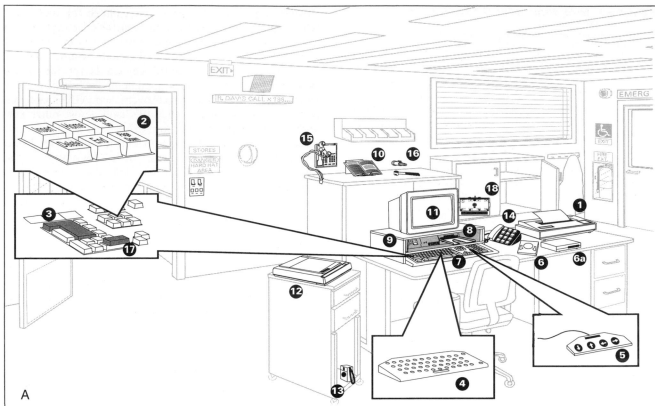

A

Incoordination

Following are modifications to Computers, Information Displays, Communication Devices, and Controls which should be considered with the input of the worker with this limitation.

Computers

❶ Provide printer paper-handling hardware, e.g., single-sheet feeder.

❷ Install enlarged key caps.

❸ Provide keycovers or keyguard (keyshield).

❹ Provide expanded keyboard.

❺ Provide keyboard emulator, remap keyboard or adjust keyboard sensitivity.

❻ Simplify input motion, e.g., mouse, joystick, trackball, light pen, touch/screen, touch-pad, scanning, direct selection, or ❻ₐ voice recognition.

❼ Eliminate simultaneous keystrokes with keylocks, sequential or "sticky-key" software, or foot pedal.

❽ Provide guides for inserting disks.

❾ Stabilize keyboard and copy stand at most convenient height and angle for access by mouthstick or headpointer.

Accelerate input with abbreviation expansion, word prediction, macros.

Suppress "auto-repeat" key feature.

Minimize disc manipulation by storing data on hard, rather than floppy disks.

Install moisture- and dust-resistant keyboard covers.

Augment hardware/software to provide environmental control.

Provide graphics software for illustrations.

B

Information Displays

❿ Provide bookstands to position documents at ideal height/angle.

⓫ Minimize document handling through microfilm and/or computer information access

⓬ "Scan" documents onto disk with optical character recognition.

Communication Devices

⓭ Provide continuous-loop tape recorder for short messages, cassette recorder for notes, dictation, etc.

⓮ Provide phone with enlarged keypad (or raised face plate/keyguard), auto-dialer .

⓯ Provide headset, speaker phone, or "gooseneck" for receiver with switch for phone cradle buttons.

Avoid need for standing while using telephone.

Controls

⓰ Limit activating force to 2 lbf.; add levers if necessary.

⓱ Provide guards or covers to avoid accidental activation.

⓲ Provide eye-gaze, eye-blink or chin/head/tongue/eyebrow/forehead/foot movement controls.

Provide remote-control electric door latches in secured areas.

Locate controls as close to body as possible, or provide adjacent handrests.

Use 3/4 - 1 1/2" round or square switch surfaces.

Provide at least 1" space between control surfaces (or separate with guards).

Avoid need for quick response.

Install alternative switches sensitive to pressure, tilt, magnetic, pneumatic, auditory, or infrared input by sip-and-puff, voice.

Note: Complete remote control systems also available as substitute for manual control.

FIGURE 24–1 Computers, information displays, communication devices, and controls: assistive modifications for workers with incoordination. *A*, Graphic illustration of a typical workstation setup for an individual with coordination problems. *B*, Key to features in *A*. (From Mueller J: The Workplace Workbook 2.0: An Illustrated Guide to Workplace Accommodation and Technology. McLean, Va, HRD Press, 1992.)

Mouse Substitution and Emulation

A mouse control is frequently used for convenience. If an individual has difficulty using a mouse, a mouse substitution or emulation might be required. Many programs (especially those written for the Windows operating environment) have equivalent keystrokes for every mouse command.

A trackball is like an upside down mouse. Rather than moving the mouse around the desktop, the user moves only the ball in a stationary holder. The trackball can be set in different positions to be more easily accessed or it may be operated by the foot or the chin. Trackballs are common, inexpensive adaptations that are 100% compatible and are available in local computer stores. Other solutions include the use of digitizers, touch screens, and head pointers. Digitizers are position-sensitive tablets on which the user provides input by using a stylus or puck. Touch screens are see-through, pressure-sensitive mats that fit over the monitor; direct pressure activates the desired area of the screen. Head pointing is an emulation that employs sensors to track the user's head position and translates the head movements to pointer positions. Digitizers, touch screens, and head pointers are more technologically complex and expensive and require additional training and support.

Output Accommodations

Just as the keyboard and the mouse are the traditional input devices for the computer, the cathode ray tube (CRT), or monitor, and the printer are the traditional output devices. Although a variety of printers and monitors are on the market, they are visual devices and are often unusable by individuals with visual deficits. Furthermore, as the software industry moves to graphical user interfaces (GUI), such as the Macintosh Finder and Microsoft Windows, the ability to deal with visual information becomes more important.

Visual limitations can sometimes be accommodated by the use of a larger monitor. Most off-the-shelf monitor screens measure 13 to 15 in. diagonally. Computer monitors as large as 21 to 25 in. may be purchased, but they can cost up to $10,000. Magnifying lenses can be attached to the front of screens to enlarge the output, but the amount of magnification that they provide is usually limited. Software programs that enlarge a portion of the screen to full size may be utilized. These programs enlarge portions of the screen 12 to 15 times normal, but the monitor only displays one section at a time. This is akin to looking at the monitor through a drinking straw: to see the whole screen, the user must move the straw across the screen and put the pieces together.

Screen readers can be used to supplement visual information. A screen reader consists of a speech synthesizer and software that converts text on the screen to speech, which is then heard by the user. Many individuals with visual deficits use screen readers as their sole source of feedback from the computer.

Graphical User Interfaces

The GUI of systems such as the Macintosh Finder and Microsoft Windows allow computer users to interact visually with the computer. Programs, commands, and document files are represented on the screen by pictures, or *icons*. The person opens documents and runs programs by using the mouse to move the icons around the screen. If a screen reader is to be used with a GUI, the graphical information must be converted into text that the speech synthesizer will recognize. Screen reader packages are designed for use with GUIs, and many individuals with visual deficits are using them effectively.

Another way around a GUI is not to use one. Many software packages are available for IBM-compatible machines that do not use a GUI. By carefully choosing software, programs can be identified for entertainment, education, and business that do not require use of the mouse or that have equivalent keystrokes for mouse functions.

Printers

The main differences between printers are print quality, ability to print graphics, and ability to print in color. Individuals using printers often have problems in seeing the printed page or in managing the paper. The most common problem is difficulty loading the paper into the printer or unloading the finished pages. Paper-loading problems can be minimized with a printer that uses continuous-feed paper. Pullout trays and top-feed printers might be considered.

Regular paper printouts can be difficult or impossible to read for individuals with visual limitations. Printing in a larger font can be a simple adaptation. For those who read Braille, there are Braille printer/embossers. Some Braille printers have the capability to produce tactile graphics. If printer noise (especially from dot matrix printers) is an issue, dome covers or insulated tiles can be used to provide a sound barrier.

COMMUNICATION TECHNOLOGIES

Augmentative Communication

Many individuals have difficulty communicating verbally. For example, persons with cerebral palsy, neuromuscular disease, traumatic brain injury, or stroke can have difficulty producing speech. Communication boards that have icons or pictures are a common method for communicating basic needs. However, for many individuals who are speech impaired, the pointer board is insufficient. The advent of computers has led to the development of computerized augmentative or alternative communication systems (AACs).

Augmentative communication devices have developed rapidly since the late 1980s. More that 250 augmentative communication hardware and software items are available. Sophisticated AAC systems can offer speech synthesis in up to ten age- and gender-appropriate voices and foreign languages. These offer access by touch, pointer, switch, and infrared scanning or even by ocular eyegaze monitors that electronically measure eye movements.[9] Word prediction software can assist a user in recognizing and predicting keystrokes, building on a dictionary of words and phrases. This can speed up the entry process and enable the user to communicate more rapidly. AAC systems for children can teach communication through play. Games, bedtime stories, prayers, descriptive concepts, basic math, and core vocabulary programs make learning and communicating fun. Stephen Hawking, who has a form of amyotrophic lateral sclerosis, dictated his best selling book *A Brief History of Time* to a personal computer adapted for single-switch scanning access with speech output through a speech synthesizer. AAC technology is complex, and evaluating a non-vocal individual for a communication system has become equally complex. The individual's expressive language skills, receptive language skills, symbol recognition skills, and functional ability to access the technology all have to be evaluated to ensure an appropriate match between the person and the device.

Telecommunications

Telephone devices for the deaf (TDD) enable individuals who are hearing-impaired, deaf, or speech-impaired to communicate by telephone. The TDD utilizes a QWERTY keyboard. The message is typed in and displayed on an LED screen while being transmitted over the telephone lines. A Braille version is available for individuals who are both deaf and blind. Computers with PC/TDD modems are also used as a means of communication. Conversations are typed in and responses received on the computer screen.

Environmental Controls

An environmental control system allows an individual with functional or sensory disabilities to independently control immediate surroundings. Usually these systems utilize a set of modules that plug into standard electrical outlets and can be used to operate lights or television, initiate or answer telephone calls, and unlock doors. Environmental control units (ECUs) are becoming a familiar tool for the able-bodied as a means of security (i.e., light activated by daylight sensors, movement, or noise). An ECU helps an individual with a disability to have a sense of freedom and independence. ECUs can activate radios, televisions, electric beds, thermostats, and telephones. They become a lifeline to emergency response teams, and can be activated by voice or touch.

ECU technology ranges from a simple commercially obtained remote control for switching lights on and off to a "smart house." The computerized house is controlled by a single unit that monitors the complete environment: it regulates the thermostats in each room for energy saving and monitors the children at play outside or visitors at the door. By way of strategically placed sensors, the system alerts home owners to such hazards as stove burners that have been left on, and continuously monitors the exterior to ensure security.

FUNDING FOR COMPUTER ASSISTIVE DEVICES

Despite the federal mandates for comprehensive consumer-responsive assistive technology and technology-related services, obtaining such devices and services remains an arduous task for both the individual user and the professional. The physician can facilitate the funding process by providing sufficient clinical information to support the written justification for the financing of computer-related technologies. The rehabilitation team should begin gathering funding information during the evaluation process, and should determine how much funding is required. It is crucial to include adequate funds to cover any necessary installation costs, training fees, and service contracts. The team should ensure that appropriate language is utilized in writing the justification. For example, if educational funding sources are requested, the justification should reflect that the equipment will assist the individual in scholastic endeavors. For Medicaid, the equipment has to be deemed medically necessary. If a vocational rehabilitation agency is to be approached for funding, the justification should clearly express that the equipment is work related. If an employer is to be approached, the justification should describe how the recommended equipment relates to the essential functions of the job. Under the Americans with Disabilities Act, reasonable accommodations are required in the workplace for qualified individuals with disabilities. Although no direct funding is available under the Act, companies have various tax relief options available for the purchase of equipment and other barrier removal activities. Table 24–6 lists some of the funding sources that may be appropriate for your patient.

Private funding sources should also be investigated. The family may need to consider its own resources; a mix-and-

TABLE 24–6   Funding Sources for Assistive Technology

Public Programs	Alternative Financing	U.S. Tax Code
Medicare	Private insurance	Medical care expense deduction
Medicaid	Private foundations	Business deductions
Individuals with Disabilities Education Act (IDEA)	Employee accommodation programs	ADA credit for small business
State grants—vocational rehabilitation	Corporate-sponsored loans	Targeted jobs tax credit
The Developmental Disabilities State grants	Community groups	Charitable contributions deduction
CHAMPUS	Religious organizations	
Workers Compensation programs	Service clubs	
The Technology Related Assistance programs	Advocacy organizations	
Social Security Administration—PASS Program	Family/friends	
Veterans benefits		

match approach is often necessary to obtain all of the required funding. Private medical insurance can be approached, as can advocacy agencies (such as the National Easter Seal Society or the Muscular Dystrophy Foundation) and community groups (such as the Lions Club or Rotary). Corporations and private foundations may help, but should usually be considered only as a last resort.

SUMMARY/FUTURE TECHNOLOGIES

Computers have changed the way we work and play and have influenced every area of our lives. The rate of increase of the processing power of computer hardware and the continuing sophistication of software is staggering. Computers that would fill wings of universities and that functioned as little more than adding machines have been replaced by technology that fits on a desk in most offices. The computational power and complex programs that can be run to perform many household and office tasks could not have been imagined 30 years ago. Computers already talk to each other; and in the future we will talk to our computers and our computers will talk back. We will travel the information superhighway using virtual reality and explore virtual worlds. Computers continue to increase in power and sophistication and lead to even more possibilities for all people. It is important that all persons, including those with disabilities, be able to access and to use computer technology.

References

1. Church G, Glennen S: The Handbook of Assistive Technology. San Diego, Singular Publishing Group, 1992.
2. Galvin J, Barnicle K, Perr A: Evaluating and choosing assistive technology. Proceedings of the Technology and People with Disabilities Conference. Northridge, California State University, 1992.
3. Jones K, Torgesen J, Sexton M: Using computer guided practice to increase decoding fluency in learning disabled children: A study using the hint and hunt I program. J Learning Disabilities 1987; 20:122–128.
4. LaPlante MP, Hendershot GE, Moss AJ: Assistive technology devices and home accessibility features: Prevalence, payment, needs and trends. Advance data from Vital and Health Statistics, No. 217. Hyattsville, Md, National Center for Health Statistics, 1992.
5. Mueller J: The Workplace Workbook 2.0: An Illustrated Guide to Workplace Accommodation and Technology. McLean, Va, HRD Press, 1992.
6. Trifiletti JK, Frith GH, Armstrong S: Microcomputers versus resource rooms for learning students with a disability: A preliminary investigation of the effects on math skills. Learning Disability Q 1984; 7:69–76.
7. Scadden L: Technology: Training awareness and needs. *In* Perlman LG, Hansen CE (eds): Technology and Employment of Persons with Disabilities: A Report of the Mary E. Switzer Memorial Seminar. Alexandria, Va, National Rehabilitation Association, 1989.
8. Scherer MJ: Living in a State of Stuck: How Assistive Technologies Affect the Lives of People with Disabilities. Cambridge, Mass, Brookline Books, 1992.
9. Vanderheiden G, Lloyd LL: Communication systems and their components. *In* Blackstone S, Ruskin D (eds): Augmentative Communication: An Introduction. Rockville, Md, ASHA Press, 1986.

Resources

American Medical Association: Primary Care for Persons with Disabilities: Guidelines for the Use of Assistive Technology. Evaluation, Referral, Prescription. Chicago, AMA, 1994. *(AMA Department of Geriatric Health (312) 464-5085.)*

Berliss JR, Borden PA, Vanderheiden GC: Trace Resource Book: Assistive Technologies for Communication, Control and Computer Access, 1992 edition. Madison, Wisc, Trace R&D Center, 1992.

Church G, Glennen S: The Handbook of Assistive Technology. San Diego, Singular Publishing Group, 1992.

Lazzaro J: Adaptive Technologies for Learning and Work Environments. Chicago, American Library Association, 1993.

Mendelsohn S: Financing Adaptive Technology: A Guide to Sources and Strategies for Blind and Visually Impaired Users. New York, Smiling Interface, 1987. *(Available in print, on audiocassette, and on disk.)*

Mendelsohn S: Tax Options and Strategies for People with Disabilities. New York, Demos Publications, 1993. *(Available in print, on audiocassette, and on disk.)*

Mueller J: The Workplace Workbook 2.0: An Illustrated Guide to Workplace Accommodation and Technology. McLean, Va, HRD Press, 1992.

Organizations/Data Bases

Job Accommodation Network (JAN). West Virginia University, 809 Allen Hall, Morgantown, WV 26506. 1-800-526-7234 (Voice/TDD)

ABLEDATA: Assistive Technology Product . Macro Systems, 8455 Colesville Rd, Suite 935, Silver Spring, MD 20910. 1-800-346-2742 (Voice/TDD)

AT&T National Special Needs Center. Suite 310, 2001 Route 46, Parsippany, NJ 07054. 1-800-233-1222 (Voice) 1-800-833-3232 (TDD)

Joint and Soft Tissue Injection Techniques

JOHN J. NICHOLAS, M.D.

The modern era of therapeutic joint injections began with Joseph Lee Hollander. Hollander, however, cited George Thorn[60] as the first physician to inject hydroxycorticosterone (17-hydroxycorticosterone) into the inflamed knee joints of patients with rheumatoid arthritis (RA), osteoarthritis, sprained knee, acute gouty arthritis, disseminated lupus erythematosus, Sjögren's syndrome, subdeltoid bursitis, and olecranon and prepatellar bursitis. Hollander and colleagues[28] subsequently reported injections of hydrocortisone acetate, 25 to 37.5 mg, into the joints of 69 patients. In six of seven measured cases, the total synovial cell count fell by 50% and the temperature within the joint fell in all cases. In a subsequent report, Hollander described the "post-injection flare," aseptic necrosis of weightbearing joints, and a frequency of infection of 1 in 15,000 injections.[27] Overall, he reported a total of 250,000 injections in 8000 patients.

BENEFITS

Many authors subsequently described the effectiveness of intra-articular (IA) steroid injections for patients with inflammatory arthritis. For example, in 1962 Stolzer et al.,[58] described 2360 injections in 589 patients. Pain relief occurred in 97% and there were no infections. Flanagan et al.,[17] in 1988, described injections of triamcinolone under fluoroscopic control into the hip joints of British patients awaiting total hip replacement. Those injected with triamcinolone obtained greater relief than those injected with bupivacaine or saline. At 1 month, nine patients were improved, one was unchanged, and two were worse. In addition to pain relief, it was asserted that function and strength were improved in muscles surrounding the injected joints. Geborek et al.,[18] in 1990, reported the results of IA injection into 11 knee joints in seven patients. They noted that extensor muscle torque increased, range of motion improved, and knee circumference diminished 7 and 14

days after injection. They also noted that removal of synovial fluid alone increased extensor muscle torque.

It has even been suggested that the benefits of the longer-acting steroid preparations have been so successful that the frequency of surgical synovectomy has decreased.[7] Stefanich,[55] in 1981, reviewed the effects and complications of IA steroid injections.

Indications

The reason for injecting joints is that IA steroids decrease inflammation. Any inflamed joint is a candidate for injection, provided there is no joint infection.[30] The use of IA steroids in osteoarthritis (minimally inflamed joints) has been debated.[46] The current consensus is that patients with osteoarthritis should have a trial of IA steroid injections. IA injections should be utilized along with all other appropriate treatments and only rarely constitute the only treatment method.

Precautions

The precautions include avoiding joint infections. Nonetheless, it has been asserted that little additional damage occurs when an infected joint is injected with steroids, although the discovery of the infection may be delayed for 24 to 48 hours.[61] In some cases, the infection may be accelerated. Proper technique (see below) diminishes the small likelihood of infecting the joint at the time of IA injection.

Many authors suggest an injection of a mixture of anesthetic and steroid. I prefer to use only the steroid, because I want to know the exact site of the needle tip to ascertain the location of the injection. The diffusion of a local anesthetic into the surrounding tissue can obscure the exact site of the needle tip. There seems to be relatively little advantage to the inclusion of anesthesia for joint or soft tissue injection as it provides at most only temporary relief.

It is not clear whether injecting the joint is beneficial to patients with a hemarthrosis. The injection of a joint in a patient taking an anticoagulant or who has a bleeding disease must be done very carefully and following a discussion of the potential harm or benefit with the hematologist. Adjacent skin infections may be a hazard and should be avoided as sites of IA injection. IA injection in immuno-compromised patients should be performed only after consultation with the attending physician.

It is generally considered that no more than three or four injections should be given to the same joint in any 12-month period in order to avoid cartilage damage or infection.[47, 48]

Chatham has described an interesting study in which 30 patients with RA were divided into those rested for 48 hours after joint injection and those who were not rested.[12] The results suggest that in an inpatient population there is no symptom difference at 48 hours for those rested or not rested after the injection. However, Chakravarty et al.[11] recently demonstrated that 1 day of complete bed rest following knee injection resulted in better walking time, CRP, perceived pain and perceived stiffness, and a decreased knee circumference than in those who did not rest.[11]

Preparations

Many preparations of steroids are available for joint injections. Their selection depends upon the association of complications and the intent of the treating physician. The preparation chosen must be designated "for intra-articular use." The preparations vary in strength, concentration, and duration of effect[3] (Table 25–1). Currently available preparations include:

Methylprednisolone acetate (Depo-Medrol, Upjohn), IA, 40 and 80 mg/mL

Triamcinolone acetonide (Kenalog, Squibb), IA, 40 mg/mL

Triamcinolone hexacetonide (Aristospan, Lederle), IA, 20 mg/mL

Betamethasone sodium phosphate and acetate (Celestone Soluspan, Schering), IA, 6 mg/mL

Prednisolone tebutate (Hydeltra-T.B.A., Merck), IA, 20 mg/mL

Prednisolone sodium phosphate (Hydeltrasol, Merck), IA, 20 mg/mL

TABLE 25–1   Relative Strengths

Duration of Action	Equivalent Glucocorticoid Dose (mg)	Glucocorticoid Potency
Short-acting		
Cortisone	25.0	0.8
Hydrocortisone	20.0	1.0
Prednisone	5.0	4.0
Prednisolone	5.0	4.0
Methylprednisolone	4.0	5.0
Intermediate-acting		
Triamcinolone	4.0	5.0
Long-acting		
Dexamethasone	0.75	30.0
Betamethasone	0.6	25.0

Blyth et al.[6] have recently demonstrated that triamcinolone hexacetonide was felt to provide greater pain relief than triamcinolone acetonide by RA patients.

Strength

The contents of a 1.0-mL vial of any of the above preparations may be injected into a joint cavity. Larger doses have been suggested for larger joints and smaller doses for smaller joints, but there are no data to substantiate the efficacy of this practice. It is important that a never-used, single vial be used to eliminate the possibility of contamination from previous withdrawal of steroid or anesthetic from the vial. It has not been shown that there are harmful side effects from any dose contained in a single 1.0-mL dose vial.

Technique

The "no touch" technique described by Hasselbacher[26] is strongly recommended. With this technique, no drapes or sterile room is required, but universal precautions require wearing gloves to prevent contact with bloodborne pathogens. The first step is for the operator to select the site of injection through the skin. The injection site is chosen based on available *bony landmarks*. Bony landmarks are usually quite stable, while soft tissue landmarks may vary from patient to patient and from time to time. Once the site has been chosen, it is carefully outlined with a marker, usually with a circle (as a target) at least 3 cm in diameter; no larger field is required. After the site has been outlined with a marker, the area is cleaned with three swipes of Betadine (povidone-iodine) and one of alcohol, taking care not to remove the landmarks. Hasselbacher recommends that "the patient's skin should not be touched with the bare finger after preparation. Identification of landmarks with ink, or impressions made on the skin with a pointed object before cleaning, will facilitate recognition of the aspiration site."[26] There are other techniques of skin preparation, but this one is my personal suggestion.[53] A 25-gauge needle is then used to inject an anesthetic into the epidermis, causing a wheal to occur. A 1.5-in. (3.8 cm) 21-gauge needle is then placed on the syringe filled with anesthetic, and the skin is entered through the wheal after approximately 30 seconds. The patient should not feel pain at this entry. The operator should stop and aspirate every 0.5 cm, and inject another small bolus of anesthetic. The patient should not perceive undue pain and should remain relaxed during the procedure. When the joint capsule is entered, the patient will experience some discomfort, but additional anesthetic should eliminate this. When the joint has been entered, the hub of the needle should be clasped with a hemostat, the syringe with anesthetic removed, and an aspirating syringe, or series of aspirating and injecting syringes, applied. If the hub of the needle is grasped for syringe exchange with the fingers, inevitably the needle shaft will be touched by the operator and contaminated and then thrust back under the skin. The hemostat is cleaner and more secure. If these precautions and equipment are used, the only possible source of contamination would be from the vials of anesthetic or steroid.

Once the joint is entered, the color and consistency of the synovial fluid is observed and a sample is removed for laboratory analysis. Examination should be performed promptly,[34] and the sample should be sent to the laboratory for white blood cell count and polarized light microscopic examination. Evaluation for the presence or absence of crystals, and Gram's stain and culture for the presence of bacteria should be performed if indicated. The operator should determine, by letting a drop of fluid drip from the end of the syringe or by palpating a sample between the fingertips, whether there is a normal consistency and viscosity to the fluid. Normal synovial fluid will stretch approximately 2.5 cm between the fingertips. The white blood cell count of the fluid may be estimated by attempting to read 0.25-in. print through a standard test tube of the fluid. If the print can be read, the fluid is probably noninflammatory. If the print cannot be read, it likely indicates inflammation or infection. Additional tests, such as the rheumatoid factor, complement, albumin, protein electrophoresis, and glucose level have not been shown to help in the diagnosis of the patient's condition or to determine whether or not the sample is infected.[51]

There are few articles describing infections following joint injections. My experience is limited to a knowledge of only three patients, one with an infected elbow and two with infected knees. Each of these joints was injected with multiple punctures through the skin in an effort to obtain specimens of joint fluid. Multiple skin punctures are to be avoided. If joint fluid is not readily obtained at the first attempt, the needle should be redirected but not removed or pulled out of the skin in order to do this. The tip of the needle should be pulled out to within a short distance of the skin, but it then should be redirected while still under the skin surface.

The use of single-dose vials of steroid preparation and anesthetic should reduce the likelihood of infection from the solutions in this relatively safe procedure.

CHOICE OF SITE

There have been many articles describing joint injection techniques. Readers are referred to Hendrix et al.[26] for a description of injection of the sacroiliac joint. The hip joint is usually injected under fluoroscopic guidance to ensure entrance into the site, especially when no synovial fluid is obtained. The temporomandibular joints are not routinely injected because of their proximity to the facial nerve, artery, and parotid gland. Spinal facet joint injections also require fluoroscopic guidance. Gray and Gottlieb,[23] Samuelson et al.,[50] Leversee,[37] and Zuckerman et al.[63] have presented reviews.

STERNOCLAVICULAR JOINT. The sternoclavicular joint cannot ordinarily be entered by a needle. The site of the injection is actually on the top or superior aspect of the joint where the clavicle attaches to the sternum. The deposit is made in the subcutaneous tissues adjacent to the joint. The bony surfaces of the sternum and clavicle may be readily palpated (Fig. 25-1A).

ACROMIOCLAVICULAR JOINT. The approach is similar to the sternoclavicular joint. Deposition of the injected steroid is made superior to the joint where the clavicle

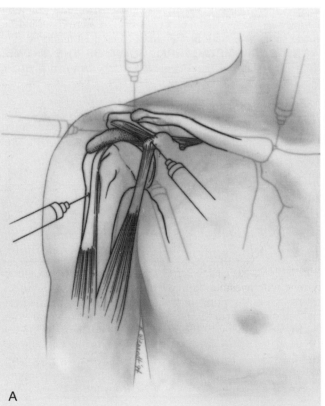
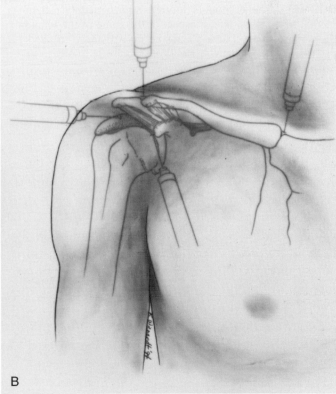

A   B

FIGURE 25-1   *A,* It is important to identify the acromioclavicular joint, the acromion, and the coracoid process as bony landmarks to aid joint injection around the shoulder. *B,* The bony bicipital groove can be palpated at the anterior aspect of the humerus.

joins the acromion, approximately 12.5 mm (0.5 in.) medial to the tip of the acromion (see Fig. 25–1A). The site is readily palpable.

LONG HEAD OF THE BICEPS TENDONS. The injection is made at the point of maximum palpable tenderness in the bicipital groove (bony landmark) in the head of the humerus (Fig. 25–1B). No attempt is made to inject the tendon sheath, but the steroid is deposited in immediate proximity to the point of tenderness.

SHORT HEAD OF THE BICEPS TENDON. Similarly, the steroid is injected at the point of greatest tenderness, which is usually right on top of the coracoid process (see Fig. 25–1B). The tendon arises from the coracoid process and clinical inflammation seems maximal at this site (bony landmark).

SHOULDER. The bony landmarks are the coracoid process and the head of the humerus (see Fig. 25–1A). A site is chosen just lateral to the coracoid process. The joint is entered either between the head of the humerus and the coracoid process or 0.5 cm superior to this site. An injection medial to the coracoid process may result in harm to the brachial plexus, subclavian artery, vein, or lung. The steroid preparation is deposited approximately 1.5 in. (3.8 cm) below the skin surface after entering directly perpendicular to the skin at the described site. Entrance into the shoulder joint from a posterior approach is less reliable because there are no good bony landmarks.

SUBACROMIAL BURSA. The subacromial bursa lies beneath the tip of the acromion (bony landmark), and the steroid is deposited approximately 1.5 cm. under the skin beneath the tip of the acromion process and superior to the head of the humerus (see Fig. 25–1A).

SUPRASPINATUS TENDON (IMPINGEMENT SYNDROME). The tendon is located approximately 2.5 cm medial to the most lateral aspect of the spine of the scapula (bony landmark). There should be no resistance to needle insertion. A tender area will be "discovered" by the point of the injecting needle.

ELBOW. The elbow joint may be entered anteriorly, but this can present a hazard to the biceps tendon, brachioradialis tendon, median nerve, radial nerve, and branches of the radial artery. A medial approach is to be avoided because of potential ulnar nerve injury, so a lateral site is generally best. The bony landmarks are the olecranon process, the head of the radius, and the lateral epicondyle. These landmarks form a triangle. The joint may be entered just anterior to the center of this triangle, and posterior to the head of the radius (Fig. 25–2). If there is considerable synovial fluid, there will be a slight bulge. The needle must be moved toward where the operator estimates the center of the joint to be (much as when performing a spinal tap). There is not much room through a bony tunnel at this site, but if bony landmarks are chosen carefully and consistently, good results are obtained.

OLECRANON BURSITIS. The olecranon bursa overlies the olecranon process of the ulna. The needle is directed into the most fluctuant part of the enlarged bursal sac.

CARPAL JOINTS. The ulnar and radial styloids are the bony landmarks for carpal joint injection. A line connecting these two bony landmarks defines the proximal row of carpal bones. Injections should not be made too far proximally. There are many carpal joints, each of which has its own synovial cavity. Injections of each should be done at the point of maximal tenderness.

DE QUERVAIN'S DISEASE. The tendons of the extensor pollicis brevis and abductor pollicis longus may be located by palpation (Fig. 25–3). The point of injection should be at the site of maximal tenderness. Entering the tendon sheath should not be attempted because of potential damage to the tendon. The deposition of steroid should be made subcutaneously in the area of maximal tenderness.

THE CARPOMETACARPAL JOINT OF THE THUMB.

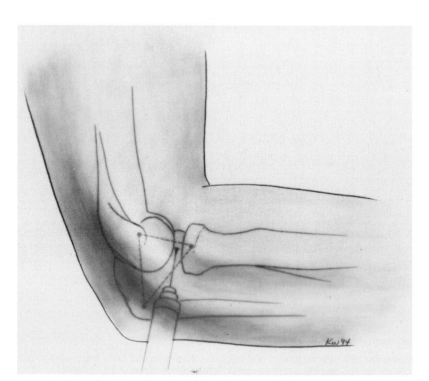

FIGURE 25–2 The site of injection at the elbow lies just inferior and posterior to the head of the radius.

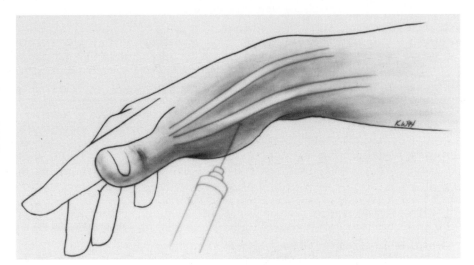

FIGURE 25–3 The tendon of the extensor pollicis brevis can be readily palpated and identified beneath the skin without the aid of a bony landmark.

The anatomical snuff box lies between the abductor pollicis longus and extensor pollicis longus, and the extensor brevis pollicis tendons of the thumb. Osteoarthritis at this site usually results in tenderness to palpation. The operator should inject the steroid at the point of tenderness, approximately 12.5 mm (0.5 in.) below the skin.

THE METACARPOPHALANGEAL JOINT OF THE THUMB AND FINGERS. This joint is more difficult to inject than one would suspect. When the fist is clenched and the knuckles protrude (bony landmark), the joint may be palpated just *distal* to the apex of the knuckle (Fig. 25–4). It can be readily palpated just beyond the bulge of the knuckle. The joint should be entered from an angle, not directly laterally or directly superiorly, in order to avoid the digital nerve, artery, and vein, as well as the extensor tendon apparatus on the superior aspect of each digit. A 25-gauge needle enters this joint readily.

DISTAL INTERPHALANGEAL AND PROXIMAL INTERPHALANGEAL JOINTS. These joints cannot readily be entered by a needle, and an effort to do so may only cause joint damage. The operator should palpate the bony landmarks in a fashion similar to the metacarpophalangeal joints, and deposit the steroid subcutaneously in the area just beyond the apex of the knuckle. This is where the joint will most likely be, and the medication will get into the joint space.

THE CARPAL TUNNEL. The boundaries of the carpal tunnel may be readily determined if the pisiform and trapezoid bones are palpated on the palmar aspect of the proximal hand (bony landmark) (Fig. 25–5). A line connecting these bony landmarks reveals the position of the transverse carpal ligament. The median nerve enters the palm just medial (ulnarward) to the trapezoid. The injection is made through the transverse carpal ligament in this area, approxi-

FIGURE 25–4 The metacarpophalangeal joint is more distal than usually thought, just beyond the bony prominence of the distal end of the metacarpal bone (the knuckle).

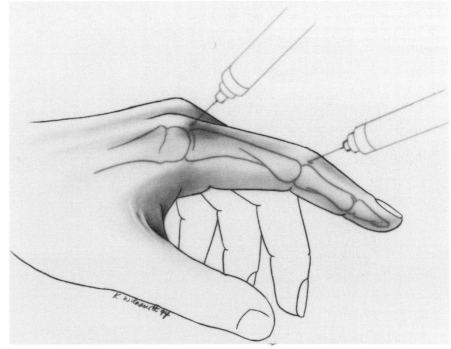

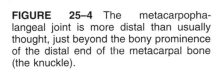

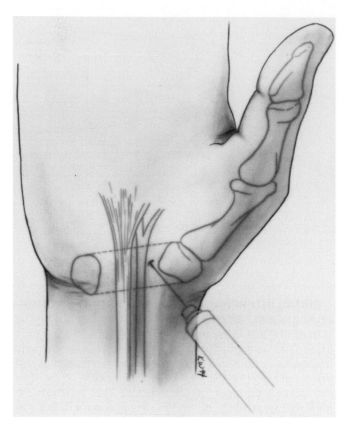

FIGURE 25–5 The boundaries of the carpal tunnel are defined by the pisiform and the trapezoid bones.

mately 6 mm below the surface of the skin. If paresthesias occur owing to being on or near the median nerve, the operator should maneuver the needle more laterally and less deep.

An alternative injection technique is to determine the site of the palmaris longus tendon and enter the skin at a point on the radial side of the tendon. The needle should be directed toward the palm of the hand in the hope of entering the carpal tunnel near the site of the median nerve entrapment.

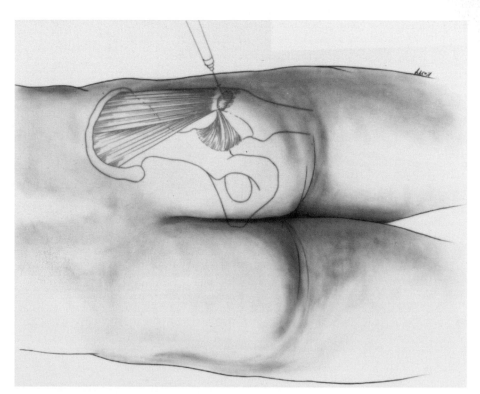

FIGURE 25–6 The bony prominence of the greater trochanter is best palpated with the patient lying on the uninvolved side.

THE HIP JOINT. The hip joint is routinely injected only under fluoroscopic control.

ISCHIAL BURSITIS. Inflammation of a bursa inferior to the ischial tuberosity can occur from persistent sitting, as in "weaver's bottom." Injection of this bursa is rarely required, but the ischial tuberosity should be palpated and injection made directly into the point of maximum tenderness.

THE GREATER TROCHANTERIC BURSA. The greater trochanteric bursa is located superiorly to the greater trochanter, which can be readily palpated through the skin (bony landmark) (Fig. 25–6). The point of maximal tenderness is usually superior, but sometimes inferior, to this bony landmark. The skin is entered using a spinal needle in most cases, because the bursa is surprisingly deep. After a depth of several inches, the tip of the needle will touch a tender area superior but not directly on top of the greater trochanter. This is the site at which to deposit the steroid.

THE SACROILIAC JOINT. The sacroiliac joint may be injected at the point of maximal tenderness, or it more certainly may be injected under fluoroscopic guidance.[27]

THE KNEE JOINT. Knee injections are generally performed poorly because most authors describe entering the lateral aspect of the knee midway between the superior and inferior margins of the patella and beneath the patella. There is very little room at this site for the operator to insert a needle between the femur and patella. Commonly the joint surfaces are engaged by the needle, causing the patient to contract the quadriceps muscle in pain and narrow the joint space even further. The recommended procedure is that the operator outline the patella with a pen, and then select a site just superior to the superior margin of the patella on the medial aspect of the knee. This site should be low enough on the medial aspect of the knee to allow direction of the needle below the quadriceps *tendon* (Fig. 25–7). This puts the medication into the suprapatellar pouch, which is contiguous with the synovial cavity. Since it lies below the quadriceps tendon, it may be readily entered without causing undue pain or contraction of the quadriceps muscle.

An alternative method is to inject the knee joint with the knee flexed, and the patient supine or sitting. In this procedure, the tibial tubercle and the patella are outlined and are connected with lines to outline the patellar tendon. The needle may be directed medially or laterally just below the superior margin of the patella toward the operator's sense of where the knee joint cavity is located. The joint may be entered without any bony contact. This is an especially advantageous site when there are osteophytes around the patella or when the patient is very obese. The disadvantage of the flexed knee technique is that only rarely can fluid be obtained from this position, apparently because the fluid migrates to a posterior position in the knee during flexion.

HOUSEMAID'S KNEE. Housemaid's knee is an inflammation of the prepatellar bursa. No bony landmarks are needed and the prepatellar bursa may be injected at the site of maximal fullness.

THE ANSERINE BURSA. The anserine bursa is located approximately 5 cm distal to the tibial joint line on the medial aspect of the tibia and somewhat posterior (bony landmark). The site for injection should be determined by palpation. The bursa is often surprisingly deep below the

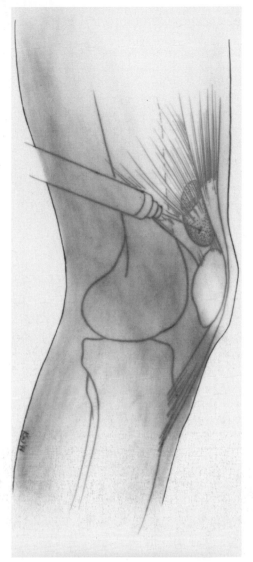

FIGURE 25–7 Palpation of the superior margin of the patella allows the operator to avoid inserting the needle between the patella and the femur.

skin, but tenderness to the tip of the needle will indicate the location of the inflamed bursa (Fig. 25–8).

THE ANKLE JOINT. The bony landmarks are the medial and lateral malleoli. A line is drawn 1 cm superior to these two structures, joining them. This line outlines the distal end of the tibia (Fig. 25–9). The patient is asked to dorsiflex the foot, and the anterior tibial and extensor communis tendons can be readily identified. The dorsalis pedis artery is beneath these structures. The operator then should select a site on either the medial or lateral aspect of the joint, so that the needle will enter beneath the landmark line at the end of the tibia, but sufficiently close to avoid the tarsal bones and tendinous structures.

THE METATARSOPHALANGEAL JOINTS. The metatarsophalangeal joints are injected from the dorsal aspect. Bony landmarks are difficult to find because of the overlying soft tissue. The patient should flex the foot, and the operator should recall that the joint is probably distal to the largest palpable part of the joint. The site chosen should

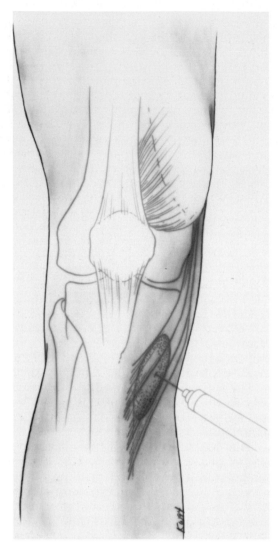

FIGURE 25-8 The anserine bursa lies medial and distal to the knee joint. An inflamed anserine bursa can often be palpated.

not be lateral or superior, but between these two planes to avoid essential structures.

MORTON'S NEUROMA. Morton's neuroma commonly occurs between the distal metatarsal bones of the second and third or third and fourth digits of the foot. The exact site can be determined by palpation of the point of maximal tenderness. The preparation is deposited through the skin of the dorsum of the foot into the tender area.

PLANTAR FASCIITIS. The inflammation occurs at the site of the attachment of the plantar fascia to the calcaneus. The exact site of inflammation may be determined by palpation. The site is approached from the plantar aspect of the foot. The injection is quite painful, and the use of fluoromethane or epidermal anesthesia may also be quite painful. Rarely does a patient ask for a second injection, although they are often quite effective. The steroid is deposited in the midline at the site of maximum tenderness.

COMPLICATIONS

A debate was held at the Heberden Society (published in 1984) concerning whether the benefits outweighed the risks of the use of IA steroids.[13] It was decided that the benefit of steroids outweighed the complications, but there are many complications which the operator should be aware of and attempt to avoid.

RARE AND UNUSUAL COMPLICATIONS. Gladman and Bombardier,[22] in 1987, reported a sickle cell crisis following IA steroid therapy for RA in two patients. Facial flushing after IA steroid injection has also been reported, but has never been observed in my experience. Gray and Gottlieb[23] reported an estimated frequency of complications following IA injections of steroids (Table 25–2).

POSTINJECTION FLARE. The postinjection flare has been clearly described by McCarty and Hogan,[40] who reproduced it by injecting mongrel dogs with various steroid preparations. The authors attributed it to the microcrystalline structure of the steroids. They and others found that prednisolone acetate and hydrocortisone acetate, but not triamcinolone acetonide, produced such flares.

PERIARTICULAR CALCIFICATIONS. Sparling et al.,[54] Gilsanz,[21] Dalinka,[14] Gerster and Fallet,[19] and McCarty[39] have all reported asymptomatic periarticular calcifications in finger joints following injections.

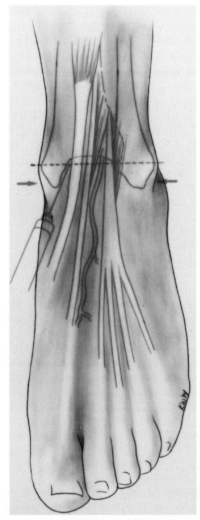

FIGURE 25-9 The medial and lateral malleoli are bony landmarks that help outline the inferior margin of the tibia or superior boundary of the tibiotalar joint.

TABLE 25–2 Prevalence of Complications Following Intra-Articular Steroid Injection

Complication	Prevalence (%)
Postinjection flare	2–5
Steroid arthropathy of weightbearing joints	0.8
Tendon rupture	<1
Facial flushing	<1
Skin changes	<1
Infection	<0.1000006
Transient paresis of injected extremity	Rare
Hypersensitivity	Rare
Asymptomatic periarticular calcification	Rare

Adapted from Gray RG, Gottlieb NL: Intra-articular corticosteroids: an updated assessment. Clin Orthop 1983; 177:235–236.

STEROID ARTHROPATHY. Following the introduction and widespread use of IA steroid injections, many authors described progression of radiological and clinical evidence of joint destruction occurring after multiple steroid injections.[20] I have seen patients who seemingly benefited greatly from IA steroid injections, with marked suppression of clinical inflammation, only to have the radiographs show a continued progression of joint destruction. Chandler and Wright[9] also described this phenomenon. It occurred in patients receiving four injections over approximately 1 year. Sweetnam et al.[59] asserted that aseptic necrosis of the hip may follow oral steroids and IA steroid injections. Steinberg et al.,[57] reported that a patient who received 22 injections into the shoulder in 24 months' time developed a Charcot-like joint. Bentley and Goodfellow[4] reported that 12 weekly injections into the left knee and 26 more weekly injections into the right knee were followed by Charcot-like disorganization of the knee joints. Further credence to the assertion of joint destruction was presented by Moskowitz and colleagues[43] who showed that triamcinolone acetonide injected into rabbit joints caused destructive changes. More recently, Parikh and colleagues[45] reported that 18 injections over a 4-month period caused a Charcot-like arthropathy of the shoulder joint.

Miller and Restifo,[41] in 1966, reviewed the literature and asserted that there was evidence to suggest that only in cases in which there had been an unusual frequency of injections could joint destruction be related to the injections. Stefanich,[55] in 1986, further reviewed this topic and agreed there was little evidence to support the concept of steroid arthropathy, other than in exceptional cases of multiple injections.

SKIN CHANGES. Skin changes may appear following intradermal, subcutaneous, or intramuscular injection of steroid preparations. Local depigmentation, scarring, and depression of the skin have been described. The hardened scar resembles a lupus skin plaque. There can be destruction of underlying hair follicles and sebaceous and sweat glands. These scars are not harmful, but certainly can be unsightly. Atrophy of the underlying subcutaneous tissues causes the scar to becomes depressed. Atrophy of underlying muscle has also been reported. Some patients feel that such atrophy on the back, shoulder areas, or hands is unsightly and highly undesirable. These complications may be avoided by using less concentrated preparations. Triamcinolone preparations may cause these complications with increased frequency.

Cassidy and Bole[8] reported skin changes in eight patients following injection of methylprednisolone acetate, triamcinolone diacetate, triamcinolone acetonide TBA, and hydrocortisone TBA. They reproduced these findings in rabbits. Dymant[16] reported skin atrophy in a 3-year-old girl following triamcinolone acetonide injection. McCarty[39] reported skin atrophy over 13 proximal interphalangeal and five metacarpophalangeal joints using triamcinolone hexacetonide. Morris[42] reported hypopigmentation and atrophy of the subcutaneous tissues following the use of triamcinolone acetonide, triamcinolone hexacetonide, and betamethasone sodium phosphate and acetate for interlesional injections of keloids. Steffey[56] reported subcutaneous gluteal atrophy following intramuscular injection of triamcinolone in 6 of 45 asthma patients, and no skin changes in 45 patients injected with methylprednisolone acetate. Abdel-Fattah[1] reported subcutaneous atrophy after injections of keloids in 8 of 144 patients following triamcinolone acetonide. Rowe[49] published a photograph of the subcutaneous atrophy which occurs with injections around the shoulder. Lemont and Hetman[36] reported linear depigmentation of the foot of a patient after IA injection of triamcinolone acetonide.

These unsightly skin lesions are said to remit after a number of years. Lund et al.[38] reported that the skin lesions improved over a period of 5 years. Their occurrence may be avoided by the selection of steroid preparation, but it is probable that they are inevitable in a small percentage of patients.

SYSTEMIC EFFECTS. IA steroids do not remain solely within the joint cavity. Serum levels can be detected shortly after injection, and suppression of the pituitary adrenal axis occurs if injections are frequently repeated. Triamcinolone hexacetonide and betamethasone sodium phosphate seem to remain within the joint cavity longer than methylprednisolone acetate, and their systemic effect is limited because of their low serum levels and release over a prolonged period of time. Aseptic necrosis and Cushing's syndrome occur concurrently with suppression of the pituitary adrenal axis if IA steroids are given frequently enough and for a prolonged period of time.[5, 15, 32, 44, 62]

TENDON RUPTURE. Ismail et al.[31] reported a patellar ligament rupture in a high jumper following injection of either hydrocortisone or triamcinolone into the area of the patellar ligament on four occasions in a 12-month period. Karpman et al.[33] reported ruptures of the extensor communis tendon of the hand, the extensor tendon of the ring finger, and the extensor tendons of the thumb and little finger, and of the long head of the biceps in four patients with RA following IA injections with prednisolone tebutate, triamcinolone hexacetonide, triamcinolone hexacetonide, and prednisolone tebutate, respectively. Although spontaneous tendon rupture can occur following trauma and RA, these rare examples illustrate a complication of IA steroids.

PHONOPHORESIS AND IONTOPHORESIS

Phonophoresis or iontophoresis has been suggested as a substitute technique for delivering adrenocorticosteroid preparations to inflamed soft tissue areas. Chantraine and colleagues[10] studied the transmission of adrenocorticosteroids by iontophoresis through cadaver skins and in the urine of rabbits after administration through shaved thighs. They found no evidence of the passage of adrenocorticosteroids through the skin. They also described 188 patients, 56% of whom said they felt better after iontophoresis of triamcinolone acetinide. They concluded that there was no evidence that iontophoresis provided transmission of adrenocorticosteroids through the skin.

Agostinucci and Powers[2] studied the effect of lidocaine hydrochloride on motor neuron excitability through the skin by iontophoresis and found that both lidocaine and placebo were effective in changing motor nerve excitability. These authors and Chantraine and co-workers concluded that electrical current may affect soft tissue inflammation and motor neuron excitability without involving the passage of any substances through the skin.

Kleinkort and Wood[35] described 285 patients with soft tissue pain and inflammation and reported a very small difference in the beneficial effect of between 1% and 10% hydrocortisone ointment with phonophoresis. They quoted Griffin and Touchstone[24, 25] who claimed hydrocortisone could penetrate 7 cm into porcine soft tissue through the skin with iontophoresis.

The actual penetration of adrenocorticosteroid beneath the skin of human subjects through the use of iontophoresis and phonophoresis has not been substantiated. It may well be that electrical current and ultrasound waves provide some analgesic or anti-inflammatory effects, however. A review by Singh and Roberts[52] is consistent with this view.

References

1. Abdel-Fattah AMA: Unusual complications of triamcinolone injected keloids: Tissue necrosis and systemic corticosteroid effects. Br J Plast Surg 1976; 29:283.
2. Agostinucci J, Powers WR: Motoneuron excitability modulation after desensitization of the skin by iontophoresis of lidocaine hydrochloride. Arch Phys Med Rehabil 1992; 73:190–104.
3. Axelrod L: Glucocorticoids. In Kelly WN, Harris ED, Ruddy S, Sledge CB (eds): Textbook of Rheumatology. Philadelphia, WB Saunders, 1993, p. 779–796.
4. Bentley G, Goodfellow JW: Disorganisation of the knees following intra-articular hydrocortisone injections. J Bone Joint Surg Br 1969; 51:498–505.
5. Bertouch JV, Meffin PJ, Sallustio BC, Brooks PM: A comparison of plasma methylprednisolone concentrations following intra-articular injection in patients with rheumatoid arthritis and osteoarthritis. Aust N Z J Med 1983; 13:538–586.
6. Blyth T, Hunter JA, Stirling A: Pain in the rheumatoid knee after steroid injection. A single-blind comparison of hydrocortisone succinate, and triamcinolone acetonide or hexacetonide. Br J Rheumatol 1994; 33:461–463.
7. Carlsson A, Lindmark B, Marsal L: Intra-articular steroids—an alternative to knee synovectomy in rheumatoid arthritis? Scand J Rheumatol 1984; 13:375–378.
8. Cassidy JJ, Bole GG: Cutaneous atrophy secondary to intra-articular corticosteroid administration. Ann Intern Med 1966; 65:1008–1018.
9. Chandler GN, Wright V: Deleterious effect of intra-articular hydrocortisone. Lancet 1958; 27:661–663.
10. Chantraine A, Ludy JP, Berger D: Is cortisone iontophoresis possible? Arch Phys Med Rehabil 1986; 67:38–40.
11. Chakravarty K, Pharoah PDP, Scott DGI: A randomized controlled study of post-injection rest following intra-articular steroid therapy for knee synovitis. Br J Rheumatol 1994; 33:464–468.
12. Chatham W, Williams G, Moreland L, et al: Intraarticular corticosteroid injections: Should we rest the joints? Arthritis Care Res 1989; 2:70–74.
13. Correspondent, Heberden Society: Intra-articular steroids. Lancet 1984; 1:385.
14. Dalinka MK, Stewart V, Bomalaski JS, et al: Periarticular calcifications in association with intra-articular corticosteroid injections. Radiology 1984; 153:615–618.
15. Derendorf H, Möllmann H, Grüner A, et al: Pharmacokinetics and pharmacodynamics of glucocorticoid suspensions after intra-articular administration. Clin Pharmacol Ther 1986; 19:313–317.
16. Dyment PG: Local atrophy following triamcinolone injection. Pediatrics 1970; 46:136–137.
17. Flanagan J, Casale FF, Thomas TL, Desai KB: Intra-articular injection for pain relief in patients awaiting hip replacement. Ann R Coll Surg Engl 1988; 70:156–157.
18. Geborek P, Månsson B, Wollheim FA, Moritz U: Intraarticular corticosteroid injection into rheumatoid arthritis knees improves extensor muscles strength. Rheumatol Int 1990; 9:265–270.
19. Gerster JC, Fallet GH: Periarticular hand hydrozyapatite deposition after corticosteroid injections. J Rheumatol 1987; 154:1156–1159.
20. Gigia PP, Brown M, Al-Obaidi S: Hydrocortisone and exercise effects on articular cartilage in rats. Arch Phys Med Rehabil 1993; 74:463–467.
21. Gilsanz V, Bernstein BH: Joint calcification following intra-articular corticosteroid therapy. Radiology 1984; 151:647–649.
22. Gladman DD, Bombardier C: Sickle cell crisis following intraarticular steroid therapy for rheumatoid arthritis. Arthritis Rheum 1987; 30:1065–1068.
23. Gray RG, Gottlieb NL: Intra-articular corticosteroids: An updated assessment. Clin Orthop 1983; 177:235–263.
24. Griffin JE, Touchstone JC: Ultrasonic movement of cortisol into pig tissue: I. Movement into skeletal muscle. Am J Phys Med 1963; 42:77–85.
25. Griffin JE, Touchstone JC: Ultrasonic movement of cortisol into pig tissue: II. Movement into paravertebral nerve. Am J Phys Med 1965; 44:20–25.
26. Hasselbacker P: Synovial fluid analysis. In Utsinger PD, Zvaifler NJ, Ehrlich GE (eds): Rheumatoid Arthritis. Philadelphia, JB Lippincott, 1985, pp 194–196.
27. Hendrix RW, Lin P-J P, Kane WJ: Simplified aspiration or injection technique for the sacro-iliac joint. J Bone Joint Surg Am 1982; 64:1249–1252.
28. Hollander JL: Intrasynovial corticosteroid therapy in arthritis. M Med J 1970; 19:62–66.
29. Hollander JL, Brown EM Jr, Jessar RA, Brown CY: Hydrocortisone and cortisone injected into arthritic joints. JAMA 1951; 147:1629–1635.
30. Intra-articular steroids, letter. Lancet 1984; 1:385.
31. Ismail AM, Balakrishnan R, Rajakumar MK: Rupture of patellar ligament after steroid infiltration. J Bone Joint Surg Br 1969; 51:503–505.
32. Jarratt MT, Spark RF, Arndt KA: The effects of intradermal steroids on the pituitary-adrenal axis and the skin. J Invest Dermatol 1974; 62:463–466.
33. Karpman RR, McComb JE, Volz RC: Tendon rupture following local steroid injection. Steroid Injection 1980; 68:169–176.
34. Kerolus G, Clayburne G, Schumacher HR Jr: Is it mandatory to examine synovial fluids promptly after arthrocentesis? Arthritis Rheum 1989; 32:271–278.
35. Kleinkort JA, Wood F: Phonophoresis with 1 percent versus 10 percent hydrocortisone. Phys Ther 1975; 55:1320–1324.
36. Lemont H, Hetman J: Cutaneous foot depigmentation following an intra-articular steroid injection. J Podiatr Med Assoc 1991; 81:606–607.
37. Leversee JH: Aspiration of joints and soft tissue injections. Primary Care 1986; 13:579–599.
38. Lund EM, Donde R, Knudsen EA: Persistent local cutaneous atrophy following corticosteroid injection for tendinitis. Rheum Rehabil 1979; 18:91–93.
39. McCarty DJ: Treatment of rheumatoid joint inflammation with triamcinolone hexacetonide. Arthritis Rheum 1972; 15:157–173.
40. McCarty DJ Jr, Hogan JM: Inflammatory reaction after intrasynovial injection of microcrystalline adrenocorticosteroid esters. Arthritis Rheum 1964; 7:359–367.
41. Miller WT, Restifo RA: Steroid arthropathy. Radiology 1966; 86:652–657.
42. Morris WJ: Undesirable side effects following intralesional corticosteroid therapy. West J Med 1972; 116:55.

43. Moskowitz RW, Davis W, Sammarco J, et al: Experimentally induced corticosteroid arthropathy. Arthritis Rheum 1970; 13:236–243.

44. O'Sullivan MM, Runfeld WR, Jones MK, Williams BD: Cushing's syndrome with suppression of the hypothalamic-pituitary-adrenal axis after intra-articular steroid injections. Ann Rheum Dis 1985; 44:561–563.

45. Parikh J, Houpt JB, Jacobs S, Fernandes BJ: Charcot's arthropathy of the shoulder following intraarticular corticosteroid injections. J Rheumatol 1993; 20:885–887.

46. Pelletier J-P, Martel-Pelletier J: The therapeutic effects of NSAID and corticosteroids in osteoarthritis: To be or not to be. J Rheumatol 1989; 16:266–269.

47. Pfenninger JL: Injections of joints and soft tissue: Part I. General guidelines. Am Fam Physician 1991; 44:1196–1202.

48. Pfenninger JL: Injections of joints and soft tissue: Part II. Guidelines for specific joints. Am Fam Physician 1991; 44:1690–1701.

49. Rowe CR: Injection technique for the shoulder and elbow. Orthop Clin North Am 1988; 19:773–777.

50. Samuelson CO Jr, Cannon GW, Ward JR: Arthrocentesis. J Fam Pract 1985; 20:179–184.

51. Shmerling RH, Delbanco TL, Tosteson ANA, Trentham DE: Synovial fluid tests. What should be ordered? JAMA 1990; 264:1009–1014.

52. Singh J, Roberts MS: Transdermal delivery of drugs by iontophoresis: A review. Drug Des Deliv 1989; 4:1–12.

53. Smith RW, Campbell MJ, O'Connell S, Cawley MID: Methods of skin preparation prior to intra-articular injection. Br J Rheumatol 1993; 32:648.

54. Sparling M, Malleson P, Wood B, Petty R: Radiographic followup of joints injected with triamcinolone hexacetonide for the management of childhood arthritis. Arthritis Rheum 1990; 33:826.

55. Stefanich RJ: Intraarticular corticosteroid in treatment of osteoarthritis. Orthop Rev 1986; 15:27–33.

56. Steffey JM: Subcutaneous atrophy following intramuscular administration of triamcinalone acetonide. Am J Dis Child 1973; 126:561–562.

57. Steinberg CLR, Duthie RB, Piva AE: Charcot-like arthropathy following intra-articular hydrocortisone. JAMA 1962; 181:145–148.

58. Stolzer BL, Eisenbeis CH Jr, Barr JH Jr, et al: Intra-articular injections of adrenocorticosteroids in patients with arthritis. Pa Med 1962; August:911–914.

59. Sweetnam DR, Mason RM, Murray RO: Steroid arthropathy of the hip. Br Med J 1960; 1:1392–1394.

60. Thorn GW: Personal communication to Joseph Lee Hollander, nd.

61. Weiss MM: Corticosteroids in rheumatoid arthritis. Semin Arthritis Rheumat 1989; 19:9–21.

62. Weiss S, Kisch ES, Fischel B: Systemic effects of intraarticular administration of triamcinolone hexacetonide. Isr J Med Sci 1983; 19:83–84.

63. Zuckerman JD, Meislin RJ, Rothberg M: Injections for joint and soft tissue disorders: When and how to use them. Geriatrics 1990; 45:45–55.

Achieving Functional Independence

CRISTINA M. MIX, O.T.R., AND
DONNA PIEPER SPECHT, P.T.

Functional independence refers to the ability to perform daily living skills without help. Independence has been described as freedom from the influence, control, or determination of another or others. Being independent includes performance of living tasks which occupy time in a manner customary to that person's sex, age, and culture.[25] Everyone, whether disabled or not, must regularly carry out certain tasks or activities to live and participate in society.[4] These activities include tasks of self-maintenance, mobility, communication, home management, leisure skills, and school, work, and play skills.[19] If a person fails to achieve functional independence in any one of these activities, the person cannot be self-sufficient and will need assistance from another person to meet daily living needs. Such dependence can affect whether the person can work, live in his or her own home, and travel.[4]

Minimizing a person's dependence on assistance from others is one of rehabilitation's most cherished goals.[11] Dependence can have a major impact on a person's quality of life. Quality of life includes those activities that a person enjoys and values as a meaningful part of life. The foundations of independent living skills begin in infancy and are refined, with nurturing, time, and opportunity, through various stages of development and mastery until functional independence is achieved. Attainment of independent living skills is generally believed to be critical to the development of a positive self-image[20] which is enhanced by the person's participation in productive and enjoyable activities.

Health professionals need to be sensitive to what persons consider to be meaningful in their lives. Everyone has goals and aspirations to fulfill during life. As health professionals, we are instrumental in assisting people whose physical or mental challenges interfere with achieving their goals. Ways in which we assist others to meet their goals include restoration of the components of function, education of patient and family in compensatory techniques, and instruction in the use of adaptive equipment.[12]

The family plays a leading role in the lives of practically all of us. In the process of assisting people, we need to include families and significant others who play a main role in the person's life. Family-centered care is a name given to the philosophies, attitudes, and approaches to care for persons with special needs and their families.[10] Family-centered care refers to a relationship between the person, family, and health care professional that places a specific emphasis on responding to the person's and family's priorities and goals.[5] Family-centered care supports families by building on the unique strengths of the family and on the strengths of individual family members. Families differ in the strategies they use to reach for their dreams; there is no single approach that is right for all families. Health professionals must respect this diversity.[10]

Some key elements in family-centered care include recognizing family strengths and individuality and respecting different methods of coping, facilitating family and professional collaboration at all levels of healthcare, and sharing complete and unbiased information with families on a continuing basis and in a supportive manner. These elements also include designing accessible healthcare systems that are flexible, culturally competent, and responsive to family-identified needs.[10] A family- or person-centered philosophy encourages and respects family involvement in decisions made for individual family members. Family members play an important role in the evaluation process, treatment program, and advocacy for the person in need of rehabilitation services.

EVALUATION

Evaluation of performance skills identifies impairments that interfere with a person achieving the goals of functional independence. Evaluation includes assessment of the patient's abilities and limitations in school, work, play,

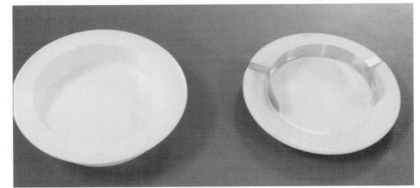

FIGURE 26–1 Scoop dish and plate with plate guard are used by pushing food against rim to scoop; it also aids as a guide.

leisure activities, mobility, self-care, and home maintenance.[19] Multiple evaluation tools and assessments exist which assist in identifying a person's abilities and limitations.

The evaluation begins with an interview with patient and family to identify the person's interests, premorbid status, and current perception of impairment. Within the evaluation, component areas of involvement which can interfere with function are assessed. These component areas include assessment of range of motion (ROM), strength, tone, sensation, balance and coordination, visual perception, and cognition. Direct observation of functional activities ensures accuracy and shows which areas of limitations are problematic.[4] Throughout the treatment phase of rehabilitation, it is important to measure patient progress according to functional outcome, which provides information of rehabilitation effectiveness, rehabilitation progress, and program efficiency. Many outcome-oriented scales exist such as the Children's Hospital Rehabilitation Independence Scale (CHRIS)[7] which is specific to pediatrics and is used at The Children's Hospital in Denver, Colorado; the Rehabilitation Institute of Chicago Functional Assessment Scale (RICFAS)[13]; and the Functional Independence Measure (FIM).[22] Centers choose the scale appropriate to their needs.

This chapter reviews the general principles involved in developing functional independent living skills underlying self-maintenance, mobility, communication, home management, leisure skills, and occupational activities. Suggested uses of adaptations and modifications to allow functional independence are included.

SELF-MAINTENANCE

Basic self-maintenance activities include feeding, upper and lower extremity dressing, and grooming and hygiene.

Feeding

The process of self-feeding involves adequate ROM, and coordination and strength sufficient to scoop and bring the hand to the mouth from a surface while grasping a utensil or cup. When coordination is difficult, stabilization of dishes may be needed and obtained from the use of nonskid mats such as Dycem. Commercially available scoop dishes or plate guards (Fig. 26–1) assist a person with functional use of one hand in stabilizing food against the raised side while scooping food. Weighted utensils and cups and swivel utensils may aid when hand control is limited. A rocker knife can help when bilateral upper extremity motor skills are impaired as with involvement such as hemiplegia. A rocker knife is used by pushing the knife down into food and rocking the knife until the food is cut. This avoids the traditional sliding method while stabilizing the food with a fork in the opposite hand (Fig. 26–2).

When grasp is weak or absent, a variety of adapted and built-up utensils, use of utensil cuffs, or a splint with utensil slots, lightweight cups or cups with handles make grasping a cup or utensil easier. A common way to build up handles includes the use of built-up foam placed over the utensil. The foam is round with a hole in the center, and comes in various widths to conform to the palm and grip (Fig. 26–3). Utensils such as knives can also be

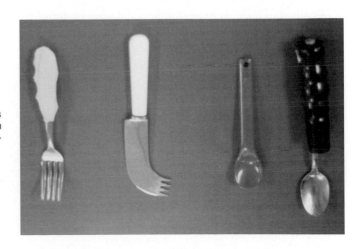

FIGURE 26–2 Adapted utensils from *left* to *right*: weighted utensils used by a person with decreased stability. Rocker knife used by an individual with functional use of one hand; spoon with plastic shallow bowl; custom made handle made of putty.

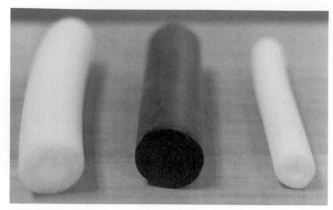

FIGURE 26–3 Built-up foam used to build up various handles (e.g., utensils, writing tools) when grasp is limited.

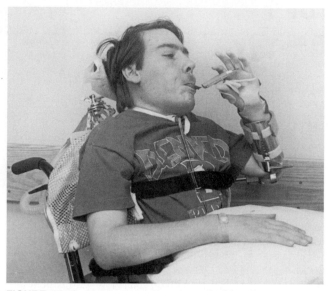

FIGURE 26–4 Mobile arm support used with a long opponens splint and vertical holder to aid in feeding: mobile arm supports and upper extremity function when shoulder or forearm strength is weak. The subject also has a long opponens splint with a utensil and a vertical holder for a spoon for feeding.

adapted with the use of orthotic material by fabricating a custom-made palmar cuff. The knife is attached to the cuffs facing down near the ulnar border of the hand with orthotic material. A sheath for the knife is often fabricated for safety when storing. Many kinds of adapted knives are also commercially available.

If ROM is limited for hand-to-mouth activity, use of long straws for drinking, long-handled and curved utensils, a sandwich holder, or use of mobile arm support or suspension slings can help (Fig. 26–4). A mobile arm support is a system which supports the forearm while assisting and maximizing motions such as shoulder flexion and extension, horizontal abduction and adduction, external and internal rotation, and elbow flexion and extension when muscle weakness exists. A person should exhibit some functional upper extremity movement in the gravity-eliminated planes mentioned above with strength in upper extremities of at least trace (Tr+) to poor (P−) for the mobile arm support to be used successfully. Electrical and mechanical feeders and elevated spoon and plate setups are also available for those persons with moderate to severe physical limitations who want to achieve independence in feeding.

Adequate oral motor skills such as sucking, lip closure to utensil, and tongue mobility are necessary for eating. Oral motor skills can be facilitated by a variety of feeding tools, such as various nipples for children when bottle-drinking, spoons made of sturdy plastic with a shallow bowl, and cups with nose cutouts or spouts (Fig. 26–5). It is important to have an optimal functional position for self-feeding and oral intake.

Dressing

Dressing involves putting on and taking off clothing, along with managing fasteners (i.e., buttons, zippers, snaps) and handling accessories such as belts and shoes. The person's usual clothing should be used when evaluating and performing dress training. Dressing requires adequate active ROM, coordination, strength, and gross mobility skills (i.e., rolling, trunk control, and sitting balance).

Frequently used modifications that allow one to perform independent dressing when limitations are present may be as simple as avoiding clothes with many fasteners or choosing loose clothing (i.e., pullover shirts and dresses, pants and shorts with elastic waistbands, no elastic at cuffs). Use of clothes with larger buttons can assist those with limited dexterity. To manage fasteners when fine motor skills are weak, button aids, zipper pulls, elastic shoelaces and Velcro are available. A button aid consists of a wire loop which hooks around the button and is then pulled through the hole. It works especially well for those with reduced manipulation and bilateral motor skills. Zipper pulls can be as simple as a loop tied to the zipper or a wire hook used to pull the zipper up. It is used primarily by those with limited

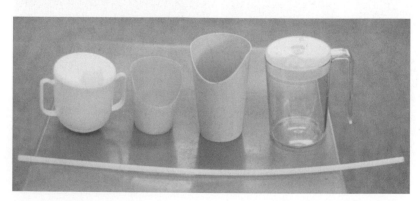

FIGURE 26–5 Various cups to assist with oral control. *Left* to *right:* tippy cup, small and large nose cut-out cup, and cup with handle and spout.

prehension. Elastic shoelaces are used similarly to regularly used cloth laces except the laces do not need to be untied or retied each time. The laces stretch as a person places the foot in the shoe, adapting to the shoe (Fig. 26–6). Although modified clothing is now commercially available, simple modifications can be made such as loops on socks to assist in pulling up when hand strength is limited, Velcro openings on pants to facilitate ease when toileting, and labeling clothes to identify front from back when perceptual or cognitive problems exist.

When reach and mobility is limited, commercially available reachers assist in retrieving items of clothing. A reacher consists of an extended stick, usually made of lightweight aluminum, with a grasping unit at the end. It is operated by squeezing the handle which activates the gripper position to open and close. Reachers come in many lengths and handle types to adapt to a person's ability to grasp (Fig. 26–7). A variety of dressing sticks, which are long sticks with a hook at the end, aid in pulling up clothing such as pants and socks. Stocking aids consist of a part that holds a sock open and is pulled up the leg via a rope attached (Fig. 26–8). The rope is long enough to reach up to the person's lap which reduces bending at the hips.

When providing recommendations for adapted dressing modifications or equipment, it is important to consider developmental age, cognitive abilities, motivation to use the equipment, and its potential to allow or impede independence (Fig. 26–9).

Grooming and Hygiene

In order to perform hygiene and grooming skills, a person must have adequate grasp to maintain a hold on appropriate tools, adequate active ROM to reach all areas of the head and body, bilateral hand function, fine and gross motor coordination, strength, trunk control, and sitting balance (Fig. 26–10).

When hand function is limited because of decreased strength or ROM, several adaptations can be used to enhance function. A utensil cuff is a palmar strap with a slot located at the palm where small items can be placed and stabilized, for example, a toothbrush. The cuffs are commercially available or can be fabricated from orthotic material or webbing. Built-up foam and Velcro straps may be used in conjunction with the toothbrush. A razor or electric

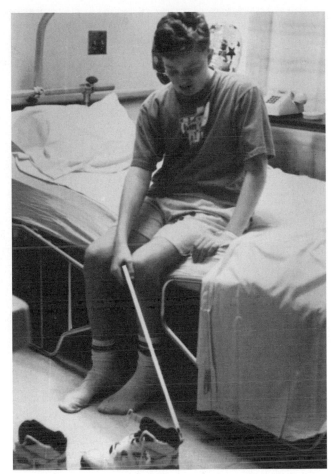

FIGURE 26–7 Reacher used to assist in picking up objects from floor. A reacher aids persons with limited lower extremity and upper extremity mobility. It is operated by squeezing the handle, which opens the tongs. The handle is released to maintain grasp.

shaver, electric toothbrushes, and Water Piks can greatly assist those with limited strength and endurance. Soap-on-a-rope and wash mitts, which hold the soap inside the mitt, assist with washing the face; a suction brush attached to the sink will aid with nail and denture care when bilateral hand function is limited; and an attachment of nail clipper and emery board to a board with Dycem or suction cups on the back may compensate for the strength necessary to pinch or hold a clipper.[8]

The adaptations discussed consider weak hand strength and incoordination. When shoulder strength is weak, long handles added to grooming tools such as brushes or combs can aid in reach. A mobile arm support or balanced forearm orthosis can also be used to allow one to work in reduced antigravity planes, maximizing motion to perform activities.

Bowel and Bladder

An important factor of hygiene is bowel and bladder care. Skills necessary to perform bowel and bladder care include having adequate upper extremity ROM, hand function, mobility, endurance, and ability to manage clothes. Therapists work closely with the patient, family, and nurses to discuss possible adaptations and positioning to allow the

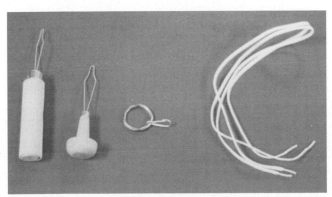

FIGURE 26–6 Fastener adaptions, *left* to *right*: button aid, knob handle button aid, zipper pull, and elastic laces.

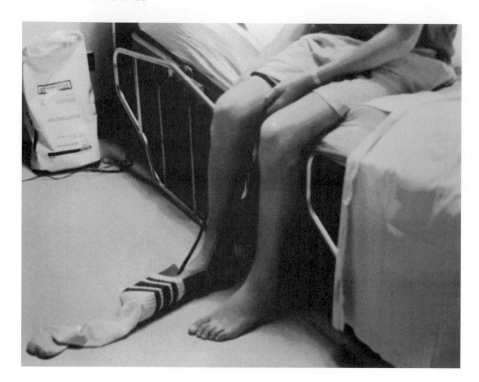

FIGURE 26–8 Stocking aid used when a person is limited in reaching down to the feet or when lower extremity mobility limits bringing the foot near to the hands. A person places stocking over sock holder, places the holder in front of foot, and pulls at rope to pull up.

patient to perform this care. Reaching aids that hold toilet tissue are available when ability to reach for dressing is impaired. Aids exist to help the patient perform bowel and bladder management. Various commode chairs, raised toilet seats, and potty chairs can be used when standard toilets make toileting difficult. Dynamic splints or catheter inserters can aid in performing catheterization. For the female, labia spreaders may aid in positioning while performing catheterization. For those using leg bags, various adapted leg bag emptiers and catheter clamps are available along with modified strapping for urinary drainage bags. Adapted

condom catheter holders can be used to secure condom catheters. Bowel care may require use of adapted suppository inserters or digital stimulators to aid those with weak hand strength or with incoordination.[14] Bowel and bladder care is discussed in detail in Chapter 28.

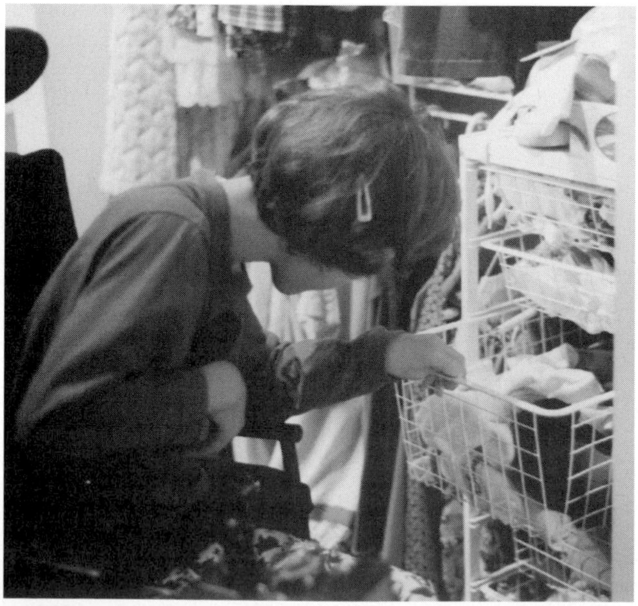

Skin Management

Another aspect of care is skin management, especially for those with absent or reduced sensation. A long-handled mirror allows one to personally perform skin inspection. Specialized timers provide an auditory reminder to perform weight shifts to assist in preventing pressure sores. The timer is placed underneath the wheelchair and beeps every 15 minutes to remind a person to perform a pressure relief.

Menstrual Care

Menstrual care can also require the use of a dynamic splint to allow handling and adequate placement of hygiene products when prehension is weak.

Bathing

Bathing can often be a complex activity since it requires that a person perform gross motor mobility skills in an environment that can be dangerous (i.e., slippery). In addition, in order to bathe, one must have adequate active ROM, fine motor coordination, and sitting balance.

Environmental adaptations that assist with bathing and safety include placement of grab bars outside and inside the bathing area, placement of nonskid strips inside the tub, provision of a handheld shower head, and automatic water temperature controls. A variety of bath chairs are available for those whose mobility and balance are impaired. The bath chairs vary depending on the person's size and motor abilities (e.g., bath ring is used for a small

FIGURE 26–9 Commercially available closet organizer with mesh basket drawers allows a person with limited hand function to easily open and close drawers.

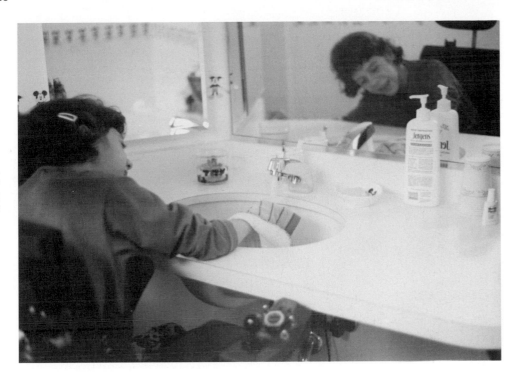

FIGURE 26–10 Sink with infrared sensor for easily turning water on and off when performing grooming and hygiene activities at the sink.

child). A wheelchair commode or shower chair is recommended for those who have a roll-in shower. Other equipment or modifications to assist those with limited reach or grasp can include a bath mitt, a long-handled brush with soap holder (including a loop or built-up handle if grasp is impaired), soap-on-a-rope, pump dispensers for shampoo, and finger ring brushes for scrubbing the hair. For those who have severe physical difficulties, inflatable bed baths and shampoo trays are available.

MOBILITY

Functional mobility is the ability to move from one position in space (whether sitting, lying down, standing, etc.) to another position in space no matter the distance between starting and ending point.[4] Functional mobility includes bed mobility, transfers, ambulation, wheelchair mobility, and driving.

Bed Mobility

Bed mobility includes rolling in bed; scooting up, down, or toward either edge of the bed; and coming to a sitting position at the edge of the bed. In order to be independent in bed mobility, a person must be able to get into bed, position or reposition oneself in bed to sleep, and get out of bed without the assistance of another person. Good head control, as well as upper extremity strength and endurance, is needed to accomplish bed mobility independently. Motor planning skills are also important for efficient and timely mobility.

Bed mobility can be a challenging and exhausting feat, depending on the person's physical or mental limitations. Some adaptations that facilitate bed mobility in terms of time efficiency and energy conservation include loops attached along the edge of the bed or bed railings. These

can help a person who has inadequate trunk strength to use the upper extremities to pull himself or herself to either side when rolling. An overhead trapeze bar can aid a person in coming to sit at the edge of the bed or help to scoot up or down in bed. A step stool placed on the floor at the edge of the bed may facilitate a person's independence when getting into and out of bed. An electric bed can raise or lower the head of the bed and assist a person in coming to sit at the edge of the bed or for positioning for sitting in bed. Electric beds, however, are most often used to raise the height of the bed to an appropriate level so care can be given without back injury to the caregiver.

Transfers

A transfer is the act of moving from one position in space a short distance to another position. Transfer ability is necessary for persons who use a wheelchair for mobility or who need to move from a sitting position on one piece of equipment or furniture to another. In order for a person to be independent in daily living tasks, independent transfers must be performed to wheelchair, bed, commode, tub, and car if a van is not adapted for the wheelchair. Children must learn to transfer from the wheelchair to the floor in order to participate in activities with other children. It is desirable that wheelchair users be adept at wheelchair-to-floor and floor-to-wheelchair transfers in case of a fall. (Sometimes a small bench can be used as an intermediate step to go halfway between the floor and the wheelchair seat.) There are many different ways in which a person can perform a transfer. Depending on the functional limitations, certain transfers can be faster and more efficient than others and might change as the person's abilities change. Some of the common methods of performing transfers are described below.

STAND-PIVOT TRANSFER. For persons who can attain and maintain standing for a short period of time, the stand-

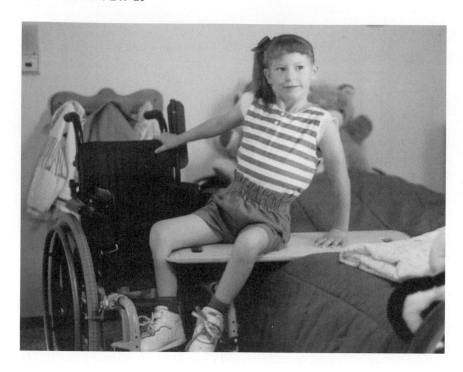

FIGURE 26–11 Sliding board transfer: the sliding board bridges the gap between the wheelchair and bed. The person uses upper extremities to scoot across the surface from the wheelchair to the bed.

pivot transfer can be the most efficient method. Adequate hip and knee extension and good sitting balance are required. In this transfer, the person rises from a seated to a standing position and pivots to the adjacent chair to sit down. A modification is the sit-pivot transfer where the person relies on good upper extremity strength and short sitting balance to push the buttocks up and lift across to another chair without coming to a standing position. The feet are usually positioned on the floor, but if the legs are too short to reach the floor, as with children, they can remain positioned on the footrests of the wheelchair or on a step stool.

SLIDING BOARD TRANSFER. Sliding boards bridge the gap between transferring surfaces.[18] The sliding board

must be positioned securely under the buttocks of the person and placed solidly on the opposite surface. Once the board is positioned securely between the surfaces, the person scoots the buttocks across the board to the new surface (Fig. 26–11). As with the sit-pivot transfer, the feet may be positioned on the floor or remain on the footrests of the wheelchair. Sliding boards are available in many shapes and sizes, and adaptations can be added according to a person's individual situation.

WHEELCHAIR-TO-FLOOR TRANSFERS. There are a variety of ways in which a person may transfer from the wheelchair to the floor. Using the forward method, the person moves the footrests to the side, and places the feet on the floor. Then the person leans forward in the wheel-

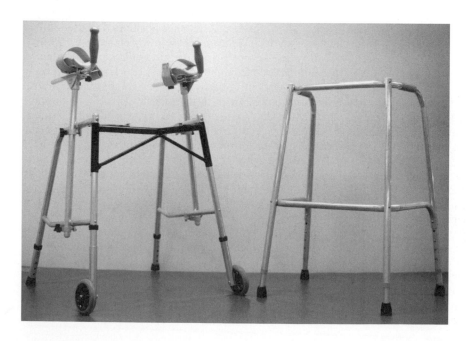

FIGURE 26–12 *Left* to *right:* rolling walker with platform attachments for a person with limited upper extremity strength and range of motion. The person's forearms rest on the pads and accept the person's weight as the lower extremities take "steps." The wheels allow the walker to be pushed forward without having to lift the walker. Standard walker: The person must have significant hand strength and range of motion to grip the walker, as well as good standing balance and upper extremity strength to lift the walker to advance it forward.

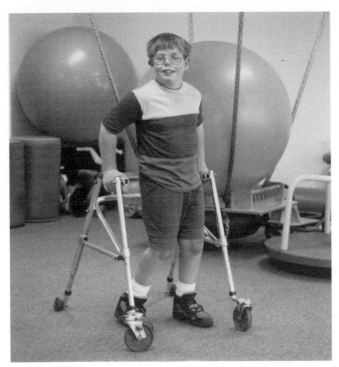

FIGURE 26–13 Reverse walker is used to facilitate extension posture with a person who tends to maintain a flexed posture while standing.

chair, places the hands on the floor, then slowly lowers himself or herself to the floor.

Pivoting to the floor is another method. With the footrests removed or placed to the side, the person scoots to the edge of the wheelchair and pivots the hips so that he or she is sitting on only one side. The hands are placed on the seat of the wheelchair. Using the upper extremities, the body is pivoted out of the wheelchair and lowered to the floor, landing in a kneeling position facing the wheelchair. The person can then lower the buttocks into a side-sitting position.

Another method of transferring from the wheelchair to the floor is used when long leg braces are worn. The person removes the footrests or swings them to the side, scoots the buttocks to the edge of the wheelchair, and extends the knees with the heels placed on the floor. Then, placing the hands on the forwardmost frame of the wheelchair, the person lowers the buttocks to the floor. This method requires good upper extremity strength and long arms for leverage to lower oneself in a controlled manner the entire distance to the floor. Children's wheelchairs, with a lower floor-to-seat height, aid in this type of transfer; however, the height of the wheelchair often is still too high for a child to perform this method of transfer.

The last two methods can be reversed to transfer from the floor back into the wheelchair. The last method is more difficult, since good upper extremity strength and leverage are important for success.

Ambulation

A person's level of functional independence can be affected by ability to ambulate. In order to ambulate, a person must have sufficient lower extremity and trunk strength, balance, coordination, and cognitive skills for safety and timing (see Chapter 5 for a discussion of gait analysis). If limitations exist in these areas, physical compensations, orthoses, and other assistive ambulation devices can be used individually or in combination to help a person be independent with ambulation.

Many physical compensations (e.g., locking the knee during the stance phase of gait, abducting the leg during the swing-through phase, or with the foot flat instead of heel-strike at initial contact) are neither energy- nor time-efficient and can be minimized through therapy programs and use of orthoses and assistive ambulation devices. There are many orthoses available to support various joints of the lower extremity that also help one to compensate for physical limitations. Chapter 17 describes the variety of lower limb orthoses that are available. It is important to remember that in order to be independent, a person must also be able to don and doff their orthotic devices.

There are a tremendous variety of assistive gait devices. In general, walkers provide the most stability and are prescribed for persons with more significantly decreased balance, coordination, or strength. Crutches provide moderate stability and canes provide the least stability. Careful assessment of a person's function allows the recommendation of the device that maximizes function and best meets the person's needs.

Figures 26–12 to 26–15 show some examples of assistive ambulation devices.

Wheelchair Mobility

For people who are unable to ambulate or are able to ambulate only short distances, using a wheelchair for mo-

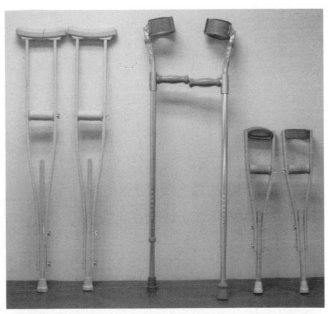

FIGURE 26–14 *Left* to *right:* axillary crutches used by individuals with good balance and coordination; length of time crutches are required is usually short. Forearm crutches have a cuff around the forearm that is open at the front or side, and are used mostly by individuals needing crutches on a long-term basis (e.g., individual with paraplegia who may require bracing with ambulation). Kenney crutches are used mostly by children who need total contact around their forearm.

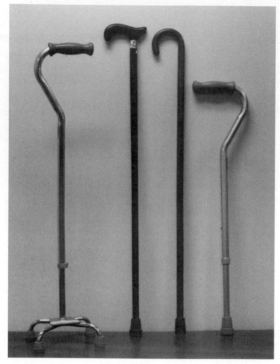

FIGURE 26–15 *Left* to *right:* quad cane and various standard canes used by individuals who need minimal assistance for balance during ambulation and who may or may not have limited use of one upper extremity. The quad cane provides more stability due to the four prongs at the base.

bility can still allow functional independence in the community. Proper positioning in the wheelchair, good sitting tolerance, strength, endurance, and cognitive skills are necessary for efficient and safe mobility in a wheelchair.

Proper positioning in the wheelchair (described in Chapter 19) helps a person to be more alert, increases comfort in, and tolerance of, the wheelchair, and allows for more efficient use of the upper extremities to propel the wheelchair or other switch access site to activate a power wheelchair. In order to propel a manual wheelchair, a person must have sufficient strength in at least one upper extremity (e.g., a person with hemiplegia operating a one-arm-drive wheelchair) or in bilateral upper extremities (e.g., a person with paraplegia) (Fig. 26–16). Lighter-weight wheelchairs, such as sports models, are easier to propel and maneuver over a variety of surfaces such as grass, curbs, and thick carpeting (Fig. 26–17). Adaptations such as lateral trunk supports for balance or quad pegs to the rims of wheels for a person with decreased hand function increase the weight of the wheelchair but are sometimes necessary to enhance a person's independence with wheelchair mobility.

As a result of advances in technology, even persons with significant limitations in upper and lower extremity function might still be able to be independent in wheelchair mobility. There are many ways to access a power wheelchair. Some examples include using a straw (sip-and-puff), proportional head controller, separate switches for directions, and joysticks. A person must understand the concepts of mobility in order to safely and efficiently drive a power wheelchair. Children as young as 2½ to 3 years old can be taught to safely operate a power wheelchair.[9] Physical and occupational therapists are an integral part of the team in helping a person decide on the best type of wheelchair to meet his or her positioning and mobility needs.

Driving

Transportation is an important aspect of a person's functional independence. Persons who are unable to drive must rely on others or on the public transportation system for transportation. All people must be properly restrained in the seat of a car, wheelchair, or in a car seat in the case of children. Harness systems can be used for people who need added trunk support.

Many people with physical limitations can drive with adaptations to the vehicle. Hand controls for driving and braking accommodate for diminished upper extremity strength. Levers and knobs can be attached to the controls for optimal function. Adaptations also vary depending on whether the person will be driving from the wheelchair or from a captain's chair in the van. Electric lifts and wheelchair tie-down systems are available for vans. Portable ramps can be used when there is a large step to enter the vehicle. Assistance can be required to set the ramp up, supervise the stability of the ramp, and for maneuvering up the ramp if strength is wanting. If a person is able to transfer from the wheelchair to the seat of the car, the wheelchair can be loaded into the back seat or onto an electric cartop carrier.

Companies that specialize in custom van modifications for disabled persons and some car dealerships can provide information regarding the latest modifications available.

COMMUNICATION

Often, patients are limited in their choice of nonverbal communication tools (i.e., writing, typing, computer, phone use, and book). The use of communication tools requires adequate fine motor strength, coordination, reach, and grasp to use the device.

Adaptations for writing tools can vary from use of built-up foam, cuffs, or mouthsticks with pens or pencils, hand splints and writing devices that support and compensate for weak hand musculature while positioning and holding the writing tool, and weighted pens for controlling coordination of movement for writing. Figures 26–18, 26–19, and 26–20 show some adaptations for writing tools. Bookholders, page turners, mouthsticks, or a head stick can help in handling books.

Typing either on a typewriter or computer can be performed by the use of typing sticks with adapted handles, splints with a slot for a typing stick (e.g., a vertical holder, pointer mouthstick, or head pointer). If coordination is impaired, keyguards and a key latch can facilitate accuracy. Alternative keyboards are also available such as the expanded keyboard or a small keyboard. Adapted switches (i.e., single-switch or sip-and-puff) can also be added for the use of a computer. Armrests, mobile arm supports, or overhead slings can be used for typing if arm strength and endurance are limited. For phone use, a telephone clip holder, dialing stick, a speaker phone with a quick dial feature, and a gooseneck to hold the receiver are available.

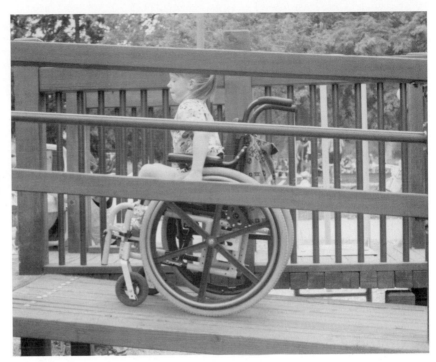

FIGURE 26–16 Good upper extremity strength is needed for self-propelling a wheelchair up a ramp.

Environmental control units and technology aids are discussed in Chapter 24.

HOME MANAGEMENT

Home management involves cooking, cleaning, and safely and appropriately using tools and appliances. Before providing recommendations it is important that the thera-pist assess the individual performing homemaking activities to determine which activities can be done safely with or without adaptations (Fig. 26–21).

It is important to educate and train the individual in energy conservation and work simplification techniques for incorporation into home management activities that the person will be returning to or is currently performing.

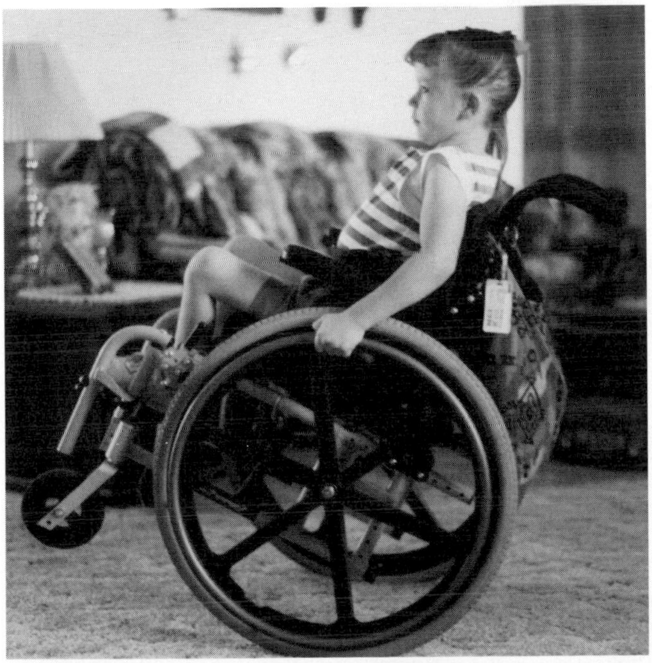

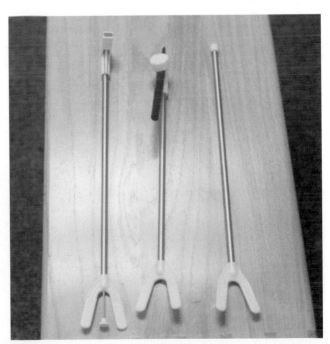

FIGURE 26–17 Demonstration of "wheelie" for ease in wheelchair mobility over obstacles or through rough terrain, such as grass or thick carpeting.

FIGURE 26–18 Various mouthsticks are used to perform different functions. *Left* to *right:* pincer mouthstick used by pushing tongue forward onto center piece, which then opens up the distal end to pick up light objects. Middle mouthstick holds writing tools from pencil to crayon. Pointer mouthstick used for turning pages and pushing forward.

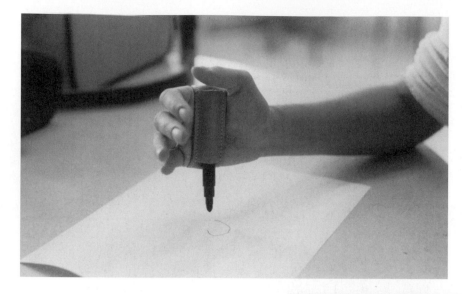

FIGURE 26–19 Utensil cuff holding a writing tool fits over the hand. It can also hold other tools such as feeding utensils and grooming tools.

FIGURE 26–20 Built-up handle made out of setting putty was conformed to person's grasp to facilitate functional tripod grasp for writing. Modifications can vary from application of foam to commercially available plastic grips.

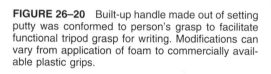

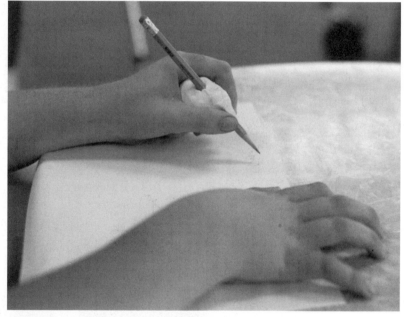

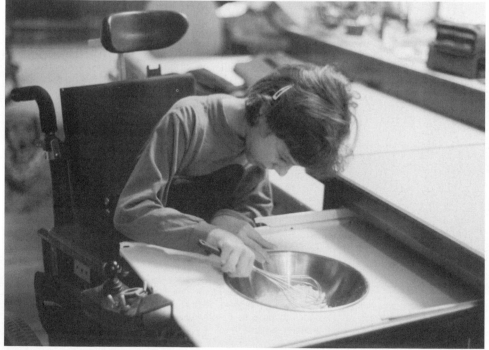

FIGURE 26–21 House with wheelchair-accessible cooking area so child with physical limitations can participate in cooking activities, such as mixing ingredients for a cake.

These tasks require gross motor mobility skills and upper extremity fine and gross motor coordination and strength. When limitations exist, environmental adaptations and assistive devices can be used in conjunction with work simplification and energy conservation techniques. Examples include reachers to retrieve items; lever-type handles to faucets, doorknobs, and appliances; adapted cooking utensils with loop Velcro handles; stabilizers such as Dycem; cutting boards with a suction cup on the bottom and prongs to hold vegetables (Fig. 26–22); use of commercially available power appliances (e.g., can opener); and use of extended handles for reach (e.g., dustpan, broom).

Home Accessibility

Many adaptations exist for performance of home management skills. Home modifications are also important to allow persons to live efficiently and successfully in their homes. Examples of modifications range from very simple

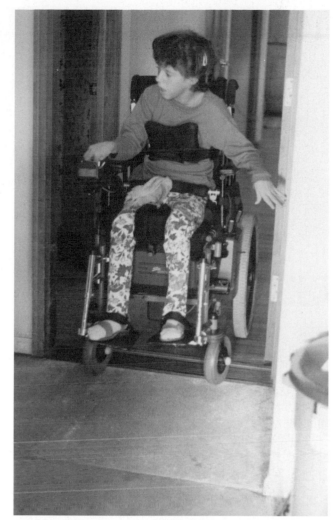

FIGURE 26–23   Ramp in residential setting· this small ramp provides accessibility over one step. Longer ramps are necessary to provide accessibility over several steps; the recommended slope of the ramp is 12 in. run for every 1 in. of rise.

ones, such as rearranging the furniture and placing commonly used items within reach, to complex ones such as widening doorways, adding a ramp (Fig. 26–23 and 26–24), and construction of a roll-in shower. A thorough home assessment by a therapist is recommended for persons who have or may have difficulty functioning within their home environment.

LEISURE SKILLS

Leisure is free, unoccupied time during which a person may indulge in rest and recreation, etc.[24] Recreational activities benefit people both physically and emotionally through enjoyment, exercise, competition, and meeting other people.[6, 20] If the person is in a rehabilitation setting, therapists can facilitate independence in leisure activities through a community reintegration program, either individually or in groups. Goals of community reintegration include performing self-maintenance, mobility skills, and problem solving in a community setting so the person can

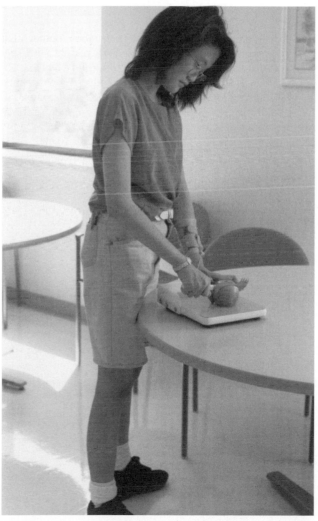

FIGURE 26–22   A rocker knife and an adapted cutting board with rubber feet, to avoid slippage of board, and prongs and edges, to hold the food, assists the person with functional use of one upper extremity. A rocker knife with fork edges cuts food by rocking down on food; the traditional sliding motion often receives stabilization from the opposite upper extremity. The fork edges are used in place of a fork, avoiding the need for two utensils.

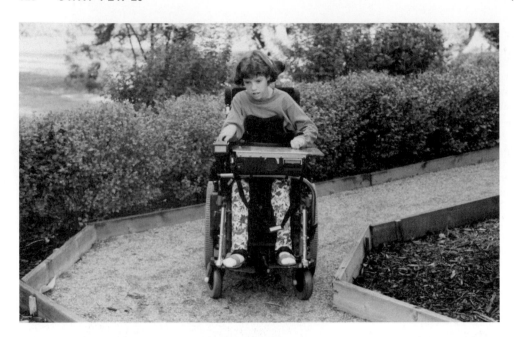

FIGURE 26–24 Specially designed walkway through yard provides accessibility outdoors when grass is an obstacle.

perform comfortably in school, work, and leisure activities in the community (Fig. 26–25). Some examples of activities which can be practiced include popping a wheelchair over a curb, reaching for items on a high or low shelf, negotiating a wheelchair at a counter to pay, practicing toileting skills in a public restroom. Exposure to various community activities facilitates comfortable functioning in social settings.

Many organizations exist throughout the country that provide programs especially designed for people with special needs. Information about these programs can be obtained from local parks and recreation departments, churches, and national organizations, which may be disability-specific (e.g., the National Head Injury Foundation). An example of an outdoor sports organization is the National Sports Center for the Disabled (NSCD) in Winter Park,

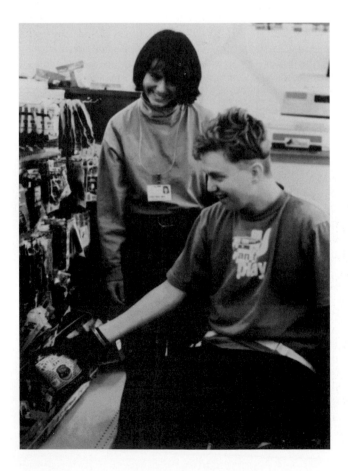

FIGURE 26–25 Problem-solving in the community: therapist facilitating independence in the community. Person is solving problem of how to reach items off the shelf in a grocery store.

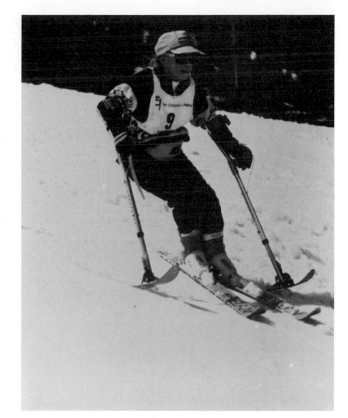

FIGURE 26–26 Outrigger skis used while skiing by a person who has difficulty shifting weight, maintaining upright stance, and maintaining balance. A person must be able to stand independently but may have difficulty with coordination.

Colorado. Activities at this center include alpine skiing, biking, hiking, white-water rafting, fishing, rock-climbing, and camping. Camps that are geared toward people with specific needs are widely available. Camps can be sports-specific[2] or include a variety of activities such as a tennis camp or a week filled with canoeing, rock-climbing, and camping.

Many adaptations exist to compensate for a person's mental limitations and physical disability. These include equipment as well as environmental modifications. Occupational and physical therapists are instrumental in helping individuals access resources, and perform task analysis and identify adaptations for participation in leisure activities.

Figures 26–26 to 26–30 illustrate some examples of adapted activities that serve as therapeutic modalities and more important, for enjoyment.

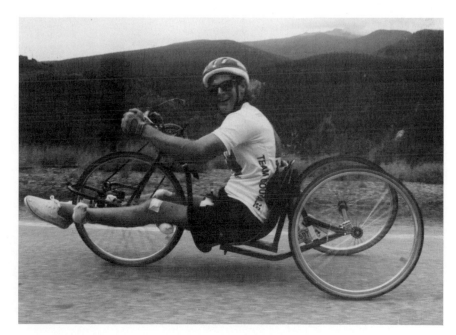

FIGURE 26–27 Bicycle adapted for a person with spinal cord injury to be propelled with upper extremities. Bars and straps support lower extremities while providing adequate seating to maintain sitting balance. (Courtesy of Steve Ackerman, American Wheelsports, Ft. Collins, Colo.)

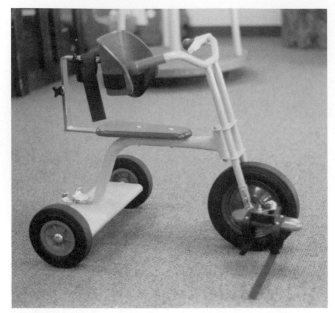

FIGURE 26–28 Tricycle adapted with footplates and straps, trunk support, and an extended seat, for children with limited balance, coordination, and strength.

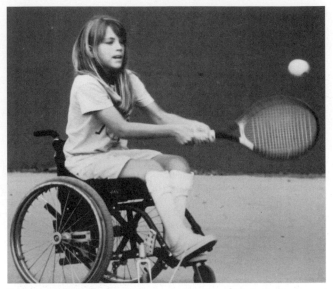

FIGURE 26–29 Many sports, such as tennis, basketball, and rugby, can be adapted for participation by a person in a wheelchair.

OCCUPATIONAL ENVIRONMENTS

Work has been described as "a behavior which is motivated by an intrinsic urge to be effective in the environment . . . influenced by cultural tradition and learned through the process of socialization."[16] Work can be a mere source of livelihood.[17, 23] Occupations are age-specific. A preschool child's occupation may be play and learning, whereas a school-age child's occupation is school activities, and play, and an adult's occupation is work and leisure activity (Fig. 26–31).

Limitations can interfere with a person's ability to perform a job. Public laws exist that have provisions that allow a person with disabilities to enter work more easily. The Americans With Disabilities Act of 1990 (ADA)[1] supports people with disabilities in competing in the workforce.[15, 21] The ADA provides persons with disabilities with civil rights protection in areas of employment, public services, transportation, public accommodation, and telecommunication. Therapists play a vital role in providing information regarding the ADA as well as in task analysis of the person's job, providing input for environmental and tool adaptations, and information on changing and problem-solving architectural barriers.

Some examples of how therapists can assist include assessment of work environments. Considerations to be taken into account for the work environment include the following:

1. Is the person able to enter and exit the work (school, play) environment?

2. Is the person able to be mobile inside the environment (i.e., access all necessary rooms)?

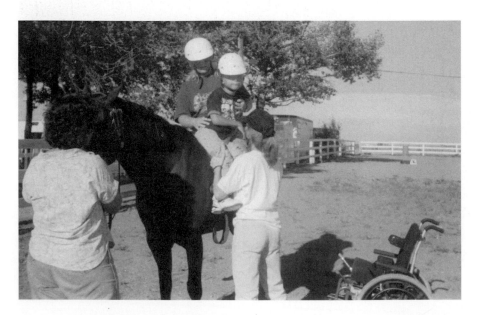

FIGURE 26–30 Therapeutic horseback riding can be used as an alternative to traditional therapy programs and as a recreational activity. Saddles can be adapted for those with decreased strength in lower extremities and trunk.

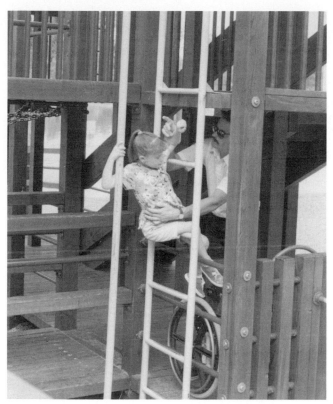

FIGURE 26–31 Parent helping child adapt to playground environment.

3. Can the person efficiently use all necessary equipment (e.g., computer, water fountain, restroom, swings) (Fig. 26–32)?

4. Can the person communicate effectively with co-workers and peers?

A variety of modifications are available that can facilitate work (school, play) access and function. The modifications vary according to the person's physical or mental limitations. Some examples of modifications that facilitate entering and exiting an environment include[1, 3]:

1. Ramps built at a ratio of 12 in. of length to 1 in. of rise

2. Wide landings at the top of ramps (5 ft × 5 ft)

3. Platforms built from sidewalks to playground equipment (Fig. 26–33)

Some examples of modifications that allow a person to be mobile inside environments include:

1. Wide doorways (36 in.)
2. Elevators
3. Ramps
4. Rearrangement of furniture or equipment (especially the restroom area)
5. Avoiding thick carpeting and throw rugs

Some examples of modifications to equipment include:

1. Computers with appropriate access (e.g., Headmaster, switches, scanning devices, etc.)

2. Lowering water fountains and providing a variety of buttons and levers to activate them

3. Handicapped-accessible swings

4. Modifications to toys (e.g., switch-activated, adapted handles, stabilizing surface)

5. Appropriate work surface (e.g., a desk or table at an appropriate height, width, length, and with space underneath)

6. Wheelchair needs to allow optimal positioning for maximum performance and interaction with the environment as well as minimizing skin and postural problems

7. Restroom facility accessible to provide functional use (e.g., grab bars and levers to flush toilet)

Some examples to foster effective communication:

1. Augmentative communication devices and telephone with adaptations

2. Proximity of student to chalkboard

3. Effective use of all communication tools (i.e., computer and all necessary software and writing tools)

Therapists are helpful in providing suggestions to teachers or employers regarding ways to allow a person to function in his or her environment.

CONCLUSION

There are many adaptations and modifications available to help a person with physical and mental limitations to achieve functional independence in the home and commu-

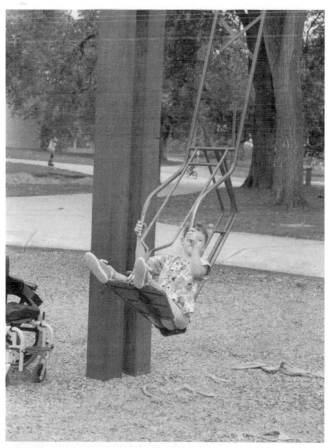

FIGURE 26–32 Adapted swing. Movement of the swing is achieved by pushing and pulling on the handles, using the arms.

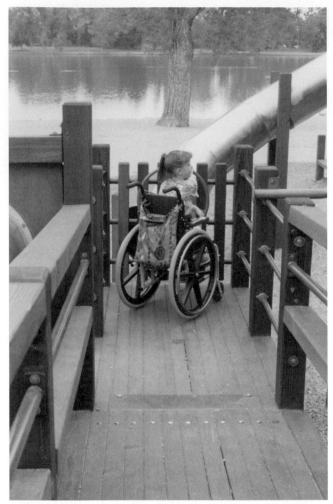

FIGURE 26–33 Playground equipment accessible by wheelchair, with platforms and ramps.

nity. It is essential that the person's developmental and cognitive level, motivation, physical abilities, and goals be considered in collaboration with patient and family before recommending any adaptations. The adaptations should enhance function without interfering with independence.

References

1. Americans with Disabilities Act of 1990. Public Law 101-336, US Code, vol 42, sec 1210.
2. American Wheelsports. 721 N. Taft Hill Road, Ft. Collins, CO 80521.
3. Architectural and Transportation Barriers Compliance Board: Americans with Disabilities Act, accessibility guidelines for buildings and facilities. Federal Register 1991; 56(July 26):35408–35453.
4. Brandstater ME: Disability: activities of daily living. *In* Basmajian JV, Kirby RL (eds): Medical Rehabilitation: A Student's Textbook. Baltimore, Williams & Wilkins, 1984, pp 246–259.
5. Breske S: When it comes to rehabilitation, family matters. Adv Phys Ther 1992; 23:4.
6. Bundy AC: Assessment of play and leisure: delineation of the problem. Am J Occup Ther 1993; 47:217–222.
7. The Children's Hospital Rehabilitation Independence Scale (CHRIS). The Children's Hospital, Denver, Department of Rehabilitation.
8. Coley IL, Procter SA: Self-maintenance activities. *In* Pratt PN, Allen AS (eds): Occupational Therapy for Children. St. Louis, Mosby–Year Book, 1989, pp 260–294.
9. Dietz JC: Functional evaluation of pediatric powered mobility devices. Arch Phys Med Rehabil 1989; 70:A-20.
10. Edelman L: Getting on Board: Training Activities to Promote the Practice of Family-Centered Care. Bethesda, Md, Association for the Care of Children's Health, 1991.
11. Fisher AG: Functional measures: Part 1. What is function, what should we measure, and how should we measure it? Am J Occup Ther 1992; 46:183–185.
12. Haley S, Baryza MJ, Webster HC: Pediatric rehabilitation and recovery of children with traumatic injuries. Pediatr Phys Ther, 1992; 4:24–30.
13. Intagliata S, Sullivan B: Development and implementation of the Rehabilitation Institute of Chicago Functional Assessment Scale. Occup Ther Pract 1991; 2:26–37.
14. Jones R: Bladder and bowel management. *In* Hill JD, Intagliata S (eds): Spinal Cord Injury: A Guide to Functional Outcomes in Occupational Therapy. Rockville, Colo, Aspen, 1986, pp 145–168.
15. Kalscheur JA: Benefits of the Americans with Disabilities Act of 1990 for children and adolescents with disabilities. Am J Occup Ther 1992; 46:419–426.
16. Kielhofner G: Health Through Occupation: Therapy and Practice in Occupational Therapy. Philadelphia, FA Davis, 1983; p 136.
17. Mills CW: The meanings of work throughout history. *In* Best F (ed): The Future of Work. Englewood Cliffs, NJ:Prentice-Hall, 1973, pp 6–13.
18. Nawoczenski DA, Rinehart ME, Duncanson P, Brown BE: Physical management. *In* Buchanan LE, Nawoczenski DA (eds): Spinal Cord Injury Concepts and Management Approaches. Baltimore, Williams & Wilkins, 1987, pp 123–184.
19. Pedretti LW: Activities of daily living. *In* Pedretti LW, Zoltan B (eds): Occupational Therapy: Practice for Physical Dysfunction. St Louis, Mosby–Year Book, 1990, pp 230–271.
20. Procter SA: Adaptations for independent living. *In* Pratt PN, Allen AS (eds): Occupational Therapy for Children. St Louis, Mosby–Year Book, 1989, pp 335–357.
21. Reed KL: History of federal legislation for persons with disabilities. Am J Occup Ther 1992; 46:397–408.
22. Uniform Data System (UDS). Functional Independence Measures (FIM). University of Newark at Buffalo. Department of Rehabilitation Medicine. Buffalo General Hospital, Buffalo.
23. Velazo CA: Work evaluations: critique of the state of the art of functional assessment of work. Am J Occup Ther 1993; 47:203–209.
24. Webster's New World Dictionary. Guralnik DB (ed), New York, William, Collins, & World, 1976; p 807.
25. Whitneck G: Quantifying handicap: a new measure of long-term rehab outcomes. Arch Phys Med Rehabil 1992; 73:519–526.

Management of Special Problems in Physical Medicine and Rehabilitation Practice

27

Rehabilitation of Patients With Swallowing Disorders

STEPHEN F. NOLL, M.D., CLAIRE E. BENDER, M.D.,
AND MARGE C. NELSON, O.T.

Dysphagia can represent yet another barrier and another loss to a person already limited in mobility or self-care. The inability to swallow without drooling, coughing, or choking robs a person of enjoyment in eating and of socialization that often accompanies eating. But more than a loss of pleasure, dysphagia also is a serious threat to a person's health from the risk of aspiration pneumonia and malnutrition. *Dysphagia*, a Greek word that means disordered eating, is difficulty in eating as a result of disruption in the swallowing process.

THE SWALLOWING PROCESS

Normal deglutition is a smooth, coordinated process that has been divided into three phases: oral, pharyngeal, and esophageal.[26, 63] Each stage is responsible for a specific function, and if they are impaired by disease, specific symptoms result (Fig. 27–1 and Table 27–1).

Early in the oral phase, the bolus is prepared and placed on the tongue; this phase requires intact lip closure, a mobile tongue, and functional muscles of mastication. Mastication not only modifies the bolus but also stimulates salivation, without which swallowing is difficult and delayed.[53] Once it is properly positioned, the bolus is propelled into the pharynx by a syringe-like action.[9] An important event that occurs simultaneously with the initiation of swallowing is the inhibition of breathing. Before the onset of swallowing, however, the airway is open. If a portion of bolus slips into the pharynx early because of poor oral control or coordination, aspiration can occur before swallowing.[63]

The pharyngeal phase is of particular importance, because without intact laryngeal protective mechanisms, aspiration is most likely to occur during this phase (Fig. 27–2). Protection from laryngeal penetration and aspiration is afforded in several ways: folding of the epiglottis over the laryngeal opening, closure of the vocal cords, and elevation

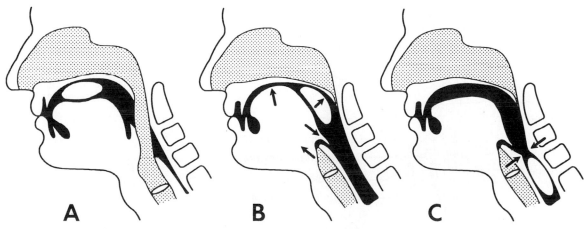

FIGURE 27–1   Three phases of normal deglutition. *A*, Oral. *B*, Pharyngeal. *C*, Esophageal.

TABLE 27–1   Stages of Deglutition

	Stage		
	Oral	*Pharyngeal*	*Esophageal*
Purpose	Bolus preparation and transport	Bolus transport without aspiration	Bolus transport with limited reflux
Requirements	Lip closure for bolus containment	Tongue elevation to prevent oral regurgitation	Coordinated peristalsis and lower esophageal sphincter relaxation for bolus transport
	Lingual control for bolus manipulation, positioning, and transport	Palatal elevation to prevent nasal regurgitation	Cricopharyngeal tonic contraction to prevent pharyngeal regurgitation
	Mastication and salivation for bolus modification	Laryngeal elevation, folding of epiglottis, and vocal cord adduction to prevent aspiration	Relaxation of lower esophageal sphincter
		Coordinated pharyngeal motility and cricopharyngeal relaxation for bolus transport	
Symptoms	Drooling	Oral/nasal regurgitation	Food sticking
	Pocketing (squirreling)	Food sticking	Heartburn
	Repeated swallowing attempts	Cough or choke	
	Head tilt	Wet, gurgling voice	

and anterior displacement of the larynx.[63] The last-listed movement positions the larynx under the base of the tongue while opening the upper esophageal sphincter by traction, increasing the diameter of the pharynx, and engulfing the bolus.[26] Bolus propulsion by the tongue and pharyngeal constrictors is also an important factor[49]; propulsion through the pharynx lasts only about 0.6 sec. If this function is slow or ineffective, there is greater laryngeal exposure to the bolus. In the normal state, the tongue, the pharyngeal palate, and a portion of the superior pharyngeal constrictors (the Passavant cushion) also close the oral and nasal cavities to prevent regurgitation.[47]

The pharynx is a shared structure for both deglutition and respiration. Of concern are potential food traps within this structure that are located near the laryngeal opening: the vallecula and pyriform sinuses (Figs. 27–2 and 27–3A).

Ordinarily, food is cleared from these spaces with repeated swallowing. Retention of food in these recesses, however, allows for spillage (penetration) into the larynx after swallowing and for possible aspiration into the tracheobronchial tree.[47, 63]

The cricopharyngeus muscle and pharyngoesophageal sphincter (PES) mechanism, called the *upper esophageal sphincter,* can also serve as a pharyngeal trap. The cricopharyngeus is unique among the pharyngeal constrictors[10] (Fig. 27–3B) and tonically contracts while other pharyngeal constrictors are at rest. The cricopharyngeus muscle, however, is only a portion of the physiological mechanism that serves as a closed portal to prevent esophageal reflux into the pharynx.[23, 33] With pharyngeal weakness, the propulsive force generated in the pharynx might not be great enough to transport the bolus past the upper esophageal sphincter.

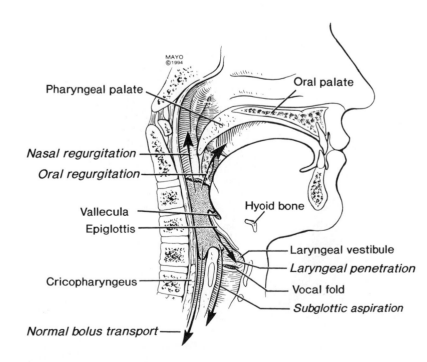

FIGURE 27–2   Perils of the pharyngeal phase: oral regurgitation, nasal regurgitation, laryngeal penetration, and subglottic aspiration. By permission of Mayo Foundation for Medical Education and Research.

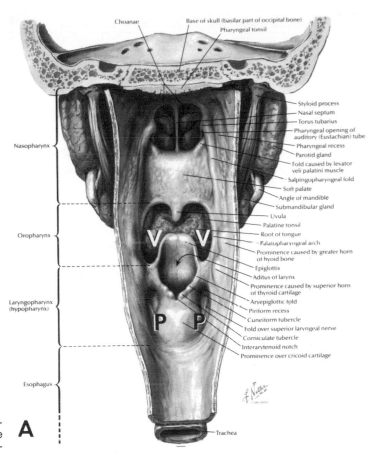

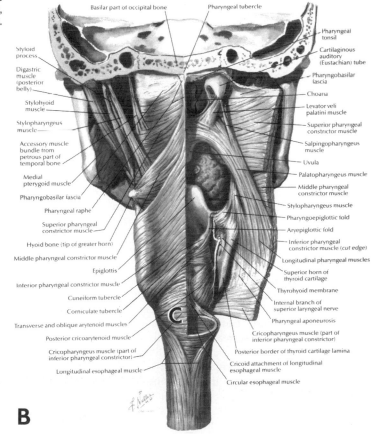

FIGURE 27–3   *A,* Pharynx: opened posterior view. *P,* Pyriform sinuses; *V,* vallecula, which sits between base of tongue and epiglottis. *B,* Muscles of pharynx: partially opened posterior view. *C,* Cricopharyngeus muscle. (From Netter FH: Atlas of Human Anatomy, plates 60 and 61. Summit, New Jersey, Pharmaceuticals Division, CIBA-GEIGY Corporation, 1989. By permission of the publisher.)

With pharyngeal incoordination, a form of dyssynergia can occur if the PES remains uninhibited and fails to relax during the swallowing process. In either of these instances, a portion of the bolus is retained in the pharynx and can result in aspiration after swallowing.[47, 63]

The esophageal phase, the last phase, is notable for being the longest phase, lasting approximately 6 to 10 sec. Peristalsis is responsible for the bolus transport through the esophagus.[26] The lower esophageal sphincter is a high-pressure zone that, like the PES, relaxes to allow peristaltic movement of the bolus distally.[53] Disorders of the esophageal phase are diagnostically problematic, because symptoms of this phase can be referred to the pharyngeal region.[47]

The organization of deglutition is neurologically highly complex, much like the process it controls. Simply stated, however, the swallowing process requires the following elements: sensory input from the peripheral and central nervous systems, a coordinating center or centers, and a subsequent motor response sent back through these systems.[26] Sensory input from the peripheral system is primarily through cranial nerves V, VII, IX, and X. Sensory receptors take on several forms, including taste, fluid, or pressure sensors.[53] The fauces, pharynx, and posterior larynx appear to be key areas from which the most effective swallowing stimuli originate.[26] Centrally, cortical and subcortical pathways modulate the swallowing threshold,[73] although the exact role of the cerebral cortex is unclear.[71] The brainstem swallowing centers receive the input, organize it into a programmed response, and transmit the response.[26, 53, 93] Swallowing is only one of the possible programmed responses from these centers; the gag is another.[26] Output from the swallowing centers is passed to nuclei of cranial nerves V, VII, IX, X, and XII, and subsequently to the muscles they innervate. In response to the output, there is also a sensory feedback system that varies depending on the swallowing phase.[73]

CLINICAL ASSESSMENT

A thorough clinical assessment, or the "bedside" evaluation, is one method to determine how the swallowing process is impaired and which stage or stages are involved (Fig. 27–4).

History

Documentation of the course of the disease and specific symptoms of dysphagia is imperative, but other information is also important.[38, 57, 81] For example, dental disorders or the presence of dentures can affect the oral phase of swallowing. A history of recurrent pneumonia raises the question of aspiration. The presence of significant cardiopulmonary disease, such as chronic obstructive lung disease or congestive heart failure, can increase morbidity from aspiration. Previous neck surgery or radiation and cervical spondylosis or ankylosis can also alter the mechanics of swallowing or limit compensatory options for treatment. A dietary history provides clues to the problem based on the types and textures of food that a person has chosen.

Examination

Cranial nerve testing (V and VII through XII) is the basis for determining physical evidence of oral or pharyngeal dysfunction and provides direct observation of lip closure, jaw closure, tongue mobility and strength, palatal elevation, and oral sensitivity. However, additional observations are necessary to unveil other impairments that can affect swallowing.[57, 72, 81] For example, the level of alertness and cognitive status can significantly impact the safety of swallowing and also the ability to learn compensatory measures. Foamy oral secretions or an altered voice quality points to pharyngeal dysfunction and possible aspiration. Testing for the gag reflex is helpful, but an absent gag does not imply the inability to swallow safely.[63]

Assessing respiratory function is essential during the evaluation for many reasons. If the breathing rate is rapid because of respiratory distress, the timing and energy of swallowing can be difficult. If there is inadequate respiratory force with a cough or with clearing the throat, the risk of aspiration is increased. Chest auscultation can uncover an unsuspected pneumonitis or evidence of obstructive lung disease. Palpating for laryngeal excursion while a patient swallows helps identify the presence or absence of a key laryngeal protective mechanism (Fig. 27–5).

One final step in evaluation (if clinically appropriate and safe) is a diagnostic feeding assessment with various food textures. This assessment allows the opportunity to observe swallowing behavior directly. The "3-oz water swallow test" has compared favorably with the video swallow in identifying aspiration.[25] The result of this test is positive if the patient's voice develops a wet, hoarse quality or if the patient coughs within 1 min after swallowing 3 oz of water.

The bedside evaluation has some predictive capabilities for determining the risk of aspiration. For example, the presence or absence of the gag or a cough has been used to identify patients with bilateral infarctions who are at greatest risk for aspiration.[41] But the bedside evaluation tends to underestimate the occurrence of aspiration, particularly in older patients, in patients with expressive aphasia, and when more than 30 days has elapsed after onset of injury.[62, 102]

Laboratory Data

Chest radiography is a simple assessment for aspiration pneumonia. No pathognomonic sign of aspiration is seen on the chest radiograph, but the presence of infiltrates in a patient at risk raises suspicion. Other routine laboratory tests are also useful. For example, the serum albumin value can be a marker for nutritional status. A low value suggests chronic nutritional insufficiency or chronic illness.[22]

TECHNICAL ASSESSMENT OF DYSPHAGIA

Radiographic Imaging

VIDEOFLUOROSCOPY. Most swallowing disorders are best evaluated with the dynamic recorded videofluoroscopy technique. Although many of the newer imaging methods (ultrasonography, computed tomography [CT], magnetic

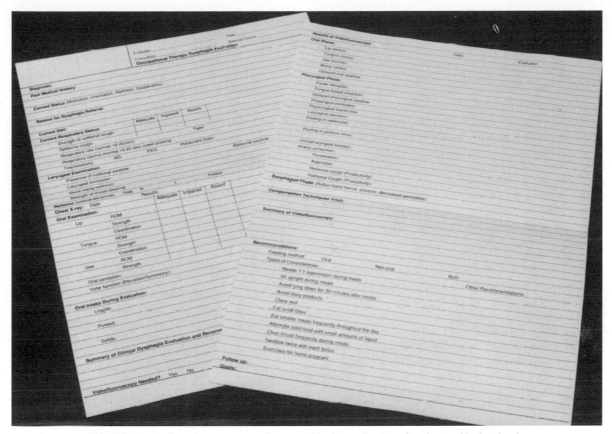

FIGURE 27-4   Sample assessment form used in the evaluation of patients with dysphagia.

FIGURE 27-5   Positioning of the hand for clinical evaluation of laryngeal elevation includes positioning the index finger immediately behind the mandible anteriorly, middle finger at the hyoid bone, third finger at the top of the thyroid cartilage, and fourth finger at the bottom of the thyroid cartilage.

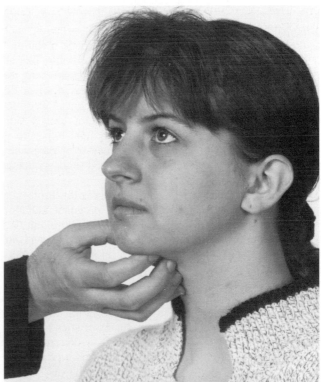

resonance imaging [MRI], scintigraphy, and endoscopy) have been used for workup, videofluoroscopic technique with the use of existing fluoroscopy systems, which are easily connected to inexpensive videotape recorders, continues to be the standard. Although this system has some loss of quality when compared with the more expensive, specialized cinefluorography systems, it is easier to use. However, radiation is still being used, and radiation exposure to the patient, fluoroscopist, and swallowing therapist exists and carries attendant risks.

Radiation Risk. X-rays (as used in videofluoroscopy and plain films) are a common form of low-dose ionizing radiation that have been associated with tissue damage, genetic injury, and cancer. The risks associated with low-dose exposures have been extrapolated downward from high-dose data; consequently, the precise risks cannot be determined. It is important to note that low levels of radiation exist in our natural environment (air, ground, and water). During any x-ray study, it is the responsibility of the clinician to keep the amount of radiation at a minimum for the patient and for all personnel in the examining room.

Radiation effects depend on the amount of radiation energy absorbed. One gray (Gy) results from the absorption of 1 joule of radiation energy in a kilogram of tissue (1 Gy = 100 rad). Levels of x-ray doses are more commonly described in millirad or rad. Another measurement is the dose equivalent (1 sievert [Sv] = 100 rem). For general purposes, 1 Sv = 1 Gy; 1 rem = 1 rad.

Radiation effects can be (1) nonstochastic (i.e., with a threshold dose that must be exceeded for effects to occur) or (2) stochastic (i.e., the biological effect is all or nothing, the probability of the effect increases with dose [but *not* its severity], and there is no threshold dose level below which the effect cannot occur).[5] An example of nonstochastic effect is lens cataract induction with a single exposure dose equivalent of 200 rem. Stochastic effects include the principal health risks of diagnostic levels of radiation, such as the potential induction of cancer and genetic mutation.

It is well recognized that the embryo and fetus, like all rapidly growing tissues, are particularly sensitive to the effects of radiation. Caution must be exercised when the patient, fluoroscopist, or therapist is pregnant. Videofluoroscopy for a swallowing evaluation does not directly radiate the pelvic region of the patient, so fetal exposure is very minimal. It is during the first trimester of pregnancy that the most severe effects can be induced (e.g., spontaneous abortion, gross organ malfunction).

Currently, the National Council on Radiation Protection and Measurements recommends that a pregnant radiation worker (therapist, fluoroscopist) not exceed 500 mrem (0.5 cSv) exposure during the entire gestation period, and not exceed 50 mrem exposure in any 1 month. With proper shielding, the pregnant female operator can safely remain within these limits.

Exposure dose to the patient during videofluoroscopy is dependent on exposure times, the technique of the fluoroscopist, the equipment, and patient characteristics (cooperativeness, size). Exposure to the patient is determined by multiplying the number of minutes (seconds) of fluoroscopy by the dose (to a particular body part) per minute. Generally, the exposure to the patient is small.

The following several key steps protect both the patient and the operators:

Minimize the duration of exposure to x-rays.

Think before you perform fluoroscopy (check the position of the patient and the equipment maintenance and handling).

Ensure x-ray beam collimation (image only the area or areas of interest).

Locate personnel at appropriate positions (Fig. 27–6).

Use lead shielding (e.g., aprons, glasses, thyroid shields).

Screen for pregnancy.

Ensure that radiation monitor badges are worn by all radiation workers, including therapists, who assist in videofluoroscopy.

The image document (the videotape) becomes part of the patient's medical record. If additional documentation is warranted, image transfer to film can be achieved, but the image is of lesser quality than that of traditional spot filming or overhead filming for a permanent record. These techniques add to the overall exposure dose to the patient during the evaluation.

Equipment. Fluoroscopy is performed with standard radiographic and fluoroscopic units with image intensification. The x-ray tube is located beneath the tabletop. A videotape recorder (½-in.) with audio recording capability is adapted to the fluoroscopy unit for audiovisual examination. To facilitate the investigation of swallowing disorders in difficult patients, we have utilized a special lightweight mobile chair (Fig. 27–7). This equipment has the following benefits[18]:

Narrow dimensions, which permit use with standard fluoroscopic units.

Rugged yet lightweight construction for ease in mobility.

Easy rotation of chair for posteroanterior and lateral viewing.

Safety features, including seatbelts, head restraints, locking wheels, and footrests.

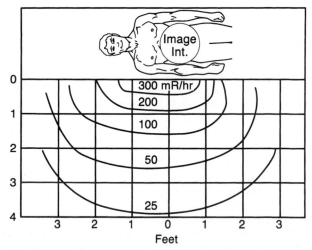

FIGURE 27–6 Radiation exposure to personnel depends on the inverse square law: intensity of beam is inversely proportional to the inverse square of the distance from the x-ray beam ($I \propto 1/d^2$).

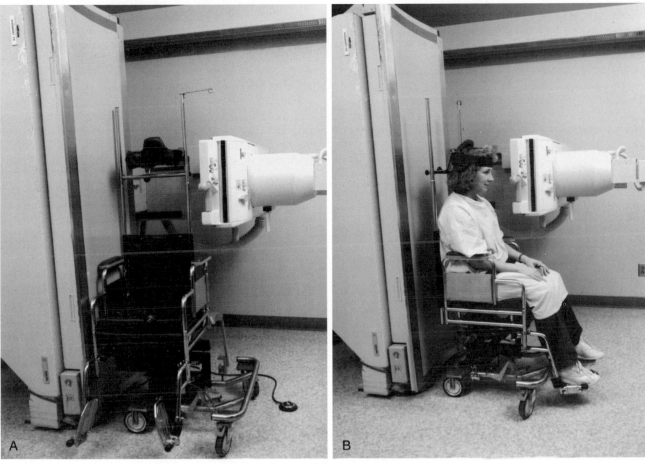

FIGURE 27-7 Lightweight chair mounted on special transporter. (Video FluoroChair is manufactured by Rehab Tech, Inc., Dayton, Ohio.) *A,* Chair positioned for lateral fluoroscopy. *B,* Chair rotated for posteroanterior fluoroscopy. Note belts for head and body restraints.

Can be modified to transportable chair for ease of patient transportation.

Procedural Guidelines. The examination is facilitated by coordinated consultation between the occupational therapist and the radiologist (fluoroscopist). The videofluoroscopic swallowing evaluation team includes the therapist, the fluoroscopist, the radiology nurse or technologist, and the patient.

The standard procedure is performed with the patient in the upright (sitting) position; posteroanterior and lateral views are obtained. Swallowing is evaluated (and documented) by simultaneous video and audio recording, and the following methods or agents are used: dry swallow, thin liquid barium, thick liquid barium, or solid barium cookie.

Individual patient needs might require that the examination be modified (such as by use of a semi-upright or a supine position instead of a sitting position).[25] The dry swallow is a screening tool to evaluate how the patient handles secretions. This can be further adapted by having the patient swallow sips of water.[34] Aspirated barium is usually well tolerated, but complications have occasionally occurred.[36] Water-soluble agents with high osmolality (such as diatrizoate meglumine [Gastrografin]) should not be used because of the risk of aspiration-induced pulmonary edema. The newer, more expensive, low-osmolar, iodinated

contrast material can be used with less risk of pulmonary or allergic reaction.

Interpretation. Diagnosis by fluoroscopy is a skill achieved through dedicated training and experience. The fluoroscopy diagnosis is recorded by the radiologist in the patient's permanent record. The entire upper gastrointestinal tract (from the mouth to the ligament of Treitz of the jejunum) should be evaluated to avoid missing an underlying disease (such as obstructing gastric carcinoma with aspiration).

There is a distinct clinical difference between the videofluoroscopic examination and the routine upper gastrointestinal series. Both examinations evaluate the gastrointestinal tract from the mouth to the small intestine. The videofluoroscopic evaluation of swallowing has *both* diagnostic and potentially therapeutic capabilities. After aspiration is diagnosed, changes in the texture of the barium meal or variations in head positioning can provide immediate feedback for treatment of a swallowing problem.[85]

Quantitative evaluation of the pharyngeal transit time (measured during fluoroscopy) can be useful for following the progress of patients with dysphagia and for evaluating the effects of remedial therapy.[44]

PLAIN FILM ANALYSIS. Plain radiographic film documentation is obtained if any abnormality is observed. Spot film analysis can be performed at the time of videofluoroscopy, or overhead films can be taken after fluoroscopy. Any variety of views (anteroposterior, posterolateral, lateral, oblique) can be obtained to document the diagnosis (Figs. 27–8 through 27–12).

ULTRASONOGRAPHY.   Ultrasonography has been used in the evaluation of swallowing.[39, 44] As with any ultrasound technique, it has advantages and disadvantages (Table 27–2). When the swallowing mechanism is evaluated, only the region of the tongue posterior to the hyoid level can be studied.[68] The major advantage is the delineation of soft tissues within this region (Fig. 27–13).

Most real-time ultrasound systems can be used to evaluate swallowing. For viewing the oropharynx, a real-time sector scanner should be used; for evaluating the larynx, a linear array system should be used. A 5-MHz transducer provides the best focal depth for both areas. Ultrasonography may be used with baseline videofluoroscopy to document aspiration and to further evaluate esophageal activity.[100]

CT AND MRI.   The major indications for cross-sectional imaging in the evaluation of patients with a swallowing disorder include the following: (1) identification and staging of a mass in the upper digestive tract and (2) diagnosis of a central or peripheral nervous system mass to explain the pathophysiology of the swallowing disorder. With the

rapid development of MRI technology, CT has taken a lesser role. MRI is noninvasive, whereas CT utilizes ionizing radiation. Speech, tongue movements, and the swallowing motion can now be studied in motion series using the fast low-angle shot magnetic resonance imaging (FLASH-MRI) tomography technique.[36]

SCINTIGRAPHY.   Nuclear medicine techniques have very limited use in the evaluation of pharyngeal swallowing disorders (such as quantification of aspiration).[96] Scintigraphy has been more useful in the quantitative and qualitative evaluation of esophageal motility disorders and gastroesophageal reflux (Fig. 27–14).[39, 104]

MANOMETRY.   Esophageal motor disorders are best evaluated with manometry.[80, 90] Manometry is time-consuming and may be uncomfortable to the patient because of the placement of a peroral multilumen catheter system. Videofluoroscopy is an excellent screening tool for the evaluation of suspected esophageal motor disorders (Fig. 27–15).

ENDOSCOPY.   Fiberoptic endoscopy has been introduced for the evaluation of oropharyngeal dysphagia.[59] This procedure is a sensitive technique for detecting premature spillage, laryngeal penetration, tracheal aspiration, and pharyngeal residue. The endoscope is passed transnasally to view the larynx and pharynx. Swallowing is directly evalu-

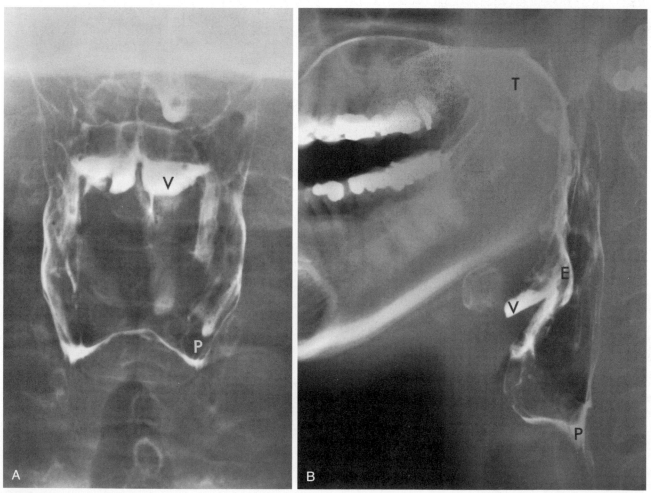

FIGURE 27–8   A, Normal posteroanterior view of pharynx. B, Normal lateral view of pharynx. E, Epiglottis; P, pyriform sinus; T, tongue; V, vallecula.

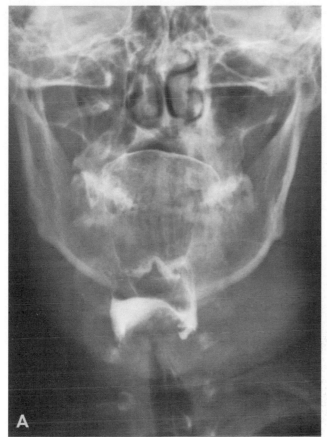

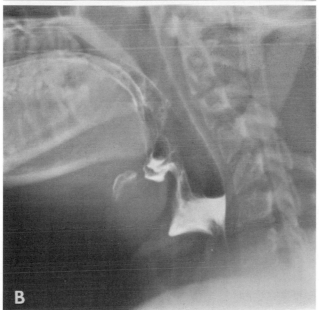

FIGURE 27–9   Pooling of barium in asymmetrically enlarged right pyriform sinus in patient who had had a stroke. No aspiration. *A,* Posteroanterior view. *B,* Lateral view.

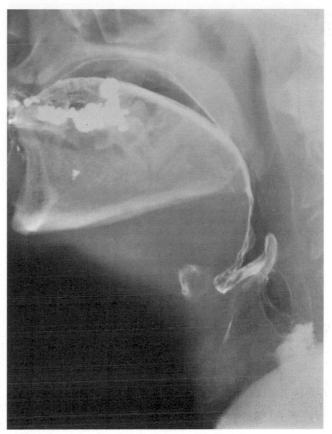

FIGURE 27–10   Lateral view, showing laryngeal penetration of barium due to poor covering of epiglottis. Calcified hyoid bone is just anterior to valleculae.

ated using measured quantities of liquid dye with blue food coloring for contrast and food (such as applesauce or bread). Although the videofluoroscopic examination remains the standard for evaluation of swallowing disorders, certain patients are more amenable to endoscopy, such as critically ill patients who are unable to tolerate any risk of aspiration, patients in intensive care units who cannot be transferred to the fluoroscopy suite, and patients who require immediate evaluation.

DYSPHAGIA IN SPECIFIC DISORDERS

Dysphagia has been reported in multiple types of disorders, and for purposes of categorization, it can be classified as neurological or nonneurological (Table 27–3). In rehabilitation medicine, the neurological swallowing disorders are more frequently encountered, and a few deserve further discussion.

Stroke

The frequency of dysphagia in association with stroke has been reported to be as high as 30% to 45%,[41, 106] and

TABLE 27–2   Advantages and Disadvantages of Ultrasonography for Evaluation of Swallowing

Advantages	Disadvantages
Noninvasive	Limited scanning region
Soft tissue delineation	Air, bone artifacts
Multiplanar imaging: sagittal, parasagittal, coronal, transverse	Missed aspirations
No contrast agent given	
Video recording	
Hard copy prints	

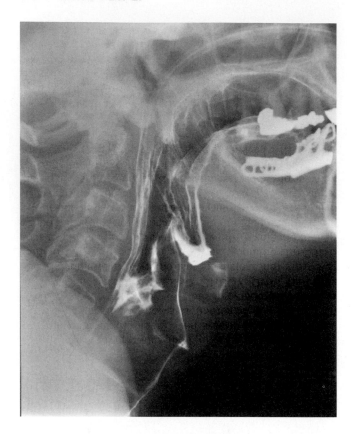

FIGURE 27–11   Tracheal aspiration of barium due to overflow of barium pooled in valleculae in patient who had had a stroke.

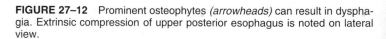

FIGURE 27–12   Prominent osteophytes *(arrowheads)* can result in dysphagia. Extrinsic compression of upper posterior esophagus is noted on lateral view.

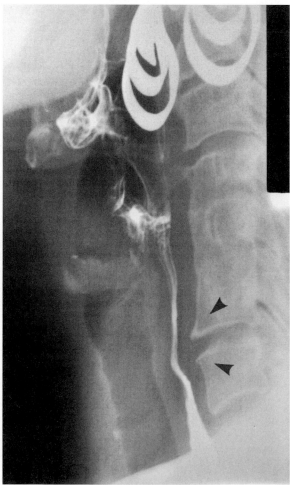

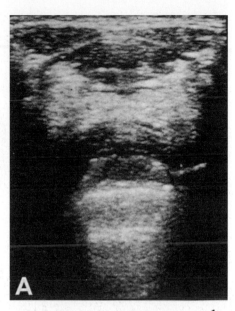

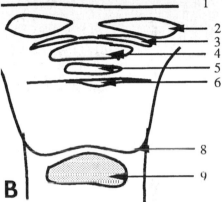

FIGURE 27-13 *A,* Ultrasound scan of coronal section of tongue during swallowing. Lateral borders of tongue are elevated to form a hollow, which contains the bolus. *B,* 1, superficial plane; 2, anterior belly of digastric muscle; 3, mylohyoid muscle; 4, geniohyoid muscle; 5, genioglossus muscle; 6, alveololingual groove; 8, superior or dorsal surface of tongue; 9, bolus. (From Maniere-Ezvan A, Duval J-M, Darnault P: Ultrasonic assessment of the anatomy and function of the tongue. Surg Radiol Anat 1993; 15[1]: 55. By permission of Springer-Verlag France.)

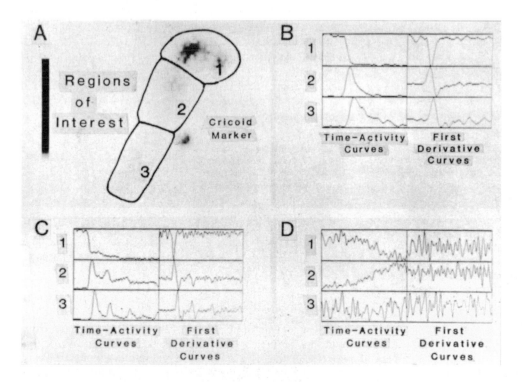

FIGURE 27-14 *A,* Scintiscan of oropharynx in which selected regions of interest have been drawn to represent the mouth (1), pharynx (2), and esophagus (3). The time-activity curves (time on horizontal axis, counts on vertical axis) that are constructed from the area of the mouth (1), pharynx (2), and esophagus (3) together with corresponding first-derivative curves are shown in *B, C,* and *D.* The peaks and nadirs correspond to peak emptying or filling rates of the respective compartments. *B,* Transit data recorded during swallowing in the control subject. *C* and *D,* Abnormal bolus transit in two patients (one with bulbar palsy and one with myasthenia gravis) manifested by major change in pattern of the time-activity and first-derivative curves. (From Holt S, Miron SD, Diaz MC, et al.: Scintigraphic measurement of oropharyngeal transit in man. Dig Dis Sci 1990; 35[10]: 1198. By permission of Plenum Publishing Corporation.)

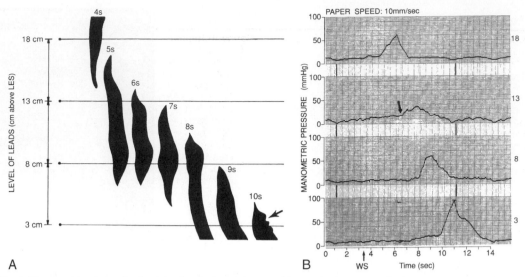

FIGURE 27–15 *A,* Temporal tracings of a 5-mL barium bolus at 1-second intervals show normal primary peristalsis at fluoroscopy. Tapered tops of the barium column correspond to the peristaltic contraction wave seen at manometry. Mild tertiary activity *(arrow)* affects tracing at 10 seconds. Numbers on vertical axis represent positions of the catheter ports. *B,* Manometric tracing of bolus in *A.* Wet swallow (WS) occurred at 3.4 seconds. Time scale is synchronous with the temporally labeled barium tracings. On the lead 13 cm above the lower esophageal sphincter (LES), peristaltic onset is at about 6.6 seconds *(arrows),* corresponding precisely to the fluoroscopic level of primary peristalsis. (From Ott DJ, Chen YM, Hewson EG, et al.: Esophageal motility: assessment with synchronous video tape fluoroscopy and manometry. Radiology 1989; 173[2]: 419. By permission of the Radiological Society of North America.)

the condition is not limited to only brainstem or bilateral infarctions. Unilateral lesions also result in dysphagia.[3, 65, 86] The most common swallowing impairments associated with stroke are reduced lingual control, reduced pharyngeal peristalsis, and a delayed swallowing reflex.[109] Aspiration is frequently associated with dysphagia in stroke, but it cannot be predicted by the imaged location of the stroke.[1] The presence of a cough or an absent gag can predict the risk of aspiration,[42] but aspiration is "silent," or without symptoms or signs, in many persons. When aspiration occurs on videofluoroscopy, the chances of pneumonia developing are significantly greater than if aspiration is not present.[91] A prolonged pharyngeal transit time also helps predict patients in whom pneumonia will develop.[45] The prognosis for oral feeding after stroke is good, and the risk for aspiration pneumonia decreases over time.[40, 42, 105]

Traumatic Brain Injury

The occurrence of dysphagia in the head-injured population has been reported to be as high as 27%. Cognitive impairment is often the most significant factor, followed by motor control difficulties.[114] Behavioral difficulties also can interfere, necessitating various behavioral strategies, such as systematic desensitization of oral hypersensitivity.[12] Drooling may present as a significant problem in this population. Several options exist for treatment, usually beginning with oral motor exercises to control oral secretions, followed by administration of drugs, such as atropine sulfate, to dry oral secretions, and, finally, surgical intervention to block oral secretions.[27]

Motor Neuron Disease

Upper and lower motor neuron dysfunction occurs commonly in a significant number of patients with motor neu-

ron disease and results in oral and pharyngeal dysphagia.[14] Because of the progressive nature of this disorder, difficult emotional and ethical issues often arise. Various treatment measures can be used in this disorder, including surgical options such as laryngeal diversion.[19]

Parkinson's Disease

Patients with Parkinson's disease can present with dysphagia and nutritional deficits, in part due to oropharyngeal motility problems.[111] On videofluoroscopic examination, oral phase dysfunction is very common, occurring in up to 92% of patients complaining of dysphagia. Aspiration is also common[103] and can be silent. Swallowing function usually improves with administration of levodopa, but improvement in parkinsonian signs does not always signify improvement in swallowing.[17]

Poliomyelitis

With careful examination, oropharyngeal function is found to be disturbed to some degree in many patients with post-polio syndrome.[101] Videofluoroscopy reveals not only neurogenic dysfunction, such as weakness of the pharyngeal constrictors, poor laryngeal elevation, and aspiration without a cough, but also structural lesions, including pharyngeal pouches, Zenker's diverticulum, and focal stenosis.[15, 46]

Multiple Sclerosis

Management of dysphagia can vary significantly over time in the patient with multiple sclerosis because of the disease course. If it is relapsing and remitting, interventions might be intermittent. If the course is progressive, more permanent compensatory measures could be necessary.[14]

TABLE 27–3 Disorders Associated with Dysphagia

Neurological	Nonneurological
Central nervous system	Structural
Vascular	Cervical osteophytes
Stroke	Goiter
Intracranial hemorrhage	Neoplasm
Motor neuron disorders	Foreign body
Progressive spinal muscular atrophy	Congenital anomalies
Progressive bulbar palsy	Vascular aneurysm or anomaly
Amyotrophic lateral sclerosis	Schatzki's ring
Infantile spinal muscular atrophy	Zenker's diverticulum
Degenerative/extrapyramidal	Esophageal webs
Parkinsonism	Esophageal dysmotility
Spinocerebellar degeneration	Gastroesophageal reflux
Olivopontocerebellar atrophy	Achalasia
Progressive supranuclear palsy	Diffuse esophageal spasm
Huntington's disease	"Nutcracker" esophagus
Alzheimer's disease	Other gastrointestinal disease
Adrenoleukodystrophy	Crohn's disease
Dystonia	Ulcerative colitis
Tardive dyskinesia	Amyloid
Immune-mediated	Rheumatologic
Multiple sclerosis	Scleroderma
Infectious	Sjögren's syndrome
Encephalitis/meningitis	Systemic lupus erythematosus
Structural	Mixed connective tissue disease
Neoplasm	Rheumatoid arthritis
Arnold-Chiari malformation	Infectious
Syringomyelia, syringobulbia	Candida
Exogenous	Herpesvirus
Traumatic brain injury	Cytomegalovirus
Drug-induced	Human immunodeficiency virus (HIV)
Peripheral nervous system	Psychiatric
Guillain-Barré syndrome	Globus
Sarcoidosis	Skin diseases
Porphyria	Mucus membrane pemphigoid
Myopathy/dystrophy	Epidermolysis bullosa dystrophica
Inflammatory myopathy (polymyositis, dermatomyositis)	Lichen planus
Metabolic myopathy (mitochondrial myopathy, dysthyroid	Psoriasis
myopathy)	Stevens-Johnson syndrome
Myotonic dystrophy	Chronic graft-vs.-host disease
Oculopharyngeal dystrophy	Metabolic
Neuromuscular junction	Hypercalcemia
Myasthenia gravis	Diabetes mellitus
Eaton-Lambert syndrome	Treatment-related
Botulism	Postoperative head and neck radiation
	Foreign device (tracheostomy tube, nasogastric tube)

Data from Brin and Younger,[11] Buchholz,[14] Buchin,[16] and Jones et al.[48]

Myasthenia Gravis

Dysphagia is unique in myasthenia, in that symptoms often resolve solely with pharmacological intervention.

Myotonic Dystrophy

Although dysphagia is not common in Duchenne muscular dystrophy, the facial and pharyngeal muscular weakness in myotonic dystrophy often results in significant dysphagia.

In addition to the neurological causes, nonneurological causes for dysphagia are important to consider in the rehabilitation setting. The patient with primarily neurological dysphagia might also have a concurrent, nonneurological cause that is aggravating the swallowing process, such as cervical osteophytes (Fig. 27–12) or Zenker's diverticulum (Fig. 27–16). The presence of pain or difficulties in swallowing solids early in the course of dysphagia raises a strong suspicion of a nonneurological cause.[57]

AGE CONSIDERATIONS IN DYSPHAGIA

Elderly Patients

Aging is not a cause of dysphagia, but changes that occur with aging or that are associated with aging can cause a predisposition to dysphagia or can aggravate the condition in an older person.[99] Some of those changes affect the oral stage, such as poor dentition, atrophy of the tongue and alveolar ridge, and diminished taste and smell sensitivity. Others can affect the pharyngeal stage, such as decreased muscle tone and increased ligamentous laxity, which impair pharyngeal clearing capabilities and limit laryngeal elevation. In addition to these changes, certain illnesses, such as stroke, parkinsonism, and hiatal hernia with gastroesophageal reflux, occur more commonly with age.[28, 31, 94, 99]

Aspiration during the swallowing process results from oral phase or combined oropharyngeal phase dysfunction

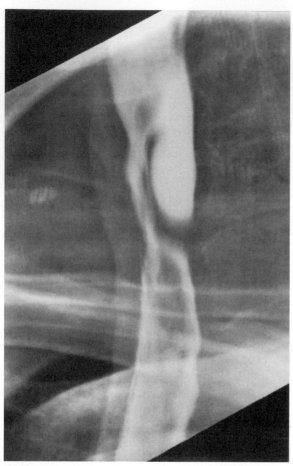

FIGURE 27–16 Lateral projection of video swallow test demonstrates large Zenker's diverticulum arising posteriorly from upper esophagus.

in the elderly as commonly as, if not more than, pharyngeal stage problems alone. Abnormalities identified on video-fluoroscopy during the oral stage include difficulties with bolus containment and poor coordination of bolus movement orally with the initiation of a swallow. Retention of the bolus in the pharynx and inadequate laryngeal protection are common defects visualized during the pharyngeal stage.[30]

Management of the elderly patient with dysphagia can involve special considerations. From a dietary standpoint, the older patient might routinely take in fewer calories and have secondary deficiencies in vitamins and minerals, particularly vitamin D, calcium, zinc, copper, and chromium.[54] From a standpoint of nutrition delivery, ethical issues may arise. For example, a mentally competent patient might not choose to accept enteral feeding despite a risk of aspiration. Such choices are often difficult for the swallowing team. More difficult are decisions about the management of an elderly patient with end-stage dementia or severe brain injury. Specific goals for treatment, clearly understood by family and team members, help alleviate ethical concerns.[92]

Young Patients

Swallowing difficulties in children result in the same medical concerns as those in adults: poor nutrition and aspiration. Certain factors make dysphagia in children unique, however.

Just as the child normally grows and develops, so too does the swallowing process. Differences between the infant and adult are most apparent in the oral phase of swallowing. *Suckling* is an early feeding behavior that consists of a rhythmic compression of the nipple by the tongue and lower jaw against the palate and upper jaw. Suckling activity is important for infants, even if it is with a nonfeeding nipple (*nonnutritive suck*).[108] With development, this behavior evolves through a series of chewing functions until about age 3 years, and becomes further coordinated by about age 6 years, when the oral phase approximates that of the adult. The pharyngeal phase in the infant is similar to that of the adult from early on, although the swallow typically occurs with greater frequency and speed in an infant.[58]

Difficulties in feeding and swallowing arise from several sources. For example, prematurity by itself can result in poor coordination of sucking and breathing, often manifested by apnea and bradycardia.[66] Neurological impairment, as occurs in cerebral palsy, is a common cause of dysphagia in the young. Affected children can exhibit findings such as the bite reflex, tongue thrust, poor trunk control, and slowness in eating.[110] The degree of swallowing difficulty typically parallels the degree of impairment in cerebral palsy, but aspiration can remain clinically hidden, even with severe disability. Videofluoroscopy documents that silent aspiration is very common in this population.[87] Coordination of deglutition and ventilation is frequently impaired and is associated with a prolonged, exhausting feeding time. Because hypoxemia can occur while a child with swallowing difficulties eats, pulse oximetry during mealtime can be useful in these situations to help direct treatment.[88]

As with the adult, gastroesophageal reflux is a common problem in very young children, and it contributes to both feeding and respiratory difficulties.[66] Gastric pH changes with age, and the lowest mean pH (1.99) occurs in the pediatric age group.[67] This low pH places the child at particular risk for aspiration-induced chemical pneumonitis.

Congenital structural lesions can interfere with the normal anatomical transport of a bolus. Multiple disorders can occur, ranging from choanal atresia, cleft lip and palate, and craniofacial syndromes, to vascular anomalies, such as a double aortic arch or an aberrant right subclavian artery.[112] With certain structural lesions, prosthetic devices or adapted feeding equipment, including modified nipples, might be necessary. A Chiari malformation is another type of structural lesion that can result in neurogenic dysphagia.[84]

Management of the pediatric patient requires a special approach. Cognitive, developmental, and behavioral issues can affect treatment options. If a child has acquired dysphagia after having learned feeding skills, treatment can be drawn from the child's prior experience. If dysphagia is congenitally acquired, feeding skills must be learned for the first time, often in the face of neurological or structural impairments.[21]

Treatment does not necessarily imply the use of feeding therapy.[74] Addressing such problems as tonal abnormalities, postural control, adverse behavior, and primitive reflexes might precede any attempt at oral feeding. When feeding does begin, it is clear from both clinical experience and videofluoroscopy that positioning and dietary makeup are important for the neurologically impaired child. Isolated oral phase dysfunction is usually best managed with feeding in a reclined position, whereas an erect position is most effective for pharyngeal phase problems.[75] In addition, children with cerebral palsy typically manage solid boluses more easily than liquid boluses, and small liquid boluses more easily than large liquid boluses.[20]

COMPLICATIONS OF DYSPHAGIA

Aspiration Pneumonia

Dysphagia is a major risk factor for aspiration pneumonia, a serious medical complication.[70] Aspiration typically occurs at the time of eating, but it can also occur at other times. Some individuals without dysphagia even aspirate during sleep.[43] Not every episode of aspiration results in pneumonia. Aspiration results in pneumonia primarily by three mechanisms: chemical injury, bacterial infection, and obstruction (Table 27–4).[4, 55, 56]

Chemical pneumonitis typically presents with acute dyspnea and hypoxemia. It develops from the burn of gastric acid present in the aspirate and implies gastric reflux. The pH and volume of the aspirate seem to be the most important determinants of whether pulmonary injury will occur. When the pH is less than approximately 2.5, there is particular concern for chemical pneumonia.[4, 107] The natural course of pneumonia is variable. Rapid improvement typically occurs over about 5 days. In other instances, improvement occurs initially, followed by a superimposed infection. Least commonly, but most worrisome, the course is fulminant, and death occurs. Treatment is supportive, with fluids and ventilation as needed. The role of steroids and antibiotics is not clearly defined in this type of aspiration pneumonia.[4]

Bacterial pneumonia typically presents with fever and sputum production over a more insidious onset. Anaerobes present in oral flora are common pathogens in community-acquired pneumonia, whereas gram-negative bacilli and *Staphylococcus aureus* become more prominent in hospital-acquired disease.[4, 32, 55, 56] This information can guide antibiotic selection in the absence of culture identification.

Aspiration of particles of food can result in airway obstruction. The right mainstem bronchus territory is typically involved, and symptoms include wheezing, coughing, choking, and respiratory distress.[55] The severity of this condition partially depends on the size of the particle aspirated. The potential for aspiration of particulate matter mandates that persons caring for any patient with dysphagia know the Heimlich maneuver. A superimposed bacterial infection can also occur in this type of aspiration as a result of obstruction of normal pulmonary drainage.[4]

In addition to specific treatment for dysphagia, measures to prevent aspiration pneumonia include elevation of the head of the bed, use of H_2-blocking agents or antacids to increase gastric pH above 2.5, and decrease in food intake before sleep.[4]

Malnutrition

Poor nutritional status has been documented as a common problem in the general hospital patient[7] as well as in patients admitted for rehabilitation.[78] Presumably, the patient with dysphagia is in a particularly high-risk category for undernutrition.[97]

As part of the dysphagia evaluation, some measure of nutritional status is useful as a baseline. Multiple measures are available, including the simple measures of percentage ideal weight and percentage weight lost. All of the measures have limitations,[95] but a recent weight loss of more than 10% to 15% and weight below 90% of ideal body weight represent significant malnutrition.[50, 52, 97] The visceral protein compartment can be measured from serum albumin and transferrin levels. Because of albumin's long half-life (20 days), the albumin value does not reflect acute nutritional deficiencies; but a level of less than 3.5 g/dL can be of nutritional concern.[22] Nitrogen balance assesses protein catabolism as well as the effects of nutritional

TABLE 27–4   Classification of Aspiration Pneumonia

Inoculum	Pulmonary Sequelae	Clinical Features	Therapy
Acid	Chemical pneumonitis	Acute dyspnea, tachypnea, tachycardia with or without cyanosis, bronchospasm, fever Sputum: pink, frothy X-ray: infiltrates in one or both lower lobes Hypoxemia	Positive-pressure breathing Intravenous fluids Tracheal suction Corticosteroids
Oropharyngeal bacteria	Bacterial infection	Usually insidious onset Cough, fever, purulent sputum X-ray: infiltrate involving dependent pulmonary segment or lobe with or without cavitation	Antibiotics
Inert fluids	Mechanical obstruction Reflex airway closure	Acute dyspnea, cyanosis with or without apnea Pulmonary edema	Tracheal suction Intermittent positive pressure breathing with oxygen and isoproterenol
Particulate matter	Mechanical obstruction	Dependent on level of obstruction, ranging from acute apnea and rapid death to irritating chronic cough with or without recurrent infections	Extraction of particulate matter

From Bartlett JG: Aspiration pneumonia. *In* Baum GL, Wolinsky E (eds): Textbook of Pulmonary Diseases, ed 5, vol 1. Boston, Little, Brown, 1994, p 593. By permission of the publisher.

intervention. Nitrogen balance is defined as the balance of input (protein intake divided by 6.25) and nitrogen output (urine urea nitrogen + 4). If the nitrogen output exceeds the input by 15 to 20 g/day, protein losses are significant.[52]

In cases of malnutrition, the daily caloric needs are traditionally determined with the Harris Benedict formula for basal energy expenditure (BEE), which takes into account weight, height, and age:

BEE for women = 655 + (9.6 × weight [kg]) + (1.8 × height [cm]) − (4.7 × age [yr])

BEE for men = 66 + (13.7 × weight [kg]) + (5 × height [cm]) − (6.8 × age [yr])

This formula was derived from healthy individuals at rest. Adjustment factors have been defined for activity and injury. General hospital patients require 120% of BEE, whereas medically stressed patients can require 150% to 200%.[22] An estimate of caloric need is typically 25 to 30 calories/kg of ideal body weight. Protein requirements are typically estimated at 1.0 to 1.5 mg/kg per day, but are increased in catabolic states and decreased in significant renal or liver disease.[52] Daily caloric counts, serial weight determinations, and monitoring of nutritional measures, such as nitrogen balance, help direct further refinement of dietary needs.

When nutritional needs can be orally only partially or not at all, enteral feeding is the usual route of choice unless there is a need to eliminate the risk of aspiration completely.[98] An initial feeding route is easily accomplished with a soft nasogastric feeding tube. If enteral feeding is prolonged, the use of a gastrostomy tube, typically placed percutaneously, is better tolerated by the patient, provides the prescribed nutrition more reliably, and results in more weight gain than the long-term use of a nasogastric feeding tube.[82] The absence of a nasogastric tube also facilitates swallowing interventions, although a nasogastric tube is not a contraindication to therapeutic feeding.[81] The absence of a nasogastric tube does not eliminate the risk of aspiration. Whether a tube placed in the jejunum affords greater protection from aspiration than a gastric tube is unclear.[60] Data from patients hospitalized for acute conditions who are enterally fed by various routes suggest that the incidence of aspiration is only 2.4 per 1000 tube-feeding days, and there is no excess mortality and only minimal morbidity. Continuous feedings by infusion pump result in the least gastric distention and might be preferable in patients at high risk for reflux aspiration.[76] Continuous feedings are also useful in patients with poor enteral motility or in persons who require hypertonic formulas. Intermittent or bolus feeding, however, is less disruptive to rehabilitation activities and to general daily living.[106]

TREATMENT MENU FOR DYSPHAGIA

Dietary Manipulation

Modification of the diet for the patient with dysphagia is a critical step in establishing a therapeutic feeding pro-

gram. If oral feedings, in some form, are determined to be appropriate, the type of food to be administered needs careful consideration. Although thin liquids can result in less pharyngeal residue, they are often difficult for the patient with a neurological disorder to manage. Liquids can be thickened with various thickening agents. These agents typically are added to, for example, hot or cold beverages or soups. A thicker consistency can be beneficial to patients who have a delayed swallow reflex because there is less tendency for the material to fall over the base of the tongue before the swallow is triggered. The patient or a family member can be instructed in the amount of the thickening agents to be added to obtain an optimal consistency.

Food can be modified to have a pureed, semisolid, or solid consistency, depending on the results of the patient's clinical or videofluoroscopic evaluation. Pureed consistencies can be used for patients who have difficulty chewing or who are unable to form a cohesive bolus because of decreased tongue function. As tongue function, chewing ability, and pharyngeal function improve, patients might tolerate advancing their food types to soft, semisolid, and regular consistencies. Many centers have adapted the "dysphagia diet" concept as a means for organizing and administering appropriate foods. The benefit of the dysphagia diet is that it links similar foods. Examples of a dysphagia diet are in the first column of Table 27–5.

As the patient demonstrates clinical or radiographic improvement, the dysphagia diet can be advanced to the next level (Table 27–5). Careful monitoring of the patient with the introduction of each new food type is important to ensure safety and to avoid the risk of aspiration. Because many patients are instructed in various compensatory techniques to be used during mealtimes, monitoring the patient

TABLE 27–5   Dysphagia Diet

Group	Initial Evaluation	Reevaluation	Reevaluation
Date			
1. Thin liquids (fruit juice, coffee, tea)			
2. Medium-thick liquids (tomato juice, sherbet, strained cream soup)			
3. Spoon-thick foods (applesauce, mashed potatoes with gravy, cooked cereal)			
4. Semisolids (ground meats with gravy, meatloaf, bananas)			
5. Foods that fall apart (plain ground meats, eggs)			
6. Sticky or bulky foods (diced/regular meats, casseroles)			
7. Mixed textures (stews, gelatin with fruit)			

during mealtime is essential. This can be done by nurses or family members after instruction by the swallowing therapist.

Oral hygiene needs careful consideration. Dried secretions can accumulate on the tongue and palate, reducing oral sensitivity and promoting growth of bacteria in the mouth.[35] Lemon-glycerin, plain swabs, or a damp washcloth can be used to remove the secretions. This step should be done before treatment or administration of food substances.

Exercise and Facilitation Techniques

Numerous exercises and methods of facilitation have been described for the patient with dysphagia. Clinical experience and anecdotes indicate the effectiveness of these techniques despite the lack of research to scientifically support their benefits. The techniques and exercises require that the patient be able to follow directions and participate in a therapy program. The indications for use of the exercises are outlined in Table 27–6.

Exercises designed to facilitate oral motor strength, range of motion, and coordination are best done frequently (5 to 10 times per day).[62] Patients and family members can be instructed by the swallowing therapist to perform the exercises between therapy sessions. The variety of exercises is limited only by the clinician's creativity.

Examples of exercises for the lips to facilitate the ability to prevent food or liquid from leaking out of the oral cavity, are as follows:

> Open mouth wide, relax, repeat
> Smile, grin, or sneer

TABLE 27–6 Indications for Exercises in Patients With Dysphagia

Clinical Diagnosis	Clinical Observation	Exercise/Technique
Decreased lip range of motion, strength, or coordination	Drooling, facial droop	Lip exercises
Decreased tongue range of motion, strength, or coordination	Inability to propel food from front to back of mouth Food pooling in sulci	Tongue exercises
Decreased jaw range of motion, strength, or coordination	Inability to chew food adequately	Jaw exercises
Weak or absent cough	Inability (or decreased ability) to produce productive cough	Respiratory exercises
Increased respiratory rate	Rapid or shallow breathing	Respiratory exercises
Decreased airway protection	Wet or "gurgly" voice Hoarse voice Coughing during the swallow	Vocal cord adduction exercises
Delayed/absent swallow reflex	Decreased laryngeal elevation during swallow Coughing before the swallow	Thermal stimulation

> Repeat "pa, pa, pa, ba, ba, ba"
> Blow through a straw, party favor, or windmill, or blow bubbles

Examples of exercises for the tongue to facilitate manipulation of the bolus and its propulsion through the oral cavity, or to aid pharyngeal swallowing abilities by improving retraction of the tongue base,[37] are as follows:

> Protrude tongue
> Push tongue into side of cheek
> Push tongue against a tongue depressor in varying directions
> Repeat "la, la, la, ta, ta, ta"

Examples of exercises for the jaw to facilitate the rotary movements required for mastication are as follows:

> Open mouth as wide as possible, relax, repeat
> Move jaw from side to side

Any of these exercises for lip, tongue, or jaw can be modified by applying manual resistance to increase strength. Increasing the speed of the exercise can help coordination.

Patients with impaired respiratory status are at increased risk for aspiration because of their inability to successfully cease respiration in order to swallow. Their inability to successfully clear penetrated or aspirated material from the airway compromises safe swallowing. Several exercises can improve respiratory strength, as follows:

> Take in a big breath, inhale deeply, and exhale slowly
> Take in a big breath. Repeat "ah, ah, ah" as long as possible
> Blow through a straw, a windmill, or party favor
> Read poems or sing a song

Vocal cord adduction exercises are performed as an attempt to strengthen weak cords and approximate them to prevent aspiration. Examples of these exercises include the following:

> Repeat "ah, ah, ah," while pushing down on a chair or pushing hands together
> Say "ah" for 5 sec while pushing down on a chair

Because these vocal cord adduction exercises create a Valsalva effect, caution is necessary when they are being performed by a patient with a cardiac disorder.

Thermal stimulation is a facilitative technique designed to increase the speed at which the swallow occurs. It can be performed with a laryngeal mirror (size 00) or a metal rod of similar size. The mirror is placed in ice for approximately 10 seconds and then placed along the area of the anterior facial arch (bilaterally) and rubbed or tapped five to eight times. After this icing procedure, the patient is asked to swallow.[62] This technique can be performed frequently throughout the day as well as before mealtimes. If oral feedings are not recommended, the therapist can use it without trials of food as a means to facilitate triggering of the swallow reflex. This technique has been found to be of clinical benefit in some patients,[24] although findings are mixed.[89] Patients might report an easier time initiating a swallow when the technique is done immediately before mealtime.

If abnormal oral reflexes (such as tongue thrust or bite

reflex) are found during the clinical evaluation, attempts should be made to inhibit them.[35] The bite reflex can be inhibited by applying sustained pressure to the tongue with a rubber seizure stick and positioning the head in an upright position with the chin tucked.[29] The tongue thrust can be inhibited by a sequence of techniques, including pressure under the chin to tongue retraction musculature, manual vibration under the tongue, and quick stretch of the tongue into protrusion to facilitate retrusion.[29]

The gag reflex can be either hypoactive or hyperactive. Although a normal gag reflex is not required for safe swallowing, attempts to normalize it are recommended. Facilitation of a hypoactive gag can be done by applying a tongue depressor, cotton-tipped swab, or quick tap or stretch to the arch of the soft palate in an upward and outward direction. A hyperactive gag can be desensitized by using firm pressure with a tongue depressor to slowly "walk" back on the tongue.[79] As the gag reflex becomes less sensitive, the tongue depressor can be advanced farther back in the mouth.

Compensatory Techniques

Various methods can be used to compensate for swallowing dysfunction (Table 27–7). The patient's head and trunk can be positioned to compensate for swallowing dysfunction. The ideal position for most patients with a neurological disorder is to be seated upright in a chair with the head in the midline, the trunk erect, and the neck slightly flexed forward. Pillows and other supports can be used to maintain trunk support and to support the limbs.

Common postural techniques used to decrease or eliminate aspiration include tilting the chin down, turning the head, or tilting the head to the right or left. As described by Logemann,[62] the chin tuck can be beneficial in that it widens the vallecular space (Fig. 27–17). In the case of aspiration due to a delayed swallow reflex, the chin tuck provides greater airway protection by allowing food substances to sit in the valleculae until the reflex is triggered.

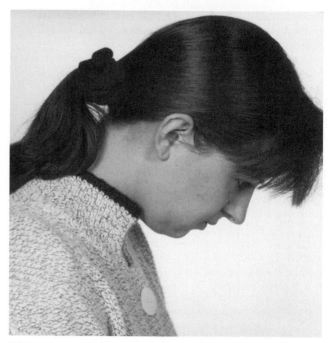

FIGURE 27–17   Positioning of the head for the chin tuck; this is used to increase protection to the airway.

Research shows that the chin tuck can be beneficial in that it decreases the space between the base of the tongue and the posterior pharyngeal wall, and so creates increased pharyngeal pressure to move the bolus through the pharyngeal region.[113]

Turning of the head to the affected side can be beneficial when decreased pharyngeal peristalsis is noted unilaterally (Fig. 27–18). This helps direct food down the stronger or

TABLE 27–7   Indications for Compensatory Techniques in Patients with Dysphagia

Clinical Diagnosis	Clinical Observations	Compensatory Technique
Delayed swallow reflex	Coughing before the swallow Aspiration	Chin tuck Supraglottic swallow
Decreased pharyngeal peristalsis (unilaterally)	Unilateral pooling in the pharyngeal region Coughing after the swallow	Turning of head to weaker side Tilting of head to stronger side
Decreased pharyngeal peristalsis	Coughing after the swallow	Effortful swallow Double swallow Alternating liquids and swallows
Decreased laryngeal closure	Coughing during or after the swallow	Chin tuck Supraglottic swallow
Decreased opening of cricopharyngeal region	Coughing after the swallow Pooling in the pyriform sinus	Mendelsohn's maneuver Turning of head to weaker side

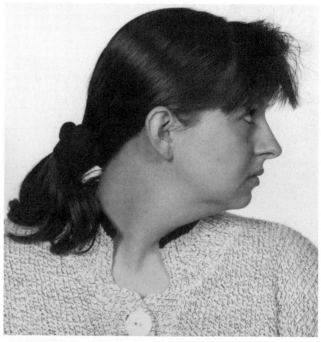

FIGURE 27–18   Turning of the head to one side; this is used to direct food down the stronger side of the pharynx.

more normal side of the pharynx. Recent work also has shown improved function of the upper esophageal sphincter with head turning.[64]

Tilting of the head to the right or left toward the stronger side can be of similar assistance in that it keeps food on the stronger side of the pharynx.[62] It also is effective for patients who have unilateral tongue weakness because it directs food toward the stronger side of the tongue. From clinical experience, these techniques can be effective for decreasing or eliminating aspiration in some, but certainly not in all, cases. The effectiveness of these techniques is best determined by viewing them on videofluoroscopy.

Other compensatory techniques include effortful swallows and double swallows. For the former, the patient swallows "hard" while eating in an attempt to help propel food through the pharyngeal cavity in a forceful and timely manner. For double swallowing, the patient swallows twice (or more if needed) after food swallows. One or both of these techniques can be beneficial for cases in which decreased pharyngeal peristalsis is noted on videofluoroscopy.

Alternating liquids and solids can be another effective technique in some cases in which decreased pharyngeal peristalsis is present. The liquid swallows help to clear any material remaining in the pharyngeal recesses.

The supraglottic swallow is a technique designed to close the airway voluntarily.[62] It incorporates closure of the vocal folds along with clearing the airway of any aspirated material after the swallow. This technique can be useful for patients who have reduced laryngeal closure. The steps of the supraglottic swallow are as follows:

1. Take a deep breath and hold it.
2. Take a bite of food or a sip of liquid.
3. Swallow.
4. Cough immediately after swallow.
5. Breathe.

This technique can be used with just one or with all consistencies of food. Because numerous steps are required, the patient must demonstrate the ability to follow and sequence the instructions.

Logemann (in a paper read at the Seminar on Evaluation and Treatment of Swallowing Disorders, Bloomington, Minn, March 28–29, 1992), also described the super supraglottic swallow, which incorporates the supraglottic swallow with the patient's bearing down on a table or pressing the hands together to create a Valsalva effect. This can assist in creating additional laryngeal closure.

The Mendelsohn maneuver is a technique designed to prolong the opening of the cricopharyngeal region.[83] The technique might be indicated for cases in which decreased laryngeal elevation and subsequent decreased cricopharyngeal opening are present. It is done by instructing the patient to swallow, to "hold" the swallow for 2 to 3 sec when the pharynx is in the uppermost stage, and then to complete the swallow and relax.[37] It is one of the few techniques that can be of assistance in working with a disorder of the cricopharyngeal region.

Biofeedback techniques have been of assistance in swallowing retraining. They can be useful for oral motor and facial exercises and for giving the patient feedback on the actual swallow.[13]

Adaptive Equipment

Numerous devices are available to assist patients who have difficulty with the motor or perceptual components of feeding. Examples include rocker knives, swivel utensils, built-up handles on utensils, scoop dishes, nonskid mats, and large-handled cups (Fig. 27–19). These devices compensate for decreased upper extremity function, including limited grasp, incoordination, decreased range of motion, hemiparesis, and hemiplegia (see Chapter 26).

Surgical Procedures

Operative intervention is another option in the treatment of dysphagia. It is particularly helpful when conservative

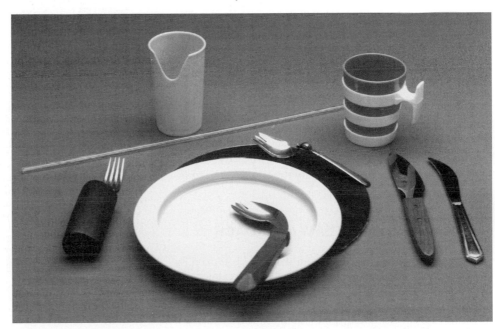

FIGURE 27–19 Adaptive equipment used to compensate for limited upper extremity function: from left to right, built-up fork, nose cut-out cup, long straw, inner lip plate, nonskid mat, offset spoon and fork, large-handled mug, and rocker knives.

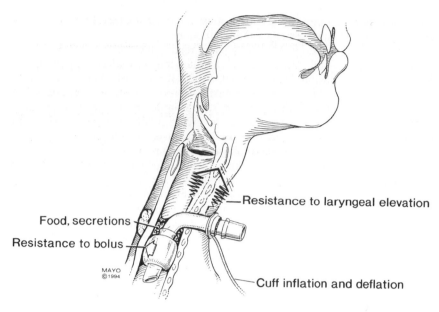

FIGURE 27–20 The swallowing impairments from a tracheostomy. (Redrawn from Nash M: Swallowing problems in the tracheotomized patient. Otolaryngol Clin North Am 1988; 21:701. By permission of Mayo Foundation for Medical Education and Research.)

Resistance to laryngeal elevation

Food, secretions

Resistance to bolus

Cuff inflation and deflation

measures have failed and swallowing difficulties arise from a focal neuromuscular disorder or obstruction.

A tracheostomy is commonly used to provide optimal pulmonary ventilation and hygiene, and it also serves as a short-term solution for airway protection from aspiration.[8] Ironically, it can also be a risk factor for aspiration. After tracheostomy, laryngeal elevation is impaired, which increases the risk of aspiration. Aspiration can also be associated with cuff inflation or deflation. The inflated cuff applies a compressive force to the esophagus and may increase resistance to the passage of a food bolus. The deflated cuff allows food or secretions that have been retained above the cuff to pass into the trachea,[77] and careful suctioning after cuff deflation is necessary (Fig. 27–20).

Cricopharyngeal myotomy is often done in patients with Zenker's diverticulum and is effective in the treatment of cricopharyngeal achalasia.[2, 6] Myotomy is not generally recommended for conditions in which a generalized failure of the swallowing process is present,[8] although it has been used successfully in neuromuscular disease.[61] Videofluoroscopy has limitations in the assessment of cricopharyngeal function, and manometry or newer study tools can be helpful in making decisions regarding myotomy.[23]

Several procedures have been devised for protection of the larynx, including vocal cord augmentation in mild aspiration and laryngeal diversion for more severe and chronic cases. Microsurgical techniques and progress with microprocessors in the application of electrical stimulation give hope that a more functional solution to severe aspiration will evolve with time.[8]

OUTCOMES OF THE TEAM APPROACH

Dysphagia is a complex symptom that can be evoked by a myriad of disorders. The assessment and treatment of this symptom and its cause often transcend one specialty or discipline. Consequently, utilization of a multidisciplinary treatment team, functioning in an interdisciplinary manner,

has become common. In the rehabilitation setting, a team frequently consists of a speech pathologist, an occupational therapist, a physiatrist, a radiologist, a dietitian, and a rehabilitation nurse with consultation from a gastroenterologist, an otolaryngologist, and other subspecialists as needed. Use of this team approach for evaluation and treatment seems to result in improved outcomes. The risk of aspiration cannot be completely eliminated, but patients managed with this approach aspirate less often than their control group counterparts,[51] and they also have greater caloric intake and weight gain.[69]

References

1. Alberts MJ, Horner J, Gray L, et al: Aspiration after stroke: Lesion analysis by brain MRI. Dysphagia 1992; 7:170.
2. Baredes S: Surgical management of swallowing disorders. Otolaryngol Clin North Am 1988; 21:711.
3. Barer DH: The natural history and functional consequences of dysphagia after hemispheric stroke. J Neurol Neurosurg Psychiatry 1989; 52:236.
4. Bartlett JG: Aspiration pneumonia. In Baum GL, Wolinksy E (eds): Textbook of Pulmonary Diseases, ed 5, vol 1. Boston, Little Brown, 1994, p 593.
5. Beck TJ, Gayler BW: Image quality and radiation levels in videofluoroscopy for swallowing studies: A review. Dysphagia 1990; 5:118.
6. Berg HM, Jacobs JB, Persky MS, et al: Cricopharyngeal myotomy: A review of surgical results in patients with cricopharyngeal achalasia of neurogenic origin. Laryngoscope 1985; 95:1337.
7. Bistrian BR, Blackburn GL, Vitale J, et al: Prevalence of malnutrition in general medical patients. JAMA 1976; 235:1567.
8. Blitzer A: Approaches to the patient with aspiration and swallowing disabilities. Dysphagia 1990; 5:129.
9. Bosma JF: Deglutition: Pharyngeal stage. Physiol Rev 1957; 37:275.
10. Bosma JF, Donner MW, Tanaka E, et al: Anatomy of the pharynx, pertinent to swallowing. Dysphagia 1986; 1:23.
11. Brin MF, Younger D: Neurologic disorders and aspiration. Otolaryngol Clin North Am 1988; 21:691.
12. Brown GE, Nordloh S, Donowitz AJ: Systematic desensitization of oral hypersensitivity in a patient with a closed head injury. Dysphagia 1992; 7:138.
13. Bryant M: Biofeedback in the treatment of a selected dysphagic patient. Dysphagia 1991; 6:140.
14. Buchholz D: Neurologic causes of dysphagia. Dysphagia 1987; 1:152.

15. Buchholz D, Jones B: Dysphagia occurring after polio. Dysphagia 1991; 6:165.

16. Buchin PJ: Swallowing disorders: Diagnosis and medical treatment. Otolaryngol Clin North Am 1988; 21:663.

17. Busmann M, Dobmeyer SM, Leeker L, et al: Swallowing abnormalities and their response to treatment in Parkinson's disease. Neurology 1989; 39:1309.

18. Cameron DC, Guy D: The design of a lightweight mobile chair for use with video fluoroscopy in the investigation of swallow disorders. Australas Radiol 1990; 34:274.

19. Carter GT, Johnson ER, Bonekat HW, et al: Laryngeal diversion in the treatment of intractable aspiration in motor neuron disease. Arch Phys Med Rehabil 1992; 73:680.

20. Casas MJ, Kenny DJ, McPherson KA: Swallowing/ventilation interactions during oral swallow in normal children and children with cerebral palsy. Dysphagia 1994; 9:40.

21. Christensen JR: Developmental approach to pediatric neurogenic dysphagia. Dysphagia 1989; 3:131.

22. Ciocon JO: Indications for tube feedings in elderly patients. Dysphagia 1990; 5:1.

23. Cook IJ: Cricopharyngeal function and dysfunction. Dysphagia 1993; 8:244.

24. de Lama Lazzara G, Lazarus C, Logemann JA: Impact of thermal stimulation on the triggering of the swallowing reflex. Dysphagia 1986; 1:73.

25. DePippo KL, Holas MA, Reding MJ: Validation of the 3-oz water swallow test for aspiration following stroke. Arch Neurol 1992; 49:1259.

26. Dodds WJ: Physiology of swallowing. Dysphagia 1989; 3:171.

27. Dworkin JP, Nadal JC: Nonsurgical treatment of drooling in a patient with closed head injury and severe dysarthria. Dysphagia 1991; 6:40.

28. Ergun GA, Miskovitz PF: Aging and the esophagus: Common pathologic conditions and their effect upon swallowing in the geriatric population. Dysphagia 1992; 7:58.

29. Farber SD: Neurorehabilitation: A Multisensory Approach. Philadelphia, WB Saunders, 1982, p 115.

30. Feinberg MJ, Ekberg O: Videofluoroscopy in elderly patients with aspiration: Importance of evaluating both oral and pharyngeal stages of deglutition. Am J Roentgenol 1991; 156:293.

31. Feinberg MJ, Knebl I, Tully J, et al: Aspiration and the elderly. Dysphagia 1990; 5:61.

32. Finegold SM: Aspiration pneumonia. Rev Infect Dis 1991; 13(Suppl 9):S737.

33. Goyal RK, Martin SB, Shapiro J, et al: The role of cricopharyngeus muscle in pharyngoesophageal disorders. Dysphagia 1993; 8:252.

34. Gray C, Sivaloganathan S, Simpkins KC: Aspiration of high-density barium contrast medium causing acute pulmonary inflammation—report of two fatal cases in elderly women with disordered swallowing. Clin Radiol 1989; 40:397.

35. Groher ME: Dysphagia: Diagnosis and Management. Butterworth, Boston, 1984.

36. Hagen R, Haase A, Matthaei D, et al: Oropharyngeale Funktionsdiagnostik mit der FLASH-MR-Tomographie. HNO 1990; 38:421.

37. Hardy E, Robinson NM: Swallowing Disorders: Treatment Manual. Bisbee, Ariz, Imaginart Communication Products, 1993.

38. Hendrix TR: Art and science of history taking in the patient with difficulty swallowing. Dysphagia 1993; 8:69.

39. Holt S, Miron SD, Diaz MC, et al: Scintigraphic measurement of oropharyngeal transit in man. Dig Dis Sci 1990; 35:1198.

40. Horner J, Buoyer FG, Alberts MJ, et al: Dysphagia following brainstem stroke: Clinical correlates and outcome. Arch Neurol 1991; 48:1170.

41. Horner J, Massey EW, Brazer SR: Aspiration in bilateral stroke patients. Neurology 1990; 40:1686.

42. Horner J, Massey EW, Riski JE, et al: Aspiration following stroke: Clinical correlates and outcome. Neurology 1988; 38:1359.

43. Huxley EJ, Viroslav J, Gray WR, et al: Pharyngeal aspiration in normal adults and patients with depressed consciousness. Am J Med 1978; 64:564.

44. Johnson ER, McKenzie SW, Rosenquist CJ, et al: Dysphagia following stroke: Quantitative evaluation of pharyngeal transit times. Arch Phys Med Rehabil 1992; 73:419.

45. Johnson ER, McKenzie SW, Sievers A: Aspiration pneumonia in stroke. Arch Phys Med Rehabil 1993; 74:973.

46. Jones B, Buchholz DW, Ravich WJ, et al: Swallowing dysfunction in the postpolio syndrome: A cinefluorographic study. Am J Roentgenol 1992; 158:283.

47. Jones B, Donner MW: How I do it: Examination of the patient with dysphagia. Dysphagia 1989; 4:162.

48. Jones B, Ravich WJ, Donner MW: Dysphagia in systemic disease. Dysphagia 1993; 8:368.

49. Kahrilas PJ: Pharyngeal structure and function. Dysphagia 1993; 8:303.

50. Kamel PL: Nutritional assessment and requirements. Dysphagia 1990; 4:189.

51. Kasprisin AT, Clumeck H, Nino-Murcia M: Efficacy of rehabilitative management of dysphagia. Dysphagia 1989; 4:48.

52. Kelly KG: Advances in perioperative nutritional support. Med Clin North Am 1993; 77:465.

53. Kennedy JG III, Kent RD: Physiological substrates of normal deglutition. Dysphagia 1988; 3:24.

54. Kerstetter JE, Holthausen BA, Fitz PA: Nutrition and nutritional requirements for the older adult. Dysphagia 1993; 8:51.

55. Khawaja IT, Buffa SD, Brandstetter RD: Aspiration pneumonia: A threat when deglutition is compromised. Postgrad Med 1992; 92:165, 173, 181.

56. Kirsch CM, Sanders A: Aspiration pneumonia: Medical management. Otolaryngol Clin North Am 1988; 21:677.

57. Koch WM: Swallowing disorders: Diagnosis and therapy. Med Clin North Am 1993; 77:571.

58. Kramer SS, Eicher PM: The evaluation of pediatric feeding abnormalities. Dysphagia 1993; 8:215.

59. Langmore SE, Schatz K, Olson N: Endoscopic and videofluoroscopic evaluations of swallowing and aspiration. Ann Otol Rhinol Laryngol 1991; 100:678.

60. Lazarus BA, Murphy JB, Culpepper L: Aspiration associated with long-term gastric versus jejunal feeding: A critical analysis of the literature. Arch Phys Med Rehabil 1990; 71:46.

61. Lindgren S, Ekberg O: Cricopharyngeal myotomy in the treatment of dysphagia. Clin Otolaryngol 1990; 15:221.

62. Logemann JA: Evaluation and Treatment of Swallowing Disorders. San Diego, College Hill Press, 1983.

63. Logemann JA: Swallowing physiology and pathophysiology. Otolaryngol Clin North Am 1988; 21:613.

64. Logemann JA, Kahrilas PJ, Kohara M, et al: The benefit of head rotation on pharyngoesophageal dysphagia. Arch Phys Med Rehabil 1989; 70:767.

65. Logemann JA, Shanahan T, Rademaker AW, et al: Oropharyngeal swallowing after stroke in the left basal ganglion/internal capsule. Dysphagia 1993; 8:230.

66. Loughlin GM: Respiratory consequences of dysfunctional swallowing and aspiration. Dysphagia 1989; 3:126.

67. Manchikanti L, Colliver JA, Marrero TC, et al: Assessment of age-related acid aspiration risk factors in pediatric adult and geriatric patients. Anesth Analg 1985; 64:11.

68. Maniere-Ezvan A, Duval JM, Darnault P: Ultrasonic assessment of the anatomy and function of the tongue. Surg Radiol Anat 1993; 15:55.

69. Martens L, Cameron T, Simonsen M: Effects of a multidisciplinary management program on neurologically impaired patients with dysphagia. Dysphagia 1990; 5:147.

70. Martin BJ, Corlew MM, Wood H, et al: The association of swallowing dysfunction and aspiration pneumonia. Dysphagia 1994; 9:1.

71. Martin RE, Sessle BJ: The role of the cerebral cortex in swallowing. Dysphagia 1993; 8:195.

72. Milazzo LS, Bouchard J, Lund DA: The swallowing process: Effects of aging and stroke. Phys Med Rehabil 1989; 3:489.

73. Miller AJ: Neurophysiological basis of swallowing. Dysphagia 1986; 1:91.

74. Morris SE: Development of oral-motor skills in the neurologically impaired child receiving non-oral feedings. Dysphagia 1989; 3:135.

75. Morton RE, Bonas R, Fourie B, et al: Videofluoroscopy in the assessment of feeding disorders of children with neurological problems. Dev Med Child Neurol 1993; 35:388.

76. Mullan H, Roubenoff RA, Roubenoff R: Risk of pulmonary aspiration among patients receiving enteral nutrition support. J Parenteral Enteral Nutr 1992; 16:160.

77. Nash M: Swallowing problems in the tracheotomized patient. Otolaryngol Clin North Am 1988; 21:701.

78. Newmark SR, Sublett D, Black J, et al: Nutritional assessment in a rehabilitation unit. Arch Phys Med Rehabil 1981; 62:279.

79. O'Sullivan N: Dysphagia Care: Team Approach With Acute and Long-Term Patients. Los Angeles, Cottage Square, 1990.

80. Ott DJ, Chen YM, Hewson EG, et al: Esophageal motility: Assessment with synchronous video tape fluoroscopy and manometry. Radiology 1989; 173:419.

81. Palmer JB, DuChane AS: Rehabilitation of swallowing disorders due to stroke. Phys Med Rehabil Clin North Am 1991; 2:529.

82. Park RH, Allison MC, Lang J, et al: Randomised comparison of percutaneous endoscopic gastrostomy and nasogastric tube feeding in patients with persisting neurological dysphagia. Br Med J 1992; 304:1406.

83. Penington GR, Krutsch JA: Swallowing disorders: Assessment and rehabilitation. Br J Hosp Med 1990; 44:17, 20, 22.

84. Pollack IF, Pang D, Kocoshis S, et al: Neurogenic dysphagia resulting from Chiari malformations. Neurosurgery 1992; 30:709.

85. Rasley A, Logemann JA, Kahrilas PJ, et al: Prevention of barium aspiration during videofluoroscopic swallowing studies: Value of change in posture. Am J Roentgenol 1993; 160:1005.

86. Robbins J, Levine RL, Maser A, et al: Swallowing after unilateral stroke of the cerebral cortex. Arch Phys Med Rehabil 1993; 74:1295.

87. Rogers B, Arvedson J, Buck G, et al: Characteristics of dysphagia in children with cerebral palsy. Dysphagia 1994; 9:69.

88. Rogers BT, Arvedson J, Msall M, et al: Hypoxemia during oral feeding of children with severe cerebral palsy. Dev Med Child Neurol 1993; 35:3.

89. Rosenbek JC, Robbins J, Fishback B, et al: Effects of thermal application on dysphagia after stroke. J Speech Hearing Res 1991; 34:1257.

90. Schima W, Stacher G, Pokieser P, et al: Esophageal motor disorders: Videofluoroscopic and manometric evaluation—prospective study in 88 symptomatic patients. Radiology 1992; 185:487.

91. Schmidt J, Holas M, Halvorson K, et al: Videofluoroscopic evidence of aspiration predicts pneumonia and death but not dehydration following stroke. Dysphagia 1994; 9:7.

92. Serradura-Russell A: Ethical dilemmas in dysphagia management and the right to a natural death. Dysphagia 1992; 7:102.

93. Sessle BJ, Henry JL: Neural mechanisms of swallowing: Neurophysiological and neurochemical studies on brain stem neurons in the solitary tract region. Dysphagia 1989; 4:61.

94. Sheth N, Diner WC: Swallowing problems in the elderly. Dysphagia 1988; 2:209.

95. Signore J, Erickson RV: Nutritional assessment of the stroke patient. Phys Med Rehabil 1989; 3:501.

96. Silver KH, Van Nostrand D, Kuhlemeier KV, et al: Scintigraphy for the detection and quantification of subglottic aspiration: Preliminary observations. Arch Phys Med Rehabil 1991; 72:902.

97. Sitzmann JV: Nutritional support of the dysphagic patient: Methods, risks, and complications of therapy. J Parenteral Enteral Nutr 1990; 14:60.

98. Sitzmann JV, Mueller R: Enteral and parenteral feeding in the dysphagic patient. Dysphagia 1988; 3:38.

99. Sonies BC: Oropharyngeal dysphagia in the elderly. Clin Geriatr Med 1992; 8:569.

100. Sonies BC: Ultrasound imaging and swallowing. *In* Jones B, Donner MW (eds): Normal and Abnormal Swallowing: Imaging in Diagnosis and Therapy. New York, Springer-Verlag, 1991, p 109.

101. Sonies BC, Dalakas MC: Dysphagia in patients with the post-polio syndrome. N Engl J Med 1991; 324:1162.

102. Splaingard ML, Hutchins B, Sulton LD, et al: Aspiration in rehabilitation patients: Videofluoroscopy vs bedside clinical assessment. Arch Phys Med Rehabil 1988; 69:637.

103. Stroudley J, Walsh M: Radiological assessment of dysphagia in Parkinson's disease. Br J Radiol 1991; 64:890.

104. Tatsch K, Schroettle W, Kirsch CM: Multiple swallow test for the quantitative and qualitative evaluation of esophageal motility disorders. J Nucl Med 1991; 32:1365.

105. Teasell RW, Bach D, McRae M: Prevalence and recovery of aspiration poststroke: A retrospective analysis. Dysphagia 1994; 9:35.

106. Teasell RW, Finestone HM, Greene-Finestone L: Dysphagia and nutrition following stroke. Phys Med Rehabil 1993; 7:89.

107. Terry PB, Fuller SD: Pulmonary consequences of aspiration. Dysphagia 1989; 3:179.

108. Tuchman DN: Cough, choke, sputter: The evaluation of the child with dysfunctional swallowing. Dysphagia 1989; 3:111.

109. Veis SL, Logemann JA: Swallowing disorders in persons with cerebrovascular accident. Arch Phys Med Rehabil 1985; 66:372.

110. Waterman ET, Koltai PJ, Downey JC, et al: Swallowing disorders in a population of children with cerebral palsy. Int J Pediatr Otorhinolaryngol 1992; 24:63.

111. Waxman MJ, Durfee D, Moore M, et al: Nutritional aspects and swallowing function of patients with Parkinson's disease. Nutr Clin Pract 1990; 5:196.

112. Weiss MH: Dysphagia in infants and children. Otolaryngol Clin North Am 1988; 21:727.

113. Welch MV, Logemann JA, Rademaker AW, et al: Changes in pharyngeal dimensions effected by chin tuck. Arch Phys Med Rehabil 1993; 74:178.

114. Winstein CJ: Neurogenic dysphagia: Frequency, progression, and outcome in adults following head injury. Phys Ther 1983; 63:1992.

28

Urinary Tract and Bowel Management in the Rehabilitation Setting

DIANA D. CARDENAS, M.D.,
MICHAEL E. MAYO, M.B.B.S., AND
JOHN C. KING, M.D.

This chapter is divided into two sections. The first section describes the neuroanatomy and the classification of the neurogenic bladder. It then focuses on methods of clinical evaluation, management, and common complications. The second section is devoted to the neurogenic bowel and provides a comparable discussion. Bladder and bowel dysfunction is commonly found in patients cared for by physiatrists. Basic knowledge of these areas is therefore important.

NEUROANATOMY

RECEPTORS. Receptors active during bladder contraction are cholinergic muscarinic (M_2) and are widely distributed in the bladder, trigone, bladder neck, and urethra. Adrenergic receptors are concentrated in the trigone, bladder neck, and urethra and are predominantly α_1. These, when active, have excitatory effects and maintain continence by contraction of the bladder neck smooth muscle. β_2-Adrenergic receptors are found in the bladder neck and also in the body of the bladder. These are inhibitory when activated and can produce relaxation at the bladder neck on the initiation of voiding and relax the bladder body to enhance storage (Fig. 28–1). In humans, however, the storage role seems to be a minor one. The striated sphincter muscle contains cholinergic nicotinic receptors. Other possible lower urinary tract transmitters have been considered to explain the fact that atropine only partially blocks cholinergic muscarinic transmission. A full discussion of this is beyond the scope of this chapter.[34]

INNERVATION. The afferent and efferent peripheral pathways are the autonomic through the pelvic (parasympathetic) and hypogastric (sympathetic) nerves and the somatic through the pudendal nerves (Fig. 28–2 and Table 28–1).

CENTRAL CONNECTIONS AND CONTROL. The reflex center for the bladder lies in the pons along with the other autonomic centers (Fig. 28–3). Not shown in Figure 28–3 is a reflex with afferent axons originating from the bladder and synapsing on the pudendal nerve nucleus at S2, S3, and S4, which allows inhibition of pelvic floor activity during voiding. Another important reflex is the local segmental innervation of the external sphincter with afferents from the urethra, sphincter, and pelvic floor and efferents in the pudendal nerve. Higher (voluntary) control over the pelvic floor is due to afferents that ascend to the sensory cortex, and descending fibers from the motor cortex descend to synapse with the pudendal motor nucleus.[9]

BLADDER FUNCTION

Urodynamic studies in both intact patients and those with neurological disease have given clinical insights into the normal and abnormal function of the lower urinary tract over the course of life.

INFANT AND YOUNG CHILD. Neonates and infants have truly reflex bladders that empty at approximately 50- to 100-mL volumes. Sometime after the first year of life, the child begins to show some awareness of bladder evacuation and can begin to delay urination for a brief period by contracting the voluntary sphincter. For normal control, the detrusor reflex has to be inhibited by the higher centers at the level of the pontine nucleus. By 5 years of age, approximately 90% of children have normal control, but the remaining 10% have a more infantile or immature pattern with

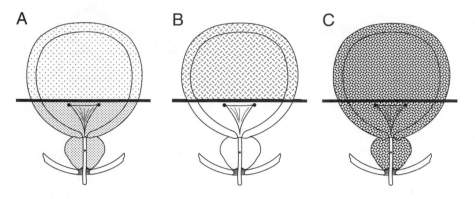

FIGURE 28–1 *A,* Distribution of the α-adrenergic receptors, with few in the dome of the bladder and more in the base of the bladder and prostate. *B,* Distribution of the β-receptors, which are largely in the dome. *C,* Distribution of the cholinergic receptors, which are widely distributed throughout the dome and the base of the bladder and the urethra.

detrusor activity between voluntary voidings that produces frequency, urgency, and occasionally urge incontinence and nocturnal enuresis. Most of these children gradually develop inhibition of the detrusor reflex by puberty.

ADULT. With bladder filling, there is only a minimal rise in intravesical pressure (accommodation) together with an increase in recruitment of activity in the pelvic floor and voluntary sphincter. Normal voiding is initiated by voluntary relaxation of the pelvic floor with subsequent release of inhibition of the detrusor reflex at the pontine level. The detrusor contraction is maintained steadily throughout voiding, and the pelvic floor remains quiescent.

ELDERLY. Frequency, urgency, and incontinence with incomplete emptying are common in the elderly. Urodynamic studies show that many elderly persons have bladder contractions during filling, producing frequency, urgency, and incontinence. During voiding, these contractions are poorly sustained and result in incomplete evacuation. Some elderly men may have prostatic obstruction, and some women may have incontinence related to impaired sphincter activity or stress incontinence. In the absence of these mechanical factors, the changes in bladder function in the elderly have been ascribed to loss of cerebral control due to minor strokes and changes in the bladder wall due to collagen deposition. The changes can also be due to polyuria secondary to reduced renal concentrating ability, diuretic use, lack of normal increase in antidiuretic hormone secretion at night, and the mobilization of lower extremity edema during sleep.

CLASSIFICATION

The neurogenic bladder has been classified in a variety of ways, beginning with the anatomical classification of

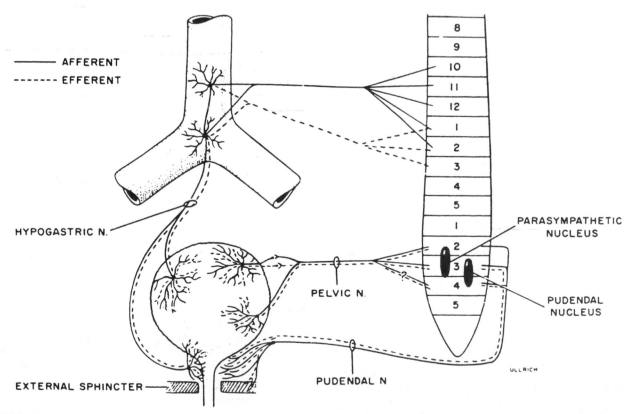

FIGURE 28–2 The diagram displays the parasympathetic, sympathetic, and somatic nerve supply to the bladder, urethra, and pelvic floor.

TABLE 28-1   Bladder Afferent Pathways

Receptor	Pelvic (Parasympathetic)	Hypogastric (Sympathetic)	Pudendal (Somatic)
Bladder wall tension	+	−	−
Bladder mucosal nociception (pain, temperature, chemical irritation)	+	+	−
Urethral mucosal sensation (pain, temperature, passage of urine)	−	−	+

Bors and Comarr.[8] The first functional classification was based on cystometric findings, and five basic groups were described: (1) reflex, (2) uninhibited, (3) autonomous, (4) motor paralytic, and (5) sensory neurogenic bladders.[49] However, this system does not take into account the function of the sphincter mechanisms, and there are a few patients in whom the detrusor reflex does not return after spinal cord injury (SCI) above the sacral outflow. There was a return to a more anatomical classification in which the neurogenic bladder was subdivided into supraspinal, suprasacral spinal, infrasacral, peripheral autonomic, and muscular lesions (Fig. 28–4). At the same time others developed functional classifications, all of which were based on conventional urodynamic evaluations and attempted to categorize the lower urinary tract according to the passive storage ability of the bladder and the activities and coordination of the detrusor and sphincter mechanisms (Table 28–2). It is common in practice to use a combination of both anatomical and functional classifications, with any known neurological lesion described in anatomical terms (e.g., supraspinal, suprasacral). Management is based on functional changes as demonstrated by conventional urodynamics.

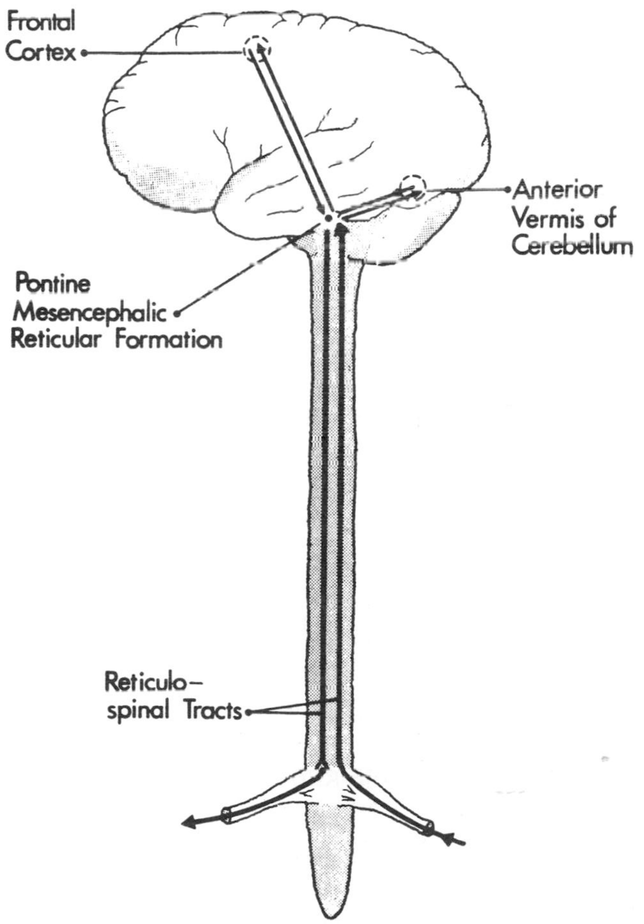

HISTORY AND PHYSICAL EXAMINATION

Although the symptoms associated with bladder neuropathological processes are often misleading and correlate poorly with objective findings, relief of symptoms is one of the patient's main concerns. It is often helpful to have the patient or attendant record fluid intake, output, and incontinence episodes over several 24-hour periods. This will show if there is excessive intake or reversed diurnal rhythm of urine production. The history should ascertain whether there were voiding symptoms prior to the putative neurological event, any premorbid conditions such as diabetes or cerebrovascular accidents, or prior urological or pelvic surgery. The neurological diagnosis, especially the level of the lesion and its completeness, is important in predicting the type of lower urinary tract dysfunction that might be expected.

Physical examination should assess mental status and confirm the neurological level (if present). The perineal sensation and pelvic floor muscle tone are particularly

FIGURE 28–3 The central connections of the bladder reflex are shown, with the afferents ascending possibly in the reticulospinal tracts or the posterior columns to the pontine mesencephalic reticular formation and the efferents running down to the sacral outflow in the reticulospinal tracts. The pontine center is largely influenced by the cortex but also by other areas of the brain, particularly the cerebellum and basal ganglia.

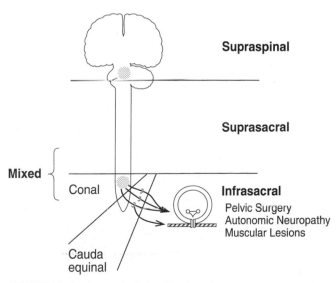

FIGURE 28–4 Anatomical classification of the neurogenic bladder.

TABLE 28–2 Functional Classification of the Neurogenic Bladder

	Bladder Factors	Outlet Factors
Failure to store	Hyperreflexia	Denervated pelvic floor
	Decreased compliance	Bladder neck descent
		Intrinsic bladder neck sphincter failure
Failure to empty	Areflexia	Detrusor-sphincter dyssynergia (striated sphincter and bladder neck)
	Hypocontractility	Nonrelaxing voluntary sphincter
		Mechanical obstruction (benign prostatic hypertrophy or stricture)

important in lower spinal cord and peripheral lesions. Reflexes are also important, but the bulbocavernosus, cremasteric, and anal reflexes are sometimes difficult to elicit, even in intact persons. The skin of the perineum, state of bladder supports, and degree of vaginal support and estrogenization in women should be assessed. The prostate in males should be evaluated, but size or consistency alone is not a good indicator of obstruction. Lastly, an assessment should be made of the patient's motivation, lifestyle, body habitus, and other physical impairments, as these factors will affect management.

DIAGNOSTIC TESTS

Indications

The extent of upper and lower urinary tract testing has to be individualized to each patient and the neurological condition. The upper tracts need evaluation if there are symptoms suggestive of pyelonephritis or prior history of renal disease. Some neurological conditions, such as cerebrovascular accidents, rarely cause upper tract involvement or only occasionally do so, as in Parkinson's disease and multiple sclerosis. For these conditions, a simple baseline screening test such as renal ultrasound is sufficient. Conditions such as those involving complete SCI and myelodysplasia need more extensive and regular upper tract surveillance using both structural and functional tests. The lower urinary tract evaluation can be quite simple and ranges from urinalysis to urine culture to measurement of postvoid residual (PVR). Full urodynamic evaluation may be necessary, especially if there is incomplete bladder emptying, incontinence, recurrent bacteriuria, or upper tract changes.

The bladder findings on urodynamics cannot be used to determine the level of neurological lesion. For example, a suprasacral neurogenic bladder from a complete spinal cord injury can remain areflexic, and a conal or cauda equinal bladder can exhibit high pressures from poor compliance. The anatomical level of the neurological lesion can guide the clinician as to the commonest pattern of bladder dysfunction, but urodynamic testing should always be performed to confirm this.

Upper Tract Tests

ULTRASOUND. This is a low-risk and relatively low-cost test for routine evaluation of the upper urinary tracts. It is not sensitive enough for acute ureteral obstruction, and in this clinical setting an excretory urogram should be performed. Ultrasound is adequate for chronic obstruction

and dilation, scarring, renal masses (both cystic and solid), and renal stones. The ureter is only seen if dilated. The bladder, if partially filled, can be evaluated for wall thickness, irregularity, and the presence of bladder stones.

PLAIN FILM OF THE URINARY TRACT—KIDNEYS, URETER, AND BLADDER (KUB). This is often combined with ultrasound to identify any possible radiopaque calculi in the line of the ureter or bladder stones not seen on ultrasound.

EXCRETORY UROGRAM OR INTRAVENOUS PYELOGRAM. The term *excretory urogram* has replaced intravenous pyelogram, as modern techniques show much more than the collecting system. Renal tomograms taken 1 to 3 min after contrast injection should show a clear nephrogram. If the serum creatinine is more than 1.5 mg/dL, or if the patient has insulin-dependent diabetes, intravenous contrast carries increased risk of contrast nephropathy. In these cases ultrasound, radioisotope renography, and possibly cystoscopy with retrograde pyelography should be considered.

CREATININE CLEARANCE. This has been the gold standard for assessing renal function and is said to approximate to glomerular filtration rate, but its accuracy depends on meticulous urine collection. In quadriplegic patients with low muscle mass and 24-hour creatinine excretion of less than 1000 mg, the calculated creatinine clearance can be too inaccurate to be clinically useful.

ISOTOPE STUDIES. The technetium 99m DMSA (dimercaptosuccinic acid) scan is still the best study for both differential function and evaluation of the functioning areas of the renal cortex. The renogram with technetium 99m MAG 3 (mertiatide) also gives information on urinary tract drainage, as well as a good assessment of differential function. In patients who might have ureteral reflux, these studies should be done with the bladder drained with an indwelling catheter.

Lower Tract Tests

URINALYSIS, CULTURE AND SENSITIVITY. These are done routinely for all patients with neurogenic bladder disease and should be repeated as often as necessary. Bacteriuria should be treated prior to any invasive tests.

POSTVOID RESIDUAL. By itself, a low PVR of less than 20% of capacity is not indicative of a "balanced" bladder as it was once defined. High intravesical pressures may be present in spite of low PVRs. The PVR is simple to obtain and clinically useful when compared with prior recordings and taken in conjunction with the bladder pressure, clinical symptoms, and the appearance of the bladder wall. A catheter insertion has been used for PVR in the past, but there are now simple ultrasound machines that can noninvasively obtain the PVR.[12]

CYSTOGRAM. This study is usually performed to test for the presence or absence of ureteral reflux, and it also shows the bladder shape and outline. The procedure is usually performed in the radiology department, often with no control over rate of filling and without any monitoring of intravesical pressure. It is often helpful in planning management to know the level of intravesical pressure at which ureteral reflux occurred. Significant bacteriuria should be treated prior to the test. Blood pressure should be monitored throughout the test in all patients with spinal cord lesions above T6 who are at risk for autonomic dysreflexia. In many cases, a full videourodynamic study, which includes fluoroscopy of the bladder and monitoring of the intravesical pressure, is more clinically useful and is described later.

CYSTOMETROGRAM (CMG). This is a filling study and gives little information about the voiding phase of bladder function. Although carbon dioxide as a filling medium is convenient with the commercially available apparatus, comparison studies using water have shown considerable variability, poor reproducibility, and the presence of artifacts due to leakage of CO_2 gas around the catheter. Hyperemia of the bladder mucosa has also been noted at cystoscopy immediately after using CO_2. An advantage of the CO_2 CMG is that any size of catheter can be employed as there is little resistance to flow and therefore no pressure artifact from the pump. Water CMGs are best done with a two-channel catheter, with one channel for filling and the other for pressure recording. A rectal pressure trace is also helpful in many patients in order to distinguish intravesical pressure variations (due to intra-abdominal transmission) from contractions of the detrusor itself. Reported filling rates vary but are usually in the range of 25 to 60 mL/min. During filling, patients are asked to suppress voiding. Normal findings are a capacity of 300 to 600 mL with an initial sensation of filling at approximately 50% of capacity. The sensation of normal fullness is said to be appreciated in the lower abdomen with a sense of urgency in the perineum. The change in volume divided by the rise in baseline pressure during filling (i.e., in the absence of a detrusor contraction) describes the bladder's compliance. This should be greater than 10 mL/cm H_2O, and 10 to 20 mL/cm is borderline if capacity is reduced. Normal persons are able to suppress detrusor contractions during this test. Any detrusor contraction, usually defined as a phasic pressure change of more than 15 cm H_2O, is abnormal. If the patient is neurologically intact, these contractions are referred to as uninhibited. If the patient has a suprasacral or supraspinal lesion, these contractions are called hyperreflexic.[2]

Although patients can be instructed to try to void at capacity, many are unable to generate a detrusor contraction. The presence of an easily obtainable involuntary detrusor contraction confirms the presence of hyperreflexia in a patient with a suprasacral or supraspinal lesion. However, the absence of a contraction does not necessarily imply true areflexia in a patient with an infrasacral lesion. The CO_2 CMG is a useful bedside test to monitor the return of a detrusor reflex in the spinal shock phase of SCI and to confirm the presence of detrusor hyperreflexia in patients with supraspinal or cerebral insult prior to starting pharmacotherapy.

SPHINCTER ELECTROMYOGRAPHY (EMG). This can be combined with the CMG or, even better, with a full multichannel videourodynamic study.[46] Recordings have been made with a variety of electrodes (monopolar and coaxial needles and surface electrodes) from the levator, perianal, or periurethral muscles. Since some authors claim there is a functional dissociation between these muscle groups, periurethral recordings are preferred. The integrated EMG is displayed on the same trace as the bladder pressure. EMG activity gradually increases as bladder capacity is reached during bladder filling and then becomes silent just prior to voiding. In complete SCI, low levels of EMG activity with no recruitment during filling is a common pattern, but as a reflex detrusor contraction occurs, EMG activity in the sphincter can increase rather than decrease. With this detrusor-sphincter dyssynergia, voiding often occurs toward the end of the detrusor contraction, as the striated sphincter relaxes more quickly than the smooth muscle of the bladder. This type of sphincter EMG does not display individual motor units and cannot be used for the evaluation of infrasacral denervation of the pelvic floor musculature (standard needle EMG is needed for this).

VIDEOURODYNAMICS. This study is designed to give the maximum information about the filling and voiding phases of lower urinary tract function, and every effort is made to make it as physiological as possible.[7] Videourodynamics is indicated in the following patients: those with incomplete spinal cord lesions with incontinence who have some ability to void and inhibit voiding voluntarily but empty incompletely; persons with mechanical obstruction (e.g., benign prostatic hyperplasia) with neuropathy; candidates for sphincterotomy to assess detrusor contraction and the presence or absence of bladder neck obstruction in addition to striated sphincter dyssynergia; those who fail to respond to pharmacotherapy; those who will undergo any surgical procedures such as augmentation, continent diversion, or placement of an artificial sphincter or a suprapubic catheter; patients who have deterioration of the upper tracts; and finally, patients who relapse frequently with symptomatic bacteriuria.

The procedure requires placement of a 7F two-channel catheter in the bladder and an 8F balloon catheter in the rectum. EMG of the sphincter is recorded along with bladder, rectal, and detrusor (bladder minus rectal) pressures. A contrast solution at 50 mL/min is used to fill the bladder, with the patient sitting or lying as appropriate. The blood pressure is recorded in patients with spinal cord lesions above T6. The bladder image is monitored intermittently with fluoroscopy, and the combined radiographic and urodynamic image is mixed on the same screen and recorded on videotape (Fig. 28–5). If the patient can sit and void during the study, a flow rate can also be recorded. Videourodynamics in children with myelodysplasia or SCI may have to be modified, and adequate clinical information can often be obtained by recording bladder pressure combined with fluoroscopy. Table 28–3 is a list of urodynamic definitions used to categorize the bladder and outlet abnormalities.

CYSTOSCOPY. The only routine indication for cystoscopy is the presence of a long-term indwelling suprapubic

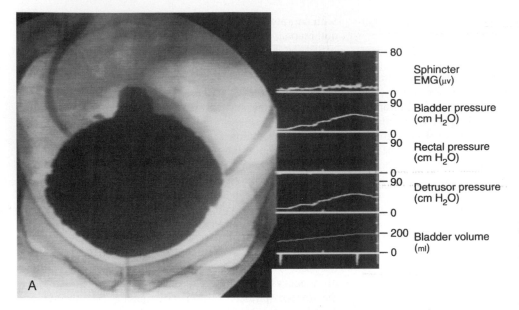

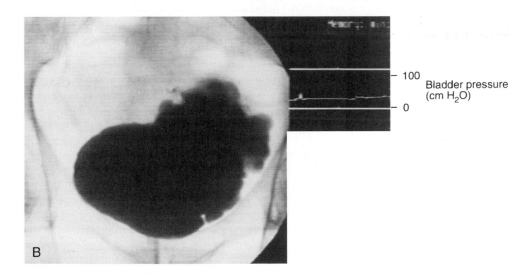

Sphincter EMG(μv)

Bladder pressure (cm H_2O)

Rectal pressure (cm H_2O)

Detrusor pressure (cm H_2O)

Bladder volume (ml)

Bladder pressure (cm H_2O)

FIGURE 28–5   *A,* A videourodynamic study showing a hyperreflexic bladder in a woman with a bilateral ureteral reflux. The detrusor pressure maximum is about 60 cm H_2O, and the rise in detrusor pressure is associated with a rise in sphincter EMG; the bladder neck stays closed. There are moderate bladder wall changes with trabeculation and a small diverticulum. *B,* A videourodynamic study showing a very irregular, asymmetrical bladder that is very noncompliant. The baseline pressure has risen to just over 30 cm H_2O and the volume of contrast in the bladder at that time is 150 mL. This gives a compliance of 5 mL per cm H_2O.

or urethral catheter, as there may be a risk of bladder tumor development.[33] This is recommended after 5 years in high-risk patients, such as smokers, or 10 years in those with no risk factors. Patients who have either gross or microscopic hematuria that cannot be clearly associated with urinary tract infection (UTI), stones, or trauma should also undergo cystoscopy after they have had an excretory urogram. Bladder stones can usually be detected on plain films or ultrasound, but persistent infection can be associated with gravel too small to be detected on imaging studies. Therefore, repeated lower tract infections may be an indication for cystoscopy.

Other Tests

LONG-TERM MONITORING.   Monitoring over 12 to 24 hours of bladder and rectal pressures with sphincter EMG is now possible with solid-state microtip transducers and miniaturized digital recorders. The patients can go about their normal daily activities and cue in any symptoms, incontinence, or voiding episodes. Studies to date indicate that reduced compliance may not be as important in upper tract decompensation as is currently believed.[68]

TRANSRECTAL OR TRANSVAGINAL ULTRASOUND. This imaging study can visualize the bladder base and posterior urethra continuously during urodynamic studies without exposing the patient to ionizing radiation. However, the bladder wall and ureteral reflux cannot be evaluated, and the rectal transducer is large and uncomfortable for patients with perianal sensation.[55]

URETHRAL PRESSURE PROFILES.   These are performed by withdrawing a measuring device (microtip transducer or perfused side-hole catheter) gradually down the urethra and measuring the centrally oriented forces. It has limited value except to determine if there is a sphincter-active area still present after a sphincterotomy.

URECHOLINE (BETHANECHOL) STIMULATION TEST. This is based on Cannon's law of denervation, which says that an end-organ becomes supersensitive to its neurotransmitter when denervated. In practice, this is used in patients with possible infrasacral lesions when the detrusor appears to be areflexic. A rise in baseline pressure of more than 20

TABLE 28–3 Urodynamic Definitions

BLADDER

Hyperreflexia	Uninhibited contractions of the detrusor during filling due to neurological disease
Hypocontractility	Unsustained contractions causing failure to empty
Areflexia	Absent contractions with attempt to void
Compliance	Change in volume divided by change in baseline pressure with filling (<10 mL/cm H_2O abnormal; 10–20 mL/cm H_2O borderline if capacity reduced)

OUTLET

Detrusor-sphincter dyssynergia

1. At bladder neck	Usually in high quadriplegic patients with autonomic hyperactivity
2. At striated sphincter	Uncoordinated pelvic floor and striated sphincter contraction with detrusor contraction during attempts to void
Nonrelaxing sphincter	Poor voluntary relaxation of voluntary sphincter in patients with areflexia attempting to void by Valsalva's maneuver
Decreased outlet resistance	Incontinence due to damage to the bladder neck or striated sphincter, pelvic floor descensus, or denervation

cm H_2O on CMG at a volume of 100 mL is positive. There are unfortunately false-positives and false-negatives, and the test is only positive in complete decentralization.

MANAGEMENT

General Principles

Bladder management has to be done in the context of the whole person. The goals are to empty the bladder not more than every 3 to 4 hours, remain continent, sleep without interference from the urinary drainage system, and avoid recurrent urinary infection or other complications. Less-than-optimal bladder management decreases the person's social, vocational, and avocational potential. The following discussion describes specific management approaches (Table 28–4).

Approaches and Rationale

Behavioral Management

TIMED VOIDING. For patients with hyperreflexia producing urgency or reflex incontinence, a timed voiding program may help by having the patient urinate before the anticipated detrusor contraction. The limitation to this is that those with dementia need continual reminding. It is also useful in patients with sphincter weakness, as the incontinence is worse when the bladder is full and timed voiding reduces the amount of urine leakage.

BLADDER STIMULATION. Various maneuvers have been tried to stimulate the bladder. Stroking or pinching the perineal skin, which is intended to cause reflex stimula-

tion, is rarely effective. Suprapubic tapping or jabbing over the bladder causes a mechanical stretch of the bladder wall and subsequent contraction. Controlled studies have shown that deeper indentation of the bladder with a jabbing technique is the most effective maneuver.[13] This can be used by SCI patients with condom catheters. It is most effective in paraplegic patients who have good upper extremity function.

VALSALVA'S AND CREDÉ'S MANEUVERS. Patients with areflexia and some denervation of the pelvic floor (infrasacral lesions) are able to void by Valsalva's maneuver or straining. This is most effective in women because the paralyzed pelvic floor descends with straining and the bladder neck opens. Over the course of time, however, the pelvic floor descent increases as the paralyzed muscles atrophy and stretch, and the patient complains of worsening stress incontinence. Credé's maneuver, usually performed by an attendant, mechanically pushes urine out of the bladder in quadriplegic patients. The abdominal wall must be relaxed to allow Credé's maneuver to be effective and

TABLE 28–4 Bladder Management Options

Failure to store	
Bladder factors	
Behavioral	Timed voids
Collecting devices	Diaper, condom catheter, indwelling catheter
CIC	With drugs to lower bladder pressure
Drugs	Anticholinergics, musculotropics, intrathecal baclofen,* calcium channel blockers*
Surgery	Augmentation, continent diversion, denervation procedures*
Outlet factors	
Behavioral	Timed voids, pelvic floor exercises
Collecting devices	Diaper, condom catheter, indwelling catheter
Drugs	α-Agonists, imipramine, estrogens
Surgery	Collagen injection, fascial sling, artificial sphincter, Teflon injection*
Failure to empty	
Bladder factors	
Behavioral	Timed voids, bladder stimulation, Valsalva's and Credé's maneuvers
Collecting devices	Indwelling catheter
CIC	
Drugs	Bethanechol
Surgery	Neurostimulation*
Outlet factors	
Behavioral	Anal stretch void
Collecting devices	Indwelling catheters
CIC	
Drugs	α-Blockers, oral striated muscle relaxant, intrathecal baclofen*
Surgery	Sphincterotomy incision, bladder neck incision, prostate resection, pudendal neurectomy,* stent sphincterotomy*
Failure of storage and emptying with nonusable urethra	
Surgery	Suprapubic catheter ± bladder neck closure, ileal conduit

*Experimental or nonstandard management.
Abbreviation: CIC, clean intermittent catheterization.

there is a theoretical risk of producing ureteral reflux by the long-term use of this method.

ANAL STRETCH VOIDING. In paraplegic patients with a spastic pelvic floor, effective voiding has been achieved by relaxing the pelvic floor by first stretching the anal sphincter and then evacuating by Valsalva's maneuver.[36] It requires transfer onto a toilet for bladder emptying, absence of anal sensation, and the ability to generate adequate intra-abdominal pressure. For these reasons it has not achieved popularity, although the technique was well described 15 years ago.

PELVIC FLOOR EXERCISES. These are effective only in female patients with stress incontinence due to pelvic floor descent. In infrasacral neuropathy, most need surgery to achieve continence.

Urine Collection Devices

EXTERNAL CONDOM CATHETERS. These are convenient and often the best management for men with quadriplegia who are unable to do self-catheterization, provided that any outflow obstruction is treated. Although attendants and family members can perform intermittent catheterization, the program often breaks down if the patient is at school or work. Bacteriuria with fever is more common in those who have intermittent catheterization done by an attendant than in those on any other bladder management program, including indwelling catheterization.[14] Problems with skin breakdown and urethral damage can occur if the condom is applied too tightly. There is also an increased risk of urinary tract infection because of poor hygiene. This is further increased in patients who have to do intermittent catheterization because of inadequate emptying but also need a condom catheter for incontinence.

INDWELLING CATHETERS. These can be either urethral or suprapubic and are typically used because other programs have failed or for patient convenience. Sphincterotomy and condom drainage, although ideal for men with quadriplegia, often fail because of inadequate detrusor contractions or because of penile skin problems. In the past, indwelling catheters have justifiably had a bad reputation, but there are recent reports that some patients with indwelling catheters do no worse than those with other methods of management.[20] This change is due to a number of factors including improved catheter materials, but good catheter care is still very important. Some of the important aspects of care include monthly catheter changes, copious fluid intake, control of hyperreflexia with medication, sterilization of the collecting bags with bleach, and avoidance of traction on the catheter. The prevalence of squamous cell carcinoma of the bladder associated with an indwelling catheter may be lower than reported.[33] Most centers continue to recommend yearly cystoscopy, cytology, and biopsy, if indicated, when the patient has had an indwelling catheter for 10 years or more, and possibly after only 5 years if there are increased risk factors such as smoking.

ADULT DIAPERS AND OTHER PROTECTIVE GARMENTS. These have improved considerably over the past few years and now have a combination of a high-absorbent gel-impregnated material that allows the lining against the patient's perineal skin to stay dry. These are commonly used in incontinent demented patients who have adequate bladder emptying.

Clean Intermittent Catheterization

Intermittent catheterization using a sterile technique was introduced by Guttman and Frankel in the 1950s[30] for management of acute SCI patients. Lapides et al in 1972[37] proposed a nonsterile but "clean" technique for the management of chronic retention and infection. The technique has since been employed extensively for neurogenic bladder disease. An intermittent catheter program requires a low-pressure bladder of adequate capacity (>300 mL) and enough outflow resistance to maintain continence with normal daily activities. If the bladder is not sufficiently areflexic and compliant, anticholinergics or musculotropics can be used. If these fail, some form of surgery, such as augmentation, can be done to achieve a low-pressure reservoir. Men with lesions at C7 and below can manage self-catheterization, but women may be unable to do so because of lower limb spasticity and the added burden of transferring to a lying position. Patients should restrict fluid intake to maintain an output of not more than 600 mL in the time period chosen. Some patients have enough sensation to be able to catheterize on demand, but most have to do so on a timed schedule. A minimum of three catheterizations per 24 hours is recommended, since longer intervals theoretically increase the risk of symptomatic bacteriuria. Most patients wash their catheters with soap and water, but if recurrent bacteriuria becomes a problem, sterilization by soaking in Cidex (a glutaral preparation) or boiling the catheters is recommended. Rarely, a completely sterile technique is used.

The most common problems with self-catheterization are symptomatic bacteriuria and urethral trauma. Occasionally, a bladder stone formed on a nidus of hair or lint is found, and patients should be warned to avoid introducing foreign material with the catheter. Urethral trauma and catheterization difficulties are usually due to sphincter spasm. This can be managed by using extra lubrication and local anesthetic urethral gel (lidocaine 2%), and sometimes a curved-tip (coudé) catheter is helpful. Repeated urethral bleeding suggests the presence of a break in the urethral mucosa or a false passage, and using an indwelling urethral catheter for a period of time may be necessary for this to resolve. Occasionally, urethroscopy and unroofing of a false passage is necessary.

Drugs

Many drugs for lower urinary tract management have been tried, and the rationale for their use has often been based on animal and organ bath experiments. Bladder management drugs in humans have generally been disappointing, with the most effective group being those that inhibit detrusor activity.

CHOLINERGIC AGENTS. The detrusor is innervated by cholinergic muscularinic (M_2) receptors. Bethanechol, a cholinergic agonist, can be helpful in detrusor areflexia by increasing detrusor activity. While a pharmacological effect can be seen with a parenteral dose when the bladder is partially innervated, oral doses are not effective at levels that can be tolerated by patients. Clinical trials using double blind control techniques have not been performed, and the use of this drug has declined.[24]

ANTICHOLINERGIC AGENTS. These have been used for many years for suppression of detrusor activity. Propantheline bromide (15–30 mg three times a day) is the prototype, and hyoscyamine (0.125–0.25 mg three or four times a day) is regaining popularity. Oxybutynin hydrochloride is a more recent preparation, which at 5 to 10 mg three times a day has similar actions but is effective mostly on the muscle cell membrane (musculotropic) rather than on anticholinergic endings. Oxybutynin in solution can be given as an intravesical instillation in patients on intermittent catheterization. It appears to be effective, although somewhat delayed serum levels result that are almost as high as with the oral route and side effects appear to be less than when given by the oral route.[47] A problem with this technique is that, at present, there is no sterile liquid form, and the 5-mg tablet has to be dissolved in sterile water. Imipramine is recommended by several authors for its presumed anticholinergic actions. It is said to be additive in its effectiveness, but not in its side effects, when combined with other agents such as oxybutynin and propantheline.

CALCIUM CHANNEL BLOCKERS. Pure calcium channel blockers, although promising in experimental preparations, do not seem to be effective inhibitors of detrusor activity in humans. Terodiline was effective and was available in Europe until recently; it was withdrawn because of its association with cardiac arrhythmias.

ADRENERGIC ANTAGONISTS. The α-adrenergic antagonist phenoxybenzamine (10–30 mg/day) has α_1- and α_2-blocking actions and has been used for inhibiting smooth muscle activity at the bladder neck and in the prostate. Newer agents with more specific α_1-blocking actions are available, such as prazosin, terazosin, and doxazosin. These are typically given at doses of 1 to 20 mg/day as tolerated. Although these agents seem to reduce the irritative symptoms in men with obstruction due to benign prostatic hyperplasia, increased emptying in patients with neurogenic voiding dysfunction has not been reported in controlled studies; beneficial effects have been reported as increasing compliance secondary to decentralization. These agents are effective in control of the vascular manifestations of autonomic dysreflexia, and phenoxybenzamine with its α_1- and α_2-blocking action may be better in this regard than the pure α_1-blocking agents.

ADRENERGIC AGONISTS. Adrenergic agonists have been used to increase urethral resistance in patients with mild stress incontinence. Anecdotally, ephedrine (25–75 mg/day) has been effective in children with myelodysplasia, but control studies are lacking and adrenergic agonists are rarely used in adults with bladder neuropathy. In humans, the β-agonists and antagonists seem to have little effect on normal or neuropathic bladder function.

ESTROGENS. Postmenopausal women have atrophy of the urethral submucosa, and this can lead to stress incontinence. Estrogen administration often restores or maintains this tissue and may be helpful in women with a partially denervated pelvic floor and stress incontinence.

MUSCLE RELAXANTS. Diazepam, dantrolene sodium, and baclofen are frequently used for skeletal muscle spasticity (see Chapter 29) but have never been shown to be effective in controlled studies in patients with detrusor striated sphincter dyssynergia. Baclofen given intrathecally by infusion pump for severe lower extremity spasticity depresses pelvic floor reflexes but also depresses the detrusor reflex.[60] This net result is a lower-pressure bladder that may empty less effectively. Since intrathecal baclofen is most often indicated in quadriplegic patients, this overall decrease in bladder emptying may not be desirable.

Surgery on the Bladder or Bladder Nerves

Bowel Procedures

AUGMENTATION. Bladder augmentation is often recommended for patients who have detrusor hyperreflexia or reduced compliance that fails to respond to anticholinergic or musculotropic drugs.[58] The patient must be motivated to continue indefinitely with clean intermittent catheterization and have adequate outflow resistance. The patient must be fully informed of the immediate surgical risks and the possible long-term sequelae of this procedure. Immediate surgical risks include prolonged intestinal ileus or obstruction, anastomotic leak with peritonitis, wound infection, and pulmonary complications such as pneumonia and emboli. All the long-term sequelae are unknown, since these procedures have only been performed over the past 20 years. The known sequelae include chronic bacteriuria, theoretical risk of neoplastic change, possible diarrhea or malabsorption from a shortened gut or decreased intestinal transit time, and hyperchloremic acidosis due to absorption of urine with secondary mobilization of skeletal calcium as a buffer.

In this procedure the bladder is opened widely and an opened and reconfigured segment of bowel is sewn in. A 20- to 30-cm segment of distal ileum is usually used, but an ileocecal segment, sigmoid, or even a wedge of stomach can be employed (Fig. 28–6). The procedure is intended to result in a 600-mL capacity low-pressure reservoir without the use of any drugs. Mucus production is the main day-to-day problem initially, especially in those with active urinary infection. With good intermittent catheterization technique and the use of bladder irrigations as necessary, this is rarely a problem after the first 3 months. Since the risk of neoplastic changes is unknown with this procedure, yearly cystoscopy should probably begin 10 to 15 years after the augmentation.

CONTINENT DIVERSION. In this procedure, bowel is used not just to increase effective bladder capacity but also to form a continent catheterizable channel that opens onto the abdominal wall. It is particularly useful in women for whom intermittent self-catheterization via the urethra is difficult or impossible because of leg spasticity, body habitus, severe urethral incontinence, or the need to transfer from a wheelchair. Men who are unable to perform intermittent catheterization because of strictures, false passages, or fistulas are also potential candidates. However, severe urethral disease in men is usually due to poor personal care, and it is inappropriate to perform these procedures on patients who cannot or will not follow through. If the patient fails to catheterize after augmentation and continent diversion, the bowel may rupture internally before overflow

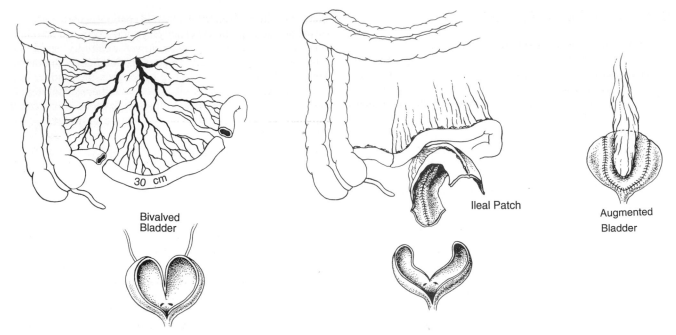

FIGURE 28–6 Augmentation cystoplasty: a 30-cm segment of small bowel is opened and reconstructed as a U-shaped patch and then sewn into the bivalved bladder.

incontinence occurs through the urethra or catheterizable channel.

The procedure involves enlarging the bladder and constructing some form of continent catheterizable channel. The terminal ileum and the ileocecal valve work well, but intussuscepted small bowel, the appendix, and a defunctioned segment of ureter have all been used. The bladder neck may require closure if there is sphincter-related incontinence.

Denervation Procedures

Denervation technique for bladder hyperreflexia, although theoretically attractive, is not used widely. The operative approaches include sectioning of the sacral nerve roots or interrupting the peripheral nerve supply near the bladder. Selective sacral rhizotomies have been attempted. The technique involves identifying the nerve root (usually S3 on one side) that carries the detrusor reflex by doing differential sacral local anesthetic blocks while monitoring the detrusor reflex by a CMG. Surgical or chemical destruction of S3 usually results in temporary areflexia. Over time the detrusor reflex reroutes through the intact sacral nerves. Bilateral S2, S3, and S4 rhizotomies permanently abolish the reflex but at the expense of loss of reflex erections and worsening of the bowel evacuation problem.[25]

Peripheral denervation of the detrusor has been attempted by transecting the detrusor above the trigone and resuturing it, or removing the paravesical ganglia via a vaginal approach, or overdistention of the bladder with the intent of damaging the intramural nerves and muscle fibers. In fact, in one clinical study in patients with complete paraplegia, the bladder was intentionally distended in the spinal shock phase with the intent of preventing the return of the bladder reflex. The prevalence of areflexia in the short term following this was 63% compared with the expected 15%.[32] None of these peripheral denervation procedures have become accepted, and long-term results of intentional overdistention of the bladder in spinal shock have not yet been reported.

Electrical Stimulation

Attempts have been made to stimulate detrusor contraction using electrodes driven by an implanted receiver conveying a stimulus generated by an external transmitter. The electrodes have been implanted on the bladder wall, pelvic nerves, sacral roots, and conus. At present, the only site being used clinically is the sacral roots and most of the reported series come from Europe.[10] The electrodes are placed on the anterior roots either intradurally or extradurally. In order to prevent spontaneous hyperreflexic contractions and antidromic reflex contractions, bilateral S2, S3, and S4 dorsal rhizotomies are usually performed. Pelvic floor contraction with anterior root stimulation will still obstruct voiding, and European centers have elected to stimulate intermittently. This leads to intermittent voiding, as the striated pelvic floor muscle relaxes more quickly than the smooth muscle detrusor. In the center developing this device in the United States, pudendal neurectomies are performed to decrease outflow resistance.[65] Adequate bladder emptying at acceptable intravesical pressures, with preservation of the bladder wall, as well as upper tract morphology and function have been reported.[10] One important disadvantage of bilateral S2, S3, and S4 rhizotomies is that reflex erections are abolished; usable erections occurring as a result of sacral root stimulation occur in less than 30% of patients. However, bowel evacuation in many patients is improved. Further refinements such as supraselective rhizotomies, with modification of stimulus parameters and electrode design, are future possibilities, but at present this technique must be considered experimental.

Surgery on the Bladder Outlet

Incontinence due to decreased outlet resistance is relatively uncommon in bladder dysfunction secondary to neurological disease and is seen in children with myelodysplasia and women with infrasacral lesions and a denervated pelvic floor. It can occur in active men with complete denervation, but this is rare. While α-adrenergic agonists may help minor incontinence, more severe leakage typically requires some form of urethral compressive procedure. The options include injection therapy into the bladder neck and urethra to increase the bulk of tissue under and around the bladder neck muscle, a fascial sling, or an artificial sphincter. Electrical stimulation of pelvic floor muscles or nerves, or muscles and nerves, via rectal, vaginal, or implanted electrodes has been tried but has not been effective enough to achieve widespread popularity.

INJECTION THERAPY. Teflon has been used for years in the urethra for certain types of stress incontinence, but its use has recently declined because of the danger of particle migration. Autologous fat and bovine collagen have been tried recently, and after one to three injections these seem to help a proportion of patients. The procedure is low in potential side effects and is especially suitable for elderly and poor-risk patients.

EXTERNAL COMPRESSIVE PROCEDURES. In the fascial sling procedure, a 2-cm strip of fascia is taken from the anterior rectus abdominus fascia or tensor fascia lata. It is wrapped around the bladder neck and fixed anteriorly to the abdominal fascia or pubic tubercle. Patients who are candidates for this procedure must have compliant low-pressure bladders. They will be unable to void by Valsalva's maneuver after a successful sling procedure and must be willing to do self-catheterization indefinitely in exchange for being continent.

The artificial urinary sphincter consists of a cuff, a pressure-regulating balloon, and a control pump. The cuff is usually implanted around the bladder neck in both sexes and less commonly around the bulbar urethra in men. The pump in the labia or scrotum allows the patient to open the cuff for voiding. Reinflation of the cuff is automatic and takes about 3 to 5 minutes. Mechanical failure, cuff erosion, and infection occur with this device. Patients can use Valsalva's maneuver to void and do not have to be on self-catheterization. In patients with myelodysplasia, although the detrusor is naturally areflexic or can be rendered so by drugs, uncontrolled hyperreflexia occurs in 10% in the first year after implantation. This probably results from activation of dormant urethrovesical reflexes. Careful follow-up is essential, and if hyperreflexia occurs, an augmentation procedure can be done secondarily.

SPHINCTEROTOMY. In male spinal cord–injured patients unable or unwilling to do self-catheterization, the use of a condom catheter is a practical alternative. As it is unusual to find a lower urinary tract that has adequate detrusor contraction and a coordinated pelvic floor in these patients, some procedure to decrease outflow resistance is usually indicated. The results are poor in patients without adequate detrusor contractions. Preoperative parameters suggested for a good outcome are low volume (<200 mL), spontaneous contraction with a quick rise time (<20 seconds), adequate amplitude (>50 cm H_2O), and an adequate duration of approximately 2 min or more. Ablation of the striated sphincter, usually by incision, is the standard procedure. It is now performed anteriorly to avoid the pudendal artery and nerve, which lie lateral to the membranous urethra (which, if damaged, can lead to impotence). Some patients also have bladder neck obstruction either because of primary hyperactivity (e.g., high quadriplegic patients) or because of total bladder wall hypertrophy, which follows striated sphincter dyssynergia. They need bladder neck ablation either by resection or by incision. In older men, prostatic obstruction from benign disease may also contribute to increased outflow resistance and require prostatic resection. The immediate morbidity from sphincterotomy is relatively high from bleeding, clot retention, and infection. The long-term results are compromised because of recurrent obstruction from stricture or recurrent dyssynergia. An implantable stainless steel stent is undergoing trial currently and should reduce morbidity and improve long-term results. This stent material is inert, and the epithelium grows through the spaces between the wires of the stent, completely covering them.[48]

Other Methods of Decreasing Outflow Resistance. Intrathecal baclofen given for severe spasticity decreases the pudendal reflexes, but the detrusor reflex and contractions are reduced as well and therefore it cannot be used as a chemical sphincterotomy. Botulinus toxin injected into the striated sphincter has also been used experimentally, but its effects last only a few months.[23]

Urinary Diversion

The use of any urinary diversion should be restricted to patients with severe urethral problems such as stricture, fistula, periurethral abscess, and intractable incontinence with perineal skin breakdown. The simplest method is to insert a suprapubic catheter and close the bladder neck. If the bladder cannot be preserved because of malignant disease, contracture, or ureteral reflux, a standard bowel conduit is recommended with removal of the bladder in most cases. Usually a 10- to 15-cm segment of small bowel is used. Since a nonrefluxing ureterointestinal anastomosis is desired, the ileocecal segment or sigmoid colon is preferred.

MANAGEMENT OF SPECIFIC DISEASES

Diseases of the Brain

Stroke

After an initial period of areflexia, stroke patients typically have hyperreflexia with frequency and urge incontinence but coordinated voiding and complete emptying (see Chapter 50). Anticholinergics and musculotropics frequently help symptomatically without affecting emptying adversely. Persistent areflexia and retention may occur with bilateral lesions. Retention in the elderly can occur due to prostatic obstruction. Videourodynamic studies are helpful in differentiating these conditions.

Parkinson's Disease

The prevalence of bladder symptoms in this disease is high (70%) (see Chapter 51). Most have frequency, urgency, and urge incontinence, and 50% complain of difficulty voiding. Evaluation shows hyperreflexia, but the contractions are poorly sustained and result in incomplete emptying. Failure to empty may also be due to bradykinesia secondary to failure of pelvic floor relaxation, the adrenergic effects of levodopa or the anticholinergic effects of other antiparkinsonian drugs.[6] Treatment is difficult because there is frequently a combination of incontinence and retention. Detrusor inhibition with drugs makes emptying worse, and α-adrenergic blockers have a marginal effect in decreasing outflow resistance.[64] Intermittent catheterization and detrusor inhibition is often the best choice, but many patients do not have sufficient upper extremity dexterity to do this independently.

Dementia, Brain Tumors, and Trauma

All of these conditions may cause hyperreflexia with reflex or urge incontinence with complete emptying. If cognitive impairment is severe, incontinence often persists in spite of detrusor inhibition. Some type of collecting device is appropriate for many of these patients (see Chapter 49).

Diseases of the Brain and Spinal Cord

Multiple sclerosis is the commonest disease in this category, with 90% of patients developing urinary manifestations in the course of their disease (see Chapter 52). The bladder symptoms usually present because of an incomplete spinal cord lesion with hyperreflexia and hypocontractility. In this situation, detrusor inhibition with drugs worsens emptying. In the rare predominantly encephalopathic variety, these agents may be useful. Multiple sclerosis patients presenting with a predominantly conal lesion have bladder areflexia. Intermittent catheterization is eventually indicated in most multiple sclerosis patients, but few are able to do this because of poor upper extremity strength and coordination. High-pressure bladders due to hyperreflexia and detrusor-sphincter dyssynergia are rare, but sphincterotomy in men is sometimes indicated.[47]

Diseases of the Spinal Cord

Injury, tumors, and vascular lesions of the spinal cord cause the majority of suprasacral neurogenic bladder problems (see Chapter 55). After a varying period of spinal shock, the detrusor reflex typically returns. With complete lesions, the center for this reflex develops in the sacral cord. Inhibitory control by the higher center is impaired, and because the long-routed detrusor reflex is interrupted, the detrusor contraction may not be completely sustained. Coordination and control of the pelvic floor are also impaired, leading to lack of voluntary contraction and relaxation. Often, in complete lesions, this causes discoordinated activity during voiding. This discoordination or detrusor-sphincter dyssynergia affects the striated voluntary sphincter, but in high complete quadriplegic patients excessive sympathetic activity may lead to detrusor–bladder neck dyssynergia as well. Incomplete lesions may produce the supraspinal pattern with urgency and adequate emptying, while patients with complete lesions have reflex incontinence and incomplete emptying due to detrusor-sphincter

dyssynergia in most cases. Some patients have hypocontractility or areflexia and retention. A truly balanced bladder with sustained detrusor contraction and coordinated pelvic floor is rare.

The onset and severity of the symptoms vary with the cause of spinal cord dysfunction, but management discussed here is in relation to SCI. An indwelling catheter is typically maintained until the patient's medical state is stable and fluid intake can be regulated to achieve a urine output of 1500 to 2000 mL/day. Intermittent sterile catheterization is then started, if possible by a dedicated "catheterization team." The patient, when able, learns self-catheterization. A sterile technique is ideal in the hospital, but a clean technique can be used when the patient is discharged home. Maximum allowable bladder volume is 600 mL. However, in some of these patients, retention of interstitial fluid in the lower extremities when upright, with subsequent mobilization and dumping at night, is frequently a problem. The use of TED hose (antiembolism stockings), recumbency early in the evening, and an extra catheterization in the middle of the night may all be necessary to manage this.

In the majority of SCI patients, the detrusor reflex returns usually within the first 6 months. Its return is often indicated by episodes of incontinence, but the presence of the detrusor reflex should be confirmed by CMG. Anticholinergics and musculotropics can be given to suppress the reflex and allow intermittent catheterization to continue. Patients with lesions at the level of C7 and below who are able to do self-catheterization can continue this in the long term. If the detrusor reflex cannot be suppressed, the patient should consider augmentation, which is still the standard method today for achieving a low-pressure reservoir if medications fail.

In male patients unable or unwilling to do self-catheterization, and for those who refuse augmentation, sphincterotomy and an external catheter are probably the best alternatives. Other options include intermittent catheterization by an attendant, although this has a greater risk of febrile UTIs.[14] Wearing an external collector can be done also, but only 15% of men with SCI have a suitable truly "balanced" bladder with coordinated voiding at low pressure. Some men with quadriplegia end up with an indwelling catheter because of sphincterotomy failure, or inadequate detrusor contractions, or skin breakdown on the penile shaft. Women using intermittent catheterization may be unable to control urinary incontinence with medications and may choose to use an indwelling catheter. A regular long-term urinary tract surveillance program (Table 28–5) should be set up for SCI patients who may, with good care, have a normal life expectancy.

Diseases of the Conus, Cauda Equina, and Peripheral Nerves

Trauma, disc disease, lumbar stenosis, arachnoiditis, and tumors are some of the mechanical lesions that may affect this region of the spinal canal. The resulting bladder is typically areflexic or noncontractile and insensate. Pelvic floor innervation is frequently affected in conal lesions, which can lead to incontinence, especially in females. In cauda equinal lesions, the nonmyelinated pelvic nerve roots

TABLE 28–5   Routine Urinary Tract Surveillance After Spinal Cord Injury

I. Initial rehabilitation admission
    Urinalysis, initial and as needed
    Urine culture and sensitivity, weekly
    IVP (this is often done 1–3 mo after SCI)
    Renal ultrasound (a baseline test)
    PVR
    CMG or urodynamics (usually no cystogram at this point)
    CrCl, 24-hr urine
II. Initial evaluations
    IVP at first annual evaluation and then every 3 yr
      (assuming all previous tests are normal)
    Urodynamics at first annual evaluation and then determined
      on individual basis (often needed annually for the first
      few years)
    Renal ultrasound and KUB for those annual evaluations in
      which no IVP/CUG is obtained
    CUG at first annual evaluation either with urodynamics or
      by radiology, then every 3 yr with IVP (usually no CUG
      with indwelling catheters)
    CrCl, 24-hr urine, annually
    PVR (by portable ultrasound or catheter) annually unless
      indwelling catheter
    Other test of renal function, as needed
III. Cytoscopy
    Generally performed in patients after 10 yr of chronic,
      continuous indwelling catheterizations (urethral or
      suprapubic) or sooner (at 5 yr) if high risk (heavy
      smoker, age >40 yr, or history of complicated UTIs) or in
      any patient with symptoms that warrant such a
      procedure.

Abbreviations: IVP, intravenous pyelography; SCI, spinal cord injury; CMG, cystometrography; PVR, postvoid residuals; CrCl, creatine clearance; KUB, kidney, ureter, bladder, plain film; CUG, cystourethrogram; UTIs, urinary tract infections.

are more easily damaged and pelvic floor innervation is usually relatively more intact than the detrusor nerve supply. Autonomic neuropathy is most common secondary to diabetes, although at times it is the result of alcohol abuse. The detrusor afferents are affected first with reduction of bladder sensation. Detrusor efferents are involved later, but because of lack of sensation, overstretching contributes to the end result, which is a noncontractile insensate bladder.

Intermittent catheterization is the initial treatment in all cases. If the pelvic floor is severely paralyzed, patients may be able to void by straining. Men may be helped by α-adrenergic blocking agents to decrease outflow resistance. Women can often empty by straining but tend to usage severe stress incontinence. These patients may be candidates for a fascial sling or artificial sphincter. Reduced bladder compliance, usually found in patients after radical pelvic surgery, does not respond well to medications, and an augmentation may be indicated, particularly if the outflow resistance is high and the upper tracts begin to dilate. Patients with diabetes can often maintain bladder function and contractility and avoid overdistention by timed voidings.

Diseases of the Spinal Cord and Conus

Myelodysplasia is the most common disease producing a mixed pattern of bladder dysfunction. Any combination of detrusor and sphincter activity can be found, but it is most common to have a hyperreflexic or noncompliant bladder, or both, with dyssynergia or a nonrelaxing sphincter.

Intermittent catheterization is used initially along with medication in infancy and childhood. In many cases, reconstructive surgery is necessary early if more conservative measures fail.

MANAGEMENT OF COMPLICATIONS

BACTERIURIA.   About one half of all hospital-acquired infections originate in the urinary tract in association with urinary catheters and other drainage devices. In patients with neurogenic bladders, UTIs are a common source of morbidity. Frequent exposure to antibiotics increases the risk of infection with antibiotic-resistant organisms, which further complicates the treatment of UTI. The diagnosis of UTI can be delayed or missed in patients with neurological disorders affecting bladder sensation. In patients with spinal cord disorders, signs and symptoms suggestive of UTI include fever, onset of urinary incontinence, increased spasticity, autonomic dysreflexia, increased sweating, cloudy and odorous urine, and malaise, lethargy, or sense of unease.[51] Unexplained signs and symptoms suggestive of UTI in the presence of pyuria warrant empirical therapy for UTI. Absence of pyuria makes the diagnosis of UTI unlikely but does not exclude it.

Asymptomatic bacteriuria is very common in patients with neurogenic bladder, especially those using intermittent or indwelling catheterization. Most authorities recommend against routine treatment of asymptomatic bacteriuria. However, the presence of significant bacteriuria with urease-producing organisms that are associated with stone formation may warrant treatment.[52]

The spectrum of uropathogens causing catheter-associated UTI is much broader than that causing uncomplicated UTI. *Escherichia coli* causes the majority of uncomplicated UTIs. *E. coli* and organisms such as species of *Proteus, Klebsiella, Pseudomonas, Serratia, Providencia,* enterococci, and staphylococci are relatively more common in patients with catheter-associated UTI.[51] Polymicrobic bacteriuria is the rule in patients with indwelling catheters.

Patients with mild-to-moderate illness can be treated with an oral fluoroquinolone such as ciprofloxacin, norfloxacin, or ofloxacin. This group of antibiotics provides coverage for most expected pathogens, including *Pseudomonas aeruginosa.* Trimethoprim-sulfamethoxazole is another commonly used antibiotic for less ill patients, but does not provide coverage for *P. aeruginosa.* It is less expensive than the fluorquinolones and may be used empirically and continued according to the results of susceptibility testing. Amoxicillin, nitrofurantoin, and sulfa drugs are poor choices for empirical therapy because of the high prevalence of resistance to these agents among uropathogens typically involved in complicated UTIs.

In more seriously ill, hospitalized patients, ampicillin plus gentamicin or imipenem plus cilastatin provides coverage against most expected pathogens, including *P. aeruginosa* and most enterococci.[11] A number of other parenteral antimicrobial agents can also be used. Patients can be switched to oral treatment after clinical improvement. At least 7 to 14 days of therapy is generally recommended, depending on the severity of the infection.[52] There are no convincing data that regimens longer than this are beneficial. Patients undergoing effective treatment for UTI with an antibiotic to which the infecting pathogen is susceptible should have a definite improvement within 24 to 48 hours. If not, a repeat urine culture and imaging studies (ultrasound or computed tomography) are indicated.

In a patient who has had UTI with high fever or hemodynamic changes suggestive of sepsis or who is having recurrent symptomatic UTIs, an excretory urogram, cystogram, or urodynamic evaluation may be indicated after successful treatment to look for correctable anatomical or functional abnormalities.

AUTONOMIC DYSREFLEXIA. Paroxysmal hypertension, sweating, piloerection, headache, and reflex bradycardia are brought on by increased stimulation into and sympathetic output from the isolated spinal cord below a complete lesion. Injuries below T6 are rarely associated with this problem. Afferent stimulation frequently arises in the bladder, and the best treatment is prevention by avoiding overdistention. If symptoms persist when the bladder has been emptied or if the blood pressure is at a dangerously high level, sublingual nifedipine 10 mg, a calcium channel blocking agent, can be given and repeated if necessary for a total of three doses. Long-term management with phenoxybenzamine (10–30 mg/day) has been used to prevent autonomic dysreflexia when all findable causes have been eliminated (see Chapter 55).

HYPERCALCIURIA AND STONES. Loss of calcium from the bones occurs in all spinal cord patients and is worse in young males. Increased urinary calcium (>200 mg/24 hours) begins about 4 weeks after injury, reaches a maximum at 16 weeks, and may persist for 12 to 18 months. Renal stone incidence in the first 9 months is approximately 1.0% to 1.5% and is due mainly to hypercalciuria. Over the next 10 years upper tract stones are found in 8%, with many of these secondary to infection. The incidence of bladder stones in the first 9 months in patients on intermittent catheterization is 2.3%. In the presence of an indwelling catheter, in spite of greater urine output, the prevalence is much higher at 8.8%.[18]

Bladder stones are effectively treated with electrohydraulic lithotripsy. Small stones and particles can be dissolved by daily bladder irrigations with 30 mL of 10% of hemiacidrin (Renacidin) solution which is left in the bladder for 30 min. Some patients with recurrent stones use this once or twice a week for prophylaxis. In patients who have ureteral reflux, it should be used with caution because of potential nephrotoxicity and absorption of magnesium. Calyceal calculi that are small (<1 cm) and asymptomatic can be followed expectantly, but 50% of these patients become symptomatic over 5 years and half of these will need some sort of invasive procedure.[26] Calculi that are growing or that are located in the renal pelvis should probably be treated before they pass into the ureter and cause obstruction (Fig. 28–7). Extracorporeal shock wave lithotripsy (ESWL) is the standard treatment. For large stones (>3 cm diameter), a percutaneous approach is preferred, as clearance of fragments is poor if patients are inactive. Ureteral stones are potentially dangerous in patients with no renal sensation. These can be managed expectantly if they pass down within 2 to 3 weeks. There is an increased risk of renal damage, as these patients with reduced sensation will not perceive continuous pain, which would normally suggest severe continuing obstruction. Obstruction and infection together will require a drainage procedure as an emergency with a percutaneous nephrostomy or a retrograde stent, and this can be followed by an endoscopic removal or ESWL later.

LOWER URINARY TRACT CHANGES. Trabeculation occurs in the majority of patients after SCI and in many cases despite appropriate management strategies. Sacculation and diverticula can occur when obstruction and high pressure are severe. If a diverticulum occurs at the ureteral hiatus, ureteral reflux is almost inevitable. Chronic infection of dilated prostatic ducts may be an important source for relapsing UTIs in men.

URETERAL REFLUX AND UPPER TRACT DILATION. Ureteral reflux or high bladder pressure in the absence of reflux can cause upper tract dilation (Fig. 28–8). Dilation without reflux is said to be due to decreased compliance, but recent data from long-term monitoring

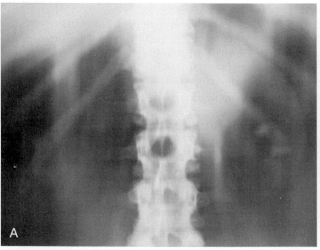 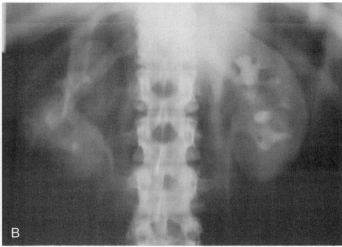

FIGURE 28–7 *A,* Tomograms of the kidneys showing partial staghorn calculi in the lower pole of the left kidney, with two smaller stones in the middle calyces. *B,* The excretory urogram shows well-preserved morphology with minimal calyectasis.

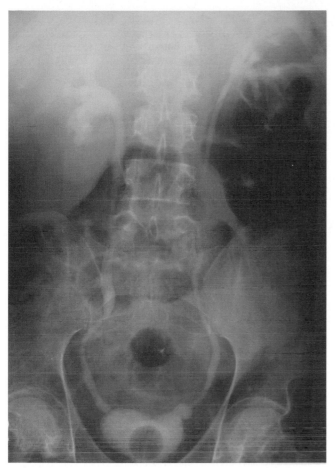

FIGURE 28–8 The 45-minute film from an excretory urogram of the patient whose urodynamic study is shown in Fig. 28–5*B*. The Foley catheter draining the bladder is clamped, and at the low bladder volume shown an obvious holdup is noted at the ureterovesical junctions on both sides, particularly the right.

suggest that baseline pressure elevations are minimal with natural rates of filling, and that increased phasic activity may be more important.[68] With reflux, or ureteral dilation without reflux, the bladder pressure should be lowered with intermittent catheterization and anticholinergics. If reflux fails to improve but the bladder pressure responds, a surgical procedure to repair the reflux can be considered. If bladder pressures do not improve, the options are to augment the bladder, or in men, to perform a sphincterotomy and rely on free drainage.

NEUROGENIC BOWEL DYSFUNCTION AND MANAGEMENT

EPIDEMIOLOGY. Neurogenic bowel dysfunction is the loss of volitional control of defecation due to neurological compromise, resulting in fecal incontinence (FI) or difficulty with evacuation (DWE). FI and fecal impaction range from 0.3% to 5.0% in the general population. DWE ranges from 10% to 50% among hospitalized or institutionalized elderly.[56, 66] While many gastrointestinal disorders can contribute to FI or DWE, disorders that impair the extrinsic (sympathetic, parasympathetic, or somatic) nervous control

of the bowel and anorectal mechanisms are more common among patients seen by physiatrists. Neurogenic bowel difficulties may be a primary disabling and handicapping feature for patients with SCI, stroke, amyotrophic lateral sclerosis, multiple sclerosis, diabetes mellitus, myelomeningocele, and muscular dystrophy.[15]

IMPACT. Satisfactory functional outcomes depend on appropriate bowel management. Fecal incontinence decreases the return-to-home rates for stroke patients.[29] Almost one third of SCI patients show worsening of bowel function 5 years beyond their injury, suggesting inadequate long-term management.[61] Nursing home costs are higher for patients with FI.[66] While restoring normal defecation may not be possible, "social continence," defined as predictable scheduled adequate defecations without incontinence at other times, is often achievable. Embarrassment and humiliation from FI frequently result in extreme vocational and social handicap. Vocational handicap and excessive institutionalization add substantial costs to the care of neurogenic bowel dysfunction. A 1983 report estimated that $8 billion per year is spent in the United States for the care of fecally incontinent institutionalized patients.[56]

BOWEL CONTINENCE

Normal Physiology

The colon serves as a reservoir for food waste until it is convenient for elimination. It serves as a storage device as long as the colonic pressure is less than that of the anal sphincter mechanism. Elimination occurs when colonic pressure exceeds that of the anal sphincter mechanism. Other functions of the colon are to reabsorb fluids (up to 30 L/day may be reabsorbed from the large and small bowel walls with typically only 100 mL water loss in feces) and gases (90% of the 7–10 L of gases produced by fermentation is absorbed rather than expelled). The colon also provides an environment for the growth of bacteria needed to assist in digestion, and also absorbs certain bacterial breakdown products.[31] The layers of the colon wall are depicted in Figure 28–9.

Key to the function of the entire gastrointestinal tract is an intrinsic bowel nervous system, the enteric nervous system (ENS). This collection of highly organized neurons is in two primary layers, the submucosal (Meissner's) and myenteric (Auerbach's) plexus. These plexus have an estimated 10 to 100 million neurons, more than those contained in the spinal cord, plus two to three glial cells per neuron, which resemble central nervous system (CNS) astrocytes, as opposed to 20 to 50 glial cells per neuron in the CNS.[28] The coordination of segment-to-segment function is largely regulated by the ENS, considered by some as a third part of the autonomic nervous system.[69] The ENS also has its own nerve-blood barrier similar to the CNS.[16]

The sympathetic and parasympathetic nervous systems seem to modulate the ENS rather than directly control the smooth muscles of the bowel.[69] The smooth muscles of the bowel have their own electromechanical automaticity which is directly modulated by the inhibitory control of the ENS.[16, 28] Sympathetic nervous system stimulation tends to promote the storage function by enhancing anal tone

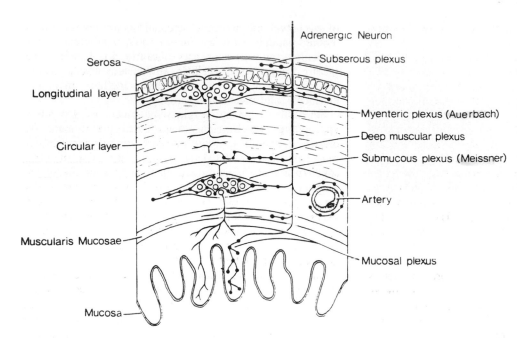

FIGURE 28–9 Diagram of a transverse section of the gut showing enteric plexus and the distribution of adrenergic neurons. Note the ganglionic plexus of Auerbach and Meissner. The deep muscular plexus contains a few ganglia, the subserosal contains an occasional ganglion, and the mucosal plexus shows none. The adrenergic fibers are all extrinsic and arise from the prevertebral sympathetic ganglia. The adrenergic fibers are distributed largely to the mesenteric, submucous, and mucosal plexus and to blood vessels. (From Goyal RK, Crist JR: Neurology of the Gut. *In* Sleisenger MH, Fordtran JS (eds): Gastrointestinal Disease: Pathophysiology, Diagnosis, Management, ed 4. Philadelphia, WB Saunders, 1989, p 34.)

and inhibiting colonic contractions, though little clinical deficit occurs from bilateral sympathectomy[19] (Fig. 28–10). Parasympathetic activity enhances colonic motility, and its loss is often associated with DWE, including impactions and functional obstructions, such as Ogilvie's pseudo-obstructive syndrome.[19]

The normal intact colon wall has a 3- to 6-Hz pattern of

slow electrical potential waves with irregularly occurring bursts of spike activity typically on the apex of these waves every 10 to 12 seconds. The spike activity is associated with development of bowel wall tension and with slow peristaltic waves of ring contractions. These ring contractions are several centimeters apart and travel at 1 to 2 mm/ sec. These waves seem to be paced from the transverse

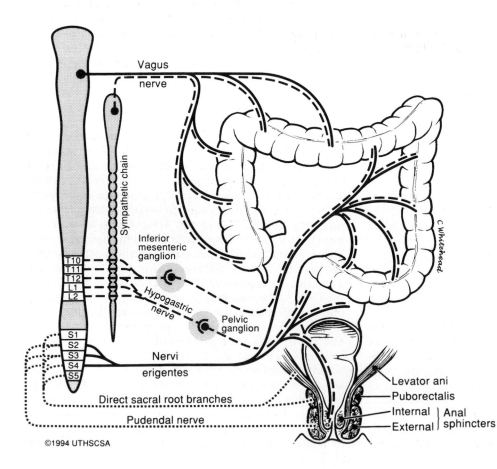

FIGURE 28–10 Neurological levels and pathways for the sympathetic, parasympathetic, and somatic nervous system innervation of the colon and anorectum. Not shown is the enteric nervous system, which travels along the bowel wall from esophagus to internal anal sphincter and forms the final common pathway to control the bowel wall smooth muscle.

©1994 UTHSCSA

colon and travel both caudad to the rectum and cephalad to the cecum.[16]

The function of the transverse and ascending colon is largely storage, with propulsion generally back toward the one-way ileocecal valve. This allows the haustral and colonic motility waves to mix and stir contents and also exposes contents to the colon wall for additional fecal liquid absorption.[16] Occasionally, these proximal traveling colonic waves reverse, especially during a giant migratory contraction (GMC) of the colon. The GMC is associated with mass movement of feces as far as one-third the length of the colon.[69] In the fasting emptied colon, GMCs occur approximately four times per day, but twice or less per day in the normal colon.[69] The GMCs origin is poorly understood but commonly occurs in response to meals, as part of the gastrocolic reflex, or to increased physical activity, though it does not seem to be under volitional control.[16]

The rectum is usually empty until just prior to defecation. Anal canal pressure is largely determined by the angulation and pressure at the anorectal junction by the puborectalis sling and the tone of the smooth muscle internal sphincter. Only about 20% of the anal canal pressure is due to the static contraction of the somatically innervated striated external sphincter.[4] The external anal sphincter and puborectalis are the only striated skeletal muscles with normal resting states of tonic contraction and consist mainly of slow-twitch fatigue-resistant type I fibers (as opposed to nonupright animals such as the cat or dog in which it consists of predominately type II fibers).[3] Anal pressure can be increased volitionally by contracting the external sphincter and puborectalis muscles. Maximum volitional squeeze pressures, however, are not as high as can be generated reflexively against Valsalva pressure. The external anal sphincter (EAS) is physically larger than the internal sphincter, and its contraction is under both reflex and volitional control, which is learned with maturation. Normal baseline reflex action of the anorectal mechanism allows spontaneous stool elimination. The EAS is innervated by the S2 to S4 roots via the pudendal nerve and the puborectalis by direct branches from the S1 to S5 roots[54] (see Fig. 28–10). The remarkable degree of learned EAS coordination allows the selective discrete passage of gas while balancing a variable mixture of solids, liquids, and gases.

Normal defecation begins with reflexes triggered by rectosigmoid distention (Fig. 28–11). A rectorectal reflex occurs in which the bowel proximal to the distending bolus contracts and the bowel wall distally relaxes, serving to propel the bolus further caudad. Reflex relaxation of the internal sphincter also occurs, which is enhanced by, but does not require, an extrinsic nerve supply. This relaxation, called the rectoanal inhibitory reflex, correlates with the urge labeled "the call to stool."[69] One may then volitionally contract the levator ani to open the proximal anal canal and relax the external sphincter and puborectalis muscles, which allows a straighter anorectal passage (see Fig. 28–11), allowing the bolus to pass. Increasing intra-abdominal pressure by squatting and Valsalva's maneuver assists this process. One may elect to defer defecation, however, by volitionally contracting the puborectalis and external anal sphincter. The internal anal sphincter relaxation reflex will subsequently fade, usually within 15 seconds, and the urge

will resolve until triggered again. The rectal wall accommodates to the bolus by decreasing its wall tension with time, resulting in less sensory input and less reflex triggering from that bolus. This is somewhat analogous to the function of the striated external urethral sphincter in volitional control of urinary voiding.

The external sphincter generally tenses in response to small rectal distentions via a spinal reflex, though reflexive relaxation of the external sphincter occurs in the presence of greater distentions. These spinal cord reflexes are centered in the conus and are augmented and modulated by higher cortical influences. When cortical control is disrupted, as by spinal cord injury, the external sphincter reflexes usually persist and allow spontaneous defecation. During sleep, colonic activity, anal tone, and protective responses to abdominal pressure elevations are all decreased, while rectal tone increases.[16, 69]

The "gastrocolic reflex" refers to increased colonic activity (GMCs and mass movements), which occurs in the first 30 to 60 minutes after a meal. This increased colonic activity appears to be modulated by both hormonal effects from release of peptides from the upper gastrointestinal tract, which increase contractility of colonic smooth musculature, and a spinal cord–mediated vescicovescical reflex.[16] Upper gastrointestinal receptor stimulation results in increased activity in the colon, probably due to reflexively increased parasympathetic efferent activity to the colon. The possibility of a purely ENS-mediated activation exists, though the small bowel and colon motor activities do not seem to be synchronized. In SCI the measured increase in colonic activity after a meal is blunted as compared to normals.[16] The gastrocolic reflex is often used therapeutically, even in SCI patients, to enhance bowel evacuation during this 30- to 60-min postprandial time frame.[1, 22] Occasionally, certain foods may serve as trigger foods that especially induce bowel evacuation shortly after consumption.

Dietary Considerations

Food choices are important when colonic transient time is prolonged, as in SCI (96 hours vs. 30 hours in normals).[3, 5, 50] Excessive fluid resorption may result in the hardening of stools and subsequent constipation. Gases and liquids are propelled 30 to 100 times faster than solids by the colon. Stools that have lost their plasticity may not be kneaded and folded by the haustra and instead may be impeded. To maintain a more fluid content, stool softeners, both docusate and food fiber, have been used. No increase in stool bulk, as would be expected with fluid retention, occurs from docusate in normals, questioning its efficacy.[3] Fiber does increase stool bulk and plasticity, especially in the more physically coarse forms, which also tend to decrease colonic pressures.[3] Control of excessive stool hardness requires higher-fiber foods in preference to lower-residual foods.

The American norm is stated to be 100 g of solid feces expelled daily or less frequently.[56] However, the high pressures involved in moving solid feces probably contribute to the 90% incidence of hemorrhoids in Americans and to premature diverticula formation and hemorrhoidal complications in more than 70% of SCI patients.[61] Constant

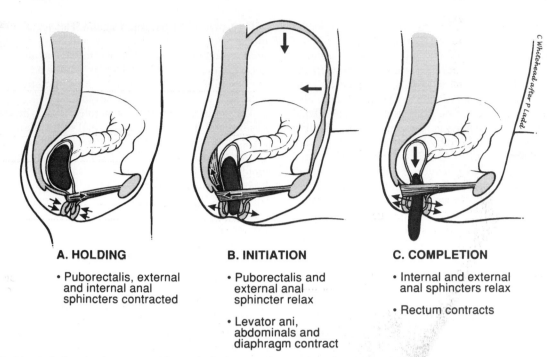

A. HOLDING

- Puborectalis, external and internal anal sphincters contracted

B. INITIATION

- Puborectalis and external anal sphincter relax

- Levator ani, abdominals and diaphragm contract

C. COMPLETION

- Internal and external anal sphincters relax

- Rectum contracts

FIGURE 28–11 *A,* Defecation is prevented by statically increased tone of the internal anal sphincter and puborectalis, as well as by the mechanical effects of the acute anorectal angle. Dynamic responses of the external anal sphincter and puborectalis to rectal distention reflexes or increased intra-abdominal pressures further impede defecation. *B,* To initiate defecation, the puborectalis and external anal sphincter relax while intra-abdominal pressure is increased by Valsalva's maneuver, which is facilitated by squatting. The levator ani helps reduce the acute anorectal angle to open the distal anal canal to receive the stool bolus. *C,* Intrarectal reflexes result in continued internal anal sphincter relaxation and rectal propulsive contractions, which help expel the bolus through the open canal. (Modified from Shiller LR: Fecal Incontinence. *In* Sleisenger MH, Fordtran JS (eds): Gastrointestinal Disease: Pathophysiology, Diagnosis, Management, ed 4. Philadelphia, WB Saunders, 1989, p 322.)

straining at stool may also contribute to peripheral neuropathic deficits in the anal sphincteric musculature. Acceptance of softer stools, from a higher-fiber diet, might help reduce these complications and is often recommended for their treatment. The longer perineal hygiene time required for softer stools may be a deterrent for some and should be discussed with patients.

A wide range of "normal" bowel patterns occur. Defecation frequencies in nonimpaired persons vary dramatically from several times per day to less than once per week. Ninety-four percent have a frequency of between three times per day and three times per week. Stool consistencies vary, from liquid to pudding, pasty, semisolid, soft-formed, medium-formed, and hard-formed. Patients rarely have an adequate vocabulary to describe this socially taboo subject. Fully appreciating an individual's premorbid "normal" bowel function is important in the planning and goal setting for a new neurogenic bowel program.

NEUROGENIC BOWEL FINDINGS

Innervation

The lower colon and anorectal mechanisms receive parasympathetic, sympathetic, and somatic innervation in addition to the intrinsic ENS (see Fig. 28–10). The neurogenic bowel loses the direct somatic sensory or motor control functions and may or may not have impaired sympathetic and parasympathetic innervation. The intrinsic ENS for most conditions remains intact. The most common excep-

tion would be cases of autonomic neuropathy from diabetes mellitus, which can involve the ENS (although this does not necessarily correlate with the severity of the polyneuropathy). The intact intrinsic ENS continues to integrate and modulate bowel function, even with the absence of autonomic and somatic nervous system input, and may be the neurological substrate for bowel habit training.

Evaluation

The history should include premorbid bowel pattern information such as defecation frequency, typical time(s) of the day, associated predefecatory activities, bowel medications and techniques or trigger foods, and stool consistency. It is important to review any premorbid gastrointestinal disease problems. The presence of gastrointestinal sensations or pain, warning sensations for defecation, sense of urgency, and ability to prevent stool loss during Valsalva activities such as laughing, sneezing, coughing, or transfers, should be noted. Excessively large-caliber hard stool can be ascertained by a history of toilet plugging.[44] The patient's goals and willingness to alter prior patterns need to be established.[35]

Physical examination begins with inspection of the anus. A patulous gaping orifice suggests a history of overdistention and trauma by a previous regimen. A normal anal-buttock contour (Fig. 28–12) suggests an intact EAS muscle mass, whereas its loss results in a flattened, fanned-out "scalloped"-appearing anal region. The patient should perform Valsalva's maneuver while the anus and perineum are observed for excessive descent.[63] Perianal cutaneous sharp stimulation normally results in a visible anal sphincter reflexive contraction. This can be checked by tugging perianal hairs or by the application of the sharp edge of a broken cotton swab stick to the perianal skin. This anocutaneous (AC) reflex should be checked in all four quadrants, as selective (especially side-to-side) deficits may occur. Sensation to pinprick is tested at the same time. A gloved lubricated finger should then be inserted through the anus until no pressure is appreciated at the fingertip. The length of the anus, where pressure is sensed, is normally 2.5 to 4.5 cm long. Where the pressure decreases marks the anorectal junction. Along the posterior wall, 1.5 to 2.5 cm from the anal verge, the puborectalis muscular sling can be palpated as a ridge that will push the finger forward upon resisting defecation. No palpable ridge or push suggests puborectalis atrophy or dysfunction. A shortened length of anal pressure zone suggests EAS muscle atrophy. With the finger in place, the bulbocavernosus (BC) reflex can be elicited by rapidly tapping or squeezing the clitoris or glans penis. Multiple random trials are needed to be certain the vesicoanal Valsalva protective reflexes are not occurring at the same time by random chance. The response can be delayed up to a few seconds. A consistent response to the stimulus indicates an intact BC reflex. Insertion of the finger in the anal canal occasionally triggers internal anal sphincter (IAS) relaxation, but more often triggers a tightening squeeze that is efferently equivalent to the BC reflex. If IAS and EAS relaxation occur, wait several seconds for tone to be restored before BC reflex testing. Ask the patient to volitionally squeeze the anus before removing the finger ("resist defecation") to check for volitional EAS and puborectalis tone and control. With the abdomen relaxed, transabdominally palpate the colon for hard stool. Palpable hard stool should not be present on the right side of the abdomen (ascending colon).

Diagnostic Testing

The history and physical examination provide most of the necessary information. The clinical cause of the neurogenic bowel dysfunction in most patients who are referred to physiatrists is readily apparent. Additional objective laboratory testing may be helpful when the cause of FI or DWE is obscure, the history appears doubtful, conservative interventions fail, or surgical interventions are contemplated. Table 28–6 lists some of the many tests available.

Upper Motor Neurogenic Bowel (UMNB)

Any supraconus disease process, from spinal cord injury to dementia, can lead to this type of bowel dysfunction. Spinal cortical pathway deficits lead to decreased ability to sense the urge to defecate. Most SCI patients, however, sense a vague discomfort when excessive rectal or colonic distention occurs, and 43% have chronic complaints of vague abdominal distention discomfort, which eases with bowel evacuation.[41, 61] These sensations are likely mediated by afferent fibers bypassing the zone of cord injury in sympathetic nerves.

Studies of rectal distention in SCI patients show the development of elevated rectosigmoid pressures as compared to normals, especially when higher or continuous filling rates are used. These increases are associated with

TABLE 28–6   Laboratory Tests of Colonic and Rectoanal Function

Test	Purpose
Colonoscopy, rectosigmoidoscopy, anoscopy	Visualize anatomy to identify lesions Limited benefit to assess function
Radiography	
Defecography	Visualize kinesiology of defecation
Barium enema	Identify structural defects; fluoroscopy time too limited to assess function in any detail
Serial radiographs of tiny radiopaque plastic beads ingested with food	Evaluate colonic transit time; useful to confirm constipation history, identify dysfunctional segments that help plan colostomy level
Manometry	
Kymography	Measure pressure and volume change by intraluminal balloons
Catheter	Measure pressures by catheter in various compartments of the bowel Manometry can assess giant migratory contractions and anal pressures; with intrarectal balloon inflation it can evaluate rectoanal inhibitory reflex
Solid-sphere retention test	Measures maximal anal resistance force to extraction of spheres of standard sizes
Rectally infused saline continence test	Quantitative reproducible assessment of liquid continence ability
Electromyography	
Traditional	Assess motor nerve supply to puborectalis, anococcygeus, levator ani, and external anal sphincter; assess sensory pelvic afferents by nerve conduction studies, bulbocavernosus reflex testing, or somatosensory evoked potentials
Intraluminal catheter	Research tool to assess colonic smooth muscle electrical potential activity

Compiled from Christensen J: The motor function of the colon. In Yamada T (ed): Textbook of Gastroenterology. Philadelphia, JB Lippincott, 1991, pp 180–196; Schiller LR: Fecal incontinence. In Sleisinger MH, Fordtran JS (eds): Gastrointestinal Disease. Philadelphia, WB Saunders, 1989, pp 317–330; Stone JM, Wolfe VA, Niro-Murcia M, Perkash I: Colostomy as treatment for complications of spinal cord injury. Arch Phys Med Rehabil 1990; 71:514–518.

increased external sphincter pressure development due to sacral reflexes and are abolished by pudendal block.[3] This form of rectal sphincter dyssynergia has unfortunately been labeled decreased colonic compliance, even though intermittent or slow filling in the rectum appears to be associated with normal bolus accommodation and pressure relaxation.[41, 53] This contrasts with the true decreased compliance found in ischemic or postinflammatory rectal bowel wall due to fibrosis, which cannot accommodate and relax regardless of flow rates.

Internal sphincter relaxation upon rectal distention occurs in SCI patients as in normals. After sufficient rectal distention the external sphincter may completely relax, resulting in expulsion of the fecal bolus. Rectal sphincter dyssynergia does not necessarily correlate with bladder sphincter dyssnergia but often results in DWE.[54] The protective vesicoanal reflex, wherein the external sphincter pressure increases in response to increased intra-abdominal pressure, is usually intact[3] (Table 28–7). Patients with UMNB also have normal or increased anal sphincter tone, intact AC and BC reflexes, a palpable puborectalis muscle sling, and normal anal verge appearance (Fig. 28–12).

Lower Motor Neurogenic Bowel (LMNB)

Polyneuropathy, conus medullaris or cauda equina lesions, pelvic surgery, delivery, or even chronic straining at stooling can impair the somatic innervation of the anal sphincter mechanism. These conditions can also produce sympathetic and parasympathetic innervation deficits. If an isolated pudendal insult has occurred, colonic transit times will be normal and FI will predominate. Colonic sluggishness can occur as a result of loss of parasympathetic

supply, adding constipation and DWE to FI difficulties. This is an especially bad combination because the large hard stool that can result from such colonic inertia can overstretch the weakened anal mechanism, resulting in a gaping, patulous, incompetent orifice. The denervation and atrophy of the EAS lead to loss of the protective vesicoanal reflex, which can result in stool soilage from the increased abdominal pressures associated with everyday activities. Rectal distention leads to the expected internal sphincter relaxation, but attenuated or absent external sphincter protective contractions result in FI or fecal smearing whenever boluses present at the rectum. The presence of a large bolus in the rectal vault can further compromise the rectoanal angulation at the pelvic floor and contribute to paradoxical liquid incontinence around a low impaction.[3]

Patients with LMNB dysfunction have decreased but present anal tone due to the smooth muscle internal sphincter. If no tone is found initially upon inserting the examin-

TABLE 28–7 Features of Colorectal Function in Normals, Upper Motor Neurogenic Bowel (UMNB), UMNB with Posterior Rhizotomy, and Lower Motor Neurogenic Bowel (LMNB)

	Normals	UMNB	UMNB and Posterior Rhizotomy	LMNB
Bowel dysfunction	Normal colon activity and defecation	Chronic intractable constipation, fecal impaction, reflex defecation ± incontinence	Chronic constipation; no reflex defecation	Chronic constipation; fecal impaction maximal in the rectum
Transit time (cecum–anus)	12–48 hr	Prolonged >72 hr	Very prolonged unless sacral nerve stimulator used	Prolonged >6 days, especially left colon
Colonic motility at rest	GMC approx. 4/24 hr	GMC may be reduced in frequency	Reduced GMC	Reduced GMC
In response to stimuli	GMC facilitated by defecation, exercise, and food ingestion	Less GMC facilitation by defecation, exercise, or food ingestion	Less GMC facilitation by defecation, exercise, or food ingestion	Less GMC facilitation by defecation, exercise, or food ingestion
Anal sphincter pressure (mm Hg)				
Resting tone	>30	>30	Normal	Reduced
Volitional squeeze	>30 (up to 1800)	Absent	Absent	Absent
Rectal compliance	Normal	Normal but sigmoid compliance decreased	Normal or increased	Rectum dilated; increased distention volume; increased compliance
Rectal balloon distention				
Effect on IAS	Normal RA inhibitory reflex	Normal RA inhibitory reflex	Normal RA inhibitory reflex	Normal RA inhibitory reflex
Effect on EAS	Causes contraction	Causes contraction	No contraction	No contraction
Sensory perception threshold	<20 mL volume	None	None	None
Stimulation of rectal contraction	Induced by balloon distention	Giant rectal contractions stimulated readily	Rectal contraction stimulation	Rectal contraction stimulation
Vesicoanal reflex	Present (>50 mm Hg)	Present	Absent	Absent
Valsalva protective reflex				
Reflex defecation	Yes	Yes	Impaired	Impaired
Perianal sensation				
Cutaneous sensation (touch, pinprick)	Normal	No sensory perception	No sensory perception	Loss of perianal and buttock sensation due to injury to sacral nerves
Anocutaneous reflex ("anal wink")	Present	Present; may be increased	Absent	Absent due to injury to afferent/efferent sacral pathways
Bulbocavernosus reflex	Present	Present; may be increased	Absent	Absent
Anal appearance	Normal	Normal	Normal	Flattened, "scalloped," due to loss of EAS bulk

Abbreviations: GMC, giant migratory contractions; IAS, internal anal sphincter; EAS, external anal sphincter; RA, rectoanal.
Modified from Banwell JG, Creaswey GH, Aggarwal AM, Mortimer JT: Management of the neurogenic bowel in patients with spinal cord injury. Urol Clin North Am 1993; 20:523; Schiller LR: Fecal incontinence. In Sleisenger MH, Fordtran JS (eds): Gastrointestinal Disease. Philadelphia, WB Saunders, 1989, pp 317–330.

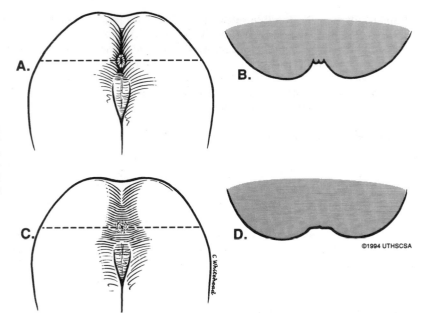

FIGURE 28–12 Upper motor neurogenic bowel presents an appearance similar to normal (*A,* rear view; *B,* profile from above). Anal contour of the lower motor neurogenic bowel (*C,* rear view; *D,* profile from above), with its atrophic external anal sphincter, shows a flattened, scalloped-appearing anal area.

ing finger, wait up to 15 seconds to allow IAS reflex relaxation to recover and restore tone. Chronic overstretching has probably occurred if tone does not return. The anal-to-buttock contour typically appears flattened and "scalloped" (see Fig. 28–12) owing to atrophy of the EAS. The AC reflex is absent or decreased (depending on the completeness of the lesion). Likewise, the BC reflex is weak if present (see Table 28–7). The anal canal is shortened (as compared to the normal 2.5–4.5 cm length) and the puborectalis muscle ridge may not be palpable. Excessive perineal descent and even rectal prolapse may occur with Valsalva's maneuver.

Management

General Principles

Neurogenic bowel dysfunction results in problems of fecal storage and elimination. Inability to volitionally inhibit spontaneous defecations leads to incontinence, while the inability to adequately empty leads to constipation and impactions. Impactions can result in paradoxical diarrhea and incontinence. Providing adequate emptying must be combined with the inhibition of spontaneous defecations except at desired times in order to achieve social continence.

Approaches and Rationale

Colonic transit time and fecal elimination are enhanced by softer stool. However, if the stool becomes too liquid, the protective angle provided by the puborectalis becomes less effective and greater external anal sphincter pressures are required to maintain continence. Neurogenic bowel resting anal pressures are usually normal to slightly decreased but are unable to develop the protective increases in EAS tone needed to control more liquid stool.[3] Some degree of stool firmness must be tolerated to prevent incontinence. To avoid incontinence upon straining, more firmness (medium-formed) is required for the weaker anal

sphincter mechanism of LMNB than for UMNB (semi-formed to soft-formed). Docusate is often used to try to increase fluid content and plasticity in the stool, though its clinical efficacy needs to be individually monitored. Fiber more consistently softens stool but also adds bulk. Bulkier stools can help stimulate the defecatory response more easily in LMNB, though less stimulus is needed in UMNB.[21, 39] The presentation of stool to the rectum triggering defecation may be more associated with GMC and mass movements than with accumulation of sufficient rectal stool to trigger reflex defecation, and this may be what is actually habituated.[56]

The frequency and specific timing to induce adequate emptying may be chosen. Regular emptying is recommended as the primary means for enhancing both elimination and decreasing incontinence between stooling. Incontinence is reduced by less stool accumulation, since stool is not presenting to the rectum between desired defecation times. Adequate emptying is accomplished by (1) making stools easier to move by means of softening, (2) adding bowel stimulant medication if needed, and (3) triggering the defecatory reflex at consistent desired times to promote habituation.

Choosing long intervals between elimination allows more fluid reabsorption, resulting in harder stools, which can worsen DWE. Since 94% of unimpaired persons defecate three or more times per week, choosing a frequency of every other day or less would seem more physiological and less likely to contribute to constipation. The desire to avoid the unpleasant task of stool elimination leads some to elect longer time intervals, but this carries the attendant risk for impaction or sphincter damage caused by larger-caliber harder stools.

Chronic oral bowel stimulant medication use been questioned because of concerns of developing the atonic "cathartic bowel" syndrome. Certain stimulants, especially in the anthroquinone family (senna, cascara, aloes), have been shown to damage myenteric neurons with chronic use.[17, 59] It has not been established whether late complications from chronic oral bowel stimulant medications occur in those with neurogenic bowel dysfunction. Approaches that appear effective initially need longer-term studies to verify continued benefits, especially since there is a high incidence of late gastrointestinal problems reported in an initially successfully managed SCI population.[61]

Triggering of defecation can be accomplished by digital stimulation, rectal stimulant suppository use, or enemas. All of these cause reflex relaxation of the IAS, and if strong enough can reflexly relax the EAS as well. This initiates the rectorectal reflex that helps to eliminate any stool that is present. The GMC and mass movement associated with the call to stool for many intact persons often occurs at consistent times, which may be trainable. If a bowel habit (consistent time or times of day when defecation typically occurs for that individual) existed premorbidly, its consistency should be encouraged by inducing defecation at similar times. Such bowel habits may be a trainable event that also enhance adequate emptying if consistent training is used. A change from the patient's usual pattern can be habituated but may take several weeks of inducing defecations at the new desired time before incontinence at the prior time subsides.[35]

Theoretically, fewer long-term complications will occur if the following are minimized: anorectal overdistention (as with enemas), anal trauma (as by manual disimpaction), and oral stimulant medication use. An accelerating enema volume required for efficacy should be a warning that chronic rectal overdistention may be leading to less responsiveness.[35] Digital stimulation to induce defecatory reflexes should be favored over manual disimpaction because the latter can easily result in inadvertent overstretching of the insensate and more delicate anal mechanisms of the neurogenic bowel. Local rectal stimulant suppositories and minienemas with bisacodyl or glycerin do not carry the same risk as oral stimulant medications and do not appear to lead to chronic inflammatory changes of the rectal mucosa.

One approach to initiating neurogenic bowel training is outlined in Table 28–8. Each step is added only after 2

weeks' consistent trial of the previous step has been ineffective. In this approach, obtaining elimination at the desired time is emphasized as the first step and usually precedes development of complete continence by several weeks. This pattern suggests enhanced responsiveness and emptying at the habituated time with apparently less responsiveness, or less rectal or stool presentation, at other times.

Bowel function is a very private matter, and patients may be reluctant to seek advice or information despite its major importance to their overall well-being and self-concept.[56] Information should be freely disseminated in order to enhance the development of healthy habits and minimize bowel complications. Bowel habituation training is more difficult to accept among those with long-established patterns of managing stool hygiene even if their current methods are ineffective in eliminating incontinence or constipation.

Intrinsic loss of the ENS, or any segment, including surgical reanastomosis, may result in loss of the rectoanal inhibitory reflex, causing DWE. Oral laxative abuse can cause dysfunction of the ENS.[17, 59] If bowel training is not accomplishing defecations at the desired times, anorectal manometry and kymography may be indicated (see Table 28–6).

When neurogenic bowel deficits are incomplete and some degree of control and sensation are present, biofeedback may offer a means of enhancing the patient's residual sensory and motor abilities. Improved sensory awareness after biofeedback training is an indicator of success. This typically requires only a few sessions, and most patients improve after just one session.[56] Among more severely impaired nonselected myelomeningocele children, biofeedback and behavioral training are equally effective in restoring continence.[56] For selected individuals with some degree of volitional EAS activation and some degree of anorectal sensation, biofeedback may be a tool to help restore not just social continence but normal defecatory control.

Surgical Options

Sacral nerve deficits interfere with the action of the puborectalis, levator ani, and EAS (see Fig. 28–10). The resulting pelvic floor descent impairs the protective puborectalis sling angle and decreases the efficacy of protective EAS contractions. Some patients have benefited from transposition of innervated gracilis, adductor longus, gluteus maximus, or free muscle graft palmaris longus to replace puborectalis function and restore the acute anorectal junction angle that this sling provides. Chronic electrical stimulation to enhance development of fatigue resistance is used with these transplants. Sensory deficits are not improved, but continence is somewhat restored with the ability to inhibit defecation if some degree of sensation remains.[43, 56]

Incomplete EAS relaxation during defecation (dyssynergia), results in a functional outlet obstruction and DWE. Prolonged descending colon transit time occurs, which does improve with an IAS and partial EAS myotomy.[19] This procedure relieves constipation in 62% of patients but results in FI in 16% and has not become a popular option.[45]

Stimulation of anterior sacral roots S2, S3, and S4 has

TABLE 28–8   Protocol for Progressive Steps in Bowel Habituation Program*

1. Bowel clean-out if stool is present in the rectal vault or palpable proximal to the descending colon, by multiple enemas or oral cathartic
2. Appropriately soft stool consistency with diet (fiber or "trigger" foods) and bulking agents (docusate)
3. Glycerin suppository 20–30 min after meal; 10 min later on toilet, limited to less than 40 min, relieving skin pressure every 10 min
4. Dulcolax suppository in place of glycerin
5. Digital stimulation—20 min post suppository every 5 min × 3
6. Timed oral medications—casanthranol–docusate sodium (Peri-Colace), senna (Senokot), bisacodyl (Dulcolax) tablets timed so that bowel movement would otherwise result 30 min to 1 hr after anticipated triggered bowel timing
7. If defecation occurs in less than 10 min after suppository insertion, transition to digital stimulation technique only; once well habituated, rarely straining alone may trigger defecations at desired time

*Steps 1–3 are initial interventions and are always followed, with steps 4–6 incorporated only as needed. At least 2 weeks' trial with proper technique is pursued before advancing to the next step.

been performed on patients for whom a stimulator was placed for micturition and by transrectal stimulation. Stimulation of S2 tends to promote nonperistaltic, low-pressure colorectal motor activity. Stimulation of S3 causes occasional high-pressure peristalic waves, especially with repetitive stimulation. Stimulation of S4 increases both rectal and anal tone.[40, 67] Electrodefecation has been obtainable by sacral root stimulation in about 50% of patients but is unpredictable.[3, 16] A reliable defecation electroprosthesis remains an elusive goal.[3] Artificial anal sphincters with a subcutaneous pump reservoir similar to urinary artificial sphincters suffer from high complication rates and poor outcomes and remain investigative.[43]

Colostomy has been shown to reduce bowel care time, especially when offered to those with chronic DWE.[62] It may be indicated when conservative medical measures and training have failed; or when intrinsic bowel deficits exist such as in Hirschsprung's disease, Chagas' disease, "cathartic colon," and when pressure ulcers or other skin lesions occur that cannot be effectively healed because of frequent soiling; or when frequent urinary tract seeding by frequent bowel impactions occurs.[62] Although diversion for pressure ulcer healing is usually anticipated to be reversed, those with neurogenic bowel often elect to maintain the colostomy even after the pressure ulcer is healed.[62] Colostomy carries a surgical risk, is cosmetically disfiguring, and is seldom necessary to achieve adequate social continence, but it remains a procedure of last resort for the treatment of FI or DWE.[3, 61]

Complications

Significant bowel complications requiring medical treatment or lifestyle alterations are reported in 27% of spinal cord–injured patients 5 years or greater beyond their injury, even though bowel management was satisfactory during the first 5 years. Over 80% of these SCI patients had bowel impactions, and 20% had chronic bowel impaction and DWE problems.[61] Impactions have been reported to be complicated by perforation or even death. Impactions have a morbidity range between 0% and 6% in the normal population, being higher in the cognitively impaired elderly.[70] Other late gastrointestinal complications reported by SCI patients include gastroesophageal reflux, premature diverticulosis, and autonomic dysreflexia.[27, 61] Morbidity from colonic perforation by enema use has also been reported.[38]

Hemorrhoids are more important when patients have intact sensation, but rectal bleeding due to hemorrhoids has been reported by 74% of SCI patients in one study.[61] Hemorrhoids develop as a result of frequent high pressures in the anorectal marginal veins and are associated with constipated hard stool passage. Stool softening is the best preventive and chronic treatment measure, but this must be balanced with maintaining continence.

An overstretched patulous noncompetent sphincter associated with rectal prolapse often is an end result of passage of very large hard stool through a weakened anorectal mechanism in LMNB. Overdistention of the weakened neurogenic anal mechanism should be avoided by use of stool softening and gentle care whenever manual disimpaction is required to avoid trauma to these denervated

structures. Although the anus can be significantly dilated to accommodate two fingers for breaking up low impactions, anorectal overdistention has been hypothesized to lead to atonic segments similar to bladder overdistention. The bowel, however, cannot be as easily decompressed and rested to allow recovery as can the bladder. The IAS is smooth muscle which will shorten and remodel to eventually regain competent closure if the overstretching can be eliminated. Unfortunately, this may require months of incontinent liquid-to-soft pasty stools, which is seldom tolerated. Should the patient require temporary colostomy for some other disease process, it may be possible, after many months, to train toward social continence with the restored sphincter. However, such patients have usually had long courses of constant soiling and often prefer to keep their colostomy and continence rather than pursue surgical reversal and training, which may not be as successful.

Autonomic dysreflexia occurs in SCI patients with lesions at or above the midthoracic region. Fecal impaction is a common and potentially dangerous cause of autonomic dysreflexia because of the substantial time that may be required for its clearance. If manual disimpaction is required, lubrication with lidocaine gel is recommended to decrease additional nociceptive sensory input from the richly innervated anal mechanism.

Bloating and abdominal distention are common complaints of patients with neurogenic bowel dysfunction. These complaints can be reduced in SCI patients by increasing the bowel program frequency. This complaint can be especially severe in those with hyperactive EAS protective responses to rectal distention, which can preclude the passing of flatus. Digital release of flatus may be required in addition to diet modification to eliminate foods that produce excessive gases. Workup should also include assessment for any contributing aerophagia.

Treatment Outcomes

Bowel habituation training in myelomeningocele children with suppository or digital stimulation, or both, resulted in 83% of compliant patients obtaining less than one incontinent stool per month.[35] The continence catheter enema, which has a distal rectal balloon to avoid immediate enema expulsion, when used daily or every other day, reduced fecal incontinence to fewer than three episodes per month in children with myelomeningocele.[57] Tobin and Brocklehurst[66] treated demented FI nursing home residents by medically constipating (with codeine) those deemed to have UMNB and giving biweekly enemas. Those diagnosed to have LMNB had their stools softened with lactulose and received weekly enemas. Fecal continence was restored in 80% of those consistently treated.[66] Although all complete SCI patients have episodic FI,[41] this is a chronic problem for only 2%.[61] DWE appears to be a progressive problem that develops 5 years or more after SCI. This is rarely reported after training in the first 4 years but occurs in 20% by a mean of 17 years after injury.[61] Gastrointestinal problems in SCI are not merely nuisances but account for 10% of SCI late mortality.[27] Patients with multiple sclerosis, parkinsonism, or muscular dystrophy have also been helped by methods to enhance bowel storage or elimination in the face of deteriorating neuromuscular and anorectal function.[3, 15] Colostomy also provides a means of achieving social continence. Colostomy complications include embarrassing gas problems, appliance loosening and leakage, and cosmetic difficulties.

Patients who develop social bowel continence can venture into public without fear of malodorous embarrassment and unpredictable social disaster that humiliates as well as requires substantial clean-up time. When such fears persist, full social and vocational reintegration is impeded. A major hurdle that many patients with neuromuscular compromise can overcome is control of the seemingly automatic neurogenic functions of defecation and bowel elimination. Such patients should not needlessly suffer owing to inadequate attention by care providers to this potentially functionally impairing and socially handicapping deficit.

References

1. Aaronson MJ, Freed MM, Burakoff R: Colonic myoelectric activity in persons with spinal cord injury. Dig Dis Sci 1985; 30:295–300.
2. Abrams P, Blaivas JG, Stanton SL, Andersen JT: Standardization of terminology of lower urinary tract function. In Krane RJ, Siroky MB (eds): Clinical Neurourology, ed 2. Boston, Little, Brown, 1991, pp 651–669.
3. Banwell JG, Creaswey GH, Aggarwal AM, Mortimer JT: Management of the neurogenic bowel in patients with spinal cord injury. Urol Clin North Am 1993; 20:517–526.
4. Bartolo DC, Read NW, Jarratt JA, et al: Differences in anal sphincter function and clinical presentation in patients with pelvic floor descent. Gastroenterology 1983; 85:68–75.
5. Beuret-Blanquart F, Weber J, Gouverneur JP, et al: Colonic transit time and anorectal manometric anomalies in 19 patients with complete transection of the spinal cord. J Auton Nerv Syst 1990; 30:199–208.
6. Berger Y, Blaivas JG, DeLa Rocha ER, Salinas JM: Urodynamic findings in Parkinson's disease. J Urol 1987; 138:836–838.
7. Blaivas JG: Videourodynamics. In Krane RJ, Siroky MB (eds.): Clinical Neurology, ed 2. Boston, Little, Brown, 1991, pp 265–274.
8. Bors E, Comarr AE: Neurological Urology. Baltimore, University Park Press, 1971.
9. Bradley WE: Physiology of the urinary bladder. In Walsh PC, Gittes RF, Perlmutter AD, Stamey TA (eds): Campbells' Urology. Philadelphia, WB Saunders, 1986, pp 129–185.
10. Brindley GS, Rushton DN: Long-term follow-up of patients with sacral anterior root stimulator implants. Paraplegia 1990; 28:469–475.
11. Cardenas DD, Hooton TM: Urinary tract infection in persons with spinal cord injury. Arch Phys Med Rehabil 1995; 76:272–280.
12. Cardenas DD, Kelly E, Krieger JN, Chapman WH: Residual urine volumes in patients with spinal cord injury: measurement with a portable ultrasound instrument. Arch Phys Med Rehabil 1988; 69:514–516.
13. Cardenas DD, Kelly E, Mayo ME: Manual stimulation of reflex voiding after spinal cord injury. Arch Phys Med Rehabil 1985; 66:459–462.
14. Cardenas DD, Mayo ME: Bacteriuria with fever after spinal cord injury. Arch Phys Med Rehabil 1987; 68:291–293.
15. Caroscio JT: Amyotrophic Lateral Sclerosis—A Guide to Patient Care. New York, Thieme, 1986, p 126.
16. Christensen J: The motor function of the colon. In Yamada T (ed): Textbook of Gastroenterology. Philadelphia, JB Lippincott, 1991, pp 180–196.
17. Cummings JH: Laxative abuse. Gut 1974; 15:758–766.
18. DeVivo MJ, Fine PR, Cutter GR, Maetz HM: The risk of renal calculi in spinal cord injury patients. J Urol 1984; 131:857–860.
19. Devroede G, Lamarche J: Functional importance of extrinsic parasympathetic innervation in the distal colon and rectum in man. Gastroenterology 1974; 66:273–280.
20. Dewire DM, Owens RS, Anderson GA, et al: A comparison of the urological complications associated with long-term management of quadriplegics with and without chronic indwelling urinary catheters. J Urol 1992; 147:1069–1072.
21. Dikenson VA: Maintenance of anal continence—a review of pelvic floor physiology. Gut 1978; 19:1163–1174.
22. Doughty DB, Jackson DB: Gastrointestinal Disorders. St Louis, Mosby–Year Book, 1993, p 268.
23. Dykstra DD, Sidi AA: Treatment of detrusor-sphincter dyssnergia with botulinum A toxin: a double-blind study. Arch Phys Med Rehabil 1990; 71:24–26.
24. Finkbeiner AE: Is bethanechol chloride clinically effective in promoting bladder emptying? A literature review. J Urol 1985; 134:443–449.
25. Gasparini ME, Schmidt RA, Tanagho EA: Selective sacral rhizotomy in the management of the reflex neuropathic bladder: a report on 17 patients with long-term follow-up. J Urol 1992; 148:1207–1210.
26. Glowacki LS, Beecroft ML, Cook RJ: The natural history of asymptomatic urolithiasis. J Urol 1992; 147:319–321.
27. Gore RM, Mintzer RA, Calenoff L: Gastrointestinal complications of spinal cord injury. Spine 1981; 6:538–544.
28. Goyal RK, Crist JR: Neurology of the gut. In Sleisenger MH, Fordtran JS (eds): Gastrointestinal Disease. Philadelphia, WB Saunders, 1989, pp 21–52.
29. Granger CV, Hamilton BB, Gresham GE, Kramer AA: The stroke rehabilitation outcome study: Part II. Relative merits of the total Barthel Index score and a four-item subscore in predicting patient outcomes. Arch Phys Med Rehabil 1989; 70:100–108.
30. Guttmann L, Frankel H: The value of intermittent catheterization in the early management of traumatic paraplegia and tetraplegia. Paraplegia 1966; 4:63–84.
31. Guyton AC: Textbook of Medical Physiology, ed 8. Philadelphia, WB Saunders, 1991, pp 731–735, 742.
32. Iwatsubo E, Komine S, Yamashita H, et al: Over-distension therapy of the bladder in paraplegic patients using self-catheterization: a preliminary study. Paraplegia 1984; 22:210–215.
33. Kaufman JM, Fam B, Jacobs SC, et al: Bladder cancer and squamous metaplasia in spinal cord injury patients. J Urol 1977; 118:967–971.
34. Kinder RB, Mundy AR: Neurotransmitters. In Krane RJ, Siroky MB (eds): Clinical Neurology, ed 2. Boston, Little, Brown, 1991, pp 83–92.
35. King JC, Currie DM, Wright E: Bowel training in spina bifida: importance of education, patient compliance, age, and anal reflexes. Arch Phys Med Rehabil 1994; 75:243–247.
36. Kiviat MD, Zimmerman TA, Donovan WH: Sphincter stretch: a new technique resulting in continence and complete voiding in paraplegics. J Urol 1975; 114:895–897.
37. Lapides J, Diokno AC, Silber SJ, Lowe BS: Clean intermittent self-catheterization in the treatment of urinary tract disease. J Urol 1972; 107:458–461.
38. Liptak GS, Reveli GM: Management of bowel dysfunction in children with spinal cord disease or injury by means of the enema continence catheter. J Pediatr 1992; 120:190–194.
39. Longo WE, Ballantyne GH, Modlin IM: The colon, anorectum, and spinal cord patient. Dis Colon Rectum 1989; 32:261–267.
40. MacDonagh RP, Sun WM, Smallwood R, et al: Control of defecation in patients with spinal injuries by stimulation of sacral anterior nerve roots. Br Med J 1990; 300:1494–1497.
41. MacDonagh RP, Sun WM, Smallwood R, et al: Anorectal function in patients with complete supraconal spinal cord lesions. Gut 1992; 33:1532–1538.
42. Madersbacher H, Jilg G: Control of detrusor hyperreflexia by the intravesical instillation of oxybutynine hydrochloride. Paraplegia 1991; 29:84–90.
43. Madoff RD, Williams JG, Caushaj PF: Fecal incontinence. N Engl J Med 1992; 326:1002–1007.
44. Martelli H, Devroede G, Arhan P, Dugay C: Some parameters of large bowel motility in normal man. Gastroenterology 1978; 75:612.
45. Martelli H, Devroede G, Arhan P, Dugay C: Mechanisms of idiopathic constipation: outlet obstruction. Gastroenterology 1978; 75:623–631.
46. Mayo ME: The value of sphincter electromyography in urodynamics. J Urol 1979; 122:357–360.
47. Mayo ME, Chetner MP: Lower urinary tract dysfunction in multiple sclerosis, Urology 1992; 34:67–70.
48. McInerney PD, Vanner TF, Harris SAB, Stephenson TP: Permanent urethral stents for detrusor sphincter dyssynergia. Br J Urol 1991; 61:291–294.
49. McLellan FC: The Neurogenic Bladder. Springfield, Ill, Thomas, 1939, pp 57–70, 116–185.
50. Menardo G, Bausano G, Corazziari E, et al: Large bowel transit in paraplegic patients. Dis Colon Rectum 1987; 30:924–928.

51. Montgomerie JZ, Chan E, Gilmore DS, Canawati HN: Low mortality among patients with spinal cord injury and bacteremia. Rev Infect Dis 1991; 13:871–876.

52. National Institute on Disability and Rehabilitation Research Consensus Statement: The prevention and management of urinary tract infections among people with spinal cord injuries. J Am Paraplegia Soc 1992; 15:194–204.

53. Nino-Murcia M, Stone JM, Chang PJ, Perkash I: Colonic transit in spinal cord-injured patients. Invest Radiol 1990; 25:109–112.

54. Pedersen E: Regulation of bladder and colon-rectum in patients with spinal lesions. J Auton Nerv Syst 1983; 7:329–338.

55. Perkash I, Friedland GW: Transrectal ultrasonography of the lower urinary tract: evaluation of bladder neck problems. Neurourol Urodynamics 1986; 5:299.

56. Schiller LR: Fecal incontinence. In Sleisenger MH, Fordtran JS (eds): Gastrointestinal Disease. Philadelphia, WB Saunders, 1989, pp 317–330.

57. Shandling B, Gilmour RF: The enema continence catheter in spina bifida: successful bowel management. J Pediatr Surg 1987; 22:271–273.

58. Sidi AA, Becher EF, Reddy PK, Dykstra DD: Augmentation enterocystoplasty for the management of voiding dysfunction in spinal cord injury patients. J Urol 1990; 143:83–85.

59. Smith B: Effect of irritant purgatives on the myenteric plexus in man and mouse. Gut 1968; 9:139–142.

60. Steers WD, Meythaler JM, Haworth C, et al: Effects of acute bolus and chronic continuous intrathecal baclofen on genitourinary dysfunction due to spinal cord pathology. J Urol 1992; 148:1849–1855.

61. Stone JM, Nino-Murcia M, Wolfe VA, Perkash I: Chronic gastrointestinal problems in spinal cord injury patients: a prospective analysis. Am J Gastroenterol 1990; 85:1114–1119.

62. Stone JM, Wolfe VA, Nino-Murcia M, Perkash I: Colostomy as treatment for complications of spinal cord injury. Arch Phys Med Rehabil 1990; 71:514–518.

63. Swash M: New concepts in the prevention of incontinence. Practitioner 1985; 229:895–899.

64. Swierzewski SJ III, Gormley EA, Belville WD, et al: The effect of terazosin on bladder function in the spinal cord injured patient. J Urol 1994; 151:951–954.

65. Tanagho EA, Schmidt RA, Orvis BR: Neural stimulation for control of voiding dysfunction: a preliminary report in 22 patients with serious neuropathic voiding disorders. J Urol 1989; 142:340–345.

66. Tobin GW, Brocklehurst JC: Faecal incontinence in residential homes for the elderly: prevalence, aetiology and management. Age Aging 1986; 15:41–46.

67. Varma JS: Autonomic influences on colorectal motility and pelvic surgery. World J Surg 1992; 16:811–819.

68. Webb RJ, Styles RA, Griffiths CJ, et al: Ambulatory monitoring of bladder pressure in low compliance neurogenic bladder dysfunction. J Urol 1992; 48:1477–1488.

69. Wingate DL, Ewart WR: The brain-gut axis. In Yamada T (ed): Textbook of Gastroenterology. Philadelphia, JB Lippincott, 1991, pp 50–60.

70. Wrenn K: Fecal impaction. N Engl J Med 1989; 321:658–666.

Management of Spasticity

RICHARD T. KATZ, M.D.

Spasticity is more difficult to characterize than to recognize and still more difficult to quantify. Occurring in a variety of central nervous system disorders, spastic hypertonia has both diagnostic and therapeutic significance. Spasticity is a diagnostic hallmark of an upper motor neuron disorder, and therapeutically it represents one of the most important impairments for those who care for patients with central nervous system disease.

The purpose of this chapter is to examine the subject of spastic hypertonia in an encyclopedic fashion. Owing to space limitations, the reader is referred to recent reviews for an extensive list of references.[42, 43, 47, 72] The references cited in the rest of this chapter were selected as representing recent information, key studies, or useful reviews. The discussion of spastic hypertonia is divided into three parts: (1) pathophysiology, (2) methods of quantifying spasticity, and (3) therapeutic management.

PATHOPHYSIOLOGY

A widely accepted definition of *spasticity* is: "a motor disorder characterized by a velocity-dependent increase in tonic stretch reflexes (muscle tone) with exaggerated tendon jerks, resulting from hyperexcitability of the stretch reflex, as one component of the upper motor neuron syndrome."[51]

Muscle tone may be defined as "the sensation of resistance felt as one manipulates a joint through a range of motion, with the subject attempting to relax."[52] Although this definition is adequate for the bedside clinical examination, a more vigorous analysis indicates that muscle tone is likely to consist of several distinct components: (1) physical inertia of the extremity, (2) mechanical-elastic characteristics of muscular and connective tissues, and (3) reflex muscle contraction (tonic stretch reflexes). As the inertia of the limb does not change after an upper motor neuron lesion, it is clear that the heightened resistance on bedside examination represents changes in the musculotendinous unit (e.g., contracture), or changes within the segmental reflex arc (hyperactive stretch reflexes), or a combination of these changes.

Mechanical Changes Intrinsic to Muscle

The intrinsic stiffness of a muscle is one contributor to muscle tone. The biomechanical stiffness of a muscle may be estimated, at least in part, by studying the tension elicited when a joint is extended a given angle at varying angular velocities. The slope of a curve relating muscle force to length (or in this case angle of joint displacement) is influenced both by the intrinsic stiffness of muscle as well as by reflex action. This response simulates the behavior of a simple spring, which generates a restoring force that is proportional to its change in length. The restoring force typically develops only after a certain amount of stretch is imposed. This initial length change is like the "slack length" of a spring, which generates resistance only when the slack is taken up. The slack length is governed by the threshold of the stretch reflex, although some springlike properties of skeletal muscle persist even when the tissue is stripped of its reflex controls.

Given that muscle normally exhibits springlike behavior, the possibility exists that an increase in the intrinsic mechanical stiffness of the muscle is responsible for spastic hypertonia. Furthermore, it is possible that this stiffness could be mediated by permanent structural changes in the mechanical properties of muscle connective tissues or could be variable in character. In either case, the changes in muscle stiffness would appear as an increase in the resistance to limb extension without a commensurate increase in muscle excitation as measured by the electromyogram (EMG).

In relation to this latter possibility, it has been proposed that *changes in the intrinsic muscle mechanical properties* (rather than stretch reflex enhancement) are largely responsible for spastic hypertonia.[20] These claims are based on EMG and tension analysis of leg muscles of hemiplegic adults and cerebral palsy children during ambulation. Abnormally high tension developed in the spastic triceps surae during passive stretch without a parallel increase in EMG activity. On the basis of these EMG findings, coupled with observations of temperature effects on muscle response, it has been argued that there is a change in the intrinsic mechanical response of muscle to stretch, akin to the "stretch activation" that is described in slow amphibian or myotonic mammalian muscle. (Stretch activation refers to a stretch-induced excitation of muscle that occurs without a change in the efferent neural command.)

Although this idea is highly interesting and provocative, these findings may be equally well explained by some form of degenerative or atrophic change in muscle structure, e.g., precipitous muscle atrophy with collagenous and elastic tissue infiltration. There are no present grounds on which to propose an anomalous change in the physiological muscle response to stretch. Moreover, this "intrinsic" muscle hypothesis does not easily account for many established findings—such as enhanced phasic muscle stretch reflexes and increased tendon jerks—which indicate that motor neuron excitability is also markedly increased.

Neural Mechanisms for Muscular Hypertonia

The most basic neural circuit contributing to spastic hypertonia is the segmental reflex arc, which consists of muscle receptors, their central connections with spinal cord neurons, and the motor neuronal output to muscle (Fig. 29–1). Within this arc, the alpha motor neuron may be likened to a final conduit for motor neuronal outflow. This outflow is the summation of a host of different synaptic and modulatory influences, including: (1) excitatory postsynaptic potentials from group Ia and II muscle spindle afferents, (2) inhibitory postsynaptic potentials from interneuronal connections from antagonistic muscles and Golgi tendon organs, and (3) presynaptic inhibition initiated by descending fiber input.[81] Presynaptic inhibition is exerted by axons which end on primary afferent nerve terminals and which reduce the ability of sensory afferents to depolarize the postsynaptic membrane. Exteroceptive (e.g., cutaneous) and interoceptive (e.g., visceral) afferent information can also provide important input into the segmental milieu. It is via these basic pathways that spinal and supraspinal influences modulate reflex behavior.

TABLE 29–1   Possible Neural Mechanisms for Spastic Hypertonia

I. Increased motor neuronal excitability
  A. Excitatory synaptic input is enhanced
    1. Segmental afferents
    2. Regional excitatory interneurons
    3. Descending pathways, i.e., lateral vestibulospinal tract
  B. Inhibitory synaptic input is reduced
    1. Renshaw cell recurrent inhibition
    2. Ia inhibitory interneurons
    3. Ib afferent fibers
  C. Changes in the intrinsic electrical properties of the neuron
    1. Changes in passive membrane electrical properties
    2. Changes in voltage-sensitive membrane conductance
II. Enhanced stretch-evoked synaptic excitation of motor neurons
  A. Gamma efferent hyperactivity
  B. Excitatory interneurons more sensitive to muscle afferent
    1. Collateral sprouting
    2. Denervation hypersensitivity
    3. Decrease in presynaptic inhibition

With the above segmental configuration in mind, there are two distinctly different ways in which the nervous system could produce an enhanced reflex response to muscle stretch. *The first is by selectively increasing motor neuronal excitability*, which is reflected as an increased motor neuronal response to a particular level of stretch-evoked synaptic input. *The second is by increasing the amount of excitatory synaptic input elicited by muscle extension.* Various mechanisms may be responsible for such changes (Table 29–1). While it is possible that both enhanced stretch-evoked motor neuronal excitability and increased synaptic input may coexist, it is useful to examine the possibilities independently.

INCREASED MOTOR NEURONAL EXCITABILITY. Alpha motor neuron hyperexcitability exists if motor neuronal recruitment or increased discharge is elicited with smaller-than-normal levels of excitatory input. An increase in motor neuronal excitability would mean that either a smaller stretch amplitude or a slower-than-usual stretch

FIGURE 29–1   The basic neural circuitry is the segmental reflex arc, which consists of muscle receptors, their central connections with spinal cord neurons, and the motor neuronal output to muscle. This outflow is the summation of a host of different synaptic and modulatory influences, including (1) excitatory postsynaptic potentials from group Ia and II muscle spindle afferents; (2) inhibitory postsynaptic potentials from interneuronal connections from antagonistic muscles and Golgi's tendon organs; and (3) presynaptic inhibition initiated by descending fiber input.

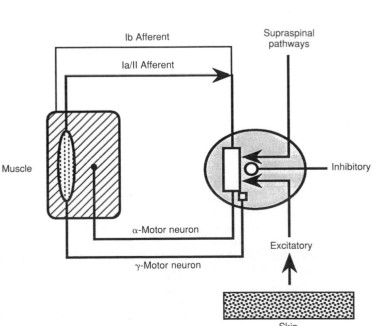

velocity would excite motor neurons. Similarly, synaptic input elicited by synchronous electrical excitation of Ia afferent fibers (H-reflex; see below) or mechanical excitation (muscle stretch reflex) would result in an augmented evoked response in the tested muscle. The evidence for enhanced motor neuronal excitability in spasticity is very strong, although the sources of such an increase are not yet clearly established.

A state of increased excitability would arise *if motor neurons are continuously more depolarized than normal*, so that they are perched close to their threshold for recruitment. Little added synaptic input would then be required to achieve activation. This increased depolarization could arise either because tonic excitatory input is enhanced (e.g., from segmental afferents, regional excitatory interneurons, or monosynaptic descending pathways such as the lateral vestibulospinal tracts) or because there is a tonic reduction of inhibitory synaptic input from regional inhibitory interneurons (such as Renshaw cell recurrent inhibition, Ia inhibitory interneurons, or Ib afferent neurons). There is substantial evidence for this type of disturbance in spasticity.

A different way that motor neurons may show increased excitability is via *change in the intrinsic electrical properties of the neurons*. This could include changes in passive membrane electrical properties (such as resistance or capacitance), or changes in the normal ionic conductance mechanisms. Both types of disturbance could have the net effect that a given synaptic current (elicited in response to stretch-induced afferent excitation) would evoke a larger-than-normal voltage change and a resulting increase in motor neuronal activity without commensurate change in stretch reflex threshold.

There is presently no convincing evidence in support of a change in the intrinsic membrane properties in chronic spastic animals. Studies supporting this concept were performed in anesthetized animals, rather than decerebrate-unanesthetized preparations, and other changes in neuronal intrinsic behavior are still quite feasible. Such changes would be expressed as alterations in voltage-sensitive membrane conductances mediated by changes in concentrations of neural modulators carried by various descending brainstem pathways. Substances such as serotonin (an indoleamine) or substance P (a peptide) may "gate" neuronal responses to transmitter-induced voltage changes, dramatically changing the way neurons respond to a given change in voltage.

For example, in the presence of serotonin, spinal motor neurons respond to a square wave depolarizing pulse with a rather prolonged depolarization which far outlasts the stimulus, and which may return to the baseline only after the application of a hyperpolarizing pulse. Changes in the intrinsic properties of the neuron would be expressed as an enhanced responsiveness of motor neurons during muscle stretch, which might appear as an abnormal and progressive increase in reflex force during muscle extension.

INCREASED STRETCH–EVOKED SYNAPTIC EXCITATION OF MOTOR NEURONS. The second way an increased motor neuronal response to stretch could arise is secondary to augmented stretch-evoked excitatory synaptic input, that is, if muscle afferent discharges in spastic patients give rise to increased excitatory synaptic current

flowing into motor neurons, either directly from muscle afferent terminals or via interposed interneurons. This increased synaptic current could arise in several ways: (1) if muscle spindle afferents showed enhanced response to stretch because of increased dynamic fusimotor bias or (2) if interposed excitatory interneurons are more responsive to muscle afferent input.

Previously, it was believed that spastic hypertonia was due to *hyperactivity of the gamma efferent fibers ("gamma spasticity"* in the older nomenclature), causing an increased sensitivity of the muscle spindle receptor to change in muscle length. This hypothesis was based on the observation that spasticity diminished when nerves were infiltrated with dilute local anesthetic at concentrations appropriate for blocking fusimotor input. Although stretch reflexes can be diminished by gamma efferent blockade, this does not prove that spasticity is due to hyperactivity within afferent limbs of the reflex arc. If this were true, blockade of gamma fibers would induce loss of tone in normal as well as abnormal muscle, since voluntary alpha motor neuronal activation is normally accompanied by significant gamma activation. To determine whether the level of gamma activity is abnormal in spastic muscle would require that the effects of gamma blockade be compared in normal and spastic muscle at equivalent levels of motor output, a prohibitively difficult experimental protocol to implement.

Another alternative is to use microneurographic recordings of spindle afferent discharge to evaluate the levels of gamma activation. Microneurography, in which a tungsten steel microelectrode is used to impale a single human nerve fiber, has also failed to confirm fusimotor hyperactivity.[31] Moreover, studies of spindle responses in monkeys after cortical ablation also failed to reveal an excess of fusimotor activity after the development of spastic hypertonia.[27] In summary, there is no present evidence to support the concept of enhanced dynamic fusimotor bias.

Three mechanisms have been proposed which may cause interposed excitatory interneurons to become more responsive to muscle afferent input: (1) *collateral sprouting*, (2) *denervation hypersensitivity*, and (3) *changes in presynaptic inhibition*. In the course of postinjury recovery, muscle afferents could undergo sprouting of their terminal branches to accommodate synaptic sites vacated by destruction of supraspinal tracts. Collateral sprouting has been observed in spinal cord and autonomic nervous systems, as well as in several specific regions of the brain. In principle, sprouting could also help explain the significant delay before spastic hypertonia appears after a spinal cord injury (SCI). However, recent investigation offers little support for the view that collateral sprouting is an important process in spinal cord reorganization following partial deafferentation.[66] Models of sprouting in the mammalian central nervous system typically require much more radical removal of afferent input to a spinal neuron than is likely to arise in most supraspinal lesions.

Secondly, synapses that lose their presynaptic terminals may become more sensitive to ambient transmitter effects. Studies utilizing chemical destruction of descending spinal cord tracts mediated by serotonin and norepinephrine lend support to the idea of denervation sensitivity as a contributing factor to spastic hypertonia. Exaggerated extensor hind limb reflexes are observed after administration of serotonergic agonists in animals whose serotonergic systems were chemically destroyed, and similarly exaggerated flexor reflexes were noted in animals with noradrenergic destruction. Histochemical studies of serotonergic and noradrenergic receptor density demonstrated a nearly complete degeneration of these receptors approximately 2 weeks after axonotomy, followed by a regeneration of terminal density to 50% to 66% of original levels after 3 to 6 months. The regeneration of these terminals suggests that surviving fibers may have produced new sprouts by the mechanisms of collateral sprouting and reinnervated the empty synaptic sites.

Finally, enhanced synaptic excitation could also arise if the level of baseline presynaptic inhibition were reduced, since this would result in a greater-than-normal release of transmitter for each incoming afferent impulse. Evidence for this has been largely based on the failure of the tonic vibration reflex (TVR) to suppress the H-reflex in the spastic patient. In this paradigm a tonic vibratory stimulus is applied to a limb, usually the lower extremity. Tonic vibratory stimuli have been shown to preferentially and repetitively splint Ia afferent fibers. They exert their inhibitory characteristics by way of an interneuron which is both excited by Ia afferent input and then acts on terminal Ia fiber arborizations. This interneuron is strongly modulated by descending pyramidal and extrapyramidal (vestibulospinal, reticulospinal, rubrospinal) tracts, so the TVR can help to elucidate the role of these descending fibers on the segmental reflex arc.

When an electrical stimulus is applied to the tibial nerve in normal subjects, the predominantly monosynaptic H-reflex is noted approximately 30 ms later in the triceps surae. This H-reflex is partially suppressed in normal subjects when the TVR is applied to the limb. The *failure* of the TVR to effectively inhibit the H-reflex in those with spasticity has been a strong argument implicating lessened presynaptic inhibition as a mechanism contributing to spastic hypertonia. Presynaptic inhibition may act by limiting the magnitude of calcium current moving into primary afferent terminals, which in turn limits neurotransmitter release.

Additional evidence for altered presynaptic mechanisms comes from a recent model in which H-reflex studies in the spastic hind limbs of a chronic spinal hemisectioned rat were found to have reduced dependence on H-reflex stimulus frequency.[73] The authors argue that frequency-dependent H-reflex reduction is related to increased presynaptic inhibition and that failure to show such reduction is an indication of a diminished presynaptic inhibition in motor neurons innervating spastic muscles. Whether the effects are indeed attributable to presynaptic inhibition or to other presynaptic phenomena, the finding does point to systematic differences in spastic-lesioned animals which may be important in mediating hind limb spasticity.

This list of possible sources of augmented reflexes is certainly incomplete, but it is already apparent that many factors may be involved. The problem of distinguishing these possibilities may appear to be insurmountable in the intact human subject; however, there are several likely differences in the patterns of mechanical and EMG response to muscle extension which should help to distinguish the broad categories of disturbance (see Threshold vs. Gain Disturbances later).

Supraspinal Mechanisms

Descending tracts contribute to spastic muscle hypertonia either via monosynaptic excitatory projections to lower motor neurons (e.g., from the corticospinal or lateral vestibulospinal tracts) or indirectly by inhibition or facilitation of interneurons within spinal reflex pathways. Operationally, the synaptic effects of descending pathways may be categorized, at least in principle, as mediating changes in the excitability of spinal motor neurons or as mediating changes in the responses of segmental reflex pathways, or both.

CHANGES IN MOTOR NEURON EXCITABILITY. It has been proposed that changes in motor neuronal excitability may be contingent primarily on changes in the "baseline" levels of depolarization of the motor neuron rather than on changes in intrinsic motor neuron properties. The increased baseline depolarization depends, in turn, on the net *tonic* excitatory synaptic input that is converging on the neuron, either from descending pathways or from segmental interneuronal input.

For example, the lateral vestibulospinal pathway is apparently very important for the development of the increased excitability in axial and extensor alpha motor neurons that characterizes spastic hypertonia, at least in supraspinal forms of spasticity. While this effect is due partly to monosynaptic input, more powerful excitatory contributions from the vestibulospinal system are almost certainly provided by local excitatory interneurons. Similarly, it is also likely that the excitation or inhibition of motor neurons mediated by descending reticulospinal fibers originating in medullary and pontine centers is mediated largely by segmental interneurons.

CHANGES IN SEGMENTAL REFLEX FUNCTION. While the activity of many descending pathways is likely to be impaired in either supraspinal or spinal injury, loss of the inhibitory effects of descending pathways (especially reticulospinal) on regional interneurons receiving input from cutaneous and muscle segmental afferents is also believed to be very important, especially in spinal forms of spasticity. This loss of inhibition may arise as a result of either direct pathway interruption (as in spinal or brainstem injury) or the loss of supraspinal facilitation of brainstem reticulospinal neurons, whose discharge may be reduced or even silenced. These reductions in descending input release a number of powerful segmental reflexes, which are normally completely suppressed.

For example, the Babinski reflex, a characteristic accompaniment of spastic hypertonia, represents a transition from the normal plantar reflex to a more diffusely organized flexion withdrawal reflex. The normal plantar reflex appears to promote postural stability by increasing the grip of the digits on the terrain and thus resembles the feline plantar cushion reflex. The Babinski reflex is a more diffusely organized flexion withdrawal reflex in which toes, ankles, and even more proximal joints are progressively flexed.

The clasp-knife reflex is a second and less common manifestation of this phenomenon of interneuronal release in spasticity. This reflex is characterized by an abrupt reduction of EMG activity and force, once a spastic muscle is stretched through a particular length. The term *clasp knife* is applied because the initial high resistance of spastic hypertonia is interrupted by the onset of inhibition, making the resistance of the hypertonic limb decline abruptly, rather like the behavior of an old-fashioned clasp knife. Although initially attributed to tendon organ action, and then to secondary spindle afferent input, recent evidence suggests that the clasp-knife reflex is a reflection of the activity of group III and IV mechanoreceptors, whose central effects become pronounced because of the reduced descending inhibition of segmental interneurons.[67] There are numerous other illustrations of alterations in reflex responsiveness that arise in supraspinal or spinal types of spasticity. Many of them are characterized by the pairing of increased flexor reflexes with the inhibition of antagonist extensors, presumably via the Ia reciprocal inhibitory interneuron. This is well illustrated by the clasp-knife reflex, in which inhibition of antigravity muscles, such as the triceps and quadriceps, is accompanied by an excitation of the opposing flexors.

To summarize, spasticity can be characterized by a combination of two major disturbances, both mediated by alterations in the balance of descending pathway activity. The first induces an increase in excitability of motor neurons innervating antigravity muscles (which are physiological extensors in the legs, and flexors in the arms), and the second changes the patterns of reflex responsiveness of many segmental reflexes, often promoting flexor muscle activity and reduced extensor activity.

PATHWAYS RESPONSIBLE FOR MODIFICATION IN DESCENDING CONTROL IN SPASTICITY. Cortex, basal ganglia, and cerebellum all provide important modulation of brainstem structures in normal motor control. Selective destruction of corticospinal tracts does not result in spastic hypertonia but rather in hypotonia and loss of fine hand movements. Interruption of extrapyramidal fibers is evidently needed before spastic hypertonia develops. Lesions of particular premotor cortical sites, specifically areas 4 and 6 of Brodmann, result in hypotonia followed by hypertonic hemiparesis. With bilateral premotor damage, spasticity is more severe.

We do not yet understand which pathways are instrumental in mediating the increase in motor neuron excitability. However, it seems likely that the alterations in segmental interneuronal responsiveness follow loss of activity in the so-called dorsal reticulospinal system. This pathway appears to require substantial facilitation from corticobulbar projections, so that extensive white matter lesions, which diminish the excitatory inflow to the brainstem, have the effect of reducing the descending inhibition of segmental interneurons.

Another, similar possibility is that descending monoaminergic systems, such as the locus ceruleus pathways, are involved in regulating the excitability of segmental circuits. These pathways may be damaged directly in spinal cord injury or may lose cortical excitatory drive, causing them to reduce their inhibitory control of segmental interneurons. This reduced inhibition may (1) release segmental interneurons, such as those subserving cutaneous or muscle-based inhibitory pathways, or (2) release excitatory interneurons, such as those receiving input from secondary spindle afferents, or both.

Upper Motor Neuron Syndrome

The wide variety of motor dysfunctions that occur in the patient with "spasticity" are not simply a result of the hypertonic changes discussed previously. The *upper motor neuron (UMN) syndrome* is a more general term used to describe patients with abnormal motor function secondary to lesions of cortical, subcortical, or spinal cord structures. Careful study of patients with UMN syndrome reveals that the patient's motor difficulties can be divided into a series of *abnormal behaviors* (positive symptoms), and *performance deficits* (negative symptoms)[81] (Table 29–2).

Positive symptoms are easily recognized in disorders of the spinal cord, as in the patient suffering from transverse myelitis or spinal cord injury. These symptoms include the exaggerated flexion reflexes addressed earlier and the related Babinski response. The release of reflexes from descending inhibitory control causes flexor or adductor spasms. Flexor spasms may become so severe as to require a paraplegic patient to be restrained to remain in the wheelchair. Hip adductor spasms cause "scissoring" of the lower extremities, limiting a patient's ability to ambulate effectively. Clonus, a cyclical hyperactivity of antagonistic muscles in response to stretch, may become so severe as to prohibit potentially functional muscle groups from performing effectively for the patient.

A final positive symptomatic component of the UMN syndrome that is frequently overlooked is the loss of precise autonomic control. A loss of upper motor neuron modulation on spinal autonomic mechanisms can result in a disorganization of autonomic function below the level of a spinal cord injury. In patients with spinal cord lesions above approximately the T6 level, seemingly innocuous sensory input can result in a potential hypertensive crisis. This hypertensive response is one component of autonomic dysreflexia, a gross nonselective "mass response." Disorganization of sympathetic activity below the level of an SCI may be responsible for autonomic dysreflexia, but mechanisms other than exaggerated sympathetic outflow may contribute as well.

Negative symptoms, or performance deficits, are more frequently observed in hemiparetic patients, such as those suffering from cerebrovascular accidents or traumatic brain injury, but may also be found in the multiple sclerosis or SCI patient. Motoric actions are often weak, and patients are easily fatigued and lacking in dexterity. Several physiological factors may contribute to these performance deficits.

TABLE 29–2   Upper Motor Neuron Syndrome

Abnormal behaviors (positive symptoms)
Reflex release phenomena
Hyperactive proprioceptive reflexes
Increased resistance to stretch
Relaxed cutaneous reflexes
Loss of precise autonomic control
Performance deficits (negative symptoms)
Decreased dexterity
Paresis/weakness
Fatigability

The *loss of orderly recruitment and rate modulation of motor neurons* within a given motor neuron pool leads to inefficient muscle activation, inducing early loss of force, augmented subject effort, and the clinical perception of weakness. High threshold motor units with rapid rates of adaptation are evidently recruited early, and these "fast-twitch" units are poorly suited to maintain sustained muscle contractions. Changes in mean motor unit discharge rates in paretic muscles may be the cause of abnormal EMG-force relationships, where surface EMG activity is augmented per unit force generated. The twitch contraction time of fast motor units has also been shown to change in hand muscles of hemiplegic limbs.

Intramuscular and surface EMG recordings from spastic patients demonstrate *disturbances of spatial selection of muscles* in hemiparetic limbs. Recordings from normal limbs during isometric torque generation at the elbow reveal an orderly spatial distribution of muscle action. Each muscle is activated over a broad angular range in a symmetrical pattern, with EMG scaling with increasing force and with the peak EMG value located at the angle of calculated maximum mechanical advantage. In contrast, spastic paretic limbs exhibit severe disturbances in the pattern of muscle activation, so that the angular range and spatial orientation are radically disturbed. For example, normal elbow flexor muscles are activated maximally in the direction of flexion. However, in the hemiparetic patient these muscles show a substantial shift in the angle of peak EMG and are maximally activated 90 or even 135 degrees away from the normal angle.[9]

The final major type of disturbance appears as *an alteration in the time course of EMG activation in agonist and antagonist muscles.* For example, in normal limbs, rapid flexion of a joint is associated with a so-called triphasic pattern of EMG activation, in which the agonist muscle is activated in two sequential bursts and the antagonist is activated in the intervening interval. In the UMN syndrome, the orderly timing is lost, so that only a portion of the triphasic pattern is expressed. In the extreme case, there is a poorly timed and ineffective *simultaneous* co-contraction of agonist and antagonist. Impaired agonist control and antagonist relaxation have been shown in various movement schemata.

Kinesiological analysis of hemiplegic ambulation offers valuable insight into abnormal motor behaviors in patients with spastic hypertonia. Spastic reflexes tested in a passive limb are not identical with those in movements actively performed by the patient. In some patients a low threshold for stretch reflex activation can be found at bedside examination in muscles that are not activated by the stretch imposed by ambulation. These studies have demonstrated that there is a wide interindividual variation in gait patterns among affected patients. However, all patients demonstrated varying degrees of (1) a lowered stretch reflex threshold, (2) inadequate muscular activation, and (3) stereotyped coactivation of muscles in primitive locomotor patterns.[49]

In summary, relief of the hypertonic "spastic" components of the UMN syndrome does not necessarily infer enhanced performance. Co-contraction of agonist and antagonist muscles, dyssynergic patterns of contraction, flexor spasms, paresis, and loss of dexterity are probably more disabling than hypertonia for the patient suffering from this motor disorder.

QUANTIFICATION OF SPASTIC HYPERTONIA

The quantification of spasticity has been a difficult and challenging problem and has been based primarily on highly observer-dependent measurements. The lack of effective measurement techniques has been quite restrictive, since quantification is necessary to evaluate various modes of treatment. For example, measurement of day-to-day torque variations for a particular joint within a given subject is likely to be extremely valuable in quantifying the effects of a therapeutic intervention such as a drug or surgical procedure.

Previous quantitative efforts have concentrated on tabulation of functional activities, EMG and biomechanical analysis of limb resistance to mechanical displacement, rectified surface EMG responses to perturbation or voluntary movement, gait analysis, and a host of electrophysiological reflex studies. Nonetheless, for a variety of reasons, no uniformly useful clinical measurements have emerged. The quantification of spasticity has been hampered by a host of complicated issues. Changes in performance due to training effects, emotional status, and various systemic factors may all hamper a detailed analysis.

Clinical Scales

A gross clinical scale to grade muscle tone from 0 (normal) to 4 (severe) was first proposed by Ashworth.[3] It offers ease of measurement but may lack temporal and interexaminer reproducibility. Moreover, scales such as the Ashworth suffer from a "clustering" effect; that is, most of the patients are grouped within the middle grades. The patient is examined in a comfortable position, usually supine, and muscle stretch reflexes and passive muscle tone are assessed bilaterally and separately for the upper and lower extremities. A modification of these scales has been created that adds an additional intermediate grade and has been shown to have high interrater reliability when testing elbow flexors[7] (Table 29–3). Although clinical scales offer only qualitative information, they have been widely used in the study of spasticity and are the present yardstick

TABLE 29–3   Clinical Scale for Spastic Hypertonia

0	No increase in tone
1	Slight increase in muscle tone, manifested by a catch and release or by minimal resistance at the end of the range of motion when the affected part(s) is moved in flexion or extension
1+	Slight increase in muscle tone, manifested by a catch, followed by minimal resistance throughout the remainder (less than half) of the range of motion
2	More marked increase in muscle tone through most of the range of motion, but affected part(s) easily moved
3	Considerable increase in muscle tone, passive movement difficult
4	Affected part(s) rigid in flexion or extension

From Bohannon RW, Smith MB: Interrater reliability on a modified Ashworth scale of muscle spasticity. Phys Ther 1987; 67:206–207.

TABLE 29–4   Fugl-Meyer Scale of Functional Return After Hemiplegia

Movement of the shoulder, elbow, forearm, and lower extremity
I   Muscle stretch reflexes can be elicited
II   Volitional movements can be performed within the dynamic flexor and extensor synergies
III   Volitional motion is performed mixing dynamic flexor and extensor synergies
IV   Volitional movements are performed with little or no synergy dependence
V   Normal muscle stretch reflexes
Wrist function≅stability, flexion, extension, circumduction
Hand function
Mass flexion, mass, extension, 5 different grasps
Coordination and speed≅assess tremor, dysmetria, speed
Finger-to-nose test, heel-to-shin test
Balance
Sit without support
Parachute reaction≅nonaffected side, affected side
Stand≅supported, unsupported
Stand on nonaffected side, affected side
Sensation≅light tough, position sense
Passive joint motion, joint pain

Modified from Katz RT, Rovai G, Brait C, Rymer WZ: Objective quantification of spastic hypertonia: Correlation with clinical findings. Arch Phys Med Rehabil 1992; 73:340.

against which newer, more exact methods must be compared.

The Fugl-Meyer scale (Table 29–4) is an accurate and objective method of assessing function (but not necessarily spastic hypertonia) in hemiplegic patients based on the natural progression of functional return.[25] Hemiplegic patients often have recurrence of muscle stretch reflexes before volitional motor action, followed by synergistic movement patterns, return of voluntary selective motor function, and finally a decrease in hyperreflexic stretch reflexes.

Motor evaluation in the upper extremity assesses move-

ment within and independent of synergistic patterns, including coordination and speed of movement. The intricate movements of the hand and wrist are assessed separately, as is the patient's ability to maintain body posture. Light touch, position sense, joint movement, and pain-free movement add critical sensory observations because they contribute to motor function. The Fugl-Meyer scale has been demonstrated to have high intratester and intertester reliability and can be completed in 10 to 20 minutes. Decline of function of the Fugl-Meyer scale has been shown to correlate closely with the severity of spastic tone.[46] Scales with similar purpose have been reported but do not appear to have any clear advantage.

Biomechanical Investigations

Biomechanical investigations attempt to quantify changes in phasic and tonic reflex activity within the limbs of spastic patients. Quantitative observations can be made of the following variables: (1) torque—the amount of force elicited by moving a limb over a specified angle; (2) threshold—that particular angle where torque or EMG starts to increase significantly during constant-velocity joint extension; and (3) EMG—electrical recordings of muscle activation, often adding rectified signal analysis of EMG from superficial muscle groups. By definition, spastic limbs demonstrate abnormal resistance to externally imposed joint movement. This resistance is augmented by increasing the angle of deflection and the rate at which the limb is moved.

Various investigators have performed biomechanical investigations such as these, utilizing either linear or sinusoidal stretch. These investigations have yielded conflicting results. Earlier studies have shown spastic hypertonia to be (1) strongly dependent upon the rate of stretch and (2) an exaggeration of dynamic (phasic) rather than static (tonic)

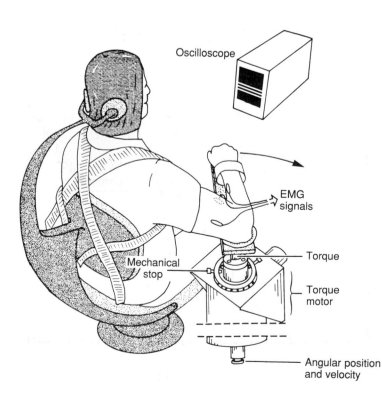

FIGURE 29–2   A diagram of a servo-controlled motorically driven device, which applies ramp and hold movements to the upper extremity. Such apparatus allows measurement of angular position and velocity in the horizontal plane. Electromyographic activity in the biceps brachialis, brachioradialis, and lateral triceps muscles can be measured with surface electrodes.

reflex output. These results are somewhat puzzling, as normal mammalian muscle spindles are only weakly dependent on the rate of stretch, and this sensitivity does not vary significantly with changes in fusimotor input.

Recent investigations suggest that the reflex response in spastic hypertonia may be quite different from what was previously believed.[54, 63, 64] These studies were carried out using a servo-controlled motorically driven device, which applied ramp and hold movements to the elbow (Fig. 29–2). EMG activity in the biceps brachialis, brachioradialis, and lateral triceps muscles was measured with surface electrodes.

NEW CONCEPTS. These studies have generated some exciting and novel concepts in the causation of spastic hypertonia. Spastic hypertonia may be the result simply of a *decrease in stretch reflex threshold*—that is, reflexes are elicited with less angular displacement of the extremity. The reflex stiffness co-varied in much the same way as that recorded in normal muscle, where reflex stiffness increases progressively with increasing background force (especially at lower force levels). The magnitude of reduction of this threshold angle proved to be inversely proportional to the clinical severity of hypertonia. This is to be expected if threshold changes were the predominant source of change in the stretch reflex response.

Secondly, there was *no preferential enhancement of dynamic over static reflex activity*. As in normal muscle, reflex torque was relatively insensitive to extension velocity. Moreover, the rather small amount of velocity dependence of force and EMG output was determined to a large extent by the velocity-related behavior of the reflex threshold rather than by the velocity-induced changes in reflex response overall. That is, the onset of the reflex was greatly advanced as stretch velocity was increased, but once activated, the response was very similar to the response in normal muscle.

Thirdly, when initial conditions were matched, stretch reflexes were similar in the hemiplegic limb and nonhemiplegic limb of hemiplegic volunteers—limb "stiffness" was quite similar when the hemiplegic and nonaffected sides were compared. In subjects that showed systematic variations in the degree of spastic hypertonia within a given recording session, the changes in tone could be attributed almost entirely to fluctuations in the angular threshold.

These findings are largely in disagreement with prevailing views about stretch reflexes in spasticity, which treat spastic hypertonia as a straightforward velocity-dependent increase in limb resistance. Why do these results differ so markedly from previous investigations?

THRESHOLD VS. GAIN DISTURBANCES. The main reason is that many earlier investigators failed to dissociate the contributions of changes in stretch reflex threshold from those of changes in reflex gain. In principle, there are two distinct parameters which may be altered in the pathological stretch reflex, and these have important implications for the neurophysiological disturbances outlined earlier (Fig. 29–3). First, the "slack length" or *threshold of the stretch reflex could be reduced*. In this scenario a smaller or slower motion is sufficient to reach the reflex threshold, which is manifested clinically as a catch point at which the resistance to manual stretch abruptly increases. Once the reflex is activated, the torque or force of the muscle increases in proportion to the increasing joint angle. Both the slope of the force-length relationship and the increase in force with a standard velocity of stretch are similar to those recorded in normal muscle.

The most likely physiological substrate for this pattern of response is simply that motor neurons are more depolarized as a result of a net increase in tonic excitatory synaptic input from descending pathways or regional interneurons, so that motor neuron recruitment takes place more readily.

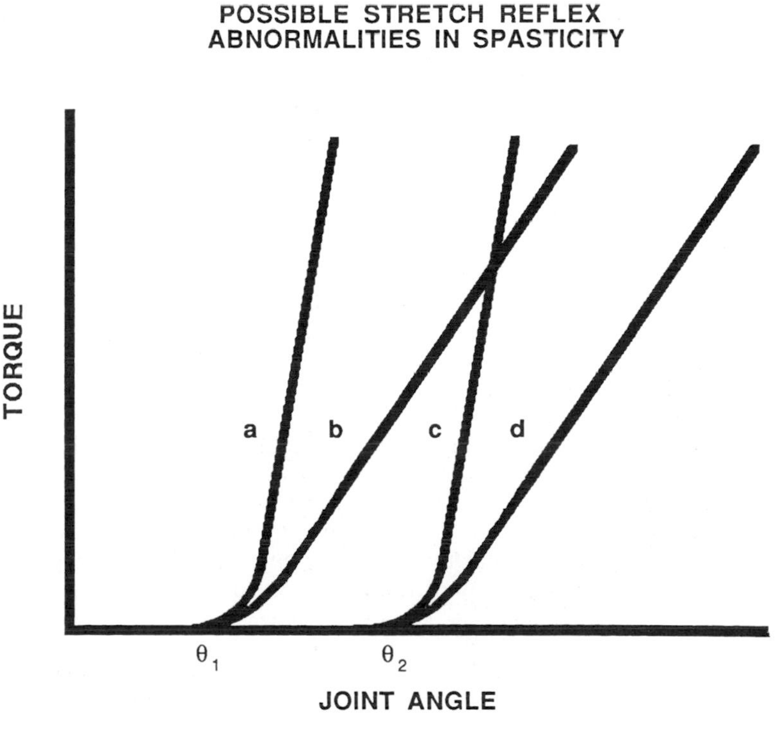

POSSIBLE STRETCH REFLEX ABNORMALITIES IN SPASTICITY

FIGURE 29–3 Possible stretch reflex abnormalities in spasticity. As a joint is extended, the torque elicited by muscle stretch begins to increase after a certain threshold angle (q) is reached. The amount of torque per unit angle, or muscle stiffness, is the slope of the curve; (q2) denotes a "normal" threshold angle; (q1) a reduced threshold for motor neuron recruitment. Curve *a* represents a state in which reduced threshold and increased stiffness exist. Curves *b* and *c* represent the case in which only reduced threshold or increased stiffness exist alone, respectively. Curve *d* represents the normal state of reflex threshold and stiffness. See text for further discussion.

There is no additional requirement for enhanced synaptic input during stretch.

The second possible disturbance of the stretch reflex is an *increase in reflex gain* characterized by an abnormal increase in reflex force with increasing extension, without substantial change in the reflex threshold angle. Expressed in quantitative terms, the angular stiffness, which is a measure of stretch reflex gain, is increased above normal.

Increased reflex gain would arise if the excitatory response to ongoing stretch were augmented because of increased gamma dynamic bias (increasing spindle afferent discharge rates), afferent terminal sprouting (increasing the number of active terminals), postsynaptic receptor hypersensitivity (increasing the impact of released transmitter), reductions in presynaptic inhibition (increasing the amount of transmitter released for each incoming action potential), or changes in intrinsic motor neuronal properties (increasing the voltage change induced by release of a given amount of transmitter).

It is conceivable, then, that changes in reflex gain and threshold can be used to distinguish between normal and spastic-hypertonic reflexes. If the reflex threshold is reduced, motor neurons are likely in a state of sustained depolarization. If reflex stiffness is enhanced, either stretch-evoked afferent input or the postsynaptic effects of that input are enhanced. If both threshold and reflex stiffness are changed, both forms of disturbance probably coexist.

To illustrate this difficulty further, the application of a stretch to a spastic muscle often gives rise to an increased torque and EMG response, which is usually interpreted as reflecting an increase in reflex gain. Such an outcome could equally well arise from a change in stretch reflex threshold. For example, if the motor neuron pool innervating a spastic muscle is depolarized by descending spinal input, the introduction of a muscle perturbation will activate motor neurons more readily. However, once activated, they would be expected to obey the usual rules for recruitment and rate regulation and would not demonstrate any increase in reflex stiffness.

EXPERIMENTAL DIFFERENTIATION OF THRESHOLD VS. GAIN DISTURBANCES. In order to dissociate gain and threshold contributions to increased muscle tone, one must establish a known level of motor neuron excitability against which the responses to increased stretch can be compared. This can be accomplished by establishing a known background force, or "preload," before the muscles are tested. Provided that the patterns of muscle and motor neuron activation are similar in spastic and normal muscles, setting muscles to the same initial force provides a means to match approximately the excitability of the motor neuron pools. Furthermore, this matching of excitability would also imply a matching of a reflex threshold, provided that afferent inflow induced by stretch is comparable in normal and spastic muscles. Even though these various assumptions are not easily confirmed at present, the failure to match neuron excitability in spastic and control muscles, even approximately, essentially eliminates any possibility for quantitative comparisons of reflex gain in spastic and normal muscles.

Other investigators have also found substantial static responses to maintained stretch in spastic patients, without stiffness that was significantly different from that of normal muscle. Rack et al.[65] found muscle stiffness in spastic patients to be set at one end of the normal range of variability. Substantial static responses to maintained stretch were found in spastic patients, without a significantly different stiffness than that of normal muscle. Knutsson[49] noted that spastic reflexes tested in passive limb movements are not identical with those actively performed by the patient. In some individuals a low threshold for stretch reflex activation can be found at bedside examination in muscles that are not activated by the stretch imposed by ambulation. Antagonistic restraint of voluntary motion, a previously mentioned component of the UMN syndrome, becomes much more dramatic as the cadence of gait increases, indicating that spastic reflex mechanisms are not uniformly operational in any particular movement.

These findings may have important implications for evaluating hypotheses about mechanisms of spastic muscular hypertonia. Once the muscle is activated, reflex stiffness and velocity sensitivity of reflex torque are essentially normal in hypertonic muscles; there is no obvious need to invoke mechanisms that require enhanced stretch-evoked synaptic input to spinal motor neurons. These include such hypotheses as enhanced gamma dynamic bias, afferent sprouting, or changes in the level of presynaptic inhibition. Rather, findings in spastic hypertonia may simply be attributed to changes in reflex threshold that are due in large part to supraspinally mediated increased background levels of depolarization of motor neurons.

Pendulum Test

A pendular model for assessment of spastic hypertonia of the quadriceps and hamstring muscle groups has been proposed and has been evaluated in supine normal and spastic patients.[75] Stiffness of the lower limb is assessed by placing the patient in a supine position with both legs extending over the edge of a table which supports the legs only as far as the distal thigh. In this way the knee joint can be easily flexed and extended. When the lower limb segment falls from a fully extended position, it sways about the vertical like a pendulum, and its movement is damped or "braked" by the viscoelastic elements of the limb (Fig. 29–4). Knee movement is assessed by an electrogoniometer and rate of movement by a tachometer. These instruments usually show sinusoidal patterns of angular motion on which a mathematical model has been created to differentiate a spastic from a normal limb.

Although easy to use, the mathematical analysis of the pendulum biomechanical model suffers from the questionable assumption that mechanical properties of knee extensor and flexor musculature are equal and that the model can be treated as a simple linear "second-order" system (in which elements can be simulated by various masses, springs, and variable resistors). In fact, muscle stiffness and viscosity vary with the level of muscle excitation and with muscle length. Moreover, the model includes no explanation for threshold and stiffness variation, which is in disagreement with data obtained from mechanical perturbations. Despite its flaws, the pendulum test may be performed on commercially available isokinetic exercise equipment, with a high correlation between trials.[46]

PRACTICAL ISSUES RELATED TO BIOMECHANICAL

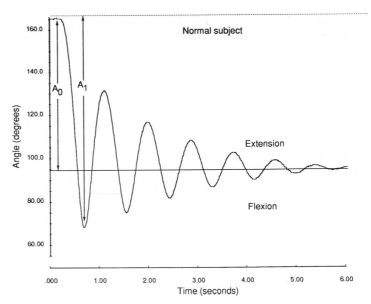

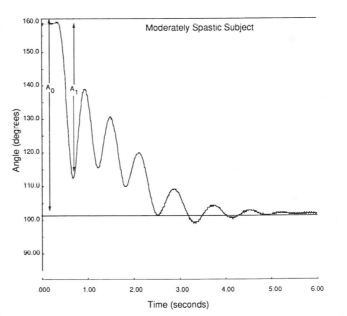

FIGURE 29–4 Pendulum test for spastic hypertonia used to assess spastic hypertonia of the quadriceps and hamstring muscle groups. Stiffness of the limb is assessed by placing the patient in a supine position with both legs extending over the edge of a table that supports them only as far as the distal thigh. A_0 represents the amplitude of the damped sinusoidal curve as it falls from the extended position to the final resting angle. A_1 represents the amplitude of the plotted waveform from full extension to its first absolute minimum. The *upper tracing* depicts a normal subject. The *lower tracing* depicts a moderately spastic subject. Notice that the initial swing from full extension (A_1) does not reach the vertical, whereas the normal subject obtains 27 degrees of flexion beyond the vertical. The marked damping of the altered sinusoidal curve is evident in the spastic subject. (From Katz RT, Rovai G, Brait C, et al: Quantification of hypertonia. Arch Phys Med Rehabil 1992; 73:343.)

QUANTIFICATION. There is *not* likely to be any useful outcome from measuring angular joint stiffness, since stiffness would not be expected to change significantly. In fact, a finding of increased joint stiffness is more likely to indicate contracture than increased stretch reflex response. The major variable that does appear to be worth measuring is the stretch reflex threshold, the angle at which reflex torque and EMG begin to increase in an initially passive muscle.

There are some unresolved difficulties with these measurements, however, which make threshold estimates less attractive as an index of the severity of spastic hypertonia. Although measuring the angle at which EMG activity begins during extension of passive muscle is an obvious possibility, estimating the onset angle of low levels of EMG is technically quite difficult, and different muscles typically show quite different reflex thresholds by EMG techniques. Although rigorous quantitative techniques are

available for EMG threshold estimation, these are not readily applied in a clinical setting.

An alternative possibility would be to estimate the reflex threshold of the various muscles using mechanical measurements. Mechanical measurements are appealing since they are likely to reflect the contributions of all relevant muscles and have an obvious clinical parallel—the catch point of the reflex response. On the other hand, they require sensitive torque recordings, which are not routinely performed in a clinical setting, as well as relatively sophisticated mathematical techniques to allow the active reflex torque to be separated from passive viscoelastic forces that arise during extension of the joint. Commercially available isokinetic systems may serve as a uniform and standard method for assessing hypertonia on a clinical basis.

A reasonable approach for mechanical quantification is simply to measure the torque at some specified joint angle, such as immediately prior to the end of a constant-velocity–

constant-amplitude ramp stretch. Since stiffness is not a reliable variable, the torque measured at a predetermined angle during a specified constant-velocity extension is closely dependent on the stretch reflex threshold. (This is because the smaller the threshold angle, the greater the angular range over which muscle stretch produces reflex excitation of spinal motor neurons.) For a given angular extension applied to muscles of one particular spastic subject, variations in torque are then directly attributable to differences in reflex threshold.

The use of torque measurements as an index of spastic hypertonia is certainly not a straightforward matter, especially since most clinicians are inexperienced with mechanical measurements of any kind. Moreover, the torque recorded in limbs of different subjects will certainly vary with limb mass, muscle bulk, and the characteristics of the individual's muscular anatomy. This implies that objective quantification of hypertonia in a diverse group of spastic subjects is unlikely to be successful, at least until we document the range of torque variation in normal passive limbs. A more immediately useful application is the assessment of day-to-day variations in the severity of spastic hypertonia within a given subject. This is because limb inertia, muscle mechanical moments, and passive viscoelastic elements remain constant over relatively long time periods, so that short-term variations in torque are legitimately attributed to changes in stretch reflex response magnitude.[46]

Electrophysiological Testing

A wide variety of electrophysiological reflex studies have been performed to assess spasticity and explore neuronal circuits within the spinal cord. While they are easily recorded, analyzed, and quantified, they have yet to be proved clinically useful. Readers are referred to other sources for a full description of these tests;[22, 44, 61] the following discussion will, I hope, provide a useful overview.

Several standard electrophysiological tests require definition. The *M-response* is a compound muscle action potential generated by maximally stimulating a peripheral nerve and recording over a muscle innervated by that nerve. The *H-reflex* is not a direct response of muscle to stimulation of its corresponding motor nerve but rather a reflex similar to (but not the same as) a muscle stretch reflex. The H-reflex is usually elicited by delivering a submaximal stimulus to the tibial nerve in the popliteal fossa and recording over the soleus muscle. The generated nerve action potential propagates up to the spinal cord and then, via a *predominantly* monosynaptic reflex arc, passes down the efferent motor axon. The H-reflex is unlike the muscle stretch reflex in that (1) the muscle spindle is bypassed, (2) the afferent volley is temporally less disperse, and (3) the tendon jerk involves significantly fewer Ib fibers. Although the H-reflex is routinely recorded in this manner, it may be similarly recorded in many normal subjects from the flexor carpi radialis upon stimulation of the median nerve and from the vastus medialis upon stimulation of the femoral nerve.

LIMITATIONS OF THE H-REFLEX. Although the H-reflex has many theoretically interesting applications, it is riddled with methodological difficulties when studying patients with central nervous system disorders.[46] For example, inexact placement of the recording electrodes allows contamination of the soleus response by gastrocnemius activity. Examination of the contribution of various deep and superficial muscles to the conventionally recorded H-reflex helps explain why amplitudes and latencies may vary significantly in studies using slightly different techniques. H-reflex studies may be influenced by changes in stimulation frequency, patient relaxation, limb position, or changes in head and neck position.[33, 34] For example, laterally tilting a human subject results in inhibition of the H-reflex ipsilateral to the tilting and facilitation of the contralateral response. The amplitude of the H-reflex and the relation between the H-reflex and the M-response change markedly with stimulus duration. H-reflexes are brought out to advantage using a stimulus duration between 0.5 and 1 ms. Studies utilizing the H-reflex to scale spasticity must be cautiously interpreted.

ELECTROPHYSIOLOGICAL TECHNIQUES UTILIZING THE H-REFLEX. A ratio of the maximal H-reflex and the M-response, or *H(max)/M(max),* has been reported to assess the excitability of the motor nucleus by determining the percentage of motor neurons activated via the H-reflex in comparison to direct activation of the motor neurons. It assumes that presynaptic inhibition via descending tracts, which synapse on the terminal arborizations of Ia afferents, remains constant. Increased H(max)/M(max) ratios have been reported in the spastic phase of hemiplegia. Following SCI the H-reflex amplitude and H(max)/M(max) ratio increase significantly over a 3-month period. There is a reduction in the H(max)/M(max) ratio following intrathecal administration of baclofen in patients with severe lower extremity spasticity due to SCI. There has been little correlation between H(max)/M(max) ratios and the severity of spastic hyperreflexia.[16, 46] Similar results have been obtained substituting a mechanically induced muscle stretch reflex for electrical activation of Ia afferent fibers, the so-called *T/M* ratio.

The effects of reciprocal innervation can be assessed, at least theoretically, by determining the effect of an anterior tibial contraction on the H-reflex. Normal reciprocal inhibitory mechanisms from contraction of the anterior calf muscle should inhibit the reflex response within the triceps surae. Facilitation of Ia interneurons by descending spinal tracts has been demonstrated in human subjects, and the loss of such descending influences may explain the loss of effectiveness of reciprocal inhibition in spastic subjects. Peroneal nerve stimulation may be substituted for voluntary contraction of the anterior tibial.

H-reflex recovery curves claim to reflect polysnaptic changes in motor neuron excitability secondary to segmental and suprasegmental mechanisms. Paired equal stimuli of the tibial nerve are applied in varying temporal arrangement. The resulting H-reflexes demonstrate various phases of inhibition and facilitation that are poorly reproducible and of unknown significance. In the hemiplegic stroke patient there is a decrease in motor neuron excitability only within the first several days, followed by an increase in excitability thereafter. The changes in motor neuron excitability have not been found to be predictive of future motor function or ultimate degree of spastic hypertonia. Similar periods of facilitation and inhibition of the H-reflex can be achieved via exteroceptive conditioning, such as stimulating the sural nerve. Alterations in these periods of facilitation and inhibition have been noted in spastic patients.

Paired H-reflex studies utilizing a collision technique may also be used to assess Renshaw cell activation and recurrent inhibition. Normally, supramaximal stimulus of a mixed nerve (e.g., tibial) will eliminate the H-reflex (e.g., in the gastrocnemius-soleus) due to antidromic cancellation of the efferent volley. However, this is not true when the supramaximal M-response is *preceded* by a conditioning electrical stimulus sufficient to generate an H-reflex. The volley of the *conditioning* H-reflex collides with the *antidromic* volley of the M-stimulus, which subsequently allows the *afferent* volley from the supramaximal stimulus to generate an H-reflex. On the basis of animal and pharmacological experiments, it has been suggested that Renshaw cells are activated by the conditioning H-discharge and that recurrent inhibition is assessed by the subsequent H-reflex.[61] This method was used to assess recurrent inhibition in spastic and control patients, and spastic patients demonstrated an increase in the second H-reflex amplitude. However, these results have been variably interpreted.

H-reflexes have also been used to assess short-latency autogenic inhibition, or Ib inhibition in human spasticity. Ib fibers from Golgi tendon organs normally project to the motor neurons of muscle from which they originate and inhibit them. Their activation results in a postsynaptic short-lasting inhibition. There is a technique in which a 1-ms conditioning stimulus is applied to the nerve to the medial head of the gastrocnemius (the gastrocnemius medialis nerve) at the lower part of the popliteal fossa.[17] This particular nerve was selected as it apparently has a considerable number of Ib projections with a relative paucity of Ia afferent fibers. The conditioning stimulus inhibits a subsequent H-reflex to varying degrees. In a study of six hemiplegic subjects, there was an inhibition of the subsequent H-reflex on the normal side, with a facilitation on the hemiplegic side. This suggests that a loss of Ib inhibition may offer an additional mechanism in the development of spastic hypertonia.

Attempts have been made to differentiate the effects of group Ia vs. group II projections on the quadriceps stretch reflex in response to stretch. On the basis of "selective" ischemic blockade of Ia fibers vs. procaine (Novocain) blockade infiltration into the muscle (which, it is argued, preferentially blocks small fibers such as group II), it has been argued that decreased inhibition from group II afferents to extensor muscles does not significantly contribute to increased stretch reflexes in spastic patients.

F WAVE. The *F wave* is similar to the H-reflex in that it reflects proximal conduction of the peripheral nervous system. It is recorded by *supramaximal stimulation* of a mixed nerve (in contrast to the submaximal stimulation in performing the H-reflex) while recording over a distal muscle innervated by that nerve. Unlike the H-reflex, the electrical potential travels antidromically to the spinal cord via motor efferents to activate motor neurons, and after an approximately 1-ms turnaround, travels orthodromically down similar motor fibers to produce a relatively small compound muscle action potential. The F wave seems to be less affected by postural changes than the H-reflex. The maximal size of the F wave as a percentage of the amplitude of the M wave (F_{av}/M) has been found to be increased in spastic patients and in those with polyneuropathy.[24]

TONIC VIBRATION REFLEX. The *tonic vibration reflex* has been used to assess the status of presynaptic inhibition. Presynaptic inhibition may act by limiting the magnitude of calcium current moving into primary afferent terminals, which in turn limits neurotransmitter release. Enhanced synaptic excitation could arise if the level of baseline presynaptic inhibition were reduced, since this would result in a greater-than-normal release of transmitter for each incoming afferent impulse.

Tonic vibration (e.g., a vibrator of frequency 100 Hz and excursion of 1 mm) preferentially stimulates Ia (but also group II) afferent nerve fibers. It exerts inhibitory characteristics by way of an interneuron which is both excited by Ia afferent input and then acts on terminal Ia fiber arborizations. This interneuron is strongly modulated by descending pyramidal and extrapyramidal (vestibulospinal, reticulospinal, rubrospinal) tracts, and so the TVR can help to elucidate the role of these descending fibers on the segmental reflex arc.

This is routinely carried out in humans by the application of a tonic vibration to the Achilles tendon, resulting in a strong discharge in triceps surae Ia fibers. Normally, this results in a depression of the soleus H-reflex. Since this depression is seen along with a motor discharge (the tonic vibration reflex), reflecting an increased excitability at the motor neuronal level, it was postulated that it was presynaptic in origin. The *failure* of tonic vibration to suppress the H-reflex in spastic patients has been cited as evidence for the loss of presynaptic inhibition in the spastic state.

The ratio of the maximal H-reflex during vibration and without vibration, $H(max)_{(vib)}/H(max)$, is increased in the spastic patient, suggesting a loss of presynaptic inhibition. Unfortunately, the tonic vibration reflex is of dubious value in the evaluation of spastic hypertonia, as there is a wide dispersion of values among patients and poor correlation with the intensity of spasticity. Also, when prolonged vibration is applied, a variety of mechanisms might contribute to suppression of the H-reflex. These include refractoriness of Ia fibers, transmitter depletion at Ia terminals, postsynaptic reciprocal Ia inhibition due to spread of vibration, activation of muscle spindles in antagonists, and postsynaptic nonreciprocal group I inhibition.

In order to address such problems, investigators have attempted to isolate presynaptic inhibition from a variety of postsynaptic components by studying the effects of the TVR during voluntary contraction of the soleus at constant torque.[37] It is suggested that the inhibitory action under these conditions should be largely presynaptic. Similarly, they found that spastic subjects showed less inhibition than controls at all levels of voluntary torque investigated.

In yet another variation, a recent technique has been developed in which a weak, brief vibration is applied over the anterior tibial tendon in the form of three brief shocks over 10 ms.[35] The resulting Ia volley results in a depression of the H-reflex similar to electrical volleys in Ia afferents of the peroneal nerve, as mentioned above. With this method in a comparison of amyotrophic lateral sclerosis and normal patients, spastic patients demonstrated a smaller presynaptic inhibition of the H-reflex than the controls.

FLEXOR WITHDRAWAL RESPONSES. The automatic

withdrawal of the lower extremity upon electrically stimulating the sole of the foot, the flexor withdrawal response, is believed to reflect global interneural activities. EMG recording from the anterior tibial muscle and other lower extremity flexors record a low-threshold early response (50–60 ms) which disappears with an upper motor neuron lesion, and a later (110–400 ms) high-threshold response. Increasing the stimulus strength decreases the latency and increases the amplitude and duration of both components. Flexor withdrawal responses have not proved to be useful because of the variability of their polysynaptic response.[15]

LUMBOSACRAL SPINAL EVOKED RESPONSES. Lumbosacral spinal evoked responses are claimed to be a reflection of presynaptic inhibition in the dorsal horn of the spinal cord. Upon submaximal stimulation of the tibial nerve, an evoked response can be most easily measured over the spinous process of T12. The evoked response routinely has three peaks: (1) an inconstant positive deflection (P1), (2) a negative deflection (S), and (3) a second larger-amplitude positive deflection (P2). Studies in multiple sclerosis patients have demonstrated a reduction of the ratio between the areas of the large positive and negative deflection (P2/S), which strongly correlated with the intensity of spasticity (as measured by the Ashworth scale). Based on previous animal work, the P2 wave is attributed to presynaptic inhibitory mechanisms, and a diminution of the P2/S ratio reflects a loss of presynaptic inhibition in the spastic patient.[18] With this technique, the administration of intrathecal baclofen in three SCI patients suppressed the P2 wave amplitude and area, while the S wave amplitude was suppressed to a lesser degree.[50]

ELECTROPHYSIOLOGICAL TESTING: COMMENTARY. Electrophysiological testing has been a fascinating tool to examine changes in spinal cord function and segmental reflexes in spastic patients. However, its weakness lies in the poor correlation between various tests as well as the etiology of the lesion, location of the lesion, and intensity of spasticity. Systematic attempts have failed to demonstrate the usefulness of four such parameters—H(max)/M(max), T(max)/M(max), H(max)$_{(vib)}$/H(max), and H-reflex recovery curves—in assessing the response to single doses of different myorelaxant drugs.[16] Diazepam clearly reinforced vibratory inhibition in spastic patients, causing the index to return to near-normal values. Baclofen did not modify vibratory inhibition at all but reduced the abnormal facilitation seen in H-reflex recovery curves of spastic patients. Unfortunately, as these scales correlate poorly with clinical severity, it is unclear what significance these changes in electrophysiological parameters reflect.

In summary, a large number of neurophysiological studies have been performed using a variety of electrophysiological techniques to assess the mechanisms as well as to quantify the severity of spastic hypertonia. Often the premises for use of these techniques are based on animal models, which may or may not be applicable to intact human subjects. Most of these studies also assess the neural circuitry of the spastic patient at rest, ignoring the biomechanical and neurophysiological features of movement. As any clinician would aptly point out, much of the disability present in a spastic patient is associated with human movement. Thus, in essence, electrophysiological studies are hampered by taking neural mechanisms out of the milieu of the behavioral motoric complex and studying them as an isolated event.

THERAPEUTIC MANAGEMENT OF SPASTIC HYPERTONIA

Before treatment of spasticity is initiated, the physician needs to address several important questions. Is there a functional impairment due to the spastic hypertonia? Is there a disturbance of gait? Do flexor spasms force the patient from his or her chair or interfere with transfers? Does the pain that can be associated with "spasms" disturb the patient's sleep? Is the lower extremity extensor tone useful to the patient in support during gait? Although stereotyped therapeutic approaches have been proposed, treatment is best individualized to the particular patient.

Good nursing care can reduce nociceptive and exteroreceptive stimuli, which can exacerbate the patient's hypertonia (Table 29–5). The avoidance of noxious stimuli is an important initial management step. This includes such measures as prompt treatment of urinary tract complications (infections, stones), prevention of pressure sores and contractures, release of tightly wrapped leg bags and clothes, proper bowel and bladder management to prevent fecal impaction and bladder distention, and deep venous thrombosis prophylaxis. Heterotopic bone has been suggested as an exacerbant of spasticity, but the prevention of this complication can be difficult (see Chapter 55).

Proper bed positioning early after SCI has been suggested as an important step in the long-term reduction of spastic hypertonia, but this assertion has never been systematically evaluated. A daily stretching program is an integral component of any management program for spastic hypertonia. A common bedside observation is that the resistance perceived as one continuously moves a limb over its range of motion progressively diminishes as one repeats the motion.

Physical Modalities

Regular range-of-motion maneuvering of a patient's limbs helps prevent contractures and can reduce the severity of spastic tone for several hours. The reason for this "carryover" of several hours is not completely clear but may be related to mechanical changes in the musculotendinous unit, as well as to plastic changes occurring within the central nervous system. These plastic events may correlate with short- and long-term modulation of synaptic efficacy associated with neurotransmitter changes on a cellular

TABLE 29–5   General Treatment Considerations

Preliminary considerations	Basic management
Functional impairment from hypertonia?	Proper bed positioning
Causes gait disturbance?	Avoid noxious stimuli
Is hypertonicity needed for standing?	Daily stretching program
Flexor spasms?	Physical measures
Painful spasms?	Therapeutic facilitation
	Topical cold/anesthesia
	Casting/splinting

level. Habituation of reflex activity has been studied in the marine snail *Aplysia californica*, which has a simple nervous system. The snail has a reflex for withdrawing its respiratory organ and siphon that is similar to the leg-flexion withdrawal reflex in humans. Repetitive activation results in a decrease in synaptic transmission, partly due to an inactivation of calcium channels in the presynaptic terminal. The decrease in calcium influx diminishes the release of neurotransmitter, probably due to the calcium-dependent exocytosis of neurotransmitter vesicles.[11, 12]

SHORT-TERM STRATEGIES. Certain interventions may be valuable as temporizing strategies when a specific goal is in mind.[13] Several schools of therapeutic exercise have suggested that reflex-inhibiting postures may temporarily decrease spastic hypertonia so that underlying movements may be unmasked. Utilizing these strategies, therapists are able to help hemiplegic and cerebral palsy patients produce voluntary movements.

Topical cold has been reported to decrease tendon reflex excitability, reduce clonus, increase range of motion of the joint, and improve power in the antagonistic muscle group. These effects can be used to facilitate improved motor function for short periods of time. Tone may be decreased very shortly after the application of ice, which is probably due to decreased sensitivity in cutaneous receptors and slowing of nerve conduction. Central factors, changes in central nervous system excitability, may take longer to occur. Thus, a therapist might apply a cold pack for 20 or more minutes to obtain maximum effect. Topical anesthesia may have similar effects.

CASTING AND SPLINTING. Casting or splinting techniques, or both, can improve the range of motion in a joint owing to hypertonic contracture, and positioning the limb in a tonic stretch has been observed to decrease reflex tone.[8] In one study, long-term, but not short-term, casting resulted in a significant decrease in both dynamic and static reflex sensitivity. Elongation of the series elastic component of the musculotendinous unit and an increase in the number of sarcomeres within muscle fibers may each have contributed to the decrease in tone.[59] Biofeedback techniques have also been observed to modulate spastic hypertonia but have not demonstrated much widespread usefulness.[4, 78]

ELECTRICAL STIMULATION. The concept of using electrical stimulation to improve patient function, or "functional electrical stimulation," has received wide medical and lay press attention (see Chapter 23). Electrical stimulation of peripheral nerves has been a potential adjunct to traditional rehabilitation therapeutics for paraplegic patients during standing, walking, and exercise training.[80] Cyclical use of electrical stimulation has been shown to decrease upper extremity contractures, improve motor activity in agonistic muscles, and reduce tone in antagonistic muscle groups of the hemiplegic and quadriplegic patient. Stimulation of the sural nerve, a flexor reflex afferent, resulted in decreased extensor tonus and increased strength of ankle dorsiflexion. The therapeutic effect may last for an hour or more after stimulation has been discontinued, perhaps as a result of neurotransmitter modulation within the segmental reflex. Peroneal nerve stimulation may suppress ankle clonus in ambulatory hemiplegic patients via reciprocal inhibition. Electrical stimulation has limited but defined applica-

tions as an ankle dorsiflexor assist during hemiplegic gait and as a hand-opening device in the hemiplegic upper extremity. Significant decrements in spastic hypertonia using cutaneous stimulation in a hemiplegic population have been demonstrated in rigorous biomechanical quantification studies to last up to 30 minutes. Recently, investigators using rectal probe stimulation to induce ejaculation in spinal cord–injured men noted a significant reduction in spasticity which lasted up to 24 hours.[32] Such reductions could arise because of changes in the effectiveness of synaptic transmission due to mechanisms such as short-term facilitation, short-term depression, long-term potentiation, and long-term depression.[19]

Spinal cord stimulation (Fig. 29–5), also known as dorsal column stimulation, was initially embraced enthusiastically in the treatment of spinal hypertonia. A short chain of stimulating electrodes is threaded into the epidural space, resting in the vicinity of the spinal cord dorsal columns. Maximal improvement depends upon finding the ideal combination of electrode placement, stimulation intensity, and stimulation frequency. A critical analysis of the beneficial effects of dorsal column stimulation has questioned its efficacy in improving motor and bladder function.[38] In a carefully performed study in which examiners were blinded as to whether stimulation was on or off, measures of joint compliance and standardized neurological examination were no better than chance in determining whether spinal cord stimulation was being received.[29]

Pharmacological Intervention

ORAL MEDICATIONS. No medication (Table 29–6) has been uniformly useful in the treatment of spastic hypertonia.[14, 45, 77] Considering the variety of problems associated with spasticity—flexor spasms in the spinal patient, dys-

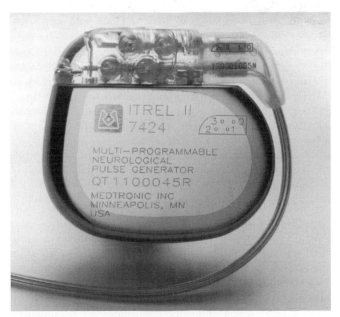

FIGURE 29–5 A subcutaneous stimulation unit can directly neuromodulate the spinal cord by threading a short chain of stimulating electrodes into the epidural space to rest beside the dorsal columns (Medtronic Itrel II Spinal Cord Stimulator). (Courtesy of Medtronic Neurological, Minneapolis.)

TABLE 29–6 Drug Treatment of Spastic Hypertonia*

Agent	Daily Dosage	Half-Life (hr)	Mechanism of Action
Baclofen	10–80+ mg	3.5	Presynaptic inhibitor by activation of γ-aminobutyric acid (GABA) B receptor
Diazepam	4–60+ mg	27–37†	Facilitates postsynaptic effects of GABA, resulting in increased presynaptic inhibition
Dantrolene	25–400 mg	8.7	Reduces calcium release, interfering with excitation-contraction coupling in skeletal muscle
Clonidine	0.1–0.4 mg (oral) 0.1–0.3 mg (patch)‡	12–16 (oral)	α₂-Adrenergic agonist

*Ketazolam, tizanidine, and progabide are not available in the United States. Baclofen and morphine can be administered intrathecally.
†Half-life of active primary metabolite is significantly longer.
‡Patch is changed weekly.

tonic posturing in the hemiplegic patient, spastic diplegia in the cerebral palsy child—it is unlikely that one agent will be beneficial to all parties. More important, all drugs have potentially serious side effects, and these negative features should be carefully weighed when beginning a patient on any drug. Continued use of a drug should be contingent on a clearly beneficial effect.

Baclofen (Lioresal) is an analog of δ-aminobutyric acid (GABA), a neurotransmitter involved in presynaptic inhibition. Baclofen does not bind to the classic GABA A receptor but rather to a recently discovered and less well-characterized B receptor. Agonism at this site inhibits calcium influx into presynaptic terminals and suppresses release of excitatory neurotransmitters. Baclofen inhibits both monosynaptic and polysynaptic reflexes and also reduces activity of the gamma efferent. Although therapeutic effects have been shown to occur when plasma levels exceeded 400 ng/mL, optimal responses have been obtained at very different plasma and cerebrospinal fluid levels. Baclofen is completely absorbed after oral administration and is eliminated predominantly by the renal route. Its half-life is approximately 3.5 hours. Baclofen readily crosses the blood-brain barrier, in contrast to GABA.

Baclofen is probably the drug of choice in spinal forms of spasticity. It has been demonstrated to be effective in reducing flexor spasms, increasing range of motion, and decreasing spastic hypertonia. Baclofen is equivalent to diazepam in efficacy but has less sedative effect. The role of baclofen in the treatment of cerebral forms of spasticity remains unsettled; it may interfere with attention and memory in brain-injured patients. Baclofen may improve bladder control by decreasing hyperreflexive contraction of the external urethral sphincter. It has been shown to be safe and effective in long-term use. Baclofen also has an anxiolytic effect, which probably contributes to its antispasticity actions.

Dosage in adults begins at approximately 5 mg orally bid or tid and may be slowly titrated upward toward a recommended maximum dose of 80 mg/day. This "recom-

mended maximum dose" may not necessarily be the most effective dose for the patient, however, and higher doses may be well tolerated by the patient and be additionally therapeutic. There is a low incidence of side effects, which include hallucinations, confusion, sedation, hypotonia, and ataxia. Sudden withdrawal of the drug can lead to seizures and hallucinations. Stereospecific L-baclofen has been shown to be more effective than the presently used racemic form in treatment of headache pain. L-Baclofen deserves evaluation for treatment of spastic hypertonia.

Safe use of baclofen has not been established in children under the age of 12 years. Its use in this age group is thus "not recommended." However, physicians have used baclofen in this age group with dosages initiated at 2.5 to 5.0 mg/day, with maximum dosages of 30 mg (children 2–7 years of age) to 60 mg (children 8 years or older).

Diazepam (Valium) facilitates the postsynaptic effects of GABA, resulting in an increase in presynaptic inhibition. It has no direct GABA-mimetic effect but exerts indirect mimetic effect only when GABA transmission is functional. In addition to its known effects in the brain, it has been shown to have an effect in patients with demonstrated spinal cord division. However, its effect in complete spinal lesions was not confirmed in one report. Diazepam has been a successful treatment for spastic hypertonia in SCI and is generally well tolerated except for its sedative effect. Diazepam is generally unsuitable in patients with brain injury because of its deleterious effects on attention and memory. Other side effects include intellectual impairment and reduced motor coordination. Evidence of abuse and addiction is rare, but true physiological addiction may occur. Withdrawal symptoms can appear if diazepam is tapered too rapidly. There is some synergistic depression of the central nervous system when administered with alcohol. Although the potential for overdose exists, the benzodiazepines have an extremely large index of safety. Dosage begins at approximately 2 mg orally bid, and may be slowly titrated up to 60 mg/day or more, in divided doses. Pediatric dosages range from 0.12 to 0.8 mg/kg/day in divided doses.

Dantrolene sodium (Dantrium) reduces muscle action potential–induced release of calcium into the sarcoplasmic reticulum, decreasing the force produced by excitation-contraction coupling. Dantrolene is the only drug which intervenes in spastic hypertonia at a "muscular" rather than a segmental reflex level. It reduces the activity of phasic stretch reflexes more than tonic ones. Dantrolene affects fast more than slow muscle fibers, and for unknown reasons seems to have little effect on smooth and cardiac muscle tissues. It is metabolized largely in the liver and eliminated in urine and bile. Its half-life is approximately 8 to 9 hours.

Dantrolene is preferred for cerebral forms of spasticity, such as hemiplegia or cerebral palsy, but may be a useful adjunct to the treatment of spinal forms of spasticity. It is less likely to cause lethargy or cognitive disturbances than baclofen or diazepam. Although dantrolene theoretically "weakens" muscles, the effects on spastic hypertonia are generally without impairment of motor performance. Its most pronounced effect is possibly the reduction in clonus and muscle spasms resulting from innocuous stimuli.

Dantrolene is mild to moderately sedative and may cause

malaise, nausea and vomiting, dizziness, and diarrhea. It has been suggested that the drug may exacerbate seizures in cerebral palsy patients. The most commonly considered side effect is that of hepatoxicity, which can occur in approximately 1% of patients. Liver function tests should be monitored periodically, and the drug can be tapered or discontinued if enzyme elevations are noted. In early reports fatal hepatitis was reported in 0.1% to 0.2% of patients treated for longer than 60 days. However, its hepatotoxic effects may have been overstated. Dosage begins at 25 mg/day and may be slowly increased up to 400 mg/day. However, clinical results are not clearly related to dose and may plateau at a dosage of 100 mg/day. Pediatric doses begin 0.5 mg/kg bid, increasing the frequency and dosage until maximum effect is reached. The maximum dosage is generally 3 mg/kg qid or less than 100 mg qid.

Tizanidine (Sirdalud) is an imidazoline derivative which has an agonistic action at central α_2-adrenergic receptor sites. It may facilitate the action of glycine, an inhibitory neurotransmitter, and prevents the release of excitatory amino acids, that is, L-glutamate and L-aspartate, from the presynaptic terminal of spinal interneurons. It reduces tonic stretch reflexes and enhances presynaptic inhibition in animals. It enhances vibratory inhibition of the H-reflex and reduces abnormal co-contraction. Tizanidine has the unusual effect of increasing the torque of spastic muscle by increasing the amplitude of the agonist EMG signal. It has been shown to be equivalent to baclofen as an antispastic agent (but may be better tolerated) in both cerebral as well as spinal forms of spasticity in divided dosages up to 36 mg/day. It has similarly been shown to be equally efficacious and better tolerated than diazepam in patients with chronic hemiplegia. Multiple sclerosis patients have shown significant benefit in several large double blind studies. Common side effects include mild hypotension, daytime sleepiness, weakness, and dry mouth. Daytime somnolence may be secondary to nighttime insomnia, which was reported more frequently by patients receiving tizanidine than by those receiving baclofen.[74a] In double blind comparative studies, tizanidine was generally found to be better tolerated than baclofen.[74a] Both tizanidine and baclofen are more effective in extensor than flexor musculature.[74a] Recently, a modified release form of tizanidine has been formulated which allows for once- or twice-daily dosing.[36] Despite recent double blinded clinical trials,[80a] the Food and Drug Administration (FDA) has presently denied approval for tizanidine as a treatment for spasticity.[23a]

Ketazolam, a benzodiazepine, has been shown to be equally effective and less sedating than diazepam in spinal forms of spasticity; it may have a similar pharmacological action. An additional benefit is that ketazolam may be administered in a single 30- to 60-mg/day dosage.[5, 6] Unfortunately, it is not presently approved for use in the United States. *Tetrazepam* (Myolastan), a benzodiazepine derivative, is reported to reduce the tonic component of spastic hypertonia with little effect on tendon hyperreflexia and no influence on muscle strength.[56] A benzodiazepine analog, *clorazepate,* is transformed into desmethyldiazepam, the major metabolite of diazepam, and has been shown to be effective in normalizing phasic but not tonic stretch reflexes.

Chlorpromazine has been applied to the treatment of hypertonia because of its α-adrenergic blocking effect. Clinical and electrophysiological studies in humans before and after administration of α- and β-blocking agents suggest descending adrenergic and noradrenergic pathways may have important modulatory effects on spastic hypertonia. However, the depression of motor function by phenothiazines is thought to be due largely to its effects upon the brainstem reticular formation. A small double blind study of *chlorpromazine with phenytoin* suggests that a combination of these drugs may be beneficial in the treatment of spastic hypertonia. Neither drug alone was as efficacious as the combination of the two, although chlorpromazine alone was nearly as effective. Phenytoin serum levels did not correlate with therapeutic effect as long as this concentration was above 7 μg/mL. The addition of phenytoin lowered the needed optimally therapeutic dose of chlorpromazine, decreasing its sedative effect.

Clonidine, an α_2-adrenergic agonist, has been used with fair success in SCI patients. Clonidine, in combination with desipramine, improved the vibratory inhibition of the H-reflex after SCI. Coactivation of antagonist muscle decreased, allowing improved locomotor function in a spastic paraparetic patient with clonidine therapy. Syncope, hypotension, and nausea and vomiting are the most common side effects. Most patients who benefit from the drug note acceptable relief with dosage of 0.1 mg bid or less.[21] Clonidine is now available in an adhesive patch (Catapres-TTS) for weeklong transdermal delivery. Initial studies have demonstrated favorable results starting with a 0.1-mg patch and titrating up to a 0.3-mg patch as needed. Adverse effects were similar to those reported with oral clonidine.[76]

Progabide, a systemically active GABA agonist at both the A and B receptors, and *THIP (tetrahydroisoxazolopyridin),* a second GABA agonist, have been proposed as possible antispasticity drugs. Electrophysiological studies suggest that progabide's likely site of action is spinal interneurons. A median dose of 24.3 mg/kg (1800 mg/day) resulted in satisfactory reduction in spastic hypertonia, tendon reflexes, and flexor spasms without a significant improvement in voluntary strength.[57] The beneficial effects of progabide in higher dosages seems to be limited by serious side effects—fever, weakness, and elevated liver enzymes.

Glycine, a neurotransmitter involved in reciprocal inhibition, has not been thoroughly investigated in the treatment of spastic hypertonia. Glycine passes the blood-brain barrier in amounts sufficient to affect reflex activity and has decreased spasticity in small groups of patients. Glycine is rapidly depleted in the spinal cord ventral gray matter after spinal cord transection, and the depletion correlates with spasticity onset in a canine model. Similarly, *threonine,* a glycine precursor, has shown potential efficacy in preliminary investigations. Although glycine levels in serum and cerebrospinal fluid did not rise after the administration of threonine, enhancement of glycinergic postsynaptic inhibition of the spinal reflex arc is the hypothesized mechanism of action. *Tetrahydrocannabinol (THC),* the active agent in marijuana, although not approved by the FDA for use as an agent in the treatment of spastic hypertonia, has occasionally been noted to decrease hypertonia. Although various other medications have been suggested in the treatment of spasticity, such as *cyclobenzaprine, carisoprodol, cyproheptadine, L-acetylcarnitine,* there is no consistent evidence to recommend their use.

EXPERIMENTAL DRUGS. GABA and glycine are *inhibitory* neurotransmitters in the central nervous system. The antispastic effects of the benzodiazepines and baclofen result from agonism at these inhibitory neurotransmitter receptor sites. Spinal *excitatory* neurotransmitters include glutamate and aspartate; antagonism at their receptor sites would provide another pharmacological option for management of spastic hypertonia. There are several types of glutamate receptors: they can be broadly categorized as the *N*-methyl-D-aspartate (NMDA) and non-NMDA types. The NMDA receptors have been implicated in excitotoxic effects after neurological injury. A prototype for an NMDA receptor antagonist is the street drug phencyclidine hydrochloride (PCP or "angel dust"). An experimental drug used to block the NMDA receptor is MK-801. As far as the non-NMDA receptor antagonists, the quinoxalinediones (specifically NBQX) have been shown to reduce hind limb extensor tone in genetically spastic rats.[74]

Vigabatrin is an experimental drug specifically designed to increase brain GABA levels by inhibiting catabolism of this neurotransmitter. It replaces GABA as a substrate for GABA transaminase, the enzyme responsible for the first step in GABA breakdown. Vigabatrin was developed as an antiepileptic agent and has shown promise in the treatment of refractory cases of epilepsy. In placebo-controlled trials vigabatrin in doses of 2 to 3 g/day improved spasticity in patients with SCI and multiple sclerosis. The most common adverse reactions were drowsiness, fatigue, and weight gain, but behavioral disturbances are reported to be uncommon.[30]

INTRATHECAL MEDICATIONS. Intrathecal administration of baclofen has been successfully attempted in the treatment of spastic hypertonia related to spinal cord dysfunction and, more recently, cerebral palsy.[1, 10, 58, 60] A pump can be planted subcutaneously in the abdominal wall, with a catheter surgically placed into the subarachnoid space. In this manner, higher dosages of these medications can be placed near the spinal cord—the desired site for action of the drug—while largely avoiding the central nervous system side effects associated with increased oral intake. The pump may be refilled on a monthly basis by transcutaneous injection. Complications include tube dysfunction (dislodgment, disconnection, kinkage, and blockage), pump failure, infection, and baclofen overdosage.

The ideal patient for intrathecal baclofen infusion with the spinal form of spasticity has either SCI or multiple sclerosis with some preserved function below the level of the lesion allowing the patient to be ambulatory.[10] The baclofen dosage is adjusted to provide maximal spasm relief while minimizing weakness. The patient should be free of active infection and decubitus ulcer. The skin over the back should be intact, and there should be an anterior abdominal wall site suitable for pump placement. Multiple abdominal procedures such as colostomies, ileal conduits, and feeding tubes must be separated from the pump site. In patients who have a potential block of cerebrospinal fluid flow, myelography may be required to ensure that there is communication between the proposed site of infusion and the source of spasticity. As pumps are expensive (approximately $6500 for the pump alone plus another $3000/year for the drug itself *plus* surgical costs), a short trial run with intrathecal baclofen via percutaneous lumbar catheter (preferably in combination with an external continuous infusion pump) is suggested. Medicare now covers the implantation of infusion pumps for spasticity.

There are two types of pump available. Infusaid Inc., Norwood, Massachusetts, manufactures a gas-powered bellows device that is purely mechanical and has no battery. Unfortunately, it can only infuse drug at a constant rate, and thus offers changes of titration of dose primarily at the time of refill. The electronic pump (Fig. 29–6) can be programmed to deliver drug several times daily via an onboard computer. It allows precise titration of drug. The computer can be adjusted by an external laptop computer equipped with a programming wand. Battery life is presently about 4 to 5 years.

Baclofen is initially infused continuously at 25 µg/day. The most common side effects are drowsiness, dizziness, nausea, hypotension, headache, and weakness. The dosage is titrated up to an average of 400 to 500 µg/day or until satisfactory reduction in spasticity has been achieved. Some authors report experience with doses as high as 1500 µg/day.[39] While dosages may escalate early in the course of intrathecal baclofen use, it generally reaches a plateau 6 months following implantation. In addition to beneficial effects on limb spasticity, intrathecal baclofen may have a beneficial effect on bladder management. Caution concerning inadvertent overdose should be exercised, as reversible coma due to baclofen toxicity has been reported. However, patients suffering from respiratory depression due to accidental intrathecal bolus injection were reversed with 2 mg physostigmine administered intravenously. The half-life of intrathecal baclofen is approximately 5 hours.

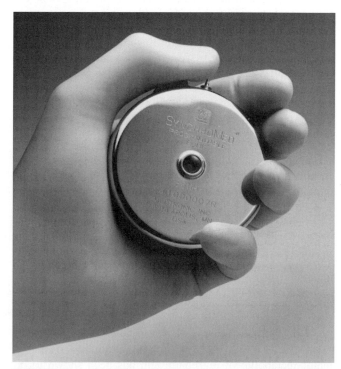

FIGURE 29–6 Intrathecal baclofen can be administered via a pump planted subcutaneously in the abdominal wall via a catheter placed into the subarachnoid space (Medtronic SynchroMed Drug Infusion Pump). (Courtesy of Medtronic Neurological, Minneapolis.)

One to 2 mg of intrathecal morphine has similarly caused a dramatic reduction in spasticity and pain in spinal cord–injured patients.[23] Patients do not seem to develop drug tolerance or lose the beneficial effect of the morphine in long-term follow-up. Despite its efficacy, intrathecal morphine is currently rarely used.

A recent trial of intrathecal baclofen pumps in 37 patients with spasticity of cerebral origin, mostly due to cerebral palsy, showed a decrease in upper and lower extremity spasticity and an improvement in hamstring motion, upper extremity function, and activities of daily living.[1]

NERVE BLOCKS.   Nerve blocks refer to the application of a chemical agent to a nerve to either temporarily or permanently impair the function of the nerve.[28] This can result in improved range of motion, lessening of clonus, increase in speed and dexterity of movement (owing to blockade of inappropriately firing antagonists), improved crawling, sitting, and standing in children, and even diminished spasticity in the contralateral extremities.

Commonly used agents include local anesthetics (e.g., lidocaine), phenol, alcohol, and botulinus toxin. Local anesthetics temporarily block conduction by interfering with the increase in permeability of sodium ions that normally occurs when the membrane is depolarized. The effects are short-lived (several hours) and are used in the assessment of the potential effect of a longer-acting nerve block or surgical procedure (see Orthopedic Procedures later). Ethyl alcohol is also a potent neurolytic agent, but it offers no particular advantage over phenol and has not been as extensively evaluated.

Two percent to 6% aqueous phenol solutions are the agents most commonly used to produce chemical neurolysis when applied to a nerve trunk or its terminal nerve fibers (motor point block).[19] Concentrations of phenol greater than 5% cause protein coagulation and necrosis of axons of all sizes. Neurolysis of motor points—actually the terminal branches of motor nerves—are often less effective by themselves, perhaps owing to the multiplicity of motor

points within a muscle. They are more appropriate when using agents that diffuse, such as botulinus toxin (see below). Nerve blocks may be quite effective and may last 3 to 6 months or more when performed using electrophysiological guidance and a Teflon-coated needle (Fig. 29–7). Gradually, axons destroyed by phenol regenerate with some increase in fibrous tissue at the site of injection.

Musculocutaneous nerve blocks can be helpful in the hemiplegic patient with severe elbow flexion contracture or in the C5 quadriplegic patient with flexor contractures due to loss of triceps function. Elbow flexion is preserved through the action of the brachioradialis muscle, which unlike other elbow flexors is innervated by the radial nerve. Median nerve blocks help relax the tightly flexed hemiplegic wrist and fingers. An obturator block decreases lower extremity scissoring during gait and facilitates hip abduction to ease personal hygiene. Hip flexor spasticity may be diminished by paravertebral block of the upper lumbar spinal nerves. Owing to the proximity of important visceral and vascular structures, lumbosacral paravertebral nerve blocks require special caution. Tibial nerve block can reduce severe equinovarus ankle posturing or painful clawing of the toes. Perineal nerve block can significantly reduce postvoid residual volumes when the external urethral sphincter is very spastic.

Because both sensory and motor nerve fibers are damaged, phenol nerve blocks can be associated with burning and discomfort. Dysesthesias and causalgia have been reported in approximately 10% of patients, so the patient should be advised of this before the block is administered. Severe persistent dysesthesias may be treated with oral steroids, transcutaneous nerve stimulation, or repetition of the phenol block. Open phenol nerve blocks are performed by a surgeon, and selected motor trunks can be blocked as they enter the muscle bulk, which leaves cutaneous sensory fibers unharmed. Presumably, the incidence of dysesthesias should also be lower using this method. Unwanted weakness may acutely complicate a phenol block but often resolves in the first hours or days after nerve block. Over-

FIGURE 29–7 Nerve blocks can be performed using a 22-gauge Teflon-coated needle with a bared bevel. The hub of the needle is connected to a stimulator, which delivers a square pulse of approximately 0.1 ms once or twice per second. Surface stimulation can be used to approximate the site of the nerve while the examiner watches for a visible twitch in the desired muscle. After the needle is inserted, the needle is gradually moved until only the minimal current (approximately 1 mA) is necessary to obtain a maximal twitch in the desired muscle(s). At this point the phenol is injected. Motor point blocks may require multiple injections into a single muscle. As commonly practiced, aspiration should be carried out before injection to avoid intravascular administration of the drug.

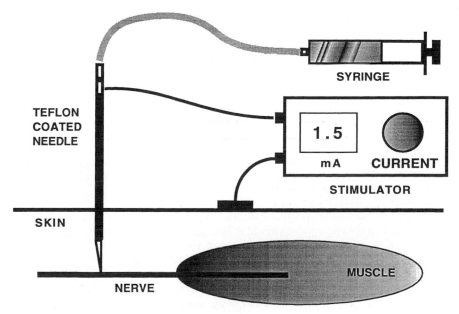

dosage with phenol can result in convulsions, central nervous system depression, and cardiovascular collapse. However, the usual dosages (e.g., 20 mL of 5% phenol) are well below the lethal range of the drug ($\geq$ 8.5 g). Venous thromboses can be a complication of phenol injection for chemical neurolysis.

Botulinus toxin has been used to diminish spasticity and is presently being evaluated in prospective clinical trials. Botulinus toxin works at the neuromuscular junction by inhibiting the release of acetylcholine.[40] It was originally developed for clinical use by an ophthalmologist treating disorders such as blepharospasm and strabismus. Its use spread to the treatment of movement disorders such as torticollis and focal dystonias and, most recently, to spastic hypertonia. Botulinus toxin injections do not require the rigorous localization of phenol injections, as the compound diffuses through muscle membranes, causing a "leaking" of the neuromuscular effect. Applications of approximately 30 to 50 units per muscle site may be attempted, with a combined limit of approximately 400 units per session.[71] Localization techniques are identical to those for phenol. Reported side effects include unwanted weakness and transient fatigue, nausea, and headache.

SPINAL BLOCKS. Intrathecal chemical neurolysis is another method of decreasing spastic hypertonia. Spinal root neurolysis may be carried out via spinal administration of 5% to 7% phenol in water or absolute alcohol, but control over affected fibers is rather imprecise. The effects of alcohol are more permanent than phenol. Patients must be carefully immobilized to allow precise layering of the neurolytic material so that damage is limited to the desired spinal roots. Complications of this procedure include urinary and fecal incontinence, paresis, paresthesias, and even death. Complication rates have varied from 1% to 10% in various series of patients.

Surgical Interventions

ORTHOPEDIC PROCEDURES. Orthopedic surgery may be a useful adjunct in the management of selected patients.[48] Surgical procedures are generally reserved for patients who have been refractory to more conservative measures, including range-of-motion maneuvers and casting. Several considerations should be addressed before surgery is considered:

1. *When was the insult to the central nervous system?* It is important to schedule surgical intervention only when the plastic changes of recovery have more or less plateaued. This may be at least 6 months after a stroke but often 12 to 24 months after a traumatic brain injury.

2. *Are the "spastic" changes dynamic or static in nature?* *Dynamic* refers to dysfunction that appears with movement, for example, scissoring of the lower extremities during ambulation in a patient with cerebral palsy. *Static* deformities are fixed contractures that are present both at rest and with movement, for example, the clenched flexed hand of the hemiplegic upper extremity. This differentiation is based on examination of the patient and can often be augmented with a diagnostic block with lidocaine or similar anesthetic. For example, a median nerve block at the elbow is useful in determining the dynamic vs. static contribution of finger and wrist flexion in the hemiplegic patient.

3. *What are the goals of surgery?* Is it to increase function (e.g., hand opening and closing or gait) or simply to increase range of motion to facilitate self-care or nursing care? For example, hip adduction can be lessened to diminish scissoring during gait in a cerebral palsy child or to facilitate perineal hygiene in a patient with traumatic brain injury.

4. *What is the residual sensory and motor function of the limb in question?* Sensory input is vital to useful function in the upper extremity and can be assessed with a variety of tools, including two-point discrimination. Residual motor function in the upper extremity can be assessed with clinical scales, a vital component of which is the degree of remaining trunk and shoulder stability. A functioning hand and wrist is useless without the ability to place them meaningfully to interact with oneself and the environment. Gait analysis with polyelectromyography is frequently used as an adjunct in planning procedures in the lower extremity. There are occasions when intervention can be rationally performed only after analysis of muscle firing during the gait cycle (e.g., see the discussion of stiff-knee gait below).

5. *What type of procedure will best restore the abnormal forces acting on muscles and joints?* Deforming forces can be eliminated with a tenotomy or neurectomy, redirected with a tendon transfer, diminished with tendon-lengthening procedures, or stabilized by a fusion procedure when soft tissue procedures alone would be inadequate (e.g., triple arthrodesis of the foot).

6. *What preexisting complications may interfere with surgery?* Preoperative plain films and bone scans are useful in assessing the patient for fractures, dislocations, arthritis, and heterotopic ossification. Care should be taken on the physical examination to assess that weakness is due to upper motor neuron insult and not undiscovered lower motor neuron injury (e.g., undiscovered brachial plexopathy or peripheral nerve injury).

Orthopedic surgery for the upper extremity (Table 29–7) may be useful in selected spastic patients.[62] The spastic posturing of the hemiplegic shoulder (adduction and internal rotation) can be treated with release of the pectoralis

TABLE 29–7   Orthopedic Intervention for the Spastic Upper Extremity

Shoulder
Adducted and internally rotated shoulder: pectoralis major and subscapularis tendon release
Painful shoulder subluxation: biceps tendon sling
Elbow
Flexor spasticity: step-cut lengthening of brachioradial, biceps, and brachial muscles
Extensor spasticity: V-Y lengthening of triceps
Wrist and hand
Flexor spasticity
Fractional lengthening of FDS and FDP
Step-cut lengthening of FPL
Overlengthening of FCR and FCU
Flexor-pronator origin release
Sublimis-to-profundus transfer
Thumb-in-palm deformity: release of thenar and adductors

Abbreviations: FDS, flexor digitorum superficialis; FDP, flexor digitorum profundus; FPL, flexor pollicis longus; FCR, flexor carpi radialis; FCU, flexor carpi ulnaris.

major and subscapularis tendons, followed by a sling and passive stretching program. Inferior subluxation is a frequent problem in the paretic shoulder. When a sling gives inadequate symptomatic or functional relief, the biceps tendon can be looped over the coracoid process of the shoulder to serve as a static sling.

Dynamic flexion deformities of the elbow can be treated by step-cut lengthening of the biceps and fractional musculotendinous lengthening of the brachial muscle. The rare patient with triceps spasticity may benefit from V-Y lengthening of the triceps (V-Y refers to the shapes of the proximal and distal end of the tendon after a V-shaped incision). Occasionally, when simple lengthening is not adequate, a more extensive release may be necessary.

When flexor spasticity is not too severe, the patient with inadequate hand opening may benefit from fractional lengthening (Fig. 29–8) of the flexor digitorum sublimis and profundus tendons combined with step-cut lengthening of the flexor pollicis longus and overlengthening of the flexor carpi radialis and flexor carpi ulnaris. Patients are splinted in neutral, with active range-of-motion training beginning on the third postoperative day. Overlengthening of the finger flexors can result in a loss of grip strength. An alternative procedure for patients with voluntary control but overpowering flexors is to perform a flexor-pronator origin release. For the nonfunctional spastic hand, the superficialis-to-profundus tendon transfer of finger flexors provides sufficient flexor tendon lengthening with preservation of a passive tether to prevent hyperextension deformity.

Procedures for hand deformities include release of the thenar and thumb adductor muscles for thumb-in-palm deformity, release of hand intrinsics, and wrist arthrodesis. While these procedures may be cosmetic, the functional improvement after these procedures in hemiplegic patients

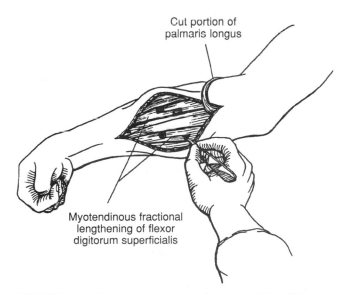

Cut portion of palmaris longus

Myotendinous fractional lengthening of flexor digitorum superficialis

FIGURE 29–8 When upper extremity flexor spasticity of the wrist and fingers is not too severe, the patient who cannot adequately open the hand may benefit from fractional lengthening of the flexor musculature. (Modified from Keenan MA, Kozin S, Berlet A: Manual of Orthopaedic Surgery for Spasticity. New York, Raven Press, 1993.)

TABLE 29–8 Orthopedic Intervention for the Spastic Lower Extremity

Functional deformities
  Limb scissoring: obturator neurectomy
  Crouched gait: iliopsoas recession, hamstring lengthening
  Stiff-knee gait: selective quadriceps release in selected patients
  Equinovarus foot: Achilles tendon lengthening, split anterior tibial tendon transfer, release of extrinsic and intrinsic toe flexors
  Spastic valgus foot: release and transfer of peroneus longus
Static deformities
  Hip adduction contracture: release of adductor longus, gracilis
  Hip flexion contracture: release of sartorius, rectus femoris, tensor fascia lata, iliopsoas, pectineus
  Hip extension: release proximal hamstrings
  Knee flexion contracture: release distal hamstrings
  Knee extension: V-Y plasty to lengthen quadriceps
  Foot: as for functional deformities; other options include release of plantar fascia and triple arthrodesis

is unclear because the patients frequently continue to carry out most activities with the uninvolved upper extremity.

There are five common dynamic clinical scenarios in the lower extremities for which surgery may be considered (Table 29–8): (1) limb scissoring, (2) crouched gait, (3) stiff-knee gait, (4) equinovarus foot, and (5) spastic valgus foot.[2]

Limb scissoring is often treated with obturator neurectomy, which improves the base of support during ambulation. If a static component complicates the picture, a hip adductor release may also be needed (see below). No immobilization or abduction splinting is needed following surgery, and early gait training with weightbearing as tolerated should follow.

Crouched gait results from spastic hip flexors with compensatory knee flexion and lumbar hyperlordosis. This results in a highly energy-inefficient gait. The iliopsoas tendon is removed from the lesser trochanter while maintaining its capsular insertions. This allows the iliopsoas to recess proximally and diminish its pull. There is no need for postoperative immobilization, and range-of-motion and gait training (weightbearing as tolerated) is initiated early. Distal hamstring lengthening may also improve the crouched gait, but care must be taken to extend the flexed knee deformity only very gradually for fear of overstretching the neurovascular bundle. Postoperatively the patient is immobilized in a long-leg cast, and the cast can be changed weekly to promote further extension. Transfers and gait training can be started once the cast is applied.

Stiff-knee gait results from inappropriate firing of the quadriceps muscle, preventing adequate knee flexion during the gait cycle. Gait analysis with EMG analysis of the various heads of the quadriceps is important so that the offending muscle groups can be selectively released (often the rectus femoris or vastus intermedius, or both). Postoperative management includes a knee immobilization splint for 5 days followed by postoperative ambulation with weight training as tolerated. Range-of-motion training and strengthening are begun approximately 5 days postoperatively.

Equinovarus foot is the most common deformity seen in the lower extremity with flexed ankle and a turned-in foot, often accompanied by excessive toe curling. The SPLATT

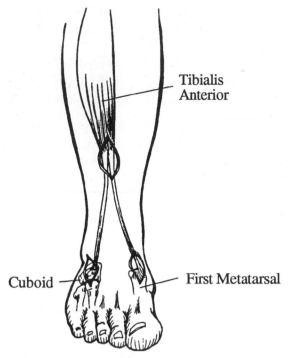

FIGURE 29–9 The SPLATT procedure helps reduce excessive supination at the subtalar joint due to the spastic tibialis anterior muscle. The tibialis anterior tendon is split along its length, and the distal end of the lateral half is tunneled into the cuboid and sometimes the third cuneiform bones. This creates an eversion force that is slightly greater than the varus pull of the remaining medial portion. (Modified from Keenan MA, Kozin S, Berlet A: Manual of Orthopaedic Surgery for Spasticity. New York, Raven Press, 1993.)

procedure—*spl*it *a*nterior *t*ibial *t*ransfer—is a procedure to help reduce excessive supination at the subtalar joint due to the spastic anterior tibial muscle (Fig. 29–9). The anterior tibial tendon is split along its length, and the distal end of the lateral half is tunneled into the third cuneiform and cuboid bones. This creates an eversion force that is slightly greater than the varus pull of the remaining medial portion. It is generally performed in combination with Achilles tendon lengthening (Fig. 29–10), often using the Hoke triple hemisection technique. Occasionally, the posterior tibial may be the offending muscle for the turned-in foot. Toe clawing or curling is often simultaneously treated with release of the intrinsic and extrinsic toe flexors. Postoperative management includes a short-leg walking cast for 6 weeks followed by a molded ankle foot orthosis for an additional 4½ months. The SPLATT, Achilles tendon lengthening, and toe flexor release are some of the most successful and rewarding procedures for the hemiplegic patient.

Valgus foot results from overactivity of the peroneus longus muscle. This may occur in concert with an equinovarus deformity during swing phase. Spastic valgus is corrected by release and transfer of the peroneus longus across the dorsum of the foot into the navicular bone. Postoperative management involves a short-leg walking cast in neutral position for 6 weeks, with immediate ambulation and weightbearing as tolerated. A molded ankle-foot orthosis (AFO) is worn for an additional 4½ months.

Static contractures in the lower extremity are treated with muscle release and lengthening. In patients with a static adductor contraction, hip adductor release (adductor longus, gracilis) is performed, followed by 4 weeks of forced abduction with casts or an abduction pillow splint. Hip flexion contracture is corrected with release of the sartorius, rectus femoris, tensor fascia lata, iliopsoas, and pectineus. Wound care is especially important in wounds near the perineum. The patient is placed prone three times a day with limited time in a seated position. Hip extension contractures (sometimes seen in patients with prolonged decerebrate posturing) may be treated by releasing the proximal hamstrings, followed by gentle hip range-of-motion exercises and sitting.

Knee flexion contractures are improved with release of

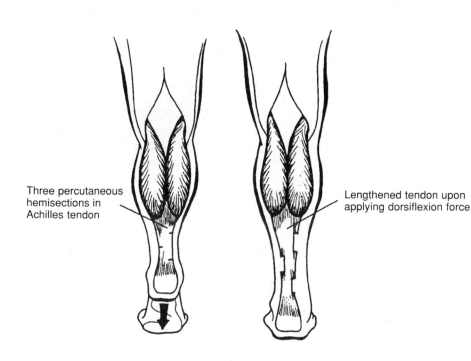

Three percutaneous hemisections in Achilles tendon

Lengthened tendon upon applying dorsiflexion force

FIGURE 29–10 The tendo-Achilles lengthening is often performed in conjunction with the SPLATT procedure using the Hoke triple hemisection technique. (Modified from Keenan MA, Kozin S, Berlet A: Manual of Orthopaedic Surgery for Spasticity. New York, Raven Press, 1993.)

the distal hamstrings. The knee is cast postoperatively and extended progressively with weekly cast changes. The extension contracture of the knee is treated with V-Y-plasty of the quadriceps tendon, followed by casting in flexion for 3 weeks. Therapy is initiated once the cast is removed. Fixed equinovarus posturing of the foot with clawing of the toes is treated as above. In addition, it may be necessary to perform a release of the plantar fascia or triple arthrodesis of the ankle, or both.

NEUROSURGICAL PROCEDURES. Rhizotomies, cutting spinal roots, may be performed for the remediation of spasticity in severe cases. Rhizotomies may be categorized as open (requiring laminectomy) or closed, complete or selective, anterior or posterior. Anterior rhizotomies are associated with severe denervation-type atrophy of all innervated muscles and may place the patient at increased risk of skin breakdown. The recent work in surgical management of spasticity focuses largely around the issue of selective posterior rhizotomy.

Selective dorsal rhizotomy (SDR), the neurosurgical ablation of a selected proportion of dorsal rootlets, has been most often performed on children with cerebral palsy.[55] While selective rhizotomy is most often carried out in the lumbosacral roots, success has also been reported for treatment of spasticity and pain in the hemiplegic upper extremity. The term "selective" refers to the sectioning of particular segmental rootlets or fascicles, generally chosen because of their abnormal neurophysiological characteristics. The preferred subjects for this procedure are young children with spastic (not athetoid, ataxic, dystonic, rigid) cerebral palsy with good motor control and some degree of forward locomotion whose function is primarily limited owing to the spastic hypertonia (Table 29-9). However, other forms of spasticity have also been treated with SDR.

The dorsal aspect of the thecal sac is exposed by laminectomy, although surgical approaches to the spine may differ. Dorsal roots are stimulated with an insulated bipolar stimulator, and responses are recorded with a polyelectromyogram (surface or intramuscular) from the ipsilateral and contralateral muscles of various myotomes. Neurophysiological assessment is used to distinguish afferent rootlets that cause "spastic" responses in muscles from

those that do not. The electrophysiological criteria for determining "abnormal" rootlets remain controversial, however. Investigators have stimulated rootlets at frequencies from 1 to 50 Hz, observing the "spread" of the evoked response to various muscle groups. Various parameters of the H-reflex—H-reflex recovery curves and ratios of initial and subsequent H-reflexes—have also been employed. It remains unclear whether the neurophysiological direction for rootlet section makes a significant difference in outcome as compared with a more random rootlet selection. Part of the problem may be related to lack of standardization of simulation and recording techniques.

The proportion of dorsal rootlets sectioned varies from 25% to 80% in different reports. Complete section of all dorsal rootlets at a given level is generally avoided to preserve sensory function. L5 and S1 are the most frequently abnormal roots. Most reports of outcome have been based on the modified Ashworth scale (discussed earlier). While most surgical series offer favorable outcomes, there is still considerable controversy whether SDR makes a significant contribution to the range of functional motor performance deficits seen in cerebral palsy. Subjective improvements have been noted in range of motion and gait, while difficulties in motor control persist. Intensive therapy appears necessary to maximize long-term functional gains. The most common unwanted postsurgical effects have included hypotonia (usually transitory) and weakness. Sensory changes, bladder dysfunction, and hip subluxation and dislocation have also been reported. There is also concern that a laminectomy in a young child may predispose to later spinal deformity. Most agree that there is great need for a randomized long-term clinical trial in the evaluation of SDR.[53]

Closed rhizotomies are performed under fluoroscopic control utilizing a radiofrequency needle to destroy nerve tissue. Although percutaneous rhizotomies are not permanent, they are highly effective in reducing spastic hypertonia in the lower extremities with minimal morbidity. Recently, microsurgical dorsal-route entry zone selective destruction has been performed for the treatment of spasticity and pain in the lower limbs.[68, 69] However, it is not clear what advantage this procedure offers over selective posterior rhizotomy.

Myelotomy, the severing of tracts in the spinal cord, has been advocated as a treatment modality in the most severe cases of spastic hypertonia.[26, 41, 70] The Bischoff myelotomy interrupts the reflex arc by lesioning the cord through the lateral funiculus on one side, extending through the middle of the cord to traverse through the gray matter on the other side. Only segmental analgesia resulted from the procedure, and all long tracts except the pyramidal tract remained intact. A modification of this procedure was the posterior longitudinal myelotomy, which similarly cut through the gray matter on each side using a T-shaped myelotome via a median sulcus approach. This improvement preserved lateral funiculus white matter tracts bilaterally. Loss of bowel and bladder function must be considered as possible complications of myelotomy. Sectioning (cordotomy) or excision (cordectomy) of portions of the cord causes severe muscle wasting, frequent voiding difficulties, and loss of erectile function and is rarely practiced.

TABLE 29-9   Favorable Selection Criteria for Selective Dorsal Rhizotomy

Pure spasticity (limited dystonia, athetosis)
Function limited primarily by spasticity
Not significantly affected by primitive reflexes or movement patterns
Absence of profound underlying weakness
Selective motor control
Some degree of spontaneous forward locomotion
Adequate truncal balance and righting responses
Spastic diplegia
History of prematurity
Age 3–8 yr
Minimal joint contractures or spine deformity
Adequate cognitive ability to participate in therapy
No significant motivational or behavioral problems
Supportive and interactive family

From MacDonald CM: Selective dorsal rhinotomy. In Katz RT (ed): Spasticity. State of the Art Reviews in Physical Medicine and Rehabilitation, Vol 8. Philadelphia, Hanley & Belfus, 1994.

SUMMARY AND CONCLUSIONS

Spastic hypertonia has been defined as "a motor disorder characterized by a velocity-dependent increase in tonic stretch reflexes (muscle tone) with exaggerated tendon jerks, resulting from hyperexcitability of the stretch reflex, as one component of the upper motor neuron syndrome."[51] Heightened muscle tone may result from changes intrinsic to the muscle or from altered reflex properties. Increased motor neuronal excitability and enhanced stretch-evoked synaptic excitation of motor neurons are mechanisms whereby stretch reflexes can be enhanced.

Two distinct parameters may be altered in the pathological stretch reflex—the "set point," or angular threshold of the stretch reflex, and the reflex "gain," the amount of force required to extend the limb in proportion to the increasing joint angle. Previous studies of spastic hypertonia may be limited by the failure to dissociate the contributions of reflex threshold and reflex gain. Recent investigations suggest that spastic hypertonia may be the result of a decrease in stretch reflex threshold without significant increase in reflex gain, as was previously believed.

Various clinical scales, biomechanical paradigms, pendulum models, and electrophysiological studies have been used to quantify spastic hypertonia. Biomechanical methods seem to correlate most closely with the clinical state. Spastic hypertonia is but one component of the upper motor neuron (UMN) syndrome, whose features also include loss of dexterity, weakness, fatigability, as well as various reflex release phenomena. These other features of the UMN syndrome may well be more disabling to the patient than the changes in muscle tone.

The functional impairment due to spasticity must be carefully assessed before any treatment is considered. Therapeutic intervention is best individualized to the particular patient. The basic principles of treatment to ameliorate spastic hypertonia are (1) avoid noxious stimuli and (2) provide frequent range-of-motion training. Therapeutic exercise, cold, or topical anesthesia may decrease reflex activity for short periods of time to facilitate minimal motor function. Casting and splinting techniques are extremely valuable in extending joint range diminished by hypertonicity.

Baclofen, diazepam, and dantrolene remain the three most commonly used pharmacological agents in the treatment of spastic hypertonia. Baclofen is generally the drug of choice for spinal cord types of spasticity, while sodium dantrolene is the only agent that acts directly on muscle tissue. Tizanidine and ketazolam, not yet available in the United States, may become significant additions to the pharmacological armamentarium. Intrathecal administration of antispastic medications allows high concentrations of drug near the site of action, which limits systemic side effects. This form of treatment is the most exciting recent development in the treatment of spastic hypertonia.

Peripheral electrical stimulation may have limited use in diminishing tone and facilitating paretic muscles. Dorsal column stimulation via electrodes within the spinal column was initially hailed as a therapeutic advance but has subsequently been shown to be minimally effective. Phenol injections provide a valuable transition between short-term and long-term treatments and offer remediation of hypertonia in selected muscle groups.

Tenotomies and tendon transfers offer significant benefit to carefully chosen patients. The SPLATT procedure, transfer of the lateral portion of the anterior tibial tendon to the lateral part of the foot, is one of the most successful rehabilitative surgeries. Hamstring tenotomies, Achilles tendon lengthening, and release of long toe flexors may all benefit selected patients with spastic hypertonia.

Surgical neurectomies can release spastic muscles in selected patient groups. Obturator neurectomies can substantially improve scissoring of gait in cerebral palsy patients. Lesions of spinal roots can decrease hypertonic reflexes; selective rhizotomies are the most invasive treatment but offer the most precise control of neural destruction. While selective dorsal rhizotomies have enjoyed a swell of enthusiasm, especially in children with cerebral palsy, their efficacy remains to be clearly defined. Closed radiofrequency rhizotomies are performed under fluoroscopic guidance but may only have temporary effect.

References

1. Albright AL, Barron WB, Fasick MP, et al: Continuous intrathecal baclofen infusion for spasticity of cerebral origin. JAMA 1993; 270:2475–2477.
2. Anmuth CJ, Esquenazi A, Keenan MAE: Lower extremity surgery for the spastic patient. *In* Katz RT (ed): Spasticity. State of the Art Reviews in Physical Medicine and Rehabilitation, vol 8. Philadelphia, Hanley & Belfus, 1994.
3. Ashworth B: Preliminary trial of carisoprodol in multiple sclerosis. Practitioner 1964; 192:540–542.
4. Basmajian JV: Biofeedback in rehabilitation: a review of principles and practices. Arch Phys Med Rehabil 1981; 62:469–475.
5. Basmajian JV, Shankardass K, Russell D: Ketazolam once daily for spasticity: double-blind cross-over study. Arch Phys Med Rehabil 1986; 67:556–557.
6. Basmajian JV, Shankardass K, Russell D, Yucel V: Ketazolam treatment for spasticity: double-blind study of a new drug. Arch Phys Med Rehabil 1984; 65:698–701.
7. Bohannon RW, Smith MB: Interrater reliability on a modified Ashworth scale of muscle spasticity. Phys Ther 1987; 67:206–207.
8. Booth BJ, Doyle M, Montgomery J: Serial casting for the management of spasticity in the head-injured adult. Phys Ther 1983; 63:1960–1966.
9. Bourbonnais D, VanDen Novin S, Carey K, Rymer WZ: Abnormal spatial patterns of elbow muscle activation in hemiparetic human subjects. Brain 1989; 112:85–102.
10. Bucholz RD: Management of intractable spasticity with intrathecal baclofen. *In* Katz RT (ed): Spasticity. State of the Art Reviews in Physical Medicine and Rehabilitation, vol 8. Philadelphia, Hanley & Belfus, 1994.
11. Castellucci VF, Carew TJ, Kandel ER: Cellular analysis of long-term habituation of the gill withdrawal reflex of *Aplysia californica*. Science 1978; 202:1306–1308.
12. Castellucci VF, Kandel ER: A quantal analysis of the synaptic depression underlying habituation of the gill-withdrawal reflex in *Aplysia*. Proc Natl Acad Sci USA 1974; 71:5004–5008.
13. Chan CWY: Some techniques for the relief of spasticity and their physiological basis. Physiother Can 1986; 38:85–89.
14. Davidoff RA: Antispasticity drugs: mechanisms of action. Ann Neurol 1985; 17:107–116.
15. Delwaide PJ: Electrophysiological testing of spastic patients: its potential usefulness and limitations. *In* Delwaide PJ, Young RR (eds): Clinical Neurophysiology in Spasticity: Contribution to Assessment and Pathophysiology. Amsterdam, Elsevier, 1985.
16. Delwaide PJ: Electrophysiological analysis of the mode of action of muscle relaxants in spasticity. Ann Neurol 1985; 17:90–95.
17. Delwaide PJ, Oliver E: Short-latency autogenic inhibition (IB inhibition) in human spasticity. J Neurol Neurosurg Psychiatry 1988; 51:1546–1550.

18. Delwaide PJ, Schoenen J, De Pasqua V: Lumbosacral spinal evoked potentials in patients with multiple sclerosis. Neurology 1985; 35:174–179.

19. DeWald JPA, Given JD: Electrical stimulation and spasticity reduction: fact or fiction. In Katz RT (ed): Spasticity. State of the Art Review in Physical Medicine and Rehabilitation, vol 8. Philadelphia, Hanley & Belfus, 1994.

20. Dietz V, Berger W: Normal and impaired regulation of muscle stiffness in gait: a new hypothesis about muscle hypertonia. Exp Neurol 1983; 79:680–687.

21. Donovan WH, Carter RE, Rossi D, Wilkerson MA: Clonidine effect on spasticity: a clinical trial. Arch Phys Med Rehabil 1988; 69:193–194.

22. Eisen A: Electromyography in disorders of muscle tone. Can J Neurol Sci 1987; 14:501–505.

23. Erickson DL, Lo J, Michaelson M: Control of intractable spasticity with intrathecal morphine sulfate. Neurosurgery 1989; 24:236–238.

23a. Fisher LM: Athena shaves plunge on rejection of drug. New York Times, March 8, 1995, p C5.

24. Fisher MA: F/M ratios in polyneuropathy and spastic hyperreflexia. Muscle Nerve 1988; 11:217–222.

25. Fugl-Meyer AR, Jaasko L, Leyman I, et al: The post-stroke hemiplegic patient: a method for evaluation of physical performance. Scand J Rehabil Med 1975; 7:13–31.

26. Gildenberg PL: Functional neurosurgery. In Schmidek HH, Sweet WH (eds): Operative Neurosurgical Techniques: Indications, Methods, and Results. New York, Grune & Stratton, 1982, pp 1163–1175.

27. Gilman S, Lieberman JS, Marco LA: Spinal mechanisms underlying the effects of unilateral ablation of areas 4 and 6 in monkeys. Brain 1974; 97:49–64.

28. Glenn M: Nerve blocks. In Katz RT (eds): Spasticity. State of the Art Reviews in Physical Medicine and Rehabilitation, vol 8. Philadelphia, Hanley & Belfus, 1994.

29. Gottlieb GL, Myklebust BM, Stefoski D, et al: Evaluation of cervical stimulation for chronic treatment of spasticity. Neurology 1985; 35:699–704.

30. Grant SM, Heel RC: Vigabatrin: a review of its pharmacodynamic and pharmacokinetic properties and therapeutic potential in epilepsy and disorders of motor control. Drugs 1991; 41:889–926.

31. Hagbarth KE: Exteroceptive, proprioceptive and sympathetic activity recorded with microelectrodes from human peripheral nerves. Mayo Clin Proc 1979; 54:353–364.

32. Halstead LS, Seager SWJ, Houston JM, et al: Relief of spasticity in SCI men and women using rectal probe electrostimulation. Paraplegia 1993; 31:715–721.

33. Hugon M: Methodology of the Hoffman reflex in man. In Desmedt JE (ed): New Developments in Electromyography and Clinical Neurophysiology, vol 3. Basel, Karger, 1973, pp 277–293.

34. Hugon M: A discussion of the methodology of the triceps surae T- and H-reflexes. In Desmedt JE (ed): New Developments in Electromyography and Clinical Neurophysiology, vol 3. Basel, Karger, 1973, pp 773–780.

35. Hultborn H, Meunier S, Morin C, Pierrot-Deseilligny E: Assessing changes in presynaptic inhibition of Ia fibers: a study in man and the cat. J Physiol (Lond) 1987; 389:729–756.

36. Hutchinson DR: Modified release tizanidine: a review. Journal Int Med Res 1989; 17:565–573.

37. Iles JF, Roberts RC: Presynaptic inhibition of monosynaptic reflexes in the lower limbs of subjects with upper motoneuron disease. J Neurol Neurosurg Psychiatry 1986; 49:937–944.

38. Illis LS, Read DJ, Sedgwick EM, Tallis RC: Spinal cord stimulation in the United Kingdom. J Neurol Neurosurg Psychiatry 1983; 46:299–304.

39. Intrathecal baclofen for spasticity. Med Lett Drugs Ther 1994; 36:21–22.

40. Jankovic J, Brin M: Therapeutic uses of botulinum toxin. N Engl J Med 1991; 324:1186–1194.

41. Kasdon DL: Controversies in the surgical management of spasticity. Clin Neurosurg 1986; 33:523–529.

42. Katz RT: Management of spasticity. Am J Phys Med Rehabil 1988; 67:108–116.

43. Katz RT (ed): Spasticity. State of the Art Reviews in Physical Medicine and Rehabilitation, vol 8. Philadelphia, Hanley & Belfus, 1994.

44. Katz RT: Electrophysiological quantification of spastic hypertonia. In Katz RT (ed): Spasticity. State of the Art Reviews in Physical Medicine and Rehabilitation, vol 8. Philadelphia, Hanley & Belfus, 1994.

45. Katz RT, Campagnolo D: Pharmacologic care of the spastic patient. In Katz RT (ed): Spasticity. State of the Art Reviews in Physical Medicine and Rehabilitation, vol 8. Philadelphia, Hanley & Belfus, 1994.

46. Katz RT, Rovai G, Brait C, Rymer WZ: Objective quantification of spastic hypertonia: correlation with clinical findings. Arch Phys Med Rehabil 1992; 73:339–347.

47. Katz RT, Rymer WZ: Spastic hypertonia: mechanisms and measurement. Arch Phys Med Rehabil 1989; 70:144–155.

48. Keenan MA, Kozin S, Berlet A: Manual of Orthopaedic Surgery for Spasticity. New York, Raven Press, 1993.

49. Knutsson E: Studies of gait control in patients with spastic paresis. In Felman RG, Young RR, Koella WP (eds): Spasticity: Disordered Motor Control. St Louis, Mosby–Year Book, 1980.

50. Kofler M, Donovan WH, Loubser PG, Beric A: Effects of intrathecal baclofen on lumbosacral and cortical somatosensory evoked potentials. Neurology 1992; 42:864–868.

51. Lance JW: Symposium synopsis. In Feldman RG, Young RR, Koella WP (eds): Spasticity: Disordered Motor Control. St Louis, Mosby–Year Book, 1980.

52. Lance JW, McLeod JG: Disordered muscle tone. In Physiological Approach to Clinical Neurology. Boston, Butterworth, 1981.

53. Landau WM, Hunt CC: Dorsal rhizotomy, a treatment of unproven efficacy. J Child Neurol 1990; 5:174–178.

54. Lee WA, Boughton A, Rymer WZ: Absence of stretch reflex gain enhancement in voluntarily activated spastic muscle. Exp Neurol 1987; 98:317–335.

55. MacDonald CM: Selective dorsal rhizotomy. In Katz RT (ed): Spasticity. State of the Art Reviews in Physical Medicine and Rehabilitation, vol 8. Philadelphia, Hanley & Belfus, 1994.

56. Milanov I: Mechanisms of tetrazepam action on spasticity. Acta Neurol Belg 1992; 92:5–15.

57. Mondrup K, Pedersen E: The clinical effect of the GABA-agonist, progabide, on spasticity. Acta Neurol Scand 1984; 69:200–206.

58. Ochs G, Struppler A, Meyerson BA, et al: Intrathecal baclofen for long-term treatment of spasticity: a multi-centre study. J Neurol Neurosurg Psychiatry 1989; 52:933–939.

59. Otis JC, Root L, Kroll MA: Measurement of plantar flexor spasticity during treatment with tone-reducing casts. J Pediatr Orthop 1985; 5:682–686.

60. Penn RD, Savoy SM, Corcos D, et al: Intrathecal baclofen for severe spinal spasticity. N Engl J Med 1989; 320:1517–1521.

61. Pierrot-Deseilligny E: Electrophysiological assessment of the spinal mechanisms underlying spasticity. Electroencephalogr Clin Neurophysiol 1990; 41(suppl):264–273.

62. Pinzur MS: Upper extremity surgery for the spastic patient. In Katz RT (ed): Spasticity. State of the Art Reviews in Physical Medicine and Rehabilitation, vol 8. Philadelphia, Hanley & Belfus, 1994.

63. Powers RK, Campbell DL, Rymer WZ: Stretch reflex dynamics in spastic elbow flexor muscles. Ann Neurol 1989; 25:32–42.

64. Powers RK, Marder-Meyer J, Rymer WZ: Quantitative relations between hypertonia and stretch reflex threshold in spastic hemiparesis. Ann Neurol 1988; 23:115–124.

65. Rack PMH, Ross HF, Thilman F: The ankle stretch reflexes in normal and spastic subjects. Brain 1984; 107:637–654.

66. Rodin BE, Sampogna SL, Kruger L: An examination of intraspinal sprouting in dorsal root axons with the tracer horseradish peroxidase. J Comp Neurol 1983; 215:187–198.

67. Rymer WZ, Houk JC, Crago PE: Mechanisms of the clasp-knife reflex studied in an animal model. Exp Brain Res 1979; 37:93–113.

68. Sindou M, Jeanmonod D: Microsurgical DREZ-otomy for the treatment of spasticity and pain in the lower limbs. Neurosurgery 1989; 24:655–670.

69. Sindou M, Keravel Y: Microsurgical procedures in the peripheral nerves and the dorsal root entry zone for the treatment of spasticity. Scand J Rehabil Med 1988; 17:139–143.

70. Sindou M, Pregelj R, Boisson D, et al: Surgical selective lesions of nerve fibers and myelotomies for modifying muscle hypertonia. In Eccles J, Dimitrijevic MR (eds): Recent Achievements in Restorative Neurology: Upper Motor Neuron Function and Dysfunction. Basel, Karger, 1985.

71. Snow BJ, Tsui JKC, Bhatt MH, et al: Treatment of spasticity with botulinum toxin: a double blind study. Ann Neurol 1990; 28:512–515.

72. Thilmann AF, Burke DJ, Rymer WZ, eds: Spasticity: Mechanisms and Management. Berlin, Springer-Verlag, 1993.

73. Thompson FJ, Reier PJ, Lucas CC, Parmer R: Altered patterns of reflex excitability subsequent to contusion injury of the rat spinal cord. J Neurophysiol 1992; 68:1473–1486.

74. Turski L, Jacobsen P, Honore T, Stephens D: Relief of experimental spasticity and anxiolytic/anticonvulsant actions of the alpha-amino-3-hydroxy-5-methyl-4-isoxazolepropionate antagonist 2,3-dihydroxy-6-nitro-7 sulfamoyl-benzo(F) quinoxaline. J Pharmacol Exp Ther 1992; 260:742–747.

74a. Wallace JD: Summary of combined clinical analysis of controlled clinical trials with tizanidine. Neurology 1994; 44(suppl 9):S60–S69.

75. Wartenberg R: Pendulousness of the legs as a diagnostic test. Neurology 1951; 1:18–24.

76. Weingarden SI, Belen JG: Clonidine transdermal system for treatment of spasticity in spinal cord injury. Arch Phys Med Rehabil 1992; 73:876–877.

77. Whyte J, Robinson KM: Pharmacologic management. *In* Glenn M, Whyte J (eds): The Practical Management of Spasticity in Children and Adults. Philadelphia, Lea & Febiger, 1990.

78. Wolf SL, Binder-MacLeod SA: Electromyographic biofeedback appli-
cations to the hemiplegic patient: changes in upper extremity neuromuscular and functional status. Phys Ther 1983; 63:1393–1413.

79. Wood KM: The use of phenol as a neurolytic agent. Pain 1978; 5:205–229.

80. Yarkony GM, Roth EJ, Cybulski G, Jaeger RJ: Neuromuscular stimulation in spinal cord injury. Arch Phys Med Rehabil 1992; 73:78–86, 195–200.

80a. Young RR (ed): Role of tizanidine in the treatment of spasticity. Neurology 1994; 44(suppl 9):S1–S80.

81. Young RR, Shahani BT: Spasticity in spinal cord injured patients. *In* Bloch RF, Basbaum M (eds): Management of Spinal Cord Injuries. Baltimore, Williams & Wilkins, 1986.

Acknowledgments

W. Zev Rymer, M.D., Ph.D., Professor of Physiology, Physical Medicine and Rehabilitation, and Biomedical Engineering at Northwestern University Medical School, Chicago, offered extensive guidance in the preparation of the sections on pathophysiology and the biomechanical quantification of spastic hypertonia.

30

Sexuality Issues in Persons With Disabilities

DIANE M.-L. GILBERT, M.D.

A virtually universal concern of rehabilitation patients, regardless of their impairment, is the impact of their disability on their sexual function and sexuality. It is not uncommon for patients, upon grasping the seriousness of their disability, to experience significant—albeit, often unexpressed—anxiety over the prospects for their sexual life. Yet, despite the ubiquity of patient sexual concerns, medical schools pay little attention to training physicians in methods of patient sexual education. As early as 1900, Lewis chided his colleagues for this oversight and urged reform: "It is, therefore, proper for medical men, in their deliberations, to take cognizance of this great factor in human life. They should know its relationship to health and happiness. They should not be deterred from its scientific investigation by false modesty or by the fear of being accused of sensationalism."[53] Ende et al.[33] noted that physicians generally report discomfort in discussing sexual issues with their patients. Teal and Athelstan[95] reported that 65% of patients with spinal cord injuries (SCIs) did not discuss sex with anyone during their acute hospitalization and that 85% did not discuss these matters with their physician. Since physiatrists value holistic functional return to independence, they are remiss when they omit this area in the rehabilitation program.

This chapter serves as an introduction to sexual functioning and sexuality in persons with disabilities and discusses new research developments. It should be noted from the outset that the emphasis in this chapter is on "sexual intercourse," defined broadly as communication involving sexual self-expression and associated pleasuring, with or without genital involvement, to which everyone is entitled (Fig. 30–1). When sexuality is viewed from this encompassing perspective, it becomes apparent what a vital part knowledge in this area plays in developing the rehabilitation team's care plan and how important it is to incorporate discussions on the subject of sexual issues in that plan. The first section concentrates on *sexual function*, with a summary of normal function and a detailed coverage of

the many changes that accompany impairments. The second section deals with the impact of impairment on the *sexuality* of the patient, with emphasis on the idea that sexuality is not confined to the performance of sex acts but rather involves a much broader concept of identity and self-

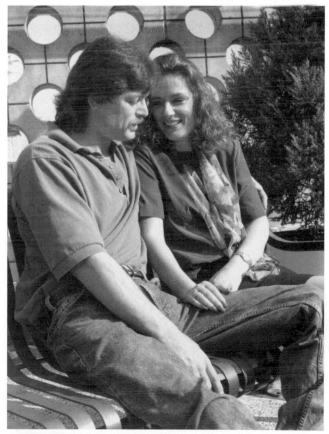

FIGURE 30–1 Sexuality is a form of communication to which all are entitled.

image. The third section is devoted to the actual interaction between the rehabilitation team and the patient with the *process of assessment and recommendation for sexual satisfaction (PARSS)*. The goal of this chapter is to familiarize any member of a rehabilitation team with the common sexual concerns faced by patients and to provide a guide to better care in this often-neglected area.

SEXUAL FUNCTION

Anatomy and Physiology

NORMAL. Masters and Johnson have described four phases of sexual response: excitement, plateau, orgasm, and resolution[58] (Table 30–1; Figs. 30–2 and 30–3). Arousal or excitement occurs at multiple levels using the various senses: vision, smell, hearing, memory, fantasy, and touch. Men's arousal pattern is more direct than women's, usually ending with climax. Women have varying patterns with prolonged plateau phases: no climax, single climax, or multiple climaxes (Fig. 30–3). Although our focus is on sexual physiological changes, sexual education must include other important issues. Knowledge of sexually transmitted diseases and their prevention, and fertility issues such as birth control, should be an integral part of the curriculum.

EXCITEMENT OR AROUSAL. The neurological components of the sexual response are summarized in Figure 30–4, while Figure 30–5 delineates the vascular anatomy. Excitement or arousal occurs in response to sexual stimulation either due to touch (reflexogenic) or imagination (psychogenic). In the male, the normal result is an erection and in the female, vaginal lubrication, swelling of the labia, and clitoral erection. This phase may last several minutes to hours.

The brain is the most important sexual organ in the body, with multiple loci responsible for sexual activity. Considering the importance of sexual function to species survival, it is not surprising that the cerebral tissue that results in erection and vaginal lubrication is related to the brain's phylogenetically oldest area, the limbic system.[43] Psychogenic stimuli can be both facilitory or inhibitory, and the degree of tactile stimulation necessary to produce reflex lubrication or erection can be diminished by psychic stimulation.[111] Libido is affected by concentrations of neurotransmitters, and is decreased by serotonin or stimulated by dopamine.[9] Libido is affected by depression and medications affecting the neurotransmitters[31] (Table 30–2).

The old acronym for sexual function was "*point and shoot*," where the *p* stands for the *p*arasympathetics required for *p*ointing or erections, while *s* stands for *s*ympathetics required for *s*hooting or ejaculation. Research demonstrates this is no longer an accurate description of the neurological innervation. Reflexogenic erections are those mediated via sensory input elicited by direct stimulation of the genital area through the sensory fibers of the dorsal nerve through the pudendal nerve to the sacral spinal cord. The sacral parasympathetic (S2–S4) response travels via the nervi erigentes to the cavernosal nerves and into the corporal trabeculae via autonomic fibers[111] (see Fig. 30–4). Psychogenic erections are believed to originate in the cerebral cortex through the different senses such as visual stimuli like movies, pictures, or fantasizing. The impulses producing psychogenic erection travel through the hypothalamic and thalamic centers to the sympathetic thoracolumbar cord and the parasympathetic sacral cord. Supraspinal mechanisms are complex and can facilitate or inhibit erections.[49, 111]

Many studies have been done documenting the type and frequency of erections in spinal cord–injured males[13] (Table 30–3). The phenomenon of psychogenic erections seen in paraplegics with reported complete lower motor neuron lesions and abolished reflexogenic erections indicated that pathways for erection from the sympathetic outflow exist.[111] An animal model using cats demonstrates the sympathetic outflow. Cats whose sacral cord was resected were still able to attain erection in the presence of female cats in estrus. There is sympathetic discharge to genitals as long as there is no disruption above L2 (T11–L2).[49] It was postulated that the erections in the 26% of patients with complete lower motor neuron lesions studied by Comarr (see Table 30–3) were possible because sympathetic nerves mediate erections.[49] This theory is supported by Whitelaw's study showing a 63% incidence of impotence after sympathectomies, although many patients were older men with vascular disease which could have explained the impotence.[49] On the other hand, Kedia et al.[46] studied young males status post retroperitoneal lymph node dissection, including bilateral sympathetic chains, and only rarely found impotence.

The sympathetic pathways involved in male erections have been intensively studied.[82] In the penile flaccid state, tonic sympathetic discharge (probably postsynaptic α-receptors) causes contraction of the smooth muscles of the penile arterioles and sinusoids which keeps blood from entering the corpora cavernosa.[1] The final common pathway for hemodynamic control in erections appears to be short adrenergic nerves, which release norepinephrine and act on β-receptors resulting in increased blood flow by modulation of corporal smooth muscle tone. The predominant theory of venous outflow occlusion is passive venoocclusion as the sinusoids dilate and the trabecular walls are forced against the tunica albuginea[5, 63] (see Fig. 30–5). There is little evidence to support the role of only *thoracolumbar* sympathetic outflow in erection development and in retrospect, the previously mentioned potent 26% in Comarr's study might have had imcomplete lesions.[49] Erections are now believed to occur only rarely with complete lower motor neuron lesions.

PLATEAU. The plateau phase can be very brief (seconds) or prolonged (minutes) and is described as a pleasurable sense of well-being.[58] A number of sexual dysfunctions can occur in this stage. With *anorgasmy* the individual does not progress further than the plateau stage. *Premature ejaculation* refers to emission or ejaculation that is accompanied by loss of erection before or immediately upon vaginal penetration.

EJACULATION. Male ejaculation requires a coordinated series of muscular and neurophysiological events, involving the sympathetics, parasympathetics, and somatic nervous supply, that cause the constituents of the ejaculate to be deposited in the posterior urethra, then evacuated through the urethra and urethral meatus in an antegrade

TABLE 30–1   Physiological Changes Seen in Men and Women During Sexual Activity

	Phases			
	I. Excitement	**II. Plateau**	**III. Orgasm**	**IV. Resolution**
Description	Occurs in response to sexual stimulation either due to touch (reflexogenic) or imagination (psychogenic) in both female and male	The high level of sexual arousal that precedes the threshold levels required to trigger orgasm	Believed to be a cortical experience; seems to be mainly dependent upon intactness of sensation associated with muscles of ejaculation	Return to prearousal state over a period of 5–15 min
Duration	May be seconds, minutes, or hours	2 min to a much more prolonged duration	10–20 sec	Depends on length of excitement phase and sensory stimulation
Cardiovascular	HR and BP increase	HR continues to increase (110–175), as does BP (SBP up 20–80 mm Hg, and DBP up 10–40 mm Hg); RR begins to rise; hyperventilation begins	HR: 110–180; BP: SBP increases 40–100 mm Hg; RR: 40	RR, HR, and BP return to normal; one third of men and women have perspiratory reaction of soles of feet, palms of hands, or entire body
FEMALE				
Skin	No change	Sexual flush: inconstant; may appear on abdomen, breasts, neck, face, thighs	No change	Flush disappears in reverse order
Breasts	Nipple erection, venous congestion, areolar enlargement	Venous pattern prominent; size may increase one fourth over resting state; areolae enlarge, impinge on nipples so they seem to disappear	No change	Return to normal
Clitoris	Glans diameter increased; shaft: variable increase in diameter; elongation occurs in only 10% of subjects	Retraction: shaft withdraws deep into swollen prepuce	No change (shaft movements continue throughout if thrusting maintained)	Shaft returns to normal position in 5–10 sec; full detumescence in 5–10 min
Labia majora	Nullipara: thin down, flatten against perineum	Nullipara: may swell if phase II unduly prolonged	No change	Nullipara: increase to normal size in 1–2 min or less; multipara: decrease to normal in 10–15 min
Labia minora	Color change: bright pink in nullipara and red in multipara; size: increase 2–3 times normal	Color change: bright red in nullipara, burgundy red in multipara; size: enlarged labia form a funnel into vaginal orifice	Proximal areas contract with contractions of lower third	Return to resting state in 5 min
Vagina	Transudate appears 10–30 sec after onset of arousal; drops of clear fluid coalesce to form a well-lubricated vaginal barrel	Copious transudate can continue to form; quantity of transudate generally increased by prolonging preorgasm stimulation	No change	Some transudate collects on floor of upper two thirds formed by its posterior wall (in supine position)
Upper two thirds	Balloons: dilates as uterus moves up, pulling anterior vaginal wall with it; fornices lengthen; rugae flatten	Further ballooning occurs, then wall relaxes in a slow tensionless manner	No change; fully ballooned-out and motionless	Cervix descends to seminal pool in 3–4 min
Lower one third	Dilation of vaginal lumen occurs; congestion of walls proceeds gradually	Maximum distention reached rapidly; contracts lumen of lower third; contraction around penis aids thrusting traction on clitoral shaft via labia and prepuce	3–15 contractions of lower third and proximal labia minora at 0.75-sec intervals	Congestion disappears in seconds (if no orgasm, congestion persists for 20–30 min)
Uterus	Ascends into false pelvis in phase I	Contractions: strong sustained contractions begin late in phase II	Contractions strong throughout orgasm; strongest with pregnancy and masturbation	Slowly returns to normal position
Rectum			Inconstant rhythmic contractions	All reactions cease within a few seconds

Table continued on following page

TABLE 30–1   Physiological Changes Seen in Men and Women During Sexual Activity *Continued*

	Phases			
	I. Excitement	**II. Plateau**	**III. Orgasm**	**IV. Resolution**
MALE				
Physiology	Coordinated interaction of nervous, arterial, venous, and sinusoidal systems[1] Need intact neuronal innervation, intact arterial supply, appropriately responsive corporal smooth muscle, and intact venous mechanics[109] Exact nature of venous control still not clear Phases of erection 1. Flaccid phase 2. Latent (filling) phase 3. Tumescent phase 4. Full erection phase 5. Skeletal or rigid erection phase (elicit BCB reflex) 6. Detumescent phase[1]	*Ejaculation*—SNS, PS, and somatic systems involved synchronously *Emission* of semen Prostatic secretions, sperm from distal vas deferens and ampulla expressed through ejaculatory ducts Traverse the prostatic urethra posteriorly and join the fructose-rich contents of the seminal vesicles Development of a pressure chamber in the posterior urethra Expulsion of ejaculate through the urethra with contractions of periurethral and pelvic floor muscles[18] *Orgasm*—the sensory appreciation of this muscle response		Back to baseline *Refractory period* Time period immediately after ejaculation when further ejaculation cannot occur but erection may occur Length of period varies and tends to increase with age
Skin	No change	Sexual flush; inconsistently appears on abdomen and spreads to chest, face, and neck; can include shoulders and forearms	Widely spread flush if present, persists	Flush disappears in reverse order of appearance
Penis	Erection within 10–30 sec	Increase in size of glans and diameter of penile shaft; deepened coronal and glans coloration	Ejaculation: marked by 3–4 major contractions at 0.8-sec intervals followed by minor contractions	Partial involution of erection in 5–10 sec with variable refractory period; complete detumescence in 5–30 min
Scrotum and testes	Elevation of testes toward perineum and tightening and lifting of scrotal sac	Marked increase in size of testes over unstimulated state due to vasocongestion	No change	Return to normal size due to loss of vasocongestion; testicular and scrotal descent within 5–30 min
Other	Inconsistent nipple erection	A preejaculate of a few drops of mucoid fluid which may contain viable sperm; this is not the ejaculate	Partial loss of voluntary muscular control along with ejaculation; rhythmic contractions of rectal sphincter may be noted	Return to quiescent state in 5–10 min

Abbreviations: HR, heart rate; BP, blood pressure; SBP, systolic blood pressure; DBP, diastolic blood pressure; RR, respiratory rate; BCB, bulbocavernosus reflex; SNS, sympathetic nervous system; PS, parasympathetic system.
Adapted from Masters WH, Johnson VE, Kolodny RC: Human Sexuality. Boston, Little, Brown, 1982.

fashion. It is generally agreed that no anatomical sphincter exists within the posterior urethra in the area of the bladder neck, but rather the neck has inherent tension in postpubertal males which is augmented during ejaculation by sympathetic input to prevent retrograde flow.[69] The tension corresponds to the sense of inevitability of ejaculation where cerebral control is minimal, described by Masters et al.[58] Emission and ejaculation are reflexive and can occur independently, and erection is not an absolute prerequisite. The emission center of the cord is T10 to L2, and Sato et al.[84] have proposed three routes for the efferent signal transmission for seminal emission from the L1 paravertebral sympathetic ganglion. They are through the hypogastric nerves, sympathetic nerve fibers through the lumbosacral sympathetic trunk, or through the spermatic nerves.[18]

Female ejaculation is not an easily quantifiable response as is the male norm, and remains a more controversial subject. When it occurs, the ejaculate has been traced to the motor response of the above and the anterior portion of the vagina (G-spot). Vaginal transudate accumulates throughout the arousal process and can give the appearance of an ejaculate.

ORGASM. Orgasm is believed to be a cortical experience of "supreme pleasure followed by a feeling of well-being and satiation."[112] It occurs in the limbic system. In the majority of men, orgasm seems to be dependent on intactness of sensation associated with the muscles of ejaculation. That orgasm can be experienced separate from ejaculation is very important in those with ejaculatory disorders. The relatively long waiting period between ejaculations for men is related to the time required to build up seminal ejaculate. Intensity of orgasms varies from person to person and often from each encounter to the next. Women have described orgasm on a continuum from

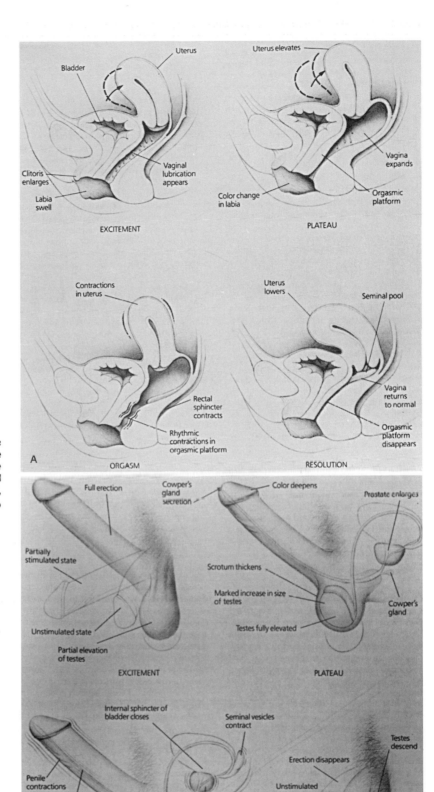

FIGURE 30–2 *A,* Internal changes in the female sexual response cycle (explained in detail in Table 30–1). *B,* External and internal changes in the male sexual response cycle (explained in detail in Table 30–1). (From Masters WH, Johnson VE, Kolodny RC: Human Sexuality Boston, Little, Brown, 1982, pp 60–61.)

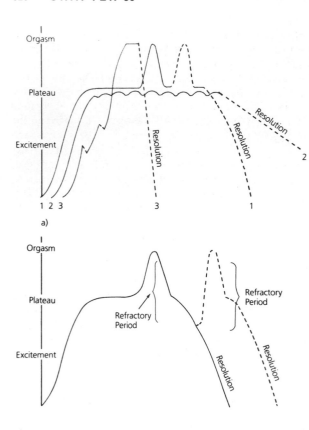

FIGURE 30–3 The sexual phases of men and women as described by Masters and Johnson: excitement, plateau, orgasm, and resolution. (From Masters WH, Johnson VE, Kolodny RC: Human Sexuality. Boston, Little, Brown, 1982, p 58.)

TABLE 30–2   Sexual Dysfunction Side Effects Associated with Medication

Medication	Gender	Type of Sexual Dysfunction
Cardiovascular agents		
Chlorothiazide	M	Impotence, failed ejaculation
Clonidine	M	Impotence in ~24%
Guanethidine	M/F	Diminished libido, dose-related
	M	Delayed ejaculation, libido impairment, potency impairment, retrograde ejaculation
Hydrochlorothiazide	M/F	Decreased erection in ~9%; in combination with β-blockers, 23%
Labetalol	M	Changes in erection, delayed tumescence, delayed ejaculation, priapism
Methyldopa	M/F	Sedation, depression, sexual dysfunction in ~32%
Prazosin	M	Priapism
Propranolol	M	Decreased potency, impotence, failed ejaculation
	M/F	Decreased libido
Reserpine	M	Impotence, failed ejaculation, dose-related in ~60%
Spironolactone	M	Gynecomastia, impotence
	F	Menstrual irregularity
Digoxin	M/F	Decreased libido and arousal
Psychotherapeutic agents		
Phenothiazine, MAO, TCA	M/F	Sedation, anticholinergic, sympatholytic
Serotonin uptake inhibitors	M/F	Decreased libido; impotence/anorgasmia
Lithium, diazepam	M/F	Sedation, decreased libido
Anxiolytics	M/F	Decreased libido/anorgasmia
Other		
Phenytoin	M/F	Decreased libido
Cimetidine	M	Impotence
Naproxen	M	Impaired ejaculation
Alcohol	M/F	Prominent libido suppression, impotence, dysfunction with orgasm, relationship problems
Tobacco	M	Impotence
Marijuana	M/F	Delayed orgasm
Cocaine, heroin	M/F	Autonomic dysfunction with excessive use

Abbreviations: MAO, monoamine oxidase inhibitor; TCA, tricyclic antidepressant.

Data from Deamer RL, Thompson JF: The role of medications in geriatric sexual function. Clin Geriatric Med 1991; 7:95–111; Murphy JB, Lipshultz LI: Abnormalities of ejaculation. Urol Clin North Am 1987; 14:583–595; Relf MV: Sexuality and the older bypass patient. Geriatr Nurs 1991; 34:294–296; Seidl A, Bullough B, Haughey B, et al: Understanding the effects of a myocardial infarction on sexual functioning: A basis for sexual counseling. Rehabil Nurs 1991; 16:255–264.

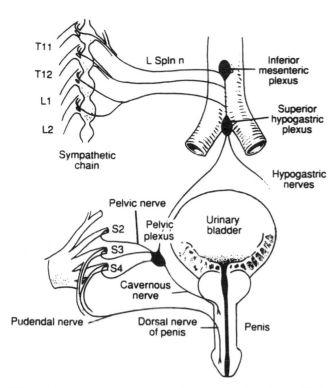

FIGURE 30–4 Summary of neurological sexual anatomy. Parasympathetic innervation: originates in the anterior divisions of spinal roots S2 to S4; preganglionic fibers enter the pelvis as the nervi erigentes or pelvic nerves course in close proximity to the hypogastric vessels, terminating in the pelvic plexus; cavernous nerve then travels to the corpora, and other fibers to the scrotum and pubis. Sympathetic innervation: T10 to L2 supply the sympathetic fibers to the penis and female genitalia; preganglionic fibers course to the superior hypogastric plexus, join the pelvic plexus via the hypogastric nerves, and travel via the cavernous nerve to the genitalia; postganglionic nerves in the hypogastric nerves travel to the vas deferens, seminal vesicle, ampulla, bladder neck, musculature of the prostate, and blood vessels of the prostate and penis. Somatic innervation: pudendal nerve is formed from the anterior divisions of S2 to S4; it supplies both sensory innervation (to penis, scrotum, and pubis) and motor innervation (to bulbocavernosus, ischiocavernosus, striated urethral sphincter, and perineal muscles). (From Melman A, Christ GJ, Hirsch MS: Anatomy and physiology of the penis. In Bennett AH (ed): Impotence: Diagnosis and Management of Erectile Dysfunction. Philadelphia, WB Saunders, 1994, p 21.)

a "mild stimulation [to] a sensation of ecstasy so overwhelming that a [woman] momentarily loses consciousness."[112] The muscles involved in orgasm produce a biphasic motor response involving sympathetic contraction of the smooth muscles of the fallopian tubes, uterus, and paraurethral glands of Skene; somatic contraction of striated pelvic floor muscles; perineum; and anal sphincter.

RESOLUTION. Resolution is the return to the prearousal physiological state usually occurring over a period of 5 to 15 minutes (see Table 30–1). Sympathetic tonic discharge resumes in the penis, resulting in contraction of the smooth muscles around the sinusoids and arterioles. Arterial blood flow is decreased and venous channels are reopened.[1] Presumably, the analogous situation occurs in the female.

NORMAL AGE-RELATED PHYSIOLOGICAL CHANGES. These occur in women most dramatically at the onset of menopause when the relative steroid deficit reduces the

rapidity and intensity of the physiological sexual response. There is a decrease in the frequency of vaginal and uterine contraction during orgasm.[38] The vaginal canal becomes thinner and shorter secondary to decreased estrogen. Lubrication diminishes or takes longer, and nonpetroleum-based lubricating jelly can be helpful. There is an increased incidence of vulvovaginitis and urethritis, atrophy of the external genitals, changes in the size of the clitoris and labia, and loss of pubic hair. These changes are greatly ameliorated in women using estrogen replacement.[56] Prolapse and stress incontinence are also seen in multiparous aging women but they can be managed well surgically. Changes seen in men are summarized in Table 30–4.[45, 85, 105]

Changes With Impairments

From a physiological point of view, normal sexual function depends on the interaction of libido and potency.[47] *Sexual dysfunction* can be defined as any sexual behavioral problem that makes sexual expression consistently unsatisfying for the individual or partner (Table 30–5).[86] Eighty percent of sexual complaints can be successfully managed in the office setting.[47] The sudden onset of disability or the more chronic issues of malaise, pain, fatigue, or stress can contribute to decreased libido.

Sixty percent of all male sexual dysfunction at a performance level is physical in origin and this dysfunction increases with age. Dysfunction is most common in patients with diabetes, circulatory changes, autonomic nervous disorders, venous leakages or arteriovenous shunting, alcoholism, or from effects of medications.[28] Sadoughi et al.[91] studied 34 males and 21 females with emphysema, arthritis, stroke, and amputation. Disability related physical limitations were the most frequently cited reasons for fear and feelings of discomfort in carrying out sexual activity, with 78% reporting a decline in frequency of sexual activity, and greater than 50% reporting a change in pattern. Thirty-six percent desired more satisfaction, and 42% believed their spouses presently desired more sexual satisfaction. Just as in spinal cord–injured patients, 50% would have liked to discuss sexual problems with a member of the hospital staff prior to discharge, preferably with a physician of the same sex.[81]

SPINAL CORD–INJURED. Spinal cord–injured patients constitute less than 5% of a typical physiatrist's practice, but much of the sexuality literature in rehabilitation has focused on this subset of patients. This is probably due to the fact that function is greatly changed in SCI patients and more than half are 15 to 25 years old (a time of great sexual awareness). The 15% of SCI patients who are female have unfortunately been largely ignored in the literature. In a recent survey of female SCI patients, only 37% indicated they had received information on sexual issues since their injury.[107] For a more detailed look at SCI, I refer the reader to the excellent reviews by Linsenmeyer and Perkash,[54] Yarkony,[111] Sipski and Alexander[87] (men), Bérard,[6] Charlifue et al.[23] (women) and Rabin.[77]

Neurological injury can affect either upper motor neurons (e.g., quadriplegia) or lower motor neurons (e.g., cauda equina). These lesions usually involve motor and sensory pathways, and the patient has to deal with motor weakness, loss of sensation, and changes in erection or

ARTERIAL SUPPLY

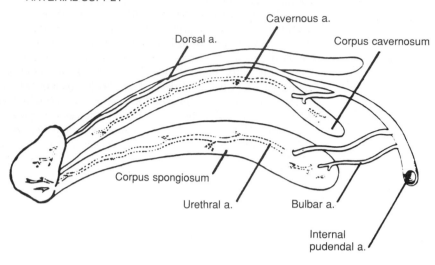

VENOUS RETURN

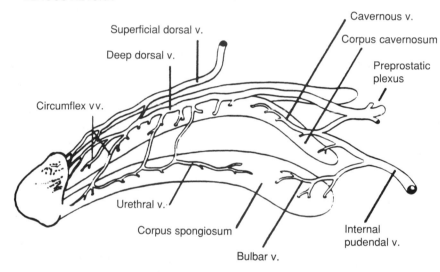

FIGURE 30–5 There are four paired *arteries*: (1) *dorsal*, which supply the glans; (2) *cavernosa* (corporal), which are responsible for tumescence; (3) *spongiosal* (ventral), which supply the spongiosa, urethral tissue, and glans; and (4) *bulbar*, which supply the Cowper's gland and proximal urethral bulb. The *venous system* is composed of the superficial, intermediate, and deep systems. (From Aboseif SR, Lue TF: Hemodynamics of penile erection. Urol Clin North Am 1988; 15:2.)

lubrication, ejaculation, orgasm, and fertility. Incomplete lesions might spare some sexual function, but genital sensation is lost with injury to the spinal cord above S2. Males with complete lower motor neuron disease involving the S2 to S4 segments (i.e., cauda equina) will have poor erectile function as the S2 to S4 reflex arc is interrupted. The motor deficits can interfere with mobility and impair social contact, both of which can affect sexual function.

After SCI, previous erogenous zones may now be insensate, which can affect the excitement phase. The demarcation between insensate and sensate skin may become the new erogenous zone. Incomplete SCI patients often have erogenous sensation in the perianal area, but cultural attitudes towards anal stimulation can prevent patients from benefiting from this erogenous area.[12] Patients must be encouraged to experiment with their bodies to learn and understand the new changes and effectively communicate their needs to their partners.

Achieving Erection. Reflexogenic erections can occur with stroking, oral stimulation, vibration, pulling pubic

hair, or a full bladder. The degree of stimulation required may decrease or increase with psychogenic stimulation. The genitals might need continuous physical stimulation to maintain their arousal. Experimentation is encouraged to discover individual stimulation techniques. Education by the staff can help prevent uncomfortable or embarrassing situations, such as when a male patient has an erection while a nurse performs a bladder catherization. Psychogenic erections can occur with incomplete lower motor neuron lesions, as previously described. The importance of a secure, private location for the patient's experimentation must be emphasized.

The results of several large studies on erectile functioning after SCI help predict what can be expected with various SCI levels. These studies should be viewed with caution since the studies generally relied on patient report[111] (see Table 30–3). Psychogenic erections are typically lost with lesions between T10 and T12 while both reflexogenic and psychogenic erections are possible with lesions between L2 and S1. Talbot[94] reported that erections (both

TABLE 30–3 Erectile Functioning After Spinal Cord Injury: Observations in Several Large Series

Study*	Subjects	Overall (%)	Reflex (%)	Psycho-genic (%)	C-T (%)	L-S (%)
Munro, 1949	84	74			83	50
Talbot, 1949	200	64	43	21	75	53
Kuhn, 1950†	25	88			88	
Talbot, 1955	208	69	49	20	75	60
Comarr, 1977‡	679	80	73	7	73§	31¶
Zeitlin, 1957	100	86			86	86

From Yarkony GM: Enhancement of sexual function and fertility in spinal cord–injured males. Am J Phys Med Rehabil 1990; 69:81–87.

*Munro D, Horne HW, Paull DP: N Engl J Med 1948; 239:903; Talbot HS: Sexual function in paraplegia. J Urol 1955; 73:91–100; Kuhn RA: Functional capacity of the isolated human spinal cord. Brain 1950; 73:1–51; Zeitlin AB, Cottrell TL, Lloyd FA: Fertil Steril 1957; 8:337.

†All T2–T12.

‡Summary of reference 13 and Comarr AE: Sexual function in patients with spinal cord injury. In Pierce PS, Nickel VH (eds): The Total Care of Spinal Cord Injury. Boston, Little, Brown, 1977, pp 171–185.

§Upper motor neuron lesions all reflexogenic.

¶Lower motor neuron lesions all psychogenic.

Abbreviations: C-T, cervicothoracic; L-S, lumbosacral.

types) are most common in males with injury levels higher than T11, and those with incomplete lesions. Kuhn[50] found that erections could always be induced if there was reflex activity (bulbocavernosus reflex) below the lesion level. There is a sharply circumscribed reflexogenic area on the penis which includes the corona of the glans and the penile frenulum.[111]

Patients should be evaluated carefully and individually to assess their deficits. The evaluation should follow the PARSS model (see later) with a thorough history and

TABLE 30–4 Normal Age-Related Physiological Changes in Men

Phase	Change
Excitement	Develop erections 2–3 times slower than younger men
	Tactile stimulation may be necessary
	Erection is not as firm, approaches full ridigity only seconds before ejaculation
Plateau	Able to maintain erection for longer period prior to ejaculation
	Less discernible nipple swelling and erection
	Testicular elevation is reduced
Ejaculation/orgasm	Ejaculation lacks the well-defined sense of impending orgasm because accessory organs fail to secrete and create the welling of semen in the prostatic urethra
	One to two expulsive contractions of the urethra occur instead of the usual four major contractions
	Seepage can occur rather than expulsion, which diminishes the sensation through the urethra
Resolution	More rapid detumescence
	Refractory period increases in length (>55 yr ~12–24 hr)

Adapted from Kaiser FE: Sexuality and impotence in the aging man. Clin Geriatr Med 1991; 7:63–71; Schiavi RC, Schreiner-Engel P, Mandeli J, et al: Healthy aging and male sexual function. Am J Psychiatry 1990; 147:766–771; Weiss JN, Mellinger BC: Sexual dysfunction in elderly men. Clin Geriatr Med 1990; 6:185–196; LoPiccolo J: Counseling and therapy for sexual problems in the elderly. Clin Geriatr Med 1991; 7:161–179.

general neurological examination. Patients with bilateral sphincterotomies have a 2% to 56% incidence of erectile dysfunction while those with the more recent anteromedian sphincterotomy approach have less than a 5% incidence.[110] Neurogenic causes of erectile dysfunction can be confirmed by testing with vasoactive substances injected into the corpora. During the period of spinal shock, which can last from a few hours to several weeks, it is impossible to predict sexual impairment. In all deliberations regarding sexual function, it is important to note that function might not return for 6 to 24 months (80% do so within 1 year of injury and another 5% recover in 2 years).[110] Aggressive (especially invasive) intervention should be limited during this time period.

Techniques to Restore Erection. Restoring erection in the SCI male may be accomplished using one of the following four options.

Intracavernous injection of vasoactive substances:[3, 83, 110] Injection into the corpora of papaverine (a nonspecific smooth muscle relaxant producing vasodilation and relaxation of the sinusoidal spaces), a combination of papaverine and phentolamine (an α-adrenergic blocker producing vasodilation), or prostaglandin E1 produces an erection. The patients are typically managed by a urologist, who carefully titrates the doses of the vasoactive substances, as there is a risk for priapism, even with small doses. This risk is increased in the SCI patient because neurogenic-based erectile dysfunction requires lower doses. The vasoactive agents are injected with a sterile technique into the lateral aspect of the base of the penile shaft, avoiding midline neurovascular structures. Hematomas are prevented by compressing the injection site for 2 to 5 minutes. Sympathomimetic agents such as phenylephrine and epinephrine can be used to treat drug-induced priapism.[3] Our institution has a policy of treating patients with injection therapy only if they comply with their bladder, bowel, and skin management.

Vacuum tumescence constriction therapy (VTCT):[70, 109] VTCT is a term used to describe the use of external devices that create a vacuum and cause an erection-like state that is maintained by a constricting band (Fig. 30–6). The flaccid penis is placed in a rigid cylinder. A pump creates the vacuum needed to fill the corpora with blood. A constricting band is placed at the base of the penis, after the cylinder is removed, to prevent blood from leaving the penis (partners may complain of a cold penis) (Fig. 30–7). This can maintain an erection for up to 30 minutes. Detumescence follows rapidly after the band is removed. The ErecAid (ErecAid Osbon Medical Systems, Augusta, Ga.), originally marketed as the Youth Equivalent Device, has been available since 1917.[111] These devices can be found in many shops that sell sex-related paraphernalia for far less cost than from a medical vendor. The constricting band prevents urinary leakage but also antegrade ejaculation. Reliability of the patients is important, since the constricting band should not be left in place longer than 30 minutes because of a risk of penile ischemia and necrosis. Patients on anticoagulant medication or those with bleeding disorders should not use VTCT.[110]

Penile prosthesis:[67] Implantable penile prostheses are available in numerous designs including fixed, semirigid (flexible), or inflatable. Semirigid prostheses can be hinged,

TABLE 30–5 Types of Sexual Dysfunction

Dysfunction	Characteristics
Decreased libido	Decline in sexual drive or desire; may be conscious or unconscious
Decreased vaginal lubrication	Reduction in lubrication fluid in vagina
Delayed orgasm	Prolonged time for orgasm to occur
Anorgasmia	Inability to achieve orgasm
Breast hyperplasia	May adversely affect self-esteem and body image, especially as adolescent
Gynecomastia	Enlargement or excessive development of male breast; may be unilateral or bilateral
Impotence	Inability to achieve or maintain erection sufficient for penetration and intercourse
Priapism	Prolonged, painful erection caused by lack of drainage of corpus cavernosum
Retarded ejaculation	Delayed ejaculation or inability to ejaculate
Retrograde ejaculation	Ejaculation into urinary bladder caused by insufficient tightening of internal urethral neck
Premature ejaculation	When emission/ejaculation is accompanied by loss of erection, before or immediately upon vaginal penetration

Adapted from Seidl A, Bullough B, Haughey B, et al: Understanding the effects of a myocardial infarction on sexual functioning: A basis for sexual counseling. Rehabil Nurs 1991; 16:255–264.

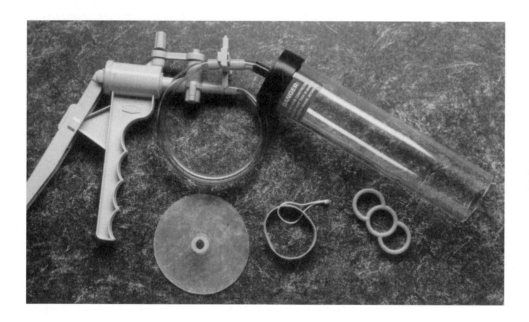

FIGURE 30–6 Assembled vacuum tumescence constriction device, with two types of constriction bands displayed.

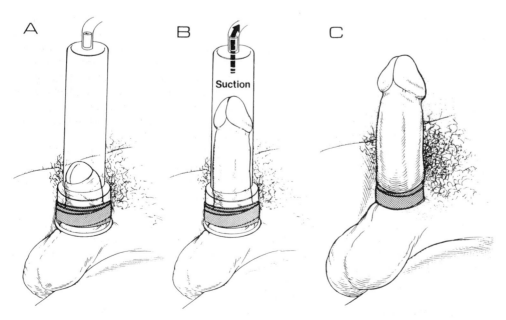

FIGURE 30–7 A, Cylinder with constriction bands around base placed over flaccid penis. B, Suction applied, creating negative pressure within cylinder and resulting in penile engorgement. C, Constriction bands guided from cylinder to base of penis. (From Witherington R: External aids for treatment of impotence. J Urol Nurs 1987; 6:10.)

malleable, or articulated. Inflatable penile prostheses can be multicomponent or self-contained (Fig. 30–8).[111] With the inflatable prosthesis, the penis is inflated to full erection by means of a pump located in the scrotum. When a valve is opened, the penis deflates. The multicomponents of the inflatable prosthesis make it more difficult and costly to insert than the fixed or flexible rods.[100] Indications for these devices in SCI patients include both erectile dysfunction and maintenance of external catheters. Their use has recently declined in SCI males. The reason for this decrease is twofold: the frequency of complications and the simpler, safer cost-effectiveness of the injection and vacuum techniques. The problem with the fixed prosthesis is that the malleable rods that are placed in the corpus callosum can sometimes cause problems such as infection and erosions, especially in the insensate. The rate of postoperative infection in the general population is 2%, but it is 7% in the SCI population. The erosion rate is as high as 11% in the SCI population, but only 1% in the general population[26, 111] (Table 30–6). An artificial penis (dildo) can be strapped on the groin to simulate a natural erection.[100]

Neuropharmacotherapy:[68] Transcutaneous nitroglycerin has been used as topical therapy for erectile dysfunction in SCI patients. It produced an erection sufficient for coitus in 25% of patients in whom papaverine injections had induced rigid erections.[91, 110] Nitroglycerin has frequent side effects including hypotension and headaches. Oral levodopa has also been used with 55% to 60% of patients reported to achieve rigid erection.[110]

Achieving Vaginal Lubrication. Much of what was said in the Achieving Erection section applies to females with respect to vaginal lubrication and engorgement. There is both reflexogenic and psychogenic lubrication. A sensation similar to that of a full bladder is described by some women with reflexogenic lubrication, while the sensation with psychogenic lubrication is often attenuated. Those with complete lesions involving T10 to T12 do not have lubrication and benefit from vaginal lubricants such as saliva, Replens, or K-Y jelly.

Coitus. *Coitus* is defined as intromission and intravaginally sustained erection. To accomplish this an erection must occur at the right time, be sufficiently hard for penetration, and last long enough to satisfy the partner.[111] Talbot[94] studied 208 SCI patients and found that only 23% of those who attained an erection were able to achieve successful coitus (see Table 30–3). It is important not to overemphasize the need for an erection in sexual relationships, and to ensure that the patients are aware that greater than 50% of well-adjusted women do not reach orgasm with vaginal stimulation alone. The "stuffing technique" can be used if the patient or his partner desire vaginal intromission.[100] Loss of lubrication in the female patient can interfere with coitus. Pelvic floor and adductor muscle spasticity can restrict penile penetration.[6] Premedication with benzodiazepines can help reduce this spasticity. Both male and female SCI patients must learn to empty their bladder and bowel prior to sexual activity and remember to void or catheterize themselves after sexual activity to lessen the chances of urinary infection. The level of concern regarding incontinence during sex is very high in both males and females.[106, 107]

Ejaculation.[4] Failure of synchronous activity involving

deposition of ejaculate constituents and antegrade evacuation through the urethra constitute *retrograde ejaculation* or *ejaculatory failure.* Retrograde ejaculation can be secondary to an abnormal state (sympathetic nervous system damage) preventing adequate closure of the bladder neck, leading to retrograde semen flow. After sexual activity, males may complain of dry ejaculate (sensation of orgasm with no expulsion of semen) or cloudy urine at the time of their next void or catherization. Ejaculatory failure also occurs in up to 90% of patients after transurethral prostatectomy (TURP).[69] The higher the spinal cord lesion the more likely the patient is to have an erection, but the less likely to have ejaculation. Twenty percent of all SCI males retain some ability to ejaculate in either antegrade or retrograde fashion. Ejaculatory failure is seen least often in those with lower lesions or incomplete lesions.[111]

Orgasm. We have previously emphasized the importance of the brain in the experience of orgasm. All the issues discussed in the sexuality section play a vital role in the patient's libido and responsiveness to the sexual experience. There is a correlation between the richness of the individual's sexual fantasy and fulfillment of sexual life, which may be even more important when genital impairments exist.[6, 76] Phantom orgasm was described by Money as an occasional culmination of vivid fantasies or dreams with no physical stimulation.[66] The brain can work independent of genitalia in the generation of erotic experience, just as the genitalia of SCI patients can work reflexively independent of the brain. Surveys of able-bodied females report that approximately 10% have never achieved orgasm and that up to 75% do not routinely achieve orgasm with penile thrusting alone.[112] It should not be surprising to find that, with SCIs, female orgasms are typically experienced differently than they were premorbidly. They are described as pleasurable feelings of intense excitement or as sudden enhancement of spasticity followed by prolonged relaxation.[37] The extragenital responses during orgasm include "headache, warm sensation, physical pleasure, and sexual excitement."[111] It is important to educate the patient that the orgasms are real, just different.[96]

If SCI males anticipate pleasurable feelings (orgasm) only if they ejaculate, they will be disappointed, as the percentage of successful ejaculation is low. Education about the importance of the mind and awareness of other body changes will enhance their sensation. Orgasms are practically nonexistent in patients with complete upper motor neuron lesions. Persons with complete lower motor neuron injuries occasionally perceive pleasurable sensation lower in the abdomen, pelvis, or thighs.

Autonomic Dysreflexia.[97] All patients with SCIs at or above T4 to T6 are at risk for autonomic dysreflexia. Patients are advised to evacuate bowel and bladder prior to sexual activity, thus avoiding incontinence and reducing the risk of autonomic dysreflexia from these stimuli. If autonomic dysreflexia occurs during sexual activity, the patient should be educated to stop, and to sit up to elevate the head (to help lower blood pressure). Medical assistance should be sought if the headache does not subside. Prophylactic medication can be used if autonomic dysreflexia is not otherwise manageable.

Male Fertility.[54] The etiology of infertility in the SCI

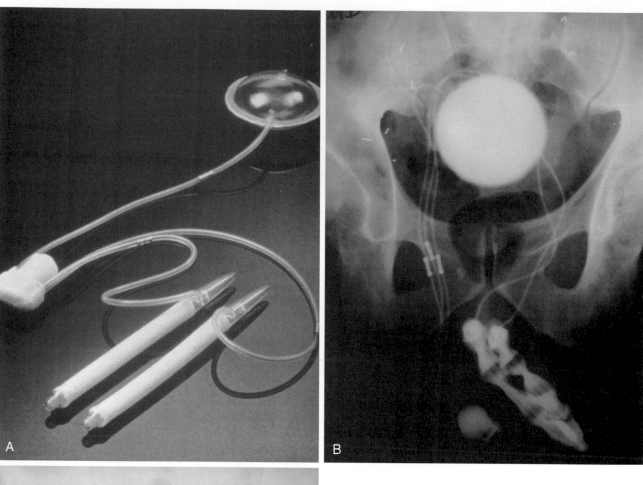

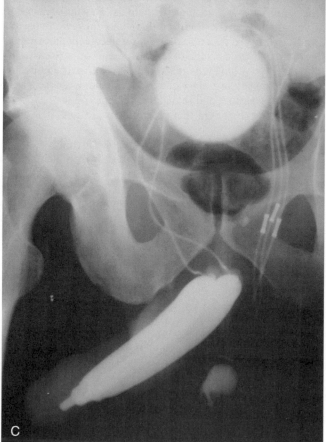

FIGURE 30–8   *A*, Inflatable prosthesis with the paired cylinders, scrotal pump, and an abdominal fluid reservoir. *B*, Three-piece inflatable prosthesis viewed by x-ray prior to full inflation. *C*, Inflatable prosthesis at full inflation.

TABLE 30–6   Complications Reported With Penile Prostheses in Spinal Cord–Injured Men

Study	Type of Prostheses	Complication	Comments
Van Arsdalen et al.	20 noninflatable	25% erosion rate	Decrease in skin problem in 70% due to maintenance of condom catheter
Rossier and Fam	36 semirigid	Removal in 19.5%, infection in 11%	
Yarkony	Semirigid	22% erosion	
	29 inflatable	8%	Minor surgical repair in 31%
Collins and Hackler	53 semirigid	33% extrusion	After reimplantation, 83% function rate
	10 inflatable	40% lost	

From Van Arsdalen KN, Klein FA, Hackler RH, et al: Penile implants in spinal cord injury patients for maintaining external appliances. J Urol 1981; 126:331–332; Rossier AB, Fam BA: Indication and results of semirigid penile prosthesis in spinal cord injury patients: Long term followup. J Urol 1984; 131:59–62; Yarkony GM: Enhancement of sexual function and fertility in spinal cord–injured males. Am J Phys Med Rehabil 1990; 69:81–87; Collins KP, Hackler RH: Complications of penile prostheses in the spinal cord injury population. J Urol 1988; 140:984–985.

population is the subject of much research. Less than 10% of SCI patients retain the ability to impregnate their partner spontaneously.[4, 37] A successful pregnancy requires the male to produce complete and adequate spermatogenesis, ductal transport of sperm, erection, emission, and ejaculation.[69] Problems arise from ejaculatory failure, obstruction of genital passages, impairment of spermatogenesis, or a combination of the these.[99]

Techniques to restore ejaculation are usually aimed at restoring fertility.[78] A review of the patient's medication and prior sexual function is required. The techniques involve stimulation of the intact neurological center below the SCI through chemical, vibratory, or transrectal electrical ejaculation.[69] These are most successful when the T10 to T11 spinal segments are intact. α-Adrenergic agonists (pseudoephrine and imipramine) are used in attempting to convert retrograde ejaculation to anterograde ejaculation. If this is not successful, harvesting and processing of the retrograde ejaculation should be attempted. One method is to have the patient void (almost completely) prior to masturbation and then collect the postejaculatory voided urine. To ensure optimal sperm survival, the second method involves washing the bladder with sperm-processing buffer, leaving 30 mL of the buffer in the bladder; masturbation; and collection of the postejaculate fluid. The ejaculate must be processed carefully to obtain a concentrated healthy sample.[18] Intrathecal physostigmine was used by Guttmann and Walsh[39] to elicit ejaculation chemically, but this lost favor because of complications, including autonomic dysreflexia. Subcutaneous physostigmine was also rejected because of its dangerous side effects.[22, 110]

Vibratory stimulation of the glans penis has been used successfully by various groups to collect semen (successful in about 50% of SCI males).[7, 16] The advantages are noninvasiveness, home use, possibility of "natural" fertilization, and that retrograde emission is less likely than with transrectal electrical stimulation. Improvement in quantity and quality of sperm with weekly use of the vibratory ejaculatory technique has been noted.[7] The disadvantages are an unpredictable response in many patients and risk of autonomic dysreflexia.[18, 110]

Transrectal electrical stimulation or electroejaculation involves stimulation of the myelinated preganglionic efferent sympathetic fibers of the hypogastric plexus to obtain seminal emission into the posterior urethra[4] (Fig. 30–9). The semen is obtained from the posterior urethra by milking the urethral bulb and by catheterization. This technique

was first introduced in humans in 1948, but until recently experience and further research were acquired mainly through veterinary use. It is currently the most common method used in the United States. Buch and Zorn[19] found that semen could be obtained from up to 90% of all patients evaluated. There appears to be a decrease in sperm motility in the semen collected by transrectal stimulation, with normal fertility seen in only 25%.[19] Electroejaculation is an office- or hospital-based procedure because of the need to monitor for autonomic dysreflexia and the anoscopy performed to evaluate the rectal mucosa. Pretreatment with sublingual nifedipine has decreased the risk of autonomic dysreflexia in both techniques.[110] Anesthesia may be required in some patients with incomplete lesions due to pain. Perkash and co-workers[72] have been successful in simplifying the equipment, lowering the current required, and therefore increasing the patient's tolerance.

Direct retrieval of sperm can be attempted from the vas deferens when the other methods have failed. Brindley[17] has studied hypogastric stimulation with implanted platinum electrodes connected to a subcutaneous radio receiver. The seminal fluid is then extracted via cannulation of the vas deferens. There have also been attempts to implant a cannula into the vas deferens and collect fluid into a subcutaneous capsule.[7]

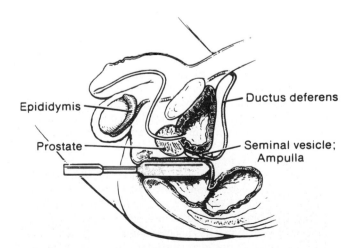

FIGURE 30–9 Sagittal view of rectal probe placement for electroejaculation. (From Buch JP: Disorders of ejaculation. *In* Bennett AH (ed): Impotence: Diagnosis and Management of Erectile Dysfunction. Philadelphia, WB Saunders, 1994, p 193.)

Fertility problems can also stem from obstructed passages of the vas deferens, epididymis, and seminiferous tubules, most likely from repeated infection involving the bladder. Duct obstruction can be treated only by surgical resection. Spermatogenesis may be impaired, resulting in a decrease in number of sperm, decrease in normal motility, and increase in abnormal morphology. Sperm contact with urine, medication, antisperm antibodies, or raised scrotal temperature may be explanations for the poor semen quality typically seen in patients with SCI.[54] The local testicular temperature is normally 2.2 °C lower than the intra-abdominal temperature, but the lifestyle of sitting with thighs together or crossed, not shifting position frequently, or wearing tight clothes can raise the temperature. Lowering the testicular temperature can reverse the maturation arrest caused by the increased temperature.[15] This emphasizes the importance of patient education. SCI men are predisposed to the development of antisperm antibodies because of blockage of ductal tracts and urinary tract infections (UTIs). It is not known what contribution antisperm antibodies make to impaired spermatogenesis.[42, 99] Weakness with marked debility is commonly associated with testicular atrophy. There are numerous articles regarding testicular biopsies in the literature, but insufficient data exist to correlate testicular abnormalities with potential contributing factors such as SCI level, urological management, history of urological complications, and medications.[54, 111] Studies seem to indicate close to normal levels of testosterone and an intact hypothalamus-pituitary-testicular axis.[111] Medications such as nitrofurantoin cause temporary spermatogenesis arrest in rats. This has been reviewed by Linsenmeyer and Perkash.[54]

As in vitro fertilization and present methods of semen collection are improved, and as even better methods are developed, the chances of an SCI male fathering a biological offspring are increased. Physiatrists must work with urologists and fertility specialists to provide the best possible opportunity to induce pregnancy. Counseling of the patient and partner is an integral part of any assisted reproductive program.

Female Fertility. Amenorrhea occurs in most women acutely after traumatic SCI, and lasts from 6 months to 1 year. The first ovulation cycle is unpredictable and therefore contraception must be considered from the beginning. There are a number of contraceptive methods that can be used[36, 103] (Table 30–7).

Although the ability to bear children is usually not affected, pregnancy presents many challenges to the SCI female.[6, 29] Self-care must be heightened to avoid the complications of UTIs, thrombophlebitis, edema of the legs, pressure ulcers, premature labor, and immobilization-induced osteoporosis.[29, 110] Repeated UTIs increase the risk of developing toxemia of pregnancy.

The uterus is innervated by T10 to T12; therefore patients with complete lesions above T10 will not appreciate uterine contractions or fetal movement. Although the discomfort of labor is not felt as in able-bodied women, the onset of labor is typically detected but as a different sensation. The contractions may be stronger, more prolonged, and more frequent, but the duration of labor is shorter than for the non-SCI women.[113] Although the abdominal muscles may be paralyzed, the uterus will contract due to

hormonal influence. Delivery of the fetus may require the use of forceps or episiotomy. Cesarean section should be performed for the same indications as with the able-bodied. Patients with lesions above T6 are at risk for autonomic dysreflexia during childbirth.[101] The treatment of choice is epidural anesthesia, as it allows continuous medication administration. Oral premedication can be tried as an alternative.

Breast-feeding may require adaptation of wheelchairs or assistance from others. Women with lesions above T6 usually experience a decrease in milk production after 6 weeks. One of the major concerns of SCI women during their pregnancy is the loss of control and sense of helplessness which develops. This is exacerbated by a decrease in level of functioning, fear of the unknown, and lack of knowledge, all of which can be addressed by a well-organized rehabilitation team.[29]

CORTICAL INVOLVEMENT. With cortical involvement, one may be required to cope with aphasia (communication), left- or right-sided neglect (disinhibition, impulsivity, poor social interaction), or apraxias (motor planning difficulty). Sexuality and sexual function are related to understanding and communication between the patient and partner, which are affected by these neurological sequelae.

Cerebrovascular accidents (CVAs) affect 600,000 persons in the United States every year. The mean age of the 400,000 who survive is 60 years. Most led an active life prior to the disability and want sexuality issues to be addressed during hospitalization. There is a general decline in sexual activity and libido in both sexes after stroke, but there is little evidence of organic causes for the sexual dysfunction.[11, 20] The co-morbidity associated with CVA, such as diabetes, hypertension, and cardiac problems, contributes to sexual dysfunction.[35] Psychological factors seem to be important in determining changes in sexual life after stroke. These factors may be a result of change in the sex role, dependence on a partner for activities of daily living, or attitudes of partners. The patient might be forced into a more passive role, but have a partner unwilling to become more aggressive or use new sexual positions.[60] The more dependent the patient is on the spouse, the more likely there will be a decrease in sexual activity.[88] The partner may fear a recurrence of the event, may resent loss of income, or may infantilize the patient. These phenomena produce dysfunction in other disabilities as well. Impairment of cutaneous sensibility, neurogenic bladder, fatigue, depression, and aphasic disorders have been found to play a role in sexual changes.[11] With the decrease in verbal communication and decrease in spontaneous touching, establishing successful "sexual intercourse" becomes more difficult. There are discrepancies in the literature regarding the incidence of arousal, ejaculation, and orgasmic dysfunction after strokes, which may be partly explained by the methodology used (most frequently questionnaires).[11, 14]

Traumatic brain injury (TBI) patients share many of the epidemiologic characteristics of SCI patients.[114] The severity of disability varies from case to case depending on the injury, premorbid status, family support, and extent of rehabilitation.[43] Therefore, the rehabilitative process must be adaptable.[10] When 19 male patients with postconcussive syndrome were studied for sexual dysfunction, (58%) reported difficulty.[48] Cerebral involvement can lead

TABLE 30–7   Female Fertility and Contraception

Type	Side Effects	Comments
Periodic abstinence or coitus interruptus	None	A woman must be well instructed in her biological rhythms to avoid unplanned pregnancy
Condoms	Decreased effectiveness if not properly used Must be reapplied for second sexual activity Taste may be offensive	Ready availability, increased acceptability, increased effectiveness Need dexterity Indwelling catheter may tear condom; therefore, lubricate Protects against sexually transmitted diseases
Foam and sponge	None	Ready availability, increased acceptability, increased effectiveness
Diaphragm/foam	Weakened pelvic muscles may not hold diaphragm in place	Requires dexterity Partner may be trained to insert the diaphragm
Intrauterine device (IUD)	May be unable to feel early signs of pelvic inflammatory disease Manual dexterity is needed to check for placement	Inserted by physician Insertion may be easier with paralysis Teach the patient to look for spotting, irregular periods, increased spasticity, fever, increased or different vaginal discharge
Oral contraceptive pill	Studies of the early use (estrogen, 50–150 μg; progestin) revealed an association with cardiovascular, thromboembolic, cerebrovascular, and thrombophlebitic disease Studies of low-dose estrogen (35 μg) and progestin suggest only individual situations of hypertension and thrombophlebitis Both are aggravated by smoking Spinal cord–injured women must be taught the warning signs of thrombophlebitis	Most common reason for unplanned pregnancy is improper dosing Need sufficient cognition and reliability as well as the manual dexterity to take pill as required
Subdermal hormonal implants (Norplant)	Has not been shown to produce thromboembolic, cerebrovascular, or cardiovascular disease Monitor for hypertension and thrombophlebitis Side effects include irregular vaginal bleeding, changes in weight, and psychic symptoms similar to menopause or premenstrual syndrome	Good option for women who do not desire children for a period of years Added benefit of reducing or totally eliminating menstrual bleeding, which can facilitate hygiene
Medroxyprogesterone acetate (Depo-Provera)	Same as above	Added benefit of reducing or totally eliminating menstrual bleeding, which can facilitate hygiene
Sterilization by tubal ligation or vasectomy	Permanent	Continue to menstruate
Therapeutic abortion		Prior to sexual activity, patient and partner should discuss family planning and options

Data from Bérard EJJ: The sexuality of spinal cord injured women: Physiology and pathophysiology: A review. Paraplegia 1989, 27:99–112; Goddard LH: Sexuality and spinal cord injury. J Neurosci Nurs 1988; 20:240–243.

to sexual disinhibition, hyposexuality, and hypersexuality (Klüver-Bucy syndrome) in that order of frequency.[115] Upper motor deficits can lead to spasticity, paresis, paralysis, heterotopic ossification, contractures, and neurogenic bowel and bladder. Cortical involvement can result in dysphasia, dysarthria, dysprosody, and oromotor apraxias, which can interfere with communication and oral sexual contact. In addition to the objective impairments listed, TBI patients may have significant personality changes that adversely affect their relationships and appear to deteriorate over time rather than improve.[71]

Multiple sclerosis is a chronic illness that affects many aspects of sexuality (often in young adults)[98, 104] (see Chapter 52).

DIABETIC NEUROPATHY. Peripheral neuropathies, such as in diabetes mellitus, have many effects on the peripheral somatic and autonomic nervous systems affecting the expression of sexuality. Diabetes mellitus is a chronic illness and affects psychological aspects of sexuality through changes in body image and control issues.[44] Within 5 years of the onset of diabetes mellitus, one third to one half of males experience some sexual dysfunction. This is usually impotence secondary to a combination of physiological (neurological and vascular) and psychological factors. The physiological factors can involve erectile problems, including the vasodilation necessary for increased arterial inflow, relaxation of muscles necessary for the spaces in the corpora cavernosa to fill, possibly the venous outflow or the sensory input that facilitates obtaining and maintaining an erection. The importance of the peripheral neuropathy was shown dramatically in a study in which 23 impotent men had a vibratory threshold that was 3 SD higher than the norm, even though vibratory sense increased dramatically after 60 years of age in 118 nonimpotent men.[102] Female diabetic patients experience sexual dysfunction with impaired lubrication, impaired sensation, increased vaginal infections leading to dyspareunia, and changes in sexual desire.[51]

VASCULAR DISEASE. Cardiovascular disease has a high prevalence in our culture, especially in men greater than 50 years old.[79] Research is now demonstrating a much higher incidence of disease than previously estimated in females. Coronary disease resulting in myocardial infarction and peripheral vascular disease leading to amputation have a significant impact on patients and their sexual functioning.[41] Vascular disease can cause a loss of the ability to maintain an erection from a "venous leakage." Medications used for treatment often interfere with libido or sexual function. For example, long-term digoxin use in men causes estradiol levels three times higher than controls, while testosterone decreases by two thirds (correlating with an increased incidence of impotence). Hypertension interferes with sexual function most directly because of the medications used to treat it (see Table 30–2). It is important to evaluate sexual function prior to initiating therapy if possible. Sexual dysfunction is one of the main reasons for noncompliance with antihypertensive medication regimens.

The frequency of sexual activity decreases dramatically after myocardial infarction or coronary bypass. Survivors of myocardial infarction often experience anxiety and depression even 1 year after insult, and their sexual concerns are frequently not adequately addressed during the acute hospitalization.[41] Energy expenditure during sexual activity is similar to that of walking on a treadmill at 3 to 4 miles/hour (5–6 METS [metabolic equivalents of oxygen consumption]).[34] The amount of energy expenditure during sexual activity has been compared to climbing two flights of stairs at a brisk rate, or climbing 20 steps in 10 seconds. It is now recommended that counselors advise patients to use their usual sexual position(s), as these are generally less stressful than learning a new position[86] (Table 30–8).

PHYSICAL DISFIGUREMENT. This includes a wide variety of diagnoses: amputations, burns, cancer, and arthritis. Often genital sexual function is not affected, but other factors affecting sexuality are severely affected. Resuming sexual activity helped those with amputations incorporate their prostheses into their body image, increased self-esteem, and facilitated rehabilitation.[61]

Oncology patients have multiple issues including body image (as in breast cancer postmastectomy) as well as the issue of mortality. Chemotherapy-induced nausea, malaise, or weakness may compromise sexual frequency.[89] Although 3% to 12% of men are impotent post TURP, appropriate counseling can result in continued satisfactory sexual relationships. Impotence occurs in 15% of prostatectomy patients, in 67% of cystoprostatectomy cases, in 15% in males less than 50 years old after abdominoperineal resection, and in 100% in males older than 70 years. Patients with an ileostomy or colostomy often have secondary erectile failure due to decreased self-esteem and depression.[105]

Arthritis is a chronic disease and as with diabetes mellitus, chronic obstructive pulmonary disease,[40] and renal disease, increased age, severity of illness, and depression are associated with decreased sexual function.[40, 55] Thirty-eight percent to 80% of patients with chronic renal failure requiring dialysis have reduced or partial erectile function, but only 20% to 55% are completely impotent.[27] Chronic diseases seen in children, such as juvenile rheumatoid arthritis, cystic fibrosis, or myelomeningocele, affect many of the sexuality issues all adolescents face.[30]

With the dramatic improvement in burn survival, attention must be directed to the quality of life for the patient. Physiological function is usually intact and the concerns are body image, self-esteem, and interpersonal relationships. Following the models described in the following pages allows for integrating sexual issues into the comprehensive, often lengthy rehabilitation of the burn patient.[108]

TERMINAL ILLNESS. When dealing with the terminally ill, physicians do not typically consider the consequences to the patient's sexuality. Patients can get mired in the grieving process and not be able to move forward to the enjoyment of their modified sexuality. Physicians view the more obvious medical problems to be more worthy of attention than sexuality. This is not the case with the majority of such patients, however, and education of both clinicians and patients can help ameliorate this discrepancy. The rehabilitation of the human immunodeficiency virus (HIV)–positive patient or the patient with acquired immunodeficiency syndrome (AIDS) underscores the importance of treating the whole patient.[52, 90]

TABLE 30–8   Patient Guidelines for Sexual Intercourse

1. Resume sexual intercourse in familiar surroundings. Strange environments add to psychological stress.
2. Provide a room with a comfortable temperature for intercourse. Extreme room temperatures and extremely hot or cold showers or baths add to heart stress.
3. Remember that foreplay is desirable and helps prepare your heart gradually for the increased activity of intercourse.
4. Use positions that are comfortable and relaxing and permit unrestricted breathing.
5. Usual positions are the most desirable because they are the least stressful.
6. If inclined, oral-genital sex causes no undue strain and may be a satisfactory means of sexual expression with appropriate attention to disease prevention.
7. Obtain rest before intercourse; morning is an ideal time for lovemaking.
8. Postpone intercourse for 3 hours after eating a heavy meal or drinking alcohol.
9. Remember that sex with someone other than your usual partner may increase stress to your heart.
10. See that clothing, if worn, is loose-fitting.
11. Take medications, such as nitroglycerin or isosorbide dinitrate, before intercourse to prevent chest pain.
12. Consider masturbation because it requires less energy than intercourse.

From Seidl A, Bullough B, Haughey B, et al: Understanding the effects of a myocardial infarction on sexual functioning: A basis for sexual counseling. Rehabil Nurs 1991; 16:255–264.

SEXUALITY

We have previously defined *sexuality* as a form of communication and sexual self-expression to which everyone is entitled. Sexuality is a "combination of sex drive, sex acts and all those aspects of personality concerned with learned communications and relationship patterns . . . rooted in the human need to relate to others, to receive and share pleasure, to love and to be loved."[80] The patient, his or her relationships, and the environment reflect the wide spectrum of beliefs and attitudes encompassed by sexuality.[25]

Sexuality is an integral part of a person's psychological makeup and self-concept. We know that psychological health can positively or negatively affect the course of rehabilitation. It should come as no surprise that impairments affect sexuality and that sexuality issues affect a patient's ability to deal with the rigors of rehabilitation.

Sexual Development

Clinicians attempting to assist patients' return to healthy sexual function must be careful not to convey their biases or prejudices to the patient. This requires being fully informed about the physiological and psychological aspects of sexuality. Of course, clinicians need to be comfortable with their own sexuality. It is incumbent upon the physiatrist to allow patients the opportunity to address sexual issues. However, it is also appropriate to refer those patients whose issues are outside one's expertise or values to a trained clinician.

Our culture abounds with myths and taboos about sexual function, performance, and expression. For example, pre- or extramarital sexual activity, masturbation, aging,[28] homosexuality, and birth control are differently defined and accepted intraculturally and cross-culturally. These form one's construction of norms that are communicated by family, educators, and peers across the life span. This is no less true for persons with disabilities and their families.

Parental attitudes toward the developing sexuality of children can be facilitative or inhibitive, affecting adult options of sexual expression.[59] These attitudes may be extremely repressive, controlling, and overprotective. Assumptions may be made by the family that a child with a disability will never marry, reproduce, or have intimate relationships.[62] A more supportive stance parallels the stance that the parent of an able-bodied child would be advised to take. Such a parent might acknowledge a "disabled child's sexuality, help the child develop a sexual identity, and respond in a neutral or positive manner when the child begins to form intimate relationships in late adolescence and early adulthood."[59]

Shielding and overprotecting children and adolescents with disabilities prevents them from experiencing the sexual banter that goes on, the verbal and nonverbal communication with another person in whom they are sexually interested. Placing these limitations on a disabled child can lead to a more socially disabled adult. Supporting the child or adolescent's participation in peer groups is critical for the development of interpersonal skills, including the socially appropriate communication skills associated with sexual development. A healthy adjustment is becoming "sexually assertive," for example, using a wheelchair or brace as an introduction to a conversation rather than allowing it to be a barrier to interactions.[59]

Myths that the elderly are asexual, or should be, pervade the culture and enforce incongruity between what many elderly persons experience and what is considered normal.[57] Elderly patients undergoing rehabilitation deserve the same consideration of their sexuality issues as younger patients.[47] The sexual interest of the elderly is affected by many factors of which clinicians should be aware. These include the following:[47]

- General health (including mental health)
- Availability of a partner and opportunity to be alone with a partner
- Personality and attitude
- Educational level
- Social status
- Degree of satisfaction with life
- The attitude of others
- Sexual beliefs, activity, interests, and practices earlier in life (especially those of the patient when between the ages of 20 and 40)

The most common sexual problem in older couples is male erectile difficulties. Disease, drug reactions, and disability can contribute to emotional upset, decreased libido, decreased erectile function, and consequently, decreased sexual activity. Fifty percent to 75% of all marriages among older persons can be affected by some sexual disability, with erectile failure reported in 20% of 60-year-olds, 27% of 70-year-olds, and 75% of 80-year-old men.[57] Some patients (mostly women) continue sexual activity for their partners rather than for self-gratification. Knowing they can still please others sexually can improve their morale and self-concept. Those most likely to discontinue all sexual activity after a disabling accident or illness are widowed or single persons.[100]

Factors Affecting Sexuality

When patients are confronted with serious illness or disability, a central task of coping is a redefinition of self that incorporates the limitations or adjustments of the illness or disabling condition.[27]

Unfortunately, because of the nature of hospitals, patients are denied privacy, and social permission for sexual questioning and exploration is withheld. Patients often share the societal negative stereotypes of disabled people as pathetic, unhappy, unproductive, and asexual.[103] Physiatrists can counteract these images by supporting patients in reconstruction of their sexual identities. In order to assist them, it is imperative that we understand not only biological but psychosocial factors affecting sexuality. These include body image, self-esteem, gender identity, and role compliance.[103] Each of these factors involves a composite of the patient's personal cognitions based on the messages construed from family, peers, culture, and, of course, from the clinicians assigned to their care. Through education, support, and normalization, physicians (especially physiatrists) and the team of rehabilitation professionals are uniquely positioned to enhance their patients' lives in each of these domains. Since the focus of rehabilitation medicine is to maintain and increase a patient's function, our practice is solution-based: relationships with patients are long term and our therapeutic stance with patients is supportive. We serve as a partner to our patients and their families by fostering their reintegration into the lifestyles that they choose. Our goal is to add life to years, not just years to life (see Figs. 30–1 and 30–10).

BODY IMAGE.   Body image is one of the most essential components of self, incorporating "feelings and attitudes toward one's own body, body parts, and body functions."[80] Prostheses, wheelchairs, scars, or adaptive equipment all have to be incorporated into a new body image.[75] If this is viewed negatively by the patient or society, a spiral of loss of confidence and body shame can result. The term "body shame" was coined by Kaufman in discussing shame associated with aging. These experiences with bodily changes are often similar to those of persons with disability. The decline in appearance, bodily function, and vitality become increasing sources of shame and frustration. This change

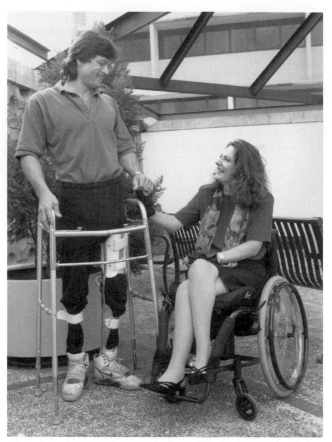

FIGURE 30–10 Factors affecting sexuality: impaired body image; decreased self-esteem; difficulty with gender identity and role; difficulty with decisions about sexuality and parenthood; personal and observed sexual experience; value system, morality, religion, prohibition, and taboos; personal, cultural, and societal attitudes; and health status and physical capabilities.[80] What was your reaction to the "romantic" portrait in Figure 30–1 vs. your reaction to this portrait? Did you make assumptions? It is easy to comprehend how the visible factors can affect sexuality, but we carry an entire host of hidden factors.

is experienced as a loss, and loss activates distress and grieving.

To illustrate the point, picture yourself with a third-degree burn covering your face, or with an eruption of Kaposi's sarcoma across your body as a result of being HIV-seropositive. Failure to accept one's body as is, in the presence of disability, can lead to feelings not only of shame but also of dissociation with one's body and perceived loss of control. Such feelings can be exacerbated in women by perceptions that their self-worth is associated with physical appearance and sexual attractiveness (a perception that is consistent with societal expectations). In addition, maintenance of hygiene and use of associated devices (catheters, ostomy bags, menstrual products) may require the assistance of another person. If a partner assists with such intimate personal care, it may be difficult for the partner and the patient to readjust to sexual intimacy. Clinicians should not assume that patients will inevitably have body image distortions or problems, but should be ready to treat them when they occur.[80]

SELF-ESTEEM. Self-esteem, the personal sense of one's inherent worth, is essential to mental health and identity. As with other components of self, self-esteem develops interactively over the course of the life span. The presence of impairments and physical disabilities can be an assault on one's self-esteem, particularly if these are perceived by the patient or significant others as a diminution of competence, attractiveness, or intrinsic value. In some patients, diminished self-esteem can exist concurrently with inadequate sexual relationships and feelings of inferiority, weakness, and helplessness.[25] Concerns about not satisfying a partner ranked number one in a study of 79 SCI males.[106] Loneliness and isolation can emerge in combination with a fear of humiliation that leads to avoidance of sexual situations.[8]

Other patients react to diminished self-esteem by displaying hypersexuality, apparently seeking assurance or validation from others that they are still attractive.[115] It is important to understand the insecurity that underlies these inappropriate displays, so as not to further undermine the patient's self-esteem with negative reactions. Physicians are often viewed by the patient as being very powerful, and should use this position to assist the team with dealing with such issues. The patient's feelings should be acknowledged, and then the patient should be redirected to a more appropriate expression (rephrasing an offensive statement, suggesting a more appropriate expression). Patients need to learn to express their needs and desires with family, partner, and clinicians. Assertiveness training has been used successfully to assist with this expression and subsequently has increased patients' self-esteem.[103] For example, in vivo and in vitro situational behavior rehearsals, essentially practice sessions, can make it easier the next time a potential real-life "sexual intercourse" occasion presents itself.

GENDER IDENTITY. One's gender identity exists at a point along a continuum of femininity and masculinity that is consistent or inconsistent with societal assumptions based on the individual's gender. Both gender identity and gender role develop in socially interactive processes. For disabled patients, gender identity can be compromised by an impairment in their ability to express their assumed gender role. How this is negotiated is greatly influenced by the patient's interaction with clinicians, family, peers, and intimate partners. Patients might test their identity by acting out an exaggeration of their assumed gender role. For example, a male who has been raised to value assertiveness, dominance, and strength, and then finds himself with quadriplegia is forced to accept a more passive physical role. He may attempt to compensate through verbal abuse of family, therapists, or nursing staff.

Literature as recent as the 1970s gave the opinion that SCI was not as devastating to women because they could continue their passive role.[96] Yet, females, particularly those who value a more traditional feminine role, are much more sensitive to their perceived loss of sexual attractiveness and perceived loss of fertility in defining their female identity.[29]

Children with disabilities encounter many unique challenges in the struggle to develop their own gender identity and role. Often these develop because parents avoid sexual subjects and limit participation in the normal sexual developmental activities, for example, dances, parties, dating, sports. Rehabilitation specialists can assist with family training and providing safe environments for social experimentation.

PROCESS OF ASSESSMENT AND RECOMMENDATION FOR SEXUAL SATISFACTION (PARSS) MODEL

History and Physical Examination

Sexuality is central to the patient's health and quality of life. Physiatrists are comfortable asking very personal questions from patients to assist with skin integrity, physical strength, bowel and bladder programs, and to reintegrate the patient's independence. However, they are frequently uncomfortable with sexual issues. This section details the processes of history taking and physical examination in the context of providing the patient maximum opportunity to voice sexual concerns. The goals of the process of assessment and recommendation for sexual satisfaction (PARSS) are to enable patients to express their concerns openly and to offer them counseling and education, whenever possible, in order to minimize sexual dysfunction and maximize sexual satisfaction[74] (Table 30–9). More than 80% of sexual complaints can be successfully managed in the office setting, but only if they are addressed[47] (see Table 30–5).

In a study of patient-physician interactions, physicians stated they did not include sexual issues in their evaluation because of lack of knowledge and training, discomfort and embarrassment, and lack of research in connection with sex and disability. Experimentally trained physicians obtained a sexual history 82% of the time, compared with 32% of the time by the untrained physicians. Many physicians assumed sexual function was not important to the patient, but without confirmation from the patient, that assumption is invalid.[33] Patients whose physician had asked sexual questions as a part of the initial history assessment thought the subject was more appropriate in an examination than those whose physician has not broached the subject.[64] All patients with impairments have some type of sexual concern, whether physiological, physical, social, or psychological.

A good example of this is in adolescents with cancer who have many concerns their peers do not.[21] History taking that includes questions about sexuality is critical to learning about their concerns.

During the initial evaluation, the physician must establish rapport and present himself or herself as approachable. Spica[92] emphasizes that "a knowledgeable, nonjudgmental clinician [nurse] with good communication skills can play an important role in enhancing a patient's quality of life through effective sexual counseling." In re-educating patients with impairments, we need to discuss not only the physiological aspects of sex but also the more subtle expression of sexuality such as caring, touching, holding, and being held.

The physiatrist should initiate these discussions with patients throughout their care. At a minimum, these topics should be broached during the screening sexual history, admission physical examination, and discharge planning sessions. Several factors facilitate the PARSS: attention to the topic throughout therapy, privacy, confidentiality, awareness of sociosexual variation with generations, and appreciation of the difficult nature of the topic for patients and many physicians. In considering outlines to clarify various clinical situations and thus to enhance positive outcomes and limit negative outcomes, a simple model is used to guide history taking. It goes beyond the traditional set of standard questions—often cold and at "arm's length"—and emphasizes the clear need to update the history and information throughout the process (PARSS).

The *ENIGMA* model is orderly and open-ended. First one should *engage* the patient in conversation providing an opening and opportunity to talk. It need not be directly sexual. The first contact may be solely with the patient, but the partner should be included as soon as the patient gives permission. *Normalize* sexual interest and activity in a matter-of-fact way that makes the subject standard and legitimate. *Inform* the patient and partner about sexual physiology and anatomy. This leads to answering questions in a more natural fashion. *Guide* the patient and his or her partner by responding in the same language and metaphors. A common error made by clinicians is to use medical terminology instead of the vernacular. *Maximize* problem-solving ability by encouraging experimentation, reading, and peer counseling. *Assess and reassess* the sexual issues at the next visit and make it an ongoing subject, not a one-time thing (Table 30–10). For example, with the SCI patient, I routinely review a problem list (skin, bowel, bladder, mobility, sexual function). By the third visit the patient is usually waiting with a sexual question, but the patient typically does not bring it up on his or her own. The pertinent physical examination, which should be performed when assessing sexual function, is described in Table 30–11. This should be a routine part of the physical examination, addressing concerns raised during the screening history.[47] After the sexual history, physical examination, and psychosocial evaluation, a diagnostic formulation should be made which delineates the sexual dysfunction, distress, and disability.[65]

Table 30–12 summarizes the findings of a Canadian SCI rehabilitation program developed in 1975, where a nonphysician specialist was trained to diagnose and treat sexual dysfunction of disabled persons in acute, rehabilita-

---

TABLE 30–9 Goals of the Process of Assessment and Recommendation for Sexual Satisfaction (PARSS)

To minimize sexual dysfunction and maximize sexual satisfaction:
  Give the patient permission to discuss sexual issues and
    establish these as legitimate concerns
  Obtain important information needed for the medical care of the
    patient:
    Insight into family and social support
    Potential risks of infection or injury
    Side effects of medication
    Functional impact on the patient's life of chronic diseases and
      disabilities
    Symptoms such as impotence, dyspareunia, and angina,
      which may lead the clinician to investigate previously
      undiagnosed medical problems
  Discovery of sexual misconceptions, anxieties, or dysfunctions
    Myths about masturbation, different sexual activities, genital
      size
    Anxiety about cardiovascular problems, performance

Adapted from Cheadle MJ: The screening sexual history: Getting to the problem. Clin Geriatric Med 1991 7:9–13.

TABLE 30–10   ENIGMA—Model of Assessment and Recommendation for Sexual Satisfaction

E—engage	*Engage* the patient in conversation providing an opening and opportunity to talk	Need not be directly sexual History of surgery, presence of other significant medical conditions Assess interpersonal skills for expression of need Is sexual partner(s) present or absent and what is current relationship to patient? If no partner, is masturbation a release option?
N—normalize	*Normalize* sexual interest and activity in a matter-of-fact way that makes the subject standard and legitimate	Open discussion acknowledging individual variations Clarify sexual concerns, preferences, interest, experience, values Clarify satisfaction with sexual functioning as well as the existence and nature of any problem with sexual functioning Leads to acceptance of self and validation of interest
I—inform	*Inform* the patient and partner about sexual physiology and anatomy, thus naturally answering their questions	Establish current sexual knowledge regarding normal body anatomy and physiological function of both patient and partner Thorough, frank but sensitive education of function and response, both physical and emotional, of the disabling condition and its effects on motor and sensory function, communication, cognition, and fertility Discuss health issues relevant to patient's sexual behavior (e.g., risk factors for human immunodeficiency virus) Re-educate about masturbation Discuss health issues relevant to patient's medications
G—guide	*Guide* the patient and partner by responding in the same language and metaphors	The clinician is a powerful role model and can set the stage by understanding the patient's language, e.g., "hard-on," for erection, "come" for experiencing orgasm Problems such as pain, spasticity, decreased endurance and bowel and bladder function may require introduction by clinician
M—maximize	*Maximize* their problem-solving ability by encouraging experimentation, reading, and peer counseling	Discuss experimentation such as masturbation, sexual aids such as vibrators, couple-play Provide list of reading, medical and lay
A—assess/reassess	*Assess and reassess* the sexual issues at the next visit and make it an ongoing subject, not a one-time thing	At each visit a checklist through the ENIGMA model should be briefly reviewed to monitor progress, hang-ups or anxiety, acceptance of each area There are frequent anxieties and misconceptions after heart attack, hysterectomy, stroke, or life-altering medical condition Discuss the patient's sexual experience since the onset of the disability Assess interpersonal and psychosocial factors that may enhance or interfere with sexual relationships

tion, and extended care settings.[65] It is reasonable to expect such a specialist would be invaluable in a general rehabilitation practice as well. Results of patients' sexual satisfaction showed a positive correlation with active, varied, and satisfying sexual relationships prior to injury, as well as with having an available interested and adventurous partner. A negative correlation was noted with anger. "Untrained professionals who attempt counseling without knowing the sexual diagnosis and without understanding of the dynamics of the sexual rehabilitation process [can do harm to the patient]."[65] The next section introduces a simple model of sexual counseling which outlines the various levels of competence for clinicians.[2]

PLISSIT Model (*Permission, Limited Information, Specific Suggestions, Intensive Therapy*)[2]

The goals of the patient-clinician interaction should be to develop trusting relationships, support gender identity, maintain body image, and teach socialization[36] (Table 30–13). The entire rehabilitation team should be particularly adept at handling the first phase, permission, and understand how to lead patients through the appropriate phases. Personal attitudes and beliefs about one's own sexuality and the expression of such attitudes and beliefs by disabled patients must be examined.

The patient's interest in sexuality often comes out in a subtle way as an expression of poor self-image, hostile humor, profanity, or sexual aggressiveness.[73] Clinicians should recognize these subtleties and respond appropriately. This might include acknowledgment of the patient's sexual need with the suggestion that it be directed toward more appropriate partners, or by setting firm limits.[93] Not all patients want sexual information, and it should not be pushed on them. Patients can use their impairment as an excuse for avoiding sexuality in their life, perhaps because of fear of rejection, failure, or unavailability of a partner. Table 30–14 lists precautions that should be followed when counseling patients. The single most important factor in improving sexual relationships between people is communication.

The PLISSIT model is simplistic and has been critiqued as providing a way for clinicians (especially physicians) to pass on their patient's sexual concerns to other clinicians. However, the rehabilitation model is interdisciplinary and the PLISSIT model provides the basis for addressing sexual issues in a comprehensive manner.[2] Counselors should have factual information about sexuality, sexual physiology and function, and changes caused by disabling conditions. This knowledge can be gained in in-service programs, professional workshops,[32] seminars, and by availing oneself of topical literature and audiovisual materials.[92] Discussing feelings, concerns, and questions with colleagues and expe-

TABLE 30-11   Suggested Physical Examination for Assessing Sexual Function

System		Examination
Mental health	Cognition	Competence to consent to sexual activity
		Judgment to make safe decisions regarding high-risk sexual activity and contraception
	Mood	Depressed
		Abusive
Neurological	Sensation	Evaluate sensate distribution
		Assess for decubitus ulcers
		*Educate regarding possible new erotic areas (insensate-sensate border)
		*Instruct patient and partner to concentrate on sensate skin
	Dysesthesia	*Positions to avoid stimulating sensitive areas
		*Techniques for desensitization
	Strength	Assess potential for touching, caressing, receiving touch
		Review positioning that allows for above
	Communication	Assess for aphasias, dysarthria
Musculoskeletal	Contractures	Assess for evidence of arthritis
		Does patient demonstrate knowledge of stretching?
		Is surgical intervention necessary?
	Spasticity	In females, evaluate adductor spasms as these may interfere with coitus
Genitalia	Hygiene	Examine for general hygiene, odors suggestive of yeast infection
		Is there need for attendant care?
	Sensation	Sensate distribution
		Evidence of reflexogenic erection or lubrication
	General	Evidence of sexually transmitted disease—condyloma, herpes
		In females, pelvic examination may need modified positioning[103]
Urological	Continence	Evidence of epididymitis
		If indwelling catheter, evidence of scrotal fistula; may wear condom over the folded catheter
		If external catheter, is there a good seal?
		If incontinent, skin breakdown
Gastrointestinal	General	Evaluate any ostomy sites
	Rectal	Assessment of anal wink, sphincter tone, voluntary control
		Assessment of bulbocavernosus reflex (manual compression of glans penis/clitoris or pulling on Foley catheter should elicit a reflex contraction of the anal sphincter)
		*Provides an opportunity to instruct patient regarding reflexogenic erection or lubrication
General	Vascular	Evidence of peripheral vascular disease or diabetes may alert clinician to presence of difficulty with erectile or lubrication function
	Cardiac	Assess for arrhythmias, pulse rate, blood pressure
	Pulmonary	Evidence of rales, shortness of breath

*Opportunities to instruct the patient.

TABLE 30-12   Role of a Sexual Healthcare Program

Clinician role	1. Patient care services—contact with family and patient, assessment, diagnosis, prognosis, treatment.
	2. In-service and professional education.
	3. Liaison with hospital community agencies—involved with national and local associations.
	4. Administration and research—statistical analysis, evaluation.
Stages of program	1. Begins on admission to acute unit as more than two thirds of patients have sexual concerns and more than half experiment with some form of genital exploration or sexual activity before discharge from acute unit. Early acknowledgment to patient and family that sexually related problems occur with spinal cord injury (SCI) but that sex life is not over.
	2. Introductory visits with the patient and family where potential problems and concerns are outlined and discussed.
	3. Assessment and diagnostic formulation, history, physical and psychosexual examination.
	4. Series of follow-up visits to clarify areas of confusion, misinformation, monitor changes, encourage experimentation. May return months or years after finding a partner.
Patient concerns	1. Sexual disabilities exist after SCI and patients want and need information about their future sexual potential.
	2. Patient concerns are often present soon after injury.[74] It is not surprising to find patients more concerned about loss of sexual function than ambulation.
	3. Concerns surface in many ways other than planned consultation.
	4. When professionals do not inquire about patient's sexual concerns, they confirm to the patient suspicions that sexual life is over.
Benefits	1. Early legitimization of sexually related concerns.
	2. Crystallization of physiological, emotional, and social capabilities and needs.
	3. Specific instructions for experimentation with various sexual alternatives.
	4. Patients not treated in the acute setting indicate long-standing sexual concerns, difficulty relating to partner, negative attitude toward sexual abilities.

Adapted from: Miller S, Szasz G, Anderson L: Sexual health care clinician in an acute spinal cord injury unit. Arch Phys Med Rehabil 1981; 62:315-320.

TABLE 30–13 PLISSIT Model for Sexual Counseling

	Goals	Responsibility	Example	References
P *permission*	Assure the patient that sexuality is a legitimate concern in the rehabilitation process.[36, 80] Provide a positive climate in which patients feel comfortable to ask questions, seek advice, and experiment. Do not expect the patient to initiate the discussion! Open the door with your questions.	Should be addressed by any team member in any discussion.	If sexual history is included as a routine part of *every* intake examination, it signals to the client that sexuality is considered an integral part of rehabilitation. The initial interaction can also serve to set the stage for further discussion and questions. "Being a good listener, attending to and acknowledging spoken or body language, asking leading questions, initiating discussion of sensitive subjects, and making observations about physical manifestations, such as reflex erections in the male client with spinal cord injury."[80] Telling people that their thoughts, feelings, and behaviors are "normal."[86]	The clinician is directed to read general textbooks and review articles.[27, 58]
LI *limited information*	Deals with the disability and its Implications for sexual health in a general fashion.[80] Used to change 'relevant attitudes and behavior. Can serve as the means for dispelling general sexual myths relating to breast and genital size, masturbation, oral-genital contact, anal intercourse.	May be provided to the patient in a private impersonal manner by way of educational material or by any comfortable team member.	This level of information is easily provided during the initial examination. While eliciting the bladder-bowel history or examining the genitalia, one can provide vital information. For example, performing the bulbocavernosus reflex can be very intimidating or embarrassing for the patient but can be an easy steppingstone to a more in-depth discussion regarding sexual function. Clients should be encouraged to seek out new areas of hypersensitivity. This information should also be provided to family and significant others.	Pamphlets or educational handouts on head injury, stroke,[60] or spinal cord injury. (Sexuality After Spinal Cord Injury: Fact Sheet No. 3. National Spinal Cord Injury Association, 1987; Male Reproductive Function After Spinal Cord Injury: Fact Sheet No. 10. National Spinal Cord Injury Association, 1988.)
SS *specific suggestions*	Patient and partner are actively assisted by staff to set and reach specific goals to address sexual concerns and dysfunctions.[80]	Rehabilitation team member knowledgeable about sexuality and the particular physical disability affecting the patient.	Therapists can assist patients with positioning for comfortable lovemaking like using the partner for a backboard, sensual ways to undress, techniques of foreplay, the use of fantasy, types of mechanical devices available, how to deal with urinal and bowel mishaps. Pipe-cleaner figures can be useful in demonstrating alternative sexual positions. "You'll have to try it and see" is not good enough. Use peer counseling.	Excellent books and videos depicting different lovemaking options. (Mooney TO, Cole TM, Chilgren RA: Sexual Options for Paraplegics and Quadriplegics. Boston, Little, Brown, 1975; Bregman S: Sexuality and the Spinal Cord Injured Woman. Minneapolis, Sister Kenny Foundation, 1975; Rabin BJ: The sensuous wheeler. Long Beach, Calif, 1980.)
IT *intensive therapy*	When is it time to refer? Psychological problems General sexual dysfunction Overall low sexual interest Primary orgasmic dysfunction Vaginismus Primary impotence Ejaculatory incompetence Destructive paraphilias	Requires assistance of a specially trained professional or professional sexual therapist, since harm may be done to the patient if a clinician is inexperienced.	"Injury is likely to magnify any sexual difficulties that the patient and the partner have (interpersonal and psychological issues) and these must be overcome before progress can be made."[100]	American Association of Sex Educators, Counselors and Therapists, 435 N. Michigan Ave., Suite 1717, Chicago, IL 60611 (312)644–0828.

Adapted from Annon JS, Robinson CH: Treatment of common male and female sexual concerns. *In* Ferguson JM, Taylor CB (eds): The Comprehensive Handbook of Behavioral Medicine, Vol 1. New York, SP Medical & Scientific Books, 1980, pp 273–296.

TABLE 30–14   Sexual Counseling Precautions

1. Do not put persons in conflict with their God.
2. Avoid extreme pressure on the patient to discuss sexuality.
3. Avoid forcing your morality and convictions on the patient.
4. Do not threaten the patient with your own sexuality.
5. Do not make sex an all-or-none sort of experience.
6. Do not assume that once the topic is discussed that you can leave it alone.
7. Do not conclude that there is only one way to convey information.
8. Be sure that the conjoint nature of sexual relationships is held paramount.
9. Do convey the notion that all relationships, including the sexual one, are a matter of compromise.

From Rieve JE: Sexuality and the adult with acquired physical disability. Nurs Clin North Am 1989; 24:265–276. Information compiled by Rieve from Hohmann GW: Sexual dysfunction associated with physical disabilities. Arch Phys Med Rehabil 1975; 56:1, and other sources.

rienced patients are methods that can be used to increase counseling competence and comfort level.[80]

CONCLUSION

Full and positive understanding and achievement of sexuality and sexual experience are accepted by most social components in both Eastern and Western civilization as a valuable, creative, recreative, and stress-releasing part of the quality of life. This can be no more true than in the health and medical processes of rehabilitation, in acquired physical or mental disabilities, and in rehabilitation of those with congenital or lifelong limitations.

The rules and religions of various social and cultural groups can add strength to or undermine the individual's sexual self-concept. When a patient is confronted by a physical or mental disability, an adequate or optimal sexual rebuilding must include not only an education of normal and modified sexual function and physiology, of acceptable options, and of ways to see his or her new physique and brain function as desirable, but also a process to expand positively sexuality and moral beliefs.

The plumbing of sexual function—the mechanics of how to make what is present work to the fullest extent—is the challenge to the physiatrist. Sexuality is a primary example of head, heart, and body interaction. Positive issues must be encouraged. Negative issues must be examined and addressed. All this must be done in the full knowledge and understanding of the patient, partner, family, and support by the rehabilitation team. Any individual therapist can rehabilitate, but in the complex area especially, it is typically best done by a well-coordinated team.

In looking at the complete individual patient, a thorough history, physical evaluation, assessment of self-concept and formation of goals must all be inculcated into sexuality rehabilitation. It must be accepted by all involved—patient included—that the acquisition of a disability requires a reexamination of the patient's sexuality. Treatment of an acquired disability should include sexual therapy.

References

1. Aboseif SR, Lue TF: Hemodynamics of penile erection. Urol Clin North Am 1988; 15:1–7.
2. Annon JS, Robinson CH: Treatment of common male and female sexual concerns. In Ferguson JM, Taylor CB (eds): The Comprehensive Handbook of Behavioral Medicine, vol 1. New York, SP Medical & Scientific Books, 1980, pp 273–296.
3. Barada JH, McKimmy RM: Vasoactive pharmacotherapy. In Bennett AH (ed): Impotence: Diagnosis and Management of Erectile Dysfunction. Philadelphia, WB Saunders, 1994, pp 229–250.
4. Bennett CJ, Seager SW, Vasher EA, et al: Sexual dysfunction and electroejaculation in men with spinal cord injury: review. J Urol 1988; 139:453–456.
5. Benson GS, McConnell J, Lipshultz LI: Neuromorphology and neuropharmacology of the human penis. An in vitro study. J Clin Invest 1980; 65:506–513.
6. Bérard EJJ: The sexuality of spinal cord injured women: Physiology and pathophysiology: a review. Paraplegia 1989; 27:99–112.
7. Beretta G, Chelo E, Zanollo A: Reproductive aspects in spinal cord injured males. Paraplegia 1989; 27:113–118.
8. Berkman AH, Weissman R, Frielich MH: Sexual adjustment of spinal cord injured veterans living in the community. Arch Phys Med Rehabil 1978; 59:29–33.
9. Bitran D, Hull EM: Pharmacological analysis of male rat sexual behavior. Neurosci Biobehav Rev 1987; 11:365–389.
10. Blackerby WF: A treatment model for sexuality disturbance following brain injury. J Head Trauma Rehabil 1990; 5:73–82.
11. Boldrini P, Basaglia N, Calanca MC: Sexual changes in hemiparetic patients. Arch Phys Med Rehabil 1991; 72:202–207.
12. Bolling RD: Prevalence, goals and complications of heterosexual anal intercourse in a gynecologic population. J Reprod Med 1977; 19:120–124.
13. Bors E, Comarr AE: Neurologic disturbances of sexual function with special reference to 529 patients with spinal cord injury. Urol Surv 1960; 10:191–222.
14. Bray GP, DeFrank RS, Wolfe TL: Sexual functioning in stroke survivors. Arch Phy Med Rehabil 1981; 62:286–288.
15. Brindley GS: Deep scrotal temperature and the effect on it of clothing, air temperature activity, posture and paraplegia. Br J Urol 1982; 54:49–55.
16. Brindley GS: The fertility of men with spinal injuries. Paraplegia 1984; 22:337–348.
17. Brindley GS: The actions of parasympathetic and sympathetic nerves in human micturition, erection and seminal emission, and their restoration in paraplegic patients by implanted electrical stimulators. Proc R Soc Lond 1988; 235:111.
18. Buch JP: Disorders of ejaculation. In Bennett AH (ed): Impotence: Diagnosis and Management of Erectile Dysfunction. Philadelphia, WB Saunders, 1994, pp 186–196.
19. Buch JP, Zorn BH: Evaluation and treatment of infertility in spinal cord injured men through rectal probe electroejaculation. J Urol 1993; 149:1350–1354.
20. Burgener S, Logan G: Sexuality concerns of the post-stroke patient. Rehabil Nurs 1989; 14:178–181.
21. Chambas K: Sexual concerns of adolescents with cancer. J Pediatr Oncol Nurs 1991; 8:165–172.
22. Chapelle PA, Blanquart F, Peuch AJ, et al: Treatment of anejaculation in the total paraplegic by subcutaneous injection of physostigmine. Paraplegia 1983; 21:30–36.
23. Charlifue SW, Gerhart KA, Menter RR, et al: Sexual issues of women with spinal cord injuries. Paraplegia 1992; 30:192–199.
24. Cheadle MJ: The screening sexual history: Getting to the problem. Clin Geriatr Med 1991; 7:9–13.
25. Chicano LA: Humanistic aspects of sexuality as related to spinal cord injury. J Neurosci Nurs 1989; 21:366–369.
26. Collins KP, Hackler RH: Complications of penile prostheses in the spinal cord injury population. J Urol 1988; 140:984–985.

27. Comfort A: Sexual Consequences of Disability. Philadelpha, GF Stickley, 1978.
28. Comfort A, Dial LK: Sexuality and aging: An overview. Clin Geriatr Med 1991; 7:1–7.
29. Craig DI: The adaptation to pregnancy of spinal cord injured women. Rehabil Nurs 1990; 15:6–9.
30. Cromer BA, Enrile B, McCoy K, et al: Knowledge, attitudes and behavior related to sexuality in adolescents with chronic disability. Dev Med Child Neurol 1990; 32:602–210.
31. Deamer RL, Thompson JF: The role of medications in geriatric sexual function. Clin Geriatr Med 1991; 7:95–111.
32. Eisenberg MG, Rustad LC: Sex education and counseling program on a spinal cord injury service. Arch Phys Med Rehabil 1976; 57:135–140.
33. Ende J, Rockwell S, Glasgow M: The sexual history in general medicine practice. Arch Intern Med 1984; 144:558–561.
34. Fletcher GF, Johnston BL, Cantwell JD: Dynamic electrocardiographic monitoring during coitus in patients postmyocardial infarction and revascularization. Circulation 1978; 57(suppl 2):204.
35. Freda M, Rubinsky H: Sexual function in the stroke survivor. Phys Med Rehabil Clin North Am 1991; 2:643–658.
36. Goddard LR: Sexuality and spinal cord injury. J Neurosci Nurs 1988: 20:240–243.
37. Griffith ER, Tomko MA, Timms RJ: Sexual function in spinal cord–injured patients: A review. Arch Phys Med Rehabil 1973; 54:539–542.
38. Gupta K: Sexual dysfunction in elderly women. Clin Geriatr Med 1990; 6:197–203.
39. Guttmann L, Walsh JJ: Prostigmin assessment test of fertility in spinal man. Paraplegia 1971; 9:39–50.
40. Hahn K: Sexuality and COPD. Rehabil Nurs 1989; 14:191–195.
41. Hamilton GA, Seidman RN: A comparison of the recovery period for women and men after an acute myocardial infarction. Heart Lung 1993; 22:308–315.
42. Hirsch IH, Sedor J, Callahan HJ, et al: Antisperm antibodies in seminal plasma of spinal cord-injured men. Urology 1992; 39:243–247.
43. Horn LJ, Zasler ND: Neuroanatomy and neurophysiology of sexual function. J Head Trauma Rehabil 1990; 5:1–13.
44. Jensen SB: Sexual relationships in couples with a diabetic partner. J Sex Marital Ther 1985; 11:259–270.
45. Kaiser FE: Sexuality and impotence in the aging man. Clin Geriatr Med 1991; 7:63–71.
46. Kedia KR, Markland C, Fraly EE: Sexual function following high retroperitoneal lymphadenectomy. J Urol 1975; 114:237.
47. Kligman EW: Office evaluation of sexual function and complaints. Clin Geriatr Med 1991; 7:15–39.
48. Kosteljanetz M, Jensen T, Norgard B, et al: Sexual and hypothalamic dysfunction in the post-concussional syndrome. Acta Neurol Scand 1981; 63:169–180.
49. Krane RJ, Siroky MB: Neurophysiology of erection. Urol Clin North Am 1981; 8:91–101.
50. Kuhn RA: Functional capacity of the isolated human spinal cord. Brain 1950; 73:1–51.
51. LeMone P: Human sexuality in adults with insulin-dependent diabetes mellitus. Image J Nurs Scholarship 1993; 25:101–105.
52. Levinson SF, O'Connell PG: Rehabilitation dimensions of AIDS: A review. Arch Phys Med Rehabil 1991; 72:690–696.
53. Lewis D: The gynecologic consideration of the sexual act. JAMA 1983; 250:222–227.
54. Linsenmeyer TA, Perkash I: Infertility in men with spinal cord injury. Arch Phys Med Rehabil 1991; 72:747–754.
55. Lipe H, Longstreth WT Jr, Bird TD, et al: Sexual function in married men with Parkinson's disease compared to married men with arthritis. Neurology 1990; 40:1347–1349.
56. LoPiccolo J: Counseling and therapy for sexual problems in the elderly. Clin Geriatr Med 1991; 7:161–179.
57. Marsiglio W, Donnelly D: Sexual relations in later life: A national study of married persons. J Gerontol 1991; 46:S338–344.
58. Masters WH, Johnson VE, Kolodny RC: Human Sexuality. Boston, Little, Brown, 1982.
59. Mayers KS: Sexual and social concerns of the disabled: A group counseling approach. Sex Disability 1978; 1:100–111.
60. McCormick GP, Riffer DJ, Thompson MM: Coital positioning for stroke afflicted couples. Rehabil Nurs 1986; 11:17–19.
61. Medhat A, Huber PM, Medhat MA: Factors that influence the level of activities in persons with lower extremity amputation. Rehabil Nurs 1990; 15:13–18.
62. Meeropol E: One of the gang: sexual development of adolescents with physical disabilities. J Pediatr Nurs 1991; 6:243–249.
63. Melman A, Christ GJ, Hirsch MS: Anatomy and physiology of the penis. In Bennett AH (ed): Impotence: Diagnosis and Management of Erectile Dysfunction. Philadelphia, WB Saunders, 1994, pp 18–30.
64. Merrill JM, Laux LF, Thornby JI: Why doctors have difficulty with sex histories. South Med J 1990; 83:613–617.
65. Miller S, Szasz G, Anderson L: Sexual health care clinician in an acute spinal cord injury unit. Arch Phys Med Rehabil 1981; 62:315–320.
66. Money J: Phantom orgasm in the dreams of paraplegic men and women. Arch Gen Psychiatry 1960; 3:373–382.
67. Montague DK, Lakin MM: Penile prostheses. In Bennett AH (ed): Impotence: Diagnosis and Management of Erectile Dysfunction. Philadelphia, WB Saunders, 1994, pp 257–295.
68. Morales A: Nonsurgical management options in impotence. Hosp Pract, 1993, March, pp 16–23.
69. Murphy JB, Lipshultz LI: Abnormalities of ejaculation. Urol Clin North Am 1987; 14:583–595.
70. Nadig PW: Vacuum therapy and other devices. In Bennett AH (ed): Impotence: Diagnosis and Management of Erectile Dysfunction. Philadelphia, WB Saunders, 1994, pp 251–256.
71. O'Carroll RE, Woodrow J, Maroun F: Psychosexual and psychosocial sequela of closed head injury. Brain Injury 1991; 5:303–313.
72. Perkash I, Martin DE, Warner H, et al: Electroejaculation in spinal cord injury patients: Simplified new equipment and technique. J Urol 1990; 143:305–307.
73. Pervin-Dixon L: Sexuality and the spinal cord injured. J Psychosoc Nurs Ment Health Surv 1988; 26:31–34.
74. Phelps G, Brown M, Chen J, et al: Sexual experience and plasma testosterone levels in male veterans after spinal cord injury. Arch Phys Med Rehabil 1983; 64:47–52.
75. Pilsecker C: Starting out: the first six months posthospital for spinal cord–injured veterans. Am J Phys Med Rehabil 1990; 69:91–95.
76. Purifoy FE, Grodsky A, Giambra LM: The relationship of sexual daydreaming to sexual activity, sexual drive, and sexual attitudes for women across the life-span. Arch Sex Behav 1992; 21:369–385.
77. Rabin BJ: The Sensuous Wheeler: Sexual Adjustment for the Spinal Cord Injured. Long Beach, Calif, Rabin, 1980.
78. Rawicki HB, Hill S: Semen retrieval in spinal cord injured men. Paraplegia 1991; 29:443–446.
79. Relf MV: Sexuality and the older bypass patient. Geriatr Nurs 1991; 34:294–296.
80. Rieve JE: Sexuality and the adult with acquired physical disability. Nurs Clin North Am 1989; 24:265–276.
81. Sadoughi W, Leshner M, Fine HL: Sexual adjustment in a chronically ill and physically disabled population: A pilot study. Arch Phys Med Rehabil 1971; 52:311–317.
82. Saenz de Tejada I, Goldstein I, Krane RJ: Local control of penile erection. Urol Clin North Am 1988; 15:9–15.
83. Sarosdy MF, Hudnall CH, Erickson DR, et al: A prospective double-blind trial of intracorporeal papaverine versus prostaglandin E1 in the treatment of impotence. J Urol 1988; 141:551–553.
84. Sato K, Kihara K, Ando M, et al: Seminal emission by electrical stimulation of the spermatic nerve and epididymis. Int J Androl 1991; 14:461.
85. Schiavi RC, Schreiner-Engel P, Mandeli J, et al: Healthy aging and male sexual function. Am J Psychiatry 1990; 147:766–771.
86. Seidl A, Bullough B, Haughey B, et al: Understanding the effects of a myocardial infarction on sexual functioning: A basis for sexual counseling. Rehabil Nurs 1991: 16:255–264.
87. Sipski ML, Alexander CJ: Sexual function and dysfunction after spinal cord injury. Phys Med Rehabil Clinics North Am 1992; 3:811–828.
88. Sjogren K: Sexuality after stroke with hemiplegia. II. With special regard to partnership adjustment and to fulfillment. Scand J Rehabil Med 1983; 15:63–69.
89. Smith DB, Babaian RJ: The effects of treatment for cancer on male fertility and sexuality. Cancer Nurs 1992; 15:271–275.
90. Smith LL, Lathrop LM: AIDS and human sexuality. Can J Public Health 1993; 84:S14–18.

91. Sonksen J, Biering-Sorensen F: Transcutaneous nitroglycerin in the treatment of erectile dysfunction in spinal cord injured. Paraplegia 1992; 30:554–557.

92. Spica MM: Sexual counseling standards for the spinal cord-injured. J Neurosci Nurs 1989; 21:56–60.

93. Stockard S: Caring for the sexually aggressive patient. Nursing 1991; 11:72–73.

94. Talbot HS: Sexual function in paraplegia. J Urol 1955; 73:91–100.

95. Teal JC, Athelstan GT: Sexuality and spinal cord injury: Some psychosocial considerations. Arch Phys Med Rehabil 1975; 56:264–268.

96. Thornton CE: Sexuality counseling of women with spinal cord injuries. Sex Disability 1979; 9:267–277.

97. Trop CS, Bennett CJ: Autonomic dysreflexia and its urological implications: A review. J Urol 1991; 146:1461–1469.

98. Valleroy ML, Kraft GH: Sexual dysfunction in multiple sclerosis. Arch Phys Med Rehabil 1984; 65:125–128.

99. VerVoort SM: Infertility in spinal-cord injured male. Urology 1987; 29:157–165.

100. Walbroehl GS: Sexuality in the handicapped. Am Fam Physician 1987; 36:129–133.

101. Wanner MB, Rageth CJ, Zäch GA: Pregnancy and autonomic hyper-reflexia in patients with spinal cord lesions. Paraplegia 1987; 25:482–490.

102. Ware CJ: Impotence and aging. Clin Geriatr Med 1989; 5:301–314.

103. Weinberg JS: Human sexuality and spinal cord injury. Nurs Clin North Am 1982; 17:407–419.

104. Weiss J: Multiple sclerosis: Will it come between us? Sexual concerns of clients and their partners. J Neurosci Nurs 1992; 24:190–193.

105. Weiss JN, Mellinger BC: Sexual dysfunction in elderly men. Clin Geriatr Med 1990; 6:185–196.

106. White MJ, Rintala DH, Hart KA, et al: Sexual activities, concerns and interests of men with spinal cord injury. Am J Phys Med Rehabil 1992; 71:225–231.

107. White MJ, Rintala DH, Hart KA, et al: Sexual activities, concerns and interests of women with spinal cord injury living in the community. Am J Phys Med Rehabil 1993; 72:372–378.

108. Whitehead TL: Sexual health promotion of the patient with burns. J Burn Care Rehabil 1993; 14:221–226.

109. Witherington R: Vacuum constriction device for management of erectile impotence. J Urol 1989; 141:320–322.

110. Yalla SV, Vickers MA, Sullivan MP, et al: Sexual dysfunction and spinal cord injury. In Bennett AH (ed): Impotence: Diagnosis and Management of Erectile Dysfunction. Philadelphia, WB Saunders, 1994, pp 175–185.

111. Yarkony GM: Enhancement of sexual function and fertility in spinal cord–injured males. Am J Phys Med Rehabil 1990; 69:81–87.

112. Yoffe E: Women and sex. Health 1994; 4:53–60.

113. Young BK, Katz M, Klein SA: Pregnancy after spinal cord injury: Altered maternal and fetal response to labor. Obstet Gynecol 1983; 62:59–62.

114. Zasler ND, Horn LJ: Rehabilitative management of sexual dysfunction. J Head Trauma Rehabil 1990; 5:14–24.

115. Zencius A, Wesolowski MD, Burke WH, et al: Managing hyper-sexual disorders in brain-injured clients. Brain Injury 1990; 4:175–181.

31

The Prevention and Management of Pressure Ulcers

RICHARD SALCIDO, M.D., DENNIS HART, M.D., AND ANN MARIE SMITH, PH.D., R.N., C.R.R.N.

Pressure ulcers have been a human affliction since antiquity. Recently, however, the overall management of pressure ulcers has gained prominence among national health care issues. Pressure ulcers primarily affect elderly, spinal cord–injured, diabetic, and mobility-impaired persons.[1, 4, 5] National consensus indicates a need for guidelines that can help providers standardize the treatment of pressure ulcers. These guidelines should improve the quality of care and help control its cost.[18, 22, 88] In response to this clear need, the Agency for Health Care Policy and Research (AHCPR) selected pressure ulcers as one of the major areas in which to develop clinical practice guidelines for prevention and treatment. The AHCPR guidelines have been developed for the management of some other diseases and reflect a national trend toward standardization of care.[18, 22, 88]

Despite advances in medicine, surgery, nursing care, and self-care education, pressure ulcers remain a major cause of morbidity and mortality, particularly for persons with impaired sensation, prolonged immobility, or advanced age.[1] Research in the area of pressure ulcers (specifically, characterization, prevention, and treatment) is important in preventing secondary complications in persons with disabilities. As the standards of acute, post-traumatic, and rehabilitation care are raised, the population of persons with lifelong functional impairments will grow and preventing secondary complications will become an increasingly prominent concern.

Attempts to develop scientifically sound modes of pressure ulcer prevention and treatment have been hampered by the lack of specific information about the etiology, pathophysiology, biochemistry, and cell biology of these lesions. In the absence of such data, myriad approaches to treatment have been, and continue to be, developed on an empirical basis. The magnitude of the cost and morbidity attributable to pressure ulcers is clearly disproportionate to the quantity of scientific information available to practitioners who face the challenge of providing care for persons with pressure ulcers.

This chapter focuses on the major clinical issues that can enable practicing physicians to approach the management and treatment of pressure ulcers systematically, assisted by the pressure ulcer prediction and prevention strategies that are based on the *AHCPR Pressure Ulcer Prevention and Treatment Guidelines*.[18, 22, 88] It is also intended to be an information resource, covering the spectrum of this important clinical problem from basic science to clinical treatment.

THE SCOPE OF THE PROBLEM

Definition

One dictionary defines an ulcer as "an inflammatory, often suppurating lesion on the skin or an internal mucosal surface of the body, as in the duodenum, resulting in necrosis of the tissue."[148] *Dorland's Medical Dictionary* describes an ulcer (Latin, *ulcus*; Greek, *heliosis*) as "a local defect or excavation on the surface of an organ or tissue which is produced by sloughing of inflammatory necrotic tissue."[50] The National Pressure Ulcer Advisory Panel (NPUAP), an independent, non-profit organization formed in 1987 and dedicated to the prevention, management, treatment, and research of pressure ulcers, defines a pressure ulcer as an area of unrelieved pressure over a defined area, usually over a bony prominence, resulting in ischemia, cell death, and tissue necrosis.[103]

Description

The taxonomic description of pressure ulcers lacks general consistency.[1, 4, 152] Textbooks refer to these lesions in various ways, usually in regard to the depth of the lesion based on macroscopic and morphological criteria (Fig. 31–1).[103] They are often referred to as *pressure sores, bed sores,* or *decubitus ulcers* (from the Latin word *decumbere,* "to lie on one's side"). Because persons at risk can develop lesions in various positions (e.g., sitting), the term "pressure ulcers" is used in this chapter.

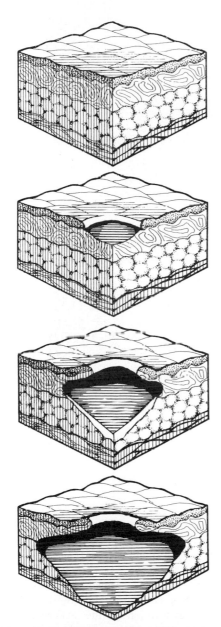

FIGURE 31–1 National Pressure Ulcer Advisory Panel (NPUAP) classification: Identification and staging of pressure ulcers. *Stage 1:* Non-blanchable erythema not resolved in 30 min; epidermis intact; reversible with intervention. *Stage 2:* Partial-thickness loss of skin involving epidermis, possibly into dermis; may appear as blisters with erythema. *Stage 3:* Full-thickness destruction through dermis into subcutaneous tissue. *Stage 4:* Deep tissue destruction through subcutaneous tissue to fascia, muscle, bone, or joint. (Used with permission from the NPUAP.)

Measurement

The most common method of monitoring the healing of pressure ulcers utilizes photography and diagrams.[152] The VistaMed wound measurement system[142] is a useful new tool to evaluate wounds quantitively. It is possible to obtain precise objective information on size, shape, outline, area, color, and surrounding tissue changes using color- and light-balanced computerized photographic image capture. Digital sub-pixel measuring techniques achieve measurements of clinician-defined image areas, such as wound edge, eschar, necrotic tissue, or granulation formation. Concise, documented measurement contributes to efficient wound treatment, management, and progress review (Fig. 31–2).[142] Numerous other devices have been used to measure the volume (volumetrics) and the dimensions of the pressure ulcer wound. A simple method is to use a measured amount of saline to infer the volume of the wound. More sophisticated radiographic techniques such as sinus x-rays, computed tomography, and magnetic resonance imaging are too expensive for routine use.[152] Developing standardized measuring techniques is necessary to provide quantitative information on wound healing and to validate research.

Common Sites of Involvement

Sites of occurrence vary in different studies and with different diagnoses.[1, 4, 5, 65–67, 103] Practitioners should vigilantly inspect the most common sites of pressure ulcer formation: the ischium (28%), the sacrum (17% to 27%), the trochanter (12% to 19%), and the heel (9% to 18%). Pressure ulcers commonly develop on the occiput of geriatric and pediatric patients who spend extended amounts of time lying supine. Patients with the secondary manifestations of osteoporosis and associated thoracic kyphosis can develop pressure ulcers over the spinous processes. Elderly and diabetic patients often have pressure ulcers of the heel.

Epidemiology

The incidence of pressure ulcers in the United States is approximately 1,000,000 per year,[70, 139] but definitive information on the epidemiology and natural history of this condition is still limited. Studies to date have been encumbered by methodological issues and variability in describing the lesions.[28, 103] The incidence in hospitalized patients ranges from 2.7%[68] to 29%[39] (prevalence, 3.5%[130] to 69%[7, 99]). Patients in critical care units run a higher risk of developing pressure ulcers, as evidenced by 33% incidence[21] and 41% prevalence.[120] Elderly patients admitted to acute care hospitals for nonelective, orthopedic procedures such as hip replacement and long bone fractures are at even greater risk for developing pressure ulcers (66% incidence).[119, 143]

In the nursing home environment, the prevalence of pressure ulcers ranges from 2.6% to 24%.[28, 116] The incidence is 25% in residents admitted from an acute care hospital,[116] and patients with pre-existing pressure ulcers showed a 26% incidence of additional pressure ulcer formation over a 6-month period. The incidence in chronic care hospitals is reported to be at 10.8%,[13] whereas 33% of those admitted to a chronic care hospital have pressure

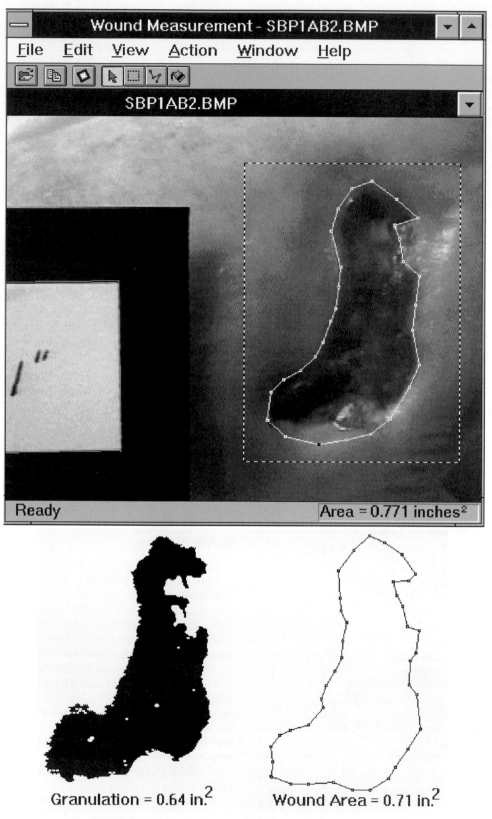

FIGURE 31–2   Force sensing array (FSA) wound measurement system.

ulcers.[23] Long-term follow-up demonstrates that the majority of ulcers healed within a year.[23, 28] Although these epidemiological studies demonstrated increased morbidity and mortality, acute hospitalization for pressure ulcers did not increase.[28] Given the current practice environment of shorter hospital stays, patients with pressure ulcers will likely receive care at alternative levels, perhaps in nursing homes and even at home.[41]

Persons with spinal cord injury (SCI) and associated co-morbidity are also at increased risk for the formation of pressure ulcers.[15] The incidence of pressure ulcers in this population ranges from 25% to as high as 66%.[65, 108] A recent study of the prevalence of pressure ulcers in community residents with SCI demonstrated that higher-level SCI lesions carried a greater risk of pressure ulcers than did lower-level lesions. Of 100 patients with pressure ulcers, 33 had pressure ulcers that were classified as stage 2 or greater. Blacks ($N = 13$) had more severe ulcers than other ethnic groups in the study.[65] Some authors speculate that darker-pigmented skin can make detection of erythema more difficult,[14] which can result in undetected grade I pressure ulcers, as prolonged non-blanching erythema is typically an early warning sign of pressure ulcer risk and development.

Economic Impact

A 1991 market study estimated that the cost in treatment and hospital stays could be as much as $6 billion a year for ulcers that develop in hospital patients alone.[146] In elderly and institutionalized populations, pressure ulcers are one of the most costly diseases to treat, adding an estimated burden to our health care system of over $1 billion worth of expenditures and an additional 2.2 million Medicare hospital days.[134] The cost of treatment ranges from $2000 to $40,000 per pressure ulcer,[18, 22, 103] depending on the stage of development.[64, 72] For reconstructive surgery, costs are estimated at $25,000 per patient.[103] These costs alone, without even considering the cost of human suffering, demonstrate the importance of pressure ulcer prevention and of cost-effective treatment practices.

Morbidity and Mortality

Pressure ulcers and the associated co-morbid factors that predispose patients to them lead to high rates of morbidity and mortality. Complications include infection, pain, depression, and even death. Approximately 60,000 people die each year from complications of pressure ulcers,[4] and pressure ulcer development has been associated with a 4.5 times greater risk of death than that for persons with the risk factors but without pressure ulcers.[135] A secondary complication, wound-related bacteremia, can increase the risk of mortality to 55%.[4, 5, 51, 94]

Generally, infection is the major complication associated with pressure ulcers. Systemic sepsis and bacteremia are life threatening, particularly in aged persons, who are often malnourished, debilitated, and immunocompromised. The offending pathological organisms in pressure ulcers can be anaerobic or aerobic. Aerobic pathogens are commonly present in all pressure ulcers,[141] whereas anaerobes tend to occur more often in larger wounds (65% in grade III and above).[113] The most common organisms isolated from

pressure ulcers are *Proteus mirabilis,* group D streptococci, *Escherichia coli, Staphylococcus* species, *Pseudomonas* species, and *Corynebacterium* organisms. Patients with bacteremia are more likely to have *Bacteroides* species in their pressure ulcers.[113] These wounds do not need to be cultured routinely unless systemic signs of infection are present (e.g., malodorous drainage, leukocytosis, fever, hypotension, increased heart rate, changes in mental status). Clinical alertness is needed because the signs commonly associated with impeding or fulminating infection are frequently absent in elderly or immunocompromised patients.

In geriatric pressure ulcer patients, bacteremia is reported to occur at the rate of 3.5 per 10,000 hospital discharges.[135] Because the mortality rate in this population approaches 50%,[94] the antibiotic treatment for wound infection or secondary bacteremia provides the appropriate spectrum of coverage that is specific to the offending organisms. Because indiscriminate use of antibiotics leads to resistant organisms and because the specific drugs of choice and antimicrobial agents change rapidly, physiatrists typically need to consult an infectious disease specialist to facilitate the management of these complex problems.

Sepsis can also occur secondary to osteomyelitis, which has been reported to occur in 26% of non-healing ulcers.[135] A more recent prospective study demonstrated that osteomyelitis was associated with non-healing grade IV pressure ulcers in 86% of the study population.[46, 47] This study utilized three-phase technetium methyl diphosphate radionuclide flow to detect early osteomyelitis.

Various tests can be used to diagnose osteomyelitis in pressure ulcer patients. Plain x-ray has sensitivity of 78% and specificity of 50%, but x ray findings often are not present early in the infection. Bone scan is more sensitive but has low specificity (50%).[11, 93] Bone biopsy has the highest specificity (96%) and sensitivity (73%).[46, 47] Using a combination of diagnostic tests (such as leukocyte count, erythrocyte sedimentation rate, plain x-rays) provided sensitivity of 89% and specificity of 88%. If all three test results are positive, the positive predictive value of this combination is 69%. If all are negative, the negative predictive value is 96%.[46, 47]

Osteomyelitis should be considered whenever an ulcer fails to heal, especially one over a bony prominence. Clinicians should also rule out other conditions associated with non-healing ulcers, such as heterotopic calcification or ossification. Most studies agree that antibiotic treatment for osteomyelitis should last 6 to 8 weeks. Surgery is needed for some cases of chronic osteomyelitis.[15] Systemic amyloidosis can result from chronic, suppurative pressure ulcers. Additional complications of pressure ulcers include spreading cellulitis, sinus tract or abscess, septic arthritis, squamous cell carcinoma in the ulcer, periurethral fistula, and heterotopic ossification. Because some of the secondary complications of pressure ulcers can preclude wound healing, they should be aggressively prevented and treated.[152]

ETIOPATHOLOGICAL FACTORS

Pressure ulcers are caused by the interaction of multiple, diverse, etiopathological factors that can be classified as *pathomechanical* or *pathophysiological.*[4, 9, 27]

TABLE 31–1   Contributing Factors to Pressure Ulcers

PATHOMECHANICAL (EXTRINSIC OR PRIMARY)
   Compression
   Maceration
   Immobility
   Pressure
   Friction
   Shear

TISSUE AT RISK

PATHOPHYSIOLOGICAL (INTRINSIC OR SECONDARY)
   Fever
   Anemia
   Infection
   Ischemia
   Hypoxemia
   Malnutrition
   Spinal cord injury
   Neurological disease
   Decreased lean body mass
   Increased metabolic demands

Pathomechanical Factors (Extrinsic or Primary; Table 31–1)

Prolonged Pressure

The most important factor in pressure ulcer development is unrelieved pressure.[83, 85] Pressure ulcers arise from prolonged tissue ischemia caused by pressure that exceeds the tissue capillary pressure. Prolonged pressure deprives tissues of oxygen and essential nutrients, owing to ischemia and hypoxia, which then causes pressure ulcers.[85] Several critical questions remain unanswered, however. How much pressure is required to produce predictable ulceration? How long must pressure be sustained to produce predictable ulceration? Which tissues are at greatest risk of ulceration?

In 1930, Landis used a microinjection method to cannulate the arteriolar limb of capillaries in human fingernail beds to study capillary blood pressure.[89] He reported an average pressure of 32 mm Hg in the arteriolar limb, 22 mm Hg in the mid-capillary bed, and 12 mm Hg on the venous side. This has been reproduced recently utilizing laser Doppler methods in an animal model[124–126] in which the mean capillary pressure was 45 mm Hg, approximating human capillary pressure. This finding is useful for future studies of this component of the pressure ulcer cascade.[124–126]

Interface Pressure

Interface pressure remains an ambiguous factor in pressure ulcer development. Defined as "perpendicular force per unit area between the body and support surface,"[103] it is commonly believed that interface pressure is affected by the stiffness and composition of the body tissue and by the geometric shape of the body being supported. Interface pressure in excess of 32 mm Hg is also thought to lead to closure of capillary beds and to result in tissue ischemia. Pressures under 32 mm Hg are assumed by many clinicians to be safe.[122]

These perceptions remain to be challenged, however. Products aimed at reducing or relieving pressure have tended to use interface pressure as the standard for judging

product efficacy.[88, 122, 124] Further investigation of the application of the "gold standard" of 32 mm Hg that resulted from Landis' work to pressure ulcer pathology is needed, particularly since the transmission of load on tissue and muscle can decrease or increase based on characteristics of the tissue at different sites.[17] Tissue can be more or less able to withstand pressure, depending on other patient characteristics.

Another area that requires more vigorous study is pressure as the primary factor in the development of pressure ulcers. For example, what helps able-bodied persons withstand extreme tissue loads in areas at risk without developing pressure ulcers? Why are persons with certain types of disease processes typically free from pressure ulcers? A few articles have noted that persons with amyotrophic lateral sclerosis (ALS) are at relatively low risk for pressure ulcers owing to changes in the skin (dermal thickening and increased collagen secondary to increased density of the collagen fibrils).[128, 117]

A recently developed hypothesis asserts that pressure overcoming capillary closing pressure leads to ischemia and reperfusion injury, notably in the muscle, which develops the lesion and eventually ulcerates. This ischemia-reperfusion mechanism ultimately leads to neutrophil-mediated inflammatory tissue destruction, most likely a free radical injury, that eventually causes pressure ulceration.[124–126]

Shear

Shear is mechanical stress directed parallel to the plane of interest. Shearing forces have been implicated as pathomechanical contributors in pressure ulcer development, especially on the sacrum. Though scientific evidence is lacking, it is logical to conclude that the angular and vertical force downward while patients are in the semiupright position in bed tends to distort the tissues and blood vessels near the sacrum, placing this region at risk for tissue breakdown (Figs. 31–3 and 31–4).[27, 117] The synergy of shear and pressure in the pathomechanical process leads to the formation of pressure ulcers.

Friction

Friction is the force of two surfaces moving across each other.[95] Friction and the increased drag coefficient caused by moving patients across bedsheets and other support surfaces can cause microscopic or macroscopic tissue trauma. *Moisture, maceration*, and *tissue breakdown* increase the surface tension of both the skin and the support surface. Moisture from sensible fluid loss or incontinence leads to maceration of tissues, which in turn makes them more susceptible to pressure, shear, and friction damage.

Immobility

Immobility is a major extrinsic factor associated with the risk and formation of pressure ulcers. Immobility in bed tends to cause pressure ulcers on the occiput, sacrum, heels, malleoli, and trochanteric regions, and wheelchair-mobile patients tend to develop pressure ulcers over the ischial tuberosity.[92] In persons with paralysis or in neurologically compromised persons, the afferent nerves are unable to

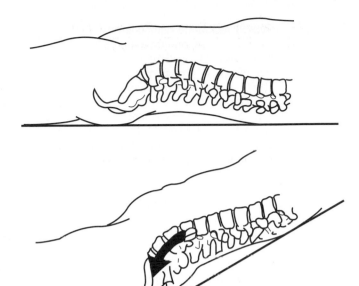

FIGURE 31–3 Shearing forces. (From Reichel SM: Shearing force as a factor in paraplegics. JAMA 1958; 166:672; with permission.)

engage the sensorimotor feedback system. As a result, early warnings of prolonged ischemia, such as discomfort, do not produce the normal adjustments in body position that intermittently relieve pressure on areas at risk.[95] Such adjustments occur instinctively in neurologically intact persons, even during sleep. Healthy subjects while asleep show some movement and change of position every 15 minutes,[35, 56] and making fewer than 20 movements per night increases the risk of developing a pressure ulcer.[12]

In a study of 40 elderly patients, nocturnal movements associated with sleep tended to decrease as the hospital stay increased.[12, 13] Analysis of periodic movements in persons at risk for pressure ulcers clearly suggests a relationship between spontaneous body movement and the development of pressure ulcers.[56] Studies using diverse measurement techniques[58] have documented pressures at specific anatomic sites that are at risk for pressure ulcers. One study utilized laser Doppler to measure local blood flow in geriatric patients at risk for pressure ulcers.[131] This study demonstrated that geriatric patients have a delayed hyperemic response to increased regional blood flow as a result of pressure applied to areas at risk. Both tissue at risk and ulcerous tissue were slower to exhibit increased blood flow as a result of a controlled local hyperthermic stimulation.[131]

Pathophysiological Factors (Intrinsic or Secondary)

These diverse elements include fever, anemia, infection, ischemia, hypoxemia, hypotension, malnutrition, spinal cord injury, neurological disease, decreased lean body

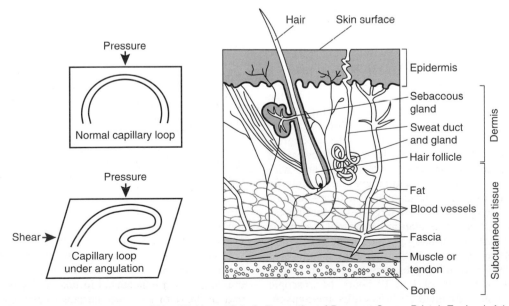

FIGURE 31–4 Prevention of pressure sores. (From Webster JG (ed): Prevention of Pressure Sores. Bristol, England, Adam Hilger, 1991.)

mass, and increased metabolic demands (see Table 31–1). Nutrition and anemia are important factors in pressure ulcer healing and prevention. The patient should have adequate nutrition, especially good protein intake and stores. Decreased lean body mass is a particular risk factor for pressure ulcers. The clinical parameters indicating good nutrition and immunocompetence are adequate calorie intake and maintenance of ideal body weight. The indirect measurements of these parameters are total lymphocyte count, transferrin level, and total albumin and protein.[25, 28–33, 52, 54]

Anemia is not only an intrinsic risk for the development of pressure ulcers,[111, 112] but patients whose hemoglobin value is below 10 have difficulty healing. Hypotension is an additional intrinsic risk factor for the formation of pressure ulcers.[19, 118] It is imperative to treat the patient's medical condition that predisposes to risk for pressure ulcers. If possible, the pathophysiological factors should be controlled in conjunction with eliminating the pathomechanical factors. If any problem is treated in isolation, this multifactorial problem will not be resolved.

A Brief Review of Pressure Ulcer Research

A monograph prepared by the Research Committee of the NPUAP suggests several research priorities for pressure ulcers: (1) outcome-focused research, (2) intervention and product efficacy studies, (3) basic research related to staging of the ulcer, (4) refinement of risk assessment methods, (5) risk-based, multi-intervention trials. Additional issues requiring investigation include cost issues, ethical decision making, guideline dissemination, public policy, and national outcome evaluations. Methodological issues, such as research design, study population, and control group use, also need further investigation.[103]

Early investigators tended to focus on pressure as the primary cause of pressure ulcers.[20, 85] Groth,[71] Kosiak,[83–85] and Dinsdale[48] were among the first investigators to explore pressure and tissue injury relationships. Groth found that pressure ulcers similar to those of humans could be produced experimentally in animals. His experiments showed that larger muscle masses withstand pressure better. He noted that effective pressure force increases toward the smaller surface. This accounts for the greater destruction of tissue at the base of the inverted cone, typified by the small area of skin redness or destruction overlying a bony prominence. This condition is frequently observed in ischial ulcers, trochanteric ulcers, and, to a lesser degree, over the sacrum. Groth also noted that generalized sepsis can result in local infection at the site of pressure, with abscess formation, extension of inflammation, thrombosis of the larger vessels, and, consequently, a larger area of tissue necrosis. He concluded that large-vessel thrombosis is not typically a cause of ulceration because of the extensive collateral circulation usually present in the skin.[71, 83, 84]

In a classic experiment, Kosiak,[83] a physiatrist, subjected dogs to accurately controlled pressures ranging from 100 to 550 mm Hg for periods of 1 to 12 hours. Microscopic examination of tissue obtained 24 hours after the application of 60 mm Hg pressure for only 1 hour showed cellular infiltration, extravasation, and hyaline degeneration. Tissues subjected to higher pressures for longer periods also showed muscle degeneration and venous thrombosis. Kosiak concluded that intense pressure of short duration was as injurious to tissues as lower pressure applied longer. In both cases, tissue ischemia led to irreversible cellular changes and, ultimately, to necrosis and ulceration. He also concluded that prolonged pressure was the direct and primary cause of pressure ulcers.[83]

Kosiak disagreed with Groth about the location and severity of skin damage, stating that it extended equally to the area under pressure instead of being most severe at the deepest part overlying the bony prominence. Kosiak concluded that skin and subcutaneous tissue provide a sling or suspension effect, which allows only a fraction of the applied pressure to be transmitted to the deep tissues.

Husain[73] reported microscopic changes in rat muscle subjected to a pressure of 100 mm Hg for as little as 1 hour. His microscopic findings were similar to those of Groth and Kosiak. Keane noted that muscle is more susceptible to pressure injury than skin and noted that the body weight is borne on superficial, weight-bearing bony prominences that are covered only with skin and superficial fascia.[80] Nola and Vistnes[105] supported Keane's ideas by documenting significant areas of muscle necrosis on histological examination of rats when pressure was applied to a transposed muscle flap over a bone. In cadaver dissections, Daniel and co-workers found that muscle is seldom interposed between bone and skin over bony prominences in normal human weightbearing positions.[44]

Dinsdale analyzed the role of pressure and friction in the production of pressure ulcers in normal and paralyzed pigs. Pressures of 160 to 1120 mm Hg were mechanically applied with friction and without friction for 3 hours. The ulcerations that were produced extended into the dermis and persisted after 24 hours. He concluded, "Friction is a factor in the pathogenesis of decubitus ulcers since it applied mechanical force in the epidermis."[48] He also concluded that a constant pressure of 70 mm Hg applied for longer than 2 hours produced irreversible tissue damage. He cautioned against blindly accepting the pressure-ischemia relationship as the only cause for ulceration, however. Dinsdale also found that minimal changes occurred with intermittent pressure relief, even at pressures of 240 mm Hg.[48]

In a more recent animal model experiment, Salcido and colleagues confirmed that muscle is more sensitive to pressure-induced ischemia than skin in anesthetized rats and noted that the association between ischemia reperfusion injury and experimentally derived pressure ulcers is evidenced by oxygen free radical–mediated tissue destruction (as studied in biopsy specimens from animal lesions).[124–126]

Clinical studies of pressure ulcers are difficult to assess, however, because they are often qualitatively based on random observation and uncontrolled studies. More fundamental approaches must be considered with respect to pressure ulcers. For example, what are the basic histological, pathological, and biochemical markers in an evolving pressure ulcer? Is it ethical to take a biopsy specimen of a human pressure ulcer for purposes of research? What are the multiple variables in the formation of pressure ulcers in the human environment?

Histology

There is a paucity of literature on the histopathological nature of decubitus ulcers, particularly in humans. Witkowski and Parish were among the first to publish on the histology of decubitus ulcers in human skin,[151] but their findings, which included vascular infiltrates, thrombosis, and edema, were not intended to represent a histopathological continuum of the evolving pressure ulcer. Husain's experiments utilized hairy rats to analyze the histological changes (primarily in the muscle) resulting from the application of pressure,[73] and Kosiak's classic work on dogs focused primarily on the epidermis.[83] Dinsdale showed that a combination of friction and pressure produced lesions in the epidermis of swine.[48]

Salcido's research team has developed an analog system to study pressure ulcers in an animal model where computer-controlled pressure was applied for 6 hours to the skin over the hip of anesthetized fuzzy rats. Interval histopathological changes seen in experimentally derived pressure ulcers have been characterized.[124–126] Histological findings included a scattering of neutrophils in the dermis and subcutaneum along the line of necrosis and patchy necrosis to the muscularis in the subdermal region. Foci of damage appeared to be associated with high concentrations of neutrophils, and lesions appeared to develop first in the muscle rather than in the dermis or epidermis. Evidence indicates that the erosion typical of pressure ulcers is mediated via a neutrophil, eosinophil, or macrophage-induced exacerbation and the appearance of vascular damage. Recurrent pressure results in increasingly severe damage to the vascular system and parenchyma consistent with an ischemia-reperfusion insult initiated through a free radical mechanism, which has implications for preventing and treating pressure ulcers.[124–126]

IDENTIFYING PATIENTS AT RISK: ASSESSMENT SCALES AND EVALUATION

The AHCPR was established in December 1989 under the Omnibus Reconciliation Act. One of the mandates of this agency through the Office of the Forum for Quality and Effectiveness of Health Care was to develop science-based guidelines for patient care whenever a problem is common and treatment is highly variable and costly. After convening a multidisciplinary panel of experts, AHCPR released guidelines for the prediction and prevention of pressure ulcers in May 1992 (Tables 31–2 and 31–3).

Pressure ulcers are preventable. They should not occur, but they continue to be one of the most pervasive and perplexing problems in managing persons who are ill, recovering from illness, or functionally impaired. Effective prevention and treatment measures depend on a comprehensive care plan, which includes scheduled turning and body repositioning.[132] The frequency and the interval between turnings seem more critical than pressure in the production of pressure ulcers. This is why nurses have adopted the practice of turning patients every 2 hours, which originated with Reswick and Rogers[18, 95, 118, 131] and is the mainstay of prevention strategies.

TABLE 31–2 AHCPR Prevention Guidelines Outline

1. The risk assessment process
   a. Complete medical history
   b. Norton (or Braden) score (see Table 31–4)
   c. Skin examination
   d. Identification of previous pressure ulcer sites
2. Prime candidates for pressure ulcers
   a. Elderly persons
   b. Chronically ill persons (cancer, stroke, diabetes)
   c. Immobile persons (due to fracture, arthritis, pain)
   d. Weak and debilitated persons
   e. Patients with altered mental status (i.e., under the effects of narcotics, anesthesia, or coma)
   f. Persons with decreased sensation and or paralysis
3. Secondary factors
   a. Illness or debilitation increases pressure ulcer formation
   b. Fever increases metabolic demands
   c. Predisposing ischemia
   d. Diaphoresis promotes skin maceration
   e. Incontinence causes skin irritation and contamination
   f. Other factors: edema, jaundice, pruritus, and xerosis (dry skin)

In view of the uncertainties about the level of pressure at which cell damage begins, and given the high incidence of ulcers occurring in persons at risk, the best advice is still to establish a regimen in which there is complete relief to all areas of the body at regular intervals.[85, 132] Various

TABLE 31–3 Rationale for Strategies to Prevent Pressure Ulcers

Skin care is paramount and must be carried out in conjunction with the following principles:
1. Pressure relief
   a. Patients should have their position shifted or turned every 2 hr
   b. Support surfaces and specialty beds require criteria for use
2. Patients can benefit from lying prone
3. Minimize shearing forces by keeping the head of the bed lower than 45 degrees
4. Air-fluidized bed
5. Wheelchair users should be taught to perform pushup exercises and to lean side to side for pressure relief
6. Pressure-relieving cushions of air, foam, gel, or a combination can be used to relieve pressure
7. Frictional relief
8. Nutritional support
   a. Nutritional history
   b. Physical examination
   c. Anthropometric measurements
   d. Laboratory studies, albumin, total lymphocyte count, transferrin level
   e. Enteral or parenteral support
   f. Vitamin therapy
9. Control of muscle spasms
   a. Involuntary muscle contractions can lead to abrasions
   b. Oral antispasticity agents are the simplest method of controlling spasticity
   c. Pressure ulcers occur more frequently in SCI patients with flaccid paralysis than in those with spasticity
10. Prevention of contractures
    a. Uncontrolled spasticity or lack of movement causes shortening of the muscles, usually the hip, knee, elbow, and ankle plantar flexors
    b. Contractures can limit the patient to only a few positions
    c. Contractures can be prevented in patients who have some mobility by encouraging ambulation and range-of-motion exercises bid

other factors clearly contribute to the formation of pressure ulcers (see Fig. 31–1).

Providers working with persons at risk need to be able to recognize skin changes that can indicate an impending breakdown. The earliest clinical evidence of damage to the skin is inflammation of the skin that blanches on application of digital pressure. This process originally presents like a hyperemic response. Unlike hyperemia, however, the inflammation persists longer, usually 30 minutes.[22] Prevention of progression to more serious damage requires immediate, complete elimination of pressure to the involved area. If we accept the proposition that pressure in excess of capillary pressure is the chief cause of pressure ulcers, then the primary prevention efforts have to be directed toward reducing or eliminating pressure over susceptible areas. Nursing strategies include prevention of prolonged pressure, elimination of shearing forces and friction, and removal of skin secretions and excretions. Additional interventions include avoiding hot water, using a mild cleansing agent that does not irritate or dry the skin, using moisturizers, using topical agents as moisture barriers, keeping the sheets dry and wrinkle free, providing adequate intake of protein and calories, and maintaining current levels of activity, mobility, and range of motion. It is also good to avoid massaging body prominences, since this practice has been associated with increased tissue breakdown and risk for the formation of pressure ulcers.[18, 22, 53, 88, 91] Positioning devices such as pillows or foam wedges should be used to prevent direct contact between bony prominences (knees, ankles). Donut-type devices should not be used because they are known to cause venous congestion and edema.[42]

Other recommendations are to avoid positioning patients directly on the trochanter, to maintain the head of the bed as low as possible, to utilize pressure-reducing devices on the bed and in the wheelchair (including various mattresses and wheelchair cushions), and to use lifting devices such as a trapeze rather than dragging the patient. Interventions should be monitored and documented. Specific details that are required include who should provide the care, how often it should be provided, and the supplies and equipment needed. How the care is to be undertaken should be individualized, written down, and readily available. Results of the interventions and the care being rendered should be documented. To ensure continuity, documentation of the plan of care should be clear, concise, and accessible to every caregiver. Patient education is of utmost importance. Patients and everyone involved in their care should have the knowledge necessary to prevent the formation of pressure ulcers.[22, 88]

Evaluation Tools

Various investigators have sought to establish the reliability and predictive validity of instruments such as the Braden scale.[20, 21] Prospective studies of these and other risk assessment tools, combined with a study of additional risk factors, are needed to refine the instrumentation, thereby permitting improvement in prediction technologies and the targeting of specific preventive interventions.

Numerous approaches and techniques have been tested to identify persons "at risk" for the formation of pressure ulcers.[22, 34] Persons at "greater risk" of developing pressure

TABLE 31–4   The Norton and Braden Scales

	Norton Scale	Braden Scale
Assessment criteria	Physical condition, mental condition, activity, mobility, incontinence (score ≤ 12 "at risk")	Activity, mobility, sensory perception, moisture, nutrition, friction, and shear
Attributes	Tested on elderly persons in hospital settings	Evaluated in diverse sites: med-surg, ICU, nursing homes
Replications	Tested extensively	Tested extensively
Reliability	Not available	Good inter-rater

ulcers often require supplemental measures beyond the usual three: (1) turning, (2) keeping the skin clean and dry, and (3) applying lotions. How is it determined if a person is at risk for formation of pressure ulcers? A person who uses a wheelchair or bed for most of the day or has impaired ability to reposition the body should be assessed for "additional factors" that increase risk for developing pressure ulcers. Research has shown that a person's general physical and mental condition, nutritional status, activity level, mobility, and degree of bowel and bladder control all affect the chances of developing pressure ulcers.[19, 24, 25, 94, 139] Patients should be assessed on admission to a unit, to a facility, or to home care and then periodically reassessed throughout their stay. A systematic risk assessment can be accomplished by using a validation risk assessment tool such as the Braden scale[19-21] or Norton scale[106, 107] (Table 31–4). Both of these instruments provide a means of predicting persons at risk for the development of pressure ulcers. No information is currently available to suggest that adaptations of these risk assessment tools or the assessment of any single risk factor or a combination of risk factors predicts risk as well as the overall scores obtained with these tools.

TREATMENT GUIDELINES

This section is based on the AHCPR guidelines for the treatment of pressure ulcers.[18] Once a pressure ulcer has developed, immediate treatment is required. Commonly used treatments over the years have included innovative mattresses, ointments, creams, solutions, dressings, ultrasound, ultraviolet heat lamps, sugar, and surgery. In choosing a treatment strategy, consideration should be given to the stage of the wound and the purpose of the treatment (protection, moisture, or removing necrotic tissue). An algorithm for assessment and treatment appears in Table 31–5.[51, 81]

TABLE 31–5   Steps in Wound Assessment and Treatment

1. Wound care can be divided into nonoperative and operative methods.
2. It is usually nonoperative for stage I and II pressure ulcers.
3. Stage III and IV lesions can require surgical intervention.
4. Some 70%–90% of pressure ulcers are superficial and heal by second intention.

Non-operative Guidelines

Solutions for Wound Cleansing

The major purpose of cleansing the wound is to decrease its "bioburden" and facilitate healing.[81, 121] Normal saline is used when no germicidal action is required. Saline solution should also be used as a rinse after other solutions are used to irrigate the wound and minimize fluid shifts within newly forming tissue. Normal saline solution also reduces the drying effects that some irrigants have on tissue.[37, 81]

Povidone-iodine is useful against bacteria, spores, fungi, and viruses. Dilution is recommended, and povidone-iodine should be discontinued when granulation occurs.[81] Laboratory data demonstrate povidone-iodine is toxic to fibroblasts in vitro, a finding that has theoretical implications for wound healing. Because povidone-iodine can affect thyroid function, it could be contraindicated for some patients.[37] Acetic acid can change the color of tissue and can mask potential suprainfection. Acetic acid (0.5%) is specifically effective against *Pseudomonas aeruginosa*, a particularly difficult and common organism in fungating lesions. Rinsing with normal saline is also recommended.[37]

Sodium hypochlorite (2.5%) is another oxidizing agent available for cleansing. Although it has some germicidal activity, it is used primarily to debride necrotic tissue. Before using it, zinc oxide should be placed around the edges of the wound to reduce the amount of irritation.[81] Normal saline should be used as a rinse after sodium hypochlorite.[37] A multitude of cleansing agents are on the market, but none has been shown to be more efficacious than the others, and expert opinion still favors normal saline.[18]

Debridement and Debriding Agents

The purpose of wound debridement is to remove necrotic tissue, eschar, and slough (the stringy yellow, green, or gray nonviable debris in an ulcer), all materials that promote infection, delay granulation, and impede healing. Accurate ulcer staging cannot be made until necrotic tissue is removed. Three debridement procedures are commonly used: (1) enzymatic debridement, (2) mechanical non-selective debridement, and (3) sharp debridement.

Enzymatic Debridement

Enzymatic debridement uses various chemical agents (proteolytic enzymes) that act by attacking collagen and liquefying necrotic wound debris without damaging granulation tissue. Proteolytic enzymes are used to chemically debride wounds. The action of these enzymes is aimed specifically at necrotic tissue.[18, 81]

Mechanical Non-selective Debridement

Mechanical non-selective debridement, in which necrotic tissue is loosened and removed, is generally accomplished by whirlpool treatments, forceful irrigation, or use of wet-to-dry dressings. Wet-to-dry dressings involve placing wet gauze into the lesion and allowing it to dry. A few hours later, when the dressing is removed, necrotic debris now adhering to it is also removed. Solutions commonly used for wet-to-dry dressings include normal saline, 0.25% acetic acid solution, and povidone-iodine solution for infected ulcers. Although the effervescent action of hydrogen peroxide results in wound debridement, it is not recommended for frequent use in pressure ulcers because it indiscriminately removes both necrotic material and fragile granulation tissue.[18] Once debridement has been completed and clean granulation tissue has been established, the use of debridement agents should be discontinued and the site should be kept clean and moist.[79] The widespread practice of using hydrogen peroxide continues, but it is not recommended for long-term use because it and other cleansing agents have been found to be toxic to fibroblasts (Table 31–6).[79, 121]

Sharp Debridement

Sharp debridement is surgical removal of the eschar and any devitalized tissue within it. Although sharp debridement is the most effective method of removing necrotic tissue, it is contraindicated in certain patients, particularly those who cannot withstand the loss of blood that can occur during the procedure. Moist, devitalized tissue supports the proliferation and growth of pathogens. The removal of this devitalized tissue is a prerequisite to new tissue growth. Sharp debridement also is indiscriminate in the removal of vital and devitalized tissue. A great deal of clinical skill and judgment are needed in surgically debriding a wound.[24, 41] Elderly and diabetic patients often have pressure ulcers of the heel that look black and escharred. Conventional wisdom encourages physicians to debride the eschar, but it is usually protective and should be left to autodebride unless an active infection dictates more aggressive measures. Surgical debridement is well-established as an approach to pressure ulcer care, but more research is needed.

Dressings for Pressure Ulcers

Transparent adhesive dressings are semipermeable and occlusive. They allow gaseous exchange and transfer of water vapor from the skin and prevent maceration of the healthy skin around the wound. They are not absorptive, they reduce the incidence of secondary infection, and they

---

TABLE 31–6   Treatment Strategies for Topical Therapy

A. Assessment for appropriate topical therapy
1. The nature of the wound surface and depth of the lesion must be evaluated.
2. Is the skin intact or covered by eschar?
3. If the epidermis is denuded, does the ulcer have a clean, granulating surface or a necrotic base?
4. Is the ulcer non-draining or draining?
5. If the wound is draining, what is the amount, color, and odor of the exudate?

B. Categories of topical products and dressings
1. Antimicrobials
2. Moisturizers
3. Emollients
4. Topical circulatory stimulants
5. Semipermeable dressings
6. Calcium alginate dressings
7. Hydrocolloid and hydrogel dressings
8. Exudate absorbers
9. Wet-to-dry dressings
10. Moist-to-dry dressings
11. Enzymes and liquid or gel film formers

eliminate the risk of traumatic removal. They do not function well on diaphoretic patients or in wounds that have significant exudate.[51, 63]

Hydrocolloid wafer dressings contain hydroactive particles that interact with wound exudate to form a gel. These dressings provide absorption of minimal to moderate amounts of exudate and keep the wound surface moist. This gel can have fibrillolytic properties that enhance wound healing, protect against secondary infection, and insulate the wound from contaminants.[51, 74]

Gel dressings are available in sheet form, in granules, and as liquid gel. All forms of gel dressings keep the wound surface moist as long as they are not allowed to dehydrate. Some gel dressings provide limited to moderate absorption; some provide insulation; some provide protection against bacterial invasion; and all provide atraumatic removal (Table 31–7).[18, 51, 86]

Calcium alginate dressings (e.g., Sorbsan)[69, 98] are semi-occlusive, highly absorbent, and easy to use. They are natural, sterile, non-woven dressings derived from brown seaweed. Calcium alginate dressings are extremely effective in treating wet (exudative) wounds and can be used on wounds that are contaminated or infected.[69]

PHYSIOLOGY OF WOUND HEALING (INFLAMMATION)

When the tissues are compromised by pressure ulcer formation, a vascular and cellular response to injury occurs. This inflammatory response serves to destroy, dilute, or sequester injurious agents and is the precursor to wound healing and repair. Local signs of this inflammatory reactive hyperemia, or non-blanching erythema, include redness, swelling, heat, and pain. The systemic indicators of infection or inflammation include elevated temperature and leukocytosis.

TABLE 31–7 Eight Major Dressing Types and Their Key Performance Characteristics

Major Dressing Categories	Key Performance Characteristic(s)
Alginates (sheets and fillers)	Exudate absorption, obliterate dead space, autolytic debridement
Foams (sheets and fillers)	Exudate absorption, obliterate dead space, autolytic debridement
Gauzes (woven and non-woven)	Obliterate dead space, moisture retention, exudate absorption, mechanical debridement
Hydrocolloids (wafers and fillers)	Occlusion, moisture retention, obliterate dead space, autolytic debridement
Hydrogels (sheets and fillers)	Moisture retention, autolytic debridement
Transparent films	Occlusion, moisture retention, autolytic debridement
Wound fillers	Obliterate dead space, exudate absorption, moisture retention, autolytic debridement
Wound pouches	Exudate control

Healing By Primary and Secondary Union

Primary Union

Wounds that are clean or surgically controlled can close by primary intention. This type of wound requires only re-epithelialization for healing, and it heals by first intention.

Secondary Union

Wounds that have some complicating factor that precludes immediate closure, such as infection or contamination, are allowed to form granulation tissue to fill the crater or gap. Such wounds typically are pressure ulcers, abscesses, or large-surface wounds. Large tissue defects fill by granulation followed by epithelialization. Wound closure occurs via wound contracture. Wound healing by secondary intention or delayed closure differs from primary closure: (1) the inflammatory response is more intense; (2) greater amounts of granulation tissue are formed when larger wounds heal; and (3) wound contraction of large-surface wounds produces a scar that is considerably smaller than the initial dimensions of the wound. Another problem encountered in wound healing is exuberant granulation, or proud flesh. This tissue protrudes above the margins of the wound and the closing defect, which precludes epithelialization. Some persons tend to form keloids, which are large, bulging, tumorous scars caused by abnormal amounts of collagen in connective tissues.

SURGICAL CONSIDERATION IN PRESSURE ULCER MANAGEMENT

Several options are available for surgical management of pressure ulcers, including direct closure, skin grafting, skin flaps, and musculocutaneous flaps. Surgical management of pressure ulcers can provide skin coverage and soft tissue coverage as well. Flaps containing muscle provide a physiological barrier to infection, eliminate dead space in the wound, and improve vascularity. Improved vascularity enhances local oxygen tension, provides extended soft tissue penetration for antibiotics, and improves total lymphocyte function.[9, 16, 36]

When considering operative repair, many other factors should be considered. These factors are perhaps best addressed by the entire team caring for the patient. The patient should be medically stable and should be able to benefit from the procedure. The patient should also participate in the decision. Operative procedures often result in blood loss and prolonged exposure to general anesthesia. The nutritional status of the patient must be considered, because good nutritional parameters are required for good wound healing and immune function. Tobacco use and smoking are associated with intrinsic factors that compromise wound healing.[62] Carbon monoxide and nicotinic acid, for example, are potent vasoconstrictors and increase blood viscosity.[114] These factors predispose tissue to excessive oxidase activity and free radical injury. Under normal conditions, the body is able to handle normal oxidative stress. With excessive stress, however, comes increased risk for pressure ulcer development and impaired wound healing.

A neutrophil-mediated free radical injury results in excessive oxidase activity, which can cause vascular damage and thrombosis leading to cell death and tissue destruction.[124–126] Factors associated with impaired healing should be corrected preoperatively. Several procedures are commonly utilized.

Direct Closure

Although direct closure is the simplest procedure, pressure ulcers considered for surgery are usually too large to close by direct, primary closure. Because these wounds are tense as a result of large soft tissue defects, direct closure can lead to wound defects, excessive wound tension, and a paucity of soft tissue coverage. Tissue expanders have recently been used to provide more skin surface and to facilitate closure.[26]

Skin Grafts

Split-thickness skin grafts can be used to repair shallow defects and pressure ulcers, but skin grafts provide only a skin barrier. When applied directly to granulating bone, skin grafts quickly erode, precluding healing. They also cause scars in the area from which the skin is harvested, and the transplanted skin is never as "tough" as normal skin.

Skin Flaps

Before the 1970s, repair using local full-thickness skin flaps was the standard surgical treatment for ulcers; today, they are typically used as alternatives to secondary repair.[127] Local skin flaps have a random vascular supply, and the tissue repair is essentially a redistribution of inadequately perfused tissue rather than a planned revascularization using specific blood vessels.

Musculocutaneous Flaps

Musculocutaneous flaps are usually the best choice for spinal cord–injured patients or when loss of muscle function does not contribute to co-morbidity. For ambulatory patients the choice is less clear, since the improved blood supply and reliability of the muscle flap must be balanced against the need to sacrifice functional muscle units.[82, 87, 144] Musculocutaneous flaps can help heal osteomyelitis and limit the damage caused by shearing, friction, and pressure.[44, 97, 140] They bring muscle and skin to the area of the defect and are probably as resistant to future pressure ulcers as the original skin.

Free Flaps

Free flaps are muscle-type flaps in which the vein and artery are disconnected at the donor site and reconnected to the vessels at the recipient site with the aid of a microscope. This is the most complex method of wound closure, and it has not yet been described in the literature for pressure ulcers.

SUPPORT SURFACES AND SPECIAL BEDS

Support surfaces have become an important and widely used modality in the treatment and prevention of pressure ulcers. There is a wide array of products on the market that claim to reduce the occurrence of pressure ulcers, though few clinical trials have been performed to evaluate the effectiveness of these products. These claims are based on studies evaluating tissue interface pressures,[2, 3, 10, 96, 115, 137] which have become standards in distinguishing pressure relief from pressure reduction. These concepts as well as device type have been used to develop a convenient classification to help select the appropriate products for pressure ulcer treatment and prevention.[38, 88] Selection of a product must be based on the patient's management plan and evaluation of an individual's risk factors for developing a pressure ulcer.[10, 138] These risk factors must be monitored and the modalities re-evaluated as the patient's condition improves or worsens. Finally, cost and service support must be evaluated.

An important focus in pressure ulcer prevention and treatment is reducing pressure over the bony prominences to below capillary closing pressure (32 mm Hg), which has become the standard threshold value for evaluating support surfaces.[2, 3, 96, 110, 129, 137] Since capillary closing pressure cannot be measured under clinical conditions, tissue interface pressure has been used to evaluate and compare products. Tissue interface pressure, an approximation of capillary closing pressure, is the force per unit area that acts perpendicularly between the body and the support surface.[38] It is measured using a pressure sensor placed between the patient and the support surface. Much of the recent research comparing the tissue interface pressures of various surfaces involves case studies on healthy human adults.[2, 3, 96, 110, 137] These experiments use various sensors, making comparisons of the findings difficult, and they do not address other etiological factors.[58] Newer technologies, including transcutaneous oxygen tension and laser Doppler blood flow, are currently being evaluated.[58, 59, 129] The FSA pressure measurement assessment system (Fig. 31–5) uses a thin, flexible mat to determine interface pressures in a clinically effective method. The Windows-based computer software visually demonstrates the pressure map in a way that is easy for clinician, patient, and support staff to understand. It is useful in patient teaching, wheelchair or cushion selection, bed positioning, and documentation enabling the clinician to track the pressure-relieving strategies chosen for each patient.[142] Currently, no clear evidence supports the adequacy of these instruments, and further studies must be undertaken.

Classification

A convenient classification system was developed in *Acute and Chronic Wounds: Nursing Management*[38] that distinguishes three types of devices: mattress overlays, mattress replacements, and specialty beds. Table 31–8 describes the selected characteristics as well as the advantages and disadvantages of separate classes of support surfaces. The mattress overlay is designed to be effective when applied directly over a mattress. Mattress replacement systems are designed for use on an existing hospital bed frame without an underlying mattress. Finally, specialty beds are entire units used in place of hospital beds.

Each type of device may be subdivided into dynamic systems, which require an energy source to alternate pres-

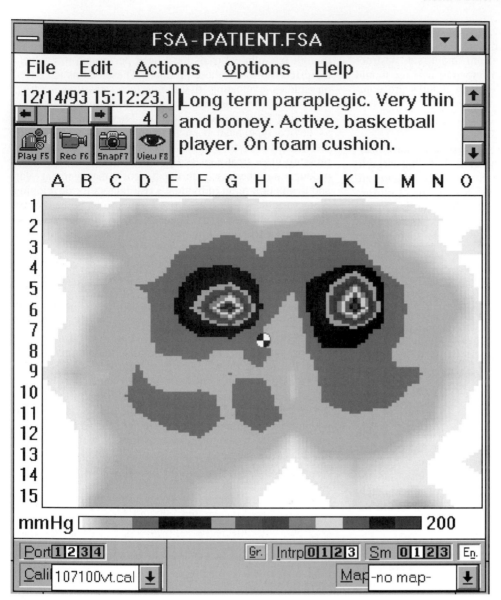

FIGURE 31–5 Force sensing array (FSA) pressure mapping.

sure points and static systems, which rely on redistribution of pressure over a large surface area and do not require an energy source. Each device may be further described as a pressure-reducing or pressure-relieving device. Pressure-relieving devices are those that consistently reduce pressure below capillary closing pressure. Pressure-reducing devices keep pressures lower than with the standard hospital bed but not consistently below capillary closing pressure. Mediums used in mattress overlays and replacements include water, gel, foam, air, and composite products. Air mattresses and overlays may be static or dynamic. Most overlays and replacement mattresses are considered pressure-reducing devices.

Specialty beds include low–air loss beds and air-fluidized beds. Low–air loss beds use separate air-filled cushions that are individually monitored to reduce pressures below capillary closing pressures. Air-fluidized therapy uses warm air forced through silicone beads to simulate a fluid environment in reducing pressures. The specialty beds are considered pressure-relieving devices. Clinical trials for pre-vention and treatment of pressure ulcers have been performed on air-fluidized and low–air loss beds.[6, 55, 61, 75] Table 31–9 describes the results of these trials. Although there is evidence that these surfaces can provide an environment in which ulcers can be prevented or improved, there is no evidence that one support surface consistently performs better than all others in all circumstances.[6, 40, 61, 77, 101, 136, 145, 150] Therefore, patients should be actively managed on an individual basis to reduce specific risk factors. Selection of a support surface is an adjunct to other therapy.

Selection of a Support Surface

It is futile to select a support surface unless the product's appropriateness can be assessed adequately beforehand. In addition to frequent, written risk assessments, a dynamic management plan for each individual should include discontinuing the use of a support surface when it is determined that a patient is no longer at risk for developing pressure ulcers.[6, 40, 77, 109, 123] Any individual thought to be at

TABLE 31–8 Advantages and Disadvantages of Support Surfaces

Surface	Advantages	Disadvantages
Static overlays		
Air	Low maintenance	Can be punctured
	Inexpensive	Require proper
	Multipatient use	inflation
	Durable	
Gel	Low maintenance	Heavy
	Easy to clean	Expensive
	Multipatient use	Little research
	Resists puncture	
Foam	Lightweight	Retains heat
	Resists puncture	Retains moisture
	No maintenance	Limited life
Water	Readily available in	Requires heater
	community	Transfers are difficult
	Easy to clean	Can leak
		Heavy
		Difficult maintenance
		Procedures difficult
Dynamic	Easy to clean	Can be damaged by
overlays	Moisture control	sharp objects
	Deflates for transfers	Noisy
	Reusable pump	Assembly required
		Requires power
Replacement	Reduced staff time	High initial cost
mattresses	Multipatient use	May not control
	Easy to clean	moisture
	Low maintenance	Loses effectiveness
Low air loss	Head and foot of bed can	Noisy
	be raised	Difficulty with transfers
	Less frequent turning	Expensive
	required	Requires energy
	Pressure relieving	source
	Reduces shear and	Restricts mobility
	friction	Skilled setup required
	Moisture control	Rental charge
Air fluidized	Reduces shear and	Expensive
	friction	Noisy
	Lowest interface pressure	Heavy
	Low moisture	Dehydration can occur
	Less frequent turning	Electrolyte imbalances
	required	can occur
		May cause
		disorientation
		Difficulty with transfers
		Hot

(Adapted from Bryant R: Acute and Chronic Wounds: Nursing Management. St Louis, Mosby–Year Book, 1992.)

risk for developing pressure ulcers should be placed on a pressure-reducing device (foam, static air, alternating air, gel, or water) when lying in bed[8, 43, 78, 149] to relieve pressure on the heels.[42, 109] For wheelchair-mobile persons, pressure-reducing devices of foam, gel, air, or a combination of these materials should be used.[45, 60, 67, 91, 115] Pressure-reducing devices should be used in addition to standard nursing care.[1, 76, 139]

Guidelines developed by the AHCPR Pressure Ulcer Panel for managing existing pressure ulcers include these:

1. Use positioning devices to raise a pressure ulcer off the support surface. If the patient is no longer at risk for developing pressure ulcers, these devices may reduce the need for pressure-reducing overlays, mattresses, and beds. Avoid using donut-type devices.[42]

2. Assess all patients with existing pressure ulcers to determine their risk for developing additional pressure ulcers. If the patient remains at risk, use a pressure-reducing surface.[20, 21, 106, 107]

3. If patients can assume a variety of positions without bearing weight on the lesion and without "bottoming out," a static support surface should be used.[40, 61, 133, 145, 150]

4. If, however, the patient cannot assume a variety of positions without bearing weight on the ulcer, if the patient fully compresses the static support surface, or if the pressure ulcer does not show evidence of healing, a dynamic surface should be used.[61]

5. Finally, if the patient has large stage III or stage IV pressure ulcers on multiple turning surfaces, a pressure-relieving product is warranted.[6, 61, 100, 102, 104, 133, 145, 150]

Currently, no perfect product exists, so it is important to tailor product selection to the patient's needs. Add to this the variation in cost and customer services associated with each product and the choices become more difficult. This demonstrates the need for written policy and procedure guidelines in each institution addressing the variables associated with product selection. It is clear that additional randomized clinical trials to distinguish efficacy are needed. Further, research needs to be continued that addresses the accuracy of tissue interface pressures in determining prevention of pressure ulcers and in advancing new technologies relating capillary closing pressure.

DISCHARGE PLANNING AND PATIENT AND CAREGIVER EDUCATION

Discharge planning begins early during hospitalization and requires an interdisciplinary approach. Knowledge of available resources facilitates smooth transitions through all levels of the continuum of care. With more care conducted in the home environment, education of the patient and caregiver in the prevention and treatment of pressure ulcers becomes increasingly important. A variety of methods can be employed to facilitate this educational process, including charts, diagrams, photographs, and videos. This comprehensive approach can positively influence the overall patient outcome.

FUTURE TRENDS IN MANAGEMENT

While we continue to strive for the ultimate treatment for pressure ulcers, we must consider the role of newer therapies such as cytokine growth factors (e.g., recombinant platelet-derived growth factors and basic fibroblast growth factors and skin equivalents).[57, 152] There is a nascent body of evidence that electrical stimulation may enhance the rate of wound healing in pressure ulcers.[90] Other exciting possibilities include free radical scavengers and special drug delivery systems used in a preventive way for areas at risk for pressure ulcers.[124–126] More research is needed, and a multitude of opportunities exist in this rapidly developing field (Table 31–10). The gaps between basic, applied, and clinical outcomes research must be closed.

TABLE 31-9   Clinical Trials on Pressure-Relief Surfaces

Study	Surface/Investigation	Result
Allman R, et al: Air-fluidized beds or conventional therapy for pressure sores. Intern Med 1987; 107:641.	Clinitron air-fluidized bed vs. Lapidus air float alternating air mattress with foam pad as conventional therapy Prospective, randomized, clinical trial of 72 acutely hospitalized patients with pressure sores.	Air-fluidized therapy showed a median improvement in total surface area of 1.2 cm^2 compared with an increase in total surface area of 0.5 cm^2 with conventional therapy. Outcomes were not significantly different for patients with small sores. For sores greater than 7.8 cm^2, air-fluidized beds showed a statistically significant improvement, with median reduction of sores of 5.3 cm^2 compared with an expansion of sores by 4.0 cm^2 on conventional therapy. Masked assessment in this group showed 63% of patients improved on air-fluidized therapy, as compared with 29% on conventional therapy. Thus, after adjusting for other factors, air-fluidized therapy was 5.6 times more likely to show improvement on masked assessment than standard therapy.
Ferrell B, et al: A randomized trial of low-air loss beds for treatment of pressure ulcers. JAMA 1993; 269:494-497.	Kin-air low air loss bed vs. 10-cm convoluted foam overlaying a regular hospital mattress Prospective, randomized clinical trial of 84 nursing home patients with pressure sores.	Rate of healing three times greater in the low air loss bed. Pressure sores are 2.5 times more likely to heal with Kin-air.
Inman KJ, et al: Clinical utility and cost-effectiveness of an air suspension bed in the prevention of pressure ulcers. JAMA 1993; 269:1193.	Kin-air low air loss bed vs. standard hospital bed Controlled, randomized, clinical trial of 100 critically ill hospital patients at risk of developing pressure ulcers. Includes cost analysis.	Of 49 of the 98 patients completing the study who were randomized to the Kin-air, 8 developed pressure sores, compared with 39 of 49 randomized to the standard bed. Treatment using the Kin-air bed showed significantly fewer patients developing single, multiple, or severe pressure ulcers. No significant difference was demonstrated with regard to resolution of the pressure ulcers. The air-suspension bed proved to provide a more clinically effective treatment less expensively through all scenarios in the sensitivity analysis (US $).

SUMMARY

Many factors influence the development and healing of pressure ulcers. Nursing plays a pivotal role in this challenging and complex process, using a multifaceted approach involving skin care, pressure relief, and nutritional support. Prevention is the key to managing pressure ulcers, and it begins with a complete medical and nursing history, risk assessment, and skin examination when the patient is admitted.[18, 19, 22] Pathomechanical and pathophysiological factors that subject the tissue at risk to potential skin breakdown should receive particular attention. Patients should be kept clean and dry and should be repositioned frequently. For patients at risk, adequate pressure relief must be provided, along with adequate nutritional support.

For patients who develop pressure ulcers, these preventive measures must be employed together with the techniques of general wound care. Non-operative wound care may involve simple topical therapy, as for pressure ulcers with unbroken skin or superficial lesions with non-draining, non-infected granulation tissue. For draining necrotic or infected lesions, treatment may also include absorption agents, calcium alginate dressings, wound coverings, debridement, and antimicrobial therapy. Other therapeutic modalities, such as whirlpool, physical therapy, and specialty beds, may also be added to the treatment regimen.

TABLE 31-10   Other Resources

Division of Communications
Agency for Health Care Policy and Research
Executive Office Center, Suite 501
2101 E Jefferson St
Rockville, MD 20852
Telephone: (301) 227-6173

National Pressure Ulcer Advisory Panel
State University of New York at Buffalo
Beck Hall
3435 Main St
Buffalo, NY 14214
Telephone: (716) 881-3558

Acknowledgments

The authors gratefully acknowledge Steve Jenkins in the Department of Physical Medicine and Rehabilitation at the University of Kentucky for his significant editorial assistance in preparing this chapter. Dr. Salcido would also like to acknowledge that his studies cited in this chapter are supported by NIH (National Heart, Lung, and Blood Institute grant P01HL36552–07; National Center for Medical Rehabilitation Research grant R01HD31426-01), the Paralyzed Veterans of America Spinal Cord Research Foundation (SCRF grant 1118), and Ethicon Inc.

References

1. Abrussezze RS: Early assessment and prevention of pressure ulcers. *In* Lee BY (ed): Chronic Ulcers of the Skin. New York, McGraw-Hill, 1985, pp 1–9.

2. Allen V, Ryan D, Murry A: Air-fluidized beds and their ability to distribute interface pressures generated between the subject and the bed surface. Physiol Meas 1993; 14:359–364.

3. Allen V, Ryan D, Murry A: Potential for bed sores due to high pressures: Influence of body sites, body position, and mattress design. Br J Clin Pract 1993; 47:195–197.

4. Allman RM: Pressure ulcers among the elderly. N Engl J Med 1989; 320:850–853.

5. Allman RM, Walker JM, Hart MK, Laprade CA: Pressure ulcers among hospital patients. Ann Intern Med 1987; 107:337–342.

6. Allman RM, Walker JM, Hart MK, et al: Air-fluidized beds or conventional therapy for pressure sores: A randomized trial. Ann Intern Med 1987; 107:641–648.

7. Ameis A, Chiarcossi A, Jimenez J: Management of pressure sores. Comparative study in medical and surgical patients. Postgrad Med 1980; 67:177–184.

8. Andersen K, Jensen O, Kvorning S, Bach E: Decubitus prophylaxis: A prospective trial on the efficiency of alternating-pressure air mattresses and water mattresses. Acta Dermatol Venereol (Stockh) 1983; 63:227–230.

9. Anthony JP, Huntsman WT, Mathes SJ: Changing trends in the management of pelvic pressure ulcers: A 12 year review. Decubitus 1992; 5:44–47, 50–51.

10. Aronovitch SA: Evaluating risk factors. A retrospective study of the use of specialty beds in the medical and surgical intensive care units of a tertiary care facility. Decubitus 1992; 5:36–42.

11. Aust JB, Page CP: Hemicorporectomy. J Surg Oncol 1985; 30:226–230.

12. Barbenel JC, Fergeson-Pell MW, Beale AQ: Monitoring the mobility in bed. Med Biol Eng Comput 1985; 23:466.

13. Barbenel JC, Jordan MM, Nicol SM, Clark MO: The incidence of pressure sores in the Greater Glasgow Health Board area. Lancet 1977; 2:548–550.

14. Basset A, Liautaud B, Ndiaye B: Dermatology of Black Skin. Oxford, Oxford University Press, 1986.

15. Basson MD, Burney RE: Defective wound healing in patients with paraplegia and quadriplegia. Surg Gynecol Obstet 1982; 155:9–12.

16. Becker H: The distally-based gluteus maximus muscle flap. Plast Reconstr Surg 1979; 63:653–656.

17. Bennett L, Lee BY: Pressure versus shear in pressure sore causation. *In* Lee BY (ed): Chronic Ulcers of the Skin. New York, McGraw-Hill, 1985, pp 39–56.

18. Bergstrom N, Bennett MA, Carlson CE, et al: Treatment of Pressure Ulcers. Clinical Practice Guideline Number 14. AHCPR Publication No. 95–0642. Rockville, MD, Agency for Health Care Policy and Research, Public Health Service, US Department of Health and Human Services, 1994.

19. Bergstrom N, Braden BJ: A prospective study of pressure sore risk among institutionalized elderly. J Am Geriatr Soc 1992; 40:747–758.

20. Bergstrom N, Braden BJ, Laguzza A, Holman V: The Braden Scale for Predicting Pressure Sore Risk. Nurs Res 1987; 36:205–210.

21. Bergstrom N, Demuth PJ, Braden BJ: A clinical trial of the Braden Scale for Predicting Pressure Sore Risk. Nurs Clin North Am 1987; 22:417–428.

22. Bergstrom N and the Panel for the Prediction and Prevention of Pressure Ulcers in Adults: Pressure Ulcers in Adults: Prediction and Prevention Clinical Practice Guideline, Number 3. AHCPR Publication No. 92–0047. Rockville, Md, Agency for Health Care Policy and Research, Public Health Service, US Department of Health and Human Services, 1992.

23. Berlowitz DR, Wilking SV: Risk factors for pressure sores. A comparison of cross-sectional and cohort-derived data. J Am Geriatr Soc 1989; 37:1043–1050.

24. Black JM, Black SB: Surgical management of pressure ulcers. Nurs Clin North Am 1987; 22:429–438.

25. Bozzetti F, Terno G, Longoni C: Parenteral hyperalimentation and wound healing. Surg Gynecol Obstet 1975; 141:712–714.

26. Braddom RL, Leadbetter MG: The use of a tissue expander to enlarge a graft for surgical treatment of a pressure ulcer in a quadraplegic. Am J Phys Med Rehabil 1989; 68:70–72.

27. Brand P: Pressure sores—the problem. *In* Kenedi R, Cowden J, Scales J (ed): Bed Sore Biomechanics. London, MacMillan Press, 1976, pp 19–23.

28. Brandeis GH, Morris JN, Nash DJ, Lipsitz LA: Epidemiology and natural history of pressure ulcers in elderly nursing home residents. JAMA 1990; 264:2905.

29. Breslow R: Nutritional status and dietary intake of patients with pressure ulcers: Review of research literature 1943 to 1989. Decubitus 1991; 4:16–21.

30. Breslow RA, Hallfrisch J, Goldberg AP: Malnutrition in tubefed nursing home patients with pressure sores. J Parenter Enter Nutr 1991; 15:663–668.

31. Breslow RA, Hallfrisch J, Guy DG, et al: The importance of dietary protein in healing pressure ulcers. J Am Geriatr Soc 1993; 41:357–362.

32. Breslow R, Hallfrisch J, Moser PB, et al: High calories and protein improve healing of pressure sores in malnourished nursing home patients. Fed Proc 1987; 46:1010.

33. Brose L: Prealbumin as a marker of nutritional status. J Burn Care Rehabil 1990; 11:372–375.

34. Brown MM, Boosinger J, Black J, Gaspar T: Nursing innovation for prevention of decubitus ulcers in long term care facilities. J Plast Reconstr Surg Nurs 1981; 1:51–55.

35. Bruce AD, Ferrell BA, Osterweil D, Christenson P: A randomized trial of low–air loss beds for treatment of pressure ulcers. JAMA 1993; 269:494–497.

36. Bruck JC, Buttenmeyer R, Grabosch A, Gruhl L: More arguments in favor of myocutaneous flaps for the treatment of pelvic pressure sores. Ann Plast Surg 1991; 26:85–88.

37. Bryant CA, Rodeheaver GT, Reem EM, et al: Search for a nontoxic surgical scrub solution for periorbital lacerations. Ann Emerg Med 1984; 13:317–321.

38. Bryant R: Acute and Chronic Wounds: Nursing Management. St Louis, Mosby–Year Book, 1992.

39. Clarke M, Kahdom HM: The nursing prevention of pressure sores in hospital and community patients. J Adv Nurs 1988; 13:365–373.

40. Conine T, Daechsel D, Lau M: The role of alternating air and silicone overlay in preventing decubitus ulcers. Int J Rehabil Res 1990; 13:57–65.

41. Cooper DM: Challenge of open wound assessment in the home setting. Progressions Develop Ostomy Wound Care 1990; 2:11–18.

42. Crewe R: Problems of rubber ring nursing cushions and a clinical survey of alternative cushions for ill patients. Care Sci Pract 1987; 5:9–11.

43. Daechsel D, Conine T: Special mattresses: Effectiveness in preventing decubitus ulcers in chronic neurologic patients. Arch Phys Med Rehabil 1985; 66:246–248.

44. Daniel RK, Hall EJ, MacLeod MK: Pressure sores: A reappraisal. Ann Plast Surg 1979; 3:53–63.

45. DeLateur B, Berni R, Hangladarom T, Giaconi R: Wheelchair cushions designed to prevent pressure sores: An evaluation. Arch Phys Med Rehabil 1976; 57:129–135.

46. Deloach ED, Christy RS, Ruf LE, et al: Osteomyelitis underlying severe pressure sores. Contemp Surg 1992; 40:25–32.

47. Deloach ED, DiBenedetto RJ, Womble L, Gilley JD: The treatment of osteomyelitis underlying pressure ulcers. Decubitus 1992; 5:32–41.

48. Dinsdale SM: Decubitus ulcers: Role of pressure and friction in causation. Arch Phys Med Rehabil 1974; 55:147–152.

49. Dolezal R, Allman R, Walker R, et al: Air-fluidized beds or conventional therapy for pressure sores—a randomized trial. Ann Intern Med 1987; 107:641–647.

50. Dorland's Illustrated Medical Dictionary, ed 25. Philadelphia, WB Saunders, 1974, p 1668.

51. Doughty D: The process of wound healing: A nursing perspective. Progressions Develop Ostomy Wound Care 1990; 2:3–12.

52. Dowding C: Pressure sores: The role of nutrition. Community Outlook 1984; 8:70.

53. Ek AC, Gustavsson G, Lewis DH: The local skin blood flow in areas at risk for pressure sores treated with massage. Scand J Rehabil Med 1985; 17:81–86.

54. Ek AC, Unosson M, Bjurulf P: The Modified Norton Scale and the nutritional state. Scand J Caring Sci 1989; 3:183–187.

55. Exton-Smith AN, Overstall PW, Wedgwood J, Wallace G: Use of the air wave system to prevent pressure sores in hospital. Lancet 1982; 1:1288–1290.

56. Exton-Smith AN, Sherwin RW: The prevention of pressure sores: The significance of spontaneous bodily movements. Lancet 1961; 2:1124.

57. Falanga V, Zitelli JA, Eaglestein WH: Wound healing. J Am Acad Dermatol 1988; 191:559–563.

58. Feldman DL, Sepka RS, Klitzman B: Tissue oxygenation and blood flow on specialized and conventional beds. Ann Plastic Surg 1993; 30:441–445.

59. Feldman DL, Sepka RS, Klitzman B: Tissue oxygenation and blood flow on specialized and conventional hospital beds. Ann Plast Surg 1993; 30:441–444.

60. Fergson-Pell M, Cochran G, Cardi M, Trachtman L: A knowledge-based program for pressure sore prevention. Ann NY Acad Sci 1986; 463:284–286.

61. Ferrell B, Osterweil D, Christenson P: A randomized trial of low–air-loss beds for treatment of pressure ulcers. JAMA 1993; 269:494–497.

62. Fincham JE: Smoking cessation: Treatment options and the pharmacist's role. Am Pharm 1992; NS32:62–70.

63. Fowler E, Papen JC: Evaluation of alginate dressing for pressure ulcers. Decubitus 1991; 4:47–52.

64. Frantz RA: Pressure ulcer costs in long-term care. Decubitus 1989; 2:59–60.

65. Fuhrer M, Garber S, Rintala D, et al: Pressure ulcers in community-resident persons with spinal cord injury: Prevalence and risk factors. Arch Phys Med Rehabil 1993; 74:1172–1177.

66. Garber S, Campion L, Krouskop T: Trochanteric pressure in spinal cord injury. Arch Phys Med Rehabil 1982; 63:549–552.

67. Garber S, Krouskop T, Carter R: A system for clinically evaluating wheelchair pressure-relief cushions. Am J Occup Ther 1978; 32:565–570.

68. Gerson LW: The incidence of pressure sores in active treatment hospitals. Int J Nurs Stud 1975; 12:201–204.

69. Gilchrist T, Martin AM: Wound treatment with Sorbsan™—an alginate fibre dressing. Biomaterials 1982; 4:317–320.

70. Gosnell DJ, Johansen J, Aryres M: Pressure ulcer incidence and severity in a community hospital. Decubitus 1992, vol 5, no. 5.

71. Groth KE: Clinical observations and experimental studies of the pathogenesis of decubitus ulcers. Acta Clin Scand 1942; 87 (suppl 76):207.

72. Hibbs P: The economics of pressure ulcer prevention. Decubitus 1989; 2:32–38.

73. Husain T: Experimental study of some pressure effects on tissues, with reference to bed sore problems. J Pathol Bacteriol 1953; 66:347.

74. Hutchinson J, McGuckin M: Occlusive dressings: A microbiologic and clinical review. J Infect Control 1990; 18:257–268.

75. Inman KJ, Sibbald WJ, Rutledge FS, Clark BJ: Clinical utility and cost-effectiveness of an air suspension bed in the prevention of pressure ulcers. JAMA 1993; 269:1139–1143.

76. International Association of Enterostomal Therapy: Dermal wounds: Pressure sores. Philosophy of the IAET. J Enterostomal Ther 1988; 15:4–17.

77. Jackson B, Chagare R, Nee N, Freeman K: The effect of a therapeutic bed on pressure ulcers: An experimental study. J Enterostomal Ther 1988; 15:220–226.

78. Jester J, Weaver V: A report of clinical investigation of various tissue support surfaces used for the prevention, early intervention and management of pressure ulcers. Ostomy Wound Manage 1990; 26:39–45.

79. Johnson AR, White AC, McNalley B: Comparison of common topical agents for wound treatment: Cytotoxicity for human fibroblast in culture. Wounds 1989; 1:186–192.

80. Keane FX: The function of the rump in relation to sitting and the Keane reciprocating wheelchair seat. Paraplegia 1978; 16:390.

81. Knauer CJ: Management of malignant fungating breast lesions. Progressions Develop Ostomy Wound Care 1990; 2:3–11.

82. Koshima I, Moriguchi T, Soeda S, et al: The gluteal perforator-based flap for repair of sacral pressure sores. Plast Reconstr Surg 1993; 91:678–683.

83. Kosiak M: Etiology and pathology of ischemic ulcers. Arch Phys Med Rehabil 1959; 40:62–69.

84. Kosiak M, Kubicek WG, Olson M, et al: Evaluation of pressure as a factor in the production of ischial ulcers. Arch Phys Med Rehabil 1958; 39:623.

85. Kosiak M: Prevention and rehabilitation of pressure ulcers. Decubitus 1991; 4:60–68.

86. Krasner D: Shifting paradigms for wound care: Dressing decisions; multidisciplinary care; effectiveness. In Portnow J (ed): Wound Care. Durable Medical Equipment Review 1994; 1:12.

87. Kroll SS, Rosenfield L: Perforator-based flaps for low posterior midline defects. Plast Reconstr Surg 1988; 81:561–566.

88. Krouskop T, Noble P, Garber S, Spencer W: The effectiveness of preventive management in reducing the occurrence of pressure sores. J Rehabil Res Dev 1983; 20:74–83.

89. Landis E: Micro-injection studies of capillary blood pressure in human skin. Heart 1930; 15:209–228.

90. Levine SP, Kett RL, Gross MD, et al: The bloodflow in the gluteus maximus in seated individuals during electrical muscular stimulation. Arch Phys Med Rehabil 1990; 71:682–686.

91. Lindan O: Etiology of decubitus ulcers: An experimental study. Arch Phys Med Rehabil 1961; 42:774–783.

92. Lloyd EE, Baker F: An examination of variables in spinal cord injury patients with pressure sores. SCI Nurs 1986; 3:19–22.

93. Longe RL: Current concepts in clinical therapeutics: Pressure sores. Clin Pharmacol 1986; 5:669–681.

94. Makelbust J: Pressure ulcers: Etiology and prevention. Nurs Clin North Am 1987; 22:360–361.

95. Makelbust J, Baron MC: The skin and wound healing. Topics Clin Nurs 1983; 5:11–22.

96. Makelbust J, Mondoux L, Sieggreen M: Pressure relief characteristics of various support surfaces used in the prevention and treatment of pressure ulcers. J Enterostomal Ther 1986; 13:85–89.

97. Mathes SJ, Feng LJ, Hunt TK: Coverage of the infected wound. Ann Surg 1983; 198:420–429.

98. McMullen D: Clinical experience with a calcium alginate dressing. Dermatol Nurs 1991; 3:216–219.

99. Meehan M: Multisite pressure ulcer prevalence survey. Decubitus 1990; 3:14–17.

100. Mulder G, Seeley J: The effectiveness of specialty beds in the treatment of severe pressure ulcers in nursing home patients: A preliminary report. Unpublished research report, 1991.

101. Munro B, Brown L, Heitman B: Pressure ulcers: One bed or another? Geriatr Nurs 1989; 10:190–192.

102. National Center for Cost Containment. National Specialized Bed Study and Other Support Surface Guidelines. Washington, DC, US Department of Veterans Affairs, 1992.

103. National Pressure Ulcer Advisory Panel: Pressure Ulcers: Incidence, Economics, Risk Assessment. Consensus Development Conference Statement. West Dundee, IL, S-N Publications, 1989.

104. Nimit K: Public health service assessment guidelines for home air-fluidized bed therapy. Health Technol Assess Rep 1989; 5:1–11.

105. Nola GT, Vistnes LM: Differential response of skin and muscle in the experimental production of pressure sores. Plast Reconstr Surg 1980; 66:728.

106. Norton D: Calculating the risk: Reflections on the Norton Scale. Decubitus 1989; 2:24–31.

107. Norton D, McLaren R, Exton-Smith A: An Investigation of Geriatric Nursing Problems in Hospital. London, Churchill Livingstone, 1975.

108. Okamoto G, Lamers J, Shurtleff D: Skin breakdown in patients with myelomeningocele. Arch Phys Med Rehabil 1983; 64:20–23.

109. Parish L, Witjiwski J: Clinitron therapy and the decubitus ulcer: Preliminary dermatologic studies. Int J Dermatol 1980; 19:517–518.

110. Patel U, Jones J, Babbs C, et al: The evaluation of five specialized support surfaces by use of a pressure-sensitive mat. Decubitus 1993; 6:28–37.

111. Perkash A, Brown M: Anemia in patients with traumatic spinal cord injury. J Am Paraplegia Soc 1986; 9:10–15.

112. Perkash A, Brown M: Anaemia in patients with traumatic spinal cord injury. Paraplegia 1982; 20:235–236.

113. Peroment M, Labbe M, Yourassowsky E, et al: Anaerobic bacteria isolated from decubitus ulcers. Infection 1973; 1:205.

114. Read RC: Presidential address. Systemic effects of smoking. Am J Surg 1984; 148:706–711.

115. Reddy N, Cochran G: Phenomenological theory underlying pressure-time relationship in decubitus ulcer formation [abstr]. Fed Proc 1979; 38:1153.

116. Reed JW: Pressure ulcers in the elderly: Prevention and treatment utilizing the team approach. Md State Med J 1981; 30:45–50.

117. Reichel S: Shearing force as a factor in decubitus ulcers in paraplegics. JAMA 1958; 166:762–763.

118. Reswick JB, Rogers JE: Experience at Rancho Los Amigos Hospital with devices and techniques to prevent pressure sores. *In* Kenedi RM, Cowden JM, Scales JT (eds): Bedsore Biomechanics. London, University Park Press, 1976, p 300.

119. Roberts BV, Goldstone LA: A survey of pressure sores in the over sixties on two orthopaedic wards. Int J Nurs Stud 1979; 16:355–364.

120. Robnett MK: The incidence of skin breakdown in a surgical intensive care unit. J Nurs Qual Assur 1986; 1:77–81.

121. Rodeheaver GT, Kurtz L, Kircher BJ, Edlich RF: Pluronic F-68: A promising new skin wound cleanser. Ann Emerg Med 1980; 9:572–576.

122. Russ GH, Motta GH: Eliminating pressure: Is less than 32 mm Hg enough for wound healing? Ostomy Wound Manage 1991; 34:60–63.

123. St. Clair M: Survey of the uses of the Pegasus airwave system in the United Kingdom. J Tissue Viabil 1992; 12:9–16.

124. Salcido R, Carney J, Fisher S, et al: A reliable animal model of pressure sore development: The role of free radicals. J Am Paraplegia Soc 1993; 16:61.

125. Salcido R, Donofrio J, Fisher S, et al: Histopathology of pressure ulcers as a result of sequential computer-controlled pressure sessions in a fuzzy rat model. Adv Wound Care 1994; 7:23–40.

126. Salcido R, Fisher S, Donofrio J, et al: An animal model and computer-controlled surface pressure delivery system for the production of pressure ulcers. J Rehabil Research Dev 1994, in press.

127. Sanchez S, Eamegdool S, Conway H: Surgical treatment of decubitus ulcers in paraplegics. Plast Reconstr Surg 1969; 43:25–28.

128. Seiitsu O, Toyokura Y, Toru M: Increased dermal collagen density in amyotrophic lateral sclerosis. J Neurol Sci 1988; 83:81–92.

129. Seiler W, Allen S, Stahelin H: Influence of the 30 degrees laterally inclined position and the 'super-soft' 3-piece mattress on skin oxygen tension on areas of maximum pressure—implications for pressure sore prevention. Gerontology 1986; 32:158–166.

130. Shannon ML, Skorga P: Pressure ulcer prevalence in two general hospitals. Decubitus 1989; 2:38–43.

131. Shubert V, Fargell B: Evaluation of the dynamic cutaneous postischemic hyperaemia and thermal response in elderly subjects and in an area at risk for pressure sores. Clin Physiol 1991; 11:169–182.

132. Smith AM, Malone JA: Preventing pressure ulcers in institutionalized elders: Assessing the effects of small, unscheduled shifts in body position. Decubitus, 1990; 3:20–24.

133. Smoot F: Clinitron bed therapy hazards [letter]. Plastic Reconstr Surg 1986; 77:165.

134. Staas WE Jr, Cioschi HM: Pressure sores: A multifaceted approach to prevention and treatment. West J Med 1991; 154:539.

135. Staas WE Jr, LaMantia JG: Decubitus ulcers and rehabilitation medicine. Int J Dermatol 1982; 21:437–444.

136. Strauss M, Gong J, Gary B, et al: The cost of home air-fluidized therapy for pressure sores: A randomized controlled trial. J Fam Pract 1991; 33:52–59.

137. Thompson-Bishop J, Mottola C: Tissue interface pressure and estimated subcutaneous pressures of 11 different pressure-reducing support surfaces. Decubitus 1992; 5:42–48.

138. University Hospital Consortium: Guidelines for the Use of Pressure Relief Devices in the Treatment and Prevention of Pressure Ulcers. Oak Brook, Ill, University Hospital Consortium Technology Advancement Center, 1990.

139. VanEtten N, Sexton P, Smith R: Development and implementation of a skin care program. Ostomy Wound Manage 1990; 27:40–54.

140. Vasconez LO, Schneider WJ, Trukiewicz MJ: Pressure sores. Curr Probl Surg 1977; 24:23.

141. Vaziri ND, Caesarior T, Mootoo K, et al: Bacterial infections in patients with chronic renal failure: Occurrence with spinal cord injury. Arch Intern Med 1982; 142:1273–1276.

142. Verg, Inc: Wound Measurement System. Verg Inc., 633 Wellington Crescent, Winnipeg, Manitoba, Canada R3M OA8.

143. Versluysen M: How elderly patients with femoral fractures develop pressure sores in hospital. Br Med J Clin Res Ed 1986; 292:1311–1313.

144. Vyas SC, Binns JH, Wilson AN: Thoracolumbar-sacral flaps in the treatment of sacral pressure sores. Plast Reconstr Surg 1980; 65:159–163.

145. Warner DE: A clinical comparison of two pressure-reducing surfaces in the management of pressure ulcers. Decubitus 1992; 5:52–64.

146. Washington Post, May 19, 1992 (Health News), page 9.

147. Watanebe S, Yamada K, Ono S: Skin changes in patients with amyotrophic lateral sclerosis: Light and electron microscopic observations. J Am Acad Dermatol 1987; 17:1006–1012.

148. Webster's New Riverside University Dictionary. Boston, Houghton Mifflin, 1984, p 1250.

149. Whitney J, Fellows B, Larson E: Do mattresses make a difference? J Gerontol Nurs 1984; 10:20–25.

150. Wiersema L, Lueckenotte A. Determination of the effectiveness of four sleep surfaces in the treatment of stage 2 and 3 pressure sores (unpublished research report). Batesville, IN, Barnes Hospital, St. Louis, and Hill Rom, 1992.

151. Witkowski JA, Parish LC: Histopathology of the decubitus ulcer. J Am Acad Dermatol 1982; 6:1014–1021.

152. Yarkony GM: Pressure ulcers: A review. Arch Phys Med Rehabil 1994; 75:908–917.

32

Cardiac Rehabilitation

**JONATHAN R. MOLDOVER, M.D., AND
MATTHEW N. BARTELS, M.D., M.P.H.**

GOALS OF CARDIAC REHABILITATION

There are two primary goals of any cardiac rehabilitation program: increasing the functional capacity of the patient, and changing the natural history of the disease to reduce morbidity and mortality. The first goal is readily attainable, as has been repeatedly demonstrated and accepted for many years. The second goal was considered questionable until relatively recently, but there are now a number of studies showing that a comprehensive program of risk factor reduction, lifestyle alteration, and exercise training can lower morbidity and mortality and even produce regression of atherosclerotic stenoses.[39, 64, 66]

EPIDEMIOLOGY OF HEART DISEASE

Cardiac disease is the leading cause of morbidity and mortality in the adult population in the United States. With increased public awareness of cardiac risk factors, better management of cardiac disease, and risk intervention by the medical community, these rates have been steadily declining. Reductions in cigarette smoking and red meat consumption, and increasing exercise have all contributed to the decrease in coronary artery disease (CAD). The major risk factors are outlined in Table 32–1. The death rate of CAD was 228.1 per 100,000 population in 1970 but had declined to 102.6 per 100,000 in 1990.

CAD is the number one cause of mortality in men aged 45 years and older, and in women aged 75 and older. CAD is the overall number one cause of death in the United States, with over 72,000 deaths in 1990. The estimated mortality cost of cardiac disease in 1990 was more than $70 billion, with an estimated 8.2 million life-years lost.[82]

Cardiac disease accounts for a large proportion of total healthcare expenditures. In 1992, cardiovascular disease was the single greatest cause of hospital admissions (3.9 million). Myocardial ischemia accounted for more than 2.1 million of these hospital admissions, and congestive heart failure (CHF) accounted for approximately 800,000 admissions. Cardiac arrhythmias cause nearly 550,000 admissions each year.

Cardiac surgery accounts for the third largest number of surgical procedures for inpatients. In 1992, more than 1 million cardiac catheterizations were performed and more than 300,000 coronary artery bypass grafts (CABGs).[37]

With new technologies, congestive heart disease patients are living longer, and more patients are surviving myocardial infarction (MI). For example, new abilities to allow patients to survive after transplant have increased the number of cardiac transplant procedures performed. In 1990, there were over 2100 heart transplants, and more than 2200 people were on the waiting list.[82]

TYPES OF HEART DISEASE

The types of heart disease that are likely to be encountered by the physiatrist practicing cardiac rehabilitation have increased in current years. "Standard" cardiac rehabilitation of the post-MI patient is still the majority of the practice, but post-CABG, post-transplant, and postvalvular surgery patients are now being referred for cardiac rehabilitation in increasing numbers. Patients with chronic CHF

TABLE 32–1 Risk Factors for Coronary Artery Disease (CAD)

Irreversible Risks	Reversible Risks
Male gender	Cigarette smoking
Family history of	Hypertension
premature CAD (before	Low HDL cholesterol
age 55 yr in a parent or	[<0.9 mmol/L (35 mg/dL)]
sibling)	Hypercholesterolemia
Past history of CAD	[>5.20 mmol/L (200 mg/dL)]
Past history of occlusive	High lipoprotein A
peripheral vascular	Abdominal obesity
disease	Hypertriglyceridemia
Past history of	[>2.8 mmol/L (250 mg/dL)]
cerebrovascular disease	Hyperinsulinemia
	Diabetes mellitus
	Sedentary lifestyle

are now also being referred for cardiac rehabilitation, as are patients with life-threatening arrhythmias.

EXERCISE PHYSIOLOGY

The clinician needs to understand the cardiac response to exercise and the effects of aerobic training in order to design a safe and effective rehabilitation program for any given patient.[59]

AEROBIC CAPACITY. *Aerobic capacity* is a physiological term used to measure the work capacity of an individual. It is represented by the maximum oxygen consumption ($\dot{V}O_2$max), usually expressed in millimeters of oxygen consumed per kilogram of body weight per minute. If the total oxygen consumption ($\dot{V}O_2$) of the exercising individual is measured and plotted against the workload (Fig. 32–1), the $\dot{V}O_2$ increases in a linear fashion until it levels off in a short plateau. This plateau represents the point at which the $\dot{V}O_2$ cannot increase further despite further increases in the workload. This is the $\dot{V}O_2$max (or aerobic capacity) of this individual. The total $\dot{V}O_2$ provides a measure of the increasing metabolic work of the peripheral skeletal muscles, not of the heart itself. The $\dot{V}O_2$ is useful as a measure of the physical work being performed. In research studies the work being performed is often expressed as a percentage of the $\dot{V}O_2$max. Since physiological responses to exercise are typically proportional to the relative workload for any individual rather than the absolute workload, using the percentage of $\dot{V}O_2$ max allows us to normalize the data for a population of subjects.

CARDIAC OUTPUT. Cardiac output (CO) increases with increasing work. In early exercise, CO increases due to augmented stroke volume via the Frank-Starling mechanism. In late exercise, CO is increased primarily through an increase in ventricular rate.[28] Plotting CO against $\dot{V}O_2$ (Fig. 32–2), we see that this increase is essentially linear. The break in the slope of the line represents a lessening of the rate of increase caused by shifts in the oxyhemoglobin dissociation curve due to increasing temperature, acidity, and carbon dioxide in the working muscles. The maximum CO is the primary determinant of the $\dot{V}O_2$max. The CO in

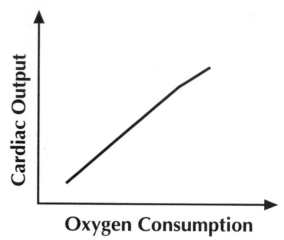

FIGURE 32–2   Relationship between cardiac output and oxygen consumption.

turn has two determinants: the heart rate and the stroke volume (SV).

HEART RATE. Heart rate (HR) increases in a linear manner when plotted against the $\dot{V}O_2$ or other measures of physical work (Fig. 32–3). The HR is limited by the person's age. Even with regular exercise there is a linear decrease in the maximum HR with age.[3] For practical purposes a person's maximum HR can be estimated by subtracting the age in years from 220.

STROKE VOLUME. Stroke volume represents the quantity of blood pumped with each heartbeat. With upright exercise it increases in a curvilinear fashion until it reaches a plateau at about 40% of the $\dot{V}O_2$max (Fig. 32–4). In the supine position the SV is close to maximal from the beginning of exercise, with increases in CO being due to increasing HR. A major determinant of SV is the diastolic filling volume, which is inversely related to the HR.

MYOCARDIAL OXYGEN CONSUMPTION. The myocardial oxygen consumption ($M\dot{V}O_2$) is the actual oxygen consumption of the heart, as opposed to the $\dot{V}O_2$, which represents the oxygen consumption of the whole body (mainly due to the work of the skeletal muscles). The

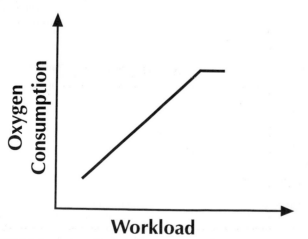

FIGURE 32–1   Relationship between oxygen consumption and intensity of work being performed.

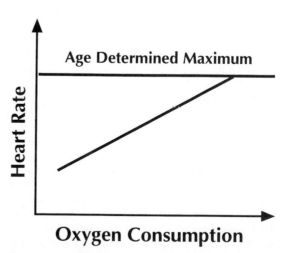

FIGURE 32–3   Relationship between heart rate and oxygen consumption.

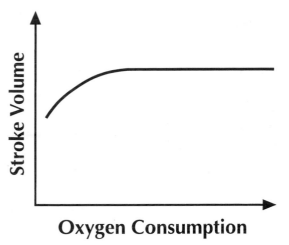

FIGURE 32–4   Relationship between stroke volume and oxygen consumption.

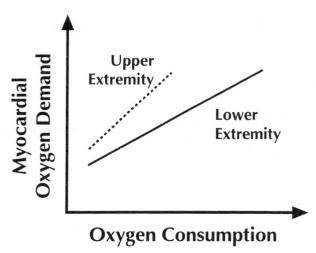

FIGURE 32–6   Comparison of the myocardial oxygen demand for upper extremity vs. lower extremity exercise.

$M\dot{V}O_2$ rises in a linear fashion when plotted against the $\dot{V}O_2$ or other measure of workload (Fig. 32–5). It is limited by the anginal threshold, if one exists, or by the $\dot{V}O_2max$ if there is no CAD. The *anginal threshold* is defined as the point where the myocardial oxygen demand exceeds the ability of the coronary circulation to meet that demand. At the anginal threshold the patient may experience typical anginal chest pain, ischemic changes on the electrocardiogram (ECG), or arrhythmias. Although the $M\dot{V}O_2$ can be measured directly with cardiac catheterization, this is rarely practicable in a clinical setting. It has been shown that the HR and systolic blood pressure (BP) correlate well with the actual $M\dot{V}O_2$ and can be used as a clinical guide. The usual measure is the rate pressure product (RPP), which is calculated by multiplying the HR by the systolic BP and dividing the product by 100.

The linear relationship between the $M\dot{V}O_2$ and the $\dot{V}O_2$ has been used to suggest that the relative cardiac stress of various activities can be compared by measuring the $\dot{V}O_2$ produced by the activities. However, it should be noted that the linear relationship only holds true for a single activity performed under identical circumstances with varying intensity (e.g., pedaling a bicycle ergometer at different workloads or walking on a treadmill at different speeds).

Activities performed with the upper extremities as opposed to the lower extremities generate a higher $M\dot{V}O_2$ at the same $\dot{V}O_2$ (Fig. 32–6). Activities performed supine as opposed to upright generate a higher $M\dot{V}O_2$ at low intensities and a lower $M\dot{V}O_2$ at higher intensities (Fig. 32–7). Activities performed under emotional stress, after smoking a cigarette, after eating, or in cold weather all generate a higher $M\dot{V}O_2$ at the same $\dot{V}O_2$ than activities performed at baseline. Activities that have an isometric component generate a higher $M\dot{V}O_2$ than a similar activity at the same $\dot{V}O_2$ without the isometric component (e.g., ambulating while gripping a cane or carrying a briefcase compared with ambulation without anything in the hands).

AEROBIC TRAINING

Aerobic training refers to an exercise program that involves dynamic exercise with large muscle groups and of a sufficient intensity, duration, and frequency to alter the cardiopulmonary response to exercise.

Principles

INTENSITY.   The *intensity* of aerobic exercise can be defined either in terms of the individual's physiological

FIGURE 32–5   Relationship between myocardial oxygen demand and total body oxygen consumption.

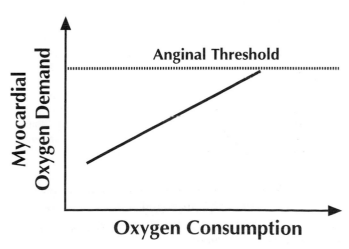

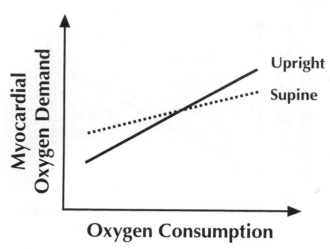

FIGURE 32–7 Comparison of the cardiac response to lower extremity exercise performed in upright and supine positions.

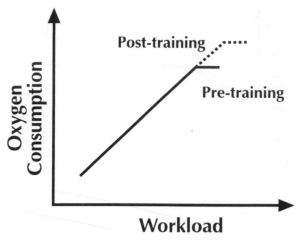

FIGURE 32–8 Effect of training on relationship between oxygen consumption and workload.

response (HR or RPP) or in terms of exercise intensity (speed or resistance setting). A typical exercise prescription might be written with a target HR to be sustained after an appropriate warmup period. The usual target HR is approximately 85% of the maximum HR achieved during a pretraining exercise tolerance test (ETT). If the individual is very frail or deconditioned, or if the limiting factor on the ETT was a dangerous arrhythmia, then an intensity as low as 60% of maximum can be prescribed and a training effect can still be expected. Alternatively, if the training exercise is to be the same as the testing exercise, then the prescription can be written in terms of the workload on a bicycle ergometer, or speed and grade on a treadmill.

DURATION. The duration of each exercise session in the typical aerobic training program is 20 to 30 min. The actual training period is preceded by a warmup phase at lower intensity and followed by a cooldown phase at a lower intensity. In general, training at a lower intensity of exercise requires a longer duration to achieve a training effect, and training at a relatively higher intensity requires a shorter duration.

FREQUENCY. Aerobic training schedules usually involve exercise 3 days a week. Programs involving exercise at lower intensities should be performed at least 5 days a week.

SPECIFICITY. A key concept in all exercise training is that of specificity of training. The changes in the cardiac response to exercise apply only to exercise with muscles that have been involved in the training program. Training with a walking program or on a bicycle does not affect the cardiac response to upper extremity work. Training a carpenter with a vigorous treadmill program does nothing to change his cardiac response to strenuous woodworking activities performed with the arms. All muscle groups that the person needs for vocational or avocational pursuits should be included in the training program.

Effects

AEROBIC CAPACITY. The defining characteristic of a successful aerobic training program is an increase in the aerobic capacity ($\dot{V}O_2max$), as shown in Figure 32–8. Note that while the $\dot{V}O_2max$ increases, there is no change in the resting $\dot{V}O_2$ or in the $\dot{V}O_2$ at any given submaximum workload. It should also be noted that the effect is only seen if both the pretest and the post-test use the same muscle groups that are used in the training program.

CARDIAC OUTPUT. The maximum CO increases with aerobic training, as seen in Figure 32–9. As with the $\dot{V}O_2$, note that while the CO at maximum exercise increases, the resting and the submaximum CO remain the same.

STROKE VOLUME. Although the CO at any given submaximum workload remains the same, there are significant changes in the way that the CO is generated. The SV is higher at rest, submaximum work, and maximum work after aerobic training (Fig. 32–10). This increase in SV is mostly due to a combination of increased blood volume and prolonged diastolic filling time.

HEART RATE. The HR following aerobic training is lower at rest and at any given submaximum workload but remains unchanged at maximum work (Fig. 32–11). As noted above, the maximum HR is determined by the person's age, not level of fitness. Of course, if the ETT is prematurely limited by a noncardiac endpoint, then one

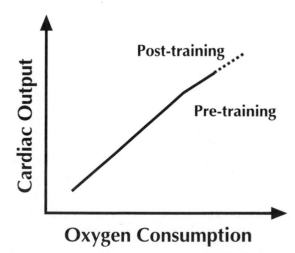

FIGURE 32–9 Effect of training on relationship between cardiac output and oxygen consumption.

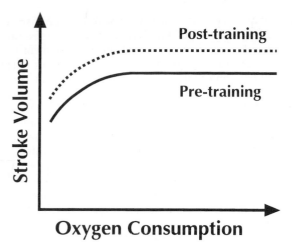

FIGURE 32–10 Effect of training on relationship between stroke volume and oxygen consumption.

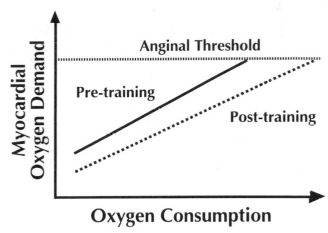

FIGURE 32–12 Effect of training on relationship between myocardial oxygen demand and oxygen consumption.

might see an increase in the maximum HR obtained during the post-test.

MYOCARDIAL OXYGEN CONSUMPTION. From the point of view of cardiac rehabilitation, it is the effect of aerobic training on the $M\dot{V}O_2$ that makes exercise training such an important part of any rehabilitation program. Note that in Figure 32–12 there is a decrease in the $M\dot{V}O_2$ at rest and at any submaximum workload, but there is no change in the maximum $M\dot{V}O_2$. The maximum level is still determined by the anginal threshold, which is not affected by aerobic conditioning. Thus, exercise training does not appear to have a significant effect on the coronary circulation. Pharmacological interventions also have an effect on resting and submaximum, but not maximum $M\dot{V}O_2$. Only angioplasty or bypass surgery can raise or eliminate the anginal threshold.

Benefits

Even though the anginal threshold is not changed by aerobic training, the change in the cardiac response to exercise is extremely beneficial. The workload that can be tolerated before the anginal threshold is reached increases

significantly. Patients can now do activities because they can perform them without overtaxing the coronary circulation. In addition, activities which could be performed before now require a lower percentage of the maximum, making them less stressful and creating a wider margin of safety between the cardiac response to that activity and the anginal threshold.

In addition to the reduced relative stress of specific activities provided by the increased physical work capacity, there is a growing body of evidence that aerobic training has a beneficial effect on the natural history of CAD that can be isolated from other lifestyle alterations. Paffenbarger et al.[66] demonstrated that beginning moderate physical activity in or after middle age resulted in a significant reduction in mortality from all causes and from CAD in particular, and that this effect was separable from the benefits of smoking cessation, BP normalization, and weight control. Hambrecht et al.[39] used quantitative coronary angiography to show that regression in artery stenosis correlated with the level of physical activity. Aerobic training is an integral part of other more comprehensive studies of lifestyle alteration which have shown regression of atherosclerotic plaques.[64]

ASSESSMENT OF CARDIAC FUNCTION

History and Physical Examination

The cardiac history and physical examination are a very important part of the evaluation of the patient with cardiac disease who is to undergo cardiac rehabilitation. The history often reveals important issues to be addressed and gives the treating physiatrist the information needed to develop and direct a rehabilitation program. Often some of the most pertinent details and important aspects of a patient's disability can be obtained from the physician-directed history as the patient establishes a relationship of trust, and the examiner can get the nuances of the history from verbal and nonverbal cues. The patient can express concerns and goals to the physician. This facilitates the patient and physician's establishing mutual goals that often result in improved compliance with the treatment program.

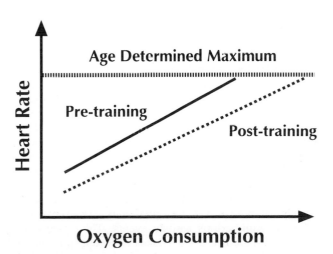

FIGURE 32–11 Effect of training on relationship between heart rate and oxygen consumption.

History

Historical information can help direct the testing and help with the interpretation of the results. The physician also has the opportunity to observe the patient's emotional state, giving further insight into the effects of the cardiac disability. Concurrent illnesses and disabilities also need to be taken into account when designing an optimal rehabilitation program, as well as in creating realistic goals and planning appropriate testing protocols. The functional history, occupational history, social history, and personal habits need to be verified, since they make a considerable contribution to the eventual outcome of the rehabilitation of the patient. It is also important to elicit data from family members, who can often substantiate the data or give additional information. This is especially true regarding information about functional limitations and disability, as well as family dynamics and the effect of disability and cardiac illness on the patient's performance in the community. Table 32–2 summarizes the key issues to address in the history. When taking the actual cardiac history, special attention should be paid to the nature of the symptoms at rest and with activity. Several important symptoms specific to the cardiac history are discussed separately below.

DYSPNEA. Shortness of breath (SOB) is often one of

TABLE 32–2   Key Issues to Address in the History of a Patient With Cardiac Disease

Key Elements of the History

FAMILY HISTORY
  Premature CAD (before age 55 yr in first-degree relative)
  Family history of familial hypercholesterolemia or hyperlipidemia
  Family history of sudden death
  Family history of arrhythmias
  Family history of Marfan disease
  Family history of hypertrophic cardiomyopathy
SOCIAL HISTORY
  Cigarette use, cigar/pipe use
  Sedentary lifestyle
  Alcohol abuse history
SYMPTOM HISTORY
  Chest pain: duration, location, character, precipitating and
    relieving factors, pain radiation
  Shortness of breath: duration, precipitating and relieving factors,
    day or night, position
  Dizziness/lightheadedness
  Syncope
  Presence of nausea/vomiting, anorexia
  Cyanosis/pallor
  Palpitations
  Edema
  Cough
  Hemoptysis
  Fatigue
FUNCTIONAL HISTORY
  Level of activity prior to cardiac event
  Present level of activity
  Exercise tolerance level
  Level of activity required at home and at work
  Level of function, stable or progressively worse
  Extent and rate of activities performed
PATIENT GOALS
  Vocational plans
  Leisure activities
  Emotional adaptation to the cardiac condition
MEDICATIONS
COMPLETE REVIEW OF SYSTEMS AND PAST MEDICAL HISTORY

the central symptoms in a patient with cardiac disease. A complete description of the dyspnea and all its features is needed to be able to make an adequate assessment of the cardiac status of the patient. Noncardiac causes of dyspnea are common, and with a good history it is often possible to differentiate cardiac SOB from other causes. Chronic SOB can be an indicator of either cardiac or pulmonary disease. The presence of chronic obstructive pulmonary disease (COPD) and restrictive lung disease can usually be deduced from the history, even if concomitant with cardiac disease. Chronic CHF, due to any of a number of causes, is the usual cardiac cause of SOB. Often, both cardiac and pulmonary problems are present in the same patient and each limits the progress that can be made in rehabilitation.

Exertional dyspnea also has a number of causes that can be differentiated with a careful history. Deconditioning is commonly encountered in patients who have been hospitalized for prolonged periods. Anxiety and hyperventilation are often characterized by facial paresthesia and a prolonged dull chest discomfort that is often relieved by sedation or exertion. In patients with resting SOB due to CHF, the SOB is classically relieved by sitting up and is worsened in the recumbent position. Paroxysmal nocturnal dyspnea (PND) is seen with the development of pulmonary congestion approximately 2 to 5 hours after onset of sleep and is relieved with sitting up, and the patient classically reports getting up to open the window for some "fresh air." Exertional dyspnea, if not of pulmonary origin, can be an anginal equivalent, with or without associated chest pain. Similarly, diastolic dysfunction of a hypertrophied left ventricle can lead to acute pulmonary edema with SOB on exertion. The patient's history can help define the diagnosis as well as contribute to the management plan for the patient.

CHEST PAIN. Chest pain, tightness, and burning are the classic symptoms in a history of a patient with CAD. These symptoms often are also seen in patients with valvular heart disease or arrhythmia. Often the history gives clues to help differentiate these causes of chest pain. The most important items to note about the chest pain history are the duration, the quality, the provocation, and the location of the pain, and any ameliorating factors (Table 32–3). The possible precipitating factors for chest pain are of particular interest to the physiatrist, as these influence the design of an appropriate therapy program and allow for assessment of the functional limitations placed on the patient by the cardiac disability.

PALPITATION. Palpitation refers to the subjective sensation of an irregular or forceful heartbeat. It is often benign but can be indicative of serious tachyarrhythmias. There are patients who are aware of every single benign premature beat and will report them by history. Some patients with more serious arrhythmias may be able to accurately report the start and end of their arrhythmias, whereas others having the same life-threatening arrhythmias might be free of palpitation.

SYNCOPE. There are numerous causes of syncope, but in a patient with CAD, this particular symptom can be associated with serious cardiac events. The syncope that occurs with a cardiac event is usually abrupt in onset, and often there is no warning or only a brief warning (with the patient feeling as if he or she were about to pass out). If

TABLE 32–3 Cardiac vs. Noncardiac Chest Pain by Symptoms

Cardiac Pain Symptoms	Noncardiac Pain Symptoms
PAIN QUALITY	
Constricting/squeezing	Dull aching
Visceral quality	Sharp, stabbing, piercing, knife-like
Burning	Muscular
Heaviness	
PAIN LOCATION	
Substernal	Left submammary area, apex of heart
Across precordium	Superficial tissues of the left chest
Neck	Right lower chest
One or both shoulders, arms	Very discrete localization possible
Intrascapular region	
One or both forearms, hands	
Epigastrium	
PAIN DURATION	
Angina, 2–10 min	<20 sec
Infarction, >20 min to 24 h	Persistent without change for >24–48 hr
PRECIPITATING AND AGGRAVATING FACTORS	
Exercise, particularly with hurrying	After completion of exercise
Excitement	With specific body positions, chest wall movement, and respiration
Cold temperature exposure	With direct palpation of chest wall
Stressful stimuli	Spontaneous
Postprandially, after heavy meal	Head and neck movement
	During fasting, with cold liquids
RELIEVING FACTORS	
Rest	Antacids
Nitroglycerin	Food
	Nonsteroidal analgesia

syncope occurs, the patient often sustains a fall and injury can occur. The event is usually brief and the patient typically has no convulsions. Syncope is a marker for such severe cardiac illnesses as aortic stenosis, idiopathic hypertrophic subaortic stenosis (IHSS), primary pulmonary hypertension, ventricular arrhythmias, reentrant arrhythmias, high-degree atrioventricular (AV) block, or sick sinus syndrome. Postural syncope can be due to autonomic dysfunction, neurological disease, vagal stimuli, or psychological stimuli. These differences can usually be determined by the history.

EDEMA. A history of peripheral edema can be an indication of CHF. With more modern techniques, often CHF can be diagnosed long before edema occurs, so the history of edema is best thought of as a marker of severe CHF. Careful history can also usually determine if the peripheral edema is due to a cause other than CHF, such as postural edema caused by prolonged sitting (e.g., in a wheelchair), liver disease, or renal disease. Unilateral edema is much more common in venous disease or lymphatic obstruction. It is useful to get a history from the patient about the onset, duration, and activities prior to the onset of edema. Edema also takes on importance in the disabled population as there are many patients who wear braces or prostheses and could have further disability due to the edema's interfering with the use of these devices.

FATIGUE. A good history can differentiate among the many causes of this common symptom. Depression, use of certain medications, physical exhaustion, and deconditioning are common noncardiac causes of fatigue in the patient with known cardiac disease. The cause of cardiac fatigue is usually heart failure with chronic low CO. This usually begins as increasing fatigue during or after an activity that previously caused no fatigue. The fatigue is typically relieved with rest and occasionally presents as a form of atypical angina.

COUGH. Cough is a symptom with many potential causes. Most often it is due to pulmonary causes or upper airway irritation, but in the case of cardiac disease it is often a symptom of CHF. The "cardiac" cough is often initiated by postural changes, especially the recumbent position. There is little or no sputum production and the cough is usually relieved by assuming an upright position. Often the coughing is nocturnal and episodic.

LIMITATIONS OF THE HISTORY. As important as the history is, it has some limitations as well. In patients with known CAD, often the data required for the design of a cardiac rehabilitation program cannot be assessed by history alone. There is the need to proceed with some form of cardiac stress testing or other techniques to permit cardiac risk assessment that cannot be done in any other way. As illustrated in Table 32–4, there are some historical features that can indicate prognosis, but true risk assessment requires the detection of subclinical features that can only be obtained through testing.

Physical Examination

The physical examination is an important part of the diagnostic evaluation of the cardiac patient. The cardiac physical examination starts with a general survey of the patient. The eyes can reveal exophthalmos (which might be a clue to thyrotoxicosis) or xanthelasma (indicating hypercholesterolemia). Remember that there are associa-

TABLE 32–4   Historical Data That Indicate Increased Cardiac Risk

Postinfection angina
Symptomatic congestive heart failure
Age >70 yr
Severe exercise limitation
Diabetes
History of hypertension, or loss of hypertension
Palpitation
Syncope
Fatigue

tions between conditions, such as ankylosis with aortic valve disease or conduction defects, and that patients with Down syndrome can have associated cardiac abnormalities. The presence of myasthenia or other neuromuscular disease on a physical examination should bring to mind the possibility of a cardiomyopathy or conduction disease.

The actual details of the cardiac examination are well described in basic physical examination textbooks. There are several findings that a physiatrist should be on the lookout for in patients who are to undergo cardiac rehabilitation. Congenital heart defects are not unusual in the disabled population, and the examination often alerts the physician to their presence.

Cardiac auscultation can be a particularly helpful part of the physical examination. A fixed splitting of the second heart sound can indicate an atrial septal defect. Aortic valve stenosis can be detected via a systolic murmur. Pulmonary hypertension typically produces a heightened second heart sound in the pulmonic valve portion. A mid-systolic click can be heard in mitral valve prolapse. The presence of a noncompliant ventricle which might be subject to diastolic dysfunction can be detected via an atrial gallop at the cardiac apex. A left ventricular gallop can be heard in patients with heart failure. Aortic valve sclerosis that is seen in many older patients results in an aortic systolic murmur. The combination of pulse contour, the nature of the splitting of the heart sounds, and the quality of the murmur can help differentiate aortic sclerosis from aortic stenosis. Pulmonary stenosis can be detected in young patients with possible cardiac anomalies, as well as in adults with valvular heart disease. IHSS can be seen in younger patients and is often difficult to differentiate on examination from aortic stenosis or mitral regurgitation. Diastolic murmurs in patients about to start a cardiac rehabilitation program can give clues to the presence of mitral stenosis, or the presence of pulmonary hypertension with pulmonary valve regurgitation. Continuous murmurs often need further investigation for the presence of a ventricular septal or atrial septal defect. The physical examination leads to a further diagnostic workup which may then avoid complications in cardiac rehabilitation.

Summary

Although the cardiac examination and history are important in the detection of cardiac disease and in the determination of prognosis, the new imaging and cardiac testing techniques offer the most reliable assessment of the patient's true cardiac status. Still, the detection of patients at risk for complications in a cardiac rehabilitation program

can often be started in the physiatrist's office with the basic history and physical examination.

Exercise Tolerance Testing

Exercise tolerance testing is an essential first step in the exercise training phase of any cardiac rehabilitation program. It is used to create an individualized exercise prescription, allowing an optimal level of training stimulus without exposing the patient to undue risk. Besides the classic exercise treadmill test, many newer techniques are now available. These tests can be used in patients with physical impairments and other challenging patients, which broadens the range of patients who can be tested. These variations in exercise testing are in the areas of methods of application of the stress and in evaluating the response of the myocardium. These new stress tests allow the physiatrist to better evaluate and rehabilitate the disabled patient with coexisting cardiac disease, as well as furnish a better assessment of the cardiac status of nonhandicapped patients.

Electrocardiographic Exercise Tolerance Testing

Although other more modern tests have taken over the diagnostic role for cardiac ischemia, the exercise stress test is still the most commonly used test to perform cardiac risk stratification and to determine functional capacity. Contraindications to exercise stress testing are summarized in Table 32–5. Some of the noncardiac contraindications can be overcome with the newer techniques of applying cardiac stress or recording methods. The basic principle of the exercise stress test is to use the physiological response to exercise to increase physiological demand on the myocardium, which increases the $M\dot{V}O_2$, which can reveal ischemic changes via the ECG.

TABLE 32–5   Contraindications to Exercise Tolerance Testing

ABSOLUTE CARDIAC CONTRAINDICATIONS TO EXERCISE TESTING
1. Unstable angina with recent chest pain
2. Untreated life-threatening cardiac arrhythmias
3. Uncompensated congestive heart failure
4. Advanced atrioventricular block
5. Acute myocarditis or pericarditis
6. Critical aortic stenosis
7. Severe hypertrophic obstructive cardiomyopathy
8. Uncontrolled hypertension
9. Acute myocardial infarction
10. Active endocarditis

ABSOLUTE NONCARDIAC CONTRAINDICATIONS TO EXERCISE TESTING
1. Acute pulmonary embolus or pulmonary infarction
2. Acute systemic illness

RELATIVE CONTRAINDICATIONS
1. Significant pulmonary hypertension
2. Significant arterial hypertension
3. Tachyarrhythmias or bradyarrhythmias
4. Moderate valvular heart disease
5. Myocardial heart disease
6. Electrolyte abnormalities
7. Left main coronary obstruction
8. Hypertrophic cardiomyopathy
9. Psychiatric disease

TABLE 32–6 Bruce Protocol*

Stage	Grade (%)	Speed (mph)	Time (min)	Total Time (min)
1	10	1.7	3	3
2	12	2.5	3	6
3	14	3.4	3	9
4	16	4.2	3	12
5	18	5.0	3+	15+

*For each stage, both the grade and the speed are increased every 3 min.

EXERCISE PROTOCOLS. Exercise protocols are normally designed with stages of 3 to 5 min in duration each, to achieve a steady-state response.[32] Usually protocols include a warmup period of low-intensity exercise and end with a cooldown period of suitable length. The exercise protocol needs to be tailored to the individual patient and should allow for testing of patients with very limited cardiac reserve as well as patients with excellent aerobic conditioning.

TREADMILL PROTOCOLS. The most commonly used treadmill protocol is the Bruce protocol[25, 31] (Table 32–6). The limitations in this protocol are in the large increases in $\dot{V}O_2$ (5 METs*) between stages and the additional cost of energy in running that occurs in Bruce stage III and above.[12(p 163)] In order to overcome some of these limitations, especially in patients with disability or limited cardiac reserve, other protocols are available. The Naughton, Weber, and Balke-Ware protocols use 1- to 2-min stages which have 1-MET increments, and these are sometimes better tolerated by patients with CHF, deconditioning, or other causes of limited exercise tolerance. The Cornell protocol is a modification of the Bruce protocol with increments in 2-min stages, allowing a better estimate of ST segment–HR measurements.[63] Table 32–7 compares the various protocols.

---

*One MET is defined as the resting metabolic rate (approximately 3.5 mL O_2/kg body weight/min).

BICYCLE ERGOMETRY. The most common alternative to treadmill protocols is bicycle ergometry. It offers several advantages, one of which is that the patient's chest and arms remain relatively stable, allowing for better ECG recording during the test. Blood pressure recording is also easier on the bicycle. The influence of the patient's weight is less, and a bicycle often takes up less room in the laboratory. Bicycle ergometry can also be done supine, which can be an advantage in some patients. Some patients have difficulty with bicycle pedaling because of incoordination or fatigue.[62] The RPP and systolic BP are greater on the bicycle at a given level of submaximum $\dot{V}O_2$ than on the treadmill. The maximum $M\dot{V}O_2$, however, is approximately 10% greater on the treadmill.[61] Table 32–8 compares the alternative tests discussed in this chapter.

In all ETTs, it is important that the patient not hold the hand rail or handlebars because the exaggerated cardiac response caused by the isometric hand grip can cause the functional capacity to be overestimated by as much as 20%.[12(p 163)]

UPPER EXTREMITY ERGOMETRY. The main advantage of this type of ETT is that it can be used in patients who have orthopedic, vascular, or neurological disabilities which do not permit them to perform the standard treadmill or bicycle test. The patients who typically get this type of testing include amputees, paraplegic patients, and patients who have arthritis or have had orthopedic procedures. The effects on physiology during upper extremity ergometry are different from those seen in treadmill exercise testing. The RPP is elevated more in upper extremity ergometry owing to a greater increase in the systolic BP than HR. This effect is thought to be due to the increase in vascular tone seen in the nonexercising vascular beds. There is also less of an increase in CO seen in subjects with upper extremity ergometry than in treadmill exercise testing.[2]

PREPARATION FOR STRESS TESTING. Although the techniques of stress testing can vary slightly from laboratory to laboratory, there are some basic rules that generally apply to all patients who undergo stress testing. Patients

TABLE 32–7 Comparison of Exercise Tolerance Testing Protocols

	Bruce	Cornell	Weber	Balke-Ware	Naughton
Time of stages	3 min	2 min	2 min	1 min	2 min
MET level	2 to >16	2 to 16	1 to 10	4 to 16	2 to 7 at 2 mph 3 to 16 at 3 mph 4 to 16 at 3,4 mph
Step changes	2 MET steps from 2 to 7 MET 3 MET steps from 7 to >16 MET	2 MET	1 MET	½ MET	1 MET
Changes grade	Yes	Yes	Yes	Yes	Yes
Range of grade	0%–20%	0%–18%	0%–15%	1%–26%	0%–17.5% at 2 mph 0%–32.5% at 3 mph 0%–26% at 4 mph
Step changes	5% from 0% to 10% 2% from 10% to 20%	5% from 0% to 10% 1% from 10% to 18%	3.5% from 0% to 10.5% (2 mph) 2.5% from 7.5% to 15% (3 mph) 14% fixed at 3.4 mph	1% from 1% to 26%	3.5% from 0% to 17.5% (2 mph) 2.5% from 0% to 32.5% (3 mph) 2% from 2% to 26% (3.4 mph)
Changes speed	Yes	Yes	Yes	No	No
Range of speed	1.7 to 5.5 mph	1.7 to 5.0 mph	1.0 to 3.4 mph	Constant 3.3 mph	2, 3, or 4 mph
Step changes	0.8 mph	0.4 mph	0.5 mph		
NYHA functional classes tested	Normal, I, II, III	Normal, I, II, III	Normal, I, II, III, IV	Normal, I, II, mild III	Normal, I, II, III

TABLE 32–8   Advantages and Disadvantages of Alternative Test Devices

Test	Bicycle Ergometry	Upper Extremity Ergometry	Treadmill	Pharmacological Agents
Advantages	Has good correlation with treadmill testing Thorax and arms remain stable Less effect of patient body weight	Useful for patients with orthopedic, vascular, or neurological conditions who cannot perform leg exercise	Readily available Well standardized Multiple protocols available Can be used for ramp protocols	Can be used in all patients, even the most deconditioned or impaired Good reliability Well standardized
Disadvantages	Patient may not be able to learn to bicycle $M\dot{V}O_2$ 6%–25% less than in treadmill exercise Greater cardiac stress (rate pressure product) for a given $\dot{V}O_2$ Bicycle takes up space in laboratory	Less increase in cardiac output than in treadmill testing Greater rate pressure product increase than in treadmill testing	Overweight, orthopedic, neurological, vascular, or arthritic patients may not be able to reach acceptable exercise levels	Not physiological Some risks involved, depending on the agent Invasive Need to have special imaging equipment and properly equipped and staffed laboratory

should not eat for at least 3 hours before a stress test and should have no caffeinated beverages for up to 24 hours before the stress test. Patients should wear comfortable, loose-fitting clothes and comfortable walking shoes. A 12-lead ECG is taken before the start of the test and a limited physical examination is performed. Supine and erect ECGs with the torso electrodes usually are also obtained to ensure that there are no changes in the ECG based solely on position changes. The patient is taught how to ambulate on the treadmill, and vital signs and ECGs are taken before, after, and at each stage of the test as well as during the recovery period.

ECG CRITERIA. The normal lead placement in cardiac stress testing is the modified 12-lead system. The hallmark of ischemia on the exercise cardiogram is ST segment depression. ST depressions of 2 mm or more in one lead is a positive test[12(p 166)] (Fig. 32–13). Not all ST depression is of cardiac origin.[12(p 168)] Other abnormalities can be seen in patients during exercise stress testing, such as ST elevation, upsloping ST segments, and variation of the R wave amplitude. ST segment elevation in a lead with an abnormal Q wave can be seen in patients with poor left ventricular function.[15] This can be seen in up to 30% of patients with anterior wall MI and 15% of patients with inferior wall MI tested within 2 weeks of MI; it decreases after 6 weeks. ST segment elevation in these Q wave leads is not a marker of cardiac ischemia.[38] In the absence of previous MI or Q wave, ST elevation is a marker of high-grade stenosis or coronary vasospasm causing transmural ischemia.

Upsloping of ST segments is a normal finding in the ECG during maximum exercise. The finding of a slowly upsloping ST segment after a 1.5-mm ST depression is an indicator of probable ischemia.[18] The changes in R wave amplitude during exercise are relatively nonspecific. When the R wave meets the criteria for left ventricular hypertrophy (LVH), ST segment response is not usable for the diagnosis of ischemia, and loss of R wave in a lead after MI reduces the prognostic use of that particular lead for ischemic changes after MI.

NON-ECG CRITERIA. In addition to the ECG, there are other clinical factors to observe during the performance of the ETT. The BP and symptoms of chest discomfort are also important. Several important pieces of information can

be determined during the stress test which are particularly useful to the physiatrist in the development and pursuit of the cardiac rehabilitation program. Among these are the maximum work capacity, the RPP, and the HR response. The BP in normal exercise increases progressively with each increasing workload. The failure of systolic BP to increase appropriately can be a sign of ischemia or of left ventricular dysfunction.[25, 31] A fall in the systolic BP with increasing load is an indication for aborting the ETT. Non-ischemic causes of fall in systolic BP in ETT include cardiomyopathy, cardiac arrhythmias, vasovagal reaction, left ventricular outflow tract obstruction, use of antihypertensive drugs, hypovolemia, and prolonged vigorous exercise. The diastolic BP does not change significantly in normal patients during exercise. A rise in diastolic BP in a stress test can be associated with ischemia.

After exercise, there should be a gradual decline in the systolic BP. In up to 3% of healthy normal adults there can be an episode of profound postexercise hypotension that is not due to CAD.[29]

Although chest pain starts after the onset of ST depression in most cases, chest pain may be the only indicator of ischemia in some patients.[53] The presence of pain with no ECG changes is often an indication that nuclear or echocardiographic testing is needed.

The maximum work capacity can be determined during the ETT and is an important prognostic measurement, as well as allowing for the determination of the maximum work that can be performed by the patient during a rehabilitation program.[9, 57, 87] A limited exercise capacity in a patient with a known cardiac disease is associated with an increased risk of cardiac events and worse prognosis. The best estimate of functional capacity is the amount of work performed or the level reached. The time the patient exercised is not as useful, as it is dependent on the test protocol used. The exercise impairment is determined by comparing the patient's performance to that in a table of normal levels adjusted for age, which is available in the literature and specific to the exercise protocol employed[85] (Table 32–9). If serial determinations of exercise capacity are to be determined, the patient needs to have exactly the same protocol, preferably administered by the same testing team to minimize variation.

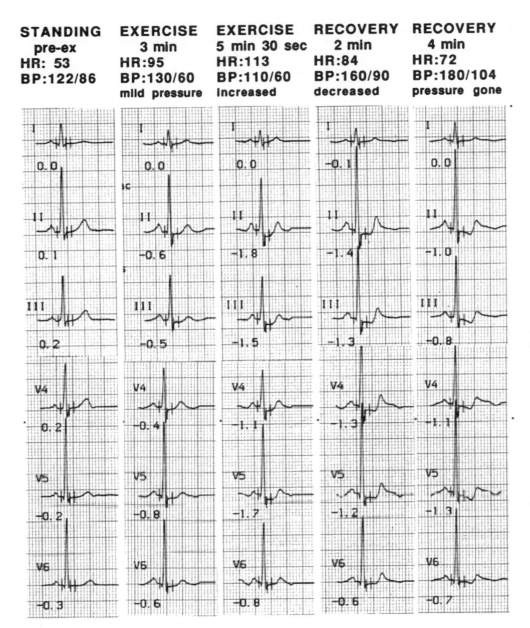

STANDING	EXERCISE	EXERCISE	RECOVERY	RECOVERY
pre-ex	3 min	5 min 30 sec	2 min	4 min
HR: 53	HR:95	HR:113	HR:84	HR:72
BP:122/86	BP:130/60	BP:110/60	BP:160/90	BP:180/104
	mild pressure	Increased	decreased	pressure gone

FIGURE 32–13 Electrocardiographic changes of ischemia during exercise testing in a 71-year-old man with exertional chest pain: progressive ST segment depression with upsloping contour is noted during exercise. The ST depression becomes horizontal during recovery with partial T wave inversion. (Courtesy of David Blood, M.D.)

Other Cardiac Stress Testing Techniques

Recently there have been numerous additions made to the procedures available for cardiac stress testing. Alternative techniques for applying cardiac stress permit the cardiac stress testing of disabled or debilitated persons as well as overcoming anxiety or poor patient effort. Newer techniques for detecting cardiac ischemia have the benefit of allowing testing in patients who previously had obstacles to assessment, such as left bundle branch block, and atypical standard ECG tests.

ECHOCARDIOGRAPHIC STRESS TESTING. Exercise echocardiography has become one of the more commonly used techniques in exercise testing. There are three basic assumptions that underlie the use of echocardiography in stress testing: (1) induction of ischemia will result in an area of left ventricular dyssynergia; (2) these regional wall motion abnormalities are specific for ischemia; (3) changes in wall motion can be accurately seen on two-dimensional echocardiography[76] (Fig. 32–14). The evidence for the first two assumptions has been long-standing, and the improvement in technique and the addition of digital echocardiography have now also made the third assumption true.[27] The exercise can be performed either on a treadmill or with a bicycle ergometer. The use of treadmill testing is limited to scanning before and after exercise, while the bicycle allows for continuous monitoring and the detection of transient ischemic changes.[24, 41] Exercise echocardiography with newer techniques and digital imaging has a diagnostic sensitivity of about 74% to 97% and specificity on the

TABLE 32–9   Examples of Some Age-Adjusted Normal Fitness Levels

Study	Predicted MET	Age Range (yr) (Mean)	Protocol
Bruce	13.7 − 0.08 (age)	NA (44.4)	Bruce
Wolthius	13 − 0.05 (age)	25–54 (37)	Balke-Ware
Morris (<54 yr old)	18.8 − 0.17 (age)	21–53 (42)	USAFSAM
Morris	18.1 − 0.17 (age)	21–89 (57)	USAFSAM
Dehn	16.2 − 0.11 (age)	40–72 (52.2)	Mixed
Froelicher	13.1 − 0.08 (age)	20–53 (NA)	Balke-Ware

Abbreviations: USAFSAM, United States Air Force School of Aerospace Medicine; NA, not applicable.

Adapted from Froelicher VF: Exercise and the Heart. St Louis, Mosby–Year Book, 1987.

order of 64% to 100%. This compares favorably with the results of stress ECG.[76] The test is particularly useful in situations in which the stress ECG is ambiguous or nondiagnostic, in women (who have a higher likelihood of a false-positive ECG test), and in those with abnormalities on their resting ECG.

NUCLEAR STRESS TESTING. Thallium 201 perfusion scintigraphy is a widely accepted modality for the detection of ischemia in CAD. It has been proved to be more accurate than the use of stress echocardiography alone.[42, 73] The imaging is typically performed in conjunction with a treadmill test.[55] It is also used with dipyridamole and adenosine pharmacological stress testing.[35, 52] Comparisons between the findings on ECG, radionuclide ventriculography, and thallium 201 scanning during exercise with a treadmill and on a bicycle ergometer have demonstrated that the diagnosis with scintigraphy is more accurate than when done by ECG alone.[7, 10]

The physiological basis behind the use of thallium 201 scintigraphy is the uptake of thallium 201 in the cardiac myocyte via the Na^+, K^+-ATPase pump. The first-pass extraction of thallium 201 from the blood is 85%, and it is continuously exchanged.[86] This means that images taken early and late after injection provide different pathophysiological data: immediate images give information about regional myocardial blood flow, while delayed images (2 to 24 hours) show distribution of the potassium pool and thus myocardial viability[12(pp 276–311)] (Fig. 32–15). Thallium 201 testing offers the advantages of the ability to image all patients regardless of habitus and can often be done in patients in whom echocardiography cannot be performed. It also can be used in both exercise and pharmacological testing. The disadvantages to thallium 201 testing lie with the test's being invasive, with the injection of a radioactive agent with a long half-life, and with the need for expensive and complex imaging equipment.[93]

Comparisons between the findings on ECG, radionuclide ventriculography, and thallium 201 scanning during exercise on a treadmill and on a bicycle ergometer have demonstrated that the diagnosis with scintigraphy is more accurate than that done by ECG alone.[7, 10] Because of the poor sensitivity of ECG recording alone with upper extremity ergometry, the test is usually performed with thallium 201 scintigraphy.[4, 5]

PHARMACOLOGICAL STRESS TESTING. Among the most common and perhaps the best types of diagnostic stress testing available for the disabled are the pharmacological stress tests. Although their usefulness for functional evaluation for exercise prescription for rehabilitation programs is questionable, they can be used for diagnosis of CAD and for risk stratification. The earliest tests used dipyridamole, but in recent years other agents have been tested and have gained acceptance. The main advantage of the use of these agents for cardiac stress testing is that a patient can be tested regardless of ability to perform adequate levels of exercise. The usual protocols call for simultaneous use of a form of cardiac imaging and follow distinct protocols.

Dipyridamole has been well studied as a pharmacological agent to induce cardiac stress, most often when used in conjunction with thallium 201 scintigraphy.[1, 52] It has been used for detection of CAD, cardiac risk stratification, and perioperative risk evaluation. There have been proposed protocols for the use of thallium 201 scintigraphy with dipyridamole and the simultaneous application of isometric hand grip or low-level exercise to increase the accuracy of those tests.[13, 17] The mechanism of action of dipyridamole is via its activity as a coronary artery vasodilator, especially of the smaller arterioles.[26] The development of ischemia in the cardiac vessels results from differential vasodilation of the cardiac arteries and arterioles. Dipyridamole causes normal vessels to dilate, causing a decrease in the vascular resistance of the coronary bed with a subsequent increase in coronary blood flow. In areas of significant CAD, the distal vessels already have a degree of vasodilation. Normal coronaries dilate, but the diseased vascular beds do not

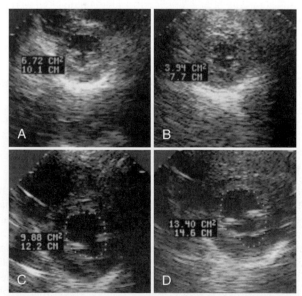

FIGURE 32–14 Echocardiographic changes of ischemia during exercise. *A,* End-systolic size of normal left ventricle at rest. *B,* Note smaller end-systolic size of the same heart during exercise. *C,* Resting end-systolic size of left ventricle of patient with coronary artery disease. *D,* Note increase in end-systolic size of ischemic ventricle during exercise. (Courtesy of ECHO Dx, Inc.)

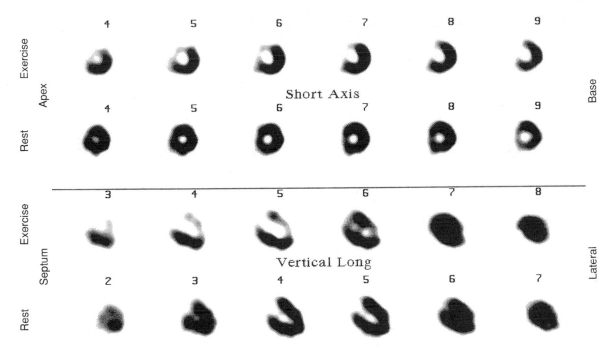

FIGURE 32–15 Exercise and redistribution myocardial perfusion SPECT scans using thallium 201: diminished thallium uptake in the septum, anterior wall, and apex of the left ventricle is seen after exercise injection of thallium 201. The thallium uptake normalizes at rest (redistribution), reflecting exercise-induced ischemia in the distribution of the left anterior descending artery. (Courtesy of David Blood, M.D.)

have the capacity to further dilate. This phenomenon is described as cardiac steal. A typical dipyridamole protocol is shown in Table 32–10. The dosage of dipyridamole in this protocol increases blood flow by three to five times the resting level. Continuous ECG and BP monitoring is done during the procedure. Initial imaging is done at 12 to 35 min followed by delayed imaging at 180 to 240 min[36] (Fig. 32 16).

The use of echocardiography with dipyridamole stress testing is gaining popularity. The same basic instructions pertain to the performance of the test, but since the sensitivity of the test with the standard dose of dipyridamole was inadequate, a "high-dose" protocol for the administration of dipyridamole was developed to increase the sensitivity.[56, 70] A positive test is one in which areas of transient asynergy arise or worsen from baseline on the echocardiogram.

Adenosine is a powerful vasodilator and causes its effects via two types of receptors in blood vessels: a vascular smooth muscle receptor and an endothelial cell receptor.[6] Dipyridamole and adenosine work similarly in the cardiac circulation and their effects are similar. The major advantage of adenosine via intravenous (IV) administration is that it has a rapid onset of action and a brief half-life of 10 to 30 sec. This short duration of action allows for repeated measurements, an advantage over dipyridamole. Adenosine raises coronary blood flow by a factor of 4.4 times, to near the maximum coronary blood flow reserve.

The mechanism of action of *dobutamine,* a synthetic catecholamine, is via the β_1-, β_2-, and α_1-adrenergic receptors. Dobutamine has strong β_1, moderate β_2, and mild α_1 stimulation.[75, 81] In the heart, β_1 stimulation leads to increased inotropy and chronotropy while α_1 stimulation causes only a mild increase in inotropy, and β_2 stimulation yields moderate coronary vasodilation. As a result, IV dobutamine causes increased SV and CO, increasing the RPP. Dobutamine also increases SV and ejection fraction, resulting in decreased end-systolic volume, decreasing wall stress and $M\dot{V}O_2$. BP usually remains relatively constant with dobutamine infusion, as β_2 stimulation decreases systemic vascular resistance and sympathetic tone decreases owing to the increased CO. The rationale for the use of dobutamine as a pharmacological stressor lies in its ability to elevate the RPP by raising both inotropy and chronotropy. Dobutamine has been shown to be relatively safe in patients with CAD, even in the perimyocardial infarction period.[20, 90]

The final determination of the best agent to test any

TABLE 32–10 Sample Dipyridamole Protocol

THALLIUM 201 IMAGING

0.142 mg/kg/min infusion intravenously over 4 min (0.568 mg/kg total dose)

Thallium imaging performed at 10 min, 4 hr, and, depending on protocol, 12–24 hr

Isometric hand grip exercises may be performed simultaneously with the infusion

Continuous ECG and vital sign monitoring is done throughout the test

ECHOCARDIOGRAPHY

High-dose protocol may be followed

0.142 mg/kg/min infusion intravenously over 4 min (0.568 mg/kg total dose), followed by 4 min of no infusion, followed by 0.142 mg/kg/min infusion intravenously over 2 min (0.282 mg/kg supplemental dose) for a total of 0.850 mg/kg over 10 min

2-Dimensional echocardiography is performed continuously throughout the infusion and for 10 min after the infusion is completed

Continuous ECG and vital sign monitoring is done throughout the test

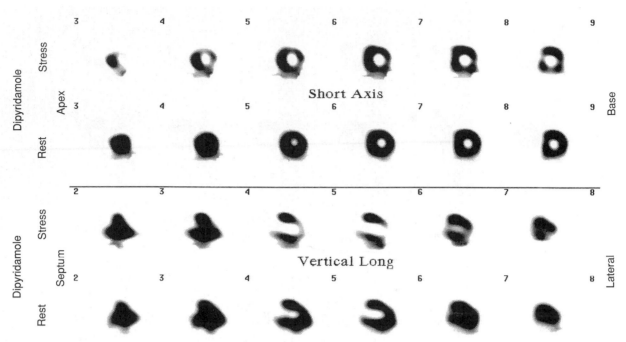

FIGURE 32–16 Pharmacological stress and redistribution myocardial perfusion SPECT scans using thallium 201: diminished thallium uptake in the anterolateral wall and apex of the left ventricle after injection of thallium 201 during dipyridamole coronary vasodilatation (stress). The thallium uptake normalizes at rest (redistribution). These findings reflect severe stenosis of a large diagonal branch of the left anterior descending artery. (Courtesy of David Blood, M.D.)

given patient still must be decided on a case-by-case basis. All of the various agents described previously have their advantages and offer the ability to test the severely disabled or deconditioned patient who might be encountered in a physiatric practice.

ISOMETRIC HAND GRIP TEST. This test uses the isometric contraction of the upper extremity with a dynamometer to provide the exercise stress. Usually, the test is performed with the patient squeezing the dynamometer at one fourth to three fourths of maximum hand strength for as long as he or she can tolerate.[25] The isometric exercise increases the RPP by increasing both HR and BP. The ejection fraction does not normally change, and some studies show that a decline of 5% in the ejection fraction can occur in some patients.[13, 69] This variation in the ejection fraction response means that some of the major imaging studies used to assess the heart for ischemia are of limited use after this type of cardiac stress, limiting its utility. In addition, since this technique does not provoke ischemia as effectively as some of the other available tests, it should be used only in selected cases.[49]

Modifications for the Physically Disabled

Exercise tolerance testing for the physically disabled is especially challenging because of the restrictions created by weakness, limb availability, balance problems, and spasticity. Echocardiographic and nuclear testing increase the sensitivity of testing performed on various exercise devices, partially compensating for the reduced workloads achieved. Devices which have been used successfully include the arm crank ergometer, an adapted Schwinn Airdyne (Fig. 32–17),[11, 50] a supine bicycle ergometer (Fig. 32–18),[58] and a wheelchair ergometer (Fig. 32–19).[33]

Assessment of Cardiac Demands of Activities

Direct assessment of the cardiac demands of various activities is technically difficult. The use of the RPP or HR gives a reasonable estimate of the relative stress on the coronary circulation by correlation with $M\dot{V}O_2$, and these numbers can be used in conjunction with the patient's ETT to judge the safety of the activity in relation to the anginal threshold. The information obtained in this manner is highly individualized but can be difficult to obtain during functional activities. The usual way around this problem is the use of tables of metabolic demands of various self-care, mobility, vocational, and avocational activities[34] (Table 32–11). These tables usually express the metabolic demands of the activities in METs (1 MET = approximately 3.5 mL O_2/kg body weight/min).

The rationale for using these tables for cardiac patients is the linear relationship between the $M\dot{V}O_2$ and the $\dot{V}O_2$, as noted above. However, the fallacy which occurs in the blind use of the tables comes from ignoring the fact that the linear relationship only holds true for a single activity performed at varying intensities under the same conditions. Knowing the MET level achieved safely on a treadmill ETT tells the clinician very little about the MET level that might be achieved during activities by the upper extremities without crossing the anginal threshold. A treadmill test cannot be used to evaluate a subject who must perform at a high MET level with the upper extremities (e.g., a carpenter). The $M\dot{V}O_2$ will also be higher for any given activity if performed under conditions of emotional or physiological stress, even though the MET level is unchanged. Although the MET tables give useful information about the relative metabolic demands of various activities, the clinician must

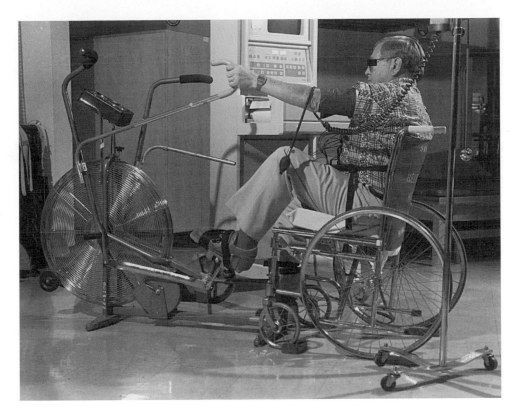

FIGURE 32–17 Exercise tolerance testing with an adapted Airdyne bicycle ergometer (Schwinn).

use them with great caution and an awareness of the physiological limitations involved.

CARDIAC REHABILITATION PROGRAMS

Risk Factor Modification

In addition to exercise training, all cardiac rehabilitation programs should emphasize patient and family education for risk factor reduction and lifestyle modification. Although in the past the goal of this part of the program was to slow the progression of the disease, recent reports by Ornish et al.,[64] with a very low fat vegetarian diet, and by Hambrecht et al.,[39] with a more vigorous exercise program

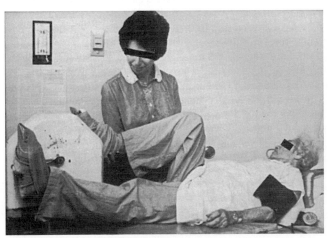

FIGURE 32–18 Exercise tolerance testing with a supine bicycle ergometer.

and less severe fat restriction, have actually shown regression of stenotic lesions. Both of these studies had control groups which had progression of the stenoses.

Smoking cessation is essential. Elevated BP should be normalized. Elevated blood lipids should be lowered, preferably by means of dietary modification. Although reduction of dietary fat from the average of 37% of caloric intake to 30% is estimated to have only limited benefit in terms of life expectancy,[14] more significant fat reduction does have clear benefit.[64] The Ornish diet consists of only 10% of caloric intake as fat. While this might not be palatable to many Americans, further studies on diets consisting of 10% to 30% intake as fat could help to find a more generally acceptable compromise.

Stress management has been recognized as an important component of these programs since Friedman first described the type A behavior pattern. In later refinements of his diagnostic criteria, he has emphasized impatience and free-floating hostility as the key elements of this behavior pattern, not ambition and competitive drive. He reports that counseling directed toward these behavior patterns can produce a significant reduction in coronary morbidity and mortality.[30] The Ornish program includes the following stress management techniques: stretching exercises, breathing techniques, meditation, progressive relaxation, and imagery.[64] A similar approach is used in Kabat-Zinn's Stress Reduction Clinic at the University of Massachusetts Medical Center.[44]

In addition to eliminating the usual medical risk factors such as smoking, hypertension, and physical inactivity, a comprehensive lifestyle modification program should provide dietary guidance for a significant reduction in dietary fat and a stress management program with ongoing individual and group counseling. The material must be presented

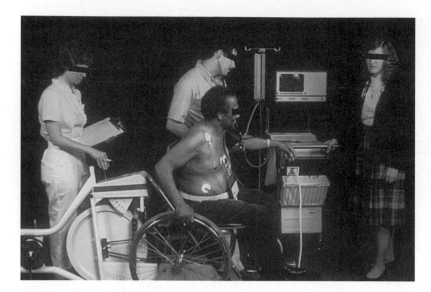

FIGURE 32–19 Exercise tolerance testing with a wheelchair ergometer. (Courtesy of Majorie King, M.D.)

in a format suitable for the patient's learning style, and material must be repeated as necessary until the patient gains mastery of the techniques. It must be remembered that these patients are under a great deal of stress related to their medical illnesses and should not be expected to assimilate major lifestyle recommendations with a single series of lectures or brochures. The material should be reviewed during the different stages of the rehabilitation programs described below.

Primary Prevention Programs

Programs designed to intervene before the clinical onset of CAD have the greatest opportunity for producing major alterations in the natural history of the disease. The program should consist of identification and modification of risk factors, dietary counseling, stress management training, and instruction in a sustainable exercise regimen. Evaluation of the long-term benefits of such a program is difficult owing to the self-selection process typically involved in entering and maintaining such a program. Based on the results reported by Paffenbarger,[66] Hambrecht,[39] and Ornish[64] and their co-workers, it would seem reasonable to expect significant benefit from the application of the same principles in this setting with little risk of harm.

TABLE 32–11   A Typical MET Table

Activity	MET
Lying quietly	1.0
Sitting at ease	1.2–1.6
Sitting writing	1.9–2.2
Standing at ease	1.4–2.0
Walking 1 mph	2.3
Standing, washing and shaving	2.5–2.6
Standing, dressing and undressing	2.3–3.3
Light housework	1.7–3.0
Heavy housework	3.0–6.0
Office work	1.3–2.5
Walking 2 mph	3.1
Light industrial work	2.0–5.0
Walking 3 mph	4.3

Rehabilitation Following Myocardial Infarction

The rehabilitation program following MI is the classic model for cardiac rehabilitation. It can be divided into four phases: (1) the acute in-hospital phase beginning in the cardiac care unit (CCU); (2) the convalescent phase continuing the program at home until a strong scar has formed on the damaged myocardium; (3) the training phase, where aerobic conditioning is used to increase the patient's physical work capacity; and (4) the maintenance phase, where the gains achieved by training are sustained by regular exercise. Patient education aimed at risk factor reduction and lifestyle modification is included during each of these phases.

ACUTE PHASE.   Early mobilization of the patient with an acute MI was introduced by Wenger.[88] Rather than the traditional 4 to 6 weeks of bed rest after acute MI (longer in some countries), this program takes the patient from bed rest in the CCU to climbing two flights of stairs in 14 days. There is a gradual daily increase in exercise intensity which progresses as long as there are no arrhythmias, congestive failure, or ischemia. Patients are monitored with ECG telemetry during each increase in exercise level. The schedule obviously has to be altered if complications occur. A Swiss study compared outcomes of two groups of patients, one mobilized early with a modified Wenger program, and the other managed with the then-accepted 6 months of rest.[8] At the end of 1 year there was no difference in mortality and morbidity between the two groups. Although there was no difference in physical work capacity between the two groups there was a significantly higher return-to-work rate in the group of patients who were mobilized early. The authors' suggestion that the difference was mostly due to an improved psychological adjustment was confirmed by later studies. A typical early mobilization protocol is outlined in Table 32–12. The goals of this phase are to progress the patient gradually and safely from the initial bed rest of the CCU to a level consistent with most activities of daily living. By mobilizing the patient early, deconditioning from excessive bed rest and psychological invalidism are reduced or eliminated. Actual exercise train-

TABLE 32–12   Summary of Wenger Early Mobilization Program

Step   1—Passive range of motion (ROM), active ankle exercise; self-feeding, orientation to program.
Step   2—Same exercise; legs dangling at side of bed.
Step   3—Active assisted ROM; sitting in chair, bedside commode; more detailed explanation of program; light recreation.
Step   4—Minimal resistance; increase sitting time; patient education; light craft activities.
Step   5—Moderate resistance; unlimited sitting, sitting for meals, seated ADL activities; continued patient education.
Step   6—Increase resistance, walking to bathroom; standing ADL; group meetings up to 1 hr.
Step   7—Standing warmup exercises, walking 100 ft at comfortable pace; tub bath; walking to group meetings.
Step   8—Increase active standing exercise, increase ambulation, walk down stairs (take elevator up); continue education program.
Step   9—Increase exercise program; review energy-conservation and pacing techniques.
Step 10—Increase exercises with light weights and increase walking distance; increase craft activities; discuss home exercise program.
Step 11—Increase duration of each activity.
Step 12—Increase walking down stairs to 2 flights; increase resistance used in exercises.
Step 13—Continue same activities.
Step 14—Walk up 1 flight of stairs and down; complete instructions for home exercise program and pacing of activities.

ing for a higher work capacity is not a goal of this phase. Educational programs for risk factor modification should be introduced at this time.

CONVALESCENT PHASE.   During the convalescent phase the goal is to maintain early mobilization and gradually increase the endurance for exercise at the same intensity used at the end of the acute phase program. This is usually walking or bicycling using a target HR taught at the end of the acute phase and known to be within the patient's safe capacity. In an uncomplicated case, this phase lasts for about 6 weeks from the time of the infarction. This allows time for a firm scar to form on the infarcted area, thereby reducing the risk of ventricular aneurysm or wall rupture.

TRAINING PHASE.   This is the actual exercise training program which most people associate with cardiac rehabilitation. It begins with a symptom-limited ETT. The test screens out patients with contraindications for exercise training, such as dangerous arrhythmias or a drop in BP with increasing exercise intensity. The results of this test are used to determine a target HR for exercise training. If the maximum HR achieved on the ETT is limited only by a relatively benign endpoint such as fatigue, musculoskeletal pain, or angina preceding ECG changes, then a target HR as high as 85% of the maximum HR can be used. If the endpoint is a serious arrhythmia or ECG changes without chest pain, then a lower target HR should be chosen. Target HRs as low as 60% of maximum can result in effective training. It is critical for patient safety that target HRs in this population be based on actual ETTs, not tables or equations estimating maximum rates from the patient's age. Monitoring with ECG telemetry is usually used with each upgrading of the exercise prescription, but continuous monitoring is not necessary for each session. The patient can

be taught to monitor HR (using the carotid pulse) or to use the Borg scale (Table 32–13).

As noted above, the improvements in the cardiac response to exercise that result from aerobic training only occur when muscles that were involved with the training are used. It is necessary to individualize each patient's program to include the muscle groups necessary for vocational and avocational goals. A generic treadmill or bicycle exercise program cannot meet everyone's needs.

The usual training program calls for three sessions a week for 6 to 8 weeks. Each session should start with a stretching program, followed by the aerobic program, which can use equipment such as treadmills, upper or lower extremity ergometers, Airdynes, rowing machines, walking, running, and calisthenics. Each exercise should have a warmup period, a training period at target HR, and a cooldown period.

MAINTENANCE PHASE.   The maintenance phase is probably the most important phase of all, because if it is neglected, the benefits of the training phase are lost within a few weeks. This part of the program needs to be addressed before the patient starts training, and a commitment to continue with the maintenance program must be obtained from the patient in order to justify the time and expense of the training program. The actual exercises included should reflect the selection of muscles trained in the preceding period and should fit within the interests and lifestyle of the individual patient. Exercise at least twice a week and preferably three times a week for at least 30 min should be considered a minimum requirement. ECG monitoring is not necessary during this phase.

Rehabilitation of the Patient With Angina Pectoris

Rehabilitation of the patient with stable angina can begin once the medical regimen has been optimized. As explained above (see Fig. 32–12), an aerobic training program results in an improved work capacity for these patients, even though there is no effect on the anginal threshold. An educational program for risk factor modification should be an integral part of the overall program. The exercise program begins with the ETT and then progresses with the training and maintenance programs as outlined above for the post-MI patient.

TABLE 32–13   The Borg Scale of Perceived Exertion

Score	Perceived Exertion
6	
7	Very very light
8	
9	Very light
10	
11	Fairly light
12	
13	Somewhat hard
14	
15	Hard
16	
17	Very hard
18	
19	Very very hard
20	

Rehabilitation Following Bypass Surgery

In the post–bypass surgery patient, cardiac rehabilitation can provide benefit by several mechanisms[43] (Table 32–14). Since patients who have just undergone CABG usually have not had a recent MI and have just been revascularized, they make excellent candidates for cardiac rehabilitation.[89] Complicating issues to remember in the post-CABG patient include the fact that the patient may have incomplete revascularization. With recent advances in surgical technique, there are now many patients with low ejection fractions who are undergoing the procedure. This means that the rehabilitation program must be individualized to each patient's needs. A symptom-limited ETT can be safely performed at 3 to 4 weeks after surgery to determine the level of exercise that a patient can tolerate.[23, 71, 84]

Cardiac rehabilitation after CABG can be thought of in two phases: the immediate postoperative period, and the later maintenance phase. The in-hospital first phase is usually in the first week or so postoperatively, as patients are typically sent home after that period of time. The initial period can be thought of in three stages: (1) intensive mobilization in the immediate postoperative period; (2) progressive ambulation and daily exercises; (3) discharge planning and exercise prescription for the maintenance stage.[43] Mobilization in the intensive care unit on postoperative day (POD) 1 includes sitting upright, active leg exercises, and mobilization out of bed. Only an unstable postoperative course or severe CHF should interfere with this early mobilization. This aggressive early intervention has several benefits, including decreasing the deleterious effects of bed rest such as deep venous thrombosis (DVT), pulmonary embolus (PE), pulmonary complications, and cardiac deconditioning.

The POD 2 to 5 program should include progressive ambulation and daily exercise. Initially, ambulation with supervision for distances of 150 to 200 feet is followed by gradually progressive ambulation until most patients are starting independent ambulation by POD 3. Monitoring with ECG telemetry is usually used during the early mobilization. In the last few days prior to discharge, the patient and physicians should develop a program that can be self-monitored at home and which allows for gradual progression to previous levels of activity.

The second stage of a program for the post-CABG patient is conducted at home for the usual patient, or in an inpatient rehabilitation center for the high-risk patient or those who need more intensive interventions and monitoring.

Each patient can be in one of three types of programs: low, moderate, or high intensity. A low-intensity program

TABLE 32–14   Benefits of Cardiac Rehabilitation After Bypass Surgery

Increased ischemic threshold
Improved left ventricular function
Increased coronary collaterals
Ameliorated serum lipids
Decreased serum catecholamines
Decreased platelet aggregation and increased fibrinolysis
Improved psychological status

is a progressive walking program with energy expenditures in the area of 2 to 4 METs, and a target HR of 65% to 75% of maximum HR. A moderate-intensity program is a progressive walk to walk-jog program from 3.0 to 6.5 METs, with target HR 70% to 80% of maximum HR. A high-intensity program is a progression from walk-jog to jogging from 5.0 to 8.5 METs, with a target HR of 75% to 85% of maximum HR. For a patient on a β-blocker the target HR is set at 20 beats per minute above the resting HR. The assignment of patients to a level of exercise is determined by both objective criteria and patient observation in the postoperative period. A submaximum stress test before discharge is an important way to evaluate physiological response to submaximum effort.[43] The inpatient program has to be tailored to the specific needs of the patient and is best designed in cooperation with the patient's cardiologist.

Rehabilitation Following Cardiac Transplantation

As the techniques of cardiac transplantation have improved, the number of patients receiving transplants has increased. Five- and 10-year survival rates are now 82% and 74%, respectively.[40] Typically, cardiac transplant patients are middle-aged, have suffered from months of preoperative invalidism, have generalized muscle weakness, and suffer from depression and anxiety. The transplant itself usually resolves the cardiac disability, but a comprehensive approach to the patient is necessary. The physiology of the post-transplant patient is somewhat different from that of the post-CABG patient. Because of the loss of vagal inhibition to the sinoatrial node, the resting HR of the denervated heart is usually near 100 beats per minute.[21] The resting tachycardia implies a small SV, and therefore, in response to light exercise, CO can be increased via the Frank-Starling mechanism. With increased exercise, the circulating catecholamine-induced chronotropic and inotropic responses increase CO.[16, 92] These patients have a blunted HR response to an incremental exercise test, with peak HRs 20% to 25% lower than those seen in age-matched controls. Resting hypertension, thought to be due to the renal effects of cyclosporine, is common.[79]

Owing to the lack of activity and the use of high-dose steroids in the perioperative period, transplant recipients usually have a 10% to 50% loss of lean body mass. This means that maximum work output and $\dot{V}O_2$max are reduced to about two thirds that of the age-matched population.[48] At submaximum exercise levels, perceived exertion, minute ventilation, and the ventilatory equivalent for oxygen are all higher than in normal persons, while $\dot{V}O_2$ is the same, implying earlier onset of anaerobic metabolism. At maximum effort transplant patients demonstrate lower work capacity, CO, HR, systolic BP, and $\dot{V}O_2$. In performing exercise testing it is important to note that the donor denervated heart cannot demonstrate ischemia through anginal pain and that dyspnea, faintness, and ECG changes are to be followed. Initially, heart transplant patients have no ECG abnormalities, but in long-standing transplants, accelerated atherosclerosis can develop and lead to cardiac ischemia.

The cardiac training regimen in transplant patients

should address their overall conditioning as well as their cardiac function. Walking, jogging, cycling, and swimming are common exercises used in the program for transplant patients. In the initial postoperative period, sitting upright, lower extremity exercises, and mobilization from the bed are encouraged. The patient is then encouraged to start ambulating, as with the post-CABG patient. At the time of discharge, after the patient has learned self-monitoring, the patient is encouraged to increase ambulation to 1 mile. The program then consists of progressively increasing distances for ambulation, with the pace designed to be at a level of 60% to 70% of peak effort for 30 to 60 min three to five times weekly.[46] The level of perceived effort, using the Borg scale (see Table 32–13), should be maintained at 13 to 14, with the level of activity increasing incrementally to stay at this level.

Other important aspects of the rehabilitation of cardiac transplant patients include the complicated medical regimen and psychological needs. Patients often also need vocational rehabilitation before being able to resume work, and a program of exercises to address generalized weakness may need to be prescribed.

The outcomes of rehabilitation in the cardiac transplant population have been generally favorable. The usual reports are of increased work output and improved exercise tolerance.[48] Some transplant patients can even resume competitive-level athletics.[47] In areas of general well-being and quality of life, a recent survey of patients after transplant demonstrated that post-transplant patients reported a quality of life on the level of cardiac arrest survivors and post-MI patients: less than that of normals, but better than that of low back pain patients. There were also significant musculoskeletal and neurological complaints (weakness, fatigue, low back pain) in this group of patients.[74] It is also hoped that the use of an exercise conditioning program, in combination with reduction of other cardiac risk factors, will help prevent the accelerated atherosclerosis which can follow transplantation.

Rehabilitation of the Patient With Cardiomyopathy

With increasingly aggressive cardiac care, the number of patients with a left ventricular ejection fraction of less than 30% has increased, and this group represents one of the fastest-growing subsets of the cardiac rehabilitation population.[67] These patients have different complications and expectations than the post-CABG or post-MI population owing to the fact that they have poor left ventricular function. They are at higher risk of sudden death and often are emotionally depressed because of their chronic cardiac disability.[19, 45, 65] Patients with heart failure demonstrate inconsistent responses to exercise.[80] Limited exercise capacity is one of the earliest findings in heart failure. The hemodynamic alterations seen with exercise do not always correlate with the overall exercise capacity.[54] The normal response to exercise is often absent. Exercise in heart failure can cause a drop in ejection fraction, a decrease in SV, and exertional hypotension, and in the worst cases, CO might not be increased sufficiently to generate a dynamic exercise response.

Low endurance and fatigue are also problems encoun-

tered with this population of patients, and after achieving a high aerobic workload, they often experience fatigue for hours to days after the session.[22] In addition, there can be concomitant factors such as atrial fibrillation, fluid overload, or medication noncompliance which decrease exercise tolerance. Despite these problems, there is documented benefit from exercise in this patient population.[22, 77] A gradual program of increasing the HR above resting level can be safe and increases oxygen extraction efficiency. Patients who have participated in cardiac rehabilitation programs have lower HRs during submaximum exercise, and increased maximum workloads.[51] The return to the ability to sustain activity at a low MET level can mean the difference between independent living and dependency.

The evaluation of the CHF patient consists of a graded ETT and can include measurements of left ventricular ejection fraction by multiple gated acquisition scanning (MUGA) or echocardiography during exercise. Unstable angina, decompensated CHF, and unstable arrhythmias are contraindications to cardiac rehabilitation. In the design of the rehabilitation program, certain aspects specific to the failure patient need to be kept in mind. Prolonged warmups and cooldowns are appropriate since these patients can increase the duration of exercise but are unable to tolerate more than a limited workload. Dynamic exercise is preferable to isometrics, and the target HR should be 10 beats per minute below any significant endpoint, such as exertional hypotension, significant dyspnea, or sustained arrhythmia seen in the pretraining exercise test.[68] The exercise program is best done initially under supervision, at least until the patient is able to self-monitor and prevent complications during exercise. Patients with severe left ventricular dysfunction will need telemetry during warmup, exercise, and cooldown. The clinical status and progress can be monitored with body weight, BP, and HR response to exercise.

CARDIAC ARRHYTHMIAS. The risk of death from cardiac arrhythmia during rehabilitation exercises is very low. From 1980 to 1984, one cardiac arrest per 112,000 patient-hours of cardiac rehabilitation was reported.[83] This means that it might be prudent to continually monitor only those patients who are at high risk (Table 32–15). For those patients with life-threatening arrhythmias, the automatic implantable cardiac defibrillator (AICD) has become much more common.[91] The modifications to the cardiac rehabilitation program in these patients are few. The AICD devices are rate-sensitive, so it is essential to ensure during the exercise stress test that this rate is not exceeded and that the HR achieved with exercise does not exceed this threshold. The support and reassurance that can be given to these patients during an exercise program is important, as anxiety of arrhythmia is a significant concern.[72]

Rehabilitation of the Patient With Valvular Heart Disease

In patients with valvular heart disease, the major problem is often deconditioning and CHF, as in the transplant population. The management of the valvular heart disease patient in CHF is essentially as outlined in the section on CHF. After surgical correction, the patient improves in cardiac fitness as measured by improved $\dot{V}O_2$.[60] Training can increase physical work capacity by 60% and decrease

TABLE 32–15 Patients at High Risk During Cardiac Rehabilitation

RISK OF ISCHEMIA

Postoperative angina
Left ventricular ejection fraction <35%
NYHA grade III or IV congestive heart failure
Ventricular tachycardia or fibrillation in the postoperative period
Systolic BP drop of 10 points or more with exercise
Excessive ventricular ectopy with exercise
Incapable of self-monitoring
Myocardial ischemia with exercise

RISK OF ARRHYTHMIA

Acute infarction within 6 wk
Active ischemia
Significant left ventricular dysfunction (LVEF <30%)
History of sustained ventricular tachycardia
History of sustained life-threatening supraventricular arrhythmia
History of sudden death, not yet stabilized on medical therapy
Initial therapy of patients with automatic implantable cardioverter defibrillator
Initial therapy of a patient with rate-adaptive cardiac pacemaker

Abbreviations: BP, blood pressure; LVEF, left ventricular ejection fraction.

perceived exertion and the RPP by 15%.[78] A complicating feature in these patients is the fact that many of them are on anticoagulation postoperatively and need to be on low-impact exercises to avoid hemarthroses and bruising. They also need special education to avoid injury.[67] The training program is similar to that followed for the post-CABG patient.

Modifications for the Physically Disabled

Little attention has been paid to the problem of cardiac rehabilitation programs for the physically disabled. The risk factor modification programs are easily adapted for any patient population. The exercise training can be accomplished with the same adapted equipment described above for modified exercise testing. The same training principles can be applied. This is an area where physiatrists can take a leadership role, as most existing programs are limited in the ability to compensate for physical handicaps.

References

1. Albro PC, Gould KL, Westcott RJ, et al: Noninvasive assessment of coronary stenoses by myocardial imaging during pharmacologic vasodilation. III. Clinical trial. Am J Cardiol 1978; 42:751.
2. Åstrand P-O, Ekblom B, Messin R, et al: Intra-arterial blood pressure during exercise with different muscle groups. J Appl Physiol 1965; 20:253.
3. Åstrand P-O, Rodahl K: Textbook of Work Physiology, ed 3. New York, McGraw-Hill, 1986.
4. Balady GJ, Weiner DA, McCabe CH, et al: Value of arm exercise testing in detecting coronary artery disease. Am J Cardiol 1985; 55:37.
5. Balady GJ, Weiner DA, Rothendler JA, et al: Arm exercise thallium imaging testing for the detection of coronary artery disease. J Am Coll Cardiol 1987; 9:84.
6. Belardinelli L, Linden J, Berne RM: The cardiac effects of adenosine. Prog Cardiovasc Dis 1989; 32:73–97.
7. Beller GA, Gibson RS: Sensitivity, specificity, and prognostic significance of non-invasive testing for occult or known coronary disease. Prog Cardiovasc Dis 1987; 29:241.
8. Bloch A, Maeder JP, Haissly JC, et al: Early mobilization after myocardial infarction. A controlled study. Am J Cardiol 1974; 34:152–157.
9. Bogaty P, Dagenais GR, Cantin B, et al: Prognosis in patients with a strongly positive exercise electrocardiogram. Am J Cardiol 1989; 64:124.
10. Borer JS, Kent KM, Bacharach SL, et al: Sensitivity, specificity and predictive accuracy of radionuclide cineangiography during exercise in patients with coronary artery disease: Comparison with electrocardiography. Circulation 1979; 60:572.
11. Bostom AG, Bates E, Mazzarella N, et al: Ergometer modification for combined arm-leg use by lower extremity amputees in cardiovascular testing and training. Arch Phys Med Rehabil 1987; 68:244–247.
12. Braunwald E (ed): Heart Disease, a Textbook of Cardiovascular Medicine. Philadelphia, WB Saunders, 1993.
13. Brown BG, Josephson MA, Peterson RB, et al: Intravenous dipyridamole combined with isometric handgrip for near maximal acute increase in coronary flow in patients with coronary artery disease. Am J Cardiol 1981; 48:1077–1085.
14. Browner WS, Westenhouse J: What if Americans ate less fat? JAMA 1991; 265:3285–3291.
15. Bruce RA, Fischer LD, Pettinger M, et al: ST segment elevation with exercise: A marker for poor ventricular function and poor prognosis. Coronary Artery Surgery Study (CASS) confirmation of Seattle Heart Watch results. Circulation 1988; 77:97.
16. Cannom DS, Rider AK, Stinson EB, et al: Electrophysiologic studies in the denervated transplanted human heart. Am J Cardiol 1975; 36:859.
17. Casale PN, Guiney TE, Strauss HW, Boucher CA: Simultaneous low level treadmill exercise and intravenous dipyridamole stress thallium imaging. Am J Cardiol 1988; 62:799–802.
18. Chaitman BR: The changing role of the exercise electrocardiogram as a diagnostic and prognostic test in chronic ischemic heart disease. J Am Coll Cardiol 1986; 8:1195.
19. Christopherson LK: Cardiac transplantation: A psychological perspective. Circulation 1987; 75:57–62.
20. Cillespie TA, Ambos HD, Sobel BE, Roberts R: Effects of dobutamine in patients with acute myocardial infarction. Am J Cardiol 1977; 39:588–594.
21. de Marneffe M, Jacobs P, Haardt R, Englert M: Variations of normal sinus node function in relation to age: Role of autonomic influence. Eur Heart J 1986; 7:662.
22. Dubach P, Froelicher VF: Cardiac rehabilitation for heart failure patients. Cardiology 1989; 76:368–373.
23. Dubach P, Froelicher V, Klein J, et al: Use of the exercise test to predict prognosis after coronary artery bypass grafting. Am J Cardiol 1989; 63:530.
24. Duchak J, Ryan T, Sawada SG, et al: Bicycle stress echocardiography for the detection of coronary artery disease (abstract). J Am Soc Echocardiogr 1990; 3:225.
25. Ellestad MH: Stress Testing, Principles and Practice, ed 3. Philadelphia, FA Davis, 1986.
26. Elliot EC: The effect of Persantine on coronary flow and cardiac dynamics. Can Med Assoc J 1961; 85:469–476.
27. Feigenbaum H: Exercise echocardiography. J Am Soc Echocardiogr 1988; 1:161–166.
28. Flamm SD, Taki J, Moore R, et al: Redistribution of regional and organ blood volume and effect on cardiac function in relation to upright exercise intensity in healthy human subjects. Circulation 1990; 18:1550.
29. Fleg JL, Lakatta EG: Prevalence and significance of post-exercise hypotension in apparently healthy subjects. Am J Cardiol 1986; 63:81.
30. Friedman M: Type A behavior: Its diagnosis, cardiovascular relation and the effect of its modification on recurrence of coronary artery disease. Am J Cardiol 1989; 64:12C–19C.
31. Froelicher VF: Exercise and the Heart. Clinical Concepts. St Louis, Mosby–Year Book, 1987.
32. Froelicher VF, Marcondes GD: Manual of Exercise Testing. St Louis, Mosby–Year Book, 1989.
33. Glaser RM, Sawka MN, Laubach LL, Suryaprasad AG: Metabolic and cardiopulmonary responses to wheelchair and bicycle ergometry. J Appl Physiol 1979; 46:1066–1070.
34. Gonzalez EG, Corcoran PJ: Energy expenditure during ambulation. In Downey JA, Myers SJ, Gonzalez EG, Lieberman JS (eds): The Physiological Basis of Rehabilitation Medicine, ed 2. Boston, Butterworth-Heinemann, 1994.
35. Gould KL: Noninvasive assessment of coronary stenoses by myocardial perfusion imaging during pharmacologic coronary vasodilation.

I. Physiologic basis and experimental vasodilation. Am J Cardiol 1978; 41:267–278.

36. Gould KL, Westcott RJ, Albro PC, Hamilton GW: Noninvasive assessment of coronary stenoses by myocardial imaging during pharmacologic coronary vasodilation. II. Clinical methodology and feasibility. Am J Cardiol 1978; 41:279–287.

37. Graves EJ: 1992 Summary: National Hospital Discharge Survey. Advance data from vital and health statistics; no. 249. Hyattsville, Md, National Center for Health Statistics, 1994.

38. Haines DE, Beller GA, Watson DD, et al: Exercise induced ST segment elevation 2-weeks after uncomplicated myocardial infarction: Contributing factors and prognostic significance. J Am Coll Cardiol 1987; 9:996.

39. Hambrecht R, Niebauer J, Marburger C, et al: Various intensities of leisure time physical activity in patients with coronary artery disease: Effects on cardiorespiratory fitness and progression of coronary atherosclerotic lesions. J Am Coll Cardiol 1993; 22:468–477.

40. Heck CF, Shumway SJ, Kaye MP: The registry of the International Society for Heart Transplantation: Sixth official report 1989. J Heart Transplant 1989; 8:271–276.

41. Heng MK, Simard M, Lake R, Udhoji VH: Exercise two dimensional echocardiography for the diagnosis of coronary artery disease. Am J Cardiol 1984; 54:502–507.

42. Iskandrian AS, Wasserman LA, Anderson GS, et al: Merits of stress thallium-201 myocardial perfusion imaging in patients with inconclusive exercise electrocardiograms: Correlation with coronary arteriograms. Am J Cardiol 1980; 46:553–558.

43. Juneau M, Geneau S, Marchand C, Brosseau R: Cardiac rehabilitation after coronary bypass surgery (review). Cardiovasc Clin 1991; 21:25–42.

44. Kabat-Zinn J: Full Catastrophe Living. New York, Delta, 1990.

45. Kannel WB, Plehn JF, Cupples LA: Cardiac failure and sudden death in the Framingham Study. Am Heart J 1988; 115:869–875.

46. Kavanagh T: Exercise training in patients after heart transplantation. Herz 1991; 16:243–250.

47. Kavanagh T, Yacoub MH, Campbell R, Mertens D: Marathon running after cardiac transplantation: A case history. J Cardiac Rehabil 1986; 6:16–20.

48. Kavanagh T, Yacoub M, Mertens DJ, et al: Cardiorespiratory responses to exercise training after orthotopic cardiac transplantation. Circulation 1988; 77:162–171.

49. Kerber RE, Miller RA, Najjar SM: Myocardial ischemic effects of isometric, dynamic, and combined exercise in coronary artery disease. Chest 1975; 67:388.

50. King ML, Guarracini M, Lennihan L, et al: Adaptive exercise testing for patients with hemiparesis. J Cardiopulmonary Rehabil 1989; 9:237–242.

51. Lee AP, Ice R, Blessey R, et al: Long-term effects of physical training in coronary patients with impaired ventricular function. Circulation 1979; 60:1519.

52. Leppo JA: Dipyridamole thallium-201 imaging: The lazy man's stress test. J Nucl Med 1989; 30:281–287.

53. McCance AJ, Forfar JC: Selective enhancement of the cardiac sympathetic response to exercise by anginal chest pain in humans. Circulation 1989; 80:1642.

54. McKirnan MD, Sullivan M, Jensen D, et al: Treadmill performance and cardiac function in selected patients with coronary heart disease. J Am Coll Cardiol 1984; 3:253–261.

55. Mahmarian JJ, Verani MS: Exercise thallium-201 perfusion scintigraphy in the assessment of coronary artery disease. Am J Cardiol 1991; 67:2D–11D.

56. Margonato A, Chierchia S, Cianflone D, et al: Limitations of dipyridamole echocardiography in effort angina pectoris. Am J Cardiol 1987; 59:225–230.

57. Mark DB, Hlatky MA, Harrel FE, et al: Exercise treadmill score for predicting prognosis in coronary artery disease. Ann Intern Med 1987; 106:793.

58. Moldover JR, Daum MC, Downey JA: Cardiac stress testing of hemiparetic patients with a supine bicycle ergometer: Preliminary study. Arch Phys Med Rehabil 1984; 65:470–473.

59. Moldover JR, Stein J: Cardiopulmonary physiology. In Downey JA, Myers SJ, Gonzalez EG, Lieberman JS (eds): The Physiological Basis of Rehabilitation Medicine, ed 2. Boston, Butterworth-Heinemann, 1994.

60. Newell JP, Kappagoda CT, Stoker JB, et al: Physical training after heart valve replacement. Br Heart J 1980; 44:638–649.

61. Niederberger M, Bruce RA, Kusumi F, Whitkanak S: Disparities in ventilatory and circulatory responses to bicycle and treadmill exercise. Br Heart J 1974; 36:377.

62. Niemeyer MG, van der Wall EE, D'Haene EG, et al: Alternative stress methods for the diagnosis of coronary artery disease. Netherlands J Med 1992; 41:284–294.

63. Okin PM, Klingfeld P: Effect of exercise protocol and lead selection on the accuracy of heart rate adjusted indices of ST-segment depression for the detection of three vessel coronary artery disease. J Electrocardiol 1989; 22:187.

64. Ornish D, Brown SE, Scherwitz LW, et al: Can lifestyle changes reverse coronary artery disease? The Lifestyle Heart Trial. Lancet 1990; 336:129–133.

65. Packer M: Sudden unexpected death in patients with congestive heart failure: A second frontier. Circulation 1985; 72:681–685.

66. Paffenbarger RS Jr, Hyde RT, Wing AL, et al: The association of changes in physical-activity level and other lifestyle characteristics with mortality among men. N Engl J Med 1993; 328:538–545.

67. Pashkow F: Rehabilitation strategies for the complex cardiac patient. Cleve Clin J Med 1991; 58:70–75.

68. Pashkow FJ: Complicating conditions. In Pashkow FJ, Pashkow P, Schafer M (eds): Successful Cardiac Rehabilitation: The Complete Guide for Building Cardiac Rehabilitation Programs. Loveland, Colo, Heart Watchers, 1988, pp 228–247.

69. Peter CA, Jones RH: Effect of isometric handgrip and dynamic exercise in left ventricular function. J Nucl Med 1980; 21:1131.

70. Picano E, Lattanzi F, Masini M, et al: High dose dipyridamole echocardiography test in effort angina pectoris. J Am Coll Cardiol 1986; 8:848–854.

71. Pollock ML, Foster C, Anholm JD, et al: Diagnostic capabilities of exercise testing soon after myocardial revascularization surgery. Cardiology 1982; 69:358.

72. Pycha C, Gulledge AD, Hutzler J, et al: Psychological response to the implantable defibrillator. Psychosomatics 1986; 27:841–845.

73. Ritchie L, Trobaugh GB, Hamilton GW, et al: Myocardial imaging with thallium-201 at rest and during exercise: Comparison with coronary arteriography and resting and stress electrocardiography. Circulation 1977; 56:66–71.

74. Rosenblum DS, Rosen ML, Pine ZM, et al: Health status and quality of life following cardiac transplantation. Arch Phys Med Rehabil 1993; 74:490–493.

75. Ruffolo RR Jr: The pharmacology of dobutamine. Am J Med Sci 1987; 294:244–248.

76. Ryan T, Feigenbaum H: Exercise echocardiography. Am J Cardiol 1992; 69:82H–89H.

77. Shabetai R: Beneficial effects of exercise training in compensated heart failure. Circulation 1988; 78:775–776.

78. Sire S: Physical training and occupational rehabilitation after aortic valve replacement. Eur Heart J 1987; 8:1215–1220.

79. Starling RC, Cody RJ: Cardiac transplant hypertension. Am J Cardiol 1990; 65:106–111.

80. Sullivan MJ, Higginbotham MB, Cobb FR: Exercise training in patients with severe left ventricular dysfunction. Circulation 1990; 81(suppl 2):II-5–II-13.

81. Tuttle RR, Mills J: Dobutamine: Development of a new catecholamine to selectively increase cardiac contractility. Circ Res 1975; 36:185–196.

82. US Bureau of the Census: Statistical Abstract of the United States: 1993, ed 113. Washington, DC, US Bureau of the Census, 1993.

83. Van Camp S, Peterson R: Cardiovascular complications of outpatient cardiac rehabilitation programs. JAMA 1986; 256:1160–1163.

84. Wainright RJ, Brennand-Roper DA, Maisey MN, et al: Exercise thallium-201 myocardial scintigraphy in the follow-up of aortocoronary bypass graft surgery. Br Heart J 1980; 43:56.

85. Wasserman K, Hansen JE, Sue DY, Whipp BJ: Principles of Exercise Testing and Interpretation. Philadelphia, Lea & Febiger, 1987.

86. Weich HF, Strauss HW, Pitt B: The extraction of thallium-201 by the myocardium. Circulation 1977; 56:188.

87. Weiner DA, Ryan TJ, McCabe CH, et al: Prognostic importance of a clinical profile and exercise test in medically treated patients with coronary artery disease. J Am Coll Cardiol 1984; 3:772.

88. Wenger NK: Physiological basis for early ambulation after myocardial infarction. Cardiovasc Clin 1978; 9:107–115.

89. Wenger NK: Rehabilitation of the coronary patient. Status 1986. Prog Cardiovasc Dis 1986; 29:181.

90. Willerson JT, Hutton I, Watson JT, et al: Influence of dobutamine on regional myocardial blood flow and ventricular performance during acute and chronic ischemia in dogs. Circulation 1976; 53:828–833.

91. Winkle RA, Mead RH, Ruder MA, et al: Long term outcome with the automatic implantable cardiac-defibrillator. J Am Coll Cardiol 1989; 13:1353–1361.

92. Yusuf S, Aikenhead J, Theodoropoulos S, et al: Mechanism of cardiac output during dynamic exercise in cardiac transplant patients (abstract). J Am Coll Cardiol 1986; 7:225A.

93. Zaret BL, Wackers FJ, Soufer R: Nuclear Cardiology. *In* Braunwald E (ed): Heart Disease, a Textbook of Cardiovascular Medicine. Philadelphia, WB Saunders, 1993.

33

Concepts in Pulmonary Rehabilitation

AUGUSTA S. ALBA, M.D.

PRINCIPLES

Statistics regarding smoking and respiratory disease with chronic airway obstruction (CAO) are shown in Table 33–1.[1, 13, 41] Restrictive pulmonary disease is most commonly caused by neuromuscular orthopedic disorders, such as spinal cord injury (SCI). The annual incidence of SCI in developed countries is 11.6 per 1 million.[31] Motor vehicle accidents alone result in 500 to 650 new SCI quadriplegic patients per year.[70] Diseases can also result in restrictive pulmonary dysfunction, such as Duchenne muscular dystrophy (DMD) which has an incidence of 21/100,000 in the United States. DMD invariably leads to respiratory insufficiency, and pulmonary assistance and rehabilitation can add years to a patient's life.

Pulmonary rehabilitation (PR)[78] is defined as a comprehensive team approach that provides patients with the ability to adapt to their chronic lung disease. It includes medical management, training in coping skills, and exercise reconditioning. Fear of dyspnea can lead to panic, which increases the work of breathing, and to progressive inactivity, which further weakens the patient. PR addresses this fear and uses exercise reconditioning to increase strength and endurance, which leads to greater tolerance of dyspnea. When exercise reconditioning is no longer possible in a progressive disorder, mechanical ventilation and lung transplants become options. The guidelines for PR when exercise reconditioning is still possible are straightforward. A candidate should have a decrease in functional capacity due to pulmonary disease; relative stability of the underlying pulmonary disease; absence of other significant diseases, including orthopedic limitations; adequate motivation to undergo a rigorous program; and a pattern of continued improvement in the course of the program.[57]

PRIMARY MODALITIES

General Medical Management

Pharmacological therapy includes vaccination against influenza and pneumococcal pneumonia, inhaled quaternary anticholinergic or β₂-agonist bronchodilators, or both, and oral theophylline. Theophylline can improve respiratory muscle endurance and provides ventilatory stimulation. Persistent airway obstruction may be an indication for a trial of oral steroid therapy. If hypoxemia is present, supplemental oxygen therapy will improve survival and quality of life.[13] Environmental and occupational pollution must be prevented and eliminated.

Chest Physical Therapy

A good understanding of pulmonary function tests (Figs. 33–1 and 33–2) and the mechanics and work of breathing in the normal and diseased states[38] is essential in planning an effective physical therapy program for persons with pulmonary disease. Breathing exercises include relaxation techniques, which then become the foundation for breathing retraining. Some of these exercises are pursed-lips breathing, head-down and bending-forward postures, slow deep breathing, diaphragmatic breathing, and localized expansion exercises or segmental breathing.[30] The other component utilized to reduce fatigue is respiratory muscle endurance training, which usually concentrates on inspiratory resistance training.

Clearance of secretions is mandatory to reduce the work of breathing and to limit infection and atelectasis. Tech-

TABLE 33–1 Statistics Regarding Smoking and Respiratory Disease

American youth, aged 12–17: 2.2 million smoke
Children under age 5: 9 million live with a smoker
Annual deaths from tobacco-related illness: 417,000
Mothers who smoke 10 or more cigarettes per day: 26,000 new cases of asthma among their children
Persons with asthma in the United States: 11.6 million
Persons with chronic bronchitis in the United States: 12 million
Persons with emphysema in the United States: 2 million
Fifth leading cause of death in North America: COPD
Only leading cause of death increasing in prevalence: COPD

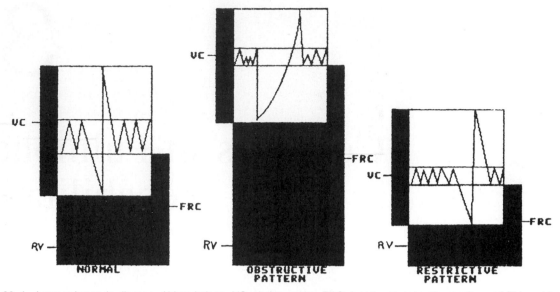

FIGURE 33–1 Lung volumes in disease. Abbreviations: VC, vital capacity; FRC, functional residual capacity; and RV, residual volume.

niques for clearing secretions are postural drainage, manual or device-induced chest percussion and vibration, incentive spirometry, and various measures that improve the ability to cough. These measures include methods to control coughing, since an uncontrolled cough can precipitate dynamic airway collapse, bronchospasm, or syncope. In a manually assisted cough, the patient's abdomen is compressed while the patient controls the depth of inspiration and the timing of opening and closing of the upper airway. Intermittent positive pressure ventilation (IPPV) or glossopharyngeal breathing (GPB) or both, are used, if needed, to increase the depth of inspiration. Similarly, in persons with an upper motor neuron lesion affecting the abdominal muscles, as in SCI with a lesion above the midthoracic level, a cough can be produced by electrical stimulation of the abdominal muscles.[46]

Positive expiratory pressure (PEP) mask therapy followed by "huff coughing" is a useful technique when other methods of raising secretions are not tolerated.[55] The patient exhales down to the functional residual capacity (FRC) through a fixed-orifice resistor, which achieves a PEP of 10 to 20 cm H_2O, for 10 to 20 breaths. The huff cough is performed with short, quick forced exhalations with the glottis open.

Autogenic drainage (AD) is a secretion clearance technique that combines variable tidal breathing at three distinct lung volume levels, controlled expiratory airflow, and huff coughing. The in-exsufflator machine (Fig. 33–3), manufactured by the J. H. Emerson Company, Cambridge, Mass., which provides a deep inspiration either through a mask or a tracheostomy attachment followed rapidly by a controlled suction, has also been shown to provide highly effective secretion removal.[7] Preliminary studies on the use of high-frequency chest compression (HFCC) have shown it to be as effective a technique as combined percussion and postural drainage in raising secretions.[85]

Exercise Conditioning

If the cardiovascular, respiratory, and neuromuscular systems have adequate reserve to undergo a program of progressive exercise, skeletal muscles on such a program can develop an increased ability to perform aerobic exercise. After training, a given level of heavy exercise results in lower levels of blood lactate. This also means that the requirement for oxygen uptake, carbon dioxide production, and ventilation for a given level of work is less. Healthy subjects must train for at least 30 min/day, 3 to 5 days per

TEST	OBSTRUCTIVE DISEASE		RESTRICTIVE DISEASE	
VC	↔	↓	↓	↓
FEV	↓	↓	↔	↓
MMF	↓	↓	↔	↓
MVV	↓	↓	↔	↓
RV	↑	↑	↓	↓
FRC	↑	↔	↓	↓
TLC	↑	↑	↓	↓

FIGURE 33–2 Typical results of disease on ventilatory function. Abbreviations: VC, vital capacity; FEV, forced expiratory volume; MMF, midmaximal flow; MVV, maximal voluntary ventilation; RV, residual volume; FRC, functional residual capacity; and TLC, total lung capacity.

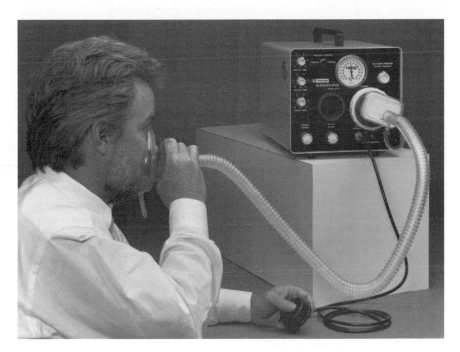

FIGURE 33–3   In-exsufflator cough machine in use with face mask.

week, for 4 to 8 weeks to achieve this effect. Whether a critical training intensity exists and how to measure it are more controversial. Moss and Make[62] recently reviewed the pulmonary response to exercise in health and disease. Once the training effect has been achieved, regular exercise must be continued or the gains will be lost.[15]

Cardiopulmonary exercise testing is necessary for the selection and evaluation of patients with chronic obstructive pulmonary disease (COPD) for exercise training. Exercise testing is carried out as a baseline measurement and as a measurement of progress. It also helps to define the cause of dyspnea, the need for supplemental oxygen, and the status of the preoperative patient.[28] After studying multiple physiological and psychosocial variables, Carlson and co-workers[14] have developed an equation which relates the peak oxygen uptake ($\dot{V}O_2$) to diffusion capacity (DCO), maximal voluntary ventilation (MVV), the peak dead space/tidal volume ratio (VD/VT), and resting minute ventilation ($\dot{V}E$). The equation is as follows: Peak $\dot{V}O_2$ (L/min) = $(0.0327 \times DCO) + (0.0040 \times MVV) - (0.0156 \times$ peak exercise VD/VT) $+ (0.0259 \times$ resting $\dot{V}E) + 0.848$; $r = .90$; SE $= 0.233$ L/min. This equation has been shown to have excellent validity, but the variability of the prediction limits its usefulness in individual patients.[14] The parameters of inspiratory vital capacity (IVC), forced expiratory volume in 1 sec (FEV₁), maximum minute ventilation ($\dot{V}Emax$), and maximum oxygen consumption ($\dot{V}O_2max$) have the greatest clinical potential for functional assessment of patients because they show the least variability over time in stable COPD patients.[63]

In a study of COPD patients with hypercapnia subjected to intensive inpatient exercise conditioning of all extremities, it has been shown that even this group with severe ventilatory impairment can benefit from exercise.[33] Ambulation distances on a 6-min walk (6 MD) doubled in a eucapnic group as well as in a group with moderate hypercapnia (partial pressure of carbon dioxide [PCO_2] = 45–54

mm Hg). They were almost doubled in a group with severe hypercapnia (PCO_2 over 54 mm Hg).

A study of 317 COPD patients with severe impairment and 32 non-COPD patients who were given a 4-week inpatient PR program showed that both groups doubled the 6 MD.[34] There was no difference among the diagnostic subgroups of the non-COPD patients. No patient had walked more than 500 ft in 6 min before the program or more than 900 ft in 6 min afterward. Another study found that patients with a greater ventilatory reserve (1 − [$\dot{V}Emax/MVV$] × 100) had more improvement in their 12-minute walk (12 MD), both with respect to distance and percentage of increase over baseline.[87]

Types of Exercise

These include lower extremity exercise training on a bicycle ergometer or treadmill, respiratory muscle training using a threshold inspiratory pressure trainer, and unsupported vs. supported arm exercise. Unsupported exercise is carried out with free weights; supported exercise is performed on the arm ergometer with the arms supported by the handgrip on the ergometer pedals. The roles of ventilatory muscle endurance exercise, of muscle rest therapy, and of nasally administered continuous positive airway pressure (CPAP) are not yet clearly defined in the management of COPD.[66]

Physiological Results of Exercise in COPD

The results of exercise from several studies[16, 24, 67, 87] are summarized in Table 33–2. It has been demonstrated that high work rates above pretraining anaerobic threshold (AT) (70 W), reduce the production of lactate at any given work rate to a considerably greater degree than a low work rate above AT.[16, 67] Simple arm elevation increases metabolic demands in COPD patients and contributes to dyspnea in patients during activities of daily living (ADL). Unsup-

TABLE 33–2 Improvements Seen in Exercise Reconditioning in Moderate COPD

IMT
    Maximal inspiratory mouth pressure ↑
    EMG fatigability of the diaphragm ↓
PR with or without IMT
    Maximal workload ↑
    ADL scores ↑
    Anxiety and depression scores ↓
    12 MD ↑
PR (cycle ergometry, 70 W)
    $\dot{V}_E$ decrease of 2.5 L/min per blood lactate decrease of 1 mEq/L
    (normal, $\dot{V}_E$ decrease of 7.2 L/min per blood lactate decrease
    of 1 mEq/L)

Abbreviations: IMT, inspiratory muscle training; EMG, electromyography; PR, pulmonary rehabilitation; ADL, activities of daily living; 12 MD, 12-minute walking distance; $\dot{V}_E$, minute volume.

ported arm exercise decreases $\dot{V}_{O_2}$ measured in the last minute of 2 min of arm elevation.[21, 59]

Patients who are hypertensive and who participate in a PR program typically show no change in the hypertension.[58] Medical treatment of the hypertension is necessary. The main hemodynamic abnormality in COPD is raised pulmonary vascular resistance and pulmonary hypertension.[69] Pulmonary hypertension worsens with the increased demand of exercise because of the absence of reserve collateral vessels. This increases afterload and reduces right ventricular ejection fraction and stroke volume, forcing cardiac output to be maintained by a relative tachycardia. Few studies have been done on the effects of PR on pulmonary hemodynamics, but those done to date have not shown significant improvement.

Exercise in Asthma

Moderate asthma is defined as asthma in which there is no pulmonary impairment during symptom-free intervals. *Severe asthma* is defined as asthma with persistent airway obstruction. Studies of young asthmatic patients in a stable state have shown that the $\dot{V}_{O_2}$max is limited in the severe asthmatic group by decreased cardiac output and stroke volume. It is hypothesized that the high tidal volume leads to decreased left ventricular performance. Aerobic training is recommended because it can decrease $\dot{V}_E$ and therefore the tidal volume for any given workload.[82] Aerobic dance is an example of this type of therapeutic exercise.[86]

Exercise in Cystic Fibrosis (CF)

An estimated 30,000 persons in the United States are affected with this hereditary autosomal recessive disorder. The basic defect is one of chloride transport, which produces a viscid mucus that inhibits the capability of the lungs to clear infection. Ultimately, the patient suffers from severe combined obstructive-restrictive pulmonary disease that leads to hypoxia, pulmonary hypertension, and death. However, the number of people with CF reaching adulthood and living productive lives is increasing by 10% per year, with the median age of survival having increased to 29.4 years.[35] These improved statistics have resulted from (1) a multidisciplinary team approach to management in accredited CF centers; (2) a better understanding of antimi-

crobial treatment, including the liberal use of aerosolized antibiotics; and (3) the recent addition of daily long-term nebulization of dornase alfa (Pulmozyme). Dornase alfa, or human recombinant deoxyribonuclease (DNase), is an enzyme capable of digesting extracellular DNA. The abnormal viscosity of the CF secretions is caused to a great extent by degenerating neutrophils which produce extracellular DNA. Thus far, the Food and Drug Administration (FDA) has approved dornase alfa for patients older than 5 years of age or with an FVC greater than 40%. With the marked reduction in viscosity, the secretions can be more readily mobilized, and the obstruction caused by the secretions alleviated.

Chest physical therapy of all pulmonary segments from one to four times daily is indicated with increased frequency during exacerbations. Such therapy cannot usually be obtained with the necessary frequency in a long-term care setting because patient/staff ratios do not permit it. The person with CF is best cared for in a home setting with personal caregivers who have been trained to deliver the therapy. Hospital nosocomial infections are also avoided in the home treatment setting.

Exercise in Disorders of Chest Wall Function

Ankylosing spondylitis, kyphoscoliosis or scoliosis, pectus excavatum, obesity, neuromuscular diseases with weakness of the respiratory bellows mechanism, and superimposed spinal curvatures are all disorders in which respiratory muscle fatigue can be reduced by ventilatory muscle training. Hornstein and co-workers[43] outlined this approach for kyphoscoliosis. Refsum and associates[68] noted that bracing, in this instance the Boston thoracic brace, can cause a marked decrease in lung volumes, and increase the energy cost of exercise while the brace is being worn. However, 6 months after removing the brace there was no persistent deterioration.

SCI patients can benefit from PR techniques. The SCI child as young as 3 years old can learn neck breathing as a form of voluntary respiration.[36] It produces enough tidal volume in children with levels as high as C2 with no diaphragmatic function, that the child can spend some time off the respirator. With some ability to breathe without aid, the child has less fear of accidental disconnection of the respirator, and can have some degree of privacy and independence in the home.

Vital capacity (VC) and $\dot{V}_E$ during exercise can be improved even in chronic quadriplegia, using resistance exercise by pedaling an arm ergometer (AE) 30 min three times a week, and by incentive spirometry for 15 min three to five times per week.[84] Incentive spirometry is a technique in which a patient trains to perform regular deep insufflations by inspiring through a hand-held apparatus which gives visual feedback of inspiratory flow.

GPB, or frog breathing (Fig. 33–4), is another technique a patient can use to perform or supplement regular deep insufflations. Like neck breathing it can also be used as an alternative form of respiration. Air is pumped into lungs by the patient using the tongue as a piston. The ball of the tongue strokes boluses of air at the rate of 100/min into the throat. The lips, soft palate, and vocal cords open and

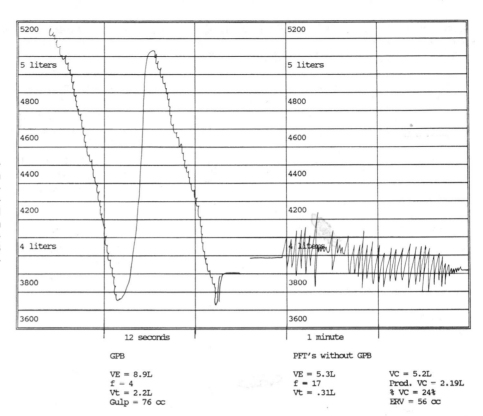

FIGURE 33–4 Glossopharyngeal breathing tracing and results compared with PFTs without GPB in a quadriplegic ventilator user with post-polio syndrome. Abbreviations: GPB, glossopharyngeal breathing; PFTs, pulmonary function tests; VE, minute ventilation; f, frequency; Gulp, volume/single GPB stroke; VT, tidal volume; and ERV, expiratory reserve volume.

GPB

VE = 8.9L
f = 4
Vt = 2.2L
Gulp = 76 cc

PFT's without GPB

VE = 5.3L   VC = 5.2L
f = 17   Prod. VC = 2.19L
Vt = .31L   % VC = 24%
                   ERV = 56 cc

close in rhythm during each stroke. The patient usually obtains a full tidal breath by stacking gulps of 60 to 90 mL over a period of 10 to 15 sec and then exhales. Full inflation of the lungs requires stacking for a period of 30 to 40 sec. Quadriplegic patients, in whom resting $\dot{V}O_2$ is approximately half-normal (150 mL/min, personal observation), are able to obtain adequate $\dot{V}E$ by this method if their lungs have no major abnormalities. This enables them to breathe without artificial ventilation for hours. If the lungs are abnormal, as in severe scoliosis, a person may only be able to frog-breathe for minutes because the $\dot{V}E$ is not adequate to prevent hypoxia. As soon as the oxygen saturation falls to 85% to 90%, the patient will typically ask for mechanical ventilatory assistance. GPB improves vocal volume and the flow of speech, allows the patient to call for help, and provides the deep breath needed for an assisted cough.

Patients with midthoracic and lower thoracic paraplegia have aerobic and anaerobic capacities that are primarily limited by available muscle mass rather than impaired cardiovascular (CV) or cardiopulmonary function.[26] A study of four subjects using AE and functional neuromuscular stimulation (FNS) of the hips and lower extremities showed mean METS (metabolic equivalents of oxygen consumption) during FNS of 4.8, during FNS + AE of 10.3, and during AE of 7.2.[26] $\dot{V}E$ and $\dot{V}O_2$ for the three midthoracic subjects were greater than 90% of those observed in sedentary normals. In only one subject, a T11 paraplegic patient, was CV limitation due to excessive lactic acid production noted.[26]

Nutrition

In acute respiratory failure a fat emulsion (Pulmocare) can be given as 20% to 30% of total daily calories to reduce carbon dioxide production and to provide a volume-concentrated source of calories in the fluid-restricted patient. Dietary fat has a lower level of carbon dioxide production per kilocalorie of energy extracted. This is evident in the respiratory quotient, which is 0.7 for fat and 1.0 for carbohydrate. Metabolic measurements of $\dot{V}O_2$ and carbon dioxide production for the intensive care setting are readily available today to assist in determining caloric needs.[61]

In 40% to 50% of persons with COPD with either chronic hypoxemia or severe airflow obstruction (FEV_1 < 35% of predicted), and in 25% of persons with moderate airflow obstruction (FEV_1 < 50% of predicted), there is depletion of body weight, of fat-free mass, and of muscle mass.[72] Persons of normal weight with COPD can demonstrate depletion of fat-free mass and show less endurance on the 12 MD than the underweight person without fat-free mass depletion. A recent study showed that persons with COPD and FEV_1 of less than 50% and PaO_2 of greater than 7.3 kPa had a strong correlation between distance walked and fat-free mass. Fat-free mass, maximal inspiratory mouth pressure, and PaO_2 accounted for 60% of the variation in the 12 MD.[71]

Mechanical Ventilation

In the patient whose respiratory status is compromised there may be alterations in the central drive for breathing, obstructive changes in the upper airway, and restrictive and obstructive changes in the lungs. These conditions can exist alone or in various and changing combinations. Assessment of the central drive for breathing and the upper airway is best done at a sleep disorders center with specialized staff and equipment for diagnosis and therapy. Portable polysomnography has allowed this valuable information to be obtained in the intensive care unit (ICU) and in the home. Certified polysomnography technologists prepare the patient with monitoring equipment. Data are collected on an electromagnetic tape recorder. Later the tape is analyzed at a central office with the assistance of a computer.

A reduction in the central drive for breathing results in central apnea. Obstruction at any site in the upper airway produces obstructive apnea. Both forms of apnea frequently coexist and are generally more severe during sleep, especially during rapid eye movement (REM) sleep, when there is the greatest degree of muscle relaxation. Mechanical ventilation is necessary when symptoms and signs of respiratory failure develop. Tobin[79] recently reviewed the current concepts in mechanical ventilation.

The type of mechanical ventilation to be used and the frequency and duration of its use is a joint decision to be made by the physician and the patient. Cost, availability, portability, and preference are factors to consider. The choice of ventilators can be confusing. However, if the basic features of ventilators are kept in mind, the prescription is readily generated (Fig. 33–5). If four basic questions can be answered, all of the other features of ventilators are readily mastered. These questions are: Does the ventilator act on the body or the airway? Does the ventilator produce a positive or negative pressure? Does the machine's pressure produce an active inspiration or an active expiration? Does the ventilator have a cycling device?

Noninvasive artificial ventilation is the use of a ventilator without an endotracheal or tracheostomy tube. There are numerous advantages to a noninvasive approach (Table 33–3). One of the most important is the avoidance of respiratory nosocomial infection. Noninvasive approaches like nasal intermittent positive-pressure ventilation (NIPPV) are now being used even in the ICU for patients in acute respiratory failure (Fig. 33–6). The concomitant use of the in-exsufflator is necessary for removal of tracheobronchial secretions.[7]

Two of the most acceptable forms of noninvasive ventilation that are used during the daytime are mouth intermittent positive-pressure ventilation (MIPPV) with a small mouthpiece held between the teeth (Fig. 33–7) and the pneumobelt (Fig. 33–8). The pneumobelt holds a bladder which when inflated produces a forced expiration. This

IPPV -

Volume respirator-Console
Pressure respirator-Console
Volume respirator-Compact
Pressure respirator-Compact
Manual ventilator (resuscitator)
Mouth to mouth, to mouth-nose,
  to tracheostomy
In-exsufflator (positive phase)
High frequency ventilation

Inspiratory muscles
  Iron Lung
  Poncho
  Cuirass
  Rocking bed-head up
  Phrenic nerve
    stimulation

GPB

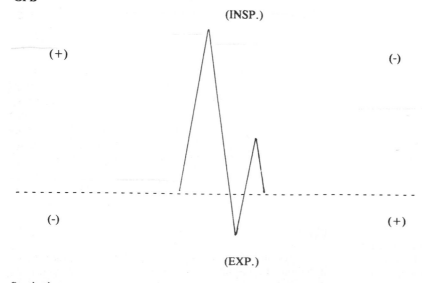

Suctioning -

Suction machine
GPB-reversed
In-exsufflator
  (negative phase)

Expiratory muscles
  Pneumobelt
  Rocking bed-head down
  Manual body
    resuscitation

FIGURE 33–5 Respiratory assistive devices superimposed on a graphic representation of the vital capacity. Abbreviations: IPPV, intermittent positive-pressure ventilation; INSP., full inspiration; GPB, glossopharyngeal breathing; EXP., Forced expiration; airway (+), ventilation by positive pressure on airway, producing inspiration; airway, (−), ventilation by negative pressure on airway, producing suctioning; body (−), ventilation by negative pressure on body, producing inspiration; body (+), ventilation by positive pressure on body, producing expiration.

TABLE 33–3   Respiratory Assistive Devices: Pros and Cons

Type	Use	Pro	Con
Airway Positive Pressure			
Intermittent positive-pressure ventilation			
Console	Bedside; generally hospital setting, acute care, via tracheostomy	Sophistication (alarms; %O$_2$)	Stationary; high cost
Compact	Long-term; generally noninvasive	Portability; generally AC/DC; lower cost	Some models bulky
Body Negative Pressure			
Iron lung	Replaces bed; long-term	Reliable; good ventilation	Weight; size; confining
Porta-Lung	Same as iron lung	Same as iron lung	Light weight; relative portability
Poncho (wrap)	In bed; long-term	Same as iron lung	May restrict upper chest expansion
Chest shell (cuirass)	In bed; rarely in wheelchair; long-term	Less confining than iron lung	Restricts upper and lateral chest expansion
Diaphragmatic pacemaker	Long-term; relatively intact phrenic nerve, diaphragm muscle, and lower lobes	Very light weight; easy operation	Surgery; initial cost very high; moves only diaphragm
Body Negative/Positive Pressure			
Rocking bed	Replaces bed; requires healthy lower lobes; "movable abdomen"; long-term	Less confining than iron lung; passive movement of body	Weight; size; moves only diaphragm
Body Positive Pressure			
Pneumobelt	Long-term; generally requires sitting position of at least 45 degrees; "movable abdomen"	Good cosmetic effect	Moves only diaphragm

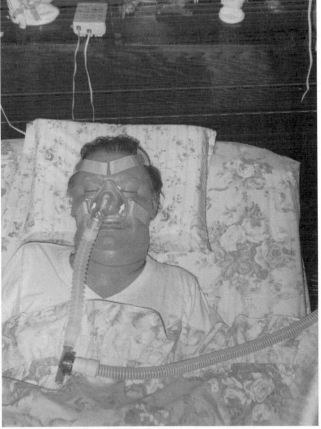

FIGURE 33–6 Nasal intermittent positive-pressure ventilation in a quadriplegic ventilator user with post-polio syndrome.

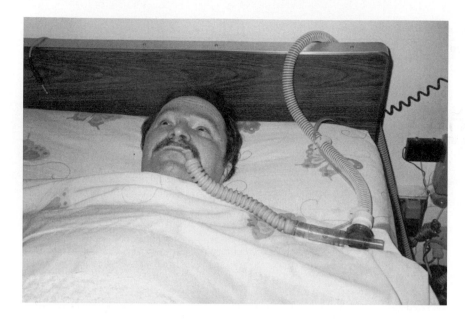

FIGURE 33–7 Mouth intermittent positive-pressure ventilation with mouthpiece in a quadriplegic ventilator user with post-polio syndrome.

expiration is followed by a passive inspiration. The inspiration may be supplemented by the use of the remaining inspiratory muscles or frog breathing, or a combination of these. MIPPV can be used at night by using a mouthpiece with a lip seal (Fig. 33–9). The patient can use a rocking bed (Fig. 33–10) or a chestpiece (Fig. 33–11) at rest or during sleep. Kirshblum and Bach[50] reported on the use of a modified rolling walker to transport a portable ventilator for those patients requiring artificial ventilation but who are still capable of ambulating.

When a decision has been made to retain a tracheostomy in a ventilator-dependent patient, a cuffless tracheostomy tube or a tube with a partially deflated cuff can generally be used.[6] Tubes without a fully inflated cuff require adequate pulmonary compliance and sufficient oropharyngeal strength for functional swallowing and articulation. If the patient has a progressive disorder, periodic monitoring with continuous overnight oximetry and capnography is indi-

cated to ensure that leakage through the nose or mouth during sleep is not excessive. When a fully inflated cuff must be used, the lowest possible cuff pressure needed to achieve a seal should be used (preferably <15 mm Hg). If the pressure exceeds the critical pressure for perfusion of the tracheal mucosa (25 mm Hg), destruction of the tracheal wall can occur. Ulceration, bleeding, perforation, loss of tracheal cartilage, localized trachiectasis or stenosis, and granulation tissue are potential complications.

Types of tracheostomy tubes include metal or disposable tubes. The disposable tubes are made of plastic or silicone. Specialized tubes include fenestrated tubes, talking tubes, and tubes for the laryngectomized person. Mason[60] recently published a comprehensive text on communication in tracheostomized and ventilator-dependent patients. There are both pneumatic and electrical devices which assist vocalization in the presence of a tracheostomy tube. Two of the talking tracheostomy tubes are the COMMUNItrach TMI

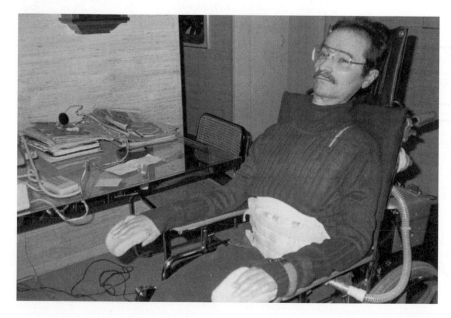

FIGURE 33–8 Pneumobelt ventilation in a quadriplegic ventilator user with post-polio syndrome.

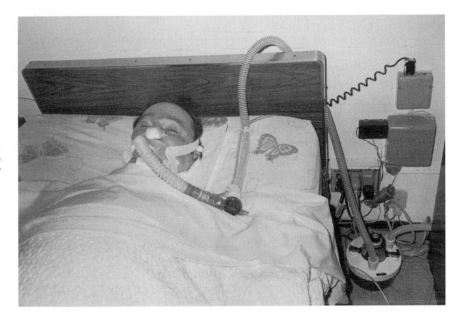

FIGURE 33–9 Mouth intermittent positive-pressure ventilation with lip seal, mouthpiece and nose taped in a quadriplegic ventilator user with post-polio syndrome.

and the Portex "Talk" tracheostomy tube. Speaking valves can be attached to the tracheostomy tube adapter. The most frequently used valve currently is the Passy-Muir. When vocalization is not possible, nonvocal communication can be provided by a manual or electronic communication system. There are numerous systems for nonvocal communication available today and the expertise of a speech pathologist should be sought in making the decision regarding the most appropriate system in each case.

In cases of advanced COPD, mechanical ventilation via a tracheostomy is often necessary for survival. More controversial, however, is the use of mechanical ventilation to reduce respiratory muscle fatigue. Celli et al.[17] found that adding external negative pressure ventilation with the use of the Emerson Pulmowrap ventilator to an in-hospital PR program did not provide any added effects on leg cycle endurance time, maximal transdiaphragmatic pressure, breathing pattern as expressed by tension time index, and sense of well-being.

Mechanical ventilation in patients with neuromusculoskeletal disorders has been facilitated in the past 15 years by the development of portable volume ventilators. In the ICU the increased sophistication of console volume ventilators, such as the Puritan-Bennett 7200 AE, has aided the survival of persons with these disorders. The critically ill patient in the ICU with sepsis and multiple organ failure can develop a primary axonal form of polyneuropathy, which delays weaning as well as overall recovery and mobilization.[73] Early diagnosis with the aid of electrodiagnostic studies facilitates the rehabilitation process.

Tetanus has to be quickly recognized in its early stage with prompt ventilator support, vigorous treatment of infection, and management of the muscle rigidity with benzodiazepines, narcotics, and neuromuscular blockers. With this regimen patients can usually be ready for rehabilitation within 4 weeks.

The halo brace is frequently used for patients with SCI if surgical stabilization has not been carried out after frac-

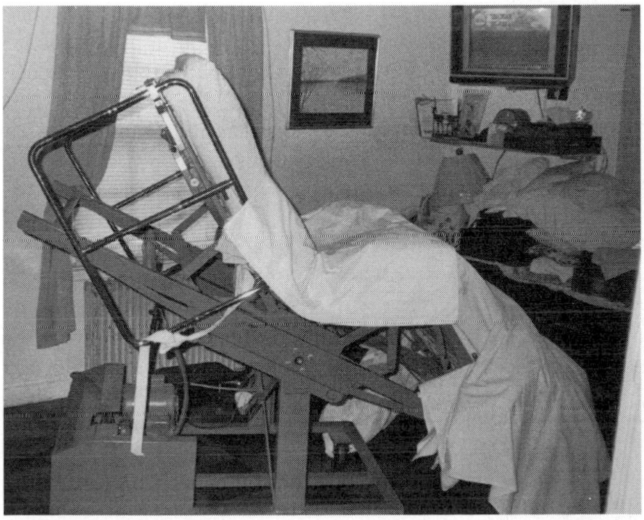

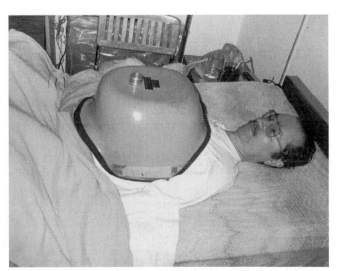

FIGURE 33–10 Rocking bed in head-up position with elevation of the head of bed.

FIGURE 33–11 Chestpiece without hose applied to a quadriplegic ventilator user with post-polio syndrome.

ture of the cervical spine.[10] The halo brace permits early patient mobilization and early admission to a rehabilitation setting. Early mobilization helps prevent the pulmonary complications associated with prolonged bed rest and paralysis, the most serious of which are atelectasis and pneumonia. Cervical spine fractures typically cause neurological injury (with the majority having quadriplegia) in as many as 30% of patients.[65] As many as 20% of such patients can have associated abdominal and chest trauma.

Persons with high and midcervical quadriplegia will invariably require mechanical ventilation during the initial hospitalization. At least one in five quadriplegics who require mechanical ventilation will be discharged on ventilator support. Persons with low quadriplegia frequently require mechanical ventilation during the acute hospitalization. Financial support for hospitalization, rehabilitation, and long-term care is a serious national health issue. Bach[5] describes conversion of high-level quadriplegic patients to noninvasive ventilatory support or providing such support from the onset as a means of simplifying care and reducing cost.

Other common neurological disorders in which long-term mechanical ventilation is used include amyotrophic lateral sclerosis (ALS), syringomyelia, multiple sclerosis, muscular dystrophies, and poliomyelitis. Bach[3] found that ALS patients can survive a mean of 4.4 (SD 3.9) years (range, 1 month to 26.5 years) using respiratory support. Survival was comparable for patients maintained at home or in chronic care facilities. The use of noninvasive respiratory aids not only simplified care but gave patients and families time for decision making regarding tracheostomy.

DMD patients, once on ventilator assistance, tend to increase its use approximately 1 hour/day/year.[23] Their average length of survival increased by 6 years with respiratory assistance.[23]

Postpoliomyelitis patients on long-term nocturnal ventilation have also been studied. Curran and Colbert[23] found that these patients showed no significant decrease in muscle strength or increase in the number of hours of nocturnal ventilation over a 12-year-period. Speier et al.,[75] in a 1986 review of an epidemic population of poliomyelitis (1952–1953), showed that 40% complained of increased weakness and 11% reported new breathing problems. Reasons for the apparent discrepancy between studies are the small number of patients studied by Curran and Colbert and the relatively short period of time during which they were studied. Postpoliomyelitis ventilator users over a period of 30 to 40 years invariably show an increase in the number of hours of assisted ventilation (personal observation). Increased weakness of oropharyngeal muscles over time can also occur with occasional new problems of swallowing and obstructive apnea.

The use of mechanical ventilation in patients post cardiac surgery is a "crutch" that can facilitate the rehabilitation process, as has been described by Sivak.[74] Gradual withdrawal and concise protocols are necessary in this program.

Weaning from mechanical ventilation is an important aspect of PR, both in terms of reduced cost and patient satisfaction. Weaning techniques include CPAP, blow-by systems or T piece, pressure support, and the use of the Passy-Muir ventilator speaking valve. The use of manual and mechanical exsufflation to clear airway secretions, and

the use of noninvasive positive airway pressure ventilatory assistance by nasal or oral interfaces speeds weaning in the patient on tracheal intermittent positive-pressure ventilation (IPPV). Lamid and associates[53] advise that weaning of the SCI patient be carried out in an SCI center where staff can alleviate anxiety and depression, enlist family support, solve problems as a team, and prevent infections. Diaphragmatic strengthening and endurance training can be used to facilitate weaning in the high quadriplegic patient in whom there is only partial involvement of the anterior horn cells of the phrenic nerve at the C3 to C5 levels.[54]

Patients on mechanical ventilation in the home or in an alternative setting benefit from those aspects of PR that promote a quality lifestyle of independence and autonomy. International conferences on PR and home mechanical ventilation have been held during the past decade. The information presented at the Third International Conference is available in summary form.[56]

It has been demonstrated that a chronic ventilator-dependent unit in an acute hospital is cost-effective.[37] Because of the multidisciplinary approach, weaning can be performed with greater success in such a unit. COPD was usually the most frequent underlying diagnosis. In the study of Gracey et al.,[37] almost 90% of the patients admitted to the unit over an 18-month period were weaned and over 70% were discharged home. A small number required nocturnal mechanical ventilation at home. Indihar[44] reported on 500 patients seen over a period of 10 years in a prolonged respiratory care unit. He found that over time a large number of patients need chronic ventilator support. The differences in these outcomes are probably due to patient selection for admission.

Diaphragmatic pacing (Fig. 33–12) is a highly sophisticated form of mechanical ventilation. It has been available in the clinical setting for over 20 years, but has attained a higher level of reliability and broader application in the past decade.[25] Cost and the risks of surgery are limiting factors in the use of pacers. Infection, failure of components, and the need to retain a tracheostomy because of obstructive sleep apnea are possible complications. Worldwide there have been over a thousand phrenic nerve implants in patients ranging from a few months old to over 80 years of age. Many of these patients have been successfully paced for more than 10 years. Diaphragmatic pacing is indicated in patients who have damage to the respiratory control centers or their pathways in the brainstem and spinal cord. The pacing system consists of an external transmitter and antenna and an implanted electrode and receiver. The transmitter produces impulses which are delivered via the external antenna loop. This loop is taped to the skin over the implanted receiver site. The working life expectancy of the receiver has recently been extended to the life of the patient and the size of the implanted receiver has been reduced by 79%. A bipolar electrode is available for use in persons who already have demand cardiac pacers. The transmitter now weighs only 0.5 kg and batteries have been improved to last 2 to 3 weeks. There is advanced warning of transmitter battery failure via a gradual decrease in tidal volume over several days. The pacer is thermal-stabilized to allow full outdoor activities while pacing.

With "customized" stimulation parameters which enable pacing with small numbers of residual fibers, the cervical

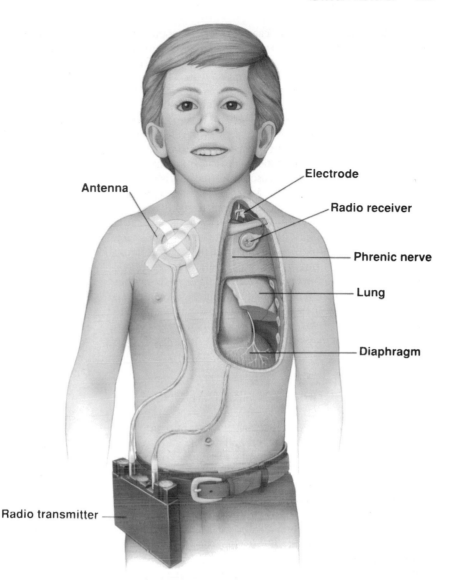

Antenna

Electrode

Radio receiver

Phrenic nerve

Lung

Diaphragm

Radio transmitter

FIGURE 33–12 Diaphragmatic pacemaker use in child with central hypoventilation syndrome.

implant in now recommended in the older child and adult. The surgery is simple and the hospitalization brief. Thoracic implants requiring bilateral thoracotomies are still done for infants. The physician can use transtelephonic monitoring (TTM) for remote assessment of stimulation effectiveness and diagnosis of problems from any telephone. The most common problems for which the pacer can be used include idiopathic central hypoventilation syndrome (CHS), or Ondine's curse; acquired CHS; and high SCI. Patients with previously intractable lesions of one or both phrenic nerves may now be candidates for diaphragm pacing. If the lesion is incomplete, special stimulus techniques permit diaphragm pacing even in cases in which transcutaneous phrenic nerve conduction studies show no response.

Krieger and associates[52] have developed a technique to reinnervate the recently denervated diaphragm by intercostal nerve-to-phrenic nerve anastomosis with implantation of a pacing electrode. This approach permits axons from intercostal motor neurons, located in the thoracic anterior horn, to grow into the diaphragm via the phrenic nerve. The phrenic nerve lies in close proximity to the intercostal nerves in the thoracic cavity. They are related in size and have similar functions.

Oxygen Therapy

Oxygen therapy (like mechanical ventilation) can be administered on a long-term basis. The physician should provide a prescription to the vendor who furnishes oxygen in the home.[77] The physician must include on the prescription the diagnostic reasons for oxygen, results of blood gas studies, type of delivery system, and specific liter flow for the patient during rest, sleep, or exertion. For the hypoxemic patient oxygen should be administered continuously to improve mortality and morbidity. Whether it should be used to improve exercise performance in the normoxemic COPD patient or to treat dyspnea is less clear. Oxygen therapy is most easily monitored by pulse oximetry during the different activity conditions of the patient.

The American Lung Association (ALA) has a newly revised edition of a leaflet for users of supplemental oxygen who fly.[83] Dialing 1-800-586-4872 connects the caller with the nearest office. Estimates of the number of supplemental oxygen users in the United States range from 600,000 to 800,000. No major airline permits an oxygen user to bring a personal tank into the cabin, but the majority supply oxygen, for a fee, to those who request it in advance and who provide a letter from their physician specifying their needs. Continental Airlines has created a medical form for the use of oxygen, which is considered a model and which is available through the ALA. The fee for oxygen is usually $50 for each leg of a trip or for each unit of oxygen used. The Americans With Disabilities Act of 1991 contains no specific references to oxygen users, but its provisions still apply. Home oxygen systems available are high-pressure compressed gas cylinders in several sizes, transfilling liquid oxygen systems with both a stationary reservoir and a portable device weighing 11 lb when full, and oxygen concentrators which require an electrical outlet. The liquid oxygen canister can provide up to 9 hours of oxygen at 2 L/min. Methods of conservation include devices that either cause the oxygen to flow only during inspiration or that store oxygen during the expiratory phase. Both as a method of conservation and for the cosmetic effect, transtracheal oxygen can be used. Nasal cannulas can be concealed in the eyeglasses.

BIOPSYCHOSOCIAL CONSIDERATIONS

These considerations for persons with pulmonary dysfunction include education of the patient and family, psychotherapy, disability evaluation, vocational counseling, and availability of resources. Education must be ongoing in all clinical settings and is the responsibility of all team members. A format should be utilized which simplifies documentation of what has been taught, and makes it readily available to the other team members. Janelli and co-workers[47] studied the effect of group teaching programs in a PR setting on the COPD patient. They found that they increased knowledge, but did not change coping strategies unless the patients were specifically taught how to incorporate appropriate strategies into their lifestyle. Psychotherapy includes the assessment of neurocognition, which can be affected by hypoxemia and hypercapnia, and of the individual's self-concept. Kersten[48] has developed a 20-item assessment tool to evaluate the patient's self-concept, and past, present, and future selves. This provides a relatively easy way to monitor subjective changes in psychological status.

Stress management includes cognitive restructuring, progressive relaxation, breathing exercises, and visual imagery. Blake and associates[8] did a study of patients with obstructive or restrictive pulmonary disease who were given a brief period of stress management in a PR clinic. Reading materials and audiotapes were used. No differences were found between the intervention recipients and a control group at 1 year except for somewhat better physical and psychosocial function in the experimental group. Biofeedback and sexual counseling are additional psychotherapeutic approaches.

Resources in the community should include financial support, home healthcare agencies with personnel trained to care for the person with respiratory disability, and support groups. Burns[11] found that support groups helped overcome the isolation, depression, and irritability associated with chronic respiratory disease. However, such groups require a large investment of time and energy on the part of volunteers and patients to be self-sustaining.

SURGICAL APPROACHES TO PULMONARY REHABILITATION

Stulbarg and colleagues[76] reported on the results of bilateral carotid body resection (BCBR) for the relief of severe dyspnea in three patients. The patients reported relief, but this occurred with a fall of $\dot{V}E$ by 25% at rest, and 39% with exercise, primarily secondary to a fall in respiratory rate. There were decreases of $\dot{V}O_2$ of 26% and of carbon dioxide output of 22% with the same external workload. Arterial blood gases deteriorated.

Lung-heart transplant for end-stage lung disease of various causes is being increasingly performed.[29] In selected patients long-term mechanical ventilatory support has not been shown to be a contraindication to lung transplantation. A program of physical training prior to surgery expedites postoperative recovery. The mortality rate for lung transplantation, both single and bilateral, is almost 15%, and significant complications can occur.[27] Survivors are typically able to return to an active lifestyle within 2 months of discharge from the hospital.

Cardiac transplant candidates waiting for a donor heart often benefit from a left ventricular assist device.[12] The device can be used up to several months prior to the transplantation. This device reverses multiorgan failure including pulmonary dysfunction, and the candidate can participate in a cardiac rehabilitation program prior to transplantation. Khaghani and co-workers[49] reported a series of 222 combined heart and lung transplants for the treatment of pulmonary vascular disease and parenchymal lung disease. Of this group, 17 had emphysema and seven of the emphysematous patients had alpha$_1$-antitrypsin deficiency. After transplantation, patients with this deficiency did not need alpha$_1$-antitrypsin augmentation or replacement therapy. Overall survival in the transplant patients was 91% at 1 year, and all survivors achieved an excellent level of rehabilitation.

LONG-TERM RESULTS OF PULMONARY REHABILITATION

Long-Term Results in COPD

Programs of PR are usually either short-term inpatient or short-term outpatient programs. The latter can be set up in a storefront setting, a community hospital, or in the physician's office. The program needs a proper team structure, adequate space, knowledge of the services to be provided, a marketing plan, and reimbursement for services.[40] Services may include medical and nutritional management, addressing of psychosocial issues, education, physical rehabilitation, recreational therapy, and occupational therapy. The way the participants define their health is a major consideration in the program because their definition typically parallels their goals.[32] If the providers of a program fail to listen to the participants, communication is not optimal and participants will likely be dissatisfied. Mall and Medeiros,[57] in a study of 101 patients in an outpatient program followed for 1 to 5 years, showed that 31.7% remained improved, 31.7% died, and 36.5% of patients became worse from either progression of the pulmonary disease or the occurrence of other disease. Of the patients who completed the program, 86% showed a better understanding of their disease and were able to tolerate an increased workload on the treadmill with lower heart and respiratory rates. Of 41 patients tested, only 11, or 25%, were able to reach a workload above anaerobic threshold.

Holle and colleagues[42] studied 44 patients with mean FEV_1 of 33% (SD 4%) predicted who completed a 6-week program of supervised treadmill training and a continued home program. Unsuspected cardiac disease was discovered during the program in nine patients (20%). Unsuspected exercise desaturation was found in 16 (36%). There was a 73% (SD 16%) improvement in aerobic capacity (METS peak [power]) and a 250% (SD 78%) improvement in endurance (METS-min [work]). A follow-up study was done on 24 subjects a year later. This group maintained 89% (SD 7%) of their peak performance. Ojanen et al.,[64] in a study of 40 COPD patients who received an intensive 3-week rehabilitation program, showed that there was immediate improvement in the patients' sense of well-being, emotional state, and respiratory symptoms, but the effects had dissipated at the 6-month follow-up. This indicates that short-term programs can be effective, but require ongoing follow-up for long-lasting benefit.

Cox et al.[22] studied 44 persons with asthma or mild COPD who participated in a 3-month comprehensive rehabilitation program and were followed for a 2-year period along with a control group. The treatment group showed improvement in endurance, decreased body fat percentage, an increase in working days, more active life, and a decrease in consumption of medical care. However, bronchial hyperreactivity, need for pulmonary drugs, degree of coughing, and sputum production were not affected. Vale and co-workers[80] evaluated 51 COPD patients who completed a 6-week outpatient rehabilitation program at ½ to 1½ years later. The group was divided into those who continued on an exercise maintenance program and those who did not. Endurance as determined on the 12 MD and quality-of-life measurements showed some loss of gains in both groups, with no difference found between the groups.

Cyclical training in 36 patients over a period of 6 years in both diaphragmatic breathing and exercise training produced a great enhancement of workload in nine (25%), some enhancement in 25 (69%), and little enhancement in two patients (6%).[18] Pulmonary hyperinflation was reduced, as demonstrated by a mean reduction in residual volume of 32%. Boyars[9] reported on the presence of all three entities of CAO—asthma, chronic bronchitis, and emphysema—in the elderly. PR had gratifying results even in this group. Corriveau et al.[20] similarly showed that improvement in a PR program was not related to the patients' age.

Van-der-Schoot and Kaptein[81] described the stabilization of respiratory symptoms in asthmatics, whose symptoms could not be otherwise controlled. The authors used interdisciplinary treatment in a high-altitude climate with low air humidity and low allergen concentration. However, 6 months later, approximately 35% of patients were readmitted to a hospital for an exacerbation. Psychological factors played a key role in the readmissions.

Long-Term Results in Pneumonia

Asauliuk[2] reviewed more than 1000 cases of acute pneumonia in young adult patients. At the time of discharge approximately 50% were normal clinically, by laboratory studies including VC measurement, and radiologically. Moderate deficits in pulmonary function tests were found in 17% before discharge. An asthenic syndrome that was retained after discharge in 30% of patients required 3 to 10 months of PR to reverse.

Long-Term Results in Neuromuscular Disorders

Koch and colleagues[51] have shown that an outpatient neuromuscular disease clinic is cost-effective. In a total of 210 patients over a 1-year period, ancillary services were utilized as follows: pulmonary (11% of patients), orthopedic (10%), social service (43%), formal occupational therapy (7%), and physical therapy (6%). Seventy percent of the annual costs of the clinic were for equipment, 11% for laboratory testing, and 8% for physician costs. The total mean per capita cost of outpatient rehabilitation in this population was $750 per year.

Bach[4] has shown that persons with SCI who are weaned despite having a significant restrictive pulmonary problem may develop ventilatory decompensation weeks to decades after weaning. Their course can be complicated by multiple pulmonary complications, including bouts of acute respiratory failure. Noninvasive mechanical ventilation is an option when ventilatory aid is needed again. Chawla[19] reported that although there has been an increased survival rate among persons with high SCI, ideal rehabilitation for those who remain paralyzed and in need of partial or complete ventilator support is frequently not available because of cost factors. This includes the cost of delivery of home care, reliable portable ventilators, phrenic nerve stimulators, environmental controls, specialized wheelchairs, and alternative communication aids.

Although disability in adductor spastic dysphonia (ASD) is limited to a severe communication disability, Harrison and co-workers[39] noted that the presence of phonatory spasm during speech can be so extreme that the use of inspiratory speech is preferable. Voice quality is poor, but it is better for the speaker and the listener than expiratory speech. Blood gas measurements showed no change during extended speaking periods.

SUMMARY

The physiatrist requires a basic knowledge of the anatomy and physiology of the respiratory system, and of exercise physiology to be able to practice PR. Patient assessment skills include proficiency in electrodiagnosis as it applies to the respiratory muscles, in particular the diaphragm (phrenic nerves), and in the interpretation of radiological studies of the lungs. The evaluation of a patient's disability, capacity for independence, and quality of life must include the respiratory system.

The practice of PR can be in a setting limited to this subspecialty, or in a broader setting where patients with neurological or musculoskeletal disabilities have pulmonary dysfunction as a co-morbidity, or as a medical complication of the disease. This includes both congenital and acquired pediatric disabilities, degenerative and demyelinating neurological disorders, stroke, traumatic brain injury, SCI, and the effects of aging.

General rehabilitative therapeutic approaches apply. Team participation and management, vocational rehabilitation, management of leisure time and of sexual disability, social integration, and psychological therapeutic methods are needed. Therapeutic exercise, including aerobic training and specific respiratory muscle strengthening, is utilized. Rehabilitation equipment includes not only appropriately prescribed wheelchairs and spinal orthoses but communication aids, portable ventilators, and oxygen.

Health policy, legislation, and regulations, including new healthcare delivery systems, must take into account the need for PR at all ages in society, from the premature infant with bronchopulmonary dysplasia, to the young athlete with exercise-induced asthma, to the octogenarian with chronic bronchitis and COPD.

References

1. American Heart Association: Heart and Stroke Facts: 1994 Statistical Supplement. Dallas, American Heart Association.
2. Asauliuk IK: The rehabilitation of young patients with a history of acute pneumonia. Vrach Delo, 1989; 7:53–55.
3. Bach, JR: Amyotrophic lateral sclerosis: Communication status and survival with ventilatory support. Am J Phys Med Rehabil 1993; 72:343–349.
4. Bach JR: Inappropriate weaning and late onset ventilatory failure of individuals with traumatic spinal cord injury. Paraplegia 1993; 31:430–438.
5. Bach JR: New approaches in the rehabilitation of the traumatic high level quadriplegic. Am J Phys Med Rehabil 1991; 70:13–19.
6. Bach JR, Alba A: Tracheostomy ventilation: A study of efficacy with deflated cuffs and cuffless tubes. Chest 1990; 97:679–683.
7. Bach J, Smith WH, Michael J, et al: Airway secretion clearance by mechanical exsufflation in post poliomyelitis ventilator assisted individuals. Arch Phys Med Rehabil 1993; 74:170–177.
8. Blake RL Jr, Vandiver TA, Braun S, et al: A randomized controlled evaluation of a psychosocial intervention in adults with chronic lung disease. Fam Med 1990; 22:365–370.
9. Boyars MS: COPD in the ambulatory elderly: Management update, Geriatrics 1988; 43:29–32, 35–37, 40.
10. Browner CM, Hadley MN, Sonntag VK, et al: Halo immobilization brace care: An innovative approach. J Neurosci Nurs 1987; 19:24–29.
11. Burns M: Outpatient pulmonary rehabilitation. A new lease on life, Postgrad Med 1989; 86:129–130.
12. Burnett CM, Duncan JM, Frazier OH, et al: Improved multiorgan function after prolonged univentricular support. Ann Thorac Surg 1993; 55:63–71.
13. Canadian Thoracic Society Workshop Group: Guidelines for the assessment and management of chronic obstructive pulmonary disease. Can Med Assoc J 1992; 147:420–428.
14. Carlson DJ, Ries AL, Kaplan RM: Prediction of maximum exercise tolerance in patients with COPD. Chest 1991; 100:307–311.
15. Casaburi R: Principles of exercise training. Chest 1992; 101(Suppl 5):263S–267S.
16. Casaburi R, Pastesio A, Loli F, et al: Reductions in exercise lactic acidosis and ventilation as a result of exercise training in patients with obstructive lung disease. Am Rev Respir Dis 1991; 143:9–18.
17. Celli B, Lee H, Criner G, et al: Controlled trial of external negative pressure ventilation in patients with severe chronic airflow obstruction. Am Rev Respir Dis 1989; 140:1251–1256.
18. Cervasini A, Satta A, Orienti S: Clinical and functional course of a group of patients with COPD under controlled medical-rehabilitative treatment over a 6-year period. Minerva Med 1987; 78:1849–1855.
19. Chawla JC: Rehabilitation of spinal cord injured patients on long term ventilation. Paraplegia 1993; 31:88–92.
20. Corriveau ML, Rosen BJ, Dolan GF: Exercise capacity following pulmonary rehabilitation in the elderly. Mo Med 1989; 86:751–756.
21. Couser JI Jr, Martinez FJ, Celli BR: Pulmonary rehabilitation that includes arm exercise reduces metabolic and ventilatory requirements for simple arm elevation. Chest 1993; 103:37–41.
22. Cox NH, Hendricks JC, Binkhorst RA, et al: A pulmonary rehabilitation program for patients with asthma and mild chronic obstructive pulmonary disease (COPD). Lung 1993; 171:235–244.
23. Curran FJ, Colbert AP: Ventilator management in Duchenne muscular dystrophy and post poliomyelitis syndrome: 12 years experience. Arch Phys Med Rehabil 1989; 70:180–185.
24. Dekhuijzen PN, Beek MM, Folgering HT, et al: Psychological changes during pulmonary rehabilitation and target-flow inspiratory muscle training in COPD patients with a ventilatory limitation during exercise. Int J Rehabil Res 1990; 13:109–117.
25. Dobelle WH, D'Angelo MS, Goetz BF, et al: 200 cases with a new breathing pacemaker dispel myths about diaphragm pacing. ASAIO J 1994; 40:M244–M252.
26. Edwards BG, Marsolais EB: Metabolic responses to arm ergometry and functional neuromuscular stimulation. J Rehabil Res Dev 1990; 27:107–114.
27. Egan TM, Westerman JH, Lambert CJ, et al: Isolated lung transplantation for end-stage lung disease: A viable therapy. Ann Thorac Surg 1992; 53:590–596.
28. Epstein SK, Celli BR: Cardiopulmonary exercise testing in patients with chronic obstructive pulmonary disease. Cleve Clin J Med 1993; 60:119–128.
29. End A, Grimm M, Mares P, et al: Successful lung transplantation in a long-term ventilator-dependent patient. Ann Thorac Surg 1993; 56:562–564.
30. Faling LJ: Pulmonary rehabilitation—physical modalities, Clin Chest Med 1986; 7:599–618.
31. Flavel H, Marshall R, Thorton A, et al: Hypoxia episodes during sleep in high tetraplegia. Arch Phys Med Rehabil 1992; 73:623–627.
32. Folden SL: Definitions of health and health goals of participants in a community-based pulmonary rehabilitation program. Public Health Nurs 1993; 10:31–35.
33. Foster S, Lopez D, Thomas HM: Pulmonary rehabilitation in COPD patients with elevated PCO_2. Am Rev Respir Dis 1988; 138:1519–1523.
34. Foster S, Thomas HM: Pulmonary rehabilitation in lung disease other than chronic obstructive pulmonary disease. Am Rev Respir Dis 1990; 141:601–604.
35. Franz MN, Cohn RC, Wachnowsky-Diakiw DM, et al: Management of children and adults with cystic fibrosis: One center's approach. Hosp Formul 1994; 29:364–378.
36. Gilgoff IS, Barras DM, Jones MS, et al: Neck breathing: A form of voluntary respiration for the spine-injured ventilator-dependent quadriplegic child. Pediatrics 1988; 82:741–745.
37. Gracey DK, Viggiano RW, Naessens JM, et al: Outcomes of patients admitted to a chronic ventilator-dependent unit in an acute care hospital. Mayo Clin Proc 1992; 67:131–136.
38. Haas F, Axen K (eds): Pulmonary Therapy and Rehabilitation. Principles and Practice, ed 2. Baltimore, Williams & Wilkins, 1991, pp 29–42.
39. Harrison GA, Davis PJ, Troughear RH, et al: Inspiratory speech as a management option for spastic dysphonia. Case study. Ann Otol Rhinol Laryngol 1992; 101:375–382.
40. Hodgkin JE: Organization of a pulmonary rehabilitation program. Clin Chest Med 1986; 7:599–618.
41. Hodgkin JG, Connors GL, Bell CW: Pulmonary Rehabilitation. Guidelines to Success, ed 2. Philadelphia, JB Lippincott, 1992, p xiii.
42. Holle RH, Williams DV, Vendree JC, et al: Increased muscle efficiency and sustained benefits in an outpatient community hospital-based pulmonary rehabilitation program. Chest 1988; 94:1161–1168.
43. Hornstein S, Inman S, Ledsome JH: Ventilatory muscle training in kyphoscoliosis. Spine 1987; 12:859–863.
44. Indihar FJ: A 10-year report of patients in a prolonged respiratory care unit. Minn Med 1991; 74:23–27.
45. Jackson, NC: Pulmonary rehabilitation for mechanically ventilated patients. Crit Care Nurs Clin North Am 1991; 3:591–600.

46. Jaeger R, Turba RM, Yarkony GM, et al: Cough in spinal cord injured patients: Comparison of three methods to produce cough. Arch Phys Med Rehabil 1993; 74:1358–1361.

47. Janelli LM, Scherer YK, Schmieder LL: Can a pulmonary health teaching program alter patients' ability to cope with COPD? Rehabil Nurs 1991; 16:199–202.

48. Kersten L: Changes in self concept during pulmonary rehabilitation, Part 1. Heart Lung 1990; 19:456–462.

49. Khaghani A, Banner N, Ozdogan E, et al: Medium-term results of combined heart and lung transplantation for emphysema. J Heart Lung Transplant 1991; 10:15–21.

50. Kirshblum SC, Bach JR: Walker modification for ventilator-assisted individuals. Case report. Am J Phys Med Rehabil 1992; 71:304–306.

51. Koch SJ, Arego DE, Bowser B: Outpatient rehabilitation for chronic neuromuscular diseases. Am J Phys Med 1986; 65:245–257.

52. Krieger AJ, Gropper MR, Adler RJ: Electrophrenic respiration after intercostal to phrenic nerve anastomosis in a patient with anterior spinal artery syndrome: Technical case report. Neurosurgery 1994, vol 35.

53. Lamid S, Ragalie GF, Welter K: Respirator-dependent quadriplegics: Problems during the weaning period. J Am Paraplegia Soc 1985; 8:33–37.

54. Lerman RM, Weiss MS: Progressive resistive exercise in weaning high quadriplegics from the ventilator. Paraplegia 1987; 25:130–135.

55. Mahlmeister MJ, Fink JB, Hoffman GL, et al: Positive-expiratory-pressure mask therapy: Theoretical and practical considerations and a review of the literature. Respir Care 1991; 36:1218–1229.

56. Make BJ: Mechanical ventilation in the home: Summary of the Third International Conference on Pulmonary Rehabilitation and Home Mechanical Ventilation. Neuromuscular Disord 1991; 1:229–230.

57. Mall RW, Medeiros M: Objective evaluation of results of a pulmonary rehabilitation program in a community hospital. Chest 1988; 94:1156–1160.

58. Marchman HB, Skolnick JL: Blood pressure changes in patients with chronic obstructive pulmonary disease and hypertension completing phase II pulmonary rehabilitation. J Ky Med Assoc 1992; 90:503–505.

59. Martinez FJ, Vogel PD, Dupont DN, et al: Supported arm exercise vs unsupported arm exercise in the rehabilitation of patients with severe chronic airflow obstruction. Chest 1993; 103:1397–1402.

60. Mason M: Speech Pathology for Tracheostomized and Ventilator Dependent Patients. Newport Beach, Calif, Voicing 1993.

61. Mlynarek M, Zarowitz BJ: Individualizing nutrition in patients with acute respiratory failure requiring mechanical ventilation. Drug Intell Clin Pharm 1987; 21:865–870.

62. Moss M, Make BJ: Pulmonary response to exercise in health and disease. Semin Respir Med 1993; 14:106–120.

63. Noseda A, Carpiaux JP, Prigogine T, et al: Lung function, maximum and sub-maximum exercise testing in COPD patients: Reproducibility over a long interval. Lung 1989; 167:24.

64. Ojanen M, Lahdensuo A, Laitinen J, et al: Psychosocial changes in patients participating in a chronic obstructive pulmonary disease rehabilitation program. Respiration 1993; 60:96–102.

65. Olesen KM, Hiller FC: Management of tetanus. Clin Pharm 1987;6:570–574.

66. Olopade CO, Beck KC, Viggiano RW, et al: Exercise limitation and pulmonary rehabilitation in chronic obstructive pulmonary disease. Mayo Clin Proc 1992; 67:144–157.

67. Patessio A, Carone M, Loli F, et al: Ventilatory and metabolic changes as a result of exercise training in COPD patients. Chest 1992; 101:274S–278S.

68. Refsum HE, Naess-Anderson CF, Lange JE: Pulmonary function and gas exchange at rest and exercise in adolescent girls with mild idiopathic scoliosis during treatment with Boston thoracic brace. Spine 1990; 15:420–423.

69. Rogers TK, Howard P: Pulmonary hemodynamics and physical training in patients with chronic obstructive pulmonary disease. Chest 1992; 101(suppl 5):289S–292S.

70. Roye WP Jr, Dunn EL, Moody JA: Cervical spinal cord injury—a public catastrophe. J Trauma 1988; 28:1260–1264.

71. Schols AM, Mostert R, Soeters PB, et al: Body composition and exercise performance in patients with chronic obstructive pulmonary disease. Thorax 1991; 46:695–699.

72. Schols AM, Soeters PB, Dingemans AM, et al: Prevalence and characteristics of nutritional depletion in patients with stable COPD eligible for pulmonary rehabilitation. Am Rev Respir Dis 1993; 147:1151–1156.

73. Seiser A, Schwartz S, Brainin M: Critical illness polyneuropathy: Clinical aspects and long-term outcome. Wien Klin Wochenschr 1992; 104:294–300.

74. Sivak ED: Management of ventilator dependency following heart surgery. Semin Thorac Cardiovasc Surg 1991; 3:53–62.

75. Speier J, Owen RR, Knapp M, et al: Occurrence of post-polio sequelae in an epidemic population. Research and clinical aspects of the late effects of poliomyelitis. 1987; 23:39–48.

76. Stulbarg MS, Winn WR, Kellett LE: Bilateral carotid body resection for the relief of dyspnea in severe chronic obstructive pulmonary disease. Physiologic and clinical observations in three patients. Chest 1989; 95:1123–1128.

77. Tiep BL: Long-term home oxygen therapy. Clin Chest Med 1990; 11:505–521.

78. Tiep BL: Reversing disability of irreversible lung disease. West J Med 1991; 154:591–597.

79. Tobin MJ: Current concepts: Mechanical ventilation. N Engl J Med 1994; 330:1056–1061.

80. Vale F, Reardon JZ, Zu-Wallack RL: The long-term benefits of outpatient pulmonary rehabilitation on exercise endurance and quality of life. Chest 1993; 103:42–45.

81. Van-der-Schoot TA, Kaptein AA: Pulmonary rehabilitation in an asthma clinic. Lung 1990; 168(suppl):495–501.

82. Varray A, Mercier J, Savy-Pacaux AM, et al: Cardiac role in exercise limitation in asthmatic subjects with special reference to disease severity. Eur Respir J 1993; 6:1011–1017.

83. Wade B: Key concerns for a safe trip. The New York Times, Jan 9, 1994, p 4.

84. Walker J, Cooney M, Norton S: Improved pulmonary function in chronic quadriplegics after pulmonary therapy and arm ergometry. Paraplegia 1989; 27:278–283.

85. Whitman J, Van Beusekom R, Olson S, et al: Preliminary evaluation of high-frequency chest compression for secretion clearance in mechanically ventilated patients. Respir Care 1993; 38:1081–1087.

86. Wolf SI, Lampl KL: Pulmonary rehabilitation: The use of aerobic dance as a therapeutic exercise for asthmatic patients. Ann Allergy 1988; 61:357–360.

87. Zu-Wallack RL, Patel K, Reardon JZ, et al: Predictors of improvement in the 12-minute walking distance following a six-week outpatient pulmonary rehabilitation program. Chest 1991; 99:805–808.

Deconditioning, Conditioning, and the Benefits of Exercise

RALPH M. BUSCHBACHER, M.D.

It has been recognized since civilization began that exercise is good for the body, whereas inactivity promotes its decline. Perhaps Maimonides said it best in his *Treatise of Hygiene* in AD 1199: "Anyone who lives a sedentary life and does not exercise, even if he eats good foods and takes care of himself according to proper medical principles—all his days will be painful ones and his strength shall wane." Physicians from ancient Greece to China to medieval Europe all espoused one form of exercise or another to treat and prevent illness and infirmity. This belief was not just held by physicians but was also the province of poets and philosophers. As John Dryden wrote: "Better to hunt in fields, for health unbought,/Than fee the doctor for a nauseous draught./The wise, for cure, on exercise depend;/God never made his work, for man to mend."

Yet somehow, in the mid- to late-1800s and earlier in this century, medicine turned its back on promoting activity and began recommending long periods of bed rest and immobilization for a variety of disorders. Hugh Owen Thomas and John Hunter were among the first to recommend (per Thomas) "enforced, uninterrupted, and prolonged" rest,[61] and in 1863 John Hilton published his book, *On the Influence of Mechanical and Physiological Rest in the Treatment of Accidents and Surgical Diseases, and of the Diagnostic Value of Pain.*[78] In it he described a series of cases successfully treated with enforced rest. Eventually, his work went through six editions and numerous printings. And although he did not see rest as a panacea, his teachings were misunderstood and misapplied and influenced several generations of physicians to view bed rest as a desirable treatment, rather than an occasionally necessary evil.

In various medical specialties, particularly in obstetrics and gynecology and in surgery, prolonged bed rest became a mainstay of treatment. It was once considered routine to prescribe a week or more of bed rest after simple back strain. When White and colleagues[166] and Mallory and others[109] noted that it took approximately 8 weeks for large myocardial infarctions to heal (5 weeks for small infarcts), they recommended at least 1 month of bed rest (2 weeks absolute) followed by 1 month of limited activity after infarction. At least 3 weeks of bed rest was advocated for even the smallest infarcts.

Clearly, much has changed since this method of treatment was considered routine. Through the pioneering efforts of Cuthbertson,[41] Dietrick and others,[45] Saltin and co-workers[135], Taylor and colleagues,[158] and many others, we have come to understand the deleterious effects of immobility. In addition, the space program has provided much information about the effects of bed rest, immobilization, and weightlessness. One by one, the outdated tenets of the past have been refuted, and today exercise is viewed as a positive mode of treatment, while bed rest is a negative. Yet even today misperceptions abound in the lay press. In a recent *U.S. News & World Report* article it was stated that "While prolonged bed rest can cause emotional and financial hardships, it doesn't have the side effects that drugs do. So doctors have believed that at least bed rest does no harm. . . ."[132]

This chapter explores the fundamental physiological changes that occur with deconditioning and examines the benefits of exercise. *Deconditioning* as a rehabilitation diagnosis is also discussed.

Many of the data presented here are the result of research in the space program. As the effects of weightlessness may not be directly applicable to the person on bed rest, every effort has been made to cite the most clinically useful references. Similarly, much of the information on the consequences of immobility, especially at the cellular level, comes from animal studies. Again, where possible, the emphasis is on appropriate human models.

CONSEQUENCES OF DISUSE

The functional capacity of the body and of the body organs depends on the previous stresses placed on the body and its organs. Within certain physiological limits the body can be trained to be stronger, quicker, more conditioned, and fit. It can also be "trained" to deteriorate. The physiological maximum potential is the upper limit on function. It cannot be altered through activity or use. With age, illness, and injury this maximal limit may decline, but this does not necessarily have to lead to a corresponding decline in functional ability. As depicted in Figure 34–1, most persons operate at a level well below their maximum. With training they can move closer to this limit. With disuse they move farther away. But as long as the limit is not lowered excessively, the person can maintain and even increase function. Thus we see persons who have had myocardial infarctions who started training afterward and who are now "in the best shape of their lives."

Obviously, such a scenario is not realistic in all cases, but in rehabilitation we strive to maximize function. Even if the physiological maximum is decreased, the person will be better off if operating at or near this (lowered) limit (see Fig. 34–1).

Bed rest, immobilization, or relative rest is unfortunately necessary in some situations. These include some acute injuries, especially fractures and dislocations, acute myo-

cardial infarction or pulmonary disease, and severe medical or surgical disorders. Yet even when rest is properly prescribed, we should be aware of its deleterious effects. The consequences of such disuse on the body organs and systems are described below (Table 34–1).

The Musculoskeletal System

The primary functions of the musculoskeletal system are to support the body, to transport the body, and to use the body to accomplish physical tasks. Obviously, it is affected by both activity and inactivity, and disorders of the system in turn affect the activity level that is possible.

Muscles

Disuse leads to muscle weakness. In the classic studies by Mueller,[121] the muscles of persons on strict bed rest lost approximately 1.0% to 1.5% of their initial strength (torque about a joint) per day (over a 2-week period with a sampling of 17 muscles tested). With cast immobilization of the upper extremity, 1.3% to 5.5% of strength was lost per day, again, over a 2-week period.[121] This corresponds to an approximately 10% to 20% loss of strength per week for

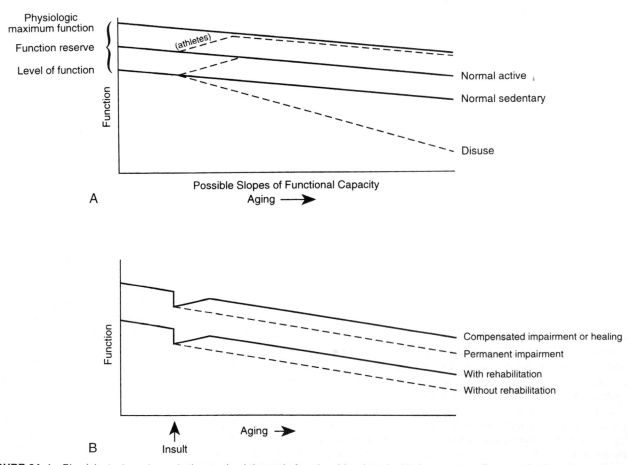

FIGURE 34–1 Physiological maximum is the maximal theoretic functional level attainable by a person. For most body systems, this value decreases somewhat with age. *A*, Athletes operate near their physiological maximum. Normal sedentary persons operate at a level below that of the normal active individual through exercise or disuse. It is possible to change the slope of the line representing a given person's physiological maximum. This will affect function regardless of the maximal attainable level. *B*, When a body system (or the whole body) sustains an insult its level of function is lowered. This might lead to a permanent impairment *(top dotted line)*. If the insult is healed or compensated for, the previous functional level can be regained. The *lines below* indicate that rehabilitation may raise a person's capacity back to the higher level. However, prolonged inactivity may permanently alter the maximum physiological potential that can be obtained.

TABLE 34–1   Major Complications of Immobility by Body System

Musculoskeletal
  Muscles
    Atrophy; decreased strength and endurance
    Contracture
    Altered electrical activity/excitation
    Weakened myotendinous junction
    Contractures
    Decreased strength of tendons and ligaments and their
      insertions on bone
  Bone
    Osteoporosis
  Joints
    Cartilage degeneration
    Fibrofatty tissue infiltration
    Synovial atrophy
    Ankylosis
Cardiovascular
  Cardiac (at rest)
    ↑ Heart rate
    ↓ Stroke volume
  Cardiac output unchanged or slightly decreased
    $\dot{V}O_2$ unchanged
    ↓ Cardiac size/volume
    ↓ Left ventricular end-diastolic volume
  Systolic/diastolic blood pressure unchanged
  Arteriovenous oxygen difference unchanged or slightly
    increased
  Cardiac (with exercise)
    ↑ Heart rate response to submaximal exercise
    Maximum heart rate unchanged
    ↓ $\dot{V}O_2$ max
    ↓ Stroke volume (submaximal/maximal)
    ↓ Cardiac output (submaximal/maximal)
    ↑ Arteriovenous oxygen difference (submaximal) (maximal is
      unchanged)
  Neurovascular
    Orthostatic intolerance
  Fluid balance
    ↓ Plasma volume
    ↓ Total blood volume
    ↓ Red blood cell mass
    Mineral and plasma protein loss (mainly isocontent)
  Blood coagulation
    ↑ Venous thrombosis
    ↓ Calf blood flow (possible)
    ↑ Blood fibrinogen
Skin
  Pressure ulcer
  Edema
  Subcutaneous bursitis

Body Composition, Metabolism, Nutrition
  ↓ Lean body mass
  ↑ Body fat
  Minerals
    Nitrogen loss
    Calcium loss
    Phosphorus loss
    Sulfur loss
    Potassium loss
Endocrine
  Impaired glucose tolerance
  Altered circadian rhythm
  Altered temperature and sweating response
  Altered regulation of parathyroid hormone, thyroid hormones,
    adrenal hormones, pituitary hormones, growth hormone,
    androgens, and plasma renin activity
Respiratory
  ↑ Forced vital capacity
  ↑ Total lung capacity (slight)
  Residual volume unchanged
  Functional residual capacity unchanged
  ↑ Respiratory rate
  Vital capacity unchanged (possibly decreases in time owing to
    contractures of chest wall)
  Maximal minute ventilation unchanged
  Possible ventilation/perfusion mismatch
  Pulmonary embolism (possible)
Genitourinary
  Diuresis
  ↑ Mineral excretion
  Difficulty voiding
  ↑ Postvoid residual volume (possible)
  ↑ Urinary tract infection (possible)
  ↑ Overflow incontinence (possible)
  ↑ Calculus formation (possible)
  ↓ Glomerular filtration rate
  ↓ Ability to concentrate urine
Gastrointestinal
  ↓ Fluid intake
  ↓ Appetite
  ↓ Bowel motility
  ↓ Gastric secretion
  Constipation (possible)
Neurological, Emotional
  Compression neuropathies
  Sensory deprivation (attention span, altered time awareness,
    hand-to-eye coordination, depression, anxiety)
  ↓ Balance
  ↓ Coordination
  Sleep disturbance
  ↑ Auditory threshold
  ↓ Visual acuity

Abbreviations: $\dot{V}O_2$, oxygen consumption; $\dot{V}O_2$ max, maximum oxygen consumption.

most persons. The loss was greatest during the first week of inactivity and gradually plateaued at a 25% loss.[121] In other studies of immobilization, up to a 40% loss of strength has been recorded.[108] In a compilation of data from other studies Greenleaf et al.[67] concluded that there is a loss of approximately 0.7% of strength per day. Mueller's studies (and most others) were performed by testing isometric strength, and this may not be as functionally relevant as other methods of testing strength and endurance. In addition, the generalizability of his results is limited because loss of strength may be different in previously sedentary vs. trained subjects.

Loss of strength varies among muscle groups. In a classic study by Dietrick et al.[45] healthy volunteers were placed on bed rest in bivalved casts from the umbilicus to the toes, with a 30- to 40-min break per day. They were immobilized in this fashion for 6 to 7 weeks. On average, the subjects lost 6.6% of their elbow flexor strength, 8.7% of their shoulder flexor strength, 13.3% of their dorsiflexor strength, and 20.8% of their plantar flexor strength. They experienced approximately a 2% loss of girth in the upper arms and forearms. Thigh circumference decreased between 2.1% and 5%, and calf circumference decreased between 5.5% and 6.3%. This corresponded to a loss of cross-sectional area of 4.2% to 10% in the thighs and 9.7% to 12.5% in the calves, a loss attributed primarily to atrophy of muscle tissue (Fig. 34–2). In more recent studies measuring muscle circumference, 1 month of bed rest caused

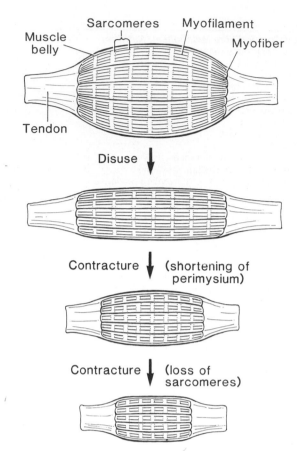

FIGURE 34–2 Progression of muscle atrophy and contracture. In early disuse, a loss of muscle mass occurs through a reduction in myofilaments (muscle cross-section). The total number of myofibers (muscle cells) is unchanged, and sarcomere number remains constant. With contracture, however, a shortening of the perimysial connective tissue, and later a loss of sarcomeres (in series), occurs.

an approximate 8% to 13% loss of cross-sectional area of selected leg muscles measured by magnetic resonance imaging[17] and quadriceps cross-sectional area declined by 27% with 4 weeks of cast immobilization as measured by computed tomography (CT).[162] Such atrophy is not necessarily to be viewed as an abnormal response. In fact, it is most likely a normal reaction to an activity level that does not require the tissues to be present; the body does not needlessly support redundant tissues.

Antigravity muscles, such as the gastrocnemius-soleus and the back muscles, appear to lose strength disproportionately, and large muscles seem to lose strength twice as quickly as smaller ones.[67] Handgrip strength is not affected by prolonged bed rest,[67, 158] though grip endurance does seem to be reduced.[67] The loss of strength may vary with different speeds of muscle contraction.[10]

It is commonly reported that type I, slow-twitch muscle fibers are more subject to immobilization atrophy than are type II, fast-twitch fibers.[10] Many of the data supporting this contention come from animal studies. Animals often have a more homogeneous fiber-type preponderance in various muscles than do humans, and these observations may not be directly applicable to humans. Nevertheless, it appears that in muscles that have been trained to have a relatively high cross-sectional area of type I fibers (such as

the antigravity muscles predominantly affected by disuse) atrophy may selectively affect these fibers.[73, 89] This preferential atrophy is most likely influenced by the location and function of the involved muscles.[77] The affected fibers degenerate and develop an increased noncontractile connective tissue content.[77, 115] The total number of fibers is unchanged.[29, 123]

Muscle fiber atrophy has been shown to begin after as little as 1 day of immobilization,[115] and in rats there are signs of decreased protein synthesis within only 6 hours.[22] Positioning is important in the development of atrophy, at least in animal studies. Stretching of the muscles seems to delay the atrophy (and may even cause growth), whereas immobilization in a shortened position promotes a more rapid deterioration (primarily due to a loss of muscle length).[11, 76, 83, 147] Immobilization has been shown to cause changes in muscle electrical activity[49] and in the myoneural junction.[125] There is also a decrease in strength of the myotendinous junction.[87]

There may be some protective effect of training before immobilization,[10, 67, 88] especially in untrained persons. Trained subjects, however, lose the most absolute muscle strength when they are immobilized.[10]

After remobilization, it may take two or more times the period of immobilization to recover muscle strength.[79] In some cases, residual deficits from a period of disuse have lasted for months or years, especially after injury or surgery.[69, 133] Consequently, it is desirable, when possible, to prevent the disuse weakening from developing. Muscle strength can be maintained by performing daily muscle contractions, though the type and amount of exercise are not known. Hettinger showed that isometric muscle strength can be maintained by performing daily isometric contractions of 10% to 20% of maximal tension for 10 sec.[121] His subjects were placed in bivalved arm casts and were otherwise free to go about their daily activities. Undoubtedly they experienced a training effect from incidental activity, and it is difficult to generalize his results to persons on bed rest. It is also unclear exactly what isotonic or isokinetic exercise is required to prevent a decline in function. Therefore, it is advisable to maintain as near normal activity as possible, even during periods of immobilization or hospitalization. In patients with casts, muscle contraction within the cast, either voluntary or through electrical stimulation, may also be beneficial.

Periarticular Soft Tissues

Contracture is an abnormal limitation of passive joint range of motion. It is usually due to a restriction of the periarticular connective tissue, but in more advanced cases also involves tendons, ligaments, muscles, and joints. If not treated, it can lead to bony ankylosis of the joint. While there are many possible causes of contractures (Table 34–2), the primary cause (and the one pertinent to this chapter) is lack of normal joint mobilization. Joints must periodically be put through their full range of motion to prevent a tightening of the surrounding soft tissues and muscles.

Ordinarily, the mobile tissues of the body are separated by thin layers of loose areolar connective tissue. This allows tendons, ligaments, muscles, and joint capsules to glide on one another during normal motion. With immobili-

TABLE 34–2   Major Causes of Joint Contracture

Muscular
    Muscle strength imbalance
    Neuromuscular disease
    Burn tracts
    Degenerative disease
    Inflammation
    Trauma
Skin, soft tissues
    Scleroderma
    Scar
    Burns
Joints
    Connective tissue disease
    Pain
    Inflammation
    Congenital disorders
    Sepsis
    Ankylosis

zation, the loose connective tissue is reorganized and is replaced by more dense material which contains a greater abundance of collagen cross-links (the type of collagen is probably unchanged).[2, 6, 52] This process can begin after as little as 1 week of immobilization[95] and is aggravated in conditions of increased collagen turnover. It is complemented by an active fibroblast-mediated contraction within these tissues.[170] It is also believed to be accelerated in the presence of superimposed local trauma, hemorrhage, impaired circulation, pre-existing degeneration, or edema.[94] Once the other soft tissues have become involved in contracture formation, the muscles may become shortened as well (see Fig. 34–2).

In the early phase of this muscular shortening, the primary contribution to the loss of length comes from the intrinsic muscle-supporting tissues, mainly the perimysium.[169] Only later does actual muscle fiber shortening occur. When it does occur, it is due to a loss of sarcomere number (in series),[11, 147, 168] mainly at the ends of the muscle fibers.[11]

As the affected body part loses normal range of motion, other parts of the body must compensate for the loss. This leads to increased stress on adjacent and distant joints.

Increased energy expenditure due to abnormal biomechanics may lead to even more immobility. Ultimately, function is lost. In addition, the abnormal range of motion makes the nursing care of bedridden patients more difficult.

A number of conditions predispose patients to contractures. Spasticity, paralysis, or muscle strength imbalance hastens the development of contractures. Amputees tend to develop contractures, mainly because of position and strength imbalances. The below-knee amputee, for instance, often sits with the knee flexed. This leads to a hip and knee flexion contracture. The above-knee amputee loses strength of the hip adductors, some of which insert below the knee. This can lead to a fixed hip flexion and abduction deformity.

In conditions of joint pain and inflammation, the patient tends to position the joint in the least painful position (to minimize intra-articular pressure). The most common such positions are flexion and external rotation of the hip, flexion of the fingers and knees, and plantar flexion of the ankles. Similar positions are taken by patients on bed rest (Fig. 34–3). They also tend to position the shoulders in internal rotation. Common joint contractures and their sequelae are described in Table 34–3.

Inactive persons, whether ill and bedridden, or sedentary by choice, eventually develop contractures. These may be mild and seemingly insignificant, but often affect the ability to reach, to take long strides, to comb one's hair, etc.

Contractures are likely to affect muscles that cross multiple joints, because stretching of only one joint or the other may not adequately stretch the entire muscle. Where and how contractures develop depend on the position of the joint and the length of time that position is maintained (as well as predisposing factors). They may be precipitated by painful conditions. For instance, a "frozen shoulder," in which the inferior axillary fold of the joint capsule is lost, often follows tendinitis, surgery, or trauma. The shoulder is particularly susceptible to loss of range of motion because of its normally great mobility. The only major contracture with little functional disability is a mild-to-moderate elbow flexion contracture. Contractures of this joint are maintained in a position of function, such as for eating.

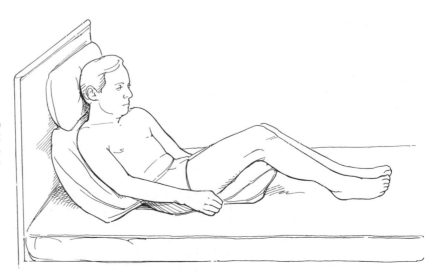

FIGURE 34–3 Common bed position and the areas susceptible to contracture: neck, flexed; shoulders, internally rotated; thorax, flexed; arms, flexed; forearms, supinated; fingers, flexed; hips, flexed; knees, flexed; and ankles, plantar flexed.

TABLE 34–3 Common Joint Contractures and Their Sequelae

Contracture	Sequelae
Hip joint flexion	Compensatory lordosis (back pain), knee flexion, short steps
Hip joint external rotation	Stiff-legged gait, excessive stress on medial knee ligaments
Knee flexion	Plantar flexion (toe-walking), crouch gait
Ankle plantar flexion	Genu recurvatum, absence of heel-strike
Shoulder flexion, adduction, and internal rotation	Cannot reach back pocket, comb hair, or reach above shoulder level
Elbow flexion	If mild, little function loss; if severe, interferes with dressing, weakens triceps position
Wrist flexion	Weakened grip
Finger flexion	Cannot open hand to grasp

TABLE 34–4 Progression of Treatment of Contractures From Least to Most Aggressive Methods

Proper positioning
Active range-of-motion exercise
Active-assisted range-of-motion exercise
Passive range-of-motion exercise
Static splinting
Dynamic splinting
Nerve/motor point blocks
Serial casting
Surgery

Elbow extension contractures are actually more limiting than flexion contractures (Fig. 34–4).

It is not clear how often the soft tissues must be passed through a complete range of motion to prevent contracture. Normal living and motion cause compound motions that most likely stretch nearly all parts of the body multiple times a day. It is commonly believed that contractures can be prevented by daily or twice-daily range-of-motion exercise. This is especially important in the hospitalized patient, in the elderly, and in arthritic joints, which are believed to develop contractures relatively rapidly.

In the presence of risk factors predisposing to contractures (such as muscle strength imbalances or paralysis), proper positioning and possibly intermittent splinting (or dynamic splinting) may be necessary. Too soft a bed may aggravate abnormal positioning and should be avoided. It is important for patients to occasionally lie prone, especially to stretch the hip joint. However, even lying prone may not stretch this joint adequately, so a pillow under the knees while in the prone position may be advisable, especially in persons who are sitting or lying for prolonged periods of time. Standing upright is also an effective stretch of the anterior hip, as well as of the posterior knee. In bed, pillows or trochanteric rolls applied to the lateral surfaces of the thighs may help prevent external rotation deformity of the legs. Proper active dorsiflexion exercise and possibly a footboard may help prevent plantar flexion contractures.

Once contractures have developed, they are treated with range-of-motion exercise (Table 34–4). Voluntary active range-of-motion exercise is preferred, but in some cases assisted range-of-motion exercise is needed. When stretching a contracted area, it is important to make sure that there is no bony block or other mechanical limitation to

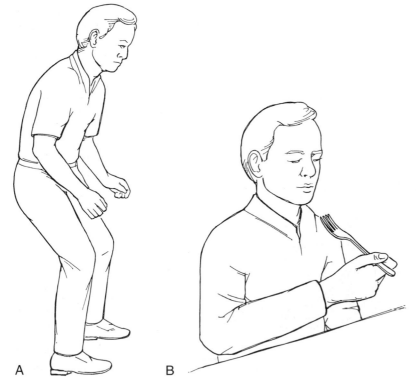

A   B

FIGURE 34–4 Similar contractures of knee *(A)*, and elbow *(B)* cause vastly different functional outcomes. In fact, the elbow contracture might be virtually unnoticed.

TABLE 34–5 Mechanical Limitations to Joint Range of Motion Which May Be Contraindications to Stretching

Bony block
Cartilage damage
Loose body in joint
Joint incongruity
Synovial thickening
Severe bony degenerative disease
Fracture
Dislocation

motion (Table 34–5). If such a condition is present, it may be a contraindication to range-of-motion exercise. In addition, it is important not to be overly aggressive when stretching. If the tissues are torn and damaged during stretching, they are more likely to develop an even thicker connective tissue barrier to normal mobility. Overly aggressive stretching may also lead to joint dislocation or damage, especially in the knee or elbow.

When manual stretching is inadequate, or in cases of advanced contractures, deep heating to the involved connective tissue may help increase range of motion.[165] In some cases, motor point or nerve blocks may be used to weaken an overpowering muscle imbalance. (This also helps to differentiate a true contracture from abnormal tone or spasticity.) In refractory cases, serial casting may be necessary. The joint is stretched maximally and a cast is applied. The process is repeated, with a cast change every 2 to 3 days to progressively stretch the connective tissues. Care must be taken not to cause pressure sores to the skin or circulatory compromise to the limb when performing the casting. If such casting still does not reduce the contracture, surgical treatment may be necessary. This may include capsular release, tenotomy, or tendon-lengthening procedures. In conditions of muscle strength imbalance, tendon transfer may be indicated as well. (Also, in conditions of muscle imbalance, strengthening of the weak muscles may be helpful.) Postsurgical contractures can often be prevented by using continuous passive range-of-motion machines.

Ligaments and Tendons

Ligaments and tendons are composed primarily of longitudinally arranged, parallel, type I collagen fibers. This gives them great strength in the direction of pull. This parallel alignment of collagen fibers is fostered by longitudinal stress applied to these connective tissues. When this stress is lacking, as during immobilization, the newly formed collagen is laid down in a haphazard array (Fig. 34–5) and the function of the structures deteriorates.[7] Immobilization causes an increase in collagen turnover,[7] a decrease in collagen mass,[2] a decrease in glycosaminoglycan and water content,[3] an increase in soft tissue stiffness,[124] and an alteration in fibroblast function.[122] In addition to a deterioration of the soft tissues themselves, there is also a loss of strength at the collagen-bone interface, with bone resorption directly below the insertion site.[91, 99, 124]

As stated earlier, longitudinal stress is required to achieve proper collagen orientation.[7] Even in the absence of weightbearing stress in the joint, movement may prevent soft tissue deterioration, although bone atrophy is not necessarily retarded.[91] It is important to continue to stress the tendons and ligaments in all persons, both healthy and ill, and as soon as is clinically feasible, in those recovering from injury or surgery. Ligaments have been shown, in a primate model, to lose up to one third of their strength in just 8 weeks of immobilization.[124] Once weakness of these tissues has developed, it takes months to years to recover.[1, 124]

Bones

Bone is normally in a state of dynamic equilibrium in which the rate of bone formation and resorption is held in balance. The ratio of formation to resorption is influenced by the stresses that the bone is subject to, in what is commonly known as Wolff's law. Weightbearing is the primary stress on most of the bones of the body, and it causes a buildup of bone. Other stressful activities in which the pull of muscles stresses the bone also increase bone mass.

Lack of stress on the bones leads to a predominance of bone resorption (osteoclastic activity), which decreases bone mass and causes osteoporosis (see Chapter 40 on osteoporosis). In rats this loss of bone mass may start to occur in as little as 30 hours after immobilization.[159] The rate of loss of bone varies with the type of disuse and by body part, with weightbearing bones being relatively more affected. During bed rest there may be an almost 1% loss

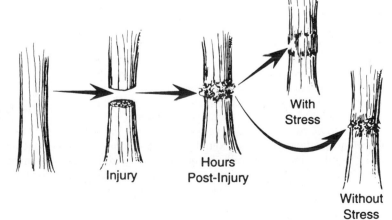

FIGURE 34–5 Normal recovery progression of a tendon after laceration. If the tendon is not stressed, the collagen scar remains unorganized instead of the fibers being arranged in parallel. Similar haphazard collagen orientation is promoted through immobilization, though weakening is not as rapid or dramatic. (From Buschbacher RM: Tissue injury and healing. *In* Buschbacher RM (ed): Musculoskeletal Disorders: A Practical Guide for Diagnosis and Rehabilitation. Stoneham, Mass, Butterworth Heinemann, 1994, p 21.)

With
Stress

Injury

Hours
Post-Injury

Without
Stress

of vertebral mineral content per week.[98, 102] With immobilization, the bone mass generally drops until it plateaus at approximately 50% of the original mass in animal models.[105, 160] In human studies of the calcaneus, losses of 25% to 45% have been documented after 30 to 36 weeks of bed rest.[48] There is a loss of 4.2% of total body calcium during this same time period.[48] The remaining bone is histologically normal, with a normal ratio of mineral to matrix, although the organization of the bone may be altered. The bone is less massive.

In addition to generalized osteoporosis, there can also be local bone loss in conditions of partial immobilization, as after casting of fractures. In persons with paralysis, osteoporosis is often severe, and fractures can occur with relatively untraumatic events such as transfer activities.

Osteoporosis is a slowly advancing disease which may show little or no outward sign of its progression until pathological fractures occur. It is not easily diagnosed radiographically, since a large loss of bone is required before it can be detected on plain films. In the early stages, special bone density measurement techniques, such as photon absorptiometry or CT scanning,[105] are needed to make the diagnosis. It commonly affects trabecular bone more than cortical bone in the early stages; later, cortical bone loss occurs as well, especially in the midcortical layer.[171]

Osteoporosis is best treated with preventive measures such as active weightbearing exercise and active muscle contraction. Exercise in bed, even if intense, may not be effective in preventing or treating the disorder.[117] In women postmenopausal estrogen supplementation is also an option, and proper calcium intake is important as well.

Proper exercise is also advocated once osteoporosis has developed (after any fractures have healed). If the osteoporosis is related to a short duration (less than 3–6 months) of immobilization, as for casting of a fracture, it is likely to be reversed nearly completely. Longer-standing disuse osteoporosis, or that due to years of sedentary living, is not as easily reversed.[117] In a study of primates immobilized for 7 months, there was evidence of renewed bone formation after 2 months of resumption of activity. Normal bone formation was seen after 6 months, but it was thought that the trabecular bone would never completely recover its normal architecture.[173] While exercise may not reverse the bone loss that has already occurred, it will slow the progression of the disorder.[98]

Immobilization hypercalcemia is a condition often associated with osteoporosis, especially in adolescent males who have had traumatic injuries. As their bones are resorbed, serum calcium levels rise. They may become symptomatic, usually 2 to 4 weeks after the immobilization began. Signs and symptoms include nausea, vomiting, abdominal pain, lethargy, muscle weakness, and anorexia. If not treated, death may occur. Treatment is with intravenous furosemide and hydration. Etidronate disodium and calcitonin may be used as well, especially in refractory cases.[114]

Heterotopic ossification is a condition of bone growth in abnormal locations, usually around joints. It is not caused by immobility, but is generally found in persons who have experienced trauma. The trauma can be neurological (such as spinal cord injury) or a direct muscle contusion. Thus it may be seen in persons immobilized because of other injuries.

Joints

During embryonic development joints are formed in response to movement. Little wonder, then, that movement is required to maintain their integrity.

The hyaline cartilage in synovial joints is not supplied by vascular blood flow. It receives its nutrition from the synovial fluid by a regular loading and unloading of pressure, which draws fluid into and out of the cartilage in a process known as imbibition. During immobilization imbibition ceases, and the cartilage is dependent on simple diffusion to obtain nutrients. This diffusion is not adequate to the needs of the cartilage and the joints begin to deteriorate.

Immobilization-induced cartilage degeneration affects both the opposing joint surfaces that are in contact with each other and those that are not. The areas in contact develop pressure necrosis and erosions.[51] The noncontact surfaces develop fissures and lose their smoothness[1, 86] (Fig. 34–6). Proteoglycan balance is altered,[16] and the cartilage becomes stiffer. As the joints attempt to repair themselves, there is a compensatory cartilage proliferation and osteophyte formation.[51] In addition, there is a fibrofatty infiltration of the joint cavity, and the synovium becomes atrophic. There is deterioration of the subchondral bone as well.[145] This is accompanied by extra-articular connective tissue contracture, which exacerbates the condition,[51] and can eventually lead to ankylosis.

These changes can occur in some joints, not only with cast immobilization but also when weightbearing is restricted.[127] As little as 2 weeks of immobilization begins the process, at least in rabbits.[55] The cause of the joint changes is believed to be an attempt to repair tissues damaged by inadequate nutrition.[51] In the early stages this degeneration may be reversible to some extent[126]; later it most likely is not.

Nevertheless, in some arthritic conditions a short period of joint immobilization is indicated and may help to reduce synovitis and pain caused by even passive range-of-motion exercise.[113] Such short-term immobilization may, however, worsen cartilage destruction,[161] and, as a rule, should be kept to a minimum.

Patients with paralysis sometimes develop knee joint effusions of unknown cause. This has been termed "benign knee joint effusion of paralysis," and is seen predominantly in persons with spinal cord injury. It may also occur in Guillain-Barré syndrome and neuromuscular diseases.[27] It has been hypothesized that these effusions are due to inadequate muscular control of the intra-articular knee joint structures, namely the meniscus and the plica. As passive range-of-motion exercise is performed, these structures are irritated and cause an effusion; thus the cause is not true immobilization but rather muscle weakness.

The Cardiovascular System

Disuse (especially bed rest) causes a number of cardiovascular adaptations that are generally deleterious. These adaptations include (1) cardiac deconditioning, (2) an impaired response to the upright position (neurovascular deconditioning), (3) changes in fluid balance, and (4) decreased ability to prevent venous thrombosis. In general, long-term inactivity is comparable to hypertension, smok-

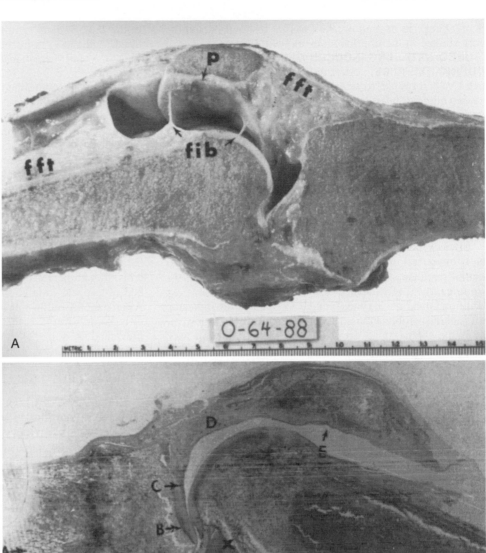

FIGURE 34–6 Cartilage degeneration with immobilization. The knees were obtained from human subjects whose knees had been immobilized and who later underwent proximal amputation. *A,* Sagittal section demonstrates fibrofatty tissue *(fft)* filling the inferior portion of the joint cavity. Fibrous septa *(fib)* extend from the femoral condyle to the patella. The articular cartilage of the patella *(p)* is irregular. *B,* There is a fibrofatty infiltration from the inferior fat pad *(D)* covering the distal pole of the patella. This has become adherent to the articular surface of the tibia *(C).* Fibrofatty tissue from the suprapatellar pouch covers the proximal patella. The posterior cruciate ligament *(x)* has been completely enveloped by fibrofatty tissue. The articular cartilage of the patella *(L)* has been compressed and replaced by fibrous connective tissue. (From Enneking WF, Horowitz M: The intra-articular effects of immobilization on the human knee. J Bone Joint Surg Am 1972; 54:973–985.)

ing, and an elevated serum cholesterol level as a risk factor for coronary heart disease.[128]

Cardiac Deconditioning

It is a common observance for athletes to develop a resting bradycardia. Elite athletes may have heart rates in the 50s. Their heart rates increase less with submaximal exercise than is the case in untrained persons, whereas their maximal heart rates are essentially unchanged. Deconditioned persons have a resting tachycardia and an abnormally high heart rate with submaximal exercise. A severely deconditioned person may reach maximal heart rate with a seemingly trivial workload.

When a normal person assumes the recumbent position a number of changes occur. First, venous return increases because there is no longer a pooling of blood in the venous system of the legs. This causes an increase in cardiac contractility and output, a decrease in heart rate, and an increase in cardiac work. There is a shift of fluid from the extravascular spaces to the intravascular circulation. This, in turn, stimulates diuresis to reduce the blood volume. Ordinarily, these effects are mild and rapidly reversible, but during periods of prolonged bed rest they progress.

DECONDITIONING-INDUCED CHANGES OCCURRING AT REST. After a period of bed rest, resting heart rate starts to rise.[45, 135, 158] It is generally believed to rise by about one-half beat per minute each day for the first 3 to 4 weeks of immobilization.[135, 158] The reason for this rise is unclear but it appears to be due to an imbalance of autonomic nervous system function.[130] Resting stroke volume is decreased for most persons,[135] while cardiac output is not changed significantly.[135, 158] Cardiac size falls by up to 11%[135, 158] and there is believed to be atrophy of the cardiac muscle.[90] Resting systolic and mean blood pressures are not changed, nor is total peripheral resistance.[35, 45, 135] There is no change in oxygen uptake ($\dot{V}O_2$) at rest and no significant change in the arteriovenous oxygen difference.[135]

DECONDITIONING-INDUCED CHANGES OCCURRING DURING EXERCISE. After prolonged bed rest the normal heart rate response to exercise is altered. Deconditioning causes a higher heart rate at any given level of submaximal exercise, although maximal heart rate is unchanged or only slightly increased.[35, 68, 135] The heart rate response to submaximal exercise may be as much as 30 to 40 beats per minute greater than expected after only 3 weeks of bed rest.[68, 135] With this faster heart rate, the diastolic filling period of the cardiac cycle is shortened and myocardial perfusion is decreased. This, along with an increase in the rate-pressure product,[35] can precipitate angina in the person with pre-existing coronary artery disease.

After deconditioning there is a decrease in stroke volume at submaximal and maximal exercise (30%).[135] Cardiac output declines slightly at submaximal exercise and more significantly (26% mean drop) at maximal exercise.[135] In addition, maximal oxygen uptake ($\dot{V}O_2max$), an indicator of general aerobic fitness, is reduced (mean, 28% lower), as is the submaximal $\dot{V}O_2$.[35, 135, 151, 158] This reduction may be related to the orthostatic intolerance described below.[35] Deconditioning also produces an increase in the arteriovenous oxygen difference with submaximal, though not with maximal, exercise.[135] There is no significant difference in total peripheral resistance. In the deconditioned person it takes longer for the heart rate to return to the resting state after a period of exercise.[45]

RECOVERY FROM DECONDITIONING EFFECTS. It is difficult to state the exact rate of recovery from cardiovascular deconditioning, because the studies to date have used different patient populations and different methods of enforcing disuse, and a number have also assessed the effects of training in the recovery period. Nevertheless, for most parameters it seems to take at least as long to recover from the disuse as it took to deteriorate. It may take up to twice as long or more (with intensive training) to reverse the decline in $\dot{V}O_2max$ caused by 20 days of bed rest in previously active subjects, but less for previously sedentary persons.[135, 155] Resting heart rate returns to near normal levels after a time period approximately equal to the duration of disuse, at least for 7 weeks of immobilization in the study of Dietrick and co-workers.[45] After 3 to 4 weeks of immobilization, heart rate recovery (after exercise) is only 50% of normal by 16 days and is again normal by 36 days.[158] Submaximal $\dot{V}O_2$ recovers to normal between 16 and 36 days. $\dot{V}O_2max$ recovers in 2 weeks after 3 to 4 weeks of immobility.[158]

Hemodynamic and Neurovascular Deconditioning

As described earlier, lying down causes a shift in blood volume to the thorax. Conversely, standing up causes blood to pool in the lower extremities. This causes an immediate drop in venous return which reduces stroke volume and cardiac output. In a normal person, immediate vasoconstriction and a rise in heart rate and systolic blood pressure compensate for these effects. The person who has been on prolonged bed rest, however, loses this adaptation and develops an orthostatic intolerance.[31, 35, 45, 158] Blood pools

in the legs, venous return drops, stroke volume is diminished, and the systolic blood pressure is not maintained. This may be due, at least in part, to an altered carotid baroreflex.[36, 37]

When a deconditioned person stands up there is an abnormally large increase in heart rate, as much as 37 beats per minute in the study of Taylor and others.[158] This is accompanied by the common signs and symptoms of orthostatic hypotension, including a feeling of lightheadedness, nausea, dizziness, sweating, pallor, tachycardia, and a drop in systolic blood pressure. In severe cases, syncope or angina may occur.

Most of the effects of neurovascular deconditioning appear to occur in the first 4 to 7 days of bed rest.[64] They may become evident in as little as 3 days of immobilization in a normal person.[31] They develop much more rapidly in the elderly and in persons with associated medical problems, though persons more conditioned before undertaking bed rest appear to have the greatest absolute deterioration. After remobilization these effects may take twice as long, or more, to reverse as they took to develop.[158] They can be prevented to some extent by exercising, even while on bed rest.[37, 64]

Fluid Balance

As described earlier, when assuming recumbency there is an immediate shift in blood volume to the thorax and a delayed shift of extravascular fluid into the circulation. This causes a compensatory diuresis, which leads to a decreased plasma volume.[65] Because red blood cell mass remains unchanged, hematocrit rises[63] and blood viscosity may be increased. Over the course of 2 to 4 weeks, red blood cell mass decreases and hematocrit begins to fall, although proportionately the loss of plasma volume is greater than the loss of red blood cells.[57, 63, 65] Later, red blood cell losses exceed plasma losses.

Plasma volume loss is approximately 13% by day 4 of bed rest and 15% by 2 weeks.[65] The decrease in plasma and blood volume continues and most likely plateaus around 70% of normal plasma volume and 60% of normal blood volume.[64, 65] It is accompanied by a proportionate loss of plasma proteins. There also appears to be an isocontent loss of albumin, creatinine, chloride, phosphorus, calcium, potassium, and glucose. Urea nitrogen, globulin, sodium, and osmotic concentrations are increased, while uric acid is decreased.[65] It is unclear what, if any, clinical significance is attached to these changes.

Thrombotic Disease

In 1899 Welch, summarizing previous work, described what is now known as Virchow's triad.[4] He thought that three factors might contribute to clot formation: (1) factors intrinsic to the blood, (2) blood vessel injury, and (3) stasis of blood flow. It is easy to appreciate that immobility causes stasis due to reduced muscular pumping of the blood out of the venous plexus of the legs, and it may reduce blood flow through the calves.[72] By increasing blood viscosity, immobility also may increase the intrinsic predisposition of the blood to clot.[64] Platelet aggregation may be stimulated,[24] and blood fibrinogen may be increased as well.[64] Therefore, disuse is a significant risk factor for developing thrombotic complications. This is often seen in patients acutely hospitalized. It is also seen in patients with paralysis, particularly in the early stages of spinal cord injury and stroke.

Prevention and Treatment of the Cardiovascular Complications of Immobility

Prevention is obviously the most effective way to deal with cardiovascular deconditioning. Avoiding prolonged bed rest and immobility is important. Even just sitting in a chair prevents a large amount of the deterioration in $\dot{V}o_2$max and orthostatic tolerance that occurs with bed rest.[20] Isometric exercises have also been shown to minimize the decline of $\dot{V}o_2$max and plasma volume.[151] Isotonic exercises reduce the decline in $\dot{V}o_2$max to a lesser extent,[151] but significantly reduce the decrease in plasma volume and the decrease in red blood cell volume.[68, 151] They have not been shown to decrease orthostatic intolerance.[19, 68] Supine exercise has been shown to help maintain $\dot{V}o_2$ but does not prevent orthostatic intolerance.[38]

Cardiovascular deconditioning can be reversed by progressively increasing activity and regaining the upright posture (as tolerated). This can initially be done with passive and active range-of-motion exercise in bed and with a tilt table. Later, more aggressive activity is promoted. Deep venous thrombosis (DVT) is obviously associated with bed rest as well as surgery, trauma, and paralysis. It may be prevented with active calf contractions to pump the blood out of the venous plexus of the legs, subcutaneous heparin, intermittent pneumatic compression of the legs, gradient pressure stockings, and in high-risk patients, with anticoagulation. Proper position, active exercise, and proper leg elevations are also used. Treatment of DVT requires anticoagulation. The most serious complication of DVT is pulmonary embolism, which needs to be prevented to reduce morbidity and mortality.

Integumentary System

Pressure ulcer formation (see also Chapter 31) is a leading health problem in immobilized or bedridden patients. It is a particular problem in persons with insensate skin or mental status deterioration. It is also a major health problem among the elderly nursing home population. Factors that predispose to development of pressure sores are listed in Table 34–6. Of these, the intrinsic risk factors cannot necessarily be modified. Other factors that cause pressure ulcers that can be modified by intervention are the position of the patient, the patient handling procedure, proper skin care, and the length of time the patient is kept in one position.

Capillary blood pressure is approximately 30 mm Hg. Sitting can cause a pressure in excess of this amount over the ischial tuberosities, whereas supine lying causes an excess of pressure over the sacrum. Such excess pressures are also found over the heels and occiput (especially in children because of their a proportionally greater head size) while supine, and over the greater trochanter while sidelying. These pressures can completely occlude the capillaries, and if sustained long enough they lead to skin necrosis. In the presence of a shear force, as when slumping in a

TABLE 34–6   Risk Factors for Developing Pressure Sores

Intrinsic
 Abnormal skin sensation
 Abnormal mental status or altered consciousness
 Advanced age
 Increased local tissue metabolic rate
 Previous pressure sore
 Muscle and skin atrophy
 Scars
 Edema
 Malnutrition
 Anemia
 Sedative medication
 Obesity
 Skin grafts
 Infection
Extrinsic
 Pressure
 Duration of pressure
 Shear force
 Skin maceration

chair or during improper patient transfers, necrosis is even more likely to occur.

Prevention of pressure ulcers is much more desirable than having to treat them. Proper turning of hospitalized patients, especially those with abnormal sensorium or sensation, the judicious use of a pressure-relieving bed when indicated, proper skin care and toileting, proper seating, and proper nutrition are all important. If pressure sores still develop, they may be treated with enzymatic, mechanical, or surgical debridement, and in severe cases may require surgical excision. It is imperative that all patients with abnormal skin sensation be taught adequate pressure relief and skin care procedures.

Other skin disorders that occur with immobilization are dependent edema and subcutaneous bursitis. The edema can generally be prevented with adequate mobilization and elevation. In some cases elastic stockings or gloves, pressure gradient compression, or massage may be indicated. Care should be taken to investigate cardiac or metabolic causes of edema. Such edema may predispose to cellulitis and should be minimized if possible.

Subcutaneous bursitis occurs when there is excessive pressure on the bursae. This commonly occurs as "housemaid's knee," a prepatellar bursitis obviously not caused by immobilization (except occasionally in a person restricted to lying prone to treat a pressure ulcer on the buttock). *Student's elbow*, an olecranon bursitis, is also due to prolonged pressure, as can be seen in students who study for prolonged periods of time with their elbows propped on armrests.

Bursitis is best treated by removing the aggravating pressure, but it may also be treated with nonsteroidal anti-inflammatory agents, percutaneous drainage, and instillation of corticosteroid. In refractory cases, surgical drainage or excision may be necessary.

Body Composition, Metabolic, and Nutritional Changes

In addition to the fluid balance changes described earlier, there are a number of metabolic and body composition changes that occur with bed rest or immobilization. There is a decrease in lean body mass and an increase in body fat content.[96, 135] In one study of 5 weeks of bed rest, lean body mass decreased by 2.3% and body fat increased by 12%.[96] Total body weight is not changed.[96, 135]

The body appears to become less efficient at storing excess calories as fat while on bed rest, because the increase in fat percentage is actually less than would be predicted by caloric intake.[96] Energy absorption from food is unchanged,[96] but appetite and water intake are lowered. Bed rest does not cause increased protein breakdown, but if dietary protein is low, total body protein synthesis is decreased.[152] There may be a decrease in basal metabolic rate,[45, 158] probably related to loss of muscle mass, though this is not evident in all studies.[64] There are also a number of changes in body minerals and metabolites seen with immobilization.

NITROGEN. Nitrogen is lost during immobilization. This loss occurs through urinary excretion and basically parallels the loss of muscle. The loss begins 5 to 6 days after the start of immobilization and peaks in the second week. When activity is resumed (after 6–7 weeks of immobility) nitrogen is still lost for another week, but by the second week excretion is normalized. Later, nitrogen excretion falls to below normal levels to recapture the amount that was lost. Maximum nitrogen retention occurs 4 weeks after resumption of activity and is back to a normal balance by around the sixth week.[45]

CALCIUM. As with all other body components calcium is normally in a dynamic equilibrium with absorption, distribution, and excretion, being balanced by the needs of the body (Fig. 34–7). During periods of disuse there is loss of this mineral. This loss parallels the loss of bone mass described above. Calcium is excreted in both urine and feces. Fecal excretion is somewhat variable and increases progressively, at least through the 6 to 7 weeks of immobility that have been studied.

Urinary calcium excretion begins to rise after 2 to 3 days of immobility. It peaks in 3 to 7 weeks[45, 48, 138] at approximately twice the normal rate of excretion.[19] It then plateaus, at least through 6 to 7 weeks. By approximately 16 weeks, excretion drops to a new plateau which is maintained at least through 36 weeks.[138] Throughout this time total body calcium is lost at a rate of about 0.5% per month.[138] This loss can be prevented to some extent by weightbearing activity, even standing.[82]

When activity is resumed, calcium excretion initially remains high, but gradually returns to normal by 3 weeks. Excretion continues to fall to reach a trough below the normal excretion level at 5 to 6 weeks, and then gradually normalizes.

PHOSPHORUS. Phosphorus loss with immobilization is primarily through the urine, although a small amount is also lost fecally. The loss begins during the first week of immobility and peaks at 2 to 3 weeks (along with nitrogen). Excretion then falls, but peaks again at 6 to 7 weeks (along with calcium). On resumption of activity, phosphorus excretion returns to normal by the third week. This is followed by less than normal excretion for weeks 3 through 5 and normalization of excretion by week 6.[45]

OTHER LOSSES. Sulfur loss during immobilization basically parallels nitrogen loss, and is believed to result from loss of muscle mass.[45]

Other minerals such as sodium, potassium, magnesium,[62] and zinc[62, 97] are also lost during immobilization. This is due in part to the loss of plasma volume, but there may also be an excess excretion. Sodium and chloride loss is greatest during early immobilization (as is plasma loss).[31] Potassium loss increases progressively through 2 to 3 weeks of bed rest,[31] and recovery of this mineral during remobilization is twice the amount that was lost.[45]

Endocrine and Receptor Function

Prolonged bed rest causes a decrease in glucose tolerance. This is primarily due to changes in peripheral muscle sensitivity to circulating insulin,[106, 153] though some adaptation is also believed to occur in the cells of the pancreas.[116] The glucose intolerance caused by bed rest can to some extent be ameliorated with both isotonic and isometric exercise.[46] Following 2 weeks of bed rest approximately 2 weeks of resumed activity is required for the glucose response to return to normal.[106]

Another immobility-induced change in endocrine function is in parathyroid hormone production. In the rat model, immobilization causes a suppression of parathyroid hormone and a decrease in intestinal calcium absorption.[172] This has been supported in human studies,[148] and is believed to be a response to the calcium released from bone resorption. In persons with immobilization hypercalcemia, however, the parathyroid hormone level may be elevated.[103]

Other immobility-induced changes may include an increase in urinary hydrocortisone excretion (at least in a

Calcium Homeostasis

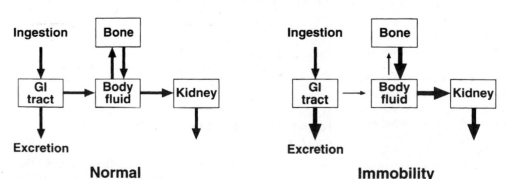

Normal

Immobility

FIGURE 34–7 Calcium homeostasis and flux. Normally the calcium balance of intake and excretion is fairly equal and changes only slowly over the course of years. With immobilization, less calcium absorption occurs from the gastrointestinal tract, accompanied by a net resorption from bone and an increased renal excretion of the mineral.

very long bed rest study),[101] increased plasma renin activity,[30, 112, 163] increased aldosterone secretion,[30, 112] altered growth hormone production,[164] and altered spermatogenesis[34] and androgen secretion.[23, 53, 163] There may be changes in adrenal[101] and pituitary function,[150, 163] though this may not be directly attributable to the immobility.[131] There is also an increased body temperature response to exercise.[64, 66] Central nervous system function and receptors may be altered, as is the circadian rhythm.[136] There appears to be no change in thyroid hormone degradation, though blood levels may be altered.[12, 53, 164, 175]

Respiratory System

There are both immediate and long-term consequences of bed rest on the respiratory system. Immediately after assuming a supine or forward-slumped position the diaphragm and intercostal muscles are restricted in their normal motion and breathing is impaired (an exception may be in spinal cord–injured patients in whom the supine position may place the diaphragm into a biomechanically advantageous position; see Chapter 55). The work of breathing is increased in the slumped or supine position owing to increased mechanical resistance. Because of blood pooling in the thorax, there is also an immediate decrease in lung volume and residual volume.

Although not proven, it is commonly held that if the recumbent position is maintained, gravity-induced changes will occur within the lungs. There is thought to be a pooling of mucus in the lower (dependent) parts of the airway, whereas the upper segments tend to dry out. This is believed to create an environment predisposing to respiratory infection, mucous plugging, and atelectasis. This situation is aggravated by a decrease in respiratory activity and an impaired cough mechanism. In addition, there may also be a mismatch between lung ventilation and perfusion.

Both Dietrick and others[45] and Saltin and co-workers[135] found no major changes in pulmonary tests after immobilization. Beckett and colleagues,[14] however, in a study of normal subjects placed on bed rest for 11 to 12 days, found that there was an increase in forced vital capacity and a small increase in total lung capacity. Residual volume and functional residual capacity were unchanged.[14] Other studies have not shown demonstrable changes in maximal ventilatory volume or maximal minute volume, at least in normal subjects on a relatively short period of bed rest.[65, 151] Convertino (and others)[35] reported that in middle-aged men exposed to 10 days of bed rest the ventilatory volume was elevated during maximal and submaximal exercise. They found that the respiratory exchange ratio was significantly increased during upright submaximal exercise. They concluded that orthostatic stress, not pulmonary function, was the main limiting factor in exercise tolerance after bed rest.[35]

With prolonged bed rest, the intercostal muscles and costal joints develop contractures, breathing becomes more shallow, and respiratory rate increases. In addition, the immobilized patient is at risk of developing pulmonary embolism due to DVT in the lower extremities.

The pulmonary deterioration induced by bed rest can be prevented to a large extent by frequent changes in position, incentive spirometry, deep breathing, coughing, and pulmonary toilet. The only definitive solution to the problem is mobilization.

Genitourinary System

Genitourinary effects of bed rest and immobility include the increased diuresis and mineral excretion described above. There are also other changes, which are primarily mechanical in nature. While one study in rats demonstrated early bladder distention and relatively rapid increase in bladder tissue growth,[8] the main problems encountered are urinary stasis and calculus formation.

Voiding is more difficult when supine, so patients tend to wait longer before emptying their bladders. There is also a lack of gravity assistance in voiding, and postvoid residual volume may be increased. This predisposes to urinary tract infection, and in severe cases, to overflow incontinence.

In addition, there may be gravity-induced urinary stasis in the renal pelves. This, together with increased calcium excretion, may increase the incidence of calculus formation, another factor predisposing to urinary tract infection. Calculus formation is especially common in patients with fractures and spinal cord injury.

Long-term consequences of immobilization may lead to a sustained (up to 9 months) decrease in glomerular filtration rate and (greater than 4 weeks) decreased ability to concentrate urine.[9]

Reproductive effects of immobility have not been studied adequately to date, but there appears to be a decrease in spermatogenesis, at least in primates.[34] Androgen secretion may be altered as well.[23, 53, 163]

The genitourinary consequences of immobility can most likely be prevented by assuming the upright posture as frequently as possible and by ambulation. Adequate fluid intake is important, and voiding while supine should be discouraged. In select cases postvoid residual volumes should be measured, and in some cases catheterization is needed.

Gastrointestinal Tract and Digestion

Bed rest causes mechanical effects on the gastrointestinal tract similar to those experienced in the genitourinary system. There is an increased risk of constipation due to decreased mobility, decreased peristalsis (possibly due to an increased adrenergic state), and decreased fluid intake. Gastrointestinal secretion decreases and "heartburn" symptoms increase.[64] There is also a decrease or loss of appetite,[64] which can lead to impairment of nutrition.

The supine position may also interfere with eructation and may increase gastroesophageal reflux. The potential embarrassment of using a bedpan often causes people to delay defecating.

Persons on bed rest should ingest adequate protein, fiber, and fluid. Stool softeners may be helpful, but enemas and laxatives should be avoided, if possible.

Neurological System, Emotions, and Intellectual Function

There are few true neurological sequelae of bed rest that affect either the central or peripheral nervous systems. Instead, there are disorders of coordination, balance, and emotions that may have a component of physiological deterioration as well as a predominant integrative component.

One potential complication of bed rest is the occurrence of compression neuropathies. Peroneal nerve compression below the fibular head and ulnar nerve compression at the retrocondylar groove are probably the most common such compression neuropathies. They are specifically due to bed rest rather than immobilization. Ulnar nerve compression was found in 23% of patients in a small study of orthopedic, neurological, neurosurgical, and rehabilitation inpatients.[33] Other compression neuropathies may occur as well, especially in obtunded patients or in those with sensory or motor deficits. They can also occur in patients who are restrained.

The integrative components of emotions and cognitive function are affected by bed rest and immobilization, most likely due to sensory deprivation and boredom. Anxiety also results from being restricted to bed.[134] Medications and "ICU [intensive care unit] psychosis" play a role as well in medically ill patients. Affected persons may experience a lowered pain threshold and a decrease in coordination[174] and balance.[50, 74, 158] They may have emotional disturbances such as depression, anxiety, withdrawal, apathy, incontinence, and sleep disturbance,[134, 174] and may even develop paranoia and dementia. Intellectual function is impaired, as is orientation and the perception of time.[144] Patients with these problems become emotionally labile, irritable, and uncooperative. They may suffer from headache, dizziness, general discomfort, nightmares, and even hallucinations, primarily because of sensory deprivation.[144, 174] They may also have a decreased visual acuity and a raised auditory threshold.[64]

DECONDITIONING AS A REHABILITATION DIAGNOSIS

There are six basic conditions causing disuse: (1) a sedentary lifestyle that is a result of personal choice; (2) bed rest that is imposed because of a medical or surgical illness; (3) medical or caregiver "neglect," with a person needlessly restricted from mobility, usually in a hospital or nursing home; (4) immobilization of the body or part of the body by casts or braces, usually after trauma or fracture; (5) disuse due to paralysis or neuromuscular disorder; and (6) disuse due to weightlessness.

Weightlessness is germane to this chapter mainly because many of the studies of immobility were performed to assess the effects of weightlessness in astronauts.

Disuse due to paralysis or weakness, as well as casts and braces used to treat an injury, can cause local, regional, or systemic complications, depending on the extent of the problem. Physical medicine and rehabilitation consultation in such patients is often typically aimed at aiding in recovery from injury, maximizing function, and preventing long-term health hazards (such as cardiovascular deconditioning).

The abundance of persons who suffer from disuse because of a sedentary lifestyle is in large part a consequence of modern life, with people relying on machines to perform their work.

Deconditioning due to bed rest is largely associated with

hospitalization or being in a nursing home. It has also in the past been seen in women in the peripartum period and in patients with back injuries. In some cases bed rest is indicated; often it is not.

Inpatient Rehabilitation Interactions

A recent survey of a large inpatient rehabilitation unit revealed that over a 6-month period, nearly 20% of admissions were for the diagnosis of deconditioning. In a consult service at a large tertiary care hospital, 21% of adult consultations were for patients with deconditioning. These patients were typically older and had a longer hospital stay with more serious medical complications than other patients who received a physical medicine and rehabilitation consult.[26]

Most of the deconditioned patients were hospitalized with a variety of medical and surgical illnesses, were treated successfully, but were left with residual weakness and other complications of immobility. These residual impairments were often more disabling than the problem for which they were admitted. These patients had what is known as *deconditioning syndrome*. They were unable to function as before, could not be returned home safely, and required a short inpatient rehabilitation stay to regain their lost independence.

Treatment of inpatients with deconditioning syndrome includes adequate sensory and intellectual stimulation, regaining an upright posture as tolerated, regaining and maintaining proper joint range of motion with active (preferred) or passive (if needed) exercise, and increasing strength and coordination with a combination of isometric, isotonic, and functional activities. In addition, all the other interventions described earlier, such as incentive spirometry, proper fluid intake, and so forth, are incorporated as well.

Prevention of deconditioning involves these same principles. In addition, it is important to allow the patient to sit upright, if possible, to "see the world." Lying in bed, staring at the ceiling, removes a normal perspective on life. It is also important that healthcare workers avoid "talking down" to the patient. Often adults are treated like children just because they are in bed and require help with their activities of daily living (ADL). Little wonder that these patients become anxious and uncooperative. Excessive use of medications is to be avoided and proper sleep-wake cycles should be fostered. Reliance on sleep medications at night in a patient who naps out of boredom during the day can promote emotional and intellectual deterioration. Proper nutrition, proper positioning and turning, and exercise are important as well. It is somewhat unclear which type of exercise is best in the immobilized patient, as studies have mainly been done on young healthy volunteers. Pending further data, it is probably reasonable to encourage a variety of isotonic, isometric, and aerobic exercises, as tolerated.

Outpatient Rehabilitation Interactions

Deconditioning in the outpatient physical medicine and rehabilitation setting centers mainly on persons who have had an injury and who have been off work long enough to develop muscle weakness and inflexibility. This may put them at risk of further injury if they return to work without proper conditioning. Such patients often benefit from a work-conditioning or work-hardening program prior to return to activity. Viewing them as "occupational athletes" is helpful, as many principles of sports rehabilitation can be incorporated into their care.

Aging vs. Disuse Effects on the Body

It is common knowledge that as we age we deteriorate to a certain extent. But aging is often compounded by disease, and it appears that disuse and aging synergistically accelerate the decline in maximal physiological capacity of virtually every body system. The increased incidence of medical illness in the elderly necessarily enforces a certain amount of disuse. Nevertheless, it is clear that active persons can prevent a large amount of the physical decline seen in aging.

THE BENEFICIAL EFFECTS OF EXERCISE

Muscle Strength and Endurance

Since strength is ultimately proportional to the cross-sectional area of muscle, muscle-building exercise increases the strength available to a person to meet the physical demands of living. Similarly, muscular endurance is enhanced by endurance training. The major benefits of exercise are summarized in Table 34–7. Chapter 20 describes the benefits of exercise in more detail. For the purposes of this chapter, it is important to remember that excessive muscle weakness, even of local or regional muscle groups, can prevent a person from leading a normal lifestyle. This is, of course, exaggerated in the elderly or otherwise impaired. Strength and endurance training will not increase the maximal physiological potential, but they can certainly increase a person's fitness and function.

Obesity

Obesity is usually defined as a state in which body weight exceeds ideal body weight by more than 20%. It is common in the United States, with up to 25% of the population being affected. Most obese persons have a long-term battle with their weight. They commonly choose to attack the problem by dieting, even though exercise may be more effective.

Regular aerobic exercise helps reduce body weight even while maintaining fat-free weight.[137] It brings about a more sustained weight loss than does dieting alone. In general, any form of aerobic exercise is beneficial for weight loss, although swimming does not seem to help decrease weight as well as walking, running, and bicycling.[70]

Hypertension

Aerobic exercise training can be valuable in the treatment of mild-to-moderate essential hypertension.[104] It may cause a decrease of up to 10 mm Hg in blood pressure[72] and appears to lower both systolic and diastolic blood pressures.[104] The blood pressure response to such exercise may also be used to screen normotensive persons for the risk of later developing elevated blood pressure.[157]

The first line of treatment for mild hypertension is usually pharmacological, but aerobic exercise and lifestyle changes such as weight loss, diet changes, and cessation of smoking are probably a better choice. Exercise alone may normalize blood pressure, but if it does not, pharmacological treatment can still be instituted at a later date. In moderate-to-severe essential hypertension, exercise should probably be combined with lifestyle changes and antihypertensive medication for first-line treatment. When exercise starts to decrease the blood pressure, lower doses of medication may be possible.

According to the American College of Sports Medicine, in normal healthy adults, aerobic exercise is recommended at 60% to 85% of the maximum heart rate, three to four times per week, for 20 to 60 min per session.[5] Since exercise at the upper limit of this level of intensity may actually worsen hypertension,[156] aerobic exercise of more moderate intensity is recommended in the hypertensive patient.[72] Such low-to-moderate intensity of training has been shown to be as effective as high-intensity training in lowering blood pressure.[104]

Isometric exercise (approximated by heavy weightlifting) is generally to be avoided in the hypertensive population, as it may increase blood pressure both during exercise and for a sustained period afterward. Isometrics may increase myocardial oxygen demand out of proportion to the physical work being performed.[47] Despite these caveats, it is not entirely clear that isometrics are harmful, and moderate weightlifting may be helpful even in patients with coronary artery disease and mild hypertension.[149] Lighter weights used for more repetitions may help the hypertensive patient gain strength with less risk. Because heart rate

TABLE 34–7   Major Benefits of Exercise

Musculoskeletal
  ↑ Muscle strength and endurance
  ↑ Bone mass
Obesity
  Sustained weight loss
Cardiovascular
  ↓ Hypertension
  Improved blood lipids
  ↑ $\dot{V}O_2$ max
  ↑ Maximal cardiac output
  ↓ Resting and submaximal heart rate
  ↑ Peripheral oxygen extraction
Endocrine
  Improved glucose tolerance
Emotional
  Improved sense of well-being
Neurological
  Improved balance and coordination
  ↑ Pain threshold
Elderly
  May help to prevent falls (improved margin of safety)
  ↑ Functional capacity
Women
  ↓ Premenstrual syndrome
  ↓ Symptoms of endometriosis
  Lessened stress of labor
Disabled
  ↑ Quality of life
  ↑ $\dot{V}O_2$ max
  ↓ Medical complications (possible)

Abbreviations: $\dot{V}O_2$ max, maximum rate of oxygen consumption.

and systolic blood pressure (and thus myocardial oxygen demand) are higher in upper extremity than in lower extremity exercise for a constant workload[118] (Fig. 34–8), caution should be exercised in prescribing upper extremity weightbearing activities. It should also be kept in mind that a variety of antihypertensive agents can alter the heart rate response to exercise as well as cause dehydration or hypokalemia.

Cardiovascular Disease

Aerobic exercise has long been used as part of cardiac rehabilitation in patients who have suffered from myocardial infarction or who have had cardiac surgery. It is also useful in helping prevent the atherosclerosis that causes so much morbidity and mortality in the Western world. The mechanism of action of exercise is not fully understood, but exercise may modify the risk factors for atherosclerosis.[110] It also appears to have both peripheral and cardiac benefits in patients with coronary artery disease.[71] As described earlier, it may reduce hypertension and obesity. It also lowers serum triglycerides and may alter serum cholesterol levels to increase the high-density/low-density lipoprotein (HDL/LDL) ratio.[71, 141, 154] In some persons, these benefits may be due to weight loss or other changes, and not directly due to the exercise. Aerobic exercise may be particularly effective at increasing the HDL_2 subfraction, which is thought to be an especially important anti-atherogenic factor. These benefits to the lipid profile appear to require a threshold amount of exercise. Superko[154] noted that jogging at least 15 miles/week is needed to produce a beneficial change in blood lipids. Haskell[75] reported that at least 1000 kcal/week must be expended to obtain these benefits. Above this level he reported a "dose-related" increase in benefit up to 4500 kcal/week, and above this a plateau. He believed that the beneficial effects on the lipid profile were evident only if accompanied by weight loss.[75] They do not appear to occur in resistance exercise.[80]

In addition to the benefits of reducing atherogenic risk

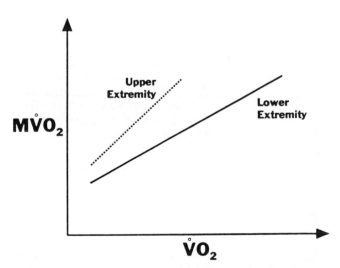

FIGURE 34–8   A comparison of the relationship between myocardial oxygen demand and total oxygen consumption for upper and lower extremity work. (From Downey JA, Myers SJ, Gonzales EG, Lieberman JS (eds): The Physiologic Basis of Rehabilitation Medicine, ed 2. Stoneham, Mass, Butterworth-Heinemann, 1994.)

factors, regular aerobic exercise helps to increase the body's aerobic endurance, as demonstrated by a higher $\dot{V}O_2$max (Fig. 34–9A). There is an increase in maximal cardiac output (Fig. 34–9B), an increase in stroke volume for a given level of $\dot{V}O_2$ (Fig. 34–9C), and an increase in peripheral oxygen extraction. Resting heart rate drops. The intensity of the exercise should most likely be moderate; high intensity is not necessarily more beneficial.[58]

Persons who regularly participate in an aerobic exercise program have an increase in life expectancy and a decreased risk of coronary artery disease.[128] They have a decreased heart rate (Fig. 34–9D) and blood pressure response to submaximal exercise, an increase in $\dot{V}O_2$max, a decreased myocardial oxygen demand for a given workload, and decreased angina for a given workload (though anginal threshold for a given myocardial oxygen demand is unchanged)[43] (Fig. 34–10). Ideally, exercise should be combined with healthy lifestyle changes and a proper diet. Such risk factor modification has been shown to reverse atherosclerosis to some extent.[167]

Diabetes

Inactivity causes a decreased peripheral sensitivity to insulin. Conversely, aerobic exercise increases the end-organ cell receptor sensitivity to insulin,[21, 93] primarily in the regions being exercised.[44] This can be an important benefit in those with non-insulin-dependent diabetes mellitus (NIDDM). It may also reduce the other risk factors for diabetes. In insulin-dependent diabetes mellitus (IDDM), exercise has little effect, except that it lowers insulin requirements by utilizing circulating glucose.

When a person is first diagnosed as having glucose intolerance or mild diabetes, exercise can be combined with diet changes as the first mode of treatment. This may obviate the need for oral hypoglycemic medication in some, although many patients will probably eventually need such medication. Exercise can also be used as part of the treatment program in patients with more severe diabetes and in gestational diabetes.[25] However, care should be taken when exercising not to cause postexercise hypoglycemia. This can be a problem in persons who exercise in the evening, as they may become hypoglycemic during sleep. Diabetics can also suffer from silent myocardial ischemia during exercise, so before initiating an exercise program they should have an appropriate cardiac screening evaluation.

Osteoporosis

As described earlier, immobility causes a loss of bone mass, primarily in the weightbearing bones. Conversely, exercise can help to maintain bone mass. In early adulthood the weightbearing exercise may help to increase bone mass, which generally peaks in the early 30s. After the fourth decade, exercise probably does not increase bone mass, but can help slow down the normal decline in bone mass with aging.

Exercise can have beneficial effects even on bones not involved in a loading stress,[42, 84] but it has its primary benefit on the bones being stressed. Intermittent bone compression appears to be more beneficial than static stress.[28] It is probably reasonable to combine weightlifting and

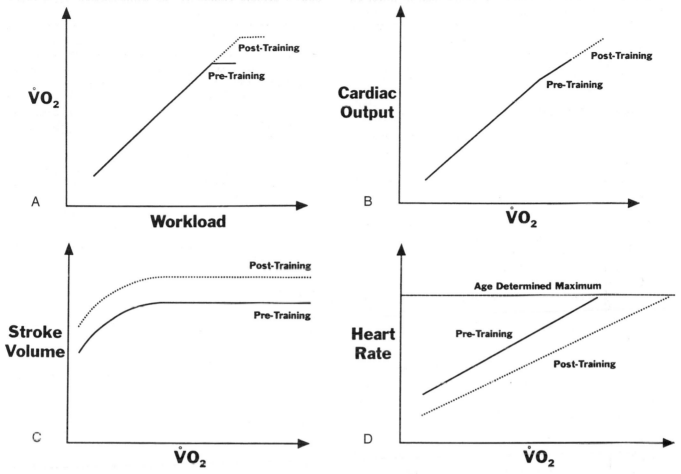

FIGURE 34–9   A, Effect of training on relationship between oxygen consumption and workload. B, Effect of training on relationship between cardiac output and oxygen consumption. C, Effect of training on relationship between stroke volume and oxygen consumption. D, Effect of training on the relationship between heart rate and oxygen consumption. (From Downey JA, Myers SJ, Gonzales EG, Lieberman JS (eds): The Physiologic Basis of Rehabilitation Medicine, ed 2. Stoneham, Mass, Butterworth-Heinemann, 1994, p 135.)

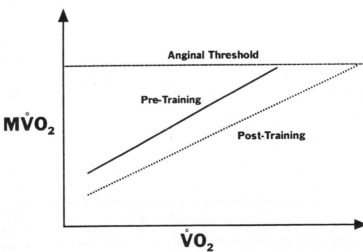

FIGURE 34–10   Effect of training on relationship between myocardial oxygen demand and total body oxygen consumption. (From Downey JA, Myers SJ, Gonzales EG, Lieberman JS (eds): The Physiologic Basis of Rehabilitation Medicine, ed 2. Stoneham, Mass, Butterworth-Heinemann, 1994, p 136.)

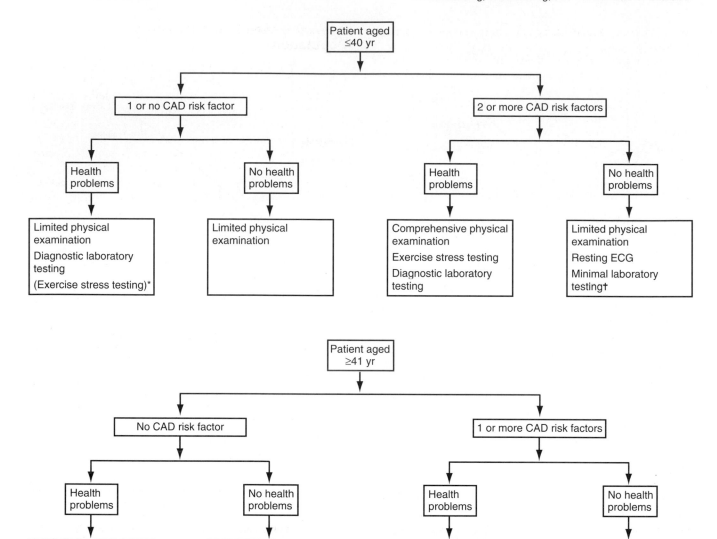

FIGURE 34-11 Preparticipation screening evaluation for persons wishing to begin an exercise program. *Risk factors* for coronary artery disease (CAD) include hypertension, smoking, diabetes, hypercholesterolemia, previous CAD, strong family history, and obesity or sedentary lifestyle. *Health problems* include cardiopulmonary disease, neurologic disease, endocrinopathy, musculosketetal disorder, psychiatric disorder, renal or hepatic disease, anemia, current drug use, and other chronic or acute diseases. Diagnostic laboratory testing can include fasting chemical survey, complete blood cell count, urinalysis, and lipid profile. Minimal laboratory testing can include a chemical survey. *Exercise stress testing is recommended if the patient has cardiopulmonary disease. †Diagnostic laboratory testing is indicated if coronary heart disease risk factors include hyperlipidemia, hyperglycemia, or hyperuricemia. (From Putukian M, McKeag D: The preparticipation physical examination. *In* Buschbacher R, Braddom RL: Sports Medicine and Rehabilitation: A Sports-Specific Approach. Philadelphia, Hanley & Belfus, 1994.)

weightbearing exercise to benefit bones not directly involved in weightbearing.

The exercises that are most beneficial for maintaining bone mass are walking and running, not swimming. The exercise should be combined with adequate calcium intake, proper diet, and treatment of hypoestrogenemia, if appropriate (in young and postmenopausal women).

Sense of Well-Being and the Pain Threshold

Regular aerobic exercise is generally believed to raise the pain threshold, probably by stimulating the release of endogenous opiates.[60, 140] It is useful in conditions such as fibromyalgia, myofascial pain syndrome, chronic pain syndrome, and back pain. It also increases the general sense of well-being and helps to reduce anxiety, depression, and neuroticism.[32, 92, 111, 119]

Balance, Coordination, and Proprioception

As described earlier, immobility decreases balance,[74] and there is some evidence to support the clinical observation that exercise improves balance.[107] In addition, proprioceptive exercise is commonly used in sports medicine to treat ankle injuries, and exercise has been shown to increase velocity of gait.[85]

There is little direct evidence that exercise specifically improves balance, proprioception, and coordination. But by promoting general fitness, strength, and health habits, it increases the functional reserve of persons going about their daily activities. This allows the fit person to better compensate for the natural stresses and potentially risky incidents that arise in normal life. In essence, it creates a buffer of safety.

Exercise in the Older Population

As most of the medical conditions described earlier are more prevalent in the elderly, exercise may be especially important in this age group. Exercise earlier in life may help prevent some of the disorders, while later in life it may slow their progression. This may be true for osteoporosis, obesity, coronary artery disease, diabetes, and hypertension. In addition, exercise can increase strength in the elderly, even in frail persons.[54] This occurs primarily through a more advantageous neural recruitment of muscles rather than hypertrophy,[120] though hypertrophy also occurs.[59] The increase in strength may help prevent falls and other injuries, and exercise appears to improve the quality of life in the elderly.[142] Before prescribing exercise in the older population, a proper screening evaluation is indicated (Fig. 34–11). A proper exercise prescription, tailored to the appropriate activity level, is important as well.

Exercise in Women

The effect of aerobic exercise on the cardiovascular endurance of women is qualitatively similar to that of men, although women do not seem to be able to attain as high a Vo_2max as men. This is due to a number of factors, including a higher body fat content, a smaller heart,[81] lower hematocrit,[40] and other, as yet unknown, factors.[146] The reaction of women to strength training is also qualitatively similar to that of men. Owing to the absence of testosterone, women are unable to build as much muscle mass as men and thus do not generally attain as great a strength. Women are especially lacking in upper body strength compared with men.[100] They do gain strength with weight training, through some hypertrophy and through neural factors such as improved recruitment.

In addition to the physiological effects just described, aerobic exercise may lessen the effects of premenstrual syndrome (PMS)[129] and endometriosis.[13, 39] It also tends to normalize the menstrual cycle, though very heavy endurance exercise may adversely affect the cycle. Exercise in moderation has been shown to be safe for women with routine pregnancies. While women should probably be counseled not to try to markedly increase their exercise load during pregnancy, moderate exercise is believed to be safe for both mother and fetus,[15, 56] and may even improve the process of labor and postlabor recovery. It is important when exercising during pregnancy to avoid dehydration and hyperthermia. Hyperthermia is a teratogen.[143]

Other beneficial effects of exercise that are particularly important in women include the slowing or prevention of osteoporosis described earlier.

Special Issues in the Disabled Population

Sports are becoming increasingly available to persons with physical impairments. This is especially true for wheelchair athletes, mainly those with paraplegia. Exercise in wheelchair athletes has been shown to increase Vo_2max, decrease cardiovascular disease and respiratory infection, improve self-image, improve psychological function, and decrease time hospitalized. These benefits come at a price, namely an increase in traumatic and overuse injuries, shoulder pain and degeneration, compression neuropathies, and bladder and skin problems. When done carefully, however, the benefits outweight the risks in most persons.[139]

References

1. Akeson WH, Amiel D, Abel MF, et al: Effects of immobilization on joints. Clin Orthop 1987; 219:28–37.
2. Akeson WH, Amiel D, Mechanic GL, et al: Collagen cross-linking alterations in joint contractures: Changes in the reducible cross-links in periarticular connective tissue collagen after nine weeks of immobilization. Connect Tissue Res 1977; 5:15–19.
3. Akeson WH, Woo SLY, Amiel D, et al: The connective tissue response to immobility: Biochemical changes in periarticular connective tissue of the immobilized rabit knee. Clin Orthop 1973; 93:356–362.
4. Allen EV, Barker NW, Hines EA Jr: Peripheral Vascular Diseases, ed 2. Philadelphia, WB Saunders, 1955, p 490.
5. American College of Sports Medicine: Guidelines for Graded Exercise Testing and Exercise Prescription. Philadelphia, Lea & Febiger, 1990.
6. Amiel D, Akeson WH, Harwood FL, Mechanic GL: The effect of immobilization on the types of collagen synthesized in periarticular connective tissue. Connect Tissue Res 1980; 8:27–32.
7. Amiel D, Woo SLY, Harwood FL, Akeson WH: The effect of immobilization on collagen turnover in connective tissue: a biochemical-biomechanical correlation. Acta Orthop Scand 1982; 53:325–332.
8. Anderson RL, Lefever FR, Francis WR, Maurer JK: Urinary and bladder responses to immobilization in male rats. Food Chem Toxicol 1990; 28:543–545.
9. Andrews PI, Rosenberg AR: Renal consequences of immobilization in children with fractured femurs. Acta Paediatr Scand 1990; 79:311–315.
10. Appell H: Muscular atrophy following immobilization. Sports Med 1990; 10:42–58.
11. Baker JH, Matsumoto DE: Adaptation of skeletal muscle to immobilization in a shortened position. Muscle Nerve. 1988; 2:231–244.
12. Balsam A, Leppo LE: Assessment of the degradation of thyroid hormones in man during bed rest. J Appl Physiol 1975; 38:216–219.
13. Barbieri RL: Etiology and epidemiology of endometriosis. Am J Obstet Gynecol 1990; 162:565–567.
14. Beckett WS, Vroman NB, Nigro D, et al: Effect of prolonged bed rest on lung volume in normal individuals. J Appl Physiol 1986; 61:919–925.
15. Beckmann CRB, Beckmann CA: Effect of a structured antepartum exercise program on pregnancy and labor outcome in primiparas. J Reprod Med 1990; 35:704–709.
16. Behrens F, Kraft EL, Oegema TR Jr: Biochemical changes in articular cartilage after joint immobilization by casting or external fixation. J Orthop Res 1989; 7:335–343.
17. Berry P, Berry I, Manelfe C: Magnetic resonance imaging evaluation of lower limb muscles during bed rest—a microgravity simulation model. Aviat Space Environ Med 1993; 64:212–218.
18. Bird AD: The effect of surgery, injury, and prolonged bed rest on calf blood flow. Aust N Z J Surg 1972; 41:374–379.
19. Birkhead NC, Blizzard JJ, Daly JW, et al: Cardiodynamic and Metabolic Effects of Prolonged Bed Rest. Ohio Aerospace Medical Research Laboratories, Wright-Patterson Air Force Base. AMRL-TDR-63-37, May 1963.
20. Birkhead NC, Blizzard JJ, Daly JW, et al: Cardiodynamic and metabolic effects of prolonged bed rest with daily recumbent or

sitting exercise and with sitting inactivity. Ohio Aerospace Medical Research Laboratories, Wright-Patterson Air Force Base, AMRL-TDR-64-61, August 1964.

21. Bjorntorp P, Krotkiewski M: Exercise treatment in diabetes mellitus. Acta Med Scand 1985; 217:3–7.

22. Booth FW, Seider MJ: Early change in skeletal muscle protein synthesis after limb immobilization of rats. J Appl Physiol 1979; 47:974–977.

23. Briggs MH, Garcia-Webb P, Cheung T: Androgens and exercise. BMJ 1973; 3:49–50.

24. Buczynski A, Kedziora J, Wachowicz B, Zolynski K: Effect of bed rest on the adenine nucleotides concentration in human blood platelets. J Physiol Pharmacol 1991; 42:389–395.

25. Bung P, Bung C, Artal R et al: Therapeutic exercise for insulin-requiring gestational diabetics: Effects on the fetus—results of a randomized prospective longitudinal study. J Perinat Med 1993; 21:125–137.

26. Buschbacher R: Unpublished results, January 1994.

27. Buschbacher R, Coplin B, Buschbacher L, McKinley W: Noninflammatory knee joint effusions in spinal cord–injured and other paralyzed patients. Am J Phys Med Rehabil 1991; 70:309–312.

28. Camay A, Tschantz P: Mechanical influences in bone remodeling: Experimental research on Wolff's law. J Biomechanics 1972; 5:173–180.

29. Cardenas DD, Stolov WC, Hardy MR: Muscle fiber number in immobilization atrophy. Arch Phys Med Rehabil 1977; 58:423–426.

30. Chaviari M, Ganguly A, Luetscher JA, Zager PG: Effect of bedrest on circadian rhythms of plasma renin, aldosterone, and cortisol. Aviat Space Environ Med 1977; 48:633–636.

31. Chobanian AV, Lille RD, Tercyak A, Blevins P: The metabolic and hemodynamic effects of prolonged bed rest in normal subjects. Circulation 1974; 49:551–559.

32. Choi PYL, Van Horn JD, Picker DE, Roberts HI: Mood changes in women after an aerobics class: A preliminary study. Health Care Women Int 1993; 14:167–177.

33. Chuman MA: Risk factors associated with ulnar nerve compression in bedridden patients. J Neurosurg Nurs 1985; 17:338–342.

34. Cockett ATK, Elbadawi A, Zemjanis R, Adey WR: The effects of immobilization on spermatogenesis in subhuman primates. Fertil Steril 1970; 21:610–614.

35. Convertino V, Hung J, Goldwater D, DeBusk RF: Cardiovascular responses to exercise in middle-aged men after 10 days of bedrest. Circulation 1982; 65:134–140.

36. Convertino VA, Doerr DF, Eckberg DL, et al: Carotid baroreflex response following 30 days exposure to simulated microgravity. Physiologist 1989; 32:S67–S68.

37. Convertino VA, Doerr DF, Guell A, Marini JF: Effects of acute exercise on attenuated vagal baroreflex function during bed rest. Aviat Space Environ Med 1992; 63:999–1003.

38. Convertino VA, Goldwater DJ, Sandler H: $\dot{V}O_2$ kinetics of constant-load exercise following bed-rest–induced deconditioning. J Appl Physiol 1984; 57:1545–1550.

39. Cramer DW, Wilson E, Stilman RJ, et al: The relation of endometriosis to menstrual characteristics, smoking, and exercise. JAMA 1986; 225:1904–1908.

40. Cureton K, Bishop P, Hutchinson P, et al: Sex difference in maximal oxygen uptake. Eur J Appl Physiol 1986; 54:656–660.

41. Cuthbertson DP: The influence of prolonged muscular rest on metabolism. Biochemistry 1929; 23:1328–1345.

42. Dalen N, Olsson E: Bone mineral content and physical activity. Acta Orthop Scand 1974; 45:170–174.

43. DeBusk RF, Hung J: Exercise conditioning soon after myocardial infarction: Effects on myocardial perfusion and ventricular function. Ann N Y Acad Sci 1982; 382:343–354.

44. Devlin JT: Effects of exercise on insulin sensitivity in humans. Diabetes Care 1992; 15 (suppl 4):1690–1693.

45. Dietrick JE, Whedon GD, Shorr E: Effects of immobilization upon various metabolic and physiologic functions of normal men. Am J Med 1948; 4:3–36.

46. Dolkas CB, Greenleaf JE: Insulin and glucose responses during bed rest with isotonic and isometric exercise. J Appl Physiol 1977; 43:1033–1038.

47. Donald KW, Lind AR, McNichol GW, et al: Cardiovascular responses to sustained (static) contractions. Circulation 1967; 20 (suppl 1):115–130.

48. Donaldson CL, Hulley SB, Vogel JM, et al: Effect of prolonged bed rest on bone mineral. Metabolism 1970; 19:1071–1084.

49. Duchateau J, Hainaut K: Effects of immobilization on contractile properties, recruitment and firing rates of human motor units. J Physiol 1990; 422:55–65.

50. Dupui P, Montoya R, Costes-Salon M, et al: Balance and gait analysis after 30 days −6° bed rest: Influence of lower-body negative-pressure sessions. Aviat Space Environ Med 1992; 63:1004–1010.

51. Enneking WF, Horowitz M: The intra-articular effects of immobilization on the human knee. J Bone Joint Surg Am 1972; 54:973–985.

52. Evans EB, Eggers GWN, Butler JK, Blumel J: Experimental immobilization and remobilization of rat knee joints. J Bone Joint Surg Am 1960; 42:737–758.

53. Farabollini F, Lupo Di Prisco C, Carli G: Changes in plasma testosterone and in its hypothalamic metabolism following immobility responses in rabbits. Physiol Behav 1978; 20:613–618.

54. Fiatarone MA, Marks EC, Ryan ND, et al: High intensity strength training in nonagenarians: Effects on skeletal muscle. JAMA 1990; 263:3029–3034.

55. Finsterbush A, Friedman B: Early changes in immobilized rabbits knee joints: A light and electron microscopic study. Clin Orthop 1973; 92:305–319.

56. Fishbein EG, Phillips M: How safe is exercise during pregnancy? J Obstet Gynecol Neonatal Nurs 1990; 19:45–49.

57. Fortney SM, Hyatt KH, Davis JE, Vogel JM: Changes in body fluid compartments during a 28-day bed rest. Aviat Space Environ Med 1991; 62:97–104.

58. Franklin BA, Gordon S, Timmis GC: Amount of exercise necessary for the patient with coronary artery disease. Am J Cardiol 1992; 69:1426–1432.

59. Frontera WR, Meredith CN, O'Reilly KP, et al: Strength conditioning in older men: Skeletal muscle hypertrophy and improved function. J Appl Physiol 1988; 64:1038–1044.

60. Fuller AK, Robinson ME: A test of exercise analgesia using signal detection theory and a within-subjects design. Percept Mot Skills 1993; 76:1299–1310.

61. Ghormley RK: The abuse of rest in bed in orthopedic surgery. JAMA 1944; 125:1085–1086.

62. Giannetta CL, Castleberry HB: Influence of bedrest and hypercapnia upon urinary mineral excretion in man. Aerospace Med 1974; 45:750–754.

63. Greenleaf JE: Energy and thermal regulation during bed rest and spaceflight. J Appl Physiol 1989; 67:507–516.

64. Greenleaf JE: Physiological responses to prolonged bed rest and fluid immersion in humans. J Appl Physiol 1984; 57:619–633.

65. Greenleaf JE, Bernauer EM, Young HL, et al: Fluid and electrolyte shifts during bed rest with isometric and isotonic exercise. J Appl Physiol 1977; 42:59–66.

66. Greenleaf JE, Reese RD: Exercise thermoregulation after 14 days of bed rest. J Appl Physiol 1980; 48:72–78.

67. Greenleaf JE, Van Beaumont W, Convertino VA, Starr JC: Handgrip and general muscular strength and endurance during prolonged bedrest with isometric and isotonic leg exercise training. Aviat Space Environ Med 1983; 54:696–700.

68. Greenleaf JE, Wade CE, Leftheriotis G: Orthostatic responses following 30-day bed rest deconditioning with isotonic and isokinetic exercise training. Aviat Space Environ Med 1989; 60:537–542.

69. Grimby G, Gustafsson E, Peterson L, Renstrom P: Quadriceps function and training after knee ligament surgery. Med Sci Sports Exerc 1980; 12:70–75.

70. Gwinup G: Weight loss without dietary restriction: Efficacy of different forms of aerobic exercise. Am J Sports Med 1987; 15:275–279.

71. Hagberg JM: Physiologic adaptations to prolonged high-intensity exercise training in patients with coronary artery disease. Med Sci Sports Exerc 1991; 23:661–667.

72. Hägberg JM, Seals DR: Exercise training and hypertension. Acta Med Scand Suppl 1986; 711:131–136.

73. Häggmark T, Eriksson E, Jansson E: Muscle fiber type changes in human skeletal muscle after injuries and immobilization. Orthopedics 1986; 9:181–185.

74. Haines RF: Effect of bed rest and exercise on body balance. J Appl Physiol 1974; 36:323–327.

75. Haskell WL: The influence of exercise training on plasma lipids

and lipoproteins in health and disease. Acta Med Scand Suppl 1986; 711:25–37.

76. Herbert RD, Balnave RJ: The effect of position of immobilization on resting length, resting stiffness, and weight of the soleus muscle of the rabbit. J Orthop Res 1993; 11:358–366.

77. Herbison GJ, Jaweed MM, Ditunno JF: Muscle fiber atrophy after cast immobilization in the rat. Arch Phys Med Rehabil 1978; 59:301–305.

78. Hilton J: On the Influence of Mechanical and Physiological Rest in the Treatment of Accidents and Surgical Diseases, and the Diagnostic Value of Pain. London, Bell & Daldy, 1863.

79. Houston ME, Bentzen H, Larsen H: Interrelationships between skeletal muscle adaptations and performance as studied by detraining and retraining. Acta Physiol Scand 1979; 105:163–170.

80. Hurley BF: Effects of resistive training on lipoprotein-lipid profiles: A comparison to aerobic exercise training. Med Sci Sports Exerc 1989; 21:689–693.

81. Hutchinson PL, Cureton K, Outz H, et al: Relationship of cardiac size to maximal oxygen uptake and body size in men and women. Int J Sports Med 1991; 12:369–373.

82. Issekuts B Jr, Blizzard JJ, Birkhead NC, Rodahl K: Effect of prolonged bed rest on urinary calcium output. J Appl Physiol 1966; 21:1013–1020.

83. Jarvinen MJ, Einola SA, Virtanen EO: Effect of the position of immobilization upon the tensile properties of the rat gastrocnemius muscle. Arch Phys Med Rehabil 1992; 73:253–257.

84. Jones HH, Priest JD, Hayes WC, et al: Humeral hypertrophy in response to exercise. J Bone Joint Surg Am 1977; 59:204–208.

85. Judge JO, Underwood M, Gennosa T: Exercise to improve gait velocity in older persons. Arch Phys Med Rehabil 1993; 74:400–406.

86. Jurvelin J, Helminen HJ, Lauritsalo S, et al: Influences of joint immobilization and running exercise on articular cartilage surfaces of young rabbits. Acta Anat 1985; 122:62–68.

87. Kannus P, Josza L, Kvist M, et al: The effect of immobilization on myotendinous junction: An ultrastructural, histochemical and immunohistochemical study. Acta Physiol Scand 1992; 144:387–394.

88. Karpakka J, Vaananen K, Orava S, Takala TES: The effects of preimmobilization training and immobilization on collagen synthesis in rat skeletal muscle. Int J Sports Med 1990; 11:484–488.

89. Kasper CE, McNulty AL, Otto AJ, Thomas DP: Alterations in skeletal muscle related to impaired physical mobility: an empirical model. Res Nurs Health 1993; 16:265–273.

90. Katsume H, Furukawa K, Azuma A, et al: Disuse atrophy of the left ventricle in chronically bedridden elderly people. Jpn Circ J 1992; 56:201–206.

91. Klein L, Heiple KG, Torzilli PA, et al: Prevention of ligament and meniscus atrophy by active joint motion in a non-weight-bearing model. J Orthop Res 1989; 7:80–85.

92. Koeppl PM, Heller J, Bleecker ER, et al: The influence of weight reduction upon the personality profiles of overweight males. J Clin Psychol 1992; 48:463–471.

93. Koivisto VA, DeFronzo RA: Exercise in the treatment of type II diabetes. Acta Endocrinol Suppl 1984; 262:107–111.

94. Kottke FJ: Deterioration of the bedfast patient. Public Health Rep 1965; 80:437–447.

95. Kottke FJ, Pauley DL, Ptak RA: The rationale for prolonged stretching for correction of shortening of connective tissue. Arch Phys Med Rehabil 1966; 47:345–352.

96. Krebs JM, Schneider VS, Evans H, et al: Energy absorption, lean body mass, and total body fat changes during 5 weeks of continuous bed rest. Aviat Space Environ Med 1990; 61:314–318.

97. Krebs JM, Schneider VS, LeBlanc AD: Zinc, copper, and nitrogen balances during bed rest and fluoride supplementation in healthy adult males. Am J Clin Nutr 1988; 47:509–514.

98. Krølner B, Toft B: Vertebral bone loss: An unheeded side effect of therapeutic bed rest. Clin Sci 1983; 64:537–540.

99. Laros GS, Tipton CM, Cooper RR: Influence of physical activity in the knees of dogs. J Bone Joint Surg Am 1971; 53:275–286.

100. Laubach LL: Comparative muscular strength of men and women: A review of the literature. Aviat Space Environ Med 1976; 47:534–542.

101. Leach CS, Hulley SB, Rambaut PC, Dietlein LF: The effect of bedrest on adrenal function. Space Life Sci 1973; 4:415–423.

102. LeBlanc AD, Schneider VS, Evans HJ, et al: Bone mineral loss and recovery after 17 weeks of bed rest. J Bone Miner Res 1990; 5:843–850.

103. Lerman S, Canterbury JM, Reiss E: Parathyroid hormone and the hypercalcemia of immobilization. J Clin Endocrinol Metab 1977; 45:425–428.

104. Levine DM, Cohen JD, Dustan HP, et al: Behavior changes and the prevention of high blood pressure. Workshop II. AHA Prevention Conference III. Behavior change and compliance: Keys to improving cardiovascular health. Circulation 1993; 88:1387–1390.

105. Li XJ, Jee WSS, Chow S, Woodbury DM: Adaptation of cancellous bone to aging and immobilization in the rat: A single photon absorptiometry and histomorphometry study. Anat Rec 1990; 227:12–24.

106. Lipman RL, Schnure JJ, Bradley EM, Lecocq FR: Impairment of peripheral glucose utilization in normal subjects by prolonged rest. J Lab Clin Med 1970; 76:221–230.

107. Lord SR, Caplan GA, Ward JA: Balance, reaction time, and muscle strength in exercising and nonexercising older women: A pilot study. Arch Phys Med Rehabil 1993; 74:837–839.

108. MacDougall JD, Elder GCB, Sale DG, et al: Effects of strength training and immobilization on human muscle fibres. Eur J Appl Physiol 1980; 43:25–34.

109. Mallory GK, White PD, Salcedo-Salgar J: The speed of healing of myocardial infarction: A study of the pathologic anatomy in seventy-two cases. Am Heart J 1939; 18:647.

110. Marti B, Suter E, Riesen WF, et al: Effects of long-term, self-monitored exercise on the serum lipoprotein and apolipoprotein profile in middle-aged men. Atherosclerosis 1990; 81:19–31.

111. Martinsen EW: Benefits of exercise for the treatment of depression. Sports Med 1990; 9:380–389.

112. Melada GA, Goldman RH, Luetscher JA, Zager PG: Hemodynamics, renal function, plasma renin, and aldosterone in man after 5 to 14 days of bedrest. Aviat Space Environ Med 1975; 46:1049–1055.

113. Merritt JL, Hunder GG: Passive range of motion, not isometric exercise, amplifies acute urate synovitis. Arch Phys Med Rehabil 1983; 64:130–131.

114. Meythaler JM, Tuel SM, Cross LL: Successful treatment of immobilization hypercalcemia using calitonin and etidronate. Arch Phys Med Rehabil 1993; 74:316–319.

115. Michelsson J, Aho HJ, Kalimo H, Haltia M: Severe degeneration of rabbit vastus intermedius muscle immobilized in shortened position. APMIS 1990; 98:336–344.

116. Mikines KJ, Dela F, Tronier B, Galbo H: Effect of 7 days of bed rest on dose-response relation between plasma glucose and insulin secretion. Am J Physiol 1989; 257:E43–E48.

117. Minare P: Immobilization osteoporosis: A review. Clin Rheumatol 8:95–103;1989.

118. Moldover JR, Downey JA: Cardiac response to exercise: Comparison of 3 ergometers. Arch Phys Med Rehabil 1983; 64:155–159.

119. Morgan WP: Affective beneficence of vigorous physical activity. Med Sci Sports Exerc 1985; 17:94–100.

120. Moritani T, deVries HA: Neural factors versus hypertrophy in the time course of muscle strength gain in young and old men. J Gerontol 1981; 36:294–297.

121. Mueller EA: Influence of training and of inactivity on muscle strength. Arch Phys Med Rehabil 1970; 51:449–462.

122. Newton PO, Woo SLY, Kitabayashi LR, et al: Ultrastructural changes in knee ligaments following immobilization. Matrix 1990; 10:314–319.

123. Nicks DN, Beneke WM, Key RM, Timson BF: Muscle fiber size and number following immobilization atrophy. J Anat 1989; 163:1–5.

124. Noyes FR: Functional properties of knee ligaments and alterations induced by immobilization. Clin Orthop 1977; 123:210–242.

125. Pachter BR, Eberstein A: Neuromuscular plasticity following limb immobilization. J Neurocytol 1984; 13:1013–1025.

126. Palmoski M, Perricore E, Brandt KD: Development and reversal of a proteoglycan aggregation defect in normal canine cartilage after immobilization. Arthritis Rheum 1979; 22:508–515.

127. Palmoski MJ, Colyer RA, Brandt KD: Joint motion in the absence of normal loading does not maintain normal articular cartilage. Arthritis Rheum 1980; 23:325–334.

128. Powell KE, Thompson PD, Caspersen CJ, Kendrick JS: Physical activity and the incidence of coronary heart disease. Annu Rev Public Health 1987; 8:253–287.

129. Prior JC, Vigna Y, Alojado N: Conditioning exercise decreases

premenstrual symptoms: A prospective controlled three month trial. Eur J Appl Physiol 1986; 55:349–355.

130. Raab W, De Paula e Silva P, Marchet H, et al: Cardiac adrenergic preponderance due to lack of physical exercise and its pathogenic implications. Am J Cardiol 1960; 5:300–320.

131. Roberts NA, Barton RN, Horan MA, White A: Adrenal function after upper femoral fracture in elderly people: Persistence of stimulation and the roles of adrenocorticotrophic hormone and immobility. Age Aging 1990; 19:304–310.

132. Rubin R: Pregnant? Go to bed. US News & World Report 61, Jan 10, 1994, p 61.

133. Rutherford OM, Jones DA, Round JM: Long-lasting unilateral muscle wasting and weakness following injury and immobilisation. Scand J Rehabil Med 1990; 22:33–37.

134. Ryback RS, Lewis OF, Lessard CS: Psychobiologic effects of prolonged bed rest (weightlessness) in young, healthy volunteers (study II). Aerospace Med 1971; 42:529–535.

135. Saltin B, Blomquist G, Mitchell JH, et al: Response to exercise after bed rest and after training. A longitudinal study of adaptive changes in oxygen transport and body composition. Circulation 1968; 38(suppl 7):VII1–VII78.

136. Samel A, Wegmann H, Vejvoda M: Response of the circadian system to 6° head-down tilt bed rest. Aviat Space Environ Med 1993; 64:50–54.

137. Saris WH: The role of exercise in the dietary treatment of obesity. Int J Obesity 1993; 17(suppl 1):S17–S21.

138. Schneider VS, McDonald J: Skeletal calcium homeostasis and countermeasures to prevent disuse osteoporosis. Calcif Tissue Int 1984; 36:S151–S154.

139. Schutz LK: The wheelchair athlete. In Buschbacher RM, Braddom RL (eds): Sports Medicine and Rehabilitation: A Sports Specific Approach. Philadelphia, Hanley & Belfus, 1994.

140. Schwarz L, Kindermann W: Changes in β-endorphin levels in response to aerobic and anaerobic exercise. Sports Med 1992; 13:25–36.

141. Seip RL, Moulin P, Cocke T, et al: Exercise training decreases plasma cholesteryl ester transfer protein. Arteriosclerosis Thromb 1993; 13:1359–1367.

142. Shephard RJ: Exercise and aging: Extending independence in older adults. Geriatrics 1993; 48:61–64.

143. Smith DW, Claren SK, Harvey MAS: Hyperthermia as a possible teratogenic agent. J Pediatr 1978; 92:878–883.

144. Smith MJ: Changes in judgement of duration with different patterns of auditory information for individuals confined to bed. Nurs Res 1975; 24:93–98.

145. Smith RL, Thomas KD, Schurman DJ, et al: Rabbit knee immobilization: Bone remodeling precedes cartilage degeneration. J Orthop Res 1992; 10:88–95.

146. Sparling PB: A metanalysis of studies comparing maximal oxygen uptake in men and women. Res Q Exerc Sport 1980; 51:542–552.

147. Spector SA, Simard CP, Fournier M, et al: Architectural alterations of rat hind-limb skeletal muscles immobilized at different lengths. Exp Neurol 1982; 76:94–110.

148. Stewart AF, Adler M, Byers CM, et al: Calcium homeostasis in immobilization: An example of resorptive hypercalciuria. N Engl J Med 306:1136–1140, 1982.

149. Stewart KJ: Weight training in coronary artery disease and hypertension. Prog Cardiovasc Dis 1992; 35:159–168.

150. Stolk JM, Harris PQ: Differentiation of adrenomedullary catecholamine synthesizing enzyme responses to repeated immobilization in hybrid rats. Life Sci 1980; 26:2099–2104.

151. Stremel RW, Convertino VA, Bernauer EM, Greenleaf JE: Cardiorespiratory deconditioning with static and dynamic leg exercise during bed rest. J Appl Physiol 1976; 41:905–909.

152. Stuart CA, Shangraw RE, Peters EJ, Wolfe RR: Effect of dietary protein on bed-rest–related changes in whole-body-protein synthesis. Am J Clin Nutr 1990; 52:509–514.

153. Stuart CA, Shangraw RE, Prince MJ, et al: Bed-rest–induced insulin resistance occurs primarily in muscle. Metabolism 1988; 37:802–806.

154. Superko HR: Exercise training, serum lipids, and lipoprotein particles: Is there a change threshold? Med Sci Sports Exerc 1991; 23:677–685.

155. Suzuki Y, Kashihara H, Katagiri A, et al: Effects of moderate physical training after 10 days horizontal bed-rest on peak $\dot{V}O_2$ and cardio-respiratory functions during submaximal supine and sitting exercise in young subjects. Physiologist 1992; 35(suppl 1):S198–S199.

156. Tanji JL: Hypertension part I: How exercise helps. Phys Sports Med 1990; 18:77–82.

157. Tanji JL, Champlin JJ, Wong GY, et al: Blood pressure recovery curves after submaximal exercise: A predictor of hypertension at ten-year follow-up. Am J Hypertens 1989; 2:135–138.

158. Taylor HL, Henschel A, Brožek J, Keys A: Effects of bed rest on cardiovascular function and work performance. J Appl Physiol 1949; 2:223–239.

159. Thompson DD, Rodan GA: Indomethacin inhibition of tenotomy-induced bone resorption in rats. J Bone Miner Res 1988; 3:409–414.

160. Uhtoff HK, Jaworski ZFG: Bone loss in response to long-term immobilization. J Bone Joint Surg Br 1978; 60:420–429.

161. van Lent P, Wilms FHA, van den Berg WB: Interaction of polymorphonuclear leucocytes with patellar cartilage of immobilised arthritic joints: A scanning electron microscopic study. Ann Rheum Dis 1989; 48:832–837.

162. Veldhuizen JW, Verstappen FTJ, Vroemen JPAM, et al: Functional and morphological adaptations following four weeks of knee immobilization. Int J Sports Med 1993; 14:283–287.

163. Vernikos J, Dallman MF, Keil LC, et al: Gender differences in endocrine responses to posture and 7 days of −6° head-down bed rest. Am J Physiol 1993; 265:E153–161.

164. Vernikos-Danellis J, Leach CS, Winget CM, et al: Changes in glucose, insulin, and growth hormone levels associated with bedrest. Aviat Space Environ Med 1976; 47:583–587.

165. Warren CJ, Lehmann JF, Koblanski JN: Elongation of rat tail tendon: Effect of load and temperature. Arch Phys Med Rehabil 1971; 52:465–474.

166. White PD, Mallory GK, Salcedo-Salgar J: The speed of healing of myocardial infarcts. In Transactions of the American Clinical and Climatological Association. Framingham, Mass, Lakeview Press, 1937, pp 97–104.

167. Whitney EJ, Ashcom TL, Hantman RK, et al: Reversibility of fixed atherosclerotic lesions with aggressive risk factor modification: Milit Med 1991; 156:422–429.

168. Williams PE: Use of intermittent stretch in the prevention of serial sarcomere loss in immobilized muscle. Ann Rheum Dis 1990; 49:316–317.

169. Williams PE, Goldspink G: Connective tissue changes in immobilized muscle. J Anat 1984; 138:343–350.

170. Wilson CJ, Dahners LE: An examination of the mechanism of ligament contracture. Clin Orthop 1988; 227:286–291.

171. Yagan R, Radivoyevitch M, Khan M: Double cortical line in the acetabular roof: A sign of disuse osteoporosis. Radiology 1987; 165:171–175.

172. Yeh JK, Aloia JF: Effect of physical activity on calcitropic hormones and calcium balance in rats. Am J Physiol 1990; 258:E263–E268.

173. Young DR, Niklowitz WJ, Brown RJ, Jee WSS: Immobilization-associated osteoporosis in primates. Bone 1986; 7:109–117.

174. Zorbas YG, Andreyev VG, Popescu LB: Fluid-electrolyte metabolism and renal function in men under hypokinesia and physical exercise. Int Urol Nephrol 1988; 20:215–223.

175. Zorbas YG, Naexu KA, Federenko YF: Blood serum biochemical changes in physically conditioned and unconditioned subjects during bed rest and chronic hyperhydration. Clin Exp Pharmacol Physiol 1992; 19:137–145.

Management of Specific Diagnoses Encountered in Physical Medicine and Rehabilitation Practice

Rehabilitation of Patients With Rheumatic Disorders

JOHN J. NICHOLAS, M.D.

The rehabilitation of patients with rheumatic diseases has changed dramatically over the last few decades. These changes have been due to new medical and surgical treatments and to economic developments that affect the provision of rehabilitation care to rheumatic disease patients.

In the late 1940s and subsequently, a classic protocol of medical, surgical, and rehabilitation care was developed to treat arthritis patients.[9, 30, 40, 82, 84, 107, 108, 114, 132, 152, 175] This treatment program provided comprehensive care in medical centers and rehabilitation hospitals, and some outpatient facilities, utilizing an almost unlimited length of stay. The treatment included the careful prescription of rest, both at home and in hospitals, various forms of exercise, the applications of casts and splints, instruction in work simplification and energy conservation, prescription of heat and cold, and many medical treatments. Improvement was noted in most cases. It was demonstrated that bed rest and casts for as long as 14 days did not permanently diminish the active range of motion of joints of patients with rheumatoid arthritis (RA).[144] It was further demonstrated that those patients with RA who had the most severely involved joints benefited most from inpatient treatment and rest.[5] Generally, inpatient care was shown to be more effective than outpatient care in providing these treatments.[103]

Various physical modalities were widely used. Studies documented patients' appreciation and acceptance, but few studies demonstrated improvement in the patient's disease or function following the application of modalities.[125]

Beginning in the 1950s, the use of adrenocorticosteroids (ACs) provided great relief from joint pain for patients with RA, but ACs were subsequently shown to frequently lead to myopathy, cataracts, gastrointestinal bleeding, osteoporosis, compression fractures, and other complications. Patients suffering from these complications were often hospitalized in rehabilitation centers so that other treatment modalities could make up for the discontinuation of the steroids.

Nowadays, ACs are rarely given in large enough doses or long enough to cause these complications. Thus, such patients are no longer admitted to rehabilitation centers. In addition, intramuscular gold, hydroxychloroquine, azathioprine, and, most recently, methotrexate, have provided better suppression of joint inflammation than was previously possible. Currently, patients with RA and other inflammatory joint diseases seem, on balance, to be doing better, with less destructive inflammation, and, therefore, to have less need to be hospitalized in an inpatient rehabilitation hospital or unit.[18]

Developments in orthopedic surgery have been highly successful. Joint replacement (arthroplasty) has provided physiatrists a whole new range of therapeutic challenges, including patients with remarkable relief from pain and new functional deficits. These patients do very well, but postoperatively many require rehabilitation care to maximize the gains from their surgical procedure. Those without complications frequently leave the hospital within their diagnosis-related group (DRG)–designated length of stay, but those with severe RA or osteoarthritis in non-operated joints or with co-morbidity (strokes, amputations, congestive heart failure, persistent pain, bilateral arthroplasties, lack of knee flexion, bone grafts, arthroplasty revision) require hospitalization on rehabilitation units (Table 35–1). As described by Opitz at the Mayo Clinic, rehabilitation of postoperative orthopedic patients has become quite frequent, and the postarthroplasty patient now is more common in many rehabilitation care settings than the patient with a stroke.[138]

Since the advent of DRG-based hospital reimbursement for Medicare patients, the acute hospital length of stay has become shorter and admissions for treatment of rheumatic diseases less frequent. It would appear that physicians in acute hospitals would be anxious to discharge patients when their DRG time has run out and that admission to a rehabilitation hospital would be quite appropriate and sought after. The Health Care Financing Administration (HCFA) has funded formal rehabilitation care for the pa-

TABLE 35–1   Indications for Comprehensive Rehabilitation After Arthroplasty Procedures*

Complex medical problems	Revision arthroplasty
Multiple joint involvement	Bone grafting
Severe contralateral joint disease	Cementless prosthesis
Stroke	Lack of knee flexion
Amputation	Slow progress
Congestive heart failure	Hemodialysis patients
Persistent pain	Fractures
Bilateral arthroplasties	Possible infections

*These medical problems are a partial list of suggested reasons to hospitalize arthroplasty patients in a comprehensive rehabilitation unit or free-standing center.

TABLE 35–2   Typical Reasons for Physiatric Consultation for Patients Hospitalized for Acute Rheumatic Disease*

Leg-length discrepancy secondary to severe ankle degeneration (heel lift)
Flexion contracture (treatment suggestions)
Metatarsalgia (footwear and appropriate modifications)
Neurogenic bladder secondary to lupus vasculitis, spinal cord involvement (catheterization schedule suggestions)
Lower extremity edema and ulcers; postphlebitis syndrome (pressure gradient stockings)
Diabetic neuropathy (ankle-foot orthoses)
Upper extremity splinting
Vertebral compression fractures (spinal jacket)
Pressure sore (treatment suggestions)
Polymyositis (aerobic training recommendations)
Severe rheumatoid arthritis (cervical collar prescription)

*Finestone catalogued the consultation problems he encountered in his practice. Experience will undoubtedly reveal other opportunities for physiatrists to provide services to rheumatic disease patients.

tients, provided they meet the criteria for admission to a DRG-exempt rehabilitation unit. A complication arose, however, in that rheumatologists and physiatrists could not submit bills for concurrent care for the same current procedural terminology code (CPT) and DRG. In the case of RA, there must be two separate CPT codes that are used to designate two separate treatment efforts. It appears that the lack of two appropriate CPT codes has led to a trend for rheumatologists to refer fewer patients to rehabilitation centers.

It is unfortunate that the current medical financing situation does not allow a better opportunity for physiatrists and rheumatologists to care for arthritis patients co-operatively. Common practice has demonstrated that there are features of the rheumatic disease patient that must be cared for by each specialist. In addition, surveys have demonstrated that rheumatologists receive relatively little education in rehabilitation techniques during their training,[80] and, conversely, physiatrists have little exposure to education in the treatment and diagnosis of rheumatic disease patients in their residency programs.[81] There currently is a project to increase the knowledge of rehabilitation treatments among rheumatology fellows, sponsored by the American College of Rheumatology.*

In the past, a classic analogy for the description of the application of treatments to rheumatic disease patients was the therapeutic pyramid.[92, 115] This analogy placed surgical treatments at the apex of the pyramid, and rehabilitation treatments at the base or at the initial onset of the disease. A more recent analogy suggests that various treatments should be added as the severity of the disease increases. In this model, rehabilitation treatments are recommended at the onset of the disease. The most recent model places the patient in the center and various treatments around the periphery.[147] Again, it is recommended that rehabilitation treatments be applied early, at the onset of the various rheumatic diseases.

Where will these treatments be performed? Certainly at the present time, inpatient rehabilitation units and free-standing rehabilitation centers have been shown to provide exemplary care.[34] In addition, Finestone has demonstrated many opportunities for the physiatrist to provide consultation and patient services to patients hospitalized in an

"acute" general hospital or on a rheumatology service (Table 35–2).[52] Alternative treatment sites include comprehensive outpatient rehabilitation facilities (CORFs), outpatient units, subacute rehabilitation units, skilled nursing facilities (SNFs), nursing homes, and home health services. Many of these provide care in a less costly setting. The physiatrist must become involved in the provision of rehabilitation services to rheumatic disease patients in these settings.

Some of the reasons to admit rheumatic disease patients to a rehabilitation unit include a marked decline in activites of daily living, inability to get around owing to steroid myopathy, the development of quadriparesis (atlantoaxial subluxation), mononeuritis multiplex (vasculitis), severe anemia, out of control inflammation, and amputations (Table 35–3).

In addition, there are circumstances under which a rheumatologist should be involved with the daily or near daily care of these patients. The rheumatologist is needed to manage medications in difficult situations, initiate disease-modifying antirheumatic drugs and help with the diagnostic dilemmas of anemia, mononeuritis multiplex, renal disease, unexplained weakness, and on occasion to solve a diagnostic dilemma (Table 35–4).

The physiatrist must determine when to hospitalize postoperative orthopedic patients in the rehabilitation unit or center. It is generally acknowledged that the patients with best results go home, but many others require admission to nursing homes or "subacute units." Some of these patients should be hospitalized for the comprehensive intensive rehabilitation services provided in a rehabilitation unit or center under such circumstances as those listed in Table 35–1. Although to date no data demonstrate a better result following hospitalization on an inpatient unit than in a nursing home for these patients, the physician must be a

*Hicks J (Chairman, Subcommittee on Curriculum, Section of Rehabilitation Rheumatology and the Subcommittee on Educational Materials, the Education Committee, American Academy of Rheumatology): Personal communication.

TABLE 35–3   Typical Reasons for Hospitalizing Rheumatic Disease Patients in a Comprehensive Rehabilitation Unit

Decline in ADL	Severe anemia
Steroid myopathy	Uncontrolled inflammation
Quadriparesis	Amputation
Vasculitis	

TABLE 35–4   Reasons for Concurrent Care by a Rheumatologist for Rheumatic Disease Patients in a Rehabilitation Unit*

Consultation of medication management
Treatment with DMARDS
Diagnostic problems:
Anemia
Vasculitis
Peripheral neuropathy
Unexplained weakness
Gastrointestinal bleeding, renal disease

*Almost any rheumatic disease patient who experiences a severe decrease in function requires consultation from a rheumatologist on admission to a comprehensive rehabilitation unit or free-standing center.

patient advocate and insist on rehabilitation unit or center admission when it is clinically clear that such an admission would provide a quicker and/or better outcome.

The effectiveness of the rehabilitation team has been demonstrated, but there must be a genuinely therapeutic team.[34] A team is not just a group of skilled persons playing the same game. There must be a coach, a captain, position players, and a clearly defined game plan. These interdisciplinary teams have traditionally been available in inpatient settings, but they can be developed for day hospital, outpatient, or home care as well.

This chapter describes the modern rehabilitation techniques that are appropriate for patients with rheumatic diseases. The reader is referred to current rheumatology textbooks for detailed information about specific rheumatic diseases and the latest diagnostic techniques. The rheumatic diseases that are most appropriately treated by rehabilitation techniques include osteoarthritis (OA), RA, ankylosing spondylitis and the other spondyloarthropathies, systemic lupus erythematosus (SLE), progressive systemic sclerosis (PSS), and dermatomyositis/polymyositis (DM/PM).

EVALUATION OF PATIENTS

Specific Historical Details

The rheumatic disease patient requires attention to details of the history and physical examination that are specific to the rheumatic diseases.[148] Before prescribing a comprehensive rehabilitation program, the physiatrist must obtain the following information:

FUNCTIONAL SCREEN.   Can the patient perform such ADL tasks as dressing, bathing, feeding, toileting hygiene and transfers, and walking (see Chapter 1)?

VOCATIONAL SCREEN.   Can the patient get into and out of a car and into and out of a parking place? Are ergonomic changes required at work, or is a different job necessary?

The items listed in Table 35–5 should be included in the initial history.

Specific Physical Findings

Physiatrists cannot evaluate and subsequently treat patients with a rheumatic disease unless they are familiar with the physical findings (Table 35–6). Further description

TABLE 35–5   Frequent Signs and Symptoms of Rheumatic Diseases and Possible Causes

Sign/Symptom	Likely Causes
Alopecia	ACS or cyclophosphamide therapy, SLE
Morning stiffness	RA, spondylitis
Morning back pain	Ankylosing spondylitis
Joint crepitus	OA, joint damage, soft tissue inflammation
Diarrhea	Ulcerative colitis with spondylitis or arthritis
Dysuria	Reiter's syndrome
Genital sores	Reiter's syndrome
"Nephritis"	SLE
Numb thumb	Carpal tunnel syndrome
Palpable purpura	Systemic cutaneous vasculitis
Photosensitivity	SLE, drugs
Pleuritis	SLE, drug-induced or spontaneous
Raynaud's phenomenon	Color changes PSS vs. CREST
	DM/PM, RA, local trauma (e.g., from tennis playing or air hammer)
Red eyes	Reiter's conjunctivitis, uveitis
Rash	Psoriasis, drug eruption (ibuprofen, d-penicillamine), SLE, drug-induced or spontaneous, rheumatic fever
Weakness on arising from chair or bathtub	DM/PM, steroid-induced proximal myopathy

of these findings is available in rheumatic disease textbooks.[148]

Physical Examination Techniques

RANGE-OF-MOTION TESTING.   In patients with rheumatic disease the range of motion (ROM) is frequently limited at one or more joints. At times, the joint surfaces

TABLE 35–6   Frequent Physical Findings in Rheumatic Disease and Possible Causes

Finding	Possible Cause
Boutonnière deformity	RA, SLE, parkinsonism, MCT disease
Metacarpophalangeal subluxation	
Ulnar deviation	
Swan-neck deformity	RA
Bouchard's nodes	PIP joint OA
Finger drop	Tendon rupture
Footdrop	Mononeuritis multiplex
Heberden's nodes	DIP joint OA
Joint effusions	Ballotte patella, "bulge sign"
Lhermitte's sign	Cervical myelopathy, also occipital paresthesias as a sign when flexed with atlanto-axal subluxation
Occipital paresthesias	
Mouth ulcers	Reiter's syndrome
Skin ulcers	Venous stasis, arteritis, pressure sores
Subcutaneous nodules	Gouty tophi, RA, rheumatic fever
Synovitis	Joint pain only vs. inflammation (place finger beneath MCP joint to detect small amounts of synovitis)
Telangiectasia	CREST syndrome
Tendon rubs	PSS
Tender points	Fibromyalgia, tendinitis, bursitis
Trigger points	Referred pain of fibromyalgia

and supporting structures are damaged so badly that the joint does not perform a normal arc of motion. The examiner should estimate the instantaneous axis of rotation to determine range of motion (ROM) and whether subluxation or dislocation is present. Both *active* and *passive* ROM are recorded for all involved joints. The examiner also records if pain limits motion or if there is a pain-free limit to the motion. Each joint having limited ROM is compared with its plain radiographs and the joints on the opposite side. Inflammation should be recorded for each joint that is abnormal. It should also be noted if a joint is swollen, deformed, hot, or unstable.

MANUAL MUSCLE TESTING. The manual muscle test cannot be performed accurately at a joint where muscle contraction causes pain. The examiner should record whether or not pain is present during muscle contraction and should estimate strength (see Chapter 1). The examiner should also take into account strength training, conditioning, sex, age, diagnosis, and degree of patient *effort* when assessing strength. Muscle weakness should be noted and whether it is distributed in a proximal, distal, lateral, or generalized pattern. It must also be taken into consideration whether muscle-affecting medications have been administered, such as ACS, lovastatin, or hydroxychloroquine.

THERAPEUTIC MODALITIES

Heat and Cold

Various methods of applying heat have been used for thousands of years to treat rheumatic disease (see Chapter 22). Most have utilized superficial heat. The mineral springs at Bath, England, for example, have been in use since the first millennium, BC. In addition, there are hot springs all over Europe and the United States that patients have visited in the hope of relieving various ailments, including arthritis. In modern times, Elkayam[45] described patients with both RA and OA who were treated in a controlled study with mineral baths and mud packs. No statistical evaluations were performed, but grip strength increased in treated subjects. Sukenik and co-workers[160] and Helliwell[77] also provided a review of spa therapy. There is no conclusive scientific evidence that spa therapy benefits patients with OA, RA, or other rheumatic diseases, but patients avail themselves of this form of treatment, with or without the advice of their physicians, and many claim improvement.

Superficial heat is more *commonly* used than deep heat for treating rheumatic conditions. It has also been felt to be more beneficial and *appropriate* than deep heat.[51] This is partly because of reported patient discomfort from deep heat and because of Harris' study, which demonstrated that heating to therapeutic levels increased the activity of synovial collagenase obtained from a rheumatoid joint.[74]

In the past it was noted that when moist superficial hot packs were applied over arthritic joints, the joint temperature fell by as much as 2.2 °F.[85] Furthermore, the use of microwave diathermy (12.2 Hz) increased the temperature at the skin surface and within the knee joint as much as 5 °F.[83] Spiegal demonstrated that heating RA patients' knee joints with diathermy at 13.56 Hz for as long as 60 minutes

did not increase pain.[156] Falconer showed that ultrasound treatment of OA knee joints did not appear to cause any improvement.[50] The recent series of studies by Weinberger and associates[170-172] has shown that, in both experimental animals and humans, diathermy at 9.15 Hz for 1 hour decreased chronic knee effusions of RA patients. They demonstrated in rabbits that zymosan synovitis was improved by this treatment. While these findings need to be confirmed, this "thermal synovectomy" seems to hold promise. Further data on the use of superficial vs. deep heat in rheumatic disease patients are both incomplete and inconclusive.[72]

There was no improvement with ultrasound or short-wave diathermy in osteoarthritic patients' knees in a study using functional capacity score and Cybex testing as end-points.[88] A long-forgotten study by Frankel showed that prolonged rest (4 weeks) and application of electric heating blankets below the waist was followed by a fall in sedimentation rate, diminution in soft tissue swelling, and improvement in ROM.[61] Mainardi demonstrated that heating the hands of patients with RA in an electric mitten raised the intra-articular temperature and did not cause radiographic evidence of progression or destruction of the joints.[111]

Pegg and Kirk and their groups described the application of ice packs to patients with RA.[98, 145] Many patients preferred cold to heat. Some thought cold produced better ROM than hot packs. Trial and patient preference should direct the prescription of heat or cold for rheumatic disease.

It is apparent from clinical observation of patients with various types of inflammatory arthritis that the application of moist heat packs, moist heating pads, hot showers, paraffin baths, and the like produces at least temporary diminution in pain and increased ability to move and exercise inflamed joints. There is no scientific evidence to demonstrate that heat improves joint erosions, nor any to suggest it further damages joints. Before exercising, superficial heat, and deep heat if available, should be applied. The dose is determined by *c*ost, *c*ustom, and *c*onvenience rather than by scientific data. For example, moist heating packs should be applied as early in the day as possible, to help relieve morning stiffness, and then repeated once or twice during the day.

Other Modalities for Treating Rheumatic Diseases

Various other modalities have been tried in the treatment of patients with rheumatic disease, and there is some scientific evidence to support their efficacy. Culic[35] treated RA patients with nylon spandex compression gloves. Patients reported feeling better after wearing the gloves, but there was little measurable change except for reduced finger circumference. These compression gloves are particularly helpful if finger stiffness is excessive. Topical counterirritant ointments have been reported by White and Sage[173, 174] to provide relief, as judged by patients. In addition, McCarthy and McCarty[116] found that topical capsaicin reduced pain of OA of the fingers as determined by a dolorimeter. It was impossible to demonstrate improvement in RA patients with capsaicin.

The use of transcutaneous electronic nerve stimulation (TENS) has been reported for many conditions (see Chapter 23). Improved wrist and hand function with TENS was reported for RA patients by Mannheimer[112, 113] and confirmed by Kumer and Redford.[101] Application of TENS to hands and wrists, however, will probably be awkward and will limit use and interfere with compliance.

TENS has also been applied for OA of the knees.[106, 163] The results were not very dramatic, but selected patients reported considerable pain relief. A recent publication reviewed the use of TENS and acupuncture for rheumatic diseases and in general found the results of treatment not very remarkable.[125]

Relief of Joint Contractures

Patients with various forms of inflammatory rheumatic diseases or OA can lose the ability to move their joints through the full ROM. Historically, such joint contractures have been a great problem, but in contemporary medicine many are now relieved by surgery (arthroplasty). The cause and treatment of these contractures were recently reviewed.[146] Adhesions across the joint surfaces *have not* been shown to be the cause. Studies (beginning with that of Ely and Mensor in 1933) in both animals and patients have shown that surgical muscle release relieves contractures in the early stage.[46] After about 2 weeks, however, capsular and pericapsular structures change and must be released to regain motion. The changes in these capsular and pericapsular structures include a loss of water and glycosaminoglycans (4% to 6% loss of water and 30% to 40% glycosaminoglycans). There was no increase in total collagen, but there was an alteration in cross-linkages and the organization of the collagen fibers, which was thought to affect the ability to glide under tension. There was ingrowth of fibrofatty connective tissue into the joint space and degenerative changes in the collagen.[3-4, 6, 7, 47, 49, 53, 71]

Contractures also affect patients with central nervous system injury, but their loss of ROM is due to lack of active motion and spasticity rather than to joint disease (see Chapters 29 and 49).[23] A review of surgical treatment of joint contractures and of surgical evaluation and treatment of joint contractures in spastic patients was recently published.[94, 95]

Many authors have reported successful treatment of contractures, usually at the knee, with casts and splints. Modalities include wedge casting,[15] casts plus traction,[41, 42] serial casting, traction, weights and exercise and manipulation under anesthesia,[149] splints for knees and wrists,[161] casts, exercise, and traction,[93] plaster casts and splints,[33] plaster spints with cuffs,[70] plaster casts, posterior splints, and a unique knee-straightening device.[75] In addition, casts have been used in an unsuccessful attempt to correct deformities of PSS.[153] Casts have been used to correct burn scar contractures[150] and elbow fractures or contractures.[154, 178] Relief of contractures through use of a constant passive motion machine (CPM) has been reported anecdotally.

When joint contractures secondary to rheumatic disorders are treated with serial casting or splinting, the results are directly related to the severity of the joint destruction as demonstrated by radiographs (the better the x-ray appearance the better the result; Table 35–7). Treatment can be provided with various materials (e.g., plaster, fiberglass, plastic). Full cylinder casts, posterior splints, and splints

TABLE 35–7   Steps in Cast Correction of Flexion Contractures

1. Assess radiographic status.
2. Cast in maximum voluntary extension.
3. Remove cast for daily hygiene.
4. Recast weekly.
5. Last 10 degrees of ROM is most difficult to achieve.
6. ROM migrates.

with cuffs have all been used successfully. The casts are applied in a position of maximum extension without excessive force and are removed for hygiene every day. At the end of 5 to 7 days, the casts or splints are replaced and more extension is noted. The last 10 degrees of extension is typically the most difficult to achieve, and often that is impossible. The total ROM usually does not change, but the ROM shifts toward the extension limits rather than the flexion limits of joint motion.[131]

APPROACHES TO SPECIFIC RHEUMATIC DISEASES

Rheumatoid Arthritis

Sir William Osler considered syphilis the prototypical disease to study. He believed that if student physicians could treat all the manifestations of syphilis, they could treat almost all medical conditions. "I often tell my students that it [syphilis] is the only disease which they are required to study thoroughly. Know syphilis in all its manifestations and relations and all other things clinical will be added unto you."[139] Similarly, if physiatrists can apply rehabilitation techniques to patients with RA, they should be able to treat the manifestations of any other of the rheumatic diseases.

RA is an inflammatory disease of joints that has some systemic manifestations. The exact cause of the inflammation is not yet known, but it is a complex hypersensitivity reaction. The inflammation causes weakening of the joint capsule, tendons, ligaments, and cartilaginous surfaces of joints. The underlying bone becomes osteoporotic and weak. The bone is also eroded, especially at the attachments of the synovial tissue to bone. These erosions are pathognomonic of RA. A number of deformities are characteristic of RA, especially in the fingers (metacarpophalangeal ulnar deviation and subluxation, boutonnière and swan-neck deformities of the proximal and distal interphalangeal joints, and ruptured finger tendons). Many of these deformities occur in other diseases as well, as they are due to weakening of the supporting tendinous and capsular structures and not to the underlying bony erosions. Whether or not erosions occur separates the deformed hands of patients with, for example, SLE or Charcot-Marie-Tooth disease (deforming non-erosive arthritis) from those with RA.[27, 39]

Rehabilitation goals for patients with RA include pain relief, increased ROM, increased strength and endurance, prevention and correction of deformities, and provision of various counseling and education services.

Pain Relief

The time-honored treatment of RA joint pain has been application of moist heat. This has been accomplished through various devices, including moist heating packs, electric mittens, hot showers, hot water, and spas. It has been demonstrated in normal subjects that hot packs provide heat (lasting about 15 minutes) to a depth of 1 to 1.5 cm.[105] The frequency of application is guided by cost, custom, and convenience, but it should be at least twice daily. Burns can occur with moist heat, and the patient must be tested for sensory deficits before moist heat is used. Additional contraindications to heat are listed in Chapter 22.

The use of microwave was thought in the past to increase synovial collagenase activity[74] and possibly cause joint destruction and was not felt to be tolerated well by patients.[51] Recently, however, Weinberger has advocated the use of "thermal synovectomy" through diathermy treatment, but this modality needs further study.[170–172]

It is also appropriate to treat joints with moist heat in preparation for ROM, stretching, and most muscle-strengthening exercises. In fact, only rarely is heat alone used for RA patients. It usually is a pain reliever, reduces stiffness, and serves as preparation to an exercise program. The joints that are most painful should be treated first. Patients should be encouraged to treat their joints at home just as in treatment centers. At least part of the treatment time in physical or occupational therapy should be used to make certain the patient knows how to use the modality at home. Moist heat treatments are no more *temporary* than non-steroidal anti-inflammatory drugs (NSAIDs), but they are more *inconvenient*.

Application of splints, mostly for wrists and knees, has been shown to relieve pain in inflamed RA joints.[96, 97, 131] Gault demonstrated that splints universally diminished the signs of inflammation in RA-involved hands as compared with signs in the opposite non-splinted hand.[62] The chief drawbacks that decrease the use of splints for pain relief are poor cosmesis and inconvenience, but patients often choose to wear them anyway. They are particularly helpful during heavy use activities.[128, 129]

Prevention and Correction of Deformities

It is possible to predict the deformities at most joints in most patients with RA (Table 35–8).[158] For example, knee deformities occur in a position of flexion. Shoulders are always in adduction contracture. Hand deformities are much less predictable.

Routine examination demonstrates whether or not there is loss of such joint motion as abduction at the shoulder, extension at the hip, knee, or wrist, or flexion of the fingers. Once a deformity has been detected, a co-operative venture between physician, therapist, and patient must be formed, to eliminate it or at least prevent it from getting worse. This requires persistent, tedious compliance on the part of the patient. Initially, application of moist heat to the joints, followed by ROM active stretching exercises, helps reduce the contracture if the inflammation is relieved or is not too severe. In more severe cases, protective splints should be applied. Joint mobilization, as described by Maigne—

TABLE 35–8   Prediction of Deformities* in Rheumatoid Arthritis

Joint	Deformity	Position of Splinting
Head and neck	Flexion, rotation	Full extension, cervical spine, chin forward
Dorsal spine	Flexion, chest flat	Full extension
Shoulder	Adduction, internal rotation	90 degrees abduction, neutral rotation
Elbow	Flexion, pronation	90 degrees flexion, 10 degrees supination
Wrist	Palmar flexion	30 degrees dorsiflexion
Thumb	Flexion	Extension, apposition
Finger	Flexion, ulnar deviation	Extension, no lateral deviation
Hips	Flexion, adduction, external rotation	Extension; in line with body; foot pointing upward
Knee	Flexion	Extension
Ankle	Plantar flexion	Right angle to leg
Foot	Valgus, spread of forefoot	No varus or valgus, upward pressure beneath second, third, and fourth metatarsal bones
Toe	Plantar flexion in phalangeal joints, flexion at metatarso-phalangeal joints	In line with plantar surface of foot

*The deformities consequent to chronic rheumatoid arthritis have not changed since Dr. Steinbrocker first recorded them, and are thus quite predictable.

From Steinbrocker O: Arthritis in Modern Practice. Philadelphia, WB Saunders, 1947.

gentle manipulation of joints past the range normally reached by active ROM exercises—probably will not benefit patients with RA.[110] Spinal and other joint manipulation (see Chapter 21) has never been shown to prevent or correct these deformities.

Knees and wrist splints are most easily fitted. They can help prevent deformities. Gerber[64] described a hindfoot orthosis for preventing further progression of pronation and valgus deformity of the foot and ankle. Several varieties of resting wrist and hand splints are available (Fig. 35–1). Molded shoe insoles of materials such as plastizote can be used in combination with "extra-depth" shoes, to provide support and spread pressure. This can relieve pain, extend walking range, and slow progression of such deformities as protruding metatarsal heads. These shoes are unattractive and costly and often have to be refitted every few years, but they can be very effective (Fig. 35–2).

The "joint preservation" and "work simplification" techniques promulgated by Cordery and colleagues are thought also to help prevent deformities.[32] Many devices are available (Fig. 35–3). The concept is that if the patient does not overstress or overuse a joint and avoids biomechanical torques that excessively bend the wrist and fingers, then these deformities can be prevented or limited.[119] Certainly, there are no serious side effects to these energy-saving techniques, which probably would benefit even able-bodied persons.

Increasing Strength and Endurance

Most patients with RA complain of fatigue, feel chronically tired, and frequently do not want to exercise. Their

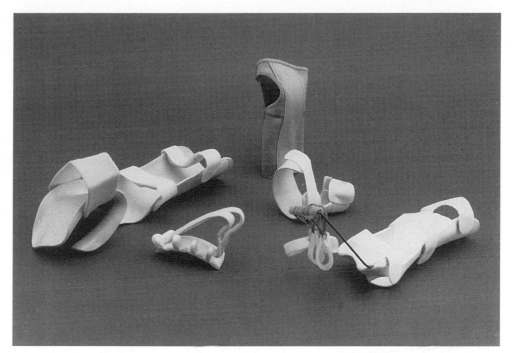

FIGURE 35-1 Molded wrist and hand splints provide pain relief and support for painful, inflamed wrists.

lack of strength and endurance has been documented.[44, 121, 137] The clinician can usually demonstrate these deficiencies, from diminished maximum oxygen consumption (Vo_2max) to decreased strength, on manual muscle testing. There are only minimal changes on microscopic examination of muscles of patients with RA, and even steroid-induced myopathy is amenable to improvement by strengthening exercises.

Exercise can also be harmful to patients with RA. A patient who has been on a shopping spree or has cleaned the house for guests is a likely candidate for both general and specific joint flareups. Many patients know this and ask for joint injections before undertaking extra work or a special activity. Multiple studies have demonstrated that patients with hemiplegia, peripheral nerve damage, and polio develop gout, RA, or OA more severely (or even unilaterally) on the *sound* side as opposed to the neurologically involved or *rested* side.[17, 66–68, 157, 164] Merritt and Hunder demonstrated in rats,[120] and Agudelo in dogs,[1] that in crystalline-induced arthritis the total synovial fluid white

cell count was increased after exercise but not after rest. Merritt and Hunder also demonstrated that isometric exercise *did not* increase the number of synovial fluid white cells or volume of fluid, whereas *passive* ROM exercises did. Other animal experiments have confirmed these findings.[69, 122]

However, because patients complained of weakness and fatigue, several investigators exercised patients with RA and discovered that both strength and endurance can be increased. Machover and Sapecky demonstrated in 1966 that the isometric strength of the quadriceps muscle improved on both the exercised side and the opposite rested side of RA patients following isometric exercise.[109] Nordimar and others[43, 134–136] demonstrated that not only can patients with RA increase their strength, but their type II muscle fibers increase in size on serial biopsy, their ADL are performed with less effort, and the Vo_2max increases. Banwell and colleagues have shown that aerobic exercise on treadmill or bicycle is followed by an increase in aerobic and ADL capacity and an enthusiastic response from their

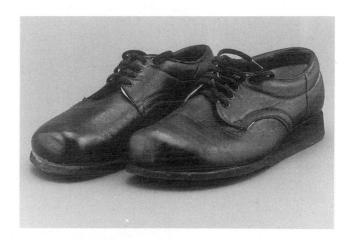

FIGURE 35-2 These extra-depth shoes accommodate cock-up toes or hallux valgus deformities and protruding metatarsal heads. They have room for custom-molded inserts.

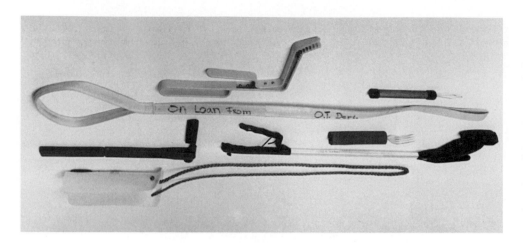

FIGURE 35–3 These devices conserve patients' energy and enable those with arthritis in the hands and arms to perform ADL more easily and competently. The *top* item is a clamp with enlarged handle for perineal care. To its *right* is a large-handled button hook. *Beneath* that is a leg lifter for arthroplasty patients. *Middle left* is a comb extender; *center*, a large-handled reacher; and *just above*, a large-handled fork. Across the *bottom* is a sock aid.

patients.[13, 73] Danneskiold-Samsøe and colleagues have demonstrated that in-water exercises increase both strength and endurance in patients with rheumatoid arthritis.[36] In all these studies, there was no report of marked increase in joint pain or signs of inflammation following exercise. While little radiographic evidence was presented, it is presumed that the radiographic changes in the exercised joints were also relatively mild. There are no long-term follow-up studies other than those of Nordimar and his group, and these showed continuing improvement without subsequent joint damage with exercise.

It should be remembered, however, that the most inflamed joints are often those that have been exercised more (especially in Nature's experiments in hemiplegia). It would seem prudent for the physician to suppress the inflammation as thoroughly as possible before prescribing exercise. The exercise should be performed under careful, controlled conditions, and the patient and the physician should both monitor the exercised joints for an increase in joint inflammation. Since long-term follow-up studies are not now available, the patient should be cautioned that moderation must be the watchword.

Psychosocial Counseling

Patients with RA may well be depressed or suffer multiple social problems, mood swings, fatigue, and frustration.[11, 31, 118, 133, 155, 159, 165] These can affect the patient's entire family. Early detection of social and interpersonal problems allows early referral for treatment.[166] Often, social service or psychological evaluation on a rehabilitation unit can solve such problems. Patients may or may not wish to accept psychotherapy or drug treatment. A trial of antidepressants and referral to a psychiatrist, however, is often in order.

A discussion of the patient's job is also pertinent. Many times, patients find that the physical demands of the work place have exceeded their capability. Minimal changes in the ergonomics of their work station, or perhaps something as simple as obtaining a permit to park closer to the work station, can prolong employment. In general, the employment rate diminishes in direct proportion to the length of time a patient has RA. This is especially true of those who perform demanding physical tasks.[127] The physician encountering a patient with early RA is well-

advised to evaluate the work situation and suggest that the patient begin training for lighter work immediately.

It is typically helpful to discuss sexual function with the patient with RA. A recent survey among upper socioeconomic, highly educated, university-associated persons described a high proportion of "dysfunction" among "normal" couples.[60] RA only makes the "normal" situation worse. It is likely that sexual difficulties can arise owing to mechanical problems and problems with medication and also "normal" dysfunction.[162, 177] Mechanical problems related to disease of the hip joint can be treated with total hip arthroplasty.[10] Other difficulties respond to a change in medication or to counseling. A frank discussion of sexual function may or may not be welcomed by RA patients,[126] but it is more likely to be accepted if a caring relationship between the patient and the practitioner has been established (see Chapter 30).

Osteoarthritis

In any one patient who has OA, only one or a few joints are usually involved. The pathological process begins with histological changes and ends in frank destruction of joint cartilage. There is an increase in the density of the bone adjacent to the joint, and bony excrescences, called *osteophytes*, can occur at the margins of the joints. OA occurs most commonly in older patients, but it can affect younger ones as well. OA is frequently associated with conditions of previous joint damage or excessive wear, or obesity, but it has not been shown to be a clear-cut result of excessive exercise.[24–26, 87, 102, 141, 142] Although OA is frequently termed *degenerative arthritis*, it can also be described as a misguided repair effort. Patients typically note pain on use or weight bearing, but sometimes after rest.

Shoulders

OA of the shoulders usually occurs in older patients and can be associated with excessive joint destruction or rotator cuff wear or rupture. Patients should be taught isometric exercises to strengthen the shoulder musculature, including the deltoid and rotator cuff muscles. Intra-articular steroid injections of the glenohumeral joint can also help. It is important to gain the patient's cooperation in trying to prevent adhesive capsulitis through active ROM exercises. The clinician must also be alert to the presence of other shoulder problems, such as biceps tendinitis, subdeltoid bursitis, and acromioclavicular arthritis, that can compound the symptoms of shoulder OA or mimic it.

Elbows

OA of the elbow occurs after trauma, joint overuse, or inflammatory joint disease. Injections often provide symptomatic relief (see Chapter 25), and full ROM is not totally necessary. The patient needs only to be able to flex the elbow sufficiently to get the hand to the mouth and face for eating and hygiene. Neoprene sleeves help diminish pain but should be removed and cleaned frequently, to avoid moisture build-up and fungal growth.

Hip

OA of the hip is common. While it can be due to congenital dislocation, previous infections, or aseptic necrosis, it is generally idiopathic. Initially, the pain may be relieved by having the patient walk with a cane in the contralateral hand.[19] Isometric gluteus medius and -maximus exercise can increase hip pain, so for some patients they are not practical. Steroids are difficult to inject into the joint without fluoroscopic guidance. Most patients now receive total hip arthroplasty for intractable hip OA. Before or after surgery a shoe lift may be required to correct leg-length discrepancies. Patients who have difficulties performing ADL or ambulation often need a rehabilitation unit or center admission to maximize recovery and function (see Table 35–1).

Knee

OA of the knee is associated with obesity in women but has not been shown to result from osteochondritis dissecans or athletic activity. Quadriceps muscle strength in patients with OA of the knees has been shown to be consistently weak, and electrical stimulation has revealed additional inhibited strength or arthrogenous inhibition.[12, 86] Intra-articular steroid injections temporarily diminish pain and may increase the ability to perform exercise, as does the application of a moist heating pad. Many braces have been manufactured for arthritis of the knee, especially OA, but they are not generally successful. The use of elastic bandages, neoprene sleeves, or canvas braces has been shown to improve proprioception about the knee and to diminish arthrogenous muscle inhibition.[12] Many patients note an increased sense of stability and strength and diminished pain with these knee orthoses.

Use of a cane or crutches helps by relieving some of the weight-bearing stress in the knee. The cane should be held in the patient's hand of choice. There is no clear evidence to demonstrate that a cane in the contralateral hand gives consistent relief of pain for osteoarthritis of the knee more frequently than one held in the ipsilateral hand.[167] Wearing shoes with soft soles such as those of Vibram diminishes knee pain in many patients with OA of the knees. Studies have demonstrated that TENS has relieved pain of OA of the knee, but the results across studies have not been consistent.[89, 106, 163]

Recent studies confirmed the previous adage that multiple-angle isometric exercises performed at the knee in-

crease strength throughout the knee ROM and relieve pain of OA. Pendergast, Fisher, and Gresham demonstrated in a series of elegant papers that patients with OA of the knee have diminished muscle strength, especially with the hip in extension. They subsequently demonstrated that, in a specially designed machine, multiple-angle isometric exercises increased muscle strength, improved ability to perform ADL, and decreased the use of analgesics. The improvement was in excess of that following the usual active exercises.[55-59]

Base of the Thumb

OA of the base of the thumb (carpometacarpal and metacarpophalangeal joints) is a common cause of pain. A thumb spica which immobilizes the two joints of the thumbs, while it is somewhat awkward and interferes with some ADL, provides consistent relief of pain (Fig. 35–4).[22]

Cervical Spine

OA of the cervical spine is common among older persons. OA of the cervical spine can cause symptoms of radiculopathy due to osteophytes impinging on nerve roots and myelopathy due to bony overgrowth causing spinal cord compression. The x-ray evidence of OA of the cervical spine is frequent, but despite this, symptoms of OA are rare. If bony osteophytes can be determined to be a cause of radiculopathy, treatment with a cervical collar to hold the neck in neutral position or flexion helps, since putting the neck in extension reduces the volume of the interforaminal space and can exacerbate symptoms. Cervical myelopathy from osteoarthritis usually requires surgical treatment (see Chapter 36).

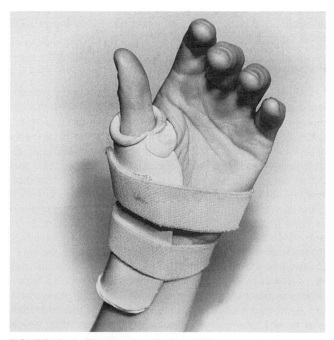

FIGURE 35–4 This thumb spica immobilizes the carpometacarpal and the metacarpophalangeal joint of the thumb while allowing fairly dexterous use of the hand.

Lumbosacral Spine and Spinal Stenosis

Spinal stenosis has been shown in recent years to be a common cause of lumbosacral polyradiculopathy and myelopathy. Epidural injections and a brace to hold the spine in slight lumbosacral flexion can provide temporary relief. NSAIDs are also helpful in many patients. Frequently, patients with a compromised spinal canal have an acute lumbar disc herniation and for a time have increased symptoms. Then, as time passes and the disc retracts, symptoms improve. Exercises have a small part to play in the treatment of this condition, but extension of the spine increases symptoms. If polyradiculopathy is significant and the patient does not wish surgery, a plastic ankle-foot orthosis for footdrop might help.

OA of the lumbosacral spine is almost universal in middle-aged to elderly persons. Myelopathy and radiculopathy, however, are rare in these patients. Symptoms of back pain in adults at an age when OA is prevalent should be carefully studied to find the exact cause, which may be cancer, infection, osteoporosis, or something else, but OA is diagnosed only by exclusion. Spinal stenosis in mature adults is usually caused by OA rather than a small spinal canal. The back pain of spinal stenosis is characteristically increased by spinal extension and relieved by flexion. It may resemble radiculopathy, especially in the L3 to L4 spinal root dermatomes. It is brought on by walking and relieved by rest, and it may occur at night if congestive heart failure is present.

Foot

Hallux valgus of the great toe and cock-up deformity of digits two through five are the most common expressions of OA in the feet. A deep–toe box shoe (extra depth) with a molded insole to accommodate dropped metatarsal heads is helpful (see Fig. 35–2). A rocker-bottom sole to compensate for a stiffened great toe (hallux rigidis) makes walking difficult and unstable. Surgical procedures are often helpful for these problems.

Psoriatic Arthritis

Psoriatic arthritis occurs in a small subgroup of patients who have psoriasis. The arthritis is characterized by tendinitis, enthesitis, and synovitis of both peripheral and spinal joints in various clinical pictures. In a recent review, Veale described 100 consecutive patients with psoriatic arthritis admitted to both inpatient and outpatient clinics who met the criteria of having at least one psoriatic skin lesion, more than 20 fingernail pits and/or onycholysis, and a rheumatoid factor titer of less than 1:80.[168] Forty-three percent of these patients had the asymmetrical oligoarthritis type, 33% had symmetrical arthritis and more bony erosions, 16% had arthritis predominantly of the distal interphalangeal joints, 4% had spondylitis, 2% had arthritis mutilans, and 2% had the synovitis-acne-pustulosis-hyperostosis-osteomyelitis syndrome. The physician must look for psoriatic lesions in all of these patients, and examination of the scalp, anal area, and umbilicus may reveal hidden psoriatic plaques.

The rehabilitation of psoriasis patients requires detailed attention to the joints most severely involved. Patients with tendinitis and synovitis of the toes should be supplied with high–toe box shoes having soft leather uppers. A heel lift and a longitudinal arch support are helpful for associated plantar fasciitis. Intra-articular injections may help individual finger joints and others. Splinting is less helpful, since the hand involvement is not symmetrical. Paraffin baths provide moist heat to inflamed fingers for pain relief. Splinting individual proximal or distal interphalangeal joints can relieve pain but does not prevent deformity in the long run.

Inflammation and pain in the costochondral joints may require individual injections and the use of superficial heat. If significant spondylitis is present with stiffness and progressive deformity, spinal extension exercises, such as walking into the corner with abducted arms and performing push-ups, should be emphasized. The spinal joint involvement in psoriatic arthritis, however, is often asymmetrical, and as a result, the spine becomes less stiff and exercises will be more successful and should be encouraged more strongly.

Ankylosing Spondylitis

Ankylosing spondylitis (AS) is inflammation of the enthesis (the tissue attaching tendons and joint capsules to bone) plus synovitis. Inflammation of the synovial joints and tendons of the spine heals by ossification, causing the spine to become progressively more rigid and stiff. The spine usually becomes stiff in flexion rather than extension, probably because of the posture of the patient. This can leave the patient unable to see straight ahead, as the face ends up facing to the floor during standing and walking. Inflammation of the uveal tract (iritis) and aortic valve disease are also common in AS. The condition is similar in some ways to Reiter's syndrome and psoriatic arthritis, but is distinguished because it is predominantly a disease of the spine.

No studies to date have demonstrated that exercises, braces, or medications preserve the flexibility of the spine or prevent stiffening. The physician's job is to keep the spine as functional as possible, despite gradual stiffening. An extension deformity of the spine is better for most purposes than extreme flexion. The physician must make certain that the spine is becoming stiff in extension rather than flexion by measuring the patient at each visit with Schober's test, measuring the distance from the patient's occiput to the wall when standing in maximum extension with heels against the wall, and measuring the expansion of the thoracic cage at the third to the fourth intercostal space.

Exercises thought to maintain the erect posture include performing push-ups and "walking into corners" with the hands on the occiput and the shoulders abducted. The patient must be constantly reminded to attempt to maintain an erect posture and to sleep on a firm mattress with the spine extended as much as possible. Kraag and co-workers[100] demonstrated that exercise therapy only twice monthly helps maintain posture, and Fisher and associates[54] found that those who exercised maintained greater aerobic capacity (though it was unrelated to chest expansion). Other individual synovial joints can be involved, and NSAIDs, other systemic medication, or intra-articular steroids may be required.

Above all, the physiatrist should join the patient with AS in the battle to maintain upright posture and not allow the patient to slip into noncompliance with daily exercises. If arthroplasty is performed it should be remembered that postoperative heterotopic ossification is very common in patients with AS as it is not in those who have RA or OA.

Scleroderma and Progressive Systemic Sclerosis

Patients with progressive systemic sclerosis (PSS) form excessive amounts of abnormal collagen, which causes thickening of the skin and difficulty moving the joints, especially those of the fingers, shoulders, and knees. Systemic involvement can occur, with the fibrosis affecting motility of the gastrointestinal tract, air exchange in the lungs, expansion or motion in the pericardium, and infiltration of muscles (myopathy) can take place, which decreases strength. The kidneys are frequently affected by a particular kind of vasculitis, and kidney disease is a leading cause of death in patients with PSS. A large percentage of PSS patients have Raynaud's phenomenon, in which blood flow to the fingers is markedly constricted on an episodic basis, and ulcers, sores, and pain can ensue. A variant of PSS called the CREST syndrome consists of subcutaneous calcinosis, Raynaud's phenomenon, esophageal dysfunction, sclerodactyly, and telangiectasia, often of the lips and fingers. These patients usually have less joint restriction.

The rehabilitation techniques for preventing joint contractures of PSS have been only partially successful but must not be ignored. Patients with myopathy or localized myopathy frequently respond to exercise therapy and diminution of ACS doses, but the creatine phosphokinase levels must be monitored. Finger function is not typically helped by splinting, but plaster casts can be used to cover painful ulcers and patients can be offered finger exercises to maintain strength.[153]

Speech pathologists and occupational therapists should become involved in treating dysphagia and can help the patient by determining appropriate swallowing techniques and food consistency (see Chapter 27). It has recently been shown that patients with scleroderma who have amputations of the lower extremities tolerate standard prostheses as well as other patients do. Appropriate prostheses, therefore, should be prescribed for all patients (see Chapter 15).[151]

Dermatomyositis/Polymyositis

Dermatomyositis/polymyositis (DM/PM) is a disease characterized by inflammation of the muscles, with or without a rash. It has been divided into five varieties by Bohan and co-workers:[20] PM in adults, DM in adults, DM/PM in adults with malignancy, childhood DM/PM, and DM/PM with collagen vascular disease. Regardless of the variety, the physiatrist is faced with a patient who has weakness, usually of the proximal muscles, though distal muscle involvement has been described. Joint disease is rare, but bony erosions have been reported. Subcutaneous calcinosis occurs frequently in children and can limit joint ROM. Weakness of the respiratory muscles and the muscles of swallowing can result in aspiration pneumonia and subsequent lung dysfunction, which has been negatively linked

to survival in this disease (see Chapters 6 and 7 for further information on myopathy diagnosis).

Preserving and increasing muscle strength are main rehabilitation goals. Hicks described a 4-week course of isometric muscle contractions, six per muscle on 6 days weekly for 6 sec each.[79] Patients who had DM/PM for less than 2 years had better results, so it was recommended that exercises be performed early in the course of DM/PM.

Escalante and others described five patients with DM/PM, persistent muscle weakness, and elevated serum muscle enzymes of less than 1 year's duration who were treated with alternating periods of exercise.[48] These consisted of functional activities plus resistive exercises (two to three sets of five to ten repetitions each), alternating with periods of functional activities only.[48] The patients had only mild increases in CPK levels following exercise. Responses were not uniform, and one patient with severe weakness did not improve. A second patient demonstrated functional improvement but little strength improvement. The third and fourth patients improved considerably, and the fifth improved remarkably. Hicks and colleagues described an additional patient with DM/PM of less than 2 years' duration who gained strength in the quadriceps and biceps without creatine phosphokinase elevations following an isometric exercise program.[78]

A dilemma frequently occurs when it must be decided whether the patient with increasing weakness has an exacerbation of DM/PM or has steroid myopathy from ACS treatment. The evaluation of serum muscle enzymes, electromyography, muscle biopsy, or a trial of steroids is often required to resolve this dilemma. Often a trial of increased oral ACS increases strength if active DM/PM is the problem.

If persistent or chronic weakness cannot be improved, the patient may require fitting with a plastic ankle-foot orthosis to stabilize the knee and ankle and prevent footdrop (see Chapter 17). In addition, assistive living devices to help with toileting, hygiene, eating, and dressing are often required (see Chapter 26). Wheelchairs or electrically powered wheeled carts are helpful for many patients (see Chapter 19). The patient with suspected dysphagia should be referred for a swallowing evaluation and proper dietary precautions taken (see Chapter 27).

It is still controversial whether or not the physician should extensively test all DM/PM patients for possible malignancy. If any suggestions of malignancy are present, consultation with the primary care physician should be enlisted and a search for occult malignancy carried out. Adults with a rash are thought most likely to have a malignancy.

Systemic Lupus Erythematosus

Systemic lupus erythematosus (SLE) is a systemic immune-mediated disorder, but one of its major manifestations is a mild but painful synovitis that resembles RA. The synovitis results in weakening of tendinous and capsular structures, so that the hands demonstrate the deformities characteristic of RA, such as ulnar deviation and subluxation of the metacarpophalangeal joints and boutonnière and swan-neck deformities of the proximal interphalangeal joints. These joint findings are termed *non-erosive deforming arthritis* or *Jaccoud's arthritis* and are not RA.[27, 39]

Because bony erosions are not a feature, the joints are not destroyed as in RA, but they can have reduced function because of the deformities. Lively splints to help hold hands and fingers in place during activities, if tolerated, can be helpful.

A second form of joint disease, avascular necrosis, occurs with increased frequency in SLE patients, independent of treatment with steroids.[99] The knees, hips, shoulders, and other joints are frequently involved. At initial diagnosis, consideration must be given to orthopedic surgery, but the pain can often be relieved by causing less weight to be distributed to the involved joint, through use of a walker, canes, crutches, or other ambulation aids.

SLE patients also have ruptures of the patellar and Achilles tendons, with or without association with ACS. Following repair and diminution of the steroid dose, muscle-strengthening exercises must be initiated. Both functional electrical stimulation and biofeedback can help to train patients to once again contract these repaired and weak muscles.

Patients with SLE also exhibit systemic involvement—wolf-like skin rash, renal failure, central and peripheral nervous system abnormalities, hematologic problems (including hemolytic anemia and idiopathic thrombocytopenic purpura) and systemic cutaneous vasculitis. Pleurisy is a frequent accompaniment of lung disease, and it has been suggested that TENS can help manage the pain of this transient phenomenon.[64] Other neurological problems can occur, such as stroke or footdrop from peripheral neuropathy.

It is clear that patients with SLE often have psychological difficulties that are probably secondary to immune-mediated insults to the central nervous system. Psychological evaluation and counseling are appropriate, and the psychological status must be considered when prescribing exercise or splints, because of potential compliance problems.

MAXIMIZING COMPLIANCE WITH TREATMENT

Treatment can be successful only if the patient complies with the treatment. Unfortunately, rehabilitation modalities, exercises, aids, and devices do little good if the patient neglects them. Patient non-compliance with treatment programs has been widely documented in the medical literature, and unfortunately has also been demonstrated in the rehabilitation literature with arthritis patients.[14, 16, 37, 76] Parker and Bender administered a questionnaire to 56 patients about a "home treatment" program and found only 54% persisted in following it at 12 months.[143] Carpenter and Davis questioned 54 patients about an exercise program and found only about half continued to follow instructions.[28] Belcon has reviewed a number of studies describing compliance with splint use (Table 35–9).[14] Compliance rates varied from 28% to 78%, and there was a wide variety of reasons for non-compliance. The non-compliance rate is so high that it is difficult to assess the actual efficacy of splint wear in these studies.

Numerous studies have described medication compliance in arthritis patients. Joyce studied 60 women with rheumatoid arthritis;[91] Geertson, Gray, and Ward studied 123 patients with RA;[63] Wright and Hopkins studied 200 rheumatic patients;[176] and Lee and Tan studied 100 patients with RA.[104] The high level of non-compliance described in these studies was attributed to lack of physician-patient interaction time, protracted waiting room periods, impersonal doctors, poor communication, preference for capsules or tablets, dislike of side effects, dislike of taking pills, forgetfulness, and amelioration of symptoms. In a study of 66 RA patients, 41 OA patients, 27 gout patients, and 14 ankylosing spondylitis patients, it was found that the more drugs patients were prescribed, the better was their compliance.[38] The highest compliance rate was 80%, for prednisone. Wasner studied 33 patients with RA and 32 with ankylosing spondylitis and found, conversely, that the more pills were prescribed, the less they complied.[169] Bond and Monson studied 81 rheumatic disease patients and found that intervention by a clinical pharmacist and nurse clinician helped educate patients and increased their compliance by solving problems.[21] Another study of 178 RA patients showed that the ones who complied tended to have more severe rheumatic disease.[140]

It is not yet possible to formulate a definitive list of

TABLE 35–9 Compliance Rates for Splinting

Subjects (N)	Study Design	Intervention or Disease Feature	Compliance Measure	Compliance Result (%)	Compliance Definition	Disease Definition	Regimen Definition	Duration of Observation
56	Cross-sectional analytic survey	Home physiotherapy	Interview	39	0	0	0	0
218	Cross-sectional analytic survey	Home physiotherapy	Interview	65	0	0	0	+
40	Cross-sectional analytic survey	ASA use	Interview + serum assay	78	+	0	0	0
		Exercise	Interview	40	+	0	0	0
		Splint wear	Interview	25	+	0	0	0
12	Time series	Exercise/visual feedback	Electronic counter	Enhancement	+	0	+	+
46	Cross-sectional analytic survey	Splinting	Weighted-index	28	+	0	0	0
36	Cross-sectional analytic survey	Splinting	Interview	50	0	0	0	0
50	Cross-sectional analytic survey	Splinting	Interview	62	+	+	0	+
66	Prospective analytic survey	Splinting	Interview	65	0	+	+	+

Key: +, presence, 0, absence of feature; ASA, acetylsalicylic acid.
Adapted from Belcon MC, et al: A critical review of compliance studies in rheumatoid arthritis. Arthritis Rheum 1984; 27:1230.

reasons why patients do not comply with exercise, splint wearing, and other modalities. It has been suggested that the physician or other health professional discuss frankly with all patients whether or not they are compliant and attempt to discover the specific reasons in each case. The use of a Compliance Card or other device that lists reasons for non-compliance can help gather appropriate information (Fig. 35–5).[125] Once the patient discloses the reason for non-compliance, there is an opportunity to rectify the situation. It is difficult for the patient to improve if a treatment program is not followed, and it is difficult for the physician to assess the efficacy or failure of a treatment program if the patient does not follow all of it.

In closing this section, I should point out that it may or may not be easier for patients to comply with physical medicine and rehabilitation treatments than with surgical or medical programs. The physiatrist, however, must be tenacious in monitoring patients' compliance, monitoring

Compliance Card

When you have difficulty following directions about your medicine, is it because you:

☐ Feel your doctor doesn't care about you,

☐ or spend enough time with you?

☐ Have not been told enough about your medicine?

☐ Worry about side effects?

☐ Think the medicine won't help enough?

☐ Forget to take it?

☐ Do not have regular reminders such as regular meal times?

☐ Do not have enough money to pay for it?

☐ Have trouble getting money for medicine from your family?

☐ Feel your family doesn't want you to take your medicine?

☐ Feel angry at your doctor and don't take his medicine?

☐ Feel angry at your spouse or family and won't take your medicine?

☐ Feel too sad/depressed to help yourself by taking your medicine?

☐ Feel overwhelmed by arthritis and just can't do anything?

© Copyright UNIVERSITY OF PITTSBURGH
1986 All Rights Reserved

FIGURE 35–5 The compliance card is to be presented to the patient to solicit possible causes of non-compliance that, then, can possibly be eliminated.

the efficacy of treatments, and making changes and adaptations where necessary. Most of the rheumatic conditions dealt with by physiatrists are chronic and persistent and require patience and persistence on the part of *both* patient and physician.

REHABILITATION AFTER ARTHROPLASTY

Arthroplasty for hips and knees has been developed to achieve high rates of success over the last few years. Success of arthroplasty at the shoulder and elbow is improving. The physiatrist should know the elements of rehabilitation following these surgical procedures, because more such patients are being admitted to rehabilitation units and centers. As we discussed previously, not every arthroplasty patient is appropriate for a comprehensive rehabilitation unit or free-standing hospital. Those who, because of pain or other reasons, are progressing very slowly, or those who have significant co-morbidity may be better off with a short stay in a comprehensive intensive setting than in a slower-going (less than 3 hours a day), more extended subacute program (see Table 35–1).

Hip

Rehabilitation following hip arthroplasty has been well described.[8, 29] The hip is an inherently stable joint, and treatment for severe osteoarthritis, avascular necrosis, and other destructive lesions of the hip joint took a giant step forward with the development of total hip arthroplasty, a procedure in which both the acetabulum and the femoral head are replaced with prosthetic devices. The gluteus medius muscle and the greater trochanter can be divided in the lateral approach, whereas the posterior approach is through the extensor and short external rotator muscles.

Ambulation can be started as early as 1 to 2 days postoperatively. The weightbearing status of the patient must be determined from the orthopedic surgeon first, however. The patient must be very careful to avoid positions of hip adduction, flexion, and internal rotation following the posterior approach, as this can lever the femoral head out of the acetabulum and "dislocate" the components. Elevated chair seats, and especially toilet seats, are recommended to prevent excessive hip flexion. Patients should be taught to avoid crossing their legs.

Ambulation following surgery is usually successful, and pain relief typically comes early. ROM exercises can be started early and gently, in an effort to prevent contraction in an internally rotated, flexed, and adducted direction. The patient should be taught stair-climbing techniques and other precautions before discharge. Resistive exercises are not begun for 6 to 8 weeks postoperatively, and a cane or walker should be used until the hip abductor muscles are strong enough so that the patient no longer limps during unassisted walking.

Patients who do well with their ADL and have minimal pain postoperatively can usually be discharged directly to home. Patients who have co-morbidity, such as arthritis of other joints, stroke, amputation, or an old restricted joint motion from fracture, usually require admission to a rehabilitation center or unit, to improve gait and ADL function.

Knee

Total knee arthroplasty is also typically quite successful now. Full weight bearing can be permitted as early as a few days postoperatively, as pain tolerance allows. In case of knee instability, revision arthroplasty, previous infection, or bone grafts, however, only partial weight bearing is allowed for 6 to 8 weeks. The patient can be placed in a constant passive motion (CPM) machine within 48 hours of the operation, for as many hours a day as tolerable. Usually, patients do not tolerate CPM at night. As the patient's passive ROM increases, the degree of flexion should be increased on the CPM machine. These devices have been shown postoperatively to decrease pain and the requirement for manipulation. They do not damage the wound and do decrease the length of hospital stay.[90, 117] Weight bearing routinely is to tolerance and is usually not a significant problem. The major problem usually is that the patient is unable to flex the knee adequately. In some centers if 90 degrees of knee flexion has not been achieved by 3 weeks, manipulation under anesthesia is done.[130] The therapist should be diligent with both active and passive assisted exercises, in an effort to get the patient to flex the knee 90 degrees or more. If there is any question about vigorous exercise interfering with the stability of the suture line or the viability of the skin over the prosthesis, the orthopedic surgeon should be consulted. Non-cemented knees (like non-cemented hips) cannot bear full weight for 6 to 8 weeks after surgery.

The goals at discharge are to have patients able to walk far enough and to flex the knee to 90 degrees or better, so they can stand and sit. Isometric or resistive exercises probably should not be started for 8 weeks after surgery. As with the total hip arthroplasty, if excessive pain, swelling, or instability occurs after exercise or under the observation of therapists or physiatrists, the orthopedic surgeon should be consulted.

Shoulder

The shoulder arthroplasty developed by Neer is usually performed to relieve pain but not to achieve additional active motion.[123] An increase of active shoulder ROM frequently does not follow surgery, but patients should be started on ROM exercise immediately. Marked flexion or abduction of the shoulder should be avoided. Internal and external rotation are performed with the elbow held at the side, and progressive resistive exercises can be performed in this range, especially at 4 weeks postoperatively. Although increased shoulder ROM is not a goal, assisted ROM exercises should be performed to achieve as reasonable a range as possible. It is hoped that the patient can reach the hand to the mouth, and even to the face or scalp for hygiene activities. Goals include a pain-free shoulder and the capability of performing facial hygiene tasks.

Elbow

The goals of surgery are to diminish pain and to allow the patient to get the hand to the mouth. Full ROM of the elbow usually is not possible after elbow arthroplasty. Immediately postoperatively, gentle exercises can be pursued, but resistive exercises should not begin until 6 to 8 weeks after surgery. CPM machines are available for the elbow, but since the joint is so near the skin surface, any stretching or tearing or blanching (to suggest loss of sufficient coverage) should be brought to the attention of the orthopedic surgeon.

SUMMARY

Arthroplasty of the hip, knee, and other joints has been developed to a high standard of skill. Unless proper postoperative rehabilitation techniques are provided, however, the patient will not gain maximum benefit. The physiatrist should understand the limits and goals the surgeon has established for the patient and supervise the exercise program so that these goals can be achieved in a reasonable time. To do this, the patient's motivation, pain tolerance or lack of it, and preoperative muscle deficits must be carefully evaluated.

References

1. Agudelo CA, Schumacher HR, Phelps P: Effect of exercise on urate crystal-induced inflammation in canine joints. Arthritis Rheum 1972; 15:609.
2. Akeson WH, Amiel D, Abel MF, et al: Effects of immobilization on joints. Clin Orthop 1987; 219:28–37.
3. Akeson WH, Amiel D, Woo SL: Immobility effect of synovial joints. The pathomechanics of joint contracture. Biorheology 1980; 17:95–110.
4. Akeson WH, Woo SL, Amiel D, et al: Value of 17β-oestradiol in prevention of contracture formation. Ann Rheum Dis 1976; 35:429–436.
5. Alexander GJM, Hortas C, Bacon PA: Bed rest, activity, and the inflammation of rheumatoid arthritis. Br J Rheumatol 1983; 22:134.
6. Amiel D, Akeson WH, Harwood FL, et al: Stress deprivation effect on metabolic turnover of the medial collateral ligament collagen. A comparison between nine- and 12-week immobilization. Clin Orthop 1983; 172:265–270.
7. Amiel D, Woo SL, Harwood FL, et al: The effect of immobilization on collagen turnover in connective tissue: A biochemical-biomechanical correlation. Acta Orthop Scand 1982; 53:325–332.
8. Aufranc OE, Harris SM, McKay SJ, Dinardo DM: Rehabilitation in revision arthroplasty. *In* Turner RH, Scheller AD (eds): Revision Hip Arthroplasty. New York, Grune & Stratton, 1982, pp 379–396.
9. Bach F: Physical medicine and the rheumatic diseases. Br J Phys Med 1947; 10:66–69.
10. Baldursson H, Brattstrom H: Sexual difficulties and total hip replacement in rheumatoid arthritis. Scand J Rheumatol 1979; 8:214–216.
11. Barem J: A review of the psychological aspects of rheumatic diseases. Semin Arthritis Rheum 1981; 11:352–361.
12. Barrett DS, Cobb AG, Bentley G: Joint proprioception in normal osteoarthritic and replaced knees. J Bone Joint Surg 1991; 73B:53–56.
13. Beals CA, Lampman RM, Banwell BF, et al: Measurement of exercise tolerance in patients with rheumatoid arthritis and osteoarthritis. J Rheumatol 1985; 12:458.
14. Belcon MC, Haynes RB, Tugwell P: A critical review of compliance studies in rheumatoid arthritis. Arthritis Rheum 1984; 27:1228.
15. Bell BT: The prevention and correction of deformities in arthritis. Med Clin North Am 1940; 24:1735–1743.
16. Blackwell B: Drug therapy—patient compliance. N Engl J Med 1973; 289:249.
17. Bland JH, Eady WM: Hemiplegia and rheumatoid arthritis. Arthritis Rheum 1968; 11:72.
18. Blocka KLN: Changing trends in the hospitalization of patients with rheumatoid arthritis and the future of the inpatient rheumatic disease unit. J Rheumatol 1994; 21:587–590.
19. Blount WP: Don't throw away the cane. J Bone Joint Surg 1956; 2:695–698.
20. Bohan PA, Peter JB: Polymyositis and dermatomyositis. N Engl J Med 1974; 292:344.

21. Bond CA, Monson R: Sustained improvement in drug documentation, compliance, and disease control—a four-year analysis of an ambulatory care model. Arch Intern Med 1984; 144:1159.

22. Bongi SM, Guidi G, Concetti A, et al: Treatment of carpo-metacarpal joint osteoarthritis by means of a personalized splint. Pain Clinic 1991; 4:119–123.

23. Botte MJ, Nickel VL, Akeson WH: Spasticity and contracture. Physiologic aspects of formation. Clin Orthop 1988; 233:7–18.

24. Bunning RD, Materson RS: A rational program of exercise for patients with osteoarthritis. Semin Arth Rheum 1991; 21:33–43.

25. Bunning RD, Materson RS: Exercise and osteoarthritis (letter to the editor). Ann Intern Med 1992; 117:697–698.

26. Burry HC: Sport, exercise and arthritis. Br J Rheumatol 1987; 26:386–388.

27. Bywaters E: Jaccoud's syndrome: Today's view. Clin Rheumatol Practice, Winter, 1986, pp 148–152.

28. Carpenter JO, Davis LJ: Medical recommendations—followed or ignored? Factors influencing compliance in arthritis. Arch Phys Med Rehabil 1976; 57:241.

29. Chandler HP: Postoperative rehabilitation of the total hip patient. In Stillwell W (ed): The Art of Total Hip Arthroplasty. New York, Grune & Stratton, 1987, pp 371–401.

30. Clark WS, Case HB, Furey JG: Rehabilitation of patients with rheumatoid arthritis. J Chron Dis 1957; 5:712–722.

31. Cobb S: Contained hostility in rheumatoid arthritis. Arthritis Rheum 1959; 2:419–425.

32. Cordery JC: Joint protection: A responsibility of the occupational therapists. Am J Occup Ther 1965; 19:285.

33. Convery FR, Conaty JP, Nickel VL: Flexion deformities of the knee in rheumatoid arthritis. Clin Orthop 1971; 74:90–93.

34. Cosgrove JL, Nicholas JJ, Barwak J, et al: The effects of a treatment team on a special unit. Am J Phys Med Rehabil 1988; 67:253.

35. Culic DD, Battaglia MC, Wichman BS, Schmid FR: Efficacy of compression gloves in rheumatoid arthritis. Am J Phys Med 1979; 58:278.

36. Danneskiold-Samsøe B, Lynsbert K, Risum T, Telling M: The effect of water exercise therapy given to patients with rheumatoid arthritis. Scand J Rehab Med 1987; 19:3.

37. Deyo RA: Compliance with therapeutic regimens in arthritis: Issues, current status, and a future agenda. Semin Arthritis Rheum 1982; 12:233.

38. Deyo RA, Inouye TS, Sullivan B: Noncompliance with arthritis drugs: Magnitude, correlates, and clinical implications. J Rheumatol 1981; 8:931.

39. Dorwart BB, Schumacher HR: Hand deformities resembling rheumatoid arthritis. Semin Arthritis Rheum 1974; 4:53–71.

40. Duthie JJR: The fundamental treatment of rheumatoid arthritis. Practitioner 1951; 166:22–32.

41. Edström G: Kinesotherapy and extension treatment in rheumatoid arthritis. Br J Phys Med 1947; 10:4–8.

42. Edström G: Rehabilitation and treatment by movement of contractures in rheumatoid arthritis. Ann Rheum Dis 1952; 2:196–203.

43. Ekblom B, Lovgren O, Alderin M, et al: Effect of short-term physical training on patients with rheumatoid arthritis I. Scand J Rheumatol 1976; 5:70.

44. Ekblom B, Lovgren O, Alderin M, et al: Physical performance in patients with rheumatoid arthritis. Scand J Rheumatol 1974; 3:121.

45. Elkayam O, Wigler I, Tishler M, et al: Effect of spa therapy in Tiberias on patients with rheumatoid arthritis and osteoarthritis. J Rheumatol 1991; 18:1799–1803.

46. Ely LW, Mensor MC: Studies on the immobilization of the normal joint. Surg Gynecol Obstet 1933; 57:212–215.

47. Enneking WF, Horowitz M: The intra-articular effects of immobilization on the human knee. J Bone Joint Surg Am 1972; 54:973–985.

48. Escalante A, Miller L, Beardmore T: Resistive exercise in the rehabilitation of polymyositis/dermatomyositis. J Rheumatol 1993; 20:1340–1344.

49. Evans EB, Eggers GWN, Butler JK, et al: Experimental immobilization and remobilization of rat knee joints. J Bone Joint Surg Am 1960; 42:737–758.

50. Falconer J, Hayes KW, Chang R: Effect of ultrasound on mobility in osteoarthritis of the knee. Arthritis Care Res 1992; 5:29–35.

51. Feibel A, Fast A. Deep heating of joints: A reconsideration. Arch Phys Med Rehabil 1976; 57:513–514.

52. Finestone HM: Rheumatology rehabilitation: The role of a physical medicine and rehabilitation liaison consultation service. Am J Phys Med Rehabil 1992; 71:191–192.

53. Finsterbush A, Friedman B: Early changes in immobilized rabbits' knee joints: A light and electron microscopic study. Clin Orthop 1973; 92:305–319.

54. Fisher LR, Dawley MIO, Holgate ST: Relation between chest expansion, pulmonary function, and exercise tolerance in patients with ankylosing spondylitis. Ann Rheum Dis 1990; 49:921.

55. Fisher NM, Gresham GE, Abrams M, et al: Quantitative effects of physical therapy on muscular and functional performance in subjects with osteoarthritis of the knees. Arch Phys Med Rehabil 1993; 74:840–847.

56. Fisher NM, Gresham G, Pendergast DR: Effects of a quantitative progressive rehabilitation program applied unilaterally to the osteoarthritic knee. Arch Phys Med Rehabil 1993; 74:1319–1326.

57. Fisher NM, Pendergast DR, Calkins EC: Maximal isometric torque of knee extension as a function of muscle length in subjects of advancing age. Arch Phys Med Rehabil 1990; 71:729–734.

58. Fisher NM, Pendergast DR, Calkins E: Muscle rehabilitation in impaired elderly nursing home residents. Arch Phys Med Rehabil 1991; 72:181–185.

59. Fisher NM, Pendergast DR, Gresham GE, Calkins E: Muscle rehabilitation: Its effect on muscular and functional performance of patients with knee osteoarthritis. Arch Phys Med Rehabil 1991; 72:367–374.

60. Frank E, Anderson C, Rubinstein D: Frequency of sexual dysfunction in "normal" couples. N Engl J Med 1978; 299:111–115.

61. Frankel E: Electric blanket treatment of rheumatoid arthritis. Lancet 1949; 2:1084.

62. Gault SJ, Spyker JM: Beneficial effect of immobilization of joints in rheumatoid and related arthritides. A splint study using sequential analysis. Arthritis Rheum 1969; 12:34–44.

63. Geertson HR, Gray RM, Ward J: Patient non-compliance within the context of seeking medical care for arthritis. J Chronic Dis 1973; 26:689.

64. Gerber LH, Hicks JE: Rehabilitation management of rheumatic diseases. In Hicks JE, Nicholas JJ, Sweazey RL (eds): Handbook of Rehabilitative Rheumatology. Atlanta, American Rheumatism Association, 1988, p 95.

65. Gerber LH, Ungt G, Horwitz S: Ankle orthosis for rheumatoid disease. Arthritis Rheum 1985; 28:547.

66. Glick L: Asymmetrical rheumatoid arthritis after poliomyelitis. Br Med J 1967; 3:26.

67. Glyn JH, Sutherland I, Walker GF, Young A: Low incidence of osteoarthritis in hip and knee after anterior poliomyelitis: A later review. Br Med J 1966; 2:739.

68. Glynn JJ, Clayton ML: Sparing effect of hemiplegia on tophaceous gout. Ann Rheum Dis 1976; 35:534.

69. Glynn LE: The chronicity of inflammation and its significance in rheumatoid arthritis. Ann Rheum Dis 1968; 27:105.

70. Guess VA: Plaster cuff-in splints to reduce knee flexion contracture in patients with chronic rheumatoid arthritis. Phys Ther 1972; 52:634–638.

71. Hall MC: Cartilage changes after experimental immobilization of the knee joint of the young rat. J Bone Joint Surg Am 1963; 45:36–44.

72. Hamilton DE, Bywaters EGL, Please NW: A controlled trial of various forms of physiotherapy in arthritis. Physiotherapy 1959; 45:139–142.

73. Harkcom TM, Lampman RM, Banwell BF, Castor CW: Therapeutic value of graded aerobic exercise training in rheumatoid arthritis. Arthritis Rheum 1985; 28:32.

74. Harris ED Jr, McCroskery PA: The incidence of temperature and fibril stability on degradation of cartilage collagen by rheumatoid synovial collagenase. N Engl J Med 1974; 290:1–6.

75. Hawkes J, Fogden J, Wright V: Straightening the knees in rheumatoid arthritis. Physiotherapy 1972; 58:226–229.

76. Haynes RB, Taylor DW, Sackett D (eds): Compliance in Health Care. Baltimore, Johns Hopkins University Press, 1979.

77. Helliwell PS: An appraisal of medicinal spa therapy for rheumatological disorders. J Roy Soc Health 1989; 109:3–7.

78. Hicks JE, Miller F, Plotz P, et al: Geometric exercise increases strength and does not produce sustained creatine phosphokinase increase in a patient with polymyositis. J Rheumatol 1993; 20:1399–1401.

79. Hicks J, Miller F, Plotz P, et al: Strength improvement without CPK

elevation in a polymyositis patient on an isometric exercise program. Arthritis Rheum 31(suppl):559, 1988.

80. Hicks J, Nicholas JJ: Rehabilitative rheumatology content in current rheumatology training programs. Arthritis Rheum 1984; 27:1076.

81. Hicks J, Nicholas JJ: Rehabilitative rheumatology content in current rehabilitation medicine training programs. Arch Phys Med Rehabil 1985; 66:631.

82. Hill D: Basic treatment in rheumatoid arthritis. Med Clin North Am 1955; 39:393–403.

83. Hollander JL, Horvath SM: The influence of physical therapy procedures on the intra-articular temperature of normal and arthritic subjects. Am J Med Sci 1949; 218:543–548.

84. Holt PJL: Management of rheumatoid arthritis. Br Med J 1969; 3:514–518.

85. Horvath SM, Hollander JL: Intra-articular temperature as a measure of joint reaction. J Clin Invest 1949; 28:469–473.

86. Hurley MV, Newham DJ: The influence of arthrogenous muscle inhibition on quadriceps rehabilitation of patients with early, unilateral osteoarthritic knees. Br J Rheumatol 1993; 32:127–131.

87. Isdale A, Helliwell PS: Athletes and osteoarthritis—is there any relationship? (Letter to the editor). Br J Rheumatol 1991; 30:67–68.

88. Jan M, Lai J: The effects of physiotherapy on osteoarthritic knees of females. J Formosan Med Assoc 1991; 90:1008–1013.

89. Jensen H, Zesler R, Christensen T: Transcutaneous electrical nerve stimulation (TNS) for painful osteoarthrosis of the knee. Int J Rehabil Res 1991; 14:356–358.

90. Johnson DP: The effect of continuous passive motion on wound-healing and joint mobility after arthroplasty. J Bone Joint Surg Am 1990; 72:421–426.

91. Joyce CRB: Patient co-operation and the sensitivity of clinical trials. J Chronic Dis 1962; 15:1025.

92. Kantor TO: Order out of chaos—the primary mission of the pyramid. J Rheumatol 1990; 17:1580.

93. Karten I, Koatz AO, McEwen C: Treatment of contractures of the knee in rheumatoid arthritis. Bull NY Acad Med 1968; 44:763–773.

94. Keenan MAE: Surgical decision making for residual limb deformities following traumatic brain injury. Orthop Rev 1988; 17:1185–1192.

95. Keenan MA, Ure K, Smith CW, et al: Hamstring release for knee flexion contractions in spastic adults. Clin Orthop 1988; 236:221–226.

96. Kelly M: The prevention of deformity in rheumatic disease. Med J Austral 1990; 2:1–8.

97. Kelly M: Rheumatoid arthritis. The active immobilization of acutely inflamed joints. NZ Med J 1961; 60:311–315.

98. Kirk JA, Kersley GD: Heat and cold in the physical treatment of rheumatoid arthritis of the knee. A controlled clinical trial. Ann Phys Med 1968; 9:270–274.

99. Klippel J, Gerber LH, Pollack L, et al: Avascular necrosis of bone in systemic lupus erythematosus. Am J Med 1979; 67:83–87.

100. Kraag G, Stokes B, Groh J, et al: The effect of comprehensive home physiotherapy and supervision on patients with ankylosing spondylitis—a randomized controlled trial. J Rheumatol 1990; 17:228.

101. Kumar VN, Redford JB: Transcutaneous nerve stimulation in rheumatoid arthritis. Arch Phys Med Rehabil 1982; 63:595–596.

102. Lane NE, Buckwalter JA: Exercise: A cause of osteoarthritis? Rheum Dis Clin North Am 1993; 19:617–633.

103. Lee P, Kennedy AC, Anderson J, Buchannan WW: Benefits of hospitalization in rheumatoid arthritis. Q J Med 1974; 43:205–214.

104. Lee P, Tan LJP: Drug compliance in outpatients with rheumatoid arthritis. Aust NZ J Med 1979; 9:274.

105. Lehmann JF, Silverman DR, Baum BA, et al: Temperature distributions in the human thigh, produced by infrared, hot pack and microwave application. Arch Phys Med Rehabil 1966; 47:291.

106. Lewis D, Lewis B, Sturrock RD: Transcutaneous electrical nerve stimulation in osteoarthrosis: A therapeutic alternative? Ann Rheum Dis 1984; 43:47–49.

107. Lowman EW, Lee P, Rusk HA: Total rehabilitation of the rheumatoid arthritic cripple. JAMA 1955; 158:1335–1344.

108. Lowman EW, Solomon WM, Hill F, Martin GM: Panel on rehabilitation in rheumatoid arthritis. GP 1955; 12:69–86.

109. Machover S, Sapecky AJ: Effect of isometric exercise on the quadriceps muscle in patients with rheumatoid arthritis. Arch Phys Med Rehabil 1966; 47:737.

110. Maigne R: Manipulations and mobilizations of the limbs. In Rogoff JB (ed): Manipulation, Traction and Massage. Baltimore, Williams & Wilkins, 1980.

111. Mainardi C, Walter JM, Spiegel PK, et al: Rheumatoid arthritis: Failure of daily heat therapy to affect its progression. Arch Phys Med Rehabil 1979; 60:390–392.

112. Mannheimer C, Carlsson C: The analgesic effect of transcutaneous electrical nerve stimulation (TNS) in patients with rheumatoid arthritis. A comparative study of different pulse patterns. Pain 1979; 6:329–334.

113. Mannheimer C, Staffan L, Carlsson CA: The effect of transcutaneous electrical nerve stimulation (TNS) on joint pain in patients with rheumatoid arthritis. Scand J Rheumatol 1978; 7:13–16.

114. Martin GM: Physical medicine in rheumatoid arthritis. Arthritis Rheum 1963; 6:177–185.

115. McCarty DJ: Treatment of rheumatoid arthritis. In McCarty DJ, Koopman WJ (eds): Arthritis and Allied Conditions, ed 12. Philadelphia, Lea & Febiger, 1993, pp 878–880.

116. McCarthy GM, McCarty DJ: Effect of topical capsaicin in the therapy of painful osteoarthritis of the hands. J Rheumatol 1992; 19:604–607.

117. McInnes J, Larson MG, Daltroy LH, et al: A controlled evaluation of continuous passive motion in patients undergoing total knee arthroplasty. JAMA 1992; 268:1423–1428.

118. Medsger AR, Robinson J: A comparative study of divorce in rheumatoid arthritis and other rheumatic disease. J Chronic Dis 1972; 25:269–275.

119. Melvin JL: Rheumatic Disease, Occupational Therapy and Rehabilitation. Philadelphia, FA Davis, 1982, pp 351–372.

120. Merritt JL, Hunder G: Passive range of motion, not isometric exercise, amplifies acute urate synovitis. Arch Phys Med Rehabil 1983; 64:130.

121. Minor MA, Hewett JE, Webel RR, et al: Exercise tolerance and disease related measures in patients with rheumatoid arthritis and osteoarthritis. J Rheumatol 1988; 15:905.

122. Murray D: Modification of experimental arthritis in rabbits by tenotomy. J Surg Res Clin Lab Invest 1966; 6:488.

123. Neer CS: Shoulder Reconstruction. Philadelphia, WB Saunders, 1990, p 498.

124. Nicholas JJ: Compliance Card. Pittsburgh, University of Pittsburgh, 1985.

125. Nicholas JJ: Physical modalities in rheumatological rehabilitation. Arch Phys Med Rehabil 1994; 75:904–1001.

126. Nicholas JJ: Unpublished data, 1982.

127. Nicholas JJ: Vocational capacity with arthritis. In Scheer SJ (ed): Medical Perspectives in Vocational Assessment of Impaired Workers. Gaithersburg, Md, Aspen, 1991, pp 101–117.

128. Nicholas JJ, Gruen H, Weiner G, et al: Splinting in rheumatoid arthritis. I. Factors affecting patient compliance. Arch Phys Med Rehabil 1983; 63:92–94.

129. Nicholas JJ, Gruen H, Weiner G, et al: Splinting in rheumatoid arthritis. II. Evaluation of Lightcast. II. Fiberglass polymer splints. Arch Phys Med Rehabil 1982; 63:95–96.

130. Nicholas JJ, Rosenberg AN: Arthritis and arthroplasty in the elderly. In Rehabilitation of the Aging and Elderly Patient. Felsenthal GF, Garrison SJ, Steinberg FU (eds): Baltimore, Williams & Wilkins, 1994, pp 101–106.

131. Nicholas JJ, Ziegler G: Cylinder splints: Their use in the treatment of arthritis of the knee. Arch Phys Med Rehabil 1977; 58:264–267.

132. Nickel VL, Kristy J, McDaniel L: Physical therapy for rheumatoid arthritis. J Am Phys Ther Assoc 1965; 45:198–204.

133. Noldofsky H, Chester WJ: Pain and mood patterns in patients with rheumatoid arthritis: A prospective study. Psychosomat Med 1970; 32:309–318.

134. Nordemar R: Physical training in rheumatoid arthritis: A controlled long term study. II. Functional capacity and general attitudes. Scand J Rheumatol 1981; 10:25.

135. Nordemar R, Berg U, Ekblom B, Edstrom L: Changes in muscle fibre size and physical performance in patients with rheumatoid arthritis after 7 months' physical training. Scand J Rheumatol 1976; 5:233.

136. Nordemar R, Edstrom L, Ekblom B: Changes in muscle fibre size and physical performance in patients with rheumatoid arthritis after short-term physical training. Scand J Rheumatol 1976; 5:70.

137. Nordesjo L, Nordgren B, Wigren A, Kolstad K: Isometric strength

and endurance in patients with severe rheumatoid arthritis or osteoarthrosis in the knee joints. Scand J Rheumatol 1983; 12:152.

138. Opitz JL: Total joint arthroplasty. Principles and guidelines for post-operative physiatric management. Mayo Clin Proc 1979; 54:602–612.

139. Osler W: Aequanimitas, with Other Addresses, ed 3. Philadelphia, Blakistons Son, 1932, pp 133–135.

140. Owen SG, Friesen WT, Roberts MS, Flux W: Determinants of compliance in rheumatoid arthritic patients assessed in their home environment. Br J Rheumatol 1985; 24:313.

141. Panush RS: Does exercise cause arthritis? Long-term consequences of exercise on the musculoskeletal system. Rheum Dis Clin North Am 1990; 16:827–838.

142. Panush RS, Brown DG: Exercise and arthritis. Sports Med 1987; 4:54–64.

143. Parker LB, Bender LF: Problem of home treatment in arthritis. Arch Phys Med Rehabil 1957; 38:392.

144. Partridge RH, Duthie JJR: Controlled trial of the effect of complete immobilization of the joints in rheumatoid arthritis. Ann Rheum Dis 1963; 22:91.

145. Pegg SMH, Littler TR, Litten EN: A trial of ice therapy and experience in chronic arthritis. Physiotherapy 1969; 55:51–56.

146. Perry J: Contractures. Clin Orthop 1987; 219:8–14.

147. Pincus T, Callahan LF: Remodelling the pyramid or remodelling paradigms concerning rheumatoid arthritis—lessons from Hodgkin's disease and coronary artery disease. J Rheumatol 1990; 17:1582.

148. Polly HF, Hunder GG: Rheumatologic Interviewing and Physical Examination of the Joints, ed 2. Philadelphia, WB Saunders, 1978, p 286.

149. Preston RL: The rehabilitation of the patient with rheumatoid arthritis. NY J Med 1955; 55:2887–2896.

150. Ridgway CL, Daugherty MB, Warden GD: Serial casting as a technique to correct burn scar contractures: A case report. J Burn Care Rehabil 1991; 12:67–72.

151. Riedy E, Steen V, Nicholas JJ: Lower extremity amputation in scleroderma. Arch Phys Med Rehabil 1992; 23:811–813.

152. Ropes MW: Conservative Treatment in Rheumatoid Arthritis. Pub. No. 293, Boston, Robert W. Lovett Memorial Unit for the Study of Crippling Diseases, Harvard Medical School, Massachusetts General Hospital, 1960.

153. Seeger MW, Furst DE: Effects of splinting in the treatment of hand contractures in progressive systemic sclerosis. Am J Occup Ther 1987; 41:1118–1121.

154. Shewring DJ, Beaudet M, Carvell JE: Reversed dynamic slings: Results of use in the treatment of post-traumatic flexion contractures of the elbow. Injury 1991; 22:400–402.

155. Spergel P, Ehrlich G, Glass D: The rheumatoid arthritic personality. Psychosomatics 1978; 19:79–86.

156. Spiegel TM, Hirschberg J, Taylor J, Paulus HE: Heating rheumatoid knees to an intra-articular temperature of 42.1 °C. Ann Rheum Dis 1987; 46:716–719.

157. Stecher RM, Karnash LJ: Heberden's nodes. VI. The effect of nerve injury upon formation of degenerative joint disease of the fingers. Am J Med Sci 1947; 213:181–190.

158. Steinbrocker O: Arthritis in Modern Practice. Philadelphia, WB Saunders, 1947, p 485.

159. Stitt FN, Frane M: Mood changes in rheumatoid arthritis. J Chronic Dis 1977; 30:135–145.

160. Sukenik S, Buskila D, Neumann L, et al: Sulphur bath and mud pack treatment for rheumatoid arthritis at the Dead Sea area. Ann Rheum Dis 1990; 49:99–102.

161. Swanson N: The prevention and correction of deformity in rheumatoid arthritis. Can Med Assoc J 1956; 75:257–261.

162. Swinburne WR: Sexual counselling for the arthritic. Clin Rheum Dis 1976; 23:639–651.

163. Taylor P, Hallett M, Flaherty L: Treatment of osteoarthritis of the knee with transcutaneous electrical nerve stimulation. Pain 1981; 11:233–240.

164. Thompson J, Bywaters EGL: Unlimited rheumatoid arthritis following hemiplegia. Ann Rheum Dis 1962; 21:370.

165. Udelman HD, Udelman D: Emotions in rheumatologic disorders. Am J Psychother 1981; 35:576–587.

166. Udelman HD, Udelman DL: Group therapy in rheumatoid arthritis patients. Am J Psychother 1978; 32:288–299.

167. Vargo MM, Robinson LR, Nicholas JJ: Contralateral vs. ipsilateral cane use: Effects on muscles crossing the knee joint. Am J Phys Med Rehabil 1992; 71:170–176.

168. Veale D, Rogers W, Fitzgerald O: Classification of clinical subsets in psoriatic arthritis. Br J Rheumatol 1994; 33:133–138.

169. Wasner C, Britton MC, Kraines RG, et al: Nonsteroidal anti-inflammatory agents in rheumatoid arthritis and ankylosing spondylitis. JAMA 1981; 246:2168.

170. Weinberger A, Abramonvici A, Fadila R, et al: The effect of local deep microwave hyperthermia on experimental zymosan-induced arthritis in rabbits. Am J Phys Med 1990; 69:239–244.

171. Weinberger A, Fadilah R, Lev A, et al: Deep heat in the treatment of inflammatory joint disease. Med Hypotheses 1988; 25:231–233.

172. Weinberger A, Fadilah R, Lev A, et al: Treatment of articular effusions with local deep microwave hyperthermia. Clin Rheumatol 1989; 8:461–466.

173. White J, Sage J: Effects of a counterirritant on muscular distress in patients with arthritis. Phys Ther 1971; 51:36–42.

174. White JR: Effects of a counterirritant on perceived pain and hand movement in patients with arthritis. Phys Ther 1973; 53:956–960.

175. Wright V: The treatment of rheumatoid arthritis. J Chron Dis 1963; 16:83–103.

176. Wright V, Hopkins R: Administration of antirheumatic drugs. Ann Rheum Dis 1978; 35:174.

177. Yoshino S: Sexual problems of women with rheumatoid arthritis. Arch Phys Med Rehabil 1981; 62:122–123.

178. Zander CL, Healy NL: Elbow flexion contractures treated with serial casts and conservative therapy. J Hand Surg 1992; 17A:694–697.

36

Assessment and Treatment of Cervical Spine Disorders

FRANCIS P. LAGATTUTA, M.D., AND
FRANK J. E. FALCO, M.D.

Cervical spine disorders have been described since ancient times. The *Papyrus* written over 4600 years ago by the Egyptian physician Imhotep, of the Third Dynasty, describes cervical sprains and dislocations.[94] Hippocrates, born about 460 BC, developed the cervical traction concept and recognized that vertebral injuries to the cervical spine resulted in paralysis. The Greek physician Paulus Aeginata (AD 625–690) was the first to perform cervical laminectomies.[1] In the second century, Galen, physician to the Roman emperor Marcus Aurelius, performed cervical surgery on gladiators.[105, 210] Galen separated the spinal cord at different cervical root levels and recorded the subsequent motor and sensory effects. In 1828, Smith[193] performed the first laminectomy in America. The term *whiplash* was introduced in 1928 by Crowe.[57]

Neck complaints are commonly encountered in clinical practice and account for multiple visits to the physician. The prevalence of neck pain with or without arm pain is approximately 13% of females and 9% of males in the general population.[129, 141] One out of every three people can recall an incident of neck pain at least once in his or her lifetime.[129] The occurrence is greater in the workplace, where 51% to 80% of laborers can recall an episode of neck and arm pain.[106, 108] The frequency of neck complaints increases with age in the workplace. In the 25- to 29-year-old age group, 25% to 30% complain of neck stiffness and 5% to 10% complain of pain radiating into the upper limb. In those over 45 years of age, 50% complain of neck stiffness and 25% to 40% complain of pain radiating into the upper limb.[107] Overall, 45% of working men experience at least one episode of neck discomfort, 23% remember at least one incident of upper limb pain, and 51% complain of both symptoms.[107]

Chronic neck pain has a statistically significant correlation with previous neck, back, or shoulder injury, work-related mental distress, and physical stress.[141] Chronic neck pain is rare in those with a high educational level, white-collar workers, and housewives.[141] There is no association between chronic neck pain and smoking.[141]

Conditions affecting the neck that can lead to pain and other associated symptoms are listed in Table 36–1. The history and physical examination are still the most important elements in making the diagnosis. Recent advances in diagnostic testing have improved the clinician's ability to make the appropriate diagnosis, as well as determine the presence or absence of serious complications.

After a review of cervical anatomy and biomechanics, this chapter outlines the clinical evaluation and treatment of cervical spine disorders. A discussion of the most common cervical spine conditions encountered in clinical practice is also presented.

ANATOMY AND BIOMECHANICS

The cervical spine is a discrete part of the axial skeleton. The neck is the most mobile portion of the spine and serves three major functions: (1) it supports and provides stability for the head; (2) it enables the head to move in all planes of motion; and (3) it protects the structures that pass through it, specifically the spinal cord, nerve roots, and vertebral artery. Restriction of these basic cervical spine functions by injury or disease can lead to impairment, disability, and handicap.

Osseous Structures

The cervical column is made up of seven vertebrae which are divided into an upper (C1–C2) and a lower (C3–C7) region (Fig. 36–1). There are distinct anatomical and functional differences between these two sections of vertebrae.[20, 54]

The C1 (atlas) and C2 (axis) are considerably different from other vertebrae in the spinal column (Fig. 36–2). The atlas is a ringlike structure without a vertebral body. There

TABLE 36–1   Disorders Affecting the Neck

Mechanical	Tumors
Cervical sprain	Benign tumors
Cervical strain	Osteochondroma
Herniated nucleus pulposus	Osteoid osteoma
Osteoarthritis	Osteoblastoma
Cervical spondylosis	Giant cell tumor
Cervical stenosis	Aneurysmal bone cyst
Rheumatologic	Hemangioma
Ankylosing spondylitis	Eosinophilic granuloma
Reiter's syndrome	Gaucher's disease
Psoriatic arthritis	Malignant tumors
Enteropathic arthritis	Multiple myeloma
Rheumatoid arthritis	Solitary plasmacytoma
Diffuse idiopathic skeletal	Chondrosarcoma
hyperostosis (DISH)	Ewing's sarcoma
Polymyalgia rheumatica	Chordoma
(PMR)	Lymphoma
Fibrositis (fibromyalgia)	Metastases
Infectious	Extradural tumors
Vertebral osteomyelitis	Epidural hemangioma
Discitis	Epidural lipoma
Herpes zoster	Meningioma
Infective endocarditis	Neurofibroma
Granulomatous process	Lymphoma
Epidural, intradural, and	Intradural tumors
subdural abscesses	Extramedullary, intradural
Retropharyngeal abscess	Neurofibroma
Acquired Immunodeficiency	Meningioma
syndrome (AIDS)	Ependymoma
Endocrinological and	Sarcoma
metabolic	Intramedullary
Osteoporosis	Ependymoma
Osteomalacia	Astrocytoma
Parathyroid disease	Arteriovenous malformations
Paget's disease	Syringomyelia
Pituitary disease	

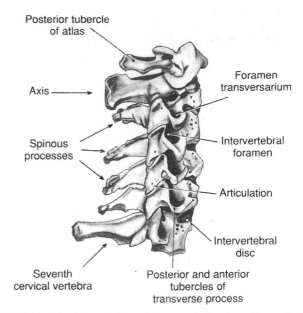

FIGURE 36–1   Lateral view of the cervical spine. (From Crafts RC: Textbook of Human Anatomy, ed 2. New York, John Wiley & Sons, 1979.)

are two lateral atlantal masses that articulate with the occipital condyles above and the axis below. The axis has a vertebral body, bifid spinous process, and an upward projecting odontoid process which is the congenitally fused body of the atlas. The odontoid articulates with the anterior arch of the atlas. This normal relationship allows for less than 3-mm separation between the anterior arch and odontoid.[215] This joint can be weakened by trauma or by disease such as rheumatoid arthritis.[19, 21, 23, 38, 39] A separation of 3 mm or more in flexion and extension is considered to be unstable and evidence of instability.[215]

The atlas and axis in combination with the cranial occiputs (C0) assist in flexion, extension, and rotation. The atlanto-occipital (C0–C1) articulation permits 10 degrees of flexion and 25 degrees of extension. The greatest amount of rotation in the cervical spine occurs at the C1 to C2 joint with 45 degrees of rotation in either direction. A few degrees of flexion-extension are also seen at the C1 to C2 joint.[67–69] A true synovial joint is located between the lateral masses of the atlas and axis between the anterior arch of the atlas and the odontoid process.

The vertebrae of the lower cervical region are similar to one another in shape and function (Fig. 36–3). The C3 to C7 vertebrae have small bodies with the longest dimension in the coronal plane. The spinous processes are bifid from C3 to C6 and C7 has the longest process, which is easily palpable on examination in most people. The cervical zygapophyseal joints are more concave than convex, as com-

pared with the thoracic and lumbar spines. Cervical facet orientation is at 45 degrees, rather than the 60 degrees in the thoracic spine or the 90 degrees in the lumbar spine. The spinous processes, transverse processes, and laminae serve as areas for muscle attachments.

At the C2 to C3 junction there is a change in the shape of the articulating joints, causing a distinct difference in function. This is a transitional area for the cervical spine where the permitted motion changes from rotation to flexion, extension, and lateral bending. There is approximately 10 degrees of flexion per segment with the greatest amount of flexion occurring at C4 to C5 and C5 to C6.[80, 133] Lateral bending occurs primarily at C3 to C4 and C4 to C5. Horizontal displacement of the vertebrae during flexion and extension greater than 3.5 mm or angular deformity greater than 11 degrees indicates spinal instability.[215]

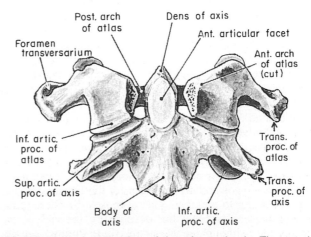

FIGURE 36–2   Anterior view of the atlas and axis. The anterior tubercle of the atlas has been removed to reveal the odontoid process of the axis. (From Crafts RC: Textbook of Human Anatomy, ed 2. New York, John Wiley & Sons, 1979.)

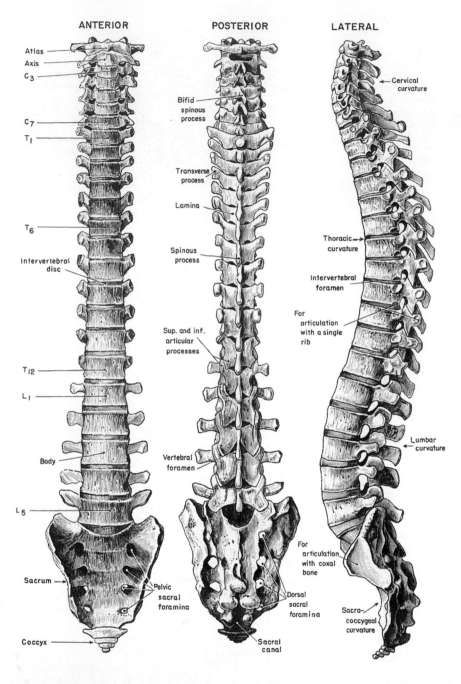

ANTERIOR POSTERIOR LATERAL

Atlas
Axis
C₃

Cervical
curvature

Bifid
spinous
process

C₇
T₁

Transverse
process

Lamina

T₆

Spinous
process

Thoracic
curvature

Intervertebral
disc

Intervertebral
foramen

Sup. and inf.
articular
processes

For
articulation
with a single
rib

T₁₂

L₁

FIGURE 36–3 Anterior, posterior, and lateral views of the entire human spine. (From Crafts RC: Textbook of Human Anatomy, ed 2. New York, John Wiley & Sons, 1979.)

Lumbar
curvature

Body

Vertebral
foramen

L₅

For
articulation
with coxal
bone

Sacrum

Pelvic
sacral
foramina

Dorsal
sacral
foramina

Sacro-
coccygeal
curvature

Coccyx

Sacral
canal

All cervical spine motions are coupled such that rotation is associated with lateral bending and vice versa. Restriction of range of motion (ROM) in a particular plane helps the clinician determine which segment is involved and especially whether it is in the upper or lower cervical spine.

The lower cervical vertebrae (C3–C7) have unique articulations called uncovertebral joints that are also known as joints of Luschka or neurocentral joints (Fig. 36–4). They arise from the posterolateral margins of the vertebral bodies and lie anterior to the exiting nerve roots.[65, 137] These joints are not present at birth, but develop by the end of the first decade. Although controversial, these "joints" are not considered true joints since they do not possess synovium.[97, 163, 168] The uncovertebral articulations are thought to develop from degenerative clefts or from fibrous tissue

resorption within the supraposterolateral margins.[97, 163, 168] These articulations can degenerate by undergoing hypertrophy and calcification with associated disc degeneration. This process can ultimately lead to encroachment on the intervertebral canal, causing nerve root or even spinal cord compression.

Soft Tissue Structures

Intervertebral discs are located in the cervical spine between the C2 and T1 vertebrae. There is no disc between C1 and C2, and only the ligaments and joint capsules resist excessive motion. The intervertebral disc provides shock absorption, accommodates movement, and separates the vertebral bodies to give height to the intervertebral foram-

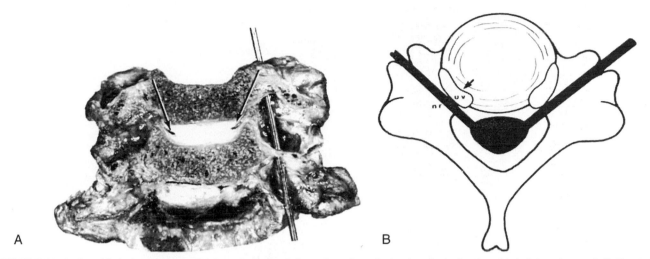

FIGURE 36–4 Luschka's (uncovertebral) joints. *A,* Coronal dissection of cervical spine displaying Luschka's joints *(arrows). B,* Proximity of uncovertebral joints to cervical nerve roots. (*A* from Parke WW: Applied anatomy of the spine. *In* Rothman RH, Simone FA (eds): The Spine, ed 3. Philadelphia, WB Saunders, 1992. *B* from Macnab I, McCulloch J: Neck Ache and Shoulder Pain. Baltimore, Williams & Wilkins, 1994.)

ina. The disc is made up of the eccentrically located nucleus pulposus and the surrounding annulus fibrosus (Fig. 36–5). Intervertebral disc degenerative changes or herniation can lead to spinal cord or nerve root injury.

There are several ligaments found at each vertebral level that give strength and stability to the cervical spine (Fig. 36–6). The transverse, alar, and accessory atlantoaxial ligaments help maintain the integrity of the odontoid and C1 articulation. The anterior (ALL) and posterior longitudinal ligaments (PLL) run along the anterior and posterior surfaces of the vertebrae and discs. They provide stability during flexion and extension. The PLL also reinforces the posterior annulus. The facet capsule ligaments, and supraspinous, interspinous, and ligamentum flavum ligaments provide flexion stability. The ligamentum nuchae spans from the occiput to the C7 spinous process and adds support to the posterior neck.

The neck muscles give support and provide movement for the cervical spine and the head. The musculature can functionally be divided into the anterior flexors and the posterior extensors. The posterior muscles are arranged with the longer groups superficial and the shorter groups closest to the vertebral column. For example, the iliocostalis and longissimus muscles span many vertebral levels and are superficial, whereas the deeply located short cervical rotators pass from only one vertebra to the next. These muscles produce extension of the spine or head, or both, when contracting bilaterally, or rotation when acting ipsilaterally. The anteriorly placed scalene and sternocleidomastoid muscles are the important flexors and additional rotators of the neck and head.

Some of the extrinsic shoulder muscles such as the trapezius, rhomboid, levator scapulae, and latissimus dorsi have attachments to the cervical spine. An injury to these structures can lead to neck pain because of this anatomical relationship.[125]

Neural Structures

The spinal cord begins at the foramen magnum and extends to approximately the L2 vertebral level. The spinal cord is about 10 mm and the vertebral canal averages 17 mm in sagittal diameter.[32, 166] The spinal canal is the widest at C3 through C5 and rapidly decreases in size to a small circular lumen throughout the thoracic area. In the cervical region, the transverse diameter of the spinal canal is almost twice that of the anteroposterior (AP) diameter. Therefore, the spinal cord has ample room to expand laterally, but has considerably less room in the AP direction.

Spinal nerves are formed by the union of the ventral motor and dorsal sensory roots (Fig. 36–7). All of the cervical nerves contain motor and sensory fibers except for the C1 nerve which only has motor fibers.[102] The first cervical nerve emerges from the vertebral canal at the atlanto-occipital junction, while the eighth nerve emerges between C7 and T1. In the cervical spine below C2, the

Posterior

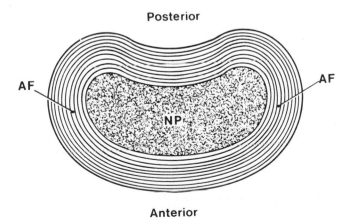

Anterior

Transverse section

FIGURE 36–5 Structural components of the intervertebral disc. NP, nucleus pulposus; AF, annulus fibrosus. (From Bogduk N, Twomey LT: Clinical Anatomy of the Lumbar Spine. New York, Churchill Livingstone, 1988.)

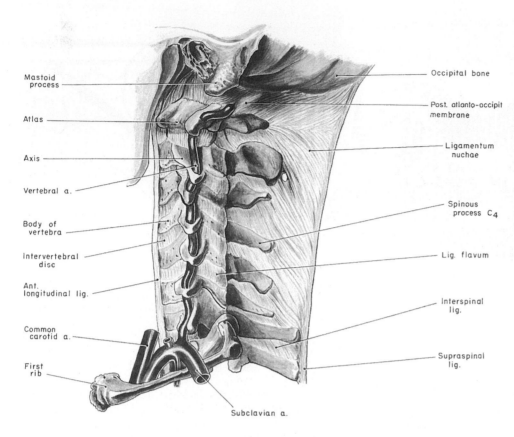

Mastoid process

Atlas

Axis

Vertebral a.

Body of vertebra

Intervertebral disc

Ant. longitudinal lig.

Common carotid a.

First rib

Subclavian a.

Occipital bone

Post. atlanto-occipit membrane

Ligamentum nuchae

Spinous process C₄

Lig. flavum

Interspinal lig.

Supraspinal lig.

FIGURE 36–6 Anatomical relationship of cervical spine ligaments to other structures in the neck. (From Crafts RC: Textbook of Human Anatomy, ed 2. New York, John Wiley & Sons, 1979, p 55.)

segmental nerves progress from the entrance of the thecal sac to the tubercles of the transverse process. The cervical nerves run over the upper border of the pedicles and slope laterally and anteroinferiorly along the upper surface of the transverse process. Cervical spinal nerves exit through the root canals dividing into anterior and posterior rami. The anterior rami supply the prevertebral and paravertebral muscles, and form the brachial plexus to provide innervation for the upper limbs. The posterior rami divide into muscular, cutaneous, and articular branches for the posterior neck structures including the postvertebral muscles.

The cervical intervertebral discs receive innervation to the outer one third of the annulus anteriorly, posteriorly, and laterally[31] (Fig. 36–8). The disc receives branches anteriorly from the vertebral nerve which accompanies the vertebral artery. The vertebral nerve is derived from the gray rami communicans of the sympathetic trunk at midcervical levels and branches of the stellate ganglion at lower cervical levels. Posterolateral innervation is provided by the sinuvertebral nerve, also known as the recurrent nerve of Luschka, which is formed by a branch of the vertebral nerve and ventral ramus at each level. The sinuvertebral

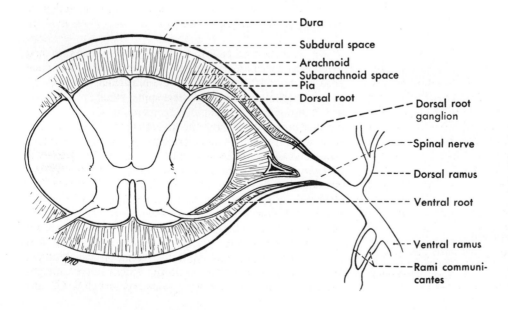

Dura

Subdural space

Arachnoid

Subarachnoid space

Pia

Dorsal root

Dorsal root ganglion

Spinal nerve

Dorsal ramus

Ventral root

Ventral ramus

Rami communicantes

FIGURE 36–7 Formation of spinal nerves from the spinal cord. (From Hollinshead WH, Jenkins DB: Functional Anatomy of the Limbs and Back, ed 5. Philadelphia, WB Saunders, 1981, p 218.)

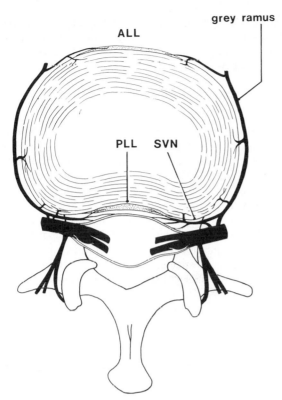

FIGURE 36–8 Nerve supply of the cervical intervertebral disc. PLL, posterior longitudinal ligament; ALL, anterior longitudinal ligament; SVN, sinovertebral nerve. (From Bogduk N, Twomey LT. Clinical Anatomy of the Lumbar Spine. New York, Churchill Livingstone, 1991, p 117.)

nerve supplies the posterior segmental disc and the disc immediately above as well as innervating the posterior longitudinal ligament, pedicle, posterior vertebral periosteum, epidural veins, and dorsal dura mater.

The cervical zygapophyseal joints are innervated by the medial branches from the posterior cervical rami. The joints from C3 and C4 to C6 and C7 are supplied by the medial branches that run above and below the joints. [21, 43, 131] The medial branch of the C3 dorsal ramus, which is the third occipital nerve, innervates the C2 and C3 joints.[21, 43, 131] The atlanto-occipital and atlantoaxial joints are respectively supplied by the C1 and C2 ventral rami.[18, 21, 131]

Pain Generators

Many structures in the neck can be potential pain generators. Pain can also be referred to the neck from other structures such as the upper limbs. Identification of the nociceptive site is important in order to make the correct diagnosis and plan the appropriate treatment.

Any structure that receives innervation can be a potential pain generator. Injury or compromise of the cervical nerves can cause radicular pain as well as weakness and sensory loss. Nerve injuries can be due to a disc herniation, an uncovertebral joint impingement, brachial plexopathy, tumor, hematoma, or infection, metabolic causes, or direct trauma.[124] Radicular symptoms include pain referred into the shoulder and beyond, sensory loss, paresthesias, and weakness.[29, 33, 77, 78, 200] There can also be injuries to the sympathetic nerves which can precipitate disorders such as

fibromyalgia.[206] Specific peripheral nerves can be injured, an example being an injury to the occipital nerve producing occipital neuralgia with headaches.[18, 126, 164]

The cervical vertebrae can also be nociceptive sources. This can be seen with cervical zygapophyseal joint injury secondary to a fracture from trauma or from osteoporosis with microscopic fractures.[20, 21, 23, 27, 136, 186, 190] Pain can originate solely from the intervertebral disc if there is disruption of the outer annular fibers.[22, 31, 47, 216]

Cervical muscles and ligaments are also potential sources of pain. The musculature can generate pain when injured from direct trauma or from the relatively common traumatic flexion-extension injuries ("whiplash").[77, 78, 111] The highly innervated ligaments can be stretched or even torn during flexion-extension injuries, resulting in pain as well.[63, 198, 199, 214]

HISTORY

The history of a patient with neck pain should have the usual format of a chief complaint, history of the present illness, past medical history, family history, social history, functional history, and occupational history and review of systems (see Chapter 1). As with most illnesses, the history provides more information about the underlying condition than any other single part of the evaluation.

Chief Complaint

Cervical conditions can present with a chief complaint involving the neck or the upper extremity. A patient may complain of upper limb pain, numbness, or weakness. There can be similar symptoms involving the lower limbs. The patient may have headaches, visual disturbances, dizziness, or jaw pain. Difficulty in performing activities of daily living (ADL), bladder dysfunction, or bowel incontinence can be the presenting concern.

History of Present Illness

The history is used to generate a differential diagnosis from a chronological account of the current disorder. Potential conditions leading to neck pain are then included or excluded with subsequent history and later confirmed by physical examination and diagnostic testing. The clinician attempts to identify the nociceptive site of any associated pain and to determine whether or not there is a serious neurological problem.[202–205] This information has a significant impact on initial management and timing of diagnostic testing.

There are many neurological symptoms associated with cervical disorders that seem unrelated to the neck, including headaches, dizziness, nausea, vomiting, upper limb paresthesias, concentration difficulties, memory disturbances, and weakness. These are important details of the history which should not be overlooked by the clinician. Limb weakness, bowel dysfunction, and bladder incontinence can indicate serious neurological compromise which warrants aggressive evaluation and treatment.[93]

The onset, duration, origin, and distribution of symptoms as well as the mechanism of injury can provide significant clues to the pathophysiology of the disorder.[114] For example, acute onset of localized posterior neck pain after a motor vehicle accident without neurological symptoms is indicative of musculoligamentous or posterior element injury. An insidious onset of slowly progressive symptoms might indicate the presence of an expanding mass or development of a systemic disease process. On the other hand, subacute onset of neck pain with discretely referred arm pain in a laborer after years of repetitive lifting is consistent with cervical radiculopathy.

Documentation of modifying activities can give additional diagnostic information. For example, the aggravation of neck and upper limb symptoms by lifting, sneezing, or coughing typically implies the presence of a disc abnormality. Radicular symptoms from foraminal stenosis usually intensify with positions that further reduce foraminal size, such as cervical extension.

The temporal relationship of symptoms also helps identify the cervical condition. For example, neck discomfort that is worse by the end of the day in an elderly person suggests a degenerative process. Pain that is worse at night is suggestive of malignancy. The presence of constitutional symptoms is very important when considering malignancy or infection.

Previous neck injuries or problems need to be documented and compared with the current disorder. This is especially important when dealing with a personal or work-related injury. The presence or absence of litigation should be noted since this has been shown to have a bearing on treatment and outcome.[9, 35, 90]

Past Medical History

The main purpose of the past medical history is to determine the presence of an existing disease process or prior surgical procedure that might have led to the present neck complaints or that could have an impact on treatment. Any history of a rheumatologic, metabolic, endocrine, or oncological process needs to be investigated as a possible cause of neck pain. Prior cervical surgery such as a fusion raises other important issues such as fusion integrity and stability as well as work limitations and treatment precautions. The presence of general medical conditions such as diabetes, chronic obstructive pulmonary disease, or coronary artery disease needs to be documented because of their potential impact on therapy and recovery. Information that can affect the prescription of medication is listed, including drug allergies or sensitivities, present medications, and gastrointestinal intolerance.

Social History

The patient's personal life, childhood experiences, social status, and cultural background all influence treatment and outcome. The tranquility of home life such as the marital relationship or disciplinary problems with children have been shown to affect recovery.[172, 206] Financial difficulties can limit treatment options or motivate conscious malingering. The loss of parents or molestation as a child can lay down psychological barriers to successful treatment, conservative or otherwise.[187] Cultural differences have been linked to pain tolerance.[107, 172, 196, 223, 224] Use of tobacco can lead to disc degeneration, presumably by affecting nutrient transport.[119, 148] Tobacco has been associated with poor

operative outcome and a decreased response to therapeutic epidural injections.[96, 103, 195] Elaboration on hobbies might identify recreational activities that should be avoided while treating the cervical disorder.

Family, Occupational, and Functional History

The clinician needs to be aware of any family history of diabetes, rheumatologic disorders, cancer, neck pain, psychological illness, or fibromyalgia. This information is important in determining the differential diagnosis. A family tradition of pain and disability can adversely affect treatment and outcome.

The current employment status is important information, especially in work-related injuries. Knowledge of the patient's job requirement and responsibilities, as well as the work environment, enables the physician to appropriately determine work status and applicable restrictions. The ergonomics of the job such as static positioning and overuse are important points regarding employment. Other nonphysical factors related to work also affect the clinical condition. An uncertain employment status and a poor perception of job security have been shown to be a risk factor for pain, as is heavy lifting.[6, 17, 59] While the studies cited were for back pain, they appear no less relevant for neck pain.

The person's quality of life with cervical disorder can be evaluated by determining if there are any restrictions on social activities or limitation on ADL. Treatment and outcome goals are then modified for each person to progress toward the return to prior recreational activities and to achieve independence in ADL.

Review of Systems

The review of systems should be similar to that for any patient, but certain aspects need to be emphasized in patients with cervical disorders. Bowel and bladder function, difficulty in sleeping, psychological problems, recent weight loss, and night sweats are all important. The clinician should inquire about any systemic or metabolic problem that could be causing the neck pain, either primarily or secondarily.

Pain Diagrams

The history is often supplemented with pain diagrams that the patient completes after instruction. The visual analog scale (VAS) and pain drawing can provide useful information to the clinician (Fig. 36–9). The VAS quantifies pain intensity by placing a point on a line that represents a continuum of pain from none to incapacitating.[109] The completed pain drawing can reveal characteristic symptom patterns consistent for particular disorders and give information regarding the patient's psychological status.[156, 173]

PHYSICAL EXAMINATION

The patient is assessed to identify any neurological deficit and to locate the pain generator site. The examination typically includes observation, inspection, ROM, neurological evaluation, palpation, and provocative maneuvers.

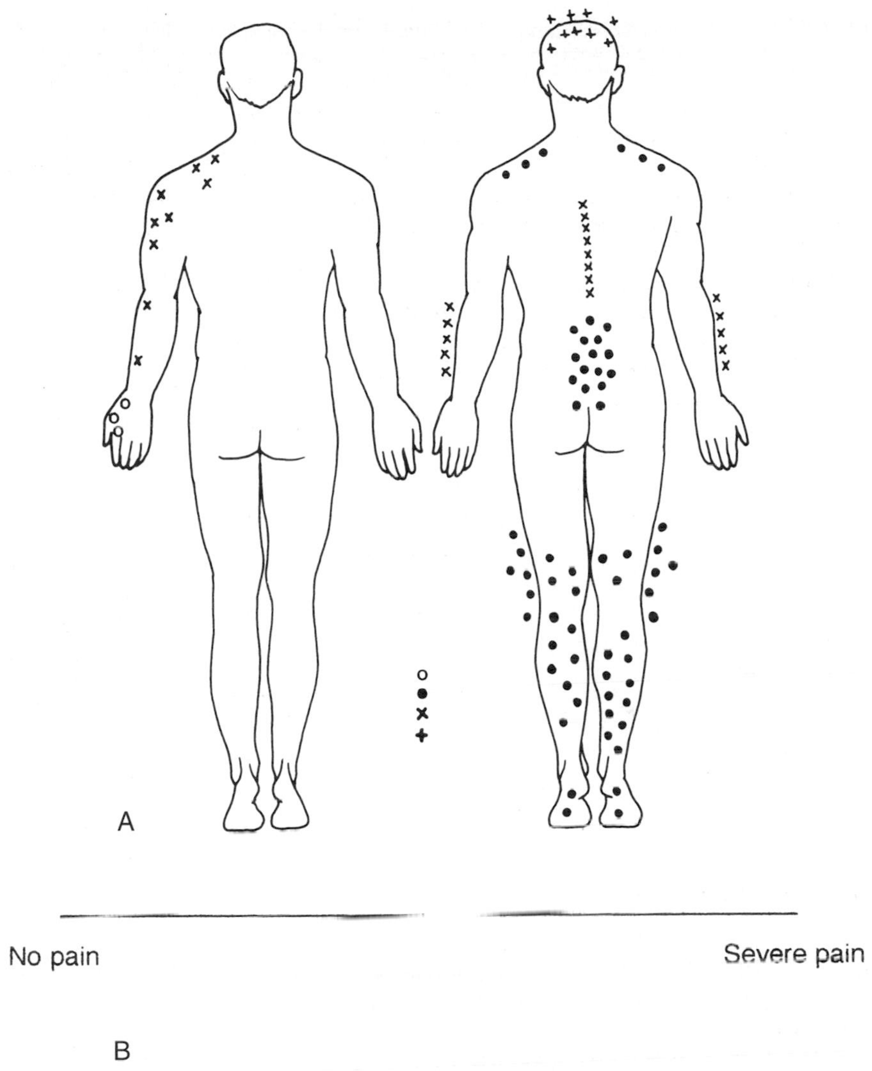

FIGURE 36–9 Pain diagrams. *A,* Pain drawing. Pain drawing on *left* represents an organic cervical radicular syndrome. Pain drawing on *right* is a diffuse nonorganic pain reaction. *Open circle,* tingling; *solid circle,* burning; *times sign,* pain; *plus sign,* numbness. *B,* Visual analogue scale. The patient is instructed to place a mark on the line that represents the intensity of the pain. (*A* from Macnab I, McCulloch J: Neck Ache and Shoulder Pain. Baltimore, Williams & Wilkins, 1994, p 138.)

No pain

Severe pain

B

Observation and Inspection

The examination begins as soon as there is patient contact. Gait, facial expressions, and body language are noted during the evaluation. These observations help identify pain behaviors and body mechanics.

The neck is surveyed for any surgical scars, erythema, lesions, or any other skin aberrations. The presence of abnormal cervical positioning is recorded such as forward posturing (camptocormia), absent cervical lordosis, kyphosis, or listing.

Range of Motion

The evaluation of cervical ROM includes flexion, extension, rotation, and lateral bending. An inclinometer is currently the most reliable instrument for documenting ROM.[122, 207] Normal ROM of the neck is 60 degrees of flexion, 75 degrees of extension, 45 degrees of lateral flexion, and 80 degrees of rotation[133] (Table 36–2). Clinical evaluation of ROM can be done without an inclinometer. The patient with normal neck ROM is able to rest the chin on the chest, look straight up at the ceiling, touch or nearly touch each ear to the shoulder, and tap the chin against

each shoulder. Patients accomplishing these movements have normal ROM. These ROM tests are reliable only if the patient does not move the shoulders, the rest of the spine, or the hips.[122]

The cervical spine is assessed for both active and passive ROM. The lack of active motion can be secondary to pain or muscle guarding. Decreased active and passive ROM can be secondary to ankylosis. The patient is asked to actively move the neck and then the examiner gently tries to passively increase the range. The neck should not be forced into a nonphysiological or painful range that can cause an increase in symptoms. ROM testing is contraindicated in the presence of spinal instability.

Neurological Evaluation

The neurological examination involves testing of the peripheral and central nervous system to determine the presence or absence of neurological deficits. Strength, muscle stretch reflexes, sensation, and reflex testing for upper motor neuron lesions are performed on every patient presenting with neck problems.

The motor examination can determine the presence of a root, trunk, or peripheral nerve injury when there is

TABLE 36–2   Cervical Spine Range of Motion at Each Segmental Level

Interspace	Combined Flexion/Extension ($\pm$ x-axis rotation)		One-Side Lateral Bending (z-axis rotation)		One-Side Axial Rotation (y-axis rotation)	
	Limits of Ranges (degrees)	Representative Angle (degrees)	Limits of Ranges (degrees)	Representative Angle (degrees)	Limits of Ranges (degrees)	Representative Angle (degrees)
Middle						
C2–C3	5–16	10	11–20	10	0–10	3
C3–C4	7–26	15	9–15	11	3–10	7
C4–C5	13–29	20	0–16	11	1–12	7
Lower						
C5–C6	13–29	20	0–16	8	2–12	7
C6–C7	6–26	17	0–17	7	2–10	6
C7–T1	4–7	9	0–17	4	0–7	2

From White AA, Panjabi MM: Biomechanics of the Spine, ed 2. Philadelphia, JB Lippincott, 1990, p 98.

involvement of motor fibers. Knowledge of the peripheral nervous system and upper limb innervation patterns allows for localization by eliciting muscle weakness in a root or peripheral nerve distribution (Table 36–3). Neck strength is tested in flexion, extension, and rotation to detect neck weakness that is typically present in myasthenia gravis, myopathy, and some rheumatologic conditions.

Reflex testing is useful in evaluating nerve root function and in localizing the lesion. While any level of reflex amplitude can be normal, hyporeflexia is consistent with lesions at the root level, plexus, or peripheral nerve, while hyperreflexia is more associated with lesions from the brain to the spinal cord. Hyporeflexia and hyperreflexia can be present together if the lesion involves both the central and peripheral nervous system. Asymmetrical hyporeflexia at a specific root level is typical of unilateral radiculopathy, whereas generalized symmetrical hyperreflexia with long tract signs is consistent with a myelopathic process.

When assessing an upper limb reflex, it is very important that the correct reflex is elicited and not an inverted reflex. An inverted reflex can occur, for example, if there is a large disc herniation. This could result in elbow flexion rather than extension when checking for the triceps reflex. The unwary clinician might note this as a normal reflex. Actually, the stimulus from the reflex at the C7 level was blocked and traveled cephalad one level to produce a biceps response.[143] This often indicates a more serious problem of myelopathy, in addition to a concurrent C7 radiculopathy.

Another significant point about muscle stretch reflex testing is that it must be established whether a decrease in

the reflex really represents a diminution. For example, a tense patient might not be able to relax, resulting in a diminished or absent reflex. Reflexes should be obtained carefully and repeated with and without facilitation. Facilitation in the upper limbs, similar to Jendrassik's maneuver for the lower limbs, is best done by asking the patient to tense muscles outside the limb. The patient can bite down hard, squeeze the knees together, or make a fist with the opposite hand. The reflex examination should include attempts to elicit pathological reflexes which typically include Babinski's and Hoffmann's tests. These testing methods are conducted to assess the integrity of the long tracts within the central nervous system. The presence of these superficial reflexes is suggestive of a central nervous system lesion such as a central cervical disc herniation, cervical spinal stenosis, or other pathologic process resulting in myelopathy.

The sensory examination is designed to test the competence of the dorsal roots.[73] Figure 36–10 shows the classic dermatomal pattern of the upper limbs. Pain, tested by pinprick, is usually the last sensory modality to be decreased and is not the most sensitive indication of sensory loss.[87] Vibration fibers are affected more often than the smaller pain fibers in a radiculopathy. Position sense is also likely to be abnormal before pain sensation. Although pain testing is more convenient, vibratory and position sense testing are likely to be the first involved in a radiculopathy.[87] The only problem with vibration is that it cannot be well localized to one dermatome. Specific patterns of sensory change must be documented and assessed to see whether these changes actually follow a dermatomal pattern. Cervical spine soft tissues also refer pain and unusual sensations into the limbs.[23, 111] These "sclerotomal" symptoms should not be confused with actual dermatomal sensory loss. Sensations referred by sclerotomal sources do not actually produce real sensory deficit.

Palpatory Examination

Palpation of the osseous structures of the anterior aspect of the neck include the hyoid bone, which should move when the patient swallows, and the thyroid cartilage. The carotid tubercles of C6 should be palpated separately. They are important structures used to identify cervical ganglion sites for sympathetic blocks. The posterior osseous struc-

TABLE 36–3   Nerve Root Levels, Peripheral Nerves, and Muscles of the Upper Limb Commonly Evaluated in the Patient With Neck Pain

Nerve Root Level	Nerve	Muscle
C5, C6	Axillary	Deltoid
C5, C6	Musculocutaneous	Biceps brachii
C5, C6	Suprascapular	Supraspinatus
	Suprascapular	Infraspinatus
C7	Radial	Triceps
	Median	Pronator teres
C8, T1	Median	Abductor pollicis brevis
	Ulnar	First dorsal interrossei

ated in the posterior neck, since it is a common site for tender points and trigger points associated with cervical trauma. The greater occipital nerves are commonly affected in flexion-extension injuries, resulting in occipital neuralgia with occipital headaches.[126] Palpation of the nerves commonly causes an increase in the patient's headache if due to occipital neuralgia. The greater occipital nerves are located at one third of the distance from the occipital protuberance to the ipsilateral mastoid process.[36] Tenderness of the ligamentum nuchae often indicates a stretched ligament resulting from a neck flexion or direct injury. Soft tissue examination of the scapular stabilizers and shoulders should be undertaken to identify trigger points and tender points.

Provocative Maneuvers

Spurling's test looks for foraminal encroachment on an inflamed cervical nerve root. The patient's head and neck are extended, laterally flexed, and held down for up to 1 min.[38, 39, 138] The sign is present if there are increased symptoms into the shoulder and into the hand in a radicular pattern.

Lhermitte's sign was first described in patients with multiple sclerosis. The patient's head is briskly flexed.[138] Electric-like pain or shock sensations shooting down through the spine as a result of this maneuver are often indicative of a spinal cord disorder. This sign is also positive in some patients with herniated cervical discs.

Adson's maneuver is a test for neurovascular compromise due to a thoracic outlet problem from a cervical rib or a tight scalenus anterior medius muscle.[138] The symptomatic arm is placed in extension and lateral rotation. The radial pulse is monitored as the patient takes a deep breath and turns the head toward the ipsilateral side. The presence of subclavian artery compression is confirmed if there is a marked diminution or absence of the radial pulse. This test is sensitive but not very specific, resulting in many false-positive findings.

Cervical spine disorders can cause difficulty with swallowing. The swallowing test assesses the patient's ability to swallow normally on command. Swallowing dysfunction can be secondary to protruding osteophytes, soft tissue swelling from hematomas, infections, or tumors located in the anterior portion of the cervical spine (see Chapter 27 for more information on swallowing dysfunction).

DIAGNOSTIC STUDIES

Imaging is an important technique in the evaluation and treatment of cervical spine problems. The clinician should remember that imaging techniques evaluate anatomy rather than function, and can have the inherent problem of false-positive or false-negative results. In the cervical magnetic resonance imaging (MRI) study of Boden et al.,[17] nearly 20% of asymptomatic subjects had demonstrable abnormalities. The physician needs to interpret diagnostic studies only in the context of each clinical case (see Chapter 11 for more information).

Radiographs

Although plain films provide limited information, they can still be useful in evaluating the cervical spine for

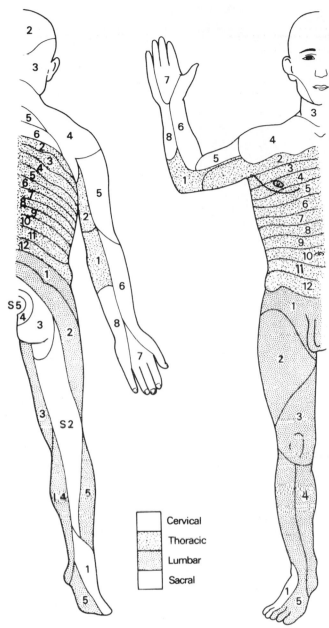

FIGURE 36-10 Dermatomal distribution of the cervical nerve roots. (From Ellis H: Clinical Anatomy: A Revision and Applied Anatomy for Clinical Students, ed 6. London, Blackwell, 1976, p 205.)

tures of the neck are examined by palpating the occiput, inion, superior nuchal line, mastoid processes, zygapophyseal joints, and the spinous processes. These structures are palpated to identify any painful sites. Cervical spine osseous structures such as the facet joints and the spinous processes can be palpated during motion to identify dysfunction in movement, especially in nonobese patients.

Soft tissue palpation is also an important part of the cervical spine examination. The sternocleidomastoid muscle is an easily palpated muscle. Lymph nodes in the region of the sternocleidomastoid can indicate infection in the oropharynx or upper respiratory tract. The consistency and size of the thyroid and parotid glands are evaluated to assess for any abnormalities. The trapezius muscle is evalu-

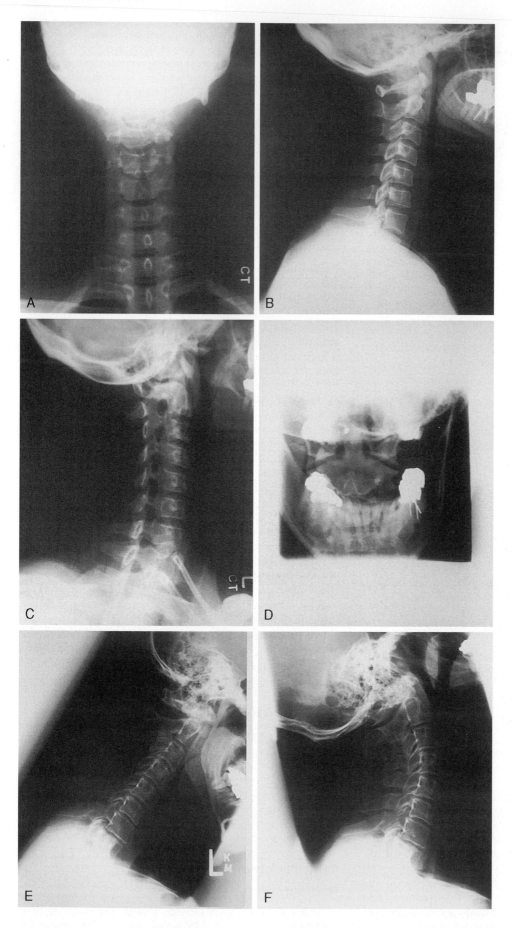

FIGURE 36–11 Complete cervical spine radiograph series. Anteroposterior (A), lateral (B), oblique (C), open-mouth (D), flexion (E), and extension (F) views.

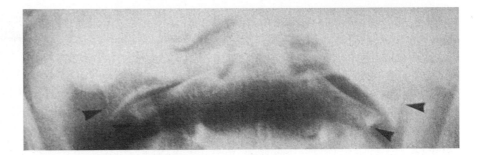

FIGURE 36–12 Open-mouth view of cervical spine demonstrating a burst fracture of the atlas (Jefferson fracture). Offsetting of the lateral masses of the atlas with those of the axis *(arrowheads)* confirms the burst fracture. (From Pavlov H, Torg JS: Roentgen examination of cervical spine injuries in the athlete. Clin Sports Med 1987; 6:761.)

chronic degenerative changes, metastatic disease, infection, spinal deformity, and stability. Cervical spine films in trauma cases typically incorporate seven views including AP, lateral, bilateral oblique, open-mouth, flexion, and extension views (Fig. 36–11). Flexion-extension views can help identify subluxations or cervical spine instability.[167] An open-mouth view is important in evaluating the status of the odontoid process and instability between the first two cervical vertebrae (Fig. 36–12). The AP view helps in the evaluation of the spine for tumors, osteophytes, and fractures. The lateral views check for stability as well as for signs of spondylosis including spurring and disc space narrowing (Fig. 36–13). Oblique views are necessary for evaluating degenerative disc disease and foraminal encroachment by osteophytes of uncovertebral joints or the facet joints[156, 179] (Fig. 36–14).

Computed Tomography and Myelography

The computed tomography (CT) scan and myelography individually or in combination continue to be important diagnostic studies in the evaluation of cervical spine problems. The CT scan is particularly helpful when a fracture of the cervical spine is suspected and should be done in trauma cases when there is any suspicion of a fracture. A myelogram followed by a CT scan is often the imaging study of choice prior to any cervical surgery.[13, 32, 106] This study provides excellent evaluation of the spinal cord and spinal canal dimensions. Nerve root impingement from disc, spur, or foraminal encroachment is best assessed in this manner. CT-myelography is superior to MRI in de-

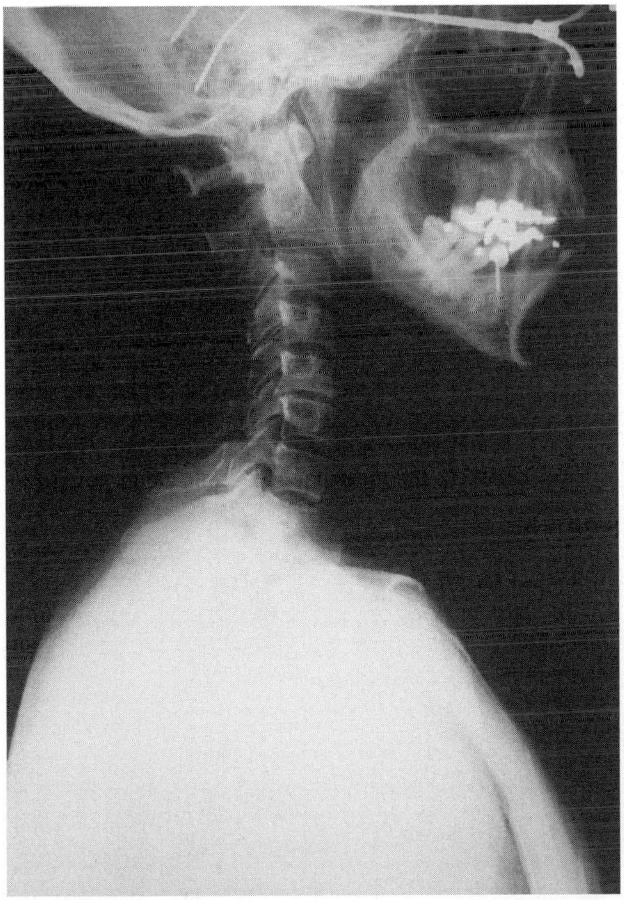

FIGURE 36–13 Lateral cervical spine radiograph revealing disc space narrowing at C5 to C6 with vertebral spurring.

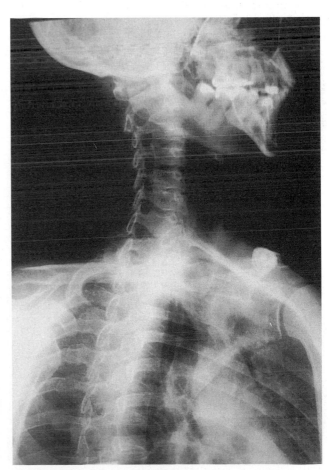

FIGURE 36–14 Oblique cervical spine radiograph showing uncovertebral spurring at the C5 to C6 intervertebral foramen, possibly encroaching on the cervical nerve root.

tecting lateral and foraminal encroachment[152, 179, 181] (Fig. 36–15). The CT-myelogram is often more expensive and has a higher morbidity than MRI.[134] Therefore, the CT-myelogram is usually not one of the initial diagnostic studies performed to evaluate the cervical spine and typically is reserved for surgical cases.

Magnetic Resonance Imaging

Magnetic resonance imaging has become the imaging technique of choice in the cervical spine when ruling out a herniated disc[58, 60, 82, 179, 182, 220] (Fig. 36–16). The major strength of MRI is the definition of soft tissue structures, including cervical discs, spinal cord, and cerebrospinal fluid, which is not possible by other imaging methods. The procedure is noninvasive and does not expose the patient to radiation.

Although MRI is widely used and provides useful information, there are some shortcomings. The test is relatively expensive, not tolerated by claustrophobic patients, requires that a patient cooperate to minimize artifact, and can have false-positive results.[17, 201] MRI is not as sensitive as the CT scan in evaluating bony structures such as spurs and bony impingements.[152, 179, 181] Persons with embedded metallic objects such as pacemakers, surgical clips, or prosthetic heart valves cannot be scanned by MRI since the powerful magnets can dislodge these items.

The MRI has to be interpreted in relation to the patient's symptoms, since many anatomical lesions on MRI are not functionally important. In the study of Boden et al.,[17] one fourth of asymptomatic subjects under the age of 40 years had at least one degenerative segment, and in those older than 40 nearly 60% had degenerative segments by MRI.[17]

Discography

Discography has remained controversial ever since its introduction in 1957 by Smith and Nichols.[194] The discomfort and invasiveness of this test make it less desirable than a cervical MRI, which provides most of the information that a discogram provides.[52] Cervical discography (Fig. 36–17) has a role in identifying the symptomatic disc(s), which can be useful in the evaluation of patients with inconclusive diagnostic tests and in the planning of cervical fusions.[216] Large disc herniations and midsagittal spinal canal diameters less than 11 mm are contraindications to discography at any level.[4]

Scintigraphy

Bone scanning is useful as a supplemental study in patients with neck pain. Scintigraphy is commonly used to rule out primary or metastatic osseous lesions, which typically display increased uptake of the radionucleotide. The scan is very sensitive in detecting these hot spots with only a 2% false-negative rate.[158] Multiple myeloma is the most frequent primary spine tumor in the adult, and the bone scan is positive in 60% of these cases.[218]

Other conditions that are detected by scintigraphy because of increased radionucleotide uptake include fractures, sacroiliitis, osteomyelitis, and discitis. Single-photon emission computed tomography (SPECT) is sometimes used for detailed evaluation of the posterior elements, such as the facet joint. Triple-phase bone scanning usually is performed in the patient with neck and upper limb pain when there is a suspicion for any condition that leads to osteopenia, such as reflex sympathetic dystrophy (RSD) or osteoporosis (see Chapter 40).

Electrodiagnostic Evaluation

Electrodiagnostic evaluation continues to be a mainstay for evaluating the cervical spine. Electrodiagnostic studies have the advantage of being relatively inexpensive as well as low in morbidity. Nerve conduction studies and electro-

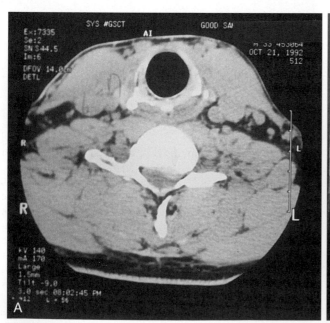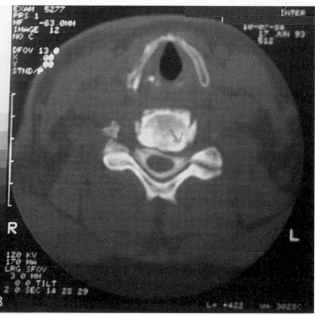

FIGURE 36–15 Cervical spine CT scan. *A,* Abnormal study demonstrating left posterolateral cervical disc herniation with nerve root impingement. *B,* Postmyelogram CT scan detailing thecal sac and nerve root compression from left posterolateral cervical disc herniation in a different patient.

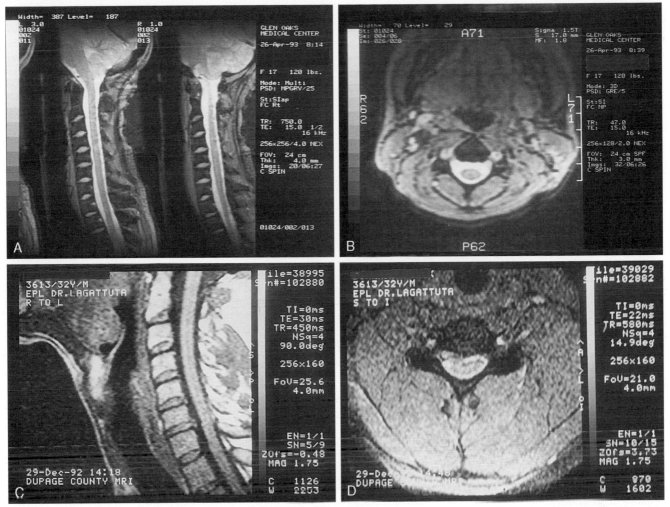

FIGURE 36–18 Cervical spine MRI. *A*, Normal sagittal image. *B*, Normal axial image. *C*, Abnormal sagittal image reveals C6 to C7 posterior disc herniation. *D*, Abnormal axial image in same patient shows right lateral projection of the posterior C6 to C7 disc herniation compromising the right C7 nerve root.

myography (EMG) provide physiological information regarding cervical nerve root and peripheral nerve function.

Acute, subacute, and chronic radicular features can be detected by needle EMG when there is involvement of motor fibers.[126, 127] Abnormal spontaneous potentials and changes in motor unit action potentials in two or more muscles innervated by the same nerve root are highly suggestive of a radiculopathy (see Table 36–3). The compound muscle action potential (CMAP) amplitude from nerve conduction studies can be helpful in determining the degree of axonotmesis. A 50% drop or more in CMAP amplitude is indicative of significant axonal loss.[113]

Ulnar nerve entrapment, carpal tunnel syndrome, and peripheral neuropathy can be confused with cervical radiculopathy.[112, 113] Electrodiagnostic testing is very helpful in diagnosing these conditions, and separating them from cervical radiculopathy.

Somatosensory evoked potentials (SEPs) are important in evaluating the sensory conduction, both peripherally and centrally. Lower limb nerve testing of such as in the tibial and peroneal nerves has been shown to be helpful in diagnosing a myelopathy by assessing spinal cord conduction. Lower limb SEPs are more sensitive than upper limb

SEPs in detecting cervical myelopathy.[219, 221] Dermatomal evoked potentials have been performed for cervical radiculopathy, but are of questionable value[185] (see Chapters 6, 7, and 8 for more detailed information on electrodiagnostic testing).

Thermography

Thermography is a noninvasive diagnostic procedure that has been used in the past for the diagnosis of many conditions. The test is based upon recording heat emission from the body using liquid crystal or infrared techniques. The sympathetic nervous system is largely responsible for the regulation of dermal circulation and maintaining skin temperature. Heat is emitted in a symmetrical fashion in the normal person. Abnormal changes in heat emission occur when there is a disturbance to the sympathetic system, as with direct nerve injury or from pain through a complex sympathetic reflex.

Thermography has typically been used to evaluate nerve root or peripheral nerve injury, reflex sympathetic dystrophy (RSD), and myofascial conditions. Although there is much controversy and skepticism today regarding the use

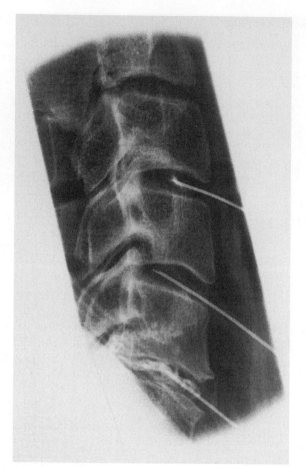

FIGURE 36–17 Cervical discogram. Lateral radiograph view showing needle placement in the C4 to C5, C5 to C6, and C6 to C7 discs. Contrast was injected into the normal C4 to C5 and abnormal C6 to C7 discs. Only a small amount of contrast could be injected into the painless C4 to C5 disc. The C6 to C7 disc revealed significant degenerative changes with spread of contrast throughout the disc. The patient's symptoms were reproduced when the C6 to C7 disc was injected during the study.

of thermography in evaluating musculoskeletal conditions, it is generally accepted as useful in the diagnosis of RSD.[208]

Sonography

Sonography is useful for evaluating many organ systems. Specific structures routinely evaluated include the peripheral vasculature, gravid uterus, heart, liver, kidneys, gallbladder, pancreas, and thyroid. A relatively new application has been to use ultrasound to evaluate the musculoskeletal system. The shoulder is the most common musculoskeletal area assessed at this time, but sonography is now also being used to evaluate the spine. Studies have demonstrated that ultrasound can document tears and inflammatory changes to ligaments.[117] Muscle inflammation has also been documented with ultrasound.[83] At this time, more research is needed to determine the clinical value of spinal and musculoskeletal ultrasound.

TREATMENT

Modalities

Physical modalities should typically be used only in the acute phase of the condition to help with pain control.

Once the patient is past the acute phase, these modalities are used only on an as-needed basis. Superficial heat modalities can relax muscles and relieve pain in many cervical disorders. On the other hand, deep heating modalities like ultrasound should be avoided in acute cervical radiculopathy, since this could increase the inflammation of a swollen nerve leading to more pain or nerve injury[132] (see Chapter 22 for more information on modalities).

Traction

Cervical traction can be helpful in relieving symptoms associated with nerve root compression. Hot packs, massage, or electrical stimulation, or any combination of these, should be done prior to traction to help relieve pain and relax the muscles.[48, 49, 51] Cervical traction can be performed using either a heavyweight intermittent or a lightweight continuous regimen.[48–50] The neck should be positioned in flexion rather than extension during traction.[51] The use of lightweight continuous home traction is less expensive and gives the patient more autonomy (see Chapter 22 for more information on traction).

Orthoses

A soft collar is recommended only in acute soft tissue neck injuries and for a short period of time, not to exceed 3 or 4 days of continuous use. There is a risk of limiting cervical ROM or losing neck strength if collars are worn continuously for longer periods of time, even though a patient can move the neck in a soft collar.[146, 149, 170] The wide part of the collar is placed posteriorly and the thin part anteriorly (Fig. 36–18) when used for radiculopathy. This allows the patient to flex the spine and open the intervertebral foramina while discouraging neck extension. The collar can also be used during certain activities for a longer period of time such as sleeping or driving. A Philadelphia collar can be used at night to give more rigid positioning. This helps prevent foraminal narrowing by keeping the neck out of extension (see Chapter 18 for more information on spinal orthoses).

Medications

Nonsteroidal anti-inflammatory drugs (NSAIDs) are the first line of pharmacological intervention in treating most cervical conditions. They provide pain relief and reduce inflammation. The patient has to have a therapeutic NSAID level in order to get an anti-inflammatory effect. NSAIDs requiring only once-a-day dosing improve compliance and increase the likelihood of reaching therapeutic levels. Decreasing inflammation is very important when treating cervical radiculopathies. Aspirin is not recommended because of the large doses needed for an anti-inflammatory effect, longer duration of action onset, gastrointestinal toxicity, and irreversible binding to cyclooxygenase. There needs to be caution when prescribing NSAIDs if there is any history of peptic ulcers, renal insufficiency, or hepatic dysfunction.

Oral steroids are used when a potent anti-inflammatory effect is needed in cervical radiculopathy, and steroid treatment is typically initiated when an inflammatory cause of the radiculopathy is suspected and there are no contraindications such as infection or peptic ulcer disease.[85, 184] The

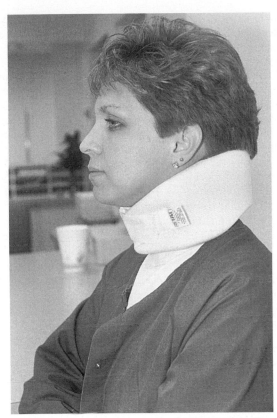

FIGURE 36–18 Cervical orthosis. Cervical soft collar with widest side posteriorly and narrowest side anteriorly.

dosage for prednisone should begin at about 70 mg/day and decrease by 10 mg/day for a total course of 280 mg. There is no documented case in the literature of avascular necrosis occurring when the total dose of prednisone or its corticosteroid equivalent is under 550 mg.[98]

Muscle relaxants, antidepressants, and narcotics are other medications prescribed for cervical disorders. Muscle relaxants should not be prescribed unless the patient absolutely cannot tolerate the pain. The only major effect of muscle relaxants is sedation (they relax muscles by relaxing the patient). Analgesics are a better choice in most cases.[64] Analgesics are typically of the narcotic type and should be used orally on a scheduled-dose basis for a short period of time. Narcotic dependency is a concern with these medications, and they should only rarely be needed for more than 6 weeks. Tricyclic antidepressants (TCAs) can help decrease pain and improve sleep. TCAs appear to decrease pain by affecting substance P and improve sleep by increasing stage IV, non-REM (non-rapid eye movement) sleep.[41, 180, 209] Unfortunately, the side effects such as dry mouth, constipation, and weight gain can limit their use in some patients.

The serotonin re-uptake inhibitor antidepressants do not have the side effects associated with TCAs and can be used in patients intolerant to the TCAs. Although the serotonin re-uptake inhibitors are not as effective as TCAs in treating pain from diabetic peripheral neuropathies,[144] their effectiveness compared with other antidepressants has not been determined for neck and back pain.

Manipulation

Spinal manipulation and mobilization are treatment modalities used to restore normal ROM and decrease pain. Although there is no clear explanation of how manipulation works, some believe that adjustments to zygapophyseal joints improve afferent signals from mechanoreceptors to the peripheral and central nervous system.[175] The normalization of afferent impulses results in improved muscle tone, decreased muscle guarding, and more effective local tissue metabolism. These physiological modifications lead to improved ROM and pain reduction.

Spinal manipulation has been shown to have beneficial short-term results in the acutely injured patient.[37, 76, 92, 100] There is no evidence that manipulation provides long-term benefits or improvement in chronic conditions, or alters the natural course of the disorder[157] (see Chapter 21 for further information on manipulation).

Stabilization

Cervicothoracic stabilization is a rehabilitation program designed to limit pain, maximize function, and prevent further injury. Stabilization includes cervical spine flexibility, posture re-education, and strengthening. This program emphasizes patient responsibility through active participation.

Restoring normal ROM and good posture is necessary to prevent repetitive microtrauma to cervical structures from poor movement patterns.[38] Full ROM is necessary to train the cervicothoracic spine in stabilization during various activities. Pain-free ROM is determined by placing the cervical spine in positions that produce and relieve symptoms. Initially, stabilization starts within the established pain-free ROM and is then applied outside this ROM as the patient's condition improves. Any soft tissue or joint restriction present is treated to help achieve normal cervical spine ROM. This is accomplished through passive ROM exercise, spine mobilization, soft tissue mobilization techniques, self-stretching, and correct posturing. The anterior and posterior neck muscles that are stretched to maintain full flexibility are listed in Table 36–4.

Postural training begins with the patient sitting or standing in front of a mirror with a therapist. The patient then

TABLE 36–4   Muscle Groups and Individual Muscles Utilized in Cervicothoracic Stabilization

Anterior Muscles	Posterior Muscles
Sternocleidomastoid	Rectus capitis posterior major
Scaleni	Rectus capitis posterior minor
Pectoralis major	Obliquus capitis inferior
Pectoralis minor	Obliquus capitis superior
Biceps (long head)	Levator scapulae
	Superior trapezius
	Latissimus dorsi
	Teres major
	Subscapularis
	Rhomboids
	Middle trapezius
	Lower trapezius
	Serratus anterior

From Sweeney T, Prentice C, Saal JA, et al: Cervicothoracic muscular stabilizing technique. Phys Med Rehabil 1990;4:339.

performs various transfer maneuvers while maintaining a "neutral spine" (correct posturing) with feedback from a mirror and the therapist. The goal is to teach the patient to maintain a neutral spine position while performing daily activities. These proprioceptive skills are implemented during strengthening exercises that will enable the patient to keep the cervical spine in a stable, pain-free, and safe position during strenuous activities.

Cervicothoracic stabilization requires training and coordination of the muscles in the neck area. The neck and shoulder girdle muscles, especially the scapular muscles, need to be individually strengthened[91, 183, 198] (see Table 36–4). The regional muscles of the cervical spine include cervical spine extensors as well as flexors, the rectus capitis anterior, rectus capitis lateralis, longissimus cervicis, and longissimus capitis. The primary thoracic stabilizers are the abdominal and lumbar paraspinal extensor muscles and latissimus dorsi muscles. The scapular muscles include the middle and lower trapezius, serratus anterior, and rhomboids. The chest wall muscles include the pectoralis major and minor muscles.

The exercises used for stabilization proceed from simple to more advanced routines (Table 36–5). A variety of isometric and isotonic resistance exercises are used to train the cervicothoracic muscles. Elastic bands, weight machines, and free weights are used in a progressive manner. The patient is instructed to maintain a neutral spine position at all times during stabilization exercises. Advanced exercises challenge the patient to maintain this position during dynamic activities. An engram is achieved through repetition which enables the patient to stabilize the cervical spine automatically.

Stabilizing the cervical spine using muscular control and enhanced proprioceptive feedback allows the patient to perform activities safely by balancing forces around the cervical spine. Conditioning and training the thorax and upper extremities help to distribute forces away from the cervical spine. The cervicothoracic spine and upper extremities cannot be trained in isolation. Successful treatment with stabilization requires that the lumbar spine and lower extremities be incorporated in the program.[198] The lumbar spine and lower extremities provide a base for the cervicothoracic area and cannot be neglected during training.

TABLE 36–5   Cervicothoracic Stabilization Exercises

	Cervicothoracic Stabilization Levels		
	I Basic	II Intermediate	III Advanced
Direct cervical stabilization exercises	Cervical active range of motion Cervical isometrics	Cervical gravity Resisted isometrics	Cervical active Range gravity resisted
Indirect cervical stabilization exercises			
Supine, head supported	Theraband chest press Bilateral arm raise Supported dying bug	Unsupported dying bug	Chest flies Bench press Incline dumbbell press
Sit	Reciprocal arm raise Unilateral arm raise Bilateral arm raise Seated row Latissimus pulldown	Swiss ball reciprocal Arm raises Chest press	Swiss ball bilateral Shoulder shrugs Supraspinatus raises

Stand	Theraband reciprocal
	Chest press
	Theraband straight
	Arm latissimus
	Pulldown
	Theraband:
	    Chest press
	    Latissimus pulldown
	Standing rowing
	Crossovers
	Triceps press
		Standing rowing
		Biceps pulldown
			Upright row
			Shoulder shrugs
			Supraspinatus raises

Flexed hip–hinge position	0–30 degrees Reciprocal arm raise Unilateral arm raise Bilateral arm raise Interscapular flies	30–60 degrees Incline prone flies Reciprocal deltoid raise Cable crossovers	60–90 degrees Bilateral anterior Deltoid raises Interscapular flies
Prone	Reciprocal arm raise Unilateral arm raise Bilateral arm raise	Quadruped Head unsupported Swiss ball bilateral Anterior deltoid raises Swiss ball prone Rowing Swiss ball prone flies	Head supported Prone flies Latissimus flies
Supine, head unsupported	Not advised for level I	Partial sit-ups Arm raises	Swiss ball chest flies Swiss ball reciprocal

From Sweeney T, Prentice C, Saal JA, et al: Cervicothoracic muscular stabilizing technique. Phys Med Rehabil 1990;4:345.

Neck School

Neck school, similar to back school, provides an opportunity to educate the cervical spine patient. Typically, a therapist, athletic trainer, or nurse instructs patients in cervical anatomy, biomechanics, pathology, and ergonomics to accomplish several goals. Patients become more familiar with their neck and typical cervical disorders. Any misconceptions or myths that a patient has about neck pain are cleared up through discussion and education. Preventive measures against further injury are incorporated by the patient in all activities.

Selective Spinal Injections

Cervical epidural, selective nerve root, facet, and sympathetic blocks can be used both diagnostically and therapeutically. These procedures can be instrumental in determining the pain generator site and allow for "aggressive conservative" treatment. Cervical epidural and selective nerve root blocks can be used when there are radicular features associated with a cervical disorder.[217] An anesthetic and steroid preparation is injected into the epidural space or along the nerve root after precise localization under fluoroscopy with radiopaque dye (Figs. 36–19 and 36–20). The anesthetic in the epidural injectant decreases or re-

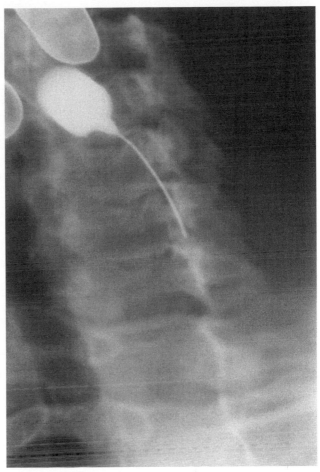

FIGURE 36–20 Cervical perisheathogram. Oblique cervical spine radiograph displaying a small amount of contrast in the C6 to C7 neuroforamen to establish proper needle position before injection of medication.

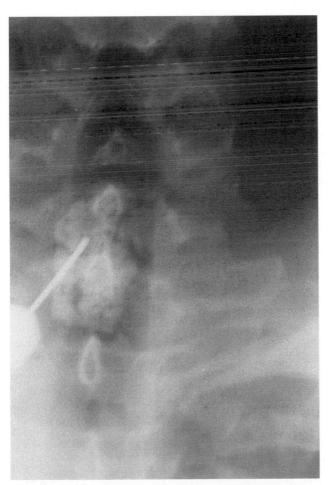

FIGURE 36–19 Cervical epidurogram. Anteroposterior cervical spine radiograph showing contrast within the epidural space and confirming correct needle placement prior to injecting medication.

solves symptoms in cases of irritation or injury to the nerve root. Long-term relief can be expected from the steroid if the pathophysiological problem is secondary to an intense inflammatory process.[20, 44, 79, 191, 211] Relief typically lasts no longer than the duration of the anesthetic if the problem is secondary to mechanical compression such as foraminal stenosis. Selective nerve root blocks are more precise than the "gunshot" approach of the epidural block and can identify the symptomatic root or roots. Cervical sympathetic blocks can be performed when sympathetic-mediated pain is suspected, as in the case of RSD.

Facet blocks are performed in one of two different ways. Either the intra-articular joint or the medial branch nerves are injected with medication (Fig. 36–21). Usually, intra-articular injections with an anesthetic and steroid are done for diagnostic and therapeutic effects when synovitis is suspected (as in osteoarthritis).[71, 104] Facet joint (medial branch) nerve blocks are diagnostic injections performed with an anesthetic, usually when there has been a mechanical injury to the posterior elements, as with whiplash-type injuries.[19, 23, 27, 38] There can be a higher diagnostic sensitivity and specificity if medial branch blocks are performed on different occasions with anesthetics having different action durations.[11] Those patients with pain relief from

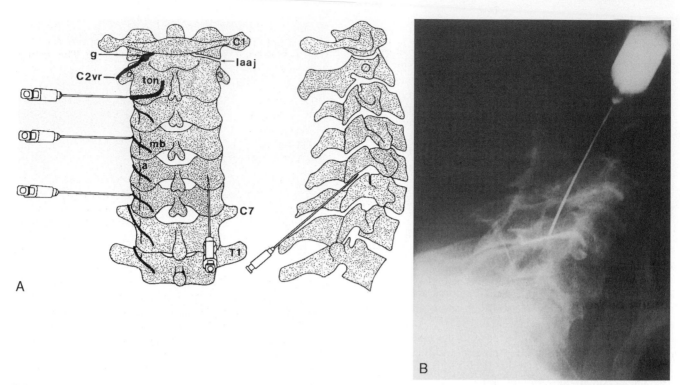

FIGURE 36–21 Cervical facet injections. *A,* Needle placement for medial branch nerve and intra-articular zygapophyseal injections. *Left,* Posterior view of cervical spine showing location of the C2 ganglion (g) behind the lateral atlantoaxial joint (laaj), the C2 ventral ramus (C2vr), location of the medial branches of the cervical dorsal rami (mb), their articular branches (a), and the third occipital nerve (ton). Needles are positioned for injection of the C4 and C6 medial branches and the third occipital nerve. The articular pillar of C7 may be obscured by the shadow of the large C7 transverse process, in which case the C7 medial branch can be located midway between the lateral convexities of the C6 to C7 and C7 to T1 zygapophyseal joints. *Right,* Lateral view of cervical spine shows course of needle in facet joint cavity of the C5 to C6 facet joint using a posterior approach. *B,* Lateral cervical radiograph demonstrates precise needle placement into the zygapophyseal joint, producing a characteristic arthrogram. The joint was entered using a lateral approach to the cervical spine. (*A* from Bogduk N: Back pain: Zygapophyseal joint blocks and epidural steroids. *In* Cousins MJ, Bridenbaugh PO (eds): Neural Blockade in Clinical Anesthesia and Pain Management, ed 2. Philadelphia, JB Lippincott, 1988, p 939.)

either intra-articular injections or medial branch blocks are considered to have a facet disorder. These patients often benefit from a medial branch nerve rhizotomy procedure.[120, 174, 192]

All of the spinal injection procedures described in this section are best done with fluoroscopic guidance and contrast dye. The major advantage of performing these procedures in this manner is proper localization of the injection.[66] Close attention to needle placement allows for more accurate injections with smaller volumes of anesthetic, which leads to more exact identification of pain generators. In addition, the use of radiopaque dye can help prevent complications by avoiding injections into structures such as the subarachnoid space or vascular system.

These injection procedures can enhance rehabilitative efforts in two ways. Identification of the pain generator allows for a more specifically designed treatment protocol, and pain relief from the procedure gives a pain-free window of opportunity for more aggressive rehabilitation.

There are risks involved with performing these procedures, including side effects from the anesthesia, the steroids themselves, and the nonionizing contrast media. Coagulation studies should be obtained prior to epidural procedures in anyone suspected of having a bleeding diathesis. Significant complications could result if bleeding occurred in the presence of relative spinal stenosis (midsagittal diameter <12 mm) where there is little room to accommodate a space-occupying lesion without spinal cord compression. There is a potential risk of seizures, vertebral artery spasm, temporary quadriparesis from the anesthetic, and respiratory arrest. Proper monitoring and emergency equipment should be present for any complications that might arise so that permanent sequelae do not follow from a temporary complication.*

Rhizotomy

Percutaneous rhizotomy procedures can be accomplished by radiofrequency electrocoagulation (hyperthermia), cryoanalgesia (hypothermia), or chemical neurolysis. Radiofrequency rhizotomy completely destroys the nerve and provides a relatively large denervation area with longer-lasting pain relief as compared with the other techniques.[3, 24, 135, 192] The duration of the relief depends on the extent of nerve destruction. Cryoanalgesia procedures provide a shorter period of pain relief compared with radiofrequency rhizotomies because the destruction of the nerve is not complete and there is a smaller area of denervation.[34, 74, 159, 188] One advantage of cryoanalgesia is that there is no risk of neuroma formation, which can occur with the radiofrequency technique.[34, 74, 159, 188] Chemical denervation is typically performed by injecting a sterile phenol prepara-

*References 14, 20, 30, 31, 44, 45, 53, 56, 62, 79, 177, 211.

tion on the facet joint nerve. This method of denervation is not as specific as the other two methods because there is little control over injection flow patterns. There is also a risk of potential complications due to the phenol spreading to nearby structures in the neck during the injection.

Percutaneous rhizotomies are usually performed in the cervical spine to denervate symptomatic facet joints identified earlier by either intra-articular or medial branch nerve injection. The facet joint is denervated by destroying the medial branch nerves that supply the joint. The facet joint nerve is localized under fluoroscopy using anatomical landmarks when performing these procedures.[25] All of these procedures have a risk of nerve root injury.

Other rhizotomy applications for cervical pain using the radiofrequency electrocoagulation technique include cervical dorsal ganglionotomy, disc annular denervation, and sympathectomy.[120]

Surgery

Surgical intervention for cervical conditions is typically felt to be indicated when there is neurological bowel or bladder dysfunction, deteriorating neurological function, or intractable pain.[139] However, a survey of the literature by Rothman et al. failed to show any convincing evidence of efficacy for these surgical indications. The majority of cervical surgeries are performed because of intractable pain, which is a subjective finding determined only by the patient. Cervical disc surgery results are best in the presence of pain that has a radicular pattern.[89, 213, 217]

Spinal Cord Stimulation

In the United States implanted spinal cord stimulation (SCS) devices are typically used in failed back surgeries and intractable causes of RSD. SCS is used as a last resort in these conditions after other means of treatment have failed. Refractory RSD involving the upper limb(s) is the condition most often treated with SCS in the cervical spine region.[128, 161] A 50% reduction in pain in half of those treated with SCS 10 years after the procedure is the best long-term pain result that can be expected from this procedure.[128, 161] Potential complications include infection, hematoma, and paralysis (see Chapter 23 for further information on electrical stimulation).

COMMON CERVICAL SYNDROMES

Cervical Sprain and Strain

Epidemiology

Sprain and strain injuries to cervical spine structures are the most commonly encountered cervical disorders. A sprain is an overstretching or tearing of ligaments or tendons, or both, secondary to joint trauma. A strain is an injury to the muscles. Whiplash injuries are the most frequent cause of cervical sprain and strain with over 1 million cases in the United States every year.[75] The typical mechanism is a hyperextension injury to the cervical spine from a rear-end motor vehicle collision.[19, 136] This condition is more common in Western societies and metropolitan areas where there is a greater concentration of automobiles. The

incidence is higher in women and in those 30 to 50 years old.[197] Approximately one third of subjects will develop neck pain within 24 hours of the injury.[189] The natural history of whiplash injuries is that 60% get better within the first year, 32% get better in the next year, and 8% have permanent problems.[10, 160, 212] Litigation, psychological factors, and personality traits may or may not have an effect on treatment outcome.[7, 90, 140, 145, 172]

Pathophysiology

Whiplash is caused by a hyperextension injury to the cervical spine typically by a rear-end automobile collision. The impact leads to cervical extension followed by flexion from elevated G forces (Fig. 36–22), causing acceleration and deceleration injuries to ligaments, facet joints, and muscle.[12, 46, 63, 186, 190] Nerve root injuries can also occur with radicular features, presumably from a stretch injury or from focal hemorrhages.[46, 116] The C2 dorsal root ganglia are vulnerable to injury between the axis and atlas vertebral arches during hyperextension, which can lead to occipital neuralgia.[26, 110] In rare instances, there can be an injury to the descending portion of the fifth cranial nerve sensory nucleus resulting in facial sensory disturbances. Temporomandibular joint injuries can also occur with whiplash injuries.[178]

Diagnosis

The history usually includes both neck pain and headaches. Symptoms can also be referred to the upper limbs (Fig. 36–23). The patient typically complains of neck fatigue, stiffness, and pain associated with movement. Pain patterns should be evaluated carefully to differentiate sclerotomal from radicular features.[71, 111, 124] Other symptoms include dizziness, lightheadedness, difficulty with concentration and memory, unusual skin sensations over the face, blurred vision, difficulty in hearing, tinnitus, and other cranial nerve problems.*

---

*References 8, 27, 33, 61, 81, 101, 164, 169, 199, 200.

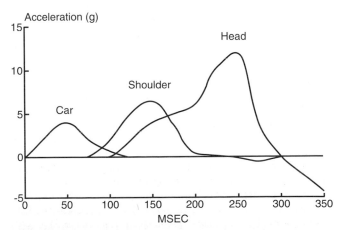

FIGURE 36–22 Idealized graph showing acceleration curves of the head, shoulders, and vehicle following a rear-end impact at 5 mph. Note that peak acceleration of the head is considerably greater than that of the car, followed by significant deceleration. (From Barnsley L, Lord S, Bogduk N: Pathophysiology of whiplash. Rev Spine 1993; 7:330.)

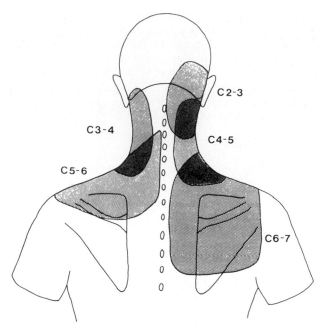

FIGURE 36–23 Pain referral from C2 to C3 through C6 to C7 facet joints. (From Dwyer A, Aprill C, Bogduk N: Cervical zygapophyseal joint pain patterns. I. A study in normal volunteers. Spine 1990; 15:456.)

The physical examination shows decreased neck ROM with poor quality of movement. Spurling's and Lhermitte's signs are typically negative. Patients frequently show tenderness to palpation in both the anterior and posterior structures of the neck. Facet joint tenderness on palpation is common with injuries to the facet joints, ligaments, or capsules.[115] The neurological examination is usually normal. Sensation abnormalities in most cases are sclerotomal rather than nondermatomal. Radicular signs are sometimes present early after injury, but usually resolve within the first 2 weeks.

Plain neck films can show loss of the normal cervical lordotic curvature. MRI and CT scans are typically normal but can reveal disc herniations, ligamentous injury, and hemorrhage.[60] Electrodiagnostic studies can help rule out radiculopathy in patients with continued pain and unusual referred limb sensations.

Treatment

Initial care involves the use of NSAIDs and analgesics to control pain. TCAs can also be used to help decrease pain and decrease sleep disturbances. There is usually no need for muscle relaxants when there is sufficient use of analgesics.

Physical therapy modalities can include mobilization, which can be effective acutely after the injury.[37, 76, 92, 100] Cervical instability in patients of all ages and vertebral insufficiency in the elderly need to be ruled out before performing mobilization. There is a risk of stroke with high-energy velocity movements.[40, 151] Massage is of great benefit in increasing circulation, decreasing pain, and facilitating the exercises that will be the mainstay of treatment. Ultrasound and electrical stimulation are also beneficial, as is postural re-education.[132] Orthotic devices should not be used continuously for more than 72 hours, since they can delay healing and lead to soft tissue tightening.[146, 149, 170]

Proper movement patterns need to be re-established within the cervical segments. Poor posture can lead to rounding of the shoulders, dorsal thoracic kyphosis, and forward head thrusting from the lower cervical spine.[38] Poor neck posture can cause microtrauma to the cervical facets, disc, ligaments and muscles.[38] This can result in bony hypertrophy, ligamentous laxity, breakdown of the disc, and facet articulations. Correct segmental movement depends on balancing the head, cervical spine, and thoracic spine. This provides optimal biomechanical balance within all three structures, and is achieved through increased cervical flexibility and proprioception. Flexibility is achieved with mobilization and self-stretching techniques. Proprioception is improved with instruction from the therapist or physician and visual feedback from a mirror. The stabilization exercises in Table 36–5 allow the muscles to self-correct the neck into proper position and posture, resulting in decreased pain and trauma to the joints.[121, 183, 198]

There is a high incidence of facet joint pain in patients with chronic neck pain and headaches.[5, 22] These patients can be identified with facet joint nerve blocks. Although intra-articular steroid injections have been shown not to provide significant relief,[13] rhizotomy of the facet joint nerves in properly identified patients can provide longer relief of symptoms.[3, 24, 135, 192] This provides an opportunity to aggressively rehabilitate these patients if they do not respond to more conservative measures.

Cervical Disc Disorders

Epidemiology

Internal disc disruption (IDD), herniated nucleus pulposus (HNP), and degenerative disc disease (DDD) are the three general types of cervical disc disorders encountered in clinical practice. The anatomical presence of these disorders in the asymptomatic population is common and degenerative disc changes are considered part of the natural aging spine process. Herniated discs are found by MRI in 10% of asymptomatic persons under 40 years old and in 5% in those older than 40 years.[17] MRI demonstrates degenerative discs in 25% of asymptomatic persons under 40 and in nearly 60% in those older than 40.[17] Younger persons tend to have herniated discs, while older persons tend to have degenerative disc changes.

Cervical radiculopathy is a relatively common consequence of an HNP (see Fig. 36–16C and D) or may be due to spurring associated with degenerative disc disease (see Fig. 36–14). A radiculopathy is any sensory, motor, or reflex abnormality secondary to nerve root injury. Although there are no data on the true incidence or prevalence of cervical radiculopathy, 51% of the adult population at some time experience neck and arm pain.[107] Job activities and smoking are other factors in addition to abnormal anatomy that predispose to the development of radiculopathy.[6, 16, 59]

Pathophysiology

Internal disc disruption is a term used to describe pathological changes of the internal structure of the disc.[55] IDD is characterized as an abnormality of the nucleus pulposus or annulus fibrosus without any external disc deformation. This disorder is believed to result from either nuclear degradation related to trauma, or isolated annular injury from a combination of cervical flexion and rotation movements.[28] Some have implicated cervical whiplash injuries as a cause of cervical IDD.[95] The outer annulus of the cervical disc is innervated and is a source of pain and pain referral.[22, 31, 216]

IDDs are generally classified into three categories based on the pathoanatomy.[17, 153] The protruding disc is described as nuclear material that penetrates asymmetrically through the annular fibers without escaping beyond the outside margin of the annulus. If nuclear material extends outside the periphery of the annulus it is called an extruded disc. A sequestered disc is an extruded disc in which a fragment of nuclear material has separated from the rest of the disc and lies in the spinal canal. Disc herniation typically occurs through a weakening of the posterolateral annulus from repetitive stress. Only rarely does herniation occur as a result of a single traumatic incident.

Cervical radiculopathy can be secondary to mechanical compression or to an intense inflammatory process.[184] In acute disc herniation, the pain is induced by chemical inflammation from proteoglycans of the nucleus pulposus as well as by any compression on the nerve root.[85, 88, 142, 147] Acute demyelination of the nerve can result from the herniation.[142]

Disc degeneration is a normal part of the aging process. Age-related cervical disc changes are indistinguishable from symptomatic degenerative discs. Degenerative disc changes on radiographic studies are simply a reflection of the natural aging process and are not necessarily indicative of a symptomatic process.

The disc begins to degenerate in the second decade of life. Circumferential tears begin in the annulus, particularly in the posterolateral aspects after recurrent strains. Several tears often consolidate to form radial tears, which eventually progress to radial fissures that extend to the nucleus. The disc then becomes completely disrupted, with tears passing through the disc. There is also loss of disc height with subsequent annular bulging at the periphery. Proteoglycans and water from nuclear degradation are lost through the fissures. Finally, the disc space becomes thin and is associated with vertebral sclerotic changes and osteophyte formation (see Fig. 36–13).

Diagnosis

Discogenic pain is typically vague and diffuse in an axial distribution. Pain referred from the disc to the arm is usually in a nondermatomal pattern. Symptoms can vary according to changes in intradiscal pressure. Activities such as lifting and Vasalva's manuever, which tend to increase disc pressure, can intensify symptoms, whereas lying supine can provide relief by decreasing intradiscal pressure. Vibration also has a tendency to exacerbate discogenic pain.

The discogenic patient on physical examination has decreased active ROM. The neurological examination is usually normal. Pain is worse with axial compression and less with distraction. Myofascial tender points or trigger points are commonly palpable.

Radicular pain is deep, dull, and achy, or sharp, burning, and electric in quality, depending on whether there is primarily motor or dorsal root involvement.[77, 78] The pain associated with radiculopathy generally follows a dermatomal or myotomal pattern in the shoulder, arm, and hand.[182, 184] The most common site of cervical radicular pain is the interscapular region, although pain can also radiate to the occiput, shoulder, or arm. Neck pain is not necessarily associated with radiculopathy and frequently can be absent. Patients with radiculopathy can have upper limb numbness or weakness in addition to pain.

The radicular patient typically displays decreased active cervical range of motion. Pain is usually worse with extension and rotation, and improved with neck flexion. There can be decreased sensation to pain, light touch, or vibration. Upper limb weakness can be present when there is significant motor root compromise, but must be differentiated from pain-related weakness. The presence of increased lower extremity reflexes or other upper motor neuron signs suggests the possibility of a myelopathy and needs an aggressive workup.

Plain films help evaluate the disc space and vertebral body height, and can reveal degenerative osseous and disc changes. Electrodiagnostic studies are helpful to evaluate for radiculopathy, or peripheral or focal neuropathy. MRI can provide an in-depth anatomical evaluation of the intervertebral discs. Clinical correlation must always be used to interpret the results of diagnostic testing and in particular anatomical studies such as imaging techniques.

Treatment

Conservative treatment is generally the same for discogenic pain with or without radiculopathy. Initially the patient is placed on NSAIDs for pain control. An oral steroid taper provides a powerful anti-inflammatory effect and can be used in treating a radiculopathy that does not initially respond to NSAIDs. Steroids should not be given concomitantly with NSAIDs or aspirin products in order to avoid gastric and other potential side effects. Most patients with DDD are elderly and NSAIDs are prescribed with caution as are any medications in this population. Muscle relaxants can be used as adjuncts to analgesics. Narcotics are used sparingly and for short periods of time.

Physical modalities are initially used for acute pain control and later used on an as-needed basis only. Cervical traction is beneficial in discogenic pain and also with radicular symptoms. Cervical spine ROM exercise is actively and passively performed to help restore normal function. As the acute episode subsides, the patient is advanced from a passive program to an active stretching and flexibility routine for the cervical spine. Strengthening and stabilization are the next part of the rehabilitation process. The patient should go through a neck school program and be independent in a home program at the time of discharge from rehabilitation. Prevention of recurrent episodes through education is very important.

Those patients who progress slowly sometimes require the use of selective spinal injection procedures. Cervical epidural and selective nerve root blocks in radiculopathy patients provide diagnostic and therapeutic benefits. An epidural block can provide enough relief to allow for an aggressive rehabilitation program. Patients with discogenic pain alone typically do not respond well to epidural procedures. In DDD patients without radicular symptoms, there can be a significant amount of segmental facet pain resulting from poor articulation mechanics due to the DDD. These patients can benefit from facet rhizotomy after an appropriate response to facet injections.

Those patients who fail with conservative treatment (including the use of spinal injection procedures) might benefit from surgery. Patients with neck pain alone and no radicular features typically do not benefit from surgery unless there is instability or myelopathic consequences. The best results of cervical disc surgery are in those patients with clear-cut radicular pain.[89, 213, 217]

Cervical Spondylosis (Osteoarthritis)

Epidemiology

Some use the terms *spondylosis* and *osteoarthritis* interchangeably whereas others define them separately. Spondylosis is described as the degenerative changes which occur to the intervertebral discs and vertebral bodies. Osteoarthritis (OA) is depicted to occur exclusively in the zygapophyseal and uncovertebral joints (which more closely resembles OA in other joints). For purposes of this chapter both terms are considered to be synonymous with a degenerative cervical spine. Factors which contribute to degenerative changes of the spine include aging, trauma, work activities, and genetics.

Degenerative changes to the cervical spine are very common with advancing age. In asymptomatic persons under the age of 40, 25% have DDD and 4% have foraminal stenosis by MRI.[17] In those over 40, almost 60% have DDD and 20% have foraminal stenosis by MRI.[17] Seventy percent of asymptomatic persons over 70 years of age have degenerative cervical spine changes in one form or another.[118, 130] Spondylitic changes can result in spinal canal, lateral recess, and foraminal stenosis. The first can result in myelopathy whereas the last two can present with radiculopathy.

Pathophysiology

Intervertebral discs lose hydration and elasticity with age, leading to cracks and fissures. The disc subsequently collapses owing to biomechanical incompetence, causing the annulus to bulge outward. The surrounding ligaments also lose their elastic properties and develop traction spurs. Uncovertebral spurring occurs as a result of the degenerative process in which the facet joints lose cartilage, become sclerotic, and develop osteophytes (see Fig. 36–14).

Acquired cervical stenosis more commonly results from degenerative changes such as spur formation, disc protrusion, ligamentum hypertrophy, or facet joint hypertrophy (Fig. 36–24). Disorders such as Paget's disease and gout can also result in cervical stenosis. Neurological sequelae from central canal stenosis typically develop when the diameter becomes less than 12 mm in the midsagittal plane.[32, 166] Spinal stenosis with myelopathic symptoms can include neurogenic bowel and bladder dysfunction, gait disturbances, impotence, and altered sexual function. Leg weakness or spasticity can also occur. Weakness and numbness can have a specific level that coincides with the location of the most severe stenosis.[143, 179] Radiculopathy can develop from degenerative changes to the joints of Luschka and facet joints, leading to lateral or foraminal stenosis.

Congenital and developmental stenosis are two other types of cervical spinal canal stenosis. Congenital stenosis is commonly due to short pedicles which cause the cervical canal to be smaller in size than normal. The average midsagittal AP diameter is 10 mm for the spinal cord and 17 mm for the spinal canal.[32, 166]

Relative stenosis is considered to be present when the diameter is less than 12 mm and absolute stenosis, when less than 10 mm.[32, 143, 166, 179] Although cervical spinal stenosis usually comes on insidiously, it can develop acutely in the presence of congenital or developmental stenosis which allows little compromise for space-occupying lesions such as an acute large central disc herniation.

Diagnosis

Cervical spondylosis can cause radicular pain due to nerve root impingement, but it can also cause cervical

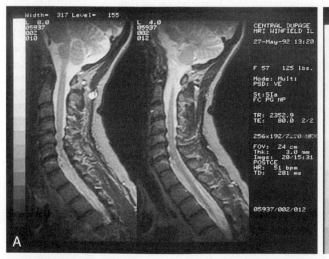
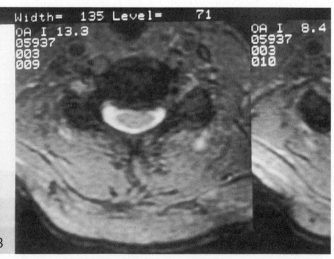

FIGURE 36–24   Cervical stenosis. Cervical MRI sagittal *(A)* and axial *(B)* views demonstrating degenerative spinal stenosis.

zygapophyseal joint pain.[171] Patients having only facet joint pain typically have pain confined to the neck and shoulder. The pain is worse with different positions and can interfere with sleep. Patients do not complain of numbness or weakness in the upper limbs. Those patients with myelopathic symptoms such as neurogenic bowel and bladder dysfunction need aggressive investigation.[15]

Physical examination typically shows decreased ROM of the cervical spine, especially with neck extension. The neurological examination concentrates on detecting long tract signs consistent with myelopathy, as well as signs of radiculopathy. Positive findings for myelopathy include hyperreflexia, Babinski's sign, and weakness at and below the involved levels. Positive signs for radiculopathy are decreased sensation, diminished reflexes, and weakness in a segmental distribution. Spurling's and Lhermitte's signs can both be present in either case.

Diagnostic testing includes cervical spine films to evaluate the uncovertebral joints, facet joints, foramen, and intervertebral disc spaces. MRI permits evaluation of the spinal canal and foramen in relation to the spinal cord, thecal sac, and nerve roots. SEP responses are delayed or of low amplitude in the presence of myelopathy. SEPs can be performed serially to evaluate the ongoing status of myelopathies. In cases of radicular symptoms, needle EMG can confirm motor nerve root involvement. CT scans and myelography are usually the imaging tests of choice to document spinal and foraminal stenosis. MRI alone is not as sensitive and can give false-positive and false-negative results.[17, 152, 179, 181]

Treatment

The treatment for cervical spondylosis pain that occurs with or without radicular features begins with NSAIDs. Analgesics can also be used in a scheduled manner and only for 6 weeks or less. TCAs can be used for pain relief and sleep dysfunction.

Physical therapy modalities in this situation can include a trial of careful traction. Orthoses are typically not worthwhile. Ultrasound, electrical stimulation, and massage can all be very helpful.[72] Mobilization such as muscle energy techniques can be of benefit.[40] Extreme mobilization can cause myelopathy and needs to be monitored closely. The exercise program is the same as for cervical radiculopathy, including flexibility, strengthening, stabilization, and aerobic conditioning.

A cervical zygapophyseal intra-articular steroid injection can be helpful in the presence of an active synovitis. The facet injections can be both diagnostic as well as therapeutic.[19, 20, 23, 27, 65, 70, 82, 99, 155] Mechanical facet pain is better evaluated with facet joint nerve blocks. Long-term relief can often be accomplished with a rhizotomy procedure. Cervical epidural block might be of benefit in cervical spondylosis, especially if there is an inflammatory component. Epidural and selective nerve root blocks can be diagnostically and therapeutically helpful in cases of radiculopathy.

Surgical referral is needed immediately when the clinical evaluation and neurodiagnostic tests are positive for myelopathy.[162] Conservative treatment is generally used when there are no myelopathic findings on clinical evaluation, even if anatomical tests show cervical stenosis.

Myofascial Pain Syndrome

Myofascial pain syndrome is discussed in detail elsewhere in this text (see Chapter 42) but deserves mention here. Myofascial pain syndrome often mimics cervical radiculopathy and cervical facet syndrome.[154] A thorough understanding of particular muscles and their referral zones is important, especially when the tests do not demonstrate clear-cut localization of the problem.[222] Myofascial pain or fibromyalgia should be investigated further as a possible cause when imaging studies are normal in a person with neck pain and referred pain into the shoulders and upper limbs.[2, 86, 123, 176]

CONCLUSION

The cervical spine is a complicated structure that can develop pathologic changes leading to pain and impairment. Success in treating cervical conditions depends upon making the correct diagnosis, providing appropriate treatment, and practicing prevention. Clinicians must establish a diagnosis, identify the pain generator, and prescribe appropriate treatment. Once the pain has decreased or resolved, treatment progresses to flexibility, strengthening, and endurance exercises. Prevention of future pain episodes is emphasized during the recovery process through proper body mechanics, posture, and exercise. Ergonomic modifications at work and at home are also important to prevent further injury.

References

1. Adams F: Paulus Aeginata, vol 2. London, Sydenham Society, 1816, pp 155–156, 193, 197.
2. The American College of Rheumatology 1990 criteria for the classification of fibromyalgia: Report of the multicenter criteria committee. Arthritis Rheum 1990;33:160–172.
3. Anderson KH, Mosdal C, Vaernet K: Percutaneous radiofrequency facet denervation in low-back and extremity pain. Acta Neurochir 1987;87:48–51.
4. Aprill CN: Diagnostic disc injection. In Frymoyer JW (ed): The Adult Spine. Principles and Practice. New York, Raven Press, 1991, pp 403–442.
5. Aprill C, Bogduk N: The prevalence of cervical zygapophyseal joint pain. A first approximation. Spine 1992;17:744–747.
6. Astrand NE: Medical, psychological, and social factors associated with back abnormalities and self reported back pain. Br J Ind Med 1987;44:327–336.
7. Awerbuch MS: Whiplash in Australia: Illness or injury? Med J Aust 1992;157:193–196.
8. Balla JI: The late whiplash syndrome. Aust N Z J Surg 1980;50:610–614.
9. Balla JI, Moraitis S: Knights in armour: A follow up study of injuries after legal settlement. Med J Aust 1970;335–361.
10. Bannister G, Gargan M: Prognosis of whiplash injuries. State Art Rev Spine 1993;7:557–570.
11. Barnsley L, Lord S, Bogduk N: Comparative local anaesthetic blocks in the diagnosis of cervical zygapophysial joint pain. Pain 1993;55:99–106.
12. Barnsley L, Lord S, Bogduk N: Pathophysiology of whiplash. State Art Rev Spine 1993;7:330.
13. Barnsley L, Lord SM, Wallis BJ: Lack of effect of intraarticular corticosteroids for chronic pain in the cervical zygapophyseal joints. N Engl J Med 1994;330:1047–1050.

14. Benzon HT: Epidural steroids for lumbosacral radiculopathy. Adv Pain Res Ther 1990;13:231.

15. Bernhardt M, Hynes R, Blune H, et al: Cervical spondylitic myelopathy. J Bone Joint Surg Am 1993;75:119–128.

16. Bigos SJ, Spengler DM, Martin NA, et al: Back injuries in industry: A retrospective study. III. Employee-related factors. Spine 1986;11:252–256.

17. Boden SD, McCowin PR, Davis DO, et al: Abnormal magnetic-resonance scans of the cervical spine in asymptomatic subjects. J Bone Joint Surg Am 1990;72:1178–1184.

18. Bogduk N: The anatomy of the occipital neuralgia. Clin Exp Neurol 1980;17:167–184.

19. Bogduk N: The anatomy and pathophysiology of whiplash. Clin Biomech 1986;1:92–101.

20. Bogduk N: Back pain: Zygapophysial joint blocks and epidural steroids. In Cousins MJ, Bridenbaugh PO (eds): Neural Blockade in Clinical Anesthesia and Pain Management, ed 2. Philadelphia, JB Lippincott, 1988, pp 935–954.

21. Bogduk N: The clinical anatomy of the cervical dorsal rami. Spine 1982;7:319–330.

22. Bogduk N, Aprill C: On the nature of neck pain, discography and cervical zygapophysial joint blocks. Pain 1993;54:213–217.

23. Bogduk N, Aprill C, Dwyer A: Cervical zygapophysial joint pain patterns II: A clinical evaluation. Spine 1990;15:458–461.

24. Bogduk N, Long DM: Percutaneous lumbar medial branch neurotomy. A modification of facet denervation. Spine 1980;5:193–201.

25. Bogduk N, Macintosh J, Marsland A: Technical limitations to the efficacy of radiofrequency neurotomy for spinal pain. Neurosurgery 1987;20:529–535.

26. Bogduk N, Marsland A: On the concept of third occipital headache. J Neurol Neurosurg Psychiatry 1986;49:775–780.

27. Bogduk N, Marsland A: The cervical zygapophysial joints as a source of neck pain. Spine 1988;13:610–617.

28. Bogduk N, Twomey LT: Clinical Anatomy of the Lumbar Spine, ed 2. New York, Churchill Livingstone, 1991.

29. Bogduk N, Valencia F: Innervation and pain patterns of the thoracic spine. In Grant R (ed): Physical Therapy of the Neck and Thoracic Spine. New York, Churchill Livingstone, 1988, pp 27–37.

30. Bogduk N, Wilson AS, Tynan W: The human lumbar dorsal rami. J Anat 1982;134:383–397.

31. Bogduk N, Windsor M, Inglis A: The innervation of the cervical intervertebral discs. Spine 1988;13:2–8.

32. Bohlman HH, Emery SE: The pathophysiology of cervical spondylosis and myelopathy. Spine 1988;13:844.

33. Braff MM, Rosner S: Symptomatology and treatment of injuries of the neck. N Y J Med 1955;55:237.

34. Brechner T: Percutaneous cryogenic neurolysis of the articular nerve of Luschka. Reg Anesth 1981;6:18–22.

35. Breck LW, Van Norman RW: Medicolegal aspects of cervical spine strains. Clin Orthop 1982; 74:124–128.

36. Brown DL: Atlas of Regional Anesthesia. Philadelphia, WB Saunders, 1992, pp 129–132.

37. Brunarski DJ: Clinical trials of spinal manipulation. J Manip Physiol Ther 1984;7:4.

38. Cailliet R: Neck and Arm Pain, ed 3. Philadelphia, FA Davis, 1991.

39. Cailliet R: Soft Tissue Pain and Disability, ed 2. Philadelphia, FA Davis, 1988.

40. Cantu R, Grodin A: Soft tissue mobilization. In Basmajian JV, Nyberg R (eds): Rational Manual Therapies. Baltimore, Williams & Wilkins, 1993, pp 199–221.

41. Carette S, McCain GA, Bell DA, et al: Evaluation of amitriptyline in primary fibrositis. A double blind, placebo control study. Arthritis Rheum 1986;29:655–659.

42. Catchlove RF, Braha R: The use of cervical epidural nerve blocks in the management of chronic head and neck pain. Can Anaesth Soc J 1984;31:188–191.

43. Cave AJE: The innervation and morphology of the cervical intertransverse muscles. J Anat 1927;71:497–515.

44. Cicala RS, Thoni K, Angel JJ: Long-term results of cervical epidural steroid injections. Clin J Pain 1989;5:10–15.

45. Cicala RS, Westbrook LL, Angel JJ: Side effects and complications of cervical epidural steroid injections. J Pain Symptom Manage 1989;4:64–66.

46. Clemens HJ, Burow K: Experimental investigation on injury mechanisms of cervical spine and frontal and rear-frontal vehicle impacts.

In Proceedings of the 16th STAPP Car Crash Conference. Warrendale, Pa, Society of Automotive Engineers, 1972, pp 76–104.

47. Cloward RB: Cervical discography: A contribution to the etiology and mechanism of neck, shoulder, and arm pain. Ann Surg 1959;150:1052.

48. Colachis S, Strohm B: Cervical traction: Relationship of traction time to varied tractive force with constant angle of pull. Arch Phys Med Rehabil 1965; 46:815.

49. Colachis SC, Strohm BR: Effect of duration of intermittent cervical traction on vertebral separation. Arch Phys Med Rehabil 1966;47:353–359.

50. Colachis SC, Strohm BR: Effect of intermittent traction on separation of lumbar vertebrae. Arch Phys Med Rehabil 1969;50:251.

51. Colachis S, Strohm B: A study of tractive forces and angle of pull on vertebral interspaces in the cervical spine. Arch Phys Med Rehabil 1965;46:820.

52. Connor PM, Darden BV: Cervical discography complications and clinical efficacy. Spine 1993;18:2035–2038.

53. Cousins MJ: Epidural neuronal blockade. In Cousins MJ, Bridenbaugh PO (eds): Neuronal Blockade in Clinical Anesthesia and Pain Management. Philadelphia, JB Lippincott, 1980, pp 183–185.

54. Crafts RC: Textbook of Human Anatomy, ed 2. New York, John Wiley & Sons, 1979.

55. Crock HV: A reappraisal of intervertebral disc lesions. Med J Aust 1970;1:983–989.

56. Cronen M, Waldman S: Cervical steroid epidural nerve blocks in the palliation of pain secondary to intractable tension-type headaches. J Pain Symptom Manage, 1990;5:379–381.

57. Crowe H: Injuries to the cervical spine. Presented at the Annual Meeting of the Western Orthopedic Association, San Francisco, 1928.

58. Czervionke L, Daniels D, Ho P, et al: Cervical neural foramina: Correlative anatomic and MR imaging study. Radiology 1988;169:753–759.

59. Damkot DK, Pope MH, Lord J, et al: The relationship between work history, work environment and low-back pain in men. Spine 1984;9:395–399.

60. Davis SJ, Teresi LM, Bradley WG, et al: Cervical spine hyperextension injuries: MR findings. Radiology 1991;180:245–251.

61. Deans GT, Magalliard JN, Kerr M: Neck sprain—A major cause of disability following car accidents. Injury 1987;18:10–12.

62. Delaney TJ, Rowlingson JC, Carron H, et al: Epidural steroid effects on nerves and meninges. Anesth Analg 1980;58:610.

63. Deng YC: Anthropomorphic dummy neck modeling and injury considerations. Accid Anal Prev 1989;21:85–100.

64. De Vries HA, Adams GM: Electromyographic comparisons of single doses of exercises and meprobamate as to effects on muscular relaxation. Am J Phys Med 1972;51:130–141.

65. Dory M: Arthrography of the cervical facet joints. Radiology 1983;148:379–382.

66. Dussault RG, Nicolet VM: Cervical facet joint arthrography. J Can Assoc Radiol 1985;36:79–80.

67. Dvorak J, Panjabi M, Gerber D, et al: Functional diagnostics of the rotary instability of the upper cervical spine: An experimental study in cadavers. Spine 1987;12:197.

68. Dvorak J, Panjabi MM, Grob D, et al: Validation of flexion extension radiographs of cervical spine. Spine 1993;18:120–127.

69. Dvorak J, Panjabi M, Novotny J, et al: In vivo flexion/extension of the normal cervical spine. J Orthop Res 1991;9:828–834.

70. Dwyer A, Aprill C, Bogduk N: Cervical zygapophyseal joint pain patterns I: A study in normal volunteers. Spine 1990;15:453–457.

71. Eisenstein SM, Parry CR: The lumbar facet arthrosis syndrome. J Bone Joint Surg Br 1987;69:3–7.

72. Eldred E, Lindsky D, Buchwald J: The effect of cooling on mammalian muscle spindles. Exp Neurol 1960;2:144–157.

73. Ellis H: Clinical Anatomy: A Revision and Applied Anatomy for Clinical Students, ed 6. London, Blackwell, 1976, p 205.

74. Evans PJD: Cryoanalgesia. The application of low temperatures to nerves to produce anaesthesia or analgesia. Anaesthesia 1981; 36:1003–1013.

75. Evans RW: Some observations on whiplash injuries. Neurol Clin 1992;10:975–997.

76. Farrell JB, Twomey LT: Acute low back pain. Comparison of two conservative treatment approaches. In Proceedings of Manipulative Therapists Association of Australia, Perth, Western Australia, 1983, p 162.

77. Feinstein B: Referred pain from paravertebral structures. *In* Buerger AA, Tobis JS (eds): Approaches to the Validation of Manipulative Therapy. Springfield, Ill, Charles C Thomas, 1977, pp 139–174.

78. Feinstein B, Langton JNK, Jameson RM, et al: Experiments on pain referred from deep somatic tissues. J Bone Joint Surg Am 1954;36:981–997.

79. Ferrante FM, Wilson SP, Jacobs C, et al: Outcome predictions after cervical epidural steroid injection. Spine 1993;18:1736–1745.

80. Fielding JW: Cineroentgenography of the normal cervical spine. J Bone Joint Surg Am 1957;39:1280–1288.

81. Fisher CM: Whiplash amnesia. Neurology 1982;32:667–668.

82. Fletcher G, Haughton V, Ho K, et al: Age-related changes in the cervical facet joints: Studies with cryomicrotomy, MR and CT. AJNR 1990;11:27–30.

83. Fornage BD, Touche DH, Segal P, et al: Ultrasonography in the evaluation of muscular trauma. J Ultrasound Med 1983;2:549–554.

84. Frankel VH: Temporomandibular joint pain syndrome following deceleration injury to the cervical spine. Bull Hosp Joint Dis 1969;26:47.

85. Franson R, Saal J: Human disc phospholipase A2 in inflammatory disease. Spine 1992;17(suppl 6):S129–S132.

86. Garvey TA, Marks MR, Wiesel SW: A prospective double-blind evaluation of trigger-point injection therapy for low-back pain. Spine 1989;14:962–964.

87. Ganong WF: Review of Medical Physiology, ed 13. Norwalk, Conn, Appleton & Lange, 1987.

88. Garfin SR, Rydevik BL, Brown RA: Compressive neuropathy of spinal nerve roots. A mechanical or biological problem? Spine 1991;16:162–165.

89. Gore D, Sepic S: Anterior cervical fusion for degenerated or protruded discs. Spine 1984;9:667.

90. Gotten N: Survey of one hundred cases of whiplash injury after settlement of litigation. JAMA 1956;162:865–867.

91. Gracovetsky S, Farfan H: The optimum spine. Spine 1986;10:543–573.

92. Hadler NM, Curtis P, Gillings DB, et al: A benefit of spinal manipulation as adjunctive therapy for acute low-back pain: A stratified controlled trial. Spine 1987;12:7.

93. Haldeman CW: Guideline factors for evaluation of neck and back injuries. Spine 1993;18:1736–1745.

94. Hamada G, Rida A: Orthopaedics and orthopaedic diseases in ancient and modern Egypt (letter). Clin Orthop 1972;89:253.

95. Hamer J, Gargan MF, Bannister GC: Whiplash injury and surgically treated cervical disc disease. Injury 1993;24:549–550.

96. Hanley EN, Shapiro DE: The development of low-back pain after excision of a lumbar disc. J Bone Joint Surg Am 1989;71:719–721.

97. Hayashi K, Yabuki T: Origin of the uncus and of Luschka's joint in the cervical spine. J Bone Joint Surg Am 1985;67:788–791.

98. Heller B: Correspondence to Francis Lagattuta, MD, regarding literature search on oral corticosteroids, April 13, 1993.

99. Hildebrandt J, Argyrakis A: Percutaneous nerve block of the cervical facets—a relatively new method in the treatment of chronic headache and neck pain. Pathological anatomical studies and clinical practice. Manual Med 1986;2:45–52.

100. Hoehler FK, Tobis JS, Buerger AA: Spinal manipulation for low back pain. JAMA 1981;245:1835

101. Hohl M: Soft tissue injuries of the neck in automobile accidents: Factors influencing prognosis. J Bone Joint Surg Am 1974;56:1675–1681.

102. Hollinshead WH, Jenkins DB: Functional Anatomy of the Limbs and Back, ed 5. Philadelphia, WB Saunders, 1981, p 218.

103. Hopwood MB, Abram S: Factors associated with failure of lumbar epidural steroids. Reg Anesth 1993;18:238–243.

104. Hove B, Gyldensted C: Cervical analgesic facet joint arthrography. Neuroradiology 1990;32:456–459.

105. Howorth B, Petrie G: Injuries to the Spine. Baltimore, Williams & Wilkins, 1964.

106. Hult L: Cervical, dorsal, and lumbar spinal syndromes. Acta Orthop Scand Suppl 1954;17:1.

107. Hult L: Frequency of symptoms for different age groups and professions. *In* Hirsch C, Zotterman Y (eds): Cervical Pain. New York, Pergamon Press, 1971, pp 17–20.

108. Hult L: The Munkford investigation. Acta Orthop Scand Suppl 1954;16:1.

109. Huskisson EC: Visual analogue scales. *In* Melzack R (ed): Pain Measurement and Assessment. New York, Raven Press, 1983, pp 33–40.

110. Hunter CR, Mayfield FH: Role of the upper cervical root in the production of pain in the head. Am J Surg 1949;78:743–749.

111. Inman VH, Saunders JB de CM: Referred pain from skeletal structures. J Nerv Ment Dis 1944;99:660–667.

112. Johnson EW: Carpal tunnel syndrome. *In* Johnson EW (ed): Practical Electromyography, ed 2. Baltimore, Williams & Wilkins, 1988, pp 187–205.

113. Johnson EW: Practical Electromyography, ed 2. Baltimore, Williams & Wilkins, 1988.

114. Johnson EW, Wolfe CV: Bifocal spectacles in the etiology of cervical radiculopathy. Arch Phys Med Rehabil 1972;53:201–205.

115. Jull G, Bogduk N, Marsland A: The accuracy of manual diagnosis for cervical zygapophysial joint pain syndromes. Med J Aust 1988;148: 233–236.

116. Kallieris D, Mattern R, Schmidt G, et al: Kinematic and spinal columnar injuries in active and passive passenger protection: Results of simulated frontal collisions. *In* Proceedings of the 1984 International Conference on Biomechanics of Impact. Bron, France, IRCOBI, 1984, pp 279–295.

117. Kaplan PA, Anderson JC, Norris MA, et al: Ultrasound of post traumtic soft tissue lesions. Radiol Clin North Am 1989;27:973–982.

118. Kellegren JH, Lawrence JS: Osteoarthritis and disk degeneration in an urban population. Ann Rheum Dis 1958;17:388–397.

119. Kelsey JL, Githens PB, O'Conner T, et al: Acute prolapsed lumbar intervertebral disc. An epidemiologic study with special reference to driving automobiles and cigarette smoking. Spine 1984;9:608–613.

120. Kline MT: Stereotactic Radiofrequency Lesions as Part of the Management of Pain. Orlando, Fla, Paul M Deutsch, 1992.

121. Knott M, Voss D: Proprioceptive Neuromuscular Facilitation: Patterns and Techniques. New York, McGraw-Hill, 1956.

122. Kottke FJ, Mundale MO: Range of mobility of the cervical spine. Arch Phys Med Rehabil 1959;40:379.

123. Kraft GH, Johnson EW, LaBan MM: The fibrositis syndrome. Arch Phys Med Rehabil 1968;49:155–162.

124. Kurz LT: The differential diagnosis of cervical radiculopathy. *In* Herkowitz HN (ed): Seminars in Spinal Surgery. Philadelphia, WB Saunders, 1989, pp 194–199.

125. Kvist M, Jarvenen M: Clinical, histochemical and biochemical features in repair of muscle and tendon injuries. Int J Sports Med 1982;3:12–14.

126. LaBan M: "Whiplash": Its evaluation and treatment. *In* Saal JA (ed): Neck and Back Pain. Phys Med Rehabil 1990;4:293–308.

127. LaBan MM: Electrodiagnosis in cervical radicular and myelopathic syndromes. *In* Herkowitz HN (ed): Seminars in Spinal Surgery. Philadelphia, WB Saunders, 1989, pp 222–228.

128. Law JD, Kirkpatrick AF: Update: Spinal cord stimulation. AJPM 1992;2:34–42.

129. Lawrence JS: Disc degeneration. Its frequency and relationship to symptoms. Ann Rheum Dis 1969;28:121.

130. Lawrence JS, Brenner JM, Bier F: Osteoarthrosis: Prevalence in the population and relationship between symptoms and x-ray changes. Ann Rheum Dis 1966;25:1–24.

131. Lazorthes G, Gaubert J: L'innervation des articulations interapophysiares vertébrales. C R Assoc Anat 1956;43:488–494.

132. Lehmann J, deLateur BJ: Diathermy and superficial heat and cold therapy. *In* Kottke EJ, Stillwell GK, Lehmann JF (eds): Krusen's Handbook of Physical Medicine and Rehabilitation. Philadelphia, WB Saunders, 1982, pp 275–350.

133. Lind B, Schlbom H, Nordwall A, et al: Normal range of motion in cervical spine. Arch Phys Med Rehabil 1989;70:692–695.

134. Lipman JC, Wang AM, Brooks ML, et al: Seizure after intrathecal administration of lopamidol. AJNR 1988;9:787–788.

135. Lora J, Long D: So-called facet denervation in the management of intractable back pain. Spine 1976;1:121–126.

136. Macnab I: Acceleration injuries of the cervical spine. J Bone Joint Surg Am 1964;46:1797–1799.

137. Macnab I, McCulloch J: Neck Ache and Shoulder Pain. Baltimore, Williams & Wilkins, 1994.

138. Magee DJ: Orthopedic Physical Assessment, ed 2. Philadelphia, WB Saunders, 1992, pp 34–70.

139. Maigne J, Deligne L: Computed tomographic follow-up study of cases of nonoperatively treated cervical intervertebral soft disc herniation. Spine 1994;19:189–191.

140. Maimaris C, Barnes MR, Allen MJ: "Whiplash injuries" of the neck: A retrospective study. Injury 1988;19:393–396.

141. Makela M, Heliovaara M, Sievers D, et al: Prevalence, determinants, and consequences of chronic neck pain in Finland. Am J Epidemiol 1991;134:1356–1367.

142. Marshall L, Trethewie E, Curtain C: Chemical irritation of nerve root in disc prolapse. Lancet 1973;320:7824.

143. Matsunaga S, Sakov T, Imamura T, Morimoto S: Dissociated motor loss in the upper extremities. Spine 1993;18:1964–1967.

144. Max MB, Lynch SA, Muir J, et al: Effects of desipramine, amitriptyline and fluoxetine on pain in diabetic neuropathy. N Engl J Med 1992;326:1250–1256.

145. Mayou R, Bryant B, Duthie R: Psychiatric consequences of road traffic accidents. BMJ 1993;307:1047–1050.

146. Mealy K, Brennan H, Fenelon GC: Early mobilization of acute whiplash injury. BMJ 1986;292:1656–1657.

147. McCarron RF, Wimpee MW, Hudkins PG: The inflammatory effect of nucleus pulposus. A possible element in the pathogenesis of low-back pain. Spine 1987;12:760–764.

148. McFadden JF: Smoking cigarettes and lumbar disc pain. A preliminary report on 400 patients. J Neurol Orthop Med Surg 1985;6:125–128.

149. McKinney LA: Early mobilization of acute sprain of the neck. BMJ 1989;299:1006–1008.

150. Miles A, Maimaris C, Finlay D, et al: The incidence and prognostic significance of radiological abnormalities in soft tissue injuries to the cervical spine. Skeletal Radiol 1988;17:493–496.

151. Miller R, Burton R: Stroke following chiropractic manipulation of the spine. JAMA 1974;229:189.

152. Modic MT, Masaryk TJ, Mulopulos GP, et al: Cervical radiculopathy: Prospective evaluation with surface coil MR imaging: CT with metrizamide and metrizamide myelography. Radiology 1986;161:753–759.

153. Modic MT, Masaryk TJ, Ross JS: Magnetic Resonance Imaging of the Spine. St Louis, Mosby–Year Book, 1990, pp 83–90.

154. Moldofsky H, Scarisbrick P, England R, et al: Musculoskeletal symptoms and non-REM sleep disturbance in patients with "fibrositis syndrome" and healthy subjects. Psychosom Med 1975;37:341–351.

155. Mooney V: Injection studies: Role in pain definition. In Frymoyer JW (ed): The Adult Spine: Principles and Practice. New York, Raven Press, 1991, pp 527–529.

156. Mooney V, Cairns D, Robertson J: A system for evaluation and treatment of chronic back disability. West J Med 1976;124:370–376.

157. Moritz U: Evaluation of manipulation and other manual therapy. Criteria for measuring the effect of treatment. Scand J Rehabil Med 1979;11:173.

158. Muroff LR: Optimizing the performance and interpretation of bone scans. Clin Nucl Med 1981;6:68–76.

159. Myers BR, Powell HC, Heckman HM, et al: Biophysical and pathological effects of cryogenic nerve lesion. Ann Neurol 1981;10:478–485.

160. Norris SH, Watt I: The prognosis of neck injuries resulting from rear-end vehicle collisions. J Bone Joint Surg Br 1983;65:608–611.

161. North RB, Kidd DH, Zahurak M, et al: Spinal cord stimulation for chronic, intractable pain: Experience over two decades. Neurosurgery 1993;32:384–395.

162. Okada Y, Ikata T, Yamada H, et al: Magnetic resonance imaging study on the results of surgery for cervical compression myelopathy. Spine 1993;18:2024–2029.

163. Orofino C, Sherman MS, Schechter D: Luschka's joint—a degenerative phenomenon. J Bone Joint Surg Am 1964;42:853–858.

164. Pand LQ: The otological aspects of whiplash injuries. Laryngoscope 1971;81:1381–1387.

165. Parke WW: Applied anatomy of the spine. In Rothman RH, Simone FA (eds): The Spine, ed 3. Philadelphia, WB Saunders, 1992, p 49.

166. Parke WW: Correlative anatomy of cervical spondylotic myelopathy. Spine 1988;13:831.

167. Pavlov H, Torg JS: Roentgen examination of cervical spine injuries in the athlete. Clin Sports Med 1987;6:761.

168. Payne EE, Spillane JD: The cervical spine. An anatomico-pathological study of 70 specimens (using a special technique) with particular reference to the problem of cervical spondylosis. Brain 1957;80:571–596.

169. Pennie B, Agambar L: Patterns of injury and recovery in whiplash. Injury 1991;22:57–59.

170. Pennie BH, Agambar LJ: Whiplash injuries. Trial of early management. J Bone Joint Surg Br 1990;72:277–279.

171. Penning L: Differences in anatomy, motion development and aging in the upper and lower cervical disk segments. Clin Biomech 1991;3:37–47.

172. Radanov BP, Stefano G, Schnidrig A, et al: Role of psychosocial stress in recovery from common whiplash. Lancet 1991;338:712–715.

173. Ransford AO, Cairns D, Mooney V: The pain drawing as an aid to the psychologic evaluation of patients with low-back pain. Spine 1976;1:127–134.

174. Rashbaum RF: Radiofrequency facet denervation. A treatment alternative in refractory low back pain with or without leg pain. Orthop Clin North Am 1983;14:569–575.

175. Roeske R: The new vertebral subluxation. J Chiropractic 1993;30:19–24.

176. Rogers EJ, Rogers R: Fibromyalgia and myofascial pain: Either, neither, or both? Orthop Rev 1989;18:1217–1224.

177. Rowlingson JC, Kirschenbaum LP: Epidural analgesic techniques in the management of cervical pain. Anesth Analg 1986;65:938–942.

178. Roydhouse RH: Torquing of the neck and jaw due to belt restraint in whiplash-type accidents. Lancet 1985;1:1341.

179. Russell E: Cervical disc disease. Radiology 1990;177:313–325.

180. Russell IJ, Bowden CL, Michlek JE, et al: Imipramine receptor density on platelets on patients with fibrositis syndrome: Correlation with disease severity and response to therapy (abstract). Arthritis Rheum 30:S63, 1987.

181. Russell E, D'Angelo C, Zimmerman R, et al: Cervical disc herniation: CT demonstration after contrast enhancement. Radiology 1984;152:703–712.

182. Rydevik B, Brown M, Lundborg G: Pathoanatomy and pathophysiology of nerve root compression. Spine 1984;9:7–15.

183. Saal JS: Flexibility training. Phys Med Rehabil 1987;1:537–554.

184. Saal JS, Saal JJ, Herzog R: The natural history of lumbar intervertebral disk extrusions treated nonoperatively. Spine 1990;15:683–686.

185. Schmid UD, Hess CW, Ludin HP: Somatosensory evoked potentials following nerve and segmental stimulation do not confirm cervical radiculopathy with sensory deficit. J Neurol Neurosurg Psychiatry 1988;51:182–187.

186. Schneider LW, Foust DR, Bowman BM, et al: Biomechanical properties of the human neck in lateral flexion. In Proceedings of the 19th STAPP Car Crash Conference. Warrendale, Pa, Society of Automotive Engineers, 1975, pp 453–485.

187. Schofferman J, Anderson D, Smith G, et al: Childhood psychological trauma and chronic low back pain. In Proceedings of the 7th Annual NASS Meeting. Boston, North American Spine Society, July 11, 1992, p 148.

188. Schuster GD: The use of cryoanalgesia in the painful facet syndrome. J Neurol Orthop Surg 1982;3:271–274.

189. Selecki BR: Whiplash. Aust Fam Phys 1984;13:243–247.

190. Severy DM, Mathewson JH, Bechtol CO: Controlled automobile rear end collisions: An investigation of related engineering and medical phenomena. Can Serv Med J 1955;11:727–759.

191. Shulman M: Treatment of neck pain with cervical epidural steroid injection. Reg Anesth 1986;11:92–94.

192. Silvers HR: Lumbar percutaneous facet rhizotomy. Spine 1990;15:36–40.

193. Smith AG: Account of a case in which portions of three dorsal vertebrae were removed for the relief of paralysis from fracture, with partial success. 1829;8:94.

194. Smith GW, Nichols P: The technic of cervical discography. Radiology 1963;68:163–165.

195. Spengler DM: Lumbar discectomy: Results with limited disc excision and selective foraminotomy. Spine 1982;7:704–706.

196. Sternbach RA, Tursky B: Ethnic differences among housewives in psychophysical and skin potential responses to electric shock. Psychophysiology 1965;1:241.

197. Su HC, Su RK: Treatment of whiplash injuries with acupuncture. Clin J Pain 1988;4:233.

198. Sweeney T, Prentice C, Saal JA, et al: Cervicothoracic muscular stabilizing technique. Phys Med Rehabil 1990;4:335–360.

199. Taylor JR, Womey T: Acute injuries to cervical joints. Spine 1993;18:1736–1745.

200. Teasell RW, McCain G: The clinical spectrum and management of whiplash injuries. In Tollison CD (ed): Painful Cervical Trauma:

Diagnosis and Rehabilitation Treatment of Neuromuscular Injuries. Baltimore, Williams & Wilkins, 1992, pp 292–318.

201. Teresi LM, Lufkin RB, Reicher MA: Asymptomatic degenerative disk disease and spondylosis of the cervical spine: MR imaging. Radiology 1987;164:83–88.

202. Torg J: The epidemiologic, biomechanical, and cinematographic analysis of football-induced cervical spine trauma and its prevention. *In* Torg JS (ed): Athletic Injuries to the Head, Neck, and Face, ed 2. St Louis, Mosby–Year Book, 1991, pp 97–111.

203. Torg J: Injuries to the cervical spine and spinal cord resulting from water sports. *In* Torg JS (ed): Athletic Injuries to the Head, Neck, and Face, ed 2. St Louis, Mosby–Year Book, 1991, pp 157–173.

204. Torg J: Trampoline-induced cervical quadriplegia. *In* Torg JS (ed): Athletic Injuries to the Head, Neck, and Face, ed 2. St Louis, Mosby–Year Book, 1991, pp 85–96.

205. Torg JS, Fay CM: Cervical spinal stenosis with cord neurapraxia and transient quadriplegia. *In* Torg JS (ed): Athletic Injuries to the Head, Neck, and Face, ed 2. St Louis, Mosby–Year Book, 1991, pp 533–552.

206. Travell JG, Simons DG: Myofascial Pain and Dysfunction—the Trigger Point Manual. Baltimore, Williams & Wilkins, 1983.

207. Tucci SM, Hicks JE, Gross EG, et al: Cervical motion assessment: A new, simple and accurate method. Arch Phys Med Rehabil 1986;67:225–230.

208. Uematsu S, Hendler N, Hungerford D, et al: Thermography and electromyography in the differential diagnosis of chronic pain syndromes and reflex sympathetic dystrophy. Electromyogr Clin Neurophysiol 1982;21:165.

209. Vaeöry H, Helle R, Förre O, et al: Elevated CSF levels of substance P in high incidence of Raynaud's phenomenon in patients with fibromyalgia: New features for diagnosis. Pain 1988;32:21–26.

210. Walker EA: A History of Neurological Surgery. New York, Hafner, 1967.

211. Warfield CA, Biber MP, Crews DA, et al: Epidural steroid injection as a treatment for cervical radiculitis. Clin J Pain 1988;4:201–204.

212. Watkinson A, Gargan MF, Bannister GC: Prognostic factors in soft tissue injuries of the cervical spine. Injury 1991;22:307–309.

213. White A, Southwick W, Deponte RJ: Relief of pain by anterior cervical spine fusion for spondylosis. J Bone Joint Surg Am 1973;55:525.

214. White AA, Panjabi MM: Biomechanics of the Spine, ed 2. Philadelphia, JB Lippincott, 1978, pp 229–235.

215. White AA, Panjabi MM: Update on the evaluation on instability of the lower cervical spine. Instr Course Lect 1987;36:513–520.

216. Whitecloud TS, Seago RA: Cervical discogenic syndrome: Results of operative intervention in patients with positive discography. Spine 1987;12:313–316.

217. Williams J, Allen M, Harkess J: Late results of cervical discectomy and interbody fusions: Some factors influencing the results. J Bone Joint Surg Am 1968;50:227.

218. Woolfenden JM, Pitt MJ, Durie BGM, et al: Comparison of bone scintigraphy and radiography in multiple myeloma. Radiology 1980;134:723–728.

219. Yiannikas C, Shahani BT, Young RR: Short-latency somatosensory-evoked potentials from radial, median, ulnar and peroneal nerve stimulation in the assessment of cervical spondylosis. Arch Neurol 1986;43:1264–1271.

220. Youssen D, Atlas S, Goldberg H, et al: Degenerative narrowing of the cervical spine neural foramina. Evaluation with high-resolution 3DFT gradient-echo MR imaging. AJNR 1991;12:229–236.

221. Yu YL, Jones SJ: Somatosensory evoked potentials in cervical spondylosis: Correlation of median, ulnar and posterior tibial nerve responses with clinical and radiological findings. Brain 1985;108:273–300.

222. Yunus MB, Kalyan-Raman UP, Kalyan-Raman K: Primary fibromyalgia syndrome and myofascial pain syndrome: Clinical features and muscle pathology. Arch Phys Med Rehabil 1988;69:451–454.

223. Zborowski M: Cultural components in responses to pain. J Soc Issues 1952;8:16.

224. Zola IK: Culture and symptoms—an analysis of patients presenting complaints. Am Soc Rev 1966;31:615.

37

Upper Limb Musculoskeletal Pain Syndromes

JEFFREY A. STRAKOWSKI, M.D.,
J. WILLIAM WIAND, D.O., AND
ERNEST W. JOHNSON, M.D.

Musculoskeletal pain syndromes of the upper limb are among the most common and challenging diagnostic and treatment problems facing the practitioner. A variety of physical problems present with a common symptom of pain. These include limitations of joint motion, soft tissue changes, and weakness, all of which can significantly compromise normal physiological function. Effective physiatric care requires an accurate diagnosis, a complete assessment of functional impairments, and an appropriate rehabilitation program. This treatment includes pain control, activity modification, and minimizing functional loss.

SHOULDER PAIN

Rotator Cuff Disease

Impingement, also called the "painful arc syndrome," is a poorly defined term that encompasses a variety of disorders that manifest as anterior shoulder pain. These disorders have in common a pathological course that includes tendinitis of the rotator cuff, which can progress to complete rupture. It ordinarily involves pain that occurs through the arc of motion as the arm is raised overhead. Impingement syndrome tends to include previously used terms such as subacromial and subdeltoid bursitis as well as rotator cuff tendinitis.

There are many entities that present with pain or decreased range of motion (ROM) of the shoulder in the differential diagnosis that need to be distinguished from rotator cuff disease. These include adhesive capsulitis, calcific tendinitis, dynamic functional instability, acromial clavicular (AC) joint degenerative disease, glenohumeral joint degenerative disease, tumors of the shoulder girdle and lung apex, crystalline and rheumatoid arthropathies, and cervical radiculopathy.[73]

A growing body of primary research and literature has led to a greater understanding of the biomechanics and etiology of rotator cuff disease which will enable improved management, both operative and nonoperative.[26, 54, 61] However, in order to have a complete understanding of these mechanisms, in-depth knowledge of the three-dimensional anatomical-spatial relationships is essential (Fig. 37–1).

There is considerable evidence in the literature supporting a multifactorial basis for the disease process of rotator cuff disease and impingement syndrome.[18, 45] Impingement itself refers to the physical process of compression and shearing of the rotator cuff tendon between the closed space of the rigid coracoacromial arch and the humeral head. Clearly, not all rotator cuff disease is a direct result of this specific extrinsic process, particularly in the elderly. Many feel that the term "impingement syndrome" fails to reflect the multiple causes and spectrum of treatment options.[4] In addition to categorizing rotator cuff disease on the basis of extrinsic vs. intrinsic causes, some utilize the division of primary and secondary impingement.[18] Primary impingement is due to the rigid coracoacromial arch (stenotic), whereas secondary impingement is defined as a relative decrease in the supraspinatus outlet caused by instability of the glenohumeral joint (nonstenotic).[45]

Stenotic Impingement

The subacromial impingement syndrome reported by Meyer[39] and Neer[43] suggests that rotator cuff degeneration and subsequent tears are produced extrinsically by the rigid coracoacromial arch. Neer states that 95% of rotator cuff tears (RCTs) are associated with extrinsic impingement[43] and describes three stages of progression (Table 37–1). Partial tears can extend to complete tears with relatively minor trauma. The stages are not discrete but occur as a continuum over time. Progression can also involve problems with the biceps tendon, subscapularis tendon, sub-

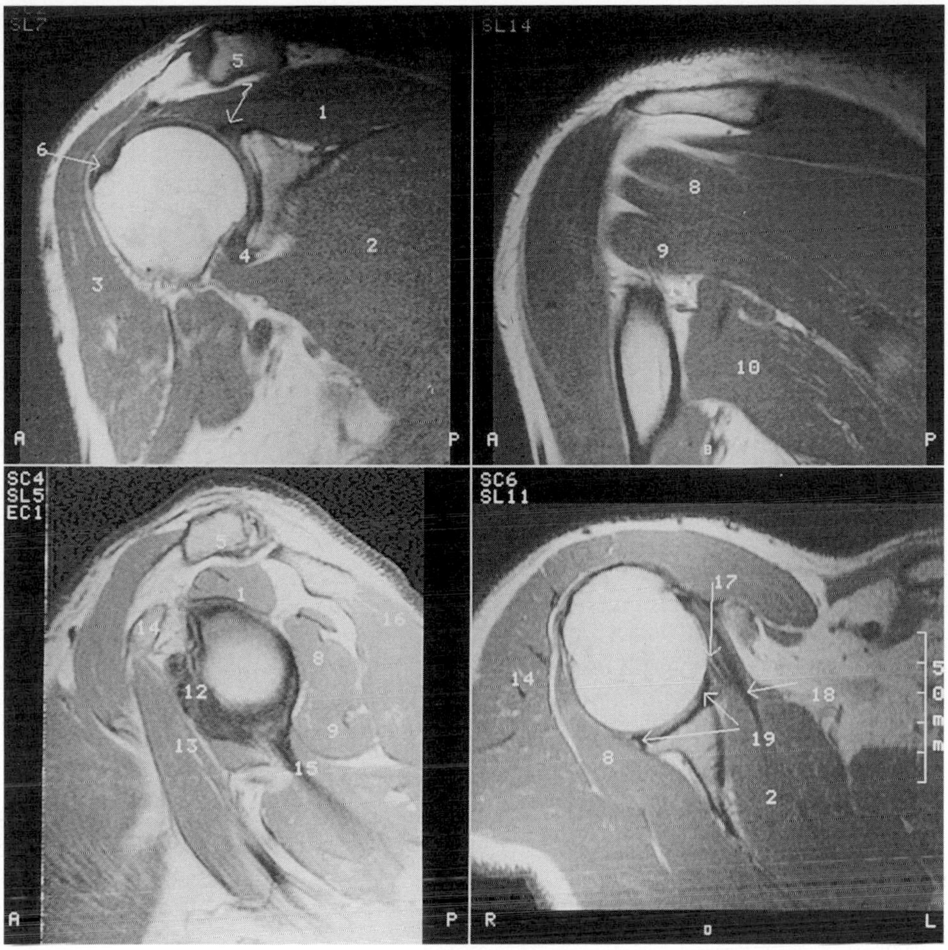

FIGURE 37–1 MRI of a normal shoulder denoting anatomical relationships. The supraspinatus muscle is shown (1), as are the subscapularis muscle (2), deltoid muscle (3), axillary recess (4), and clavicle (5). Also demonstrated is the normal cuff insertion (6), infraspinatus muscle (8), teres minor muscle (9), and latissimus dorsi muscle (10), as well as the coracobrachialis (12), the short head of the biceps muscle (13), and the subscapularis tendon (19).

acromial bursa, acromioclavicular joint, and glenohumeral joint.

Virtually all complete RCTs manifest as distal midsubstance tears. Bone-tendon junction disruptions occur but are less common.[18] Acute cuff avulsion injuries are also rare in the shoulder.

There are a number of relationships and variations which contribute to the diminution of available space for the rotator cuff tendon and result in stenosis. In addition to the rigid bony structures of the humeral head, anterior third of the acromion, and AC joint, the coracoacromial ligament constitutes the anterior third of the coracoacromial arch and also contributes to the confinement of the tendon in a fixed space.

Variations in shape and orientation of the acromion significantly affect the stenosis and subsequently the impingement originally described by Neer and by Morrison and Bigliani[42] (Fig. 37–2). They include the flat (type I), smoothed curve (type II), and angled curve (hook) (type III). It was noted[42] that the "hook-type" acromion was present more frequently in patients with a complete RCT.

Impingement can also lead to tendinitis and rupture of the long head of the biceps tendon. Neer showed that the functional arc of elevation of the shoulder is forward, not lateral, and that the impingement occurs predominantly against the anterior edge of the acromion and the coracoacromial ligament (CAL).[43] Poorly healed greater tuberosity fractures and a thickened CAL can also contribute to stenosis.

Nonstenotic Impingement

Rotator cuff disease is not always due to stenosis and can reflect other etiologies.[4] Subdeltoid bursitis is a common cause of anterior shoulder pain. It develops frequently in throwing athletes and is usually associated with the acceleration phase of throwing. Direct palpation over the subdeltoid bursa to localize the area of tenderness is essential for the diagnosis (Fig. 37–3). It ordinarily responds well to rest, ice, and anti-inflammatory medications. In refractory cases, a local steroid injection into the subdeltoid bursa might be necessary.

Occasionally, subdeltoid adhesions develop. These typi-

TABLE 37–1   The Stages of Rotator Cuff Disease

Stage I: Rotator cuff inflammation—edema and hemorrhage
Stage II: Progression to tendinitis—fibrosis and tendinitis
Stage III: Partial or full-thickness tear—tendon degeneration and rupture
Stage IIIA: Tears <1 cm in length
Stage IIIB: Tears >1 cm in length
Stage IV: Multiple tendon tears

Data from Neer CS: Anterior acromioplasty for chronic impingement syndrome in the shoulder. A preliminary report. J Bone Joint Surg Am 1972; 54:41–50.

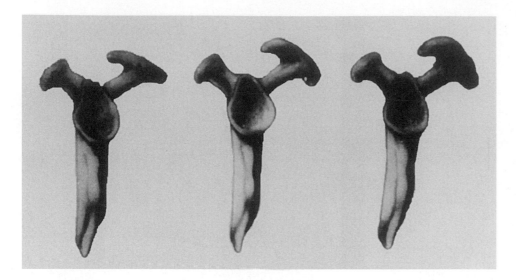

FIGURE 37–2 Acromial variation. *Left to right*, Type I Bigliani, flat acromion; type II, gentle anterior curve; type III, marked hooking. In addition, the acromion can be upsloping, horizontal, or downsloping.

cally present as limited ROM resulting from repetitive mechanotrauma, chronic bursal inflammation, crystalline disease, and rheumatologic causes. These causes are primarily manifested in external rotation and should be suspected when chronicity, loss of motion, and calcific deposits are present.

Primary glenohumeral instability should also be considered when evaluating rotator cuff disease. Abnormal excursion of the shoulder joint owing to laxity results in fatigue and traction on the shoulder girdle musculature.[27] The resulting muscular dysfunction can allow even greater humeral head motion, including proximal migration of the head under the coracoacromial arch, which subsequently leads to the development of impingement and cuff disease. These patients are often younger (less than 35 years old) and involved in throwing or repetitive overhead activities such as tennis, swimming, and baseball. Recurrent anterior subluxation is occasionally seen with the overhead phase

of throwing.[28] The clinical signs and symptoms of instability are discussed elsewhere in this chapter. The difficulty with instability associated with rotator cuff disease is that the often dramatic signs of rotator cuff disease can obscure the more subtle signs of instability. Every effort should be made to identify shoulder instability as a component of the shoulder disease, particularly in younger patients and in those with persistent symptoms, despite what would be otherwise considered adequate treatment. Imprecise diagnosis can lead to unnecessary and unsuccessful repeated injections and even, occasionally, acromioplasties.

Persons who frequently perform overhead activities can place enormous stress on the dynamic and static stabilizers of their shoulders. Over time, repetitive stresses of this nature can lead to microtrauma of the glenohumeral ligaments with eventual attenuation of these structures. Without the normal function of these static stabilizers, a pattern of mild instability can develop, placing further demands on the dynamic stabilizers of the rotator cuff.[18, 54]

Anterior shoulder pain and impingement syndrome can also result from adhesive capsulitis (discussed elsewhere) at any time during its course. Exclusion of the many other causes of adhesive capsulitis is needed before attributing the pain to this disease process.

It has also been demonstrated that scapular stabilizers are important factors in humeral head control. The relationship of the scapulohumeral complex and its reliance on glenohumeral stabilization has been discussed by Kibler and Chandler.[18] They describe a test called the lateral scapular slide. With this they measured the distance between the medial border of the scapula and the spinous processes and found that this distance was increased in the symptomatic group of throwing athletes, suggesting scapulothoracic instability. The muscle groups most specifically involved in this include the trapezius, rhomboids, and serratus anterior. Deficiencies in strength or flexibility of these muscles can affect the synchrony of scapular motion. This disruption of the normal scapulohumeral rhythm due to abnormal motion on the chest wall leads to excessive stress on the glenohumeral joint. This can then lead to impingement of the rotator cuff underneath the coracoacromial arch and is an important consideration

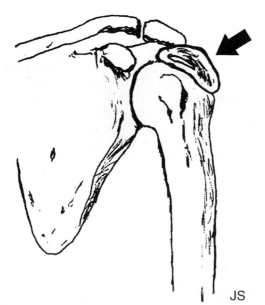

JS

FIGURE 37–3 Representation of the anatomical position of the subdeltoid bursa.

when designing an exercise program, particularly for throwing athletes.

Contrary to the extrinsic stress theories proposed by Meyer and Neer, Codman,[11] in 1934, suggested an intrinsic theory of rotator cuff disease. He postulated that initial intrinsic ischemic degenerative changes within the cuff itself lead to tears. He proposed the concept of the "critical zone" near the insertion of the supraspinatus tendon.[11] Nirschl[48] described "angiofibroblastic hyperplasia" as the initial change in the cuff that leads to more permanent change. Uhthoff,[68] in 1987, showed in a study of cadaveric specimens that the majority of cuff tears begin on the articular side and proposed that the extrinsic findings were actually a secondary process. This has since been confirmed in additional studies.[4] The severity of the degenerative acromial changes seems to correlate with the severity of the rotator cuff disease in these specimens. Despite considerable controversy, there is often no evidence of extrinsic factors in persons with rotator cuff disease.[51]

Several investigators have discussed the implications of the rotator cuff vascular supply in primary disease. The rotator cuff musculature is richly supplied by the suprascapular, anterior and posterior circumflex humeral, and axillary arteries. Despite this there are hypovascular zones in the rotator cuff tendons which are believed to coincide with commonly observed areas of degeneration, such as the area at the humeral insertion.[58] These areas may play an important role in the development of tendon degeneration and inability to heal. If the injury outstrips the blood supply, progression occurs.

Rathbun and Macnab[58] also found that a distinct and characteristic vascular pattern can be related to the position of the arm. By injecting micro-opaque spheres into the subclavian artery supplying the rotator cuff, they found the vessels supplying the supraspinatus tendon completely filled while the shoulder was in the abducted position, but had a constant area of avascularity extending from 1 cm proximal directly to the point of insertion into the greater tuberosity with the shoulder in the adducted position. Similar studies showed that the intracapsular portion of the biceps tendon has a similar avascular zone as it passes over the head of the humerus.[20]

The differential diagnosis of clinical conditions that can resemble primary rotator cuff disease is extensive (Table 37–2). Acute traumatic bursitis usually results from a direct blow to the cuff resulting in hemorrhage and edema. This is ordinarily a self-limiting condition which resolves with appropriate rest and time. It can occasionally initiate a continuing impingement syndrome. The temporal relationship to trauma and the physical findings suggest the diagnosis. Instability should be distinguished from primary rotator cuff disease.

With primary AC joint disease a history of previous trauma is ordinarily present in addition to findings restricted primarily to the AC joint itself. Physical findings include tenderness and reproduction of pain with forcible adduction and internal rotation of the humerus. This finding can be mistaken for subacromial impingement.

Cervical radiculopathy is discussed elsewhere in this text. It can frequently be distinguished from rotator cuff dysfunction by posterior shoulder pain; pain extending below the elbow; or weakness, sensory loss, and reflex changes.

Calcific tendinitis is believed to represent a separate pathological process. Calcification is seldom seen with degenerative rotator cuff disease and its presence radiologically can generally preclude the diagnosis of impingement syndrome, although occasionally capsular ruptures into the bursa result in calcification.

Diagnosis

A thorough comprehensive history is essential for accurately identifying the disease process. Age, occupation, avocation, and the presence of systemic disease can all suggest the appropriate diagnosis. Medical conditions such as diabetes mellitus, arthritides, crystalline disease, cervical spine disorders, and neuromuscular disease are all important variables for diagnosis and appropriate treatment. Previous treatment history, including specific type, duration, and degree of response, offer important insights into the specific cause and management planning.

Although the clinical picture of rotator cuff disease is more of a continuum, Hawkins and Kennedy[20] described characteristic signs and symptoms which correlate with the stage of disease (Table 37–3). Frequent findings in patients with stage I disease include persons, ordinarily under 25 years of age, who complain of a "toothache-like" discomfort which radiates laterally to the middle of the arm. It may, however, include persons of virtually any age. Point tenderness is noted over the greater tuberosity and occasionally over the anterior acromion and CAL. Pain is often induced with flexion and abduction to 90 degrees.

The classic "impingement test" has been described as pain as the examiner flexes the shoulder anteriorly while stabilizing the scapula to prevent scapulothoracic compensation.[73] This maneuver, when positive, reproduces pain and apprehension as it jams the greater tuberosity against the anteroinferior surface of the acromion. This may be the most reliable physical sign in establishing the diagnosis. Internal rotation of the shoulder in this forward flexed position typically accentuates the discomfort (Fig. 37–4). An injection of 10 mL of 1% lidocaine directly into the subacromial bursa often eliminates or reduces pain and helps to confirm the diagnosis.

TABLE 37–2 Conditions with Clinical Appearances Potentially Similar to Primary Rotator Cuff Disease

Acute traumatic bursitis
Instability
Primary acromioclavicular disease
Cervical radiculopathy
Arthritides of the glenohumeral joint
Calcific tendinitis
Adhesive capsulitis

TABLE 37–3 Clinical Stages of Rotator Cuff Disease

Stage I:	Minimal pain with activity; no weakness and no loss of motion
Stage II:	Marked tendinitis with pain and no loss of motion
Stage III:	Pain and weakness (cuff tear)

Data from Hawkins RJ, Kennedy JC: Impingement syndrome in athletes. Am J Sports Med 1980; 8:151–157.

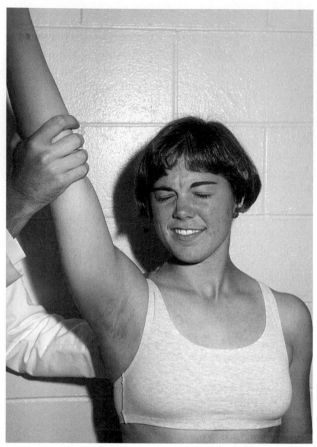

FIGURE 37–4 An illustration of positioning for the impingement test. The scapula is stabilized posteriorly while the arm is elevated, taking the shoulder through its range of forward flexion. Reproducible pain with apprehension, including grimacing, is characteristic of the positive impingement sign.

Stage II disease is most frequently seen in the 25- to 40-year-old age group, but can occur at any age. Pain is described as "toothache-like" and increases with overhead activities. It is often worse at night and frequently limits sleep. It may progress to limit the daytime activities that accentuate the discomfort. The tenderness is more severe than in stage I and can secondarily involve the AC joint. ROM often becomes painful and difficult at this stage. There can be a particularly painful "catching sensation" as the arm is brought down from the abducted position. This is believed by some to represent catching of the scar under the impingement area.[20]

Stage III disease is ordinarily seen in patients over 40 years of age. This is usually associated with a long history of intermittent or progressive shoulder problems, including the signs and symptoms seen in stages I and II. Symptoms are usually worse with overhead activity and at night. These patients typically exhibit weakness secondary to pain. Decreased ROM and shoulder "stiffness" are also noted.

Complete rotator cuff tendon rupture may demonstrate little change from previous clinical findings of an earlier stage, or there may be a dramatic clinical change from an acute event that finally causes rupture, such as the sudden inability to elevate the arm. However, there is virtually always the presence of a long history of shoulder problems

in these patients. Complete or partial tears occur at an average age of 50. Several signs indicative of full-thickness RCTs have been described.[20] These include infraspinatus and supraspinatus wasting; tenderness over the greater tuberosity and anterior acromion; AC joint tenderness; painful arc of motion at 90 degrees of abduction or forward flexion; passive greater than active ROM, particularly in abduction and external rotation; and weakness of abduction and external rotation.

Plain film evaluation is the first step in radiological imaging of the shoulder. It is most sensitive for osseous lesions, including fractures, metastatic lesions, and developmental or degenerative variations. Plain films most often have positive findings in stage III disease, which includes sclerosis and osteophyte formation on the anteroinferior acromion and greater tuberosity (which also might demonstrate cystic degeneration). Degeneration of the AC joint with osteophyte formation can be present, as well as a reduced distance between the acromion and humeral head. Osteolysis presents as demineralization of the distal clavicle and widening of the AC joint. Plain films, however, have limited usefulness in the detection of abnormal calcification and soft tissue disease. Whereas calcific bursitis and tendinitis often have radiographic manifestations, most soft tissue lesions of the shoulder do not.

Although ultrasonography is used in some select centers for rotator cuff disease, most centers in the United States have limited experience with this modality and there is difficulty with reproducibility.[16, 50]

Arthrography has limited usefulness for rotator cuff disease. It provides good sensitivity only for complete tears or high-grade partial undersurface tears. In full-thickness tears, the contrast leaks through the defect and can be seen lying outside the cuff, ordinarily adjacent to the undersurface of the acromion (Fig. 37–5). Arthrograms are ordinarily negative in partial-thickness tears or earlier stages of degeneration. Obvious drawbacks to the use of this imaging modality are that approximately 70% of tears are partial and that the bursal surface is more commonly involved than the undersurface.[26] Further lowering sensitivity are situations in which a complete tear is partially fibrosed or healed. Another limitation is the inability to distinguish muscle disorders by arthrography.

The primary role of nuclear medicine is characterizing patterns of disease in patients with known or suspected malignancies or arthritides. Its high sensitivity but low specificity limits its role in the evaluation of monoarticular disease. Magnetic resonance imaging (MRI) is quickly becoming the primary imaging modality of choice. It offers three-dimensional capabilities, providing more specific characterization of incomplete tears and three-dimensional characterization of complete tears (Fig. 37–6) and offering important information on the status of muscle groups. Examples of this are the identification of ganglia in the spinoglenoid fossa and the location of focal suprascapular nerve palsies (Fig. 37–7).

Treatment

Precise etiological diagnosis is the foundation for appropriate and effective treatment. Whereas surgically enlarging the coracoacromial space through partial acromioplasty and

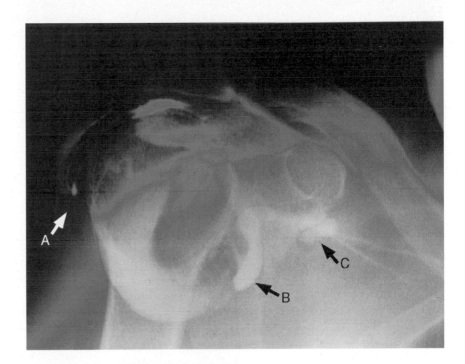

FIGURE 37–5 A contrast arthrogram demonstrating contrast in the subacromial/subdeltoid bursa *(A)*, denoting a complete tear, a normal axillary pouch *(B)*, and subcoracoid bursa *(C)*.

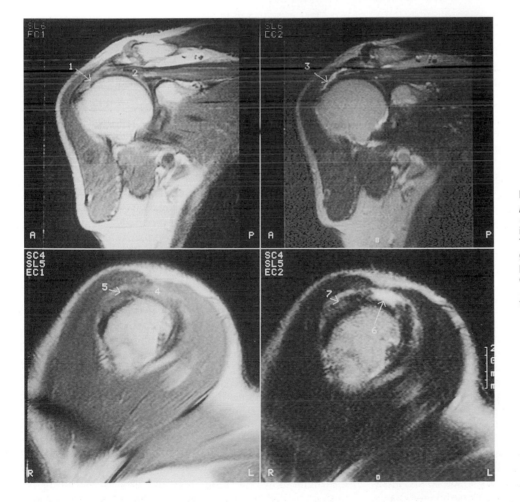

FIGURE 37–6 T1-weighted *(left panels)* and matching T2-weighted *(right panels)* MRI studies illustrating a full-thickness rotator cuff tear. The coronal images demonstrate gray signal in the supraspinatus portion of the cuff *(1)*, retracted tendon *(2)*, and fluid in the distal tear *(3)*. The sagittal images show the torn cuff *(4 and 6)* and viable cuff *(5 and 7)*.

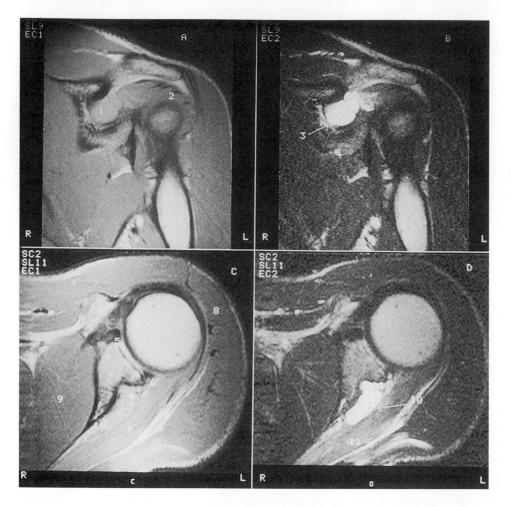

FIGURE 37–7 MRI studies of a carpenter with a ganglion in the spinoglenoid fossa. *A,* Posterior coronal T1 image with fluid in the fossa *(1)* and black cuff *(2)*. *B,* T2 image with the ganglion *(3)* becoming bright. *C,* Axial T1 image showing intermediate signal ganglion *(4)*, anterior *(5)* and posterior *(6)* labrum, and the infraspinatus *(7)*, deltoid *(8)*, and subscapularis *(9)* muscles. *D,* T2 image with the bright-signal ganglion *(10)*. The relative bright signal in the infraspinatus *(10)* is due to changes resulting from denervation.

CAL lysis provides symptomatic relief in some patients, recent trends have emphasized the importance of physiatric rehabilitation of the dynamic stabilizers as the most effective therapeutic modality. The physiatric treatment should be individualized for each patient. Many of the early rehabilitation techniques employed are similar for all patients, with the goal of promoting healing and returning the physiological motion and normal scapulothoracic rhythm of the shoulder girdle. The training techniques to be employed beyond this point are specific to the goals and demands of the individual patient (throwing athlete, laborer, sedentary person).

Primary prevention should be considered an integral part of the treatment of rotator cuff disease. Education of persons at risk can do much to circumvent the development of rotator cuff disease. Athletes, particularly those involved in throwing and overhead sports, as well as laborers with repetitive shoulder stress, should be instructed in proper warmup techniques, specific strengthening techniques, and warning signs of early impingement.

Tailoring an appropriate therapeutic prescription requires understanding of the patient's stage of rotator cuff disease. Most stage I disease is reversible.[45] The cornerstone of treatment at this stage includes modalities such as ice, alteration of activity, anti-inflammatory medications, therapeutic exercises for strengthening the dynamic stabilizers, and rarely, use of intra-articular steroids. Anti-inflammatory measures are taken to reduce cuff edema and hemorrhage.

Local ice massage for 10 to 20 min is indicated following activity that exacerbates symptoms. Ultrasound heating can be helpful. An ultrasound regimen for the supraspinatus tendon is 1.2 to 1.5 W/cm^2 for 8 min/day for 10 days. Total joint rest is to be avoided in favor of symptom-limited activity and specific therapeutic exercises.

A technique suggested to correct deficiencies in strength, flexibility, and coordination is proprioceptive neuromuscular facilitation (PNF).[18] This is performed by selective exercise patterns ordinarily led by a therapist. The neurophysiological basis for this is believed to involve the stretch reflex. This facilitates or inhibits agonist and antagonist muscle groups in a rate-dependent fashion and attempts to redevelop normal scapulohumeral rhythm with joint distraction and compression techniques. The effectiveness of this technique can be dependent upon the experience of the therapist.

Following symptomatic relief, a program of active exercise is initiated with the goal of strengthening both the internal and external shoulder rotators in the nonabducted position.

The supraspinatus is strengthened by asking the patient to move the hand from the straight adducted position to abduction at approximately 90 degrees, with the hand in the thumb-down position after the arm is placed in a position of 30 degrees anterior to the straight abducted position (Fig. 37–8).

These can be initially performed with just the weight of

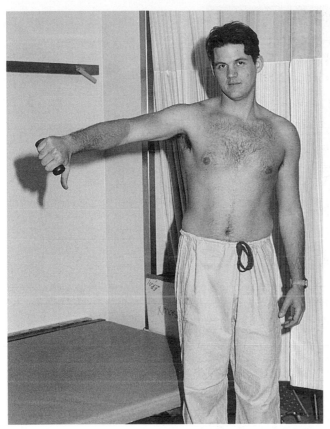

FIGURE 37–8   Demonstration of supraspinatus strengthening. The shoulder is abducted in the scapular plane with resistance while in internal rotation.

the hand, with eventual progression by adding weights (ordinarily 2.5–10 lb). Isotonic strengthening of the rotator cuff has also been found to be useful. The basic goal of rotator cuff strengthening is to regain its function as a humeral head stabilizer. This can reduce the degree of impingement and accelerate the return to pain-free activities. Strengthening of the scapulothoracic musculature can provide clinical improvement. One third of shoulder abduction is scapular rotation in origin. With an increased scapulothoracic component of shoulder motion, there is a more favorable positioning of the scapula and acromion to alleviate tendon impingement. The strength and flexibility of all of the muscles involved in the dynamic stabilization of the humerus should be continually assessed as the rehabilitation process ensues. This includes the deltoid and biceps, as well as the rotator cuff and scapulothoracic muscles.

The use of intra-articular steroids is controversial because of the well-known risks to the tendon structure,[69] which include collagen necrosis, weakness, and possible rupture. Repetitive injections increase these risks. Selective use of a well-performed single injection in the subacromial space, however, has been shown to hasten the recovery process by reducing pain and inflammation, allowing more rapid advancement to an exercise program.

Current treatment trends limit the role of surgical decompression to symptomatic relief of pain, primarily in elderly patients with a more advanced stage of disease. Widespread, indiscriminate surgical decompression in early stages of disease fails to acknowledge the current pathophysiological understanding of the disease process. Early-stage patients who are refractory to appropriate physiatric treatment protocols need to be reconsidered to ensure accurate diagnosis. Further diagnostic modalities such as MRI, electromyography (EMG), and arthroscopy should be considered in order that any unsuspected disorder can be diagnosed and addressed. Meyers[40] believed that spurs on the undersurface of the clavicle or acromion should be removed.

Conservative treatment protocols of stage II and III disease are the same as that for stage I. Surgical decompression is entertained in stage II and III patients who fail to respond to appropriate physiatric treatment protocols. Some believe that a general principle in the absence of a cuff tear is to consider surgery if pain has persisted for more than 1 year. The purpose of decompression by anterior acromioplasty and CAL release, with preservation of the deltoid by reattachment and repair of the cuff, is to reduce or eliminate impingement pain, improve function, and prevent recurrence. In successful surgical decompression, the anterior inferior acromial edge, undersurface of the AC joint, and the CAL are surgically modified.

Bicipital Tendinitis

Bicipital tendinitis is an inflammation of the long head of the biceps where the tendon passes through the bicipital groove (Fig. 37–9). Although often a manifestation of progressive cuff disease, particularly in the elderly, it is also frequently seen in younger persons as the result of chronic repetitive motion. Recurrent subluxation of the long head of the biceps tendon is also a consideration, particularly in throwing athletes. It has also been theorized that the long head of the biceps tendon plays a role in controlling superior subluxation of the humeral head,[1] which can contribute to secondary impingement.

Bicipital tendinitis as a manifestation of repetitive motion disorders is seen most often as an occupational disorder in laborers and others who use frequent overhead motions. There can be a spectrum from acute myositis and tenosynovitis to chronic tendinopathy, which may or may not be calcified.

Although less common, recurrent subluxation can lead to bicipital tendinitis. It occurs most frequently when the muscular tension is at a maximum, as during the cocking phases of throwing when the shoulder goes from extremes of external rotation into internal rotation. Persons who are most predisposed to this include those with congenitally shallow or post-traumatic bicipital grooves. These medial subluxations can be palpated by the examiner with a finger placed over the bicipital groove.

Inflammation of the intracapsular portion of the biceps tendon is a frequent manifestation of stage II and III rotator cuff disease. It is often seen with associated cuff tendinitis. Its anatomical location close to the supraspinatus and subscapularis tendon predisposes it to the inflammatory and degenerative processes of severe rotator cuff disease. This is particularly true in the elderly, who after a complete tear place undue strain on the bicipital tendon, as its role is increased in controlling superior subluxation of the humeral head. This contributes to a form of "secondary impinge-

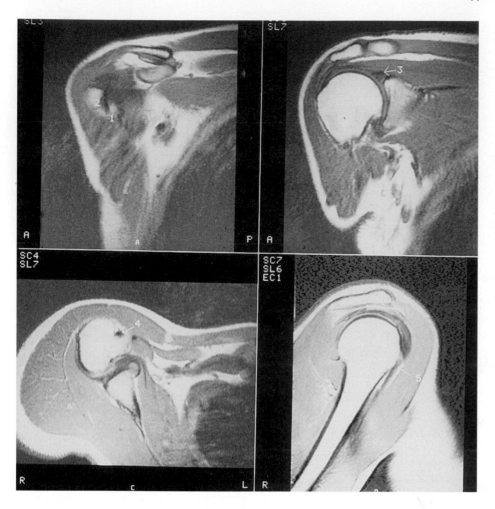

FIGURE 37–9 The spatial anatomical relationships of the long head of the biceps are demonstrated on MRI. The position in its groove *(1)* is shown on coronal section in close proximity to the greater tuberosity *(2)*. Its insertion site is also shown on the coronal *(3)*, axial *(4)*, and sagittal *(5)* views.

ment."[1] This is the most frequent cause of a complete bicipital tendon rupture in the elderly.

Diagnosis

Patients often present with anterior shoulder pain and palpable tenderness of the biceps tendon in the bicipital groove. The bicipital groove can be palpated by internally rotating the humerus 30 degrees with the patient in the supine position. The groove will be located directly anterior.

Other diagnostic tests include pain with straight arm raising, (performed with resisted forward flexion of the humerus at approximately 80 degrees with the elbow extended) or resisted supination of the forearm. Pain with both of these maneuvers occurs in the area of the bicipital groove. Complete ruptures are often apparent with inspection and palpation of the biceps muscle (Fig. 37–10).

Treatment

The treatment of patients with an intact tendon is physiatric therapy similar to that described for rotator cuff disease. Emphasis is placed on the dynamic stabilizers of the shoulder, primarily with the use of progressive resistance exercises of the internal and external shoulder rotators. Use of a Theraband is a convenient means of achieving this (Fig. 37–11). The use of nonsteroidal anti-inflammatory

drugs (NSAIDs), heat and cold modalities, and activity modification are also essential components of the treatment plan. Ultrasound over the relatively superficial biceps tendon can be useful in reducing pain, and should be administered at a dosage of 0.8 to 1.2 W/cm^2 for 8 min/day for 10 days. Steroids should not be injected into the bicipital groove because of the possibility of promoting eventual tendon rupture.[69, 73] In light of the importance of the biceps tendon as a dynamic stabilizer of the glenohumeral joint, indiscriminate surgical transfer for chronic biceps tendinitis should be avoided.

Biceps Rupture

In a younger person, violent trauma is ordinarily required to create a tear of the biceps brachii at the musculotendinous junction, a circumstance often requiring surgical repair (see Fig. 37–10). In most, and particularly in persons over 40 years of age, biceps rupture occurs in the intraarticular area and is frequently associated with rotator cuff disease and often even a full-thickness tear of the rotator cuff. Neer reported that in a population of 300 cuff tears in older people, one third had biceps involvement.[45] It most frequently manifests as a partial or complete avulsion of its insertion from the superior rim of the anterior labrum.

Instability

The shoulder joint has the greatest ROM of any joint in the body. Stability has been sacrificed for ROM. Instability

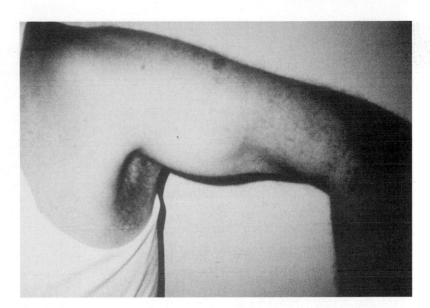

FIGURE 37–10 Distal biceps tendon rupture in a 38-year-old man. The biceps muscle has migrated proximally.

of the shoulder is essentially defined as excessive translation of the humeral head on the glenoid, and subsequent labral disease.

Although instability can be a result of congenital syndromes such as Marfan or Ehlers-Danlos syndrome, it is seen most frequently post trauma or in chronic degenerative fatigue syndromes. As the dynamic stabilizers fatigue or fail, the glenohumeral labral complex (static stabilizers) is stretched or torn. The most common, by far, is traumatic anterior dislocation with labral injury, the "Bankhart complex" (see Fig. 37–13*B*). Less common, and more frequently associated with overuse syndromes, are posterior subluxations (so-called Bennett lesions) and multidirectional instability (MDI).[17]

Diagnosis

Diagnosis requires detecting a range of problems from obvious dislocation to subtle MDI associated with fatigue. A thorough medical history is essential for properly identifying the disorder and its cause. A history of trauma, recurrent dislocation, chronic overuse, and multijoint instability can assist with properly identifying the disorder. Other problems such as nerve palsies, radiculopathies, or glenohumeral fractures should be considered and pursued if the history is suggestive.

Physical examination in these cases is often insensitive or inaccurate. The dynamic stabilization of this joint and the effect of fatigue are critical elements in the development of instability, which might not be adequately evaluated at rest or under anesthesia. Instability in throwers is often difficult for the examiner to accurately assess, including distinguishing between anterior and posterior instability. Both can be seen in the same phase of throwing, and both present with pain.

When examining the shoulder, visual inspection for gross bony deformity and muscle wasting should be performed. The shoulder should be palpated for glenohumeral relationships, and evaluation of the AC joint and coracoclavicular relationships should also be routinely performed to rule out AC separation or focal bone or muscle trauma. The shoulder should be taken through its full ROM both actively and passively and limitation in any plane noted.

Specific tests for instability include the Lachman's and relocation tests.[4] To perform Lachman's test, the examiner places the patient in a supine position on the table and abducts the shoulder to 90 degrees with external rotation. An anterior force is then applied to the humeral head. A positive test demonstrates excessive anterior translation, which can be associated with pain (Fig. 37–12*A*).

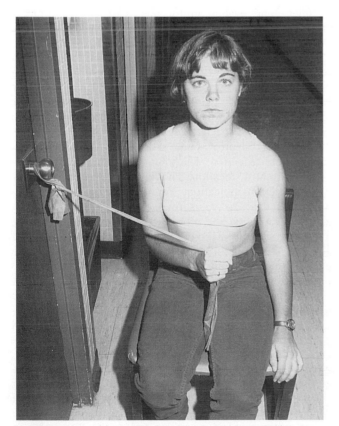

FIGURE 37–11 The use of a Theraband is a convenient method of performing internal and external rotation resistance exercises.

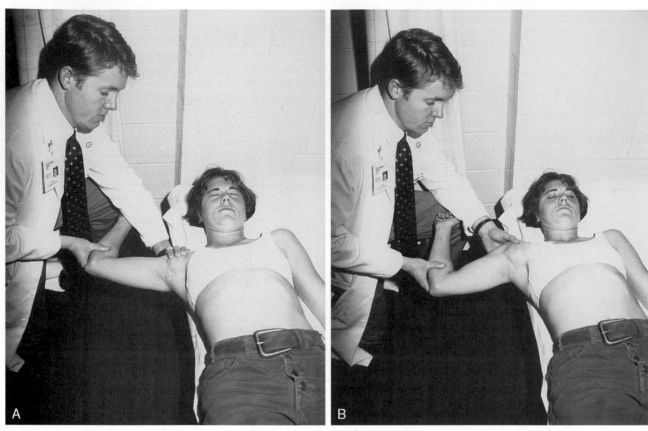

FIGURE 37-12   Demonstration of the Lachman test *(A)* and relocation test *(B)* for shoulder instability.

The positioning is the same for the relocation test, with the patient placed in the supine position and the shoulder abducted and externally rotated. Posterior force is then placed on the humerus to reduce the subluxation of anterior glenohumeral instability (Fig. 37–12*B*). The most important factor in both tests is the presence of apprehension when the arm is abducted and externally rotated.

Radiography plays an even greater role in the evaluation of instability than in rotator cuff disease. Plain film evaluation of the shoulder, in internal and external rotation, is complemented with an axillary projection. These will often demonstrate the anterior labral injuries of the Bankhart complex and show the "notchlike" defect on the superior greater tuberosity (Hill-Sachs lesion) characteristic of anterior dislocations. Also evaluated are joint surfaces that provide clues of chronic degenerative glenohumeral disease (Fig. 37–13).

When the workup is inconclusive, traditionally the next level of testing has involved the arthrogram with computed tomography (CT). Although invasive, this test provides valuable information on the labrum, glenoid, and humeral head. Increasingly, however, MRI is replacing the invasive procedure. In addition to the information offered with the arthrogram-CT, MRI provides a noninvasive additional evaluation of rotator cuff, impingement, and occasionally nerve palsies (Figs. 37–13, 37–14, and 37–15).

Treatment

The initial management of an acute shoulder dislocation is by reduction. A thorough identification of the mechanism of injury and evaluation for neurovascular compromise should be performed prior to initiating the reduction. Axillary nerve palsies are common with anterior dislocations. Closed reduction for acute dislocations is frequently performed in emergency room settings. There are multiple techniques for performing this, but it is most important that it be performed with gentle steady pressure to avoid further injury. Contraindications to closed reduction include severe osteoporosis or suspected fracture.

A thorough neurovascular examination should be performed post reduction. The joint is then protected to prevent recurrent dislocation. This is accomplished primarily with activity modification. Younger persons, particularly those less than 20 years of age, are less likely to get adhesive capsulitis and more predisposed to redislocation. Therefore, immobilization of the shoulder is better tolerated and indicated for a longer period of time than in a more elderly patient. Use of a sling for approximately 6 weeks[72] is more appropriate for a younger patient than the 2-week time period used for patients over the age of 40. Isometric exercises are begun within days following an acute dislocation. The rehabilitation program begins with active assisted exercises for increasing ROM. Progressive resistance exercises are then incorporated to strengthen the dynamic stabilizers of the shoulder (as previously described). Emphasis is also placed on the periscapular musculature, including the rhomboids, trapezius, and serratus anterior, to improve control of scapular motion. Acute surgical intervention for an initial dislocation is rare unless the dislocation is accompanied by a complete RCT.

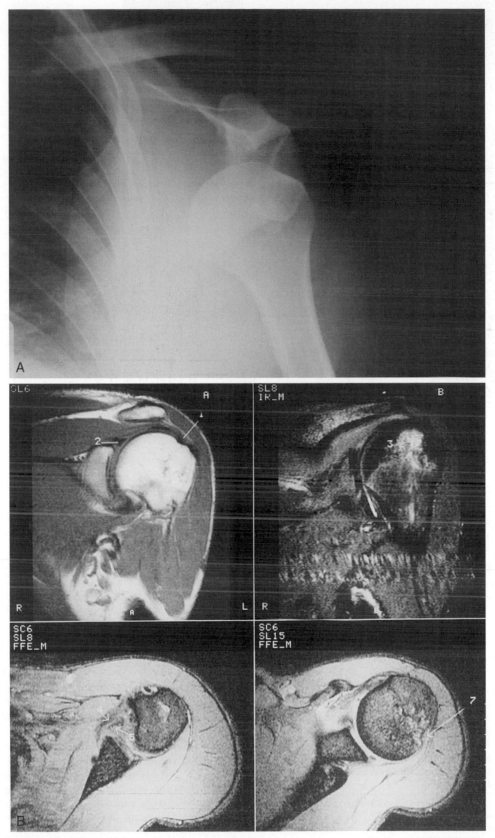

FIGURE 37–13   Radiological series of an acute shoulder dislocation in a 42-year-old man. *A,* The anterior dislocation is easily recognizable on plain film. *B,* The MRI demonstrates a normal rotator cuff *(1)* and superior labrum *(2).* The bone compression characteristic of Hill-Sachs lesions are well demonstrated on the water-weighted images *(3* and *7).* Also seen is the avulsed labral-capsular complex of the Bankhart lesion *(4* and *5).*

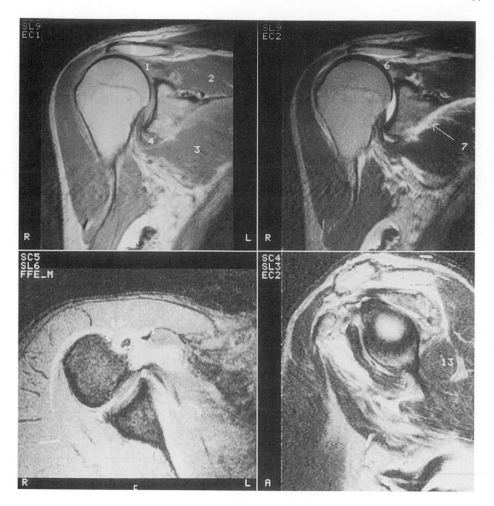

FIGURE 37–14 MRI studies of an elderly patient with an anterior dislocation. *A,* Coronal T1 image demonstrating the torn end of the supraspinatus tendon *(1),* muscle belly of the supraspinatus *(2),* subscapularis muscle *(3),* inferior axillary recess *(4),* and clavicle *(5). B,* T2 image showing the torn cuff end *(6)* and edema or blood beneath the subscapularis muscle *(7). C,* Axial gradient echo image illustrating the torn subscapularis tendon *(8)* (displaced into the anterior joint space), edematous subscapularis muscle *(9),* long head of the biceps tendon *(10),* and torn transverse ligament *(11). D,* Axillary image demonstrating edema/blood *(12)* in the supraspinatus, infraspinatus, and subscapularis *(14).* This is contrasted to the normal lower signal seen in normal muscle *(13).*

Hemiplegic Shoulder Pain

Shoulder pain is a frequent complication of hemiplegia. Its presence can compromise rehabilitation efforts. Unfortunately, it is a syndrome that is not completely understood and is somewhat controversial. Although the presentation is variable and symptoms may appear anywhere in the first year, they ordinarily appear within the first few weeks after a stroke or other neurological insult. It is more frequently associated with spastic than flaccid hemiplegia, but it may be seen in both.[55, 70]

The overall function, including stability and flexibility of the shoulder, depends less on the movement of the humeral head in the glenoid cavity than on the musculotendinous sleeve that surrounds it. Impairment of these neuromuscular components in the situation of hemiplegia or tetraplegia, therefore, greatly disrupts the usual functioning

TABLE 37–4 Factors Cited for the Multifactorial Basis of Hemiplegic Shoulder Pain

Rotator cuff and biceps tendon disease
Anteroinferior subluxation
Spasticity
Capsular constriction
Suprascapular neuropathy
Reflex sympathetic dystrophy
Ganglia
Hemineglect

of this poorly balanced joint. There is considerable controversy regarding the precise cause of this common problem, but it most likely is multifactorial. Contributing factors are included in Table 37–4.[19, 30, 35, 36, 55, 59]

Anteroinferior subluxation is the most frequently cited concomitant condition in patients with hemiplegia who have shoulder pain. Although it is seen more frequently in flaccid shoulders, it is more often associated with shoulder pain in conditions with spasticity.[70]

Diagnosis

Through physical examination, the maximal site of tenderness can often be located near the subacromial space. The degree of subluxation should be evaluated, but a valid, standardized method of measuring this has not been adequately developed.[57]

The radiographic evaluation is similar to the protocols previously described for rotator cuff disease and instability. Three-phase bone scanning is often utilized if shoulder-hand syndrome or reflex sympathetic dystrophy (RSD) is being considered. Electrodiagnosis can also be helpful in ruling out peripheral nerve compromise, radiculopathy, or plexopathy.

Treatment

The management of patients with hemiplegic shoulder pain is frequently difficult and often unsatisfactory. A pri-

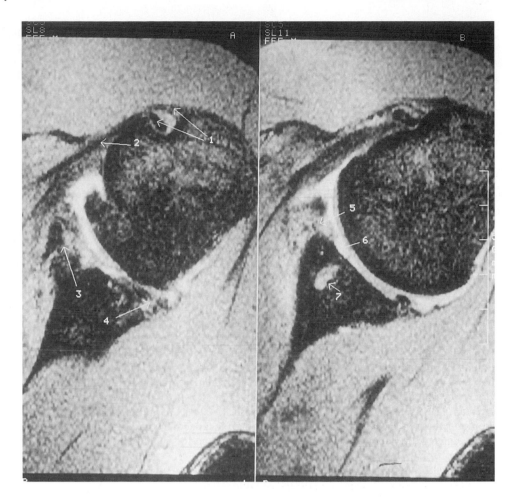

FIGURE 37–15 Two axial-gradient echo images in a patient with multidirectional instability. The long head of the biceps tendon in the intertuberculous groove *(1)* is shown with the bridging transverse ligament. The subscapularis tendon *(2)* inserting on the lesser tuberosity is shown. The Bankhart complex *(3)* of anterior band of the inferior glenohumeral ligament avulsion with labral tear is demonstrated, as is posterior fragmentation *(4)*, similar to posterior or Bennett equivalent. A displaced, fragmented anterior labrum is also seen *(5)* along with high-grade chondromalacia, with bright fluid replacing the adjoining gray hyaline *(6)*, and subchondral cyst *(7)*.

mary consideration for treatment should be combating spasticity if present, as this can play an important role. Strategies should begin with the onset of shoulder plegia with the goal of prevention. Commonly used medications include baclofen, dantrolene sodium, and diazepam, for which each patient should be evaluated individually. Heat and cold modalities can also be helpful, as can lidocaine or phenol motor point blocks.

Proper positioning should begin early. The shoulder should be positioned in abduction and external rotation while in bed. Gentle, passive ROM exercises should be instituted early. Subluxation frequently occurs in the shoulder that is flaccid. An axillary cushion, attached with a harness bandage, can be used to correct the subluxation while sitting or standing. A hemi-sling or wheelchair arm support can also serve this function. The use of the hemi-sling has been questioned by some authors.[24] Regardless, any material used should be one that is easily manipulated by the patient with the unaffected hand. An axillary cushion or hemi-sling may also be utilized for correcting subluxation in patients with spasticity, but caution must be used, as these devices may increase the spasticity or contribute to an elbow flexion contracture.

Adhesive Capsulitis

Adhesive capsulitis, also referred to as frozen shoulder, is an abnormality which ordinarily develops gradually, with increasing pain and decreasing ROM. This occurs particu-

larly in glenohumeral internal and external rotation as well as abduction. There are three clinical phases in the classic description of adhesive capsulitis, which include pain, progressive stiffness, and then a phase of gradual improvement with return of motion. The most commonly identified predisposing factor for adhesive capsulitis is a period of immobility of the shoulder,[23] but other clinical conditions are associated (Table 37–5).

Neviaser[46] describes adhesive capsulitis as a distinct entity with four identifiable stages that are distinct arthroscopically. Stage I is clinically similar to early impingement syndrome and is often confused with rotator cuff disease. The motion is restricted little if at all at this stage. Arthroscopy at this stage shows an erythematous fibrinous pannus over the synovium, primarily around the dependent fold. The articular cartilage is normal in this condition. Treatment protocols for this entity, such as that utilized for rotator cuff disease, often fail. Inappropriate acromial arch

TABLE 37–5 Predisposing Factors for the Development of Adhesive Capsulitis

Immobility
Age between 40 and 60 yr
Female
Diabetes
Thyroid disease
Humeral lesions
Personality disorder

decompression often accelerates the disease process owing to postoperative immobility.

Stage II is characterized by pain with associated loss of motion in all planes. Arthroscopically, the synovium appears red, thickened, and inflamed. Adhesions across the dependent fold may be seen. There is loss of the space between the humeral head and glenoid as well as between the humeral head and biceps tendon.

Stage III is characterized by the transition from inflammatory synovitis to chronic fibrosis as well as a markedly decreased size of the dependent fold. There is complete obliteration of the space between the humeral head, glenoid, and biceps tendon.

There is no longer synovitis present in stage IV. The dependent fold has become severely contracted by this stage, and clinically the shoulder motion is severely limited.

Diagnosis

An adequate history is essential for evaluation of the painful and stiff shoulder. Bilaterality can suggest an underlying systemic disorder (see Table 38–5). The differential diagnosis includes hemarthrosis, aseptic necrosis of the humeral head, infection (to be strongly considered in the elderly or immunocompromised), RCT, and anterior capsular tear. The usual history is the insidious onset of a stiff painful shoulder. The pain is ordinarily poorly localized but frequently most intense at the posterior and superior aspects of the shoulder.

Initially, the motion limitation may appear secondary to guarding from pain, but eventually, measurable limitation in both active and passive ROM in different planes is demonstrated. The patient often attempts to overcome the restricted glenohumeral movement with the use of accessory muscles and excessive compensatory scapular rotation. In normal scapulohumeral rhythm there is a 2:1 ratio of movement of the humerus to the scapula during 180 degrees of abduction. Of this 180 degrees, 120 degrees occurs at the glenohumeral joint and 60 degrees at the scapulothoracic joint.[62] This normal ratio is frequently disrupted in adhesive capsulitis because of excessive compensatory scapular rotation. The incorporation of accessory muscle strain can lead to additional painful cervical and shoulder musculature. Tenderness over the AC joint and biceps tendon is frequently associated.

Radiographs are of limited value in diagnosing adhesive capsulitis. The findings are inconsistent and nonspecific. Often mild degenerative changes of the glenohumeral joint and AC joint are seen as well as osteopenia. Bone scans have been studied and have been found to have limited usefulness.[3]

Although the diagnosis is ordinarily made clinically, if in doubt, it can be confirmed by an arthrogram. This may demonstrate loss of the ordinarily loose dependent fold of the joint and a dramatic decrease in the volume of contrast material that can be injected. A reduction of the normal 25 to 35 mL of joint volume to under 10 mL is seen.[46] An irregular joint outline with incomplete filling of the axillary fold, subacromial bursa, and biceps tendon sheath is frequently seen. The pain can often be reproduced by distention of the joint and relieved by withdrawing some of the

contrast fluid. The findings at athrography are not useful for prognosis or staging, however. Subacromial injection with 10 mL of lidocaine can be used to differentiate adhesive capsulitis from rotator cuff disease, as previously described. The role of arthroscopic evaluation in this condition is unclear. Although arthroscopy was used to develop the staging system by Neviaser, this is not considered a standard diagnostic procedure for this condition, and its role is limited to the detection of other possible shoulder disorders.

Treatment

There is some disagreement in the literature regarding the natural course of adhesive capsulitis. Some report it a self-limited condition that will improve spontaneously over a 1- to 2-year period.[5, 21, 36] Others think there is a significant subset of patients who will develop, without adequate treatment, persistent symptoms and disability. Irrespective of this opinion, few people can accept a full year of significant disability, and therefore aggressive treatment is warranted to accelerate recovery.

When the diagnosis has been established, the treatment goal is to control pain to facilitate progressive ROM. NSAIDs, analgesics, heat modalities, and intensive physical therapy are utilized with progression to a home exercise program. The emphasis of the therapy is passive stretching of the shoulder capsular contracture in all planes of motion. Although many modalities have demonstrated limited efficacy, including transcutaneous electrical nerve stimulation (TENS), pulley traction, corticosteroid injections, ice, and heat, most show limited value in altering the course of the disease[23, 60] when used by themselves. However, most of their value is in reducing pain in the primary stages to facilitate increased ROM.

The use of corticosteroid injections, although a popular technique, has little supportive literature to demonstrate its efficacy. Accurate location of the glenohumeral joint with the injecting needle is a problem with severe contracture. Rizk and colleagues[60] showed no significant difference in outcome between the use of lidocaine and steroid injections, but there was improved temporary pain relief with the use of steroid. The same study also demonstrated no significant difference in either intrabursal or intra-articular injection. Although one to two steroid injections may have a beneficial effect early in the course of rehabilitation, repeated injections are to be discouraged and can have an adverse effect on tissue healing.

Codman's exercises are the most frequently used for improving ROM. Efficacy can be increased with the use of wrist weights. These exercises can be easily performed by the patient at home after proper instruction (Fig. 37–16).

Some advocate the use of distention arthrography or infiltration brisement. With this technique, a combination of local anesthetic and saline is injected into the glenohumeral joint to produce hydraulic distention of the capsule and lysis of adhesions. This is ordinarily performed under general anesthesia. Many authors have reported good results.[23]

Manipulation under anesthesia is considered if the patient has poor progress with the therapy program. Manipulation is performed with forced abduction of the humerus

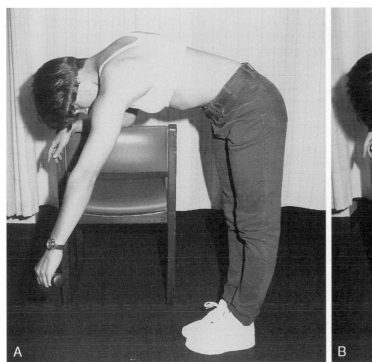
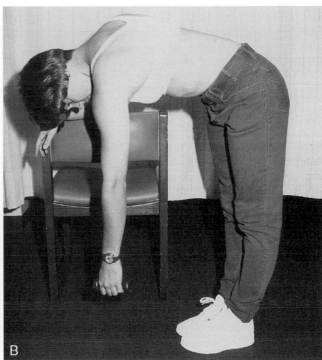

FIGURE 37–16   *A* and *B*, Demonstration of Codman's pendulum exercises. The patient uses the body to range the passive-dependent upper limb.

while fixing the scapula. This is performed with the shoulder in pure glenohumeral abduction because most of the contracture and capsular adhesions are in the dependent fold.[46] The goal is to obtain ROM as close to that of the normal opposite shoulder as possible. Physiatric care should begin the same day of the procedure with attention to positioning in bed. The patient is placed in bed with the arm restrained to maintain abduction of 90 degrees and external rotation as far as that obtained during the manipulation. Emphasis is placed on performing ROM of internal and external rotation with abduction maintained at 90 degrees as well as increasing elevation and flexion. For the next few days the arm is maintained above 90 degrees to avoid approximation of the dependent fold edges. After this, the arm is allowed down only for short periods, primarily to perform pendulum exercises. During this period the patient should sleep in a sling that maintains the arm in the abducted position as well as participate in a formal daily physical therapy program and a home exercise program. Proper patient education and close follow-up in the home setting are essential to ensure success.

Posterior capsulitis is a common cause of posterior shoulder pain. The posterior capsule can go through repeated microtrauma and tearing during the follow-through phase of throwing. This condition can remain inflamed, become calcific, and result in decreased internal rotation of the shoulder. This is frequently associated with inflammation of the long head of the triceps tendon at its attachment to the inferior glenoid rim. It may respond to a single steroid injection. This should be performed with the patient in the prone position with the arm hanging off the table in 90 degrees of shoulder flexion.

ELBOW PAIN

Lateral

Lateral Epicondylitis

Lateral epicondylitis is a common clinical condition frequently referred to as tennis elbow. A significant number of people who participate in tennis are afflicted with this ailment at one time or another.[49] The vast majority of patients seen with this condition, however, are manual laborers, office workers, or homemakers who engage in repetitive manual activities.

There is considerable controversy in the literature regarding the precise cause as well as pathological changes that occur in lateral epicondylitis. A widely accepted belief is that an inflammatory lesion with degeneration occurs at the insertion of the extensor tendons, primarily the extensor carpi radialis brevis (ECRB), with eventual fibrous adherence to the capsule[47] (Fig. 37–17). This is an area where Sharpey's fibers enter the periosteum on the lateral epicondyle of the humerus. Also closely involved is the origin of the superficial part of the supinator, which is in very close proximity to the origin of the ECRB at the lateral epicondyle, as well as the elbow joint capsule. Other muscles that are thought to possibly contribute are the extensor carpi radialis longus and the extensor digitorum communis, which originate in close proximity. Continued inflammation and fraying occur at this area with ongoing repetitive use of the wrist extensors. Hypervascularity, granulation tissue, and fibrosis in the extensor aponeurosis and in the subaponeurotic space of the elbow can develop as well as contracture of the anterolateral elbow capsule.[7]

Lateral epicondylitis usually occurs in persons over 35

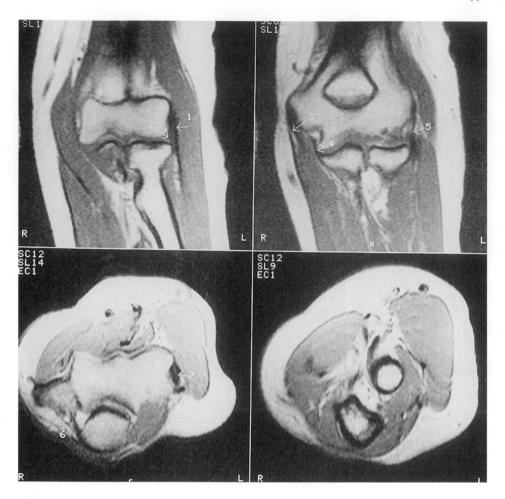

FIGURE 37–17 MRI series depicting the anatomical relationships about the elbow. The coronal views demonstrate the common extensor tendon (1), the lateral collateral ligament (2), the common flexor tendon (3), and the medial collateral ligament (4). The biceps insertion in shown on the axial view (8).

years old. Patients often present with a history of chronic activity involving repetitive flexion-extension of the wrist or pronation-supination of the forearm. However, in many instances, no predisposing event is established. The onset may be gradual or sudden.

In tennis players, it is believed that an incorrect tennis stroke can lead to the development of lateral epicondylitis. Poor technique can produce excessive stress on the forearm muscles and tendons and ligaments around the elbow joint.[25] The backhand is the most common stroke that elicits symptoms. When performed with the arm in full pronation and the trunk leaning backward at the point of impact, further stress is produced on the elbow extensors, as compared with a high-quality backhand with the forearm in mid-pronation and the trunk leaning forward[48] (Fig. 37–18).

On examination there is tenderness over the lateral epicondyle, usually at the origin of the ECRB. There is increased pain with resisted wrist extension, which is greater with a straight elbow. Pain can be maximally reproduced by having the patient make a fist, pronate the forearm, and radially deviate the wrist while performing this maneuver.

The middle finger test can also be performed. This involves resisting the extension of the proximal interphalangeal joint of digit 3. This produces stress on the extensor digitorum and ECRB and is considered positive if pain is elicited over the lateral epicondyle.

Routine anteroposterior (AP) and lateral radiographs are

of little help with this condition. Oblique views of the lateral epicondyle may show irregularity or punctate calcification around the origin of the ECRB. EMG is not helpful in the evaluation of lateral epicondylitis, except in identifying entrapment neuropathies.

Primary in treatment of this condition is decreasing repetitive stress. Avoidance of painful activities, particularly repetitive wrist flexion-extension and forearm pronation-supination, is important. For athletes or laborers in whom complete elimination is not a reasonable option, activity modification should be developed to minimize stress on the lateral epicondyle. An example of this is stroke modification in tennis players, as already discussed. Equipment modification can also provide benefit. In tennis, the proper handle size should be ensured (usually enlarging it) and the string tension should be reduced.

Anti-inflammatory medication can be a useful adjunct to reducing inflammation when initiating therapy. Heat modalities such as hot packs, short-wave diathermy, or heat lamps may provide symptomatic relief. Ultrasound can be applied directly to the inflamed area at the lateral epicondyle at 1.5 to 2.0 W/cm^2 in a continuous fashion once or twice a day for up to 10 days. Ice is useful to minimize the inflammatory response and should be applied after the inciting activity. An injection of steroid and xylocaine can be useful for temporary relief and confirmation of the diagnosis. This is injected directly over the point of maximal tenderness with care not to enter the tendon itself.

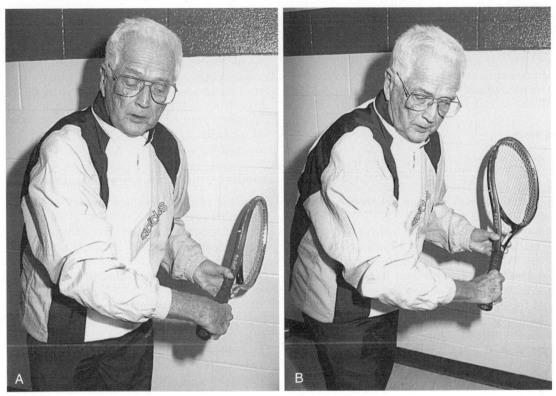

FIGURE 37–18   *A*, Demonstration of incorrect tennis form. Note the flexed and pronated wrist, improper forward lean, and lead with the elbow. This position places greater stress on the extensor mechanism with ball strike. *B*, Proper tennis form, with a straight wrist and appropriate body positioning.

Forearm bands (lateral elbow counterforce braces) have become popular in recent years (Fig. 37–19). The purpose is to prevent full muscular forearm expansion and alleviate tension on the attachment site at the lateral epicondyle.

Proper exercise is probably the most significant intervention for producing long-term benefit. We suggest a technique of using 10 repetitive maximum (10 RM) of the wrist extensors with the elbow flexed to 90 degrees, and then repeated with the elbow extended to 180 degrees. One set of 10 is done with the elbow extended to 180 degrees and the wrist over the end of a table and one set with the elbow flexed to 90 degrees. The specific technique is the slow wrist extension followed by slowly allowing the wrist into full flexion. The eccentric, or lengthening, contraction as the weight is lowered is perhaps the most important. The RM weight is determined by experimentation. It ordinarily should start with 6 to 10 lbs and increase gradually each week. This series of exercises should continue for 4 to 8 weeks. The exercises should be performed both at morning and at night. The weights can be dumbbells or another

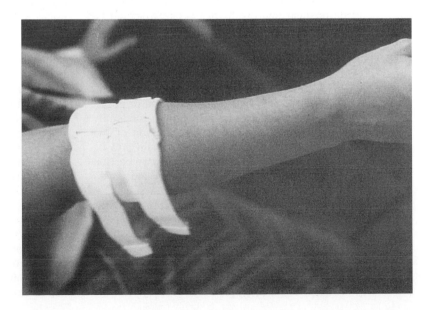

FIGURE 37–19   "Tennis elbow" band.

form of improvised weights. Discomfort might increase during the first week or two, but continuation can be facilitated by appropriate use of heat modalities and a short course of NSAIDs (10 days).

Many operative procedures have been described for this condition. Lateral extensor release is considered by some to be the surgical procedure of choice.[71]

Bone Trauma

Osteochodritis dissecans of the capitellum is commonly seen in patients younger than 25 years who present with joint pain and occasional locking. Plain films often demonstrate fragmentation of the capitellum associated with an elbow effusion.

Similarly, a history of trauma, often a direct blow or fall on an extended arm with the elbow locked, may lead to suspicion of an occult radial head fracture. Direct palpable tenderness is seen with the thumb over the radial head as the forearm is moved through pronation and supination.

Avulsion of the distal biceps tendon at the elbow is an uncommon injury. It is ordinarily without a prerupture syndrome and it is usually due to a single, acute event, often a traumatic or heavy lifting episode with the elbow flexed to 90 degrees.

Medial

Medial Epicondylitis

Pain localized to the medial aspect of the elbow suggests other diagnostic entities often related to valgus distraction forces on the medial joint structures. Medial epicondylitis, also known as "pitcher's elbow" or "golfer's elbow," develops as a result of a medial stress overload on the flexor musculature and medial collateral ligament (MCL) at the elbow. It is seen frequently in the skeletally immature, primarily in 9- to 15-year-old boys, as a physeal injury, as a result of throwing stresses (i.e., little leaguer's elbow).[48]

Critical components of the history include an acute onset or exacerbation of symptoms, which may suggest an MCL tear, epiphyseal fracture, or flexor tendon tear, whereas an insidious onset is more typical of medial epicondylitis. Bony spurring or ulnar neuropathy at the elbow should be considered in cases of chronic progression. Identification of detailed activity patterns and their relationship to pain is necessary, not only to assist with the diagnosis but also for appropriate long-term management.

The specific site of tenderness should be identified on physical examination to rule out triceps insertion or posterior elbow injury. The characteristic pain can be elicited by stressing the flexor tendons with resisted flexion at the wrist or forced wrist extension. The elbow should also be evaluated for limited or excessive ROM, in comparison with the uninjured side, as well as examined for laxity with varus and valgus stress.

Avulsion fractures and osteochondral defects are often identified using a standard series of AP, lateral, and oblique plain radiographs. Physeal separation in adolescents is difficult to identify and may require comparison views of the noninjured elbow or the use of higher-technology imaging.

Treatment for this entity is essentially the same as that previously described for lateral epicondylitis, only with the emphasis on the strengthening of the flexor muscles of the forearm as well as the use of modalities for pain relief.

Common flexor tendon avulsions are rare, whereas chronic tendinopathy is frequently seen with repetitive motion disorders. Chronic flexor tendinopathy typically presents in a manner similar to medial epicondylitis. These are difficult to distinguish clinically. The point of maximal tenderness may be located more distally, although this is not a reliable sign. MRI can be used to gain a more precise anatomical localization.

Medial Collateral Ligament Trauma

Medial collateral ligament rupture is seen in skeletally mature throwers, and is believe to be due to excessive valgus force on the medial compartment. The late-cocking and acceleration phases of throwing produce the most significant stress on this area.[33] Flexor and pronator muscle tears, as well as ulnar neuropathy, may also be associated with MCL rupture.

MCL damage ordinarily presents with a history of chronic and repetitive trauma and pain but can be a result of an acute injury. On examination, valgus instability is invariably present. This should be determined by gently applying valgus stress to the medial aspect of the elbow while flexing the elbow to 25 degrees and externally rotating the humerus[41] (Fig. 37–20).

The ligament is most frequently torn off at the medial aspect of the coronoid process, and therefore the palpable tenderness is more severe on the ulnar aspect than the humeral side of the MCL. Ecchymosis may be present in an acute rupture.

Treatment consists of rest, ice, and a short course of NSAIDs until swelling and inflammation subside. Pain should be resolved and full ROM should be attained prior to gradually resuming throwing activities. This can require 6 weeks to 3 months. Patients who have been refractory to treatment beyond 6 months may be considered surgical candidates for ligament repair.

Posterior

Olecranon Bursitis

The olecranon bursa is one of the most frequently inflamed bursae in the human body and is seen very commonly in athletes involved in contact sports and in laborers[10] (Fig. 37–21). Of the bursae around the elbow that are labeled in Figure 37–21, inflammation of the superficial olecranon bursa is the most frequently seen. It can present as acute, chronic, or infectious.

Acute bursitis tends to occur as a result of a direct blow or prolonged pressure on the area. Tenderness and distention of the bursa is noted on physical examination. This must be differentiated from cellulitis. Tendinitis; acute arthritis, including crystalline arthropathies; and ligamentous injury are also included in the differential diagnosis. Joint motion is ordinarily not limited with olecranon bursitis, unless extreme flexion causes increased skin tension over the painful, swollen bursa. Treatment involves primarily prevention of recurrence and may consist of elbow pads or other appropriate covering, especially in athletes. Aspiration can be considered if the bursa is severely dis-

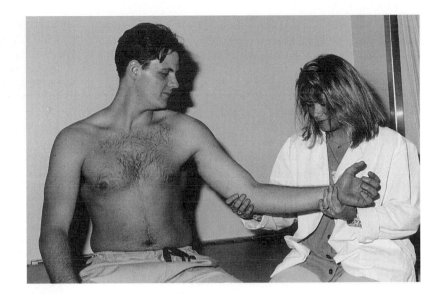

FIGURE 37-20 Evaluation for valgus instability.

tended and painful. Compression and cold packs can be applied in the first 72 hours to minimize bleeding into the area. Beyond this period, heat can be applied to hasten resorption of the bursal fluid.

Chronic olecranon bursitis occurs from repeated traumatic episodes and results in thickening and fibrosis of the bursal lining. This is seen commonly as an occupational disorder resulting from repeated traumatic exposures. Many cases present after an acute traumatic episode superimposed upon a more chronic inflammation. Examination findings are similar to those seen in acute trauma, but fibrous trabeculation of the bursal sac may often be palpated. Aspiration is frequently indicated and should be followed by a compressive dressing to minimize the tendency of the bursa to refill. Steroid injections are not indicated for acute bursitis as they tend to inhibit the

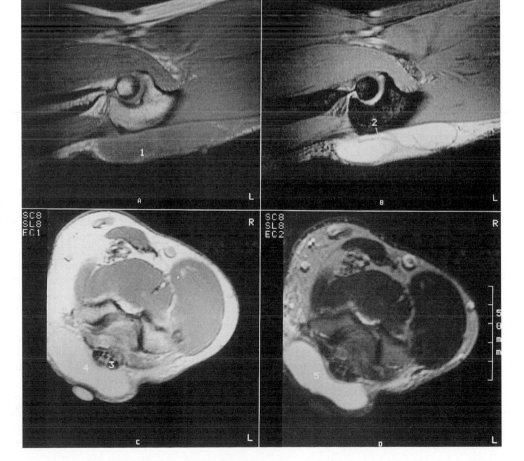

FIGURE 37-21 MRI series in a patient with olecranon bursitis. The sagittal views demonstrate the distended olecranon bursa in both the T1-weighted *(1)* and T2-weighted *(2)* images. The triceps tendon *(3)* is seen in the axial view, and the olecranon bursa is re-demonstrated *(4* and *5).*

normal protective mechanisms against infection. They have only limited success in chronic bursitis. Surgical removal of the bursa is an option in severe refractory or chronic bursitis.

Septic bursitis is diagnosed with aspiration.[22] It should be suspected with the presentation of warmth and erythema. Septic fluid may appear purulent or bloody. The fluid should be sent for Gram's stain, crystal determination, cell count, and culture. Septic joint fluid shows a predominance of polymorphonuclear cells, whereas mononuclear cells tend to predominate in nonseptic fluid. The most common infectious organism is *Staphylococcus aureus*. Treatment involves appropriate antibiotics.

Triceps Tendinitis

Another common cause of posterior elbow pain is triceps tendinitis.[48] This is seen frequently in persons involved in activities with rapid elbow extension, such as throwers and fly fisherman, and repetitive in motion occupations, such as carpentry. This is managed similarly to the lateral and medial epicondylitides, with the hallmark of treatment involving reduction of inflammation and activity modification.

WRIST PAIN

De Quervain's Tenosynovitis

In 1895 de Quervain[14] originally noted a condition of stenosing tenosynovitis. He described five women who exhibited pain and swelling of the tendon sheath of the

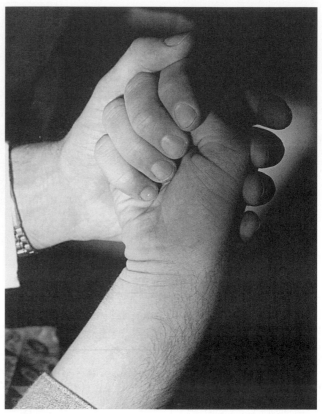

FIGURE 37–23 Demonstration of Finkelstein's test. The wrist is forced into ulnar deviation with the thumb flexed and abducted. Pain is exacerbated in a positive test.

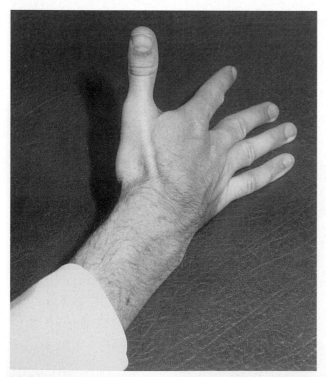

FIGURE 37–22 Demonstration of the surface anatomy of the "anatomical snuff-box." The dorsal aspect is the extensor pollicis longus tendon, and the volar is the extensor pollicis brevis tendon in close proximity to the abductor pollicis longus tendon.

abductor pollicis longus (APL) and extensor pollicis brevis (EPB) muscles near the area of the radial styloid at the wrist. He noted that there was localized thickening of the tendon sheath in that area, which he attributed to increased friction at that point.

This syndrome has become widely recognized and is called, appropriately enough, de Quervain's tenosynovitis. In this condition, swelling and palpable tenderness of the APL and EPB tendon sheaths at the lateral border of the "anatomical snuff-box" are noted as characteristically described (Fig. 37–22).

This disorder of the first dorsal compartment is often associated with a history of rapid repetitive movements of occupational and avocational stresses and less commonly with rheumatoid arthritis. The diagnosis is confirmed by localized tenderness and a positive Finkelstein's test (Fig. 37–23). In the absence of a history of predisposing activities, rheumatoid arthritis should be considered, with appropriate serological and rheumatologic testing.

The primary focus of treatment in this condition is the reduction of inflammation. This involves activity alteration, which can include the use of splinting in severe cases, NSAIDs, and local steroid injection into the tendon sheath. Surgical release of the tendon sheaths is considered in severe refractory cases.

Acute and Occult Wrist Injuries

Acute wrist injuries with their attendant osseous, ligamentous, and tendinous manifestations usually present to emergency medicine or orthopedic specialists. Physiatrists are often involved when undiagnosed pain persists more than 4 to 6 weeks, at which time subtle fractures and their complications have to be included in the differential diagnosis. Repeat plain radiographs or use of bone scanning can often detect occult bony pathologic changes. Complications of radial fractures (Colles') typically present at this time and are the most commonly seen wrist injuries of this nature.

Scaphoid Injuries

The scaphoid is the most commonly injured carpal bone.[9] It transfers axial loads from the distal radius to the distal carpal row. A common mechanism of injury involves a direct fall on an outstretched arm with a dorsiflexed wrist. The degree of dorsiflexion and the amount of radial or ulnar deviation influence the specific site of fracture (distal, waist, proximal).

The diagnosis of a scaphoid fracture is made from the classic traumatic history described, in the presence of pain and tenderness over its location at the anatomical snuffbox. There is ordinarily little outward visible evidence of this fracture. Plain radiographs with AP, lateral, and radial and ulnar oblique views should be obtained if this fracture is suspected (Fig. 37–24B). Views that stress the carpal bones should be obtained to evaluate for scapholunate dissociation if the problem has been long-standing. A bone scan should be considered in patients with negative radiographs but for whom there remains a strong clinical suspicion of bone trauma.

The patient with negative x-ray films who displays a classic history and physical findings should nonetheless be placed in a short arm-thumb spica cast and re-evaluated in 2 weeks. Meticulous follow-up for this condition is imperative in light of the high incidence of scaphoid non-union that occurs following fracture.

Understanding anatomical considerations such as fracture pattern and blood supply are essential for appropriate management. Non-union occurs in increasing frequency

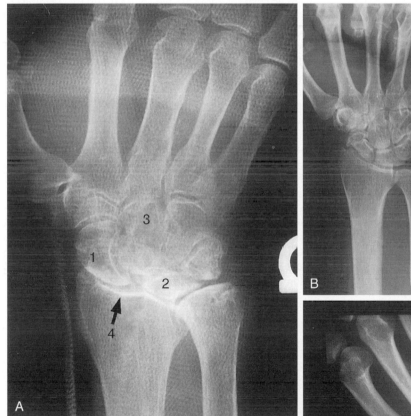
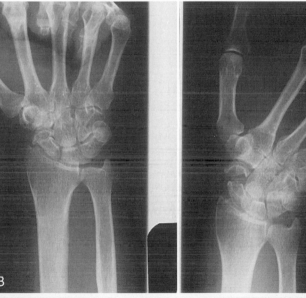
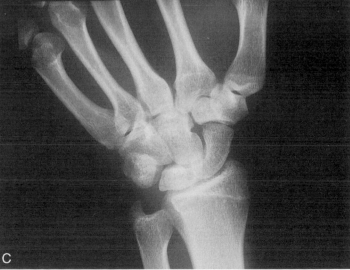

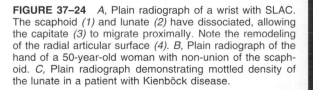

FIGURE 37–24 *A,* Plain radiograph of a wrist with SLAC. The scaphoid *(1)* and lunate *(2)* have dissociated, allowing the capitate *(3)* to migrate proximally. Note the remodeling of the radial articular surface *(4). B,* Plain radiograph of the hand of a 50-year-old woman with non-union of the scaphoid. *C,* Plain radiograph demonstrating mottled density of the lunate in a patient with Kienböck disease.

based on the location of the fracture from distal to proximal. This correlates directly with the degree of blood supply, which is quite variable throughout the length of the scaphoid.

Nondisplaced fractures in the distal third, which has an excellent blood supply, frequently heal effectively within a 6-week period with proper immobilization. Fractures in the middle third or the waist of the scaphoid are reported to have up to a 30% incidence of non-union despite adequate immobilization. Non-union can occur in as high as 90% of patients with fracture in the proximal third of the scaphoid, which has the poorest blood supply.[9] Scaphoid non-union can be relatively asymptomatic but is associated with a high incidence of the late development of osteoarthritis or carpal collapse.[38] The fracture can be treated with pulsed electromagnetic stimulation to promote healing if it is less than 5 years old, relatively asymptomatic, and there is an absence of significant degenerative changes. Surgical intervention for open reduction and internal fixation, including possible bone grafting, is considered in patients with long-term symptomatology or degenerative carpal changes.[12]

Kienböck Disease

Another common source of occult bone pain was first described by Kienböck in 1910.[31] Kienböck disease presents as wrist pain with sclerosis and collapse of the lunate secondary to avascular necrosis (Fig. 37–24C).

The precise cause of this condition is not well understood, but it is most common in the dominant wrist in 15- to 40-year-old males, most of whom give a history of preceding trauma. Surgical treatment is indicated when satisfactory relief of pain is not obtained with conservative management.[34]

Osteoarthritis of the Carpometacarpal Joint of the Thumb

Another common source of pain about the wrist and hand occurs at the carpometacarpal joint of the thumb. It is the most frequent site of osteoarthritis in the upper limb and commonly the most disabling, particularly in persons over 60 years old.

Scapholunate Advanced Collapse

The most common form of chronic wrist arthritis is scapholunate advanced collapse. This is a post-traumatic rotary subluxation that causes the scaphoid and lunate to separate and the capitate to migrate proximally. The ensuing impingement and osteoarthritic change may result in neuropathies and extensive arthropathic changes. This entity is readily determined on plain radiographs (Fig. 37–24A).

Other focal pain syndromes of the wrist are often associated with the presence of ganglia, intercarpal ligament tears, and failed carpal tunnel surgery.

HAND PAIN

Dupuytren's Contracture

Fibrous contracture of the palmar fascia leading to flexion contractures of the fingers was originally described by Clive in 1808. This subsequently became known as Dupuytren's contracture after the surgeon who described the first operation for its treatment.[8] The cause is unknown. The condition is more prevalent in men than women and is seen most frequently in the fifth to seventh decade. It is often unilateral but can present bilaterally as well. It most frequently involves the fourth or fifth digit.

Thickening of the palmar fascia is the hallmark of this condition (Fig. 37–25). As the fascia thickens progressively, the penetrating nutrient arteries are compromised, leading to further thickening, contracture, and atrophy of the overlying skin.

A classification system proposed by Shaw[8, 65] distinguishes the progression of a nodule of the palmar fascia (stage I), to a nodule with involvement of the skin (stage II), to subsequent flexion contractures of one or more fingers (stage III), to the final stage (stage IV) with fixed tendon and joint contractures.

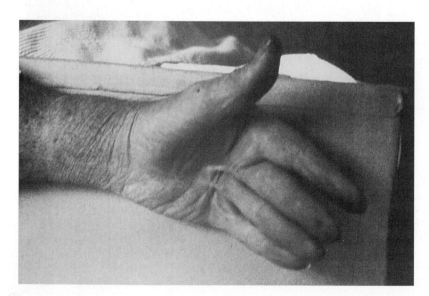

FIGURE 37–25 Hand of a 63-year-old man with Dupuytren's contracture.

Failure to establish the proper diagnosis can lead to inappropriate attempts at progressive stretching, which are typically of no benefit. Continued extensor stress may cause progression of the syndrome. Surgical release is the treatment of choice. However, it might only be indicated with severe digital contracture.

Gamekeeper's (Skier's) Thumb

Gamekeeper's thumb is characterized by an injury to the ulnar collateral ligament and insertion of the adductor pollicis. It is seen frequently in skiers and is associated with resultant instability. It can occur with acute trauma or develop gradually with acute stress. This condition is identified on physical examination by swelling and tenderness over the metacarpophalangeal joint of the thumb, pain with passive motion, and weakness in pinch. It can occasionally be identified radiographically. Surgical repair is typically the treatment of choice.

Trigger Finger

Acute or chronic inflammation and flexor tendinitis can result in a disproportion between the flexor tendon and its sheath. Subsequent constriction at the pulley near the level of the metacarpal head is associated with painful snapping of the flexor tendons. This condition is called trigger finger, or stenosing tenovaginitis.

Treatment consists of a local steroid injection, which can be repeated once if the condition is refractory. Splinting following the injections can also be beneficial. Highly resistant cases may require surgery. Complications such as postoperative bowstringing, painful scarring, and digital nerve injuries can occur.

Mallet Finger

Mallet finger occurs as a result of a tear of the extensor tendon from its attachment on the distal phalanx. This is usually due to an acute flexion injury when the extensor tendon is taut. In the majority of cases, the tendon itself is torn from the insertion, but a significant percentage sustains a bone avulsion.

Conservative treatment includes immobilization of the distal phalanx in hyperextension with the middle phalanx in flexion for approximately 6 to 10 weeks. Surgical repair is considered if functional recovery is inadequate.

Raynaud's Phenomenon

Vasomotor instability, often triggered by cold or stress, results in a syndrome of pain, a burning sensation, cyanosis, numbness, and swelling of the upper extremities. This is referred to as Raynaud's phenomenon, and is believed to be a result of increased sympathetic response to stress.

It is ordinarily bilateral and is most frequently seen in women in their 40s. The classic appearance of color changes from white to blue to red is often observed. This occurs as sudden pallor of the fingers, progressing to cyanosis, and eventually hyperemia with reflex dilation. Although most frequently seen alone (primary), it can occasionally be the first clinical sign of scleroderma, other collagen-vascular disorders, or vasculitides (secondary)

Management of this condition consists of patient reassurance and avoidance of precipitating factors such as a cold environment and handling cold objects. Nicotine is a known precipitant and smoking should be discontinued. Biofeedback has been reported to be effective in many patients.[64] Medical management with β-blockers or sympathectomies can be considered but produce inconsistent results.

HETEROTOPIC OSSIFICATION

The abnormal formation of mature lamellar bone in soft tissue is called heterotopic ossification (HO). This is characterized by a matrix and crystalline form of true bone, which develops outside the confines of normal periosteum and with a distinct vascular supply. There are multiple precipitating factors which include neurological insult, burns, direct trauma, or surgery, as well as hereditary disorders. In neurogenic diseases, such as spinal cord injury, it typically develops below the level of the lesion.

Its development is initiated by a nonspecific inflammatory phase with symptoms generally beginning 1 to 3 months after the inciting event. Osteoid deposition follows the inflammatory phase.

Diagnosis

In the upper limb, HO is most often seen in the shoulder and elbow. It is generally characterized by swelling, moderate pain, joint limitation, localized warmth, tenderness, and, occasionally, low-grade fever. Elevated alkaline phosphatase levels may be present early in this condition.[32] The specificity is increased if the levels are fractionated. Radiological studies performed early in the course of the disease often are normal, with calcifications appearing later. Bone scanning is more sensitive early in the process and shows increased uptake prior to any findings on plain films. This reflects the increased vascularity and ongoing calcium deposition.

Treatment

Treatment consists of the use of ROM exercises to maintain joint function as the ectopic bone matures. Modalities for pain relief and the use of NSAIDs for their anti-inflammatory effect, with indomethacin (Indocin) being the most studied,[63] are useful to help facilitate this. Etidronate disodium (Didronel) has been extensively described for use early in the course of the disease to minimize eventual ossification. Its long-term benefit remains in doubt.[6] Criteria for its use include early recognition prior to ossification being evident on plain films. Its detractors believe its use, at best, merely delays the inevitable ossification.

Although the prophylactic perioperative use of local radiation treatment can be effective for prevention of the process,[2] its indications and uses are complex and controversial and beyond the scope of this discussion.

Surgical removal in the acute phases prior to the completion of the ossification process is contraindicated. Aggressive recurrence is likely if surgical intervention is premature. Bone scanning should be performed to ensure no active process is ongoing. Fractionated alkaline phosphatase levels can also contribute helpful information.

REFLEX SYMPATHETIC DYSTROPHY

Reflex sympathetic dystrophy (RSD) is a syndrome involving a chronic painful condition of the upper limb associated with neurovascular disturbance and dystrophic changes of the skin and bones. There is painful impairment of the shoulder and swelling and tenderness of the hand. Typically the elbow is spared. Other names that have been given to this constellation of signs and symptoms include Sudeck's atrophy, causalgia, and shoulder-hand syndrome.

This syndrome is attributed to autonomic, particularly sympathetic, instability. The appearance of this condition in common physiatric practice is high. RSD is believed to be present in up to 10% to 15% of all patients with hemiplegia and painful shoulders.[13] Common predisposing events, other than a neurological insult such as stroke, often initiate the formation of RSD and include trauma of all severities, thoracic surgery, cervical radiculopathy, and myocardial infarction. A substantial number of these syndromes develop without any known precipitating event.[67] A psychological basis or predisposition for the development of this condition is possible but not well-substantiated in the literature.[37, 52]

The disease process ordinarily progresses through different stages. Stage I typically lasts a few weeks to 6 months and is characterized by significant pain and increased blood flow with resultant pitting edema, redness, and warmth. Reduced ROM often begins to develop at this stage and is related, in part, to pain inhibition. Hyperhydrosis may begin. The skin can be hyperesthetic and tender. The development of osteoporosis is thought to begin at this stage but is usually not detectable on plain films.

Stage II typically lasts 3 to 6 months following stage I. The edema is often less predominant and is described as brawny or spreading. However, pain and further impairment of ROM are prominent features. There is a decreased blood flow and lowered temperature of the extremity. Hair and nail growth is diminished at this stage, and hyperhydrosis persists. Atrophy of muscle and the subcutaneous tissue develops. X-ray examination may reveal localized patchy osteoporosis as well as periarticular thickening. A "causalgia personality" has been described[15] and can be a feature at this stage.

Stage III can persist for additional months. This stage is characterized by less pain but progression to irreversible changes of atrophic soft tissue, muscle atrophy, severe loss of motion, and extensive osteoporosis. The skin appears smooth and glossy and is dry and cool. Other common features include coarse hair and ridged nails.

Diagnosis

The diagnosis is ordinarily made on a clinical basis, primarily with the use of the history and observation and the physical signs outlined above. The patient typically presents with a history of pain out of proportion to the injury. It ordinarily extends beyond the confines of dermatomal patterns. Descriptions such as burning, numbness, and tingling are often used. The patient is evaluated for swelling, dystrophic changes, muscle atrophy, and tenderness (Fig. 37–26).

Radiological evaluation can be helpful. However, changes may not be seen on plain films until the later stages of the disease, ordinarily after 3 months. Triple-phase bone scan can show increased uptake in the involved limb early in the process, possibly reflecting increased blood flow from localized bone turnover due to sympathetic vasoconstriction.[56] This is most significantly seen in the carpal and metacarpal joints in the hand. The findings do not, however, correlate accurately with the degree of vasomotor disturbances.

Treatment

A large majority of patients respond to systemic corticosteroids instituted in the acute phase of the disease. This underscores the importance of early recognition. Prednisone is used most frequently in doses up to 100 mg/day or 1 mg/kg, and tapered over 2 weeks. In the face of relapse, this treatment can be repeated. A wide range of drug interventions have been suggested and include NSAIDs, anticonvulsants, tricyclic antidepressants, β-blockers, calcium channel blockers, calcitonin, and even topical cap-

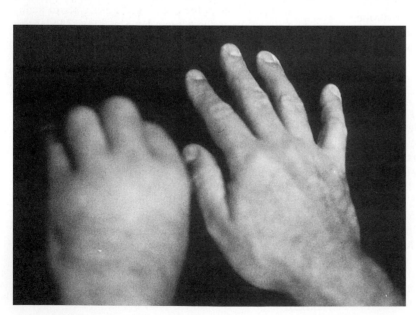

FIGURE 37–26 Reflex sympathetic dystrophy in the left hand of a 52-year-old man. Edema and dystrophic changes of the affected extremity are noted.

saicin. Although occasionally beneficial, typically disappointing or inconsistent results are obtained with these.

Graded activities are encouraged to facilitate a "desensitization" of the hypersensitive tissues. Aggressive activity to "overload" the painful input is the basic treatment for this condition.[29] Isotoner gloves are also beneficial for this purpose. Other techniques of desensitization include increasingly vigorous massage. Use of contrast baths has been also shown to be beneficial for this purpose. Reduction in distal edema can also occur with use of these modalities. Some have reported symptomatic improvement with the use of ultrasound,[53] but the mechanism is not clear. Other modalities that have been reported to be beneficial for providing symptomatic relief include TENS, paraffin baths, and pneumatic pumps.

The use of a local anesthetic block of the second or third sympathetic ganglia can often confirm the diagnosis as well as provide symptomatic relief. Other clinical signs reflecting response to injection include improvement in cyanosis and a rise in temperature of the affected limb of 1°C. Temporary procedures sometimes utilized other than stellate ganglia blockade include Bier block and peripheral nerve blocks. Sympathectomy is utilized when the chemical blocks have been effective but transient.

Following invasive procedures, emphasis must be placed on aggressive, progressive activity with the affected limb for optimal results. Early recognition is critical for intervention prior to the development of trophic changes seen in phase II and III. After this time, the prognosis for satisfactory recovery is poor.[66]

References

1. Andrews JR, Broussard TS, Carson WG: Arthroscopy of the shoulder in the management of partial tears of the rotator cuff: A preliminary report. Arthroscopy 1985;1:117.
2. Ayers DC, Evarts CM, Parkinson JR: The prevention of heterotopic ossification in high risk patients by low dose radiation after total hip arthroplasty. J Bone Joint Surg Am 1986;68:1423.
3. Binder AI, Bulgen DY, Hazelman BL, et al: Frozen shoulder: An arthrographic and radionuclide scan assessment. Ann Rheum Dis 1984;43:365–369.
4. Beach WR, Caspari RB: Arthroscopic management of rotator cuff disease. Orthopedics 1993;16:1007–1015.
5. Bulgen DY, Binder AI, Hazelman BL, et al: Frozen shoulder: Prospective clinical study with an evaluation of three treatment regimens. Ann Rheum Dis 1984;43:353–360.
6. Buschbacher R: Heterotopic ossification: A review. Crit Rev Phys Rehabil Med 1992;4:199–213.
7. Cabot A: Tennis elbow, a curable affliction. Orthop Rev 1987;16:69–73.
8. Cailliet R: Hand Pain and Impairment, ed 4. Cailliet Pain Series. Philadelphia, FA Davis, 1994, pp 179–182.
9. Calandra JJ, Goldner RD, Hardaker WT: Scaphoid fractures: Assessment and treatment. Orthopedics 1992;15:931–938.
10. Canoso JJ: Idiopathic or traumatic olecranon bursitis. Arthritis Rheum 1977;20:1213–1216.
11. Codman EA: The shoulder. Rupture of the Supraspinatus Tendon and Lesions in or About the Subacromial Bursa. Boston, Thomas Todd, 1934, pp 65–177.
12. Cooney WP, Dobyns MD, Linscheid RL: Nonunion of the scaphoid: Analysis of the results from bone grafting. J Hand Surg 1980;5:343–354.
13. Davis SW, Petrillo CR, Eichberg RD, et al: Shoulder-hand syndrome in a hemiplegic population: A 5-year retrospective study. Arch Phys Med Rehabil 1977;58:353–356.
14. de Quervain F: Ueber eine Form von chronischer Tendovaginitis. Cor-VI Schweiz Aerzte 1895;25:389–394.
15. DeGood DE, Cundiff GW, Adams LE, Shutty MS Jr: A psychosocial

and behavioral comparison of reflex sympathetic dystrophy, low back pain, and headache patients. Pain 1993;54:317–322.
16. Drakeford MK, Quinn MJ, Simpson SL, Pettine KA: A comparative study of ultrasonography and arthrography in evaluation of the rotator cuff. Clin Orthop 1990;253:118–122.
17. Fischbach TJ, Seeger LL: Magnetic resonance imaging of glenohumeral instability. Top Magn Reson Imaging 1994;6:121–132.
18. Fu FH, Harner CD, Klein AH: Shoulder impingement syndrome: A critical review. Clin Orthop 1991;269:162–173.
19. Hakuno A, Sashika H, Ohkawa T, Itoh R: Arthrographic findings in hemiplegic shoulders. Arch Phys Med Rehabil 1984;65:706–711.
20. Hawkins RJ, Kennedy JC: Impingement syndrome in athletes. Am J Sports Med 1980;8:151–157.
21. Hazelman BL: The painful stiff shoulder. Rheumatol Rehabil 1972;11:413–421.
22. Ho G, Tice AD, Kaplan SR: Septic bursitis in the prepatellar and olecranon bursae. Ann Intern Med 1978;89:21–27.
23. Hulstyn MJ, Weiss AC: Adhesive capsulitis of the shoulder. Orthop Rev 1993;22:425–432.
24. Hurd MM, Farrell KH, Waylonis GW: Shoulder sling for hemiplegia: Friend or foe? Arch Phys Med Rehabil 1974;55:519–522.
25. Ilfeld FW: Can stroke modification relieve tennis elbow? Clin Orthop 1992;276:182–186.
26. Itoi E, Tabata S: Conservative treatment of rotator cuff tears. Clin Orthop 1992;275:165–173.
27. Jobe FW: Impingement problems in the athlete. Instruct Course Lect 1989;38:205–209.
28. Jobe FW, Jobe CM: Painful athletic injuries of the shoulder. Clin Orthop 1983;173:117–124.
29. Johnson EW, Pannozzo AN: Management of shoulder-hand syndrome. JAMA 1966;195:108–110.
30. Joynt RL: The source of shoulder pain in hemiplegia. Arch Phys Med Rehabil 1992;73:409–413.
31. Kienböck R: Über traumatische Malazie des Mondbeins und ihre Folgezustände: Entartungsformen und Kompressionsfrakturen. Fortschr Geb Rontgenstr 1910;16:78–103.
32. Kim SW, Charter RA, Chai CJ, et al: Serum alkaline phosphatase and inorganic phosphorus value in spinal cord injury patients with heterotopic ossification. Paraplegia 1990;28:441–447.
33. King JW, Brelsford JH, Tullos HS: Analysis of the pitching arm of the professional baseball pitcher. Clin Orthop 1969;67.116.
34. Kuschner SH, Brien WW, Bindiger A, Sherman R: Review of treatment results for Kienböck's disease. Orthop Rev 1992;21:717–728.
35. Lee KH, Khunadorn F: Painful shoulder in hemiplegic patients: Study of the suprascapular nerve. Arch Phys Med Rehabil 1986;67:818–820.
36. Lee M, Haq AM, Wright V, et al: Periarthritis of the shoulder: A controlled trial of physiotherapy. Physiotherapy 1973;59:312–315.
37. Lynch ME: Psychological aspects of reflex sympathetic dystrophy: A review of the adult and pediatric literature. Pain 1992;49:337–347.
38. Mack GR, Boss MJ, Gelberman RH, Yu E: The natural history of scaphoid nonunion. J Bone Joint Surg Am 1984;66:504–509.
39. Meyer AW: The minute anatomy of attrition lesions. J Bone Joint Surg Am 1931;13:341–360.
40. Meyers JF: Arthroscopic management of the impingement syndrome in rotator cuff tears. Sports Med 1989;2:243–260.
41. Morrey BF, An KN: Stability of the elbow joint: A biomechanical assessment. Am J Sports Med 1984;12:315–319.
42. Morrison DS, Bigliani LU: Variations in acromial shape and its effect on rotator cuff tears. In The Shoulder. Tokyo, Professional Postgraduate Services 1987, pp 213–214.
43. Neer CS: Anterior acromioplasty for chronic impingement syndrome in the shoulder. A preliminary report. J Bone Joint Surg Am 1972;54:41–50.
44. Neer CS: Shoulder Reconstruction. Philadelphia, WB Saunders, 1990, pp 422–427.
45. Neer CS: Impingement lesions. Clin Orthop 1983;173:70–77.
46. Neviaser TJ: Adhesive capsulitis. Orthop Clin North Am 1987;18:439–443.
47. Neviaser TJ, Neviaser RJ, Neviaser JS, Ain BR: Lateral epicondylitis: Results of outpatient surgery and immediate motion. Contemp Orthop 1985;11:43–46.
48. Nirschl RP: Prevention and treatment of elbow and shoulder injuries in the tennis player. Clin Sports Med 1988;7:289–308.
49. Nirschl RP, Pettrone FA: Tennis elbow—The surgical treatment of lateral epicondylitis. J Bone Joint Surg Am 1979;61:832–839.

50. Olive RJ, Marsh HO: Ultrasonography of rotator cuff tears. Clin Orthop 1992;282:110–113.
51. Ozaki J, Fujimoto S, Nakagawa Y, et al: Tears of the rotator cuff of the shoulder associated with pathological changes in the acromion: A study in cadavers. J Bone Joint Surg Am 1988;70:1224.
52. Pak TJ, Martin GM, Nagness JL, Kavanaugh GJ: Reflex sympathetic dystrophy: Review of 140 cases. Minn Med 1970;53:507–512.
53. Portwood MM, Lieberman JS, Taylor RG: Ultrasound treatment of reflex sympathetic dystrophy. Arch Phys Med Rehabil 1987;68:116–118.
54. Post M, Silver R, Singh M: Rotator cuff tear, diagnosis and treatment. Clin Orthop 1983;173:78–91.
55. Poulin de Courval L, Barsauskas A, Berenbaum B, et al: Painful shoulder in the hemiplegic and unilateral neglect. Arch Phys Med Rehabil 1990;71:673–676.
56. Pollock FE Jr, Koman LA, Smith BP, et al: Patterns of microvascular response associated with reflex sympathetic dystrophy of the hand and wrist. J Hand Surg Am 1993;18:848–852.
57. Prevost R, Arsenault AB, Dutil E, et al: Shoulder subluxation in hemiplegia: A radiologic correlational study. Arch Phys Med Rehabil 1987;68:782–785.
58. Rathbun JB, Macnab I: The microvascular pattern of the rotator cuff. J Bone Joint Surg Br 1970;52:540–553.
59. Rizk TE, Christopher RP, Pinals RS, et al: Arthrographic studies in painful hemiplegic shoulders. Arch Phys Med Rehabil 1984;65:254–256.
60. Rizk TE, Pinals RS, Talaiver AS: Corticosteroid injections in adhesive capsulitis: Investigation of their value and site. Arch Phys Med Rehabil 1991;72:20–22.
61. Rockwood CA, Lyons FR: Shoulder impingement syndrome: Diagnosis, radiographic evaluation, and treatment with a modified Neer acromioplasty. J Bone Joint Surg Am 1993;75:409–424.
62. Rowe C: The Shoulder. New York, Churchill Livingstone, 1988.
63. Schmidt SA, Kjaersgaard-Anderson P, Pedersen NW, et al: The use of indomethacin to prevent the formation of heterotopic bone after total hip replacement. J Bone Joint Surg Am 1988;6:834–838.
64. Sedlacek K: Biofeedback treatment of primary Raynaud's disease. *In* Basmajian JV (ed): Biofeedback: Principles and Practice for Clinicians. 3rd ed. Baltimore, Williams & Wilkins, 1989.
65. Shaw MH: Treatment of Dupuytren's contracture. Br J Plast Surg 1951;4:218–223.
66. Steinbrocker O: The shoulder-hand syndrome: Present perspective. Arch Phys Med 1968;49:388.
67. Subbarao J, Stillwell GK: Reflex sympathetic dystrophy syndrome of the upper extremity: Analysis of total outcome of management of 125 cases. Arch Phys Med Rehabil 1981;62:549–554.
68. Uhthoff HK, Loehr J, Sarkar K: The pathogenesis of rotator cuff tears. *In* The Shoulder. Tokyo, Tokyo Professional Postgraduate Services, 1987, p 211.
69. Unverferth LJ, Olix ML: The effect of local steroid injections on tendon. J Sports Med 1973;1:31–37.
70. Van Ouwenaller C, Laplace PM, Chantraine A: Painful shoulder in hemiplegia. Arch Phys Med Rehabil 1986;6:23–36.
71. Verhaar J, Walenkamp G, Kester A, et al: Lateral extensor release for tennis elbow. J Bone Joint Surg Am 1993;75:1034–1043.
72. Warner J, Caborn DN: Overview of shoulder instability. Crit Rev Phys Rehabil Med 1992;4:145–198.
73. Zuckerman JD, Mirabello SC, Newman D: The painful shoulder: part II. Intrinsic disorders and impingement syndrome. Am Fam Physician 1991;43:497–512.

Musculoskeletal Disorders of the Lower Limbs

JEFFREY L. YOUNG, M.D., M.A.,
NICHOLAS K. OLSEN, D.O., AND
JOEL M. PRESS, M.D.

The overwhelming majority of musculoskeletal problems can be solved nonsurgically. However, in order for aggressive conservative treatment to be successful, the physician coordinating patient care must have the skills to make an accurate diagnosis, generate a logical differential diagnosis, and formulate a precise rehabilitation program. The physician should also be able to recognize when surgery is the best way to restore function. Acquiring a working knowledge of all the musculoskeletal ailments involving the hips, thighs, knees, lower legs, ankles, and feet is a formidable task, and cannot be achieved in a single chapter. The purpose of this chapter is not to be encyclopedic, but to provide the foundation for assessing a variety of musculoskeletal problems in the lower limbs, emphasizing those injuries which arise from repetitive musculotendinous overload.

MUSCULOSKELETAL HISTORY

A careful history is required to identify the diagnosis and mechanism of injury (see Chapter 1). The following is an overview of basic questions which need to be asked of the patient presenting with a musculoskeletal injury of the lower limbs.

CHRONOLOGY OF THE INJURY. When did the pain first appear? Was the onset of pain sudden or gradual? Has this happened before?

MECHANISM OF INJURY. Was trauma involved? Was the foot planted or in the air at the time of injury? Did the foot invert or evert? Was there a valgus or varus moment at the knee or was there a sense of rotational strain? Did the patient feel or hear a "pop" or a "snap?" Was there sudden inability to bear full body weight? A noncontact injury of the knee occurring with the foot planted, and accompanied by a valgus moment, rotation, and a pop, is classic for an acute disruption of the anterior cruciate ligament (ACL). A noncontact nonweightbearing injury in the posterior thigh occurring with the hip flexed, the knee extended, and accompanied by a pop suggests a hamstring tear.

NATURE OF THE PAIN. Is the pain constant or intermittent? What makes it more tolerable and what exacerbates it? Is it associated with weightbearing? If so, how soon does the pain occur after beginning activity? Is the pain highly localized or does it radiate to or from another area? Is the pain associated with inflammation? Pain associated with compartmental syndromes is often less apparent at rest and at the onset of exercise, but becomes worse after a relatively consistent amount of activity. Pain from a fracture is present at rest or provoked by minimal activity. Achy anterior knee pain worsened by squatting or prolonged sitting (i.e., the "theater sign") alerts the clinician to patellofemoral joint dysfunction, while anterior knee pain aggravated by maintaining full knee extension suggests infrapatellar fat pad irritation.[22, 29] A "pulled" calf muscle during a tennis match usually reflects musculotendinous overload of the medial gastrocnemius, while calf pain unassociated with exertion but worsened with forward spine flexion suggests lumbosacral radiculopathy. Tendinitis demonstrates the cardinal signs of inflammation (redness, swelling, and increased warmth) within a painful tendon. Tendinosis is painful, but lacks signs of inflammation.[79]

INJURY INVENTORY. How many other injuries have been sustained? What were the locations? Were they managed nonsurgically or surgically? The current injury is often preceded by a previous injury to that area which did not undergo proper rehabilitation.

AGE CONSIDERATIONS. The differential diagnosis of distal Achilles tendon pain in the skeletally immature runner must include calcaneal apophysitis (Sever's disease).

In the elderly runner it is much more likely to involve pathological changes within the tendon itself.[9, 10] Hip pain in the young athlete should raise suspicion of a femoral stress fracture or traction apophysitis, while the same symptoms in the elderly runner can indicate fracture or symptomatic spinal stenosis.[9, 10]

EXERCISE HABITS. How much does the patient exercise? Has there been a sudden increase in frequency, intensity, or duration of workouts? Does the patient routinely stretch before and after exercising? The patient who trains intensely every day of the week without varying the muscle groups exercised and who does not stretch is an obvious candidate for both musculotendinous overload and overtraining.

EQUIPMENT. What type of shoes does the patient use? How often are new pairs purchased and old pairs discarded? Does the patient wear shoe orthotic inserts? When were the inserts originally constructed and for what purpose? These questions help provide insight into potential errors of training and biomechanical imbalances. Shoes or inserts which have broken down and no longer serve their original intent are commonly seen and easily corrected problems. The reader is referred to articles by Subotnick[129] and Newell and Bramwell[98, 99] for excellent reviews of evaluating the foot and the role of foot orthoses. Orthotic devices are especially useful when placed to correct biomechanical imbalances that are not correctable by specific stretching and strengthening programs. In one survey study of 347 symptomatic runners whose average training was approximately 40 miles/week, 75% reported marked improvement or resolution of their symptoms with the use of the orthotic inserts.[51]

EXERCISE ENVIRONMENT. Where does the patient typically train? Does the runner train on a level dirt path, on a banked concrete surface, on a treadmill, or on a flat circular track? Poor running course selection can create imbalances at the level of the foot and ankle which are transmitted up the biomechanical chain to the more proximal structures. For example, running on a banked surface causes pronation of the "uphill" foot, which stresses the medial ankle, and creates a knee valgus force, hip abduction, and elevation of that hemipelvis. The "downhill" foot supinates more, which stresses the lateral ankle, and creates a knee varus force, hip adduction, and lowering of that hemipelvis.[21, 113]

REVIEW OF SYSTEMS. Is there a nonmusculoskeletal process contributing to the current problem? Does the middle-aged club tennis pro who presents with calf pain have signs of vascular claudication? Is the young female runner who presents with pelvic stress fractures amenorrheic and exhibiting signs of disordered body image? What medications are being used? Are anabolic steroids being taken? Has the patient been using narcotics for pain relief? Although the major focus of this chapter is musculoskeletal, other factors which can weigh heavily on the runner's overall health should be identified.

FUNCTION. How has this injury affected this person's life? Is the patient still working? Is this person still capable of performing all activities of daily living independently?

COPING SKILLS. Can this person tolerate relative or complete rest? How will this person react if true rest is required for an undetermined amount of time? Are there secondary gain issues at hand, and is there reason to be concerned about this patient developing a chronic pain problem? In taking a more holistic approach to the person with a musculoskeletal injury, input from a psychologist or psychiatrist can be essential to successful rehabilitation.

PHYSICAL EXAMINATION

Establishing a diagnosis-specific rehabilitation program requires a thorough physical examination. It is critical to adhere to the concept of the kinetic chain and to recognize that biomechanical dysfunction in one body region is capable of causing "injury at a distance." Consequently, it should be routine to examine the low back, hip, knee, and ankle regions in virtually all patients presenting with lower extremity complaints. The following section serves as an overview of the basic components of a physical examination. More specific tests are discussed within the region-specific problem sections.

The patient is evaluated during rest and ambulation. The examination at rest helps identify such entities as limb length discrepancy, scoliosis, excessive lordosis, pelvic asymmetry, genu varum or valgum, tibial torsion, side-to-side differences in muscle bulk, static ankle-foot deformities, blisters and calluses, and visible evidence of inflammation. The walking examination reveals signs of foot pronation or supination, early heel rise from a tight gastrocnemius-soleus complex, increased knee valgum or varum, and hip abductor weakness (*Trendelenburg's sign*). More subtle gluteus medius weakness can be discerned by having the patient walk with hands on hips, and watching the rise and fall of the elbows. The elbow contralateral to the weaker gluteus medius muscle will dip more during midstance.

For running athletes, video analysis of treadmill running at varying speeds with and without shoes and with and without orthotic devices is recommended. This enables the clinician to identify more subtle biomechanical imbalances, as well as flaws in running style. Video recordings are not only a useful diagnostic aid but also a vehicle for patient education. The recording and projecting system should be capable of high resolution when played at normal, fast-forward, or slow-motion speeds.

At the level of the ankle and foot, the following examination maneuvers are considered to be the minimum: palpation of the Achilles tendon, and origin and insertions of the plantar fascia; assessment of talar, subtalar, and midtarsal joint motion; and evaluation of laxity in the lateral and medial ligaments of the ankle. In cases where excessive pronation is identified, the *navicular drop test* is added. If the measured vertical descent of the navicular exceeds 1.5 cm when going from a position in which the entire foot is just touching the floor to one of full weightbearing on that side, there is considered to be excessive pronation.[122] Goniometric measurement of the subtalar joint to check for deviation from the normal 2:1 ratio of inversion to eversion through a 45-degree range and evaluation of the forefoot for presence of varus or valgus also aid in detecting areas of tightness which need stretching or regions of connective tissue laxity in need of orthotic devices for protection, stability, and support.[98]

At the level of the knee, assessment of range of motion is followed by evaluation of patellar position, patellar mobility, patellar tracking, and retropatellar pain. The Q angle (Fig. 38–1) is usually in the range of 10 to 15 degrees and considered to be excessive if over 20 degrees.[19, 21, 77, 90, 113] Hypermobility of the patella, external tibial torsion, increased Q angle, femoral neck anteversion, a broad pelvis, and pes planus with pronation in combination form the "malalignment syndrome," which is associated with medial knee pain.[19, 67, 85, 113] Assessment of the collateral and cruciate ligaments and menisci is also routine. Ober's test (Fig. 38–2) is used to evaluate tightness of the tensor fascia lata (TFL). In instances where an iliotibial band (ITB) friction syndrome is suspected, the *ITB (Noble) compression test* can be used.[100] In cases of anterior knee pain, the examination focuses on patellar orientation (internal or external rotation, the presence of patella baja or alta), defects in the medial or lateral retinacula, apprehension, increased laxity or pain with patellar mobilization, evidence of poor patellar tracking within the trochlea, retropatellar crepitus, and the presence of vastus medialis obliquus (VMO) atrophy.

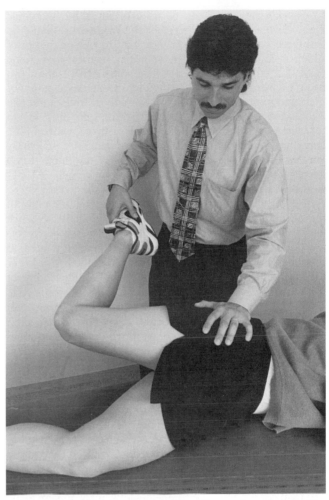

FIGURE 38–2   Ober's test. The patient lies on the untested side, with the lower (untested) leg maintained in mild to moderate hip and knee flexion for otability. The clinician extends and abducts the patient's upper thigh while maintaining the pelvis in a neutral position. The test leg is then slowly lowered.

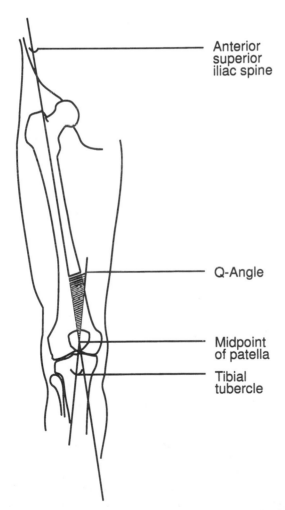

Anterior
superior
iliac spine

Q-Angle

Midpoint
of patella

Tibial
tubercle

FIGURE 38–1   The Q angle: the angle formed between the line of pull of the quadriceps and the center line of the patellar tendon *(hatched area)*. A line is drawn from the anterior superior iliac spine through midpoint of the patella, and a second line is drawn through the midaxis of the patella to the tibial tubercle for determination.

The hip and pelvic region must be evaluated for the presence of tight hip flexors, hip extensors, rotators, and adductors, as loss of mobility in this region can be a factor in development of the patient's injury.[106, 136] The Thomas test consists of having the patient bring both knees up to the chest and then trying to let just one leg descend to a flat lying position on the examination table. If the leg cannot assume this position, or if the spine must be arched in order to do so, it is indicative of hip flexor tightness.[61] Stabilizing the pelvis with one hand while attempting a straight leg raise with the other hand gives a sense of hamstring tightness as retrotilting of the pelvis begins to occur once "maximum" hamstring length is approached. External rotator tightness can be checked by internally rotating the hip while the hip and knee are flexed and the patient is lying supine. Adductor tightness can be assessed by the examiner's trying to abduct one of the patient's legs while the patient lies supine, holding the other knee to the chest. If the adductors are tight, instead of just the leg abducting, the entire body appears to pivot and rotate about the pelvis. Placing the hip in flexion plus abduction and external rotation (Patrick's test) stresses the hip joint itself.

Gaenslen's maneuver can be used to stress the sacroiliac joint. Certain bony prominences and landmarks should be assessed for tenderness—the greater trochanter, posterior superior iliac spine (PSIS), anterior superior iliac spine (ASIS), and posterior inferior iliac spine (PIIS). They also need to be checked for symmetry in the evaluation of malrotation of the sacroiliac joint or pelvis. In addition, the ASIS is a fixed landmark typically used in limb length measurement. Although minor leg length inequalities (i.e., less than ¼ in.) are typically unimportant in a sedentary person, they can have profound effect in an athlete. Limb length inequalities have been estimated to have three times as much of an effect on the runner as on the walker.[128]

A quick but effective screen of the back incorporates all the observations from the lower body segments as, once again, the concept of the kinetic chain must not be forgotten. Lumbosacral spine motion is intimately related to motion at the level of the hip and pelvis. Tightness of lower extremity muscles attaching to the pelvis can interfere with the normally smooth combination of spine flexion–pelvic rotation and spine extension–pelvic derotation (lumbopelvic rhythm), observed during trunk flexion and extension.[25] During spine flexion and extension, it is essential to identify the major motion segments; 80% to 90% of the motion in the lumbosacral spine should be at L4 to L5 and L5 to S1.[25] Migration of the motion up toward the thoracolumbar junction, altered tone of the paraspinal muscles, and lack of a "springing sensation" in the lower spine during anterior glides (placement and release of pressure along the spine while the patient is in a relaxed prone-lying position) suggest spinal segmental dysfunction. Abdominal muscle weakness and weakness of the muscles attaching to the thoracolumbar fascia further indicate that the spine is in need of conditioning.[117] Many persons who appear to be otherwise highly fit from constant aerobic exercise fail to perform regular exercise that promotes conditioning of the supportive musculature of their spine. In the young runner with back pain, provocative tests such as extending the spine while standing on one leg help identify active posterior element irritation or symptomatic spondylolysis.

A brief neurological examination is recommended regardless of whether the patient appears to present with a neurogenic problem or not. The elderly patient with "hip pain" can have unrecognized spinal stenosis. The young runner with a chronic "hamstring strain" can have an unrecognized S1 radiculopathy.[12] Cutaneous nerve injuries need to be considered as well. Careful evaluation of a persistently painful ankle which appears to have healed from an inversion sprain may reveal ongoing irritation of the superficial peroneal nerve. Persistent medial leg pain in the presence of a negative bone scan may be related to saphenous nerve irritation rather than to shin splints.

The person's shoes should be inspected for signs of breakdown. Wearing away of the leather along the distal toecap region can imply subtle anterior tibial weakness. Excessive medial or lateral wear may indicate increased pronation or supination, respectively. Matching up regions of wear on the shoe with regions on the foot (a blister or callus) may convince the patient that new shoes are needed. As a general rule, when correction of mild pronation or supination is to be attempted with footwear, pronation control is achieved better with a straight board-lasted shoe

with good rearfoot control. The supinator does better with a flexible and curve-lasted shoe.[21, 51, 128]

INJURY ANALYSIS AND REHABILITATION

Proper rehabilitation requires a thorough understanding of applied anatomy, biomechanics, and the kinetic chain. The effects of a musculoskeletal injury are rarely, if ever, confined to a single joint, and rehabilitation programs must consider the alterations in anatomy and biomechanics that have occurred proximal, distal, and contralateral to the site of acute injury. The physician must also be able to recognize the adaptations that have occurred in response to errors of training, particularly those induced by chronic musculotendinous overload. This section details a "template" for rehabilitation of musculotendinous overload injuries. Application of the template to specific lower extremity musculoskeletal problems follows.

STEP 1. *Establish an accurate diagnosis.* Inherent to this task is recognizing how muscle overload injuries and tendon injuries present. The vicious circle model for analysis of musculotendinous injury induced by repetitive overload is presented in Figure 38–3. To aid those unfamiliar with this model, some clarification of the terminology is provided:

Tissue injury complex—the area of actual tissue disruption[72–75, 108]

Clinical symptom complex—the symptoms associated with the dysfunction and injury[72–75, 108]

Tissue overload complex—the tissue group being subjected to tensile overload[72–75, 108]

Functional biomechanical deficit—inflexibilities or muscle strength imbalances that create altered mechanics[72–75, 108]

Functional adaptation complex—functional substitutions used by the patient in order to try to maintain activity[72–75, 108]

When the musculotendinous unit is subjected to tensile overload, damage occurs at a cellular level. This typically produces symptoms of pain, dysfunction, and instability, and also impairs athletic performance.[72–74] If the extent of that overload is small (microtear) and nutrition and healing time are adequate, activities can be safely resumed. However, if the injury is not adequately treated and is allowed to progress (macrotear), healing is accompanied by development of scar tissue, with the development of subclinical adaptations such as loss of flexibility and loss of strength, or strength imbalances.[72–74] This leads to further decrements in performance and biomechanical substitutions which perpetuate this "negative-feedback vicious circle" (Fig. 38–3B), creating the chance for more overload and injury.[72–74] Muscle injury can therefore present as acute or chronic injury, as exacerbation of a chronic injury, or as a subclinical injury.[74] Muscle "strain"-type injuries typically manifest themselves microscopically as a zone of myonecrosis confined to within 500 μm of the myotendinous junction.[110] Tendon injuries present as either an acute inflammatory process superimposed upon acute or chronic injury (tendinitis) or as a product of maladaptation and intratendinous

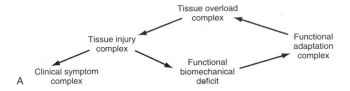

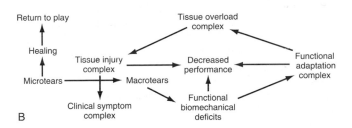

FIGURE 38–3 *A* and *B*, Model for vicious cycle of musculotendinous overload. (See text for details.)

degeneration unaccompanied by mediators of inflammation (tendinosis).[74, 79] In tendinitis, the immediate treatment goal is relief of symptoms, while in tendinosis the immediate goal is restoration of function.[74] Identification of the components of musculotendinous injury within the vicious circle facilitates understanding the functional consequences of the injury which need to be addressed in the rehabilitation program.

STEP 2. *Acute management.* Efforts are directed toward minimizing the effects of inflammation and controlling pain. The PRICE principle (*p*rotection, *r*elative rest, *i*ce, *c*ompression, and *e*levation) is followed. This is usually a period for judicious use of anti-inflammatory medications and pain-relieving modalities.[57, 74, 108, 113, 139]

STEP 3. *Initial rehabilitation.* This phase continues to focus on promotion of proper healing. Restoration of motion helps to reduce the effects of immobilization, with controlled tensile loading promoting ordered collagen growth and alignment. Identification of correctable biomechanical imbalances is initiated. Many rehabilitation programs fail by not progressing beyond this step.

STEP 4. *Correction of imbalances.* Development of symmetrical motion and symmetrical strength are goals. When the patient is pain-free, and when nearly full concentric strength has been achieved, it is essential that an eccentric strengthening program be initiated. This is a critical step in developing a musculotendinous unit which is less likely to fail in the face of future tensile stresses. One must also understand the difference between *closed kinetic chain* (CKC) and *open kinetic chain* (OKC) exercises. If, for instance, during knee flexion or extension, the foot is allowed to move freely through space, the system is called "open." In an OKC system, the hamstrings are predominant in flexion while extension is dominated by the quadriceps. During CKC exercise for the lower limbs, the foot is kept immobile or maintains contact with a ground reactive force, and there is the creation of a multiarticular closed chain. Rather than the near isolation of the large muscle groups seen during OKC exercises, performance of CKC knee flexion and extension results in "coactivation" of both hamstrings and quadriceps groups.[38, 121] Examples of CKC exercises are leg presses or partial squats (Fig. 38–4). These types of exercises

strengthen agonist and antagonist simultaneously via co-contraction, and are more physiological for lower limb sporting activities such as running. An OKC knee extension is shown in Figure 38–5. Identification of flaws in exercise technique and training practices are initiated if the patient is capable of full weightbearing under controlled conditions. Alternative aerobic conditioning exercises are encouraged. Other than local icing, modalities are rarely indicated during this phase.

STEP 5. *Return to normal function.* Cross-training, aqua training, and the use of alternative conditioning schemes give way to a gradual increase in activity specific training and eventual resumption of full activity. Endurance performance, power, and agility should be restored to baseline.

Injuries About the Hip

Applied Anatomy and Biomechanics

The hip is functionally constructed to provide stable weightbearing through a wide variety of lower limb movements. The hip joint encounters forces equivalent to more than three times body weight during walking, and nearly five times body weight during running.[116]

The femoral head approximates two thirds of a sphere and is contained within the deep acetabular fossa (ball-and-socket joint). Containment of the femoral head is enhanced by a fibrocartilaginous labrum at the outer rim of the acetabulum. The majority of the hip joint's stability

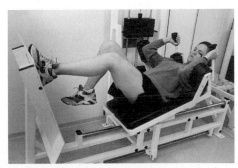

FIGURE 38–4 Example of a closed kinetic chain knee extension.

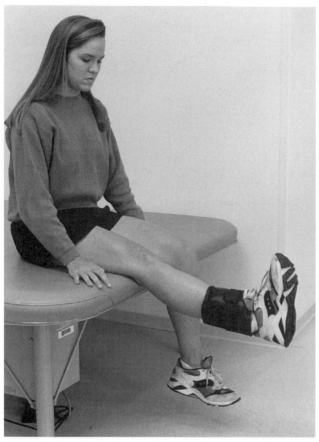

FIGURE 38–5   Example of an open kinetic chain knee extension.

comes from the articular capsule of the joint itself rather than the surrounding musculature. The primary stabilizers of the hip consist of a very strong synovial capsule reinforced by three ligaments arising from the bony components of the pelvis. The iliofemoral ligament, also called the *Y ligament of Bigelow*, arises from the AIIS and divides, forming two femoral insertions at the greater trochanter and on the anterior femur inferior to the intertrochanteric line. This ligament resembles an inverted Y and restrains hyperextension at the hip.[59] Two additional ligamentous supports include the pubofemoral (which checks abduction and extension of the femur) and ischiofemoral (which checks extension) ligaments. The spiral direction of the ligaments also serves to limit internal rotation of the femur as all three get wrapped tighter with medial femoral rotation. Functioning as a group, they contribute to hip stability by restraining extension, abduction, and internal rotation of the femur. The hip joint is consequently the least stable in flexion, adduction, and external rotation (the most frequent position of hip dislocation).[137]

The mature femoral neck is angled at 120 to 130 degrees to the central axis, and is positioned in approximately 15 degrees of anteversion (medial femoral torsion). An increase in the neck-shaft angle is termed *coxa valga*, whereas a decrease is referred to as *coxa vara*.

The vascular supply to the femoral head and neck is somewhat tenuous. In the center of the head there is a slight flattening, called the *fovea*, where the ligamentum teres attaches. The femoral head receives vascularity from a small artery within the ligamentum teres, and through the medial and lateral circumflex arteries, which pierce the capsule. This architecture renders the vascular supply vulnerable to disruption during dislocation (loss of flow to the head through the ligamentum teres) and fracture (interference with flow through the circumflex vessels).

Some of the key muscles surrounding the hip joint include the piriformis, gluteus maximus, and gemelli. The piriformis runs from the anterior sacrum through the greater sciatic foramen and inserts on the greater trochanter and functions as an external rotator. The gluteus maximus has its origins at the posterolateral sacrum, sacrotuberous ligament, and posterior ilium, and inserts on the iliotibial tract and gluteal tuberosity. It functions as a hip and spine extensor and as a hip external rotator. The gemelli are short muscles that run from the ischial spine to the greater trochanter and function as minor external rotators. The majority of neurovascular structures emerging from the sciatic foramen exit inferior to the piriformis muscle (the superior gluteal nerve and artery exit above), creating a potential point of entrapment or irritation.

Specific Problems in the Hip Region

PIRIFORMIS SYNDROME.   This is both an underrecognized yet overdiagnosed phenomenon. As mentioned previously, there is the potential for sciatic nerve entrapment beneath the piriformis as the nerve exits the sciatic foramen. In Agur's review[3] of 640 limbs, the tibial and peroneal divisions passed beneath the muscle 87% of the time. In slightly over 12% the peroneal division passed through the muscle, and in less than 1% of the cases the peroneal division emerged above the piriformis.[3] Sciatic nerve compression by this muscle leads to complaints of dysesthesias down the posterior thigh and often into the calf or foot. Buttock pain and tenderness through the piriformis can be found. Side-to-side comparisons of piriformis tightness (i.e., allowable internal rotation of the hips) should be made either with the person in a prone-lying position with the hips adducted and knees flexed to 90 degrees, or in a supine lie with 60 degrees of hip flexion and slight hip adduction while introducing the internal rotation stress.[46] Electrodiagnostic testing can reveal involvement of tibial and peroneal innervated muscles, with sparing of superior and inferior gluteal nerve–innervated structures and absence of abnormal electromyographic activity in the paraspinal musculature. Magnetic resonance imaging (MRI) can demonstrate injury or edema within the piriformis muscle, but this is rarely a necessary procedure.

The clinical symptom complex in piriformis syndrome consists of buttock (and possibly leg pain) and dysesthesias aggravated by sitting or lower limb exertion.[15] The tissue injury complex is comprised of myotendinous breakdown within the piriformis and possible focal demyelination within the tibial and peroneal divisions of the sciatic nerve. The structures within the tissue overload complex are the piriformis, gluteal muscles, gemelli, quadratus lumborum, and sacroiliac ligaments and the sciatic nerve. The functional biomechanical deficits include a tight piriformis and external rotators, hip abductor weakness, sacroiliac joint hypomobility, and lower lumbar spine dysfunction.[15, 46] Functional adaptations consist of ambulating with an externally rotated thigh, shortened stride length, and functional limb length shortening. Rehabilitation efforts are geared toward stretching of the piriformis and associated external rotators and careful evaluation of the sacrum and pelvis for other imbalances that need correction. Although many patients have tenderness, tightness, or pain in the region of the piriformis, it is essential to be sure that a lumbar spine–based problem with secondary referral to the piriformis is not being missed.

SNAPPING HIP SYNDROME. This is associated with a variety of extra-articular and intra-articular phenomena. The most common cause appears to be the snapping or popping of the ITB across the greater trochanter, although involvement of the iliopsoas tendon snapping over the iliopectineal eminence can also be seen.[46, 95, 111] Less commonly, loose bodies, labral tears, and osteochondritis dissecans can be intra-articular sources of the snap. Treatment typically consists of muscle rebalancing with stretching and myofascial release to promote return of muscles and tendons to normal length.[46] Correction should take only a few weeks. Should symptoms persist despite an adequate stretching program, evaluation of intra-articular pathological changes by computed tomography (CT), MRI, or arthroscopy is recommended.[111]

TROCHANTERIC BURSITIS. This is commonly seen in the elderly population and manifests as pain in the lateral thigh during ambulation and decreased tolerance for lying on the affected side. The trochanteric bursa lies beneath the tendon of the gluteus maximus and is located posterolateral to the trochanter. Patients may describe a pseudoradicular pattern with the pain extending down the lateral aspect of the lower extremity and into the buttock.[132] The clinical symptoms can be elicited by placing the lower extremity in external rotation and abduction. Direct palpation or deep pressure applied posterior and superior to the greater trochanter will reproduce the pain.[119] Functional biomechanical deficits consist of shortening of the TFL, rectus femoris, and the hamstrings, and weakness of the adductors.[108] Functional adaptations include increased hip external rotation with an altered gait or running pattern.[108] Treatment should be geared toward restoration of flexibility and strength imbalances. Injecting the bursa with corticosteroid and anesthetic can be helpful if the flexibility and conditioning exercises are unsuccessful.[105] Hip pain that persists despite comprehensive rehabilitation and injection therapy should alert the physician to alternative sources of pain including the lumbar spine and adjacent joints throughout the kinetic chain.[28, 134]

ISCHIAL BURSITIS. The ischial bursa lies between the ischial tuberosity and the gluteus maximus. Irritation of this bursa is not common. Classically, *ischial bursitis* (tailor's or weaver's bottom) occurs with friction and trauma after prolonged sitting on a hard surface. It can also be seen in adolescent runners, often in conjunction with ischial apophysitis. Pain can be aggravated during uphill running. The pain is distributed down the posterior aspect of the thigh and occurs with activation of the hamstring muscles. Initial treatment approaches involve modification of the patient's activity, such as a decrease in the duration and frequency of running. If an alternative to running includes cycling, the patient should be advised to avoid the use of toe clips, which increase activation of the ham-

strings. When the cause is prolonged sitting, the patient's workstation should be modified to allow for activities to be conducted in a standing position and a cushion should be used during sitting. Ice and nonsteroidal anti-inflammatory drugs (NSAIDs) are helpful in controlling symptoms. The adolescent athlete may require a radiological series to screen for callus formation secondary to ischial apophysitis if the pain does not resolve with conservative measures. Corticosteroid injections can be helpful in cases of persistent pain. The use of fluoroscopy to demonstrate a bursogram reduces the possibility of improper needle location and avoids unnecessary repeat injections.

AVASCULAR NECROSIS OF THE FEMORAL HEAD. Most clinicians have little difficulty determining if an overt hip fracture has occurred, but often neglect to aggressively evaluate the patient with groin (hip joint) pain and negative plain films. As discussed previously, the blood supply to the femoral head is fragile and subject to compromise with hip dislocation or femoral neck fracture. Disruption of this supply can have catastrophic results. There should be a high index of suspicion for *avascular necrosis* (AVN) of the femoral head if initial plain radiographs are negative, but the hip is painful with joint loading, and an external source of pain, such as a lumbar radiculopathy, cannot be identified. Although a bone scan can show a stress reaction within days, MRI scanning is preferable. MRI is sensitive to the early signs of AVN, and also provides information about the integrity of the bony cortex (necrosis and surrounding edema can be clearly seen in Fig. 38–6). As bone death occurs the plain films show destruction of the femoral head, but onset of treatment this late in the course is sure to have a poor outcome. If the MRI shows evidence of necrosis, immediate surgical consultation and nonweightbearing status are recommended.

Specific Problems in the Thigh

The thigh consists of the heavily muscled region about the shaft of the femur. The structures in this region are extremely vulnerable to both tensile overload and direct trauma. The majority of thigh injuries adhere to the overload vicious circle as previously described.

Anterior Thigh

RELEVANT ANATOMY AND BIOMECHANICS. The majority of the mass of the anterior thigh is formed by the quadriceps muscle group (Fig. 38–7). All of these muscles are innervated by the femoral nerve (L2–L4). The vastus lateralis, vastus intermedius, and vastus medialis all have their origin along the shaft of the femur and insert on the proximal patellar pole (via the quadriceps tendon), and therefore act solely as knee extensors. The fourth muscle of this group, the rectus femoris, originates at the anterior inferior iliac spine, and acts as both a hip flexor and knee extensor. The vastus medialis obliquus is often thought of as part of the quadriceps group, but it functionally does not act like the other four muscles. The sartorius, which is also less commonly involved in disorders of the thigh than the knee, has its origin at the ASIS and terminates at the pes anserinus along the inferomedial knee.

The quadriceps is capable of providing explosive forces, such as those necessary for jumping, vertical leaping, and

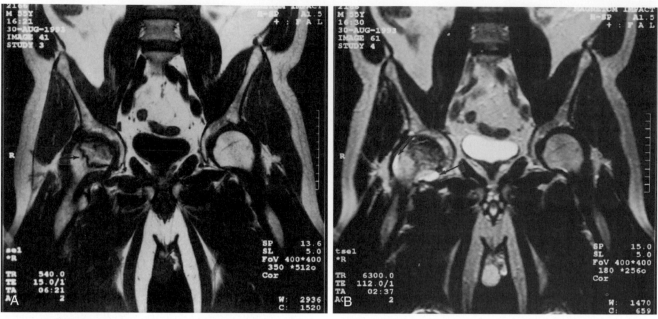

FIGURE 38–6 Avascular necrosis of the femoral head. *A,* T1-weighted image. *B,* Edema present on T2-weighted image.

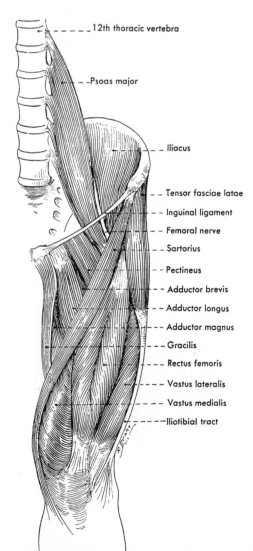

12th thoracic vertebra

Psoas major

Iliacus

Tensor fasciae latae

Inguinal ligament

Femoral nerve

Sartorius

Pectineus

Adductor brevis

Adductor longus

Adductor magnus

Gracilis

Rectus femoris

Vastus lateralis

Vastus medialis

Iliotibial tract

FIGURE 38–7 Muscles of the anterior and medial thigh. (From Hollinshead WH, Jenkins DB: Functional Anatomy of the Limbs and Back, ed 5. Philadelphia, WB Saunders, 1981.)

kicking. It is also essential in its role as a shock attenuator during landing from jumps and in the control of knee flexion during the single-leg loading response and early stance phase of the gait cycle. The rectus femoris, along with the iliopsoas, also serves to initiate forward motion of the femur during early swing phase.

Anterior thigh injuries typically occur by either of two mechanisms: tensile overloading of the musculotendinous unit with induction of a "strain," or high-velocity compressive forces resulting in a "contusion." Persons particularly prone to anterior thigh injuries include football, soccer, and rugby players.

QUADRICEPS STRAINS.   Strain injuries are graded as follows:

1. First degree (mild)—an overstretch with minimal disruption of musculotendinous unit integrity. There is probably less than 5% fiber disruption, and the patient experiences soreness with motion but has only minimal strength loss.[68, 139, 141]

2. Second degree (moderate)—an actual (although incomplete) muscle tear. There is intramuscular bleeding with hematoma formation and muscle strength is clearly compromised.[68, 139, 141]

3. Third degree (severe)—a complete rupture. Muscle function is essentially lost. Avulsion injuries are included in this category.

Of the quadriceps group, the rectus femoris is the most commonly affected.[84] The *Ely's test* (passive flexion of the knee with the patient prone) is useful for isolation of the rectus. A tight rectus induces elevation of the ipsilateral hemipelvis as maximum allowable knee flexion is approached, as the hip-flexing component of the rectus femoris is blocked.

The signs and symptoms vary depending on the severity of the injury. Lower-grade injuries are more apparent with deep palpation and passive stretch of muscle while higher-grade injuries are accompanied by swelling, discoloration, and in the case of total rupture, a palpable mass in the zone of muscle injury.

Functional biomechanical deficits and other factors that can increase risk of quadriceps strain include tightness or weakness of the quadriceps musculature, hamstring tightness, lack of sufficient warmup or stretching prior to exercise, previous injury without rehabilitation, and overtraining.

The functional adaptations that persist when the return to activity is too early include greater reliance on the unaffected leg for upward propulsion in jumping activities, shortened running stride with reduced hip flexion, and reduced running velocity. Occasionally the patient tries to maintain an externally rotated femur so the adductor group can be used to advance the thigh.

Acute rehabilitation follows the PRICE principle. Ice is generally preferable to heat, and interferential current can be useful as an adjunct in pain control.[139] The early use of NSAIDs in high-degree strains should be weighed carefully as antiplatelet activities can increase local bleeding. However, the role of NSAIDs as modifiers of the inflammatory response to acute injury make them extremely valuable in the acute management of all first- and most second-degree strains.

Initial rehabilitation includes pain-limited stretching to achieve progressive increases in muscle length. Proper technique must be emphasized, and the patient should be instructed to continue to maintain the stretching program on a long-term basis. The vastus muscles can be stretched by flexing the knee at any hip angle, but the rectus femoris is stretched only if the hip is in a neutral or extended position. An example of a combined hip flexor and knee extensor stretch is shown in Figure 38–8.

Strengthening should be initiated only after range of motion is pain-free and complete. The progression should be from either isometric or low-resistance dynamic contractions to full-range progressive resistance exercises (PREs). The PRE regimen should include both concentric and eventually eccentric exercise, and care should be taken to ensure that movements are smooth and without muscle substitutions. Eccentric work against maximal or supramaximal loads should be avoided early in the rehabilitation program to lessen the likelihood of further structural damage. Aerobic conditioning can be maintained initially by upper body ergometry, swimming with a pull buoy between the legs, or via tri-limb exercise with the affected limb kept at rest. When full range of motion is achieved, stationary two-legged bicycling, skiing, or rowing can be attempted. Full-weightbearing exercises with axial loading of the affected limb (treadmill, stair climber, etc.) are gradually added, with eventual progression to faster-paced activities, agility drills, and finally, sport-specific training when applicable.

QUADRICEPS TENDON RUPTURE.   This represents an extreme form of overload to the quadriceps and is often the end result of repeated strain injuries.[44, 77] In contrast to quadriceps strains, which are more common in younger

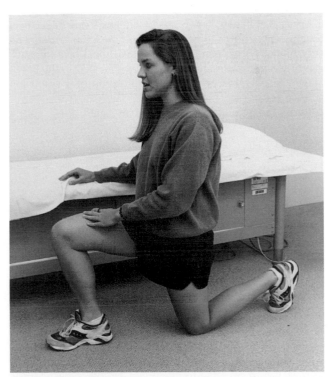

FIGURE 38–8   Stretching of the hip flexors. To obtain additional stretch for the knee extensors, the patient must grab the ankle and increase the knee flexion angle. Note that the spine must maintain a neutral position to avoid the development of lumbar injury.

athletes, tendon ruptures tend to occur in older athletes. As with strains, the rectus femoris is the most vulnerable of the quadriceps group.[104] A typical presentation is a 40-year-old basketball player landing off balance and on one leg, with sudden giving way and pain, and rapid development of a palpable defect at the site of injury. This is often at the site of tendon insertion at the proximal patellar pole.[77, 113] Incomplete tears can be treated conservatively with initial splinting and use of crutches for protected weightbearing. The patient must be warned that without full rehabilitation and reconditioning of the remaining muscles there is a great chance that there will be residual strength deficits. Complete tears require surgical repair.

QUADRICEPS CONTUSIONS. These are characterized by capillary rupture, edema, inflammation, and infiltrative bleeding. The severity of the contusion is proportional to the extent of blood vessel breakdown and muscle crush. The more relaxed the quadriceps is at the time of impact, the greater the ultimate injury.[77] Clinical grading of the contusion is related to the available passive, pain-free knee flexion 12 to 24 hours post injury. Flexion of less than 45 degrees usually indicates a severe injury; 45 to 90 degrees, a moderate injury; and greater than 90 degrees flexion, a mild injury.[64, 113, 115]

It is important to begin treatment with PRICE as close to the time of injury as possible. The thigh and lower leg should be wrapped or strapped into maximally tolerated knee flexion (Fig. 38–9). Crutch walking is advised. As with strains, NSAIDs are used judiciously. Attempted aspiration of the hematoma is not recommended, particularly since blood is usually clotting by the time the physician examines the injury. Corticosteroid and proteolytic enzyme injections probably do more harm than good. Steroid injections theoretically weaken already stressed connective tissue fibers and collagen, while use of enzymes has never been conclusively shown to be of benefit.[18, 103] Ice is perhaps the only modality that can be used safely. Local heating, short wave, and ultrasound have all been implicated in the development of the least desirable complication of a contusion, myositis ossificans traumatica.[8, 18, 53, 97, 135, 139, 141]

Early rehabilitation focuses on re-establishing normal

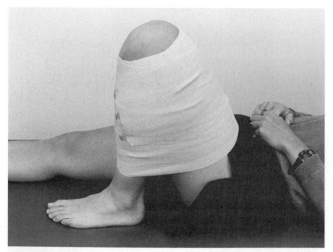

FIGURE 38–9 Compressive dressing applied to the thigh following an acute quadriceps contusion. Note the knee is kept in maximally tolerated flexion.

pain-free range through a progressive stretching program. Aerobic conditioning is started as soon as possible, with upper body or tri-limbed exercises. As knee flexion returns to normal, isometrics and then CKC strengthening of the knee flexors and extensors are instituted. Criteria for resumption of full activity include minimal thigh tenderness, as well as symmetrical range of motion and quadriceps strength. If the patient participates in a contact sport, the use of custom-molded protective padding is recommended.[139] When using off-the-shelf type of padding, it is important to be sure that the entire front of the thigh is covered. The recovery time for contusive injuries varies greatly. Although recovery from most mild injuries takes less than 2 weeks, there is considerable overlap in healing times between mild, moderate, and severe injuries, with one study reporting a range of 2 to 60 days of disability.[115]

MYOSITIS OSSIFICANS TRAUMATICA. One of the most vexing complications of contusive injuries is *myositis ossificans traumatica* (MOT) or the formation of non-neoplastic cartilage or bone in connective tissue.[18] MOT is the most common type of extraskeletal bone-forming lesion.[1, 18, 139] It is most common in football and rugby, but has been reported in hockey, soccer, baseball, wrestling, and martial arts.[8, 115, 135, 139] The quadriceps is the most common site of involvement. Initial symptoms, which are nonspecific, include local pain, warmth, and tenderness. This usually progresses to a soft tissue swelling and ultimately to a discrete mass with an associated loss of range of motion at the surrounding joints.[18, 139] MOT develops rapidly and can be evident within 3 weeks on plain films.[1] Even earlier detection is possible with three-phase bone scan or ultrasonography.[76, 92]

MOT tends to stabilize in size within 3 to 6 months, and there is great likelihood of spontaneous resorption, particularly when the MOT is near the muscle belly and not lying near the tendon.[77, 82] In Jackson's series of 71 patients with MOT, 69 recovered without residual symptoms.[66]

Recommended treatment following detection of MOT is adherence to the PRICE principle, with immobilization of the affected area while it is overtly inflamed to facilitate the natural sequence of resorption. Prophylactic use of diphosphonates does not seem warranted given the risks, the expense, and the low likelihood of a persisting lesion. The use of NSAIDs such as indomethacin is common among clinicians, but this has not been conclusively shown to halt the progression of the lesion. Follow-up radiographs showing corticated MOT borders, and "cold" bone scans are useful in determining if the lesion has become "mature." Activity is gradually increased after maturity has been determined. On rare occasions, surgical excision of a mature MOT lesion is necessary. This should generally be reserved for those patients with pain and loss of range of motion persisting 6 to 12 months after the lesion has matured.

ACUTE COMPARTMENT SYNDROME. Far less common than the above entities is an *acute compartment syndrome* of the anterior thigh. Patients present with a palpably tense thigh and exhibit decreased sensation in the front of the thigh or the saphenous distribution, or both; pain; pallor; and a progressive loss of quadriceps strength.[7, 139] A key symptom is pain that is seemingly disproportionate to the injury. The athlete might also report that the leg feels better in a dependent position. In any event, if a compartment syndrome is suspected, surgical consultation is necessary. Intracompartmental pressure measurements should be made, and when over 40 mm Hg, fasciotomy is typically necessary.

Medial Thigh

RELEVANT ANATOMY AND BIOMECHANICS. The majority of the medial thigh musculature is composed of the adductor group. The adductor longus, adductor brevis, and adductor magnus all originate along the ischiopubic ramus and insert along the linea aspera of the femur (see Fig. 38–7). The adductor brevis and longus, which are more anteriorly situated, can function as weak hip flexors. The large, posteriorly positioned adductor magnus can "double" as an accessory hamstring. The gracilis shares the same origin as the other adductors but crosses the medial knee joint, where it meets the sartorius and the semimembranosus as part of the pes anserinus. The obturator externus is a minor muscle that runs from the obturator foramen to the greater trochanter. All the adductor muscles are innervated by the obturator nerve (L2–L4). The posterior portion of the adductor magnus, in keeping with its role as an accessory hamstring, has tibial innervation as well.

The adductor muscles function as pelvic stabilizers, femoral rotators, and femoral accelerators during the gait cycle. Their peak electromyographic activity occurs shortly after heel-strike and in mid-stance to late stance.

ADDUCTOR STRAIN. Adductor injuries are relatively common in soccer and other kicking sports, horseback riding, gymnastics, and ice hockey. The most common of the medial thigh injuries is *adductor strain* due to tensile overload. The adductor longus and magnus are the most frequently affected.[141] High-grade strains can result from sudden femoral abduction in external rotation (i.e., a placekickers' plant leg slipping on a muddy field so that the kicking leg is subjected to a sudden abduction force), or from repetitive forceful adduction as when hockey players or roller bladers push off and shift weight from one leg to the other to propel themselves forward.[93, 123]

In adductor strain, the clinical symptom complex typically consists of medial thigh and groin pain that is worsened by abduction. The tissue injury complex and overloaded structures include the musculotendinous units of the adductor muscles. Associated biomechanical deficits which can precede the acute event include loss of adductor and psoas flexibility, loss of external rotation of the femur, hamstring tightness and weakness, and gluteus medius weakness. Functional adaptations to injury include shortened stride with less crossover, and an attempt to maintain a relatively internally rotated position of the femur (which accentuates the gluteus weakness).

Acute management involves application of the PRICE principle with use of NSAIDs as needed. Interferential current can be a useful adjunct in pain management as well. With high-degree strains, any attempt to advance the femur forward can induce pain and the patient should be provided with crutches for ambulation. Spica wraps with elastic bandage can be of benefit early on to remind the patient not to suddenly abduct or flex the thigh. Some athletes continue to use the spica wrap throughout the entire rehabilitation process. If a complete disruption of the adductor longus has occurred, surgical consultation to evaluate the possibility of repair is highly recommended.

Initial rehabilitation emphasizes establishment of a stretching program for the adductor group. Adductor stretching after injury can be quite painful and the stretching should be kept within a pain-free zone. The gluteal muscles and external rotators of the thigh need to be stretched as well since loss of external rotation and anterior hip capsular tightness frequently coexist with adductor inflexibility.

Correction of imbalances begins with the stretching outlined above and progresses to more aggressive adductor stretching. Using a partner to help stretch in the manner shown in Figure 38–10 or via a "contract-relax" method (a proprioceptive neuromuscular facilitation technique) helps to achieve greater gains. "Butterfly" stretches can be used for self-stretching of the adductors. (The person sits on the floor with the soles of the feet together, knees flexed, and with the hips externally rotated and abducted. Downward pressure is the applied along the inside of the

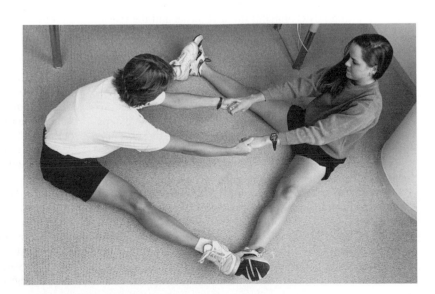

FIGURE 38–10 Assisted adductor stretch.

thigh until a pulling sensation is felt within the adductor group.) This last technique will not provide a good adductor stretch unless the anterior hip capsule has previously been mobilized. Strengthening of all muscles about the hip is necessary, particularly the external rotators, which usually have been working through a limited range prior to the stretching program. Isometrics and then elastic or rubber tubing for dynamic strengthening can be used early on for adductor strengthening. It can be 1 to 3 weeks before the patient is able to safely tolerate higher-resistance weights or aggressive CKC strengthening exercises, particularly in the high-grade strains.

OSTEITIS PUBIS. When pain in the groin or symphysis pubis region persists beyond a month, the diagnosis of *osteitis pubis* should be considered. Inflammation in the symphysis generally results from repetitive microtrauma or persistently abnormal mechanics. During mid-stance, when the unsupported hemipelvis attempts to drop, the symphysis encounters increased shear forces from the pull of the adductors below and the rectus abdominis above. Runners and cross-country skiers who abruptly increase their mileage (and who have weak gluteal muscles) are prone to this problem. Definitive diagnosis is made with radiographs or bone scan. Typical radiographic findings include periosteal reaction, demineralization, and sclerosis along the pubis, although these may not be present for 2 to 3 weeks.[77, 124] A bone scan can be positive earlier. The treatment of choice for osteitis pubis is rest for 1½ to 2 months with avoidance of lower extremity exercise. Upper extremity conditioning is emphasized, and resumption of a lower extremity rehabilitation and conditioning program is permitted only when there is no tenderness to palpation and hip abduction is pain-free.

Posterior Thigh

RELEVANT ANATOMY AND BIOMECHANICS. The bulk of the posterior thigh is comprised of the hamstrings group (Fig. 38–11). The long head of the biceps femoris, semimembranosus, and semitendinosus all arise from the ischial tuberosity. The short head of the biceps arises from the linea aspera of the femur. The semimembranosus and semitendinosus descend medially with the membranosus, inserting on the posteromedial tibial condyle and the tendinosus, meeting the gracilis and sartorius at the anteromedial tibia. The long and short heads of the biceps become confluent as they descend and both insert laterally along the proximal fibula. All except the short head function as hip extensors and knee flexors. The short head is a knee flexor only. The semimembranosus and semitendinosus are also internal rotators of the flexed knee, whereas the biceps can act as an external rotator. All of these muscles are innervated by the tibial division of the sciatic nerve (L5–S1) except for the short head of the biceps which receives peroneal innervation. The hamstrings are critical for control of swing phase deceleration, control of knee rotation, and, via CKC mechanisms, prevention of knee buckling at heel-strike.

HAMSTRING STRAINS. These are among the most common of all thigh injuries. The short head of the biceps is the most frequently involved.[55, 113] This has been theorized to be due to its different innervation from the other

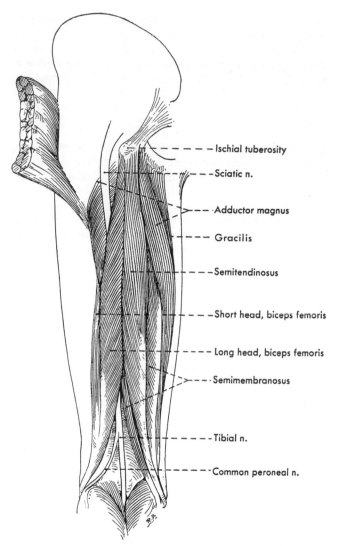

FIGURE 38–11 Muscles of the posterior thigh. (From Hollinshead WH, Jenkins DB: Functional Anatomy of the Limbs and Back, ed 5. Philadelphia, WB Saunders, 1981.)

hamstrings, which potentially results in asynchronous firing at high recruitment frequencies.[2, 23, 77, 113] Injuries are more likely to occur at higher running speeds. The higher the running speed, the less time spent in stance phase. This shorter interval subjects the hamstrings to greater angular velocities and increased eccentric (decelerating) forces at the time of heel-strike and initial loading of that limb. The remaining hamstrings, being two-joint muscles, are vulnerable to injury under conditions of extreme hip flexion combined with knee extension. Hurdlers and football punters are at risk for this type of injury mechanism.

The clinical symptom complex generally consists of pain in the proximal thigh with the onset associated with a popping sensation in the posterior thigh. By the time of examination, there may be a palpable mass, presence of ecchymosis, and extreme tenderness over the injured site. The musculotendinous junctions of the hamstrings are the primary site of tissue injury. These junctions occur throughout the gross length of these muscles and it should not surprise the examiner to find a focal site anywhere along the length of the muscle. As with other strains, eccentric overload is the major mechanism of injury.

Functional biomechanical deficits include decreased knee extension, reduced hamstring-to-quadriceps strength ratio (normally about 0.6), and increased hip flexion.[55, 108, 140] Pre-existing conditions which accentuate these deficits include insufficient warmup, poor muscle coordination, fatigue, and other muscle strength and flexibility imbalances. These should be looked for and corrected since the recurrence rate of this type of injury is high. The functional adaptations in response to the injury or previous subclinical injury include shortened walking or running stride length.[108, 140]

Acute management consists of PRICE, cane or crutch walking (especially with the higher-grade injuries), NSAIDs, and gentle passive stretching as tolerated. Isometric and dynamic strengthening begins only when the patient is pain-free. For full stretching of the hamstrings, the hip must be flexed with maintenance of complete knee extension. Stretching should be performed in a supine position, and a towel can be used to facilitate this stretching maneuver (Fig. 38–12). Rehabilitation can proceed more rapidly once full muscle length is achieved. Aerobic conditioning exercises include bicycling without toe clips (which reduces the role of the hamstrings), upper body ergometry, kayaking, and swimming breaststroke, or with a pull buoy between the thighs. Resumption of activity is allowed when motion is restored and pain-free, strength is at least 90% of the uninjured side, and the hamstrings/quadriceps strength ratio has normalized.[113, 139, 140] The use of a neoprene thigh sleeve to keep muscles warm when active may also be helpful upon return to sport.

Lateral Thigh

RELEVANT ANATOMY AND BIOMECHANICS. The primary lateral thigh structure subject to injury is the tensor fascia. The TFL has its origin at the ASIS and becomes part of the ITB inserting into Gerdy's tubercle on the anterolateral tibia. It functions as a hip flexor and internal rotator of the hip. Innervation is provided by the superior gluteal nerve (mainly L5 fibers). The gluteus medius and minimus are also innervated by the superior gluteal nerve. They originate from the lateral ilium and insert on the greater trochanter. Owing to their wide origin and fan-shaped structure, they not only function as the major hip abductors but also play a role in hip rotation, flexion, and extension.

The most common problems related to the TFL are related to inflexibility. It is not a structure frequently contused or strained. Tightness of the TFL has been associated with a number of clinical entities including snapping hip (see above), ITB syndrome (see below), patellofemoral pain, and lumbar spine dysfunction. TFL tightness is usually seen in conjunction with gluteal muscle inflexibility and weakness. TFL shortening can be demonstrated via *Ober's test* (see Fig. 38–2). Failure of the thigh to resume an adducted or neutral position easily while the hip is in extension indicates a tight TFL.

TFL tightness responds reasonably well to a stretching program, but these are difficult stretches for the patient to learn without careful instruction. Stretches may be done initially with a therapist simulating the Ober's test position (Fig. 38–13), or the patient can perform a self-stretch as demonstrated in Figure 38–14.

MERALGIA PARESTHETICA. This consists of pain and dysesthesias in the lateral thigh typically caused by entrapment of the lateral femoral cutaneous nerve (L2–L3) underneath the inguinal ligament. Less likely sites of entrapment are within the TFL, or after it emerges from the psoas muscle. Abdominal distention from pregnancy or obesity, wearing a tight lumbar corset, and sudden hip hyperextension are all potential sources of irritation of this nerve.[34, 39, 69] Treatments include weight reduction, avoidance of binding clothing, local injection of anesthetic agents at the level of the inguinal ligament, and oral medications such as amitriptyline and carbamazepine (Tegretol).

Disorders of the Knee

Applied Anatomy and Biomechanics

The knee should not be viewed as a simple "hinged joint." The knee proper actually consists of three joints, the

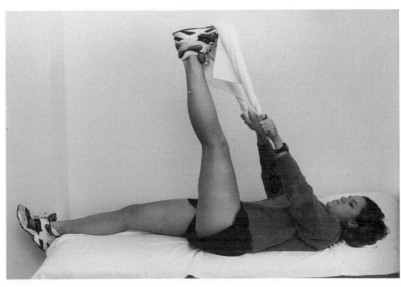

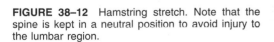

FIGURE 38–12 Hamstring stretch. Note that the spine is kept in a neutral position to avoid injury to the lumbar region.

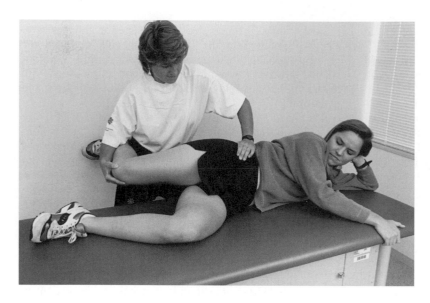

FIGURE 38–13 Assisted tensor fascia lata stretch with patellar stabilization. Note that the therapist can influence the moment acting through the patellofemoral joint.

tibiofemoral, patellofemoral, and the tibiofibular. Actions at these joints are determined by local forces and by events occurring above at the hip, pelvis, and thigh, and below at the levels of the leg, ankle, and foot. Knee joint structures are frequently injured because of muscular imbalances and mechanical flaws existing elsewhere along the kinetic chain.

Integrity of the knee is maintained via a complex system of static and dynamic restraints. The knee joint is envel-

oped by an extensive synovial capsule. The capsule is an important secondary restraint to joint destruction and can be injured in combination with high-grade damage to the primary ligamentous structures. The capsule is confluent with expansions of the patellar tendon anteriorly, the ITB laterally, and the semimembranosus tendon and the deep fibers of the tibial collateral ligament medially. Laterally, the fibular collateral ligament remains separate from the synovium. On the posteromedial corner, the capsule is reinforced by the blending of the semimembranosus and the oblique popliteal ligament. Near the fibula, the posterior capsule forms the arcuate ligament below which the popliteus enters the knee.

The primary static restraints to tibiofemoral translatory motion are the cruciate ligaments. Each cruciate ligament is described by its attachment to the tibial plateau. The anterior cruciate ligament (ACL) arises lateral and anterior to the tibial spine, and its fascicles fan out to form a broad-based attachment to the posteromedial aspect of the lateral femoral condyle. There are two primary groups of fascicles—the anteromedial bundle, which is taut in knee flexion, and the larger posterolateral band, which tightens in extension.[87] Functionally, the ACL prevents forward translation of the tibial plateau relative to the femur and aids in rotational control.

The posterior cruciate ligament (PCL) arises between the posterior junction of the tibial condyles and attaches to the lateral aspect of the medial femoral condyle. The PCL is comprised of an anterior band and a smaller posterior bundle.[87] The PCL prevents forward translation of the femur on the tibial condyles and provides secondary rotational stability. Both cruciate ligaments are intra-articular, but extrasynovial structures.

The menisci are cartilaginous structures which assist the motion of the femoral condyles at the tibiofemoral joint. They deepen the articular surfaces, provide a thin layer of lubrication, and assist in shock absorption. The menisci also guide the femur through a rolling and gliding type of motion combined with rotation and limit extremes of flexion and extension. They have been shown to transmit approximately 50% of weightbearing moments in extension

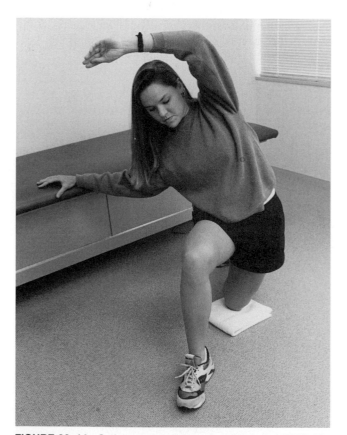

FIGURE 38–14 Self-stretching of the tensor fascia lata (TFL). The patient is stretching the left TFL.

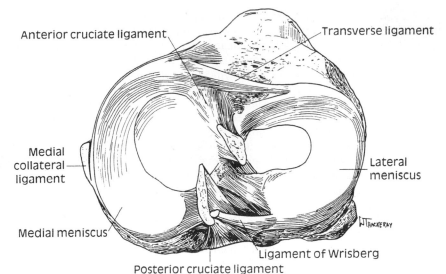

FIGURE 38–15 Attachments of menisci and ligaments at the level of the tibial plateau. (From Warren R, Arnoczky SP, Wickiewicz TL: Anatomy of the knee. *In* Nicholas JA, Hershman EB (eds): The Lower Extremity and Spine in Sports Medicine. St Louis, Mosby–Year Book, 1991.)

and 85% in flexion.[4, 43] Viewed from above, (Fig. 38–15) the menisci approximate incomplete circles, open at their central borders. The medial meniscus is firmly attached to the medial collateral ligament and the synovial capsule, while the lateral meniscus has a less significant bond to the capsule and is separate from the collateral ligament. This strong medial anchor restricts the mobility of the medial meniscus and might account for the high frequency of injuries in the posterior horn. Meniscal vascular support consists of a capillary plexus located in the thicker, peripheral one third.[11] Centrally, the meniscus is thinner and relies on the synovial fluid for diffusion of nutrients.

The two collateral ligaments control valgus and varus moments acting at the knee and help limit rotation of the tibia.[37] The medial collateral ligament (MCL) consists of superficial and deep layers separated by a bursa. Superiorly, the ligament arises from the medial epicondyle and is anchored in the medial proximal tibia with its deep layer attaching to the meniscal periphery. The lateral collateral ligament (LCL) courses from the lateral femoral condyle to the fibula, free of the meniscus and the synovial capsule.

The patellofemoral joint is essentially a soft tissue joint under the control of numerous muscular and fascial structures. The patella is the centerpiece of all the static and dynamic stabilizing forces about the patellofemoral joint (Fig. 38–16) The extensor mechanism consists of the quad-

FIGURE 38–16 Forces about the patella. (From Striazk AM, Stroberg AJ: Knee injuries in the skeletally immature athlete. *In* Nicholas JA, Hershman EB (eds): The Lower Extremity and Spine in Sports Medicine. St Louis, Mosby–Year Book, 1991.)

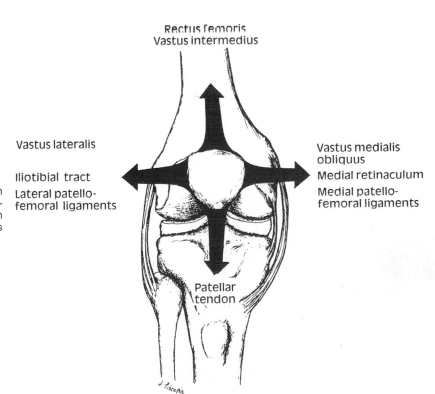

riceps group, the patella, and the quadriceps and patellar tendons. The hamstrings act as antagonists to the anterior group. The iliotibial tract, lateral retinaculum, and patellofemoral ligaments provide a laterally directed pull, while the vastus medialis obliquus (VMO), medial retinaculum, and medial patellofemoral ligaments pull medially. These stabilizing forces, by compressing the patella against the femur, create a patellofemoral joint reaction force (PFJRF). The PFJRF becomes greater with increases in quadriceps tension and with increased knee flexion (Fig. 38–17). The approximate PFJRFs for walking, ascending stairs, and squatting approximate 0.5, 3.3, and 6 to 7 times body weight respectively.[41] The patellofemoral joint reaction stress (PFJRS) refers to the PFJRF per unit contact area. A large PFJRF distributed over a large contact area produces a relatively lesser degree of articular stress. A large PFJRF over a smaller area yields high articular stresses and heightens the chances of subchondral degenerative changes. The amount of patellofemoral contact area changes with knee flexion, as demonstrated in Figure 38–18. From full extension through the first 10 to 20 degrees of flexion, little contact occurs. Trochlear engagement then begins, with the inferior margin of both medial and lateral facets sharing the load.[62] Between 20 and 90 degrees of flexion, there is increased proximal patellar and lateral edge contact, and over 90 degrees the odd facet makes contact.[62] The patellofemoral contact areas are the greatest in the mid-range (30–90 degrees).

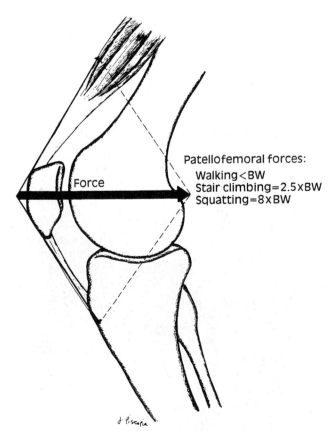

FIGURE 38–17   Patellofemoral joint reaction forces during different activities. (From Striazk AM, Stroberg AJ: Knee injuries in the skeletally immature athlete. *In* Nicholas JA, Hershman EB (eds): The Lower Extremity and Spine in Sports Medicine. St Louis, Mosby-Year Book, 1991.)

Specific Problems in the Knee

PATELLOFEMORAL PAIN SYNDROME.   This is the most common knee problem in outpatient physical medicine and rehabilitation (PM&R) practice. It is also cited as the most common knee problem in runners.[109] The differential diagnosis of anterior knee pain includes, but is not restricted to, infrapatellar bursitis, synovial plica, patellar tendinitis, quadriceps tendinitis, Osgood-Schlatter syndrome, osteochondritis dissecans, patellofemoral tracking disorder, and meniscal disorders. Factors that predispose to patellofemoral pain include the presence of patella alta, increased Q angle, femoral anteversion, and excessive pronation.[58, 91] The clinician should look for all of these as well as attempt to mobilize the patella superiorly, inferiorly, medially, and laterally to uncover any soft tissue restrictions.

The clinical symptom complex consists of pain, crepitation, and, occasionally, swelling, all typically worsened by prolonged knee flexion. The previously mentioned theater sign may also be present. Pain with knee extension should alert the clinician to the possibility of infrapatellar fat pad impingement between the inferior pole of the patella and the femoral condyle. The tissue injury complex consists of the patellar cartilage and synovium, and the insertion site of the patellar tendon.[108] Functional biomechanical deficits include all the factors above and below the knee joint which contribute to abnormal tracking. These factors include (1) medial quadriceps insufficiency, (2) inflexibility of the lateral retinacula, ITB, hamstrings, and gastrocnemius muscles (all of which either increase effective knee flexion or cause lateral tracking of the patella), (3) gluteus medius and hip external rotator weakness (leading to increased medial rotation of the femur and furthering stress on the patellofemoral joint), (4) imbalance of hip internal and external rotators (leading to increased torque at the knee) and (5) excessive pronation.[108] Tightness of the lateral retinacula and ITB creates excessive lateral tilt of the patella as demonstrated in Figure 38–19.

The functional adaptation complex consists of knee flexion contracture (loss of terminal extension), lateral patellar tracking, and altered stride to avoid full loading of the knee. The overloaded structures include the patellar tendon and lateral retinaculum locally, the hip external rotators, the medial longitudinal arch of the foot, and synovium about the first metatarsophalangeal joint (from excessive pronation and uneven load bearing at the foot).

Following acute management, problems with the malalignment syndrome should be corrected. Consideration is given to fitting the runner with foot orthotic devices to correct pronation, but only if biomechanical deficits persist after achieving full flexibility of the gastrocnemius-soleus complex, hamstrings, ITB, and VMO, and strength training has been taking place. Taping of the patella to simulate proper patellar alignment accompanied by neuromuscular re-education of the knee musculature (McConnell technique) can also be beneficial.[58, 91] McConnell has reported improvement rates of better than 90% with her technique.[58, 91] Critics of her program have pointed to the lack of data showing change in patellar position as measured radiographically, but the clinically observed improvement rates and reduction in pain scale ratings even among those

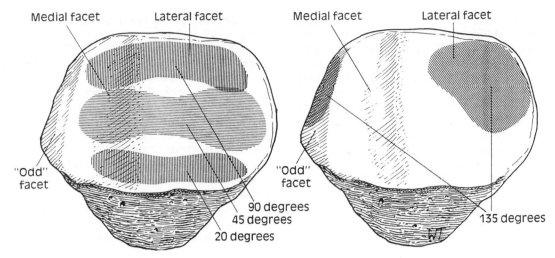

FIGURE 38–18 Areas of patellar contact at different knee flexion angles. Note that the odd facet does not effectively encounter forces until deep knee flexion. (From Warren R, Arnoczky SP, Wickiewicz TL: Anatomy of the knee. *In* Nicholas JA, Hershman EB (eds): The Lower Extremity and Spine in Sports Medicine. St Louis, Mosby–Year Book, 1991.)

without radiological improvement are far more compelling. A dynamic strengthening exercise for the hip stabilizers and the adductor magnus–VMO complex is demonstrated in Figure 38–20. Patellar stabilizing braces can be considered but should not be the first plan of attack. Strengthening of the quadriceps mechanism is typically performed in the last 30 degrees of knee extension, but the selectivity of strengthening only the VMO is debatable.[47] Recent work by Steinkamp et al.[125] indicates that the best method to strengthen the quadriceps group while incurring the least PFJRFs and PFJRS is via short-arc (<45 degrees flexion to extension) CKC exercises. Adductor squeezes, and CKC short-arc knee extension exercises also help with VMO training.

THE ITB SYNDROME.   The iliotibial band is the extension of the TFL that extends down the lateral leg to insert into Gerdy's tubercle along the lateral tibia. The *ITB syndrome* is associated with painful sensation as the ITB slides back and forth over the lateral femoral condyle as the knee flexes and extends.[94, 100, 130] Running on beveled surfaces, limb length discrepancies, tibia vara, hyperpronation, and ITB contracture are all associated risk factors.[94, 130] The Noble compression test is a useful maneuver when an ITB

friction syndrome is suspected. With the patient supine, and after positioning the knee in 90 degrees of flexion, the examiner presses on or just proximal to the lateral epicondyle. The knee is then gradually extended. Pain occurring at about 30 degrees (as the ITB crosses the bony prominence) is a positive finding.[100]

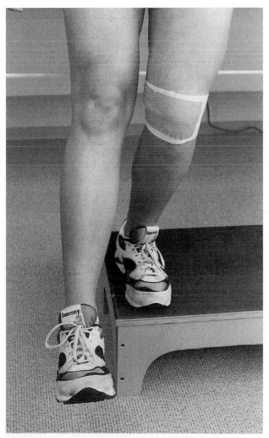

FIGURE 38–20 Patellofemoral rehabilitation. McConnell taping of the patient's knee is combined with dynamic gluteal and adductor strengthening as the patient slowly steps down.

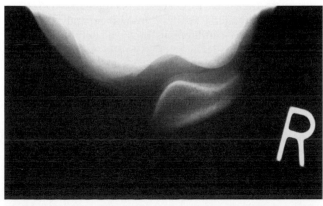

FIGURE 38–19 Sunrise view of the patella demonstrating lateral patellar tilt with elevation of the medial patellar border.

The tissue injury complex is typically the ITB over the femoral condyle or at Gerdy's tubercle. The clinical symptom complex consists of localized pain over the lateral femoral condyle, worsened with running. The functional biomechanical deficit is the inflexible ITB, while the functional adaptation complex consists of functional pronation of the foot, external rotation at the hip, internal rotation of the lower leg, and lateral patellar tracking.[108]

Rehabilitation of ITB syndrome consists of attempts to stretch the ITB, hip flexors, and gluteus maximus. Correction of foot pronation is needed and the runner should discontinue running or run only on level surfaces. Swimming and stationary ski machines can help maintain fitness. Strengthening of the hip adductors, gluteus maximus, and TFL is emphasized. The adductors counter the pull of the tight ITB and the other muscles which give rise to the ITB (gluteus maximus and TFL) and must be strengthened to avoid overuse.[108] Symptoms can take up to 2 to 6 months to resolve.[130] Occasionally, local injection of a combination of anesthetic agent and corticosteroid placed in the region of the lateral femoral condyle is helpful.[108]

PES ANSERINUS BURSITIS. The anserine bursa separates the three conjoined tendons of the pes anserinus (semitendinosus, sartorius, and gracilis muscles) from the MCL and the tibia. *Pes anserinus bursitis* is commonly seen in women with heavy thighs and osteoarthritis of the knees. The bursa can also become inflamed after direct trauma in athletes, especially soccer players. Patients complain of pain inferior to the anteromedial surface of the knee with ascension of stairs. The examiner can reproduce the symptoms by moving the knee in flexion and extension while internally rotating the leg. Palpation localizes the pain to the anserine bursa. Steroid injection is typically quite effective in reducing the inflammatory symptoms. The athlete at risk for direct trauma can benefit from padded protection around the knee. The rehabilitation program should emphasize stretching of the medial hamstrings and adductor muscles.

PREPATELLAR BURSITIS. Prepatellar bursitis, colloquially referred to as housemaid's knee, is often the result of frequent kneeling, producing an effusion of the subcutaneous bursa at the anterior surface of the patella. The patient rarely complains of pain, unless direct pressure is applied to the bursa. Occupational modifications should include patient education, avoidance of kneeling, and the use of kneepads when pressure must be applied to the patella. Rehabilitation should correct flexibility deficits in the quadriceps, hamstrings, and triceps surae, while the swelling is reduced with the application of ice.[105]

Acute Ligamentous Injuries of the Knee

Primary and secondary restraints of the knee are frequently injured in occupational and recreational activities. It is beyond the scope of this chapter to provide a detailed description of all the surgical and nonsurgical management schemes for collateral and cruciate ligament injuries. However, regardless of surgical or nonsurgical routes of treatment, the patient will benefit from a rehabilitation program that emphasizes maximizing function at the lowest cost. Once an acceptable level of function has been achieved, the patient should be directed to continue a maintenance program to prevent reinjury. There is no single best "cookbook" recipe for success; what is presented here is but one rehabilitation scheme.

ANTERIOR CRUCIATE LIGAMENT INJURIES. Partial or complete disruption of the ACL can be a disabling event for the athlete or worker. Frequently the patient describes an audible snap or pop while the lower limb undergoes hyperextension or rotational strain. The injury is painful and an acute hemarthrosis usually develops in the first hours following the insult. It is common to damage additional restraints of the knee at the same time. If the patient complains of "locking" or "clicking" and there is an associated restriction of range of motion, the clinician should be suspicious of an associated meniscal tear. An accurate diagnosis should be established to include each structure damaged, so an appropriate treatment plan can be initiated.

Examination should begin with the uninvolved lower limb and progress to include all the joints in the kinetic chain on the involved extremity. Functional limitations should be observed in standing, during ambulation, and in the squatting position. Palpation should localize tenderness and grade any effusion present. Careful examination for range-of-motion deficits is needed, using the uninvolved limb for comparison. Limitation of full extension can be seen with capsular distention, but this also raises the possibility of a meniscal tear. Loss of ACL integrity can be demonstrated with *Lachman's maneuver*.[52] As demonstrated in Figure 38–21, the examiner attempts to introduce anterior tibial translation while the limb is kept in 15 to 20 degrees of knee flexion. Complete tears of the ACL reveal significant anterior tibial translation and a loss of a distinctive end feel. A partial tear will maintain a "soft" end feel, but tibial translation will be greater than on the uninvolved side. Quantification of the tibial translation can be done with the use of an arthrometer. The *anterior drawer test* (Fig. 38–22), although technically easier for many clinicians to perform than Lachman's test, has significant limitations. For one, in this position, the hamstrings are at a mechanical advantage, and tibial translation will not be appreciated if there is any degree of hamstring activity. For another, an associated meniscal tear can act like a "door jam" and provide a block to tibial motion in this position. Finally, if there is a PCL tear, a false-positive drawer might ensue as the tibia is actually being brought back to its proper position from a position of tibial "sag" rather than truly being translated forward. The *pivot-shift test* further indicates anterolateral rotatory instability, and represents increased risk for cartilaginous injury acutely or at a later date.[37, 45, 83] The reader is referred to the work of Losee et al.[83] for a detailed explanation of this test. MRI is excellent for visualizing the disrupted ACL, as well as for assessing the presence of other coexisting injuries (Fig. 38–23).

Acute treatment includes aggressive reduction of joint swelling, either via Cryocuff compression or aspiration of the hemarthrosis. Even if surgical reconstruction is planned, there is evidence to suggest that early (within the first 3 weeks) repair is not advisable owing to an increased chance of developing graft arthrofibrosis.[120] An appropriate "prehabilitation" should be initiated after the injury and continued until surgery or entry into an aggressive nonsurgical rehabilitation program. Isometric co-contractions of patient can cycle on a stationary bike without resistance to facilitate motion as well. Once the swelling is controlled and extension is achieved, the next goal is re-establishment of a normal gait pattern. Crutch walking progresses from two crutches with partial weightbearing to one crutch and then none by the end of the first month. By this time most patients no longer need the immobilizer. CKC exercises to promote strengthening of the lower extremity are initiated. CKC exercises are theoretically preferable over the OKC type because of their reported lessening of tibiofemoral shear forces.[121] However, even with CKC exercises, hyperextension and dynamic pivot shifting must be avoided. Leg presses, bicycles, and stair climbers may be used safely. Arm ergometry and tri-limbed exercises are useful in maintaining cardiovascular fitness during this period. By the end of the first month, the bony plugs from the graft should be healed and fixed into the surrounding tibial and femoral tunnels constructed at the time of surgery.[37] The goals of the first month are summarized in Table 38–1.

During the weeks that follow, the program emphasizes further increases in range of motion, restoration of baseline strength in both hamstring and quadriceps groups, and progression to functional activities.[37, 121] Exercises to develop appropriate strength and flexibility in hip abduction, adduction, extension, and flexion are essential for maintaining control of the affected limb. Cardiovascular efforts are continued on a stationary bike, and the position of the

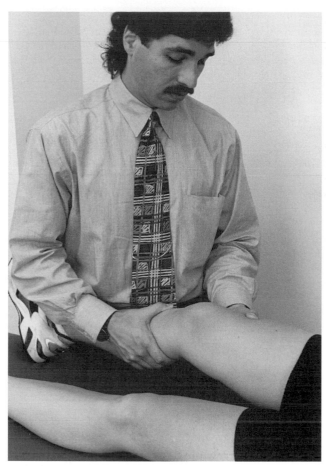

FIGURE 38–21   The Lachman maneuver. (See text for details.)

the quadriceps and hamstrings with protected weightbearing as tolerated are encouraged early on. Hyperextension of the knee should be avoided.

When reconstruction is performed, a number of materials and techniques can be used. The most common is the patellar tendon autograft with the middle third of the patellar tendon being used. The bone-patellar-bone graft offers excellent fixation and has been shown to be stronger than the original ACL.[37, 101] Following reconstruction, safe restoration of motion and weightbearing is emphasized. During the immediate postoperative period continuous passive motion (CPM) can be utilized, even at home (with the patient being instructed on correct use of the device prior to hospital discharge). In order to maximize the patient's compliance, it is necessary to provide adequate pain relief in the immediate postoperative period. Controlling the effusion with compression, ice, and elevation is the first step. Electrical stimulation of the quadriceps to help prevent atrophy can be considered. Soft tissue mobilization about the patella should be employed to restore patellar mobility and lessen the chance of adhesion formation.

It is important to gain full extension at the tibiofemoral joint during the first week to avoid a persistent "extension block." Weightbearing is done in extension while wearing an immobilizer. If swelling and other soft tissue restrictions preclude immediate extension, it can be helpful to have the patient lie prone with a towel beneath the knee while wearing an ankle weight to provide a passive stretch. The

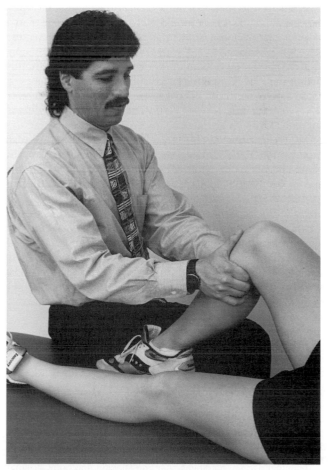

FIGURE 38–22   The anterior drawer test. (See text for details.)

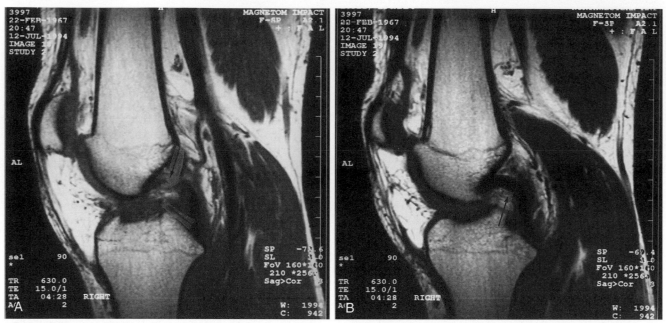

FIGURE 38–23   *A*, Disruption of the anterior cruciate ligament (ACL) viewed on sagittal MRI. *B*, The posterior cruciate ligament (PCL) is seen to be intact in the next view.

seat should be adjusted to avoid knee hyperextension. As the patient gains proprioceptive and muscular control of the lower extremity, progression to a cross-country ski machine, stair climber, or slide board is encouraged. Hyperextension at the knee should be avoided, and the entire kinetic chain should show the proper synergistic pattern for each exercise to avoid unnecessary stresses at the reconstructed knee. Reviewing proprioceptive neurofacilitation patterning can be helpful in restoring proper mechanics in these functional skills. During the second to third month, the rehabilitation program should include unidirectional jogging. Once thigh circumference approximates the size of the uninvolved limb (typically by the fourth to sixth month), functional bracing with a derotation brace may be considered. The brace provides some mechanical restraint and probably enhances proprioceptive feedback as well.[14]

Agility drills include jumping rope, lateral shuffling around cones, figure-of-8 drills, and carioca. When the quadriceps, hamstrings, and primary movers of the hip show strength that is 90% or better in comparison with the uninvolved limb, and there is no evidence of clinical pivot shifting, the patient can return to full sporting and occupational activities. Although isokinetic testing provides some level of objectivity, functional ability is our preferred method to measure the effectiveness of a successful rehabilitation program and return to full activity.

Some patients elect to pursue a nonoperative course. The exercise program is virtually identical to that following surgery, but the use of a functional brace is instituted earlier to protect the tibiofemoral joint and the menisci from potential damage. Patients who are candidates for nonoperative management include those not motivated for postsurgical rehabilitation, those who want to modify their lifestyle to accommodate the ligamentous injury, those who do not have any other associated ligamentous or meniscal injuries, and those whose lifestyle is already sedentary.[102] There are individuals who, through aggressive exercise, can often return to high levels of athletic competition without surgery. Unfortunately, at the time of injury, it is difficult to predict which patients will gain this successful outcome. Under any circumstance, the success of a nonoperative treatment requires both hard work and extensive patient education.[101]

POSTERIOR CRUCIATE LIGAMENT INJURIES.   Acute *tears of the PCL* are not as common as ACL injuries. Isolated PCL injury occurs with direct trauma forcing the tibia posteriorly (as when the knee hits a car dashboard during an automobile accident), a fall on a flexed knee, or from knee hyperflexion.[35] Unlike ACL injuries, the patient's symptoms can be vague. There is less pain, less restriction of motion, and, generally, less hemarthrosis.[35] Visual inspection will demonstrate posterior tibial translation with a positive "sag sign." The *reverse Lachman's test* (directing the tibia posteriorly while the knee is in approximately 15–20 degrees of flexion) is positive. Roentgenographic examination should be completed to exclude a bony avulsion from the tibial insertion of the PCL. Presence of an avulsed bony fragment requires immediate surgical fixation. MRI can clearly demonstrate the presence of the PCL injury.

TABLE 38–1   **Rehabilitation Goals After Anterior Cruciate Ligament Reconstruction—Weeks 0–4**

1. Control pain to maximize effort in rehabilitation
2. Rapidly reduce effusion
3. Avoid development of extension block
4. Improve flexion to 90 degrees by weeks 3–4
5. Promote wound healing and mobilize adhesions
6. Activate quadriceps mechanism
7. Begin closed kinetic chain exercises
8. Maintain general cardiovascular conditioning and body strength

Treatment of isolated injury to the PCL remains controversial. Most studies have shown good functional outcomes with nonoperative treatment and aggressive rehabilitation.[32, 42, 107, 133] Since there are relatively few reports with long-term follow-up, patients treated conservatively should be monitored for premature tibiofemoral joint degeneration due to instability. Frequently, PCL insufficiency is accompanied by other ligamentous, meniscal, or capsular damage and might necessitate surgical reconstruction[114] to manage joint instability. The MCL and the oblique popliteal ligament are commonly injured in conjunction with the PCL.

The treatment plan should be congruent with the patient's preinjury lifestyle, functional goals, and motivation for postoperative rehabilitation. Whether or not the patient undergoes surgery, it is essential to reduce the effusion and regain full range of motion as the patient reestablishes neuromuscular control to normalize gait. Exercises should initially focus on CKC strengthening of the quadriceps and then progress to include the musculature of the hip and the hamstrings. As strength returns and atrophy is reduced, the patient should begin sport-specific agility drills and be able to return to full activity at approximately 2 months post injury.

MEDIAL COLLATERAL LIGAMENT INJURIES. MCL injuries are quite common and are seen in direct trauma or as overuse syndromes. Swimmers who use the breaststroke undergo repeated valgus strain and can develop irritation of the MCL. There are three grades of damage and the first two, mild and moderate injuries, have good functional results with a nonsurgical approach and appropriate rehabilitation.

Grade I (mild) MCL strains demonstrate pain with palpation, but there is no evidence of valgus instability. Treatment is based on the type of injury and the demands of the patient's activity. In the case of a traumatic injury, pain and inflammation should be controlled with cryotherapy and possibly a limited course of NSAIDs. The patient should be placed in a locked brace for the first few days and then progressed to a hinge brace. A strengthening and flexibility program should be employed to stabilize the knee and limit further injury. Athletes attempting a return to sports can wear the hinged brace for 1 to 2 months following injury.

Grade II (moderate) injuries to the MCL are characterized by inability to fully extend the knee because of pain and inflammation. The extracapsular fibers of the MCL are ruptured. There is mild-to-moderate instability with a valgus stress applied in knee flexion and there is swelling and hemorrhage. When implementing a treatment plan it is important to recall that the ligament tightens in extension and is most relaxed in flexion. Therefore, a knee orthosis should restrict the last 20 to 30 degrees of extension for the first week while the effusion is reduced with the application of ice and compression. After the first week, a limited arc of motion (i.e., 20–75 degrees) is permitted. Early mobilization is encouraged within pain-free limits, and range of motion should be regained over a 3- to 4-week period. Full weightbearing in a brace that allows full flexion and extension begins near the end of the first month. Strengthening of the hip girdle and knee stabilizers are integrated into the rehabilitation program as the effusion is reduced and there is no exacerbation of pain. After 4 to 5 weeks the patient should be advanced to agility drills and sport-specific activities that include lateral movements. Return-to-play criteria include 90% strength or better, minimal or no thigh atrophy, and no inhibition during agility drills.[37]

Severe grade III MCL tears demonstrate instability to valgus stress in both knee flexion and extension. Hemarthrosis usually develops within a few hours owing to rupture of both the deep and superficial fibers. Treatment for grade III insufficiency remains controversial. It is essential that the knee be examined to rule out associated meniscal or cruciate ligament damage, which increases the chance that surgical repair is needed. It has been reported that isolated rupture of the MCL can undergo nonoperative treatment similar to that for a grade II tear.[54, 63, 118] Conversely, Kannus[70] reported deterioration of the knee after long-term follow-up of nonoperative treatment. However, closer review of this work reveals that one third of his population with insufficiency of the MCL also had a Lachman's maneuver of at least grade II, which could account for some of the unsatisfactory results with nonoperative care. Although the decision for surgical care remains controversial, the development of an appropriate treatment plan should focus on the patient's preinjury demands and motivation to return to biomechanically stressful activities. In the case of a young, aggressive person wanting to return to previous activities, surgical reconstruction with appropriate postoperative rehabilitation might be warranted. For patients who are able to modify their lifestyle, a nonoperative approach can achieve satisfactory functional results.

LATERAL COLLATERAL LIGAMENT INJURIES. The treatment program for *isolated LCL injuries* is similar to the nonoperative approach described for the MCL. However, the vulnerability of the peroneal nerve at the level of the fibular head must be kept in mind. The peroneal nerve can be injured during the initial trauma or can be subjected to pressure with improper taping or bracing or frozen during cryotherapy. Grade III injuries are often associated with capsular or cruciate ligament insufficiency giving rise to a rotational instability as well. These combination injuries require surgical reconstruction to avoid later degeneration of the joint and allow return to more demanding activities.[36]

MENISCAL LESIONS. These are common in both sport and industry. Tears in the semilunar cartilages are most common in the posterior horn of the medial meniscus. Injury usually follows forceful rotation of the lower extremity, while the foot is firmly placed on the ground. An effusion usually develops within 24 to 48 hours, in contrast to the rapid development of hemarthrosis seen in an acute ligament rupture. Damage may range from a small peripheral tear to a larger bucket-handle tear presenting with intense pain. The patient may describe a sensation of giving way or mechanical locking. Clinical examination often reveals tenderness on palpation of the joint line. *McMurray's test* (Fig. 38–24) is performed with varying degrees of tibial internal and external rotation combined with valgus or varus moment, while the limb is moved from full flexion to extension. The test is positive if a "click" is produced or if pain is reproduced. Care must be taken to not be fooled by clicking from within the patellofemoral joint or the pseudomeniscal clicking pro-

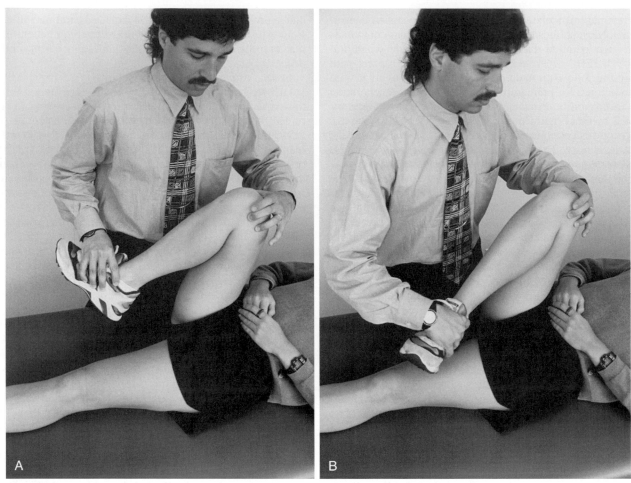

FIGURE 38–24 *A* and *B*, McMurray's test. The knee is brought in and out of flexion with internal and external rotatory loading. The examiner's fingers are on the joint line.

duced by a plica. The posterior meniscus can be further loaded by having the patient attempt to squat or by the examiner taking the knee into deep flexion and introducing rotation. Intermittent locking can be a subtle sign or be more obvious in the case of a large bucket-handle tear. MRI can be used to demonstrate a meniscal tear, but if mechanical symptoms exist, arthroscopy is probably the diagnostic test of choice. Arthroscopic evaluation is required when range of motion is severely limited, or if the knee joint is locked. Locking can be observed with osteochondral lesions, cruciate ligament rupture, bony avulsions, or meniscal impingement.

Treatment of meniscal lesions is dependent on the severity of the injury to the meniscus and the possibility of combined damage. In the absence of a locked knee, a period of observation to allow for pain control and reduction of the effusion can help delineate the most appropriate treatment. The presence of associated ligamentous tears or inability to bear weight after 2 to 3 days suggests the need for arthroscopic evaluation. If the patient is able to regain full joint motion, reduction of swelling, and full strength (and high-intensity athletic competition is not planned), a nonoperative approach can be successful.

The surgical approach to meniscal tear management has changed significantly in the last 15 to 20 years. Total meniscectomy is no longer an acceptable treatment, and

efforts are geared toward preserving as much of the cartilage as possible. The degenerative effects of meniscectomy described by Fairbanks[40] include joint space narrowing, ridging, and squaring of the condyles. Preservation of the meniscus reduces the development of such degenerative changes.[31, 81, 86] Currently, efforts are made to repair the meniscus when possible and to remove as little of the meniscus as possible.[96]

For the nonsurgically treated patient, early rehabilitation consists of pain and swelling reduction with institution of hamstring and ITB stretching and short-arc CKC activities. Swimming pool–based exercise can facilitate recovery and allow the patient to maintain endurance. Use of a cane or crutches to unload the affected side is strongly recommended. Once symptoms are reduced, the intensity of the program is increased, but activities involving loading with rotation are avoided.

For the surgically treated patient, postoperative rehabilitation depends on the complexity of the repair. Once pain-free range of motion has been established, and there is no joint line tenderness, the patient should return to full weightbearing. Too early a return to weightbearing activities or overaggressive strengthening can induce effusion and an exacerbation of pain. If this occurs the program should be modified and the patient returned to a partial weightbearing status. Deep squatting should be avoided during the first 6 months.[43] Progressive strengthening should focus on the quadriceps and hamstrings, and include the entire lower extremity.

OSTEOCHONDRITIS DISSECANS. This is a lesion of subchondral bone with or without articular cartilage involvement.[50] In the knee, the most common site for a subchondral lesion occurs at the interior portion of the medial femoral condyle. Lesions in the lateral condyle and in the patellar articular cartilage occur with less frequency. Chondral flaps and chondral loose bodies may also be present.[20, 27] Patients experience intermittent mechanical symptoms with or without pain. An effusion may be present. X-ray films should include a tunnel view to evaluate the intracondylar notch. CT is helpful in evaluating the bony lesions, while MRI can provide a more accurate view of the articular cartilage. Treatment is based on the staging of the lesion, and the patient's symptoms.[50] Arthroscopic evaluation is indicated when there is separation of the lesion from the femur, mechanical locking, or chronic pain and effusion.

The Leg

Relevant Anatomy and Biomechanics

The tibia and fibula and associated structures make up the leg. All muscles are innervated by the tibial or peroneal nerves. The crural structures are encased in a tight connective tissue fascia, with separation of the muscles of this region into four compartments. The anterior compartment consists of the anterior tibial, extensor hallucis longus, extensor digitorum, peroneus tertius, and deep peroneal nerve. The lateral consists of the peroneus longus and brevis muscles, and the superficial peroneal nerve. The superficial posterior compartment consists of the gastrocnemius-soleus complex, plantaris, and sural nerve. The deep posterior compartment includes the posterior tibialis, flexor digitorum longus, flexor hallucis longus, and posterior tibial vessels and nerve. The gastrocnemius-soleus complex blends distally into the Achilles tendon, the most powerful plantar flexor group. The anterior tibial muscle functions as a dorsiflexor and invertor, the posterior tibial muscle as a forefoot flexor and invertor, while the peroneus longus and brevis muscles serve as the only major evertors and provide some plantar flexion as well.

ACHILLES TENDINITIS (TENDINOSIS). This is perhaps the most common injury of the lower leg. Repeated episodes of microtrauma result in the development of microtearing of the tendon in the region of least vascularity, approximately 2 to 6 cm above the tendon insertion.[79, 108] Excessive pronation, tight heel cords, and rearfoot or forefoot varus can all induce this.[108] Overtraining, a single excessively strenuous workout, and hill running can create this problem as well. It is important to recognize that while the majority of patients feel they have an acute inflammatory problem (tendinitis), they actually have a chronic problem (tendinosis), in which asymptomatic intratendinous degeneration has been occurring over time.[73] This can lead to frank rupture of the tendon.

The tissue injury complex is generally confined to the myotendinous junction of the Achilles tendon. In more chronic cases, this can extend throughout the midsubstance of the tendon. The clinical symptom complex is pain located typically 6 to 8 cm proximal to the insertion on the calcaneus that is worsened by dorsiflexion.[108] The functional biomechanical deficits consist of weak dorsiflexors and tight plantar flexors, while the functional adaptation complex includes increased knee flexion and increased pronation (both particularly influenced by the tight gastrocnemius which crosses both knee and ankle joints).

The rehabilitation program is initiated with the PRICE principle and anti-inflammatory medications. The tendon is never injected. Heel lifts often provide some relief in early rehabilitation, but should not be used indefinitely (this promotes shortening of the heel cord). Ultrasound can be useful in chronic cases if loosening of old, scarred connective tissue is needed and stretching is difficult.[108] Reduction in weightbearing activity is mandatory. These patients are good candidates for aquatic-based conditioning. As pain is reduced, the patients should go through a gradual program of first concentric and ultimately eccentric strengthening of the plantar flexors. If the pain continues despite all the above measures, an MRI study of the Achilles tendon can help identify previously undetected partial tendon tears, musculotendinous tears, retrocalcaneal bursitis, or stress fractures.[73, 74, 108]

STRESS FRACTURES. A *stress fracture* is defined as a partial or complete fracture of a bone that results from that bony region's inability to withstand a repetitively applied subthreshold and nonviolent mechanical stress.[90] Persons most at risk are those who have asymmetrical limb lengths, who pronate excessively, or who run on rigid surfaces.[33, 90] Common sites of stress fractures in runners include the tibia, fibula, navicular bone, metatarsals, and femur.[33, 90] The tibia is the most common site (34%), followed by the fibula (24%), metatarsals (20%), and femur (14%).[90] Pain that is relatively well localized is a major clinical feature.[90] Pain produced over the suspected fracture site with application of a vibrating tuning fork onto the affected area or with percussion of the bone away from the affected site can also suggest stress fracture.[117, 140] Because they frequently do not produce a full cortical defect, stress fractures are difficult to detect by routine radiographs[17] early in their course. Bone scans are recommended in cases of increased clinical suspicion when the plain film study is negative.[17] An example of a fibular stress fracture in a runner that did not show up on plain films is shown in Figure 38–25.

Local bone represents the tissue injury complex. The clinical symptom complex consists of localized pain tending to worsen with a reproducible amount of activity, and which is relieved by rest.[108] The functional biomechanical deficits and adaptations are dictated by the site of fracture.

During rehabilitation of a stress fracture, the first principle is to stay below the level of activity that induces symptoms. Running on dry land is prohibited until an adequate amount of time for healing has passed; this is approximately 3 weeks for the fibula, 4 to 8 weeks for the tibia (although considerably longer if the tibial plateau has been affected), and months (with limited weightbearing) for the neck of the femur.[90, 108] In the past, athletes with stress fractures were primarily restricted to alternative forms of aerobic exercises such as swimming and bicycling, which were of general conditioning value, but were not particularly specific to running. In recent years, aqua

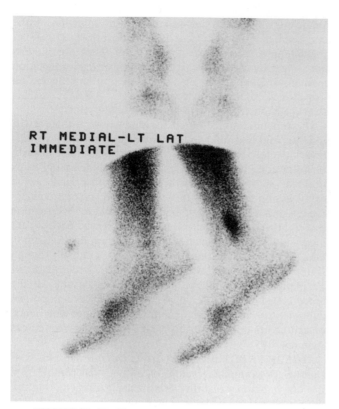

RT MEDIAL–LT LAT
IMMEDIATE

FIGURE 38–25   Bone scan, revealing a stress fracture.

running has become available. During aqua running, the runner dons an inflatable vest and is placed into the deep end of the pool so that the feet are not in contact with the bottom. The athlete is then tethered to a side of the pool and begins to "run." The viscosity and drag of the water provide resistance proportional to the effort, while the buoyancy effect maintains nonweightbearing conditions.[131] This is an excellent way to maintain condition while still protecting the injured area.

COMPARTMENT SYNDROMES.   In *dynamic compartment syndromes* of the leg, elevated tissue pressures in any of the four compartments transiently reduce the capillary perfusion below the level needed for tissue viability. The anterior compartment is most frequently affected. Dysesthesias in the distribution of the deep peroneal nerve, foreleg pain, dorsiflexor weakness, and hypoperfusion ensue. The syndrome can be confirmed with intracompartmental pressure measurements.[89, 128] Postexertional MRIs can also be of value.[6] Although fasciotomy is often seen as the definitive treatment for this problem, there is recent evidence that cycling produces lower anterior compartment pressures than does running, implying that for those athletes willing to modify their training regimens, an alternative to surgery, with maintenance of fitness, is possible.[16]

BURSAL SYNDROMES.   The retrocalcaneal, subtendinous bursa lies between the posterior surface of the calcaneus and the tendon of the triceps surae. Inflammation of the bursa can result from training errors, as in a runner who increases mileage too rapidly, and from ill-fitting shoes, which can create excessive pressure in the heel counter region. Discomfort occurs when the examiner places the thumb and index finger on the anterior edges of

the Achilles tendon and applies pressure. Footwear modification is an important first step. Symptoms are controlled with ice and anti-inflammatory medications. As the pain is resolving, the patient should stretch the triceps surae complex daily to avoid recurrence. Injections into the bursa are done only with caution, as corticosteroids can weaken the Achilles tendon, increasing the risk for tendon rupture.

Subcutaneous bursitis, or Achilles bursitis, involves the bursa lying subcutaneous to the posterior surface of the Achilles tendon. The patient develops midline swelling where the upper edge of the heel counter comes in contact with the heel cord. Subcutaneous bursitis is commonly seen in women who wear high heels that apply direct pressure on the bursa. The mainstay of treatment is to change the patient's shoes. Ice and anti-inflammatory medications help provide symptomatic relief.

Ankle Injuries

Ankle injuries are probably the most common sports-related injury and one of the most frequently seen musculoskeletal problems presenting to the outpatient physiatrist's office. Inversion sprains alone account for at least 85% of the isolated ankle injuries.[24, 30, 56, 126] As with many of the entities previously discussed, without appropriate rehabilitation there is great likelihood for recurrent injury.

Relevant Anatomy and Biomechanics

The ankle can be described as a hinge joint with a mortise (the tibia and fibula) and tenon (talus). The distal tibia forms the medial malleolus, while the fibula, which extends further distally, forms the lateral malleolus. There is approximately 20 degrees of ankle dorsiflexion and 50 degrees of available plantar flexion under normal conditions. Both the talar and tibiofibular joint are widest anteriorly, so the joint has its maximum osteological stability in dorsiflexion (when the wide portion of the talus becomes wedged into the narrower portion of the mortise) and minimal osteological stability in plantar flexion. The joint is obliquely placed relative to the knee joint axis and the line of progression, creating an external tibial torsion of approximately 20 degrees. The subtalar (talocalcaneal) and midtarsal (talonavicular and calcaneocuboid) joints both permit the additional motions of inversion and eversion, and influence hindfoot-to-midfoot load transfer.

The critical ligamentous structures on the lateral side include the posterior talofibular ligament (PTFL), anterior talofibular ligament (ATFL), and the calcaneofibular ligament (CFL) (Fig. 38–26A). Of the three lateral ligaments, the PTFL is the strongest and the ATFL is the weakest. On the medial side the deltoid ligament is composed of the anterior tibiotalar, posterior tibiotalar, tibionavicular, and tibiocalcaneal ligaments (Fig. 38–26B). Anterolaterally, between the fibula and the tibia, is the tibiofibular syndesmosis. The lateral ligaments tend to check inversion and stabilize against posterior talar displacement while the medial complex guards against eversion injuries. The hinge motion of the talar joint has a direct effect on the tautness of the LCLs. Dorsiflexion promotes ATFL laxity and CFL tautness, whereas plantar flexion results in ATFL tautness and CFL laxity. The PTFL is the restraint against posterior displacement. Inversion sprains typically occur when the

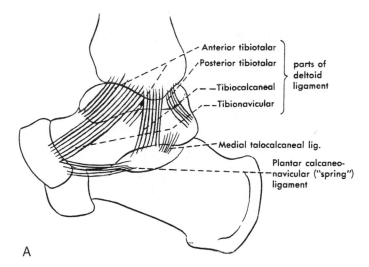

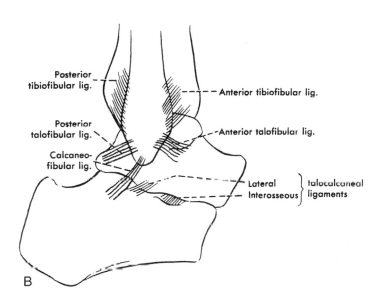

FIGURE 38–26 *A*, Medial ligaments of the ankle. *B*, Lateral ligaments of the ankle. (From Hollinshead WH, Jenkins DB: Functional Anatomy of the Limbs and Back, ed 5. Philadelphia, WB Saunders, 1981.)

ankle is plantar-flexed, so the ATFL is the most vulnerable of the lateral ligaments. The broadness of the medial malleolus, the angle of the mortise, and the toughness of the deltoid complex provide much greater restriction to extremes of eversion than do the lateral structures to extremes of inversion, so medial injuries are far less frequent. Muscular structures about the ankle that provide additional support include the peroneus longus and brevis laterally, the anterior tibial dorsally, the posterior tibial, flexor digitorum longus, and flexor hallucis longus medially, and the gastrocnemius-soleus complex posteriorly. Peripheral nerves vulnerable to injury in this region include the sural (laterally), deep and superficial peroneals (dorsolaterally), and saphenous (dorsomedially). The distal tibial nerve may be damaged with medial ankle injury or compressed in the region of the tarsal tunnel.

Mechanisms of Injury

Ankle sprains typically occur when the foot and ankle are plantar-flexed. The ATFL is generally the first structure injured with a combined inversion–plantar flexion stress.

The CFL is the second structure injured as the inversion stress increases. For the PTFL to become injured, either inversion must continue further or some posterior displacement of the talus must occur.[112] Inversion in neutral dorsiflexion primarily stresses the CFL. The deltoid ligament is injured with eversion stress. Addition of any rotatory stress to the above, or inversion in dorsiflexion leads to syndesmosis injury.[112, 113]

Classes of Injury

When ligaments endure injury, the most common site along the ligament tends to be within the midsubstance of the ligament.[112] Tears which occur closer to the insertion are often accompanied by avulsion fractures. More violent forces will be associated with multiligamentous injury or fractures of bones about the ankle mortise. Each ligament is graded separately. The following system combines the categorization of a number of authors[13, 26, 71, 112]:

Grade I (mild)—minor ligamentous disruption (essentially a stretch) with maintenance of integrity and no signs of instability.

Grade II (moderate)—near complete disruption with macroscopic tearing and swelling. There is a moderate amount of functional loss such as difficulty with toe-walking and there is mild or moderate instability.

Grade III (severe)—complete ligamentous rupture with obvious swelling, discoloration, and tenderness. There is significant functional loss with limited range of motion due to swelling, limited weightbearing tolerance due to pain, and reduced stability due to the ligamentous disruption.

The mechanism and consequences of the acute ankle injury can be obtained from the history and physical examination. Sensation of a tear or pop with a "rolling over" of the ankle are highly suggestive of an ATFL or CFL tear. Anteriorly based pain and inability to bear weight following the patient's foot "getting stuck" while the leg continued to rotate suggests syndesmosis injury.

The examination should be done in a methodical manner. The fibular head region is palpated to detect defects and tenderness suggestive of fracture and for irritability over the peroneal nerve. The fibular shaft is percussed throughout its length to identify possible fracture sites. The distal tibia and fibula, and the talar dome region are similarly inspected for overt fracture. The foot must not be ignored since metatarsal fractures (e.g., the Jones fracture of the fifth metatarsal) often accompany higher-grade sprains. Points of maximal tenderness are commonly elicited over the ATFL and CFL. Careful deep palpation underneath the distal lateral malleolus can reveal a defect consistent with complete CFL tear. A complete sensory examination and light percussion over the superficial nerves are important to identify stretch injuries which can cause superimposed dyesthetic pain. Examination of the injured ankle proper should be preceded by examination of the uninjured side. This gives a sense of the "baseline" examination for the examiner and helps put a patient a bit more at ease.

The *anterior drawer test* is the hallmark test for integrity of the ATFL. The patient's calf muscles should be relaxed and the foot should be in approximately 10 degrees of plantar flexion. The calcaneus is grasped firmly and drawn forward while the tibia is pushed posteriorly with the other hand (Fig. 38–27). Under normal conditions, the translation of the talus is no more than 4 mm.[112, 113] A drawer of more than 8 mm is indicative of at least an ATFL tear.[49, 112, 113]

The *talar tilt* (inversion) test is more sensitive for CFL tears. The lower leg is held firmly by one hand while applying an inversion stress to the talus and calcaneus with the other hand. Separation of the surface of the talus from the tibia (i.e., a tilting) is considered a positive test. The ankle should be kept in neutral during this maneuver, since plantar flexion stresses the ATFL.

The *clunk* (side-to-side) test is a gross assessment of mortise widening, as when there is a tibiofibular ligament complex injury. Grasping the calcaneus with one hand, and surrounding the distal third of the tibia and fibula with the other, the examiner attempts to move the talus from side to side. A "clunk" or "thud" is felt as the talus hits the tibia or fibula. Care must be taken not to allow inversion or eversion to occur during this maneuver, or a false-positive result will be obtained.

When there is true tibiofibular diastasis due to complete

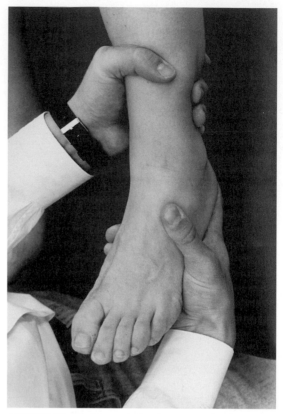

FIGURE 38–27 The anterior drawer test for the ankle.

syndesmosis injury, the *squeeze test* can be helpful. Proximal compression of the tibia and fibula together produces pain at the level of the interosseous membrane.[60] Diastasis compromises load bearing at the ankle joint severely and requires surgical consultation.

The *eversion test* assesses the integrity of the deltoid ligament complex. The lower tibia is grasped in one hand and the heel in the other. If the tibiotalar joint widens medially with eversion stress, the test is positive.

If a sprain is felt to be grade 2 or more, x-ray films should be obtained to rule out a coexisting fracture. Standard views include an anteroposterior, a lateral, and a "mortise" view, taken with the lower leg in 20 degrees of internal rotation. The mortise view is necessary to fully evaluate the talar dome surface as well as to adequately examine the distal tibial and fibular surfaces. If the mortise is not disrupted, the distances between the lateral talus and fibula and between the medial talus and the tibia are equal.[112] A medial clear space (the distance between the medial tibia border and the talus border) of greater than 5 mm suggests deltoid ligament injury, while 5 mm or more distance between the medial fibular cortex and the incisura fibularis of the talus indicates a syndesmosis tear.[80]

When examining radiographs of the ankle it is important to remember the "ring concept."[49] When the mortise is viewed directly, the lateral malleolus, the tibial plafond superiorly, the medial malleolus, and the talus inferiorly form a ring which is held together by the lateral and medial ligaments and the syndesmosis (Fig. 38–28). Disruption of any of these support structures tends to alter the shape of the ring. Furthermore, if the ring is deformed on one side

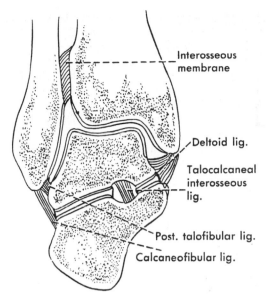

FIGURE 38–28   The "ring" of the ankle. (See text for details.)

Interosseous membrane

Deltoid lig.

Talocalcaneal interosseous lig.

Post. talofibular lig.

Calcaneofibular lig.

(i.e., a distal fibular fracture), one must always look for a coexisting injury somewhere else along the ring (i.e., a deltoid ligament injury with widening of the medial mortise).

Occasionally "stress views" of the ankle are performed.[48] These can be helpful in determining completeness of a ligamentous tear, or more important, determining the presence of avulsed fragments of bone. Traction forces are applied to the ankle to promote a tilt or drawer effect and comparisons are made between injured and uninjured sides for asymmetry. For the "tilt stress," the angle between the talar dome and tibial plafond is measured. Although controversy exists as to the exact angle constituting a significant widening, lateral opening of more than 10 degrees suggests either a CFL or ATFL injury, while greater than 20 degrees is highly suggestive of a combined CFL and ATFL injury.[30, 112, 113]

There are many types of fractures associated with ankle sprains, and it is beyond the scope of this chapter to discuss them all. The *spiral fracture of the distal fibula* is one of the most common fractures of the ankle region. When seen, the proximal fibula must also be examined as forces may have been transmitted up the interosseous membrane. The *Jones fracture* is an avulsion fracture at the base of the fifth metatarsal associated with inversion sprain and pulling of the peroneus brevis. *Osteochondral talar dome fractures* may follow almost any type of ankle injury and should be considered in "slow-healing" cases and where the region over the talus is tender. *Mortise disruption* follows syndesmosis or deltoid ligament injury; the ring of the mortise should immediately be inspected for evidence of bimalleolar (or trimalleolar) fractures.[30, 77, 112, 113] With the exception of the nondisplaced Jones fracture, all of these problems may require surgical consultation.

Ankle Rehabilitation

Acute treatment of all sprains includes icing and compressive wrapping of the injured site (tissue injury complex). Cryocuffs are particularly helpful in minimizing the amount of postinjury swelling, which will facilitate the rehabilitation process. Early mobilization of the sprained but nonfractured ankle is the preferred treatment. The ankle should be protected with elastic support, air stirrup splints, lace-up braces, or plastic-molded supports. Casting of the uncomplicated sprain actually slows recovery, even in grade 3 sprains.[24, 65, 71] Crutches are only used when gait is affected enough to increase the chance of further injury or when pain precludes full weightbearing. Ankle pumping, "writing the alphabet" with the feet, and stretching of the gastrocnemius-soleus complex (tightness is a typical accompanying biomechanical deficit) can all be started during this period. During the next phase, strengthening of the evertors, invertors, plantar flexors, and dorsiflexors can be performed dynamically with elastic tubing, and then via heel raises and partial squats. Hip abductor muscle strengthening should be included as well. Balance boards are an essential part of the rehabilitation, as these help with proprioceptive retraining as well as strengthening (Fig. 38–29). Bicycle exercise is a safe way to maintain or increase endurance without subjecting the ankle to excessive stress. As the patient progresses, more dynamic training is introduced including slide board, figure-of-8 running drills, hexagon drills, and carioca drills. Good functional tests to determine readiness to return to activity include "shuttle runs" and single-leg hopping wherewith side-to-side comparisons for hop height or time to cover a given distance can be made. In our experience, the majority of sprains treated in this manner are ready to return to activity within 1 to 3 weeks. The use of postrehabilitation bracing is not mandatory, but athletes in higher-risk sports such as

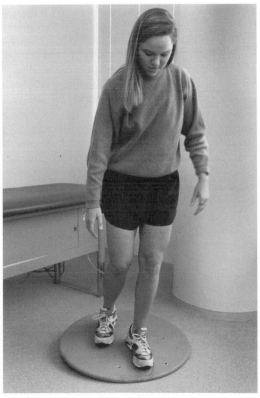

FIGURE 38–29   Dynamic ankle rehabilitation with a balance board.

basketball, soccer, and football might elect to use high-top shoes, lace-up braces, or taping for injury prophylaxis.

Foot Injuries

PLANTAR FASCIITIS. This consists of traction-induced microtears of the plantar fascia and its associated structures at the insertion on the calcaneus.[78] Ordinarily, the fascia tightens passively with toe extension, creating a stiffer midfoot with arch elevation. This "windlass effect" and the transition from pronation to supination are critical for transforming the foot from a deformable structure suited for surface accommodation and shock absorption to one that is rigid and suited for use as a lever during the attempt to push off the ground. Limited ankle dorsiflexion, excessive pronation, and a tight gastrocnemius-soleus complex all increase the chance of developing plantar fasciitis because prolonged pronation during the stance phase decreases the chances of achieving the rigid, closed, packed midtarsal joint needed to push off the ground. This subjects other medial support structures such as the plantar fascia to increased tensile forces and excessive overload. The patient with plantar fasciitis typically presents with progressively worsening pain during exertion and dreads taking the first step out of bed in the morning. It is worth noting that although plantar fasciitis is usually seen in persons with high or normal arches, it can also be seen in the person with flat feet.

Symptoms of plantar fasciitis consist of point tenderness along the medial fascia, inability to run, and a painful first step of the morning.[75] The functional biomechanical deficits include decreased plantar flexor flexibility and strength, and functional pronation.[75] Functional adaptations include attempted inversion to reduce medial structure overload and, in the case of runners, forefoot running with a choppy stride.[75, 108]

Acute management consists of the PRICE principle and use of anti-inflammatory medications as needed. Ice massage is a particularly useful modality. If the diagnosis is clear, radiographs are not needed. If they are obtained, it is important to realize that heel spurs on the calcaneus are a common radiographic finding (up to 30% of the asymptomatic population) and are likely to represent repetitive plantar ligament traction rather than a site of true pathological changes.[108] Similarly, spurs may not be found in patients with profound symptoms. Consideration is given to steroid injection into the calcaneal attachment, although this is rarely our approach.[108, 140] Arch supports, counterforce taping, and heel pads may be helpful.[75, 108] The critical measures are stretching of the gastrocnemius-soleus complex, hamstrings, and plantar fascia and foot intrinsic strengthening, not merely supporting the longitudinal arch.[75, 108] Chronic cases can take up to 3 to 4 months to resolve. For any person with this problem, formulation of a temporary alternative training program such as rowing, swimming, or aqua running can maintain fitness without delaying healing of the plantar fasciitis.

CALCANEAL BURSITIS. This often develops in elderly patients with a calcified spur subjecting the bursa to trauma after prolonged walking or running. Evaluation of the footwear often reveals poor shock-absorbing capacity. Selecting the appropriate walking or running shoes supple-

mented with a heel cup is often enough to relieve the symptoms. Restoration of normal flexibility and strengthening of the foot intrinsics can help prevent recurring symptoms. Athletes should be encouraged to change running shoes every 200 to 300 miles owing to the midsole break-down that occurs after this amount of wear.[140]

MORTON'S NEUROMA. This represents the entrapment of interdigital nerves in the foot. The structure most often implicated is the transverse metatarsal ligament, but surrounding bursal structures may also cause local irritation.[5] The neuromas are most frequently found between the third and second interspaces. Patients complain of an aching forefoot, with at times lancinating pain confined to the foot. It is exacerbated by wearing tight shoes, high heels, and athletic activities requiring repetitive forefoot weightbearing (i.e., bicycling, step aerobics). Patients obtain almost immediate relief when they take their shoes off and often prefer to walk barefoot. During physical examination, grasping the foot in one hand and squeezing the metatarsals together will reproduce the symptoms. Along with this maneuver, the examiner must examine each metatarsal ray individually to be sure that the pain is not coming directly from the shaft of the metatarsals. If there is even the slightest question of there being an overt fracture or a stress fracture, radiographs or a bone scan should be obtained. Intermediate-to-long-term relief may be obtained with footwear modification (increased width), orthotic inserts, and corticosteroid injection. For those who do not respond to conservative measures, neuroma excision may provide relief.[88]

References

1. Ackerman L, Ramamurthy S, Jablokow V, et al: Case report 488. Skeletal Radiol 1988; 17:310–314.
2. Agre JC: Hamstring injuries: Proposed aetiologic factors, prevention and treatment. Sports Med 1985; 2:21–33.
3. Agur AMR: Grant's Atlas of Anatomy, ed 9. Baltimore, Williams & Wilkins, 1991.
4. Ahmed AM, Burke DL: In vitro measurement of static pressure distribution in synovial joints in the tibial surface of the knee. J Biomech Eng 1983; 105:216–225.
5. Alexander IJ, Johnson KA, Parr JW: Morton's neuroma: A review of current concepts. Orthopedics 1987; 10:103–106.
6. Amendola A, Rorabeck CH, Vellet D: The use of magnetic resonance imaging in exertional compartment syndromes. Am J Sports Med 1990; 18:29–34.
7. An HS, Simpson JM, Gale S, et al: Acute anterior compartment syndrome in the thigh: A case report and review of the literature. J Orthop Trauma 1987; 1:180–182.
8. Antao NA: Myositis of the hip in a professional soccer player: A case report. Am J Sports Med 1988; 16:82–83.
9. Apple DF Jr: Adolescent runners. Clin Sports Med 1985; 4:641–655.
10. Apple DF Jr: End stage running problems. Clin Sports Med 1985; 4:657–670.
11. Arnoczky SP, Warren RF: Microvasculature of the human meniscus. Am J Sports Med 1982; 10:90–95.
12. Bach DK, Green DS, Jensen GM, et al: A comparison of muscular tightness in runners and nonrunners and the relation of muscular tightness to low back pain in runners. J Orthop Sports Phys Ther 1985; 6:315–323.
13. Balduni FC, Vegso JJ, Torg JS, et al: Management and rehabilitation of ligamentous injuries to the ankle. Sports Med 1987; 4:364–380.
14. Barrack RL, Skinner HB, Buckley SL: Proprioception in the anterior cruciate deficient knee. Am J Sports Med 1989; 17:1–6.
15. Barton PM: Piriformis syndrome: A rational approach to management. Pain 1991; 47:345–352.
16. Bechham SG, Grana WA, Buckley P, et al: A comparison of anterior

compartment pressures in competitive runners and cyclists. Am J Sports Med 1993; 21:36–40.

17. Belkin SC: Stress fractures in athletes. Orthop Clin North Am 1980; 11:735–742.

18. Booth DW, Westers BM: The management of athletes with myositis ossificans traumatica. Can J Sports Sci 1989; 14:10–16.

19. Bourne MH, Hazel WA, Scott SG, et al: Anterior knee pain. Mayo Clin Proc 1988; 63:482–491.

20. Bradley J, Dandy DJ: Osteochondritis dissecans and other lesions of the femoral condyles. J Bone Joint Surg Am 1983; 65:193.

21. Brody DM: Running injuries. Clinical Symp 1987; 39:2–36.

22. Brukner P, Khan K: Clinical Sports Medicine. Sydney, Australia, McGraw-Hill, 1993, p 522.

23. Burkett LN: Causative factors in hamstring strains. Med Sci Sports Exerc 1970; 2:39–42.

24. Buschbacher R: The use and abuse of ankle supports in sports injuries. J Back Musculoskeletal Rehabil 1993; 3:57–68.

25. Cailliet R: Low Back Pain Syndrome. Philadelphia, FA Davis, 1989.

26. Chapman MW: Part II. Sprains of the ankle. Instruct Course Lect 1975; 24:294–308.

27. Clanton TO, Delee JC: Osteochondritis dissecans: History, pathophysiology and current treatment concepts. Clin Orthop 1982; 167:50.

28. Collee G, Dijkmans BAC, Vandenbroucke JD, et al: Greater trochanteric pain syndrome (trochanteric bursitis) in low back pain. Scand J Rheumatol 1991; 20:262–266.

29. Cox JS: Patellofemoral problems in runners. Clin Sports Med 1985; 4:699–715.

30. Cox JS: Surgical and nonsurgical treatment of acute ankle sprains. Clin Orthop 1985; 198:118–126.

31. Cox JS, Nye CE, Schaeffer WW, et al: The degenerative effects of partial and total resection of the medial meniscus in dogs' knees. Clin Orthop 1975; 109:178–183.

32. Cross MJ, Powell JF: Long-term follow up of posterior cruciate ligament rupture: A study of 116 cases. Am J Sports Med 1984; 12:292–297.

33. Daffner RH: Stress fractures: Current concepts. Skeletal Radiol 1978; 2:221–229.

34. Deal CL, Canoso JJ: Meralgia paresthetica and large abdomens. Ann Intern Med 1982; 96:787–788.

35. Delee JC, Bergfeld JA, Drez D Jr, et al: The posterior cruciate ligament. In Delee JC, Drez D Jr (eds): Orthopaedic Sports Medicine. Philadelphia, WB Saunders, 1994, pp 1374–1400.

36. Delee JC, Riley MB, Rockwood CA: Acute straight lateral instability of the knee. Am J Sports Med 1983; 11:404.

37. Dillingham MF, King WD, Gamburd RS: Rehabilitation of the knee following anterior cruciate ligament and medial collateral ligament injuries. Phys Med Rehabil Clin North Am 1994; 5:175–194.

38. Draganich LF, Jaeger RJ, Kralj AR: Coactivation of the hamstrings and quadriceps during extension of the knee. J Bone Joint Surg Am 1989; 71:1075–1081.

39. Ecker AD, Woltman HW: Meralgia paresthetica: a report of 150 cases. JAMA 1938; 110:1650–1652.

40. Fairbanks TJ: Knee joint changes after meniscectomy. J Bone Joint Surg Br 1948; 30:664–670.

41. Ficat RP, Hungerford DS: Disorders of the Patellofemoral Joint. Baltimore, William & Wilkins, 1977.

42. Fowler PJ, Messieh SS: Isolated posterior cruciate ligament injuries in athletes. Am J Sports Med 1987; 15:553–557.

43. Fu FH, Baratz M: Meniscal injuries. In Delee JC, Drez D Jr (eds): Orthopaedic Sports Medicine. Philadelphia, WB Saunders, 1994, pp 1146–1248.

44. Funk FJ Jr: Injuries of the extensor mechanism of the knee. Athletic Training 1975; 10:141–145.

45. Galway RD, Beaupre A, MacIntosh DL: Pivot shift: A clinical sign of symptomatic anterior cruciate ligament insufficiency. J Bone Joint Surg Br 1972; 54:763.

46. Geraci MC: Rehabilitation of pelvis hip and thigh injuries in sports. Phys Med Rehabil Clin North Am 1994; 5:157–174.

47. Grabiner MD, Koh TJ, Draganich LF: Neuromechanics of the patellofemoral joint. Med Sci Sports Exerc 1994; 26:10–21.

48. Grace DL: Lateral ankle ligament injuries. Inversion and anterior stress radiography. Clin Orthop 1984; 183:153–156.

49. Grana WA: Acute ankle injuries. In Renstrom PAFH (ed): Clinical Practice of Sports Injury Prevention and Care. London, Blackwell, 1994, pp 217–227.

50. Green W, Banks H: Oteochondritis in children. J Bone Joint Surg Am 1958; 14:26.

51. Gross ML, Dalvin LB, Evanski PM: Effectiveness of orthotic shoe inserts in the long distance runner. Am J Sports Med 1991; 19:409–412.

52. Gurtler RA, Stine R, Torg JS: Lachman test revisited. Contemp Orthop 1990; 20:145–154.

53. Hait G, Boswick JA Jr, Stone NH: Heterotopic bone formation secondary to trauma (myositis ossificans traumatica): An unusual case and a review of current concepts. J Trauma 1970; 10:405–411.

54. Hastings DE: The non-operative management of collateral ligament injuries of the knee joint. Clin Orthop 1980; 147:22–28.

55. Heiser TM, Weber J, Sullivan G, et al: Prophylaxis and management of hamstring injuries in intercollegiate football players. Am J Sports Med 1984; 12:368–370.

56. Henry J: Lateral ligament tears of the ankle, 1–6 years after follow up: study of 202 ankles. Orthop Rev 1983; 10:31–39.

57. Herring SA, Kibler WB: Rehabilitation. In Cantu RC, Micheli LJ (eds): ACSM's Guidelines For the Team Physician. Philadelphia, Lea & Febiger, 1991, pp 191–195.

58. Hilyard A: Recent developments in the management of patellofemoral pain: The McConnell programme. Physiotherapy 1990; 76:559–565.

59. Hollinshead WH, Jenkins DB: Functional Anatomy of the Limbs and Back, ed 5. Philadelphia, WB Saunders, 1981.

60. Hopkinson WJ, St. Pierre P, Ryan JB et al: Syndesmosis sprains of the ankle. Foot Ankle 1990; 10:325–330.

61. Hoppenfeld S: Physical Examination of the Spine and Extremities. Norwalk, Conn, Appelton-Century-Crofts, 1976.

62. Hungerford DS, Barry M: Biomechanics of the patellofemoral joint. Clin Orthop 1979; 144:9–15.

63. Indelicato PA: Non-operative treatment of complete tears of the medial collateral ligament of the knee. J Bone Joint Surg Am 1983; 65:323–329.

64. Jackson DW: Managing myositis ossificans in the young athlete. Phys Sports Med 1975; 3:56–61.

65. Jackson DW, Ashley RL, Powell JW: Ankle sprains in young athletes. Relation of severity and disability. Clin Orthop 1974; 101:201–215.

66. Jackson DW, Feagin JA: Quadriceps contusions in young athletes: Relation of severity of injury to treatment and prognosis. J Bone Joint Surg Am 1973; 53.95–105.

67. James SL, Bates BT, Osterning LR: Injuries to runners. Am J Sports Med 1978; 6:40–50.

68. Jarvinen M: Muscle injuries. In Renstrom PAFH (ed): Clinical Practice of Sports Injury Prevention and Care. London, Blackwell, 1994, pp 115–124.

69. Jones RK: Meralgia paresthetica as a cause of leg discomfort. Can Med Assoc J 1974; 111:541–542.

70. Kannus P: Long-term results of conservatively treated medial collateral ligament injuries of the knee joint. Clin Orthop 1988; 226:103–112.

71. Kannus P, Renstrom P: Treatment for acute tears of the lateral ligaments of the ankle. J Bone Joint Surg Am 1991; 73:305–312.

72. Kibler WB: Clinical aspects of muscle injury. Med Sci Sports Exerc 1990; 22:450–452.

73. Kibler WB, Chandler TJ, Pace BK: Principles of rehabilitation after chronic tendon injuries. Clin Sports Med 1992; 11:661–671.

74. Kibler WB, Chandler TJ, Stracener ES: Musculoskeletal adaptations and injuries due to overtraining. Exerc Sports Sci Rev 1992; 20:99–26.

75. Kibler WB, Goldberg C, Chandler TJ: Functional biomechanical deficits in running athletes with plantar fasciitis. Am J Sports Med 1991; 19:66–71.

76. Kirkpatrick JS, Koman LA, Rovere GD: The role of ultrasound in the early diagnosis of myositis ossificans: A case report. Am J Sports Med 1987; 15:179–181.

77. Kuland DN: The Injured Athlete, ed 2. Philadelphia, JB Lippincott, 1988, pp 428–453.

78. Kwong PK, Kay D, Voner RT, White MW: Plantar fasciitis: Mechanics and pathomechanics of treatment. Clin Sports Med 1988; 7:119–127.

79. Leadbetter WB: Cell-matrix response in tendon injury. Clin Sports Med 1992; 11:533–578.

80. Leeds HC, Ehrlich MG: Instability of the distal tibiofibular syndes-

mosis after bimalleolar and trimalleolar ankle fractures. J Bone Joint Surg Am 1984; 66:490–503.

81. Levy M, Torzilli PA, Warren RF: The effect of medial meniscectomy on anterior-posterior motion of the knee. J Bone Joint Surg Am 1982; 64:883–888.

82. Lipscomb AB, Thomas ED, Johnston RK: Treatment of myositis ossificans traumatica in athletes. Am J Sports Med 1976; 4:111–120.

83. Losee RE, Johnson TR, Southwick WO: Anterior subluxation of the lateral tibial plateau: A diagnostic test and operative repair. J Bone Joint Surg Am 1978; 60:1015.

84. Lotke PA: Soft tissue lesions affecting the hip joints. In Tronzo R (ed): Surgery of the Hip Joint. New York, Springer-Verlag, 1973, pp 368–377.

85. Lutter LD: The knee and running. Clin Sports Med 1985; 4:685–698.

86. Lynch MA, Henning CE, Glick KR: Knee joint surface changes: Long term follow-up of meniscus tear treatment in stable anterior cruciate ligament reconstructions. Clin Orthop 1983; 172:148–153.

87. Main WK, Scott NW: Knee anatomy. In Scott NW (ed): Ligament and Extensor Mechanism Injuries of the Knee: Diagnosis and Treatment. St Louis, Mosby–Year Book, 1991, pp 17–18.

88. Mann RA, Reynolds JC: Interdigital neuroma: A critical clinical analysis. Foot Ankle 1984; 3:238–243.

89. Matsen FA, Winquist RA, Krugmire RB: Diagnosis and management of compartmental syndromes. J Bone Joint Surg Am 1980; 62:286–291.

90. McBryde AM: Stress fractures in runners. Clin Sports Med 1985; 4:737–752.

91. McConnell J: The management of chondromalacia patellae: A long term solution. Aust J Physiother 1986; 32:215–219.

92. Mellerowicz H, Stelling E, Kefenbaum A: Diagnostic ultrasound in the athlete's locomotor system. Br J Sport Med 1990; 24:31–39.

93. Merrifield HH, Cowan RF: Ice hockey groin pulls. Am J Sports Med 1973; 1:41–42.

94. Messier SP, Pittala KA: Etiologic factors associated with selected running injuries. Med Sci Sports Exerc 1988; 20:501–505.

95. Micheli LJ: Overuse injuries in children's sports: The growth factor. Orthop Clin North Am 1983; 14:337–361.

96. Miller MD, Ritchie JR, Harner CD: Meniscus surgery: Indications for repair. Operative Tech Sports Med 1994; 2:164–171.

97. Nalley J, Jay MS, Durant RH: Myositis ossificans in an adolescent following sports injury. Adolesc Health Care 1985; 6:460–462.

98. Newell SG: Functional neutral orthoses and shoe modifications. Phys Med Rehabil Clin North Am 1992; 3:193–222.

99. Newell SG, Bramwell ST: Overuse injuries to the knee in runners. Phys Sports Med 1984; 12:81–92.

100. Noble CA: Iliotibial band friction syndrome in runners. Am J Sports Med 1980; 8:232–234.

101. Noyes FR, Butler DL, Paulos LE, et al: Inter-articular cruciate reconstruction. Perspectives on graft strength, vascularization, and immediate motion after replacement. Clin Orthop 1983; 172:710–717.

102. Noyes FR, Matthews DS, Moor PK, et al: The symptomatic anterior cruciate deficient knee. II: The results of rehabilitation activity modification and counseling on functional disability. J Bone Joint Surg Am 1983; 65:163–174.

103. O'Brien M: Functional anatomy and physiology of tendons. Clin Sports Med 1992; 11:505–520.

104. O'Donoghue DH: Treatment of Injuries to Athletes, ed 4. Philadelphia, WB Saunders, 1984, pp 433–444.

105. Olsen NK, Press JP, Young JL: Bursal injections. In Lennard TA (ed): Physiatric Procedures in Clinical Practice. Philadelphia, Hanley & Belfus, 1995, pp 36–43.

106. O'Toole ML: Prevention and treatment of injuries to runners. Med Sci Sports Exerc 1992; 24:S360–S363.

107. Parolie JM, Bergfeld JA: Long term results of nonoperative treatment of isolated posterior cruciate ligament injuries in the athlete. Am J Sports Med 1986; 14:35–38.

108. Press JM, Herring SA, Kibler WB: Rehabilitation of Muculoskeletal Disorders. United States Army Publication, in press.

109. Putnam CA, Kozey JW: Substantive issues in running. In Vaughn CL (ed): Biomechanics of Sport. Boca Raton, Fla, CRC Press, 1989, pp 2–33.

110. Reddy AS, Reedy MK, Seaber AV, et al: Restriction of the injury response following an acute muscle strain. Med Sci Sports Exerc 1993; 25:321–327.

111. Renstrom PAFH: Groin and hip injuries. In Renstrom PAFH (ed): Clinical Practice of Sports Injury Prevention and Care. London, Blackwell, 1994, pp 97–114.

112. Renstrom PAFH, Kannus P: Injuries of the foot and ankle. In Delee JC, Drez D Jr (eds): Orthopedic Sports Medicine Philadelphia, WB Saunders, 1994, pp 1705–1767.

113. Roy S, Irvin R: Sports Medicine: Prevention, Evaluation, Management and Rehabilitation. Englewood Cliffs, NJ, Prentice-Hall, 1983, pp 299–305.

114. Rubinstein RA Jr, Shelbourne DK: Diagnosis of posterior cruciate ligament injuries and indications for nonoperative and operative treatment. Operative Tech Sports Med 1993; 1:99–103.

115. Ryan JB, Wheeler JH, Hopkinson WJ, et al: Quadriceps contusions (West Point update). Am J Sports Med 1991; 19:299–304.

116. Rydell N: Biomechanics of the hip joint. Clin Orthop 1973; 92:6–19.

117. Saal JA: Rehabilitation of sports related lumbar spine injuries. Phys Med Rehabil 1987; 1:613–638.

118. Sandberg R, Balkfors B, Nilsson B, et al: Operative versus non-operative treatment of recent injuries to the ligaments of the knee. J Bone Joint Surg Am 1987; 69:1120–1126.

119. Schumacher RH: Primer on the Rheumatic Diseases. Atlanta, Arthritis Foundation, 1988, pp 263–274.

120. Shelbourne KD, Nitz P: Arthrofibrosis in acute anterior cruciate ligament reconstruction: The effect of timing of reconstruction and rehabilitation. Am J Sports Med 1991; 19:332–335.

121. Shelbourne KD, Wilckens JH, Mollabashy A, et al: Accelerated rehabilitation after acute anterior cruciate ligament reconstruction. Am J Sports Med 1990; 18:292–299.

122. Shuster R: Children's foot survey. J Podiatr Soc N Y 1956; 17:13.

123. Sim FH, Scott SG: Injuries of the hip and pelvis in athletes: Anatomy and function. In Nicholas JA, Hershman EB (eds): The Lower Extremity and Spine in Sports Medicine. St Louis, Mosby–Year Book, 1986, pp 1119–1169.

124. Sim FH, Simonet WT, Scott SG: Ice hockey injuries: Causes, treatments, and prevention. J Musculoskeletal Med 1989; 6:15–44.

125. Steinkamp LA, Dillingham MF, Markel MD, et al: Biomechanical considerations in patellofemoral joint rehabilitation. Am J Sports Med 1993; 21:438–444.

126. Stormont DM, Morrey B, An K, et al: Stability of the loaded ankle. Am J Sports Med 1985; 13:295–303.

127. Striazk AM, Stroberg AJ: Knee injuries in the skeletally immature athlete. In Nicholas JA, Hershman EB (eds): The Lower Extremity and Spine in Sports Medicine. St Louis, Mosby–Year Book, 1991.

128. Styf J: Diagnosis of exercise-induced pain in the anterior aspect of the leg. Am J Sports Med 1988; 16:165–169.

129. Subotnick SI: The biomechanics of running. Sports Med 1985; 2:144–153.

130. Sutker AN, Barber FA, Jackson DW, Pagliano JW: Iliotibial band syndrome in distance runners. Sports Med 1985; 5:447–451.

131. Svedenhag J, Seger J: Running on land and in water: Comparative exercise physiology. Med Sci Sports Exerc 1992; 24:1155–1160.

132. Swezey RL: Pseudo-radiculopathy in subacute trochanteric bursitis of the subgluteus maximus bursa. Arch Phys Med Rehabil 1976; 57:387–390.

133. Tietjens BB: Posterior cruciate ligament injuries. J Bone Joint Surg Br 1985; 59:15–19.

134. Traycoff RB: "Pseudotrochanteric bursitis": The differential diagnosis of lateral hip pain. J Rheumatol 1991; 12:1810–1812.

135. Tredget T, Godberson CV, Bose B: Myositis ossificans due to hockey injury. Can Med Assoc J 1977; 116:65–66.

136. Van Mechelen W, Hlobil H, Zijlstra WP, et al: Is range of motion at the hip and ankle joint related to running injuries? Int J Sports Med 1992; 13:605–610.

137. Walsh ZT, Micheli L: Hip dislocation in a high school football player. Phys Sports Med 1989; 17:112–115.

138. Warren R, Arnoczky SP, Wickiewicz TL: Anatomy of the knee. In Nicholas JA, Hershman EB (eds): The Lower Extremity and Spine in Sports Medicine. St Louis, Mosby–Year Book, 1991.

139. Young JL, Laskowski ER, Rock M: Thigh injuries in athletes. Mayo Clin Proc 1993; 68:1099–1106.

140. Young JL, Press JM: Rehabilitation of Running Injuries. In Buschbacher R, Braddom R (eds): Sports Medicine and Rehabilitation: A Sports Specific Approach. Philadelphia, Hanley & Belfus, 1994.

141. Zarins B, Ciullo JV: Acute muscle and tendon injuries in athletes. Clin Sports Med 1983; 3:167–182.

Low Back Pain and Disorders of the Lumbar Spine

MEHRSHEED SINAKI, M.D., M.S., AND
BAHRAM MOKRI, M.D.

EPIDEMIOLOGY OF BACK PAIN

In the industrialized world, low back pain is second only to headache as a cause of pain. It is the leading cause of expenditure for Workers' Compensation. Although it is often a self-limiting symptom, it costs at least $16 billion a year[59, 140] and disables 5.4 million Americans.[48, 52]

According to estimates of the U.S. Census Bureau, 1.8 million Americans were unable to work at some time during 1984 to 1985 because of low back pain. One study reported that 2% of all U.S. workers have a compensable back injury each year. Another study[148] suggested that 25 million Americans lost 1 or more days of work annually because of low back pain. About 2% of workers each year submit claims for disability due to low back pain.

Low back pain is a symptom that can be caused by various disease entities and can be affected by various psychosocial factors. Furthermore, in the absence of specific anatomical and pathological findings, the pain is not objectively verifiable. Thus, the application of the science of epidemiology to the subject of low back pain is difficult. The available survey studies have to be analyzed with attention to several factors, including the presence or absence of specific anatomical change or pathological process, whether the pain is severe or trivial, whether the report of pain is through questionnaires or through direct evaluation of the patient, whether the patient is referring to low back pain or to spine pain in general, and the accuracy of the patient's report (a pre-employment health survey typically does not reveal the same incidence rate of low back pain as does an anonymous survey).

Fifty percent to 80% of adults will have low back pain at some time in their lives.[18, 19, 65, 66, 72, 73, 78] In 1985, the Nuprin Pain Report,[148] conducted through telephone interviews of 1254 Americans, revealed that 56% of the adult population had some low back pain in the year preceding the survey, and 3% of them had had low back pain for more than 1 month. The U.S. population in 1985 was approximately 180 million, and one can conclude from this study that approximately 100 million persons had some low back pain and 6 million had low back pain for more than 1 month during that year.[85] In a study conducted in Finland,[65, 66] about 75% of both men and women reported having had at least one episode of low back pain, 45% recalled at least six episodes of low back pain, and 18% reported having low back pain in the previous month. Prevalence was greatest in the 55- to 64-year age group.

Current studies[20, 53, 121, 141, 115] suggest a lifetime rate of low back pain of about 60% to 90% and an annual rate of about 5%. The overall incidence is equal in men and women, but women report more low back pain after age 60 years.[20] This difference is likely due to the development of osteoporosis in women. Only 1% of patients with acute low back pain have lumbar radiculopathy. This rate is probably even lower for those with chronic low back pain. Lumbar radiculopathies often occur in patients during the fourth and fifth decades of life. The average age of patients who undergo lumbar laminectomy and diskectomy is 42 years.[52, 141]

Risk Factors

Epidemiological studies also point to certain risk factors that influence the incidence or prevalence of low back pain. These can be divided into two major groups: occupational and patient-related.[121]

Occupational Factors

Hard labor and heavy exertions have been claimed as the cause of pain by more than 60% of patients with low back pain.[21, 121, 124] Lifting, pulling and pushing, twisting, slipping, sitting for an extended period, and exposure to prolonged vibration, in isolation or in various combinations, have been attributed to development of low back pain. Persons who view their occupations as boring, repetitious, or dissatisfying may also report a higher rate of low back pain.[5, 151]

Patient-Related Factors

Age

The likelihood of development of low back pain gradually increases up until approximately 55 years of age.[12, 18, 19]

Sex

Men and women have similar risks of low back pain up until age 60 years. Thereafter, women are at greater risk, probably because of the development of osteoporosis.

Anthropometric Factors

There are no strong correlations among height, weight, body build, and low back pain. However, there is a higher risk of low back pain in very obese persons[76] and possibly in tall persons.[18, 79, 82, 147]

Postural Factors

The effect of scoliosis on spine pain is discussed in Chapter 18. The role of other postural changes such as kyphosis, increased or decreased lumbar lordosis, and discrepancy in the length of the lower limbs in the production of back pain has been subject to controversy. Although these factors might contribute to back pain in some patients, no generally accepted hard evidence exists of a true association.

Spine Mobility

Most subjects with low back pain have at least some limitation of range of motion of the lumbar spine. One study[18] found more pronounced reduction of flexibility of the lumbar spine in subjects who went on to experience recurrence of low back pain during the year after the examination.

Muscle Strength

Several studies[1, 2, 16, 17, 64, 93, 104, 110, 111, 117, 125] have shown decreased strength of abdominal and spinal muscles in patients with low back pain. Some studies[131] have shown comparatively weaker extensors, whereas others[18, 122] have shown comparatively weaker flexors.

Physical Fitness

A study on Los Angeles firefighters found that physical fitness and conditioning had a preventive effect on low back injuries. Another study[16] found no difference in the rate of recovery from acute low back pain with improved physical fitness. A recent study[118] found no correlation between cardiovascular physical fitness and back strength in a group of healthy, normal women aged 29 to 40 years.

Smoking

Persons who smoke seem to have an increased likelihood of development of low back pain.[35, 65, 66] Smoking is known to increase the incidence of osteoporosis.

Psychosocial Factors

Depression, anxiety, hypochondriasis, hysteria, alcoholism, divorce, chronic headaches, and other factors have been reported with higher frequency in patients with chronic low back pain.[54] Whether these are the cause or the result of the low back pain is unclear.

Most adults in the United States will have low back pain at some time in their lives. As it stands, low back pain is the most frequent cause of lost work days in the United States, surpassing the combination of acquired immunodeficiency syndrome (AIDS), cancer, and stroke as a cause of disability among persons of working age.

Etiology

Various disease entities can cause low back pain. The causes of low back pain are many, most of which can be categorized according to the classification provided in Table 39–1. Some of the common entities are listed with each classification. Several of these disease entities are discussed later in the chapter.

ANATOMY AND KINESIOLOGY OF THE LUMBAR SPINE

The vertebrae increase in size distally in the spine. Vertebrae are most massive in the lumbar region, which constitutes 25% of the height of the entire vertebral column. The "shock absorbers" of the spine are the intervertebral discs. In young persons, they constitute 25% of the height of the spine, but this percentage decreases significantly with age, as the discs lose water and collapse. The orientation of the facet joints varies at different levels of the spine. The superior and inferior articular facets are in frontal planes in the mid-thoracic regions. The lumbar facets are almost in sagittal planes, allowing the facet joints to glide anteroposteriorly and facilitating most of the flexion and extension movements of the lower spine. The contribution from thoracic vertebral segments to these movements is negligible. Seventy-five percent of lumbar flexion and extension occurs in the lumbosacral joint, 20% at L4 to L5, and the remaining 5% at the other levels.

The lumbar vertebrae are composed mainly of cancellous bone that is susceptible to collapse under trauma or from osteoporosis. The thin but dense cortical layer may proliferate with aging at the sites of ligamentous attachments and lead to osteophyte formation. The vertebral body is attached to the neural arch, which is composed of pedicles, superior and inferior facet joints, and the lamina (Fig. 39–1). The superior facet joint is smaller than the inferior one. It has a concave cartilaginous articular surface and forms the roof of the lateral recess. This is where the nerve root leaves the central canal to enter the neural foramen. Pedicles form the floor and the roof of the neural foramina. The laminae unite posteriorly to complete the neural arch.

TABLE 39–1   Causes of Low Back Pain

Cause	Common Diseases
1. Degenerative	Degenerative joint disease (DJD), osteoarthritis, lumbar spondylolysis Facet joint disease, facet DJD Degenerative spondylolisthesis Degenerative disc disease Diffuse idiopathic skeletal hyperostosis
2. Inflammatory (noninfectious)	Spondyloarthropathies (ankylosing spondylitis) Rheumatoid arthritis
3. Infectious	Pyogenic vertebral spondylitis Intervertebral disc infection Epidural abscess
4. Metabolic	Osteoporosis or osteopenia Paget's disease of bone

5. Neoplastic	Benign
	    Spinal (benign bony tumors of spine)
	    Intraspinal (meningiomas, neurofibromas, neurilemomas, low-grade ependymomas)
	Malignant
	    Spinal (malignant bony or soft tissue tumors, metastasis)
	    Intraspinal (metastasis, high-grade ependymomas, astrocytomas, meningeal carcinomatosis)

6. Traumatic	Fractures or dislocations Sprains (lumbar, lumbosacral, sacroiliac)
7. Congenital or developmental	Dysplastic spondylolisthesis Scoliosis
8. Musculoskeletal	Acute or chronic lumbar strain Mechanical low back pain Myofascial pain syndromes Fibromyalgia, tension myalgia Tension myalgia of the pelvic floor, coccygodynia Postural abnormalities, pregnancy
9. Viscerogenic	Upper genitourinary disorders Retroperitoneal disorders (often neoplastic)
10. Vascular	Abdominal aortic aneurysm or dissection Renal artery thrombosis or dissection Stagnation of venous blood (nocturnal back pain of pregnancy)
11. Psychogenic	Compensation neurosis Conversion disorder
12. Postoperative and multiply operated on back	

They protect the neural elements and are the sites of paraspinal muscle attachments. However, the laminae contribute little to the stability of the spinal column, and unilateral fracture or surgical removal of the laminae (laminectomy) does not cause spinal instability. The pedicle facet complex normally bears only 20% of the intervertebral vertical load; the remaining 80% is absorbed by the intervertebral disc.[102] The posterior longitudinal ligament extends along the posterior aspects of vertebral bodies and is attached to the lumbar discs and vertebral body margins. This ligament is not attached to the periosteum; a potential space is thus left between the ligament and periosteum that can expand with purulent material, tumor, or hematoma. The posterior longitudinal ligament, along with the anterior longitudinal ligament, helps maintain the axial stability of the vertebral column.[77, 156]

Intervertebral discs are remnants of the notocord that act as cushions between vertebral bodies and are composed of fibrocartilaginous elements. The nucleus pulposus is an ovoid, yellowish, gelatinous, and paracentrally located middle portion of the disc made of mucoprotein. This is surrounded by a firm, concentric meshwork of collagenous fibers called the *annulus fibrosus*. The lumbar disc is normally thicker anteriorly, a shape that partly explains the normal lumbar lordosis. Tiny blood vessels enter and exit the disc in the early decades of life, but these are obliterated during the first three decades. Thereafter, the disc nutrition is supported only through the lymphatics and by extracellular fluid osmosis. This lack of support may be responsible, at least in part, for loss of water from discs with advancing age. The water content of a disc in young persons is 88%, but it is reduced to less than 70% in the elderly.[68]

Functionally, the spine is composed of a series of mechanical units. Each unit consists of an anterior segment (two adjacent vertebral bodies and the intervertebral discs between them) and a posterior segment (neural arches). The anterior segment is primarily the weightbearing and shock-absorbing component, whereas the posterior segment protects the neural structures and directs movements of the units in flexion and extension. The amount of force exerted on the spine can vary depending on the type of activity and posture. Figure 39–2 demonstrates relative changes in

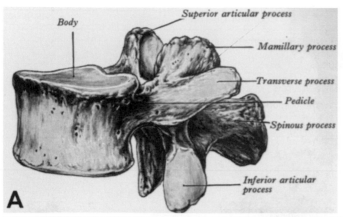

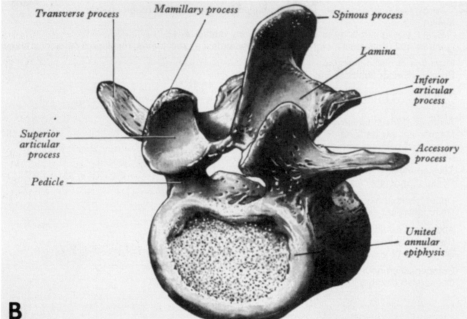

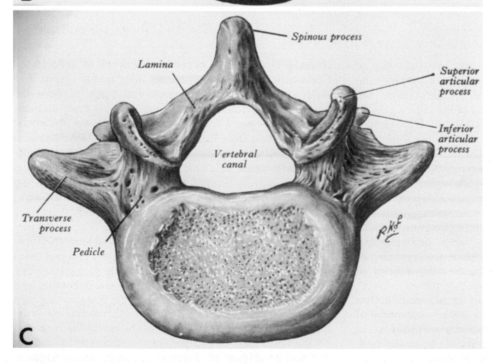

FIGURE 39–1 Lumbar vertebra. *A,* Left lateral aspect. *B,* Posterosuperior aspect, viewed obliquely from the left side. *C,* Superior aspect of the fifth lumbar vertebra. (From Williams PL, Warwick R: Gray's Anatomy, ed 36. Edinburgh, Churchill Livingstone, 1980, p 277. By permission of Longman Group.)

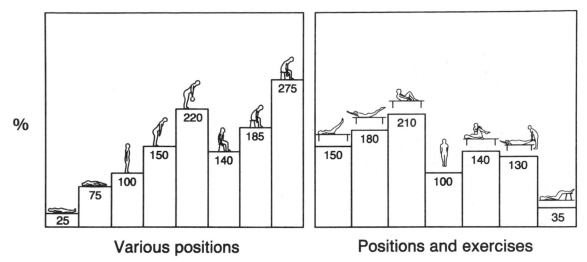

Various positions   ## Positions and exercises

FIGURE 39–2 *Left*, Relative change in pressure (or load) in the third lumbar disc in various positions in living subjects. *Right*, Relative change in pressure (or load) in the third lumbar disc during various muscle strengthening exercises in living subjects. Neutral erect posture is considered 100% in the figures; other positions and activities are calculated in relationship to this. (From Nachemson AL: The lumbar spine: An orthopaedic challenge. Spine 1976; 1:59. By permission of Harper & Row.)

L3 disc pressures in various positions and during various muscle strengthening exercises.[105, 106]

MUSCLES SUPPORTING THE SPINE AND THEIR FUNCTION

Muscle Groups

Four groups of muscles provide support to the spine: the extensors, the flexors, the lateral flexors, and the rotators of the spine. Normally, the extensors and rotators are the main supportive muscles of the spine.[13, 126] The massive musculotendinous bulk over the upper sacral and lower lumbar vertebrae is the origin of the erector spinae muscles, which extend the vertebral column. Deep to the erector spinae lie the semispinalis muscles (Fig. 39–3). The interspinal muscles are between spinous processes. The main role of the back muscles in erect posture is to resist gravity. When a movement of the spine is initiated, and once the vertebral column is bent far enough in any direction, the muscles of the back that resist this movement must actively contract to provide smooth and controlled movements and also to prevent falling. Some muscles that have no vertebral attachments also participate in movements of the spine. The abdominal muscles are the significant flexors and lateral flexors of the trunk and also participate in rotation.

Normal Posture

In normal posture, the line of gravity passes from C1 to C7 vertebral bodies to T10 and the lumbosacral junction and passes through the common axis of the hip joint or slightly behind it. It passes in front of the sacroiliac articulation and knee joint and then in front of the ankle joint. An increase in lumbar lordosis causes an increase in pelvic inclination, which can produce a protrusion of the abdominal wall. If pelvic inclination is reduced through flattening of the lumbar curve, the line of gravity is shifted forward. Any shift from standard alignment of the spine requires increased muscular activity to maintain posture as close to the line of gravity as possible. Posture is maintained through backward and forward swaying of the line of gravity. Normally, this sway has only a limited range.[142] Therefore, in comparison with other postural changes, normal posture requires the least amount of paraspinal muscular recruitment.

EVALUATION OF THE PATIENT WITH LOW BACK PAIN

Clinical Evaluation

History

At the very least, the following information should be gathered:

Mode of onset of low back pain (abrupt or insidious).

Provoking, aggravating, and relieving factors.

Effect of posture, inactivity, exertion, and rest.

Effect of cough, sneeze, or strain on the low back pain, especially if these cause pain down the lower limbs.

Presence or absence of pain at night and interference with sleep.

Course—whether the pain has been progressive, decreasing, fluctuating, or episodic.

History of similar or different back or lower limb pains.

Associated limb symptoms (pain, paresthesias, numbness, weakness, atrophy, cramps, fasciculations).

Presence or absence of urinary frequency, urgency, or retention; bowel or bladder incontinence; or constipation

History of lumbar surgery (such as laminectomy or fusion).

Types of treatments implemented, medications used, and the effects of these medications on the symptoms.

Presence or absence of litigation or compensation issues.

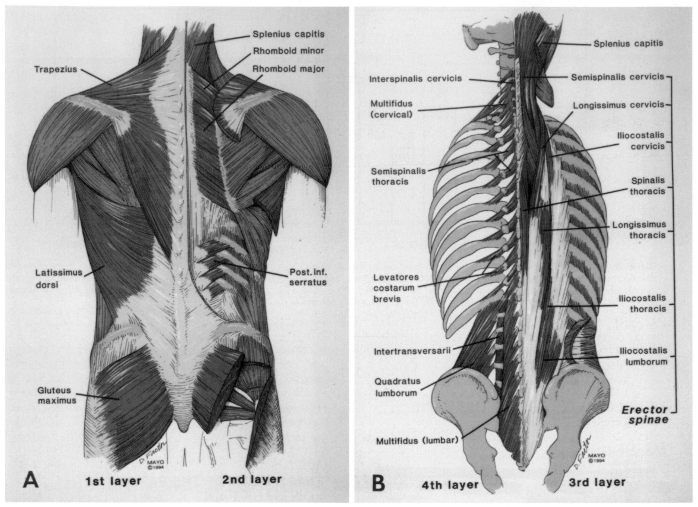

FIGURE 39–3   Muscle anatomy of spine. *A*, First and second layers. *Abbreviation:* Post. inf., posterior inferior. *B*, Third and fourth layers. (By permission of Mayo Foundation.)

Examination

Inspection

Look for deformities, paraspinal spasm, birthmarks, unusual hair growth, listing to one side, corkscrew deformity, decrease or increase in lordosis, presence of scoliosis, muscular atrophy, or asymmetries.

Palpation and Percussion

Determine whether there are tender or trigger points, local tenderness or pain on percussion, spasm, or tightness of the paraspinal muscles. Observe the patient's reaction to pain, whether there is a "touch-me-not" withdrawal to palpation or touch.

Range of Motion

Range of motion should be determined for flexion, extension, lateral bending, and rotation. Values for normal range of motion of the lumbar spine are as follows: flexion, 40 degrees; extension, 15 degrees; lateral bending, 30 degrees; lateral rotation, 40 degrees to each side. Several techniques and instruments can be used for measurement

of range of motion of the spine. These range from simple and inexpensive methods to the use of expensive and complicated machines:

TAPE MEASURE METHOD. Originally described by Schober,[130] this method is a simple and practical way to determine the amount of flexion of the lumbar spine. A line is drawn that connects the "dimples of Venus." Then, two marks are made along a line that perpendicularly bisects the first line. One mark is 5 cm below and the other 10 cm above the point of bisection, with the distance between these two marks being 15 cm. The patient is then asked to bend forward maximally. The measured distance beyond the original 15 cm gives an estimate of the degree of spinal flexion (Fig. 39–4).[67]

INCLINOMETERS. These were initially introduced by Asmussen and Heebøll-Nielsen[7] for measuring spinal motions and later were further developed by Loebl[84] (Fig. 39–5). This method fails to separate hip motion from spine motion. It is also subject to variability with the subject's effort.[92]

Various electronic and computerized gadgets are available for measurement of spinal range of motion, and many of them also measure muscle strength.

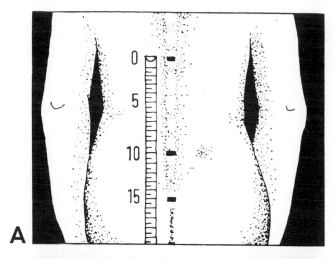

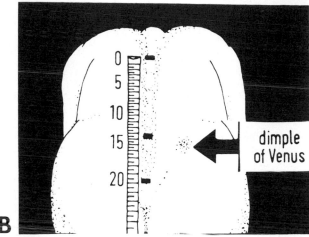

FIGURE 39–4 Modified Schober method to measure anterior flexion. *Top*, Position 1: placing of skin marks. *Bottom*, Position 2: distraction of upper and lower marks on anterior flexion. (From Helliwell P, Moll J, Wright V: Measurement of spinal movement and function. *In* Jayson M (ed): The Lumbar Spine and Back Pain, ed 4. New York, Churchill Livingstone, 1992, pp 173–205. By permission of the publisher.)

The representative rotations for flexion and extension, lateral bending, and axial rotation are shown in Figure 39-6. This is a composite of what Panjabi et al.,[116] on the basis of their studies and extensive review of the literature, consider to be the most representative values for rotation at different levels of the spine in the traditional planes of motion.

Neurological Examination

This is a very important part of the evaluation of patients with low back pain.[34]

Gait, Station, and Coordination

Gait is a complex activity that depends on the integration of several neural mechanisms, but it can also be affected by disturbed posture, disorders of joints, pain, or functional overtone. One should look for antalgic gait, footdrop, and functional or hysterical features. The patient should do toe-walking, heel-walking, and tandem gait. It should be determined whether the patient can stand on either foot or can squat and rise. Alternate motion rates are to be done rapidly and regularly. They depend on an intact sensory motor system. These can also be affected by pain, diseases of joints, insufficient effort, poor cooperation, and functional factors.

Muscle Stretch Reflexes

An increase, decrease, or absence of muscle stretch reflexes should be recorded. Neither a decrease nor an increase of these reflexes in itself can be interpreted as definitely abnormal. Neurologically normal persons can have exaggerated, diminished, or even absent reflexes. A patient's reflexes must be compared with other muscle stretch reflexes, particularly of the corresponding opposite side. Reflex asymmetry, however, is most often significant.

Muscle Bulk

Inspect for muscle atrophy. Comparison of the circumference of the lower limbs, determined with a tape measure, at different levels (such as mid-calf level) is sometimes useful. One should also look for muscle fasciculations.

Muscle Strength

It is important to determine whether the muscle weakness is genuine or whether it is a giving-way as the result of pain, functional factors, or poor effort. It should be noted whether the distribution of the weakness corresponds to a single root or multiple roots or to a peripheral nerve or plexus, or whether the weakness is of upper motor neuron type.

Sensory Examination

This is the least reliable part of the neurological examination. It should be done at the end of the examination, when the examiner typically already has some impression about the disorder affecting the patient. Asking the patient to outline areas of sensory loss may help orient the examiner and save time. The nature of the sensory tests should be carefully explained to the patient. Determine whether the reported sensory changes are consistent and reproducible, and whether they follow anatomical dermatomal patterns (although they may be noted in only part of a dermatome).

Straight-Leg Raising Test

At least one of the variations of this test should be done in all cases. The test (also called the Lasègue test) is done with the patient supine in bed or on an examining table. The relaxed lower limb in extension is gently and gradually elevated, and the patient is instructed to inform the examiner when the pain occurs and also to report the location of the pain. Sometimes, if the patient is sitting on an examining table or a chair (and, therefore, the hips and knees are flexed, each at about 90 degrees), gently bringing the knee into extension often produces the same type of pain as does the straight-leg raising test in a patient with L5 or S1 radiculopathy. Sometimes elevation of the asymptomatic lower extremity causes pain in the symptomatic

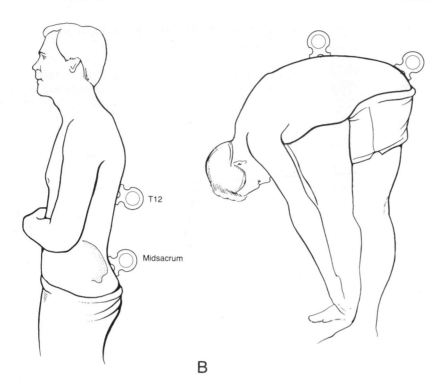

FIGURE 39–5 Loebl measurements. *A,* Double-inclinometer method: zero starting position. The inclinometers are aligned over T12 and the sacrum and their gauges are set at 0 degrees. *B,* The subject positions the spine in maximal flexion. The degrees recorded on the sacral inclinometer are subtracted from the degrees recorded on the inclinometer positioned over the T12 spinous process. (From Greene WB, Heckman JD: The Clinical Measurement of Joint Motion. Rosemont, Ill, American Academy of Orthopaedic Surgeons, 1994, p 86. By permission of the Academy.)

A   B

side ("well-leg" or crossed straight-leg raising sign). This is often a reliable sign of root irritation.

The fabere test, an acronym for *f*lexion, *ab*duction, *exter*nal *r*otation, and *e*xtension, is done to look for any associated hip disease. It is also known as Patrick's test.

Diagnostic Studies

Plain Radiography

Despite the increasing availability and use of computed tomography (CT) and magnetic resonance imaging (MRI), plain radiography is still useful as a quick and less costly screening study. It is helpful for detecting fractures, dislocations, degenerative joint disease, spondylolisthesis, narrowing of intervertebral disc space, and many bony diseases and tumors of the spine. Oblique views are helpful for visualizing the neural foramina. Flexion and extension views are useful for studying subluxations and stability. Changes of degenerative joint disease are fairly common, especially in persons past middle age. Therefore, this finding may not necessarily explain the patient's symptoms.

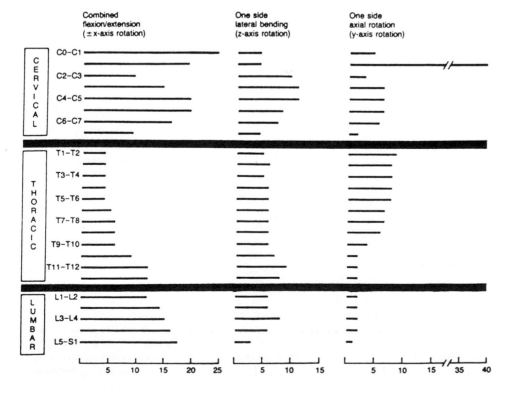

FIGURE 39–6 Representative values for rotation at different levels of the spine in traditional planes of motion. (From Panjabi MM, Hult JE, Crisco JJ III, et al: Biomechanical studies in cadaveric spines. *In* Jayson MIV (ed): The Lumbar Spine and Back Pain, ed 4. New York, Churchill Livingstone, 1992, pp 133–155. By permission of the publisher.)

Clinical judgment is required to determine any causal relationship[88] (Fig. 39–7).

Radioisotope Bone Scanning

Radioisotope scanning is a valuable test for screening the entire or a large part of the skeleton. It is useful for the detection of tumors, particularly bony metastases. Gallium scanning is used if infection is suspected.

CT and MRI

Both CT and MRI are useful for detecting disc disease, herniated or extruded disc, or tumors (vertebral, epidural, meningeal, intradural, or cord). Overall, MRI (especially with gadolinium enhancement) is superior to CT. MRI can image the entire lumbar spine in a single scanning session and shows the soft tissues better than CT. It is an excellent method for detecting epidural, intradural, and some of the intra-axial spinal cord lesions, such as tumor, cyst, or even demyelinating plaques. CT can define or demonstrate bony lesions better.

Myelography

The use of CT and, especially, MRI has decreased the use of myelography. This test is, however, still used by many surgeons before a final decision is made regarding lumbar surgery. CT-myelography has added to the accuracy of the test by detecting more subtle intraspinal lesions. CT-myelography remains the most accurate imaging method for the diagnosis of disc herniations and extrusions.

Electromyography

Electrodiagnostic studies are useful for detecting neurogenic changes and denervation, as well as the extent of these changes and the level of involvement. Unlike imaging studies, electrodiagnostic studies provide physiological information (see Chapters 6, 7, and 8).

SOME COMMONLY ENCOUNTERED PAINFUL DISORDERS OF THE SPINE

Mechanical Low Back Pain

Mechanical low back pain is a descriptive term commonly used for non-discogenic back pain that is provoked by physical activity and relieved by rest. It does not point to a single or particular cause. Although sometimes overused, the term is practically useful. This type of pain is often due to stress or strain to the back muscles, tendons, and ligaments and is usually attributed to strenuous daily activities, heavy lifting, or prolonged standing or sitting. Mechanical low back pain is often a chronic, dull, aching pain of varying intensity that affects the lower spine and might spread to the buttocks. The pain often progressively worsens during the day because daily physical activities such as bending, twisting, lifting, prolonged sitting, and standing often aggravate the pain. There are no associated neurological symptoms or signs, nor a cough or sneeze effect on the lower limbs.[97]

Deconditioning and decompensation can also cause a mechanical type of low back pain. Indeed, this decompensation syndrome is one of the most common causes of low back pain. The onset is often insidious, the patients are usually obese and display manifestations of chronic inactivity, and the back and abdominal muscles are weak. These patients demonstrate much difficulty or even inability in performing a sit-up, a hook-lying sit-up, a leg lift for 10 sec at 30 degrees, a prone torso lift for 10 sec, a prone leg lift for 10 sec, or one slow toe touch in the standing position. Patients with deconditioning or decompensation syndrome fail at least one of these maneuvers and often fail several of them. Overall, for the management of mechanical low back pain, correction of static or dynamic postural abnormalities is helpful. An exercise program consisting of abdominal and back strengthening exercise is necessary, and patients often improve quickly (Fig. 39–8).

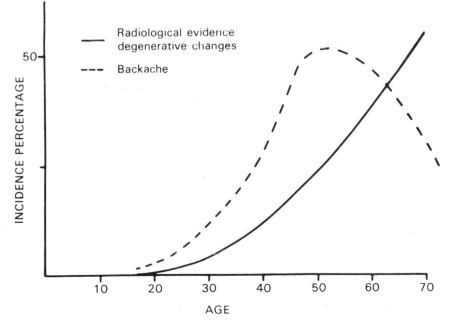

FIGURE 39–7 Incidence of radiologically demonstrable degenerative changes in lumbar spine and back pain with age. Although changes in lumbar spine increase with age, maximal incidence of back pain has a peak at age 45 years, and thereafter tends to decline. (From Macnab I: Backache. Baltimore, Williams & Wilkins, 1977, p 90. By permission of the publisher.)

Radiological evidence degenerative changes

- - - Backache

INCIDENCE PERCENTAGE

50—

AGE

10   20   30   40   50   60   70

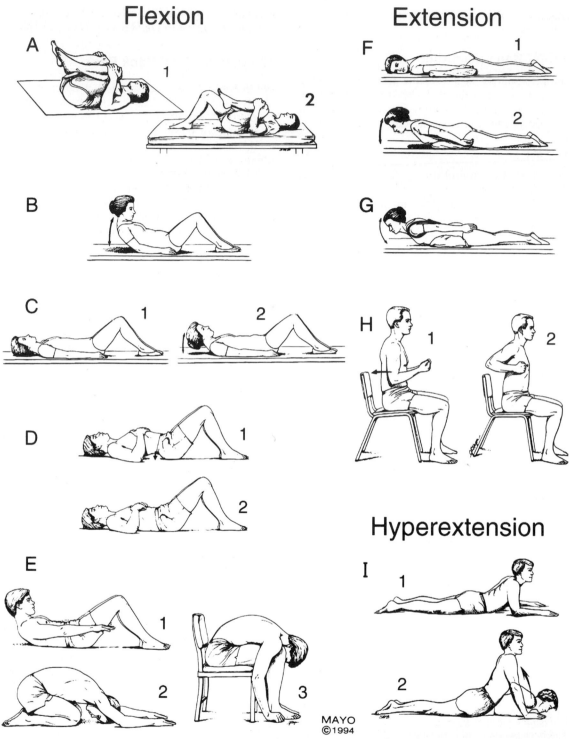

FIGURE 39–8 Back strengthening exercises. *A–E,* Flexion exercises. *A,* Knee to chest–both knees *(1)* or one knee at a time to avoid strain *(2). B,* Isotonic abdominal strengthening. *C,* Isometric abdominal strengthening. *D,* Pelvic tilt to reduce lumbar lordosis. *E,* Flexion exercises for spondylolisthesis. *F–I,* Extension exercises. *F,* In prone position with pillow under abdomen (avoid hyperextension). *G,* To increase the effect of back extension strengthening, weight is added (Posture Training Support, developed by M. Sinaki). *H,* Extension from sitting position. *I,* Prone passive extension—on elbows *(1)* or hyperextension *(2).* (*A,* From Low Back Stretches, handout no. MC 1899/R39, Mayo Foundation for Medical Education and Research, 1990. By permission of Mayo Foundation for Medical Education and Research. *B, C,* and *F,* From Sinaki M: Exercise and physical therapy. *In* Riggs BL, Melton LJ III (eds): Etiology, Diagnosis, and Management. New York, Raven Press, 1988, pp 457–479. By permission of Mayo Foundation. *E1* and *E3,* From Sinaki M, Lutness MP, Ilstrup DM, et al: Lumbar spondylolisthesis: Retrospective comparison and 3-year follow-up of two conservative treatment programs. Arch Phys Med Rehabil 1989; 70:594. By permission of Mayo Foundation. *E2* and *H,* From Sinaki M: Metabolic bone disease. *In* Sinaki M (ed): Basic Clinical Rehabilitation Medicine, ed 2. St Louis, Mosby–Year Book, 1993, pp 209–236. By permission of Mayo Foundation. *G,* From PTS: Posture Training Support, brochure no. Q255. Jackson, Mich, Camp International, 1990. By permission of Mayo Foundation. *I,* From Low Back Extension Exercises, handout no. MC 2032/R789. Mayo Foundation for Medical Education and Research, 1989. By permission of Mayo Foundation for Medical Education and Research.)

Degenerative Joint Disease

Degenerative joint disease (DJD) occurs with aging and can begin during the third decade of life.[42] Lumbar DJD can remain asymptomatic. If the disease is symptomatic, the associated pain is centered in the lower back and is often increased with movement of the spine. Stiffness, morning stiffness, and stiffness after having been in one position for an extended period are common. Range of motion of the spine may be limited. Pain is often relieved by rest. Hypertrophic changes and spurs can compress nerve roots and cause additional radicular pain. Radiographs, particularly after the early stages, are diagnostic. Improvement of spinal muscle support through proper strengthening exercises can alleviate pain. Improvement and provision of proper static and dynamic posture principles, such as bending one knee during prolonged standing (such as by placing one foot on a low stool), provide pain relief and decrease the risk of further strain (Fig. 39–9). When muscle support is poor, the application of an elastic support to control pain is advisable. The back support can be used for 6 weeks while attempts are made to improve the strength of the supporting muscles. The use of the back support enables the patient to be more mobile and prevents prolonged immobility due to pain. Exercises include abdominal and back muscle strengthening (preferably isometric exercises).

Degenerative Disease of Facet Joint

Degenerative arthritis of the facet joints results in localized spine pain, which is often episodic, that sometimes extends to the limb and can mimic radicular pain. The onset of each attack is usually abrupt. Range of motion, especially with extension, is often limited. In some cases, facet joint DJD, more diffuse DJD, and even degenerative disc disease may coexist. Pain is increased with activity and relieved by rest. Surgery is rarely indicated. Nonsteroidal anti-inflammatory drugs often help, and manipulation can at times give dramatic relief. Some patients may benefit from facet joint injection. Spontaneous improvement is not unusual. Most patients can achieve relief of pain to a tolerable level with a carefully adjusted program of weight control, rest, analgesics, or nonsteroidal anti-inflammatory medications. Back pain in patients with degenerative disease of facet joints can be induced with lumbar extension maneuvers. Conservative treatment is directed toward reducing the hyperextension. Improvement of abdominal muscle strength and isometric contraction of the quadratus lumborum with pelvic tilt exercises place the sacrum in a more vertical position. If flexion contractures of the hips are present, they need to be reduced through Thomas stretch maneuvers.

Patients with facet joint pain are instructed to avoid sleeping in the prone position. When bending over a wash basin, slightly elevating one foot by placing it on a low stool with the knee bent can decrease lumbar strain (see Fig. 39–9A). In general, the objective of exercise is to develop the supportive muscles of the lumbosacral spine. The properly prescribed exercises are performed once or twice a day (see Fig. 39–8A–D). The maximal effect of strengthening exercises appears in 6 weeks.[100] After 6 weeks, exercises may be performed three times per week

to maintain the achieved level of strength. In cases of severe low back pain, application of a lumbosacral support can decrease pain and improve compliance with the exercise program. However, prolonged use of a back support (more than 3 weeks) is discouraged because muscle disuse can result.

Lumbar Disc Syndrome and Lumbosacral Radiculopathies

Lumbar disc syndrome is a common cause of acute, chronic, or recurrent low back pain,[52, 132] particularly in young to middle-aged men, but it also occurs in women, older persons, and even adolescents, especially if they are involved in strenuous physical activity. Overall, the mean age of the patient with lumbar disc herniation is the early 40s. Disc herniation may occur in the midline, but it often occurs to one side. Pain may be unilateral, bilateral, or bilateral but more prominent on one side. The cause is usually a flexion injury. Repetitive injury results in degeneration of the posterior longitudinal ligaments and annulus fibrosus.

Irritation or compression of an adjacent nerve root may occur, as is often the case with laterally extruded ("squeezed toothpaste") disc herniations (Figs. 39–10 and 39–11). Different degrees and types of disc herniation may occur. Macnab's classification is useful, and it indeed correlates well with MRI findings:[91, 153]

BULGING DISC. A bulge and convexity of disc beyond the adjacent vertebral disc margins, but with intact annulus fibrosus and Sharpey's fibers (Fig. 39–12A).

PROLAPSED DISC. The disc herniates posteriorly through an incomplete defect in the annulus fibrosus (see Fig. 39–12B).

EXTRUDED DISC. The disc herniates posteriorly through a complete defect in the annulus fibrosus (see Fig. 39–12C).

SEQUESTERED DISC. Part of nucleus pulposus is extruded through a complete defect in annulus fibrosus and has lost continuity with the present nucleus pulposus (see Fig. 39–12D).

The pain often radiates into the buttock, the posterior thigh, and lateral calf or to lateral or medial malleoli (in cases of L5 or S1 radiculopathies). This pain follows the path of the sciatic nerve and is often referred to as *sciatica*. The pain radiates to the anterior thigh in L3 or L4 radiculopathies. When the disc is extruded, the low back pain is sometimes decreased or even relieved, but the radicular limb symptoms become more prominent. About 5% to 10% of patients with root lesions do not have associated back pain. In these cases, a mononeuropathy (such as sciatica, femoral neuropathy, or obturator neuropathy) or a lumbosacral plexus lesion has to be ruled out. Diabetic lumbar polyradiculopathy sometimes is also part of the differential diagnosis.

The most common levels of lumbar disc protrusion, herniation, or extrusion, in decreasing order of frequency, are L5 to S1, L4 to L5, L3 to L4, and L2 to L3. Therefore, the most common lumbosacral radiculopathies related to lumbar disc herniation are L3, L4, L5, and S1 radiculopathies. Lower lumbar and S1 radiculopathies are usually a result of degeneration or herniation of intervertebral

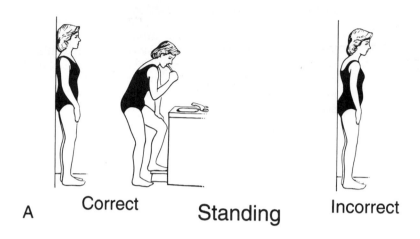

A   Correct   Standing   Incorrect

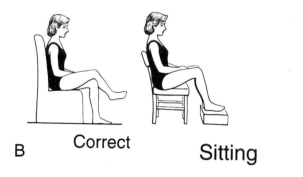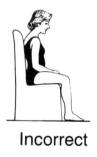

B   Correct   Sitting   Incorrect

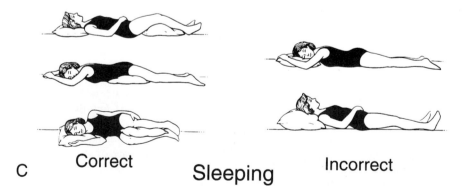

C   Correct   Sleeping   Incorrect

FIGURE 39–9 *A–I,* Static and dynamic correct and incorrect postures (developed by M. Sinaki). (By permission of Mayo Foundation.)

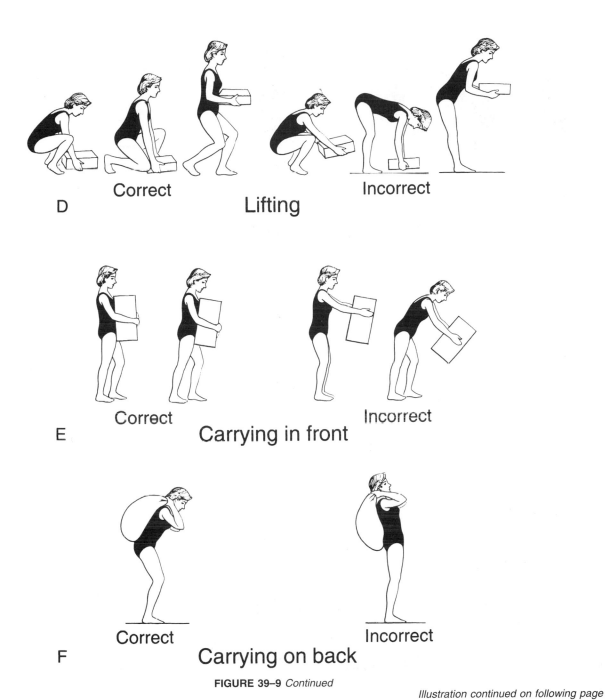

D   Correct   Lifting   Incorrect

E   Correct   Carrying in front   Incorrect

F   Correct   Carrying on back   Incorrect

FIGURE 39–9 *Continued*

Illustration continued on following page

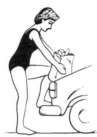
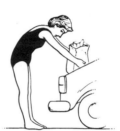

Correct Incorrect

G Driving

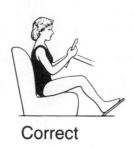

Correct Incorrect

H Loading/unloading car trunk

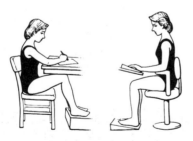
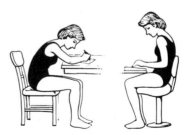

Correct Incorrect

I Working at a desk (seated)

MAYO
©1994

FIGURE 39–9 *Continued*

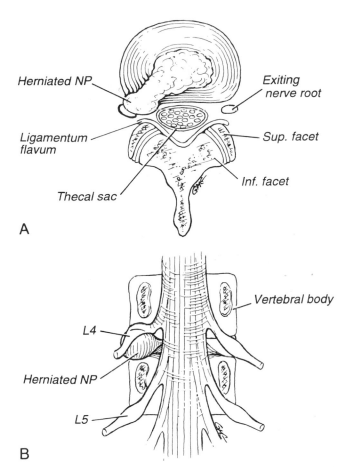

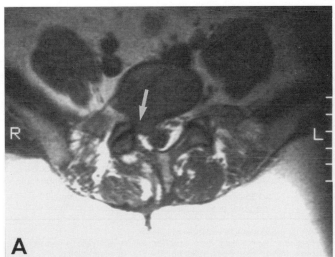 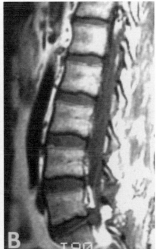

FIGURE 39–10 Lateral disc herniation. *A* and *B,* Lateral disc herniation impinges exiting nerve root, causing radicular symptoms. *Abbreviations:* Inf., inferior; NP, nucleus pulposus; Sup., superior. (From Vanderburgh DF, Kelly WM: Radiographic assessment of discogenic disease of the spine. Neurosurg Clin North Am 1993; 4:13.)

discs[43, 86, 141] and are usually unilateral. Midline disc protrusion may cause low back pain but no significant radiculopathy. Large midline disc herniations can cause bilateral radiculopathies or cauda equina syndrome severe enough to produce sphincter problems. Upper lumbar radiculopathies are less commonly caused by disc disease. When upper lumbar radiculopathy is evaluated, other etiologic factors, particularly neoplastic disease, should be ruled out.

Examination of the back often shows paraspinal muscle spasm, loss of lumbar lordosis, listing of the spine away from the side of root pain, limitation of motions of the lumbar spine with "corkscrew phenomenon" on flexion and straightening, positive straight-leg raising test, and, sometimes, crossed straight-leg raising sign in cases of L5 or S1 radiculopathies. The chin-chest maneuver may cause low back pain because of upward traction on the cord and lower nerve roots. Dorsiflexion of the foot may also cause stretching of the sciatic nerve and, therefore, stretching of the attached tendon nerve root, leading to pain. The same findings may be noted when the patient tries to perform heel-walking or tries to bend forward. Coughing, sneezing, or straining causes an increase in abdominal pressure leading to distention of epidural and intervertebral veins. These distentions directly compress and put traction on the nerve roots and cause pain, particularly radiation down the involved lower extremity.

When radiculopathy occurs, several features, including distribution of pain, reflex changes, distribution of weakness, and sensory alterations, provide reliable information that enables the clinician to localize the level of disc protrusion or root irritation. Changes in these features as they pertain to each lumbar and sacral nerve root are outlined in Table 39–2.[98]

Laboratory Tests for Lumbosacral Radiculopathies

MRI has become a major diagnostic tool in the diagnosis of herniated lumbar discs (Fig. 39–13). It is also very useful for demonstrating several non-discogenic entities that may cause root lesions or enter in the differential diagnosis, including bone disease, vertebral or epidural intraspinal tumors, scar tissue formations, infections, and even some forms of meningeal disease. However, some herniated discs may be missed by MRI.

Myelography still maintains much of its significance.

FIGURE 39–11 Recurrent extruded L5 disc, as seen on axial *(A)* and sagittal *(B)* images. Extrusion of disc to the right is well seen on axial image *(arrow in A).*

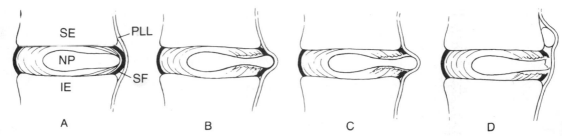

FIGURE 39–12 Classifications of disc herniation. *A,* Bulging annulus fibrosus. *B,* Prolapse. *C,* Extrusion. *D,* Sequestration. *Abbreviations:* IE, inferior end-plate; NP, nucleus pulposus; PLL, posterior longitudinal ligament; SE, superior end-plate; SF, Sharpey's fibers. (From Vanderburgh DF, Kelly WM: Radiographic assessment of discogenic disease of the spine. Neurosurg Clin North Am 1993; 4:13.)

When coupled with CT (CT-myelography), it is still the most accurate imaging test for documentation of herniated discs (Fig. 39–14). Electromyography is very helpful for localizing the level of involvement, determining whether root involvement is single or multiple, and differentiating a multiple root from a plexus lesion.[160]

Treatment

Most patients with discogenic low back pain respond to conservative management. Studies by Saal and Saal[128] and others[39] have shown that most patients with herniated lumbar disc can be treated nonsurgically. The principles of conservative management of back pain are addressed at the end of the chapter.

Operation is considered when definite radiculopathy and neurological deficits are present, especially when they are persistent or progressive. However, in the spectrum of discogenic low back pain, patients in this group are a definite minority. Progressive and significant neurological deficits justify early surgical intervention. Large midline disc protrusions with cauda equina syndrome require urgent treatment and decompression. The success of surgical treatment is greatest when there are bona fide objective neurological deficits. With proper patient selection, about two-thirds have excellent results, and half of the remaining one-third have improvement to some extent. However, in many patients with lumbar disc syndrome, the major difficulty is low back pain with only mild, slight, or no evidence of radiculopathy. Most of these patients respond to conservative management. Lumbar laminectomy and diskectomy for the sole complaint of low back pain are often unjustified.[132]

TABLE 39–2 **Clinical Features of Lumbosacral Radiculopathies**

Root	Distribution of Pain	Paresthesias or Sensory Loss	Weakness	Decreased or Absent Reflexes
L1	Lower abdomen, groin, or upper anterior medial thigh	Lower abdomen, inguinal region	Iliopsoas ($\pm$)	Hypogastric and cremasteric
L2	Groin, anterior or medial thigh	Anterior and medial thigh	Iliopsoas or adductors of thigh or both	
L3	Anterior thigh or knee	Anterior thigh and knee	Quadriceps and thigh adductors	Quadriceps
L4	Can extend below knee, often to inner leg or medial malleolus	Inner leg	Quadriceps and thigh adductors and tibialis anterior ($\pm$)	Quadriceps and medial hamstring
L5	Posterolateral thigh, lateral calf to dorsum of foot	Outer leg and dorsum of foot to great toe	Tibialis anterior, toe extensors, and extensor hallucis longus (therefore impaired heel-walking), hamstrings, perinei, and tibialis posterior, gluteus medius	Medial hamstring; ankle jerk often normal, sometimes decreased but not absent because only L5 root lesion
S1	Posterior thigh, calf, and lateral malleolus	Posterior leg, lateral foot, last two toes	Gastrocnemius-soleus and toe flexors (therefore impaired toe-walking), hamstring, gluteus maximus	Ankle jerk and lateral hamstring
S2	Posterior thigh and occasionally calf	Variable posterior thigh and saddle area	Intrinsic foot muscles ($\pm$), rectal sphincter ($\pm$)	Anal
S3 to S4	Buttock and upper posterior thigh or perianal region	Saddle and perineal area, perianal area	Rectal sphincter	Anal

Abbreviation: $\pm$, weakess may or may not be present due to variability of innervation.
From Mokri B, Sinaki M: Lumbar disk syndrome, lumbosacral radiculopathies, lumbar spondylosis and stenosis, spondylolisthesis. *In* Sinaki M (ed): Basic Clinical Rehabilitation Medicine, ed 2. St Louis, Mosby–Year Book, 1993, pp 503–513. By permission of Mayo Foundation.

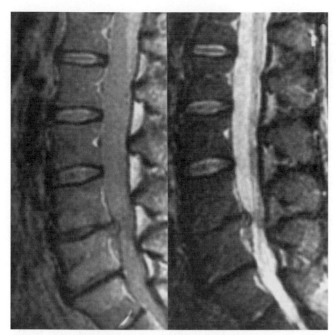

FIGURE 39–13 Magnetic resonance imaging scan of lumbar spine. T1-weighted *(left)* and T2-weighted *(right)* sagittal images demonstrate extruded L1 disc. (From Mokri B, Sinaki M: Lumbar disc syndrome, lumbosacral radiculopathies, lumbar spondylosis and stenosis, spondylolisthesis. *In* Sinaki M (ed): Basic Clinical Rehabilitation Medicine, ed 2. St Louis, Mosby–Year Book, 1993, pp 503–513. By permission of Mayo Foundation.)

The standard surgical procedure is open laminectomy and diskectomy. When there is spondylitic encroachment, facetectomy and foraminectomy might be necessary, and when there is instability, spinal fusion might be needed.

Microdiskectomy

Microdiskectomy is a generic term without a specific definition and essentially means the use of an operative microscope to accomplish posterior approaches for removal of a herniated lumbar disc through the smallest possible skin incision.[74] The skin incision is usually about 2 cm long. Long-term results from microdiskectomy are not necessarily better than those from standard operation. The initial concerns regarding increased risk of infection with the use of a microscope do not seem to be substantiated by the subsequent experience. The recurrence rate after microdiskectomy is higher than that after standard operation. Proponents of this technique argue that this increase possibly is related to earlier return of the patients to higher levels of activity. As minimally invasive surgical procedures are gaining momentum, an increase in microdiskectomy can be expected.

Percutaneous Lumbar Diskectomy

This is another procedure used to treat lumbar disc herniations less invasively and to reduce morbidity.[90] The technique has been claimed to be effective for treating patients with small to moderate-sized, well-contained disc herniation who show clinical and imaging evidence of nerve root compression. A nucleotome is guided into the disc space with precise radiographic control. The disc material is then aspirated, and because the disc is avascular, the aspirated contents should be essentially free of blood. The claimed advantages are use of local anesthesia, minimal tissue disruption, performance on an outpatient basis, earlier return to usual activities, and minimizing the possibility of development of epidural fibrosis and scarring. Misplacement of the probe and serious neurological and vascular complications are feared sequelae. The rate of

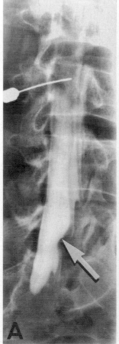
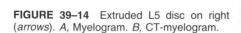
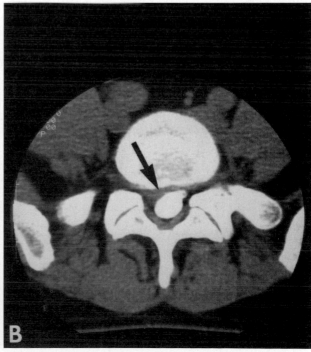

FIGURE 39–14 Extruded L5 disc on right *(arrows)*. *A,* Myelogram. *B,* CT-myelogram.

recurrent symptoms may be high because of missed disc fragments and because of collapse of disc space and exacerbation of spondylitic nerve root compression.[49] The potential for effective treatment with this technique may prove to be limited.

Chemonucleolysis

The efficacy of chemonucleolysis is inferior to that of open diskectomy. Furthermore, it is associated with a significant incidence of anaphylaxis. In a study of 151 patients with L4 to L5 or L5 to S1 disc herniations who were evenly divided between treatment with open diskectomy or chemonucleolysis,[152] 22% of the chemonucleolysis group and 0% of the diskectomy group had increased radicular pain. Twenty-five percent of the chemonucleolysis group required open diskectomy as the result of treatment failure. The resolution of pain in patients who have chemonucleolysis may be related to prolonged inactivity after the procedure and during convalescence.

In a search for less invasive techniques, investigators have utilized laser fiberoptics passing through small-gauge needles to vaporize the herniated discs. More experience is required to determine the practical validity and efficacy of these approaches compared with more established approaches. They may present some of the same problems and limitations associated with percutaneous diskectomy.

Post-traumatic Compression Fracture

Post-traumatic compression fracture usually results from compressive flexion trauma. It can also occur spontaneously in patients with osteoporosis, osteomalacia, multiple myeloma, hyperparathyroidism, and metastatic cancer. The upper lumbar spine or the middle to lower thoracic spine is most commonly affected. The pain usually is present immediately after the fracture and is often localized. There may be accompanying paraspinal muscle spasm, and the range of motion of the related level of the spine is limited. Plain radiography, CT, MRI, or bone scanning may be needed to establish the diagnosis.

Sedative rehabilitative measures, especially in the acute phase, including application of cold for the first 24 to 48 hours, analgesics, and muscle relaxants, are often necessary. The pain can be managed with use of a back support, such as a thoracolumbar support that functions on the basis of three-point contact. For provision of extension in cases of thoracic compression fractures, the three points of contact are the base of the sternum, the symphysis pubis, and the lumbar spine, as in the Jewett brace (Fig. 39–15) (see Chapter 18). When therapeutic exercises are to be prescribed, extension rather than flexion exercises should be utilized.[138] Flexion exercises can increase the incidence of vertebral body wedging and compression fractures (see Fig. 39–8C and D). Extension exercises are

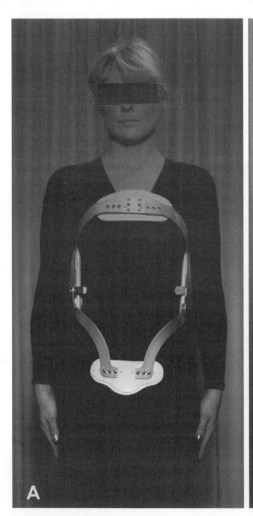
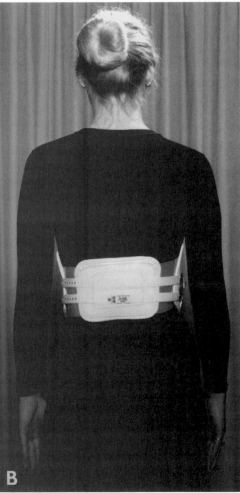

FIGURE 39–15 Jewett brace, used to prevent lumbar and thoracic flexion when patient has acute pain due to recent compression fracture of spine. Proper fitting requires proper contact at base of sternum and over pubic bone. *A,* Anterior view. *B,* Posterior view. (From Sinaki M: Exercise and physical therapy. *In* Riggs BL, Melton LJ III (eds): Osteoporosis: Etiology, Diagnosis, and Management. New York, Raven Press, 1988, pp 457–479. By permission of Mayo Foundation.)

effective for strengthening back muscles at any age (see Fig. 39–8F–H).[133, 134, 136]

Spondylolysis and Spondylolisthesis

General Considerations

Spondylolysis refers to a bony defect in the pars interarticularis. Bilateral spondylolysis of the lumbar spine may lead to anterior slipping of the vertebral body on its adjacent vertebra and cause spondylolisthesis (in Greek, "spondylo" means *vertebra*, and "olisthesis" means *sliding on a slippery surface*).[14] Even in the absence of all soft tissue attachments, spondylolisthesis does not occur unless there is a defect of the pars interarticularis or unless the pars is elongated.[4, 23, 69, 108, 109, 161] Newman,[109] Wiltse,[161] and Wiltse and associates[162] described five types of spondylolisthesis. These include (1) dysplastic, (2) isthmic, (3) degenerative, (4) traumatic, and (5) pathological (Table 39–3). To these categories, a sixth category is sometimes added: postsurgical or iatrogenic spondylolisthesis.

Symptoms and Signs

Spondylolysis or spondylolisthesis may cause back pain. However, the presence of a pars defect (spondylolysis) or even spondylolisthesis in a patient with back pain does not necessarily indicate a cause-and-effect relationship (Fig. 39–16). Spondylolisthesis is two to four times more common in males. Pars defect is at L5 in 67% of persons, L4 in 15% to 30%, and L3 in 2%. It is rare in the cervical region. In patients with back pain and spondylolisthesis, the back pain is more likely to be due to the pars defect if the patient is younger than 25 years. A pars defect is an uncommon cause of back pain in patients older than 40 years. Pain is common in children and adolescents who have spondylolysis and spondylolisthesis. Spondylolisthesis can also cause compression of nerve roots and lead

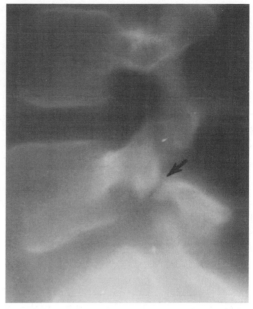

FIGURE 39–16 Incidental finding of unilateral spondylolysis in a 24-year-old woman with Ewing's sarcoma *(arrow)*.

to radicular pain or neurological deficits in the lower extremities. By creating narrowing of the spinal canal, it can cause pseudoclaudication or compression of the cauda equina and even lead to sphincter or sexual dysfunction. The lumbar lordosis is often exaggerated in patients with spondylolisthesis, and range of motion of the lumbar spine may be limited. Scoliosis and rotation of the pelvis may be noted. The hamstrings may be tight and, when standing, patients may hold their knees slightly flexed. The frequency of pars defects (spondylolysis) in children is about 4.5% (in adolescents it is about 6%), but increases to 12% in gymnasts. In children, the most common types are dysplastic and isthmic (Fig. 39–17).[14] Strenuous athletic activity in children may lead to fracture of a congenitally weak pars intra-articularis.

Radiographic and Imaging Studies

The defect in the pars intra-articularis, known as *spondylolysis*, is often visible on lateral lumbosacral radiographs and can be noted as a break in the neck of the "Scottie-dog" on oblique views of the lumbar spine (Fig. 39–18). Radioisotope bone scan may show increased activity on one or both sides.[87] Sometimes, a single photon emission computed tomography (SPECT) scan shows a pars defect that is not apparent on radiographs or bone scans.[14]

Spondylolisthesis is graded according to Meyerding's classification[96] as grades 1 to 4, depending on the degree of displacement (Fig. 39–19). In advanced cases of displacement, L5 slips completely off S1. Flexion and extension views of the lumbosacral spine are obtained to determine any segmental instability. Evaluation of patients with root symptoms, neurological deficits, or pseudoclaudication calls for further studies such as CT, MRI, myelography, and electrodiagnostic testing.

Treatment

In post-traumatic cases of spondylolisthesis, after healing of the fracture and resolution of the pain, provision of

TABLE 39–3   Classification of Spondylolisthesis

Type	Criteria
I	*Dysplastic:* The only truly congenital form of spondylolisthesis. The defect is a congenital dysplasia in the superior sacral facet or inferior L5 facet that allows L5 on S1 subluxation.
II	*Isthmic:* Defect (spondylosis) in pars interarticularis; the most common form of spondylolisthesis; typically involves L5 to S1.
	a. Lytic type, probably a fatigue fracture with hereditary predisposition.
	b. Elongated (attenuated) but intact pars, similar to type IIa, but the fatigue fractures have healed, resulting in elongated but intact pars.
	c. Acute fracture or pars due to trauma.
III	*Degenerative:* Secondary to degenerative changes at the disc and facet joints, most frequent at L4 to L5 followed by L3 to L4.
IV	*Traumatic:* Due to fracture of posterior elements other than pars (fractures of facet joints, lamina, pedicles).
V	*Pathological:* Due to pathological changes in posterior elements as a result of malignancy, primary bone disease, or infection.

From Mokri B, Sinaki M: Painful disorders of the spine and back pain syndromes. *In* Sinaki M (ed): Basic Clinical Rehabilitation Medicine, ed 2. St Louis, Mosby–Year Book, 1993, pp 489–502. By permission of Mayo Foundation.

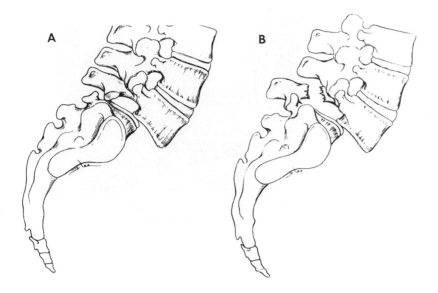

FIGURE 39–17 Dysplastic and isthmic spondylolisthesis. *A,* Dysplastic congenital spondylolisthesis. Note that neural arch of L5 is intact, although somewhat elongated. The primary defect is a deficiency in the development of the superior sacral facet, allowing anterior slippage of L5 on S1. *B,* Isthmic spondylolisthesis. Note that anterior slippage of L5 on S1 occurs because of a defect in the pars interarticularis. (From Hensinger RN: Spondylolysis and spondylolisthesis: Part I. Spondylolysis and spondylolisthesis in children. Instr Course Lect 1983; 32:132.)

immobilization for 10 to 12 weeks with application of a custom-made body jacket is the recommended treatment. In cases of chronic back pain, the patient should be instructed in abdominal muscle strengthening, lumbar flexion exercises, and static and dynamic body mechanics. In cases of persistent pain, the application of a lumbosacral brace or corset is recommended. In children, once the symptoms resolve, normal activities can be resumed, although a return to vigorous spine-bending athletic activities (such as gymnastics or football) is controversial.

For grades 1 and 2 spondylolisthesis (Fig. 39–20) and in older patients, nonsurgical treatment is recommended.[58] The physical therapeutic procedures consist of application of heat and massage for reduction of pain and stiffness. Special attention can be given to reducing the tightness of the hip flexors, hamstrings, and Achilles tendons. A program of stretching exercises is recommended. During stretching of the back and lower extremities, flexion of one hip (related knee) at a time helps reduce the strain on the lumbar spine (Fig. 39–21).

In a study to determine the efficacy of conservative management of lumbar spondylolisthesis, two groups of subjects were compared.[137] One group followed a back flexion exercise program (see Fig. 39–8*A–D*, *E1,* and *E3*), and the other group performed extension exercises (see Fig. 39–8*F1* and *F2*). At the end of 3 years, 62% of the flexion group considered themselves recovered, whereas none in the extension group did so. The goals of an exercise program should be reduction of lumbar lordosis through stretching of the lumbar paraspinal muscles and other tight structures and strengthening of lumbar flexors (see Fig. 39–8*C1, C2, D1, D2,* and *E2*). Strengthening of abdominal muscles is also of significant benefit. In cases of severe weakness of the abdominal muscles and poor response to strengthening (often seen with significant obesity or previous abdominal operations), application of an elastic lumbosacral support can decrease pain until other measures (such as weight loss or improvement of posture) contribute to reduction of pain.[137]

Spondylolisthesis can become more symptomatic during the advanced months of pregnancy. In such cases, application of an abdominal pregnancy support may help significantly. Flexion exercises are also effective for conservative management of spondylolisthesis in children.[119] In some cases, severe osteoporosis of the spine occurs with degenerative changes of ligamentous structures and spondylolisthesis. In these instances, a therapeutic exercise program that combines dynamic and static posturing along with isometric strengthening of spinal flexors and extensors without inducing strain on the osteoporotic spine has been shown to be helpful.[135]

In younger patients or persons who are involved in heavy physical jobs or strenuous sports activities, and when severe symptomatic slips with neurological symptoms or deficits are present, surgical treatment should be considered. Surgical management includes fusion of the unstable segment. Patients with advanced spondylolisthesis beyond grade 2 may require surgical intervention to decrease the

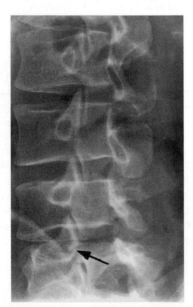

FIGURE 39–18 Radiograph from 26-year-old man with low back pain lateralizing somewhat to left side; unilateral spondylolysis at L5 on the right *(arrow).*

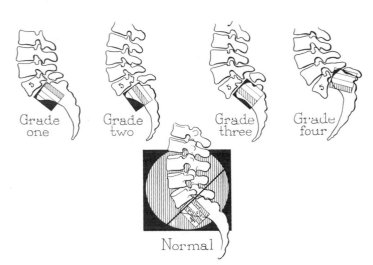

FIGURE 39–19 Meyerding's classification. The degree of subluxation is divided into four groups: grade 1, slipping on the vertebra less than one-fourth the distance of the lumbosacral angle; grade 2, less than half; grade 3, less than three-fourths; and grade 4, more than three-fourths. (From Mokri B, Sinaki M: Painful disorders of the spine and back pain syndromes. *In* Sinaki M (ed): Basic Clinical Rehabilitation Medicine, ed 2. St Louis, Mosby–Year Book, 1993, pp 489–502. By permission of Mayo Foundation.)

symptoms.[31] Adolescents who have spondylolisthesis of grade 2 or more have a greater risk for progression of the defect.[23] In these patients, serial evaluations must be done to monitor the progress of the listhesis. Once patients experience symptoms of spondylolisthesis, they should not perform heavy work or participate in high-performance, competitive sports. The patients should restrict activities such as heavy lifting, repetitive flexion of the spine, or strenuous pulling activities. Segmental fusion results in relief of pain but does not warrant resumption of strenuous activity, and surgical intervention should not be undertaken for this expectation.

Lumbar Spinal Stenosis

Stenosis of the lumbar spine may involve the central canal at a single level or multiple levels and may jeopardize the cauda equina. Sometimes the stenosis involves only the lateral recess or root canal at single or multiple levels and jeopardizes one or more nerve roots. At times, a combination of both may be present. Lumbar spinal stenosis clinically leads to the syndrome of neurogenic claudication (pseudoclaudication). When the stenosis is limited to the lateral recess or root canal, the lateral recess syndrome of root claudication (a variant of spinal stenosis) is produced. Sometimes the two syndromes coexist, but one usually dominates the clinical picture.

Pathophysiology

Spinal stenosis may be congenital, developmental, or acquired[38, 123] (Table 39–4). Because degenerative joint disease is the most common cause of spinal stenosis, the

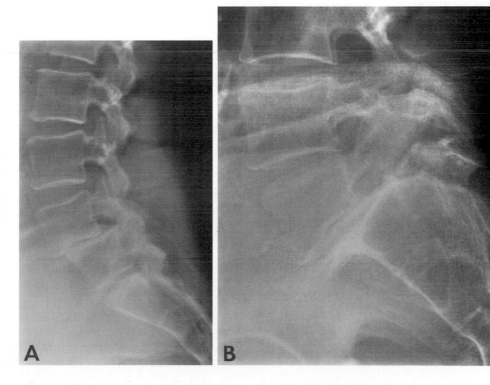

FIGURE 39–20 Grades 1 and 2 spondylolisthesis. *A,* Grade 1. Degenerative disc disease at L4 interspace with anterior subluxation of L4 on L5 due to facet joint degenerative joint disease. *B,* Grade 2, L5 on S1.

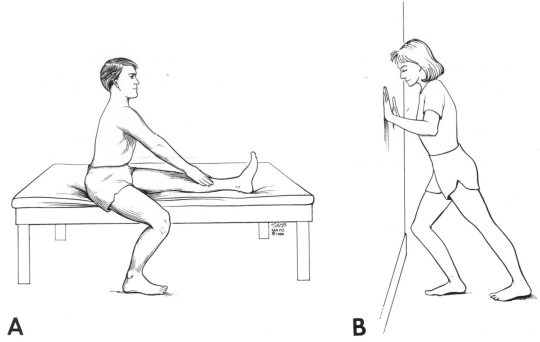

A　　　　　　　　　　　　　　　　　　**B**

FIGURE 39–21　*A,* Hamstring stretches. For a single-leg stretch, the back is kept straight and the patient leans forward until a gentle stretch is felt behind the knee. *B,* Stretches for Achilles tendons. Patient stands at arm's length from wall with palms flat against the wall. Involved leg is kept back with knee straight and heel flat on floor. Hold for 5 to 20 minutes as needed or as tolerated for each exercise. (From Mokri B, Sinaki M: Painful disorders of the spine and back pain syndromes. *In* Sinaki M (ed): Basic Clinical Rehabilitation Medicine, ed 2. St Louis, Mosby–Year Book, 1993, pp 489–502. By permission of Mayo Foundation).

resulting clinical syndromes occur most commonly after middle age.

Degenerative disc disease and narrowing of the intervertebral spaces, spur formation, ligamentous hypertrophy, facet hypertrophy, and subluxation all contribute to the decreased caliber of the central spinal canal, lateral recess, and root canal. Development of degenerative spondylolisthesis and subluxations may further compromise the central spinal canal.[164] With gradual increase in stenosis, gait endurance is gradually decreased. The caliber of the central spinal canal varies; some persons have congenitally narrow canals and are predisposed to symptoms.

Clinical Manifestations

Lumbar spinal stenosis clinically manifests as pseudo-claudication (neurogenic claudication), with unilateral or

TABLE 39–4　**Different Forms of Spinal Stenosis**

I. Primary
　A. Congenital
　B. Developmental (various forms of dwarfism)
II. Secondary
　A. Degenerative spondylolysis (with or without spondylolisthesis)
　B. Late sequelae of fracture
　C. Late sequelae of infection
　D. Systemic bone disease (Paget's disease of bone)
III. Mixed
　A. Spinal stenosis due to degenerative joint disease in an individual with a congenitally narrow spinal canal

From Postacchini F: Lumbar Spinal Stenosis. New York, Springer-Verlag, 1989, p 54. By permission of the publisher.

bilateral discomfort in the buttocks, thighs, or legs. Symptoms are produced by standing or walking and are relieved within a few minutes by sitting, lying down, or adopting a posture of flexion at the waist. The symptoms can include pain, numbness or paresthesias, or weakness. Combinations of these frequently exist, and low back pain may also be present. The waist-flexion posture is achieved by such maneuvers as backing up to a wall and leaning forward, or leaning forward on a shopping cart or a church pew.[63]

The anteroposterior diameter of the lumbar spinal canal is increased during flexion because of separation of the laminae and consequent decrease in the thickness of the ligamenta flava. At the same time, as the result of stretching of the posterior aspect of the annulus, particularly in young patients, the bulge of the disc toward the spinal canal is decreased. Lumbar flexion also leads to an increase in the caliber of the intervertebral foramina. The opposite occurs with extension of the lumbar spine (Fig. 39–22).

It is assumed that compression of the roots or cauda leads to ischemic changes in these neural structures and to the development of neurological symptoms. These are reversed when the compression is alleviated and adequate circulation is restored.

Patients frequently prefer to walk in a stooped manner rather than with a straight, erect posture, in distinction to patients with vascular claudication. For the former patients, walking uphill (waist-flexion posture) may be easier than walking downhill (straight, erect posture). In some patients, pain and discomfort are worsened by lying supine with the lower limbs extended, and they are relieved by elevating the knees or by lying on one side in a fetal position.

Symptoms are bilateral in more than two-thirds of pa-

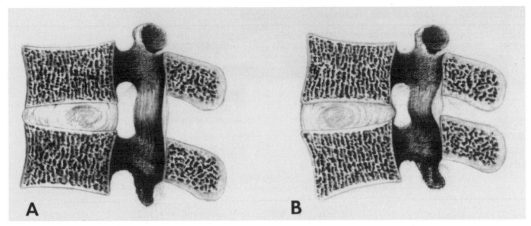

FIGURE 39–22 Functional changes of vertebral canal in spinal flexion and extension. *A,* In flexion, spinal canal lengthens and increases in width in sagittal plane, due both to separation of the luminae and the consequent decrease in thickness of the ligamenta flava and to distention of the posterior annulus fibrosus. *B,* Opposite changes occur in extension. (From Postacchini F: Lumbar Spinal Stenosis. New York, Springer-Verlag, 1989, p 41. By permission of the publisher.)

tients, but a significant asymmetry often exists. The low back pain that is present in two-thirds of patients is typically mild and non-discogenic and has essentially the same features as low back pain associated with lumbar spinal degenerative joint disease.

Absence or decrease in muscle stretch reflexes is noted in about 50% of patients. Weakness can be detected in about 40% of patients. This is usually mild, unilateral, and often in the distribution of L5 or S1 roots.

The clinical features of lateral recess syndrome and root claudication are different from those of central canal stenosis.[28] Patients usually report a unilateral intense sciatic pain (L5 or S1 root irritation) that is provoked by standing or walking and is relieved by sitting, lying down, or flexing the lumbar spine. Neurological deficits, if present, are mild. The straight-leg raising test is usually negative.[44] There is little or no low back pain.

Differentiation of Vascular Claudication From Neurogenic Claudication

Vascular claudication occurs when exertion of the lower limb muscles results in energy consumption that exceeds the amount that can be provided by the circulation. Walking (especially fast or uphill), climbing stairs, or riding a bicycle (regular or stationary) induces the pain. This pain is relieved when exercise is discontinued, and low back pain and frank neurological symptoms are not present. Overall, in vascular claudication, the lower limb pain is relieved by rest. The limb pain resulting from spinal stenosis (pseudo-claudication) is relieved only when the spine is flexed or when the patient sits down. Some of the factors that are useful for differentiating vascular from neurogenic claudication are listed in Table 39–5.

Laboratory Tests

Electromyography

Electromyographic abnormalities are noted in more than 90% of patients and are more frequent than the abnormalities detected on neurological examination. Findings include

evidence of denervation in the distribution of a single root or multiple roots, often bilaterally.[63]

Plain Radiography

Most patients have degenerative joint or disc disease with or without spondylolisthesis. In some patients, the lumbar spinal canal appears congenitally narrow. In certain congenital syndromes, such as achondroplastic dwarfism, spinal stenosis can be significant.

Myelography and Imaging Studies

Myelography shows complete or partial obstruction to the flow of contrast at one or more levels (Figs. 39–23 and 39–24). CT and MRI show stenosis of the central canal, lateral recess, root canal, or a combination of these. CT-myelography is a very accurate test for evaluation of stenosis of these regions.[26, 27, 163]

Levels of stenosis (in decreasing order of frequency) are L4 to L5 (55%), L3 to L4 (44%), L2 to L3 (26%), L5 to S1 (14%), and T12 to L1 (3%).[123]

Treatment

The natural history of pseudoclaudication is not entirely clear. The symptoms of canal stenosis either remain unchanged or gradually worsen. The symptoms of root claudication are thought to either remain unchanged or perhaps gradually improve in some patients, but in an unpredictable time frame. Many patients, however, experience marked reduction in their activities and seek a solution. For cases in which progressive neurological deficits occur, surgical decompression should be seriously considered.[41]

Conservative Management

Reduction of lumbar lordosis is effective for reducing lumbar stenosis. Exercises that are aimed at strengthening the abdominal muscles and lumbar flexors are helpful. For patients in whom it is not possible to strengthen the abdominal muscles or in those with a protuberant abdomen and extensive body weight, an elastic abdominal binder is rec-

TABLE 39–5   Differentiation of Vascular and Neurogenic Claudication

Factor	Neurogenic Claudication (Pseudoclaudication)	Vascular Claudication	Pitfalls and Remarks
Low back pain	Frequently present	Absent	Sometimes, coincidental degenerative joint disease can be present in patients with vascular claudication
Effect of standing	Provokes symptoms	Does not provoke symptoms	
Direction of radiation of pain in lower limbs	Usually downward	Usually upward	
Sensory symptoms	Present in 66% of patients	Absent	Some patients with vascular claudication can have distal sensory symptoms due to ischemic or diabetic neuropathy
Muscle weakness	Present in more than 40% of patients	Absent	
Reflex changes	Present in about 50% of patients	Absent	In older patients, especially if there is associated neuropathy, reflexes may be decreased or absent
Arterial pulses	Normal	Decreased or absent	In older patients, pulses may be reduced
Arterial bruits	Absent	Frequently present	
Effect of rest while standing	Does not relieve symptoms	Relieves symptoms	
Walking uphill	Symptoms produced later	Symptoms produced earlier	
Walking downhill	Symptoms produced earlier	Symptoms produced later	
Bicycling (stationary or regular)	Does not provoke symptoms	Provokes symptoms	

From Mokri B, Sinaki M: Lumbar disk syndrome, lumbosacral radiculopathies, lumbar spondylosis and stenosis, spondylolisthesis. *In* Sinaki M (ed): Basic Clinical Rehabilitation Medicine, ed 2. St Louis, Mosby–Year Book, 1993, pp 503–513. By permission of Mayo Foundation.

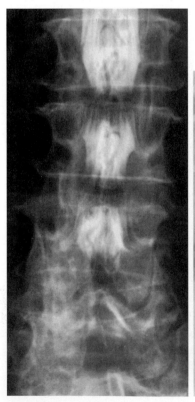
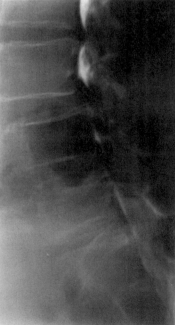

FIGURE 39–23 Lumbar myelograms. Anteroposterior *(left)* and lateral *(right)* views demonstrate multiple lumbar stenosis. (From Mokri B, Sinaki M: Lumbar disc syndrome, lumbosacral radiculopathies, lumbar spondylosis and stenosis, spondylolisthesis. *In* Sinaki M (ed): Basic Clinical Rehabilitation Medicine, ed 2. St Louis, Mosby–Year Book, 1993, pp 503–513. By permission of Mayo Foundation.)

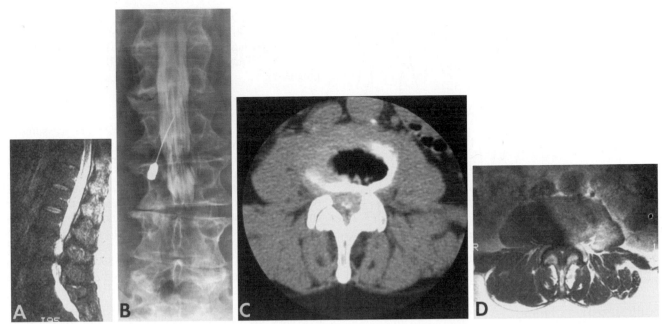

FIGURE 39–24 Lumbar spinal stenosis in a 73-year-old man. A very tight central canal stenosis is seen at L3 to L4 interspace and a moderate stenosis at L2 to L3 interspace, as noted in the sagittal T2-weighted MRI (A) and in the myelogram (B), which shows block to the flow of contrast dye at L3 to L4. CT-myelogram at this level shows a very tight canal (C), and axial T2-weighted MRI shows only a tiny cerebrospinal fluid signal (D).

ommended. A program consisting of knee-to-chest exercises, pelvic tilt, and standing against a wall while attempting to contract the lumbar flexors to decrease lumbar lordosis may be beneficial. Patients should be instructed to avoid exercises that result in hyperextension of the spine. Nonsteroidal anti-inflammatory drugs can help in managing the pain, particularly pain related to the associated degenerative joint disease.

Surgical Management

When patients are properly selected, decompressive single-level or multilevel laminectomy, with or without foraminotomies, alleviates manifestations of pseudoclaudication in most patients. However, the effect of this surgery on any associated low back pain is often less satisfactory. When low back pain rather than pseudoclaudication is the dominant feature, the expectations for an overall good recovery should be less. Although the patients with low back pain may obtain relief from the symptoms of pseudoclaudication, they may still continue to suffer from the pain.

Overall, the more pronounced the degree of spinal canal compromise and neural compression, the better the chance of obtaining a good surgical result. When long-standing and pronounced neurogenic atrophy and weakness have developed, patients may get relief from the leg pain resulting from the pseudoclaudication, but they typically have only a partial or negligible recovery of the muscle weakness and atrophy.[38]

Low Back Pain in Pregnancy

In 50% to 90% of pregnant women, low back pain develops at some point during pregnancy.[15, 45, 46, 115, 127] The back pain in 10% to 33% of these women is severe enough to reduce their activities of daily living significantly and, frequently, to require bedrest. The prevalence of low back pain during pregnancy increases 5% for every 5 years of the pregnant woman's age. Other than age, such factors as heavy labor, smoking, parity, and a previous history of low back pain have been cited as risk factors for back pain during pregnancy.[15, 114, 146] Alternatively, several studies[45–47, 127] have not found any correlation between the development of back pain during pregnancy and age, race, parity, occupation, baby's weight, mother's pre-pregnancy weight, weight gain during pregnancy, exercise habits, or sleeping posture.

Low back pain is frequent in pregnancy, and women with a history of back pain often fear that pregnancy will activate or aggravate their back pain. Physicians are apprehensive about treating pregnant patients who have back pain because of the fear of interfering with the pregnancy or adversely affecting the fetus.

Clinical Manifestations

Pregnant women obviously are not immune to the back pains of various causes that can develop in others. Additionally, they frequently also have back pains directly related to pregnancy. Essentially, four types of pain can be recognized: (1) nocturnal back pain, which occurs in more than one-third of patients; (2) low dorsal pain (Fig. 39–25A); (3) lumbar pain, which may or may not extend to one or both lower limbs (Fig. 39–25B); and (4) sacroiliac region pain (Fig. 39–25C).

Nocturnal back pain of pregnancy occurs 1 to 2 hours after lying down and is thought to be related to stagnation of venous blood in the vertebral venous plexus due to return of fluid of dependent edema of pregnancy to the circulation during recumbency on one hand, and the venous

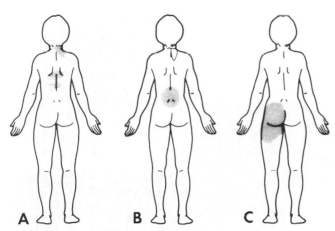

FIGURE 39–25 Areas of back pain during pregnancy. *A,* Low dorsal pain. *B,* Lumbar pain, which may or may not extend to both lower extremities. *C,* Sacroiliac region pain. (From Ostgaard HC, Andersson GBJ, Karlsson K: Prevalence of back pain in pregnancy. Spine 1991; 16:549.)

blockage caused by pressure of the fetus on the vena cava on the other.

Sacroiliac pain is probably the most common type of back pain in pregnancy.[15, 30, 129] It may be unilateral or bilateral, may extend to the upper thigh, and may not be substantially relieved by lying down. Normally, the sacroiliac joint moves only minimally. During pregnancy, the production of relaxin (a hormone secreted by the corpus luteum) leads to articular laxity that can result in sacroiliac inflammation, pain, and discomfort.

The other low dorsal and lumbar pains of pregnancy have mechanical features, are increased by physical activity, and are decreased by rest. The leg pain and radicular symptoms that may accompany the low back pain of pregnancy are frequently caused by the direct pressure of the gravid uterus on components of the lumbosacral plexus. These cases actually are lumbosacral plexopathies or proximal sciatic neuropathies rather than true radiculopathies.

The back pain of pregnancy may not disappear with delivery, and in 20% to 25% of cases the pain may linger for some time.

Other causes of low back pain, such as herniated lumbar disc, tumors, and infections, can occur in pregnant women just as in the nonpregnant population. Pregnancy may induce a remission of rheumatoid arthritis, with frequent flareups after delivery.

Prophylaxis

Measures that prevent low back pain are less effective during pregnancy. The options are few but can be helpful. These include (1) reducing the load on the spine by appropriate changes in lifestyle and work environment, especially in women with a past history of back pain or back pain with previous pregnancies; (2) avoidance of excessive weight gain during pregnancy; and (3) educating the patient regarding proper posture to decrease lumbar lordosis; proper techniques for lifting, working positions, and resting positions (Fig. 39–26); and techniques for avoidance of aggravating factors. Pregnancy back supports and exercise instructions for abdominal muscle and pelvic floor contrac-

tion (see Fig. 39–8*D*), lateral bending, and rotational trunk exercises performed in a standing position may be helpful. Sit-ups requiring a supine position and Valsalva's maneuver should be avoided, particularly after the fourth month of pregnancy.[3]

Treatment

In most cases, when pregnant women are reassured of the benign nature of the back pain, they find the discomfort tolerable and typically manage the problem symptomatically by rest and modification of their activities. For more bothersome low back pain, application of an abdominal pregnancy support with shoulder suspenders, physical therapy, and massage may help. For pain in the sacroiliac region, a trochanteric belt or a sacroiliac corset may offer reasonably good relief.[15, 40] Severe sacroiliac pain may require a period of bed rest (see Fig. 39–26) and physical therapy consisting of application of cold or superficial heat and sedative massage. Nocturnal pain of pregnancy may be difficult to manage. The use of venous support stockings to reduce the dependent edema during the waking hours and proper posturing at night may help. Acetaminophen is the analgesic of choice for management of low back pain during pregnancy.[24] Nonsteroidal agents are relatively contraindicated, and aspirin may increase the incidence of fetal intracranial hemorrhage in premature infants.[9] Medication for back pain in pregnancy should be used only as a last resort, with the approval of the obstetrician and with the informed consent of the patient.

Paget's Disease

Paget's disease of bone is a rather common disease, particularly in elderly patients. It is marked by focal disturbance of bone architecture due to abnormally increased osteoblastic activity. It may involve a single bone (monostotic) or several bones (polyostotic), including the pelvis or vertebral bones. The alkaline phosphatase level is typically elevated, except in some early, limited, or monostotic forms. The disease may be asymptomatic or may cause focal pain. Involvement of the posterior pelvis or lumbar spine causes low back pain in some patients. Malignant transformation of Paget's lesion can occur, but this is uncommon. The lesions should be differentiated from those of hyperparathyroidism, fibrous dysplasia, myeloma, and metastatic tumors, particularly metastases from prostate cancer. The involved vertebral bone typically shows gener-

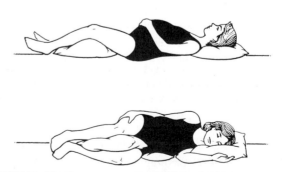

FIGURE 39–26 Proper positioning through use of cushions in bed helps decrease patient's nocturnal discomforts during pregnancy.

Back Pain

Mechanical (Non-discogenic) → Stress/strain of back muscles
"Decompensated Sd"   Tendons
                            Ligaments

- Chronic   dull/aching +/- → buttocks
- Worse = <u>sitting</u> (prolonged)/bending, twisting lifting
         <u>Standing</u>
- ↑insidious   Obese | Tx | Correction of Posture
                             Exercise
          prolonged use back support (>3 wks) →
                             mm. disuse

DJD   LBP → "Stiffness"   hypertrophic Δ's/spurs. | Dx | X Rays

- Relieved by <u>Rest</u> | Tx | posture Δ's
                            Exercises → Spinal Support
     prevent immobility by tx pain   (6wks) Elastic Support if weak

Facet Joints   Localized Spine Pain   ↓hypertext
                                       | Tx | NSAIDs
- Episodic (+/- → Limb)   • Abrupt   • manipulation
- ↓ ROM Extension   • pain ↑ w/activity ↓ w/rest   • facet injection
                                      • wt Loss
                           (DSE) Exercises x 6wks

Radiculopathy (Macnab)   Bulge → beyond disc margin (Annulus/Sharpey's intact)
                 <u>Prolapse</u> → posteriorly incomplete annulus defect
                 <u>Extruded</u> → " " complete defect Annulus
                 <u>SEQUESTERED</u> → HNP detaches

Comp. Fx   upper L/low T spine • immediate • Localized

- paraspinal mm. Spasm   Sedative Cold, Analgesia/mm. relaxants

PRIMACOR®
milrinone lactate injection

alized enlargement and increased width. There is increased trabeculation (corduroy pattern), and a thickened rim of cortex may cause a picture-frame appearance. Dense sclerosis of vertebral bodies may give a pattern of "ivory vertebrae" and may simulate osteoblastic metastases. The involved area shows significant uptake on radioisotope bone scan, but MRI may be surprisingly unremarkable.

Treatment is needed only in symptomatic cases. Aspirin or nonsteroidal agents can reduce the pain. In active disease and when the pain is clearly related to the Paget's disease and not to other conditions (degenerative joint or degenerative disc disease), treatment with etidronate sodium (5 to 10 mg/kg/day orally for 6 months) can be considered. Continuous treatment with etidronate can result in side effects of osteomalacia with increased bone fractures and pain. Consequently, drug holiday periods of 3 to 6 months should be interspersed between the treatment courses. Calcitonin is also effective but has to be given subcutaneously or intramuscularly. Ambulatory assistive devices (cane, walker) reduce the accompanying weightbearing pain. For associated focal muscle pain with tenderness, application of superficial heat and massage can be helpful.[139]

Low Back Pain Due to Neoplastic Disease

Primary spinal cord tumors such as astrocytomas, and particularly spinal ependymomas, can cause low back pain. Extramedullary intraspinal tumors such as meningiomas or neurilemomas, as well as primary tumors of the vertebral bones (whether benign or malignant), can also cause low back pain. The most common neoplastic diseases causing low back pain are the metastatic spinal or epidural cancers (multiple myeloma and malignant lymphomas included) (Figs. 39–27 through 39–32). The low back pain related to neoplastic disease can be steady or may be provoked by physical activity or change in posture. However, one of the hallmarks of cancer pain is pain at rest, particularly nocturnal pain.

With advances in radiation therapy and chemotherapy, patients with primary malignant tumors are living longer; as a result, metastases, such as spinal epidural metastases, have more time to develop. Spinal cord compression due to metastatic cancer is found in about 5% to 10% of patients with bony metastases. At the lumbar and low dorsal level, most of these are also associated with low back pain. The tumors that most frequently metastasize to the spine include cancers of the lung, prostate, breast, kidney, and colon, and malignant melanoma, myeloma, and lymphoma. Sometimes spinal metastasis is the first clinical manifestation of the cancer.

Radiation is the palliative treatment of choice (often 3000 cGy in 10 fractions). In cases of cord compromise, in addition to the radiation therapy, high-dose dexamethasone is also often administered (with a subsequent quick tapering of dose). Such treatments do not necessarily prolong survival, but they are effective for relieving pain and lessening neurological deficits and disability. In selected cases, surgical decompression or even corpectomy has been considered. Imaging studies, particularly MRI, are helpful for detection of spinal and epidural metastases, for de-

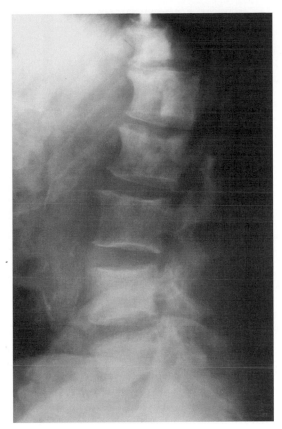

FIGURE 39–27 Spinal metastases with osteoblastic features in a 63-year-old man with prostatic cancer.

termining the field of radiation therapy, and for post-treatment follow-up.

Analgesic medications are often required, particularly for the acute pain. Proper bracing and spinal immobilization and support should be provided if they help to decrease the pain or if there is a suggestion of spinal instability. Application of a spinal orthosis to decrease the pain due to weightbearing increases the patient's ability for ambulatory activities and reduces the risks of bone loss and muscle

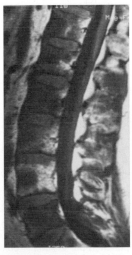

FIGURE 39–28 Multiple metastases to lumbar spine in a 66-year-old man with prostate cancer.

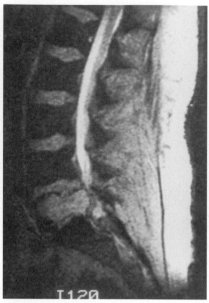

FIGURE 39–29 Metastatic carcinoma involving L5, with epidural extension, compressing the thecal sac and cauda equina.

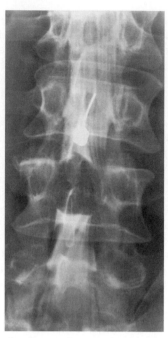

FIGURE 39–31 Lumbar myelogram showing intraspinal neurilemoma. A sharply circumscribed, round myelographic defect is displacing elements of the cauda equina. Note the cuplike upper and lower margins of the defect with concavity facing the tumor.

atrophy caused by immobility. Participation in physical activities often improves the patient's feeling of well-being. Ambulatory assistive devices such as a wheeled walker can also reduce weightbearing pain.

Ankylosing Spondylitis

Ankylosing spondylitis is a chronic inflammatory seronegative rheumatic spondyloarthropathy that affects skele-

tal and extraskeletal tissues. It mainly affects the spine and invariably involves the sacroiliac joints. Eighty percent to 90% of patients are HLA-B27–positive. The prevalence is about 1 per 1000 in the white population. Males predominate, but the frequently stated ratio of 10:1 is definitely

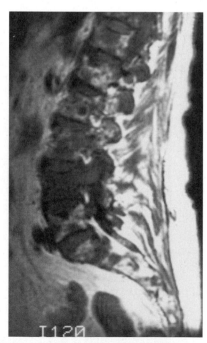

FIGURE 39–30 Extensive involvement of vertebrae in multiple myeloma; marrow replacement by infiltrating cells, deossification, and destructive and punched-out lesions. Pedicles that are so frequently involved in metastatic disease are often spared in multiple myeloma (pedicles lack red marrow).

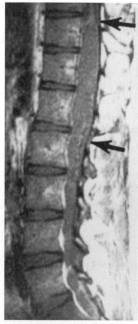

FIGURE 39–32 Magnetic resonance imaging scan of spine, demonstrating large fusiform tumor extending from T10 to L3 *(arrows)* in a 30-year-old man. Tumor was found to be a low-grade ependymoma. This patient had had unexplained low back pain for several years before neurological deficits began to appear.

less.[158] Although the true ratio is unknown, a ratio of 3:1 is more realistic. The disease often is milder in females and frequently presents with involvement of one of the appendicular joints before the appearance of sacroiliitis. The disease usually begins at age 20 to 35 years. Sacroiliitis is usually the first manifestation, presenting as unilateral or bilateral low back pain of insidious onset. Classically, significant morning stiffness and pain in the lower back are noted. These symptoms typically improve with activity during the day and return after rest or immobility. Many patients are awakened from sleep because of pain and stiffness of the lower back. To get relief, they often have to get up and move around. Pain may extend to the buttocks and posterior thighs. Lumbar lordosis may be lost (Fig. 39–33). Recurrent iritis, aortitis, and carditis are some of the peripheral manifestations of the disease.[6, 80] Cauda equina syndrome may occur in long-standing cases.[11]

The diagnosis must be confirmed by radiography. The earliest radiographic findings are almost invariably in the sacroiliac joints and include blurring of the margins of the lower two-thirds of these joints, especially on the iliac side, and widening of the joint space. With advance of sacroili-

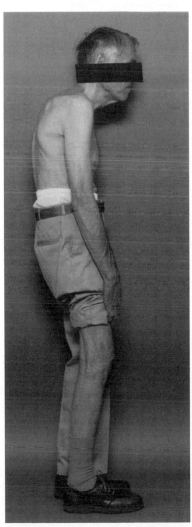

FIGURE 39–33 Ankylosing spondylitis; kyphotic posturing with contractures of hamstrings and hip flexors from compensating to maintain erect posture.

itis, increase in erosions and joint space destruction, and progression of sclerosis, total ankylosis and obliteration of the joint may finally occur. Early changes in the lumbar spine include squaring of the lumbar vertebral body and demineralization and spotty ligamentous calcification. In advanced cases with diffuse paraspinal ligamentous calcification, the classic picture of "bamboo spine" is produced. This change occurs only in a minority of patients and takes many years to develop; therefore, in reality, it has no value in early diagnosis of the disease. Myelography and CT, especially in long-standing ankylosing spondylitis with cauda equina syndrome, show characteristic enlargement of the cul de sac, enlarged and often multiloculated dorsal arachnoid diverticula, and erosion of laminae and spinous processes. These changes can be clearly seen with MRI (Fig. 39–34).

The prognosis is variable. *Osteitis condensans ilii*, a benign condition in women, should be differentiated from ankylosing spondylitis. It is particularly common in postpartum women, and the lesions likely develop as a result of mechanical strain placed on the sacroiliac joint during pregnancy. The radiographic features that differentiate the typical osteitis condensans ilii from ankylosing spondylitis include preservation of the sacroiliac joint and confinement of the sclerotic changes to the iliac side of the joint. Overall, women have less severe spinal disease but may have more peripheral joint involvement. The prognosis is less favorable in patients with refractory iliitis. Overall, most patients have mild disease and can lead full and productive lives.

Conservative treatment is the basis of management of patients with ankylosing spondylitis. Nonsteroidal anti-inflammatory medications can help diminish the pain and stiffness. Surgical intervention (such as extension osteotomies for excessive thoracic and cervical kyphosis) only very rarely becomes necessary.

Evaluation should include periodic measurements (in centimeters) of height, chest expansion, and C7 to S1 spinal flexion. A back extension exercise program (see Figs. 39–8F1, F2, H1, and H2 and 39–21), deep-breathing exercises, posture training, range of motion of the proximal joints (shoulders and hips), range-of-motion exercises to the cervical spine (if possible), and stretching exercises for the pectorals, hamstrings, Achilles tendons, hip flexors, and low back are important and should be included in the overall management program. The patient needs to have periodic measurement of height. Flexed posture needs to be avoided on the job, while driving, and during rest. Application of heat and massage before exercise can facilitate pain relief. Evaluation of chest expansion through periodic measurement of chest circumference at the level of T5 with a tape measure is recommended (this value is usually more than 5 to 7 cm). If chest expansion is reduced to less than 5 cm, respiratory function tests and encouragement for the patient to improve diaphragmatic breathing are recommended. Again, every effort should be made to avoid flexed posture because there is no cure for subsequent fusion in a flexed position. Certain assistive devices facilitate daily activities despite limited spine motion. These include prism glasses, reachers, and wide-angle rear view mirrors for the car. Activities that may unduly strain the spine (such as contact sports, motorcycle riding,

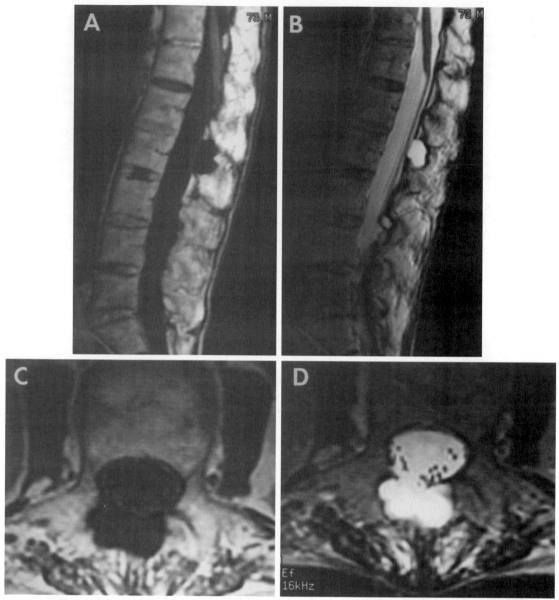

FIGURE 39–34 Ankylosing spondylitis associated with cauda equina syndrome in a 73-year-old man. Magnetic resonance imaging scans of lumbar and lower thoracic spine: sagittal T1 *(A)* and T2 *(B)* images and axial T1- *(C)* and T2-weighted *(D)* images. Note multiple arachnoid diverticula in lower thoracic and upper lumbar canal, deviation of conus medullaris, and straightening of spine.

jumping) should be avoided because they could result in vertebral fractures.

Diffuse Idiopathic Skeletal Hyperostosis (DISH)

Described by Forestier and Rotes-Querol in 1950,[50] Forestier's disease, also known as ankylosing hyperostosis, is a fairly common non-deforming, ossifying disease that occurs in elderly and middle-aged patients, particularly men. Ossification occurs along the anterior and lateral spinal ligaments without disc narrowing, apophyseal joint ankylosis, sacroiliac joint erosions, sclerosis, fusion, or vertebral body marginal sclerosis.[150] The ossification may also involve peripheral muscular tenderness at insertions. Any level of the spine may be involved, but thoracic involvement is more common, followed by involvement of

the lumbar region. The involvement may be unilateral. The condition may be asymptomatic or cause stiffness, pain, and some limitation of motion, but significant functional inability is rare. Management is conservative; nonsteroidal agents may also be helpful. Application of infrared heat and massage decrease the accompanying myalgias and stiffness.

Pyogenic Vertebral Spondylitis

This condition includes infectious discitis (intervertebral disc infection) and infectious vertebral osteomyelitis. Although these may occur postoperatively, the focus here is on childhood and adult pyogenic infectious spondylitis that occurs without a history of spinal surgery. These cause low back pain and enter into the differential diagnosis of back pain. The mechanism is from a contiguous infection or by hematogenous or lymphatic seeding from a remote site.[8, 32, 57, 62, 70, 75, 95, 99] Common sources of infection are pneumonia; urinary tract, cutaneous, and dental infections; and abdominal surgery. The source of infections is not apparent in more than one-third of cases.[8, 95] It is more common in patients with diabetes, malignancy, renal failure, alcoholism, and AIDS; in intravenous drug abusers; and in immunocompromised patients. Thoracic and lumbar spines are more frequently involved, but back pain is more common with lumbar spine involvement because the thoracic cage splints the spine and can mute the localized back pain.[113] The most common infectious agent is *Staphylococcus aureus*, but other bacteria, especially gram-negative agents and anaerobes, have been implicated.[29, 60, 155] Pyogenic vertebral spondylitis may become associated with spinal epidural abscess, which may cause compression of the spinal cord or cauda equina and create a surgical emergency.

The clinical features are often different in children and adults. In children, the onset is often abrupt, with fever, malaise, back pain, and spine tenderness. The diagnosis is typically not difficult.[113] In adults, the onset is more gradual; there is little or no fever and malaise is generally absent. Point tenderness is evident at the involved site, but in a small percentage of patients, back pain may not be evident, and it can take up to 3 months to reach a diagnosis.[143, 144] The erythrocyte sedimentation rate is usually elevated, but leukocytosis is more evident in acute cases (therefore, it is generally noted in children and might not be evident in adults).

Radiographic and Imaging Findings

Radiographic abnormalities significantly lag behind the actual pathological changes that are taking place. The radiographic findings include narrowing of intervertebral disc space in discitis, loss of definition and destruction of the cortical margins of the vertebral bodies facing the disc, bone loss and rarefaction, vertebral body collapse, and gibbus formation (Fig. 39–35).

Myelography does not directly visualize epidural abscesses but demonstrates the associated mass effect on the thecal sac and neural structures. Myelography also carries the risk of introducing the infection to the spinal subarachnoid space and creating meningitis.

CT may show the pathological alterations, including the epidural abscesses, although they may appear isodense or hypodense compared with the adjacent musculature. CT can also visualize paravertebral soft tissue components of the infectious process. The presence of an epidural mass centered on an intervertebral disc is a helpful CT feature that differentiates the process from a neoplastic cause. MRI is clearly superior to CT for evaluation of epidural abscesses and paraspinal masses. Its ability to image long segments of the spinal canal in multiple planes allows delineation of the pathological process.[154, 159] MRI is more sensitive than plain films or CT for diagnosis of discitis and osteomyelitis.[56]

Treatment

The infection should be treated with antibiotics. Ideally, the diagnosis is established before development of neurological deficits. In general, nonsurgical therapy is considered for patients without neurological deficits. Surgery for decompression and drainage of pus should be considered when pressure effects and neurological deficits develop. Undue delays should be avoided, because the chances of full recovery diminish with progression of neurological impairment. Childhood disc space infection often responds well to antibiotics and immobilization with application of a rigid orthosis for 6 to 12 weeks.

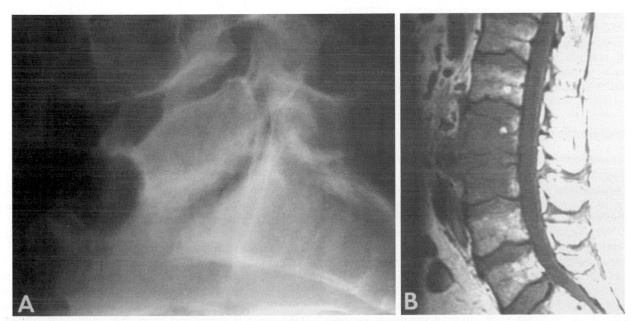

FIGURE 39–35 Pyogenic vertebral osteomyelitis and intravertebral disc infection. *A,* Radiograph of lumbar spine in a patient with L5 to S1 intervertebral disc infection. Note narrowing of the disc space and irregularities of the adjacent end-plates associated with reactive sclerosis. *B,* Magnetic resonance imaging scan of lumbar and lower thoracic spine of another patient, demonstrating involvement of L2 to L3 intervertebral disc, especially anteriorly, and involvement of adjacent vertebral bodies and soft tissues anterior to these vertebrae.

BACK PAIN IN CHILDREN

Back pain is relatively common in children, particularly in active adolescents, and is generally benign and self-limited. Sometimes the back pain in childhood can have a more significant or even serious cause, such as discogenic disease, congenital disorders, inflammatory disease, infection, or tumor.

Lumbar Disc Disease

About 1% of children presenting with low back pain have lumbar disc disease. Two percent of all operations on lumbar discs are in children.[55, 89] Overall, lumbar disc disease is an uncommon condition in children, and the vast majority of the patients are 10 years or older. Practically all patients have back pain, and 90% have radicular symptoms; in about 50% of the patients, the radicular symptoms develop sometimes after establishment of the low back pain. The straight-leg raising test is frequently positive, and neurological deficits are noted in more than half of the patients.[22, 33, 61, 149, 165] Despite a trial of conservative measures, more than 60% of patients need surgery. In 95% of the cases, the involved disc is at L4 to L5 and L5 to S1. A history of trauma is more commonly elicited in adolescents with lumbar disc disease than in adults. A family history of lumbar disc disease is 5 to 7 times more common in children and adolescents than in adults. Results of surgical therapy are encouraging. The cure rate is about 90% to 95%. It is not uncommon for children who have undergone treatment for lumbar disc disease to have disc disease at a different level in the future.

Scheuermann's Disease

Scheuermann's disease is another cause of low back pain in adolescents. It is more frequent in boys and is characterized by herniation of a disc through the end-plate into the vertebral body. Osteochondritis of the upper and lower vertebral end-plates and trauma may play a role. Some patients have marfanoid features, and a familial tendency is present in some. The back pain typically responds to rest and immobilization through application of a proper spinal orthosis.

Spondylosis and Spondylolisthesis

In the pediatric age group, spondylosis and spondylolisthesis are the most common causes of back pain associated with structural change. Spondylosis is likely related to injury to the pars interarticularis.[157] Older children and adolescents are more frequently affected than younger ones. In acute cases, a pars fracture may actually heal with immobilization for 10 to 12 weeks in a plaster body jacket. Restriction of activity and occasional bracing aid in resolution of the pain. In chronic cases, instructions in back care, abdominal muscle strengthening, and stretching of paraspinal muscles, hip flexors, hamstrings, and Achilles tendons are helpful. After resolution of symptoms, normal activities can be resumed, but a return to vigorous athletic events involving the spine (such as gymnastics and football) is controversial.[120]

Congenital Diseases

With modern neuroimaging techniques, congenital spine and spinal cord problems and dysraphic anomalies are relatively easily detected in children with back pain. About 10% of patients have more than one spinal lesion, and imaging of the entire spine is therefore prudent.

Infections

Infectious vertebral osteomyelitis and discitis have been addressed, and the differences in various features of these entities in adults and children have been outlined.

Tumor

Nocturnal pain, pain at rest, and pain on awakening are symptoms that may draw attention to tumors of the spinal column. Metastatic tumors of the spine may occur, but in contrast to the case in adults, they are uncommon in children. The most frequent tumors of the spinal column in children include osteoid osteoma, osteoblastoma, histiocytosis X, and aneurysmal bone cyst. The pain of osteoid osteoma is typically nocturnal and responds to aspirin. Osteoblastoma has features similar to those of osteoid osteoma, but it is usually of larger size. Histiocytosis X may cause vertebral body collapse.[89]

CONSERVATIVE MANAGEMENT OF BACK PAIN: GENERAL CONSIDERATIONS

Conservative treatment of back pain traditionally has included rest, avoidance of stressful activities, use of back supports in some cases, and exercise. We prefer to divide the conservative management of back pain into two categories: (1) management of acute low back pain syndromes and (2) management of chronic low back pain syndromes.

Acute Low Back Pain Syndromes

Acute back pain is usually accompanied by anxiety and fear of possible debilitating causes. Conservative treatment is indicated for each case of acute back pain (Table 39–6). However, this option should at times be modified by other factors, such as the accompanying neurological loss, repeated hospitalization, and economic hardship imposed on the patient by the situation.

Acute back pain is most commonly related to a traumatic injury or a mechanical strain that is beyond the biomechanical competence of low back structures. As in any acute injury, the contributing factors to pain are not only the injury to the structures involved but also the soft tissue edema at the location.

As in any acute injury, cold packs decrease edema and should be applied immediately after injury. The patient is encouraged to comply with physical therapy measures, such as application of cold packs during the first 48 hours after strain or sprain and, thereafter, application of heat or cold to the area for pain relief. Heat is applied to the lower back through an infrared heat lamp or an electric heating pad for 20 to 35 minutes (continuous heat application is

TABLE 39–6 Some Causes of Acute Low Back Pain and Their Treatment

Cause	Treatment
Musculoskeletal	
Muscle strain or ligamentous sprain	Symptomatic treatment (bed rest, corset, cold [first 48 hr]/ heat, massage)
Herniated disc	
Nonprogressive	Conservative treatment, injection
Progressive neurological signs	Laminectomy and disc excision
Traumatic fracture	
Stable	Spinal orthoses, analgesics
Unstable	Fusion, bone graft, or instrumentation
Inflammatory disease (acute spondyloarthropathies)	Conservative management, treatment of underlying disease
Infections (pyogenic, vertebral spondylitis, intervertebral disc infection)	Immobilization, antibiotics, surgery and drainage of pus if pressure effect and neurological deficits are present
Compression fracture (osteopenia, osteoporosis)	Bed rest (2–3 days), back support, simple analgesics, teatment of underlying disease
Degenerative joint disease with or without facet abnormality	Conservative treatment Posture instructions Back support
Malignancy, pathological compression fractures	Radiation therapy, usually high-dose dexamethasone at onset if cord compromise is present; orthosis for stabilization; surgical decompression and stabilization in selected cases

not recommended).[83] Application of light stroking massage can decrease the superficial soft tissue edema induced by the use of heat and also provide more relaxation to the paraspinal muscles. The practice of manipulation in an attempt to reposition the displaced spine is controversial.

For acute discogenic disorders, the use of simple analgesics every 4 to 6 hours is also helpful. Adequate analgesia with acetaminophen, nonsteroidal anti-inflammatory drugs, or a short course of sedative muscle relaxants or even synthetic opiates may be recommended. Simple sedatives are given to reduce muscle spasm even further. In severe cases, the use of narcotics may be necessary for a short time (1 week to 10 days). Only minor concern of addiction is present with short-term use of narcotics, and the benefits surpass the risks. It is better to avoid codeine and its derivatives because constipation induced by these agents aggravates back pain as a result of straining and elevation of intraspinal pressure.

In the acute stage of back pain it is helpful to provide support for the spine during weightbearing and ambulatory activities to decrease pain related to paraspinal muscle co-contraction. As has been demonstrated through measurement of pressure of the intervertebral discs during different positions of the spine,[105] flexing the hips and the knees with the patient in a supine or a lateral position can decrease the intervertebral pressure (see Fig. 39–2). This position reduces the lumbar lordotic curve and opens the posterior intervertebral disc interspaces. A firm mattress with a soft

top-layer covering is required for any prolonged immobilization in bed.

The optimal duration of bed rest is uncertain, and for many patients without neuromotor deficits, 2 days of bed rest may suffice without any significant difference on clinical outcome.[36] Therefore, a period of bed rest for 2 to 3 days is helpful and does not result in excessive bone loss or debilitation. The duration of bed rest varies from a few days to 2 weeks before the acute symptoms subside. Prolonged bed rest is not recommended. In a reported study[81] of 34 adults who were hospitalized for low back pain and required therapeutic bed rest, the lumbar spine bone mineral content decreased about 0.9% per week, as assessed with dual photon absorptiometry.

Patients benefit from the application of a well-fitted spinal orthosis during the acute stage. Depending on the extent or severity of injury, the back support may consist of an elastic lumbosacral corset or a rigid support in the form of a brace or a plaster cast that is applied before the patient is allowed to start ambulatory activities. During recumbency the support is removed. The reduction of motion in the lumbar spine can be achieved only if the support is extended from the lower thoracic spine to the greater trochanteric areas.[10] This reduction of mobility in the involved area significantly decreases the pain and reduces the duration of bed rest required. Restriction of back motion results in weakness of the low back supportive muscles; therefore, prolonged use of a back support is discouraged. It should be discarded as soon as low back pain symptoms have subsided. Scientific studies of spinal orthoses and functional units of the spine have suggested that muscle atrophy, accelerated osteopenia, and osteoarthritic changes result from use of rigid orthoses.[51, 107, 112] These studies were based on long-term use of orthotics in patients with spinal cord injury who used body jackets or halopelvic fixation devices. Performing isometric strengthening exercises in conjunction with application of a back support reduces the effect of immobility on muscles. A progressive, nonstrenuous back strengthening exercise program should be started as soon as tolerated by the patient. This is initiated with isometric exercises and may be advanced to flexion or extension or combined exercise programs. By the end of 6 weeks, the effects of a muscle strengthening course should be evident.[100] When the patient is pain-free, normal daily activities may be gradually resumed. Recreational and athletic activities may have to be curtailed. If slight recurrence of low back pain or sciatica is noticed, the back support can be reapplied and periodic bed rest is ordered.

Treatment of acute back sprain (defined as soft tissue injury of an otherwise normal back) should permit the patient to return to normal activities within 2 to 4 weeks. Often, busy professional patients return to work in 1 to 2 weeks. Patients involved in occupations that require heavy manual labor are usually able to return to work by 6 weeks after injury and should be encouraged to do so. Mild symptoms may persist while the patient is applying physical therapy measures. Hyperextension exercises, such as the McKenzie program, have also been advocated[37] for the management of herniated disc and, in some cases, seem to be helpful. Although hyperextension exercises may be beneficial in some instances for treatment of low back pain, we have not had favorable results. The McKenzie exercises are *hyperextension* exercises, which should not be confused with the *spinal extension* exercises that are prescribed for osteoporotic back pain.

Repetition of acute episodes of back pain associated with progressive disc degeneration, localized instability, and degenerative arthritis may result in prolonged immobility. In selected cases, spinal manipulation can result in immediate relief of pain after the first treatment. In a randomized trial,[71] patients were selected for randomization after eligibility was established through inclusion criteria. One group received manipulation therapy and the other group received soft tissue massage. The outcome was not significantly different between the two groups, and both groups showed substantial improvement.

Chronic Low Back Pain Syndromes

Back pain that has been present for more than 6 months is chronic and usually is accompanied by changes in the patient's lifestyle and behavior. The longer the pain has been present, the more resistive it becomes to therapeutic intervention. Table 39–7 lists some common causes of chronic low back pain and their management. For patients who are unable to perform any back strengthening exercises because of chronic pain, transcutaneous electrical nerve stimulation (TENS) can be tried in an attempt to control the pain and enable the patient to proceed with exercises.

In a controlled trial[94] of the effect of low-frequency electrical stimulation of back extensor muscles, a significant improvement in the back strength was demonstrated. One study[101] has shown that, overall, patients with acute back pain who complained of pain over a wider area of the body were highly anxious, had a lower activity level, and had more tendency for chronic pain syndrome. After careful evaluation of the patient's physical status, assessment of the patient's environment, work incentive and disability status, and financial loss or gain is mandatory. The multidisciplinary evaluation and approach is very helpful.

PREVENTIVE MEASURES AND BACK SCHOOLS

Episodes of acute low back pain usually subside within a few days to 3 months.[25] Low back pain becomes problematic in many patients in whom it is recurrent. Prevention of recurrence is of major importance in the management of low back pain syndromes.

During the acute phase, the patient should be instructed in proper positioning techniques to decrease low back pain during dynamic or static posturing and to avoid reinjury. At this stage, pain is managed with the use of sedative physical therapeutic measures and analgesics. Meanwhile, the patient should be introduced to progressive isometric exercise programs to improve muscular support of the spine. Provision of a back education program (back school) very early in the patient's treatment program is helpful. Back school programs may vary from small classes (six to eight patients) with a physical therapist instructor to one-on-one instruction with either a physician or physical thera-

TABLE 39–7   Some Causes of Chronic Low Back Pain and Treatment

Cause	Treatment
Osteoarthritis; degenerative joint disease (DJD)	Improve muscular back support
Lumbar spondylosis	Corset
Diffuse idiopathic skeletal hyperostosis, Forestier's disease	Weight loss Improve posture
Facet pain syndrome	Avoid lumbar hyperextension
Facet DJD	Improve muscular support
	Consider injection
	Dynamic, static posture principles
Spondylolisthesis	
Stable	Flexion exercise program
	Spinal orthosis
	Activity precautions
Progressive neurological deficit	Decompression and fusion
Spinal stenosis	Spinal flexion exercises
Pseudoclaudication	Weight reduction
Lateral recess syndrome	Correction of posture
	Decompression
Metabolic bone disease	Isometric back extension program
Osteopenia	Treat underlying disease
Osteoporosis	Avoid heavy lifting (5 to 10 lb)
Paget's disease	Weightbearing exercise program
Malignancy (multiple myeloma, metastatic)	
Stable spine	Conservative treatment
	Orthosis
	Gait-assistive devices
	Wheelchair
	Avoid strenuous activities
	Radiation therapy with or without steroids
Unstable spine	Surgical stabilization and orthotics
Chronic inflammatory disease (ankylosing spondylitis, chronic spondyloarthropathies)	Conservative treatment
	Nonsteroidal agents
	Back extension and stretching exercises
	Deep breathing exercises
Fibromyalgia	Conservative treatment
	Biofeedback
	Relaxation
	Correction of posture
Chronic pain syndrome	Multidisciplinary behavioral approach
	Psychological testing (MMPI*)
	Stretching
	Stress management to consider antidepressants
	Electromyographic biofeedback

*Minnesota Multiphasic Personality Inventory.

pist. Back schools are often supported by companies who provide back education programs for their employees. Typically, employees' performances are videotaped before participation in the back school. A back program, including audiovisual presentation, is then set up to meet the specific needs of the employees' jobs. The objective of any preventive or therapeutic rehabilitation program is to teach patients how to help themselves. They are taught how to be "kind to one's back." Figure 39-9 demonstrates correct and incorrect postures that should be provided as preliminary training for an individual.

Patients with low back pain should be instructed in basic body mechanics and the following measures:

1. If prolonged sitting is required for an occupation, one should get up every 20 minutes. In addition, to decrease strain on the low back during sitting, the patient can be instructed to perform pelvic tilt exercises, to sit with knees bent and one or both feet slightly elevated on a footrest, and to support the low back with a small cushion (see Fig. 39–9B and I).

2. For driving a car, the seat should be brought close to the steering wheel so that the knees are slightly higher than the hips (see Fig. 39–9G). In the presence of lumbar degenerative disc disease, getting out of the car frequently (every 20 to 30 mintues) to stretch is helpful.

3. Before coughing or sneezing, the stomach muscles should be tightened.

4. Begin a progressive low back isometric strengthening exercise program and perform stretching exercises to increase flexibility for performing daily activities.

5. Forward bending increases intradiscal pressure.[103] Therefore, certain precautions such as kneeling when trying to pick an object up from the floor (see Fig. 39–9D) or when making a bed are advisable to decrease intradiscal pressure.

6. To decrease low back strain when getting into bed, one should sit on the edge of the bed, turn and roll slightly to one hip, bring the knees up with the feet hanging over the edge of the bed, and slowly recline, pushing up with the arms on the bed to support the body during this procedure. For getting out of bed, one needs to reverse this sequence.

In more advanced programs, the patient's physical status is evaluated, including range of motion of the spine and measurement of body weight and back and upper and lower extremity strengths. For postmenopausal women who are involved in heavy physical labor, it is wise to keep in mind the biomechanical competence of the spine to avoid spinal compression fractures due to involutional osteopenia or osteoporosis. When avoidance of heavy lifting is not possible, provision of a rigid dorsolumbar support is recommended.

In summary, every effort should be made to prevent low back pain or to avoid its recurrence through education and instruction in proper body mechanics.

Acknowledgment

Supported in part by a research grant from the Donaldson Trust. The authors would like to thank LeAnn Stee and the Section of Publications for service, John Hagen for the illustrations, and Sandy Fitzgerald for secretarial assistance.

References

1. Addison R, Schultz A: Trunk strengths in patients seeking hospitalization for chronic low-back disorders. Spine 1980; 5:539.
2. Alston W, Carlson KE, Feldman DJ, et al: A quantitative study of muscle factors in the chronic low back syndrome. J Am Geriatr Soc 1966; 14:1041.
3. American College of Obstetricians and Gynecologists: Pregnancy and the postnatal period. In ACOG Home Exercise Program. Chicago, ACOG, 1985, pp 1–5.
4. Amundson G, Edwards CC, Garfin SR: Spondylolisthesis. In Rothman RH, Simeone FA (eds): The Spine, ed 3, vol. 1. Philadelphia, WB Saunders, 1992, pp 913–969.
5. Andersson GBJ, Svensson H-O, Odén A: The intensity of work recovery in low back pain. Spine 1983; 8:880.
6. Arnett FC: Seronegative spondyloarthropathies. Bull Rheum Dis 1987; 37(1):1.
7. Asmussen E, Heebøll-Nielsen K: Posture, mobility and strength of the back in boys 7 to 16 years old. Acta Orthop Scand 1959; 28:174.
8. Baker AS, Ojemann RG, Swartz MN, et al: Spinal epidural abscess. N Engl J Med 1975; 293:463.
9. Barron WM: Medical evaluation of the pregnant patient requiring nonobstetric surgery. Clin Perinatol 1985; 12:481.
10. Bartelink DL: The role of abdominal pressure in relieving the pressure on the lumbar intervertebral discs. J Bone Joint Surg Br 1957; 39:718.
11. Bartleson JD, Cohen MD, Harrington TM, et al: Cauda equina syndrome secondary to long-standing ankylosing spondylitis. Ann Neurol 1983; 14:662.
12. Battie MC, Bigos SJ, Fisher LD, et al: Anthropometric and clinical measures as predictors of back pain complaints in industry: A prospective study. J Spinal Disord 1990; 3:195.
13. Beimborn DS, Morrissey MC: A review of the literature related to trunk muscle performance. Spine 1988; 13:655.
14. Bell GR: Spondylolisthesis. In Hardy RW (ed): Lumbar Disc Disease, ed 2. New York, Raven Press, 1993, pp 209–223.
15. Berg G, Hammar M, Möller-Nielson J, et al: Low back pain during pregnancy. Obstet Gynecol 1988; 71:71.
16. Bergquist-Ullman M, Larsson U: Acute low back pain in industry: A controlled prospective study with special reference to therapy and confounding factors. Acta Orthop Scand Suppl 1977; 170:1.
17. Berkson M, Schultz A, Nachemson A, et al: Voluntary strengths of male adults with acute low back syndromes. Clin Orthop 1977; 129:84.
18. Biering-Sørensen F: Low back trouble in a general population of 30-, 40-, 50-, and 60-year old men and women: Study design, representativeness and basic results. Dan Med Bull 1982; 29:289.
19. Biering-Sørensen F: A prospective study of low back pain in a general population: I. Occurrence, recurrence and aetiology. Scand J Rehabil Med 1983; 15:71.
20. Biering-Sørensen F: Physical measurements as risk indicators for low back trouble over a 1-year period. Spine 1984; 9:106.
21. Boden SD, Davis DO, Dina TS, et al: Abnormal magnetic-resonance scans of the lumbar spine in asymptomatic subjects. J Bone Joint Surg Am 1990; 72:403.
22. Børgesen SE, Vang PS: Herniation of the lumbar intervertebral disk in children and adolescents. Acta Orthop Scand 1974; 45:540.
23. Boxall D, Bradford DS, Winter RB, et al: Management of severe spondylolisthesis in children and adolescents. J Bone Joint Surg Am 1979; 61:479.
24. Briggs GG, Freeman RK, Yaffe SJ: Drugs in Pregnancy and Lactation: A Reference Guide to Fetal and Neonatal Risk. Baltimore, Williams & Wilkins, 1990.
25. Cailliet R: Low Back Pain Syndrome, ed 4. Philadelphia, FA Davis, 1988.
26. Carrera GF, Haughton VM, Syvertsen A, et al: Computed tomography of the lumbar facet joints. Radiology 1980; 134:145.
27. Carrera GF, Williams AL, Haughton VM: Computed tomography in sciatica. Radiology 1980; 137:433.
28. Ciric I, Mikhael MA, Tarkington JA, et al: The lateral recess syndrome: A variant of spinal stenosis. J Neurosurg 1980; 53:433.
29. Collert S: Osteomyelitis of the spine. Acta Orthop Scand 1977; 48:283.
30. Daly JM, Frame PS, Rapoza PA: Sacroiliac subluxation: A common, treatable cause of low-back pain in pregnancy. Fam Pract Res J 1991; 11:149.
31. Dandy DJ, Shannon MJ: Lumbo-sacral subluxation (group I spondylolisthesis). J Bone Joint Surg Br 1971; 53:578.
32. Danner RL, Hartman BJ: Update of spinal epidural abscess: Thirty-five cases and review of the literature. Rev Infect Dis 1987; 9:265.
33. DeOrio JK, Bianco AJ Jr: Lumbar disc excision in children and adolescents. J Bone Joint Surg Am 1982; 64:991.
34. Department of Neurology, Mayo Clinic and Mayo Foundation: Clinical Examinations in Neurology, ed 6. St Louis, Mosby–Year Book, 1991.

35. Deyo RA, Bass JE: Lifestyle and low-back pain: The influence of smoking and obesity. Spine 1989; 14:501.

36. Deyo RA, Diehl AK, Rosenthal M: How many days of bed rest for acute low back pain? A randomized clinical trial. N Engl J Med 1986; 315:1064.

37. Dimaggio A, Mooney V: The McKenzie program: Exercise effective against back pain. J Musculoskeletal Med 1987; 4:63.

38. Duvoisin RC, Yahr MD: Compressive spinal cord and root syndromes in achondroplastic dwarfs. Neurology 1962; 12:202.

39. Ellenberg MR, Ross ML, Honet JC, et al: Prospective evaluation of the course of disc herniations in patients with proven radiculopathy. Arch Phys Med Rehabil 1993; 74:3.

40. Epstein JA (moderator): Treatment of low back pain and sciatic syndromes during pregnancy. NY State J Med 1959; 59:1757.

41. Epstein JA, Epstein NE: Lumbar spondylosis and spinal stenosis. In Wilkins RH, Rengachary SS (eds): Neurosurgery, vol 3. New York, McGraw-Hill, 1985, pp 2272–2278.

42. Fahrni WH: Conservative treatment of lumbar disc degeneration: Our primary responsibility. Orthop Clin North Am 1975; 6:93.

43. Falconer MA, McGeorge M, Begg AC: Observations on cause and mechanism of symptom-production in sciatica and low-back pain. J Neurol Neurosurg Psychiatry 1948; 11:13.

44. Fast A: Low back disorders: Conservative management. Arch Phys Med Rehabil 1988; 69:880.

45. Fast A, Shapiro D, Ducommun EJ, et al: Low-back pain in pregnancy. Spine 1987; 12:368.

46. Fast A, Weiss L, Ducommun EJ, et al: Low-back pain in pregnancy: Abdominal muscles, sit-up performance, and back pain. Spine 1990; 15:28.

47. Fast A, Weiss L, Parikh S, et al: Night backache in pregnancy: Hypothetical pathophysiological mechanisms. Am J Phys Med Rehabil 1989; 68:227.

48. Feller BA: Prevalence of Selected Impairment, United States, 1977, Hyattsville, Md, DHHS publication (PHS) 81-1562. US Department of Health and Human Services, Public Health Service, Office of Health Research and Technology, National Center for Health Statistics, Washington DC, 1981.

49. Fischer DK, Simpson RK Jr, Baskin DS: Spinal spondylosis and disc disease. In Evans RW, Baskin DS, Yatsu FM (eds): Prognosis of Neurological Disorders. New York, Oxford University Press, 1992, pp 335–351.

50. Forestier J, Rotes-Querol J: Senile ankylosing hyperostosis of the spine. Ann Rheum Dis 1950; 9:321.

51. Freehafer AA: Orthotics in spinal cord injuries. In Bunch W (ed): Atlas of Orthotics: Biomechanical Principles and Application, ed 2. St. Louis, Mosby–Year Book, 1985, pp 287–296.

52. Frymoyer JW: Back pain and sciatica. N Engl J Med 1988; 318:291.

53. Frymoyer JW, Pope MH, Clements JH, et al: Risk factors in low-back pain: An epidemiological survey. J Bone Joint Surg Am 1983; 65:213.

54. Frymoyer JW, Rosen JC, Clements J, et al: Psychologic factors in low-back-pain disability. Clin Orthop 1985; 195:178.

55. Garrido E: Lumbar disc herniation in the pediatric patient. Neurosurg Clin North Am 1993; 4:149.

56. Gellin BG, Weingarten K, Gamache FW Jr, et al: Epidural abscess. In Scheld WM, Whitley RJ, Durack DT (eds): Infections of the Central Nervous System. New York, Raven Press, 1991, pp 499–514.

57. Gilmour WN: Acute haematogenous osteomyelitis. J Bone Joint Surg Br 1962; 44:841.

58. Gramse RR, Sinaki M, Ilstrup DM: Lumbar spondylolisthesis: A rational approach to conservative treatment. Mayo Clin Proc 1980; 55:681.

59. Grazier KL, Holbrook TL, Kelsey JL, et al (eds): The Frequency of Occurrence, Impact and Cost of Selected Musculoskeletal Conditions in the United States. Chicago, American Academy of Orthopaedic Surgeons, 1984.

60. Griffiths HED, Jones DM: Pyogenic infection of the spine: A review of 28 cases. J Bone Joint Surg Br 1971; 53:383.

61. Grobler LJ, Simmons EH, Barrington TW: Intervertebral disc herniation in the adolescent. Spine 1979; 4:267.

62. Hakin RN, Burt AA, Cook JB: Acute spinal epidural abscess. Paraplegia 1979; 17:330.

63. Hall S, Bartleson JD, Onofrio BM, et al: Lumbar spinal stenosis: Clinical features, diagnostic procedures, and results of surgical treatment in 68 patients. Ann Intern Med 1985; 103:271.

64. Hasue M, Fujiwara M, Kikuchi S: A new method of quantitative measurement of abdominal and back muscle strength. Spine 1980; 5:143.

65. Heliövaara M: Risk factors for low back pain and sciatica. Ann Med 1989; 21:257.

66. Heliövaara M, Sievers K, Maatela J, et al: Descriptive epidemiology and public health aspects of low back pain. Ann Med 1989; 21:327.

67. Helliwell P, Moll J, Wright V: Measurement of spinal movement and function. In Jayson MIV (ed): The Lumbar Spine and Back Pain, ed 4. New York, Churchill Livingstone, 1992, pp 173–205.

68. Hendry NGC: The hydration of the nucleus pulposus and its relation to intervertebral disc derangement. J Bone Joint Surg Br 1958; 40:132.

69. Hensinger RN: Spondylolisis and spondylolisthesis in children. Instr Course Lect 1983; 32:132.

70. Heusner AP: Nontuberculous spinal epidural infections. N Engl J Med 1948; 239:845.

71. Hoehler FK, Tobis JS, Buerger AA: Spinal manipulation for low back pain. JAMA 1981; 245:1835.

72. Holt EP Jr: The question of lumbar discography. J Bone Joint Surg Am 1968; 50:720.

73. Horal J: The clinical appearance of low back disorders in the city of Gothenberg, Sweden: Comparisons of incapacitated probands with matched controls. Acta Orthop Scand Suppl 1969; 118:1.

74. Hudgins WR: Microdiscectomy. In Hardy RW Jr (ed): Lumbar Disc Disease, ed 2. New York, Raven Press, 1993, pp 139–145.

75. Hulme A, Dott NM: Spinal epidural abscess. Br Med J 1954; 1:64.

76. Ikata T: Statistical and dynamic studies of lesions due to overloading on the spine. Shikoku Acta Med 1965; 40:262.

77. Jenkins DB: Hollinshead's Functional Anatomy of the Limbs and Back, ed 6. Philadelphia, WB Saunders, 1991.

78. Kellgren JH, Lawrence JS: Osteo-arthrosis and disk degeneration in an urban population. Ann Rheum Dis 1958; 17:388.

79. Kelsey JL: An epidemiological study of the relationship between occupations and acute herniated lumbar intervertebral discs. Int J Epidemiol 1975; 4:197.

80. Khan MA: An overview of clinical spectrum and heterogeneity of spondyloarthropathies. Rheum Dis Clin North Am 1992; 18:1.

81. Krølner B, Toft B: Vertebral bone loss: An unheeded side effect of therapeutic bed rest. Clin Sci 1983; 64:537.

82. Lawrence JS, Molyneux MK, Dingwall-Fordyce I: Rheumatism in foundary workers. Br J Indust Med 1966; 23:42.

83. Lehmann JF, De Lateur BJ: Diathermy and superficial heat, laser, and cold therapy. In Kottke FJ, Lehmann JF: Krusen's Handbook of Physical Medicine and Rehabilitation, ed 4. Philadelphia, WB Saunders, 1990, pp 283–367.

84. Loebl WY: Measurement of spinal posture and range of spinal movement. Ann Phys Med 1967; 9:103.

85. Loeser JD, Volinn E: Epidemiology of low back pain. Neurosurg Clin North Am 1991; 2:713.

86. Love JG, Walsh MN: Protruded intervertebral disks: Report of 100 cases in which operation was performed. JAMA 1938; 111:396.

87. Lowe J, Schachner E, Hirschberg E, et al: Significance of bone scintigraphy in symptomatic spondylolysis. Spine 1984; 9:653.

88. Macnab I, McCulloch J: Backache, ed 2. Baltimore, Williams & Wilkins, 1990, p 120.

89. Mapstone TB: Back pain in children. In Hardy RW Jr (ed): Lumbar Disc Disease, ed 2. New York, Raven Press, 1993, pp 255–259.

90. Maroon JC, Onik G, Quigley M, et al: Automated percutaneous lumbar discectomy: Indications, technique, and results. In Hardy RW Jr (ed): Lumbar Disc Disease, ed 2. New York, Raven Press, 1993, pp 147–153.

91. Masaryk TJ, Ross JS, Modic MT, et al: High-resolution MR imaging of sequestered lumbar intervertebral disks. Am J Roentgenol 1988; 150:1155.

92. Mayer TG, Tencer AF, Kristoferson S, et al: Use of noninvasive techniques for quantification of spinal range-of-motion in normal subjects and chronic low-back dysfunction patients. Spine 1984; 9:588.

93. McNeill T, Warwick D, Andersson G, et al: Trunk strengths in attempted flexion, extension, and lateral bending in healthy subjects and patients with low-back disorders. Spine 1980; 5:529.

94. McQuain MT, Sinaki M, Shibley LD, et al: Effect of electrical stimulation on lumbar paraspinal muscles. Spine 1993; 18:1787.

95. Menelaus MG: Discitis: An inflammation affecting the intervertebral discs in children. J Bone Joint Surg Br 1964; 46:16.

96. Meyerding HW: Spondylolisthesis. Proc Staff Meet Mayo Clin 1934; 9:666.

97. Mokri B, Sinaki M: Painful disorders of the spine and back pain syndromes. *In* Sinaki M (ed): Basic Clinical Rehabilitation Medicine, ed 2. St Louis, Mosby–Year Book, 1993, pp 489–502.

98. Mokri B, Sinaki M: Lumbar disk syndromes, lumbosacral radiculopathies, lumbar spondylosis and stenosis, spondylolisthesis. *In* Sinaki M (ed): Basic Clinical Rehabilitation Medicine, ed 2. St Louis, Mosby–Year Book, 1993, pp 503–513.

99. Mooney RP, Hockberger RS: Spinal epidural abscess: A rapidly progressive disease. Ann Emerg Med 1987; 16:1168.

100. Müller EA: Influence of training and of inactivity on muscle strength. Arch Phys Med Rehabil 1970; 51:449.

101. Murphy KA, Cornish RD: Prediction of chronicity in acute low back pain. Arch Phys Med Rehabil 1984; 65:334.

102. Nachemson A: Lumbar intradiscal pressure: Experimental studies on post-mortem material. Acta Orthop Scand Suppl 1960; 43:1.

103. Nachemson A, Elfström G: Intravital dynamic pressure measurements in lumbar discs: A study of common movements, maneuvers and exercises. Scand J Rehabil Med Suppl 1970; 1:1.

104. Nachemson A, Lindh M: Measurement of abdominal and back muscle strength with and without low back pain. Scand J Rehabil Med 1969; 1:60.

105. Nachemson AL: The lumbar spine: An orthopaedic challenge. Spine 1976; 1:59.

106. Nachemson AL: Disc pressure measurements. Spine 1981; 6:93.

107. Nachemson AL: Orthotic treatment for injuries and diseases of the spinal column. Phys Med Rehabil 1987; 1:11.

108. Neugebauer FL: A new contribution to the history and etiology of spondylolisthesis. Select Monogr, 8°, Lond, 1888, pp 1–64.

109. Newman PH: The etiology of spondylolisthesis. J Bone Joint Surg Br 1963; 45:39.

110. Nordgren B, Schéle R, Linroth K: Evaluation and prediction of back pain during military field service. Scand J Rehabil Med 1980; 12:1.

111. Nummi J, Järvinen T, Stambej U, et al: Diminished dynamic performance capacity of back and abdominal muscles in concrete reinforcement workers. Scand J Work Environ Health 1978; 4 Suppl 1:39.

112. O'Brien JP: The halo-pelvic apparatus: A clinical, bio engineering and anatomical study. Acta Orthop Scand Suppl 1975; 163:1.

113. Onofrio BM: Spine and intraspinal infections. *In* Horwitz NH, Rizzoli HV (eds): Postoperative Complications of Extracranial Neurological Surgery. Baltimore, Williams & Wilkins, 1987, pp 169–206.

114. Ostgaard HC, Andersson GBJ: Previous back pain and risk of developing back pain in a future pregnancy. Spine 1991; 16:432.

115. Ostgaard HC, Andersson GBJ, Karlsson K: Prevalence of back pain in pregnancy. Spine 1991; 16:549.

116. Panjabi MM, Hult JE, Crisco JJ III, et al: Biomechanical studies in cadaveric spines. *In* Jayson MIV (ed): The Lumbar Spine and Back Pain, ed 4. New York, Churchill Livingstone, 1992, pp 133–155.

117. Pedersen OF, Petersen R, Staffeldt ES: Back pain and isometric back muscle strength of workers in a Danish factory. Scand J Rehabil Med 1975; 7:125.

118. Petrie RS, Sinaki M, Squires RW, et al: Physical activity, but not aerobic capacity, correlates with back strength in healthy premenopausal women from 29 to 40 years of age. Mayo Clin Proc 1993; 68:738.

119. Plucinski T, Sinaki M, Currier B, et al: Sports and spondylolisthesis in children. *In* Proceedings of Advances in Idiopathic Low Back Pain Congress, Nov 27–28, 1992. Vienna, Blackwell Scientific Publications, June 1993.

120. Plucinski T, Sinaki M, Rizzo T, et al: Spondylolisthesis in children: Surgery, symptoms and physical findings. *In* Official Program of the Spring Meeting of the Association of Academic Physiatrists, Naples, Fla, January 1994.

121. Pope MH: Risk indicators in low back pain. Ann Med 1989; 21:387.

122. Pope MH, Wilder DG, Stokes IAF, et al: Biomechanical testing as an aid to decision making in low-back pain patients. Spine 1979; 4:135.

123. Postacchini F: Lumbar Spinal Stenosis. New York, Springer-Verlag, 1989.

124. Riihimäki H, Tola S, Videman T, et al: Low-back pain and occupation: A cross-sectional questionnaire study of men in machine operating, dynamic physical work, and sedentary work. Spine 1989; 14:204.

125. Rowe ML: Preliminary statistical study of low back pain. J Occup Med 1963; 5:336.

126. Rudins A, Sinaki M, Miller JL, et al: Significance of back extensors versus back flexors in trunkal support (abstract). Arch Phys Med Rehabil 1991; 72:824.

127. Rumgee JL: Low back pain during pregnancy. Orthopedics 1993; 16:1339.

128. Saal JA, Saal JS: Nonoperative treatment of herniated lumbar intervertebral disc with radiculopathy: An outcome study. Spine 1989; 14:431.

129. Sands RX: Backache of pregnancy: A method of treatment. Obstet Gynecol 1958; 12:670.

130. Schober P: Ledenwirbelsäule and Kreuzschmerzen. Munchen Med Wchnschr 1937; 84:336.

131. Schultz A, Andersson G, Örtengren R, et al: Loads on the lumbar spine: Validation of a biomechanical analysis by measurements of intradiscal pressures and myoelectric signals. J Bone Joint Surg Am 1982; 64:713.

132. Simeone FA: Lumbar disk disease. *In* Wilkins RH, Rengachary SS (eds): Neurosurgery, vol 3. New York, McGraw-Hill, 1985, pp 2250–2259.

133. Sinaki M: Exercise and physical therapy. *In* Riggs BL, Melton LJ III (eds): Osteoporosis: Etiology, Diagnosis, and Management. New York, Raven Press, 1988, pp 457–479.

134. Sinaki M (ed): Basic Clinical Rehabilitation Medicine, ed 2. St Louis, Mosby–Year Book, 1993, pp 209–236.

135. Sinaki M, Chan C, Plucinski T, et al: Spondylolisthesis of the osteoporotic spine. *In* Proceedings of the Fourth International Symposium on Osteoporosis and Consensus Development Conference. Hong Kong, March 27–April 2, 1993, p 106.

136. Sinaki M, Grubbs NC: Back strengthening exercises: Quantitative evaluation of their efficacy for women aged 40 to 65 years. Arch Phys Med Rehabil 1989; 70:16.

137. Sinaki M, Lutness MP, Ilstrup DM, et al: Lumbar spondylolisthesis: Retrospective comparison and 3-year follow-up of two conservative treatment programs. Arch Phys Med Rehabil 1989; 70:584.

138. Sinaki M, Mikkelsen BA: Postmenopausal spinal osteoporosis: Flexion versus extension exercises. Arch Phys Med Rehabil 1984; 65:593.

139. Sinaki M, Nicholas JJ: Metabolic bone diseases and aging. *In* Felsenthal G, Garrison SJ, Steinberg FU (eds): Rehabilitation of the Aging and Elderly Patient. Philadelphia, Williams & Wilkins, 1994, pp 107–122.

140. Snook SH: Low back pain in industry. *In* White AA III, Gordon SL (eds): American Academy of Orthopedic Surgeons: Symposium on Idiopathic Low Back Pain. St Louis, Mosby–Year Book, 1982, pp 23–38.

141. Spangfort EV: The lumbar disc herniation: A computer-aided analysis of 2,504 operations. Acta Orthop Scand Suppl 1972; 142:1.

142. Steindler A: Kinesiology of the Human Body Under Normal and Pathological Conditions. Springfield, Ill, Charles C Thomas, 1965.

143. Stern WE, Balch RE: Surgical aspects of nonspecific inflammatory and suppurative disease of the vertebral column. Am J Surg 1966; 112:314.

144. Stone DB, Bonfiglio M: Pyogenic vertebral osteomyelitis: A diagnostic pitfall for the internist. Arch Intern Med 1963; 112:491.

145. Svensson H-O, Andersson GBJ: Low-back pain in 40- to 47-year-old men: Work history and work environment factors. Spine 1983; 8:272.

146. Svensson H-O, Andersson GBJ, Hagstad A, et al: The relationship of low-back pain to pregnancy and gynecologic factors. Spine 1990; 15:371.

147. Tauber J: An unorthodox look at backaches. J Occup Med 1970; 12:128.

148. Taylor H, Curran NM: The Nuprin Pain Report. New York, Louis Harris & Associates, 1985.

149. Turner PG, Green JH, Galasko CSB: Back pain in childhood. Spine 1989; 14:812.

150. Utsinger PD, Resnick D, Shapiro R: Diffuse skeletal abnormalities in Forestier disease. Arch Intern Med 1976; 136:763.

151. Vällfors B: Acute, subacute and chronic low back pain: Clinical symptoms, absenteeism and working environment. Scand J Rehabil Med Suppl 1985; 11:1.

152. Van Alphen HAM, Braakman R, Bezemer PD, et al: Chemonucleolysis versus discectomy: A randomized multicenter trial. J Neurosurg 1989; 70:869.

153. Vanderburgh DF, Kelly WM: Radiographic assessment of discogenic disease of the spine. Neurosurg Clin North Am 1993; 4:13.

154. Wagner DK, Varkey B, Sheth NK, et al: Epidural abscess, vertebral destruction, and paraplegia caused by extending infection from an aspergilloma. Am J Med 1985; 78:518.

155. Waldvogel FA, Medoff G, Swartz MN: Osteomyelitis: A review of clinical features, therapeutic considerations and unusual aspects. N Engl J Med 1970; 282:316.

156. Weinstein PR: Anatomy of the lumbar spine. *In* Hardy RW Jr (ed): Lumbar Disk Disease, ed 2. New York, Raven Press, 1993, pp 5–11.

157. Weir MR, Smith DS: Stress reaction of the pars interarticularis leading to spondylolysis: A cause of adolescent low back pain. J Adolesc Health Care 1989; 10:573.

158. Weisman MH: Spondyloarthropathies. *In* Stein JH (ed): Internal Medicine, ed 4. St Louis, Mosby–Year Book, 1994, pp 2454–2462.

159. Whelan MA, Naidich DP, Post JD, et al: Computed tomography of spinal tuberculosis. J Comput Assist Tomogr 1983; 7:25.

160. Wilbourn AJ: The value and limitations of electromyographic examination in the diagnosis of lumbosacral radiculopathy. *In* Hardy RW Jr (ed). Lumbar Disc Disease. New York, Raven Press, 1982, pp 65–109.

161. Wiltse LL: Common problems of the lumbar spine: Spondylolisthesis and its treatment. J Continuing Educ Orthop 1979; 7:13.

162. Wiltse LL, Newman PH, Macnab I: Classification of spondylolysis and spondylolisthesis. Clin Orthop 1976; 117:23.

163. Witt I, Vestergaard A, Rosenklint A: A comparative analysis of x-ray findings of the lumbar spine in patients with and without lumbar pain. Spine 1984; 9:298.

164. Yong-Hing K, Kirkaldy-Willis WH: The pathophysiology of degenerative disease of the lumbar spine. Orthop Clin North Am 1983; 14:491.

165. Zamani M, MacEwen GD: Herniation of the lumbar disc in children and adolescents. J Pediatr Orthop 1982; 2:528.

Osteoporosis: Its Prevention and Treatment

VELIMIR MATKOVIC, M.D., Ph.D.,
SAM C. COLACHIS III, M.D., AND
JASMINKA Z. ILICH, Ph.D., R.D.

With increases in life expectancy and in the number of elderly people, bone loss and fractures are becoming more common in the United States and throughout the world. The problems associated with bone loss and aging are not only medical; there are also social, cultural, and economic ramifications that affect the life of a community or a nation. By the middle of the next century, there will be up to 100 million people over the age of 55 years in the United States. As a consequence, an epidemic of bone fractures among the elderly should be expected. In many countries, even now most of the orthopedic beds are occupied by hip fracture patients, and total expenses for the community are enormous. Whereas osteoporosis is the major underlying cause of fractures of the long bones, neuromuscular instability in elderly people is an important contributor to the fall that usually produces the fracture. In this context, the benefit of exercise and maintenance of physical fitness would not only contribute to the prevention of bone loss but also improve protective responses in muscle strength over the entire body, thereby leading to a reduction in the incidence of fractures. Based on this, specialists in physical medicine and rehabilitation should be more and more involved in the prevention program for, and chronic care of, the osteoporotic population.

DEFINITION

Osteoporosis is a bone disease characterized by a reduction of bone tissue relative to the volume of anatomical bone which increases susceptibility to fracture. Current understanding of osteoporosis indicates that the disease is present when bone mass lies more than 2 SD below the mean of young adults of the same sex. All women and men become osteoporotic if they live long enough. Whether a bone breaks depends on the relationship between the sever-

ity of the trauma and the strength of the bone; what osteoporosis does is increase the fracture risk, not cause the fracture.[93] Fracture risk rises as bone density falls. The chemical composition of osteoporotic bone is considered to be normal. The skeleton is composed of a mineral component, calcium hydroxyapatite (60%), and organic material, mainly collagen (40%). In osteoporosis, the bone is of normal size but contains less bone tissue without change in the ratio of mineral component to organic material (Fig. 40–1). In osteomalacia, for example, the amount of bone can be normal or even increased, but it has reduced mineral content. In some patients, osteoporosis and osteomalacia coexist, and in those cases, the ash content of bone and the amount of bone tissue per unit volume are reduced.

CLASSIFICATION

Osteoporosis can be classified according to localization in the skeleton and according to etiology. Localized osteoporosis affects part of the skeleton; generalized osteoporosis affects, to a greater or lesser extent, different parts of the whole skeleton. Both types of osteoporosis can further be classified into primary and secondary osteoporosis (Table 40–1). The causative agent in primary osteoporosis usually is not fully known; in secondary osteoporosis the predisposing factor, either local or systemic, is always present. Finally, generalized osteoporosis can further be classified according to the age of onset of clinical signs: juvenile or idiopathic and involutional osteoporosis. Juvenile osteoporosis affects children and adolescents of both sexes; idiopathic osteoporosis affects premenopausal women and middle-aged men. Involutional osteoporosis, which is discussed in this chapter, is by far the most common form of osteoporosis and includes postmenopausal women (i.e., type I) and aging-associated osteoporosis (i.e.,

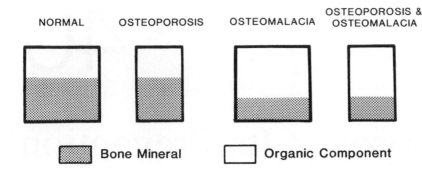

FIGURE 40–1 Diagrammatic representation of normal, osteoporotic, and osteomalacic bone.

type II), previously termed *senile osteoporosis.* Type I osteoporosis affects postmenopausal women between the ages of 50 and 65 years, and type II osteoporosis affects people over the age of 70 years.[114]

EPIDEMIOLOGY

Primary involutional osteoporosis is the most common form of osteoporosis. It begins in middle life and becomes increasingly more common with advancing age. We now recognize the three main sites of fracture associated with bone loss: spine, wrist, and hip. The epidemiology of spinal osteoporosis is difficult, because vertebral fractures can occur without symptoms, but about 8% of women will have a spinal fracture by 80 years of age. A vertebral fracture may involve a partial vertebral deformity (e.g., partial loss of height of the anterior edge or middle section of the vertebral body), or complete collapse of the vertebral body. In the United States approximately half a million cases of vertebral fractures occur each year in patients with spinal osteoporosis. The majority of patients with compression fracture syndrome are postmenopausal women, aged 50 to 70 years, and as such these fractures are associated with type I osteoporosis.[22]

The incidence of wrist fractures starts to rise immediately after menopause with a cumulative prevalence of about 15% by the age of 80. The incidence of wrist fracture is about 172,000 cases each year. Wrist fractures are the result of moderate trauma and occur during rapid postmenopausal bone loss and are associated with type I osteoporosis. These fractures are very uncommon among men (Fig. 40–2); the female-to-male ratio is 5:1. Only about 18% of forearm fractures result in hospitalization, and most patients require no rehabilitation services. These fractures are rarely fatal and cause much less disability than do the other two osteoporotic syndromes.[77]

Hip fractures tend to occur later in life with a cumulative prevalence of about 6% by the age of 80 (Fig. 40–3). There is 20 to 25 years' delay in time between the peak incidence of wrist fractures and hip fractures (Fig. 40–4). Hip fractures are twice as common in women as in men, but the female/male ratio is not as high as for wrist and vertebral compression fractures (Fig. 40–5). The majority of patients with hip fractures sustain the fractures after moderate trauma, and those patients also tend to have less cortical bone. Approximately 200,000 hip fracture cases occur every year in the United States. Adult white women who live to age 80 have a 15% lifetime risk of suffering a hip fracture. In contrast, a white male who has a 75-year life expectancy has only a 5% lifetime risk of hip fracture. An 80-year-old woman typically has an average of 9 years of remaining life expectancy, and still has about a 50% chance of suffering a hip fracture before she dies. Hip fractures are associated not only with high morbidity but also with high mortality. About 12% to 30% of patients with hip fractures die within 1 year after the accident. In the majority of cases, death occurs within the first 3 months after the trauma. Advanced age, presence of chronic illness, and disability are responsible for this. Hip fractures are associated with type II or senile osteoporosis. They are more common among whites and Asians than blacks. The reason for this could be the difference in the peak bone mass level among these groups, as well as the level of physical activity in the population.[22, 77]

The majority of patients with hip fractures are referred from nursing homes. The presence of vitamin D deficiency and secondary hyperparathyroidism could be a contributing factor to the rising incidence of these fractures among elderly people.[17, 77] Recent studies fail to show consistent differences in bone mass, measured at a number of skeletal sites, in patients with hip fractures compared with controls. The most likely explanation is that as bone mass declines, the risk of fractures increases. Another hypothesis is that the primary cause of hip fractures in the elderly is impaired balance, resulting in falls, rather than reduced bone mass. A normal neuromuscular response that protects the skeleton against trauma and subsequent fractures is possibly abnormal in those patients. Based on this, public health measures should be directed not only at prevention of bone loss but also at the prevention of falls. A third explanation could

TABLE 40–1 Classification of Osteoporosis

Generalized osteoporosis	Primary	Juvenile
		Idiopathic (type I and type II)
		Involutional
	Secondary	Metabolic
		Connective tissue disease
		Bone marrow disease
		Immobilization
		Drugs
Localized osteoporosis	Primary	Transient regional
		Reflex sympathetic dystrophy
	Secondary	Immobilization
		Inflammation
		Tumors
		Necrosis

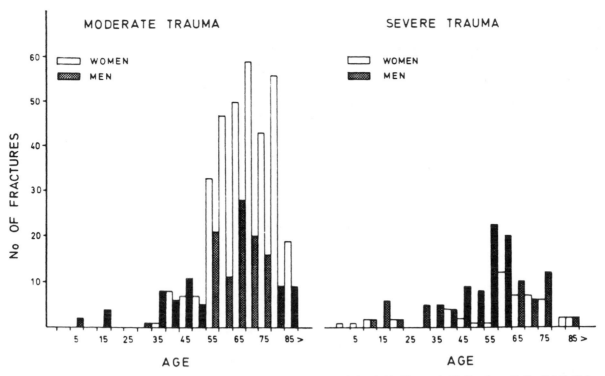

FIGURE 40–2 Annual wrist fracture rates according to age and sex. (From Matkovic V, Ciganovic M, Tominac C, Kostial K: Osteoporosis and epidemiology of fractures in Croatia: An international comparison. Henry Ford Hosp Med J, 1980; 28:116–126.)

be that a hip fracture is a result of the summation of multiple microfractures secondary to the abnormality in tissue repair and bone turnover.[21]

PATHOGENESIS

The human skeleton reaches a peak bone mass between late adolescence and the early 30s. Thereafter, bone loss occurs, gradually resulting in increased fracture risk with minimal or moderate trauma. It seems logical, then, to conclude that the main determinants of osteoporosis are the peak bone mass level reached at skeletal maturity and the subsequent rate of bone loss. Besides the bone mass level, the abnormality in microstructure and bone tissue repair could lead to bone fragility and change in bone quality, which can contribute to the overall incidence of fractures among the elderly. Each determinant of osteoporosis will be considered separately.

Peak Bone Mass

Peak bone mass is generally defined as the highest level of bone mass achieved as a result of normal growth. Peak bone mass is important because, together with age-related loss later on, it is one of the two principal factors determining bone mass late in life (and hence one of the factors determining resistance or susceptibility to fracture).[82] Men have more bone mass than women, and blacks have heavier skeletons than whites.[134] As a direct consequence of this, fractures occur less frequently in the male and black populations.[77] The timing of peak bone mass has been consid-

ered by various authors to occur from ages as early as 17 to 18 years to as late as 35 years. In some reports, peak bone mass is considered to last for only a brief moment before the decline or age-related loss begins, while in others the peak bone mass is maintained for several years. Our recent study shows that both patterns are correct, but for different skeletal regions (Fig. 40–6). Bone mass and bone mineral density were measured in 265 premenopausal white females, aged 8 to 50 years, at the spine (anteroposterior and lateral), proximal femur, radius shaft, distal forearm, and the whole body (TB), using dual x-ray absorptiometry and single photon absorptiometry. True density of the vertebral body (g/cm³) was estimated as well. The results showed that most of the bone mass at multiple skeletal locations is accumulated by late adolescence (Table 40–2). This is particularly notable for bone mineral density (BMD) of the proximal femur and the vertebral body. Bone mass, or bone mineral content (BMC), of the other regions of interest is either no different in women between the age of 18 and onset of menopause or it is maximal in 50 year-old women, indicating slow but permanent bone accumulation continuing at some sites up to the time of menopause. This gain in bone mass in premenopausal adult women is probably the result of continuous periosteal expansion with age. It is interesting to note that true density of the vertebral body does not change very much during this age period.[82] Since rapid skeletal mineral acquisition at all sites occurs relatively early in life, the exogenous factors which might optimize peak bone mass need to be more precisely identified and characterized within the scope of the primary prevention of osteoporosis.

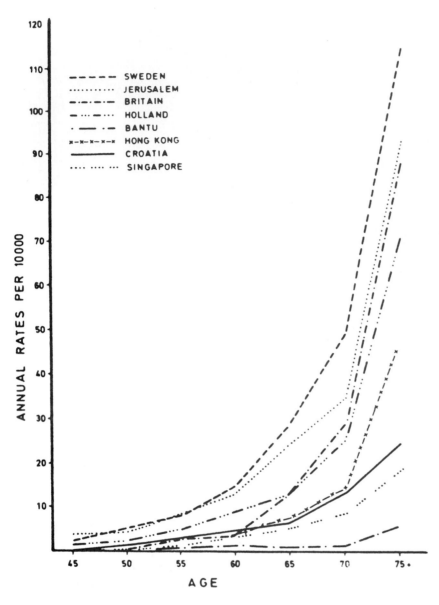

FIGURE 40–3 International comparison of the incidence of hip fractures among women. (From Matkovic V, Ciganovic M, Tominac C, Kostial K: Osteoporosis and epidemiology of fractures in Croatia: An international comparison. Henry Ford Hosp Med J 1980; 28:116–126).

Rate of Bone Loss

After peak bone mass has been reached, bone loss begins and persists until age 85 to 90 years. Lifetime losses range from 20% to 30% for males and up to 45% to 50% for females. Loss of bone with advancing age is a universal phenomenon present in almost every population studied so far, and the rate of bone loss seems to be equal among different populations. Bone loss begins earlier and proceeds more rapidly in females than in males, with an accelerated phase in postmenopausal years (Fig. 40–7). The rate of age-related bone loss is about 0.5% to 1.0% per year in both sexes. It increases in women in the immediate postmenopausal period to approximately 2% to 3% per year for 3 to 15 years after menopause. This accelerated bone loss in females is attributed to the loss of estrogen function and is responsible for the development of type I osteoporosis (and associated wrist and compression fractures of the spine).[115] The female/male ratio for the incidence of involutional osteoporosis between the ages of 50

and 70 is 5:1. This is a direct reflection of the rapid postmenopausal bone loss in females, which is two to four times higher in comparison to males.[114] After the age of 70, the rate of bone loss declines similarly for both sexes. The female/male ratio for the incidence of involutional osteoporosis and hip fractures after the age of 70 is 2:1.[77] This phase of bone loss is considered to be related to the aging process. Since men do not have menopause, the aging process is considered to be the only reason for the bone loss in men.[112, 113]

Menopause is associated with clear-cut changes in the metabolism of estrogens and calcium, which subsequently reflect the loss of bone that begins at menopause. It was initially believed that estrogen deficiency predisposes bone tissue to the action of parathyroid hormone (PTH).[48] It now appears that estrogen effects at the bone tissue level are mediated by cytokines (i.e., interleukin-6) secreted by the bone marrow stromal cells. Estrogens inhibit secretion of interleukin-6, and interleukin-6 contributes to the recruitment of osteoclasts from monocyte cell line.[58]

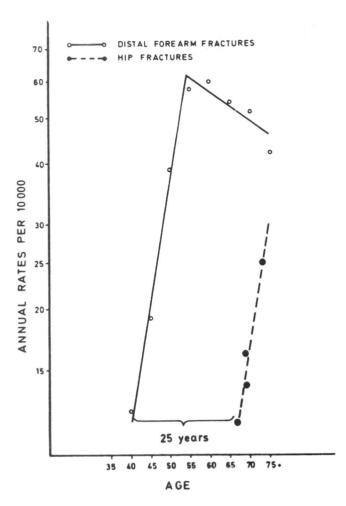

FIGURE 40–4 Annual wrist and hip fracture rates for women in Croatia; semilogarithmic presentation. Note the interval between the peak incidence of type I osteoporosis (wrist fractures) and type II osteoporosis (hip fractures). (From Matkovic V, Ciganovic M, Tominac C, Kostial K: Osteoporosis and epidemiology of fractures in Croatia: An international comparison. Henry Ford Hosp Med J 1980; 28:116–126.)

Menopause is associated with a profound fall in plasma estradiol, the main estrogen secreted by ovaries during the premenopausal period. Depending upon the phase of the menstrual cycle, the plasma range in premenopausal women is between 100 and 1000 pmol/L. During the postmenopausal period, the levels fall below 60 pmol/L. Plasma estrone levels are also decreased during menopause. Plasma estrone levels in premenopausal women are about 150 to 600 pmol/L, and between 50 and 250 pmol/L in the postmenopausal period. In the premenopausal period, one half of plasma estrone levels are derived from the ovaries and one half from the adrenal glands. After cessation of ovarian function, the main source of estrogens in the postmenopausal period is the adrenal glands, and estrone then becomes the main circulating estrogen (derived from androstenedione by peripheral conversion, presumably in the fat tissue).[20]

This abrupt fall in the secretion of estrogens is followed by a rise in plasma gonadotropins, particularly follicle-stimulating hormone (FSH). There is also a decline in adrenal androstenedione production with age. This decline suggests the existence of an adrenopause, which might further contribute to the estrogen deficiency status and influence the rate of bone loss.

Bone Turnover

Creation of peak bone mass, as well as bone loss, is the ultimate event of bone remodeling mediated by bone cells throughout our lifetime. Exchange of bone tissue, which allows bone growth and skeletal development, is usually called bone modeling. The net bone tissue balance during bone modeling is positive (i.e., formation exceeds resorption) until cessation of growth and formation of peak bone mass. During late adolescence, after growth is being completed and peak bone mass and density are being reached, the exchange of bone tissue is called bone remodeling. Bone tissue is being remodeled internally without significant change in the shape of the bone as an organ. During the process of aging, bone remodeling creates negative net bone tissue balance wherein bone resorption exceeds formation.[39]

The main cellular constituents responsible for bone remodeling are well-differentiated osteoclasts, which resorb the microscopic quantum of bone tissue, and osteoblasts, which repair the resorption-mediated defect. The osteoclasts and osteoblasts are coupled together in a basic multicellular unit (BMU). Cortical bone undergoes remodeling through a BMU represented in a haversian system. Trabecular bone undergoes remodeling within a BMU called a trabecular osteon. A typical bone remodeling sequence in a trabecular bone is represented in Figure 40–8. The local remodeling cycle begins with activation of quiescent cells at the bone surface. Remodeling stimuli (i.e., hormones, local tissue factors, physical forces) influence lining cells to contract and to expose bone surface, which then attracts osteoclasts. Osteoclasts originate from bone marrow mono-

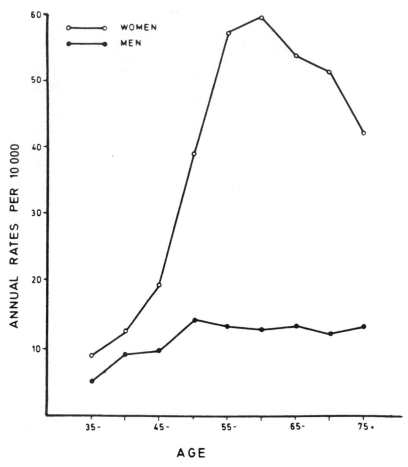

FIGURE 40–5 Annual distribution of hip fractures in men and women according to age and type of trauma. Data for population of Zagreb, Croatia (approximately 1 million people). (From Matkovic V, Ciganovic M, Tominac C, Kostial K: Osteoporosis and epidemiology of fractures in Croatia: An international comparison. Henry Ford Hosp Med J 1980; 28:116–126.)

cytes and migrate to the exposed bone surface to resorb a packet or quantum of bone. A resorption site can be identified histologically by the presence of a cutting cone in cortical bone or a resorption cavity (Howship's lacuna) on endosteal and trabecular bone surfaces. After resorption is completed, osteoblasts that originate from bone marrow mesenchymal cells invade the area and start to synthesize new bone matrix. Biochemically this is reflected in serum bone alkaline phosphatase, which originates from osteoblasts. Subsequently bone matrix becomes mineralized. Some osteoblasts are being incorporated into newly formed bone and become osteocytes. When resorptive cavity is repaired, bone remodeling ceases, and bone surface becomes quiescent again.

The entire remodeling cycle from activation to complete repair lasts about 3 months with about 2 million remodeling units active throughout the human skeleton at any one time. The resorption and formation in a remodeling cycle are coupled with bone resorption being followed by bone formation. At skeletal maturity, between the period of peak bone mass formation and menopause, bone loss is negligible, and bone formation is equal to or slightly less than bone resorption with a net bone balance of zero or slightly less than zero. During aging, bone formation cannot keep up with bone resorption (i.e., uncoupling between formation and resorption), with the creation of negative bone balance ultimately leading to osteoporosis.

The main functions of the bone remodeling process are the repair of skeletal microfractures and the release of calcium into the circulation as a part of the homeostatic control mechanism. During constant stress, every material is susceptible to fatigue fracture. Since the main role of the skeleton is to support the body and, as such, it is constantly being stressed, the development of microfractures (fatigue fractures) is probably a normal event. In normal situations, when the stress is relatively short, these microfractures heal quickly through the process of bone remodeling. If stress lasts long enough, multiple microfractures can develop, which ultimately could result in a bone fracture (e.g., typical march fractures of the metatarsal bones in runners and soldiers). The speculation is that with aging the ability of bone tissue to repair microdamage (i.e., trabecular perforation) is not sufficient, which could contribute to the development of different fracture syndromes by changing the quality of the bone.

Microfractures have been described in the proximal part of the femur as well as in the spine. Inability of bone tissue to repair microdamage can explain occurrence of fractures due to moderate trauma in patients who have normal bone mass in comparison to age-and-sex–matched controls.[6, 37, 38, 97–101]

RISK FACTORS

There are many factors that influence acquisition and maintenance of peak bone mass as well as the rate of bone loss. They all eventually can determine who is at risk of

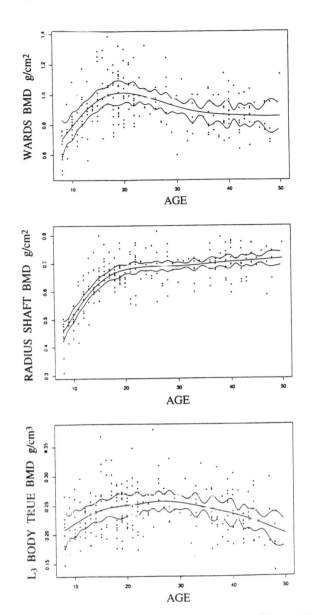

FIGURE 40–6   Cubic splines with 95% pointwise confidence interval for various bone mass–profiles. From *top* to *bottom:* Ward's bone mineral density (BMD) profile; BMD of the radius; and true density of the vertebral body. (From Matkovic V, Jelic T, Wardlaw GM, et al: Timing of peak bone mass in Caucasian females and its implications for the prevention of osteoporosis. Inference from a cross-sectional model. J Clin Invest 1994; 93:799–808.)

osteoporosis. Risk factors can be divided into endogenous and exogenous in origin (Table 40–3).

Genetics

Bone mass acquired at maturity is an important determinant of bone mass at any given subsequent time. Prevalence of osteoporosis is low in groups with a high peak bone mass; such sex and ethnic groups include men vs. women and blacks vs. whites, as previously explained. According to the international studies of bone mass among different population groups, it seems that the rate of bone loss is the same among different ethnic groups. It is likely that the racial differences in the incidence of osteoporosis reflect

differences in peak bone mass rather than in rates of bone loss. Several twin studies also suggested that bone mass is under genetic influence.[105, 126] It was suggested recently that heredity influences acquisition of bone mass rather than rate of bone loss.[19] Because the mother and father probably contribute equally to the acquisition of bone mass by the child, as we have shown, screening should include both parents.[78] There is a higher genetic linkage for body size parameters than for body density.[78] This linkage indicates that the petite body habitus should be at greater risk for the development of osteoporosis.[123] It has also been known for quite some time that osteoporosis might be familial and family history should be a part of a screening process.[124, 135]

Morrison and co-workers[88] recently found that a single gene might influence the risk of osteoporosis, suggesting a way to identify people vulnerable to the bone-weakening disease while they are young enough to take preventive steps. The investigators showed that common allelic variants in the gene encoding the vitamin D receptor (VDR) can be used to predict differences in bone density, accounting for up to 75% of the total genetic effect on bone density in healthy people. The receptor gene comes in two versions, dubbed *b* and *B*. The research linked the *b* version to higher BMD. Humans inherit one version of this gene from each parent, and their combined inheritance can be described as *bb*, *Bb*, or *BB*. In 21 of 22 healthy white monozygotic twin pairs who differed in their inheritance, researchers found spinal bone densities were higher in the twins with more *b* versions. The genotype associated with lower bone density (*BB*) was overrepresented in postmenopausal women with bone density more than 2 SD below values in young normal women. This indicates that the *bb* genotype is more common in persons with higher peak bone mass whereas the *BB* genotype dominates in subjects with lower peak bone mass. Distribution of the alleles in whites in Australia is approximately as follows: 50% *Bb*, 15% *BB*, 33% *bb*.

The biochemical basis of the VDR gene effect on bone density is uncertain and needs further investigation. The active hormonal form of vitamin D (calcitriol) is the central regulator of bone and calcium homeostasis, modulating calcium absorption in the gut, bone formation, recruitment and function of osteoclasts, PTH production, and renal vitamin D activation. The VDR, acting through vitamin D response elements, is therefore a good candidate for being a prime regulator of bone and calcium homeostasis and bone density. Functionally distinct VDR alleles might contribute to the differences in bone and calcium homeostasis and ultimately bone mass between different populations.[88, 89]

The interaction between genetic factors and environment is still not delineated. One of the reasons black people have denser skeletons is due to more favorable calcium economy in the body (less calcium excretion in the urine). Blacks also have a greater resistance to the bone-resorptive effects of PTH and 1,25-dihydroxyvitamin D (1,25(OH)$_2$D).[138] This resistance may allow them to accumulate more bone during growth. The exact distribution of various alleles in different populations is not yet known.[88]

Gonadal Hormones

Premature menopause that is either idiopathic or surgically induced can be considered a risk factor for early bone

TABLE 40–2   Age of the Inflection Point for Various Bone Parameters with Estimates of Bone Variable at the Inflection Point and r-Squared of Each Model

Region of Interest	n	r^2	Inflection Point Age (yr)*	Estimate of Bone Variable
Height	234	.692	16.25 ± 0.04	162.8 cm
TB BMC	231	.624	18.33 ± 0.07	2432 g
TB BMD	231	.587	18.70 ± 0.08	1.11 g/cm²
Skull BMD	231	.642	21.77 ± 0.12	2.29 g/cm²
Femoral neck BMD	232	.425	17.23 ± 0.07	1.04 g/cm²
Ward's BMD	232	.328	18.49 ± 0.09	1.02 g/cm²
Trochanter BMD	232	.229	16.72 ± 0.12	0.86 g/cm²
L2–L4 BMC	231	.657	18.79 ± 0.07	48.05 g
L2–L4 BMD	231	.630	18.45 ± 0.07	1.18 g/cm²
L3 Body volume	228	.583	19.18 ± 0.10	16.46 cm³
L3 Body BMC	229	.482	20.02 ± 0.10	4.20 g
L3 Body—lateral BMD	229	.274	23.97 ± 0.19	0.77 g/cm²
L3 Body—mid BMD	229	.237	23.15 ± 0.24	0.73 g/cm²
L3 Body—true BMD	227	.131	27.18 ± 0.06	0.257 g/cm³
Radius BMD	223	.673	17.82 ± 0.07	0.65 g/cm²
Wrist BMD	222	.407	22.32 ± 0.18	0.34 g/cm²

*Mean ± SE.
Abbreviations: TB, total body; BMC, bone mineral content; BMD, bone mineral density.
From Matkovic V, Jelic T, Wardlaw GM, et al: Timing of peak bone mass in Caucasian females and its implications for the prevention of osteoporosis. Inference from a cross-sectional model. J Clin Invest 1994; 93:799–808.

loss. A woman who undergoes oophorectomy at the age of 40 years (normal expected age of menopause is 50) should have bone mass 10 years later at the same level as a non-oophorectomized woman at age 60. Late menarche is also associated with a lower-than-average BMC. Prolonged amenorrhea secondary to such things as excessive physical exercise in young female athletes or heavy cigarette smoking with depressed estrogen levels in postmenopausal women can cause osteoporosis. Excessive physical exercise, which leads to hormonal abnormalities, and heavy smoking can be considered risk factors for the development of osteoporosis through interference with adequate plasma estrogen levels.[31, 57]

Women who have been taking oral contraceptives have slightly denser bones.[63] Parity and lactation seem to have no adverse effect on bone mass. Bone loss induced by lactation seems to be a transient or self-limiting condition.[130]

Nutrition

Among nutritional factors, low calcium, low vitamin D, high protein, high phosphate, and caffeine intakes have been considered to be risk factors for the development of osteoporosis. These factors can influence peak bone mass formation and the subsequent rate of bone loss.

Calcium is an essential threshold nutrient.[79] An intake threshold applies to the level below which skeletal accumulation is a function of intake, and above which skeletal accumulation is constant, irrespective of further increases in intake. This indicates that retained calcium below the threshold level cannot saturate the skeletal mass, while maximal saturation can be achieved at the threshold level and above. This type of threshold behavior is consistent with current models of bone growth, in which the bone modeling and remodeling process would be predicted to tear down existing bone if calcium intake were insufficient to meet the demands of growth. However, at fully adequate intakes, bone deposited would depend not upon intake but upon what was programmed into the growth process; hence further increases in intake would not result in further skeletal retention. Below a certain threshold level of dietary calcium intake, young persons will not be able to reach genetically predetermined peak bone mass, while adults will be losing bone tissue at a faster rate than is necessary. Adequate calcium intake above a certain threshold level is therefore absolutely required for bone health during skeletal growth and consolidation, as well as for prevention of

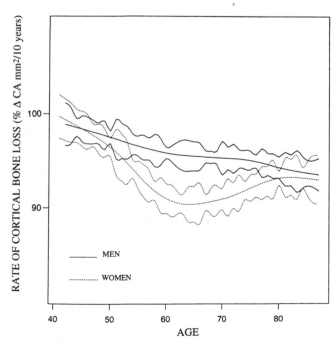

FIGURE 40–7 Age-related rate of cortical bone loss in men and women. (Adapted from Matkovic V, Dekanic D, Kostial K: The rate of cortical bone loss according to age, sex, and calcium intake. J Bone Miner Res 1988; 3:S80.)

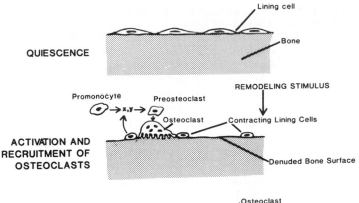

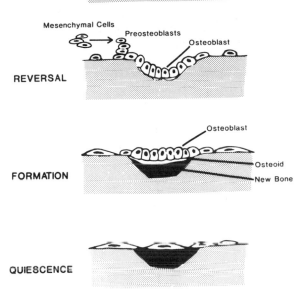

FIGURE 40–8 Bone remodeling sequence at trabecular bone surface.

excessive bone loss with advancing age. Calcium intake thresholds with corresponding threshold balances were recently reported for growing individuals[79] (Table 40–4).

The influence of calcium on peak bone mass was first shown in an epidemiological study conducted in high- and low-calcium regions in Croatia. In this study, metacarpal cortical bone mass was measured in two rural populations who had different calcium intakes over their lifetimes, primarily because of a variation in dairy product consumption. Both men and women from the high-calcium region had higher bone mass than corresponding populations from the low-calcium district. This was true throughout the age

TABLE 40–3   Risk Factors for Osteoporosis

Endogenous	Exogenous
Genetic factors	Nutrition
White and Asian	Low calcium intake
Petite body habitus	High phosphorus intake
Family history	High protein intake
Age	High sodium intake
Advanced	Lifestyle factors
Sex	Smoking
Female	High caffeine intake
Loss of ovarian function	Inactivity
Premature menopause	Immobilization
Amenorrhea	Medications
	Glucocorticoids
	Thyroid hormones

TABLE 40–4   Recommended Daily Allowances (RDAs) for Calcium, and Calcium Intake Thresholds and Balances for Growing Individuals

Age Group (yr)	Current RDA (mg/day, male/female)	Threshold Intake (mg/day)	Threshold Balance (mg/day)
0–1	500	1090	+503
2–8	800	1390	+246
9–17	800/1200	1480	+396
18–30	1200/800	957	+114

From Matkovic V, Heaney RP: Calcium balance during human growth: Evidence for threshold behavior. Am J Clin Nutr 1992; 55:992–996.

range of 30 to 75+ years. Both populations seemed to lose bone mass with age at the same rate. The men in the high-calcium district had as much bone mass at 70 as did men in the low-calcium region at age 30 (Fig. 40–9). Figure 40–10 shows a different rate of hip fractures among two populations of men with different calcium intakes. Although this was a cross-sectional study, it suggested the importance of adequate calcium intake during skeletal formation, from childhood up to 30 years of age.[83] Similar results were recently found in a study conducted in China.[53] Calcium has also protective effects on bone mass in postmenopausal women and the elderly as well. Other studies conducted in adults also indicate that calcium behaves as a threshold agent.[25, 111] Below a certain level of calcium intake (~500 mg/day) bone loss is more pronounced and therefore extra calcium is needed to prevent this decline. Immediately after menopause (1–5 years) estrogen withdrawal seems to have more profound influence on bone mass which cannot be easily overcome by dietary manipulation. The study of Chapuy et al.[17] indicates that calcium and vitamin D can stabilize bone mass in the very elderly and even reduce the risk of nonvertebral fractures. Calcium intake of about 1200 mg/day is necessary.

Vitamin D deficiency can cause rickets in children and calcium malabsorption and osteomalacia in adults. Vitamin D deficiency can be the result of either inadequate exposure to sunlight or inadequate dietary intake of vitamin D. In elderly patients, however, low plasma $1,25(OH)_2D$ levels could also be due to impaired 1α-hydroxylation by the aging kidney. It was reported that a substantial number of patients in England with hip fractures have osteomalacia and that this disease can contribute to the incidence of hip fractures.[1] Vitamin D deficiency can also cause myopathy,

which can further contribute to the hip fracture incidence through increased risk of falling secondary to neuromuscular instability. Vitamin D is very important for calcium absorption from the diet. It facilitates active transport by inducing the formation of calcium-binding protein in intestinal mucosal cells. This function is particularly important for adaptation to low intakes. However, passive transport occurs by other means, not as well elucidated, and is not dependent on vitamin D. The proportion of absorption by the two mechanisms varies with intake and is not well characterized; at high calcium intakes it is likely that active transport contributes relatively little to the total absorbed load. Nevertheless, vitamin D status can influence absorptive performance and influence calcium requirement. Vitamin D status commonly deteriorates in the elderly, whose plasma 25-hydroxyvitamin D (25(OH)D) levels are generally lower than in young adults. In a recent study among elderly women, vitamin D therapy increased calcium economy in the body which led to the stabilization of bone mass and fracture prevention.[47, 133]

Phosphorus is also very important for bone health. Phosphate makes roughly half of the weight of bone mineral and therefore must be present in adequate quantities in the diet, both to mineralize and to maintain the skeleton. Phosphorus is present in relatively adequate quantities in the American diet, and most of the recent concern of the nutrition community has centered around whether its presence in the diet might be excessive, with consequent development of secondary hyperparathyroidism which could potentiate bone loss. High phosphate intake and an abnormally low calcium-to-phosphate ratio (i.e., 1:6) was implicated in the development of osteoporosis and secondary hyperparathyroidism in laboratory animals. This has

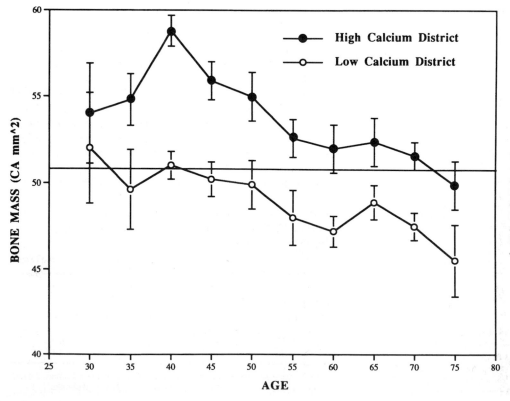

FIGURE 40–9 Bone density (metacarpal cortical area/total area) among two populations of men with lifetime difference in calcium intake. (Adapted from Matkovic V, Kostial K, Simonovic I, et al: Bone status and fracture rates in two regions of Yugoslavia. Am J Clin Nutr 1979; 32:540–549.)

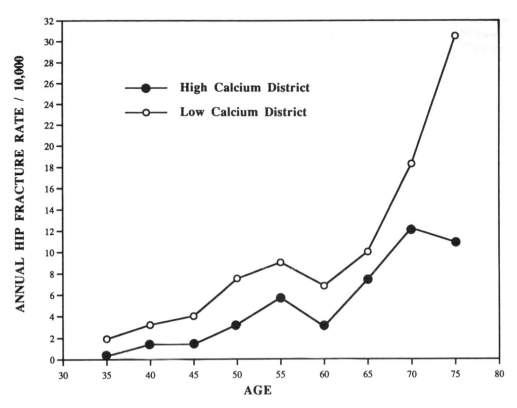

FIGURE 40–10 Hip fracture rates among two populations of men, with lifetime difference in calcium intake. (Adapted from Matkovic V, Kostial K, Simonovic I, et al: Bone status and fracture rates in two regions of Yugoslavia. Am J Clin Nutr 1979; 32:540–549.)

not been rigorously studied in humans, but it has been suggested that excessive consumption of phosphate through soft drinks could be a risk factor for the development of osteoporosis.[47, 67]

Sodium seems to be one of the most important determinants of urinary calcium excretion, both in adults[94] and in children (Fig. 40–11). Higher sodium intake leads to higher urinary calcium loss. Sodium intake increases obligatory calcium loss in the urine which disturbs calcium equilibrium and increases dietary calcium requirements.

Vitamin K is an essential cofactor for the formation

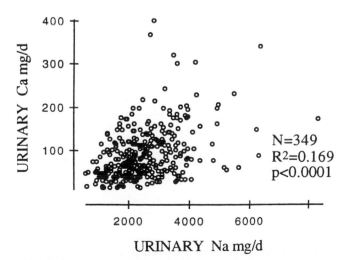

FIGURE 40–11 The relationship between urinary calcium and sodium excretion in adolescent females. (Adapted from Ilich JZ, Tzagournis MA, Hseih LC, et al: Determinants of urinary calcium excretion in young females. J Bone Miner Res 1993; 8:S252.)

of γ-carboxyglutamic acid (Gla) residues in proteins. Gla residues have a high affinity for calcium ions and, therefore, all Gla-containing proteins are Ca^{2+}-binding ones. The role of Gla-containing proteins in bone (osteocalcin) is not well understood. A possibility is that they help regulate calcium deposition in the bone. Arguments for this hypothesis come from in vitro experiments which show that these proteins strongly inhibit the precipitation of calcium salts and growth of hydroxyapatite crystals. Moreover, preliminary clinical observations indicate that administration of vitamin K could reduce urinary calcium loss and even reduce the rate of postmenopausal bone loss. Low vitamin K plasma levels were found in osteoporotic patients with vertebral compression and hip fractures.[47, 52]

Protein-caloric malnutrition during childhood can cause growth retardation and decreased formation of cortical bone, and therefore can interfere with peak bone mass formation. Several studies have documented that a state of malnutrition or undernutrition is often observed in elderly osteoporotic patients with hip fractures. Many of those patients have reduced serum albumin levels and they definitely could benefit from protein supplementation. On the other hand, excessive protein intake and increase in protein consumption above the recommended allowance level can be associated with hypercalciuria and hyperparathyroidism. This in turn could lead to a decrease in bone mass. Although information about the mechanism between excessive protein intake (>120 g/day) and bone loss is still poorly understood, a primary decrease in tubular reabsorption of calcium could be the initiating event.[47, 62] Despite these findings, there is evidence for the beneficial effect of protein intake and supplementation within recommended levels. Excessive caffeine consumption can also contribute to increased calcium excretion in the urine and potentiate negative calcium balance and increase calcium requirements.[51]

Alcoholism is probably a risk factor of greater relative importance than has been commonly recognized. The prevalence of significant alcohol abuse in the adult U.S. population ranges between 8% and 16%. It was demonstrated several years ago that bone mass is seriously depleted in both male and female alcoholics. Defective osteoblastic function rather than increased bone resorption has been reported in patients with alcoholism. Compression fractures in elderly men strongly indicate chronic alcohol consumption.[27, 122]

Physical Activity

The incidence of osteoporosis is higher in the Western hemisphere and this could be partially due to the relative lack of physical activity in the population.[15] The bone loss that occurs with prolonged immobilization suggests also that physical exercise might help to prevent osteoporosis[29] (see Chapter 34). Bone density, at least in cortical bone, is higher in athletes than in their nonathletic counterparts. Increased total body calcium and vertebral BMC have been reported after moderate exercise in patients with postmenopausal osteoporosis.[2, 91, 125] All of this indicates that daily weightbearing activity is essential to skeletal health. Mechanical weightbearing stress is probably the most important exogenous factor affecting bone development and peak bone mass formation, as well as the maintenance and integrity of bone mass later on through its action on bone remodeling.

A hundred years ago, the famous Berlin anatomist Julius Wolff was the first to recognize the relationship between mechanical stress and bone remodeling. In his publication "The Law of Bone Transformation," which was published in 1892, Wolff stated: "Every change in the function of bone is followed by definite changes in internal architecture and external confirmation according to mathematical law." He indicated that form follows function.[61] Almost 100 years since this discovery, we still do not know the mechanisms that lead to increased bone formation and increased bone density secondary to increased level of stress. Bone contains hydroxyapatite crystals with charged surfaces surrounded by water that behave as an electrolyte solution creating electrical potential under mechanical stress. It has been suggested that these electrical fields influence bone growth and that endogenous piezoelectricity generated by stress could be involved in osteoblastic stimulation and new bone formation.[9] It was also suggested recently that increased plasma levels of calcitonin found during acute physical exercise could be involved in the process as well.[4] Daily physical exercise contributes to the prevention of osteoporosis, not only by increasing bone mass but also by improving neuromuscular function and coordination, thereby decreasing falls that can cause hip fractures. In prior studies, persons with hip fractures were significantly less active than normal controls.[8, 60, 121]

CLINICAL FEATURES

The main clinical signs and symptoms of osteoporosis are back pain, spinal kyphosis, loss of height, and multiple fractures, usually of the vertebrae, wrists, and hips. Back pain is the most common symptom in patients with compression fracture syndrome. Fractures of the vertebrae can be spontaneous, but often occur after some ordinary activity such as bending or lifting. Pain can be mild or severe and can last for days or weeks before subsiding. After multiple compression fractures have occurred, chronic pain may develop in association with spinal deformity and progressive dorsal kyphosis, also known as dowager's hump. Multiple wedge-type compressions are responsible for the development of dorsal kyphosis. Associated loin pain is common in spinal osteoporosis with vertebral compression fractures and kyphosis, and results from bruising of the ribs over the iliac crests.

Compression fractures are most commonly located between the end of the thoracic spine and the beginning of the lumbar spine (T8–L3). The majority of patients with spinal osteoporosis later in life (i.e., type II osteoporosis) have asymptomatic vertebral compression that can be detected only by radiographic examination. Loss of body height or the development of kyphosis can be the only sign of multiple vertebral fractures. Discomfort, debility, and sometimes depression secondary to the constant fear of hip fracture may accompany thoracic shortening. Activities of daily living may be restricted. Loss of skin thickness (indicating loss of collagen mass), constipation, and abdominal bloating are also frequent signs of the disease. In spite of the patient's multiple vertebral compressions, the incidence of spinal cord trauma is negligible.

Wrist fractures are usually the result of moderate trauma or a fall from a standing position. They tend to occur outside the house and are more frequent during the winter months. Sometimes reflex sympathetic dystrophy, or Sudeck's bone atrophy, will develop after the wrist fracture and immobilization in a plastic cast.

Hip fractures are another important clinical manifestation of osteoporosis. Patients with hip fractures are more likely to be elderly and female than are patients with vertebral fractures. The majority of hip fractures occur at home after moderate trauma. The majority of patients have a tendency to fall backward or to the side as a result of a balance problem. In most cases the fall precedes the fracture, but in some cases a sudden increase in movement causes a fracture which then provokes a fall. Fractures occur either in the neck of the femur or at the intertrochanteric region. Patients with hip fractures tend to be debilitated as the result of multiple chronic diseases and intake of multiple medications, including psychotropic drugs. Fractures tend to promote fear of loss of independent living, fear of additional falls and fractures, and consequent depression.

DIAGNOSTIC PROCEDURES

The diagnostic approach includes medical history, physical examination, anthropometry, blood and urine chemistry, metabolic studies, bone mass measurements, and bone biopsy (Table 40–5).

Medical History and Physical Examination

The medical history is an essential part of the diagnostic workup and screening of osteoporosis in the general popu-

TABLE 40–5   Diagnostic Workup of the Patient with Metabolic Bone Disease

Medical history	
Physical examination	
Anthropometry	Total height, sitting height, arm span, weight, body composition (DXA, bioelectric impedance)
Dietary interview	
CBC, urinalysis	
Blood chemistry, general	Ca, Ca²⁺, P, Mg, creatinine, electrolytes, ASTT, GGT, albumin, total serum proteins
Parathyroid function	Intact PTH, nephrogenous cAMP, TmP/GFR
Vitamin D status	$25(OH)D_3$, $1,25(OH)_2D_3$
Markers of bone formation	Osteocalcin (serum), total serum alkaline phosphatase, bone alkaline phosphatase
Markers of bone resorption	Fasting urine Ca/creatinine ratio, fasting urine OHPr/creatinine ratio, urinary pyridinoline cross-links, urinary N-telopeptide, TRAP
24-hr urine sample	CA, P, Na, creatinine, OHPr, free cortisol
Metabolic studies	Calcium balance, absorption, kinetics
Bone mass measurements	X-ray, radiogrammetry, DXA, CT, neutron activation, UTV, triple-phase bone scan
Bone histomorphometry	Static and dynamic (tetracycline labeling)

Abbreviations: DXA, dual x-ray absorptiometry; CBC, complete blood count; AST, aspartate aminotransferase; GGT, δ-glutamyltranspeptidase; PTH, parathyroid hormone; cAMP, cyclic adenosine monophosphate; TmP/GFR, maximum tubular reabsorption of phosphate; OHPr, hydroxyproline; TRAP, tartrate-resistant acid phosphatase; CT, computed tomography; UTV, ultrasound transmission velocity.

lation. The medical history should include questions pertinent to bone mass maintenance and bone loss including the risk factors previously mentioned. Part of the medical history should also be a nutritional evaluation by dietary interview (i.e., dietary recalls) to obtain adequate assessment of protein, calcium, phosphate, and vitamin D consumption, as well as coffee and alcohol intake. Dietary history should be taken by a skilled nutritionist. Information about lifestyle is essential as well.

The physical examination is a very important part of the diagnostic process. Previously described signs and symptoms of the disease should be ascertained. Basic anthropometry should include total height, sitting height, arm span, and body weight. Loss of height is one of the features of osteoporosis and is primarily due to compression fractures of the spine and kyphosis. The ratio of sitting height to total height is abnormal in the osteoporotic population. Sometimes elderly patients cannot recall their height of 20 to 30 years earlier; measurement of arm span or tibial length could help in this regard. There is a good correlation between total height and arm span, as well as total height and tibial length. The discrepancy between arm span and

current height could provide some estimate of the degree of height loss. This applies primarily when studying a group of people rather then when studying the dynamics of height loss in one individual. As weight has a protective effect on bone tissue (direct stress to the bone and/or more favorable estrogen metabolism in the fat tissue), it is highly unlikely to find obese women with compression fractures secondary to generalized primary osteoporosis. Weight and height measurements are also important for calculation of body surface area necessary for metabolic study.

Blood and Urine Chemistry

A complete blood count as well as urinalysis should be a part of the general screening. Low hemoglobin or anemia can be present in diseases that also affect the skeleton and are responsible for the development of secondary osteoporosis (e.g., multiple myeloma, sickle cell disease, and others). Examination of urinary sediment can indicate the presence of chronic renal disease and kidney stones.

Blood chemistry should include measurement of plasma calcium, ionized calcium, serum phosphate, creatinine, albumin, and total protein as well as electrolytes and calcium-regulating hormones. Plasma calcium is usually normal in patients with primary involutional osteoporosis, and any abnormality in blood calcium could indicate the presence of some other metabolic bone disorder such as hyperparathyroidism, osteomalacia, metastatic bone disease, and others. If ionized calcium is not available, plasma calcium should be corrected for albumin or total protein.[102] Albumin is not only helpful for the evaluation of blood calcium but also can indicate malnutrition. Low albumin values were found in debilitated patients with hip fractures and such values suggest protein malnutrition. Serum phosphate is borderline-high in postmenopausal women secondary to suppression of parathyroid function and increased tubular reabsorption of phosphate. Serum phosphate is low in patients with osteomalacia, primary hyperparathyroidism, and phosphate diabetes (i.e., vitamin D resistance). Serum creatinine is essential not only for baseline renal function but also for expression of various indices of tubular reabsorption of calcium, phosphate, and cyclic adenosine monophosphate (cAMP). Determination of 25(OH)D levels could help in distinguishing patients with osteomalacia secondary to nutritional deficiency. Low 25(OH)D levels may be found in patients with hip fractures as well as in nursing home residents. Determination of $1,25(OH)_2D$ is not essential in routine clinical practice except when patients are part of the research protocols. Determination of PTH could help in screening for primary hyperparathyroidism or in patients with mild secondary hyperparathyroidism. Another screening test for parathyroid bone disease is the determination of nephrogenous cAMP based on blood and 2-hour fasting urine measurements. The cAMP of renal origin is under PTH influence and therefore serves as a biological marker of PTH activity on renal tubules as well as of maximum tubular reabsorption of phosphate (TmP/GFR).[11, 12]

Urine tests should include 2-hour fasting urine tests (after 10–12 hours' overnight fast) as well as the collection of 24-hour urine for determination of calcium, creatine, phosphate, sodium, hydroxyproline (OHPr), and collagen cross-links. Patients with osteoporosis usually have a normal excretion of calcium during 24 hours. Any type of hypocalciuria (i.e., <70 mg Ca per 24 hours) could indicate the presence of malabsorption and osteomalacia, while hypercalciuria (i.e., >300 mg Ca per 24 hours) could indicate the presence of excessive bone resorption secondary to destructive bone disease or a hyperabsorptive state. The calcium/creatinine ratio in fasting urine is usually high in patients with postmenopausal osteoporosis (i.e., type I) as well as in other conditions in which bone resorption is higher than normal. It serves also as a bone turnover index. When the calcium absorption process is completed, fasting urine tests reflect overnight changes in the skeleton and therefore indicate input of calcium from bone to extracellular fluid.[92]

Biochemical Markers of Bone Turnover

Bone turnover indices are biochemical markers of the bone remodeling process. Some markers indicate bone resorption (i.e., calcium/creatinine ratio in fasting urine, hydroxyproline/creatinine ratio in fasting urine, collagen cross-links, tartrate-resistant acid phosphatase [TRAP]), while others indicate bone formation (i.e., serum alkaline phosphatase and serum osteocalcin, also called bone GLA protein or BGP). As bone resorption is coupled with bone formation, the indices of resorption correlate highly with indices of bone formation, and both reflect bone turnover status.

Calcium/creatinine ratio reflects bone resorption after an overnight fast, as previously explained. OHPr is a product of collagen metabolism. Urine collection over 24 hours requires a collagen-free diet but this is not necessary for urine testing after an overnight fast. Values tend to be elevated in fast bone losers. Very high values are characteristics of growth and in patients with primary hyperparathyroidism, Paget's disease of bone, and in renal osteodystrophy. Urinary hydroxylysylpyridinoline (HP, pyridinoline) and lysylpyridinoline (LP, deoxypyridinoline) are nonreducible cross-links that stabilize the collagen chains within the extracellular matrix. Pyridinoline is present in bone and cartilage matrix and in minute amounts in some other connective tissues. Significant amounts of LP are found only in bone collagen. Pyridinoline and deoxypyridinoline are likely to be released from bone tissue matrix during osteoclastic bone resorption. As both cross-links result from post-translational modification of collagen, they cannot be reutilized for synthesis. Both are excreted in the urine in free (~40%) and in peptide-bound form (~60%) and the total amount can be measured by fluorimetry in hydrolyzed urine or by immunoassay.[26] Recently, Hanson and colleagues[45] identified and characterized the N-telopeptide cross-linking domain of bone type I collagen (NTx). This discovery has provided a marker of bone collagen with greater specificity than the pyridinoline cross-links. These particular peptides are derived only from mature bone collagen. NTx seems to be the most promising marker for monitoring bone resorption in individual subjects.[45] Plasma TRAP is secreted by the osteoclasts and can serve as another potential marker of bone resorption.[87] Development of a new immunoassay using monoclonal antibodies directed against the bone TRAP should facilitate its clinical

use. Alkaline phosphatase originates from osteoblasts and tends to be normal in patients with osteoporosis or slightly elevated when bone turnover increases, as in postmenopausal women or in the very elderly. If alkaline phosphatase is highly abnormal, it can indicate acute fracture, Paget's disease, osteomalacia, renal osteodystrophy, or primary hyperparathyroidism. Bone alkaline phosphatase is heat-labile and therefore can be distinguished from liver enzyme. If isoenzyme is not available, screening the liver function with γ-glutamyl transpeptidase (GGT) could help in the differentiation of the origin of isolated elevations in total alkaline phosphatase. Alkaline phosphatase is also high during growth and declines after puberty, similar to the excretion of OHPr in urine.

Osteocalcin is a protein that contains Gla. This is a calcium-binding vitamin K–dependent protein. It originates from bone cell synthesis rather than from bone matrix degradation and therefore reflects bone formation.[107] Osteocalcin is elevated in postmenopausal osteoporosis with high bone turnover and generally follows the other markers.[13]

Metabolic Studies

Calcium balance, calcium kinetics, and calcium absorption are considered to be a part of the research protocol. Calcium balance technique measures calcium input and output from the body. A continuous fecal marker has to be used to correct calcium excretion in the stool. Calcium balance is positive during bone modeling and is negative during the period of bone loss. Calcium balance technique has been considered the dominant method for the determination of calcium requirements in humans. This technique assesses calcium metabolism, but is not without errors, is time-consuming, requires hospitalization in a metabolic ward, and does not provide information regarding the calcium content of the skeleton. With the recent development of the dual x-ray absorptiometry (DXA) method, it is now possible to measure total skeletal mineral accretion (38% is Ca) with higher precision and accuracy. This method can assess calcium needs during growth, particularly with regard to the threshold calcium intake and peak bone mass. In a recent study, we used both methods to measure skeletal calcium accretion during growth as related to dietary calcium, and found a good correlation between the two methods[80] (Fig. 40–12).

Bone Mass Measurements

There are currently several methods available to study skeletal pathological processes and bone mass. These range from classic skeletal radiology to new sophisticated techniques with excellent precision and accuracy suitable for mass screening of osteoporosis in the general population. Standard radiographs are essential for the diagnosis of osteoporotic fractures of the spine, wrist, hip, or other bones. However, these radiographs are insufficient for the study of bone loss and for determining the risk of fractures. At least 30% of bone mineral has to be lost before changes are seen on classic bone radiographs.

DXA allows measurements of bone mineral in the axial skeleton (i.e., L1–L4), peripheral skeleton (i.e., forearm, hips), and the whole body (Fig. 40–13). Bone mass is usually expressed in terms of BMC (grams) and areal BMD

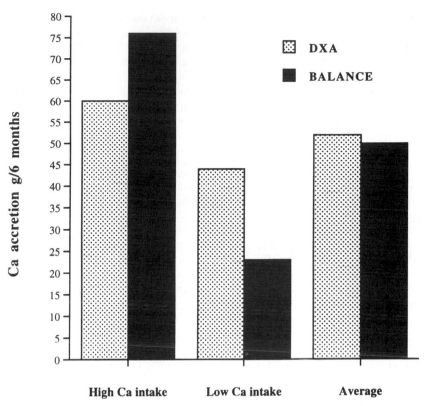

FIGURE 40–12 Comparison of skeletal calcium accretion (grams in 180 days) in 26 adolescent girls by dual x-ray absorptiometry of the total body and 2-week calcium balance study with prediction over 6 months. (Adapted from Matkovic V, Hseih L, Andon MB, Ilich JZ: Skeletal calcium accretion as determined by balance technique and dual energy x-ray absorptiometry of the total body. J Bone Miner Res 1993; 8:S253.)

in grams per square centimeter. As we are dealing with areal density (g/cm^2) and not with true density (g/cm^3), the method cannot completely correct for the effect of bone size. The DXA technique requires a relatively short measurement time of 5 to 15 min, provides good image detail, has excellent measurement precision (i.e., <1% error), and is associated with low radiation exposure (i.e., 1–3 mrem). Two types of x ray-based systems are considered: the K-edge filtered system, which operates at a fixed kilovoltage and uses filter materials having K-edges to create two peaks in their output spectra, and the switched-kV system, which uses conventional filter material but alternates between two different kilovoltages for sequential dual-energy measurements.[85, 128, 131]

Clinical indications for measuring BMD in the skeleton by DXA include (1) screening postmenopausal women who are going to take estrogens; (2) screening for low bone mass in persons with major risk factors; (3) establishing the diagnosis of osteoporosis in mild cases with minimal bone loss and some vertebral deformities; (4) determining the severity of bone loss in newly diagnosed osteoporotic patients with vertebral fractures so that the most appropriate therapy can be selected; (5) monitoring efficiency of a new medication in a research trial; and (6) evaluating the degree of bone loss and the effect of treatment in other metabolic bone disorders like osteomalacia, renal osteodystrophy, parathyroid bone disease, and others.[59, 116]

Computed tomography (CT) of the spine is currently the

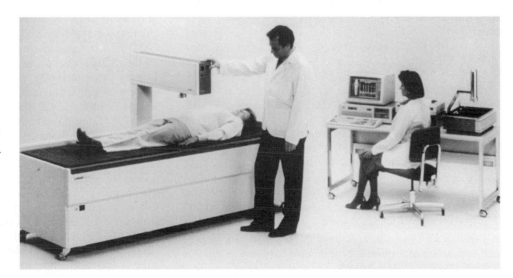

FIGURE 40–13 Dual x-ray absorptiometry equipment. (Courtesy of Dr. Richard Mazess, Lunar Corp., Wisconsin.)

only technique that allows the radiologist to record the true density of the interior trabecular portions of bones separately from their cortex. CT scans are widely available but are expensive and involve doses of radiation in the 200- to 1000-mrem range. Such scans are not convenient for mass screening in osteoporosis.[14] Magnetic resonance imaging (MRI) helps to evaluate the spinal cord in patients with severe osteoporosis and kyphosis (Fig. 40–14).

Bone Histomorphometry

A bone biopsy is an invasive procedure performed usually on the iliac crest for the purpose of analysis of bone tissue, bone cells, and bone turnover dynamics. A bone biopsy can be done as an outpatient procedure and is associated with minimal discomfort and risk to the patient.[108] An intact bone cylinder with cortical and trabecular parts can be obtained from the ilium using a special bone biopsy trephine. The specimen must be prestained in Villanueva osteochrome stain and then embedded in hard plastic (i.e., methyl methacrylate). The bone has to be cut in the undecalcified state with a heavy-duty microtome to preserve cellular and structural details. Only an experienced histomorphometrist can assess the structural and dynamic changes. It is believed that the iliac crest bone biopsy reveals the same pathophysiological changes found in the axial skeleton. Bone biopsy in osteoporotic patients reveals thin cortices and reduction in the number of trabecular profiles.

Before the biopsy, two separate courses of tetracycline are administered to the patient. Since tetracycline chelates amorphous calcium phosphate crystals, it is bound at the site of mineralization (i.e., active calcification) and can be detected by fluorescence under ultraviolet light. Patients usually take the tetracycline in a dose of 250 mg three times a day for 3 days, and then 11 days off with a repeated course for another 3-day period. The bone biopsy is usually

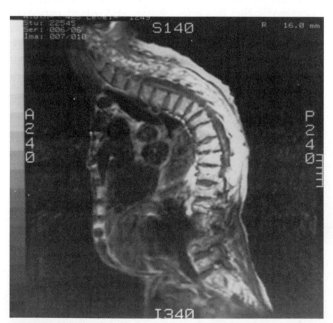

FIGURE 40–14 Magnetic resonance image of the spine of a patient with severe osteoporosis. Note multiple compression fractures and well-preserved spinal column.

done after the fourth day from the last dose. By measuring the distance between the two tetracycline labels, it is possible to calculate the mineral apposition rate, from which the bone formation rate can be derived. Bone cells, resorption, and formation samples can be measured and create a basis of bone histomorphometry.

Histomorphometric analysis of the iliac crest bone biopsies suggests that postmenopausal osteoporosis is a heterogeneous disorder with a spectrum of bone remodeling activity that ranges from accelerated to reduced bone turnover.[86] Some physicians consider bone biopsy to be a necessary part of the workup so that therapy for the underlying disorder can be adjusted to the fundamental pathophysiological process.[64] Bone biopsy should not generally be used to establish the diagnosis of osteoporosis. The indications for bone biopsy are to determine the presence of osteoporosis in a relatively young patient, to rule out osteomalacia or parathyroid bone disease, or to monitor the effect of treatment in a special research protocol.

PREVENTION

Factors that can increase peak bone mass (i.e., primary prevention) and reduce the rate of postmenopausal bone loss (i.e., secondary prevention) are ideal agents for the prevention of osteoporosis in the general population. Those agents include nutritional factors (i.e., calcium), estrogens, and weightbearing exercises. Elimination of risk factors that contribute to the incidence of falls among the elderly should also be considered as a part of the global prevention program for the reduction of the number of fractures in the population.

Primary Prevention

Adequate calcium intake is certainly essential for bone growth and development.[75, 81] The recommended dietary allowances (RDA) for calcium are 1200 mg/day for adolescents and pregnant women, and 800 mg/day for children and young adults. Recent studies indicate that RDA for calcium should be much higher for growing persons.[75, 79, 81] A recent 3-year clinical trial in monozygotic prepubertal twins living in the United States showed that supplementation of one group of twins with a highly absorbable form of calcium (i.e., calcium citrate-malate) significantly increased BMD of the forearm (5.1%), spine (2.8%), and proximal femur (3.2%), relative to the control twins (Fig. 40–15).[60] Dietary calcium intake in this study averaged about 900 mg/day. Supplementation of 1000 mg/day, after adjusting for noncompliance (27%), gave the supplemented twins an average calcium intake of 1612 mg/day, far above the saturation intake level. It would seem that, based on these metabolic and bone mass studies, a higher RDA for calcium for this age group ought to be considered.[75] Calcium needs are greater during adolescence (ages 9–17 years) than in either childhood or young adulthood when comparing the maximal calcium retention in the body. This results from the high velocity of growth during the peak of puberty as well as skeletal consolidation by late adolescence. These skeletal parameters combined exert a major influence on calcium requirements during adolescence. Puberty is an

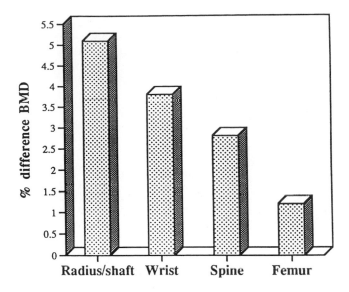

Prepubertal twins (22 pairs)

FIGURE 40–15 Percent change (g/cm² for 3 years) in bone mineral areal density for several skeletal locations in prepubertal identical twins. (Adapted from Johnston CC Jr, Miller JZ, Slemenda CW, et al: Calcium supplementation and increases in bone mineral density in children. N Engl J Med 1992; 327:82–87.)

intensely anabolic period, with increases in height and weight, alterations in body composition resulting from increased lean body mass, changes in the quantity and distribution of body fat, and enlargement of many organ systems besides the skeleton.[76, 78, 79, 81]

Surveys in the United States reveal that adolescent girls are less likely to meet the current recommended dietary levels for calcium than are teenaged boys, whose intake is higher and comes closer to achieving recommended intakes. By contrast, calcium intake in girls starts to decline at the time of the puberty. The ratio of calcium intake and the potential for maximal calcium retention is lowest for adolescent girls, indicating a status of relative calcium deficiency. During adolescence, the average maximal calcium retention is close to 400 mg/day at the intake threshold of about 1500 mg/day.

Matkovic, et al.[78] recently showed that calcium intake (from milk or supplements) above the threshold standard of 1640 mg/day was associated with a more positive calcium balance and a trend toward an increased gain in BMD in three out of four skeletal sites. The studies of Lloyd et al.[71] and Chan et al.[16] point in the same direction. Teenaged girls in the study of Lloyd et al. were supplemented with 300 mg extra calcium, and despite total intakes far below the threshold level, there was still an appreciable gain in bone mass.[71] Figure 40–16 shows bone mass accumulation over a 6-month period in two groups of adolescent girls supplemented with different amounts of calcium (below and above calcium intake threshold for this age group).

Secondary Prevention

Estrogens can effectively treat symptoms associated with menopause, such as vasomotor flushes, sweating, and dyspareunia. Estrogens are also effective agents in the prevention of postmenopausal bone loss. If treatment can be initiated early enough, estrogens can practically keep bone mass at the same level and prevent bone loss and the incidence of fractures later on[34, 54, 70, 139] (Fig. 40–17).

Guidelines for estrogen therapy are as follows: (1) Estrogen therapy can be considered for the prevention of osteoporosis in postmenopausal women who are at high risk for developing the disease. (2) low-dose estrogens can be used effectively to prevent bone loss (0.625 mg) during 3 weeks out of 4. During the fourth week, progestin (10 mg of medroxyprogesterone) could be used, which would reduce the incidence of cancer of the uterus. (3) Patients on estrogen therapy should undergo annual gynecological examinations, including mammography and breast examinations. (4) Estrogen therapy should be continued for at least 10 to 20 years beyond the onset of postmenopausal symptoms. If women have bilateral oophorectomy at an earlier age, they should continue treatment for a relatively longer period of time.[137]

The exact mechanism of estrogen action at the bone level has recently been attributed to the suppression of interleukin-6 secretion and inhibition of osteoclast recruitment.[58] The action does block bone resorption and improves calcium absorption in the gastrointestinal system. Estrogen receptors have been found recently in osteoblasts, but the meaning of this is still unknown.[32] In addition to its protective effects at the skeletal level, estrogens have been implicated in the prevention of myocardial infarction. Contraindications to estrogen use are estrogen-dependent malignacies (e.g., breast or uterine cancer), thrombophlebitis and other disorders of increased coagulability, and certainly unexplained vaginal bleeding. Cancer of the uterus is the main risk associated with estrogen treatment. Estrogen increases the risk of endometrial cancer three to eight times. This increase in the incidence of cancer is diminished with cyclic or continuous progestin treatment. In addition to cancer prevention, progestins may have a beneficial effect on bone that is independent of estrogens.[137] Anti-estrogenic compounds (e.g., tamoxifen, taramifen) used in breast cancer treatment might be a new line of medications used to treat osteoporosis. They behave like estrogens at the bone tissue level and antiestrogens at the breast cancer cellular level.[73]

Not only can adequate calcium intake at or above the threshold intake level contribute to peak bone mass formation with subsequent reduction in the incidence of osteoporosis in the population but such intake can also partially suppress postmenopausal cortical bone loss.[5, 25, 111, 118] Adequate calcium intake in the postmenopausal period can also reduce the requirement for estrogen supplementation to a minimum of 0.325 mg.[35] The recommended dietary requirement for calcium for postmenopausal women and the elderly should be above 1200 mg/day. Calcium can be obtained either through natural dietary sources or from calcium supplements. The main dietary sources of calcium are milk and dairy products. One 200-mL glass of milk has about 250 mg of calcium. The most common and least expensive calcium supplement is calcium carbonate, but probably the best bioavailability is from calcium citrate or calcium citrate-malate.[90] The bioavailability of calcium from calcium carbonate among elderly patients with achlorhydria is decreased.[109]

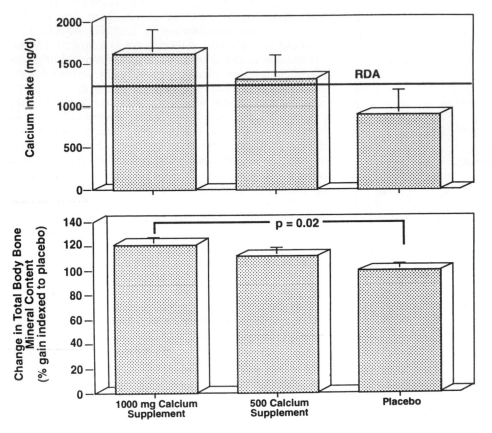

FIGURE 40–16 Bone mass accumulation over a 6-month period in two groups of adolescent girls given supplements of different amounts of calcium (below and above calcium intake threshold for this age group [~1500 mg/day]). Note that the current RDA for calcium may not be enough. (From Andon MB, Lloyd T, Matkovic V: Supplementation trials with calcium citrate malate: Evidence in favor of increasing the calcium RDA during childhood and adolescence. J Nutr 1994; 124:1412–1417.)

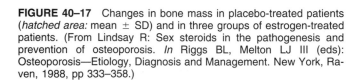

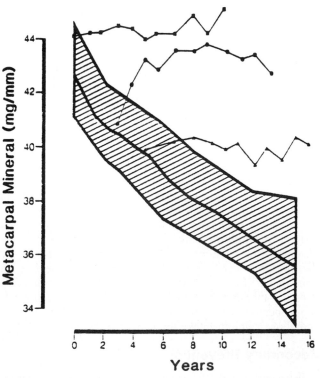

FIGURE 40–17 Changes in bone mass in placebo-treated patients (*hatched area:* mean ± SD) and in three groups of estrogen-treated patients. (From Lindsay R: Sex steroids in the pathogenesis and prevention of osteoporosis. *In* Riggs BL, Melton LJ III (eds): Osteoporosis—Etiology, Diagnosis and Management. New York, Raven, 1988, pp 333–358.)

For most adults, cutaneous vitamin D synthesis mediated by sun exposure, as well as a balanced diet, assures adequate vitamin D nutrition. There is no clear-cut evidence that vitamin D either contributes to peak bone mass formation or effectively reduces the rate of bone loss. There is no question, however, that adequate vitamin D intake is important for calcium absorption. Housebound or nutritionally deprived elderly people are particularly susceptible to vitamin D deficiency and may develop signs and symptoms of osteomalacia. The RDA for vitamin D is 400 IU/day although the current trend is to increase this to the range between 500 and 1000 IU/day.[119]

Weightbearing exercise can increase bone density and strength during growth and maturation and reduce bone loss with advancing age. Accumulated data so far indicate that exercise over many years can contribute to greater bone density. Recent studies suggest that even relatively short-term (i.e., 10–12 months) weightbearing exercise programs can enhance vertebral bone density among elderly people. Until further information is available about type, duration, and frequency of weightbearing exercise, walking three to four times weekly is a reasonable recommendation. Swimming does not satisfy weightbearing requirements and may not have the same effect on bones as walking or running.[3, 23, 66, 106, 127]

In an attempt to prevent fractures, one must design measures that aim at the prevention of falls, which increase with aging. The main factors leading to the tendency to fall are decline in vision or hearing, generalized decrease in muscle strength and coordination, loss of balance, presence of multiple chronic diseases, common use of sedatives, and consumption of alcohol. There are also numerous environmental hazards that contribute to the tendency to fall. Increasing home safety should be a part of the overall prevention program. The aim is to eliminate all factors that contribute to an unsafe home, and improvements should include the following: optimal lighting, elimination of slippery floor surfaces, and adequate hand supports in key home areas. Home visits by occupational therapists are the most efficient way of initiating improvements in home safety among the geriatric population. There are several ongoing clinical trials evaluating the efficacy of hip protection pads for the prevention of hip fractures in the very elderly.

TREATMENT OF OSTEOPOROSIS

Medical Therapy of Spinal Osteoporosis

Along with estrogens, calcitonin is the only pharmacological agent now approved in the United States for the treatment of osteoporosis. Calcitonin is a 32-amino acid protein produced by thyroid C cells. Several studies have demonstrated that calcitonin therapy decreases the rate of bone loss in osteoporotic patients. This was proved by DXA or single photon absorptiometry, as well as whole-body calcium analysis. Calcitonin works through the inhibition of bone resorption. The main disadvantage of calcitonin treatment is that it has to be given parenterally (subcutaneously). The usual dose is 50 to 100 IU/day, or every other day. Flushing and local irritation are common side effects.[44]

Sodium fluoride is the only agent known to increase bone mass. It stimulates bone formation independently of BMU function. The Food and Drug Administration (FDA), however, still has not approved sodium fluoride for general use owing to the lack of anti-fracture efficacy.[56, 113] In one epidemiological study a higher prevalence of fractures was found in regions with a higher fluoride content in the drinking water.[129] In a recently published study, when the dose of fluoride did not exceed 50 mg/day and the slow-release form was used, BMD of the spine went up about 5% with a reduction in the fracture rate of about 50%.[96] Calcium supplements should be added as well (i.e., 1000 mg Ca per day). The main side effects of sodium fluoride are nausea, gastrointestinal bleeding, and joint pains, all of which are dose-dependent.[24]

In 1979, Frost proposed coherence, or ADFR, therapy for osteoporosis (ADFR, *a*ctivate, *d*epress, *f*ree, *r*epeat).[36, 40] The basic principle of treatment is the sequential and intermittent administration of drugs that will bring into synchronization the bone areas that are otherwise in random phases of bone turnover. According to the ADFR theory, the remodeling process is first pharmacologically *activated* by an agent that initiates osteoclastic activity, then *depressed* with a second agent, and finally followed by a period *free* from treatment to allow osteoblasts to fill in the resorptive cavity. The cycle can then be *repeated* according to life cycles of bone cell lines. The agent used to activate BMUs is PTH (1–34 peptide) or oral phosphate as an indirect activator (i.e., secondary hyperparathyroidism). Etidronate disodium (diphosphonate) was used to suppress bone resorption. This treatment gave some excellent preliminary results in patients with spinal osteoporosis and seems to be promising.[132, 136] There are several ongoing clinical trials using second-generation diphosphonates as antiresorbing agents to prevent postmenopausal bone loss in elderly women, with positive preliminary results.[46, 110]

It has been shown that anabolic steroids (e.g., stanozolol) can prevent bone loss or actually increase bone mass. Unfortunately, they are associated with masculinization, with toxic liver effects if used orally, and with abnormality in lipid metabolism that can promote atherogenesis. The dose used was 2 mg three times daily for 3 weeks out of 4. They are not approved by the FDA for osteoporosis therapy.[18]

Rehabilitation of Patient with Spinal Osteoporosis

If a patient needs treatment for osteoporosis it indicates that bone has already been lost to the point of developing fractures. Acute compression fracture in the spine creates pain that lasts about 1 to 2 weeks and sometimes requires bed rest. Oral analgesics on a regular schedule can be initiated. Sometimes the application of local heat or cold can be of help. A transcutaneous electrical nerve stimulation (TENS) unit might also help in the treatment of chronic back pain secondary to spinal osteoporosis of the type II variety. After a 2-week period, ambulation should be initiated if possible. In some cases, a thoracic orthosis (perhaps the rigid shell type) should be prescribed. The main reason for the application of a thoracic orthosis is to prevent further fracture by limiting motion in the spine.

The period of time a patient should wear a spinal orthosis is still unknown. There is some evidence that spinal fracture can contribute to immobilization and that immobilization can further contribute to bone loss.[50] Therefore, back braces should not be prescribed for a long period of time. Lying on a flat surface for 30 min/day with a bath towel below the lumbar spine would help correct kyphosis and the loin pain that is the result of severe kyphosis.

Rehabilitation of Patient After Hip Fracture

The main goal is to prevent hip fractures rather than to treat the disease. When a fracture develops, the most common methods of treatment are internal fixation or Austin-Moore hemiarthroplasty. Sometimes debilitated patients who are at high risk for surgery require treatment by bed rest and traction, but they are at increased risk for developing pulmonary embolism, pneumonia, and pressure sores. The mortality in this group is substantially higher; therefore early operative management that increases mobility is widely practiced. After surgery, movement should begin relatively soon, when patients have recovered from anesthesia and all tubes and drains have been removed. Complications of surgical procedures are non-union, avascular necrosis, and infection, as well as failure of the device. Usually patients with hip fractures want to be able to enjoy quiet living, to be able to sit (90 degrees of hip flexion), to stand and walk (with some extension of the hips if possible), and to perform all kinds of activities of daily living. A much greater hip range of motion is desirable but not essential. To improve muscle strength, patients have to be encouraged to practice sitting, standing, and walking. The quadriceps, hamstrings, and gluteal muscles are the most important ones to increase and maintain strength. Adequate nutritional support is also essential in the rehabilitation program. Many patients with hip fractures are malnourished with low serum albumin levels indicating poor nutritional status. If osteomalacia is discovered, vitamin D therapy should be initiated.

SECONDARY OSTEOPOROSIS

There are many systemic and metabolic diseases that can cause bone loss in the whole skeleton (Table 40–6). These include Cushing's syndrome, hypogonadism, hyperthyroidism, and primary hyperparathyroidism. Hyperparathyroidism can cause excessive bone resorption and bone fractures, but currently with biochemical and other mass screening procedures (i.e., blood calcium), parathyroid bone disease is usually detected at a very early stage and bone fractures are uncommon. It is rare to see patients with hyperparathyroidism and compression fractures of the spine, because those patients primarily suffer from cortical bone loss.

Osteogenesis imperfecta of adult onset can sometimes mimic osteoporosis, but patients tend to have more fractures and they are relatively younger. Some of them have typical clinical features of the disease such as blue sclerae. Multiple myeloma is a relatively common condition that can mimic osteoporosis and should be ruled out by performing protein electrophoresis.

TABLE 40–6   Secondary Causes of Osteoporosis

Hormonal and metabolic disorders
   Hypogonadism
   Cushing's syndrome
   Hyperthyroidism
   Hyperparathyroidism
   Homocystinuria
Connective tissue disorders
   Osteogenesis imperfecta
   Ehlers-Danlos syndrome
Bone marrow diseases
   Multiple myeloma
Lymphoproliferative diseases
Mastocytosis
Immobilization/weightlessness
Medications
   Glucocorticoids
   Thyroid hormone (excessive dose)
   Long-term heparin therapy

Corticosteroid-Induced Osteoporosis

The most common form of secondary osteoporosis is corticosteroid-induced osteoporosis. It has long been recognized that supraphysiological doses of corticosteroids cause severe bone loss predominantly in trabecular bone, which is metabolically more active than cortical bone. As a result, compression deformities of the vertebrae, as well as pelvic bones, are very common. Corticosteroids decrease bone formation rate by depressing osteoblast function, but also increase bone resorption manifested by an increase in osteoclast number and resorption sites. There is a speculation that bone resorption activity is mediated by PTH because parathyroidectomy abolishes the osteoclastic response to steroids in laboratory animals. Malabsorption of calcium is another feature of corticosteroid therapy. It can cause secondary hyperparathyroidism and potentiate negative calcium balance. The exact mechanism of this is still unknown, but some data suggest that steroids might directly impair vitamin D metabolism or synthesis of carrier protein responsible for calcium transport in the gut. Discontinuous steroid therapy should be encouraged because recent animal studies suggest that alternate-day steroid application can produce less severe bone loss than daily treatments. The treatments also should be aimed at correcting calcium malabsorption and correcting secondary hyperparathyroidism. The patient should take vitamin D, 50,000 units three times weekly, as well as 500 to 1000 mg/day of calcium. Recent clinical trials with a new heterocyclic glucocorticoid, deflazacort, revealed that this steroid contains systemic anti-inflammatory potency that is equivalent to prednisone with relatively less adverse effect on calcium metabolism. In recent clinical studies, deflazacort did not induce to the full extent the metabolic features of secondary hyperparathyroidism. The study suggested that the skeletal effects of prednisone therapy are mediated, at least in part, by increased PTH activity and that deflazacort is less potent in this regard.[43, 74, 120]

Osteoporosis of Immobilization

Complete immobilization of the whole body or of an extremity leads to osteoporosis, either generalized or local. This condition was first described in patients who were immobilized for fractures, paraplegic patients, poliomyelitis patients, hemiplegic patients, and even normal subjects who volunteered to stay in bed for long periods of time.[29, 30, 95] Bone loss can be detected by classic radiological methods within 3 months of the onset of immobilization. The affected bone never recovers completely, even after the full restoration of movement. Studies using newer techniques of bone mass measurements, including single photon absorptiometry, dual photon absorptiometry of the spine, and histomorphometry of the iliac crest, showed that bone loss proceeds at about 4% per month during the initial phase of bed rest. Nonweightbearing bones such as the radius and bones of the hand demineralize at a much lower rate than do the weightbearing parts of the skeleton. This high degree of bone loss (4%) could be expected to be seen normally only in postmenopausal women over the 12-month period.

Patients with diffuse osteoporosis secondary to immobilization can lose up to 30% to 40% of their total bone over a relatively short period of time, which is almost the same as the loss in patients with primary involutional osteoporosis over a lifetime. After a substantial amount of bone has been lost, the rate of bone loss subsides, as in osteoporosis of the aging. Subjects with high initial bone mass lose more bone than those who start with less bone so that all immobilized patients eventually end up with much the same bone mass. PTH has been implicated in the pathogenesis of bone resorption secondary to immobilization, but PTH activity is being suppressed during the phase of acute immobilization secondary to increased level of blood calcium in extracellular fluid. Histological examination reveals a predominant number of osteoclastic bone resorption sites. Bone trabeculae become thin, but by about the fifth week of immobilization the bone tissue reaches a new steady state.

The main clinical presentation of bone loss due to immobilization is certainly the fracture. Bone that is osteoporotic from immobilization is more likely to fracture than normal bone, and it is therefore common for a fracture that has been treated by immobilization to be complicated by further fractures of the same limb when immobilization ceases. Usually, an osteoporotic limb does not cause tenderness, pain, or any other symptom except when fractured.

The abnormality in calcium metabolism is directly proportional to the amount of bone tissue immobilized. Similarly, in terms of BMUs, the abnormality is directly proportional to a number of those units present at a time in the immobilized bone. Patients in whom one extremity is paralyzed usually do not develop hypercalciuria or hypercalcemia, but quadriplegic patients, in general, develop significant hypercalciuria and mild hypercalcemia. This is more pronounced in young patients who became paralyzed during the bone modeling period than among the elderly. Also, it is well known that patients with Paget's disease develop hypercalcemia upon bed rest for any reason. The main explanation for this is the number of activated BMUs present in the immobilized skeleton. Normally, up to 2 million BMUs are working at a time, but this number is substantially higher in growing persons and in patients with Paget's disease. After acute immobilization, particularly in young persons, urine calcium can be increased for several weeks and may reach 600 to 800 mg/day before it returns

to normal. This hypercalciuria is not regularly reversed by mobilization of the patient.[104] Plasma calcium also rises, but malignant hypercalcemia is relatively rare (i.e., blood calcium >14 mg/100 mL). In the majority of patients, plasma calcium is within the normal range or is borderline-high. Plasma phosphate tends to be high with evidence of increased tubular absorption of phosphate. This probably indicates PTH suppression secondary to elevation in blood calcium despite a belief that PTH might be necessary for bone resorption. Immobilization could increase the sensitivity of bone to PTH action, but other local tissue factors might be involved. Hypercalciuria could facilitate kidney stone formation, but even in paraplegic patients the incidence of renal stones is not very high.[65] Kinetic studies show that during acute immobilization, the rate of bone resorption is two to three times higher than in normal persons.[49] Bone formation in this stage is also slightly elevated but cannot compensate for the rate of bone resorption. There is an imbalance in the coupling between bone formation and resorption. During the chronic phase, patients are back in calcium equilibrium and resorption; formation rates are close to normal.[49] This is also a time period when a substantial amount of bone tissue has been lost and the rate of bone loss declines.

So far, there is no satisfactory treatment for this type of osteoporosis. High calcium intake certainly is contradicted in patients who develop hypercalcemia because this can aggravate the symptoms of elevated blood calcium and can further increase calcium excretion in the urine leading to kidney stone formation. Phosphate, diphosphonates, and thiazide diuretics have been given in the hope of reducing the bone loss resulting from bed rest.[72] Several of these have diminished hypercalciuria, but none has been shown to reduce bone loss as judged by photon absorptiometry. Some studies indicated that passive movement on a tilting table could reduce urinary calcium, but other studies have suggested that active muscular action is required to counteract the resorption process.

Early mobilization of disabled patients certainly might help in reversing the trend of bone loss and substantially decrease the incidence of osteoporosis in this population (see Chapter 34).

LOCALIZED OSTEOPOROSIS

Among the localized osteoporotic conditions, the most common are reflex sympathetic dystrophy (Sudeck's bone atrophy) and transient regional osteoporosis.

Reflex Sympathetic Dystrophy

Reflex sympathetic dystrophy is a clinical entity with numerous synonyms that all describe a disorder of either the upper or lower extremities characterized by neuromuscular disturbances and dystrophic changes of the skin, subcutaneous tissues, bones, and joints. The disease is also known as the shoulder-hand syndrome in the upper limb or post-traumatic osteoporosis (Sudeck's bone atrophy). The main clinical characteristics of this condition are local pain and tenderness, swelling, decreased range of motion, increased redness and vasomotor instability, trophic skin changes, and localized osteoporosis.

The disease usually goes through different stages. Stage I (acute form) lasts a few weeks to 6 months. The patients have pain, decreased range of motion, and redness in the involved extremity. The skin may be hyperesthetic and tender. At this point it is not possible to see evidence of osteoporosis based on radiographic examination. Stage II follows and lasts another 3 to 6 months. The swelling decreases, but stiffness and decreased range of motion become more pronounced. There is also atrophy of subcutaneous tissue and muscles. Early signs of contractures are seen as well. An x-ray film usually shows localized patchy osteoporosis. In stage III, which lasts for months and goes on to irreversible alterations, the features are progressive atrophy of skin, muscle, bone, and joints. Pain may be decreased but there is a severe reduction in the range of motion. At this time, blood flow to the extremity is diminished, as is the skin temperature. Radiography shows diffuse osteoporosis with spotted decalcification. During the stage of bone resorption and skeletal demineralization, increased numbers of osteoclasts can be seen lining the resorption holes. This indicates that there might be bone resorption mediated by osteoclasts. Biochemical stimuli that trigger bone resorption are not known.

The majority of patients with reflex sympathetic dystrophy have had trauma as the initiating cause, cerebrovascular accident with hemiplegia, myocardial infarction, or cervical disc disease. In some cases the disease begins without any underlying recognizable cause. For almost a century, this condition has been attributed to an abnormality in sympathetic nerve discharge.

Diagnosis of reflex sympathetic dystrophy is usually made by clinical observation. A bone scan could be helpful because it can show increased uptake in the involved extremity. For the hand, this means increased uptake in carpal and metacarpal joints. In the later stage of the disease and after 3 months, radiographic changes in the form of cortical subperiosteal resorption can be seen. Bone density analysis using single photon absorptiometry also reveals a substantial amount of bone loss.[10, 33, 41, 69, 103]

In the acute phase, the majority of patients respond to systemic corticosteroids. Usually larger doses up to 100 mg/day are started and tapered over a 10-day to 2-week period. Sometimes nonsteroidal anti-inflammatory agents or local application of heat is of help. Recently, a few European studies showed beneficial effects of intravenous diphosphonates as well as application of calcitonin treatment of more chronic bone atrophy.[28] Intravenous diphosphonates probably block bone resorption by adsorption to calcium phosphate crystals. Calcitonin blocks bone resorption and treats the pain secondary to endogenous secretion of endorphins in the brain.[42] Stellate ganglion blocks may also be helpful.

Transient Regional Osteoporosis

This is a relatively uncommon condition. The disease is characterized by localized migratory osteoporosis involving one of several joints with predominance of hip involvement. The disease is usually self-limiting and lasts up to 6 to 9 months. The diagnosis is based on clinical observations, radiographic changes, and increased radioisotope uptake on the bone scan. The diagnosis is also one of exclusion. Conditions such as osteomyelitis, collagen disorders (e.g., rheumatoid arthritis), and cancer metastasis must be ruled out. The cause of this condition is not known. There is a possibility that this is also a form of reflex sympathetic dystrophy.[7, 68]

Management of transient regional osteoporosis is determined by the severity of pain and disability with the goal of maintaining some use of the involved part until the disease resolves spontaneously. Some patients respond to nonsteroidal anti-inflammatory agents or other pain medications. Use of oral corticosteroids has been rapidly effective in the majority of patients. Again, relatively large doses are started and tapered over a 7- to 10-day period. Physical therapy measures should be consistent with joint protection with slow initiation of gradual ambulation.

Acknowledgments

This work was supported in part by research grants NIH RO1 AR40736, NIH-GCRC MOI-RR00034, and NRICGP/USDA 92-37200-7586.

References

1. Aaron JE, Gallagher JC, Anderson J, Nordin BEC: Frequency of osteomalacia and osteoporosis in fractures of the proximal femur. *Lancet* 1974; 1:229–233.
2. Aloia JF, Cohn SH, Bab T, et al: Skeletal mass and bony composition in marathon runners. *Metabolism* 1978; 27:1793–1796.
3. Aloia JF, Cohn SH, Ostuni JA, et al: Prevention of involutional bone loss by exercise. *Ann Intern Med* 1978; 89:356–358.
4. Aloia JF, Ransulo P, Deftos L, et al: Exercise-induced hypercalcemia and the calciotropic hormones. J Lab Clin Med 1985; 106:229–232.
5. Aloia JF, Vaswani A, Yeh JK, et al: Calcium supplementation with and without hormone replacement therapy to prevent postmenopausal bone loss. Ann Intern Med 1994; 120:97–103.
6. Arlot M, Edouard C, Meunier PJ, et al: Impaired osteoblast function in osteoporosis: Comparison between calcium balance and dynamic histomorphometry. BMJ 1984; 289:517–520.
7. Arnstein RA: Regional osteoporosis. Orthop Clin North Am 1972; 3:585–600.
8. Astrom J, Ahnquist S, Beertema J, Jonsson B: Physical activity in women sustaining fracture of the neck of the femur. J Bone Joint Surg Br 1987; 69:381–383.
9. Bassett CAL: Biologic significance of piezo-electricity. Calcif Tissue Res 1968; 1:252–272.
10. Bekerman C, Genant HK, Hoffer PB, et al: Radionuclide imaging of the bones and joints of the hand. Radiology 1975; 118:653–659.
11. Bijvoet OLM: Kidney function in calcium and phosphate metabolism. *In* Avioli LV, Krane SM (eds): Metabolic Bone Disease, vol 1. New York, Academic Press, 1977.
12. Broadus A, Mahaffey JE, Bartter FC, Neer RM: Nephrogenous cyclic AMP as a parathyroid function test. J Clin Invest 1977; 60:771–783.
13. Brown JP, Malaval L, Chapuy MC, et al: Serum BGP: A specific marker for bone formation in postmenopausal osteoporosis. Lancet 1984; 1:1091–1093.
14. Cann CE: Quantitative CT for determination of bone mineral density: A review. Radiology 1988; 166:509–522.
15. Chalmers J, Ho CK: Geographical variations in senile osteoporosis. J Bone Joint Surg Br 1970; 52:667–675.
16. Chan GM, Hoffman K, McMurray M: The effect of dietary calcium supplementation on pubertal girls growth and bone mineral status. J Bone Miner Res 1991; 6S:625.
17. Chapuy MC, Arlot ME, Duboeuf F, et al: Vitamin D and calcium to prevent hip fractures in elderly women. N Engl J Med 1992; 327:1637–1642.
18. Chesnut CH, Ivey JL, Gruber HE, et al: Stanozolol in postmenopausal osteoporosis: Therapeutic efficacy and possible mechanism of action. Metabolism 1983; 32:571–580.
19. Christian JC, Slemenda C, Johnston CC: Heritability of adult bone density and the loss of bone mass in aging male twins. J Bone Miner Res 1988; 3:587S.

20. Crilly RG, Francis FM, Nordin BC: Steroid hormones, aging and bone. Clin Endocrinol Metab 1981; 10:115–139.

21. Cummings S: Are patients with hip fractures more osteoporotic? Am J Med 1985; 78:487–494.

22. Cummings SR, Kelsey JL, Nevitt MC, O'Dowd KJ: Epidemiology of osteoporosis and osteoporotic fractures. Epidemiol Rev 1985; 7:178–208.

23. Dalsky GP, Stocke KS, Ehsani A, et al: Weight bearing exercise training and lumbar spine bone mineral content in postmenopausal women. Ann Intern Med 1988; 108:824–828.

24. Dambacher MA, Ittner J, Ruegsegger P: Long term fluoride therapy of postmenopausal osteoporosis. Bone 1986; 7:199–205.

25. Dawson-Hughes B, Dallal GE, Krall EA, et al: A controlled trial of the effect of calcium supplementation on bone density in postmenopausal women. N Engl J Med 1990; 323:878–883.

26. Delmas PD: Markers of bone formation and resorption. *In* Favus MJ (ed): Primer on the Metabolic Bone Diseases and Disorders of Mineral Metabolism, ed 2. New York, Raven Press, 1993, pp 108–112.

27. DeVernejoul MC, Bielakoff J, Herve J, et al: Evidence for defective osteoblastic function. A role for alcohol and tobacco consumption in osteoporosis in middle age men. Clin Orthop 1983; 179:107–115.

28. Devogelaer JP, Dall'Armellino S, Huaux JP, Nagant deDeuxchaisnes C: Dramatic improvement of intractable reflex sympathetic dystrophy syndrome by intravenous infusions of the second generation bifosphonate APD. J Bone Miner Res 1988, 3:213S.

29. Dietnck JE, Whedon GD, Shorr E: Effects of immobilization upon various metabolic and physiologic functions of normal men. Am J Med 1948; 4:3–36.

30. Donaldson CL, Hulley SB, Vogel JM, et al: Effect of prolonged bed rest on bone mineral. Metabolism 1970; 19:1071–1084.

31. Drinkwater BL, Nilson K, Chesnut CH, et al: Bone mineral content of amenorrheic and eumenorrheic athletes. N Engl J Med 1984; 311:277–281.

32. Eriksen EF, Berg NJ, Graham ML, et al: Evidence of estrogen receptors in human bone cells. J Bone Miner Res 1987; 2:238S.

33. Escobar PL: Reflex sympathetic dystrophy. Orthop Rev 1986; 15:41–46.

34. Ettinger B, Genant HK, Cann CE: Long term oestrogen replacement therapy prevents bone loss and fractures. Ann Intern Med 1985; 102:319–324.

35. Ettinger B, Genant HK, Cann CE: Postmenopausal bone loss is prevented by treatment with low-dosage estrogen with calcium. Ann Intern Med 1987; 106:40–45.

36. Frost HM: The ADFR concept revisited, editorial. Calcif Tissue Int 1984; 36:349–353.

37. Frost HM: Bone Remodeling and Its Relationship to Metabolic Bone Disease. Springfield, Ill, Charles C Thomas, 1973.

38. Frost HM: Mechanical microdamage, bone remodeling, and osteoporosis: A review. *In* DeLuca HE, Frost HM, Jee WSS, et al (eds): Osteoporosis: Recent Advances in Pathogenesis and Treatment. Baltimore. University Park Press, 1981, pp 185–190.

39. Frost HM: Tetracycline based histological analysis of bone remodeling. Calcif Tissue Res 1969; 3:221–237.

40. Frost HM: Treatment of osteoporosis by manipulation of coherent bone cell populations. Clin Orthop 1979; 143:227–244.

41. Genant HK, Kozin F, Bekerman C, et al: The reflex sympathetic dystrophy syndrome. Radiology 1975; 117:21–32.

42. Gennari C, Bocchi L, Orso CA, et al: The analgesic effect of calcitonin in active Paget's disease of bone and in metastatic bone disease. Orthopedics 1984; 7:1449–1452.

43. Gennari C, Imbimbo B, Montagnani M, et al: Effects of prednisone and deflazacort on mineral metabolism and parathyroid hormone activity in humans. Calcif Tissue Int 1984; 36:245–252.

44. Gruber HE, Ivey JL, Baylink DJ, et al: Long term calcitonin therapy in postmenopausal osteoporosis. Metabolism 1984; 33:295–303.

45. Hanson DA, Weis MAE, Bollen AM, et al: A specific immunoassay for monitoring human bone resorption: Quantitation of type I collagen cross-linked N-telopeptides in urine. J Bone Miner Res 1992; 7:1251–1258.

46. Harris ST, Gertz BJ, Genant HK, et al: The effect of short term treatment with alendronate on vertebral density and biochemical markers of bone remodeling in early postmenopausal women. J Clin Endocrinol Metab 1993; 76:1399–1406.

47. Heaney RP: Calcium intake and bone health in the adult. A critical review of recent investigations. Clin Appl Nutr 1992; 2:10–29.

48. Heaney RP: A unified concept of osteoporosis. Am J Med 1965; 39:877–880.

49. Heaney RP: Radiocalcium metabolism in disuse osteoporosis in man. Am J Med 1962; 33:188–200.

50. Heaney RP, Avioli LV, Chesnut C, et al: Is bone the cause of osteoporotic fracture or its consequence? J Bone Miner Res 1988; 3:79S.

51. Heaney RP, Recker RR: Effect of nitrogen, phosphorus, and caffeine on calcium balance in women. J Lab Clin Med 1982; 99:46–55.

52. Hodges SJ, Pilkington MJ, Stamp TCB, et al: Depressed levels of circulating menaquinones in patients with osteoporotic fractures of the spine and femoral neck. Bone 1991; 12:387–389.

53. Hu JF, Zhao XH, Jia JB, et al: Dietary calcium and bone density among middle-aged and elderly women in China. Am J Clin Nutr 1993; 58:219–227.

54. Hutchinson TA, Polansky SM, Feinstein AR: Postmenopausal estrogens protect against fractures of hip and distal radius. Lancet 1979; 2:705–709.

55. Ilich JZ, Tzagournis MA, Hsieh LC, et al: Determinants of urinary calcium excretion in young females. J Bone Miner Res 1993; 8:S252.

56. Jacobsen SJ, Goldberg J, Miles TP, et al: Regional variation in the incidence of hip fracture. JAMA 1990; 264:500–502.

57. Jensen J, Christiansen C, Rodbro P: Cigarette smoking, serum estrogens and bone loss during hormone replacement therapy early after menopause. N Engl J Med 1985; 313:973–975.

58. Jilca RL, Hangoc G, Girasole G, et al: Increased osteoclast development after estrogen loss: Mediation by interleukin-6. Science 1992; 257:88–91.

59. Johnston CC, Melton LJ: Bone density measurement and the management of osteoporosis. *In* Favus MJ (ed): Primer on the Metabolic Bone Diseases and Disorders of Mineral Metabolism, ed 2. New York, Raven Press, 1993, pp 137–146.

60. Johnston CC Jr, Miller JZ, Slemenda CW, et al: Calcium supplementation and increases in bone mineral density in children. N Engl J Med 1992; 327:82–87.

61. Kaplan FS: Osteoporosis. Clin Symp 1983; 35:5.

62. Kim Y, Linkswiler H: Effect of level of protein intake on calcium metabolism and on parathyroid and reuse function in the adult human male. J Nutr 1979; 109:399–404.

63. Kleerekoper M, Brienza R, Schultz L, Johnson C: Oral contraceptive use may protect against low bone mass. Arch Intern Med 1991; 151:1971–1976.

64. Kleerekoper M, Frame B, Villanueva RA, et al: Treatment of osteoporosis with sodium fluoride alternating with calcium and vitamin D. *In* DeLuca HF, Frost HM, Jee W, et al (eds): Osteoporosis: Recent Advances in Pathogenesis and Treatment. Baltimore, University Park Press, 1981, pp 441–448.

65. Kohli A, Latnid S: Risk factors for renal stone formation in patients with spinal cord injury. Br J Urol 1986; 58:588–591.

66. Krolner B, Toft B, Pors Nielson S, Tondevold E: Physical exercise as prophylaxis against involutional vertebral bone loss: A controlled trial. Clin Sci 1983; 64:541–546.

67. Krook L, Whalen JP, Lesser GV, Lutwak L: Human periodontal disease and osteoporosis. Cornell Vet 1972; 62:32–52.

68. Lakhampal S, Ginsberg WW, Luthra H, Hunoler GG: Transient regional osteoporosis. Ann Intern Med 1987; 106:144–450.

69. Lenggenhager K: Sudeck's osteodystrophy. Minn Med 1971; 54:967–972.

70. Lindsay R, Hart DM, Forrest C, Baird C: Prevention of spinal osteoporosis in oophorectomized women. Lancet 1980; 2:1151–1154.

71. Lloyd T, Andon MB, Rollings N, et al: Calcium supplementation and bone mineral density in adolescent girls. JAMA 1993; 270:841–844.

72. Lockwood DR, Vogel JM, Schneider VS, Hulley SF: The effect of the diphosphonate EHDP on bone metabolism during prolonged bed rest. J Clin Endocrinol Metab 1975; 41:533–561.

73. Love RR, Mazess RB, Barden HS, et al: Effects of tamoxifen on bone mineral density in postmenopausal women with breast cancer. N Engl J Med 1992; 326:852–856.

74. Lukert BP, Raisz LG: Glucocorticoid-induced osteoporosis: Pathogenesis and management. Ann Intern Med 1990; 112:352–364.

75. Matkovic V: Calcium intake and peak bone mass, editorial. N Engl J Med 1992; 327:119–120.

76. Matkovic V: Calcium metabolism and calcium requirements during

skeletal modeling and consolidation of bone mass. Am J Clin Nutr 1991; 54:245S–260S.

77. Matkovic V, Ciganovic M, Tominac C, Kostial K: Osteoporosis and epidemiology of fractures in Croatia: An international comparison. Henry Ford Hosp Med J 1980; 28:116–126.

78. Matkovic VD, Fontana C, Tominac P, et al: Factors which influence peak bone mass formation: A study of calcium balance and the inheritance of bone mass in adolescent females. Am J Clin Nutr 1990; 52:878–888.

79. Matkovic V, Heaney RP: Calcium balance during human growth: Evidence for threshold behavior. Am J Clin Nutr 1992; 55:992–996.

80. Matkovic V, Hsieh L, Andon MB, Ilich JZ: Skeletal calcium accretion as determined by balance technique and dual energy x-ray absorptiometry of the total body. J Bone Miner Res 1993; 8:S253.

81. Matkovic V, Ilich JZ: Calcium requirements during growth: Are the current standards adequate? Nutr Rev 1993; 51:171–180.

82. Matkovic V, Jelic T, Wardlaw GM, et al: Timing of peak bone mass in Caucasian females and its implications for the prevention of osteoporosis. Inference from a cross-sectional model. J Clin Invest 1994; 93:799–808.

83. Matkovic V, Kostial K, Simonovic I, et al: Bone status and fracture rates in two regions of Yugoslavia. Am J Clin Nutr 1979; 32:540–549.

84. Matkovic V, Kostial K, Simonovic I, et al: Influence of calcium intake, age and sex on bone. Calcif Tissue Res 1977; 22S:393–396.

85. Mazess RB: The noninvasive measurement of skeletal mass. In Peck WA (ed): Bone and Mineral Research Annual 1. Amsterdam, Excerpt Medica, 1983, pp 223–279.

86. Meunier PJ, Sellami S, Briancon D, Edouard C: Histological heterogeneity of apparently idiopathic osteoporosis. In DeLuca HF, Frost HM, Jee WSS (eds): Osteoporosis: Recent Advances in Pathogenesis and Treatment. Baltimore, University Park Press, 1980, p 321.

87. Minkin C: Bone acid phosphatase: Tartrate-resistant acid phosphatase as a marker of osteoclast function. Calcif Tissue Int 1982; 34:285–290.

88. Morrison NA, Qi JC, Tokita A, et al: Prediction of bone density from vitamin D receptor alleles. Nature 1994; 367:284–287.

89. Morrison NA, Yeoman R, Kelly PJ, Eisman JA: Contribution of trans-acting factor alleles to normal physiological variability: Vitamin D receptor gene polymorphism and circulating osteocalcin. Proc Natl Acad Sci USA 1992; 89:6665–6669.

90. Nicar MJ, Pak CYC: Calcium absorption from calcium carbonate and calcium citrate. J Clin Endocrinol Metab 1985; 61:391–393.

91. Nilsson BE, Westlin NE: Bone density in athletes. Clin Orthop 1971; 77:179–182.

92. Nordin BEC: Assessment of calcium excretion from the urinary calcium creatinine ratio. Lancet 1959; 2:368.

93. Nordin BEC: The definition and diagnosis of osteoporosis. Calcif Tissue Int 1987; 40:57–58.

94. Nordin BEC, Need AG, Morris HA, Horowitz M: The nature and significance of the relationship between urinary sodium and urinary calcium in women. J Nutr 1993; 123:1615–1622.

95. Osteoporosis and activity. Lancet 1983; 2:1365–1366.

96. Pak CYC, Sakhaee K, Piziak V, et al: Slow-release sodium fluoride in the management of postmenopausal osteoporosis. A randomized controlled trial. Ann Intern Med 1994; 120:625–632.

97. Parfitt AM: The action of parathyroid hormone on bone. Metabolism 1976; 25:809–844.

98. Parfitt AM: The cellular basis of bone remodeling: The quantum concept reexamined in light of recent advances in the cell biology of bone. Calcif Tissue Int 1984; 36:37.

99. Parfitt AM: Quantum concept of bone remodeling and turnover: Implications for the pathogenesis of osteoporosis. Calcif Tissue Int 1979; 28:1–5.

100. Parfitt AM: Trabecular bone architecture in pathogenesis and prevention of fracture. Am J Med 1987; 82:68–72.

101. Parfitt AM, Mathews C, Rao D, et al: Impaired osteoblast function in metabolic bone disease. In DeLuca HF, Frost HM, Jee WSS, et al (eds): Osteoporosis—Recent Advances in Pathogenesis and Treatment. Baltimore, University Park Press. 1981, pp 321–330.

102. Payne RB, Little AJ, Williams RB, Milner JR: Interpretation of serum calcium in patients with abnormal serum proteins. Br Med J 1973; 4:643–646.

103. Plewes LW: Sudeck's atrophy in the hand. J Bone Joint Surg Br 1956; 38:195–203.

104. Plum F, Dunning MF: The effect of therapeutic mobilization on hypercalciuria following acute poliomyelitis. Arch Intern Med 1958; 101:528–536.

105. Pocock NA, Eisman JA, Hopper JL, et al: Genetic determinants of bone mass in adults: A twin study. J Clin Invest 1987; 80:706–710.

106. Pocock NA, Eisman JA, Yeates MG, et al: Physical fitness is a major determinant of femoral neck and lumbar spine bone mineral density. J Clin Invest 1986; 78:618–621.

107. Price PA, Parthemore JG, Deftos J: New biochemical marker for bone metabolism. Measurement by radioimmunoassay of bone GLA protein in the plasma of normal subjects and patients with bone disease. J Clin Invest 1980; 66:878–883.

108. Rao SD, Matkovic V, Duncan H: Transiliac bone biopsy. Complications and diagnostic value. Henry Ford Hosp Med J 1980; 8:112–115.

109. Recker RR: Calcium absorption and achlorhydria. N Engl J Med 1985; 313:70–73.

110. Reginster JY, Deroisy R, Denis D, et al: Prevention of postmenopausal bone loss by tiludronate. Lancet 1989; 2:1469–1471.

111. Reid IR, Ames RW, Evans MC, et al: Effect of calcium supplementation on bone loss in postmenopausal women. N Engl J Med 1993; 328:460–464.

112. Riggs BL, Wahner H, Dunn W, et al: Differential changes in bone mineral density of the appendicular and axial skeleton with aging: Relationship to spinal osteoporosis. J Clin Invest 1981; 67:328–335.

113. Riggs BL, Hodgson SF, O'Fallon WM, et al: Effect of fluoride treatment on the fracture rate in postmenopausal women with osteoporosis. N Engl J Med 1990; 322:802–809.

114. Riggs BL, Melton LF: Involutional osteoporosis. N Engl J Med 1986; 314:1676–1677.

115. Riggs BL, Peck WA, Bell NH: Physician's Resource Manual on Osteoporosis: A Decision-Making Guide, ed 2. Washington, DC, National Osteoporosis Foundation, 1991, pp 1–38.

116. Riggs BL, Wahner HW: Bone densitometry and clinical decision-making in osteoporosis, editorial. Ann Intern Med 1988; 108:293–295.

117. Riggs BL, Wahner HW, Melton LJ, et al: Rates of bone loss in the appendicular and axial skeletons of women. J Clin Invest 1986; 77:1487–1491.

118. Riis B, Thomsen K, Christiansen C: Does calcium supplementation prevent postmenopausal bone loss? A double-blind, controlled study. N Engl J Med 1987; 316:173–177.

119. Salamone LM, Dallal GE, Zantos D, et al: Contributions of vitamin D intake and seasonal sunlight exposure to plasma 25-hydroxyvitamin D concentration in elderly women. Am J Clin Nutr 1993; 58:80–86.

120. Sambrook PN, Birmingham J, Kelly PJ, et al: Prevention of corticosteroid induced osteoporosis: A comparison of calcium, calcitriol, and calcitonin. N Engl J Med 1993; 328:1747–1752.

121. Sandler RB: Muscle strength and skeletal competence: Implications for early prophylaxis. Calcif Tissue Int 1988; 42:281–283.

122. Saville PD: Changes in bone mass with age and alcoholism. J Bone Joint Surg Am 1965; 47:492–499.

123. Saville PD: Observations on 80 women with osteoporotic spine fractures. In Barzel U (ed): Osteoporosis. New York, Grune & Stratton, 1970.

124. Seeman E, Bach L, Cooper M: Bone mass in offspring of patients with osteoporosis. N Engl J Med 1989; 320:554–558.

125. Sinaki M, McPhee MC, Hodgson SF, et al: Relationship between bone mineral density of spine and strength of back extensors in healthy postmenopausal women. Mayo Clin Proc 1986; 61:116–122.

126. Smith D, Nancy W, Won Kang K, et al: Genetic factors in determining bone mass. J Clin Invest 1973; 52:2800–2808.

127. Snow-Harter C, Whalen R, Myburgh K, et al: Bone mineral density, muscle strength, and recreational exercise in men. J Bone Miner Res 1992; 7:1291–1296.

128. Sorenson JA, Hanson JA, Mazess RB: Precision and accuracy of dual energy x-ray absorptiometry. J Bone Miner Res 1988; 3:230S.

129. Sowers MFR, Clark MC, Jannausch ML, Wallace RB: A prospective study of bone mineral content and fracture in communities with differential fluoride exposure. Am J Epidemiol 1991; 133:649–660.

130. Sowers MF, Corton G, Shapiro B, et al: Bone density and bone turnover with long-term lactation. JAMA 1993; 269:3130–3135.

131. Stein JA, Waltham MA, Lazewatsdy JL, Hochberg AM: Dual energy x-ray bone densitometer incorporating an internal reference system. Radiology 1987; 165P:313.

132. Storm T, Thamsborg G, Steiniche T, et al: Effect of intermittent cyclical etidronate therapy on bone mass and fracture rate in women with postmenopausal osteoporosis. N Engl J Med 1990; 322:1265–1271.

133. Tilyard MW, Spears GFS, Thomson J, Dovey S: Treatment of postmenopausal osteoporosis with calcitriol or calcium. N Engl J Med 1992; 326:357–362.

134. Trotter M, Hixon B: Sequential changes in weight, density, and percentage ash weight of human skeletons from an early fetal period through old age. Anat Rec 1974; 179:1–18.

135. Tylavsky FA, Bortz AD, Hancock RL, Anderson JJB: Familial resemblance of radial bone mass between premenopausal mothers and their college-age daughters. Calcif Tissue Int 1989; 45:265–272.

136. Watts NB, Harris ST, Genant HK, et al: Intermittent cyclical etidronate treatment of postmenopausal osteoporosis. N Engl J Med 1990; 323:73–79.

137. Weinstein MC: Estrogen use in postmenopausal women—costs, risks, and benefits. N Engl J Med 1980; 303:308–316.

138. Weinstein RS, Bell NH: Diminished rates of bone formation in normal black adults. N Engl J Med 1988; 319:1698–1701.

139. Weiss NS, Ure CL, Ballard JH, et al: Decreased risk of fractures of the hip and lower forearm with postmenopausal use of estrogen. N Engl J Med 1980; 303:1195–1198.

Chronic Pain Syndromes: Evaluation and Treatment

**MARTIN GRABOIS, M.D.,
MICHAEL T. McCANN, M.D.,
DONNA SCHRAMM, M.D.,
ALEXANDER STRAJA, M.D.,
AND KEVIN SMITH, M.D.**

Chronic pain is difficult and frustrating to manage, and patients who experience it are often viewed as being undesirable.[31] We in the field of physical medicine and rehabilitation, however, frequently work with these patients. The approach we advocate for these patients is one that is interdisciplinary and comprehensive.

This chapter covers the basic principles of chronic pain, the concept of pain clinics, the evaluation and treatment of chronic pain, and the results to be expected with appropriate treatment.

DEFINITION

Perhaps the best way to define chronic pain is to compare and contrast it with acute pain (Table 41–1). Chronic pain syndrome is an abnormal condition in which pain is no longer a symptom of tissue injury, but in which pain and pain behavior become the primary disease processes.[79] Chronic pain syndrome is distinct from chronically or intermittently painful disease in which the patient experiences pain but manifests function and behavior appropriate to the degree of tissue injury. In chronic pain syndrome, subjective and behavioral manifestations of pain persist beyond objective evidence of tissue injury. Chronically painful conditions can lead to chronic pain syndrome, but not all persons with chronically painful conditions manifest chronic pain behavior and disability. Some of the conditions that can cause chronic pain are listed in Table 41–2.[4, 84]

In chronic pain the original causes are often blurred by subsequent complications of multiple procedures, compensation factors, medication dependency, inactivity, and psychosocial behavior changes[10] (Fig. 41–1). The Brena and

Chapman model (Fig. 41–2) takes into account the chronicity and behavioral components in a nociceptive spectrum.[13]

EPIDEMIOLOGY

Bonica[10] distinguishes chronic pain from chronic pain syndrome. From knowledge about the incidence of chronically painful disease, he extrapolates the number of persons who develop chronic pain syndrome and estimates that one third of all Americans have a chronically painful condition (including headache, back pain, and degenerative joint disease). Of these persons he notes that 50% to 60% are partially or totally disabled by pain, either transiently or permanently.[10] It is estimated that annually in the United States approximately $79 billion is spent on healthcare, Workers' Compensation, and litigation, and 40 million visits to the doctor are due to chronically painful conditions.[10]

TABLE 41–1 Acute vs. Chronic Pain

Acute	Chronic
Physicians trained in evaluation and diagnosis	Physician typically less interested and less trained
Short evaluation and treatment course	Long evaluation and treatment course
Pain is a biological symptom	Pain is a disease
Pain plus anxiety	Pain plus depression
Medications as needed	Non-narcotic analgesics, antidepressants preferred
Little addiction concern	Polyaddiction concern
Diagnosis straightforward	Diagnosis complex
Cure likely	Cure usually not achieved

Adapted from Grabois M: Chronic pain. Evaluation and treatment. *In* Goodgold J (ed): Rehabilitation Medicine. St Louis, Mosby–Year Book, 1988.

TABLE 41–2   Diagnoses Characterized by Intermittent, Recurrent, or Chronic Pain

Afferent Loss Syndromes
Diabetic mononeuropathy
Diabetic polyneuropathy
Nerve root avulsion
Central poststroke pain
Phantom pain
Postherpetic neuralgia
Ramsey-Hunt syndrome of the
    seventh cranial nerve
 	
Headache
Classic migraine
Common migraine
Complicated migraine
Cluster headache
Ophthalmoplegic migraine
Hemiplegic migraine
Lower-half headache (atypical
    facial neuralgia)
Tension
Combined
Psychogenic
Nonmigrainous vascular
Dialysis headache
Hypertension headache
Rheumatoid atlantoaxial arthritis
    headache
Traction headache
Temporomandibular joint
    headache
Vasculitic
Cranial neuralgic
Post-traumatic
Ocular headache
Tolosa-Hunt syndrome
 	
Causalgia
Causalgia
Sympathetic dystrophy
 	
Low Back Pain
Psychosomatic
Psychogenic
Modified behavior with or without
    organic disease
Low back pain with radiation to
    leg
	Low Back Pain Continued
	Mechanical low back pain
	Bilateral radicular pain
	Facet arthropathy
	Metabolic disorders (rare)
	Osteoarthritis
	Fibrositis
	Myofascial pain
	Extra-articular pain sources
	
	Failed Back Syndrome
	Persistent disc herniation
	Lateral stenosis
	Central stenosis
	Arachnoiditis
	Epidural fibrosis
	Instability
	
	***Erectile Dysfunction and Male
	Genital Pain***
	Referred pain from kidney or
	    ureter
	Referred pain from kidney,
	    ureter, psoas, retroperitoneal
	    mass, cauda mass
	Bladder obstruction
	Prostatic causes
	Prostatic inflammation
	Prostatodynia
	Urethral pain
	Urethral stricture, infection
	Testicular causes
	Testicular trauma or infection
	Testicular cancer
	Testicular torsion
	Intermittent testicular torsion
	Torsion of testicular appendage
	Testicular pain of polyarthritis
	    nodosa
	Epididymo-orchitis
	Orchialgia with negative
	    examination
	Cellulitis of the scrotum
	Varicocele
	Phimosis and paraphimosis
	Peyronie's disease
	Penile prosthesis pain
	Priapism, balanitis, penile cancer
		***Erectile Dysfunction and Male
		    Genital Pain*** Continued
		Penile pain after vasectomy
		Anal fistula
		Pelvic floor tension myalgia
		Scar entrapment of ilioinguinal
		    nerve
		Illioinguinal, genitofemoral,
		    iliohypogastric neuralgia
		
		Painful Neuropathies
		Guillian-Barré syndrome
		Chronic inflammatory
		    demyelinating neuropathy
		Porphyric polyneuropathy
		Alcoholic polyneuropathy
		Toxic, drug-related neuropathy
		AIDS sensory neuropathy
		Diabetic polyneuropathy
		Mononeuritis multiplex
		Cryoglobulin neuropathy
		Brachial neuritis
		Lateral femoral cutaneous
		    entrapment
		Other entrapment neuropathies
		Amyloidosis
		Tic douloureux (trigeminal
		    neuralgia)
		Glossopharyngeal neuralgia
		Dorsal root ganglionopathy
		
		Facial Pain
		Trigeminal neuralgia
		Glossopharyngeal neuralgia
		Nervus intermedius neuralgia
		    (Ramsey-Hunt syndrome)
		Sphenopalatine neuralgia
		Paratrigeminal neuralgia
		Vidian
		Atypical face pain
		Sinus disease
		Carotiditis
		Hyoid bone syndrome
		Temporal tendonitis
		Temporomandibular dysfunction
		    pain syndrome
			Joint Pain
			Rheumatoid arthritis
			Other systemic inflammatory
			    disease
			Autoimmune disorders
			Rheumatic fever
			Infectious arthritis
			    Granulomatous
			Crystal arthritides
			
			***Painful Metabolic Bone
			Disease***
			Osteomalacia
			Osteoporosis
			Hyperparathyroidism
			Renal osteodystrophy
			Paget's disease
			
			Cancer Pain
			
			Cervical Spine Pain
			Spinal cord compression
			Extrinsic spinal cord
			    compression
			Osteoarthritis
			Cervical spondylosis
			Cervical radiculitis
			Syringomyelia
			Cervical trauma
			Rheumatic atlantoaxial
			Ankylosis spondylitis infection
			
			Gynecological Pain
			Ectopic pregnancy
			Uterine causes: dysmenorrhea
			Adenomyosis
			Benign tumors: leiomyoma
			Malignant tumors
			Ovarian causes: inflammatory,
			    infectious
			Follicular cyst
			Corpus luteum cyst
			Theca-luteum cyst
			Ovarian malignancy
			Endometriosis
			Chronic pelvic congestion

Adapted from Aronoff GM: Evaluation and Treatment of Chronic Pain. Baltimore, Williams & Wilkins, 1992; Tollison CD, Satterthwaite JR, Tollison JW: Handbook of Pain Management. Baltimore, Williams & Wilkins, 1994.

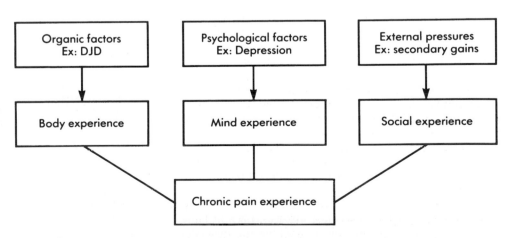

FIGURE 41–1   Chronic pain: interaction of organic, psychological, and social factors. *Abbreviation*: Ex, example. (From Grabois M: Chronic pain. Evaluation and treatment. *In* Goodgold J (ed): Rehabilitation Medicine. St Louis, Mosby–Year Book, 1988.)

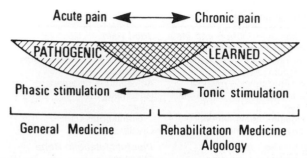

FIGURE 41-2   Nociceptive spectrum. (From Brena SF, Chapman SL: Management of Patients with Chronic Pain. New York, SP Medical & Scientific Books, 1983.)

Data on the disability, handicap, and social impact associated with low back pain and headache are available, but the chronicity of these conditions is not clear. Aronoff[4] studied the personal and social impact of back pain: 80% of all persons at some time experience low back pain severe enough to interfere with activity. Back pain annually accounts for expenditures of $14 billion per year, 19 million visits to the doctor, and half of all workers' compensation cases. Approximately 10 million Americans are disabled by chronic low back pain and 250 million workdays are lost per year.[43] Ten million people seek treatment each year for back pain, and it is the most common cause of disability in those under the age of 45 years.[84] Bonica notes that headache has a higher incidence, disables more persons, and causes more lost workdays than low back pain, but that low back pain produces higher medical costs.[10]

ETIOLOGY

Chronic pain can be caused by ongoing pathological processes (e.g., arthritis), chronic nervous system dysfunction (e.g., phantom limb pain), or a combination of both processes. The patient's perception of the pain is modified by psychological, social, and environmental factors to yield the presenting complaint. The evaluation of a chronic pain patient should be focused on defining the pain sources as either nociceptive, neuropathic, or neuropsychological,[23] while recognizing potential modifiers of the complaints.

In an effort to optimize the care of patients with chronic pain, the International Association for the Study of Pain (IASP) Subcommittee on Taxonomy has developed a scheme for the coding of chronic pain syndromes.[60] Codification of chronic pain presentations should enhance communication between treating physicians and provide direction to research efforts in this field.

As can be seen from a review of the diagnoses, they are separated into somatic, neuropathic, and psychological etiologies. The IASP classification system further defines five axes based on (1) the anatomical region affected, (2) systemic etiology, (3) temporal characteristics, (4) intensity, and (5) initiating etiology of these diseases. Each of these factors plays an important role in defining the treatment plan.

Somatic

For a somatic structure to be a source of pain it must be innervated. If a patient has degenerative disc changes that do not affect the annulus fibrosus, they will usually be painless because the outer annulus is the only portion of the disc that is innervated in adults.[36, 50]

Since nerve endings are stimulated by either mechanical or chemical irritation, any pathological process producing chronic stretching of connective tissues or inflammation of these innervated structures can lead to chronic somatic pain. This is usually manifest as aching, dull, or throbbing pain. Examples of this include rheumatoid arthritis, vertebral facet disease, and fibromyalgia.[54, 55]

Neuropathic

Neuropathic pain results from alterations in nerve structure or function with or without associated deafferentation.[48] It is characteristically described as burning, shooting, or electrical in nature and is not associated with any ongoing nociceptive process. Trauma to or disease of the peripheral nerves can lead to chronic neuropathic pain.[48] This may be the result of neuromas, phantom pain, causalgia,[17] or other sympathetically maintained pain syndromes.[17, 37, 89] Spinal cord injury or dorsal root ganglion injury can lead to various deafferentation pain syndromes, with pain being experienced in an area of sensory loss.[50] Chronic postlaminectomy back pain can, in some cases, be due to immobilization of dorsal root ganglia by scar tissue. Because of their mechanical sensitivity, the dorsal root ganglia can initiate high-frequency pain signals when stretched. This can perpetuate radicular-type pain.[48]

Thalamic infarcts can cause "central pain"[52] and postherpetic neuralgia can result from inflammatory injury with resultant deafferentation of the dorsal root ganglia and dorsal horn.[46] Metabolic derangements, as seen in diabetes, alcoholism, amyloidosis, and hypothyroidism, can lead to painful peripheral neuropathies.

Psychological

Psychogenic pain is often referred as a somatization disorder. The cause lies in an underlying emotional disturbance or stressor that often goes unrecognized by the patient. While the pain can present in any area of the body, the most common forms are tension headaches, angina-like symptoms, colitis, nonspecific vaginal pain, and myofascial pain involving the shoulders and upper and lower extremities.[79]

THE CHRONIC PAIN MANAGEMENT PROGRAM

Swanson and colleagues[80] remarked that when pain becomes chronic, it increases in complexity and the patient becomes more resistant to treatment. It is widely accepted that continuation of the sequential outpatient-inpatient approach of the medical model is not successful for the typical chronic pain patient.[34]

Since chronic pain syndrome is a complex problem with medical and psychosocial aspects, it requires a comprehen-

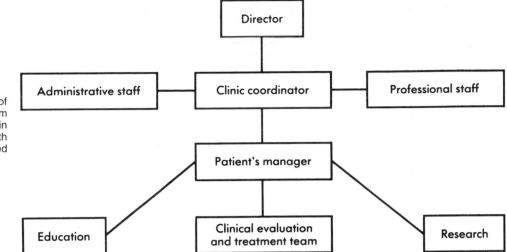

FIGURE 41–3 Organization of multidisciplinary pain clinic. (From Grabois M: Pain clinics: Role in rehabilitation of patients with chronic pain. Ann Acad Med 1983; 12:428.)

sive and interdisciplinary approach to evaluation and treatment.[34] Chronic pain syndrome should be considered similar in scope to such disabilities as alcoholism, stroke, and spinal cord injury, if the patient is to reach the highest functional goals possible within medical and psychological limitations.[32] Pain programs have attempted to accomplish this outcome by an interdisciplinary and comprehensive approach to evaluating and treating patients with chronic pain.[31]

Programs for chronic pain management, like those for physical medicine and rehabilitation, are relatively new developments and began during World War II.[33] Originated by Alexander and popularized by Bonica,[11] these programs have multiplied in recent years and now number in the thousands.

Ideally, a pain clinic should be comprehensive and interdisciplinary and offer a wide range of treatment techniques.[31] In the organization of a typical pain clinic (Fig. 41–3), the director provides overall leadership and the coordinator is responsible for day-to-day management. The patient's case manager is the attending physician.

The clinical team regularly evaluates patients, sets goals, treats patients, and evaluates treatment outcomes (Table 41–3). The team members typically include a physician, psychologist, physical therapist, vocational counselor, occupational therapist, social services counselor, pharmacist, dietician, and nurse. Some programs use other professionals such as kinesiotherapists, exercise physiologists, and so forth. Other medical subspecialists are usually available on a consultative basis. They attend regular team conferences that select patients to be accepted for treatment and monitor their progress.[31] The physician leads the team, coordinates the program, and provides overall medical management. The psychosocial-vocational team, consisting of the psychologist, social worker, and vocational counselor, provides leadership in the evaluation and treatment of the behavioral changes that are a result of chronic pain, and appropriate vocational intervention.[31]

The therapy team members typically consist of nursing, pharmacy, dietary, physical therapy, and occupational therapy personnel, and provide daily therapy to control medication levels, modulate the pain level, and increase patient activity.[1] The flow-chart of patient care in a typical pain management program is depicted in Figure 41–4.

Referrals are typically accepted from medical and nonmedical sources. An appropriate history must be supplied, and the patient should complete a pain evaluation form.

TABLE 41–3   Chronic Pain Management Team

Core Personnel	Consultant Personnel
Physician	Medical subspecialists
Psychologist	Anesthesiologist
Physical therapist	Neurosurgeon
Occupational therapist	Physical medicine and rehabilitation
Social services counselor	professional
Rehabilitation nurse	Psychiatrist
Vocational counselor	Recreational therapist
Pharmacist	Biomedical engineer
Dietitian	

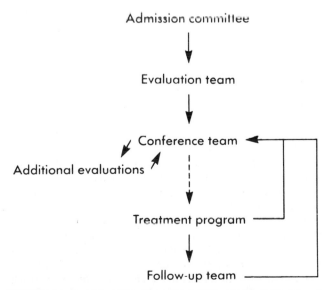

FIGURE 41–4 Pain clinic: flow chart. (From Grabois M: Chronic pain: Evaluation and treatment. *In* Goodgold J (ed): Rehabilitation Medicine. St Louis, Mosby–Year Book, 1988.)

The most appropriate patients are those chronic pain patients who are motivated to participate in the program, who do not have secondary gain issues that might inhibit improvement, and who accept the concepts and goals of the program.[31]

CLINICAL EVALUATION

Patients referred for chronic pain treatment usually have been seen by a number of specialists, and have had numerous diagnostic tests and therapeutic procedures, all without obtaining the results they anticipated or expected. They may have been labeled as "professional patients" or failures of the medical system. It is important to obtain a complete history and physical examination to assess the factors contributing to the patient's complaints, and to assess the impact of the pain on the patient's functional capacity. Searching for a single cause to explain all of the patient's symptoms, after this has already been tried by numerous other specialists, is usually nonfutile. It can, in fact, be counterproductive because it reinforces the patient's perception that "there's something seriously wrong with me and they just can't figure out what it is."

History

The history should focus on the time course, intensity, and location of the pain. The functional state of the patient prior to the onset of the problem should be established, as it is usually unrealistic to obtain improvement beyond this level. Reactions to diagnostic and therapeutic interventions should be noted, as they can be predictors of responses to future treatment. Have iatrogenic problems resulted from inappropriate or unnecessary procedures? Is there a past history of substance abuse or addictive behavior (a negative prognostic indicator)? What are the patient's relationships with family, friends, and co-workers? What exacerbates and what relieves the pain? Is litigation a factor to be considered? All responses to prior and current medications should be noted.

Physical Examination

A complete physical examination should be done, focusing on the neurological and musculoskeletal systems. The cranial nerves should be assessed, and exteroceptive sensations of pain, temperature, and touch documented. Anatomical patterns of pain and sensory loss often provide clues to the level of a lesion or to the lack of an organic basis for the complaint. For example, loss of light touch in a hand and arm, but retained ability to identify objects and perform fine motor movements (which require intact sensory input), suggest a functional overlay, malingering or somatization.

While motor system examination can be limited by pain, the assessment of strength, muscle bulk, and muscle tone should provide valuable diagnostic clues. Autonomic dysfunction such as vasomotor instability can be assessed by comparison of skin temperature, perspiration, and hair and nail changes in the extremities. These abnormalities can be signs of ongoing sympathetic overactivity, especially if localized to painful areas. Changes in reflex responses can be one of the earliest signs of central nervous system (CNS) dysfunction, and reflex testing is often one of the most objective parts of the neurological examination of pain patients. In addition to these standard evaluation techniques, it is important to use other assessment and diagnostic tests as indicated, bearing in mind that endless repetition of tests is generally not very likely to turn up a previously undiagnosed problem.

DIAGNOSTIC TESTING

Diagnostic testing should be undertaken with care in patients with chronic pain syndromes. Careful review of old records can save time and expense by preventing repetition of prior inconclusive or negative studies. Testing should always be based on clinical findings or changes in examination. If symptoms have remained static since the last evaluation, then the likelihood of finding a change in a diagnostic test is low.

Laboratory Tests

Chronic pain states usually do not produce distinct laboratory findings apart from any underlying disease. Routine monitoring for drug effects is performed for patients taking anticonvulsants or other medications known to have adverse effects on specific organ systems. Urine or blood screening is a routine part of any drug detoxification program. Evaluation and treatment of specific connective tissue syndromes require routine monitoring of laboratory indicators such as the erythrocyte sedimentation rate to assess the response to therapeutic interventions.

Imaging Studies

Radiographic studies are used extensively in the evaluation of patients with chronic pain because of their relative simplicity and lack of invasiveness. Magnetic resonance imaging, computed tomography, and plain radiographs are generally a part of every chronic pain patient's workup. They rarely must be repeated, and for the most part these patients have already been adequately diagnosed and treated on the medical model before referral to the chronic pain program. Occasionally, other tests, such as electrodiagnostic studies, bone scanning, or even thermography, are indicated (Table 41–4).

PSYCHOLOGICAL EVALUATION

The perception of chronic pain is influenced by psychological factors and chronic pain in turn influences psychological functioning. A psychological evaluation is useful in all cases in which pain causes significant impairment in psychological, vocational, or social functioning.[62] The goal of the psychological evaluation is to determine what emotional, cognitive, behavioral, social, or vocational factors are affecting the patient's perception or amount of the pain being experienced. While it is true that patients with primary psychiatric disease can present with complaints of chronic pain that are largely untenable (i.e., psychogenic

TABLE 41–4 Imaging Studies Commonly Utilized in Chronic Pain Syndrome Patients

Imaging Study	Comment
Spinal plain films	Low specificity and predictive value
Computed tomogram (with myelography)	Demonstrates over 90% of herniated disks, but can have false-positives
Magnetic resonance imaging	Excellent soft tissue and disc images
Thermography	Can be used for confirmation of autonomic dysfunction in conditions such as reflex sympathetic dystrophy
Electromyography and nerve conduction studies	Objectively assess severity, location, and extent of nerve and muscular lesions
Bone scan	One of the few imaging techniques that detects physiological changes
Three-phase bone scan	Sensitive and specific for reflex sympathetic dystrophy

pain), the use of the psychological evaluation solely for the purpose of determining a cause (i.e., organic vs. psychogenic) for a complaint of chronic pain is problematic (Table 41–5). Turk and Rudy[87] ask the following questions to illustrate the problems with this unidimensional approach:

1. What medical evidence has to be present before we say there is in fact an organic basis for a pain complaint?

2. Are all medical and diagnostic procedures 100% effective at identifying all sources of physical *pathology* likely to cause the pain reported by the patient?

3. Are there other factors beyond psychopathology which could influence the perception of pain?

4. Is it possible that the psychological difficulties expressed by the patient are a result of their pain?

5. Could there be individual differences other than psychological ones which could account for the differences expressed in pain reports?

6. Is it possible for a psychiatric problem and a pain condition to coexist in the same patient?

TABLE 41–5 Appropriate and Inappropriate Uses of Psychological Assessment

Appropriate Uses	Inappropriate Uses
To determine specific psychological and behavioral contributions to a patient's pain and concomitant behaviors, disability, and suffering	To determine if pain is organic or functional (i.e., real or psychogenic)
To determine appropriate treatment strategies	To detect malingerers
To provide essential information on particular aspects of a patient's psychosocial background and current situation that may be affecting the pain problem	To justify dumping of more difficult patients

Adapted from Turk DC: Psychological assessment of patients with persistent pain: I. Traditional views. Pain Manage 1990; 3:167–172.

These questions illustrate the need to conceptualize chronic pain beyond the unidimensional organic vs. psychogenic distinction and toward a broader and more comprehensive scheme. Practitioners should be sensitive to the multifaceted aspects of chronic pain, and not confuse the emotional consequences of pain with causation when no readily apparent medical explanation is available. Often, a person without a readily diagnosable organic cause of pain is treated as if "it's all in his head" by medical personnel. The patient can react to this by dramatization and symptom magnification in an attempt to convince the clinician that the pain is real. This cycle typically worsens with each specialist the patient sees.

Once the patient has been referred to a chronic pain program, it is important to prepare him or her for psychological evaluation. Many patients with chronic pain are defensive and concerned that a referral to a psychologist or psychiatrist implies that they are "crazy" or that their pain complaint is not accepted. Providing information to the patient to minimize this misunderstanding and defensiveness facilitates compliance and a more effective evaluation. The patient should know that the psychological evaluation and the use of psychological interventions in no way imply that the pain is not "real." Providing the patient with information about the process of evaluation and testing can also prove helpful (Table 41–6).

There are a wide variety of instruments used in clinical settings to assess pain patients on different dimensions, including pain intensity, pain sensation, psychopathology, coping strategies, beliefs, behaviors, and social functioning. The primary components of the initial psychological evaluation include the clinical interview(s) with the patient and family members, health questionnaires, pain inventories (e.g., McGill Pain Questionnaire, Multidimensional Pain Inventory), and measures of psychological and behavioral dysfunction (e.g., Minnesota Multiphasic Personality Inventory [MMPI], Symptom Checklist–90, Beck Depression Inventory, State-Trait Anxiety Inventory). Turk and Melzack[86] have published an excellent review of pain assessment instruments.

For the initial clinical interview, many clinicians utilize a structured interview format. At a minimum, a pain-specific inventory (e.g., McGill Pain Questionnaire, Multidimensional Pain Inventory) and a general measure of psychopathology (i.e., MMPI-II, Personality Assessment Inventory) are needed to assess patients with chronic pain. The conceptualizing of pain is multidimensional and necessarily requires more than one type of assessment instrument

TABLE 41–6 Guidelines for Psychological Services Referral

Clearly identify nonmedical consultants
Acknowledge that problem is legitimate
Provide a positive rationale for referral
Inform other staff of rationale
Avoid making cynical comments about referral
Let patient know if referral is routine
Personalize the referral
Inform patient that referral does not imply transfer

Adapted from Cameron R, Shepel LF: The process of psychological consultation in pain management. *In* Holzman AD, Turk DC (eds): Pain Management: A Handbook of Psychological Treatment Approaches. New York, Pergamon Press, 1986.

and approach.[74] The psychological evaluation of patients with chronic pain should be conducted by clinicians who are sensitive to, and knowledgeable about, the psychological aspects of chronic pain.

PAIN MEASUREMENT

Pain measurement is vital to the evaluation of treatment techniques.[69] Without adequate methods of measurement, pain treatments will continue to be adopted for use without proper scientific evaluation.[69] Cost-effectiveness is becoming more important in pain rehabilitation, and scientifically established and proven assessment techniques are vital in determining the treatment techniques that are the least invasive, least extensive, and least expensive.

Measurement of induced acute pain is easier than measurement of chronic pain.[31] In laboratory-induced acute pain there are minimal emotional or cognitive factors, and the quantity of the pain stimulus is easily controlled. In the measurement and assessment of chronic pain, unfortunately, there is no generally accepted laboratory model. A clear linear relationship between the quantity of noxious input and the intensity of pain experience is not apparent in chronic pain. It is difficult to capture what is a personal and private sensory experience. Many times all we have are the patients' words, their recollections of the experience, and the behavior exhibited when they have the pain experience.[31] In a very real sense all pain is "in the head" and measuring it objectively is difficult. A pain scale should meet a few basic criteria, including ease of administration and scoring, potential for accurate use by a variety of healthcare professionals, high interrater reliability, and validity.[31]

Sternbach and co-workers[79] noted that pain is a complex experience, and evidence confirming its presence involves several dimensions that depend on changing states and that are continuously influenced by a multitude of extrinsic and intrinsic stimuli. Fordyce[27] described four main components of pain: (1) nociception, (2) sensation, (3) suffering, and (4) behavioral reactions.

Using the concepts of Sternach et al. and Fordyce, three components of chronic pain measurement are noted: (1) the subjective, (2) the physiological, and (3) the behavioral. The interaction between these components is dynamic and involves a balanced appraisal of sensory input and the degree to which this is modulated by psychological factors (including other determinants of verbal and overt behavior).

The subjective component of chronic pain measurement is reflected in rating scales, questionnaires, and diary cards. The visual analog scale (1–10) is the most commonly used rating scale.

Questionnaires have gained wide acceptance, with the McGill Pain Questionnaire being the most popular.[56] It evaluates three major classes of word descriptions—sensory, affective, and evaluative—that patients use to specify their subjective pain experience. It has a built-in intensity scale. Multiple reports in the literature have evaluated this method of pain measurement, and it has been used extensively in clinical evaluation and treatment trials. Melzack[57] and others believe it provides a quantity of information that can be treated statistically, and that it is sufficiently

sensitive to detect differences in effectiveness among pain relief treatments. Although physiological techniques such as measurement of cortical evoked potentials, muscle tension, vasodilation, heart rate, and blood pressure have a firm scientific basis in the measurement of acute pain in the laboratory, they have not been scientifically evaluated in the clinical (or chronic) pain setting.

Behavioral measurements of pain, as advocated by Fordyce,[28] are logical techniques for measuring pain, since people in pain must engage in behavior indicative of their state. Most behavior measurement techniques use three categories of behavior: (1) somatic intervention, (2) impaired functional capacity, and (3) pain complaints. The University of Alabama Behavioral Measurement of Pain Scale is based on 10 behaviors such as vocalization and the frequency of intensity of these expressions.[71] Although interobserver reliability is good, many trained observers and many observations are needed to obtain accurate and valid information.

Clearly, there is at present no ideal method for evaluating and measuring chronic pain and the effectiveness of treatment techniques. Those measurements that reflect subjective, physiological and behavioral components with independent and direct monitoring are the most appropriate.[31] Reading[69] noted that behavioral indices may assume greater importance as chronicity increases, since the question of how much the patient is able to do rather than how much it hurts may be the more important question in a chronic pain management setting. This is especially true when considering the cost-effectiveness of pain management programs, since functional outcome is often more important to third-party payers than perceived level of pain.[69]

TREATMENT

Goals

The cause of the chronic pain syndrome should be determined from a medical and psychosocial point of view and the location of "pain generators" should be noted. Attempts to decrease or eliminate the "pain generators" are important and should be carried out first, followed by consideration of other treatment options. Table 41–7 describes a classification for pain patients as well as potential treatment options in patients with chronic pain syndrome.

The Fordyce model of behavioral modification is useful in patients with chronic pain syndrome.[48] The goal in these patients is not to "cure the pain" but to interrupt the pain behavioral reinforcement cycle by rewarding healthy behavior and setting appropriate goals that the patient must achieve. These goals are to reduce medication use, modulate pain response, increase activity, and modify pain behaviors.[32]

Behavioral Treatment

Behavioral treatments of chronic pain are based on an operant model of pain. Fordyce's operant model emphasizes the behavioral expression of pain.[26] So-called pain behaviors are those overt expressions of pain that a person who is suffering might exhibit (i.e., limping, grimacing, moaning, lying down). This model focuses on the environ-

TABLE 41–7   Classification of the Chronic Nonmalignant Pain Patient With Examples and Treatment Strategies

Class	Symptoms	Objective Findings	Social and Vocational Components	Example	Treatment Strategies
IA	High	High correlation	High	Rheumatoid arthritis	Behavior modification approach with emphasis on medication and modalities
IB	High	High correlation	Low	Rheumatoid arthritis	Medication and modalities approach
IIA	High	Low correlation	High	Musculoskeletal/low back pain	Behavioral modification approach
IIB	High	Low correlation	Low	Musculoskeletal/low back pain	Modalities

mental reinforcers which perpetuate pain behaviors. For example, family members can reinforce pain behaviors by providing attention or allowing the patient to avoid physical activity. Likewise, the Worker's Compensation system can reinforce pain behaviors by providing financial rewards for pain behaviors and continued disability. Physicians and therapists can reinforce pain behavior as well, and the old adage that "the squeaky wheel gets the grease" certainly holds true for these patients.

The performance of pain behaviors (Table 41–8) during the acute phase of the illness may be appropriate and adaptive. However, if these behaviors persist for an extended period of time, they become detrimental to long-term recovery. This is particularly true for decreased activity, which can lead to generalized deconditioning and decreased flexibility.

In the behavioral model, the treatment approach emphasizes the manipulation of environmental factors.[47] The goal is to extinguish pain behaviors and reinforce "wellness" behaviors. Under the behavioral model of pain management, the use of pain medications on an as-needed basis is seen as inappropriate. Exercising up to the point of increased pain is also viewed as reinforcing pain behavior. In contrast, scheduling medications on a time contingent basis and exercising on a quota system are viewed as reinforcing wellness behavior. By changing the medication regime to a time-contingent schedule, the reinforcement value of pain medications is reduced. This method maximizes medicinal pain coverage while minimizing the risk of the patient developing tolerance and dependence (physical and psychological) on the drug.

Similarly, when exercise quotas are established, pain no longer serves as a signal to stop the activity. Termination of the exercise occurs only after the quota is reached and completion of the activity becomes the reward. This pacing

TABLE 41–8   Pain Behaviors

Sighing: obvious exaggerated exhalation of breath
Grimacing: obvious facial expression of pain
Rubbing: touching, holding, rubbing affected area
Bracing: stationary position in which fully extended limb supports and maintains abnormal weight distribution
Guarding: abnormally stiff or rigid movement while shifting from one position to another

Adapted from Keefe FJ, Bloch AR: Development of an observation method for assessing pain behavior in chronic low back pain patients. Behav Ther 1982; 13:363–375.

model can be utilized in treatment settings to modify behaviors that serve to perpetuate a cycle of continued behavioral dysfunction.

More recent developments in the theory and practice of pain management have led to the development of the cognitive-behavioral approach.[67] In contrast to the behavioral approach, which emphasizes only the environmental factors, the cognitive-behavioral model of pain management emphasizes the reciprocal interaction between the individual and the environmental factors. The primary assumption from the cognitive-behavioral perspective is that the individual has learned maladaptive ways of thinking, feeling, and behaving. A further assumption is that interventions designed to change any one of these factors will also change the others. The primary components of cognitive-behavioral interventional for chronic pain are education, skills acquisition, cognitive-behavioral rehearsal, and generalization.[64] This model of pain management has gained broad recognition and practice, and initial research on the efficacy of this approach has been promising.

Pharmacological Management

Nonopioid analgesics can be subdivided into aspirin-like drugs (nonsteroidal anti-inflammatory drugs, [NSAIDs]) and acetaminophen. NSAIDs have analgesic, antipyretic, anti-inflammatory, and antithrombotic actions. Inhibition of prostaglandin synthesis appears to explain their analgesic, antithrombotic, and antipyretic actions, while interference with neutrophil function might account for their anti-inflammatory properties. These medications are well-absorbed, but demonstrate an analgesic ceiling. Gastropathy is the most common side effect and may be neutrophil- or prostaglandin-mediated.[90] Renal complications include the nephrotic syndrome and interstitial nephritis, which are reversible. Irreversible papillary necrosis can occur, but is exceedingly rare.[92] NSAIDs should be used cautiously or avoided in patients with a past history of peptic ulcer disease or with decreased renal function.

Acetaminophen's analgesic properties are equipotent with aspirin. While it is antipyretic, it is not anti-inflammatory and does not affect platelet function. Doses exceeding 4 to 6 g/day can be hepatotoxic, and caution should be taken when using combination medications that contain this amount of acetaminophen.

Opioid analgesics are generally not indicated for the treatment of nonmalignant chronic pain.[93] While efficacy without dependence has been reported for opioid treatment of somatic pain,[25] opioid use for sympathetic pain and other chronic neuropathic pain disorders has been shown to have poor efficacy.[2] For chronic somatic pain, opioids have improved efficacy, but dependence and tolerance remain a problem in some patients. Chronic malignant pain of somatic origin can be treated effectively with long-term opioid management.

It should be noted that caffeine can increase the analgesic effects of aspirin-like drugs in the treatment of headaches and other pain syndromes.[45]

Several adjuvant medications have independent analgesic effects or enhance the effects of opioids. Tricyclic antidepressants have been shown in controlled trials to have analgesic effects independent of their antidepressant properties.[53, 91] They have also been shown in laboratory animals to enhance the effects of opioid analgesics with an efficacy 70 times that of aspirin.[77] These effects were not reversed with naloxone. They were reversed by central serotonin depletion, implicating serotonin reuptake blockade as an analgesic mechanism.[84] Amitriptyline is the best studied of the tricyclics, but its anticholinergic side effects (dry mouth, sedation, blurred vision, urinary retention, constipation, or delirium) can make this drug undesirable. Doses required to achieve analgesic effects are below those needed to relieve depression (usually in a range of 10–100 mg).[12, 21] It can be given at nighttime to take advantage of its sedative properties to normalize sleep patterns and thus improve compliance. Caution should be taken in patients with hypertension or coronary artery disease, since amitriptyline can cause a precipitous rise in blood pressure.

Benzodiazepines are useful in relieving anxiety, but they have no intrinsic analgesic properties. Long-term use can lead to dependence and withdrawal effects, including seizures, muscle cramps, and dysphoria. If given in combination with opioids, they can potentiate respiratory depression, even in small doses.

Steroids, in bolus dose, have been shown to be effective in the treatment of reflex sympathetic dystrophy[42] and can also be effective in the treatment of other neuropathic-related pain.[25] Side effects with long-term use include Cushing's syndrome, weight gain, myopathy, psychosis, and gastrointestinal bleeding. Steroids should not be used in conjunction with NSAIDs. Abrupt withdrawal of steroids after long-term use can precipitate an addisonian crisis with nausea, vomiting, hypotension, and hypoglycemia.

The anticonvulsants carbamazepine, phenytoin, and valproic acid can also be effective in the treatment of neuropathic pain. Carbamazapine has been useful in the treatment of trigeminal neuralgia,[14, 81] post-traumatic neuropathies,[82] and phantom limb pain.[20] Side effects that require routine monitoring with these medications include bone marrow suppression and hepatotoxicity.

Clonidine, an α_2-adrenergic agonist, has been shown to enhance the effects of opioids[94] and has independent analgesic properties when administered intrathecally.[19] Potential side effects of clonidine include orthostatic hypotension and rebound hypertension upon withdrawal.

Medication Management Philosophy

Physicians have a long history of prescribing, and patients have a long history of using, inappropriate medications (Fig. 41–5), particularly narcotic medications. Studies

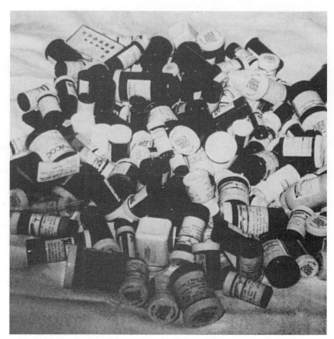

FIGURE 41–5 Medication usage of chronic pain patient over 1-year period.

show that patients are usually inadequately treated for acute pain syndromes and overtreated for chronic ones.[70] In addition, some physicians mistakenly believe that giving medication on an as-needed basis rather than on a scheduled dosage results in less addiction. Physicians also tend to incorrectly label patients who respond to a placebo as having a nonorganic type of pain.

The goal of pharmacological management of a patient with chronic pain is to moderate or eliminate the use of narcotics, tranquilizers, and hypnotic medications.[31] This approach usually requires detoxification in an in-hospital or day program. No injectable medications are allowed and patients are switched to an oral preparation as soon as possible. Initially, patients are usually allowed to take their oral medications on an as-needed basis, but with strict record keeping. No new narcotics, tranquilizers, or hypnotic drugs should be prescribed. Once the daily baseline requirement for the patient is obtained over a few days, a "pain cocktail" approach is used on a time-contingent basis (Table 41–9).

The pain cocktail typically consists of methadone or a similar preparation in a dose equivalent to the currently used narcotic medication. It is mixed with a masking vehicle such as cherry syrup. The patient is fully informed in advance that the drug will gradually be withdrawn, but is not told the daily dose of the active ingredient. The cocktail is given at the dosage and on the time schedule the patient demonstrated in the daily requirement. Gradual reduction of the active ingredient with an equal increase in the masking vehicle is carried out over 3 to 6 weeks. Decrements are made slowly so as not to elicit withdrawal signs and symptoms. Eventually the patient is receiving only the masking vehicle, and the cocktail is discontinued. Figure 41–6 compares the pain cocktail approach with the medication-as-needed method. This cocktail approach of gradual

TABLE 41–9   Sample Pain Cocktail Regimen

Inpatient Days		Pain Cocktail Format
1–6	*Baseline:*	Patient reports preadmission pattern of "one or two of the 50-mg tablets of Demerol [meperidine] two or three times a day, as needed, at home."
		Physician orders to nurse: "May have Demerol, *prn* pain, not to exceed three 50-mg tablets q3h. Carefully record amount taken."
		Analysis of baseline data: Patient averaged 600 mg of Demerol/24 hr, averaging of 3- to 4-hr intervals between requests.
7–9 *First cocktail*		
	℞ *to pharmacist:*	Demerol, 1920 mg
		Bevisol, Plebex, or other liquid B complex, 12 mL; cherry syrup qs 240 mL
	Sig:	Pain cocktail, 10 mL po q3h, day and night, *not prn*
	Nursing order:	Pain cocktail, 10 mL po q3h, day and night, *not prn*
		Since the contents of the pain cocktail are not on the label, a copy of the prescription must be kept in a separate pain cocktail book.
10–12		Decrease each daily total by 64 mg, to 1/10 of original amount. A 3-day ℞ is decreased by 64 × 3 or 192 mg.
	℞ *to pharmacist:*	Demerol, 1728 mg
		Bevisol, Plebex, or other liquid B complex, 12 mL; cherry syrup qs 240 mL
	Sig:	Pain cocktail, 10 mL po q3h, day and night, *not prn*
	Nursing order:	Pain cocktail, 10 mL po q3h, day and night, *not prn*
13–15	℞ *to pharmacist:*	Demerol, 1536 mg
		Bevisol, Plebex, or other liquid B complex, 12 mL; cherry syrup qs 240 ml
	Sig:	Pain cocktail, 10 mL po q3h, day and night, *not prn*
	Nursing order:	Pain cocktail, 10 mL po q3h, day and night, *not prn*
16–18	℞ *to pharmacist:*	Demerol, 1344 mg
		Bevisol, Plebex, or other liquid B complex, 12 mL; cherry syrup qs 240 mL
	Sig:	Pain cocktail, 10 mL po q3h, day and night, *not prn*
	Nursing order:	Pain cocktail, 10 mL po q3h, day and night, *not prn*
19–21	℞ *to pharmacist:*	Demerol, 1152 mg
		Bevisol, Plebex, or other liquid B complex, 12 mL; cherry syrup qs 240 mL
	Sig:	Pain cocktail, 10 mL po q3h, day and night, *not prn*
	Nursing order:	Pain cocktail, 10 mL po q3h, day and night, *not prn*
22–24	℞ *to pharmacist:*	Demerol 960 mg
		Bevisol, Plebex, or other liquid B complex, 12 mL; cherry syrup qs 240 ml
	Sig:	Pain cocktail, 10 mL po q3h, day and night, *not prn*
	Nursing order:	Pain cocktail, 10 mL po q3h, day and night, *not prn*
37–39	℞ *to pharmacist:*	Demerol, 0 mg
		Bevisol, Plebex, or other liquid B complex, 12 mL; cherry syrup qs 240 mL
	Sig:	Pain cocktail, 10 mL po q3h, day and night, *not prn*
	Nursing order:	Pain cocktail, 10 ml po q3h, day and night, *not prn*

(Maintain patient on vehicle for 2–10 days; if all is going well, inform patient and ask if continuation of vehicle is desired.)

Modified from Fordyce WE: Behavioral Methods for Chronic Pain and Illness. St Louis, Mosby–Year Book, 1979.

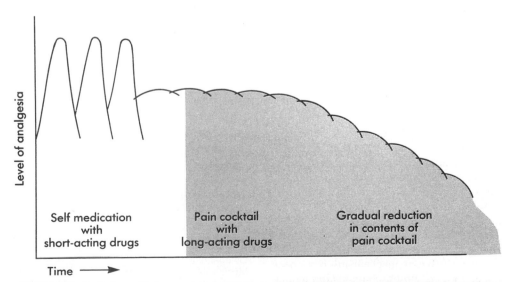

FIGURE 41–6 Pain cocktail approach: comparison of as-needed and around-the-clock approaches.

TABLE 4–10   Pharmacological and Nonpharmacological Pain Interventions

Pharmacological Interventions	Nonpharmacological Interventions
NSAIDs	Behavior modifiers
Antidepressants (TCAs)	Relaxation
Anticonvulsants	Biofeedback
Carbamazepine	Guided visual imagery
Phenytoin (Dilantin)	Music therapy
Invasive pain modulators	Distraction
Spinal opioids	Hypnosis
Peripheral nerve stimulators	Pain modulators
Dorsal column stimulators	TENS
Epidural and deep brain	Acupuncture
stimulators	Conditioning exercises
Invasive pain relievers	Stretching/flexibility
Sympathetic nerve blocks	Myofascial release
Epidural anesthetics/steroids	Spray and stretch
Root sleeve injections	
Trigger point injections	

Abbreviations: NSAIDs, nonsteroidal anti-inflammatory drugs; *TCAs,* tricyclic antidepressants; *TENS,* transcutaneous electrical nerve stimulation.

withdrawal can also be used for tranquilizers and hypnotics as well as for narcotic medications. Kanner[39] believes that judiciously used antidepressants, particularly the tricyclic antidepressants, lead to a smoother treatment course for the patient with chronic pain.

Pain Modulation

The complete eradication of chronic pain is rarely achieved and is not the goal of most interventions. The goal is the modification of pain to a more tolerable level. A comprehensive pain management program utilizes an array of modalities to accomplish this goal. Nonpharmacological methods are usually adjunctive therapies and do not necessarily substitute for pharmacological interventions.[66] For the chronic pain population, the optimal techniques are those that can be used by the patient in the home setting, are active rather than passive, and can be used for the shortest time possible or gradually weaned.[58] Transcutaneous electrical nerve stimulation (TENS), biofeedback, and thermal modalities fulfill these criteria. Table 41–10 lists commonly used pharmacological and nonpharmacological pain-modulating interventions.

Pain modulation techniques take advantage of the body's endogenous pain-modulating abilities first postulated and implied by the gate theory of pain of Melzack and Wall.[58] This theory supports the observation that a direct correlation does not always exist between the extent of organic injury and the expression of pain.[88] Melzack and Wall proposed that pain information was modulated at the level of the "target cell" in the substantia gelatinosa, or laminae II and III of the dorsal horn, by afferent information from A delta and C sensory fibers[58] (see Chapter 46). This "gating" effect on the target cell modulates input before it evokes pain perception.[25] Since the description of the gate theory, modulation events higher in the neuroaxis and modulation by descending or efferent mechanisms have been proposed. Basbaum and Fields[5] proposed that pain modulation occurs at the periaqueductal gray area of the midbrain by descending efferent tracts. The modulation of pain infor-

mation and pain perception occurs at multiple sites along the neuroaxis and by afferent and efferent pathways.

The pain modulation network can be activated by the administration of spinal opiates. It can also be activated by electrical stimulation (transcutaneously or percutaneously) to peripheral nerves, or epidurally at the level of the spinal cord or brain.[44]

Transcutaneous Electrical Nerve Stimulation

TENS at rates of 50 to 100 Hz produces analgesia that is not reversible by naloxone.[65] Stimulation of large myelinated fibers presumably blocks nociceptive transmission at the level of the spinothalamic tract cell bodies.[58] TENS can produce neuromodulation by three routes: (1) presynaptic inhibition of the spinal cord, (2) direct inhibition on an excited, abnormally firing nerve, or (3) restoration of afferent input.[29]

TENS is helpful in the treatment of many painful conditions[44, 61, 66] (Table 41–11). A recent blinded and controlled trial of TENS and exercise showed a significant benefit only in the exercise group.[18] However, double blinded, controlled trials of TENS have shown it to be of significant benefit in the treatment of rheumatoid arthritis and osteoarthritis.[1, 75, 83] Proponents of TENS recommend its use early in a pain treatment program.[51] The patients who respond best to TENS typically have neurogenic or musculoskeletal pain, as opposed to psychogenic pain. Best results are obtained in those who receive it early in their course.

The patient should learn to apply the TENS electrodes over or near the area of pain with the dipole parallel to major nerve trunks.[44] Patients should understand that they have to determine by trial and error the optimal electrode placement and stimulus intensity, and the therapist or physician should encourage the patient to adjust the unit. TENS variables that can be adjusted include amplitude, rate, pulse width, and location of the electrodes.[63] There is no current research to support the use of one mode of TENS over another (e.g., conventional, burst, modulated, brief-intense, acupuncture-like, strength-duration).[30] Adverse reactions to TENS are infrequent; the most common is skin hypersensitivity.[44] TENS should be avoided over the carotid sinus, in patients with demand-type pacemakers, and during pregnancy.

Heat and Cold

The use of hot and cold modalities which the patient can safely use at home should be encouraged. The use of devices or treatments that require the help of other persons or professional settings, such as ultrasound or massage, are

TABLE 41–11   Indications for Transcutaneous Electrical Nerve Stimulation

Musculoskeletal Pain	Neurogenic Pain
Rheumatoid arthritis pain	Deafferentated pain syndromes
Osteoarthritis pain	(phantom limb)
Myofascial pain	Sympathetically mediated pain
Dysmenorrhea	Tension headache
Visceral pain	Acute postoperative pain

best reserved for acute pain syndromes or intermittently painful chronic conditions.

Biofeedback

Relaxation training and biofeedback are behavioral treatment methods which have been successfully used to treat a wide variety of pain syndromes, including myofascial and sympathetically maintained pain syndromes.[24, 30, 49, 85] There are several relaxation techniques that are used for chronic pain. The two most commonly utilized are autogenic training[73] and progressive muscle relaxation.[87] Biofeedback is simply a system which utilizes instrumentation to provide feedback on a variety of physiological responses (e.g., hand temperature, muscle tension, sweat gland activity) to facilitate relaxation and enhance self-regulation. Relaxation training and biofeedback are thought to be equally effective.[74] Repeated practice and experience with relaxation techniques is important to ensure effectiveness.

Anesthetic Treatments

Anesthetic techniques are part of the therapeutic armamentarium used in the management of chronic pain. Some of these techniques are especially helpful when used as diagnostic or prognostic procedures. They can be powerful tools when used intelligently for chronic pain, especially in the context of a multidisciplinary approach. They also play a role in the prevention of the chronic pain syndrome. The most commonly used anesthetic techniques are listed in Table 41–12.

Nerve blocks (see also Chapter 25) can be used as diagnostic, prognostic, or therapeutic procedures. Neural blockade is done by injecting a local anesthetic onto the nerves, which interrupts the sensory and nociceptive pathways. Diagnostic blocks are used to determine the source of pain, the afferent nerve pathway involved, and as a tool for differential diagnosis. Prognostic blocks are used to weigh the effects of prolonged afferent interruption. They are used before neuroblative or neurolytic procedures. Therapeutic blocks are performed with local anesthetics or with neurolytic agents.

Sympathetic nerve blocks are some of the more effective therapeutic tools in dealing with chronic pain. These blocks can be used for diagnostic, prognostic, and especially for therapeutic purposes. The sympathetic chain can be blocked in many locations, including the stellate ganglia, thoracic ganglia, celiac plexus, splanchnic nerves, lumbar plexus, hypogastric plexus, and even the impar ganglion. When dealing with sympathetically maintained pain, a series of sympathetic blocks or neurolytic sympathetic blocks, or both, can be an effective therapeutic approach.

Chemoneurolysis

Chemoneurolysis is another very effective method of pain control. The injection of neurolytic agents interferes with the transmission of pain stimuli along the pain pathways for prolonged periods of time. Chemoneurolysis is done with agents such as alcohol, phenol, ammonium sulfate, and chlorocresal. The most frequently used agent today is phenol. Chemoneurolysis can be done intrathecally, intraepidurally, at the level of the plexus, or in peripheral nerves. Sympathetic chemoneurolysis is frequently used for the treatment of sympathetically maintained pain as well as for the control of cancer pain. Somatic neurolytic techniques are used for the control of cancer pain and chronic noncancer pain. Trigeminal neuralgia in particular typically responds well to chemoneurolysis.

Cryoneurolysis

Another neurolytic technique is cryoneurolysis or cryoanalgesia. The tip of a cryoprobe is frozen in nitrous oxide and then applied to the target nerve. Following the cryolesioning there is a second-degree axonal lesion, with subsequent recovery of function due to nerve regrowth in approximately 2 to 3 months.

Radiofrequency Thermocoagulation

Radiofrequency thermocoagulation is a neurolytic method using heat. It is used in chronic pain for a variety of conditions such as trigeminal neuralgia, facet syndrome, sympatholysis, etc. Radiofrequency thermocoagulation has advantages over chemoneurolysis because it allows better control over the extent of the lesion and its intensity. The risk of inducing deafferentation that can complicate the pain is negligible.

Steroid Injections

Local injections of corticosteroids have been widely used for the treatment of chronic pain.[3, 7, 15, 41] Injections of steroids such as triamcinolone (Kenalog) in the epidural

TABLE 41–12 Commonly Utilized Anesthetic Treatments in Chronic Pain Syndrome

Treatment	Use/Comment
Nerve blocks	As diagnostic, prognostic, or therapeutic procedures
Diagnostic blocks	To ascertain source of pain, nerve pathway, or as tools for differential diagnosis
Prognostic blocks	Before neuroablative or neurolytic procedures to assess their possible effects
Therapeutic blocks	Can be performed with local anesthetics or with neurolytic agents
Trigger point injections	Treatment of myofascial pain
Facet or zygapophyseal blocks	Diagnostic or therapeutic
Epidural blocks	Useful especially when prolonged analgesia might be required for physical therapy, not for days but for weeks
Spinal blocks	Differential pain diagnosis
Neurolytic, epidural, and spinal techniques	Specific indications for the treatment of some intractable chronic pain syndromes
Sympathetic nerve blocks	Effective therapeutic tools in dealing with sympathetically maintained pain
Chemoneurolysis	Very effective in treatment of sympathetically maintained pain and cancer or noncancer chronic pain
Cryoneurolysis/ cryoanalgesia	

space, onto peripheral nerves, into articulations, and elsewhere have been successfully used for many years in patients with nerve root irritations, joint disorders, and other pathologic conditions.[6] The use of corticosteroids has continued despite criticism.[40]

Lidocaine Challenge

Peripheral neuropathies respond well at times to the oral use of carbamazepine (Tegretol) or antiarrhythmic agents structurally similar to lidocaine, such as mexiletine (Mexitil)[16] and tocainide (Tonocard). The potential usefulness of a treatment with mexiletine can be assessed by performing a lidocaine challenge. Lidocaine is perfused over 2 hours while monitoring the patient's cardiorespiratory function. If the patient tolerates the infusion and experiences pain relief, treatment with mexiletine has a good chance of being successful.

Spinal Injection and Stimulation

Spinal narcotics are now used extensively for the management of chronic cancer pain or noncancer pain in selected patients. Opioids can be administered via an epidural or intrathecal catheter. The opioid delivery systems can be fully implantable or use external pumps. Most experts favor the fully implantable system using a programmable infusion pump. There are many considerations that should be reviewed in making the choice of the system, including cost-effectiveness, and patient life expectancy. If the patient's life expectancy is over 3 to 5 months, the programmable fully implantable system is usually preferable and more cost-effective than other systems.

Spinal Cord Stimulation

Spinal cord stimulation is used in the patient in whom all or almost all other therapeutic approaches have failed. It has been used successfully in "sympathetic maintained pain" and in "failed back syndromes," especially when the pain is radicular rather than axial. Patients with conditions limited to major peripheral nerves, especially those with causalgia, can benefit from peripheral nerve stimulation.[68]

Increasing Activity Level

Therapeutic exercises are intended to improve physical condition and functional capacities. They also indirectly provide pain relief and a better quality of life.

Patients with chronic pain conditions tend to reduce or discontinue their activities because of fear of increased pain or harm. This can result in joint stiffness, decreased endurance, decreased muscle strength, muscle wasting, and even a general state of decompensation. The aim of therapeutic exercises for these patients should be reconditioning, improved muscle strength and length, and attainment of optimal joint range of motion.

Appropriate exercises that are specific for the pain area (e.g., Williams's flexion exercises for low back pain), and general conditioning exercises such as bicycling, walking, and swimming are usually indicated. Fordyce[26] noted that appropriate exercise in a behavior modification program must be relevant to the patient's pain and limitations, and quantifiable, visible, and accessible. The patient's baseline

exercise level is determined by asking the patient to exercise to tolerance (until pain, weakness, or fatigue necessitates stopping) over a few days.[76] Once the baseline has been established, the initial exercise goal is set within the patient's tolerance and then gradually increased, with new goals being set every few days (Fig. 41–7). Rewards and reinforcement are given for accomplishing the established goals without demonstrating pain behavior. In some patients, however, it is necessary to reduce excessive activity levels by teaching them to pace themselves more appropriately.

Psychosocial Interventions

Recent evidence suggests that the use of psychological modalities in conjunction with medical interventions and physical therapy increases the effectiveness of the treatment program. A wide variety of interventions are available to improve the psychological functioning of the chronic pain patient. Psychological treatments of chronic pain include psychoeducation, psychotherapy, biofeedback and relaxation training, and vocational counseling. Cognitive-behavioral approaches to chronic pain rely heavily on skills training and psychoeducational interventions.[8, 35] Group psychotherapy has been used successfully to enhance the functioning of patients in a pain rehabilitation program.[38] Individual[86] and family therapy[9, 56] are other interventions frequently used with chronic pain patients to treat underlying psychosocial stresses. Recently a compelling case has been made for including family members and significant others in the evaluation and treatment process.[59]

Relaxation training and biofeedback are behavioral treatment methods which have been successfully used to treat a wide variety of pain syndromes, including myofascial and sympathetically maintained pain syndromes.[49, 73, 78, 85] There are several relaxation techniques which can be used for chronic pain, the two most common being autogenic

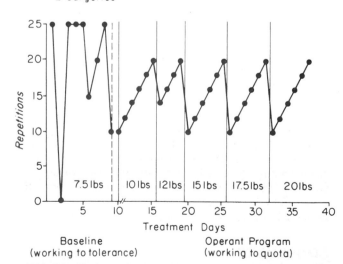

FIGURE 41–7 Behavioral modification approach to exercise. (From Fordyce WE: Behavioral Methods for Chronic Pain and Illness. St Louis, Mosby–Year Book, 1976.)

training[72] and progressive muscle relaxation.[87] Biofeedback is simply a system which utilizes instrumentation to provide feedback on a variety of physiological responses (e.g., hand temperature, muscle tension, sweat gland activity) to facilitate relaxation and enhance self-regulation of physical processes. Repeated practice and experience by the patient with relaxation techniques is important to ensure effectiveness.[87]

Vocational Rehabilitation

Vocational counseling is an important component of the psychological approach to chronic pain. Each patient is evaluated to determine work history, educational background, vocational skills and abilities, and motivation to return to work. The vocational counselor can determine whether past work skills and current aptitudes can be transferred to alternative occupations if necessary. The vocational counselor works with the patient regarding legal rights and obligations for each state (e.g., workers' compensation), and helps the patient set realistic vocational goals. They also help the patient to improve overall vocational functioning.

The modern approach to the treatment of chronic pain is multidisciplinary. Typical programs combine physical therapy interventions with behavioral and psychological approaches. These consist of the components mentioned above, of education, relaxation training, and cognitive-behavioral techniques in both group and individual formats. Vocational counseling is used to reduce functional impairment and disability, improve coping strategies, enhance effective use of pain medications, and decrease use of healthcare resources. The exact structure of the pain management program varies according to the setting and the type of population served.

RESULTS

The results of the pain management program must be measured in objective and quantifiable terms. These outcome measurements include use of medication, walking distance, strength, flexibility, sitting tolerance, pain behaviors, vocational placement, and use of healthcare resources.[31] When comparing one program with another, it is important to evaluate each program in terms of types of patients accepted, types of treatments offered, criteria for improvement, and follow-up time. "Ideal" pain rehabilitation candidates can achieve an 80% to 90% success rate. As the incidence of psychosocial problems and secondary gain issues increases, however, this rate drops to 40% to 50%. With major psychiatric or secondary gains, the success rate drops to 20% or less.[33] Steig and co-workers[78] devised a limited but useful model for determining and demonstrating the cost-benefit ratio of a pain management program. The cost to the insurance carrier of supporting the patient now and in the future is compared with the cost of the pain management program.

CONCLUSION

Patients with chronic pain syndrome are typically difficult and frustrating to manage. These patients combine traditional clinical problems with psychosocial, vocational, and behavioral issues. The "pain clinic" concept, which utilizes a comprehensive, multidisciplinary approach with knowledgeable personnel devoted to treating chronic pain syndrome, is most appropriate for evaluation and treatment of these patients. The evaluation should consist of an independent history and physical examination with emphasis on the pain experience, past evaluations, and past treatment(s). The psychosocial, vocational, and behavior aspects of the pain experience need an independent evaluation through interviews and psychological testing. Medical diagnostic tests should be reviewed and ordered or reordered only if considered absolutely necessary to complete the evaluation.

The treatment of the patient with chronic pain syndrome should emphasize four components: (1) modification of medication, (2) modification of pain, (3) increase in activity, and (4) treatment of psychosocial and vocational issues. "Pain generators" should be identified and treated, if possible. The Fordyce model of behavioral modification[27] is an appropriate one to consider in organizing and carrying out a treatment program for patients with chronic pain syndrome. With appropriate evaluation and treatment, patients with chronic pain syndrome can achieve reasonable success in improving their quality of life.

References

1. Abelson K, Langley GB, Sheppeard H, et al: Transcutaneous electrical nerve stimulation in rheumatoid arthritis. N Z Med J 1983; 96:156–161.
2. Arner S, Meyerson BA: Lack of analgesic effect of opioid on neuropathic and idiopathic forms of pain. Pain 1988; 33:11–23.
3. Arnhoff FN, Triplett HB, Pokorney B: Follow up status of patients treated with nerve block for low back pain. Anesthesiology 1977; 46:170–178.
4. Aronoff GM: Evaluation and Treatment of Chronic Pain. Baltimore, Williams & Wilkins, 1992.
5. Basbaum AI, Fields HL: Endogenous pain control mechanism. Review and hypothesis. Ann Neurol 1978; 4:451–455.
6. Benzon HT: Epidural steroid injections for low back pain and lumbosacral radiculopathy. Pain 1986; 24:277–295.
7. Benzon HT: Epidural steroids. In Raj P (ed): Practical Management of Pain, ed 2. St Louis, Mosby–Year Book 1992.
8. Blanchard EB: The use of temperature biofeedback in the treatment of chronic pain due to causalgia. J Behav Med 1979; 4:183–188.
9. Blumenthal SM: Vocational rehabilitation with the industrially injured worker. J Hand Surg Am 1987; 12:926–930.
10. Bonica JJ: General considerations of chronic pain. In Bonica JJ (ed): The Management of Pain, vol 1. Philadelphia, Lea & Febiger, 1990.
11. Bonica JJ: Preface. In Ng LKY (ed): New Approaches to Treatment of Chronic Pain: A Review of Multidisciplinary Pain Clinics and Pain Centers. National Institute on Drug Abuse Research Monograph 36, Rockville, Md, 1981.
12. Botney M, Field H: Amitriptyline potentiates morphine analgesia by a direct action on the central nervous system. Ann Neurol 1983; 13: 160–164.
13. Brena SF: Pain control facilities: Root, organization and function. In Brena SF, Chapman SL (eds): Management of Patients With Chronic Pain. New York, Spectrum, 1983.
14. Dalessio DJ: Management of the cranial neuralgias and atypical facial pain. Clin J Pain 1989; 5:55–59.
15. Davidson JT, Robin GC: Epidural injections in the lumbosaciatic syndrome. Br J Anaesth 1961; 33:595–598.
16. Dejgard A, Peterson P, Kastrup J: Mexiletine for treatment of chronic painful diabetic neuropathy. Lancet 1988; 1:9–11.
17. Devor M: Nerve pathophysiology and mechanisms of pain in causalgia. J Auton Nerv Syst 1983; 7:371–384.
18. Deyo RA, Walsh NE, Martin DC, et al: A controlled trial of transcuta-

neous electrical nerve stimulation and exercise for chronic low back pain. N Engl J Med 1990; 322:1627–1634.

19. Eisenach JC, Lysak SZ, Niscomi CM: Epidural clonidine analgesia following surgery: Phase 1. Anesthesiology 1989; 71:640–646.

20. Elliott F, Little A: Carbamazepine for phantom-limb phenomena. N Engl J Med 1976; 295:678.

21. Feinmann C: Pain relief by antidepressants: Possible modes of action. Pain 1985; 23:1–8.

22. Fine PG: The nociceptive system and persistent pain syndromes. Probl Anesth 1990; 4:452–456.

23. Fishman PS: Retrograde changes in the corticospinal tract of posttraumatic paraplegics. Arch Neurol 1987; 44:1082 1084.

24. Flor H, Turk DC, Rudy TE: Pain and families II: Assessment and treatment. Pain 1987; 30:29–45.

25. Foley KM: Adjuvant analgesic drugs in cancer pain management. In Aronoff GM (ed): Evaluation and Treatment of Chronic Pain. Baltimore, Urban & Schwartzenberg, 1985.

26. Fordyce W: Behavioral Methods for Chronic Pain and Illness. St Louis, Mosby–Year Book, 1976.

27. Fordyce WE: The validity of pain behavior measurement. In Melzack R (ed): Pain Measurement and Assessment. New York, Raven Press, 1983.

28. Fordyce WE, Lansky D, Calsyn DA, et al: Pain measurement and pain behavior. Pain 1984; 18:53–69.

29. Frampton V: Transcutaneous electrical nerve stimulation and chronic pain. In Wells PE, Frampton V, Borosher D (eds): Pain Management in Physical Therapy. Norwalk, Conn, Appleton & Lange, 1988.

30. Getto CJ, Heaton RK, Lehman RA: PSPI: A standardized approach to the evaluation of psychosocial factors in chronic pain. Adv Pain Res Ther 1985; 5:885–889.

31. Grabois M: Chronic pain. Evaluation and treatment. In Goodgold J (ed): Rehabilitation Medicine. St Louis, Mosby–Year Book, 1988.

32. Grabois M: Comprehensive evaluation and management of patients with chronic pain. Cardiovasc Res Center Bull 1981; 19:113–117.

33. Grabois M: Pain clinics: Role in rehabilitation of patients with chronic pain. Ann Acad Med Singapore 1983; 12:428–433.

34. Greehott JD, Sternbach: RA: Conjoint treatment of chronic pain. Adv Neurol 1974; 4:595–603.

35. Hathaway SR, McKinley JC: Minnesota Multiphasic Personality Inventory Manual. New York, Psychological Corp, 1976.

36. Jackson HC, Winkelman RK, Bickel WH: Nerve endings in the human lumbar spinal column and related structures. J Bone & Joint Surg Am 1966; 48:1272–1281.

37. Jensen TS: Phantom pain and related phenomena after amputation. In Wall P, Melzack R (eds): Textbook on Pain. London, Churchill Livingstone, 1989.

38. Kanfer FH, Karoly P: The psychological self-management: Abiding issues and tentative directions. In Karoly P, Kanfer FH (eds): Self-Management and Behavior Change. Elmsford, NY, Pergamon Press, 1982.

39. Kanner R: Psychotrophic drugs in the management of pain. Curr Concepts Pain 1983; 1:11.

40. Keepes ER, Duncalf D: Treatment of backache with spinal injections of local anesthetics, spinal and systemic steroids. A review. Pain 1985; 22:33–47.

41. Kelman K: Epidural injection therapy for sciatic pain. Am J Surg 1980; 64:183–190.

42. Kozin F, McCarthy DJ, Sims J, Genant H: The reflex sympathetic dystrophy syndrome, I. Clinical and histologic studies: Evidence for bilaterality, response to corticosteroids and articular involvement. Am J Med 1976; 60:321–331.

43. Kriegler JS, Ashenberg ZS: Management of chronic low back pain. A comprehensive approach. Semin Neurol 1987; 7:303–312.

44. Landau B, Levy RM: Neuromodulation techniques for medically refractory pain. Annu Rev Med 1993; 44:279–287.

45. Laska EM, Sunshine A, Mueller F, et al: Caffeine as an analgesic adjuvant. JAMA 1984; 251:1711–1718.

46. Loeser JD: Herpes zoster and post-herpetic neuralgia. Pain 1986; 25:149–164.

47. Loeser JD: Pain after amputation. In Bonica JJ (ed): The Management of Pain. Philadelphia, Lea & Febiger, 1990.

48. Loeser JD: Pain due to nerve injury. Spine 1985; 10:232–235.

49. Love AW, Peck CL: The MMPI and psychological factors in low back pain. A review. Pain 1987; 28:1–12.

50. Malinsky J: The ontogenetic development of nerve terminations in the intervertebral discs of man. Acta Anat 1959; 38:96–113.

51. Mannheimer JS, et al: Pain and TENS in pain management. In Mannheimer JS, Lampe GN (eds): Clinical Transcutaneous Electrical Nerve Stimulation. Philadelphia, FA Davis, 1984.

52. Mauguiere F, Desmedt JE: Thalamic pain syndrome of Dejerine-Roussy: Differentiation of four subtypes assisted by somatosensory evoked potentials data. Arch Neurol 1988; 34:1312–1320.

53. Max MB, Culnane M, Schafer SC, et al: Amitriptyline relieves diabetic neuropathy pain in patients with normal or depressed mood. Neurology 1987; 37:589–596.

54. McCain GA, Scudds RA: The concept of primary fibromyalgia (fibrositis): Clinical value, relation and significance to other chronic musculoskeletal pain syndromes. Pain 1988; 33:273–287.

55. McCall IW, Park WM, O'Brien JP: Induced pain referral from posterior lumbar spinal elements in normal subjects. Spine 1979; 4:441–446.

56. Melzack R: The McGill Pain Questionnaire. In Melzack R (ed): Pain Measurement and Assessment. New York, Raven Press, 1983.

57. Melzack R: Measurement of the dimensions of pain experience. In Bram EV (ed): Pain Measurement in Man: Neurophysiological Correlates of Pain. New York, Elsevier, 1984.

58. Melzack R, Wall PD: Pain mechanism. A new theory. Science 1965; 150:971–979.

59. Merskey H: Traditional individual psychotherapy and psychopharmacotherapy. In Holman AD, Turk DC (eds): Pain Management: A Handbook of Psychological Treatment Approaches. New York, Pergamon Press, 1986.

60. Merskey H, Bogduk N: Classification of Chronic Pain, ed 2. Seattle, IASP Press, 1994.

61. Meyer GA, et al: Causalgia treated by selective large fiber stimulation of peripheral nerve. Brain 1972; 95:163–168.

62. Morey LC: Personality Assessment Inventory Professional Manual. Odessa, Fla, Psychological Assessment Resources, 1991.

63. Nolan MF: Selected problems in the use of transcutaneous electrical nerve stimulation for pain control. An appraisal with proposed solutions. Phys Ther 1988; 68:1694.

64. Norris PA, Fahrion SL: Autogenic biofeedback in psychophysiological therapy and stress management. In Woolfold RL, Sherer PM (eds): Principles and Practice of Stress Management. New York, Guilford Press, 1984.

65. North RB: Electrical stimulation for pain relief. Transcutaneous peripheral nerve, spinal cord and deep brain stimulation. In Swerdlow M, Charlton JE (eds): Relief of Intractable Pain. Amsterdam, Elsevier, 1989.

66. Owens MK: Literature review of non-pharmacologic methods for the treatment of chronic pain. Holistic Nurs Pract 1991; 6:24–31.

67. Pincus T, Callahan LF, Bardley LA, et al: Elevated MMPR scores for hypochondriasis, depression and hysteria in patients with rheumatoid arthritis reflect disease rather than psychological status. Arthritis Rheum 1986; 29:1456–1466.

68. Racz G, Lewis R, Laros G, et al: Electrical stimulation analgesia. In Raj P (ed): Practical Management of Pain, ed 2. St Louis, Mosby–Year Book, 1992.

69. Reading AE: Testing pain mechanisms in persons with pain. In Wall PD, Melzack R (eds): Textbook of Pain. New York, Churchill Livingston, 1984.

70. Reuler J, Girard D, Nardone D: The chronic pain syndrome: Misconceptions and management. Ann Intern Med 1980; 93:588–596.

71. Richards JS, Nepormuceno C, Riles M, Suer Z: Assessing pain behavior: The UAB pain behavior scale. Pain 1982; 14:393–398.

72. Robinson ME, Cassisi JE, O'Connor PD, MacMillan M: Lumbar EMG during exercise: Chronic low back pain patients versus controls. J Spinal Disord 1992; 5:8–15.

73. Rook JC, Pesch RN, Keeler EC: Chronic pain and the questionable use of the Minnesota Multiphasic Personality Inventory. Arch Phys Med Rehabil 1981; 62:373–376.

74. Silver BV, Blanchard EB: Biofeedback and relaxation training in the treatment of psychophysiological disorders: Or, are the machines really necessary? J Behav Med 1978; 1:217–239.

75. Smith CR, Lewith GT, Machin D: TNS and osteoarthritic pain. Preliminary study to establish a controlled method of assessing transcutaneous nerve stimulation as a treatment for the pain caused by osteoarthritis of the knee. Physiotherapy 1983; 69:266–268.

76. Smythe HA: Problems with the MMPI. J Rheumatol 1984; 11:417–418.

77. Spiegel K, Kalb R, Pasternak GW: Analgesic activity of tricyclic antidepressants. Ann Neurol 1983; 13:462–465.

78. Steig RL, Williams RC, Gallagher LA: Multidisciplinary pain treatment centers. J Occup Med 1981; 23:94–102.

79. Sternbach RA: Psychophysiological pain syndromes: *In* Bonica JJ (ed): The Management of Pain. Philadelphia, Lea & Febiger, 1990.

80. Swanson DW, Floreen AC, Swenson WM: Programs for managing chronic pain. II. Short term results. Mayo Clin Proc 1979; 51:409–411.

81. Sweet WH: The treatment of trigeminal neuralgia. N Engl J Med 1986; 315:174–177.

82. Swerdlow M: Anticonvulsant drugs and chronic pain. Clin Neuropharmacol 1984; 7:51–55.

83. Taylor P, Hallett M, Flaherty L: Treatment of osteoarthritis of the knee with transcutaneous electrical nerve stimulation. Pain 1981; 11:233–240.

84. Tollison CD, Satterthwaite JR, Tollison JW: Handbook of Pain Management. Baltimore, Williams & Wilkins, 1994.

85. Turk DC, Flor H, Rudy TE: Pain and families I: Etiology, maintenance, and psychosocial impact. Pain 1987; 30:3–27.

86. Turk DC, Melzack R: Handbook of Pain Assessment. New York, Guilford, 1992.

87. Turk DC, Rudy TE: A cognitive-behavioral perspective on chronic pain: Beyond the scalpel and syringe. *In* Tollison CD (ed): Handbook of Chronic Pain Management. Baltimore, Williams & Wilkins, 1989.

88. Van Dalfsen PJ, Syrjala KL: Psychologic strategies in acute pain management. Crit Care Clin 1990; 6:421–431.

89. Wall PD, Gutnik M: Properties of afferent nerve impulses originating from a neuroma. Nature 1974; 248:740–743.

90. Wallace JL, Granger DN: Pathogenesis of NSAID gastropathy: Are neutrophils the culprits? TiPS 1992; 13:129–131.

91. Watson CP, Evans RJ, Reed K, et al: Amitriptyline versus placebo in post-herpetic neuralgia. Neurology 1982; 32:671–673.

92. Whelton A, Hamilton CW: Nonsteroidal anti-inflammatory drugs: effects on kidney function. J Clin Pharmacol 1991; 31:588–598.

93. Wilson P: Pain mechanisms: Anatomy and physiology. *In* Raj P (ed): Practical Management of Pain. St Louis, Mosby–Year Book, 1992.

94. Yaksh TL: The principles behind the use of spinal narcotics. Clin Anesth 1983; 1:219–232.

The Diagnosis and Treatment of Muscle Pain Syndromes

JEFFREY M. THOMPSON, M.D.

Muscle pain is a universal human experience. The muscle pain syndromes, however, have yet to achieve universal acceptance in the medical community. Muscles make up 40% of the mass of the human body. The forces muscles generate and the mechanical stresses they are subjected to are tremendous. It is not surprising, therefore, that many causes of muscle pain exist (Table 42–1). Those disorders with obvious pathological or laboratory findings are fairly easily defined and are well established as diagnostic entities. The muscle pain syndromes described in this chapter remain controversial largely because of the lack of such objective findings.

More than in most areas of medicine, a complete understanding of the muscle pain syndromes requires review of their derivations (Fig. 42–1) (the serious student of history is referred to two excellent and comprehensive reviews of the origins of muscle pain syndromes—one focusing on the concept of "fibrositis"[66] and the other addressing muscle pain syndromes in general[71]). After a quick look at the history of muscle pain, this chapter discusses the basic science of muscle nociception, outlines the proposed mechanisms for pain generation in general, examines the concept of muscle dysfunction, and addresses the diagnosis and treatment of the most common muscle pain syndromes.

HISTORICAL REVIEW

Early German Literature—Myelogelosis

The medical world did not distinguish between joint pain (rheumatism) and muscle pain (muscular rheumatism) until the early 1700s.[71] In Germany physicians focused on the presence of hardenings or nodules within painful muscles. The popularity of massage as a diagnostic and therapeutic tool likely heightened awareness of these nodules,

although a special technique of palpation was often necessary to identify the characteristic hardenings. Physicians blamed a change in the "colloidal state" of muscle cytoplasm for these nodules, thus giving rise to the term "myelogelosis." This term is still in use today and refers to localized muscle pain associated with a poorly characterized pathological area within the muscle (the tender point or nodule).

In Germany and Scandinavia the mainstay of treatment for muscle pain associated with nodules was massage with the goal of breaking up the muscle hardenings. Massage types ranged from "decongestive" to a technique called *Gelotripsie,* a traumatic massage involving beating the nodules with a stick.[71] The less frightening forms of massage remained the major form of physical therapy treatment for muscle pain syndromes well into this century.[48]

Early British Literature—The Concept of Fibrositis

In Great Britain, physicians identified nonarticular rheumatism as a disorder of connective tissue rather than muscle. In 1815, William Balfour of Edinburgh described nodules in rheumatic muscles. He ascribed the nodules to the products of inflammation in the connective tissue—edema and exudate—rather than to the German theory of a change in the muscle cytoplasm. In the 1850s, Thomas Inman proposed that nodules resulted from neuromuscular dysfunction manifest by local hypertonus or spasm. However, researchers found that these nodules persist under anesthesia and after death, which cast some doubt on any theories involving nervous action.

Many physicians had trouble finding nodules in patients with muscular rheumatism while others reported finding them in asymptomatic persons. Such discrepancies lowered the status of the nodule as a diagnostic sign. In 1824, Balfour described tender points in muscular rheumatism as

TABLE 42–1   Causes of Muscle Pain

Causes of Focal Muscle Pain	Causes of Generalized Muscle Pain
WITH SWELLING OR INDURATION	WITH MUSCLE WEAKNESS
Neoplasm	Inflammation (polymyositis, dermatomyositis)
Trauma (hematoma)	Infection
Ruptured tendon	Toxoplasmosis
Ruptured Baker's cyst	Trichinosis
Thrombophlebitis	Toxic myopathy (influenza or other viral infections,
Infection	leptospirosis, gram-negative infections, toxic shock
Streptococcal myositis	syndrome, Kawasaki's syndrome)
Gas gangrene	Poliomyelitis
Pyomyositis	Toxic and metabolic disorders
Trichinosis, hydatid cysts, sparganosis	Acute alcoholic myopathy
Painful leg weakness in children with influenza	Hypophosphatemia
Inflammation	Potassium deficiency
Localized nodular myositis	Total parenteral nutrition (essential fatty acid deficiency)
Proliferative myositis	Necrotic myopathy stemming from carcinoma
Pseudomalignant myositis ossificans	Hypothyroid myopathy
Eosinophilic faciitis	Drugs (ϵ-aminocaproic acid, clofibrate, emetine)
Sarcoidosis (nodular form)	Carnitine palmityltransferase deficiency
Ischemia	Amyloidosis
Muscle necrosis following relief of large artery occlusion	Bone pain and myopathy (osteomalacia, hyperparathyroidism)
Diabetes (infarction of thigh muscle)	Acute polyneuropathy (Guillain-Barré syndrome, porphyria)
Embolism (marantic endocarditis)	WITHOUT MUSCLE WEAKNESS
Azotemic hyperparathyroidism (muscle and skin necrosis)	Polymyalgia rheumatica
Toxic and metabolic disorders	Muscle pain-fasciculation syndrome
Acute alcoholic myopathy	Myalgia in infection or fever
Myoglobinuria in drug-induced coma	Myalgia in collagen-vascular disease
Exertional muscle damage	Steroid withdrawal
Normal persons (e.g., military recruits)	Hypothyroidism
Metabolic myopathies	Primary fibromyalgia (fibrositis)
Motor unit hyperactivity states (stiff-man syndrome, tetanus,	Fabry disease
strychnine poisoning)	Parkinsonism
NO SWELLING OR INDURATION	
Exertional myalgia	
Normal persons	
Vascular insufficiency (intermittent claudication)	
Metabolic myopathies	
Acute brachial neuritis	
Ischemic mononeuropathy	
Parkinsonism	
Resting leg pain of obscure cause	
Growing pains	
Restless legs	
Painful legs and moving toes	
Idiopathic leg pain	

Adapted from Layzer RB: Muscle pain, cramps, and fatigue. *In* Engel AG, Banker BQ (eds): Myology. New York, McGraw-Hill, 1986, pp 1907–1922.

distinct from nodules,[66] but the tender points were often found in locations typical for nodules. In 1841, Valleix hypothesized that these pain points arose from the pressure of diseased tissue on nerves. This began the shift from the nodule to the tender point as the primary diagnostic feature in muscle pain syndromes.

In 1904, Sir William Gowers wrote a paper in which he speculated on the etiology of "lumbago" (lumbar area muscular rheumatism).[30] He noted the frequent association of "sciatica" (posterior thigh pain) with lumbago and reasoned that, since sciatica was inflammatory in origin (according to the prevailing theory at that time), then lumbago too must be an inflammatory disorder. He generalized this logic to all soft tissue rheumatism and called it "fibrositis."

Also in 1904, Ralph Stockman[80] at the University of Glasgow published pathological studies of nodules he had excised from painful muscle. He described "edematous fibrous tissue" and although no leukocytes were seen, he labeled these nodules as inflammatory. This seemed to confirm Gowers' "fibrositis" hypothesis and served to combine the German-Scandinavian concept of the painful nodule with the British concept of inflamed connective tissue. Unfortunately, the concept of inflamed connective tissue dominated thinking about muscle pain syndromes for decades to come despite a dearth of corroborating studies.

Over the course of time, the lack of clear diagnostic criteria allowed fibrositis to be used as the label for a wide variety of pain disorders. The vast majority of the early literature dealt with localized or regional muscle pain usually secondary to trauma. In a 1943 review, Slocumb[74] at the Mayo Clinic stated that "fibrositis can affect any part of the body" and listed the various anatomical types as follows: intramuscular, periarticular, tendinous, bursal, perineural, and panniculitis. Slocumb and many others found only normal tissue on biopsy of palpable nodules, discrediting the notion of inflammation as the cause of pain in fibrositis. Many clinicians began to realize that the term "fibrositis" was a misnomer, but its widespread use and the lack of an alternative mechanism to explain muscle pain syndromes has allowed the term to survive to this day.

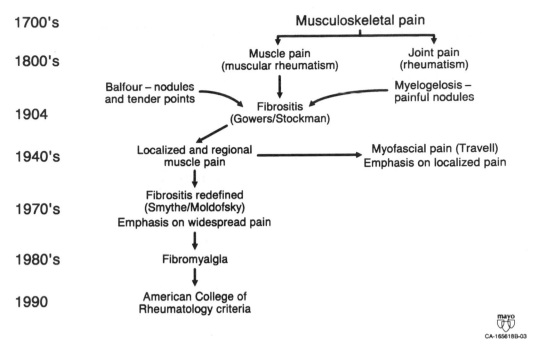

FIGURE 42–1 Muscle pain syndrome family tree—a simplified timeline depicting the derivation of two of the muscle pain syndromes (fibromyalgia and myofascial pain syndrome).

Early Theories of Etiology

As noted above, when nodules were believed to be the characteristic feature of "muscular rheumatism," theories of etiology focused on explaining their presence (products of inflammation, changes in muscle cytoplasm, local muscle spasm). As tender points became a more important diagnostic feature, theories of etiology were required to explain these points and their tendency to refer pain to distant sites. Examiners found tender points over muscles or their insertions with a consistent predilection for certain sites. Most authors invoked various reflex mechanisms to explain these findings.

J. H. Kellgren,[10, 41] expanding on work done by Sir Thomas Lewis, investigated experimentally produced muscle pain by injecting 1 to 3 mL of 6% saline into various muscles. He concluded that (1) pain from muscle is very diffuse (whereas fascia gives rise to sharply localized pain); (2) the pain has a predictable distribution for a given muscle that varies only slightly from person to person; (3) the distribution of pain generally follows a segmental pattern but differs from the segmental innervation of the skin; (4) a stimulus can cause pain that spreads over several segments; and (5) the referred pain is perceived as coming from deep structures, not the skin (Fig. 42–2).

Kellgren postulated that pain impulses from the muscle and these "deep structures" traveled a common pathway in the central nervous system (CNS) and that pain from one might be confused with pain from the other. This explained many of the findings in muscular rheumatism but not what initiated the muscle pain (presumably not surreptitious saline injections).

In 1945 and 1946, Kelly[42, 43] published two reports that attempted to explain many of the features common to fibrositis. He described his reflex theory for fibrositis as follows. Impulses from tissue injury (either somatic or visceral) travel to the CNS where they have direct connections with other cells in the CNS. Impulses from the other cells travel antidromically and cause pain in the "myalgic spot" (tender point). These myalgic spots then produce their own impulses which, again via CNS connections and antidromic spread, travel to the areas of referred pain. Kelly believed that an underlying increased excitability of the nervous system (brought about by stress or illness)

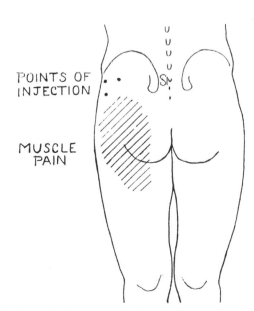

FIGURE 42–2 Kellgren's depiction of referred muscle pain after injection of 6% saline. (From Kellgren JH: On the distribution of pain arising from deep somatic structures with charts of segmental pain areas. Clin Sci 1939; 4:35–46.)

facilitated the development of myalgic spots. The "antidromic spread" described by Kelly has never been shown to exist, however.

As the 20th century wore on, fibrositis came to be increasingly identified with chronic widespread pain and less so with localized muscle pain (at least among rheumatologists).

The Redefinition of Fibrositis

In the early 1970s, the concept of fibrositis was redefined, largely through the efforts of Hugh Smythe and Harvey Moldofsky. In 1972, Smythe's chapter on fibrositis in a major rheumatology text[76] emphasized chronic, widespread pain and the presence of multiple tender points. The concepts of local muscle trauma and referral of pain to distant sites, central to Kelly's description of fibrositis, were hardly mentioned. In 1977, Smythe together with Moldofsky[78] wrote an influential paper further refining the "fibrositis syndrome" to include nonrestorative sleep and tenderness at 12 of 14 specific sites. Thus fibrositis came to be defined by rheumatologists as a chronic systemic disorder. Palpatory findings such as nodules or taut muscle bands, prominent features in the early history of soft tissue rheumatism, were left out entirely.

The Concept of Myofascial Pain

About the same time that Kelly[42, 43] wrote about fibrositis, Janet Travell formulated a theory for the cause of localized muscle pain.[11] She described the sometimes insidious onset of localized muscle spasm which led to muscle pain and, through a reflex vicious circle, to more spasm and pain. Travell uses "spasm" to describe muscle hyperactivity or guarding. Trauma was believed to be the most common cause—often such subtle trauma that the "spasm" might develop over several days before becoming evident as pain. Chronic muscular strain was deemed an equally important causative factor, often brought on by fast movements or "hurry at work." Other causes described by Travell included chilling of the body, visceral disease, and psychogenic factors. She found that the pain often radiated to distant sites from "trigger points" within the muscle (so named because they cause effects at a distance, as does the trigger of a gun). Travell advocated "local block therapy" including trigger point injections and cooling with ethyl chloride spray to interrupt the pain-spasm cycle. The various manifestations of localized muscle pain described by Travell became known as the "myofascial pain syndromes" and attracted a fervent following.

PHYSIOLOGY OF MUSCLE PAIN

Muscle pain is so common one would think its physiological basis would be well delineated. Such is not the case. Although much has been learned through extensive experimentation in both animals and humans, the exact mechanism of muscle pain and the nature of stimuli adequate to cause it remain a mystery. Nevertheless, an understanding of what is known about muscle nociception is essential to the understanding of the muscle pain syndromes.

Interestingly, the massive muscle tissue damage found in Duchenne muscular dystrophy is pain-free, yet a single sprint to first base by an unconditioned weekend athlete can result in several days of muscle pain. Obviously, simple muscle cell damage is not the stimulus for muscle pain. Mechanical damage to the connective tissue surrounding muscle cells or changes in the chemical milieu, or both, are the prime candidates for the role of muscle pain stimulators. The interaction of these stimuli with the nerve fibers purported to subserve nociception has been the topic of extensive research, well described in several reviews.[15, 53, 55, 56] The essentials are highlighted in this section.

Classification of Nociceptors

The small-diameter slowly conducting (less than 30 m/sec) afferent fibers transmit the pain signals from muscle. These include the thin myelinated group III fibers (A delta fibers) and the unmyelinated group IV fibers (C fibers).[55] In a typical nerve to a locomotor muscle, two thirds of the fibers are unmyclinated with 50% of these being sensory nerves. In turn, 43% of these sensory nerves are nociceptive.[55] Thus muscles are richly supplied with pain-sensing fibers. All of these group IV fibers begin as free nerve endings, mostly near the wall of muscle arterioles and in the surrounding connective tissue.[55] This location may explain why vascular changes (ischemia) greatly affect muscle pain (see below). Muscle sensory fibers terminate in laminae I and V of the dorsal horn, whereas skin sensory fibers terminate mostly in laminae II to IV.[55]

The group III and IV afferent fibers can be classified functionally as well. Those responding only to mechanical stimuli in the range that would cause tissue damage are termed high-threshold mechanosensitive (HTM). Those that respond to weak mechanical stimuli are called low-threshold mechanosensitive (LTM).[56] The HTM receptors are most likely the true muscle nociceptors. Mense and coworkers delineated the properties of these muscle nociceptors in an elegant series of experiments on the cat gastrocnemius muscle.[55] They functionally defined the receptive fields of nociceptor units and then subjected them to various other stimuli while recording the activity of the nociceptive unit. It became clear that these pain receptors could be activated in multiple ways. One receptor type was activated only during ischemic muscle contractions. It was postulated that these fibers transmit the pain of claudication.[56]

Mechanisms of Nociceptor Activation and Sensitization

The most potent stimulator of muscle nociceptors identified to date is bradykinin.[55] Damaged tissue releases this nonopeptide in response to lowered pH, ischemia, or blood clotting. It is likely that it is directly responsible for the muscle pain that accompanies inflammation and muscle strain (as in the weekend athlete).

The indirect effects of bradykinin can play an equally important role, however (Fig. 42–3). At lower concentrations bradykinin "sensitizes" nociceptors without activating them and lowers the threshold to mechanical stimuli of some HTM receptors. The bradykinin-sensitized HTM receptors can be activated by even gentle pressure, which

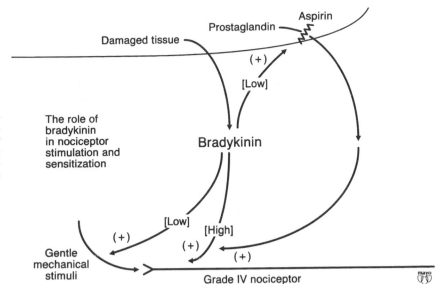

FIGURE 42–3 The role of bradykinin in nociceptor stimulation and sensitization. Bradykinin is released by damaged tissue. The arrow labeled *(high)* depicts its influence at high concentrations. The arrows labeled *(low)* depicts its influence at low concentrations. The (+) signifies activation or facilitation.

may explain the tenderness of damaged (or maybe even undamaged) muscle.[55] Bradykinin also causes the release of prostaglandins from tissue cells which in turn sensitizes nociceptors to the effects of bradykinin leading to a positive feedback loop. Aspirin, by blocking prostaglandin production, interrupts this self-perpetuating loop and thereby blocks much of the nociceptive activating effects of bradykinin. Increased temperature and lowered pH lead to sensitization of nociceptors as well, and may partially explain the beneficial effects of therapeutic cold on inflammatory pain.

Hypoxia and epinephrine also activate muscle nociceptors.[55] Nociceptors in damaged tissue are the most sensitive to activation by epinephrine, which may indicate one mechanism by which the sympathetic nervous system affects the pain experience. Other activators of nociceptors include serotonin and potassium ions.

Spinal Mechanisms of Muscle Pain

Stimulation of muscle nociceptors is only one step in the very complex physiological system that subserves the experience of muscle pain. There are several mechanisms at the spinal level that further influence muscle nociception. These include convergence of peripheral input on dorsal horn neurons, descending inhibition of the dorsal horn, distribution of muscle afferents over several spinal segments, and neuroplasticity.

Neurons that receive input from nociceptors in muscle and other deep structures are located in laminae I and IV to VI in the dorsal horn. Dorsal horn cells that receive input only from muscle nociceptors are extremely rare. The vast majority of cells that respond to stimulation of muscle nociceptors respond to skin stimulation as well.[55] In fact, these cells often respond to stimulation of several "receptive fields" located both deep and on the skin (Fig. 42–4). This convergence of several receptive fields from the periphery on a single dorsal horn cell explains the poorly localized nature of muscle pain and other deep sensations, affirming the theories of Kellgren noted above.

These convergent dorsal horn cells are also under strong tonic descending inhibition which preferentially inhibits the input from deep structures, further decreasing the accuracy of localization.

Another cause of the poor localization of muscle pain could be the distribution of afferents from a specific muscle over several spinal segments.[56] This, combined with the multiple deep receptive fields found for many dorsal horn neurons, could explain the spread or referral of muscle pain to other areas. Strong stimulation of distal motor nerve fascicles leads to deep cramping pain not only in the muscles innervated by that nerve but also in other muscles innervated at the same root level.[53] This "radicular pattern" of pain referral does not follow the cutaneous distribution of the nerve roots, confirming Kellgren's observation that referred muscle pain follows a myotome rather than a dermatome.

Neuroplasticity at the spinal level refers to the finding that dorsal horn cells can have long-lasting changes in their response characteristics and morphology after a triggering stimulus.[55] Bradykinin stimulation of skeletal muscle in animals lowers the threshold to mechanical stimuli of the injected receptive field and increases the size of this field. It also causes a prolonged lowering of the threshold in other receptive fields. Researchers believe this results from a sensitization of the dorsal horn neuron by a neuropeptide (such as substance P) released from the spinal terminals of muscle afferents. In a rat model, substance P unmasked previously ineffective dorsal horn synaptic connections. Some of these unmasked connections might include afferents from low-threshold mechanosensitive receptors, allowing these low-threshold receptors to activate nociceptive cells in the dorsal horn.[55] In this way, strong activation of muscle nociceptors could release substance P at their dorsal horn terminals, thereby inducing such changes in the dorsal horn neurons. The unmasking of previously ineffective connections to allow non-nociceptive nerve fibers to activate nociceptive dorsal horn cells may explain allodynia—the perception of pain caused by nonpainful stimuli.

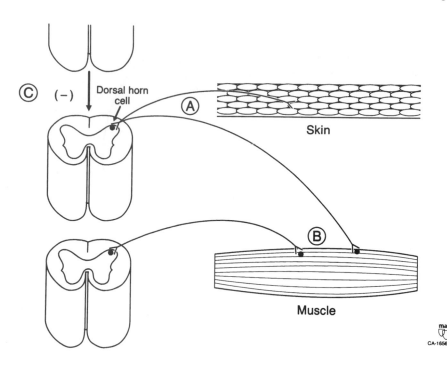

FIGURE 42–4 Spinal mechanisms of nociception. *A,* Convergence of deep and skin nociceptors on a single dorsal horn neuron. *B,* Afferents from one muscle can spread over several spinal segments. *C,* Descending inhibitory pathways also terminate on nociceptive dorsal horn cells.

Supraspinal Mechanisms of Muscle Pain

Little knowledge exists about the processing of muscle nociception at the subcortical and cortical levels of the brain, although the thalamic nuclei and somatosensory cortex are apparently involved to some degree. Cutaneous pain and muscle pain may well be processed in different areas since some patients with thalamic lesions have insensate skin but perceive the deep pain of saline injections.[55]

Evidence also exists for both inhibiting and facilitating pathways from supraspinal structures affecting the dorsal horn.[56] Serotonin appears to be one of the major neurotransmitters of the inhibitory system. Dysfunction of these central pain mechanisms forms the basis of at least one theory of widespread muscle pain.

The Concept of Motor Dysfunction

"Motor dysfunction" is a vague term used by practitioners of manual medicine. Examples of motor dysfunction include contractures, "tight" muscles, muscle "spasm," and incoordination of muscle firing patterns (including co-contraction). Most clinicians dealing with muscle pain patients describe various degrees of muscle "spasm," including the common finding of the patient who moves en bloc because of axial muscle pain. According to the manual medicine literature, this motor dysfunction leads to muscle overuse and microtrauma, which in turn lead to muscle pain. At least one study found that manual medicine to correct the motor dysfunction relieves the pain with a success rate similar to that found with traditional physical therapy.[45]

Demonstration of muscle dysfunction is largely subjective, relying on palpation and often subtle deficiencies of range of motion. Recently, dynamic surface electromyographic (EMG) monitoring has been used to more objectively measure motor dysfunction. One application of this technique monitors the activity of an individual muscle and its contralateral counterpart (e.g., right and left sternocleidomastoid) while the subject performs symmetrical movements (flex and extend, turn right and left). The "dysfunctioning" muscle often has a higher level of activity or does not return to baseline at the end of a movement[47] (Fig. 42–5A and B).

Surface EMG monitoring has also demonstrated a decrease in the number and length of pauses in EMG activity between contractions[17, 18] and higher activity during a functional task or during contraction of distant muscles.[22] In a prospective study, workers who had fewer "gaps" in their EMG activity developed localized muscle pain in the monitored muscle.[86] This implies that lack of rest between contractions leads to muscle pain. Sleep disturbance further disrupts the muscles' ability to "rest."[16]

Treatment of motor dysfunction involves restoration of normal length and tension relationships in muscle and normal range of motion around joints. Surface EMG biofeedback is a common and often effective way to accomplish the neuromuscular re-education required to treat disordered muscle firing patterns. This typically involves teaching the patient to achieve muscular relaxation at rest and to eventually maintain this relaxation without feedback. Another common strategy teaches the patient to work for symmetry of EMG activity in paired muscles by increasing activation in the "hypoactive" muscle. Pain relief often coincides with resumption of EMG symmetry.

MUSCLE PAIN SYNDROMES

Table 42–1 lists the many causes of muscle pain. The muscle pain syndromes are those entities that have muscle pain as a major component but do not have an established cause and therefore do not qualify as diseases. The following are descriptions of the most common muscle pain

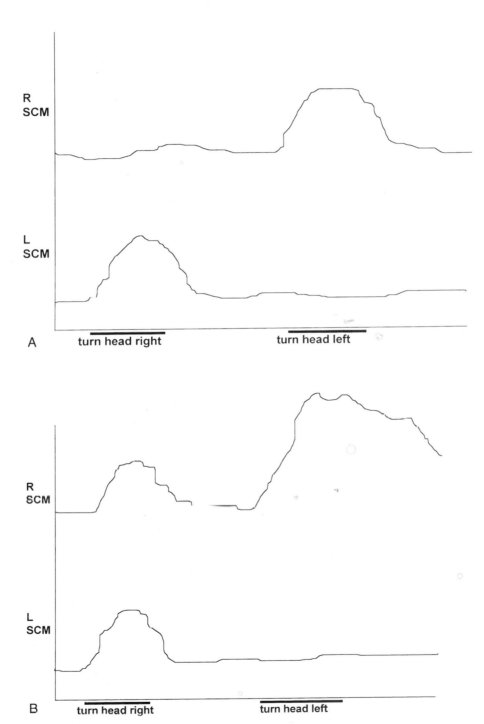

FIGURE 42–5 Surface EMG recording from the right and left sternocleidomastoid (SCM) in a subject without neck pain showing normal reciprocal activation *(A)*, and in a subject with neck pain showing "dysfunction" of the right SCM *(B)*. Note the excessive activation and the failure of the right SCM to return to baseline after the movement. (The lines under the graphs labeled "turn head right" and "turn head left" depict the duration of the respective movements.)

syndromes, roughly ordered from localized to more generalized, systemic disorders.

Postexercise Muscle Soreness

Most people experience postexercise muscle soreness at one time or another. However, its cause is still not fully understood. Clinically, the pain is most common following unaccustomed exercise using untrained muscles and peaks 24 to 48 hours after the exercise. Serum muscle enzymes reach their peak at about the same time.[50] Eccentric (lengthening) contractions provoke this pain much more efficiently than concentric (shortening) contractions. A few weeks of training can reduce or prevent this type of muscle soreness.

The cause of postexercise muscle pain may be a clue to muscle pain in general. Unfortunately, it remains an enigma. With eccentric exercise (e.g., going downstairs), the external forces acting on the muscle are greater than the forces generated by the muscle itself. These external forces are spread over a smaller percentage of motor units, leading to damage in the muscle fibers and connective tissue.[55] The release of nociceptor-sensitizing substances during repair of this damage may lead to the delayed muscle soreness. The pain probably is not caused by the mechanical muscle fiber damage directly, since serum enzyme levels do not rise immediately. Since type I (oxidative) fibers are preferentially damaged, and since training can have a protective effect, disordered metabolism is probably a contributing component.[50] The strengthening that occurs during the first few weeks of training is attributed to neural factors such as coordination of motor unit firing. This, along with motor learning, could explain how training of similar duration protects against postexercise muscle soreness.

Treatment of postexercise muscle soreness is simple and effective. Rest and a more gradual approach to exercise cures most patients. Nonsteroidal anti-inflammatory drugs do not help, which eliminates prostaglandin from contention as a sensitizing agent.

Overuse Syndromes

The terms "overuse injury" and "repetitive strain injury" encompass a wide variety of musculoskeletal pain problems. Nerve entrapments, stress fractures, tendinitis and bursitis, and muscle pain have all been labeled overuse injuries. These are covered in more detail in Chapter 44 (occupational rehabilitation) and in Chapters 37 and 38 (upper and lower limb musculoskeletal disorders). This section focuses briefly on the place of overuse injuries in the spectrum of muscle pain.

In contrast to postexercise muscle pain, overuse muscle pain often occurs in well-trained muscles. Overuse pain arises from the repetitive use of a muscle, not from a single bout of exercise. These injuries are most common in athletes, musicians, and factory-line workers, where precise repetition of motor tasks is frequently a requirement for success.

The cause of overuse muscle pain is thought to be microtrauma that outpaces the capacity of the muscle for repair. Edwards[16] describes the final common pathway of muscle pain beginning with an excessive force per muscle fiber leading to hypoxia, acidosis, and metabolic depletion,

followed by calcium-mediated cellular damage. In laborers, continued use of fatigued muscles causes mechanical damage that is directly related to the heaviness of the work. Again, eccentric work seems to subject small numbers of muscle fibers to excessive loads.

Many occupations, however, require precise manipulations, leading to excessive contraction of the proximal stabilizers that is unrelated to the heaviness of the task. The forces required to perform the task are not large enough to overload the muscles and cause damage. Rather, the conflict of motor control between the postural stabilizers and the muscles needed for precise manipulation or movement leads to the fiber damage.[16]

The combination of mental stress and precise manipulations experienced by musicians can lead to occupational cramps believed to be of central origin (focal dystonia). These cramps may be just an extreme example of the muscle pain that can occur with disordered motor planning. They occur more commonly early in the career of the artist, before the smooth, seemingly effortless motor patterns are established.[16]

Incoordination of movements and co-contraction of agonist-antagonists are often seen in the context of muscle pain. An example is the trapezius myalgia found in factory workers (see the discussion of motor dysfunction, above).

Myofascial Pain Syndromes

The myofascial pain syndromes owe their ever-widening acceptance (if not their existence) to the pioneering work of Travell[11] and her later collaboration with Simons.[84] In 1983, they combined their clinical experience in a detailed description of the multiple pain syndromes attributed to this disorder.[84] In doing so, they further defined the major clinical components characteristic of myofascial pain, the most important being the trigger point, the "taut band," and the local "twitch" response.

The Trigger Point

As noted earlier, the trigger point got its name from its propensity to cause pain at a distant site. These points play a central role in the definition of myofascial pain syndromes and appear in predictable locations, usually in the midportion or belly of the affected muscle. Flat palpation of a relaxed muscle under passive stretch best locates these small (less than 1 cm^2) discrete tender spots (Fig. 42–6). Sustained pressure (10 sec) or penetration by a needle usually causes a referral of pain into the "zone of reference" typical of that muscle. There may or may not be a palpable nodule at the site. Often the trigger point is located within a taut band in a muscle with decreased range of motion.

The significance of these trigger points is not clear. Some researchers believe they arise from localized areas of muscle trauma, but biopsy studies show mostly normal muscle. Uncontrolled studies have found nonspecific changes suggestive of localized ischemia (ragged red fibers, decreased adenosine triphosphate [ATP]).[95, 96] Others believe these findings are secondary to a local "energy crisis" in the muscle. Such an energy crisis is postulated to cause release of substances which sensitize nociceptors to respond to innocuous pressure.[35]

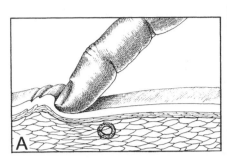
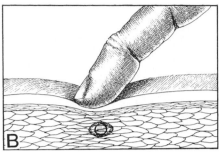
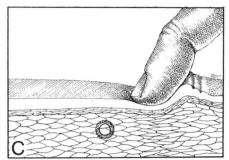

FIGURE 42–6 Cross-sectional schematic drawing of the technique of flat palpation of a trigger point. The dark ring represents a taut band and the circle within it is the trigger point. *A,* Skin is pushed to one side to begin palpation. *B,* Fingertip sliding across the muscle fibers to feel the taut band rolling beneath it. *C,* Skin pushed to other side at completion of "snapping" palpation (see also Fig. 42–7). (From Travell JG, Simons DG: Myofascial pain and dysfunction: The trigger point manual. Baltimore, Williams & Wilkins, 1983.)

A recent study using monopolar needle EMG found spontaneous electrical activity on penetration of trapezius trigger points.[37] The electrical activity was usually of low amplitude and was accompanied by aching pain in the same referral pattern as that found with sustained pressure on the trigger point. The electrical activity described is identical to that attributed to "end-plate noise" during routine EMG. The authors theorized that spontaneous activity from the muscle spindle is being recorded.[37] Sustained activity in the intrafusal fibers of the muscle spindle (due to sympathetic activity) is thought to bring about an increase in the resting tone of the muscle. Pain is attributed to damage to the spindle capsule. On the other hand, the researchers may have recorded only end-plate noise. Others, using similar techniques,[15] have found no such activity attributable to trigger points.

The inter- and intratester reliability of the trigger point examination has not been adequately investigated. In fact, in one pilot study, even expert examiners varied widely in trigger point count.[91] Less well-trained examiners performed even more poorly.[62] Pressure algometers improve the objectivity of the examination and may be useful in clinical studies or in documenting response to treatment[14, 21, 64] (although the relationship between the number and sensitivity of trigger points and disease severity has not been established).

Thermography is another tool used for documentation of trigger points. However, in a blinded study, patients without trigger points had as many hot spots as those with trigger points.[81] Whether trigger points differ from the tender points of fibromyalgia remains unclear. Rheumatologists generally do not apply sustained pressure to or needle tender points, and are therefore not likely to elicit the major differentiating feature—referred pain. There is likely a large amount of overlap between the two types of points.

The Taut Band

Trigger points are characteristically found within taut bands of muscle. The taut band is a shortened group of muscle fibers and can be best palpated by sliding the skin and subcutaneous tissues perpendicularly across the fibers of the muscle. These bands are electrically silent and therefore not due to "spasm." Localized contracture of a few muscle fibers is one proposed mechanism. Today's taut bands may be identical to the fibrositic nodules of the early muscle pain literature. Once the taut band is found, palpation along it will lead to the most tender point—the trigger point. "Snapping palpation" of the band gives rise to another cardinal sign of myofascial pain, the local twitch response (Fig. 42–7).

The Local Twitch Response

When one "snaps" the taut band containing a trigger point, a transient contraction of the band's muscle fibers occurs. This sign is diagnostically important as noted below, but its pathophysiological significance is unclear. EMG studies document electrical activity during the twitch[23] that is not blocked by total motor and sensory anesthesia. Needling of a trigger point also produces a twitch response. The technique of snapping palpation requires significant skill and its validity as a diagnostic sign has not been established.

Clinical and Research Criteria

The first international symposium on myofascial pain and fibromyalgia was held in 1989. It marked one of the first meetings of the principal proponents of the two major muscle pain syndromes. In the proceedings of that symposium, Simons[72] listed the clinical criteria for diagnosis of myofascial pain syndrome (Table 42–2). The required features include regional pain, referred pain or disturbed sensation in a predicted location, a taut band, a tender point along the taut band, and restricted range of motion. One of three "minor criteria" must also be present: (1) pain complaint reproduced by pressure on the tender spot, (2) a local twitch response, or (3) relief of the pain by stretching or injecting. At the same time Simons listed research criteria for the identification of trigger points. To qualify, the point must be exquisitely tender, located in a taut band of a muscle with restricted range of motion, refer pain when pressed or needled, and exhibit a twitch response when needled.

These criteria are obviously derived from many years of clinical experience, but their validity has not been tested. Simons suggests that, in the absence of a gold standard, these criteria should be tested against clinical expert opinion. Four such experts found taut bands and twitch responses with equal frequency in fibromyalgia patients, my-

Taut (palpable) bands in muscle

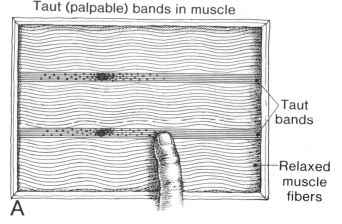

Local twitch response

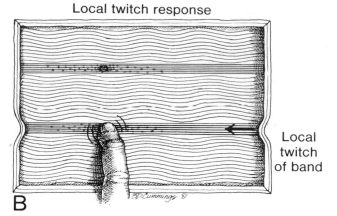

FIGURE 42–7   Schematic drawing of taut bands and myofascial trigger points. *A,* Straight lines represent the cord-like taut band of muscle within normal, relaxed muscle *(wavy lines).* The density of the stippling within the taut band corresponds to the degree of tenderness to palpation. The most tender spot *(dark ring)* is the trigger point. *B,* Rolling the taut band under the fingertip at the trigger point (snapping palpation) often produces a "local twitch response" with shortening of the band of muscle. (From Travell JG, Simons DG: Myofascial pain and dysfunction: The trigger point manual. Baltimore, Williams & Wilkins, 1983.)

ofascial pain patients, and controls. The experts also differed significantly among themselves in their determinations of trigger point count, taut bands, and twitch responses.[91] Although these criteria can be clinically useful as guidelines, they likely will not show enough validity for strict diagnostic criteria.

Pathophysiology

The myofascial pain syndromes remain largely a clinical construct based more on case studies, anecdote, and clinical experience than basic science. The application of EMG to the study of myofascial pain forced a redefinition of the syndrome. Since EMG studies failed to find "spasm" in the involved muscles,[46] the spasm-pain-spasm theory was

TABLE 42–2   Clinical Criteria for the Diagnosis of Myofascial Pain Syndrome Caused by Active Trigger Points

To make the clinical diagnosis of myofascial pain syndrome, the findings should include five major criteria and at least one of three minor criteria. The five *major criteria* include the following:

1. Regional pain complaint.
2. Pain complaint or altered sensation in the expected distribution of referred pain from a myofascial trigger point.
3. Taut band palpable in an accessible muscle.
4. Exquisite spot tenderness at one point along the length of the taut band.
5. Some degree of restricted range of motion, when measurable.

The three *minor criteria* include the following:

1. Reproduction of clinical pain complaint, or altered sensation, by pressure on the tender spot.
2. Elicitation of a local twitch response by transverse snapping palpation at the tender spot or by needle insertion into the tender spot in the taut band.
3. Pain alleviated by elongating (stretching) the muscle or by injecting the tender spot (trigger point).

Note: Additional symptoms such as weather sensitivity, sleep disturbance, and depression are often present but are not diagnostic because they may be attributable to chronic severe pain perpetuated by multiple mechanical and/or systemic perpetuating factors.

From Simons AG: Muscular pain syndromes. *In* Fricton JR, Awad EA (eds): Advances in Pain Research and Therapy, vol 17: Myofascial Pain and Fibromyalgia. New York, Raven Press, 1990, p 18.

abandoned. In its place Travell and Simons[84] combined facts of muscle physiology with some conjecture and arrived at the following sequence: acute muscle strain → tissue damage in a very localized area of muscle → tears in the sarcoplasmic reticulum → free calcium ions → sustained contraction → increased strain on vulnerable areas of muscle → free calcium ions, etc.

Travell and Simons further proposed that the free calcium ions plus ATP leads to sustained contraction of fibers causing a hypermetabolic state locally and local vasoconstriction (possibly via the sympathetic nervous system). Local vasoconstriction causes local ischemia, which, combined with increased energy demands, leads to the histological changes mentioned above.

Travell and Simons postulated that depletion of ATP leads to a contracture state with electrical silence (as in McArdle's disease or rigor mortis). In addition, the tissue damage releases serotonin, histamine, and kinins, which also lead to local ischemia as well as nerve sensitization.[84]

Even with the difficulties outlined above, the myofascial pain syndromes remain a useful clinical paradigm, often leading to successful treatment of muscle pain problems. They are also very common. Thirty percent of patients attending a general medical clinic with the chief complaint of pain were found to have myofascial pain.[73] Several of the most common single muscle syndromes are presented in Figures 42–8 through 42–13. Shown are the locations of trigger points (Fig. 42–14) and the pattern of referred pain.

Chronic Regional Myofascial Syndromes

The single muscle myofascial pain syndromes are usually acute and follow an episode of muscle overload. In some cases, the pain persists and spreads to other, usually synergistic, muscles. This is referred to as a chronic regional myofascial syndrome.[72] Many perpetuating factors encourage transformation to a more widespread muscle pain problem. Mechanical factors include postural stress, muscle imbalances, and skeletal asymmetries. These can put additional stress on surrounding muscles leading to spread of dysfunction and pain. Systemic perpetuating fac-

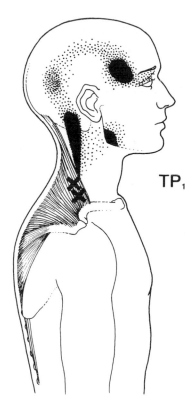

FIGURE 42–8 Location (*X*s) and referred pain pattern for the most common trapezius trigger point, referred to as trigger point 1 (TP1). *Dark areas* show the main pattern of pain referral; *stippling* maps the spillover areas. (From Travell JG, Simons DG: Myofascial pain and dysfunction: The trigger point manual. Baltimore, Williams & Wilkins, 1983.)

tors purportedly include anything jeopardizing the energy supply to muscle (i.e., anemia, endocrine imbalances, low thyroid function, vitamin deficiencies).[81] Chronic regional myofascial syndromes are conceptually close to the "malignant, metastasizing fibromyalgia" referred to by Bennett.[2]

Fibromyalgia

The Search for a Definition

As mentioned earlier, Smythe and Moldofsky redefined fibrositis to include only the widespread form of muscle pain. Table 42–3 lists their criteria, which include widespread aching for 3 months, 12 of 14 tender points, and disturbed sleep, along with several other attempts at a definition for widespread muscle pain.

Yunus[97] further refined Smythe's original criteria with the addition of commonly found associated symptoms. He reduced the required number of tender points to five and allowed as few as three tender points if five of the minor criteria were present. A later update allowed as few as 2 of 14 tender points.[93] He also changed the name from fibrositis to fibromyalgia (borrowing from Hench) because of the lack of inflammation. Most subsequent studies have used the Yunus criteria to define fibromyalgia, allowing for the inclusion of regional and even localized muscle pain. Recognizing the problem the Yunus criteria posed when trying to differentiate fibromyalgia from myofascial pain

and other localized muscle pain syndromes, Wolfe[89] raised the tender point count to 7 of 14. He also eliminated associated symptoms and modulating factors from the definition because they did not improve the sensitivity of the criteria.[89]

In 1990, the Multicenter Criteria Committee of the American College of Rheumatology (ACR 90) published its criteria for classification of fibromyalgia[92] (Table 42–4). Once again, the emphasis is placed on the widespread nature of fibromyalgia with the requirement of 11 of 18 tender points.

Prevalence and Epidemiology

Few epidemiological studies have used the ACR 90 criteria. Nevertheless fibromyalgia is common in the community, found in 2% to 4% of the general population.[88] Widespread pain as defined by the ACR 90 criteria is found in 11.2% of the adult population of northern England.[13] Eight percent of general medical patients meet previous definitions of fibromyalgia[7] as do about 15% to 20% of rheumatology clinic patients, making fibromyalgia the third most common diagnosis made by rheumatologists.[90, 97] Women make up 73% to 90% of those diagnosed with fibromyalgia,[5, 88] although this may represent a selection bias. Regardless of the definition, fibromyalgia appears to be a very common entity.

Throughout all of the definitions the major clinical fea-

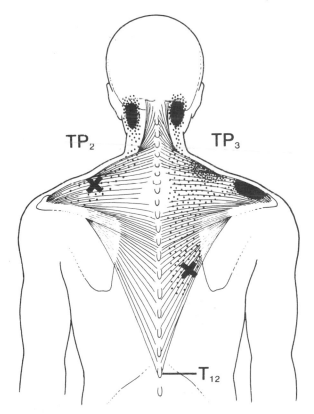

FIGURE 42–9 Locations (*X*s) and referred pain patterns of trigger point 2 (TP2), in the left upper trapezius, and trigger point 3 (TP3), in the right lower trapezius. (Conventions are as in Fig. 42–8.) (From Travell JG, Simons DG: Myofascial pain and dysfunction: The trigger point manual. Baltimore, Williams & Wilkins, 1983.)

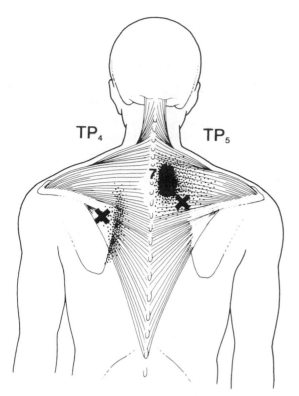

FIGURE 42–10 Locations (*X*s) and referred pain patterns of trigger point 4 (TP4) in the left lower trapezius, and trigger point 5 (TP5) in the right middle trapezius. (Conventions are as in Fig. 42–8.) (From Travell JG, Simons DG: Myofascial pain and dysfunction: The trigger point manual. Baltimore, Williams & Wilkins, 1983.)

tures of fibromyalgia have remained relatively constant but with varying degrees of emphasis. The best way to differentiate patients with fibromyalgia appears to be by widespread pain and high tender point count. Other important features include sleep disturbance, fatigue, headaches, irritable bowel syndrome, and paresthesias.

Clinical Features

Widespread Pain and Tenderness

Widespread pain of 3 months' duration is required for the diagnosis of fibromyalgia and is defined as pain both above and below the waist, on both the right and left sides of the body, along with axial pain (low back pain is considered below the waist).[92] As noted above, this may include greater than 10% of the population, making the tender point count very important in the diagnosis of fibromyalgia. The point count required was set at 11 to maximize the specificity of the classification for study purposes. Many of those with fewer points are also likely to have fibromyalgia. How low the count should be allowed to go is a matter of debate.

The reliability of the tender point count is somewhat better established than is the trigger point examination. In the study mentioned earlier the fibromyalgia experts were fairly consistent in the point count—largely owing to the predetermined examination sites and the sole requirement of tenderness.[91] The test-retest and interrater reliability of the tender point examination using a pressure algometer was quite good (.85 generalizability coefficient), but the points were marked ahead of time.[85] Even so, the two examiners differed significantly at the most common tender point site—the upper trapezius.

The sites in the ACR 90 criteria were chosen based on their utility in separating fibromyalgia patients from those with other painful conditions. It is implied that they are discrete points of tenderness. A study of 75 unilateral points found 19 that best discriminated between patients and controls.[70] Only three of the ACR 90 points were included in the 19 best points. The significant tender points clustered in regions—the anterior shoulder, anterior chest, scapula, and medial knee—suggesting that tenderness in a region may be more useful clinically than tenderness at specific points.

Three interpretations, singly or in combination, are pos-

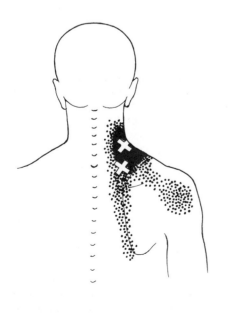

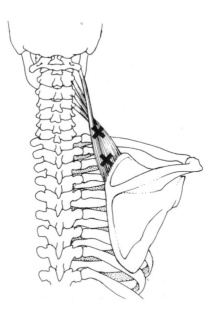

FIGURE 42–11 Trigger points (*X*s) of the right levator scapulae muscle. The *dark area* shows the pattern of referred pain and the *stippling* locates the spillover zone. (From Travell JG, Simons DG: Myofascial pain and dysfunction: The trigger point manual. Baltimore, Williams & Wilkins, 1983.)

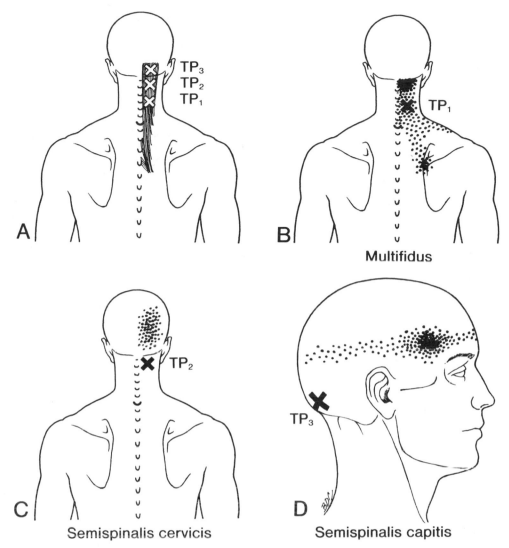

FIGURE 42–12 *A,* Trigger point locations (XS) in the medial posterior cervical muscles. *B,* The most common posterior cervical trigger point (TP1) lies deep at the C4 or C5 level. It is thought to lie in the multifidi or rotator muscles, and these muscles may entrap the greater occipital nerve. The *stippling* indicates the pattern of referred pain. *C,* Trigger point in the semispinalis cervicus (TP2). *D,* The uppermost trigger point in the semispinalis capitis (TP3). (From Travell JG, Simons DG: Myofascial pain and dysfunction: The trigger point manual. Baltimore, Williams & Wilkins, 1983.)

sible regarding tender points: (1) they represent specific areas of pathologic change; (2) they identify multiple regions of pain; or (3) they signify a generalized increase in tenderness. This has implications for the etiology of fibromyalgia. Those who have found increased tenderness at tender points but no difference between patients and controls at usually nontender control sites favor a peripheral mechanism for the production of pain.[7] Those who have found a generalized increase in sensitivity to pressure proclaim the importance of central modulating factors as a cause of increased pain in fibromyalgia.[31, 70]

Sleep Disturbance

Almost all descriptions of fibromyalgia include poor sleep as a feature. In 1975, Moldofsky and associates[59] proposed the term "non-restorative sleep syndrome" to replace fibrositis. They studied 10 patients with the diagno-

sis of fibrositis and found that seven had intrusion of alpha rhythms into stage 4 delta sleep. At one time, and even recently,[5] the alpha-delta sleep pattern was thought to be diagnostic, and possibly the cause of fibromyalgia.[60] This alpha-delta sleep pattern was originally described by Hauri and Hawkins[33] and correlates with subjective fatigue. The presence of poor sleep in the diagnostic criteria used for patient selection in the study of Moldofsky et al. likely influenced the results since fibromyalgia patients that claim to be good sleepers do not differ from controls in alpha-delta sleep.[36] Other investigators have been unable to confirm the correlation of alpha-delta sleep with fibrositis (fibromyalgia).[26] The finding is very nonspecific and can be found in any chronically painful condition.[32]

Nonetheless, disturbed sleep is common in fibromyalgia, with reports of incidence ranging from 60% to 90%.[28] Patients with myofascial pain have similar degrees of sleep disturbance,[69] with the incidence of sleep disturbance

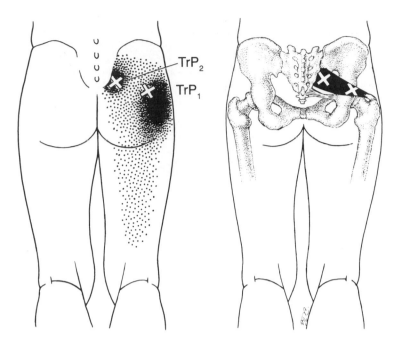

FIGURE 42–13 Locations of trigger points (Xs) in the piriformis muscle. The lateral X marks the most common location within the piriformis. The *dark area* shows the pattern of referred pain and the *stippling* locates the spill-over zone. (From Travell JG, Simons DG: Myofascial pain and dysfunction: The trigger point manual. Baltimore, Williams & Wilkins, 1983.)

correlating better with duration of pain than with diagnosis.[39]

Associated Symptoms

Multiple associated features commonly appear in reports of fibromyalgia. The most common are fatigue (75%–100%), stiffness (75%–90%), subjective swelling (30%–

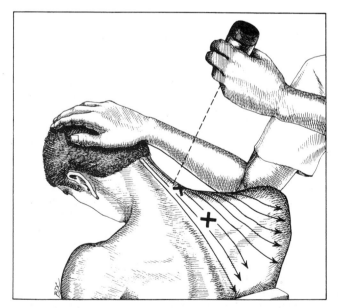

FIGURE 42–14 Technique of "spray and stretch" treatment for right levator scapulae trigger points (Xs). The *arrows* indicate the direction and pattern of the vapocoolant spray. During the "distraction" of the spray, the operator presses the patient's head forward and to the opposite side while using the elbow to press the patient's shoulder down and back. Similar techniques are applied to most other trigger points. The key ingredient is the prolonged stretch of the affected muscle. (From Travell JG, Simons DG: Myofascial pain and dysfunction: The trigger point manual. Baltimore, Williams & Wilkins, 1983.)

100%), tension-type headache (45%–75%), anxiety (40%–70%), and irritable bowel syndrome (35%–50%).[39] Other common features include aggravation of symptoms by cold, humidity, change of weather, and physical activity. The frequency of these features in regional and localized muscle pain syndromes and other chronic pain syndromes remains unclear. The prevalence of many of these features likely increases as the number of regions involved with pain increases and as the pain becomes more chronic.

Psychological Aspects

Partly because of the high number of somatic complaints voiced by patients with fibromyalgia, many clinicians view the patients as psychologically disturbed. In fact, one clinician refers to the disorder as a "psychophysiologic" state.[87] Many early studies reporting psychopathological findings used the Minnesota Multiphasic Personality Inventory (MMPI), which is poorly suited to the study of patients with pain.[77] Although some studies find no difference between fibromyalgia patients and controls using other standardized tests (Beck Depression Inventory, Spielberger State and Trait Anxiety Inventory, SCL-90-R),[8] or DSM-III (*Diagnostic and Statistical Manual of Mental Disorders*) diagnoses,[1] a review concluded that psychological disturbance is associated with fibromyalgia syndrome.[6] The majority of fibromyalgia patients do not have an active psychiatric disorder, but there is a greater prevalence of major depression and panic disorder.[38, 61] It may well be that the psychological aspects of fibromyalgia simply result from chronic pain and its effect on central pain modulation systems.[4, 49, 65]

Another view is that patients with a primary psychiatric disorder and symptoms of fibromyalgia represent one end of the spectrum of fibromyalgia disorders.[61] In these patients the symptoms of fibromyalgia wax and wane with the psychiatric disorder and with psychosocial stressors. A particularly difficult differentiation is that between fibro-

TABLE 42–3   Reported Diagnostic Features of Muscle Pain Syndromes

Feature	Fibrositis (Smythe[70])	Nonrestorative Sleep (Moldofsky[60])	Fibromyalgia		
			Wolfe[89]	Yunus et al.[97]	1990 ACR[92]
Widespread aching (3 mo)	X	X	X	X	X
Tender points (no.)	X (12/14)	X	X (7+)	X (5+)	X (11/18)
Skin roll tenderness	X	—	—	—	—
Disturbed sleep	X	X	—	X	—
Normal x-ray and laboratory findings	X	X	X	X	—
"Type A" personality	X	—	—	—	—
Relief with heat	—	X	—	—	—
Dermatographia	—	X	—	—	—
Emotional distress	—	X	—	X	—
Effects of weather	—	X	—	X	—
No trauma or rheumatic disease	—	—	—	X	—
Relief with physical activity	—	—	—	X	—
Irritable bowel syndrome	—	—	—	X	—

myalgia and somatization disorder or somatoform pain disorder. Both of these require the presence of multiple symptoms or pain without causative organic pathological findings, or that the complaint or impairment be out of proportion to the physical findings. As muscle pain persists

TABLE 42–4   The American College of Rheumatology 1990 Criteria for Classification of Fibromyalgia*

1. History of widespread pain
   Definition: Pain is considered widespread when all the following are present—pain in the left side of the body, pain in the right side of the body, pain above the waist, and pain below the waist. In addition, axial skeletal pain (cervical spine, anterior chest, thoracic spine, or low back) must be present. In this definition, shoulder and buttock pain is considered as pain for each involved side. "Low back" pain is considered lower segment pain.
2. Pain in 11 of 18 tender point sites on digital palpation
   Definition: On digital palpation, pain must be present in at least 11 of the following 18 tender point sites:
     Occiput—Bilateral, at the suboccipital muscle insertions
     Low cervical—Bilateral, at the anterior aspects of the intertransverse spaces at C5 to C7
     Trapezius—Bilateral, at the midpoint of the upper border
     Supraspinatus—Bilateral, at origins, above the scapular spine near the medial border
     Second rib—Bilateral, at the second costochondral junctions, just lateral to the junctions on upper surfaces
     Lateral epicondyle—Bilateral, 2 cm distal to the epicondyles
     Gluteal—Bilateral, in upper outer quadrants of buttocks in anterior fold of muscle
     Greater trochanter—Bilateral, posterior to the trochanteric prominence
     Knee—Bilateral, at the medial fat pad proximal to the joint line
   Digital palpation should be performed with an approximate force of 4 kg
   For a tender point to be considered "positive," the subject must state that the palpation was painful. "Tender" is not to be considered "painful."

*For classification purposes, patients will be said to have fibromyalgia if both criteria are satisfied. Widespread pain must have been present for at least 3 mo. The presence of a second clinical disorder does not exclude the diagnosis of fibromyalgia.
From Wolfe F, Smythe HA, Yunus MB, et al: The American College of Rheumatology 1990 criteria for the classification of fibromyalgia. Arthritis Rheum 1990; 33:160–172.

and becomes more widespread, the incidence of these psychiatric disorders increases.

Pathophysiology-Proposed Mechanisms

The pathophysiology of fibromyalgia remains a mystery. The few abnormalities found in various studies tend to be nonspecific and lend themselves to various interpretations. These have been combined liberally with conjecture to arrive at the leading theories of pathophysiology. The theories can be divided into three groups based on the location of the proposed mechanism: (1) primarily central, (2) a combination of central and peripheral, or (3) primarily peripheral.

One "central mechanism" theory hypothesizes that fibromyalgia is a variation of an affective disorder.[38] This is based primarily on the frequent co-morbidity of fibromyalgia with major depression, migraine, irritable bowel syndrome, chronic fatigue syndrome, and panic disorder—all of which are thought to share a common pathophysiology. No causal link exists between the disorders, but rather an underlying abnormality exists that is necessary but not sufficient for these disorders to occur. This predisposition (genetic?) combines with environmental factors to produce the particular disorder.

Another "central" theory identifies the alpha electroencephalographic (EEG) sleep anomaly as the root cause of fibromyalgia.[58, 59] Anything that disrupts sleep—an emotionally stressful event, sleep apnea, or flulike illness—can cause the alpha sleep anomaly. The sleep disorder in turn alters the brain chemistry of substances associated with both sleep arousal and pain modulation, such as serotonin and substance P.

Yunus[94] adds peripheral modulation to aberrant central pain mechanisms, combining central with peripheral components (Fig. 42–15). He blames "central neurohormonal dysfunction" for a functional deficiency of inhibitory neural transmitters or overactivity of excitatory neurotransmitters. Decreased serotonin is one possible mechanism. Peripheral factors such as microtrauma and referred pain are thought to play a minor role. The presence of a generalized decrease in pain tolerance points to the importance of central factors. The "central neurohormonal dysfunction"

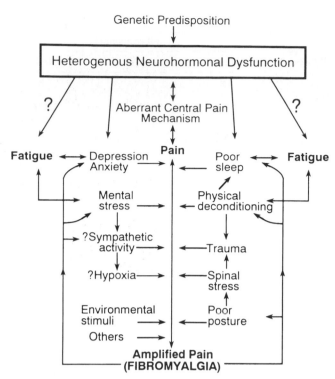

FIGURE 42–15 The pathophysiology of fibromyalgia according to Yunus. The primary defect is thought to be a poorly characterized central "neurohormonal dysfunction," which leads to an "aberrant central pain mechanism." Pain is amplified by numerous factors, including many in the periphery (trauma, hypoxia), leading to fibromyalgia. (From Yunus MB: Towards a model of pathophysiology of fibromyalgia: Aberrant central pain mechanisms with peripheral modulation. J Rheumatol 1992; 19:846–850.)

may be triggered by nonspecific stress from trauma, viral infection, or mental stress.

Smythe,[75, 79] on the other hand, favors the pre-eminence of peripheral factors such as mechanical problems in neck and low back areas as the primary cause of fibromyalgia. Local injury leads to sleep disturbance, fatigue, more pain, stiffness, and deconditioning. In regional pain the local mechanical factors predominate. Centrally acting modulating factors (along with poor sleep, deconditioning) become more important as the pain becomes more widespread.

Others point to the presence of the tender point as evidence for a predominant peripheral mechanism. Bennett,[2, 3] borrowing from the myofascial pain syndrome model, proposes that muscle microtrauma leads to activation of muscle nociceptors and is the initial event in the pathogenesis of fibromyalgia. A genetic and acquired (through alpha sleep anomaly and its effect on the hypothalamic-pituitary axis) predisposition to muscle microtrauma at low levels of exertion leads to muscle pain with eccentric contractions. The pain leads to inactivity and deconditioning which perpetuates the microtrauma. Elements of central pain enhancement also play a role (Fig. 42–16).

Another prominent theory focuses on localized ischemia due to disturbed microcirculation.[34, 35] This theory relies on the interpretation of the equivocal findings on muscle biopsy mentioned above (ragged red fibers). One study found abnormal tissue oxygenation over trigger points,[51] but this

has not been replicated. Discrete muscle tension caused by gamma reflexes, emotional stress, or insufficient relaxation combine with the disturbed microcirculation to cause muscle pain. To explain widespread pain at rest, characteristic of fibromyalgia, this theory invokes disturbed pain modulation in the CNS.

Myofascial Pain Syndrome vs. Fibromyalgia

Although fibromyalgia and myofascial pain syndrome have many similarities, most investigators maintain that they are two distinct entities. In general, myofascial pain is thought to be a local or regional problem due to acute muscle trauma, whereas fibromyalgia is a widespread pain problem affecting more than just muscle and has systemic features. The presence of taut bands, referred pain, and twitch responses is often cited to differentiate myofascial pain. As noted above, these have not been shown to be reliable findings, even in the hands of experts.[62, 91] The distinction becomes more artificial when one considers that fibromyalgia can begin as a localized pain disorder and later become widespread and that persistent myofascial pain syndromes can involve multiple sites and cause systemic symptoms.[2, 89]

Myofascial pain and fibromyalgia might be labels for the two extremes of a single disorder.[39] Bennett[2] proposed that they could well have the same pathogenic mechanism. In its simplest form, a myofascial pain syndrome consists of the acute onset of pain in one muscle after trauma to that muscle. It is more than the generalized ache of a muscle after exertion but less than the obvious trauma of a muscle strain. Under the right conditions, trigger points can develop in nearby muscles until widespread chronic pain involves multiple muscle sites associated with systemic features such as disturbed sleep, generalized fatigue, and anxiety, the characteristic features of fibromyalgia. At what point did the disorder change from myofascial pain to fibromyalgia? Is fibromyalgia myofascial pain plus chronic pain syndrome? Is myofascial pain simply localized fibromyalgia? These are questions yet to be answered.

Chronic Fatigue Syndrome

Chronic fatigue syndrome (CFS) has recently emerged as a popular diagnostic label for "a centuries-old disorder of fatigue and multiple somatic complaints."[44] It has also been termed "yuppie flu" by the lay press. Because it shares many features with fibromyalgia—including the lack of objective physical or laboratory abnormalities—Goldenberg[27] classified CFS as a subset of fibromyalgia. Others believe the two conditions may well be the same disorder.[38]

The 1987 Centers for Disease Control and Prevention (CDC) definition of CFS included fatigue of at least 6 months' duration in the absence of a known cause, and the presence of 8 of 11 symptoms that included sleep disturbance, muscle pain, postexertional fatigue, and migratory myalgias[44] (Table 42–5). The large number of symptoms required tended to select patients with psychiatric disorders. Because of this, the CDC criteria were modified to specifically exclude patients with psychoses and substance abuse.[67] The criteria also excluded many patients with what

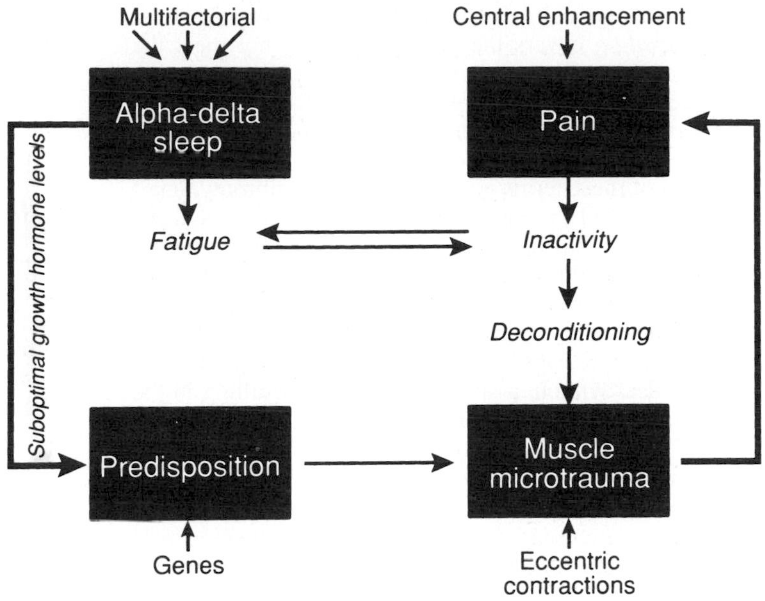

FIGURE 42–16 The pathophysiology of fibromyalgia according to Bennett. Muscle microtrauma is thought to be the primary event leading to muscle pain. Central factors play a role in enhancing the pain and in predisposing the individual to muscle microtrauma, creating several feedback loops as shown. (From Bennett RM: Fibromyalgia and the facts: Sense or nonsense. Rheum Dis Clin North Am 1993; 19:45–59.)

were thought to be overlap syndromes. These confounding syndromes were made inclusion criteria and included fibromyalgia, nonpsychotic depression, somatoform disorders, and generalized anxiety disorder. In a general medical practice, 21% met the definition of CFS.[44] Twenty-six percent of CFS patients met the criteria for fibromyalgia and

TABLE 42–5   Centers for Disease Control's Case Definition of the Chronic Fatigue Syndrome (CFS)

A case of CFS must fulfill both major criteria as well as either eight symptom criteria or six symptom criteria plus two physical criteria.

MAJOR CRITERIA
1. New onset of fatigue lasting 6 mo reducing activity to <50%
2. Other conditions producing fatigue must be ruled out

MINOR CRITERIA
Symptom Criteria—beginning at or after onset of fatigue and persisting or recurring for at least 6 mo
1. Low-grade fever, temperature of 37.5 °C–38.6 °C (99.5 °F–101.5 °F) orally or chills
2. Sore throat
3. Painful cervical or axillary lymph nodes
4. Generalized muscle weakness
5. Muscle pain
6. Postexertional fatigue lasting 24 hr
7. Headache
8. Migratory arthralgias
9. Neuropsychological complaints (photophobia, transient visual scotomata, forgetfulness, excessive irritability, confusion, difficulty thinking, inability to concentrate, or depression)
10. Sleep disturbance
11. Acute onset of symptoms over a few hours to a few days

Physical Criteria—documented by a physician twice, at least 1 mo apart
1. Low-grade fever, temperature of 37.6 °C–38.6 °C (99.7 °F–101.5 °F) orally or 37.8 °C–38.8 °C (100.0 °F–101.8 °F) rectally
2. Nonexudative pharyngitis
3. Palpable cervical or axillary lymph nodes up to 2 cm in diameter

Adapted from Klonoff DC: Chronic fatigue syndrome. Clin Infect Dis 1992; 15:812–823.

70% to 80% were women. As in fibromyalgia, there is a high lifetime incidence of major depression (46%–75%) and somatization disorder,[52] with current depression found in up to 42%.[25]

The cause of CFS is unknown. It most commonly begins suddenly after an infectious-like illness but no link to any specific pathogen has been established. Initial findings in support of such a role for Epstein-Barr virus, cocksackie B virus, and the human herpesvirus 6 have all been contradicted in more recent studies.[25, 52]

There continues to be some discussion as to whether CFS is an organic or psychiatric illness. It is likely a combination of the two, with a link between organic and psychiatric factors similar to that found in chronic pain. In both, the symptoms and functional deficits are out of proportion to the identifiable pathologic findings. In CFS, an underlying hyperresponsive immune system might provide the organic half of the link. Inappropriate release of cytokines in response to certain infections can cause CFS symptoms. Psychiatric disturbance (depression) could magnify this deranged immune response.[44]

The recommended treatment of CFS is very similar to the treatment for fibromyalgia (see below). Gantz and Holmes[24] recommend (1) exclusion of other conditions, (2) reassurance about the benign nature of the disorder, (3) use of antidepressants to treat both the depression and the sleep disorder, if present, (4) a graduated exercise program, (5) stress reduction, and (6) use of counseling and support groups.

Tension Myalgia

Starting about 1950, patients at the Mayo Clinic presenting with multiple areas of muscle pain and high levels of psychological tension or stress received the diagnosis "tension myalgia."[82] The use of the term grew as the term "fibrositis" and its incorrect implication of inflammation fell out of favor. Over the years the application of the diagnosis evolved to the point where it is now used to describe the spectrum of muscle pain syndromes from localized to regional to generalized. In this way the term *tension myalgia* covers the patients who do not meet the strict criteria for fibromyalgia or myofascial pain, that is, the majority. With the recent resurgence of interest in muscle pain disorders nationally and the more widespread use of the terms *fibromyalgia* and *myofascial pain* (and the expansion of these terms to cover "localized fibromyalgia" and "generalized myofascial pain"), use of the diagnosis tension myalgia has declined. The concept of a continuum of muscle pain disorders remains, however, and tension myalgia remains a useful paradigm.

The major utility of the term tension myalgia lies in patient education. Most patients have seen multiple healthcare providers without a specific diagnosis, resulting in the often less than subtle implication that it is "all in their head." They are concerned that something has been overlooked and that they may have cancer or some other debilitating disease. This situation often adds to the already stressful fact of chronic pain. Receiving a definite diagnosis and an understandable explanation for their symptoms allays these fears and is the first step in successful treatment.

"Myalgia" refers to the most characteristic symptom—local, regional, or widespread muscle pain, including pain at musculotendinous junctions and muscle attachments. "Tension" has two connotations. First, it suggests that a common finding (and possibly a causative factor) is muscle under tension, whether it be from "spasm," postural stress, overuse, or disordered motor sequencing. As mentioned above, there have been mixed findings in EMG studies of muscle pain syndromes. Some find no activity in muscles at rest,[46] whereas others find increased activity.[10, 20] Needle EMG of painful muscles can be silent when surface EMG reveals increased activity over the same muscles in the relaxed seated position. The presence or absence of "spasm" is not significant. Rather, these patients misuse their muscles by habitually co-contracting them, by failing to fully relax them, by overusing them, by subjecting them to unrelenting postural stress, or by a combination of these. This misuse ties in with the concept of motor dysfunction mentioned above.

Second, the word *tension* suggests that psychological tension or stress may play a major role, especially in patients with more widespread pain. When the diagnosis is presented in this way, patients more willingly accept the possibility of psychological influences on their muscle pain disorder and are more likely to take the necessary steps to address them. This also allows the physician to acknowledge that a psychological disturbance is not the primary cause.

Diagnostic Approach to Muscle Pain Syndromes

The approach to the diagnosis of muscle pain is fairly straightforward (Table 42–6). Despite a lengthy differential diagnosis (see Table 42–1), distinguishing these entities is seldom difficult in clinical practice. One difficulty can arise, however, if tension myalgia and another chronic disorder, such as rheumatoid arthritis, are present. In these cases, tension myalgia may be confused with a flare of the underlying disorder resulting in unnecessary treatments and medications.

TABLE 42–6   Suggested Laboratory Workup for Muscle Pain

Erythrocyte sedimentation rate
Serum creatine kinase
Complete blood count
Thyroid function tests
Also consider:
Electomyography
Rheumatoid factor
Antinuclear antibody
Muscle biopsy

A study of 109 consecutive patients referred with a chief complaint of muscle pain found a specific diagnosis in only one third of the patients.[57] The majority of the rest likely had tension myalgia (fibromyalgia, myofascial pain syndrome). The most useful laboratory screening tests were the erythrocyte sedimentation rate and serum creatine kinase activity. An abnormal result on either test prompted further evaluation with EMG and muscle biopsy. The initial evaluation should also include a complete blood count, thyroid function tests, and perhaps tests for rheumatoid factor and antinuclear antibody.[28, 82]

As with most diagnoses in medicine, the most important aspect is a complete history and careful physical examination, in this case emphasizing the musculoskeletal and neurological components. Points to remember include the following: the pain of tension myalgia is within or over muscles or their attachments, not in the joints; the results of the neurological examination, including strength, sensation, and reflexes, are normal, as are results of the joint examination; and laboratory findings, including those noted above, are within normal limits.

Treatment of Muscle Pain Syndromes

Specific treatment usually follows specific delineation of pathophysiology. Along with the multiple theories of etiology for muscle pain syndromes come multiple, mostly unproven, methods of treatment. This section describes one approach to treatment, combining what little has been shown to be useful with what appears empirically to be useful (Fig. 42–17).

The first step in treatment is establishing the diagnosis with the patient and spending the time to help the patient understand what the diagnosis is and is not (see Tension Myalgia, above). Such education and reassurance takes time but may put an end to the constant "doctor shopping" and help the patient focus on self-management of his or her disorder.

Elimination of Contributing Factors

The next step in treatment is the elimination of contributing factors. Travell and Simons[84] reported a host of perpetuating factors for myofascial pain syndrome including various vitamin deficiencies. A good diet is certainly important, including plenty of B vitamin sources. However, more common contributing factors include poor posture and poor body mechanics, which should be corrected to eliminate unnecessary muscle use. Anatomical variations such as a leg-length discrepancy should also be sought and corrected.

Vocational and avocational muscle overuse is a common

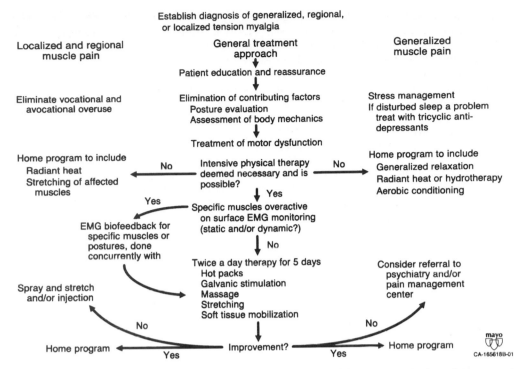

FIGURE 42–17   Treatment algorithm for tension myalgia (myofascial pain/fibromyalgia). The *central column* lists approaches useful in both localized and generalized muscle pain problems. The approaches more specific to generalized muscle pain (fibromyalgia) are in the *right column*, and the approaches more specific for localized muscle pain (myofascial pain syndromes) are in the *left column*.

contributing factor and must be specifically pursued. This more commonly appears with the more localized forms of muscle pain. Even so, patients with widespread pain benefit from principles such as frequent breaks for stretching and changes of position or task. It is important to specifically ask about hobbies, sports, daily tasks, and sleeping position. An ergonomic evaluation of the workplace is often valuable.

The more chronic and widespread the muscle pain syndrome, the more likely that psychological stress plays a role. Instruction in stress management techniques can be useful but if a major psychopathological disorder is suspected, formal psychiatric evaluation may be warranted. Often the more involved patients benefit from the cognitive-behavioral treatment approach[63] used in comprehensive pain management centers (see Chapter 41).

Poor sleep is another feature found more often in the more chronic cases. If present, it often responds to low-dose tricyclic antidepressant medications (e.g., amitriptyline 10–25 mg nightly). This is one of the few treatments shown to be useful for the reduction of pain and improvement of sleep in double blind controlled studies of patients with widespread muscle pain.[9, 29, 68] Whether these medications help in the absence of sleep disturbance remains unclear. Be sure to explain the rationale of treatment so the patient is not put off by being placed on an antidepressant.

Treatment of Motor Dysfunction

The next major category of treatment addresses the problem of motor dysfunction. This often requires specific physical therapy. The goals of treatment are to decrease pain, restore normal range of motion, restore normal neuromuscular functioning, and improve fitness.

Reducing pain will increase the patient's confidence in the treatment plan. It is also a necessary prerequisite to establishing normal motor function. One method combines hot packs and high-voltage "galvanic" stimulation to the most symptomatic area. This can be followed by deep sedative massage or gentle soft tissue mobilization. The use of these passive modalities should be limited to the early treatment phase to avoid patient dependence and the persistent notion that something must be done *to* them in order to get "fixed."

A general stretching program with special emphasis on muscle groups found to be "tight" on examination is a basic part of treatment. The patient should learn to do this several times a day. Using heat before gentle prolonged stretching may improve its effectiveness and lessen its discomfort.

The goal of neuromuscular re-education lies in restoring normal resting tone and fluid movement without co-contraction of agonists and antagonists. Surface EMG biofeedback over specific areas can be helpful, especially with the postural muscles, which often function subconsciously. Multiple muscle sites can be quickly sampled by "scanning" with hand-held post-style electrodes.[12, 83] Areas of increased activity are targeted for specific relaxation exercises. Attached surface electrodes give information about the activity of muscles in dynamic situations. This type of biofeedback helps train patients to eliminate co-contraction, and teaches them to return their muscles to electrical silence after contraction. This resting state is often missing in patients with muscle pain.[18, 86]

A short, intense course of biofeedback training (e.g., twice a day for 1 week) is often necessary in chronic, more widespread muscle pain. Since it is difficult to relearn correct motor function after prolonged dysfunction, low-intensity biofeedback (three times a week) is likely of little utility, but this has not been studied. More acute, localized muscle pain likely will not require this labor-intensive, and therefore costly, intervention.

Once pain has been reduced and motor dysfunction minimized, a very graduated aerobic fitness program can be instituted. Again, the extent and chronicity of the muscle pain problem parallels the need for this treatment step. A controlled study of widespread muscle pain patients found an aerobic program more beneficial than stretching alone.[54] It is important to stress a very gradual return to activity to avoid fatigue and increased muscle pain. I instruct patients to start at a level that seems ridiculously easy and slowly advance from there.

Local Treatments

Localized and regional muscle pain syndromes often respond to specific localized therapies. None of these have been proved effective in adequately controlled studies. Many practitioners have great success employing them, however.

Spray and stretch is the mainstay of myofascial pain syndrome treatment (see Fig. 42–14).[84] The vapocoolant spray is used to reflexively relax the muscle to allow an adequate stretch. One maintains a sweeping pattern of spray in the direction of the muscle fibers as the muscle is passively stretched by the patient or the clinician's free hand. The coolant spray serves to distract the patient and possibly relax the treated muscle to allow for a more effective stretch. The prolonged stretch is the key element and is what provides pain relief through an as yet unknown mechanism.

The second most commonly used treatment for localized muscle pain is injection. Some practitioners simply inject the general area of the most intense pain. Others take great care in locating the "trigger point," watching for the "twitch response" on entering it with the needle. Dry needling appears to work as well as any other type but most physicians use a local anesthetic for the sake of patient comfort. The addition of corticosteroids to the injection has many advocates but likely adds little but cost to the procedure. This has not been well studied, however. Proponents of injection focus on finding the primary trigger point, which, when treated successfully, leads to resolution of many of the secondary trigger points. Treating only the secondary points without finding the primary point is one reason for treatment failure.

Even less well studied is the use of ischemic compression to treat trigger points.[84] The theory is that sustained pressure over the pathological area induces increased blood flow on release of pressure with hyperemia of the skin. This in turn reverses the assumed localized ischemia in the underlying muscle. The digitally applied pressure lasts for about 1 min at gradually increasing pressure as tolerated up to 30 lbs.

Medications

Both amitriptyline and cyclobenzaprine have provided short-term relief in controlled studies of fibromyalgia patients[29] as noted above in the discussion of contributing factors. Anti-inflammatory agents (including corticosteroids) and analgesics are generally not useful[9, 29] and should be avoided.

The most important component of any treatment approach is the patient. The ultimate goal is to educate patients and provide them with the means to manage their own muscle pain disorder, eliminating dependence on (and overutilization of) healthcare providers.

References

1. Ahles TA, Kahn SA, Yunus MB, et al: Psychiatric status of patients with primary fibromyalgia, patients with rheumatoid arthritis, and subjects without pain. Am J Psychiatry 1991; 148:1721–1726.
2. Bennett RM: Myofascial pain syndromes and the fibromyalgia syndrome: A comparative analysis. In Fricton JR, Awad EA (eds): Advances in Pain Research and Therapy, vol 17: Myofascial Pain and Fibromyalgia. New York, Raven Press, 1990, pp 43–65.
3. Bennett RM: Fibromyalgia and the facts: Sense or nonsense. Rheum Dis Clin North Am 1993; 19:45–59.
4. Birnie DJ, Knipping AA, vanRijswijk MII, et al: Psychological aspects of fibromyalgia compared with chronic and nonchronic pain. J Rheumatol 1991; 18:1845–1848.
5. Boissevain MD, McCain GA: Toward an integrated understanding of fibromyalgia syndrome. I. Medical and pathophysiological aspects. Pain 1991; 45:227–238.
6. Boissevain MD McCain GA: Toward an integrated understanding of fibromyalgia syndrome. II. Psychological and phenomenological aspects. Pain 1991; 45:239–248.
7. Campbell SM, Clark S, Tindall EA, et al: Clinical characteristics of fibrositis. I. A "blinded" controlled study of symptoms and tender points. Arthritis Rheum 1983; 26:817–824.
8. Clark S, Campbell SM, Forehand ME, et al: Clinical characteristics of fibrositis. A "blinded" controlled study using standard psychological tests. Arthritis Rheum 1985; 28:132–137.
9. Clark S, Tindall E, Bennett RM: A double blind crossover trial of prednisone versus placebo in the treatment of fibrositis. J Rheumatol 1985; 12:980–983.
10. Cobb CR, deVries HA, Urban RT, et al: Electrical activity in muscle pain. Am J Phys Med 1975; 54:80–87.
11. Conferences on therapy: Treatment of painful disorders of skeletal muscles. N Y State J Med 1948; 48:2050–2059.
12. Cram JR, Steger JC: Muscle scanning and the diagnosis of chronic pain. Biofeedback Self Regul 1983; 8:229–241.
13. Croft P, Rigby AS, Boswell R, et al: The prevalence of chronic widespread pain in the general population. J Rheumatol 1993; 20:710–713.
14. Delaney GA, McKee AC: Inter- and intra-rater reliability of the pressure threshold meter in measurement of myofascial trigger point sensitivity. Am J Phys Med Rehabil 1993; 72:136–139.
15. Dunnette MR, Rodriquez AA, Agre JC, et al: Needle electromyographic evaluation of patients with myofascial or fibromyalgic pain. Am J Phys Med Rehabil 1991; 70:154–156.
16. Edwards RHT: Hypotheses of peripheral and central mechanisms underlying occupational muscle pain and injury. Eur J Appl Physiol 1988; 57: 275–281.
17. Elert JE, Rantapaa-Dahlqvist SB, Almay B, Eisemann M: Muscle endurance, muscle tension and personality traits in patients with muscle or joint pain—a pilot study. J Rheumatol 1993; 20:1550–1556.
18. Elert JE, Rantapaa-Dahlqvist SB, Henriksson-Larsen K, Gerdle B: Increased EMG activity during short pauses in patients with primary fibromyalgia. Scand J Rheumatol 1989; 18:321–323.
19. Elert JE, Rantapaa-Dahlqvist SB, Henriksson-Larsen K, et al: Muscle performance, electromyography and fibre type composition in fibromyalgia and work-related myalgia. Scand J Rheumatol 1992; 21:28–34.
20. Elliott FA: Tender muscles in sciatica: Electromyographic studies. Lancet 1944; 1:47–49.
21. Fischer AA: Documentation of myofascial trigger points. Arch Phys Med Rehabil 1988; 69:286–291.
22. Fowler RS, Kraft GH: Tension perception in patients having pain associated with chronic muscle tension. Arch Phys Med Rehabil 1974; 55:28–30.

23. Fricton JR, Auvinen MD, Dykstra D, Schiffman E: Myofascial pain syndrome: Electromyographic changes associated with local twitch response. Arch Phys Med Rehabil 1985; 66:314–317.

24. Gantz NM, Holmes GP: Treatment of patients with chronic fatigue syndrome. Drugs 1989; 38:855–862.

25. Gold D, Bowden R, Sixby J, et al: Chronic fatigue: A prospective clinical and virologic study. JAMA 1990; 264:48–53.

26. Golden H, Weber SM, Bergen D: Sleep studies in patients with fibrositis syndrome, abstract. Arthritis Rheum 1983; 26 (suppl):S32.

27. Goldenberg DL: Fibromyalgia, chronic fatigue syndrome, and myofascial pain syndrome. Curr Opin Rheumatol 1991; 3:247–258.

28. Goldenberg DL: Fibromyalgia syndrome: An emerging but controversial condition. JAMA 1987; 257:2782–2787.

29. Goldenberg DL, Felson DT, Dinerman H: A randomized, controlled trial of amitriptyline and naproxen in the treatment of patients with fibromyalgia. Arthritis Rheum 1986; 29:1371–1377.

30. Gowers WR: Lumbago: Its lessons and analogues. BMJ 1904; 1:117–121.

31. Granges G, Littlejohn G: Pressure pain threshold in pain-free subjects, in patients with chronic regional pain syndromes, and in patients with fibromyalgia syndrome. Arthritis Rheum 1993; 36:642–646.

32. Hauri P: Personal communication, February 1994.

33. Hauri P, Hawkins DR: Alpha-delta sleep. Electroencephalogr Clin Neurophysiol 1973; 34:233.

34. Henriksson KG: Pathogenesis of fibromyalgia. J Musculoskeletal Pain 1993; 1:3–16.

35. Henriksson KG, Bengtsson A: Fibromyalgia—a clinical entity? Can J Physiol Pharmacol 1991; 69:672–677.

36. Horne JA, Shackell BS: Alpha-like EEG activity in non-REM sleep and the fibromyalgia (fibrositis) syndrome. Electroencephalogr Clin Neurophysiol 1991; 79:271–276.

37. Hubbard DR, Berkoff GM: Myofascial trigger points show spontaneous needle activity. Spine 1993; 18:1803–1807.

38. Hudson JI, Goldenberg DL, Pope HG, et al: Comorbidity of fibromyalgia with medical and psychiatric disorders. Am J Med 1992; 92:363–367.

39. Jacobsen S, Petersen IS, Danneskiold-Samsoe B: Clinical features of patients with chronic muscle pain—with special reference to fibromyalgia. Scand J Rheumatol 1993; 22:69–76.

40. Kellgren JH: Observations on referred pain arising from muscle. Clin Sci 1938; 3:174–190.

41. Kellgren JH: On the distribution of pain arising from deep somatic structures with charts of segmental pain areas. Clin Sci 1939; 4.35–46.

42. Kelly M: The nature of fibrositis. Part I. The myalgic lesion and its secondary effects: A reflex theory. Ann Rheum Dis 1945; 5:1–7.

43. Kelly M: The nature of fibrositis. Part II. A study of the causation of the myalgic lesion (rheumatic, traumatic, infective). Ann Rheum Dis 1946; 5:69–77.

44. Klonoff DC: Chronic fatigue syndrome. Clin Infect Dis 1992; 15:812–823.

45. Koes BW, Bouter LM, van Mameren H, et al: The effectiveness of manual therapy, physiotherapy, and treatment by the general practitioner for nonspecific back and neck complaints. Spine 1992; 17:28–35.

46. Kraft GH, Johnson EW, LaBan MM: The fibrositis syndrome. Arch Phys Med Rehabil 1968; 49:155–162.

47. Kravitz E, Moore ME, Glaros A: Paralumbar muscle activity in chronic low back pain. Arch Phys Med Rehabil 1981; 62:172–176.

48. Krusen FH: Physical therapy of fibrositis. Arch Phys Ther 1937; 18:687–697, 722.

49. Kuch K, Cox B, Evans R, et al: To what extent do anxiety and depression interact with chronic pain? Can J Psychiatry 1993; 38:36–38.

50. Layzer RB: Muscle pain, cramps, and fatigue. In Engel AG, Banker BQ (eds): Myology. New York, 1986, McGraw-Hill, pp 1907–1922.

51. Lund N, Bengtsson A, Thorborg P: Muscle tissue oxygen pressure in primary fibromyalgia. Scand J Rheumatol 1986; 15:165–173.

52. Manu P, Lane TJ, Matthews DA: The pathophysiology of chronic fatigue syndrome: Confirmations, contradictions and conjectures. Int J Psychiatry Med 1992; 22:397–408.

53. Marchettini P: Muscle pain: Animal and human experimental and clinical studies. Muscle Nerve 1993; 16:1033–1039.

54. McCain GA: Role of physical fitness training in fibrositis/fibromyalgia syndrome. Am J Med 1986; 81(suppl 3A):73–77.

55. Mense S: Nociception from skeletal muscle in relation to clinical muscle pain. Pain 1993; 54:241–289.

56. Mense S: Physiology of nociception in muscle. In Fricton JR, Awad EA (eds): Advances in Pain Research and Therapy, vol 17. Myofascial Pain and Fibromyalgia. New York, Raven Press, 1990, pp 67–85.

57. Mills KR, Edwards RHT: Investigative stategies for muscle pain. J Neurol Sci 1983; 58:73.

58. Moldofsky H: Sleep-wake physiology and fibromyalgia. In Fricton JR, Awad EA (eds): Advances in Pain Research and Therapy, vol 17: Myofascial Pain and Fibromyalgia. New York, Raven Press, 1990, pp 227–238.

59. Moldofsky H, Scarisbrick P, England R, Smythe H: Musculoskeletal symptoms and non-REM sleep disturbance in patients with "fibrositis syndrome" and healthy subjects. Psychosom Med 1975; 37:341–351.

60. Moldofsky H, Warsh JJ: Plasma tryptophan and musculoskeletal pain in non-articular rheumatism ("fibrositis syndrome"). Pain 1978; 5:65–71.

61. Mufson M, Regestein QR: The spectrum of fibromyalgia disorders, editorial. Arthritis Rheum 1993; 36:647–650.

62. Nice DA, Riddle DL, Lamb RL, et al: Intertester reliability of judgements of the presence of trigger points in patients with low back pain. Arch Phys Med Rehabil 1992; 73:893–898.

63. Nielson WR, Walker C, McCain GA: Cognitive behavioral treatment of fibromyalgia syndrome: Preliminary findings. J Rheumatol 1992; 19:98–103.

64. Reeves JL, Jaeger B, Graff-Redford SB: The reliability of the pressure algometer as a measure of myofascial trigger point sensitivity. Pain 1986; 24:313–321.

65. Reilly PA, Littlejohn GO: Fibrositis/fibromyalgia syndrome: The key to the puzzle of chronic pain. Med J Aust 1990; 152:226–228.

66. Reynolds MD: The development of the concept of fibrositis. J Hist Med Allied Sci 1983; 38:5–35.

67. Schluederbeg A, Straus SE, Peterson P, et al: Chronic fatigue syndrome research: Definition and medical outcome assessment. Ann Intern Med 1992; 117:325–331.

68. Scudds RA, McCain GA, Rollman GB, et al: Improvements in pain responsiveness in patients with fibrositis after successful treatment with amitriptyline. J Rheumatol 1989; 16(suppl 19):98–103.

69. Scudds RA, Trachsel LC, Luckhurst BJ, Percy JS: A comparative study of pain, sleep quality and pain responsiveness in fibrositis and myofascial pain syndrome. J Rheumatol 1989; 16(suppl 19):120–126.

70. Simms RW, Goldenberg DL, Felson DT, et al: Tenderness in 75 anatomic sites: Distinguishing fibromyalgia patients from controls. Arthritis Rheum 1988; 31:182–187.

71. Simons DG: Muscle pain syndromes (in two parts). Am J Phys Med 1975; 54:289–311. 1976, 55:15–42.

72. Simons DG: Muscular pain syndromes. In Fricton JR, Awad EA: Advances in Pain Research and Therapy, vol 17: Myofascial Pain and Fibromyalgia. New York, Raven Press, 1990, pp 1–41.

73. Skootsky SA, Jaeger B, Oye RK: Prevalence of myofascial pain in general internal medicine practice. West J Med 1989; 151:157–160.

74. Slocumb CH: Fibrositis. Clinics 1943; 2:169–178.

75. Smythe HA: Links between fibromyalgia and myofascial pain syndromes, editorial. J Rheumatol 1992; 19:842–843.

76. Smythe HA: Non-articular rheumatism and the fibrositis syndrome. In Hollander JL, McCarty DJ Jr (eds): Arthritis and Allied Conditions, ed 8. Philadelphia, Lea & Febiger, 1972, pp 874–884.

77. Smythe HA: Problems with the MMPI, editorial. J Rheumatol 1984; 11:417–418.

78. Smythe HA, Moldofsky H: Two contributions to understanding of the "fibrositis" syndrome. Bull Rheum Dis 1977; 28:928.

79. Smythe HA, Sheon RP: Fibrositis/fibromyalgia: A difference of opinion. Bull Rheum Dis 1990; 39:1–3.

80. Stockman R: The causes, pathology, and treatment of chronic rheumatism. Edingurgh Med J 1904; 15:107–116.

81. Swerdlow B, Dieter JNI: An evaluation of the sensitivity and specificity of medical thermography for the documentation of myofascial trigger points. Pain 1992; 48:205–213.

82. Thompson JM: Tension myalgia as a diagnosis at the Mayo Clinic and its relationship to fibrositis, fibromyalgia, and myofascial pain syndrome. Mayo Clin Proc 1991; 65:1237–1248.

83. Thompson JM, Madson TJ, Erickson RP: EMG muscle scanning: Comparison to attached surface electrodes. Biofeedback Self Regul 1991; 16:167–179.

84. Travell JG, Simons DG: Myofascial pain and dysfunction: The trigger point manual. Baltimore, Williams & Wilkins, 1983.

85. Tunks E, Crook J, Norman G, et al: Tender points in fibromyalgia. Pain 1988; 34:11–19.

86. Veierstad KB, Westgaard RH, Andersen P: Electromyographic evaluation of muscular work pattern as a predictor of trapezius myalgia. Scand J Work Environ Health 1993; 19:284–290.

87. Weinberger LM: Fibrositis, letter. West J Med 1981; 135:425.

88. Wolfe F: The epidemiology of fibromyalgia. J Musculoskeletal Pain 1993; 1:137–148.

89. Wolfe F: Fibrositis, fibromyalgia, and musculoskeletal disease: The current status of the fibrositis syndrome. Arch Phys Med Rehabil 1988; 69:527–531.

90. Wolfe F, Cathey MA: Prevalence of primary and secondary fibrositis. J Rheumatol 1983; 10:965–968.

91. Wolfe F, Simons DG, Fricton J, et al: The fibromyalgia and myofascial pain syndromes: A preliminary study of tender points and trigger points in persons with fibromyalgia, myofascial pain syndrome and no disease. J Rheumatol 1992; 19:944–951.

92. Wolfe F, Smythe HA, Yunus MB, et al: The American College of Rheumatology 1990 criteria for the classification of fibromyalgia. Arthritis Rheum 1990; 33:160–172.

93. Yunus MB: Diagnosis, etiology and management of fibromyalgia syndrome: An update. Compr Ther 1988; 14:8–20.

94. Yunus MB: Towards a model of pathophysiology of fibromyalgia: Aberrant central pain mechanisms with peripheral modulation. J Rheumatol 1992; 19:846–850.

95. Yunus MB, Kalyan-Raman UP: Muscle biopsy findings in primary fibromyalgia and other forms of nonarticular rheumatism. Rheum Dis North Am 1989; 15:115–134.

96. Yunus MB, Kalyan-Raman UP, Kalyan-Raman K: Primary fibromyalgia syndrome and myofascial pain syndrome: Clinical features and muscle pathology. Arch Phys Med Rehabil 1988; 69:451–454.

97. Yunus MB, Masi AT, Calabro JJ, et al: Primary fibromyalgia (fibrositis): Clinical study of 50 patients with matched normal controls. Semin Arthritis Rheum 1981; 11:151–171.

43

Concepts in Sports Medicine

EDWARD R. LASKOWSKI, M.D.

Kraus and Conroy[77] estimated that 3 to 5 million sports-related injuries were treated in the United States in 1984. Many medical specialties now include sports medicine as a practice domain, for example, internal medicine, family practice, pediatrics, emergency medicine, orthopedics, and physical medicine and rehabilitation. Physiatrists are in a unique position to be important providers of care for musculoskeletal sports injuries. Because most sports injuries are musculoskeletal and do not require surgical treatment, appropriate care is best provided by someone who understands the anatomy, biomechanics, kinesiology, and rehabilitation principles related to a particular sport and injury. Physiatrists have the most comprehensive training and background in each of these realms. Furthermore, the physiatric focus on a team concept of medical care is perfectly suited to the interdisciplinary care often required in sports medicine. For example, for any given sport, the team might include athletic trainers, physical therapists, coaches, team owners, a sports psychologist, physicians, and, of course, athletes. Physiatric training provides much experience in the leadership and effective coordination necessary for these multidisciplinary team members to function for the maximum benefit of the patient. In essence, physiatrists are ideally suited for the practice of sports medicine, and sports medicine is becoming an increasingly popular part of residency and post-residency training.[46]

Physiatrists are also well equipped to address the sport-specific and disability-specific requirements of physically challenged athletes. The Americans with Disabilities Act (ADA) mandates equal opportunity for sports and recreation for persons with physical disabilities. The use of sports and conditioning-training exercises to prepare for sports is an excellent way of continuing therapeutic exercise. Unique considerations with respect to physically challenged athletes are considered later in this chapter.

GENERAL CONCEPTS OF THE MUSCULOSKELETAL SYSTEM

Muscle

A detailed description of the anatomy and structure of muscle fibers is beyond the scope of this chapter. However,

it is important to understand the mechanism and ramifications of muscle injury. Muscle injury can occur from direct macrotrauma, tissue invasion (via laceration), and repetitive microtrauma (overuse).[91] Failure often occurs when a muscle reaches overload at the myotendinous junction.[10, 55] During the healing process of a muscle injury–and after the inflammatory phase subsides and tissue healing, repair, and remodeling occur–concomitant changes take place in muscle function unless appropriate treatment is undertaken. Deficits in absolute strength, strength balance (i.e., agonist vs. antagonist muscle groups), flexibility, and proprioception (via cutaneous, muscle, and joint receptors) can occur.[71, 131] If treatment is not initiated, these deficits are likely to predispose the patient to further injury at the same site or at a distal site in the kinetic chain. The *kinetic chain*, which is referred to frequently in this chapter, can be thought of as the linked system of muscles, joints, and body segments involved in a particular biomechanical movement or task. Often, the site of pain may not be the actual origin of the problem; thus, the patient should be carefully evaluated for biomechanical, strength, and/or flexibility problems, both proximal and distal to the site of injury.

Tendons

Tendons connect muscle to bone. Their primary function is to transmit muscle force to the osseous skeleton, with minimal change in their inherent length. Tendons consist of densely packed collagen fibers that have a high tensile strength. The fibers are arranged in parallel with one another and are oriented toward the tensile pull of the muscle.[7] Herring and Nilson[62] and Barfred[22] indicated that tendons can be damaged if (1) a force is applied rapidly and obliquely through the tendon, (2) the tendon is under tension before the load is applied, (3) the musculotendinous group is stretched, (4) the attached muscle is maximally contracted, or (5) the tendinous structure itself is weak in comparison with the muscle.

Basically, tendon healing occurs in three phases. The first 48 to 72 hours of healing is known as the *inflammatory phase* and is characterized by an influx of vasoactive substances, chemotactic factors, and degradative enzymes.[121] The second phase is reparative and entails collagen production. The collagen fibers laid down during this phase have little strength because they occur in a random, haphazard pattern. During the final phase of healing, the mechanical strength of the healing tendon increases with the maturation and remodeling of fiber architecture. This increase in strength occurs along the direction of muscle force. The latter principle is crucial in injury rehabilitation—it is the basis for early mobilization and is the reason that soft tissue is not immobilized for a prolonged period unless absolutely dictated by the injury. The tensile strength of the scar tissue is not optimum unless specific and gradually applied stressors are placed on the healing tissue.[4, 5, 117, 137, 138]

It is important to note that beyond the acute inflammation and repair response, chronic repetitive microtrauma to the tendon can lead to a condition of degenerative change and damage. This pathological condition has been called *tendinosis*.[80] Conditions in which tendinosis is common include plantar fasciitis, lateral epicondylitis, patellar tendinitis, and Achilles tendinitis.[33, 79, 113] In tendinosis, cell degeneration and tissue changes, rather than an active inflammatory response, are the principal causes of pain and dysfunction. Thus, tendinosis requires complete analysis of kinetic chain function, including flexibility, muscle balance, and proximal and distal mechanics and kinesiology, rather than mere control of inflammation. "Weak links" in kinetic chain biomechanics and function must be corrected to avoid repetitive tissue stress and damage. In addition, prolonged use of nonsteroidal anti-inflammatory drugs in a tendinosis condition must seriously be questioned.

Ligaments

Ligaments consist of dense connective tissue and connect bone to bone. They have a mechanical stabilizing effect on joints. Ligaments contain proprioceptive afferents that provide feedback to the musculoskeletal system. Injuries to ligaments usually result from a large overload force. As with tendons, early motion is important to maximize tensile strength of a healing ligament.[6, 101] Continued research is needed on the time course of revascularization and recovery of strength in various ligaments after injury. With respect to patellar tendon grafts used for anterior cruciate ligament reconstruction, it is theorized that the graft tissue revascularizes more quickly with controlled stress, becoming stronger through hypertrophy during revascularization and, thus, reducing the likelihood of complications.[124]

The neuromuscular role of ligaments should not be ignored. It has been emphasized that in addition to the role of ligaments in mechanical restraint, their role in neurosensory function may be just as important.[24, 146] Palmer[103] was perhaps the first to propose that ligaments supply the central nervous system with input that enables neuromuscular control of the knee joint. Cohen and Cohen[36] coined the term *arthrokinetic reflex* and suggested that the knee joint capsule is the origin of protective afferent input and that co-contraction of the quadriceps and hamstring muscles is necessary for knee joint stability. Abbott and colleagues[1] stated that ligaments are the first link in the kinetic chain and provide rich sensory input to the central nervous system. Recent studies seem to indicate that when an injury occurs to the passive mechanical constraint system, new demands are placed on the dynamic restraints because of a loss of afferent feedback. Retraining of dynamic stability becomes a key to adaptation and complete rehabilitation.

Bursae

Bursae are sacs formed by two layers of synovial tissue. The sacs usually contain a thin layer of synovial fluid. Bursae are located at sites of friction between tendon and bone. Often, they can communicate with an adjacent synovial sac. With overuse or repetitive trauma, bursae can be injured by friction or external pressure. They also can become inflamed through the degeneration and calcification of an overlying tendon (e.g., subacromial bursitis due to calcific supraspinatus tendinitis). The response of bursae to injury usually consists of inflammation, with resultant effusion and thickening of the bursal wall.

GENERAL CONCEPTS OF THE CARDIOVASCULAR SYSTEM

The importance of maintaining appropriate cardiovascular conditioning during sports participation and injury rehabilitation is well known. The deleterious effects of bed rest and activity limitation have been well documented. Complications of inactivity include cardiovascular and musculoskeletal deconditioning, bone loss, orthostatic hypertension, deep venous thrombosis, contracture, and pressure ulceration[25, 93, 111, 125] (see Chapter 34). A 50% reduction in gains of aerobic capacity due to exercise has been shown in only 4 to 12 weeks of "detraining."[54, 70, 116] Convertino,[37] Saltin,[120] and Taylor[134] and their colleagues have shown decrements in aerobic capacity and related cardiovascular variables when subjects stay at bed rest for an extended period. Oxygen uptake decreases, as do cardiac output, stroke volume, and heart volume. In any musculoskeletal sports injury, the principle of "relative rest" applies. This principle dictates that the injured body part should be "rested" and protected from further trauma or injury, while the remaining muscle mass is used to provide appropriate stress to the cardiovascular system for maintaining optimal aerobic conditioning (see Chapter 32). In addition, strength training should continue in uninvolved body parts. "Crossover" training effects have been documented in the rested limb when the contralateral limb is exercised.[97]

INJURY PREVENTION AND PRE-REHABILITATION

The origin of the term "pre-rehabilitation" or *prehabilitation (prehab)*, which has become popular in recent years, is unclear. The term refers to rehabilitative exercises that are performed preoperatively to enhance the postoperative outcome. Theoretically, pre-rehabilitation can enhance the neuromuscular engram and hasten motor learning of the rehabilitative program after the surgical procedure. In addi-

TABLE 43–1   Main Components of a Preventive Exercise Program

Flexibility
Strength training
Aerobic training
Analysis of kinetic chain functions
Sport-specific and higher level skills
Practical training program

tion, pre-rehabilitation can refer to exercises that are used to prevent injury or to prevent previously delineated biomechanical or kinetic chain deficits from contributing to musculoskeletal injury. Currently, the scientific support for the role of exercise in injury prevention is minimal, and prospective studies about whether a specific exercise program is truly protective or preventive for a specific injury do not exist.

The six main components of a hypothetical preventive exercise program are listed in Table 43–1. They include flexibility, strength training, aerobic training, analysis of kinetic chain function, sport-specific and higher level skills training, and the incorporation of these elements into a practical training program.

Flexibility

Historically, emphasis has been placed on an appropriate and comprehensive stretching program to reduce injuries.

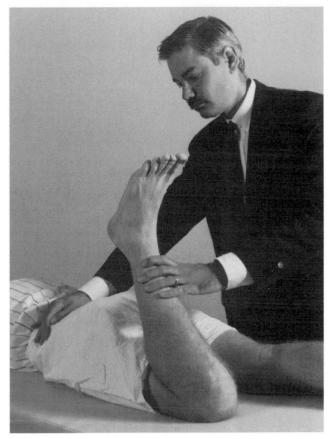

FIGURE 43–2   Ely test for evaluating tightness of the rectus femoris.

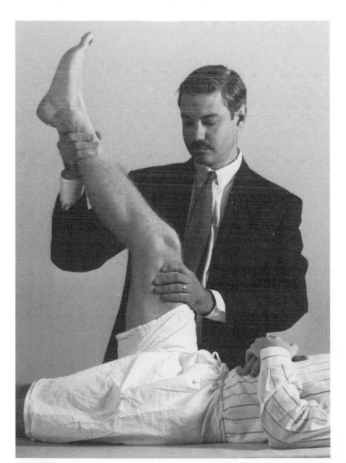

FIGURE 43–1   The popliteal angle is an objective measure of hamstring tightness. This angle is measured while the hip is flexed at 90 degrees.

Data that indicate a direct association between objective measures of flexibility and either increased or decreased risk of musculoskeletal injury are few. In order to accurately study this issue, it is important to document and follow discrete objective measures of specific muscle tightness.

Muscles that cross two joints can have an especially powerful impact on kinetic chain function. Tightness of these muscles can have more wide-ranging sequelae than for muscles crossing only one joint. In the lower extremities, hamstring flexibility can be measured objectively by measuring the popliteal angle (Fig. 43–1). In performing this test, the hip must first be flexed to 90 degrees; the knee is then gradually extended toward full extension. Performing only a straight-leg raise can give a false impression of adequate hamstring flexibility, because the proximal hamstrings will not be "hooked" around the ischial tuberosity if the leg is directly elevated without the hip first being flexed.

Quadriceps flexibility (specifically, the rectus femoris) can be measured with the Ely test (Fig. 43 2), and the distance from the buttock to the heel can be recorded to gauge improvement as the flexibility program progresses. Flexibility of the Achilles tendon can be gauged by measuring the degree of dorsiflexion that can be attained with the foot in a partially supinated position (Fig. 43–3). Iliotibial band tightness can be measured with the Ober test (Fig. 43–4), although there is no reliable objective measurement for this maneuver.

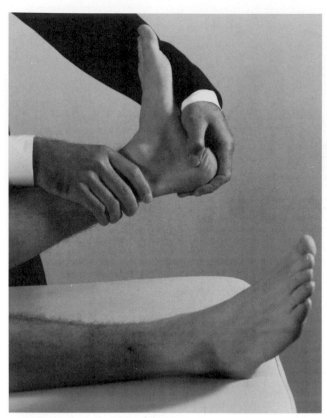

FIGURE 43–3 Testing foot dorsiflexion as a measure of tightness of the Achilles tendon. Note that the examiner's forearm keeps the subject's heel in partial supination.

In the upper extremities, range of motion at the wrists and elbows can be measured goniometrically. With respect to the shoulder, external and internal rotation have special significance (discussed later) and should be measured bilaterally.

Asymmetry, rather than "perfect" geometry, may be the most important clinical aspect of flexibility, especially after an injury. One of the most important predictors of future injury is a history of past injury, and any flexibility deficit

and asymmetry can contribute to increased risk of musculoskeletal injury or reinjury. Even without previous injury, stretching can help physiologically to prevent injury in many ways. Janda and associates[67] have shown that tight and inflexible muscles can act like an effusion and have an inhibitory effect on antagonist muscle groups. This inhibitory effect probably occurs through the afferent proprioceptive arc, and preparticipation stretching might decrease facilitation of muscle spindle afferents and assist the facilitation of Golgi tendon organs.[44] In addition, Noonan and colleagues[100] have shown that stretching can increase the temperature of the tendon, which can have a protective effect via increased skeletal muscle tensile strength. Proper stretching technique is crucial, because both the positioning of the body during the stretch and the duration of hold are important in maximizing the result of the stretch. For example, a common mistake in the gastrocnemius-soleus stretch occurs when the patient externally rotates the rear foot (Fig. 43–5). This takes the vector of stretch off the main bulk of the Achilles tendon.

It is recommended that stretches be held for at least 30 seconds to achieve maximum "creep" of the tissue. This probably is much longer than most people are accustomed to holding a stretch; thus, it is advisable for the novice to look at the second hand of a watch or to use a stop watch to make sure that the stretch is held for an adequate time. Ideally, the stretch should be performed before and after the competition or exercise period. If stretching is going to be done only once, it should be *after* the exercise session. Lehmann and associates[83] have shown in an animal model that the percentage increase in tendon length is greater when the tendon is stretched at a temperature of 45 °C than at 25 °C (Fig. 43–6). After a session of exercise, increased deep muscle blood flow can increase tissue temperature far greater than superficial heat can. Jogging for even a short time can increase tissue temperature and aid in facilitating stretches.[88]

There are also age-specific and sport-specific stretching concerns. For example, specific muscle tightness (i.e., quadriceps) during adolescence can have an impact on growth-related musculoskeletal problems, such as Osgood-

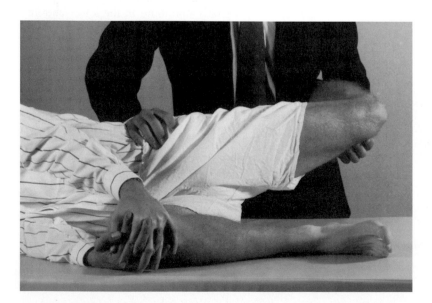

FIGURE 43–4 In Ober's test, the hip is passively extended with the pelvis in a neutral position to ensure that the tensor fascia lata passes over the greater trochanter.

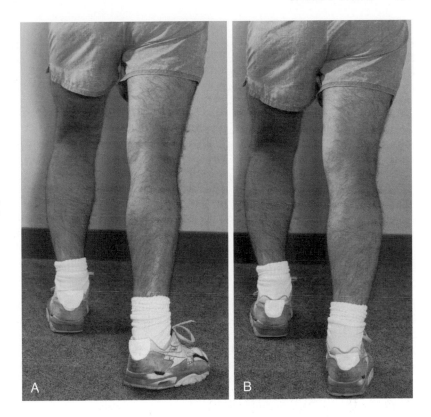

FIGURE 43–5 Technique for gastrocnemius-soleus stretch. *A,* Incorrect technique. Note externally rotated and elevated foot. *B,* Correct technique.

Schlatter disease. More concentrated stretching on two-joint muscles (such as the hamstrings, hip flexors, and rectus femoris) is important during this stage. Older adults have specific flexibility concerns with respect to posture and biomechanics. Hamstring and hip flexor flexibility are particularly important as a person ages. Also, stretching specific to the biomechanics and kinesiology of each sport is important, especially when a person is involved in multiple sports. For example, a cyclist can develop tight rectus

femoris muscles during the summer, which could affect sports activity in the fall, such as cross-country running and volleyball.

Preventive Strength Training

The role of strength training in preventing injury depends primarily on two mechanisms. First, a stronger muscle is able to absorb more tensile loading and force before break-

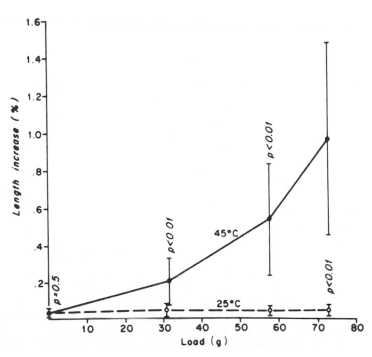

FIGURE 43–6 Percentage increase in tendon length as function of load (in grams) at 45 °C and at 25 °C. (From Lehmann JF, Massock AJ, Warren CG, et al: Effect of therapeutic temperatures on tendon extensibility. Arch Phys Med Rehabil 1970; 51:481. By permission of the American Congress of Rehabilitation Medicine and the American Academy of Physical Medicine and Rehabilitation.)

down occurs either in the muscle itself or at the musculo-tendinous junction.[21] Second, it is important clinically to address any relative muscle weakness, asymmetry, or imbalance (discussion follows).[29] Some examples of muscle deficiency that lead to musculoskeletal problems include weakness of the oblique fibers of the vastus medialis and patellofemoral pain, weakness of the scapular stabilizers and shoulder pain or dysfunction, and weakness of abdominal muscles and back or lower extremity (or both) problems.

Aerobic Training

Aerobic exercise can be a key component of a preventive musculoskeletal exercise program. The cardiovascular "protective" effects of aerobic exercise are well known, and for endurance athletes, aerobic exercise is essential in improving maximum oxygen uptake ($\dot{V}O_2$ max).[13, 19, 26, 61, 89, 123] Less well delineated are the benefits of aerobic exercise that can accrue to the musculoskeletal system. Documented muscle effects of aerobic exercise include increased capillary density, increased number of mitochondria and mitochrondrial oxidative enzymes, improved usage of free fatty acids, and increased percentage of type 2A muscle fibers (i.e., the fibers capable of adapting to endurance or short-burst activities).[2, 15, 38, 39, 64, 65, 99, 106] These alterations in skeletal muscle with aerobic training favor improvement in the "lactate threshold," or onset of blood lactate accumulation. This is favorable for endurance sports because muscle fatigue is lessened, but these alterations can also favor and enhance musculoskeletal performance.

Decreased muscular fatigue could lead to a decrease in the number of musculoskeletal injuries. Nygaard and colleagues[102] have shown that in the vastus lateralis muscle there is an average 50% decrement of glycogen on day 5 as compared with day 1 of consecutive daily alpine skiing. These authors also noted that most skiing injuries occur toward the end of the ski week and at the end of a ski day, and are likely related to muscle fatigue caused by glycogen depletion. Generally, endurance athletes use fats more efficiently and effectively during exercise and in essence are able to "spare glycogen."[89] This occurs in part because endurance athletes accumulate less lactic acid via the above mechanisms than untrained persons at the same work output.

Aerobic exercise could be an essential component of training to prevent early musculoskeletal fatigue; this might help prevent injury. Increased capillary density also helps combat the relative ischemia of a tight muscle group, perhaps contributing to earlier washout of lactic acid. Strength training can negate some of the beneficial effects of increased capillary density,[19, 39, 89, 132, 135] and a regular aerobic component can help balance this seemingly counterproductive effect.

With respect to sport-specific upper extremity training for exercises or sports that primarily use the arms (e.g., swimming and kayaking), the onset of lactate accumulation occurs earlier during arm exercise than during leg exercise.[108, 109] When subjects pursue endurance training with the arms, they have less accumulation of lactate and higher values of maximum oxygen consumption.[27]

For sports specificity, for decreasing fatigue, and for avoiding musculoskeletal injury, aerobic training should be considered an essential component of the exercise prescription. Of course, sport-specific training orients most of the work toward the predominant energy system that the sport requires. The energy systems include ATP-phosphocreatinine, anaerobic, and aerobic systems.

ATP-PHOSPHOCREATININE ENERGY SYSTEM. The ATP-phosphocreatinine system provides for explosive power and is extremely short-lived (5 to 10 sec).[61] Training in this system helps to improve speed and quickness. This system can be enhanced through plyometric-type activities that stress muscle power (discussion follows). Lower-weight, higher-repetition weight training that emphasizes speed and explosiveness of movement contribute to enhancing this energy system.

ANAEROBIC ENERGY SYSTEM. Intermediate-duration (60 to 90 sec) power comes from the anaerobic energy system (glycolysis).[61] Training of this system improves speed endurance. Exercises that enhance this energy system include 220- and 440-yard sprints, stair runs, and interval training on a bicycle or with in-line skates. Training of this type enables high-speed, high-intensity activity to be sustained over short periods of time.

AEROBIC ENERGY SYSTEM. Aerobic training enables sustained intervals of higher intensity exercise and quicker recovery between exercise sessions. It also allows more frequent periods of high-intensity exercise.[61] In aerobically fit persons, the transport of oxygen to the tissues and muscles is more efficient and recovery from a strenuous day of sport or exercise is quicker.

Kinetic Chain Function

The importance of analyzing kinetic chain mechanics cannot be overstated. Attending only to the local area of pain and treating this area exclusively can contribute to perpetuation of symptoms. For example, lateral epicondylitis (tennis elbow) is manifested as tenderness to palpation at the lateral epicondyle and forearm extensor muscle mass. This area can be iced and anti-inflammatory medication can be given, but if the biomechanical deficits of suboptimal wrist or shoulder strength, flexibility, or mechanics are not addressed, and potential problems with sports equipment (such as high tension of the strings in a graphite racquet) are not considered, the problem will continue. Another frequent example is shoulder pain in a baseball pitcher. Local modalities and shoulder exercises can be attempted for pain relief, but unless the biomechanics of the throwing motion are analyzed to ensure that kinetic chain function is normal, the problem might not be entirely addressed. For example, a pitcher might "open up" early during delivery, increasing the force load and stress on the shoulder and elbow. Furthermore, the spine and proper spine mechanics and function are essential for effectively transmitting ground reaction force into the upper extremities, and the scapular stabilizer muscles are important in ensuring that the humeral head maintains its center of rotation in the glenoid fossa during the throw.

With respect to overuse and macrotraumatic musculoskeletal injuries, a therapeutic intervention must occur to make the person "different" before he or she returns to the sport or activity that originally caused the problem. This "different" transformation occurs during rehabilitation, as suggested by Gray.[59] The injured tissue must be modified to deal more effectively with the loads and mechanics of the sport or activity and be reintegrated into the functional kinetic chain through a logical progression of sport-specific exercises. Gray[59] coined the term "integrated isolation" to describe the importance of understanding the site of injury, tightness, malalignment, or strength deficit, and how integration of this region into the kinetic chain can contribute to excessive loading, overuse, or injury.

There are many ways of incorporating kinetic chain exercises that occur in a proprioceptively enriched environment and that can be specific for integration of various upper extremity and lower extremity biomechanical movements. Various functional upper extremity and lower extremity exercises entail the use of multiple joints and muscle co-contraction (Fig. 43–7). These exercises are sport- and life-specific and use muscle groups in a coordinated fashion rather than in an isolated one.

Building on the concept of "integrated isolation," Gray[59] pointed out that we probably should stretch in a kinetic chain fashion because this is the way that the tissue is normally used. Isolated stretches can help to heal and to modify tissue at the site of injury, but true functional stretch can occur only when the tissue is incorporated into the kinetic chain (Fig. 43–8).

Sport-Specific Higher Level Skills

Before a person returns to a sport after an injury or before participating in a sport, sport- and position-specific skills are necessary to ensure that the skills related to a sport are performed with the greatest facility and dexterity. In essence, one should not "play a sport to get in shape," but rather should "get in shape to play a sport." These exercises include higher-order gait and coordination exercises, plyometrics, and sport-specific drills. In addition to sports specificity, position specificity is important. The job description for a lineman on a football team is different from that for a wide receiver; similarly, each of these jobs requires a specific exercise program.

Incorporation of Components into Training Program

None of the components of injury prevention and pre-rehabilitation mentioned previously are effective unless they can be incorporated into an individual or group training program. Education is essential and can be incorporated on three levels. The person should receive information from the sports medicine team (e.g., physician, physical therapist, athletic trainer, coach, and others, as applicable). At local and regional levels, high school and college sports programs can have considerable impact by implementing the above elements into their programs. On a national level, organizations such as the American College of Sports Medicine and the Physiatric Association of Spine, Sports, and Occupational Rehabilitation can contribute by formulating consensus and position statements.

EXTRINSIC CONTRIBUTORS TO INJURY AND SUBOPTIMAL SPORTS PERFORMANCE

The major factors that contribute to injury can be grouped into extrinsic and intrinsic factors. Extrinsic factors consist primarily of elements external to a person, whereas intrinsic factors are related to a person's anatomical and biomechanical characteristics.

Extrinsic factors that can contribute to injury or suboptimal sports performance are listed in Table 43–2.

Conditioning and Preparation

It is important to analyze an athlete's training history (e.g., the types of terrain on a runner's running route, the volume of training, and the intensity of training). The *terrible too's*—"too much, too soon, too fast, and too hard"—contribute to many overuse injuries. The classic example is medial tibial stress syndrome seen in springtime high school track participants.[98] These athletes usually progress from winter sports and activities that do not require sustained long-duration running or impact loading into training and competition that suddenly demand sustained high-impact exercise. Also, it is important to ensure that sport-specific conditioning and sport preparation have taken place.

Climate, Fluids, and Hydration

Climatic extremes can be a factor in thermal injuries. The importance of adequate hydration and fluid replacement should be stressed for persons competing in endurance events. In hot conditions, water loss from the skin and lungs can be greater than 2 L/hour. Because water constitutes most of the fluid that is lost in events lasting less than 90 minutes, water replacement is the best mode of restoring fluid status. Carbohydrate supplementation can be helpful during exercise that lasts longer than 90 minutes.[40]

Kinesiology of the Sport

Understanding the kinesiology of the sport and sports task is important for optimal performance and efficiency. For example, physiatrists should understand the basic mechanics of the throwing motion to assess the kinetic chain function of a baseball pitcher. This is true for every sport-specific movement. Each sport places unique kinesiological and biomechanical stresses on the components of the kinetic chain that are involved in performing the sport. If training focuses on optimizing the mechanics of the sport, injuries may be prevented. Often, a video camera recording can help delineate the components of the kinetic chain.

TABLE 43–2 Contributors to Injury: Extrinsic Factors

Training errors—conditioning and preparation
Climate
Nutrition and hydration
Kinesiology of the sport
Epidemiology
Equipment
Playing field

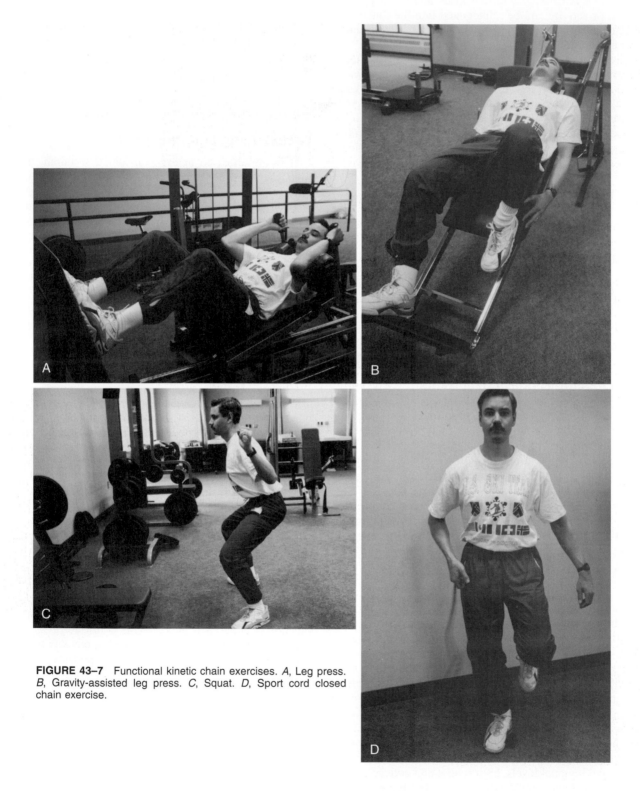

FIGURE 43–7 Functional kinetic chain exercises. *A*, Leg press. *B*, Gravity-assisted leg press. *C*, Squat. *D*, Sport cord closed chain exercise.

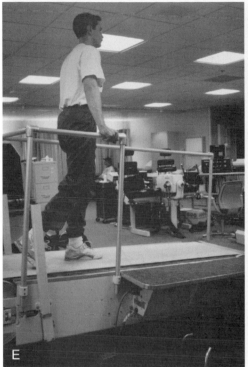

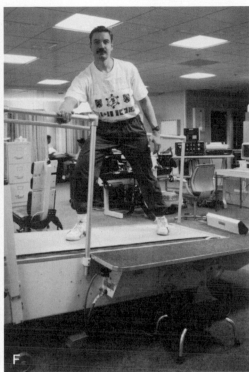

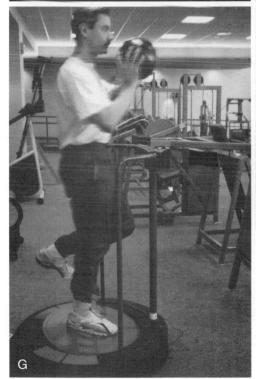

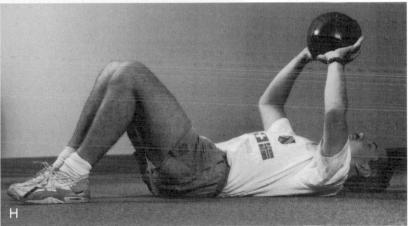

FIGURE 43–7 *Continued   E,* Retrowalking. *F,* Lateral walking. *G,* Combined upper and lower extremity exercises (proprioceptively enriched). *H,* Upper extremity medicine ball.

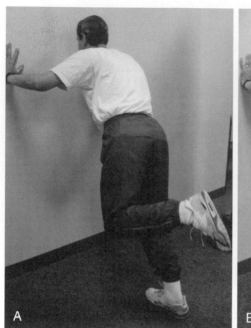
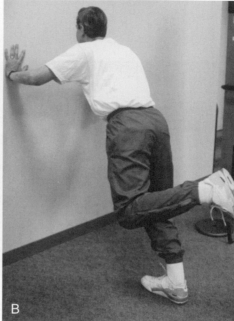
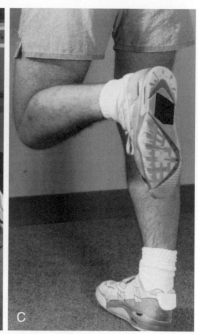

FIGURE 43–8 Stretching of Achilles tendon in kinetic chain. *A*, Pronated position. *B*, Supinated position. *C*, Close-up of supinated kinetic chain stretch.

Epidemiology

Certain sports have an inherent risk and predispose to injury of specific parts of the body, and each sport has certain risk factors that pretraining can help to minimize. The seemingly innocuous and frequently prescribed step aerobic exercise was found by one study to cause time loss because of injury in a large percentage of persons.[114] This is likely because the exercise made apparent previously unmanifested anatomical, biomechanical, strength, or flexibility problems as the kinetic chain was stressed. It is important to identify injuries that are specific for a sport or activity and to maximize the kinetic chain function related to the particular part of the body at risk.

Equipment

Equipment can have a significant role in injury. For example, appropriate release settings for ski binding and binding maintenance are essential to protect a skier in the event of a fall. Inadequate release settings increase the risk of injury many times.[75]

Playing Field

The playing field should be considered an extrinsic contributor to injury. Various artificial turf surfaces can alter foot and lower limb torque, and certain injuries (e.g., "turf toe" in football) seem to be more prevalent on artificial surfaces. However, every surface has a unique effect on transmitting reaction force up through the lower extemities. The composition of the playing surface should be considered in relation to the particular sport training and game requirements. For example, cross-country runners should not be trained exclusively on concrete surfaces.

INTRINSIC CONTRIBUTORS TO INJURY AND SUBOPTIMAL SPORTS PERFORMANCE

The intrinsic contributors to injury are listed in Table 43–3. Malalignments and anatomical variations such as excessive forefoot pronation, cavus foot, varus/valgus malalignment, excessive tibial torsion, excessive leg-length discrepancy (more than 2 cm), and excessive femoral anteversion can contribute to numerous biomechanical problems that can cause injury. Orthotic interventions, such as supports to preserve the longitudinal arch of the foot, can help to optimize foot biomechanics and to improve the distribution of force throughout the lower extremity. In addition, adequate shock absorption can help reduce the incidence of overuse injury in such sports as running.[95, 122]

Ensuring symmetrical and sport-specific flexibility is important, as is maintaining balanced muscle group strength. Signs of incomplete or improper rehabilitation from a previous injury, such as strength asymmetries or deficits, flexibility asymmetries, or a poor aerobic base, should be addressed. For example, it previously was believed that the relative lack of internal rotation of the shoulder in many tennis players was acceptable, and that it resulted from "resetting the thermostat." Essentially, this lack of internal

TABLE 43–3 Contributors to Injury: Intrinsic Factors

Malalignment
Leg-length discrepancy
Poor flexibility
Muscle weakness
Muscle imbalance
Decreased neuromuscular skills
Kinetic chain dysfunction

rotation was assumed to be adequately compensated for by excessive external rotation. This assumption is incorrect. Internal rotation deficits have been found over time to predispose to shoulder and rotator cuff injury.[30, 31] Muscle imbalances can also prove problematic, as evidenced in the shoulder muscles. Many persons concentrate heavily on anterior shoulder exercises (such as the bench press and pectoral strengthening) during strength training. If the scapular stabilizers (primarily serratus anterior, latissimus dorsi, trapezius, and rhomboids) are neglected, an imbalance results that can place the rotator cuff at risk.

Lack of appropriate neuromuscular skills for a particular sport or position within a sport can contribute to an increased risk of injury. There have been many instances of players injured after a change in position (e.g., José Canseco) or during competition at a high level in a sport outside their field. Also, if an athlete returns to competition after an injury before sport-specific skills are gained, the risk of reinjury is increased.

Generalized ligamentous laxity is often discussed as an independent risk factor for musculoskeletal injury. No study clearly validates this assumption, however, and laxity may in some instances protect from injury. Asymmetry is again a more likely contributor to injury, and if preinjury range is not reestablished, the immediate area and related kinetic chain components are at risk.

Gait, stance, and the biomechanics of a particular sport movement should be examined for possible dysfunction of the kinetic chain. It is important to look at static and dynamic alignment as well as at function. In a case of suspected patellofemoral pain, not only should the knee be thoroughly examined with the patient supine, but patellofemoral tracking and of the oblique portion of the vastus medialis activation should be assessed with the patient in weight-bearing and squatting positions.

Principles of sports psychology are important in injury prevention because they can help a person to focus his or her concentration. They also provide techniques for relaxation and stress management. Neuromuscular engrams and motor learning can be facilitated through the use of such techniques as imagery.

GENERAL PRINCIPLES OF MUSCULOSKELETAL REHABILITATION

Assessment of Injury

Most musculoskeletal injuries can be divided into two broad categories: (1) acute and (2) subacute, or chronic. Acute injuries are often related to a breach of integrity of the muscular system, such as bone fracture or ligamentous disruption. The range of severity is broad and includes everything from a mild inversion ankle sprain to a devastating spinal cord injury. For this reason, the diagnostic acumen of an evaluator should be wide-ranging. The evaluator must be capable of recognizing the signs and symptoms of a neurological problem. It is equally important to know the indications for and use of spinal stabilization and transport techniques to prevent spinal cord injury.[139, 141] Indications for surgical referral must be based on objective criteria.

The age of the patient must be considered when an injury is evaluated. For example, a high school football player who has vague left-sided abdominal pain after being tackled and has a history of viral illness should be thoroughly evaluated for splenic involvement due to possible mononucleosis. Similarly, older athletes should be evaluated in the context of concurrent medical problems such as cardiac disease, respiratory compromise, or severe degenerative changes.

Subacute or chronic injury can usually be thought of as repetitive damage to or overuse of the musculoskeletal system. Examples are the repetitive microtrauma sustained by the forearm extensor muscle mass and tendon group in lateral epicondylitis (tennis elbow) and by the tibia in medial tibial stress syndrome (shin splints). Treatment of these injuries typically involves the principle of "relative rest," in which the injured body part is protected from further trauma and then gradually rehabilitated to normal function. During the treatment, aerobic fitness is maintained by using other, noninjured parts of the body.

Treatment

The basic principles of rehabilitation after musculoskeletal injury include pain reduction by means of various modalities (i.e., ice, superficial and deep heat, interferential current) and appropriately prescribed medications, restoration of range of motion and flexibility, therapeutic strengthening, and maximization of sport-specific agility, coordination, and proprioception before return to sports. Another basic principle is the use of relative rest to maintain aerobic conditioning and cardiovascular fitness.

Relative Rest

A significant decrease in aerobic capacity can occur in as short a time as 4 weeks of detraining.[54, 70, 116] The principle of relative rest means that the injured part of the body is rested and protected from further trauma or injury, while the remaining muscle mass is used to provide appropriate stress to the cardiovascular system for maintaining optimal aerobic conditioning. The injured part should be protected by a brace, cast, or limited weight-bearing status. The patient may need to be instructed about the appropriate use of crutches or a cane. Initially, the injured part should be rested, with no movement beyond a pain-free range. Strength training should continue in the uninjured parts of the body because crossover training effects occur in the rested limb when the contralateral limb is exercised.[97]

Relative rest of an injured part of the body is achieved with splinting, bracing, taping, or specialized adaptive equipment that permits performance of aerobic exercise. (Aerobic exercise is defined by the American College of Sports Medicine as any exercise that uses large muscle groups, can be maintained continuously, is rhythmic and aerobic in nature, and lasts from 20 to 60 minutes.[12]) A resting hand splint (prescribed for a person with wrist pain from carpal tunnel syndrome or elbow pain due to lateral epicondylitis) and an elbow hyperextension block brace (which can be used for a person who is recovering from an elbow dislocation) permit the aerobic component of training to be continued while the injured part is rehabilitated. Any lower extremity injury can be protected while the upper extremities and possibly even the noninvolved

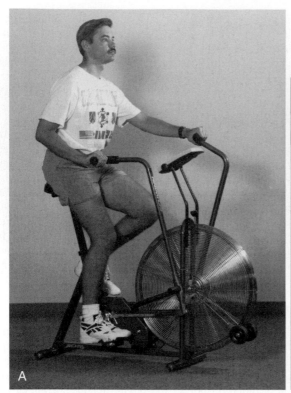

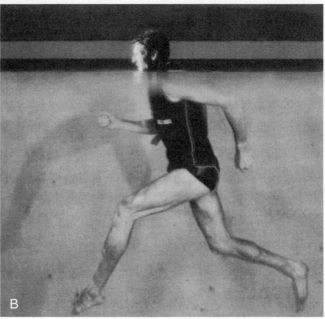

FIGURE 43–9 *A,* Resistance bicycle (Airdyne) enables exercise of upper and lower extremity muscles. *B,* Wet-vest running. (*B* from McWaters G: Aquatic rehabilitation. *In* Andrews JR, Harrelson GL (eds): Physical Rehabilitation of the Injured Athlete. Philadelphia, WB Saunders, 1991, pp 473–503. By permission of Bioenergetics Inc., Pelham, Al (1–800–938–8378).)

lower limb are used in the aerobic program. Exercise of the contralateral limb can be continued by use of devices such as resistance bicycles that provide for both upper extremity and lower extremity movement for bi- and tri-limb work (Fig. 43–9A). Wet-vest running (running in deep water with a buoyancy vest to keep the head above water) is also an effective method of non–weight-bearing training (Fig. 43–9B). The resistance of the water contributes to strengthening of the lower limb and to aerobic fitness. Similar benefits with minimal weight-bearing stress can be achieved by walking in water that is only waist deep.

Pain Relief and Inflammation Control

The initial goals of the treatment of a sports injury should be to limit as much as possible the extent of the initial injury, to aid healing, and to provide for early institution of rehabilitation measures. The mainstay of early treatment (i.e., 24 to 48 hours after the injury) follows the principles of PRICE, as listed in Table 43–4.

Ice is efficacious for decreasing pain and swelling by producing local vasoconstriction. Ice packs can safely be applied for 20 minutes of every hour. For focal injuries,

ice massage is easy to apply and it can be particularly time effective. Also, compression around the injured area helps to limit swelling and enhances comfort and earlier range of motion. Physiologically, this can improve outcome, because early tensile stress to tissue causes more linear collagen formation and enables stronger tensile strength. If compression initially is instituted with elastic wraps (e.g., Ace bandages), rewrapping should be performed every 4 hours to ensure appropriate compression. The elastic wrap should first be stretched to its fullest extent and then be reduced to two-thirds of this length, to provide appropriate tension during wrapping and to prevent circulatory compromise. Alternative means of compression include elastic fabric, which can be customized to fit the injured body part, and neoprene sleeves. Compression and cold can be applied simultaneously with an intermittent pneumatic compression pump (Fig. 43–10). The injured extremity should be raised to a level higher than the heart to facilitate venous return.

Use of superficial ice (acute and chronic) and heat (subacute and chronic) modalities are likely to continue to be the mainstays of pain relief because of the low risk of complications, the ease of application, and the therapeutic efficacy. Also, ultrasound treatment, short-wave diathermy, interferential current, and transcutaneous electric nerve stimulation can be used safely with the usual precautions and with appropriate prescription (see Chapters 22 and 23). Physiatrists need to ensure appropriate selection of therapeutic modalities to avoid misuse and abuse. For example, ultrasound treatment is most effective at sites with the greatest change in absorption characteristics of the

TABLE 43–4   PRICE Principles

P:	protection
R:	relative rest
I:	ice
C:	compression
E:	elevation

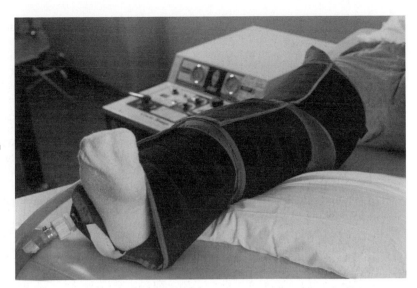

FIGURE 43–10 Intermittent pneumatic compression pump applies cold and compression simultaneously.

tissue, such as at the interface of bone and soft tissue. In these regions, the temperature may increase more than 5 °C.[81, 82] Ultrasound treatment is inappropriate and ineffective for use with diffuse and uniformly absorptive tissue, for example, the lumbar paraspinal muscle mass.

Other modalities such as electrical stimulation are often applied inappropriately to a wide range of musculoskeletal injuries. The clinical efficacy of electrical stimulation, apart from its neuromuscular reeducation value, has not been validated, and in this era of cost-containment and outcome efficacy, its random, widespread use has been questioned.

Overuse Injury

Early treatment of an overuse injury is slightly different from that of an acute injury. Because significant swelling usually is not a permanent component, a compression garment or elevation may not be needed. However, protection and ice are essential. The activity that contributed to the microtrauma must be avoided or at least greatly modified, especially with respect to frequency. Patients must be educated about appropriate biomechanical and kinesiological principles of the sport-related movement. Ice can be an effective method of pain control, but heat might be especially beneficial. Heat can be delivered as superficial heat or deeper heat at the bone-tendon interface (ultrasound treatment). Heat causes blood vessel dilatation, provides pain relief, and can help decrease muscle tightness. Heat can be used in combination with gentle prolonged stretching to increase range of motion by promoting collagen extensibility.[83] General and muscle-specific relaxation and stretching techniques can help diminish muscle tightness and enhance whole body relaxation. Massage techniques, appropriately used, can be a beneficial adjunct, and cross fiber or friction massage can be used to help mobilize contracted scar tissue.

Biofeedback is effective for reeducating the patient regarding the kinesthetic sensation of achieving and maintaining relaxation in a particular muscle. This can be helpful in cases of painful muscle splinting that are refractory to other treatment. Biofeedback can also enhance activation of a specifically inhibited muscle group and, in tandem with functional electrical stimulation, can be effective in neuromuscular reeducation. For example, the effort of the quadriceps (particularly the oblique portion of the vastus medialis) can be inhibited up to 60% by a small (20 mL) knee effusion.[47] This inhibition can cause deactivation of the neuromuscular pathway and a relative shutdown of the muscle group because of nociceptive stimuli. Pain affects the afferent neuromuscular arc by causing neural inhibition that hinders muscle activation ("deafferentation"). Athletes might find it difficult, if not impossible, to produce a voluntary contraction of the oblique portion of the vastus medialis in such circumstances. Electrical stimulation can help athletes regain kinesthetic awareness of a particular muscle group, and biofeedback can verify voluntary activation and be effective in learning to enhance selective muscle use. The latter program is particularly efficacious in entities such as patellofemoral pain, in which an afferent nociceptive stimulus causes neuromuscular inhibition of the oblique portion of the vastus medialis.

Whether nonsteroidal anti-inflammatory drugs have any direct effect on the rehabilitative course is unclear. However, if used initially and for a short time, these drugs can assist in starting the rehabilitation process by decreasing the level of pain. Pain can be a great inhibitor, and muscle co-contraction and substitution are just two of the suboptimal biomechanical effects that can result from "going through the pain." Long-term use of nonsteroidal anti-inflammatory drugs is not advisable for either able-bodied or physically challenged athletes, and special care must be taken for those with spinal cord injury because they are particularly vulnerable to renal injury. For those who have been taking nonsteroidal anti-inflammatory drugs for a long time, it is often the case that a specific etiologic problem (e.g., biomechanical deficit, flexibility or strength deficit, or asymmetry) has not been correctly identified.

Range of Motion and Flexibility

Before strength training can begin, range of motion must be maximized. Muscles are mechanically most efficient when they can shorten and lengthen maximally, especially during isotonic exercise.[111] Depending on the injury, range of motion might need to be protected, passive, or limited in the initial stages, but should progress to full range as tolerated. Joint motion provides nutrition to articular cartilage through hydrostatic pressure. It also prevents the formation of soft tissue contractures and provides proprioceptive joint and muscle feedback.[4] To achieve full range of motion, gentle terminal stretching might be necessary, especially after treatment with superficial heat or ultrasound. During the healing process, specific stresses must be applied to the tissue by range of motion and stretching to promote linear alignment of collagen.[56] Collagen produced in this manner is more effective with respect to load-bearing and has greater tensile strength.[33, 79, 113] Without stress, collagen fibers tend to be arranged in a chaotic fashion.

Stretching in combination with a strengthening program that emphasizes muscle balance is essential in athletic rehabilitation. Because of different levels of weakness and dysfunction, many persons have a relative dominance of one muscle group over another. Dominance of an agonist over a weakened or nonfunctioning antagonist group can produce contracture and joint dysfunction. Dominance of one muscle group can result from strength imbalances, for example, greater development of anterior shoulder muscle groups than of posterior shoulder muscle groups.[73] This pattern is often seen in baseball pitchers and in persons who stress the anterior muscle groups in weight training (pectorals, anterior deltoid, and biceps). Thus, the important posterior shoulder group and scapular stabilization musculature (rhomboids, serratus anterior, latissimus dorsi, and trapezius) are neglected. Consequently, relative tightness of the anterior capsule occurs; in conjunction with the relative weakness of the posterior group, this can predispose a person to shoulder problems.[71] This unbalanced system creates a potential for overuse and stress at the weak link (i.e., the point of imbalance). The entire kinetic chain mechanics must be assessed in relation to the particular task or movement of a sport.

Strength Training

After full or nearly full pain-free motion is achieved, strength training can begin. The strength that is gained in the first few weeks is due to the neural effect of enhanced synchronization and recruitment of motor units.[96] Muscle fiber hypertrophy does not occur until after 2 to 4 weeks or more of strengthening exercise.[97] The more efficient use of muscle provided by strengthening exercises has a positive effect on early return of function and performance. The various types of strength training include isometric, isotonic, isokinetic, resistance band, variable resistance, plyometric, and kinetic chain exercise (see Chapter 20).

Isometric

Isometric, or equal length, exercise is essentially a static muscular contraction. In essence, both ends of the muscle are fixed, with no motion in the muscle as a result of the contraction. It entails exerting a maximal force against a relatively immovable object, with no appreciable change in muscle length. No mechanical work is performed during the contraction; thus, the energy is dissipated as heat.

The most effective way for performing isometric exer-

cise to gain strength has not been clearly defined.[20] Hettinger[63] showed strength gains of 5% per week with one 6-sec contraction per day at 67% maximal effort. He later concluded that maximal contractions produced better results. Clarke[34] stated that the best results were obtained with maximal contractions held for 6 sec, five to ten times per day. According to Atha,[20] isometric contraction should be "near maximal, long enough for total fiber recruitment, and repeated several times per day." The problem with incorporating this advice into practical strength training is obvious.

Among the problems with isometric training is that the strength gains are specific to the angle of the joint.[58] Furthermore, isometric training does not change the ability of a muscle to exert force rapidly, and it provides little stimulus for hypertrophy or endurance in dynamic activity. Thus, isometric training is not a functional type of exercise. Nevertheless, isometric exercise does protect the joint from undue stress, and it creates less inflammatory response in the joint than does isotonic exercise.[92] Isometric exercise can prepare the muscle for functional kinetic chain strengthening at a later stage. Currently, its main use in sports medicine is to limit atrophy in muscles that cannot be used isotonically because immobilization in a splint or cast.

Isotonic

Isotonic, or equal tension, exercise ideally consists of constant muscle contraction with constantly applied tension. Isotonic exercise is dynamic in nature and occurs when the muscle contraction itself is used to move a joint that ultimately moves a load through a range of motion. Initially the load might be no more than the weight of the limb, with later progression to resistance exercises. Isotonic strength depends on the contractile force and mechanics of movement about a joint (Fig. 43–11).[144] The muscle is not contracting at constant capacity or a specific percentage thereof throughout the entire range of motion; for this reason, the term *isotonic* technically is not accurate, because equal tension is not exerted throughout the joint range of motion. Isotonic exercise can further be divided into concentric and eccentric components. Concentric contractions entail the loading of the muscle while it is shortening, whereas eccentric contractions load the muscle while it is lengthening. An example of each type occurs in a biceps curl: lifting the weight is a concentric contraction and lowering it slowly is an eccentric contraction.

The traditional belief is that eccentric exercise is more likely to cause muscle damage. Asmussen[18] demonstrated that eccentric exercise resulted in muscle soreness 24 to 48 hours after exercise. Others have shown that eccentric exercise produces muscle soreness; however, the soreness dissipates after 1 week.[76] Clarkson and Ebbeling[35] pointed out that an increase in plasma levels of creatine kinase seems unrelated to the development of muscle soreness, loss of strength after exercise, fitness level of the subject, or lean body weight. According to Evans and Cannon,[51] this exercise-induced skeletal muscle "damage" causes a release of intracellular proteins, delayed-onset muscle soreness, and an increase in turnover of skeletal muscle protein. These adaptations appear to be integral to the

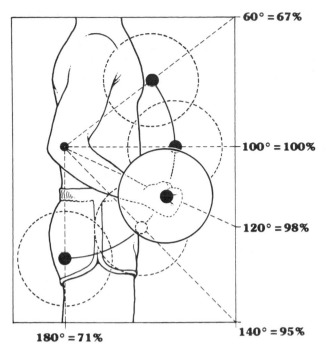

60° = 67%

100° = 100%

120° = 98%

180° = 71%   **140° = 95%**

FIGURE 43–11 Percentage of force production as a muscle moves through its range of motion. (From Wilmore JH, Costill DL: Training for Sport and Activity: The Physiological Basis of the Conditioning Process, ed 3. Dubuque, William C Brown, 1988. By permission of publisher.)

repair of the damaged muscle. Also, they may be essential for hypertrophy, because chronic exercise causes adaptations in skeletal muscle that result in an increased capacity of oxidative metabolism. The repair of damaged muscle resulting in the hypertrophy seen in eccentric exercise might be a mechanism for protection against further exercise-induced damage.[51] Eccentric exercise might offer an opportunity to delineate signals and modulators during repair of damaged muscle. Much might be learned about the response to and adaptation of muscle to chronic exercise by further investigation of this topic.

Isokinetic

Isokinetic, or equal speed, exercise was introduced by Perrine.[110] It allows maximal force production through full range of motion (e.g., Cybex machines; Ronkonkoma, NY) (Fig. 43–12). Isokinetic exercise consists of exercising at a predetermined constant velocity of joint motion. Isokinetic strength is the maximal torque that can be developed at any given velocity of contraction.[45] This type of exercise provides objective information about peak muscle torque, power, and endurance at reproducible velocities. Side-to-side data for comparison with an uninjured limb is easily obtained.

The velocities that can be achieved with isokinetic equipment are greater than those attained with traditional weight-training equipment. Yet, these velocities are much slower than those of certain sports movements (e.g., a maximum of 300 degrees/second on a machine compared with 7000 degrees/second in the overhand throwing motion).[105] This type of exercise for strength training purposes is also non-functional because only one joint and one muscle system

are used at maximal contraction. Isokinetic exercise does not approximate the way that a limb is used either during a sport or in activities of daily living.

Although objective data are obtained, athletes still must regain agility, coordination, and sport-specific skills before returning to competition. It is preferable to rely on isokinetic measurements as a rough estimate of progression and rehabilitation but use more functional testing for return-to-play criteria. Isokinetic exercise can cause increased patellofemoral shear and compression forces and is contraindicated early on in knees with a reconstructed anterior cruciate ligament.[107, 129] This type of exercise can excessively load the secondary restraints in knees with a deficient anterior cruciate ligament.[60]

Resistance Band

Resistance band exercise usually involves the use of a progressive resistance band (e.g., Theraband) that provides gradually increasing resistance when stretched. The band can be used in multiple planes of motion. Also, it can be used to simulate functional and sport-specific activities, such as the throwing motion of a baseball pitcher (Fig. 43–13) or the kicking motion of a soccer player. This type of functional exercise is preferred to isolated exercise for the upper and lower extremities because it uses muscles in more of the complex and diagonal/spiral movement planes that sport movements require. The apparatus is inexpensive and easily portable. Particularly for the upper extremities, manual resistance strengthening is a variation on resistance band strengthening and is a way of providing carefully graded resistance in multiple dynamic movement planes (Fig. 43–14). Therapists can adjust the applied resistance according to the patient's pain and limitations of range of motion and strength.

Variable Resistance

Variable resistance training means that the resistance is altered through the use of cams or pulleys in an attempt to match the force-producing capability of the muscle

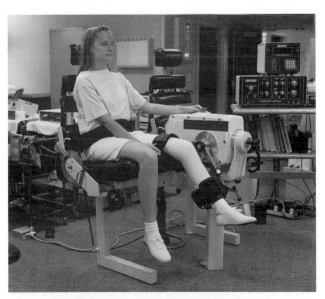

FIGURE 43–12 Isokinetic exercise machine.

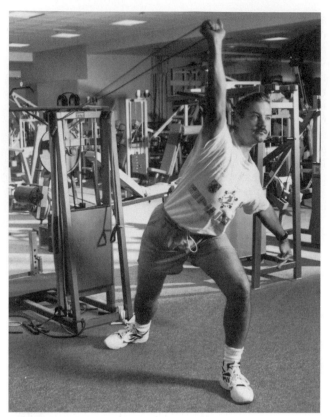

FIGURE 43–13 Resistance band exercise for "pitching-specific" strengthening.

entire range of motion. It is an isolated and nonfunctional exercise and does not stimulate associated proximal and distal components of the kinetic chain. Velocity and acceleration are variables in this type of exercise training, which is more useful for isolated strengthening than for sport-specific training.

Plyometric Exercise

Plyometric exercises emphasize speed and power. They consist of concentric muscle contractions after a previous stretch of the same muscle groups. Theoretically, this helps provide neuromuscular facilitation, releases neural inhibition, and enables stronger and more forceful muscle contractions.[32, 140, 145] Plyometric exercises contain both eccentric and concentric components and load both the elastic and the contractile elements of a muscle. Examples of higher-level plyometrics include jumping rapidly onto and off of different-sized boxes, jumping back and forth over a low object (Fig. 43–16), and performing specified weight-training maneuvers such as the "power clean." The power clean maneuver involves lifting a barbell from the ground in a rapid fashion, using coordinated kinetic chain movements of the lower extremities, trunk, and upper extremities. These exercises should be performed on an appropriate surface (e.g., grass rather than concrete), under careful supervision, and with an adequate foundation of strength in the muscle groups used. The high-speed, high-impact nature of advanced-level plyometrics theoretically creates a greater potential for injury. Nevertheless, they are an

throughout the full range of motion (e.g., Cybex or Nautilus machines) (Fig. 43–15). This training attempts to compensate for the previously mentioned practical inability of a muscle to contract at a constant capacity throughout the

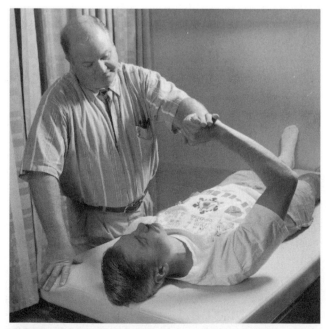

FIGURE 43–14 Manual resistance strengthening. The therapist provides resistance in functional planes of movement.

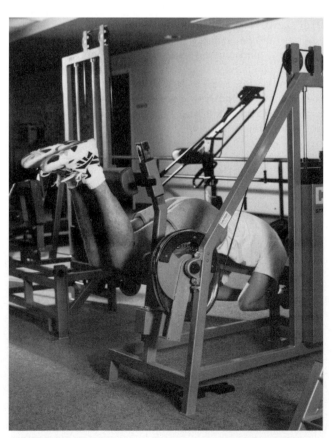

FIGURE 43–15 Variable resistance strength training equipment.

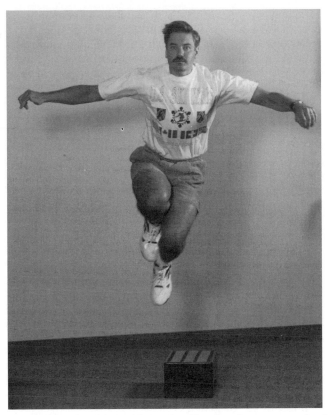

FIGURE 43–16 Side-to-side low-level box jumping, an example of plyometric exercise.

essential component in developing the speed and explosiveness necessary for many sports.

Low-level plyometrics (e.g., skipping, hopscotch variations, high stepping) can be performed safely by most persons. In my opinion, plyometrics are the most neglected segments of exercises in sports medicine and in rehabilitation in general. Very few sport biomechanical movements cannot be aided by plyometric training. Currently, baseball pitchers and basketball and volleyball players are finding significant benefit from such power training.

Power is work performed over time:

$$Power = (force \times distance)/time$$

and enhancement of power has implications for many areas in rehabilitation. For example, an elderly person not only needs to use lower extremity hip and knee muscle group strength to get up from a chair but also needs to use that strength over a specific period of time to be successful in the transfer. Muscle "power" also is needed when a person tries to cross the street before the light turns red. Lifting and strength training to improve power should emphasize lighter to more moderate weights and higher repetitions, using speed and explosiveness of movement as the main points of emphasis in the exercise.

Kinetic Chain Exercise

The concept and terminology of kinetic chain exercise were originally introduced by Steindler.[130] The term *closed kinetic chain* has become popular in recent years. Steindler

pointed out that link system segment connections are considered closed if both ends are connected to an immovable framework, preventing translation of either proximal or distal joint centers. A true closed kinetic chain exists only during isometric exercise, because by definition neither the proximal nor the distal segments can move in a closed system. Steindler explained that there are two specific kinetic chain environments. An open kinetic chain exists when the peripheral joint of the extremity can move freely, and a closed kinetic chain exists when the foot or hand meets resistance.

Closed chain exercises can be thought of as exercises in which the distal extremity remains fixed while multiple proximal joints move in a functional manner with contraction of both agonists and antagonists for stabilization (see Fig. 43–7). Examples of such exercise are squats (for the lower extremities) and push-ups (for the upper extremities). These movements entail triarticular motion of either the upper or lower extremities as opposed to movement around a single joint, which occurs with such open kinetic chain exercises as isolated leg extension. Closed chain exercises are more function-based and sport-specific for the lower extremities than exercises that isolate a specific muscle group. For example, squats involve co-contraction and use the quadriceps, hamstring, and gastrocnemius-soleus muscle groups in a functional manner similar to that used in many sports and general activities (e.g., getting up from a chair). If properly performed, squats also provide considerable joint and ligament safety. They are one of the primary exercises in rehabilitation of the anterior cruciate ligament.[86] Because co-contraction is a stabilizing factor, shear force and compression force at the knees are diminished with closed chain as compared with open chain exercise.[22a, 85, 104] Recent work, however, suggests that previous analytical models of anterior cruciate ligament strain may be limited, and maximum strain values may not be significantly different when comparing open and closed chain exercise.[52a] Closed kinetic chain exercise should certainly be the predominant type of exercise for the lower extremities in sports medicine and in rehabilitation in general; however, there is still room for appropriate use of open kinetic chain exercise, especially in the intermediate phase of "bulking up" a severely atrophied muscle before more functional closed chain work is attempted (or along with low-weight closed chain work that emphasizes proper technique and mechanics).

With respect to the current discussion about open kinetic chain exercise, Shelbourne and Nitz[124] report that reconstruction grafts of the anterior cruciate ligament did not stretch out with early, full-range, open chain quadriceps resistive early exercise. The graft may revascularize more quickly with open chain exercise, and because ligaments respond to tensile stress through hypertrophy, the graft may become stronger during the revascularization period.[48] Shelbourne and Nitz[124] claimed that the number of complications decreased with open chain exercise. Others have noted a decreased incidence of joint stiffness, patellofemoral pain, and muscle atrophy and an early return of quadriceps strength.[48] Furthermore, compliance may be improved and return to sports or work may be more rapid. For the upper extremities, open kinetic chain exercises are essential before return to sport because these exercises are similar to the limb movements used in most sports (e.g., the throwing motion).

As with any exercise and rehabilitative measure, no single protocol or exercise can be applied to all persons and to all situations. All of the previously mentioned exercises should be in the armamentarium of physiatrists who prescribe therapeutic exercise, and further research is needed to validate specific exercise applications (see Chapter 20).

AGILITY, PROPRIOCEPTION, AND SPORT-SPECIFIC SKILLS

Athletes should work to regain optimal agility and coordination either after strength has been maximized or in tandem with strength training. In many injuries, a muscle, tendon, or ligament and a joint are "detuned," and the proprioceptive feedback that the muscle or joint capsule normally provides is disrupted. Mechanoreceptors, muscle spindles, and Golgi tendon organs can be affected to various degrees. Examples of exercises that help regain this function include wobble board exercises, which help maximize balance and refine coordinating movements of lower extremity muscles, especially at the ankle (Fig. 43–17). Ankle group muscles are retrained to make the minute postural adjustments that are required for a person to maintain balance and remain upright. Knee proprioception can

be better maximized with both standing and supine exercises involving a pediatric ball and knee-specific movements (Fig. 43–18). If lower extremity ambulation has been hindered by the injury, therapy should focus on higher order gait activities, including carioca or crossover walking, and balance activities specific to the athlete's sport. For example, a football halfback could practice timed runs in tires or in a rope-maze course.

Evidence strongly supports specificity in training. Sale and MacDougall[119] state that training should simulate the movement desired as closely as possible with respect to anatomical movement pattern, velocity, and type and force of contraction. Exercise gains are specific to the type and pattern of movement addressed by training,[136] the velocity of training,[41] and the range of motion and angle at which training occurs.[58] Thorough knowledge of an athlete's sport and kinesiological demand is essential in designing an appropriate rehabilitation program for return to sports. Also essential is functional testing of these skills before competition. An athlete might have followed a comprehensive and thorough program of exercise, but rehabilitation is incomplete unless exercises specific to the sport and the athlete's position in the sport can be performed maximally and without pain or loss of function. These exercises also must be reprogrammed, and general exercises alone do not suffice. The ultimate goal is for an athlete to be at maximal strength and agility to maximize performance and to prevent recurrence of injury.

PROPRIOCEPTION

One of the new frontiers in musculoskeletal medicine is the further development and expansion of knowledge about the afferent sensory pathway for movement, or proprioception. The term *proprioception* is controversial because of lack of agreement on a definition.[16, 17, 49, 112, 129] Consensus has not been reached about the location of the key afferent receptors that trigger dynamic joint stability. Currently, the important receptors are thought to be cutaneous receptors, joint capsule receptors, muscle receptors, and receptors in ligaments. With injury there is a diminution of function of the afferent-efferent pathway in addition to the mechanical constraint disruption. Retraining of this dynamic stability is one of the essential factors in successful adaptation to injury. It is just as important as strength training, because the dynamic stability system must be challenged in order to improve the pathways and to ensure total joint stability. Research programs are currently under way to objectively delineate the neuromuscular gains achieved by a proprioceptively enriched rehabilitation program, such as the regular use of a wobble board for ankle sprains.

YOUTH SPORTS MEDICINE CONSIDERATIONS

Resistance training in young athletes must be used judiciously before closure of the growth plates occurs. These areas of growth are relatively weak in comparison with the surrounding ligamentous and fibrous supports, and if this "weak link" is injured, bony deformity and unequal

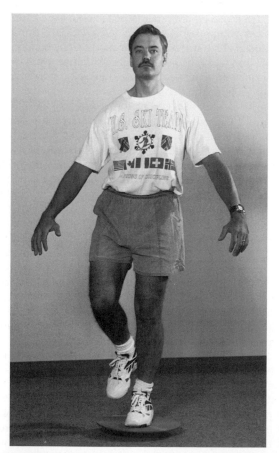

FIGURE 43–17 Wobble board exercise to enhance dynamic ankle stability.

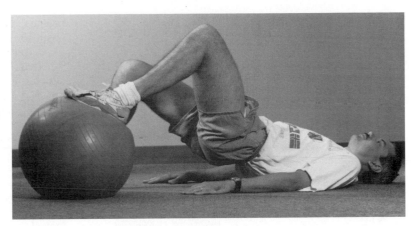

FIGURE 43–18 Supine knee-specific proprioceptive exercises with a pediatric ball.

growth can result.[115] Proper technique prevents these problems by not overloading any bone or muscle and joint complex. In this regard, prepubescent weight lifters should be encouraged to emphasize lower weight and higher repetitions, with impeccable technique, instead of trying to see how much weight they can lift. During periods of rapid growth, strength training should be decreased and flexibility exercises should be emphasized.[94] Nevertheless, strength training can be beneficial, and increased strength can be achieved in prepubescent children without an appreciable increase in muscle mass,[142] likely through improved synchronization in the recruitment of motor units.[118]

The preparticipation examination for school sports is an excellent opportunity for physicians to help prevent injury in young athletes. Musculoskeletal and cardiovascular concerns are two areas in which intervention and identification of problems can contribute to reducing morbidity and, possibly, mortality. Several excellent publications can be consulted concerning the preparticipation evaluation.[11, 50, 72, 90]

UNIQUE CONSIDERATIONS FOR PHYSICALLY CHALLENGED ATHLETES

It is estimated that 2 to 3 million athletes with physical and mental disabilities participate in organized athletic activities in the United States.[23, 42] The importance of understanding the requirements and nature of the sports of physically challenged athletes cannot be overemphasized. Most sports for physically challenged persons have assimilated the rules and regulations of sports for able-bodied persons, with minimal exceptions; however, some sports are unique to the physically challenged and warrant further investigation by the medical professional to optimize training and injury rehabilitation programs. The groups that make up the Committee on Sports for the Disabled, a standing committee of the United States Olympic Committee, are excellent resources with respect to sports for physically challenged persons and participation requirements. These groups include the American Athletic Association for the Deaf, the Dwarf Athletic Association of America, Disabled Sports USA (DS/USA), National Wheelchair Athletic Association, Special Olympics, United States Association of Blind Athletes, and the United States Cerebral Palsy Athletic Association.

Individuals who treat and advise physically challenged athletes should understand how the adaptive equipment required for the sport may affect injury risk. New aerodynamic body positions in wheelchair racing can increase the risk of pressure sores, and if the splash guards on high-performance wheelchairs are not adjusted properly, they can cause skin breakdown (Fig. 43–19). With respect to downhill snow skiing, monoskiers can risk skin breakdown if seating positions create too much ischial shear. Amputees may require special residual limb protectors or warmers (or both) if tissue blood flow is compromised. They may also need padding when downhill skiing. Athletes with cerebral palsy, multiple sclerosis, or spasticity require special containment provided by straps to enable more isolated limb movement, especially during resistance training. Wheelchair road racers benefit greatly from the use of gloves and from wearing friction-reducing material on the biceps and triceps regions of the arms and on the chest wall region of the axilla. The latter is necessary because of incidental contact with or intentional pressure on the wheels (e.g., for braking) with the axillary region.[87]

Equipment may also have an impact on the physiological benefits gained from exercise. Kinzer and Convertino[74] showed that a greater accumulation of fluid in the legs of paraplegic persons decreased cardiac preload and diminished the central cardiovascular training response. Wearing appropriately fitting compressive garments on the lower extremities during exercise can enhance the cardiovascular training effect.

Another external factor is the environment, which can pose risk of thermal injury to physically challenged athletes. Guidelines have been established for safe participation in sports in hot and humid environments.[14] In addition, wind-chill charts provide information about limits on outdoor exposure time during cold weather. The main group of athletes who need to use extra caution during temperature extremes are those with spinal cord injuries, especially with lesions above the T8 level. In these persons autoregulation is impaired, and the body temperature tends to equalize with that of the ambient environmental temperature. Athletes with ischemia or vascular dysfunction and those who are insensate are also at risk in a cold environment, and frequent skin checks are necessary to ensure that no skin damage occurs.

One of the key concepts in rehabilitation of physically challenged athletes, as in rehabilitation of able-bodied ath-

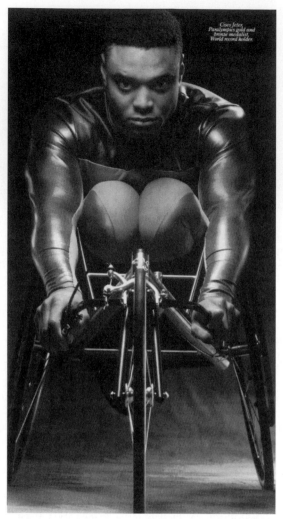

Cisco Jeter, Paralympics gold and bronze medalist, World record holder.

FIGURE 43-19 Aerodynamic wheelchair positioning. (From Sports 'N Spokes. 18:3, March/Apr 1993. By permission of Hall's Wheels.)

letes, is appropriate training and injury prevention measures. Because shoulder injuries and carpal tunnel syndrome[9] seem to be prevalent among persons using wheelchairs, prophylactic programs of rotator cuff strengthening, scapular stabilization, and shoulder muscle endurance should be implemented early in conjunction with wrist stretches, wrist strengthening, and appropriate use of ice for inflammation control. It is essential to understand the biomechanics of a sport and the kinetic chain as they apply to a person's physical disability. Whiting and associates[143] showed that members of the U.S. men's water polo team throw the ball in the water with half of the velocity with which they can throw on land. This principle should be remembered for an athlete who is unable to make full use of ground reaction force because of a disability. Also, trunk restriction causes a significant reduction in the velocity of throwing a ball.[8] In compensating for these deficiencies, other components of the kinetic chain should not be overused or misused biomechanically. Joints and muscle groups that are proximal and distal to the injury must be examined and treated to ensure that they are as biomechanically correct as possible with respect to flexibility, strength,

balance, and kinesiological movement patterns. The kinetic chain for each athlete varies depending on functional ability, and it must be uniquely applied to the specific sport.

An aerobic exercise program for physically challenged athletes is essential. Numerous studies have shown that physical training can markedly enhance cardiovascular and aerobic fitness in those with spinal cord injury,[43, 57, 66] postpolio sequelae,[69, 78] traumatic brain injury,[68] or amputation.[3] The effects of exercises that use the arms only can translate into improved endurance for wheelchair propulsion, making it easier to complete activities of daily living, including school and work.[47] It appears that many of the same metabolic benefits can be derived from arm exercises as from lower extremity exercises. Taylor and colleagues[133] showed that slow twitch fiber area increased with arm ergometer training, and Skrinar and associates[126] showed that glycogen utilization has the same pattern in the upper arm muscles of wheelchair athletes as in the legs of able-bodied athletes.

SPORTS PSYCHOLOGY

Physicians, athletic trainers, physical therapists, and coaches are the most visible members of the sports medicine team. Recently, the sports counselor or sports psychologist has had a larger presence as a member of the treatment team. Sports medicine professionals should be aware that the response of an athlete to injury can differ from that of other patients, and early identification and treatment of concurrent psychological issues by appropriate professionals often facilitate rehabilitation and maintenance of health. Many studies suggest that severe depression, tension, and anger are common among seriously injured athletes.[28, 127] As early as 1969, Little[84] found that about 75% of athletes who had symptoms of depression and anxiety had a preceding injury or illness. These symptoms were present in only 11% of nonathletes with injuries. This raises interesting questions about appropriate intervention to minimize psychological trauma and participation time lost due to injury. Many techniques have been advocated to provide psychological assistance and to facilitate rehabilitation, including visualization, relaxation, goal-setting, prioritization, and elimination of negative thoughts. However, there are not sufficient data to judge the effectiveness of any of these methods. Flint[53] suggested that modeling, or observational learning, could be a prime method for dealing with emotions that are detrimental to the recovery process. Athletes learn motor skills and social behaviors from coaches and teachers who use modeling as an instructional tool. Pride, determination, and hard work are intangible qualities possessed by many athletes, and during rehabilitation, these attributes can be used to help overcome injury.

Reinstilling self-confidence is another key aspect of the rehabilitation process. It has been shown by Smith and colleagues[128] that perceived severity of injury is often a major determinant of postinjury depression. Even though the physiological damage might not be severe, athletes who perceive an injury as serious are likely to experience more intense depression and to have a slower recovery than those who do not perceive an injury as serious. Three aspects of self-confidence that influence the recovery process have been suggested by Fisher:[52] competence, control, and commitment. Treatment programs that encompass these three elements are likely to increase compliance and outcome success. Athletes should believe that they will be able to resume competitive sports, take command of their rehabilitation, and commit time and effort to the sometimes long and arduous rehabilitation process.

Strategies for performance enhancement and stress management are ways in which sports psychology professionals can help to improve focus in competition and to maximize physical execution. Visualization and imagery also can be used in training to enhance neuromuscular engrams and to assist in rehabilitation. For example, an ice skater with a tibial stress fracture can substitute for the lack of ice time and training and augment alternative conditioning by observing videotapes that depict specific jumps and routines. This approach can expedite a return to competition because routines can be memorized and incorporated into a neuromuscular engram that might ultimately facilitate training on the ice. Control of pain can also be enhanced by imagery and relaxation techniques.

For optimal rehabilitation, athletes need the services of a multidisciplinary team that functions in an interdisciplinary manner. Each contributor plays an important role in helping an injured athlete to resume sports activities and to return to other activities of daily living.

References

1. Abbott LC, Saunders JB, Bost FC, et al: Injuries to the ligaments of the knee joint. J Bone Joint Surg 1944; 26:503.

2. Acevedo EO, Goldfarb AH: Increased training intensity effects on plasma lactate, ventilatory threshold, and endurance. Med Sci Sports Exerc 1989; 21:563.

3. Adler JC, Mazzarella N, Puzsier L, et al: Treadmill training program for a bilateral below-knee amputee patient with cardiopulmonary disease. Arch Phys Med Rehabil 1987; 68:858.

4. Akeson WH: An experimental study of joint stiffness. J Bone Joint Surg Am 1961; 43:1022.

5. Akeson WH, Amiel D, LaViolette D: The connective-tissue response to immobility: A study of the chondroitin-4 and 6-sulfate and dermatan sulfate changes in periarticular connective tissue of control and immobilized knees of dogs. Clin Orthop 1967; 51:183.

6. Akeson WH, Woo SL, Amiel D, et al: The connective tissue response to immobility: Biochemical changes in periarticular connective tissue of the immobilized rabbit knee. Clin Orthop 1973; 93:356.

7. Akeson WH, Woo SL-Y, Amiel D, et al: The biology of ligaments. In Hunter LY, Funk FJ Jr (eds): Rehabilitation of the Injured Knee. St Louis, Mosby–Year Book, 1984, pp 93–148.

8. Alexander RM: Optimum timing of muscle activation for simple models of throwing. J Theor Biol 1991; 150:349.

9. Aljure J, Eltorai I, Bradley WE, et al: Carpal tunnel syndrome in paraplegic patients. Paraplegia 1985; 23:182.

10. Almekinders LC, Garrett WE Jr, Seaber AV: Pathophysiologic response to muscle tears and stretching injuries. Trans Orthop Res Soc 1984; 9:307.

11. American Academy of Pediatrics Committee on Sports Medicine: Recommendations for participation in competitive sports. Pediatrics 1988; 81:737.

12. American College of Sports Medicine: The recommended quantity and quality of exercise for developing and maintaining cardiorespiratory and muscular fitness in healthy adults. The Official Position Papers of the American College of Sports Medicine. Indianapolis, 1990.

13. American College of Sports Medicine: Guidelines for Exercise Testing and Prescription, ed 4. Philadelphia, Lea & Febiger, 1991.

14. American College of Sports Medicine position stand on the prevention of thermal injuries during distance running. Med Sci Sports Exerc 1987; 19:529.

15. Andersen P, Henriksson J: Training induced changes in the sub-groups of human type II skeletal muscle fibres. Acta Physiol Scand 1977; 99:123.

16. Andersson S, Stener B: Experimental evaluation of the hypothesis of ligamento-muscular protective reflexes: II. A study in cat using the medial collateral ligament of the knee joint. Acta Physiol Scand 1959; 48(suppl 166):27.

17. Andrew BL: The sensory innervation of the medial ligament of the knee joint. J Physiol 1954; 123:241.

18. Asmussen E: Positive and negative muscular work. Acta Physiol Scand 1953; 28:364.

19. Åstrand P-O, Rodahl K: Textbook of Work Physiology. New York, McGraw-Hill, 1986.

20. Atha J: Strengthening muscle. Exerc Sport Sci Rev 1981; 9:1.

21. Baker BE: Prevention of ligament injuries to the knee. Exerc Sport Sci Rev 1990; 18:291.

22. Barfred T: Experimental rupture of the Achilles tendon: Comparison of various types of experimental rupture in rats. Acta Orthop Scand 1971; 42:528.

22a. Beynnon BD, Fleming BC, Johnson RJ, et al: Anterior cruciate ligament strain behavior during rehabilitation exercises in vivo. Am J Sports Med 1995; 23:24.

23. Birrer RB: The Special Olympics: An injury overview. Phys Sports Med April 1984; 12:95.

24. Brand RA: Knee ligaments: A new view. J Biomech Eng 1986; 108:106.

25. Brooks GA, Fahey TD: Exercise Physiology: Human Bioenergetics and Its Application. New York, Wiley, 1984.

26. Brooks GA, Fahey TD: Fundamentals of Human Performance. New York, Macmillan, 1987.

27. Cerretelli P, Pendergast D, Paganelli WC, et al: Effects of specific muscle training on $\dot{V}O_2$ on-reponse and early blood lactate. J Appl Physiol 1979; 47:761.

28. Chan CS, Grossman HY: Psychological effects of running loss on consistent runners. Percept Mot Skills 1988; 66:875.

29. Chandler TJ, Kibler WB: A biomechanical approach to the prevention, treatment and rehabilitation of plantar fasciitis. Sports Med 1993; 15:344

30. Chandler TJ, Kibler WB, Kiser AM, et al: Shoulder strength, power, and endurance in college tennis players. Am J Sports Med 1992; 20:455.

31. Chandler TJ, Kibler WB, Uhl TL, et al: Flexibility comparisons of junior elite tennis players to other athletes. Am J Sports Med 1990; 18:134.

32. Chu DA: Jumping Into Plyometrics. Champaign, Ill, Leisure Press, 1992, pp 1–11.

33. Clancy WJ Jr: Tendinitis and plantar fasciitis in runners. In D'Ambrosia RD, Drez D Jr (eds): Prevention and Treatment of Running Injuries. Thorofare, NJ, Slack, 1989, pp 121–131.

34. Clarke DH: Adaptations in strength and muscular endurance resulting from exercise. Exerc Sport Sci Rev 1973; 1:73.

35. Clarkson PM, Ebbeling C: Investigation of serum creatine kinase variability after muscle-damaging exercise. Clin Sci 1988; 75:257.

36. Cohen LA, Cohen ML: Arthrokinetic reflex of the knee. Am J Physiol 1956; 184:433.

37. Convertino V, Hung J, Goldwater D, et al: Cardiovascular responses to exercise in middle-aged men after 10 days of bedrest. Circulation 1982; 65:134.

38. Costill DL, Daniels J, Evans W, et al: Skeletal muscle enzymes and fiber composition in male and female track athletes. J Appl Physiol 1976; 40:149.

39. Costill DL, Fink WJ, Pollock ML: Muscle fiber composition and enzyme activities of elite distance runners. Med Sci Sports 1976; 8:96.

40. Coyle EF, Coggan AR, Hemmert MK, et al: Muscle glycogen utilization during prolonged strenuous exercise when fed carbohydrate. J Appl Physiol 1986; 61:165.

41. Coyle EF, Feiring DC, Rotkis TC, et al: Specificity of power improvements through slow and fast isokinetic training. J Appl Physiol 1981; 51:1437.

42. Curtis KA, Dillon DA: Survey of wheelchair athletic injuries: Common patterns and prevention. Paraplegia 1985; 23:170.

43. Davis G, Plyley MJ, Shephard RJ: Gains of cardiorespiratory fitness with arm-crank training in spinally disabled men. Can J Sport Sci 1991; 16:64.

44. Day RW, Wildermuth BP: Proprioceptive training in the rehabilita-

tion of lower extremity injuries. Adv Sports Med Fitness 1988; 1:241.

45. de Lateur BJ, Lehmann JF: Strengthening exercise. *In* Leek JC, Gershwin ME, Fowler WM Jr (eds): Principles of Physical Medicine and Rehabilitation in the Musculoskeletal Diseases. Orlando, Fla, Grune & Stratton, 1986, pp 25–60.

46. DeLisa JA: Academic physiatry: trends, opportunities and challenges. Am J Phys Med Rehabil 1993; 72:113.

47. DiCarlo SE: Effect of arm ergometry training on wheelchair propulsion endurance of individuals with quadriplegia. Phys Ther 1988; 68:40.

48. Dillingham MF, King WD, Gamburd RS: Rehabilitation of the knee following anterior cruciate ligament and medial collateral ligament injuries. Phys Med Rehabil Clin North Am 1994; 5:175.

49. Ekholm J, Eklund G, Skoglund S: On the reflex effects from the knee joint of the cat. Acta Physiol Scand 1960; 50:167.

50. Epstein SE, Maron BJ: Sudden death and the competitive athlete: Perspectives on preparticipation screening studies. J Am Coll Cardiol 1986; 7:220.

51. Evans WJ, Cannon JG: The metabolic effects of exercise-induced muscle damage. Exerc Sport Sci Rev 1991; 19:99.

52. Fisher AC: Adherence to sports injury rehabilitation programmes. Sports Med 1990; 9:151.

52a. Fleming BC, Beynnon BD, Peura GD, et al: Anterior cruciate ligament strain during an open and a closed kinetic chain exercise: An in vivo study. Orthopoedic Research Society Transactions, 41st Annual Meeting, February 13–16, 1995, Orlando, Fla, p 631.

53. Flint FA: Seeing helps believing: Modeling in injury rehabilitation. *In* Pargman D (ed): Psychological Basis of Sport Injuries. Morgantown, W Va, Fitness Information Technology, 1992, pp 183–198.

54. Fringer MN, Stull GA: Changes in cardiorespiratory parameters during periods of training and detraining in young adult females. Med Sci Sports 1974; 6:20.

55. Garrett WE Jr: Muscle strain injuries: Clinical and basic aspects. Med Sci Sports Exerc 1990; 22:436.

56. Gelberman RH, Woo SL, Lothringer K, et al: Effects of early intermittent passive mobilization on healing canine flexor tendons. J Hand Surg Am 1982; 7:170.

57. Glaser RM: Arm exercise training for wheelchair users. Med Sci Sports Exerc 1989; 21 (suppl 5):S149.

58. Graves JE, Pollock ML, Jones AE, et al: Specificity of limited range of motion variable resistance training. Med Sci Sports Exerc 1989; 21:84.

59. Gray GW: Chain Reaction. Adrian, Mich, Wynn Marketing, 1991, pp 80–98.

60. Grood ES, Suntay WJ, Noyes FR, et al: Biomechanics of the knee-extension exercise: Effect of cutting the anterior cruciate ligament. J Bone Joint Surg Am 1984; 66:725.

61. Guyton AC: Textbook of Medical Physiology, ed 8. Philadelphia, WB Saunders, 1991.

62. Herring SA, Nilson KL: Introduction to overuse injuries. Clin Sports Med 1987; 6:225.

63. Hettinger T: Physiology of Strength. Springfield, Ill, Charles C Thomas, 1961.

64. Hickson RC, Heusner WW, Van Huss WD: Skeletal muscle enzyme alterations after sprint and endurance training. J Appl Physiol 1976; 40:868.

65. Hickson RC, Rennie MJ, Conlee RK, et al: Effects of increased plasma fatty acids on glycogen utilization and endurance. J Appl Physiol 1977; 43:829.

66. Hooker SP, Wells CL: Aerobic power of competitive paraplegic road racers. Paraplegia 1992; 30:428.

67. Janda DH, Wojtys EM, Hankin FM, et al: A three-phase analysis of the prevention of recreational softball injuries. Am J Sports Med 1990; 18:632.

68. Jankowski LW, Sullivan SJ: Aerobic and neuromuscular training: Effect on the capacity, efficiency, and fatigability of patients with traumatic brain injuries. Arch Phys Med Rehabil 1990; 71:500.

69. Jones DR, Speier J, Canine K, et al: Cardiorespiratory responses to aerobic training by patients with postpoliomyelitis sequelae. JAMA 1989; 261:3255.

70. Kendrick ZV, Pollock ML, Hickman TN, et al: Effects of training and detraining on cardiovascular efficiency. Am Corrective Therap J 1971; 25:79.

71. Kibler WB: Concepts and exercise rehabilitation. *In* Leadbetter WB, Buckwalter JA, Gordon SL (eds): Sports-Induced Inflammation: Clinical and Basic Science Concepts. Park Ridge, Ill, American Academy of Orthopaedic Surgeons, 1990, pp 759–771.

72. Kibler WB: The Sport Preparticipation Fitness Examination. Champaign, Ill, Human Kinetics Books, 1990.

73. Kibler WB: The role of the scapula in the throwing motion. Contemp Orthop 1991; 22:525.

74. Kinzer SM, Convertino VA: Role of leg vasculature in the cardiovascular response to arm work in wheelchair-dependent populations. Clin Physiol 1989; 9:525.

75. Kok G, Bouter LM: On the importance of planned health education: Prevention of ski injury as an example. Am J Sports Med 1990; 18:600.

76. Komi PV, Buskirk ER: Effect of eccentric and concentric muscle conditioning on tension and electrical activity of human muscle. Ergonomics 1972; 15:417.

77. Kraus JF, Conroy C: Mortality and morbidity from injuries in sports and recreation. Annu Rev Pub Health 1984; 5:163.

78. Kriz JL, Jones DR, Speier JL, et al: Cardiorespiratory responses to upper extremity aerobic training by postpolio subjects. Arch Phys Med Rehabil 1992; 73:49.

79. Leach RE, Paul GR: Running injuries of the knee. *In* D'Ambrosia RD, Drez D Jr (eds): Prevention and Treatment of Running Injuries. Thorofare, NJ, Slack, 1989, pp 98–119.

80. Leadbetter WB: Physiology of tissue repair. *In* Athletic Training and Sports Medicine. Park Ridge, Ill, American Academy of Orthopedic Surgeons, 1991, pp 43–55.

81. Lehmann JF, DeLateur BJ, Stonebridge JB, et al: Therapeutic temperature distribution produced by ultrasound as modified by dosage and volume of tissue exposed. Arch Phys Med Rehabil 1967; 48:662.

82. Lehmann JF, DeLateur BJ, Warren CG, et al: Heating of joint structures by ultrasound. Arch Phys Med Rehabil 1968; 49:28.

83. Lehmann JF, Masock AJ, Warren CG, et al: Effect of therapeutic temperatures on tendon extensibility. Arch Phys Med Rehabil 1970; 51:481.

84. Little JC: The athlete's neurosis—a deprivation crisis. Acta Psychiatr Scand 1969; 45:187.

85. Lutz GE, Palmitier RA, An KN, et al: Comparison of tibiofemoral joint forces during open-kinetic-chain and closed-kinetic-chain exercises. J Bone Joint Surg 1993; 75:732.

86. Lutz GE, Stuart MJ, Sim FH, et al: Rehabilitative techniques for athletes after reconstruction of the anterior cruciate ligament. Mayo Clin Proc 1990; 65:1322.

87. Mangus BC: Sports injuries, the disabled athlete, and the athletic trainer. Athletic Training 1987; 22:305.

88. Martin BJ, Robinson S, Wiegman DL, et al: Effect of warm-up on metabolic responses to strenuous exercise. Med Sci Sports 1975; 7:146.

89. McArdle WD, Katch FI, Katch VL: Exercise Physiology: Energy, Nutrition, and Human Performance, ed 3. Philadelphia, Lea & Febiger, 1991.

90. McKeag DB: Preseason physical examination for the prevention of sports injuries. Sports Med 1985; 2:413.

91. McMaster PE: Tendon and muscle ruptures: Clinical and experimental studies on the causes and location of subcutaneous ruptures. J Bone Joint Surg 1933; 15:705.

92. Merritt JL, Hunder GG: Passive range of motion, not isometric exercise, amplifies acute urate synovitis. Arch Phys Med Rehabil 1983; 64:130.

93. Micheli LJ: Thromboembolic complications of cast immobilization for injuries of the lower extremities. Clin Orthop 1975; 108:191.

94. Micheli LJ: Overuse injuries in children's sports: The growth factor. Orthop Clin North Am 1983; 14:337.

95. Milgrom C, Finestone A, Shlamkovitch N, et al: Prevention of overuse injuries of the foot by improved shoe shock attenuation: A randomized prospective study. Clin Orthop 1992; 281:189.

96. Milner-Brown HS, Stein RB, Yemm R: The orderly recruitment of human motor units during voluntary isometric contractions. J Physiol 1973; 230:359.

97. Moritani T, deVries HA: Neural factors versus hypertrophy in the time course of muscle strength gain. Am J Phys Med 1979; 58:115.

98. Mubarak SJ, Gould RN, Lee YF, et al: The medial tibial stress syndrome: A cause of shin splints. Am J Sports Med 1982; 10:201.

99. Noakes TD: Implications of exercise testing for prediction of athletic

performance: A contemporary perspective. Med Sci Sports Exerc 1988; 20:319.

100. Noonan TJ, Best TM, Seaber AV, et al: Thermal effects on skeletal muscle tensile behavior. Am J Sports Med 1993; 21:517.

101. Noyes FR: Functional properties of knee ligaments and alterations induced by immobilization: A correlative biomechanical and histological study in primates. Clin Orthop 1977; 123:210.

102. Nygaard E, Andersen P, Nilsson P, et al: Glycogen depletion pattern and lactate accumulation in leg muscles during recreational downhill skiing. Eur J Appl Physiol 1978; 38:261.

103. Palmer I: Plastic surgery of ligaments of the knee. Acta Chir Scand 1944; 91:37.

104. Palmitier RA, An KN, Scott SG, et al: Kinetic chain exercise in knee rehabilitation. Sports Med 1991; 11:402.

105. Pappas AM, Zawacki RM, Sullivan TJ: Biomechanics of baseball pitching: A preliminary report. Am J Sports Med 1985; 13:216.

106. Pate RR, Branch JD: Training for endurance sport. Med Sci Sports Exerc 1992; 24 (suppl 9):S340.

107. Paulos L, Noyes FR, Grood E, et al: Knee rehabilitation after anterior cruciate ligament reconstruction and repair. Am J Sports Med 1981; 9:140.

108. Pendergast DR: Cardiovascular, respiratory, and metabolic responses to upper body exercise. Med Sci Sports Exerc 1989; 21 (suppl 5):S121.

109. Pendergast D, Cerretelli P, Rennie DW: Aerobic and glycolytic metabolism in arm exercise. J Appl Physiol 1979; 47:754.

110. Perrine JJ: Isokinetic exercise and the mechanical energy potentials of muscle. J Health Phys Educ Rec 1968; 39:40.

111. Pollock ML, Wilmore JH: Exercise in Health and Disease, ed 2. Phildadelphia, WB Saunders, 1990.

112. Pope DF, Cole KJ, Brand RA: Physiologic loading of the anterior cruciate ligament does not activate quadriceps or hamstrings in the anesthetized cat. Am J Sports Med 1990; 18:595.

113. Puddu G, Ippolito E, Postacchini F: A classification of Achilles tendon disease. Am J Sports Med 1976; 4:145.

114. Requa RK, DeAvilla LN, Garrick JG: Injuries in recreational adult fitness activities. Am J Sports Med 1993; 21:461.

115. Rians CB, Weltman A, Cahill BR, et al: Strength training for prepubescent males: Is it safe? Am J Sports Med 1987; 15:483.

116. Roskamm H: Optimum patterns of exercise for healthy adults. Can Med Assoc J 1967; 96.895.

117. Saal JA: General principles and guidelines for rehabilitation of the injured athlete. Phys Med Rehabil Clin North Am Nov 1987; 1:523.

118. Sale DG: Neural adaptation to resistance training. Med Sci Sports Exerc 1988; 20 (suppl 5):S135.

119. Sale D, MacDougall D: Specificity in strength training: A review for the coach and athlete. In Science Periodical on Research and Technology in Sport. Ottawa, Canada, The Coaching Association of Canada, March 1981.

120. Saltin B, Blomqvist G, Mitchell JH, et al: Response to exercise after bed rest and after training. Circulation 1968; 38 (suppl 5):VIII.

121. Schumacher HR Jr: Primer on the Rheumatic Diseases, ed 9. Atlanta, Arthritis Foundation, 1988, pp 24–30.

122. Schwellnus MP, Jordaan G, Noakes TD: Prevention of common overuse injuries by the use of shock absorbing insoles: A prospective study. Am J Sports Med 1990; 18:636.

123. Sharkey BJ: Training for sport. In Cantu RC, Micheli LJ (eds):

124. Shelbourne KD, Nitz P: Accelerated rehabilitation after anterior cruciate ligament reconstruction. Am J Sports Med 1990; 18:292.

125. Shephard RJ: Physiology and Biochemistry of Exercise. New York, Praeger, 1982.

126. Skrinar GS, Evans WJ, Ornstein LJ, et al: Glycogen utilization in wheelchair-dependent athletes. Int J Sports Med 1982; 3:215.

127. Smith AM, Scott SG, O'Fallon WM, et al: Emotional responses of athletes to injury. Mayo Clin Proc 1990; 65:38.

128. Smith AM, Stuart MJ, Wiese-Bjornstal DM, et al: Competitive athletes: Preinjury and postinjury mood state and self-esteem. Mayo Clin Proc 1993; 68:939.

129. Solomonow M, Baratta R, Zhou BH, et al: The synergistic action of the anterior cruciate ligament and thigh muscles in maintaining joint stability. Am J Sports Med 1987; 15:207.

130. Steindler A: Kinesiology of the Human Body Under Normal and Pathological Conditions. Springfield, Ill, Charles C Thomas, 1973, p 63.

131. Stone MH: Muscle conditioning and muscle injuries. Med Sci Sports Exerc 1990; 22:457.

132. Stone MH, Wilson GD: Resistive training and selected effects. Med Clin North Am 1985; 69:109.

133. Taylor AW, McDonell E, Brassard L: The effects of an arm ergometer training programme on wheelchair subjects. Paraplegia 1986; 24:105.

134. Taylor HL, Henschel A, Brožek J, et al: Effects of bed rest on cardiovascular function and work performance. J Appl Physiol 1949; 2:223.

135. Tesch PA: Skeletal muscle adaptations consequent to long-term heavy resistance exercise. Med Sci Sports Exerc 1988; 20 (suppl 5):S132.

136. Thorstensson A, Sjodin B, Karlsson J: Enzyme activities and muscle strength after "sprint training" in man. Acta Physiol Scand 1975; 94:313.

137. Tipton CM, James SL, Mergner W, et al: Influence of exercise on strength of medial collateral knee ligaments of dogs. Am J Physiol 1970; 218:894.

138. Tipton CM, Schild RJ, Tomanek RJ: Influence of physical activity on the strength of knee ligaments in rats. Am J Physiol 1967; 212:783.

139. Torg JS: Problems and prevention. In Torg JS (ed): Athletic Injuries to the Head, Neck, and Face. St Louis, Mosby–Year Book, 1982, pp 3 13

140. Verkoshanski Y: Perspectives in the improvement of speed-strength preparation of jumpers. Track and Field 1966; 9:11.

141. Watkins RG, Dillin WM: Cervical spine and spinal cord injuries. In Fu FH, Stone DA (eds): Sports Injuries: Mechanisms, Prevention, Treatment. Baltimore, Williams & Wilkins, 1994, pp 855–876.

142. Webb DR: Strength training in children and adolescents. Pediatr Clin North Am 1990; 37:1187.

143. Whiting WC, Puffer JC, Finerman GA, et al: Three-dimensional cinematographic analysis of water polo throwing in elite performers. Am J Sports Med 1985; 13:95.

144. Wilmore JH, Costill DL: Training for Sport and Activity: The Physiological Basis of the Conditioning Process, ed 3. Dubuque, William C Brown, 1988.

145. Wilt F: Plyometrics: What it is—how it works. Athlet J 1975; 55:89.

146. Wroble RR, Brand RA: Function of knee ligaments: A historical review of two perspectives. Iowa Orthop 1988; J8:67.

ACSM's Guidelines for the Team Physician. Philadelphia, Lea & Febiger, 1991, pp 34–47.

44

Occupational Rehabilitation

JOHN A. SCHUCHMANN, M.D.

Prior to the 1700s, most workers toiled at home in small shops or at agricultural enterprises. Work was performed with crude hand tools rather than machines. Rural life was the norm, with fewer than 10% of Europeans living in cities. In the 1700s and 1800s, the development of automated machinery and factories dramatically changed the way in which people lived and worked. The industrial revolution began in Great Britain in the 1700s and spread to North America in the early 1800s. Industrialization dramatically increased production of many types of goods, but also brought about many changes for workers.

Industrialization required the relocation of many workers into towns and cities. Previously skilled workers and craftsmen were often relegated to tedious, degrading jobs. Workers were required to produce at the "machine rate" rather than at their own pace. They were often required to work long hours for meager wages. The profit motive encouraged industrialists to search for even more rapid methods of production. Industrialists were often hard-working and demanded the same from their employees.

By 1900, nearly 10 million Americans lived in poverty, and a 10-hour, 6-day work week was common. Little attention was paid to worker safety, and industrial accidents and deaths were common.

Unionization of labor, which began between 1860 and 1900, developed as a means of trying to balance the demands on the worker and to ensure adequate compensation, reasonable working hours, and safe, adequate working conditions.[33, 64]

The labor movement was often stormy and violent, but ultimately conditions for the worker began to improve. Still, the injured worker in the early 1900s had little recourse or compensation. Injured workers had to use the courts to recover any damages from employers. They had to prove both that the employer was negligent and that the employer's negligence resulted in their injury. With employer defenses such as "assumption of risk" and "contributory negligence," workers usually fared poorly; 80% of cases were lost or the injured person uncompensated.[2]

Around 1910, there came a recognition that industrialization benefited the whole country. Injury and even death, however, were still inevitable components of even the most progressive and sophisticated industrial activities. Workers' Compensation programs were begun as a means of providing wage replacement and medical care for injured workers. New York was the first state to adopt compulsory Workers' Compensation in 1910. That law was later found unconstitutional. In 1911, Wisconsin passed the first workers' compensation act that remained effective. States gradually enacted Workers' Compensation plans; in 1948, Mississippi was the final state to pass such a plan.[2]

Despite major advances in industrial technology and safety, work today still poses considerable risk of injury.[19, 28, 39, 51, 58] In 1989, there were 6,576,000 occupational injuries and illnesses in the United States. More than 3,073,000 cases resulted in approximately 57,000,000 lost work days. The rate of occupational injuries and illnesses was 8.6 per 100 full-time workers.

Nine industries reported at least 100,000 injury cases each. These included the following industries: (1) motor vehicle manufacturing, (2) eating and drinking establishments, (3) wholesale grocery stores, (4) retail grocery stores, (5) hospitals, (6) trucking and over-the-road carriers, (7) nursing and personal care facilities, (8) department stores, and (9) hotels and motels. These industries accounted for more than one-fourth of all injury cases reported nationwide. In 1988, an estimated $30.8 billion was paid in Workers' Compensation benefits, with this figure increasing at a rate of more than 12% per year.[2]

A sampling of studies indicates that work injuries are certainly not unique to the United States but are universal throughout the world.[15, 20, 24, 25, 29, 34, 36, 44]

Industrial injuries are costly because of lost productivity and lost sales by the industry and lost wages by the worker. Health care costs and costs for retraining and replacing workers add to the loss. These costs are ultimately reflected in higher-priced products for the consumer. With current profit margins already slim and health care costs rising rapidly, more and more industries and businesses are becoming proactive rather than reactive in trying to prevent and minimize the impact of injuries on their overall operations and profitability.

A shortage exists throughout the United States of physicians trained to comprehensively evaluate and treat the complex neuromusculoskeletal problems often seen in injured workers. Many physicians in the field of physical medicine and rehabilitation are becoming involved in the early evaluation, treatment, and rehabilitation of workers to help them recover and return to the work site. The physiatrist possesses skills to help enhance the injured worker's physical function. Often, a team effort is required to ensure a successful outcome of return to work. The physiatrist's team orientation and training in neuromusculoskeletal disorders provides an excellent background to spearhead industrial rehabilitation efforts. The physiatrist is also able to evaluate and quantify any residual impairment once the worker has reached maximum medical improvement.

OVERVIEW OF COMMON MEDICAL PROBLEMS SEEN IN A REHABILITATIVE INDUSTRIAL PRACTICE

Low Back Pain

Low back pain is a major expense to industry owing to lost productivity, high medical costs, and compensation payments. Low back pain is so frequent in our society that 70% to 80% of persons will complain of low back pain at some time in their lives.[42] Low back pain is second only to upper respiratory illnesses as the most common cause of time missed from work. More than 7 million workers are injured on the job each year.[59] Chronic low back pain has a major economic and personal impact, as it is the leading cause of disability for individuals between the ages of 19 and 45 years.[30] On any given day, nearly 6.5 million persons in the United States are receiving treatment for low back pain. The National Safety Council estimated that 370,000 disabling work-related back injuries occurred in the United States in 1991, at a cost of approximately $50 billion. Liberty Mutual Insurance Co. Workers' Compensation claims indicated a mean cost of $6807, with a median cost of $391. The large spread in costs was due to the fact that 25% of cases consumed 95% of the costs.[61]

Lost work days attributable to low back pain have been reported to be 1400 lost days per 1000 workers.[41] Low back pain is most prevalent in heavy industry. About 50% to 80% of workers in heavy industry admit to having suffered from back pain in the past 12 years.[65] The low back injury rate has been found to be about 3 to 5 per 1000 employees per year in light industries, compared to 200 per 1000 employees per year in heavy industries.

Despite advances in automation, humans are still required by many industries to perform much manual material handling. Stresses on the spine vary depending on the lifting techniques utilized as well as on the load handled. Improper handling of work materials can precipitate back injuries. Overuse can also result in muscular fatigue and lead to a possible back injury. Repetitive vibratory stresses on the back, from such activities as driving vehicles to using vibrating tools such as jackhammers, can produce microtrauma.

Only 1% to 2% of patients with low back pain usually require surgical treatment.[37, 38] About 90% of patients with extruded lumbar discs have good to excellent outcomes with nonoperative management, with return-to-work rates of more than 90%.[52] Overall, about 90% of patients with low back pain improve with minimal or no medical intervention. A small percentage of cases, however, become chronic, leading to disability associated with increased medical expenses and compensation costs. Recurrence of low back pain is also quite common, with a recurrence rate of approximately 70%. (See Chapter 39 for additional low back pain information.)

Cumulative Trauma Disorders

Cumulative trauma disorders, also referred to as *repetitive motion disorders*, *repetition strain injuries*, or *occupational overuse injuries*, are gaining more attention throughout industry and in the healthcare sector.[18, 48] They do not represent a new entity or type of disorder, but they acknowledge that overuse may be a causative factor. Cumulative trauma disorders have been increasing at a rapid rate throughout the United States to the extent that they now account for greater than 50% of all Workers' Compensation claims[48] (Fig. 44–1). The increase in these problems is thought to be due to a number of potential causes (Table 44–1).

A variety of tissues can be affected by cumulative trauma disorders (Table 44–2). Many clinical problems fall under the category of cumulative trauma disorder, including muscle strains, tendinitis, bursitis, ligamentous injuries, compression neuropathies, fractures, cartilage damage, and disc disease. The musculotendinous unit is most often affected by cumulative trauma disorders. This is due to the relatively poor blood supply at the bone-tendon interface, which produces delayed, incomplete, or partial healing.

In cumulative trauma disorders, repetitive motion and stress lead to microtrauma of the tissue. An acute inflammatory response ensues that can become chronic. Chronic inflammation can lead to even further tissue damage. The common etiological feature of these disorders is that repetitive trauma occurs at a pace that outstrips the tissue's ability to heal itself. Usually these cumulative trauma disorders develop slowly and gradually over many weeks, months, or years.

A number of factors and job activities have been implicated as etiological and aggravating factors for development of cumulative trauma disorders.[48] Some of these are included in Table 44–3.

In the workplace, upper extremity cumulative trauma disorders far outstrip lower extremity disorders. Some of the more common cumulative trauma disorders seen in clinical practice are included in Table 44–4.

Workers complaining of chronic muscle soreness may be providing early warning signs of the development of cumulative trauma disorders. Often, workers are sore and stiff the first week or two after beginning a job as a result of new physical demands. In most cases, physical conditioning occurs and the soreness subsides. In other cases, prolonged persistence of symptoms may indicate that tissues are not able to adapt to the stress. Continuation of the activity could lead to tissue damage and the development of a cumulative trauma disorder.

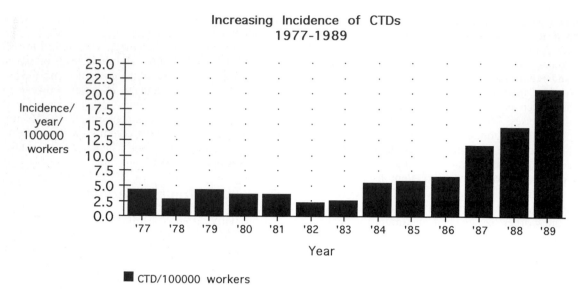

FIGURE 44–1 Increasing incidence of cumulative trauma disorders (CTDs) in industry. (Adapted from US Bureau of Labor Statistics: Reports on Survey of Occupational Injuries and Illnesses in 1977–1989. Washington, DC, Bureau of Labor, 1990.)

PREVENTION

Back Injury

On-the-job back injuries are extremely expensive to industry.[59] Krusen and Ford[32] noted that individuals receiving Workers' Compensation for back injuries demonstrated 33% less objective evidence of impairment, received nearly twice as many physical therapy treatments, and experienced long-term improvement in 44% fewer cases compared with similar patients not receiving compensation.

Sander and Meyers[53] also showed that railroad workers hurt on the job were off of work much longer than those who were hurt during off-duty hours. Workers with lumbosacral strains averaged 14.9 months off of work when hurt on the job, but only 3.6 months off of work when hurt on off-duty hours. Those who required surgery returned to work more quickly if the injury was sustained during off-duty time (4.4 vs. 9.3 months from the time of surgery).

As industries became aware of the cost of acute and chronic back injuries, attempts were made to help lessen the incidence of back injuries in industry.[10, 23, 60]

X-Ray Screening

Initial attempts were focused on lumbar spine x-rays. Individuals were required to obtain pre-employment lumbar spine x-rays, and if abnormalities were detected, employment was denied. This was a widespread practice in indus-

try until additional evidence brought this practice into question. It was subsequently discovered that, in general, no definite correlation existed between an abnormality seen on a lumbar x-ray and the chance of an individual's sustaining an on-the-job back injury.[21] The only radiographic abnormalities that seemed to have any predictive effect were spondylolysis and spondylolisthesis when found in individuals who performed very strenuous jobs. This abnormality is not seen sufficiently often in the general population (about 5% to 6%) to justify routine back x-rays.[35] Osteophytes were not found to correlate with back pain. With the advent of CT and MRI scanning it has been shown that disc abnormalities can be seen in 30% to 50% or more of asymptomatic individuals.[5, 46, 62] The use of pre-employment or preplacement spine radiographic studies is now in disrepute.

Education: The Back School Approach

Most individuals learn how to lift by trial and error. Proper lifting is something that must be taught. In the past, industries oriented workers to specific job requirements but did not always teach the worker how to properly lift and how to use the back. Now many industries are realizing that an investment in a "back school" can help to decrease on-the-job back injuries.

A back school program that is effective incorporates individual or small group instruction along with actual practice and skill development. Items actually lifted at work are used for training, and the worker is coached and reinforced in proper lifting techniques. It is also essential

TABLE 44–1 Causative Factors for Increase in Cumulative Trauma Disorders

More repetitive and faster-paced jobs
Job dissatisfaction
Increased awareness of signs and symptoms by employees, employers, and medical and legal professionals
Improved accuracy in identifying and reporting cumulative trauma disorders
Compensation coverage by Workers' Compensation carriers

TABLE 44–2 Tissues Often Involved With Cumulative Trauma Disorders

Muscles	Peripheral nerves
Tendons	Bones
Bursae	Cartilage
Ligaments	Intervertebral discs

TABLE 44–3 Sampling of Etiologic and/or Aggravating Factors and Jobs for Cumulative Trauma Disorders

ACTIVITIES
  Forceful grasping
  Highly repetitive work
  Activities causing rapid or extreme joint movements
  Overhead work
  Maintaining static work positions for prolonged times

OCCUPATIONS
  Assembly line worker
  Carpenter
  Butcher
  Typist/data entry worker
  Cashier
  Driver
  Factory worker performing repetitive activity
  Food preparer
  Postal worker
  Musician
  Electrician
  Professional athlete

TOOLS AND EQUIPMENT
  Repetitive assembly lines, on which worker performs at
    "machine pace"
  Undampened pneumatic tools
  Hammers
  Screwdrivers
  Pliers
  Scissors
  Knives
  Keyboards
  Musical instruments
  Use of gloves

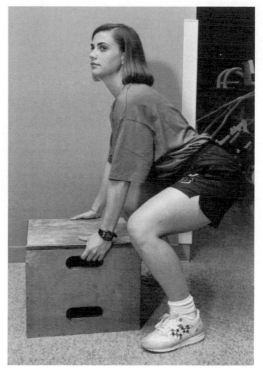

FIGURE 44–2 Proper lifting technique with the back in a neutral position.

to teach supervisory personnel proper lifting and handling techniques so that they can reinforce the use of these practices by their workers. If management doesn't fully support the training, it is not likely to decrease the number of injuries.

Generally, the preferable lifting technique requires the worker to get directly in front of and as close to the load as feasible. The worker is taught to squat while keeping the shoulders back and the low back in a neutral position with the lumbar lordosis maintained. Loads should be held close to the body to decrease stress on the low back. Footing should be secure, and the lift should be performed in a slow and controlled fashion.[17]

Jobs that require repetitive lifting by bending forward at the waist place much more stress on the back than do similar manual materials-handling jobs that allow proper squatting and lifting postures. Proper and improper lifting techniques are illustrated in Figures 44–2 and 44–3.

Workers often revert to poor lifting techniques because

their quadriceps are proportionally weak and they fatigue with repetitive squatting. The back school education can also emphasize the value of quadriceps exercises, such as the wall slide exercise (Fig. 44–4).

TABLE 44–4 Common Cumulative Trauma Disorders Related to Work Activities

Tendinitis and tenosynovitis at wrist and in forearm
Epicondylitis
Rotator cuff tendinitis and shoulder bursitis
Myofascial syndromes
Hand-arm vibration syndrome
Median nerve—carpal tunnel syndrome, nerve trauma in palm
Ulnar nerve compression—elbow, hand or wrist
Thoracic outlet syndrome

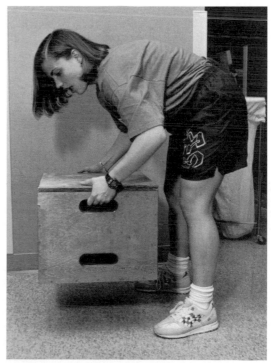

FIGURE 44–3 Faulty lifting technique with the back in a forward flexed posture.

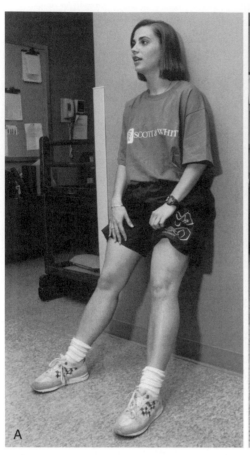
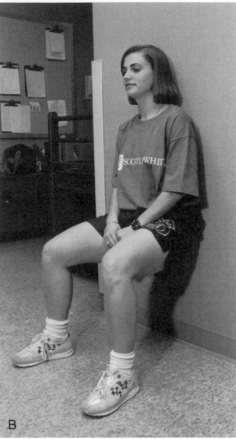

FIGURES 44–4 *A* and *B*, The wall slide exercise is excellent for strengthening the quadriceps and hip extensors. These important muscles facilitate lifting with proper technique when they have adequate strength and endurance. The worker is instructed to gradually increase the time interval maintained in the squatted down position.

Healthy lifestyle choices such as proper diet and avoidance of drugs, alcohol, and tobacco, and the value of regular exercise can be reinforced at the back school educational programs.

Cost savings and fewer injuries after educational programs can occur. Back school education was provided to a plastics-related manufacturer with 800 employees and to a woodworking firm with 400 employees. The workers were followed up for 2 years. Direct compensation and medical cost savings were 74% and 80%, respectively, whereas the incidence of back injuries decreased by 49% and 68%, respectively.[55] Much of the success was due to extensive education of management and their subsequent positive reinforcement of the program.

Evaluation and Enhancement of Strength, Flexibility, and Fitness

It is not surprising that x-rays are not of great predictive value in determining the risk of development of back injuries. Radiographs give a view of the static anatomy of the back but show nothing about actual strength, flexibility, and functional use of the back. To try to obtain better indicators of back strength and function, additional studies have been undertaken to determine if a correlation exists between fitness and risk of back injury. It was hypothesized that a more fit worker would be less likely to be injured on the job. Cady and colleagues[8] assessed fitness in 1652 firefighters. Flexibility, isometric lifting strength, and aerobic capacity on a bicycle ergometer were measured. Indi-

viduals were grouped according to fitness into thirds: least fit, middle fit, and most fit. Back injury rates varied dependent on fitness, with the rate for the least fit group being 7.1%, the middle fit group 3.2%, and the most fit group 0.8%.

Keyserling and others[31] also performed isometric strength tests on workers at a tire and rubber plant. The study showed an injury rate in the group hired after a screening strength test to be one-third that in the group hired without undergoing strength testing. Isometric strength testing was shown to be safe, but has now been replaced in many facilities with job-specific testing that measures the ability to safely perform specific job tasks. A criticism of isometric strength testing as an employment screening tool is that it is considered by some to be discriminatory against women, older individuals, and persons with disabilities.

Some industries, especially those that require much physical work, are now realizing the importance of continually emphasizing physical fitness in their work force. The military services have for many years realized the necessity of soldiers' maintaining physical fitness and "combat readiness." Regular physical training and periodic fitness evaluations are a regular part of military life. Other professions, such as police and firefighters, have also emphasized fitness in their workers. Cady and others[9] showed that a program to enhance firefighter fitness was rewarded by higher measurements of fitness (physical work capacity, strength, and flexibility) as well as by lower injury rates and Workers' Compensation costs.

Other interventions, such as flexibility programs, have been utilized to try to improve performance on the job and to subsequently decrease injuries. In firefighters, the flexibility program of Hilyer and colleagues[27] was shown to help reduce the severity and cost of musculoskeletal injuries.

Some industries have established their own completely staffed fitness centers. Smaller industries typically find it more feasible and cost-effective to encourage the use of existing community facilities and programs.

Ergonomic Assessment and Intervention

Often, injuries occur because a worker is mismatched with a job. For example, a physically deconditioned worker could be placed in a job that is very strenuous and demanding. Without adequate conditioning and training, that individual might be at a higher risk of injury. Physiatrists are often called on to help industries better understand specific physical requirements and demands of jobs to help ensure a better employee-job fit.

Ergonomics, or human factors engineering,[49, 50, 54] refers to the study of the "fit" between the worker, the job tasks, the tools and equipment used, and the work environment. The goal is to enhance the match between the worker's physical, emotional, and mental capabilities and the job. An ideal match should lessen the incidence of work injuries and errors, reduce the worker's fatigue and physical stress, and enhance overall productivity.

Lifting is often implicated as a factor that contributes to the development of low back pain. Jobs should be analyzed ergonomically to determine the amount and frequency of lifting required. Postures utilized by workers on the job should be noted. Other factors to be considered include the following: (1) What are the size and the shape of the objects lifted? (2) Can the worker get a firm grasp on the object? (3) Is twisting required along with the lifting? (4) What speed of lifting is required to keep up with the expected productivity? (5) Does awkward placement of bins (or other equipment) require the worker to forward flex the spine into a position that creates a higher back injury risk?

Other work factors should be assessed, such as amount of pushing or pulling. Are handles present that allow pushing and pulling in a biomechanically favorable position? If a wheeled cart is pulled or pushed, are wheels sufficiently maintained and large enough to allow smooth movement and to easily clear obstacles such as irregularities in the workplace floor?

Proper lifting and materials handling techniques might be impossible to utilize in certain circumstances. In these cases, an assessment should be performed to ascertain whether the load can be subdivided into lighter loads, whether a mechanical lifting device can be utilized, whether loads can be positioned to allow lifting without concomitant spine rotation, or whether help from another individual can produce a safer lift. The pace of lifting should also be sufficiently slow and deliberate to allow for the use of good biomechanics.[17]

Low back pain is also common in workers, such as secretaries and drivers, who have sedentary occupations. Properly fitting and supportive seating is essential to mini-

mize stress on the back. Industries have traditionally purchased furniture in bulk: one-size-fits-all. Now many industries are realizing that workers come in all sizes and shapes. The purchase of higher-quality seating is often a prudent investment. Chairs can be properly fitted and adjusted to meet the specific needs of the workers who will occupy them up to 8 or more hours/day.

Analysis of specific jobs is essential to ascertain the physical requirements and demands necessary for successful performance of the job. Job descriptions that actually quantitate amount and frequency of lifting, pushing, pulling, climbing, stooping, and squatting are helpful when trying to make a successful fit between a prospective worker and a specific job. Dynamometers and push-pull gauges can be helpful in assessing jobs, and occupational or physical therapists can often be helpful resources in establishing job descriptions and in evaluating specific job tasks.

Lumbar Support Orthoses

Lumbar support orthoses are widely marketed to industry as aids to help decrease the incidence of low back injuries. Studies validating the efficacy of back supports are meager at this time.[47] There might be some value in using back supports to prevent initial back injuries, but their across-the-board use for all workers in manual industries has not yet been substantiated to decrease overall injuries, injury severity, or overall cost per injury.[40]

Back supports can serve several useful functions. They are visible reminders of the need to lift properly. They also provide an increase in intra-abdominal pressure when properly fitted and worn, and they can help lessen intradiscal pressure during lifting. It appears that lumbar supports can be of some value, but that they are secondary in importance to comprehensive training of the worker in appropriate body mechanics and to ergonomic analysis and modification of the job, if necessary, to enhance safety.

Preplacement Screening: ADA Approach

The Americans with Disabilities Act (ADA) (Public Law 101–336)[1, 56] became effective on July 26, 1992. This act changed the way in which job placement could be legally performed. Under this act, an employer can require an employee to undergo *job-specific* preplacement testing only after a job offer has been made to the prospective employee. This preplacement examination can test the ability to safely perform the *usual tasks* of the specific job. The goal of the testing is to ensure that the employee is physically and emotionally capable of performing the job so as to not endanger himself or herself or other employees. If the employee is unable to successfully perform the testing due to some functional limitation, the industry is obliged to determine if job accommodations could reasonably be implemented that would allow the successful performance of the required job tasks.

The goal of the preplacement testing should be to assess for the presence and severity of:

1. Stable impairments that could affect job performance and safety. (For example, an amputee or paraplegic has a stable impairment. The examination should determine

whether this employee can safely perform the job duties with the impairment.)

2. Impairments that could be worsened or aggravated by the job requirements. (For example, an individual with stage II spondylolisthesis would be at a higher risk of back re-injury in a job that requires frequent repetitive bending and heavy lifting.)

3. Progressive conditions that would ultimately require job reassignment to a more sedentary occupation. (For example, an individual with ankylosing spondylitis would have limited ability to perform heavy labor and bending and would ultimately require placement in a more sedentary and less vigorous position.)

4. Intermittent problems that would impair performance safety. (For example, these might include such things as a history of a seizure disorder in an individual with a previous head injury. If seizure control is less than complete, placement considerations need to be taken to ensure safety of the employee and co-workers.)

Preplacement examinations cannot be performed randomly. If they are used, the following requirements must be fulfilled:

1. All new employees for the same job must be examined with the same tests.

2. Results from the medical preplacement examination must be treated as a medical record and must be maintained confidentially.

3. Supervisors and managers may be informed about any specific accommodations or work restrictions that will be necessary for the worker's safety and success on the job.

4. Any investigation about a disability or impairment must be "job-related and consistent with business necessity."

5. Future risk considerations cannot be considered when determining whether the individual can perform the specific offered job.

Ideally, preplacement testing should help to place an employee in a specific job in which the employee has the physical and emotional ability to successfully and safely complete the assigned work tasks. Proper placement should help ensure a healthy and contented worker and a safer more positive work site.

Cumulative Trauma Disorders

Cumulative trauma disorders such as tendinitis, bursitis, muscle strains, and peripheral nerve compression are usually the result of repetitive stresses applied to the body at sufficient force and/or frequency to slowly and progressively lead to tissue damage. Injuries can be treated and improvements will occur; however, if the worker is reassigned to the same job, recurrence is likely.

Cumulative trauma disorders should be actively sought out in industry and specific jobs that are found to be of high risk for producing injury should be thoroughly analyzed to determine whether ergonomic changes can be made to enhance job tolerance and safety for the worker. Site visits and job analyses may be very helpful in pinpointing specific job modifications or job rotations that could be implemented to lessen risk to the workers. At-risk jobs might require such factors as excessive force, rapid speed (often machine paced), uncomfortable and poorly fitting tools, awkward working postures, or excessive joint motion. At times, ergonomic tools designed for the worker and the specific job can help decrease risk of injury (Fig. 44–5). Handle sizes about 1.5 in. (3.75 cm) in diameter often aid comfort. Comfortable, cushioned and adequate-length grips can be useful. Vibratory and oscillating tools might require vibration dampening. Alteration in the work posture and job rotation can also help to facilitate safer job performance. Job rotation allows the worker to perform different work tasks, often utilizing different muscle groups, and can help minimize tissue overuse and prevent the development of cumulative trauma disorders.[50]

EVALUATION OF THE INJURED WORKER

Despite the best efforts of many industries on safety awareness and preventive programs, accidents occur. Appropriate early intervention and treatment that is seamlessly integrated with a system to efficiently and thoroughly manage and rehabilitate more chronic and persistent injuries can help to minimize lost time and productivity and help to prevent the development of chronic disability.

The Detailed History

An injury or accident on the job is often an emotionally charged event for employee and employer alike. The attitude and response that the injured worker perceives at the time of injury is vitally important. Occasionally, in the "heat of the battle," things are said by one or both parties that affect the long-term outcome. Is the worker treated with kindness and compassion or is he or she treated abruptly, with accusations or insinuations that the worker was to blame for the accident? The initial response, when handled properly, can help to develop a cooperative relationship between the worker and the employer. When handled poorly, the initial response can distance the employee from the employer and result in an adversarial relationship.

It is very important for the examining physiatrist to obtain a complete history of the accident from the worker. A description of the overall job tasks and requirements is helpful as is a detailed history of what happened at the time of the accident. The outline presented in Table 44–5 can be helpful when taking the history of the injury. By obtaining a thorough initial history, the physiatrist can obtain a more complete picture of the accident and the job, as well as of the initial response to the injury.

The physician is often asked by the Workers' Compensation carrier to respond to a number of questions to help determine whether a work-related problem really did occur.[48] These often include the following:

1. Do the history and physical findings clearly support that this is a work-related illness or injury?

2. Is there consistency between the history of the illness or injury and the clinical findings and diagnosis?

3. Was there sufficient job-related exposure to provide a clear cause-and-effect relationship between the work activities and the clinical presentation?

4. Are any other pre-existing problems or causative

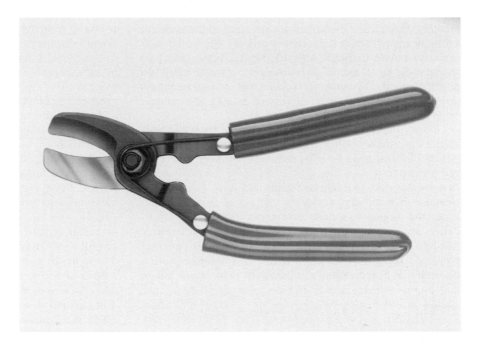

FIGURE 44–5 Ergonomic cutter features a cushioned and contoured grip with spring opening. It is designed to reduce local pressure on the hand and fatigue. (Courtesy of Torvaal Ergonomic Power Curve Tools, Chagrin Falls, Ohio.)

factors present that could lead to the development of this clinical problem?

Some workers are seen soon after the accident, but others are not seen for evaluation for weeks, months, or even years after the accident. In these more chronic cases, it is important to extend the history to include additional information (Table 44–6).

It is important to realize that the worker's perception of and satisfaction with the job may strongly influence the initial injury as well as the recovery and the return to work. Workers who "hardly ever" enjoyed their job tasks were 2.5 times more likely to report a back injury than workers who "almost always" enjoyed their jobs.[4]

It is helpful to assess the individual's current lifestyle and plans for the future. What is his or her typical day? Is the individual passive and inactive or is there evidence that efforts are being made to stay active and productive? If he or she is not working now, are plans being formulated for

the future that include a return to some type of reasonable, productive employment? What is the worker's outlook for the future? Does the worker see hope for the future or despair? Some workers focus on keeping productive, taking the necessary steps to return to work, and maintaining favorable relationships with their employers. Others, however, blame the employer for all of their problems and take a passive or even a passive-aggressive role in returning to any meaningful productivity. Also important is whether any litigation is pending because this often slows down recovery and limits response to treatment.

Concurrent Medical or Psychological Illnesses

The evaluation should include assessment of the worker's overall health. Pre-existing problems are occa-

TABLE 44–5 Important Historical Facts to Ascertain from the Initial Interview

1. Ask the worker to describe the accident in detail.
2. What was the worker's position/posture at the time of the accident?
3. If the injury occurred during lifting, was there twisting or turning associated with the lifting motion?
4. What was being handled at the time? (weight, size, shape, frequency)
5. Did a slip, fall, or other unusual event occur?
6. What was the worker's footing like?
7. Is this the worker's usual job, or were these new tasks?
8. How long has the worker been on this specific job?
9. Have other workers had injuries on this job?
10. Is there any problem with the equipment being utilized on the job?
11. At what time of day and what day of week did the accident occur?
12. Was anyone else injured?
13. What was the initial response by management to the injury?

TABLE 44–6 Important Areas to Assess With Chronic Injuries

1. Describe the initial medical examination and treatment. What did the worker understand the diagnosis to be? What was the response to initial treatment? Was there any attempt to return to work? What happened if a return was attempted?
2. If improvement did not occur, what other testing, treatments, and physicians have been involved? Has surgery been performed? If so, how many operations, and how effective were they in providing relief?
3. Has the worker been involved in rehabilitative efforts such as active physical therapy, work conditioning, or work hardening?
4. Does the worker have a job to return to? What is the worker's current relationship with the employer? Does the employer seem willing to accept the worker back on the job?
5. How is the worker currently spending a typical day? How much time does the worker spend in bed every day? In front of the television? Does the worker get out of the house regularly? Does the worker participate in hobbies and recreation?
6. Does the worker participate in any regular exercise? This includes specific exercises to correct the condition as well as general exercises to improve overall aerobic fitness. What is the worker's estimate of his or her own level of physical fitness?

sionally present that could have contributed to the accident or injury or will affect the recovery process. Medical conditions, including diabetes, arthritis, heart disease, and pulmonary disease, should be considered. Occasionally, an accident occurs because of such factors as leg weakness due to diabetic neuropathy or loss of balance due to pain in an arthritic joint.

Obesity can also occasionally be a significant factor if its presence makes it difficult to use proper body mechanics during physical tasks or if its presence prolongs the recovery period.

It is important to evaluate for use of drugs, alcohol, and tobacco. Injuries and accidents can occur from working under the influence of these substances. Prescription medication overuse should also be considered. The worker may fall into such overuse gradually. The worker has pain and therefore takes medications. With time, tolerance often develops and medication use increases, with more potent and more frequent medications being taken. Tobacco use should also be addressed, as current studies[3, 26,45] show a correlation between tobacco use and back pain, disc degeneration, and slower healing.

Physical Examination

A meticulous physical examination is essential to be sure that the condition is thoroughly assessed and that important findings are not overlooked. Evaluating workers while they are in street clothes is often difficult. Range of motion measurements can be compromised by tight-fitting clothes. Palpation can be difficult when working around clothing. Important findings such as winging of a scapula, muscle atrophy, or pertinent scars and rashes can be easily overlooked if the patient is not undressed. It is best to have workers disrobe and to utilize gowns that allow adequate exposure of the primary areas of symptomatology.

A general assessment of the worker's health, as well as a thorough assessment of the neuromusculoskeletal system, should be performed. While the patient is standing, it is useful to assess the freedom and smoothness of movement. How much pain behavior is present? Is the patient able to walk on toes and heels, to squat, and to forward flex and touch the toes? At times, ability to hop on one foot or to run in place provides useful information.

The amount of spine mobility and flexibility should be assessed, including forward flexion, extension, lateral bending, and rotation. Do any specific movements aggravate the symptoms? Leg-length inequalities or spinal deformities should be considered.

Palpation is helpful to evaluate for any areas of local tenderness (trigger points or local areas of injury), widespread tenderness, or even no tenderness. If tenderness is discovered, it should be mapped out as well as possible to find the triggering tissue or source of pain (e.g., muscle, tendon, ligament, joint).

For shoulder and shoulder girdle problems, it is essential to observe the shoulder region from the back. Is there any scapular winging with either forward flexion or abduction of the upper extremities, with and without resistance? Is pain produced at any point in the arc of motion? Are the shoulders symmetrical? Is any atrophy present? These findings are often overlooked if patients are evaluated only from the front while they are seated in a chair. (For additional information, see Chapter 37.)

Upper and lower extremity range of motion often need to be assessed, as does cervical motion (see Chapter 1). Limitation of motion should be noted as well as pain produced with movement.

A systematic evaluation of upper and lower extremity strength is useful to pinpoint areas of pathological weakness. Areas of muscle atrophy, either focal and localized or generalized, should be noted. True organic weakness results in a smooth "give-way" during muscle testing. Muscle "give-way" in a ratchety pattern suggests a possible functional component to the symptomatology. Occasionally, this ratchety response occurs despite the presence of actual organic disease, and the examiner needs to be careful to not overlook other potentially significant findings during the examination.

Measurement of grip is often helpful during the evaluation. A hand-held dynamometer can be utilized to assess grip strength in various positions. Normally grip is strongest in the dominant upper extremity by about 5 to 10 lb and is greater in the mid-position of grip, being weaker with either a narrow or wide grip. These data can be useful in assessing the amount of weakness present as well as in following progress during treatment. Multiple trials allow assessment of inconsistencies that can be useful in determining the amount of effort the patient is giving.

Sensation should also be addressed to assess whether deficits follow specific peripheral nerve, nerve root, or neuropathic patterns. Sensory deficits that incorporate the whole leg or the whole arm often suggest the presence of a nonphysiological, functional sensory deficit. Occasionally, vibratory sensation measured with a tuning fork can be evaluated to help determine the validity of otherwise questionable sensory findings. Finding a right-to-left difference in vibratory sensation in a midline bone such as the skull or sternum strongly suggests a functional, nonorganic deficit.

Muscle stretch reflexes need to be evaluated to assess integrity of the reflex arc. Straight-leg raising can be measured in both the sitting and supine positions. Also, special tests such as Tinel's sign, Phalen's wrist flexion test, Spurling's test, Finkelstein's test, Patrick's test, and tests for thoracic outlet syndrome can provide possibly helpful information, but these findings also need to be evaluated cautiously and in light of the remainder of the physical and historical findings.

The examiner needs to continually analyze the findings as the examination progresses. Findings should be reassessed several times during the examination using a variety of techniques to ensure consistency. Injured workers can occasionally demonstrate the syndrome of "symptom magnification," with inconsistencies in findings being common in these examinations. Tests such as those described by Waddell and co-workers[57] (Table 44–7) can help to differentiate nonorganic from organically mediated physical findings. Other findings, such as the presence of dirt under the nails and calluses on the hands, should be noted. Exaggerated pain behavior may indicate some degree of symptom magnification by the patient. Pain behavior and inconsistencies are important to recognize to ensure that the patient is not medically overevaluated or subjected to potentially risky tests or treatments. Also, identifying

TABLE 44-7   Nonorganic Findings in the Low Back Evaluation: Waddell's Signs

1. Tenderness of the skin to light pinch over a widespread area
2. Deep tenderness in a nonanatomical distribution
3. Reproduction of back pain with axial loading by pressing down on the worker's head while he or she is standing
4. Reproduction of back pain when the shoulders and pelvis are rotated together as a unit
5. Inconsistencies between straight leg testing done when the worker is otherwise distracted vs. that done when worker is aware of the test being performed
6. "Give-way" weakness in a widespread and nonanatomical pattern
7. Inconsistent and nonanatomical sensory deficits
8. Overreaction (disproportionate verbalization, facial expression, muscle tension and tremor, collapsing, or sweating) during the examination

Adapted from Waddell G, McCulloch JA, Kummel E, Verner RM: Nonorganic physical signs in low-back pain. Spine 1980; 5:117–125.

functional issues allows for the institution of appropriate psychologically and behaviorally based intervention.

Appropriate testing, including x-rays, CT or MRI scans, radioisotopic bone scanning, laboratory testing, or electrodiagnostic testing can also be useful in confirming the diagnosis. These tests should not be used in "shotgun" fashion, but should be used for specific indications, and their overuse should be avoided.

Diagnosis

After the evaluation is completed, a working diagnosis should be formulated and explained to the worker in clear and understandable terms. It is important to try to avoid emotionally charged words such as "ruptured" disc or "degenerative" arthritis, which might frighten the worker. The overall prognosis and treatment plan should be clearly provided to the worker. In low back pain, for example, it should be explained that the vast majority of back problems improve with nonoperative measures, and that only a small percentage (about 5% to 10% of cases, in which definite disc herniation and persistent sciatica are present) require surgical intervention.[13, 16] Approximate time frames for treatment and return to work should be provided to the patient and are also helpful for the employer and insurer.

TREATMENT

In working with injured workers, it is necessary to have access to a spectrum of treatment approaches to meet the needs of the specific individual worker. Some workers respond to acute treatment quite readily and return to work quickly. Others have more protracted courses of recovery and require organized reconditioning efforts to achieve the status of being "fit for duty." Still others may not have jobs to return to and require more comprehensive programs with specific vocational planning and rehabilitation emphases. Last, some workers are resistant to virtually all routine methods of treatment and can be best served by a chronic pain approach. (See Chapter 41 for more information.)

Early Intervention

Early treatment of the injured worker occurs in a number of settings including (1) a clinic on-site at the industry, (2) the company physician's office, (3) an occupational medicine clinic, (4) a minor emergency clinic, or (5) the emergency department of a hospital. The goals of early intervention are accurate diagnosis and appropriate treatment to facilitate the worker's return to work as soon as possible, in a manner consistent with safety. The worker needs to be seen promptly after the injury and followed up closely with scheduled, short-interval follow-up appointments. In some instances, even daily appointments are appropriate. It is important that the worker does not "get lost in the system."

Pain is the major symptom of most acute injuries and is usually reflective of some degree of tissue damage. Early treatment for an acute injury is focused on control of pain and tissue damage. Often a sports medicine orientation using the RICE treatment approach (*rest, ice, compression, elevation*) can be initially helpful. Rest should be limited in duration for most musculoskeletal injuries, with 2 days of bed rest often being preferable to 7 days of bed rest for back injuries.[12] Specific rest of an injured part for other injuries can be provided with appropriate casts, splints, or braces. Prolonged bed rest or immobilization can perpetuate disability by enhancing deconditioning.[22] Appropriate analgesics can help control pain, as can physical modalities such as heat, cold, transcutaneous electrical nerve stimulation (TENS) units, massage, and gentle stretching. Physical modalities are often underutilized for acute treatment. They have advantages over medications in that they are often more effective and safer, with fewer side effects.

During the phase of early intervention, it is often possible and desirable to provide treatment while the worker is still performing "light duty" or a modified job. As long as the medical outcome will not be compromised and no further tissue damage will occur, it is usually best to try to facilitate early return to work. This helps to avoid both physical and mental deconditioning.

As acute symptoms subside, use of medications and physical modalities should decrease. The worker should be instructed in specific flexibility and strengthening exercises to perform to help improve conditioning and lessen the chance of recurrence. A common reason for recurrence is that the acute symptoms were treated and improved, but the underlying factors that produced the injury in the first place were not addressed. At times, the worker was in a deconditioned state prior to the injury and had inadequate strength and endurance to do the specific job tasks in a safe manner. Identification of this pre-existing deconditioning gives the physician an opportunity to recondition the worker more extensively and then to return a worker to the workplace in better condition than he or she was in prior to the injury. In other instances, the job could be poorly designed or the worker might be utilizing poor biomechanics in the performance of the job tasks. Prior to returning the worker to work, it is helpful to fully understand the worker's job. Intervention at this time with ergonomic modifications or additional worker training in proper biomechanics could be helpful in avoiding recurrence of the injury.

Any identified problems with drug and alcohol overuse should be addressed with referral to appropriate treatment programs. Cessation of smoking should also be encouraged, as current studies[3, 26, 45] show a correlation between back pain, disc degeneration, slower healing, and tobacco use. Education and stopping smoking strategies can be helpful.

In general, about 80% to 85% of workers with acute problems experience improvement and return to productive work. In others, symptoms persist longer than expected and progress into a subacute phase. With these workers, it is important to intensify treatment efforts. Often, persistent stiffness or weakness prolongs the symptoms. A structured and regularly scheduled therapy program focused around reconditioning can be helpful in overcoming the residual symptoms.

Chronic Treatment

A smaller percentage of workers (about 10%)[7] still has pain complaints and physical disability that prevents return to work after the completion of acute and subacute care. These workers may be candidates for more highly structured treatment programs, such as work conditioning, work hardening, vocational rehabilitation, or chronic pain therapy.

It is well recognized that the longer workers are off of the job, the more difficult it becomes to return them to work (regardless of the type of impairment). There is about a 50% chance of return to work when a worker is off for 6 months, with the rate dropping to 25% when the worker is off for 1 year. After being off of work for 2 years, the return-to-work rate is minimal unless a worker is highly motivated and is in a comprehensive rehabilitation program.

When cases enter the chronic stage, the initial injury is often resolved, but the worker may be left with chronic weakness and deconditioning as well as inflexibility and poor endurance. Weeks or even months of inactivity have likely occurred. In addition to being physically deconditioned, the worker is psychologically deconditioned. The worker has been removed from the role of being a productive worker and does not have to get up and be ready for work by a certain hour each day. The worker does not have to perform work tasks regularly and may even be relieved of normal responsibilities at home. The worker usually is much more sedentary at home, and physical deconditioning and weight gain often occur. It is common for such workers to let other positive health habits deteriorate, and they begin smoking more, drinking more, and taking more medications than they were taking prior to the injury. Prolonged absence from work can also be reinforced by a number of factors[11, 59] (Table 44–8). Such an individual may be a candidate for a more intense program of work conditioning, work hardening, chronic pain treatment, or structured vocational rehabilitation.

Work Conditioning: A Sports Medicine Approach

Work conditioning (Fig. 44–6) is a program of progressive structured reconditioning to prepare the worker for return to the job. These programs are often provided by physical and occupational therapists in coordination with the primary physician, the employer, and the injured worker. The essential criteria for inclusion in a work conditioning program are that the worker has a job to return to

TABLE 44–8   Factors Inhibiting Return to Work

Relief from responsibility
  Responsibility of getting up and going to work for a job that may not be enjoyed in the first place
  Relief from other jobs and chores at home and in the community because of illness or injury
Attention and support from family and friends
Financial rewards, such as disability income
Use of the illness as a tool of control in the family and against the employer
Progressive deconditioning—both physical and psychological—from being off of work
Adversarial relationship between the employer and employee
Unwillingness of the employer to make reasonable accommodations or to consider temporary light-duty work for the employee

and that the employer is willing to accept the worker back on the job.

The treatment focus for work conditioning shifts further away from passive modalities and medications into more active rehabilitation and physical restoration. This stage of care is often best presented to the worker as a sports medicine model of treatment. For example, an injured athlete may require a period of rest after an acute injury. After the period of rest is completed, it is often necessary to return the athlete to the training room to restore fitness prior to return to competition. The worker might be considered to be an "occupational athlete," as many workers perform vigorous repetitive physical activities on a daily basis. Restoring fitness is often necessary prior to safe return to the job.

Having a job description is helpful in understanding the specific physical requirements of job performance. Even more useful are job site visits (Table 44–9) if they can be arranged. These allow direct inspection of the specific job performed by the worker. By understanding the job clearly, a specific physical reconditioning program can be developed to most efficiently prepare the worker for return to the job. A job that primarily involves upper body strength or flexibility would have different conditioning goals than would a job that requires much squatting or bending. Also, evaluation of the job and job site can help enhance the injured worker's confidence in the rehabilitative team. The worker and rehabilitative staff should have a common understanding of the job and its requirements. They can speak a common language about the job, the equipment utilized, and the work environment.

Communicating with the worker's employer during job site visits can help to overcome obstacles to returning the employee to the job. Management can outline whether light duty is available and, if so, what specific light duty tasks are available. Employers can also be educated about the value of light duty programs and about how they can return the worker back to productivity earlier while helping to minimize injury-related compensation costs.[14]

Work conditioning often begins on a three- to five-times-a-week schedule. The fitness level and work capacity of the worker are periodically assessed. When the worker is sufficiently conditioned to meet the requirements of light duty, the worker is usually returned to the job, and arrangements are made to continue conditioning until the worker

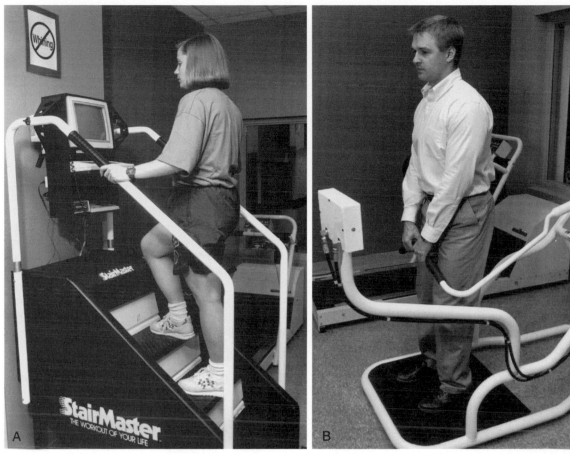

FIGURES 44–6   *A* and *B*, Work conditioning focuses on enhancing general aerobic fitness as well as on strengthening specific muscle groups that are used regularly in work activities

has maximally improved or has met the requirements for returning to the original job

In work conditioning, workers are usually treated over relatively short time frames, such as 3 to 6 weeks. The outcome is that the vast majority of workers return to their

TABLE 44–9   The Job Site Analysis: Things to Observe

THE JOB
1. Objects handled (weight, size, shape, surface texture, presence or absence of handles)
2. Frequency of physical tasks (lifts per hour, objects handled per time period)
3. Positions and postures that must be utilized to successfully perform the job
4. Tools used (handle size, weight, vibration, position of use)
5. Layout of work site (height of workbench, arrangement of tools utilized)

THE WORK ENVIRONMENT
1. Amount of lighting present (type and intensity of lighting, windows, color of walls, ceiling)
2. Temperature of the facility
3. Amount of noise present—are hearing protectors available and used if excess noise present?
4. Cleanliness of floor surface. Note any spills, greasy spots, clutter, obstacles present on floor that could lead to stumbles and falls
5. General ambience of the facility—pleasant, relaxed, clean, organized, and orderly or hurried, hostile, hectic, and cluttered

jobs at the completion of the program.[7] In addition to improving physical fitness, the worker's confidence about being able to successfully perform the job requirements is enhanced with these programs.

Work Hardening

Workers who have been off of work for protracted periods of time, such as 3 months or more, may require a more comprehensive program than can be provided by work conditioning. These individuals are often even more deconditioned than those treated in the work conditioning program. If these individuals have a job to return to, they might well benefit from a work hardening program. Work hardening programs focus on physical conditioning but also address psychological issues and vocational issues that often interfere with return to the job.

Success is facilitated if the work hardening team has a complete understanding of the worker's job and work conditions. This allows the provision of an appropriate program of reconditioning and work simulation for the worker. Work hardening (Figs. 44–7 through 44–10) usually incorporates general as well as job-related physical conditioning. The general conditioning is quite similar to that provided by the work conditioning program. To be most successful the conditioning should focus on areas of weakness as well as on areas that require additional

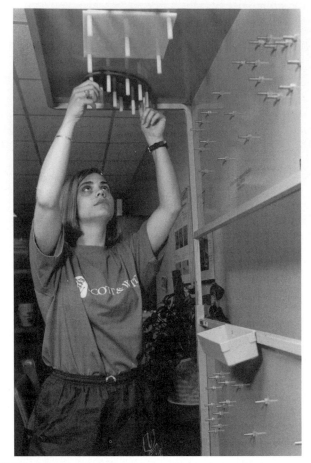

FIGURE 44–7 Work hardening continues to emphasize generalized conditioning, but it also simulates usual work activities. A job involving overhead tasks could require the redevelopment of strength, endurance, and flexibility. Work simulation helps to redevelop these abilities.

4. Assertiveness training.
5. Interpersonal skills to facilitate conflict avoidance and resolution.
6. Healthy lifestyle.

Psychological counseling can help the worker to overcome fears and anxieties about returning to work. Addressing possible unresolved anger about the injury is also important, as is evaluating for the presence of depression or other psychopathological conditions.

The work hardening team usually consists of the physician, the physical therapist, the occupational therapist, the psychologist, the vocational counselor, the exercise physiologist, and other specialists as needed, such as ergonomists and industrial engineers.

The cost of these programs is relatively high, but well-organized programs often have favorable success rates. Return-to-work rates of about 80% to 85% occur with programs that carefully select their clients.[7] Individuals selected for these programs should be motivated to return to work, should have jobs available, and should be free of overwhelming psychological or secondary gain issues that can undermine progress.

Vocational Rehabilitation

If at all possible, it is preferable to try to assist the injured worker to obtain reinstatement with the previous

conditioning to enable the worker to successfully meet the job requirements.

In addition, work hardening programs incorporate job-specific work simulation activities into the program. If the worker is required to lift boxes, for example, the program includes lifting boxes. If the worker uses a specific tool in a certain position, the program tries to simulate this activity.

The program also tries to simulate actual work conditions. The worker is often required to clock in and out daily. To minimize the worker's perception of illness and sickness, the program is often housed in a warehouse or other "worklike" setting, rather than in a medical clinic or hospital. The treatment duration usually lasts for a half-day or whole day for up to 6 weeks.[7]

The goal is to progressively increase exercise tolerance and work activities until they simulate a typical day on the job. The program strives to enhance both physical capabilities and work skills, as well as to psychologically readjust the worker to the role of being a productive employee again. Education is an important part of the program, and should encompass such areas as the following:

1. Proper use of the body to avoid re-injury.
2. Proper pacing on the job.
3. Relaxation and stress management skills.

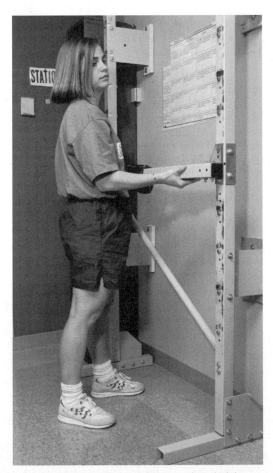

FIGURE 44–8 Lifting graded weights to various heights can simulate manual materials handling, as in stocking shelves or working in a warehouse.

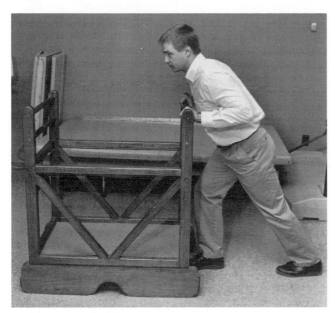

FIGURE 44–9 Simulated pushing can prepare workers for jobs requiring pushing of carts, skids, boxes, or other materials.

employer in some capacity. If the employee had a favorable work history with the employer, it is usually much easier to work with that employer rather than to go out and try to find a totally new job. Close communication between the worker, the employer, and the rehabilitation team can help to promote this goal and help to avoid misunder-

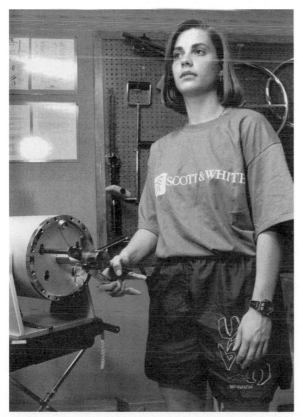

FIGURE 44–10 Use of a work simulator helps to develop strength and tolerance during the repetitive use of hand tools.

standings that can inhibit the employer's willingness to accept the worker back on the job. The case manager can play a vital role in promoting this communication and facilitating return to the job.

Many injured workers return to former jobs after appropriate medical treatment and rehabilitation. Unfortunately, other workers may not have the option to return to their former jobs. This may be the case for a number of reasons, such as the worker's inability to physically meet the job demands despite rehabilitative measures, poor worker-job match that would increase the risk of reinjury, lack of desire on the worker's part to return to the former job, or lack of willingness on the former employer's part to accept the worker back on the job. With no available job to return to, a more comprehensive vocational rehabilitation approach may be needed. Many individuals have limited work skills and educational levels. They might have little knowledge of the marketplace, of what jobs are available, or even of how to apply for a job.

Initially, a thorough assessment of the individual is in order. It is helpful to survey areas of interest and aptitude to help ascertain the appropriate vocational possibilities. Psychological testing can be helpful to determine aptitude for specific vocations as well as for various levels of vocational or educational training (e.g., vocational school, junior college, college). Physical evaluation is helpful to determine the individual's work capacity and whether this level can be enhanced with physical reconditioning programs such as work conditioning.

The vocational counselor should be familiar with job options in the geographic area and be able to assist the individual with formulating a reasonable plan for vocational rehabilitation. Vocational counseling can be provided by individual rehabilitation facilities and, in many instances, the resources of the state vocational rehabilitation services can be called on to assist with the vocational rehabilitation effort.

In formulating a vocational rehabilitation plan an individual might need to consider specific job adaptations or modifications to enable success in the work force. The prospective worker with a physical impairment, such as a previous head injury or a spinal cord injury, might need ergonomic adaptations, such as modification of the worktable or tools or special seating, for successful performance of the job. Assistive equipment such as lifts, hoists, and adapted control panels can occasionally help the worker maintain acceptable productivity and safety.

Job coaching and education are important for the individual who has been out of the work force for some time. The prospective worker might need coaching on:

1. How to fill out a job application.
2. How to prepare a resume.
3. How to dress for and act at a job interview as well as on the job.
4. How to deal with authority figures and co-workers effectively.
5. How to deal with stress or conflict in the work situation.
6. How to manage finances.

Vocational rehabilitation is a team effort. The vocational counselor usually coordinates the effort, with assistance being provided by physicians, psychologists and neuropsychologists, physical and occupational therapists, ergonomists, industrial engineers, employers, and educational facilities as needed.

The vocational rehabilitation process can be difficult, but with a motivated individual, a return to gainful employment is often possible.

Chronic Pain Treatment

Some individuals with work-related injuries develop chronic pain syndrome. Sometimes the pain reflects chronic pain induced by the original injury, or it can be an aftermath of the treatment efforts. For example, chronic pain due to arachnoiditis can develop after back surgery. In otherwise psychologically well-adjusted individuals, chronic pain can sometimes be treated effectively by use of the traditional medical model of care. Treatment modalities such as physical therapy, epidural blocks, TENS, or even implanted stimulators or pumps can be helpful and allow increased activity and productivity.

Many other individuals have chronic pain but no specific medical condition that can be readily treated or cured. Psychological factors such as depression, somatization, hypochondriasis, or passive-dependency may be present; overuse of medications, alcohol and tobacco, and medical and surgical services may also be pertinent factors. Other secondary gain issues are frequently prominent. In such cases, individuals seem to have disability far in excess of any actual organic pathological findings that are present.[63] Such patients also are usually physically deconditioned and live sedentary lifestyles. Return to work is not the initial priority with these individuals. Initial pain management efforts often revolve around medication detoxification, psychological counseling, and progressive reconditioning. Such patients may do best in an interdisciplinary program that is focused on the treatment of chronic pain syndrome. If the chronic pain program proves to be a success, patients might later qualify for one of the programs more strictly focused on preparation for returning to the work force, such as work conditioning or vocational rehabilitation. (For further information on chronic pain and chronic pain syndrome, see Chapter 41.)

WRAPPING IT UP: RETURN-TO-WORK ISSUES

Case Management

Case management can play a useful role in assisting the worker and the treatment team during the treatment process. A case manager—employed by the rehabilitation facility, the employer, an insurance carrier, or even the physician—can communicate with the health care team, the insurer, the employer, and the worker to ensure that smooth, unhindered communications take place. This communication facilitates the worker's rehabilitative program.

The case manager assesses job availability with the current employer and investigates the existence of light-duty alternatives. The case manager communicates with the insurer to be sure that prompt coverage is provided for the necessary diagnostic, therapeutic, and rehabilitative efforts

and to be certain that the insurer fully understands the proposed program, expected outcome, and time frames.

The case manager can also be valuable in maintaining lines of communication with the worker to help prevent any misunderstandings about diagnosis, treatment plans, and return-to-work options. The case manager can help ensure that the worker does not get "lost in the system." The case manager can monitor attendance by the injured worker at appropriate therapy sessions and help ensure compliance if nonattendance occurs. Through efforts at case management, many cases have successful resolution through the worker's return to productive work in a reasonable time frame.

Functional Capacity Evaluation

After completion of medical treatment, the physician is often required to make a determination about whether the worker is capable of returning to the full-duty job or if specific limitations in performance remain. In the medical office, this is often a difficult determination, as most medical offices are not set up in a way that enables testing of the worker's abilities. Often, the physician "eyeballs" the worker and makes an estimate or asks the worker if he or she thinks the job can be performed safely. A better approach is to assess the worker with a functional capacity evaluation.

Functional capacity evaluations are typically performed by physical or occupational therapists. The therapist needs the worker's specific job description to individualize the testing and then methodically tests the worker with actual or simulated job tasks to determine the worker's capabilities for performing the required job tasks. Such physical skills as lifting, bending, pushing, pulling, stooping, and carrying are measured. Assessments should include measures of strength, flexibility, and endurance factors—muscular as well as aerobic—that are also involved in the routine performance of the specific job in question.

During performance of the work capacity evaluation it is helpful to learn from the worker the amount of energy and effort being expended. The Rating of Perceived Exertion Scale (Table 44–10) outlined by Borg[6] can be useful to make this determination.

If return to light duty is a possibility, the functional capacity evaluation can be useful in outlining the worker's capabilities as well as his or her restrictions.

TABLE 44–10   Rating of Perceived Exertion

0	Nothing at all
0.5	Very weak, just noticeable
1	Very weak
2	Weak (light effort)
3	Moderate
4	Somewhat strong
5	Strong (heavy effort)
6	
7	Very strong
8	
9	
10	Very, very strong
>10	Maximal effort

From Borg GAV: Psychophysical bases of perceived exertion. Med Sci Sports Exerc 1982; 14:377–381.

A comprehensive report is prepared for the referring physician and is extremely useful when communicating with the employer about job abilities and limitations. The work capacity evaluation helps ensure that the worker-job fit is appropriate to help reduce the risk of reinjury.

Impairment Evaluation

After treatment is completed, and the patient's progress has plateaued and is not expected to change further, it is concluded that the maximum medical improvement (MMI) has been achieved. Under Workers' Compensation programs in many states, an impairment evaluation must be performed when the worker reaches this plateau. (See Chapter 10 for more information on impairment rating.)

Litigation Resolution

After completion of treatment, it is very important to document any residual impairment. Specific limitation of motion, sensory deficit, or muscle weakness is important to note in case the worker becomes involved in litigation about the injuries. Thorough documentation of the initial encounter is important, as is documentation of diagnostic procedures and their results, working diagnoses, treatments rendered, response to treatment, and patient compliance and participation in the treatment program.

If litigation occurs, the physician might be called as a factual or expert witness. Documenting the case carefully as it progresses is extremely helpful in the establishment of credibility and in accurate representation of the facts, which contribute to a fair and equitable outcome for the injured worker as well as for the employer and compensation carrier.

OPPORTUNITIES FOR THE FUTURE

In the 1990s, the cost of health care is being viewed as a national problem ("crisis" by some). Various measures are being promoted to "fix" the system. Capitated, managed care plans are becoming more common around the country. With capitated care, the health provider receives a fixed amount of funding for each individual cared for under the plan. Under capitated systems, the more services provided to each individual, the less capital is available to the health care provider to meet expenses and to invest in new technology. With a capitated system, there is a natural tendency to enhance the emphasis on prevention—keeping people well, avoiding injuries, and keeping them out of hospitals. The emphasis shifts from treating episodes of illness to meeting individuals' health care needs over their lifetimes. There will be a continuum of prevention and care, rather than illness-based episodic care. Communities need to realize that they have a responsibility to be active participants, rather than passive observers, in promoting health in their communities. Currently some communities as well as some industries are addressing these issues by limiting smoking and sponsoring health promotion programs such as blood pressure screenings, cholesterol screening, drug and alcohol testing and treatment, and fitness promotion.

Physical medicine and rehabilitation has for many years been active in physical restoration and physical fitness enhancement as well as in development of various programs for injury prevention—from back schools to ergonomic analyses of specific jobs or industries. In the future, physical medicine and rehabilitation should play a strong role in helping to enhance worker fitness, to prevent injuries, to enhance job safety, and to restore workers back to full function in an expedient and cost-effective manner. Providers of care will need to develop seamless programs that provide the appropriate level and intensity of care for the injured worker at the most reasonable cost. Outcome analysis will be essential for quantifying success of various programs and for helping insurers, employers, and others decide where to use their scarce financial resources to provide acceptable, high-quality programs to the widest range of injured workers.

References

1. Americans with Disabilities Act. Federal Register P.L. 101–336, (July 26) 1990, pp 327–378.
2. Babitsky S, Sewall HD: Understanding the AMA Guides in Workers' Compensation. New York, John Wiley & Sons, 1992.
3. Battie MC, Videman T, Gill K, et al: Smoking and lumbar intervertebral disc degeneration: An MRI study of identical twins. Spine 1991; 16:1015–1021.
4. Bigos SJ, Battie M, Spengler DM, et al: A prospective study of work perceptions and psychosocial factors affecting the report of back injury. Spine 1991; 16:1–6.
5. Boden SD, Davis DO, Dina TS, et al: Abnormal magnetic-resonance scans of the lumbar spine in asymptomatic subjects. J Bone Joint Surg Am 1990; 72:403–408.
6. Borg GAV: Psychophysical bases of perceived exertion. Med Sci Sports Exerc 1982; 14:377–381.
7. Braddom RL: Industrial rehabilitation—an overview. Phys Med Rehabil Clin North Am 1992; 3:499–511.
8. Cady LD, Bischoff DP, O'Connell ER, et al: Strength and fitness and subsequent back injuries in firefighters. J Occup Med 1979; 21:269–272.
9. Cady L, Thomas P, Karawasky R: Increasing health and physical fitness of firefighters. J Occup Med 1985; 27:110–114.
10. Daltroy LH, Larson MG, Wright EA, et al: A case-control study of risk factors for industrial low back injury: Implications for primary and secondary prevention programs. Am J Ind Med 1991; 20:505–515.
11. Derebery VJ, Tullis WH: Delayed recovery in the patient with a work compensable injury. J Occup Med 1983; 25:829–835.
12. Deyo RA, Diehl AK, Rosenthal M: How many days of bed rest for acute low back pain? N Engl J Med 1986; 315:1064–1070.
13. Deyo RA, Loeser JD, Bigos SJ: Herniated lumbar intervertebral disc. Ann Intern Med 1990; 112:598–603.
14. Dolney WP: Restricted work-activity programs minimize injury compensation cost. Occup Health Saf 1992; 61:75, 89.
15. Doyle Y, Conroy R: The spectrum of farming accidents seen in Irish general practice: A 1-year survey. Fam Pract 1989; 6:38–41.
16. Ellenberg MR, Ross ML, Honet JC, et al: Prospective evaluation of the course of disc herniations in patients with proven radiculopathy. Arch Phys Med Rehabil 1993; 74:3–8.
17. Erdil M, Dickerson OB, Chaffin DB: Biomechanics of manual materials handling and low-back pain. In Zenz C, Dickerson OB, Horvath EP (eds): Occupational Medicine, ed 3. St Louis, Mosby–Year Book, 1994, pp 239–257.
18. Erdil M, Dickerson OB, Glackin E: Cumulative trauma disorders of the upper extremity. In Zenz C, Dickerson OB, Horvath EP (eds): Occupational Medicine, ed 3. St Louis, Mosby–Year Book, 1994, pp 48–64.
19. Feldstein A, Vollmer W, Valanis B: Evaluating the patient-handling tasks of nurses. J Occup Med 1990; 32:1009–1013.
20. Frumkin H, Camara VM: Occupational health and safety in Brazil. Am J Public Health 1991; 81:1619–1624.
21. Gibson ES, Martin JE, Terry CW: Incidence of low back pain and pre-placement X-ray screening. J Occup Med 1980; 22:515–519.

22. Gogia PP, Schneider VS, LeBlanc AD, et al: Bed rest effect on extremity muscle torque in healthy men. Arch Phys Med Rehabil 1988; 69:1030–1032.

23. Graveling RA: The prevention of back pain from manual handling. Ann Occup Hyg 1991; 35:427–432.

24. Gutierrez-Fisac JL, Regidor E, Ronda E: Occupational accidents and alcohol consumption in Spain. Int J Epidemiol 1992; 21:1114–1120.

25. Harker C, Matheson AB, Ross JAS, et al: Occupational accidents presenting to the accident and emergency department. Arch Emerg Med 1992; 9:185–189.

26. Heliovaara M, Makela M, Knekt P, et al: Determinants of sciatica and low-back pain. Spine 1991; 16:608–614.

27. Hilyer JC, Brown KC, Sirles AT, et al: A flexibility intervention to reduce the incidence and severity of joint injuries among municipal firefighters. J Occup Med 1990; 32:631–637.

28. Howell E, Brown K, Atkins J: Trauma in the workplace. AAOHN J 1990; 38:467–474.

29. Jansson B, Eriksson C-G: Accident involvement and attitudes towards hazards and countermeasures in a Swedish rural population. Scand J Soc Med 1990; 18:139–142.

30. Kelsey JL, White AA: Epidemiology and impact of low-back pain. Spine 1980; 5:133–142.

31. Keyserling WM, Herrin GD, Chaffin DB: Isometric strength testing as a means of controlling medical incidents on strenuous jobs. J Occup Med 1980; 22:332–336.

32. Krusen EM, Ford DE: Compensation factor in low back injuries. JAMA 1958; 166:1128–1133.

33. Lampard EE: Industrial revolution. In The World Book Encyclopedia, vol 10. Chicago, World Book, 1985, p 186–195.

34. Low I, Holz A: Approach to risk reduction in manufacturing firms in Australia. Occup Med 1993; 43:43–46.

35. Magora A, Schwartz A: Relation between low back pain and X-ray changes. Scand J Rehabil Med 1980; 12:47–52.

36. Mathur N, Sharma KKR, Tiwari VK: Orthopaedic industrial injuries. J Indian Med Assoc 1990; 88:153–154.

37. Mayer TC, Gatchel RJ, Mager H, et al: A prospective 2-year study of functional restoration in industrial low back injury: An objective assessment procedure. JAMA 1987; 258:1763–1767.

38. McKenzie RA: Prophylaxis in recurrent low back pain. N Z Med J 1979; 89:22–23.

39. Merchant JA: Agricultural injuries. Occup Med 1991; 6:529–539.

40. Mitchell LV, Lawler FH, Bowen D, et al: Effectiveness and cost-effectiveness of employer-issued back belts in areas of high risk for back injury. J Occup Med 1994; 36:90–94.

41. Nachemson A: Work for all. Clin Orthop 1983; 179:77–82.

42. Nachemson AL: Advances in low-back pain. Clin Orthop 1985; 200:266–278.

43. Novak RD, Smolensky MH, Fairchild EJ, et al: Shiftwork and industrial injuries at a chemical plant in southeast Texas. Chronobiol Int 1990; 7:155–164.

44. Novek J, Yassi A, Spiegel J: Mechanization, the labor process, and injury risks in the Canadian meat packing industry. Intl J Health Serv 1990; 20:281–296.

45. O'Conner FG, Marlowe SS: Low back pain in military basic trainees. Spine 1993; 18:1351–1354.

46. Paajanen H, Erkintalo M, Kuusela T, et al: Magnetic resonance study of disc degeneration in young low-back pain patients. Spine 1989; 14:982–985.

47. Perry GF: Lumbar support belts in occupational medicine forum. J Occup Med 1992; 34:679–680.

48. Rempel DM, Harrison RJ, Barnhart S: Work-related cumulative trauma disorders of the upper extremity. JAMA 1992; 267:838–842.

49. Rodgers SH, Eggleton EM: Ergonomic Design for People at Work, vol 1. New York, Van Nostrand Reinhold, 1983.

50. Rodgers SH, Kenworthy DA, Eggleton EM: Ergonomic Design for People at Work, vol 2. New York, Van Nostrand Reinhold, 1986.

51. Ruckert A, Rohmert W, Pressel G: Ergonomic research study on aircraft luggage handling. Ergonomics 1992; 35:997–1012.

52. Saal JA, Saal JS: Nonoperative treatment of herniated lumbar intervertebral disc with radiculopathy—an outcome study. Spine 1989; 14:431–437.

53. Sander RA, Meyers JE: The relationship of disability to compensation status in railroad workers. Spine 1986; 11:141–143.

54. Scheer SJ: Ergonomics. Phys Med Rehabil Clin North Am 1992; 3:599–614.

55. Schuchmann JA: Low back pain: A comprehensive approach. Compr Ther 1988; 14:14–18.

56. Verville RE: The Americans with Disabilities Act: An analysis. Arch Phys Med Rehabil 1990; 71:1010–1013.

57. Waddell G, McCulloch JA, Kummel E, Venner RM: Nonorganic physical signs in low-back pain. Spine 1980; 5:117–125.

58. Waller JA, Payne SR, Skelly JM: Disability, direct cost, and payment issues in injuries involving woodworking and wood-related construction. Accid Anal Prev 1990; 22:351–360.

59. Walsh NE, Dumitru D: Compensation and low back pain. PMR 1991; 5:223–236.

60. Walsh NE, Schwartz R: Prevention of back injury in the work place. Phys Med Rehabil Clin North Am 1992; 3:553–561.

61. Webster B, Snook SH: The cost of compensable low back pain. J Occup Med 1990; 32:13–15.

62. Weinreb JC, Wolbarsht LB, Cohen JM, et al: Prevalence of lumbosacral intervertebral disk abnormalities on MR images in pregnant and asymptomatic nonpregnant women. Radiology 1989; 170:125–128.

63. Werneke MW, Harris DE, Lichter RL: Clinical effectiveness of behavioral signs for screening chronic low-back pain patients in a work-oriented physical rehabilitation program. Spine 1993; 18:2412–2418.

64. Williams TH, Current RN, Freidel F: A History of the United States, ed 2. New York, Knopf, 1965, pp 86–94.

65. Yu T, Roht LH, Wise RA, et al: Low-back pain in industry. J Occup Med 1984; 26:517–524.

Rehabilitation Concepts in Motor Neuron Diseases

JAMES C. AGRE, M.D., PH.D., AND
DENNIS J. MATTHEWS, M.D.

This chapter focuses on the rehabilitation of patients with *motor neuron diseases*, defined as diseases or conditions that produce dysfunction of the motor neurons, which then result in weakness and muscle wasting. These include diseases or conditions that affect the upper (corticobulbar and corticospinal) motor neurons, the bulbar and spinal lower motor neurons, or both.

Patients who have diseases or conditions affecting the motor neurons often benefit from rehabilitative care. As with all diseases and disorders, the management of the patient with a motor neuron disease begins with a complete evaluation in order to establish as precise a diagnosis as possible. This allows the rehabilitation professional to determine the prognosis for progression or improvement of the disorder and assists in the determination of the best course of therapeutic intervention.

There are a number of textbooks and chapters which review these neuromuscular disorders in greater detail.* It is not the purpose of this chapter to provide all of the features of each disorder. Rather, the chapter briefly highlights these disorders, including their epidemiology, genetics, clinical features, and pathology, which should be of assistance to the treating clinician. The main focus is to outline the rehabilitation issues involved in treating patients with these disorders and diseases.

CLASSIFICATION OF MOTOR NEURON DISEASES

Motor neuron diseases can be classified in a number of ways. The following classification is based on the location of pathophysiological involvement of these diseases and disorders as described in much greater detail by Hudson[59] (Table 45–1).

---

*References 18, 19, 33, 41, 59, 68, 80, 87, 123, 129, 131.

Upper Motor Neuron Disorders

Primary Lateral Sclerosis

Primary lateral sclerosis (PLS) is a rare, nonfamilial, slowly progressive corticobulbar and corticospinal tract disease of unknown cause.[59] In a review of 19 cases, Hudson reported the age of onset from 20 to 60 years with an equal incidence in men and women.[59]

CLINICAL FEATURES. The onset of spasticity is usually noted in the lower limbs in this disorder, although occasionally spasticity is first noted in the upper limbs or the bulbar musculature. As the disorder progresses, spasticity is found in all limbs and the bulbar musculature. Urinary incontinence can also occur, but usually not until late in the course. Survival is usually two to three or more decades. Spastic dysphagia can be life-threatening in these

TABLE 45–1 The Motor Neuron Diseases

Upper motor neuron disorders
Primary lateral sclerosis
Tropical spastic paraparesis
Lathyrism
Epidemic spastic paraparesis
Familial (hereditary) spastic paraplegia
Combined upper and lower motor neuron disorders
Amyotrophic lateral sclerosis (ALS)
Familial ALS
Western Pacific ALS–parkinsonism dementia complex
Groote Eylandt motor neuron disease
Postencephalitic (encephalitis lethargica) ALS
Juvenile inclusion body ALS
Disorders of the lower motor neuron
Spinal (bulbospinal muscular) atrophies
Monoclonal gammopathy and motor neuron disease
Cancer and motor neuron disease
Poliomyelitis and post-polio syndrome

Modified from Hudson AJ: The motor neuron diseases and related disorders. In Joynt RJ (ed): Clinical Neurology, vol 4. Philadelphia, JB Lippincott, 1991, pp 1–35.

patients. On physical examination, no signs of lower motor neuron dysfunction, such as muscle atrophy or fasciculations, are found. Electromyographic (EMG) examination of these patients does not reveal denervation. These findings differentiate this disorder from classic amyotrophic lateral sclerosis (ALS).[59]

PATHOLOGY. The pathogenesis of PLS is unknown. Pathological findings include a reduced number or absence of Betz's cells in the primary motor cortex or precentral gyri accompanied by degeneration of the corticospinal pathways while other structures are spared.[59]

Tropical Spastic Paraparesis

Tropical spastic paraparesis (TSP) is found in clusters in the tropics (in particular the Seychelles; Tumaco, Colombia; and the West Indies) as well as in Central and South America, India, Africa, and Japan.[59, 108] All races are vulnerable to the disease, although it is primarily found in the black population. The disease is primarily found in adults and the incidence is approximately equal in males and females.[59] Details of the disease are described elsewhere.[59]

Lathyrism

Lathyrism is an upper motor neuron disorder produced by excessive consumption of the chickling pea (*Lathyrus sativus*) or its close relatives. The toxic agent thought to cause this disorder is β-*N*-oxalylamino-L-alanine (BOAA). This is an agonist of the excitatory neurotransmitter glutamate.[59, 119] Lathyrism is endemic to the Indian subcontinent, as the chickling pea is used as an emergency food in times of drought or flooding. The disease is more common in men, who are also more severely affected by the disorder.[79] The age of onset of the disorder ranges from 2 to 70 years in both sexes and is commonly seen in males between the ages of 5 and 40 and in females between the ages of 6 and 20.[59] Details of the disease are described elsewhere.[59]

Epidemic Spastic Paraparesis

Epidemic spastic paraparesis is clinically similar to tropical spastic paraparesis, but is considered to be etiologically different as the disorder affects children as well as adults and because the patients are seronegative for human T-cell lymphotropic virus type 1 (HTLV-1).[109] The etiologic factor involved is unknown, but it may be infective or nutritional. Details of the disease are described elsewhere.[59]

Familial (Hereditary) Spastic Paraplegia

Familial spastic paraplegia can be transmitted as an autosomal dominant, occasionally as an autosomal recessive, and very rarely as an X-linked recessive syndrome.[59] The disorder can appear at any age, but usually occurs in childhood or early adult life.

CLINICAL FEATURES. The onset of familial spastic paraplegia is accompanied by complaints of stiffness and unsteadiness of the legs and gradually results in a spastic paraplegia. Muscular atrophy has been reported in some cases of familial spastic paraplegia, often in only one or two members of a large pedigree, and has been identified as a motor neuron and not a primary myopathic disorder.[59]

PATHOLOGY. The pathogenesis of familial spastic paraplegia is unknown. The pathological findings in this disease, reflecting its genetic transmission, are diverse. Symmetrical bilateral degeneration of the pyramidal pathway, spinocerebellar tract, and fasciculus gracilis has been reported in this disorder.[59, 114] In the amyotrophic form of this disorder, a severe loss of anterior horn cells, particularly in the cervical and lumbar areas, has been reported.[43, 59]

Combined Upper and Lower Motor Neuron Disorders

Classic Amyotrophic Lateral Sclerosis

Amyotrophic lateral sclerosis is the benchmark of the motor neuron disorders. ALS encompasses two conditions, progressive bulbar palsy and progressive muscular atrophy, which differ only in their site of onset.[59] Progressive bulbar palsy initially affects the bulbar motor neurons while progressive muscular atrophy initially affects the spinal motor neurons. These two diseases tend to overlap the longer the patient survives.

EPIDEMIOLOGY. The classic form of ALS is so called because it is the most prevalent motor neuron disease and because it was one of the first to be recognized.[59] The incidence of this disease is approximately 1.6 to 2.4 cases per 100,000 population, but varies with age.[59] As reported by Hudson and colleagues, the average incidence of ALS in southwestern Ontario was 1.6 per 100,000 population, but increased from the third (0.2/100,000 population) to the eighth decade of life (7.4/100,000 population).[59, 60] The average age at time of diagnosis in this study was 62 years.[59] The average survival from time of diagnosis is approximately 2.5 years, but varies with age. Survival is reported to be somewhat shorter for patients over the age of 50.[59] The male-to-female ratio varies from 1.2 to 1.6 to 1.[59]

CLINICAL FEATURES. Most patients with classic ALS complain of weakness. At the time of the initial examination lower motor neuron signs of atrophy, weakness, and fasciculations are frequently noted. In addition to these signs, muscle stretch reflexes can be depressed in regions where there is primarily lower motor neuron involvement or where atrophy is so advanced that upper motor neuron signs cannot be demonstrated. Otherwise, it is common to find brisk muscle stretch reflexes in areas of muscle atrophy.[59] Occasionally, the patient presents only with mild spasticity, suggesting a purely upper motor neuron disorder. The most notable of these cases are patients who present initially with spastic dysarthria or facies or both with no detectable lower motor neuron signs.[59] Muscle cramping is also a frequent complaint.

The most striking feature of ALS in general is the focal, and often asymmetrical, onset of weakness, which then spreads from the initial site to adjacent areas of the body.[59] Spasticity can be very disabling and can produce significant deformities of the hand.[59] Spasticity and clonus can make ambulation difficult. Except for constipation due to poor nutritional intake or inactivity, the bowel and bladder are spared in this disease. Sensation is generally spared, although subtle symptoms and signs of sensory involvement, complaints of paresthesias, and the finding of decreased vibratory sense can be found in up to 25% of patients.[59, 89] A small percentage of individuals with classic ALS also show signs of dementia (about 3.5%) or parkinsonism (about 1.5%).[58–60, 76]

PATHOLOGY. The pathogenesis of classic ALS is unknown. Characteristic pathological findings in classic ALS include degeneration or complete loss of motor neurons in the brainstem and spinal cord areas corresponding to the muscle atrophy and degeneration of the large pyramidal neurons in the primary motor cortex and of the pyramidal tracts.[59] Onuf's nucleus (controlling the striated muscles of the pelvic floor and the bowel and bladder sphincters) is preserved.[59]

Familial Amyotrophic Lateral Sclerosis

Familial ALS is clinically identical to classic ALS except for a somewhat younger average age of onset. From a review of the world literature and inclusion of their own cases, Strong and colleagues[122] reported a mean age at time of diagnosis of 46 years in familial ALS. They also found a bimodal distribution of survival in these patients with peaks of survival at 2 years and 12 years from the time of initial diagnosis. The pattern of inheritance is reported to be autosomal dominant,[115] but a recessively inherited form of chronic juvenile ALS has been reported.[13]

CLINICAL FEATURES. The clinical features of familial ALS are similar to those of classic ALS.[59]

PATHOLOGY. The pathogenesis of familial ALS is unknown. In addition to the degenerative changes in the pyramidal pathways and the lower motor neurons, as found in classic ALS, familial cases of ALS also show degenerative changes in the middle zones of the posterior columns, dorsal spinocerebellar tract, and the dorsal nucleus of Clarke.[59]

Western Pacific Amyotrophic Lateral Sclerosis–Parkinsonism Dementia Complex

The combination of ALS, parkinsonism, and dementia (ALS-PD complex) is found in a high incidence in some small populations in the western Pacific (as in the islands of Guam, Rota, and Tinian of the Mariana Islands).[59] These islands have a distinctive population, which is unlike the population of other island groups in their geographical vicinity.

EPIDEMIOLOGY. The pathogenesis of western Pacific ALS is unknown, but several hypotheses have been made, including the lack of calcium in soil and water leading to secondary hyperparathyroidism and subsequently to neuronal damage,[39] a toxic substance in the cycad seed (used as food and medicine) causing neuronal damage,[118] or that it is a sequel to encephalitis lethargica, which was pandemic in the 1920s.[61] Although neither of the last two hypotheses has been proved, both are supported by the significant decline in incidence of ALS on Guam from 50 to less than 5 cases per 100,000 population from the mid-1950s to the mid-1980s.[107]

CLINICAL FEATURES. The clinical features of western Pacific ALS are the same as classic ALS; however, the ALS-PD complex adds the symptoms and signs of parkinsonism and dementia.[59]

PATHOLOGY. The pathological findings in western Pacific ALS are the same as for classic ALS but in addition have neurofibrillary changes in certain neurons.[59]

Groote Eylandt Motor Neuron Disease

This is a very rare disorder that affects Australian aborigines and is found on Groote Eylandt in the Gulf of Carpentaria.[59]

Postencephalitic (Encephalitis Lethargica) Amyotrophic Lateral Sclerosis

The epidemic of encephalitis lethargica peaked in 1920 and 1924 and some of those who survived developed ALS.[59] The average interval between the acute encephalitis and onset of ALS was 10 years, but in some cases ALS occurred up to 30 years later.[59]

Juvenile Inclusion Body Amyotrophic Lateral Sclerosis

Juvenile inclusion body ALS is a rare condition that is clinically identical to classic ALS, except that it affects persons between the ages of 12 and 16 years.[59] The duration of the illness is also somewhat shorter than classic ALS, with survival between 1 and 1½ years from time of diagnosis.

Lower Motor Neuron Disorders

Infantile Forms of Spinal or Bulbospinal Muscular Atrophies

Acute Infantile Spinal Muscular Atrophy (Werdnig-Hoffmann Disease, Type I Spinal Muscular Atrophy, Acute Proximal Hereditary Motor Neuropathy)

The chronic form of this disease was first described by Werdnig[130] and by Hoffmann.[56] It is an autosomal recessive disorder[68] with an estimated incidence ranging from 1 in 15,000 to 1 in 25,000 live births.[96] The disease is already manifest in one third of the children by the time of birth through decreased fetal movements or by congenital arthrogryposis.[98] The diagnosis is usually made by the age of 3 months and certainly by the age of 6 months. The average survival from time of diagnosis is 6 to 9 months and survival does not exceed 3 years.[22, 95]

CLINICAL FEATURES. The clinical picture is dominated by severe hypotonia and weakness. There are resultant delays in motor milestones. At the time of birth the baby is usually floppy (hypotonic) with generalized weakness and absence of reflexes. Feeding difficulty and poor breathing are soon readily apparent. Progressive muscle weakness, atrophy of the trunk and limbs, hypotonia, and feeding difficulties are the primary clinical features.[68] The infants characteristically lie motionless with the lower limbs abducted in the frog-leg position.[68] The face often lacks expression with an open mouth due to facial muscle weakness.[18] Intercostal muscle paralysis is evident and fasciculations are present. Fasciculations of the tongue are almost pathognomonic for the disease.[18] The cause of death is typically respiratory failure.[59]

PATHOLOGY. The pathogenesis of acute infantile spinal muscular atrophy is unknown. Severe loss of motor neurons throughout the brainstem and spinal cord is the primary pathological finding.[59]

Chronic Infantile Spinal Muscular Atrophy (Chronic Werdnig-Hoffmann Disease, Type II Spinal Muscular Atrophy, Chronic Proximal Hereditary Motor Neuropathy)

The chronic form of Werdnig-Hoffmann disease is much more slowly progressive than the acute form of this disease. This actually was the form of the disease initially described by Werdnig and Hoffmann.[56, 59, 130] Clinical signs indicative of this disease are usually present by the age of 3 years, but occasionally occur as early as 3 months of age.[95] This disease has variable progression and the median age of death is about 12 years,[59] with some individuals surviving into the third decade.[18] This disease is autosomal recessive[68] and the gene for chronic spinal muscular atrophy has been found on chromosome 5q.[85]

CLINICAL FEATURES. Weakness and atrophy are predominantly proximal with the lower limbs being more involved initially than the upper limbs. Muscle stretch reflexes are reduced or absent. Sensation is normal. Owing to the gradually progressive weakness, scoliosis, thoracic deformities, and equinus deformities of the feet usually develop as the disease progresses.[59]

PATHOLOGY. The pathogenesis of chronic infantile spinal muscular atrophy is unknown. The pathological findings are the same as for the acute infantile form.[59]

Juvenile and Adult Forms of Spinal or Bulbospinal Muscular Atrophies

Juvenile and Adult Proximal Spinal Muscular Atrophy (Kugelberg-Welander Disease, Type III Spinal Muscular Atrophy, Recessive Proximal Hereditary Motor Neuropathy; Type IV Spinal Muscular Atrophy, [Juvenile] Dominant Proximal Hereditary Motor Neuropathy; Type V Spinal Muscular Atrophy, [Adult] Dominant Proximal Hereditary Motor Neuropathy)

The juvenile and adult forms of spinal muscular atrophy (Kugelberg-Welander disease) are characterized by slowly progressive weakness and atrophy of the proximal limb and girdle musculature.[74] It is genetically transmitted, usually as an autosomal recessive disorder (type III proximal hereditary motor neuropathy), but also can be autosomal dominant (type IV juvenile and type V adult proximal hereditary motor neuropathy).[9, 59, 126] The clinical onset of the disease can occur anytime between childhood and the seventh decade of life,[59] but is usually between the age of 2 and 17 years.[123] The duration is also quite variable, ranging from 2 to more than 40 years.[42] It occurs predominantly in males.[59]

CLINICAL FEATURES. Both the juvenile and adult forms of proximal spinal muscular atrophy begin with symmetrical atrophy and weakness of the pelvic girdle and proximal lower limbs. This is followed by involvement of the shoulder girdles and upper arms. The leg and forearm musculature is affected later. Fasciculations are noted in about half the cases. Dysphagia and dysarthria can occur late in the disease and are usually mild.[59]

PATHOLOGY. The pathogenesis of juvenile and adult proximal spinal muscular atrophy is presently unknown. Owing to the chronicity of this disorder, the muscle biopsy shows a pattern similar to that found in primary myopathy with the presence of both atrophic and hypertrophic fibers. Postmortem studies have shown a loss of spinal motor neurons, but no degeneration of the corticospinal tract.[59]

Bulbar Disease of Childhood (Fazio-Londe Disease and Brown-Vialetto-van Laere Syndrome)

There are two forms of progressive bulbar paralysis of childhood: Fazio-Londe disease and Brown-Vialetto-van Laere syndrome. Both cause a slowly progressive weakness of the muscles of the face, tongue, and pharynx.[59] Most cases of Fazio-Londe disease were described between 1876 and 1925. The age of onset ranged from 2 to 12 years and duration was reported as short as 9 months to no longer than 8 years.[59] Inheritance appears to be autosomal recessive.[44] In the Brown-Vialetto-van Laere syndrome the first symptom is bilateral deafness, which occurs between the age of 18 months and 31 years (average onset at 12 years of age).[44] Cranial nerve palsies usually appear about 4 to 5 years later. Survival may exceed two decades after onset. Inheritance is reported to be autosomal recessive.[44, 59]

CLINICAL FEATURES. Most reported cases describe only bulbar weakness, although a few cases have also involved the limbs.[40] In Fazio-Londe disease all of the bulbar motor neurons are affected.[44, 59] In Brown-Vialetto-van Laere syndrome cranial nerves VII through XII are affected in almost all cases while cranial nerves III, V, and VI can be affected.[59]

PATHOLOGY. The pathogenesis of bulbar disease of childhood is unknown. Postmortem findings show a loss of motor neurons of the oculomotor, trochlear, abducens, facial, vagus, and hypoglossal nerves.[44]

Distal Spinal Muscular Atrophy (Distal Hereditary Motor Neuropathy)

Distal spinal muscular atrophy is also known as the "spinal form of Charcot-Marie-Tooth disease" and "distal hereditary motor neuropathy."[59] There are a number of different forms of distal spinal muscular atrophy with different inheritance patterns: (1) autosomal recessive juvenile mild (onset between 2 and 10 years of age) and juvenile severe (onset between 4 months and 20 years) and (2) autosomal dominant in the juvenile (onset between 2 and 20 years) and in the adult (onset between 20 and 40 years).[52, 59, 83, 97] The majority of the cases reported, however, are sporadic and a recessive inheritance is suspected.[59] Life expectancy is normal except in some severe juvenile cases.[59]

CLINICAL FEATURES. Weakness and atrophy are most often initially noted distally in the legs, especially in the anterior tibial and peroneal muscles.[59] Usually the upper limbs are spared, but rarely are predominantly affected.[53] Leg weakness in severe cases can also involve the thigh musculature.[59] Sensory examination and motor and sensory nerve conduction velocities are normal.[59]

PATHOLOGY. The pathogenesis of distal spinal muscular atrophy is unknown. Other than findings of neurogenic muscular atrophy, the pathology of this entity has not been explored.[59]

Adult Forms of Bulbar and Bulbospinal Muscular Atrophies

Scapuloperoneal (Facioscapuloperoneal) Muscular Atrophy

Scapuloperoneal muscular atrophy has an autosomal dominant inheritance. The atrophy begins between 30 and 50 years of age. The disease is slow in its progression. Patients do not become incapacitated until at least 10 to 20 years after its onset and have a normal life expectancy.[59]

CLINICAL FEATURES. Weakness and atrophy begin in the muscles of the legs, but the intrinsic muscles of the feet are spared.[59] Several years later the shoulder girdle musculature and later yet the musculature of the thigh, pelvic girdle, upper arm, neck, and face become affected.[59] At this stage the disorder appears similar to facioscapuloperoneal muscular dystrophy, but in the latter disorder the shoulder girdle musculature is affected first. In some cases dysphonia or dysphagia occurs.[59] There are no upper motor neuron or sensory findings on physical examination, but the EMG reveals fibrillation potentials and fasciculations.

PATHOLOGY. The pathogenesis of scapuloperoneal muscular atrophy is unknown. Other than findings consistent with chronic denervation, the pathology of this entity has not been explored.[59]

Chronic Bulbospinal Muscular Atrophy of Late Onset

Two families have been described in which a slowly progressive proximal spinal and bulbar muscular atrophy began between the third and sixth decade of life. Only males were affected, consistent with an X-linked recessive inheritance.[59, 67, 112] This disorder, also known as Kennedy's disease, has assumed importance because of the recognition of a specific chromosomal defect.[38] Studies using DNA probes have shown that this disorder is indeed an X-linked recessive rather than an autosomal defect with sex-limited expression, and the gene defect is localized to the proximal long arm of the X chromosome.[38] Life expectancy is normal.[59]

CLINICAL FEATURES. Muscular weakness and atrophy are first noticed about the shoulder and pelvic girdle musculature. Distal muscular weakness becomes detectable later, but is never as severe as in the proximal musculature. Bulbar changes, including dysarthria, dysphagia, and atrophy of the tongue, appear later. Bowel and bladder function are preserved, sensory examination is normal, and no evidence of upper motor neuron involvement is present.[59] EMG shows potentials consistent with denervation.

PATHOLOGY. The pathogenesis of chronic bulbospinal muscular atrophy of late onset is unknown. A postmortem examination of one case revealed loss of motor neurons and neurogenic atrophy of skeletal muscle. No other spinal cord degenerative changes were found.[59]

Monomelic (Segmental) Spinal Muscular Atrophy

Monomelic spinal muscular atrophy is not an inherited disorder. It has been reported to occur primarily in the Far East, most notably in India, Japan, and Malaysia.[55, 128] It occurs primarily in male juveniles or young adults and is segmental in its distribution. Often it only affects a portion of one limb such as the forearm and hand, shoulder and upper arm, or thigh.[59] The corresponding contralateral limb may also be affected. It is insidiously progressive over a period of 1 to 3 years and almost always remains focal. Cranial nerves, upper motor neurons, bowel, bladder, and sensory systems are spared.[66] The pathogenesis is unknown. The spinal (bulbospinal) muscular atrophies are summarized in Tables 45–2, 45–3, and 45–4.

Monoclonal Gammopathy and Motor Neuron Disease

Motor neuron disease can occur in association with paraproteinemia.[59] A number of patients are reported with IgG or IgM monoclonal gammopathy who have only lower motor neuron findings[93, 100, 110] and others who have combined lower and upper motor neuron signs identical with those of ALS.[12, 20, 23, 73, 111] In the patients with exclusively lower motor neuron findings, diffuse muscle weakness and atrophy are seen. The time from onset of disease to death ranges from months to years.[59] The patients with both upper and lower motor neuron signs showed all of the signs of classic ALS including nonsymmetrical muscle atrophy, fasciculation, and upper motor neuron findings.[59] The time from onset of disease to death ranged from 9 months to 4 years.[59]

Cancer and Motor Neuron Disease

The possibility of motor neuron disease occurring as an effect of cancer is difficult to evaluate at the present time because of the many other explanations for neurological signs such as metastases to the nervous system and meninges, cachexia, and other factors.[59] However, there are reports of individuals who had apparent motor neuron disease related to cancer or lymphoma.[17, 21, 46, 59, 113, 133]

TABLE 45–2   Spinal (Bulbospinal) Muscular Atrophies

Infantile
  Acute infantile spinal muscular atrophy (Werdnig-Hoffmann disease, type I spinal muscular atrophy, acute proximal hereditary motor neuropathy)
  Chronic infantile spinal muscular atrophy (Werdnig-Hoffmann disease, type II spinal muscular atrophy, chronic proximal hereditary motor neuropathy)
Juvenile and adult
  Juvenile and adult proximal spinal muscular atrophy (Kugelberg-Welander disease, type III spinal muscular atrophy, recessive proximal hereditary motor neuropathy; type IV spinal muscular atrophy, [juvenile] dominant proximal hereditary motor neuropathy; type V spinal muscular atrophy, [adult] dominant proximal hereditary motor neuropathy)
  Bulbar disease of childhood (Fazio-Londe disease, Brown-Vialetto–van Laere syndrome)
  Distal spinal muscular atrophy (distal hereditary motor neuropathy)
Adult
  Scapuloperoneal (facioscapuloperoneal) muscular atrophy
  Chronic bulbospinal muscular atrophy of late onset
  Monomelic (segmental) spinal muscular atrophy

Modified from Hudson AJ: The motor neuron diseases and related disorders: In Joynt RJ (ed): Clinical Neurology, vol 4. Philadelphia, JB Lippincott, 1991, pp 1–35.

TABLE 45–3 Spinal (Bulbospinal) Muscular Atrophies of Infancy and Childhood

Disease	Age of Onset	Weakness Distribution	Sit	Stand	Walk	Course
Werdnig-Hoffmann disease						
Type I	< 2 mo	Proximal legs abducted; face, fingers, toes normal	–	–	–	Usually die by age 2–3 yr
Type II	2–12 mo	Proximal thigh and hip muscles	+	+	–	Most die during first decade; some live through second decade
Kugelberg-Welander disease	2–17 yr (mean: 9 yr)	Normal early development; shoulder and hip girdle atrophy (Gowers' sign frequently present)	+	+	May walk for 20–40 yr after onset	

Symbols: +, ability present; –, ability not present.
Modified from Swaiman KF: Anterior horn cell and cranial motor neuron disease. *In* Swaiman KF (ed): Pediatric Neurology. Principles and Practice, vol 2. St Louis, Mosby–Year Book, 1989, pp 1083–1103.

Acute Poliomyelitis

Acute poliomyelitis occurs as a result of a generalized viral infection that has an affinity for motor neurons. The virus is a single-stranded RNA enterovirus (picornavirus) and is comprised of three antigenically distinguishable viruses.[86] Acute poliomyelitis is presently very rare in the United States. It can occur in severely immunocompromised persons or in persons who did not receive the vaccination, and were exposed to someone who recently received the oral vaccine, which has the live, attenuated virus. Although there is a worldwide attempt to eradicate poliomyelitis, acute poliomyelitis still occurs in needy countries with poor healthcare delivery systems.

The virus usually enters the body via the oral route. It replicates in the lymphoid tissues of the pharynx and the intestine. It then spreads to the regional lymphoid tissues and a viremia can follow, leading to a nonspecific illness.[69] Viremia is the most accepted mechanism for direct nervous system exposure to the virus. The reason for the selective vulnerability of certain cells, such as the motor neurons, to the poliomyelitis virus is unknown, but may be related to specific receptors on their cell membranes.[102]

The poliovirus is an extremely infectious agent, but only a fraction of those infected have symptoms.[69] The disease progresses to central nervous system involvement and paresis or paralysis in 1% to 2% of cases, while in 90% to 95% of cases the infection is inapparent, and in 4% to 8% of cases only a nonspecific illness is noted.[57] With death of the motor neurons, wallerian degeneration occurs, and the muscle fibers associated with those neurons become "orphaned," resulting in motor weakness.

In histological studies of motor neurons of monkeys with acute paralytic poliomyelitis, nearly all (96%–97%) of the motor neurons of severely paralyzed limbs were affected by the virus during the acute infection.[16] About one half of these motor neurons died during the early convalescent period, and the other half survived. A good correlation was found between the proportion of destroyed motor neurons and the severity of paralysis.[15]

Clinical Features

The incubation period is from 1 to 2 weeks.[57, 102] The onset is usually accompanied by malaise, muscle aches, and low-grade fever, which lasts from 1 to 3 days. These may cease and no further symptoms occur. Alternatively, a symptom-free period may follow, only to be followed by recurrence of systemic symptoms.[69]

The potentially paralytic illness is characterized by fever, generalized headache, and neck and back stiffness. The illness may regress or may proceed with the appearance of paralysis by the second to fifth day from onset. Muscle soreness and a sensation of tightness are present, as well as shooting pains and hyperesthesia.[69] Sensory loss is rare.[101] The weakness appears and evolves over hours to a few days. The lumbar area is more frequently involved than the cervical area or the cranial nerves.[69] Severe bulbar involvement is seen in 10% to 15% of cases.[69] Atrophy of the involved muscle groups appears within the first week. Autonomic dysfunction with cardiac arrhythmia, hypertension, hyperhidrosis, urinary retention, and constipation can occur.[82] Changes in mental status ranging from anxiety to stupor can occur and are attributed to reticular formation or hypothalamic involvement.[11]

Mortality is usually the result of bulbar or respiratory involvement. Survivors commonly gradually recover muscle function in muscles not completely paralyzed, and some ultimately have minimal or no residua. Improvements begin in the first weeks, but can continue for several years after the acute illness.[2, 49] The mechanisms of recovery include both resolution of dysfunction of partially damaged motor neurons as well as reinnervation of denervated muscle fibers by surviving motor units.

Post-Polio Syndrome

A number of reports document the complaints registered by poliomyelitis survivors. The onset of these complaints is often several decades after the acute poliomyelitis illness. In particular, new musculoskeletal and neuromuscular

TABLE 45–4   Spinal (Bulbospinal) Muscular Atrophies (SMA), Hereditary Motor Neuropathies (HMN)

Distribution and Type	Synonyms	Inheritance	Age of Onset	Age Unable to Walk	Life Expectancy
Proximal					
Type I Acute infantile	Werdnig-Hoffmann disease, SMA type I, acute proximal HMN	AR	In utero to 6 mo	Never able to walk	7–18 mo
Type II Chronic childhood	Chronic Werdnig-Hoffmann disease, SMA type II, chronic proximal HMN	AR (some new dominant mutants)	3 mo–15 yr	Median ~ 12 yr (never to 5th decade)	18 mo–40 yr
Type III Juvenile, adult	Kugelberg-Welander disease, SMA type III, recessive proximal HMN	AR	15–60 yr	Rarely > 50 yr	Normal
Type IV Juvenile onset	SMA type IV, juvenile dominant proximal HMN	AD	6 mo–5 yr (rarely up to 15 yr)	Rare	Probably normal
Type V Adult onset	SMA type V, adult dominant proximal HMN	AD	25–65 yr	? 10 yr after diagnosis	20 yr after diagnosis
Bulbospinal					
	X-linked spinal and bulbar muscular atrophy	XLR	15–60 yr (usually 20–40 yr)	? 50+ yr	Minimally limited
Distal					
Type I Juvenile onset	Spinal form of Charcot-Marie-Tooth disease (CMTD)	AD	2–20 yr	Rare	Normal
Type II Adult onset	Spinal form of CMTD	AD	20–40 yr	Rare	Normal
Type III Mild juvenile	Spinal form of CMTD	AR	2–10 yr	Rare	Normal
Type IV Severe juvenile	Spinal form of CMTD	AR	4 mo–20 yr	~30 yr	?
Type V Upper limb predominance	—	AD	5–20 yr (Some sporadic)	Never	Normal
Scapuloperoneal					
Type I	—	AD	4–70 yr	? 50+ yr	? Reduced
Type II	—	AR	2–5 yr	?	?
Facioscapulohumoral		AD	Before 20 yr	?	?
Oculopharyngeal		AD	30–40 yr	?	?
Bulbar					
Type I With deafness	Brown Vialetto van Laere syndrome	AR	Before 20 yr (? males earlier)	—	20–40 yr (? males earlier)
Type II Without deafness	Fazio-Londe disease, progressive bulbar palsy of childhood	AR	1–12 yr		50% within 18 mo of onset

Abbreviations: *AR*, autosomal recessive; *AD*, autosomal dominant; *XLR*, X-linked recessive.
Modified from Harding AE: Inherited neuronal atrophy and degeneration predominantly of lower motor neurons. *In* Dyck PJ, Thomas PK, Lambert EH, Bunge R (eds): Peripheral Neuropathy, pt 2. Philadelphia, WB Saunders, 1984, pp 1537–1556.

symptoms are acknowledged by these patients.[5, 24, 26, 27, 48–51] Table 45–5 lists the most frequent new health and activities of daily living (ADL) problems of post-polio patients, whether they were seen in a post-polio clinic[5, 49] or had responded to a national survey.[48] The most prevalent new health-related complaints were fatigue, muscle or joint pain, and weakness. The most prevalent new ADL complaints were difficulties with walking and stair climbing. Fatigue was described by many (43% in one survey) as though they were "hitting the wall."[48] Of this group, 68% acknowledged that this phenomenon occurred on a daily basis. Most commonly, this "wall" was experienced in the mid- to late afternoon. Fortunately, for almost all patients it could be ameliorated or aborted by increasing rest time, napping, or reducing the overall level of activity during the day.[48]

The typical post-polio patient seen in a post-polio clinic had the acute poliomyelitis illness in childhood (average age of onset between 5 and 10 years), had gradually improving function over a period of 5 to 8 years after the acute illness, remained clinically stable for 25 to 30 years, and then noted the onset of new health or ADL problems beginning 5 to 8 years before coming into a post-polio clinic for evaluation.[5, 26, 49]

TABLE 45–5   New Health Problems and New Problems in Activities of Daily Living (ADL) in Post-Polio Patients

Symptom	Study		
	Halstead and Rossi[48] (n = 539)	Halstead and Rossi[49] (n = 132)	Agre et al.[5] (n = 79)
New health problems			
Fatigue	87%	89%	86%
Muscle pain	80%	71%	86%
Joint pain	79%	71%	77%
Weakness			
Previously affected muscles	87%	69%	80%
Previously unaffected muscles	77%	50%	53%
Cold intolerance	—	29%	56%
Atrophy	—	28%	39%
New ADL problems			
Walking	85%	64%	—
Stair climbing	83%	61%	67%
Dressing	62%	17%	16%

The percentage of post-polio survivors experiencing new symptoms that can be related to their previous poliomyelitis illness is not precisely known. The Sister Kenny Institute study reported that 41% of their post-polio respondents to a questionnaire complained of progressive problems.[117] A Mayo Clinic study reported that approximately 25% of their cohort of 125 survivors were experiencing the late effects of poliomyelitis.[24] In an epidemiological study of 551 poliomyelitis survivors in Allegheny County, Pennsylvania, it was reported that 28.5% of the patients acknowledged post-polio syndrome.[104] It can be estimated from these reports that approximately one fourth to one third of persons who had acute poliomyelitis in the past may be experiencing post-polio syndrome at the present time. This proportion may well increase as these persons age.

A number of terms have been used to describe the problems about which some poliomyelitis survivors complain many years after their acute illness. Such terms as "late-onset postpoliomyelitis progressive muscular atrophy," "late progressive postpoliomyelitis muscular atrophy," "late postpoliomyelitis muscular atrophy," "progressive postpolio atrophy," and "progressive postpoliomyelitis muscular atrophy" have been used.[14, 27–29, 75] Since there are no empirical research data to indicate progressive atrophy or rapid decline in strength, the term "post-polio syndrome" better describes the complaints and findings of polio survivors and does not make unfounded presumptions.

Post-polio syndrome is essentially a diagnosis by exclusion.[49] A good definition of *post-polio syndrome* has been given by Halstead and Rossi and is based on five criteria:

(1) A confirmed history of paralytic polio; (2) partial to fairly complete neurologic and functional recovery; (3) a period of neurologic and functional stability of at least 15 years duration; (4) the onset of two or more of the following health problems since achieving a period of stability: unaccustomed fatigue, muscle and/or joint pain, new weak-

ness in muscles previously affected and/or unaffected, functional loss, cold intolerance, new atrophy; and (5) no other medical diagnosis to explain these health problems.[49]

A great concern for many post-polio patients is apprehension about potential future loss of strength and function. A number of possible pathophysiological and functional etiologies have been suggested to explain the reason for progressive loss of muscle strength in poliomyelitis survivors, including premature aging of motor neurons damaged by the poliovirus, premature aging of the motor neurons due to the increased metabolic demand, loss of muscle fibers within the surviving motor units, death of motor neurons due to the normal aging process, disuse weakness, overuse weakness, or weight gain.[6, 65]

Although the development of late-onset weakness in poliomyelitis survivors was first reported over a century ago,[25, 105] at the present time there is little objective evidence in the literature to indicate that the rate of loss in strength is greater than that expected as a result of the normal aging process. In several papers the determination of progressive loss in strength was made by patient report and not by longitudinal studies using valid and reliable measures. The three reports in the refereed literature that used valid and reliable measures for determination of strength in poliomyelitis survivors did not find any loss in strength.[3, 90, 91] However, one of these studies only assessed six patients over a time span of 400 to 2100 days,[91] another study assessed the strength in 34 post-polio subjects over only 1 year, and the third study assessed only seven patients over a 3-year period.[90] With only a few subjects in two of the studies and considering the short duration of the other study, it is not surprising that none of the studies detected any significant loss in strength.

Preliminary analyses from unpublished research from the laboratory of one of the authors (J.C.A.), with yearly follow-up over a 5-year period, showed that both stable and unstable post-polio patients lost strength in the quadriceps femoris muscle, but not in the biceps humerus. The rate of loss of strength in the quadriceps, however, was no greater than that found in control (non-polio) subjects.

Although a number of plausible hypothetical reasons have been suggested to explain a more rapid decline in strength in poliomyelitis survivors, there is no empirical evidence to date to indicate that the loss of strength is directly related to poliomyelitis and it may instead be a reflection of the aging process in persons with impaired function.

EVALUATION OF THE PATIENT WITH MOTOR NEURON DISEASE

History

The initial phase in the management of a patient with a motor neuron disorder is, of course, to establish the diagnosis, which allows the clinician to better determine the progression of the disorder. Obtaining a detailed history is the first step in this process. The major complaints of the patients and their parents (in the case of childhood diseases) should be noted. The pattern of weakness can be helpful in determining the specific motor neuron disease.

It can be difficult at times to distinguish between some of the motor neuron disorders, muscular dystrophies, and neuropathies. A careful history is essential in this regard. In general, patients with neuropathic disorders usually give a history of distal rather than proximal weakness, often accompanied by sensory abnormalities (which are rare in the motor neuron disorders). It can be difficult, however, to separate the muscular dystrophies from the motor neuron disorders by history alone.

Significant elements to be obtained during the history include the age of onset of difficulties and the rate of progression of the disorder. The distribution of the weakness is also an important clue. The patient with distal weakness will, for instance, have difficulty in holding objects. The patient with proximal lower limb weakness may have difficulty arising from a chair, whereas a patient with proximal upper limb weakness may have difficulty placing an object upon a shelf. Muscle pain is very common in inflammatory neuropathies and myopathies, but is uncommon in motor neuron disorders (except for acute poliomyelitis, where it is usually seen). A careful family history is also important because a number of the motor neuron disorders are genetically transmitted. The history is very important in learning about the patient's social environment, such as support from family and friends. This is perhaps the most important factor in determining whether the patient will be able to live at home or need institutional care. Assessing the patient's living environment is also important in determining the assistive devices that might be needed to preserve function and independence.

Physical Examination

Visual inspection usually reveals areas of significant muscular atrophy, muscular hypertrophy (which can be found in some of the muscular dystrophies), and fasciculations. Visual inspection for atrophy assists in determining whether the disease involvement is greater in the proximal or the distal limb musculature. Palpation of the limbs can reveal the muscle tenderness that is found in inflammatory myopathies, but which is rare in motor neuron diseases other than acute poliomyelitis.

The sensory examination detects any sensory loss, which is very rare in motor neuron diseases, but common in the neuropathic disorders. Muscle stretch reflexes can be increased in the upper motor neuron disorders or in the combined upper and lower motor neuron disorders, but are reduced to absent in the lower motor neuron disorders. In the combined upper and lower motor neuron disorders, the muscle stretch reflexes can be increased or decreased, depending on the associated muscular weakness and atrophy. In the presence of significant weakness, the upper motor neuron component can be difficult to detect. Manual muscle testing demonstrates the level of residual muscle function and shows the distribution of the weakness (whether proximal, distal, or asymmetrical). Residual strength assessment allows for an estimation of residual functional capabilities and what assistive devices might be most helpful in improving or maintaining function.

Assessment of range of motion allows for the detection of contractures. It is important to determine passive range of motion in these patients as muscle weakness can sig-

nificantly limit active range of motion. Contractures can significantly limit the patient's functional abilities. For instance, mild flexion contractures of the elbows do not result in significant disability, but slight flexion contractures of the hips or knees can preclude ambulation in the patient with weak hip or knee extensor musculature.[63, 127]

A thorough functional assessment of the patient allows the rehabilitation team to determine the patient's present level of functional abilities including the patient's abilities to be mobile in bed, to transfer, to ambulate with or without assistive devices or be mobile in a wheelchair, and to perform all of the usual ADL (see Chapter 1). This also allows the rehabilitation team to determine what assistive devices would help the patient be most functional and independent, now and in the future as the disorder progresses.

Laboratory Evaluation

In the evaluation of a patient suspected of having a motor neuron disease, it is important to carefully investigate laboratory studies to rule out other potentially remedial causes of motor neuron disorder.

Electrodiagnosis

Electrodiagnostic testing is an important part of the evaluation of the patient suspected of having a motor neuron disease. Nerve conduction studies can confirm the presence or absence of peripheral neuropathy (see Chapters 7 and 8).[125] The EMG can be of assistance is differentiating neuropathy and myopathy,[125] and in the determination of loss of motor neurons, the amount of denervation, and the presence of collateral reinnervation.[8, 30, 131] An additional important role for EMG is to determine the muscle most appropriate for muscle biopsy. Because trauma to the muscle from the EMG needle can produce histological changes in the muscle that make interpretation difficult, it has been recommended that the EMG be limited to one side of the body. Because these disorders are usually symmetrical, an appropriate muscle from the other side of the body can then be recommended for the biopsy.[125]

Muscle Biopsy

The best muscle for biopsy depends on the experience of the clinician. The EMG can help to select a muscle that is definitely involved, but not so severely involved that it represents only end-stage disease, which would limit its diagnostic utility. The muscle biopsy can confirm whether the muscle is normal or abnormal and help classify the abnormal muscle as myopathic or neuropathic in origin.[125] The muscle biopsy can also be of significance in determining whether the disorder is an inflammatory myopathy, since most inflammatory myopathies are amenable to treatment.[125]

Other Laboratory Evaluations

Depending on the clinical presentation of the patient, the clinical laboratory investigation of the patient can consist of a number of other evaluations including serum protein electrophoresis (looking for evidence of monoclonal gammopathy or paraproteinemia), anti-acetylcholine receptor antibodies (looking for evidence of myasthenia gravis), various antiviral antibody titers (such as HLTV-1 and human immunodeficiency virus [HIV]), serum hexosaminidase A determination (looking for GM_2 gangliosidosis), anti-GM_1 and GD_{1a} ganglioside IgM antibodies (which may be elevated in ALS and motor neuropathy), endocrine tests (looking for such disorders as diabetes mellitus or thyrotoxicosis), metabolic and blood cell (looking for amyotrophic choreic acanthocytosis) studies, serum creatine kinase (usually normal in the motor neuron diseases but often elevated in myopathies), and heavy metal analysis of the urine (looking for such problems as lead and mercury intoxication).[59, 87] The spinal fluid evaluation of patients with motor neuron diseases is usually normal; any elevation of the spinal fluid protein above 80 mg/dL should lead the clinician to suspect another disorder.[132]

GENERAL PRINCIPLES OF REHABILITATION MANAGEMENT

Specific treatment for the pathophysiological processes in motor neuron disease is lacking at the present time. The best approach currently is prevention, by vaccination for the viral diseases, education to prevent toxic exposures, and genetic counseling for the hereditary diseases. Overall management should be divided into (1) prospective care and (2) expectant care.[99] The rehabilitation team should assist the patient in maximizing function and independence for as long as is possible.

Prospective care includes all the usual measures provided to all people regardless of their health status and includes such things as vaccinations and health screening tests.[99] Expectant care includes anticipation of complications that might be expected during the course of the patient's motor neuron disease. Aggressive measures can be taken to prevent or minimize these complications and maximize the patient's function and independence for as long as possible.[99] The expected complications include pain, muscle tightness, deformities of bones and joints, weakness, impaired ventilation, and impaired functional abilities.[99]

Pain

Pain is not usually a major problem in motor neuron diseases except for acute poliomyelitis. Patients with acute poliomyelitis complain of severe muscle pain.[70] Control of pain can usually be accomplished by both physical treatments as well as pharmacological treatment. The use of hot packs, especially the Kenny hot packs (made from woolen blankets), applied at 5-min intervals for 20 min, have been found to be useful in the acute stages.[70] Heat treatments along with stretching are useful in the acute stages to control pain as well as to maintain range of motion.[70] Salicylates or other nonsteroidal anti-inflammatory medications can also be helpful. Narcotic analgesics should be used sparingly because of potential respiratory depression. For neuritic pain, the tricyclic antidepressant medications, such as amitriptyline or carbamazepine, can be used.[99] The combination of physical treatment and nonsteroidal anti-inflammatory medication usually adequately controls the pain.

Muscle Tightness

Soft tissue contractures can occur at all stages in motor neuron disease. Muscles that span two joints are often the first to become tight, usually with the joint in the flexed position[99] (contracture; Table 45–6). Physical treatment includes passive, active-assistive, and active stretching, depending on the condition of the patient, usually after the application of superficial heat. A heated pool allows heat treatment and exercise to be combined.[99] Appropriate positioning also facilitates prolonged stretching and prevents deformity.[72, 78] Bracing to aid in the prevention of contractures requires careful assessment of kinesiological factors. When preventing or correcting shortening of a muscle that spans two joints, be certain that the muscles are stretched at both joints that they cross.[99]

Spasticity

In some motor neuron diseases, considerable spasticity can occur. This is treated similarly to the treatment of spasticity in other conditions (see Chapter 29).

Deformity

Malalignment of body segments leads to contracture and deformity.[72] Care must be taken in the prospective treatment of patients with motor neuron disease to prevent or minimize the development of contracture or deformity.[99] As briefly described above, appropriate stretching, bracing, and positioning help prevent contractures.

Care must also be taken in the prescription of equipment provided to patients to prevent contracture and progressive deformity wherever possible. Children are often placed in large wheelchairs to allow for growth, but such positioning does not properly support the child and can lead to contracture and subsequent deformity. For instance, a child sitting in a large wheelchair with a sling-type seat frequently results in the child sitting in the wheelchair with one hip higher than the other, with the hips internally rotated and adducted, and leaning on one elbow for support[99] (Fig. 45–1A). This postural asymmetry leads to contracture and to subsequent deformity. The minimal wheelchair prescription should include a firm seat, with adequate lumbar, truncal, and arm support (Fig. 45–1B). Deformities can be prevented or minimized by the avoidance of malalignment by appropriate stretching, positioning, and bracing. If malalignments are fixed or rapidly advancing, they can be treated by aggressive stretching with serial casts or dynamic bracing or both, and in some instances by surgical intervention.[99]

TABLE 45–6   **Frequent Areas of Soft Tissue Tightness**

Neck flexion	Hip flexion
Shoulder adduction	Hip internal rotation
Elbow flexion	Knee flexion
Forearm pronation	Ankle plantar flexion
Finger adduction	Foot inversion
Finger extension	

From Pease WS, Johnson EW: Rehabilitation management of diseases of the motor unit. *In* Kottke FJ, Lehmann JF (eds): Krusen's Handbook of Physical Medicine and Rehabilitation, ed 4. Philadelphia, WB Saunders, 1990, pp 754–764.

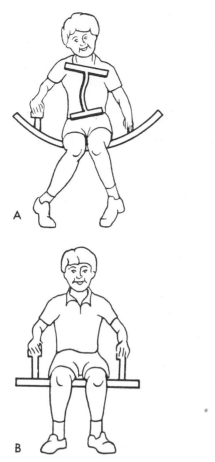

FIGURE 45–1 *A,* Wide hammock seat promotes deformity. *B,* Proper positioning includes a firm seat and correct arm height.

Management of Scoliosis

Prevention and management of scoliosis is one of the major rehabilitation goals in the management of neuromuscular disease. Abnormal spinal curvature occurs with increasing age and with advancing disability. The incidence and rate of progression of scoliosis varies with the type of disorder. The majority of children with motor neuron disease develop a collapsing, paralytic type of scoliosis. Initially, paraspinal muscular weakness is usually symmetrical, and if the child is still ambulatory, the development of scoliosis is uncommon. Once the weakness progresses sufficiently to prevent ambulation, scoliosis develops rapidly. Prevention and reduction of scoliosis is important because it affects sitting tolerance with associated skin and pressure relief problems, along with a concomitant decrease in pulmonary function.

The initial approach to scoliosis management is to prescribe the most appropriate wheelchair for the individual child (see Chapter 19). The wheelchair must be measured for each child, after assessing the child's physical, social, and vocational-educational needs. The child must maintain a symmetrical sitting posture with adequate upper and lower extremity support. The sling seat should be avoided because it permits asymmetrical pelvic rotation. The pelvis provides the base of support for the spine and any pelvic asymmetry permits the development of scoliosis. A solid foam-padded seat cushion can be used to level the pelvis during sitting in the early stages.

An erect spine is necessary for proper sitting balance and a variety of orthoses have been developed to manage the scoliosis curve from 20 to 40 degrees. Children tolerate the sitting support orthosis or the thoracolumbar orthosis well, until the curve reaches more than 40 degrees.[81] Once the curve is more than 40 degrees, a relatively rapid progression continues that generally cannot be managed orthotically.

Surgical stabilization of the spine has been advocated in a number of neuromuscular disorders.[121, 124] Various segmental instrumental and fusion techniques have been described. Postoperative complications are primarily pulmonary. It is believed that the earlier the spine is stabilized, the less likely are the secondary pulmonary and cardiac complications[106] (see Chapter 18).

Weakness

Motor weakness is a presenting problem for all motor neuron diseases, but it varies considerably in its presentation and location. Proximal weakness interferes with such activities as gait, transfers, and gross motor movements, while distal weakness interferes with more fine motor skills. Treatment of weakness, however, might include strengthening exercises, if prescribed judiciously and followed carefully. Although not well studied, it appears that vigorous, fatiguing progressive resistive exercise is contraindicated in most motor neuron diseases, as such exercise can lead to overuse weakness.[54, 125] Low-intensity, nonfatiguing exercise, however, may be quite beneficial for maintenance or improvement in muscle strength, (as has recently been demonstrated in several studies on post-polio patients),[4, 34–37] and cardiorespiratory fitness.[45, 64]

Respiratory Assistance

When motor weakness or deformity sufficiently limits the patient's ability to ventilate, mechanical ventilatory assistive devices are needed to allow for adequate ventilation. Early signs and symptoms of hypoxia include difficulty with sleeping, nighttime dyspnea, nightmares, and somnolence during the day.[10, 120] As these signs appear, appropriately prescribed ventilatory aids (such as a cuirass or plastic wrap) enhance gas exchange in the recumbent position.[120] In the later stages of motor neuron disease, oral positive pressure ventilation, pneumobelt, or cuirass ventilators can be used throughout the day, energized by the wheelchair battery. Tracheostomy is rarely needed and its use is somewhat controversial. While noninvasive management is preferable, tracheostomy may be useful if the patient has a severe scoliosis or if control of aspiration is a major problem[7, 99, 120] (see Chapter 33).

Functional Ability

The primary goals of the rehabilitation team in treating a patient with motor neuron disease are to assist the patient in the maintenance of function, independence, and quality of life for as long as possible. This entails a coordinated effort by the entire rehabilitation team in prospective and expectant care of the patient (and family). Appropriate preventive and therapeutic interventions for the treatment of pain, soft tissue tightness, deformity, scoliosis management, motor weakness, and respiratory dysfunction can minimize complications and maximize the patient's ability to function. Functional training for locomotion, dressing, eating, and other ADL are practiced as developmentally appropriate[99] (see Chapter 26).

Assistive devices, substitution training, and selective surgical procedures (such as tendon transfers, releases, and arthrodeses) all represent management techniques that can be judiciously applied to improve the patient's ability to function.[99] Figure 45–2 demonstrates the utility of a knee-ankle-foot orthosis (KAFO) and cane in a post-polio patient who was seen in the clinic with complaints of left knee pain and fatigability while ambulating. The use of the KAFO and cane not only stabilized the patient's painful, unstable left knee (the patient had a 25-degree valgus deformity and a 30-degree hyperextension deformity) but also reduced the patient's energy expenditure of ambulation. With use of the KAFO and cane, energy expenditure while ambulating was reduced by over 25%. In addition, this patient accepted the use of a motorized scooter for longer distances, which helped save energy in the performance of daily activities.

TREATMENT OF THE PATIENT WITH MOTOR NEURON DISEASE

As described earlier, motor neuron diseases include a number of disorders of the upper motor neuron, lower motor neuron, or both the upper and lower motor neurons.

The success of the rehabilitation process depends on the active involvement of the patient. The treatment of two different syndromes or disease entities, post-polio syndrome and ALS, will be briefly discussed as examples of treatment for the patient with a motor neuron disease.

Treatment of Post-Polio Syndrome

The post-polio syndrome appears to be primarily related to overactivity and overuse in individuals with significant neuromuscular impairment attributable to their original poliomyelitis illness. Frequent clinical diagnoses made in these patients include muscle pain related to such factors as overactivity, muscle pain related to overuse or myofascial pain, joint pain related to arthritis, or mechanical problems in joints not well protected owing to weakened musculature. The treatment for any particular patient, of course, depends upon the evaluation of that individual's situation. Fatigue is a very common complaint of post-polio patients. As mentioned above, many patients describe this phenomenon as "hitting the wall."[48] The cause for this complaint is unknown, and may be central in origin in at least some patients. Regardless of the cause, however, it has been reported that most post-polio patients have found that their complaint of fatigue was significantly reduced by increasing rest time, napping, or reducing the overall level of activity during the day.[48] Table 45–7 lists some of the more common interventions and recommendations made for post-polio patients as a result of their clinical evaluation. Most patients currently are getting many of the recommended treatments shown in the table. For instance, a large majority of patients in the two studies cited in the table

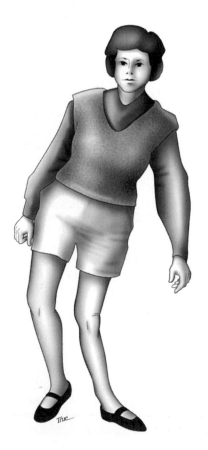
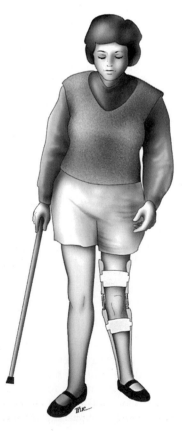

FIGURE 45–2   Post-polio patient ambulating without *(left)* and with *(right)* a knee-ankle-foot orthosis and cane.

TABLE 45–7   Common Clinical Interventions and Recommendations Made to Post-Polio Patients (Percentage of Patients Given the Recommendation)

	Halstead and Rossi[49] (n = 132)	Agre et al.[5] (n = 79)
New or modified aids*	87%	—
Energy conservation techniques	64%	73%
Change in exercise program	64%	—
Change in orthoses	52%	34%
Weight loss	52%	27%
New/modified wheelchair	26%	—
Gentle exercise program		
Aerobic exercise	—	23%
Stretching exercises	—	46%
Strengthening exercises	—	43%

*Durable products used to improve posture, diminish pain, and enhance comfort. These include corsets, lumbar rolls, neck pillows, wheelchair positioners, canes, and crutches.

were given advice or prescriptions regarding the type and amount of exercise, weight loss, and level of activity. Almost all were counseled on the need to reduce stress in their lives—both physical and emotional.[49] The use of new or modified aids (such as corsets, lumbar rolls, neck pillows, wheelchair positioners, canes, and crutches), energy conservation techniques, or the use of new orthotic devices enhances the patient's ability to function and minimizes overuse problems.[5, 49] Psychological counseling or participation in a post-polio support group to learn new coping skills was also recommended for many patients.[5]

Compliance with clinical recommendations made after physiatric evaluation for post-polio patients appears to be very helpful. For instance, Agre and colleagues[5] found that 78% of patients seen in follow-up reported an improvement in their symptoms. Improvements were noted in terms of decreased muscle and joint pain, decreased level of fatigue, improved gait pattern (with use of an orthosis or cane), and improved coping abilities. In those patients not reporting improvement, none were compliant with the recommendations made. Peach and Olejnik[94] also reported on the effects of treatment compliance in 77 patients seen in a post-polio clinic. These patients were divided into three groups based

upon degree of compliance with clinical recommendations: compliers (n = 30), partial compliers (n = 32), and non-compliers (n = 15). Symptom status at the time of follow-up (an average of over 2 years from the time of the initial evaluation) is shown in Table 45–8. In general, a significant proportion of patients in the complier group noted resolution or improvement in their symptoms. Most of the partial complier group noted improvement or no change in their symptoms, and only in the non-complier group did the majority note no change or worsening of their symptoms. The complier group had an increase in muscle strength, as measured by manual muscle testing, at an annualized rate of +0.6%. On the other hand, the partial complier group had a loss in muscle strength at an annualized rate of −1.3%, and the non-complier group had a loss in muscle strength at an annualized rate of −2.0%. It appears that patients who completely comply with clinical recommendations and successfully control the factors responsible for the neuromuscular overuse do not lose muscle strength and note an improvement in their symptoms.

The role of exercise in the patient with post-polio syndrome has been somewhat controversial. Early reports of exercise in post-polio patients have yielded conflicting results. Some studies showed that muscle-strengthening exercises were beneficial,[32, 47, 92] whereas other reports indicated that vigorous exercise or activity was detrimental.[62, 71, 77, 88] It appears that a key difference between these studies was the intensity of the exercise program. It appears most probable that the exercise regimens in the studies reporting deleterious effects were too vigorous for the patients and subsequently led to overuse problems. Four recent studies have been conducted on muscle-strengthening exercise,[4, 34–36] two studies on general exercise or aerobic fitness training,[45, 64] one on efficiency of movement,[31] and one on aquatic exercise[103] in post-polio patients. These studies have shown that judicious exercise can improve muscle strength, cardiorespiratory fitness, and the efficiency of ambulation in post-polio patients. These benefits occur when the patient's exercise program avoids excessive fatigue, muscle pain, and joint pain.

The difficulty in prescribing an exercise program for the post-polio patient has to do with the uniqueness of each patient. The physician needs to recognize each patient's

TABLE 45–8   Symptom Status of Post-Polio Patients at Time of Follow-up

		Resolved	Improved	Unchanged	Increased
Complier group (n = 30)					
Weakness	(n = 23)	17%	83%	0%	0%
Fatigue	(n = 28)	4%	96%	0%	0%
Muscle pain	(n = 25)	28%	72%	0%	0%
Joint pain	(n = 17)	41%	53%	6%	0%
Partial complier group (n = 32)					
Weakness	(n = 29)	0%	79%	21%	0%
Fatigue	(n = 31)	0%	68%	29%	3%
Muscle pain	(n = 32)	3%	88%	9%	0%
Joint pain	(n = 24)	4%	83%	13%	0%
Non-complier group (n = 15)					
Weakness	(n = 14)	0%	0%	64%	36%
Fatigue	(n = 14)	0%	0%	64%	36%
Muscle pain	(n = 14)	0%	14%	57%	29%
Joint pain	(n = 11)	0%	0%	82%	18%

From Peach PE, Olejnik S: Effect of treatment and non-compliance on post-polio sequelae. Orthopedics 1991; 14:1199–1203.

particular circumstances, including the location and degree of muscle weakness and the location and degree of subsequent arthropathy or arthralgia. It is important to remember that muscle weakness from poliomyelitis is often asymmetrical and scattered, and the weakness of different muscles can vary considerably. It is important to protect the weakened muscles and affected joints of post-polio patients from overuse during exercise. At the same time, the patient needs to exercise those body areas that can tolerate exercise so that function is not reduced as a result of disuse. At present, it appears that muscles with antigravity or greater strength on manual muscle testing[84] can tolerate strengthening exercises.[4, 34–37] Swimming and aquatic exercise may prove to be one of the best types of exercise in these persons as the buoyancy of the water reduces the effect of gravity on the patient's joints and limbs, protecting them from overuse. At present, it appears that judicious exercise in the appropriate post-polio patient (the patient who can exercise and avoid undue fatigue, muscle pain, and joint pain) is an important adjuvant in the patient's overall therapeutic program.[1]

Treatment of Amyotrophic Lateral Sclerosis

The progression of ALS is known to be quite variable. It may be rapidly progressive or slowly progressive, with the patient surviving 15 to 20 years after the initial diagnosis is made. The rehabilitation treatment program of the patient with ALS is described elsewhere in more detail.[116] Briefly, most patients with ALS go through three phases.

In the first phase, the patient is independent. This phase can be separated into three distinct stages. In the first stage, the patient is ambulatory, independent in ADL, and has mild weakness or clumsiness. Treatment at this time includes encouraging the patient to perform range-of-motion exercises and strengthening exercises of the unaffected musculature to compensate for the weakened muscles. Strenuous exercise, however, is discouraged as it might lead to increased fatigue and disability. Psychological support is also very important at this stage. In the second stage, the patient is still ambulatory with moderate selective weakness and slightly decreased independence in the performance of ADL (e.g., difficulty with climbing stairs, raising arms overhead, or buttoning clothing). Treatment at this stage includes substituting Velcro closures for buttons, encouraging the use of ankle-foot orthoses, wrist-and-thumb splints, and encouraging selective strengthening for unaffected muscles and stretching exercises to avoid contractures. Patients are advised to avoid overuse and fatigue. In the third stage, the patient is still ambulatory, but becomes easily fatigued with long-distance ambulation; has severe selective weakness in the ankles, wrists, and hands; and has a moderate decrease in independence in ADL. Treatment in this stage is designed to keep the patient independent for as long as possible. Deep breathing exercises should be added in this stage and the patient should receive an appropriate wheelchair or motorized scooter for longer-distance mobility.

In the second phase, the patient is partially independent. This phase can be divided into two separate stages. In the fourth stage, the patient is no longer ambulatory and is confined to a wheelchair. The patient has severe weakness in the lower limbs with or without the accompaniment of spasticity. The patient has moderate upper limb weakness, but is able to perform many ADL independently or with partial assistance. The patient may have shoulder pain due to weakness about the shoulder girdle musculature and may have edema of the hand. Treatment at this time includes supporting the shoulder and using heat and massage for shoulder pain. Anti-edema preventive measures should be utilized. Passive range-of-motion exercises and stretching should be performed to prevent contracture. The patient should be encouraged to perform isometric exercises of the few remaining uninvolved muscles. In the fifth stage, the patient's strength continues to decline. The patient has severe lower limb weakness and moderate-to-severe upper limb weakness. The patient progressively needs more and more assistance with all ADL. The patient needs assistance in transferring into and out of the wheelchair. Decubitus ulceration may also occur as a result of immobility and pressure. Treatment at this stage includes continuing with range-of-motion and stretching exercises to avoid contracture formation. The patient's family should be encouraged to learn proper transfer and positioning principles. Modifications of the home environment are needed to aid the patient's mobility and independence. Use of a water mattress may be helpful in preventing decubitus ulcer formation.

In the third phase, the patient is totally dependent. The patient is essentially bedridden and is completely dependent in all ADL. Treatment includes continuance of range-of-motion and stretching exercises to prevent the formation of contractures. For dysphagia, a soft diet may be helpful; otherwise the patient may require tube feeding. For accumulation of saliva, the use of suction, medications, or surgery to decrease salivary flow may be helpful. For dysarthria, the use of palatal lifts or electronic speech amplification may be helpful. For breathing difficulty, the airway will need to be carefully monitored and cleared as needed. Tracheostomy or respirator use may be required. During this phase, the physical ability of the family to care for the patient at home needs to be considered.

SUMMARY

The overall aim in the treatment of a patient with a motor neuron disease is to prolong functional abilities, independence, and quality of life for as long as possible. A coordinated effort by the rehabilitation team to maintain mobility, prevent deformity, maintain or improve strength, and manage respiratory dysfunction can minimize complications and maximize function. Functional training, the use of assistive devices, and judicious surgical procedures may also be used.

Acknowledgment

We thank Donald W. Mulder, M.D., Emeritus Professor of Neurology, the Mayo Medical School, for reviewing this chapter and providing useful suggestions for revision.

References

1. Agre JC: The role of exercise in the patient with post-polio syndrome. Ann N Y Acad Sci, in press, 1994.

2. Agre JC, Rodriquez AA: Neuromuscular function: Comparison of symptomatic and asymptomatic polio subjects to control subjects. Arch Phys Med Rehabil 1990; 71:545–551.

3. Agre JC, Rodriquez AA: Neuromuscular function in polio survivors at one-year follow-up. Arch Phys Med Rehabil 1991; 72:7–10.

4. Agre JC, Harmon RL, Carr JT, et al: Nonfatiguing muscle strengthening exercise can safely increase strength in post-polio patients. Med Sci Sports Exerc 1993; 25(suppl):S134.

5. Agre JC, Rodriquez AA, Sperling KB: Symptoms and clinical impressions of patients seen in a postpolio clinic. Arch Phys Med Rehabil 1989; 70:367–370.

6. Agre JC, Rodriquez AA, Tafel JA: Late effects of polio: Critical review of the literature on neuromuscular function. Arch Phys Med Rehabil 1991; 72:923–931.

7. Alexander MA, Johnson EW, Petty J, Stauch D: Mechanical ventilation of patients with late stage Duchenne muscular dystrophy: Management at home. Arch Phys Med Rehabil 1979; 60:289.

8. American Association of Electrodiagnostic Medicine: 1990 AAEM Course C: Motor Neuron Diseases. Rochester, Minn, American Association of Electrodiagnostic Medicine, 1990, pp 1–42.

9. Armstrong RM, Fogelson MH, Silberberg DH: Familial proximal spinal muscular atrophy. Arch Neurol 1966; 14:208–212.

10. Bach JR, O'Brien J, Krotenberg R, Alba AS: Management of end stage respiratory failure in Duchenne muscular dystrophy. Muscle Nerve 1987; 10:177–182.

11. Baker AB, Cornwell S, Brown IA: Poliomyelitis. VI. The hypothalamus. Arch Neurol Psychiatry 1952; 68:16.

12. Bauer M, Bergström R, Ritter B, et al: Macroglobulinemia, Waldenström and motor neuron syndrome. Acta Neurol Scand 1977; 55:245–250.

13. Ben Hamida M, Hentati F, Ben Hamida C: Hereditary motor system diseases (chronic juvenile amyotrophic lateral sclerosis. Brain 1990; 113:347–363.

14. Block HS, Wilbourn AJ: Progressive post-polio atrophy: The EMG findings, abstract. Neurology 1986; 36(suppl 1):137.

15. Bodian D: Pathologic anatomy. In Poliomyelitis: Transactions of the First International Poliomyelitis Conference. Philadelphia, JB Lippincott, 1949.

16. Bodian D: The virus, the nerve cell, and paralysis: Study of experimental poliomyelitis in the spinal cord. Bull Johns Hopkins Hosp 1948; 83:1–73.

17. Brain WR, Croft PB, Wilkinson M: Motor neurone disease as a manifestation of neoplasm (with a note on the course of classical motor neurone disease). Brain 1965; 88:479–500.

18. Brett EM, Lake BD: Neuromuscular disorders: I. Primary muscle disease and anterior horn cell disorders. In Brett EM (ed): Paediatric Neurology, ed 2. New York, Churchill Livingstone, 1991, pp 53–115.

19. Brooke MH: A Clinician's View of Neuromuscular Diseases, ed 2. Baltimore, Williams & Wilkins, 1986.

20. Brownell B, Oppenheimer DR, Hughes JT: The central nervous system in motor neurone disease. J Neurol Neurosurg Psychiatry 1970; 33:338–357.

21. Buchanan DS, Malamud N: Motor neuron disease with renal cell carcinoma and postoperative neurologic remission. A clinicopathologic report. Neurology 1973; 23:891–894.

22. Byers RK, Banker BQ: Infantile muscular atrophy. Arch Neurol 1961; 5:140–164.

23. Chazot G, Berger B, Carrier H, et al: Manifestations neurologiques des gammapathies monoclonales. Formes neurologiques pures—Études en immunofluorescence. Rev Neurol 1976; 132:195–212.

24. Codd MB, Mulder DW, Kurland LT, et al: Poliomyelitis in Rochester, Minnesota, 1935–1955: Epidemiology and long-term sequelae: A preliminary report. In Halstead LS, Wiechers DO (eds): Late Effects of Poliomyelitis. Miami, Symposia Foundation, 1985, pp 121–134.

25. Cornil Lepine: Sur un cas de paralysie générale spinale antérieure subaiguë, suivi d'autopsie. Gaz Med Fr (Paris) 1875; 4:127–129.

26. Cosgrove JL, Alexander MA, Kitts EL, et al: Late effects of poliomyelitis. Arch Phys Med Rehabil 1987; 68:4–7.

27. Dalakas MB, Elder G, Hallat M, et al: A long-term follow-up study of patients with post-poliomyelitis neuromuscular symptoms. N Engl J Med 1986; 314:959–963.

28. Dalakas MC, Sever JL, Fletcher M, et al: Neuromuscular symptoms in patients with old poliomyelitis: Clinical, virological and immunological studies. In Halstead LS, Wiechers DO (eds): Late Effects of Poliomyelitis. Miami, Symposia Foundation, 1985, pp 73–90.

29. Dalakas MC, Sever JL, Madden DL, et al: Late post-poliomyelitis muscular atrophy: Clinical, virological and immunological studies. Rev Infect Dis 1984; 6(suppl 2):S562–567.

30. Daube JR: Electrophysiologic studies in the diagnosis and prognosis of motor neuron diseases. Neurol Clin 1985; 3:473–493.

31. Dean E, Ross J: Effect of modified aerobic training on movement energetics in polio survivors. Orthopedics 1991; 14:1243–1246.

32. DeLorme TL, Schwab RS, Watkins AL: The response of the quadriceps femoris to progressive resistance exercises in poliomyelitis patients. J Bone Joint Surg Am 1948; 30:834–847.

33. De Vivo DC, Hays AP: Disorders of the neuromuscular system. In Fishman MA (ed): Pediatric Neurology. Orlando, Fla, Grune & Stratton, 1986, pp 111–135.

34. Einarsson G: Muscle conditioning in late poliomyelitis. Arch Phys Med Rehabil 1991; 72:11–14.

35. Einarsson G, Grimby G: Strengthening exercise program in postpolio subjects. In Halstead LS, Wiechers DO (eds): Research and Clinical Aspects of the Late Effects of Poliomyelitis. White Plains, NY, March of Dimes Birth Defects Foundation, 1987, pp 275–283.

36. Feldman RM, Soskolne CL: The use of nonfatiguing strengthening exercises in post-polio syndrome. In Halstead LS, Wiechers DO (eds): Research and Clinical Aspects of the Late Effects of Poliomyelitis. White Plains, NY, March of Dimes Birth Defects Foundation, 1987, pp 335–341.

37. Fillyaw MJ, Badger GJ, Goodwin GD, et al: The effects of long-term non-fatiguing resistance exercise in subjects with post-polio syndrome. Orthopedics 1991; 14:1253–1256.

38. Fischbeck KH, Ionasescu V, Ritter AW, et al: Localization of the gene for X-linked spinal muscular atrophy. Neurology 1986; 36:1595–1598.

39. Gajdusek DC: Foci of motor neuron disease in high incidence in isolated populations of East Asia and the western Pacific. In Rowland LP (ed): Human Motor Neuron Diseases. New York, Raven Press, 1982, pp 363–393.

40. Gallai V, Hockaday JM, Hughes JT, et al: Ponto-bulbar palsy with deafness (Brown-Vialetto-van Laere syndrome). A report on 3 cases. J Neurol Sci 1981; 45:259–275.

41. Gamstrop I, Sarnat HB (eds): Progressive Spinal Muscular Atrophies. New York, Raven Press, 1984.

42. Gardner-Medwin D, Hudgson P, Walton JN: Benign spinal muscular atrophy arising in childhood and adolescence. J Neurol Sci 1967; 5:121–158.

43. Gilman S, Romanul FCA: Hereditary dystonic paraplegia with amyotrophy and mental deficiency: Clinical and neuropathological characteristics. In Vinken PJ, Bruyn GW (eds): Handbook of Clinical Neurology, Fazio-Londe Disease. pt 2. Amsterdam, North-Holland, 1975, pp 445–465.

44. Gomez MR: Progressive bulbar paralysis of childhood. In Vinken PJ, Bruyn GW (eds): Handbook of Clinical Neurology. Fazio-Londe Disease, pt 2. Amsterdam, North-Holland, 1975, pp 103–109.

45. Grimby G, Einarsson G: Post-polio management. CRC Crit Rev Phys Med Rehabil 1991; 2:189–200.

46. Gritzman MCD, Fritz VU, Perkins S, et al: Motor neuron disease associated with carcinoma. A report of 2 cases. S Afr Med J 1983; 63:288–291.

47. Gurwitsch AD: Intensive graduated exercises in early infantile paralysis. Arch Phys Med 1950; 31:213–218.

48. Halstead LS, Rossi CD: New problems in old polio patients: results of a survey of 539 polio survivors. Orthopedics 1985; 8:845–850.

49. Halstead LS, Rossi CD: Post-polio syndrome: Clinical experience with 132 consecutive outpatients. In Halstead LS, Wiechers DO (eds): Research and Clinical Aspects of the Late Effects of Poliomyelitis. White Plains, NY, March of Dimes Birth Defects Foundation, 1987, pp 13–26.

50. Halstead LS, Wiechers DO (eds): Late Effects of Poliomyelitis. Miami, Symposia Foundation, 1985.

51. Halstead LS, Wiechers DO (eds): Research and Clinical Aspects of the Late Effects of Poliomyelitis. White Plains, NY, March of Dimes Birth Defects Foundation, 1987.

52. Harding AE: Inherited neuronal atrophy and degeneration predominantly of lower motor neurons. In Dyck PJ, Thomas PK, Lambert EH, Bunge R (eds): Peripheral Neuropathy, pt 2. Philadelphia, WB Saunders, 1984, pp 1537–1556.

53. Harding AE, Thomas PK: Hereditary distal spinal muscular atrophy. A report of 34 cases and a review of the literature. J Neurol Sci 1980; 45:337–348.

54. Herbison GJ, Jaweed MM, Ditunno JF, Jr: Exercise therapies in peripheral neuropathies. Arch Phys Med Rehabil 1983; 64:201–205.

55. Hirayama K, Tomonaga M, Kitano K, et al: Focal cervical poliopathy causing juvenile muscular atrophy of distal upper extremity: A pathological study. J Neurol Neurosurg Psychiatry 1987; 50:285–290.

56. Hoffmann J: Über chronische spinale Muskelatrophie im Kindesalter, auf familiärer Basis. Dtsch Z Nervenheilk 1893; 3:427–470.

57. Horstmann DM: Epidemiology of poliomyelitis and allied diseases—1963. Yale J Biol Med 1963; 36:5–26.

58. Hudson AJ: Amyotrophic lateral sclerosis and its association with dementia, parkinsonism and other neurological disorders: A review. Brain 1981; 104:217–247.

59. Hudson AJ: The motor neuron diseases and related disorders. In Joynt RJ (ed): Clinical Neurology, vol 4. Philadelphia, JB Lippincott, 1991, pp 1–35.

60. Hudson AJ, Davenport A, Hader WJ: The incidence of amyotrophic lateral sclerosis in southwestern Ontario, Canada. Neurology 1986; 36:1524–1528.

61. Hudson AJ, Rice GPA: Similarities of Guamanian ALS/PD to postencephalitic parkinsonism/ALS: Possible viral cause. Can J Neurol Sci 1990; 17:427–433.

62. Hyman G: Poliomyelitis. Lancet 1953; 1:852.

63. Johnson EW: Pathokinesiology of Duchenne muscular dystrophy: Implications for management. Arch Phys Med Rehabil 1977; 58:4–7.

64. Jones DR, Speier J, Canine K, et al: Cardiorespiratory responses to aerobic training by patients with postpoliomyelitis sequelae. JAMA 1989; 261:3255–3258.

65. Jubelt B, Cashman NR: Neurological manifestations of the postpolio syndrome. CRC Crit Rev Clin Neurobiol 1987; 3:199–220.

66. Kaeser HE: Scapuloperoneal muscular atrophy. Brain 1965; 88:407–418.

67. Kennedy WR, Alter M, Sung JH: Progressive proximal spinal and bulbar muscular atrophy of late onset. A sex-linked recessive trait. Neurology 1968; 18:671–680.

68. Kimura J: Electrodiagnosis in Diseases of Nerve and Muscle: Principles and Practice, ed 2. Philadelphia, FA Davis, 1989, pp 429–446.

69. Kincaid JC: Myelitis and myelopathy. In Joynt RJ (ed): Clinical Neurology, vol 4. Philadelphia, JB Lippincott, 1991, pp 1–36.

70. Knapp ME: The contribution of Sister Elizabeth Kenny to treatment of poliomyelitis. Arch Phys Med Rehabil 1955; 36:510–517.

71. Knowlton GC, Bennett RL: Overwork. Arch Phys Med Rehabil 1957; 38:18–20.

72. Kottke FJ: Therapeutic exercise to maintain mobility. In Kottke FJ, Lehmann JF (eds): Krusen's Handbook of Physical Medicine and Rehabilitation, ed 4. Philadelphia, WB Saunders, pp 436–451.

73. Krieger C, Melmed C: Amyotrophic lateral sclerosis and paraproteinemia. Neurology 1982; 32:896–898.

74. Kugelberg E, Welander L: Heredofamilial juvenile muscular atrophy simulating muscular dystrophy. Arch Neurol Psychiatry 1956; 75:500–509.

75. Kurent JE, Brooks BR, Madden DL, et al: CSF viral antibodies: Evaluation in amyotrophic lateral sclerosis and late-onset postpoliomyelitis progressive muscular atrophy. Arch Neurol 1979; 36:269–273.

76. Kurtzke JF, Beebe GW: Epidemiology of amyotrophic lateral sclerosis. 1. A case-control comparison based on ALS deaths. Neurology 1980; 30:453–462.

77. Lovett RW: The treatment of infantile paralysis: Preliminary report, based on a study of the Vermont epidemic of 1914. JAMA 1915; 64:2118–2123.

78. Lowenthal M, Tobis JS: Contractures in chronic neurologic disease. Arch Phys Med Rehabil 1957; 38:640–645.

79. Ludolph AC, Hugon J, Dwivedi MP, et al: Studies on the aetiology and pathogenesis of motor neuron diseases. 1. Lathyrism: Clinical findings in established cases. Brain 1987; 110:149–165.

80. Maloney FP, Burks JS, Ringel SP (eds): Interdisciplinary Rehabilitation of Multiple Sclerosis and Neuromuscular Disorders. Philadelphia, JB Lippincott, 1985.

81. Matthews DJ, Stempien LM: Orthopedic management of the disabled child. In Sinaki M (ed): Basic Clinical Rehabilitation Medicine. St Louis, Mosby–Year Book, 1993, pp 399–411.

82. McDowell FH, Plum F: Arterial hypertension associated with acute anterior poliomyelitis. N Engl J Med 1951; 245:241.

83. McLeod JG, Prineas JW: Distal type of chronic spinal muscular atrophy. Clinical, electrophysiological and pathological studies. Brain 1971; 94:703–714.

84. Medical Research Council: Aids to the Examination of the Peripheral Nervous System, ed 2. rev. War Memorandum No. 7. London, HMSO. 1943.

85. Melki J, Abdelhak S, Sheth P, et al: Gene for chronic proximal spinal muscular atrophies maps to chromosome 5q. Science 1990; 344:767–768.

86. Melnick JL, Agol VI, Bachrach HL, et al: Picornaviridae. Intervirology 1974; 4:303–316.

87. Menkes JH: Textbook of Child Neurology, ed 4. Philadelphia, Lea & Febiger, 1990, pp 675–721.

88. Mitchell GP: Poliomyelitis and exercise. Lancet 1953; 2:90–91.

89. Mulder DW, Bushek W, Spring E, et al: Motor neuron disease (ALS): Evaluation of detection thresholds of cutaneous sensation. Neurology 1983; 33:1625–1627.

90. Munin MC, Jaweed MM, Staas WE, et al: Poliomyelitis muscle weakness: A prospective study of quadriceps strength. Arch Phys Med Rehabil 1991; 72:729–733.

91. Munsat TL, Andres P, Thibideau L: Preliminary observations on long-term muscle force changes in the post-polio syndrome. In Halstead LS, Wiechers DO (eds): Research and Clinical Aspects of the Late Effects of Poliomyelitis. White Plains, NY, March of Dimes Birth Defects Foundation, 1987, pp 329–334.

92. Müller EA, Bechmann H: Die Trainierbarkeit von Kindern mit gelähmten Muskeln durch isometrische Kontraktionen. Z Orthop 1966; 102:139–145.

93. Parry GJ, Holtz SJ, Ben-Zeev D, et al: Gammopathy with proximal motor axonopathy simulating motor neuron disease. Neurology 1986; 36:273–276.

94. Peach PE, Olejnik S: Effect of treatment and noncompliance on post-polio sequelae. Orthopedics 1991; 14:1199–1203.

95. Pearn JH: Genetics of the spinal muscular atrophies. In Gamstrop I, Sarnat HB (eds): Progressive Spinal Muscular Atrophies. New York, Raven Press, 1984, pp 19–30.

96. Pearn JH, Carter CO, Wilson J: The genetic identify of acute infantile spinal muscular atrophy. Brain 1973; 96:463–470.

97. Pearn JH, Hudgson P: Distal spinal muscular atrophy. A clinical and genetic study of 8 kindreds. J Neurol Sci 1979; 43:183–191.

98. Pearn JH, Wilson J: Acute Werdnig-Hoffmann disease: Acute infantile spinal muscular atrophy. Arch Dis Child 1973; 48:425–430.

99. Pease WS, Johnson EW: Rehabilitation management of diseases of the motor unit. In Kottke FJ, Lehmann JF (eds): Krusen's Handbook of Physical Medicine and Rehabilitation, ed 4. Philadelphia, WB Saunders, 1990, pp 754–764.

100. Peters HA, Clatanoff DV: Spinal muscular atrophies secondary to macroglobulinemia. Reversal of symptoms with chlorambucil therapy. Neurology 1968; 18:101–108.

101. Plum F: Sensory loss with poliomyelitis. Neurology 1956; 6:166.

102. Price RW, Plum F: Poliomyelitis. In Vinken PJ, Bruyn GW (eds): Handbook of Clinical Neurology, vol 34. Amsterdam, North-Holland, 1978, p 93.

103. Prins JH, Hartung GH, Merritt DJ, et al: Effect of aquatic exercise training in persons with poliomyelitis disability. Sports Med Training Rehabil 1994; 5:29–39.

104. Ramlov J, Alexander M, LaPorte R, et al: Epidemiology of post-polio syndrome. Am J Epidemiol 1992; 136:769–786.

105. Raymond M (with contribution by Charcot JM): Paralysie essentiele de l'enfance: atrophie musculaire consecutive. Gaz Med Fr (Paris) 1875; 4:225.

106. Rideau Y, Glovon B, Delaubier A: The treatment of scoliosis in Duchenne muscular dystrophy. Muscle Nerve 1984; 7:281–286.

107. Rodgers-Johnson P, Garruto RM, Yanagihara R, et al: Amyotrophic lateral sclerosis and parkinsonism—dementia on Guam: A 30-year evaluation of clinical and neuropathic trends. Neurology 1986; 36:7–13.

108. Román GC: The neuroepidemiology of tropical spastic paraparesis. Ann Neurol 1988; 23(suppl):S113–S120.

109. Rosling H, Gessain A, de The G, et al: Tropical and epidemic spastic parapareses are different. Lancet 1988; 1:1222–1223.

110. Rowland LP, Defendini R, Sherman W, et al: Macroglobulinemia with peripheral neuropathy simulating motor neuron disease. Ann Neurol 1982; 11:532–536.

111. Rudnicki S, Chad DA, Drachman DA, et al: Motor neuron disease and paraproteinemia. Neurology 1987; 37:335–337.

112. Schoenen J, Delwaide PJ, Legros JJ, et al: Motoneuropathie héréditaire: La forme proximale de l'adulte liéé au sexe (ou maladie de Kennedy). J Neurol Sci 1979; 41:343–357.

113. Schold SC, Cho E-S, Somasundaram M, et al: Subacute motor neuronopathy: A remote effect of lymphoma. Ann Neurol 1979; 5:271–287.

114. Schwarz GA, Liu C-N: Hereditary (familial) spastic paraplegia. Arch Neurol 1956; 75:144–156.

115. Siddique T, Figlewicz DA, Pericak-Vance MA, et al: Linkage of a gene causing familial amyotrophic lateral sclerosis to chromosome 21 and evidence of genetic-locus heterogeneity. N Engl J Med 1991; 324:1381–1384.

116. Sinaki M: Exercise and rehabilitation measures in amyotrophic lateral sclerosis. In Tsubaki T, Yase Y (eds): Excerpta Medica International Congress Series 769. Amsterdam, Elsevier, 1988, pp 343–368.

117. Speier JL, Owen RR, Knapp M, Canine JK: Occurrence of postpolio sequelae in an epidemic population. In Halstead LS, Wiechers DO (eds): Research and Clinical Aspects of the Late Effects of Poliomyelitis. White Plains, NY, March of Dimes Birth Defects Foundation, 1987, pp 39–48.

118. Spencer PS, Nunn PB, Hugon J, et al: Guam amyotrophic lateral sclerosis-parkinsonism-dementia linked to a plant excitant neurotoxin. Science 1987; 237:517–522.

119. Spencer PS, Nunn PB, Hugon J, et al: Motorneurone disease on Guam: Possible role of a food neurotoxin. Lancet 1986; 1:965.

120. Splaingard ML, Frates RC, Jefferson LS, et al: Home negative pressure ventilation: Report of 20 years of experience in patients with neuromuscular disease. Arch Phys Med Rehabil 1985; 66:239–242.

121. Staheli CT: Common orthopedic problems. Pediatr Clin North Am 1986; 33:269–280.

122. Strong MJ, Hudson AJ, Alvord WG: Familial amyotrophic lateral sclerosis, 1850–1989: A statistical analysis of the world literature. Can J Neurol Sci 1991; 18:45–58.

123. Swaiman KF: Anterior horn cell and cranial motor neuron disease. In Swaiman KF (ed): Pediatric Neurology. Principles and Practice, vol 2. St Louis, Mosby–Year Book, 1989, pp 1083–1103.

124. Tachdjiam MO: Scoliosis. In Tachdjiam MO (ed): Pediatric Orthopedics. Philadelphia, WB Saunders, 1990, pp 2265–2378.

125. Taylor RG, Lieberman JS: Rehabilitation of the patient with diseases affecting the motor unit. In DeLisa JA (ed): Rehabilitation Medicine Principles and Practice. Philadelphia, JB Lippincott, 1988, pp 811–820.

126. Tsukagoshi H, Sugita H, Furukawa T, et al: Kugelberg-Welander syndrome with dominant inheritance. Arch Neurol 1966; 14:378–381.

127. Vignos PJ: Physical models of rehabilitation in neuromuscular disease. Muscle Nerve 1983; 6:323–338.

128. Virmani V, Mohan PK: Non-familial, spinal segmental muscular atrophy in juvenile and young subjects. Acta Neurol Scand 1985; 72:336–340.

129. Walton J: Disorders of Voluntary Muscle. London, Churchill Livingstone, 1981.

130. Werdnig G: Zwei frühinfantile hereditäre Fälle von progressiver Muskelatrophie unter dem Bilde der Dystrophie, aber auf neurotischer Grundlage. Arch Psychiatr Nervenkrankheiten 1891; 22:437–480.

131. Wiechers DO, Warmolts JR: Anterior horn cell diseases. In Johnson EW (ed): Practical Electromyography. Baltimore, Williams & Wilkins, 1981, pp 135–154.

132. Windebank AJ, Mulder DW: Motor neuron disease in adults. In Engel AG, Franzini-Armstrong C (eds): Myology. New York, McGraw-Hill, 1994, pp 1854–1869.

133. Younger DS, Rowland LP, Latov N, et al: Lymphoma, motor neuron diseases, and amyotrophic lateral sclerosis. Ann Neurol 1991; 29:78–86.

46

Rehabilitation of Patients With Peripheral Neuropathies

LOIS BUSCHBACHER, M.D.

Peripheral neuropathy includes any disorder of the peripheral nervous system involving either the axon or the myelin sheath. In some cases, both are affected, especially in the later stages of disease progression.

Peripheral neuropathies can be localized or generalized, proximal or distal. They can be due to compression, metabolic derangements, infection, inflammation, or autoimmune phenomena. Usually they are generalized and produce diffuse peripheral weakness, impaired sensation, and hyporeflexia. Since many diseases cause similar neuropathies, the exact cause requires a thorough history and physical examination, electrodiagnostic studies, laboratory studies, and in some cases, a biopsy.

NERVE ANATOMY AND PHYSIOLOGY

The peripheral nervous system begins as the neurons leave the brain and spinal cord. Peripheral nerves can have both afferent and efferent neurons. Figure 46–1 depicts the afferent and efferent tracts as they exit the spinal cord and

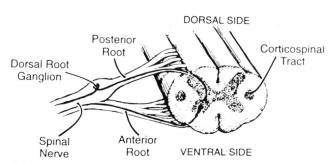

FIGURE 46–1 Cross-sectional segment of the spinal cord depicting afferent and efferent nerve roots, which combine to form a peripheral nerve. (From Buschbacher RM: Basic tissue organization and function. *In* Buschbacher RM (ed): Musculoskeletal Disorders: A Practical Guide for Diagnosis and Rehabilitation. Stoneham, Mass, Butterworth-Heinemann, 1994, p 17.)

join to form a spinal nerve. There are 12 cranial nerves and 31 spinal nerves, which together form the peripheral nervous system (Fig. 46–2). In the cervical and lumbosacral spine, these nerves intermingle with one another to form plexus (Fig. 46–3).

Each spinal nerve innervates a characteristic sensory area (dermatome) (Fig. 46–4) and muscle group (myotome) (Table 46–1). The peripheral nerves also innervate a characteristic set of muscles (see Table 46–1) as well as skin (Fig. 46–5). Knowledge of the usual paths of innervation is useful in determining the specific nerve or nerve root level of involvement. Individual patients do not always follow the usual innervation patterns, but variations are usually minor.

Each peripheral nerve is surrounded by an outer connective tissue sheath called the epineurium, which protects the nerve from compression. Inside the epineurium the nerve fibers are arranged in bundles or fascicles which are surrounded by a perineurium. The perineurium is the primary strengthening connective tissue of the nerve and also acts as a diffusion barrier. Nerve fibers may intermingle and cross from one fascicle to another along the course of the nerve. Each individual nerve fiber is surrounded by a membrane called the endoneurium[77] (Fig. 46–6).

The nerve roots are more vulnerable to injury than the rest of the peripheral nerve. This is because the roots lack perineurial and epineurial protection, the fibers are less "slack," and they are supported by less collagen.[77]

Axons are the long cellular processes of both motor and sensory nerves. They have an excitable membrane which causes an electrical current to propagate along the nerve to communicate with distal parts of the body, either to transmit sensory information or to activate the muscles and glands. Each segment of the axon must reach a threshold of electrical excitation, called depolarization, to propagate the impulse. The axonal membrane in isolation would lose current to the surrounding extracellular fluid. To counteract this and to increase the speed of nerve conduction, all

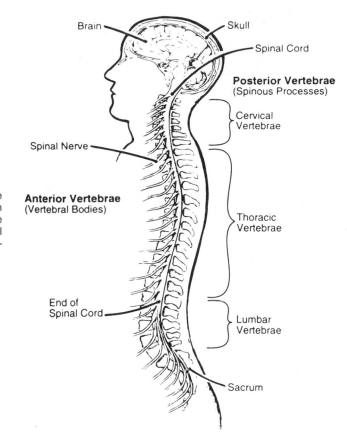

FIGURE 46–2 The central and peripheral nervous systems. Twelve cranial and 31 spinal nerves exit the brain and spinal cord to form the peripheral nervous system. (From Buschbacher RM: Basic tissue organization and function. *In* Buschbacher RM (ed): Musculoskeletal Disorders: A Practical Guide for Diagnosis and Rehabilitation. Stoneham, Mass, Butterworth-Heinemann, 1994, p 17.)

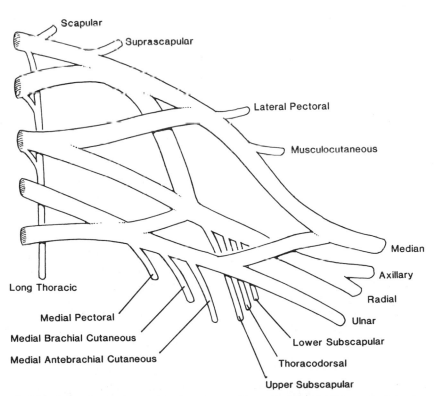

FIGURE 46–3 The brachial plexus. Ventral branches of the spinal nerves from C5 through T1 intermingle to form the peripheral nerves of the upper limb. (From Buschbacher RM: Basic tissue organization and function. *In* Buschbacher RM (ed): Musculoskeletal Disorders: A Practical Guide for Diagnosis and Rehabilitation. Stoneham, Mass, Butterworth-Heinemann, 1994, p 18.)

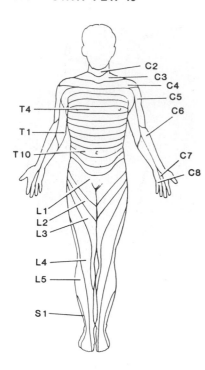

FIGURE 46–4 Dermatomal innervation pattern of the spinal nerves. Each spinal nerve goes on to provide sensation to a band of skin. This is done through a variety of peripheral nerves and is remarkably constant. (From Buschbacher RM: The musculoskeletal examination. *In* Buschbacher RM (ed): Musculoskeletal Disorders: A Practical Guide for Diagnosis and Rehabilitation. Stoneham, Mass, Butterworth-Heinemann, 1994, p 88.)

TABLE 46–1   Common Spinal Nerve Level and Peripheral Nerve Innervation Patterns of Common Muscle Groups

	Major Cranial Nerve (CN) or Spinal Nerve Level	Peripheral Nerve
Upper Extremity		
Shoulder muscles		
Elevators	CN XI, C4, C5	Spinal accessory nerve; posterior branches of spinal nerves
Protractors	C5–C7	Long thoracic nerve; pectoral nerves
Retractors	C5–C8	Dorsal scapular nerve; spinal accessory nerve; thoracodorsal nerve
Upward rotators	CN XI, C5, C6	Long thoracic nerve; spinal accessory nerve
Downward rotators	C6–C8	Thoracodorsal nerve; pectoral nerves
Abductors	C5, C6	Axillary and suprascapular nerves
Extensors	C6–C8	Thoracodorsal, axillary, and pectoral nerves
Flexors	C5, C6	Axillary, musculocutaneous, and pectoral nerves
Internal rotators	C5, C6	Pectoral nerves; thoracodorsal and subscapular nerves
External rotators	C5, C6	Axillary and suprascapular nerves
Elbow flexors	C5, C6	Musculocutaneous nerve
Elbow extensors	C7	Radial nerve
Wrist extensors	C6, C7	Radial nerve
Wrist flexors	C7, C8	Median and ulnar nerves
Finger extensors	C7	Radial nerve
Finger flexors	C7, C8	Median and ulnar nerves
Intrinsic hand muscles	T1	Ulnar and median (thumb) nerves
Trunk and Back		
Abdominal muscles	T7–T12	Segmental innervation
Back muscles	C2–C5	Segmental innervation
Lower Extremity		
Hip flexors	T12, L1, L2	Lumbosacral plexus
Hip extensors	L5, S1, S2	Inferior gluteal nerve
Hip abductors	L4, L5, S1	Superior gluteal nerve
Hip adductors	L2–L4	Obturator nerve
Knee flexors	L5, S1	Sciatic nerve
Knee extensors	L2–L4	Femoral nerve
Foot dorsiflexors	L4, L5	Deep peroneal nerves
Foot plantarflexors	S1	Tibial nerve
Foot inverters	L4	Deep peroneal and tibial nerves
Foot everters	L5, S1	Superficial peroneal nerve

Modified from Buschbacher RM: Musculoskeletal Disorders: A Practical Guide for Diagnosis and Rehabilitation. Stoneham, Mass, Butterworth-Heinemann, 1994, p 87.

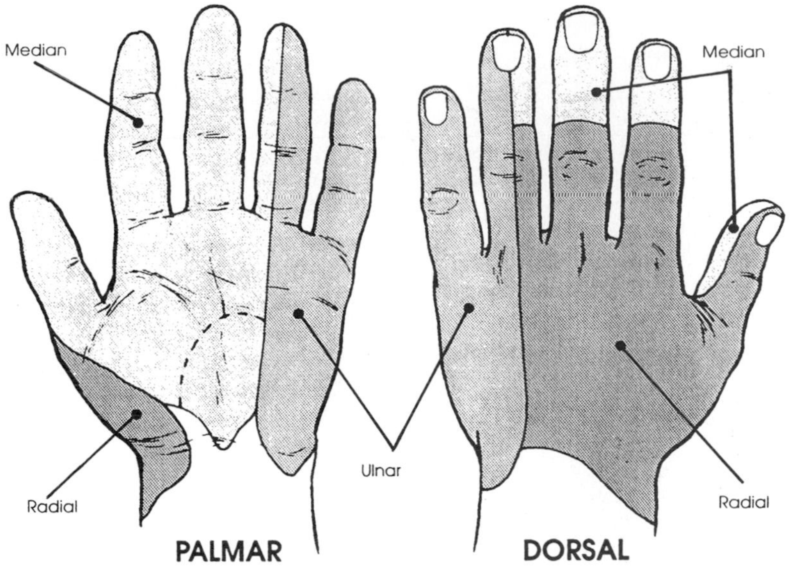

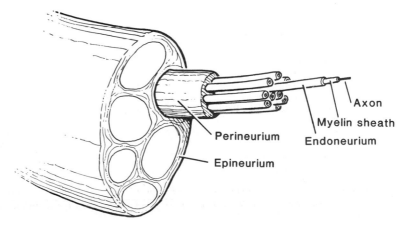

FIGURE 46–5 A sample of peripheral nerve patterns of innervation from the hand. Although overlap may occur with the dermatomal pattern, knowledge of both systems helps the examiner to distinguish spinal from peripheral nerve pathological features. (From McNeil BE, Buschbacher RM: Wrist and hand. *In* Buschbacher RM (ed): Musculoskeletal Disorders: A Practical Guide for Diagnosis and Rehabilitation. Stoneham, Mass, Butterworth-Heinemann, 1994, p 175.)

PALMAR   **DORSAL**

axons are surrounded by an insulating layer of myelin (see Chapter 6). Some axons share myelin with other axons and are poorly insulated. They are commonly called "unmyelinated fibers" and are reserved for functions that do not require rapid transmission through the body. Other axons are surrounded by individual sheaths of the Schwann cells (Fig. 46–7). They are more effectively insulated, and transmit impulses much more rapidly. Between individual Schwann cells are internodal segments known as the nodes of Ranvier. These nodes depolarize while the intervening myelinated segments tend not to, and allow the nerve impulse to "jump" from one node to another in what is called saltatory propagation. Such propagation allows fast impulse transmission with minimal energy expenditure. These axons carry information which must be rapidly disseminated and are commonly called "myelinated fibers."

The fibers that must transmit impulses rapidly are, in general, larger in diameter, since larger fibers have less electrical resistance. There is a wide array of fibers of varying diameters and degrees of myelination. Larger fibers tend to be myelinated. Table 46–2 is a common classification scheme for all nerve fibers. Table 46–3 is an alternative classification system for sensory fibers only. Both classification schemes are in widespread use.

TYPES OF NEUROPATHY

Peripheral neuropathies are divided into two major categories, demyelination and axonopathy, depending on whether they primarily affect the axon or the myelin sheath.[53]

Demyelination occurs when the myelin sheath is disturbed. Guillain-Barré syndrome (GBS) and Dejerine-Sottas syndrome are examples of diseases that predominantly cause demyelination. The interruption of the myelin sheath causes a slowing in nerve conduction. This slowing can be localized (as in a focal neuropathy like carpal tunnel syndrome) or generalized (as in GBS).

Axonopathy can be caused by toxic or metabolic derangements, by trauma, compression, traction, or by transection. If the damage is severe enough to block nerve conduction, nerve conduction studies show a decrease in amplitude of the resulting motor unit action potential (MUAP) (see Chapter 6).

CLASSIFICATION SYSTEMS

Localized nerve injuries can be classified by degree of severity. There are two main classification schemes: the

FIGURE 46–6 The internal anatomy of a nerve. The surrounding structure is called the *epineurium*. Internally, the nerve fibers are arranged in bundles, or fasciculi, surrounded by a perineurium. Each individual nerve fiber is enveloped by a sheath of myelin and an endoneurium. (From Buschbacher RM: Basic tissue organization and function. *In* Buschbacher RM (ed): Musculoskeletal Disorders: A Practical Guide for Diagnosis and Rehabilitation. Stoneham, Mass, Butterworth-Heinemann, 1994, p 17.)

Axon
Myelin sheath
Endoneurium
Perineurium
Epineurium

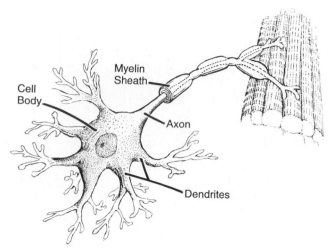

FIGURE 46–7 Schematic representation of a motor nerve from a cell body to the muscle it innervates. The nerve fiber is surrounded by myelin from the Schwann cells. (From Buschbacher RM: Basic tissue organization and function. *In* Buschbacher RM (ed): Musculoskeletal Disorders: A Practical Guide for Diagnosis and Rehabilitation. Stoneham, Mass, Butterworth-Heinemann, 1994, p 16.)

TABLE 46–3   Numerical Classification Sometimes Used for Sensory Neurons

No.		Origin	Fiber Type
I			
	a	Muscle spindle, annulospiral ending	Aα
	b	Golgi tendon organ	Aα
II		Muscle spindle, flower-spray ending; tough, pressure	Aβ
III		Pain and temperature receptors; some touch receptors	Aδ
IV		Pain and other receptors	Dorsal root C

From Ganong WF: Review of Medical Physiology, ed 13. East Norwalk, Conn, Appleton & Lange, 1987.

Seddon system[72] and the Sunderland system[77] (Table 46–4). The Sunderland system is an expansion on Seddon's divisions. Both are in common usage.

Seddon's Classification

Seddon proposed categorizing localized nerve injury into three divisions: (1) neurapraxia, (2) axonotmesis, and (3) neurotmesis.[72]

Neurapraxia

Neurapraxia is due to localized damage to the nerve that does not cause axonal death. It is often caused by nerve compression. It is characterized clinically by decreased vibratory and proprioceptive sensation and occasionally by decreased touch. Pain perception is seldom affected. Motor loss and paresthesias commonly result from neurapraxia. In neurapraxia impulse conduction is interrupted across the site of injury, but the damage is not severe enough to cause axonal death and wallerian degeneration. In mild cases, as when a leg "falls asleep," the neurapraxia is due most likely to transient ischemia.[56, 63] In more severe cases such as "Saturday night palsy," there can be a compression

injury to the myelin.[60] This causes a localized axonal conduction block, but as the myelin recovers, the conduction across the affected segment is restored. Such recovery of motor and sensory function can take from seconds to 6 months.[72]

Axonotmesis

Axonotmesis is an injury of the axon which causes axonal death and subsequent wallerian degeneration distal to the site of injury. The epineurium, perineurium, endoneurium, and Schwann cells remain intact. In Seddon's study,[72] these injuries most often occurred secondary to closed fractures or dislocations. Compressive injuries caused 18% of the axonotmetic injuries. Sensory, motor, and sudomotor function are all affected. The time course and completeness of recovery depend on the location of the injury and the age and condition of the patient. In general, axons regenerate at a rate of approximately 1.5 to 2.00 mm/day.[14] The more proximal the insult, the longer it takes to recover distal function. If the recovery is delayed excessively, the tract (endoneurial sheath) which the axon regrows into may deteriorate permanently and recovery may never be complete.[77] Wallerian regeneration is faster in younger patients, and is slower in patients with metabolic conditions such as diabetes mellitus.

Neurotmesis

This most severe injury in Seddon's classification is a complete nerve transection involving the axon as well as the supportive structures, although on gross inspection the

TABLE 46–2   Nerve Fiber Types in Mammalian Nerve

Fiber Type	Function	Fiber Diameter (μm)	Conduction Velocity (m/sec)	Spike Duration (ms)	Absolute Refractory Period (ms)
A					
α	Proprioception; somatic motor	12–20	70–120		
β	Touch, pressure	5–12	30–70	0.4–0.5	0.4–1
γ	Motor to muscle spindles	3–6	15–30		
δ	Pain, temperature, touch	2–5	12–30		
B	Preganglionic autonomic	<3	3–15	1.2	1.2
C					
Dorsal root	Pain, reflex responses	0.4–1.2	0.5–2	2	2
Sympathetic	Postganglionic sympathetics	0.3–1.3	0.7–2.3	2	2

From Ganong WF: Review of Medical Physiology, ed 13. East Norwalk, Conn, Appleton & Lange, 1987.

TABLE 46–4   The Seddon and Sunderland Classification Systems

Seddon[72]	Sunderland[77]	Description
Neurapraxia	First-degree injury	Focal conduction block; axons remain intact
Axonotmesis	Second-degree injury	Axonal damage and wallerian degeneration; intact supporting structures
Neurotmesis	Third-degree injury	Interruption of axon and endoneurium
	Fourth-degree injury	Interruption of perineurium and endoneurium
	Fifth-degree injury	All supporting structures and axon damaged

nerve may appear intact. These injuries have a poor prognosis, as axonal regrowth is problematic owing to discontinuity of the neural tube. Neuroma formation is common and surgical excision of the damaged segment with reanastomosis may be indicated.

Sunderland's Classification

Sunderlund expanded on Seddon's initial work and described five degrees of injury.[77] The third- through fifth-degree injuries are basically subcategories of Seddon's neurotmesis.

First-Degree Injury

First-degree injury is a focal conduction block in which the axon remains intact. This is essentially the same as neurapraxia.

Second-Degree Injury

As in Seddon's axonotmesis, the axon in a second-degree injury is damaged with subsequent distal wallerian degeneration. The supportive structures of the nerve, including the endoneurium, remain intact. The prognosis for nerve recovery is good since the nerve can grow down its original endoneurial tube.

Third-Degree Injury

In third-degree injury the axon and the endoneurium are both disrupted. The perineurium remains intact, but within the fascicle there is hemorrhage, edema, and subsequent fibrosis. The axon tips do not always follow their original pathway, but can grow into the distal endoneurial tubes randomly. Fibrosis can block their regrowth entirely. In general, the more proximal the level of injury, the less the likelihood of normal reinnervation reaching the end-organ. The functional outcome of regrowth (rerouting) depends to some extent on whether the fibers within the fasciculus share a similar common function. For example, a motor nerve is nonfunctional if it grows down to a sensory end-organ. As a rule, recovery is less complete than in second-degree injuries.

When axons regrow into different endoneurial tubes, they reach different end-organs. This process is called synkinesis, and it results in aberrant innervation.[78] For instance, in Bell's palsy, cranial nerve VII fibers, which previously innervated the salivary glands, may be rerouted to the tear glands, causing the salivating patient to experience "crocodile tears."[79] Similarly, proximal brachial plexus injury can cause fibers from the phrenic nerve to be rerouted so that during respiration the arm muscles might contract.[78]

Fourth-Degree Injury

Both the perineurium and endoneurium as well as the axon are damaged in a fourth-degree injury. This allows recovering axons to sprout outside of their fascicles, which can lead to neuroma formation. Surgery is usually required to remove the damaged segment and reattach the healthy ends.

Fifth-Degree Injury

All supporting structures as well as the axon are damaged in a fifth-degree injury. Recovery depends on the mechanism of injury. Nerve lacerations can be treated with surgery and outcome may be good, whereas injuries from stretch or compression have a poorer prognosis.

ETIOLOGY OF NEUROPATHY

There is a wide array of neuropathic disorders, which are usually categorized by etiology. These etiologies include hereditary (Table 46–5), toxic (Table 46–6), those associated with diseases and inflammatory processes (Table 46–7), idiopathic (Table 46–8), entrapment (Table 46–9), nutritional (Table 46–10) and those secondary to infectious processes (Table 46–11; Figs. 46–9 and 46–10).

While such a classification system allows for a labeling framework, it does little to help diagnose and treat individual patients. What follows is a more practical clinical approach.

TABLE 46–5   Hereditary Peripheral Neuropathies

> Charcot-Marie-Tooth disease (hereditary motor sensory neuropathy [HMSN] types I and II)
> Dejerine-Sottas disease (HMSN type III)
> Refsum's disease (HMSN type IV)
> Neuropathies associated with
>   Spinocerebellar degeneration (HMSN type V)
>   Optic atrophy (HMSN type VI)
>   Retinitis pigmentosa (HMSN type VII)
> Friedreich's ataxia
> Pressure-sensitive hereditary neuropathy
> Acute intermittent porphyria
> Familial amyloid neuropathy
> Fabry's disease
> Hereditary sensory neuropathy
> Giant axonal neuropathies
> Lipoprotein neuropathies
> Roussy-Lévy syndrome
> Riley-Day syndrome
> Pelizaeus-Merzbacher disease
> Metachromatic leukodystrophy
> Krabbe's leukodystrophy
> Tangier disease

TABLE 46–6   Toxic Peripheral Neuropathies

DRUGS	HEAVY METALS
Amiodarone	Antimony
Chloramphenicol	Arsenic
Corticosteroids	Gold
Dapsone	Lead
Diphenylhydantoin	Mercury
Disulfiram	Thallium
Halogenated hydroxyquinolones	ORGANIC COMPOUNDS
Heroin	Acrylamide
Hydralazine	Carbon disulfide
Isoniazid	Dichlorophenoxyacetic
Lysergide (LSD)	acid
Misonidazole	Ethyl alcohol
Nitrofurantoin	Ethylene oxide
Pyridoxine	Methylbutyl ketone
Sodium cyanate	Triorthocresyl phosphate
Tetanus toxoid	
Thalidomide	

Evaluation of the Patient With Peripheral Neuropathy

History

As with any disease process the physician must take a careful history to assess the patient with peripheral neuropathy. Was the onset sudden or gradual? Is the progression rapid or slow? Is there sensory or motor involvement? Or both? Is the primary involvement distal or proximal, symmetrical or asymmetrical, focal or generalized? Is there pain involvement? Does the patient have any associated diseases? An in-depth family and social history is useful, particularly if there have been familial occurrences or toxic exposures.

Physical Examination

Sensory Examination

All sensory modalities should be tested, including pinprick, light touch, proprioception, vibration, graphesthesia,

TABLE 46–7   Diseases Associated with Peripheral Neuropathy

Alcoholism
Amyloidosis
Benign monoclonal gammopathy (IgG, IgA, IgM)
Chronic liver disease
Chronic obstructive pulmonary disease
Cryoglobulinemia
Diabetes mellitus
   Distal symmetrical neuropathy
   Autonomic neuropathy
   Proximal asymmetrical painful motor neuropathy
   Cranial mononeuropathies
Giant cell arteritis
Gout
Hypothyroidism
Necrotizing angiopathy
Neuropathies in malignant diseases
   Lymphomas—focal and systemic
   Multiple myeloma
   Bronchogenic carcinoma
   Tumors of the ovary, testes, penis, stomach, or oral cavity
   Meningeal carcinomatosis
   Oat cell carcinoma
   Osteosclerotic myeloma

TABLE 46–8   Idiopathic Neuropathies

Brachial neuritis (Parsonage-Turner syndrome)
Chronic inflammatory polyradiculopathy
Chronic relapsing polyneuropathy
Fisher syndrome
Acute inflammatory demyelinating polyradiculoneuropathy
   (Guillain-Barré syndrome)
Steroid-responsive polyneuropathy

and temperature. If these are preserved, it is unlikely that a significant sensory deficit is present.

If sensory deficits are detected, the extent and pattern of the loss should be determined. This can both help to chart the progression of the disease, as well as identify patients who need to be counseled about protecting insensate or dysesthetic skin.

Motor Examination

Normal patients vary widely in their strength, both for reasons of their absolute muscle mass and because of varying motivation, understanding, and cooperation. Pain can also prevent a patient from exerting full muscle force (pain inhibition of function). Muscle strength should be graded by the make-and-break system and with functional tests (see Chapter 1).

Reflex Testing

Muscle stretch reflex (MSR) testing, also known as deep tendon reflex (DTR) testing, causes a rapid stretch of the muscle which activates the muscle spindle fibers and causes a reflex contraction. This gives an indication of the state of the afferent and efferent fibers to the muscle as well as the local spinal cord level and descending central nervous system (CNS) control (see Chapter 1). In peripheral neuropathy the MSRs are usually depressed, especially distally. The patient must be relaxed, as an overly tense muscle will not respond to a tendon tap. Patients with bulky muscles may appear not to have reflexes because the heavy tendons

TABLE 46–9   Common Peripheral Nerve Injury and Entrapment Syndromes

Nerve	Entrapment
Radial nerve	At the radial groove of the humerus (Saturday night palsy)
	Posterior interosseous nerve syndrome
Ulnar nerve	At the olecranon groove
	Tardy ulnar palsy
	Cubital tunnel syndrome
	Injury at the wrist (may be at the canal of Guyon)
Median nerve	At the supracondylar ligament of Struthers (at elbow)
	Pronator teres syndrome
	Carpal tunnel syndrome
	Anterior interosseous syndrome
Sciatic nerve	Injection palsy—injury to lateral division
	Injury to medial division
	Complete injury
Femoral nerve	Above or below the inguinal ligament
Peroneal nerve	At head of fibula
Tibial nerve	Tarsal tunnel syndrome

TABLE 46–10   Nutritional Neuropathies

Beriberi or pellagra—thiamine (vitamin B₁) deficiency
Riboflavin (vitamin B₂) deficiency
Pyridoxine (vitamin B₆) deficiency
Pernicious anemia (vitamin B₁₂ deficiency)
Protein or calorie deficiency in children

and muscles are not stretched adequately by the usual hammer-strike technique and for these patients a heavier hammer should be used.

When the reflex is difficult to elicit, a facilitation technique should be used. Jendrassik's maneuver has the patient interlock the fingers and pull against them. This distracts the patient and removes suprasegmental inhibitory influences on the reflex. Other distracting techniques such as clenching the teeth or squeezing the eyelids can also be effective. The Queen's square hammer is heavier and can elicit reflexes which at times are not obtainable by the usual "hatchet"-style hammers. Reflexes are graded on a scale from 0 to 4+.

Superficial skin reflexes may also be evaluated. They are elicited by stroking the skin rather than by striking a tendon. They include such normal reflexes as the abdominal and cremasteric reflexes. The presence of Babinski's, palmomental, grasp, suck, or glabellar reflex is usually considered abnormal in an adult. Abnormal superficial reflexes are usually signs of upper motor neuron disorders and are typically not present in peripheral neuropathy. Their presence can help differentiate a central from a peripheral condition.

Electrodiagnostic Examination in Peripheral Neuropathy

Nerve Conduction Studies

Nerve conduction studies (NCS) are the most helpful part of the electrodiagnostic examination for peripheral nerve disorders (Table 46–12). These studies determine the conduction velocity of the nerve as well as the amplitude of the propagated electrical waveform. In motor nerves, the NCS also provide distal latency information.[54] Both motor and sensory nerves are evaluated by NCS.

The insulating layer of myelin can be impaired through thinning of the myelin sheath or through deterioration of the internodal segments.[53] When the internode is damaged, the electrical current "leaks," delaying depolarization. The time required for the next node to reach threshold is increased. This causes an overall slowing in the nerve conduction velocity and changes in other NCS parameters.

In severe demyelination the impulse may fail to excite the subsequent node, resulting in a conduction block. The

TABLE 46–11   Infectious Causes of Peripheral Neuropathy

Cytomegalovirus in human immunodeficiency virus (HIV) infection
Diphtheria
Herpes zoster
Leprosy
Rabies

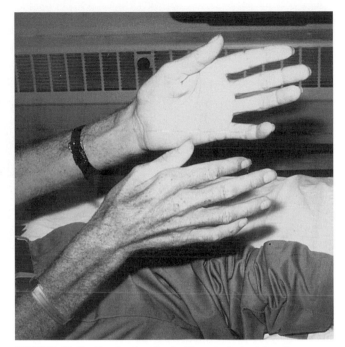

FIGURE 46–8   Hands of patient with arsenic peripheral neuropathy.

conduction velocity is typically moderately to severely slowed, and the distal latency is prolonged, while the amplitude of the evoked responses is relatively preserved. These waveforms usually display a temporal dispersion. If conduction block is present in some fibers of a nerve, the amplitude of the evoked response is reduced (see Chapters 6, 7, and 8).

In diseases where axonal degeneration predominates, the conduction velocity generally remains normal or only slightly decreased. If the larger (faster) nerve fibers are predominantly involved there may be more significant slowing. More typical of axonopathy, however, is a reduction in amplitude of the evoked responses. This is due to the fact that as some of the fibers die, they no longer contribute to the amplitude of these responses.[50] This is especially true when recording directly from nerves. When

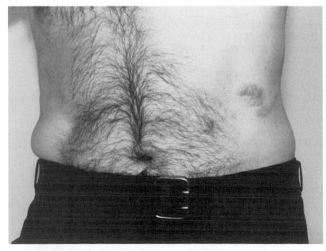

FIGURE 46–9   Patient with acute shingles (herpes zoster).

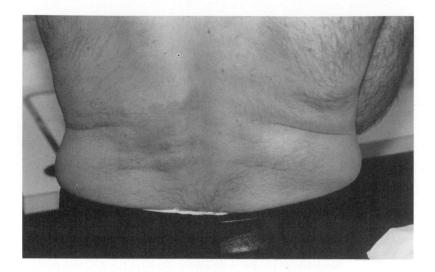

FIGURE 46–10 Patient with acute shingles (herpes zoster).

recording from the muscles, the remaining (fewer) axons may continue to innervate a constant number of muscle fibers (through reinnervation) and the evoked muscle response may be maintained well into the disease process. Temporal dispersion is usually minimal until well into the disease process, both with nerve- and muscle-recording techniques.

Many peripheral neuropathies involve a component of both axonal degeneration and demyelination, and the resultant findings on nerve conduction studies suggest a mixed picture. There is slowed conduction and temporal dispersion, as well as decreased amplitude of the recorded responses (see Chapters 6, 7, and 8).

Electromyography

The electromyograph (EMG) needle records the electrical activity of muscle fibers. Since denervated muscle fibers display characteristic abnormalities in the needle examination (see Table 46–12), this part of the examination is useful in determining the extent of such loss and in localizing the nerve lesions. It can also aid in determining the time course of the disease to some extent, as it helps in analyzing the process of reinnervation. It is less useful in evaluating purely demyelinating lesions, as the muscle fibers retain their innervation in these disorders.

In mild peripheral neuropathy the EMG findings are generally minimal. The most affected muscles (usually distal ones) show the most obvious EMG findings. In mildly affected muscles the changes include increased polyphasicity of the MUAPs. In more severe neuropathies there is muscle membrane instability. As reinnervation progresses, polyphasic motor units of prolonged duration and high amplitude are seen. Demyelination typically causes little abnormal muscle membrane irritability, and fibrillation potentials and positive sharp waves are only occasionally seen[53] (see Chapters 6, 7, and 8).

COMMON COMPLICATIONS OF PERIPHERAL NEUROPATHY

Muscle weakness, sensory loss, and autonomic problems commonly occur in patients with peripheral neuropathies. Muscle weakness can lead to joint contractures and muscle shortening. Sensory loss can result in more frequent and severe injuries to insensate areas. Autonomic problems can affect many functions, including heart rate, blood pressure, and sweating, as well as cause gastroparesis, neurogenic bladder, and impotence.

Muscle Weakness

Joint contractures and muscle shortening are associated with muscle weakness. They can be prevented with daily range-of-motion (ROM) and muscle-stretching exercises. Depending on the degree of weakness this exercise can be passive, active-assistive, or active. When in bed or at rest, proper positioning and splinting, if needed, are essential.

TABLE 46–12 Typical Electrodiagnostic Findings in the General Categories of Neuropathy*

Type	Motor Nerve Conduction Velocities	Amplitude of MUAP	Amplitude of Sensory Action Potential	EMG Findings
Hereditary	↓	NL/↓	↓	Usually denervation potentials
Toxic	NL/↓	NL/↓	NL/↓	Usually denervation potentials
Associated with disease	↓	↓	↓	Usually denervation potentials
Idiopathic	↓	↓	↓	Variable
Entrapment	↓	NL/↓	NL/↓	Variable; usually NL
Infectious	NL/slight ↓	Slight ↓	↓	Denervation potentials
Nutritional	↓	Slight ↓	↓	Denervation potentials

*Exceptions are common.
Abbreviations: MUAP, motor unit action potential; EMG, electromyography; NL, within normal limits.

A program of gentle strengthening, which can include isometric, isotonic, isokinetic, manual-resistive, and progressive-resistive exercise, should be carefully tailored to the patient (see Chapter 20). While improvement of strength is desirable, the muscles should not be overworked, as this can result in paradoxical weakening (overwork weakness).[7, 42] Orthoses should be appropriately prescribed for the patient to increase function and aid in positioning. In the patient who is at bed rest or cognitively compromised, careful positioning is indicated to prevent injury to the peripheral nerves. Peripheral nerves can be compressed between bony prominences and the bed. Injury to the ulnar nerve at the elbow and compression of the common peroneal nerve at the head of the fibula are the injuries most commonly seen (see Chapter 8).

Sensory Loss

When protective sensation is compromised, patients should carefully examine the anesthetic or dysesthetic areas daily. Owing to their being the most distal body part, the feet are most commonly affected by loss of sensation in neuropathy. The patient may traumatize the skin and cause skin breakdown and ulceration. Repetitive joint trauma can lead to the development of neuroarthropathic (Charcot's) joints. In either case the prescription of extradepth or custom-molded shoes may be indicated. A Plastizote shoe insert helps to prevent foot trauma and ulcers (see Chapters 17 and 56).

In addition to careful daily skin examination, the patient should be instructed in thorough, gentle cleaning and soaking techniques. This should be followed by application of a lubricant to help the foot resist fissuring and scaling. Such preventive care is much easier than treating a skin breakdown. Patients should be sure to rest and protect their skin at the earliest sign of trauma. Waiting too long to treat can lead to irreversible sequelae, which can ultimately result in amputation.

Autonomic Dysfunction

Autonomic problems are seen in a variety of peripheral neuropathies, but are perhaps most commonly associated with diabetes mellitus and Guillain-Barré syndrome. Cardiovascular symptoms can include orthostatic intolerance or cardiac arrhythmias. Genitourinary symptoms include a flaccid bladder and male impotence. Gastrointestinal symptoms can affect any part of the gastrointestinal tract and include vomiting, dysphagia, diarrhea, constipation, and many other problems. Sweating abnormalities are seen with autonomic involvement as well.

The autonomic dysfunction in GBS can be life-threatening. These patients should have cardiac monitoring with close observation for dysrhythmias and postural hypotension in the early phases of their disease.

REHABILITATION MANAGEMENT OF THE MORE COMMON PERIPHERAL NEUROPATHIES

The following is a discussion of the rehabilitation management of several representative disorders. This list is not all-inclusive, but the principles described can readily be adapted to other, similar disorders.

Diabetic Neuropathies

Both insulin-dependent (IDDM) and non-insulin-dependent diabetes mellitus (NIDDM) can cause neuropathies. These are subdivided into whether they are symmetrical or asymmetrical (Figs. 46–11 to 46–13). The symmetrical group are polyneuropathies and include (1) a primarily sensory peripheral neuropathy, the most common of the diabetic neuropathies (acroneuropathy); (2) autonomic peripheral neuropathy, which is often seen in conjunction with the sensory form; (3) acute painful neuropathy; (4) subclinical neuropathy; and (5) proximal lower extremity motor neuropathy, also known by the less descriptive term *diabetic amyotrophy*.

The asymmetrical neuropathies include (1) neuropathy of individual nerves (mononeuropathy); (2) some painful neuropathies; (3) truncal neuropathy or radiculopathy; and (4) entrapment neuropathies. Some cases of proximal lower extremity motor neuropathy are also asymmetrical. It can easily be appreciated that the diabetic neuropathies can also be caused by other diseases, and every neuropathy in a diabetic patient should be separately evaluated and not automatically diagnosed as a diabetic neuropathy. Diabetes

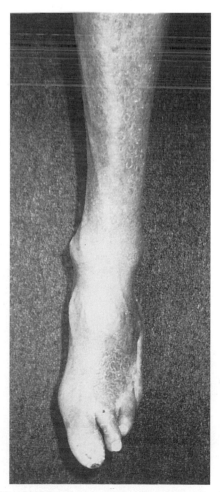

FIGURE 46–11 Typical appearance of a foot with changes of diabetic peripheral neuropathy and peripheral vascular disease.

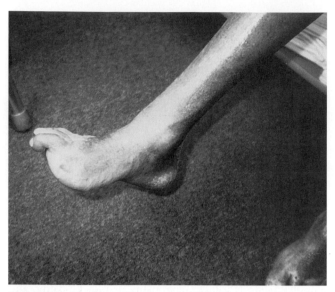

FIGURE 46–12 Foot with changes of diabetic peripheral neuropathy and peripheral vascular disease.

predisposes the patient to other neuropathies, especially focal neuropathies such as carpal tunnel syndrome.

SYMMETRICAL PERIPHERAL NEUROPATHY IN DIABETES. The initial symptoms of diabetic symmetrical polyneuropathy are usually sensory. They include burning, itching, and a "pins-and-needles sensation." On physical examination the greatest abnormalities are in light touch and vibration, with preservation of conscious proprioception until late in the course. Patients complain of muscle cramping or tightness, especially at night. They also present with hypoesthesia or analgesia. Many patients have not noticed their "painless neuropathy" because of its gradual onset. The symptoms begin in the toes and progress proximally over the course of months to years. The longest nerves are affected first. Eventually the fingers and hands become involved, giving the typical stocking-and-glove distribution.[68]

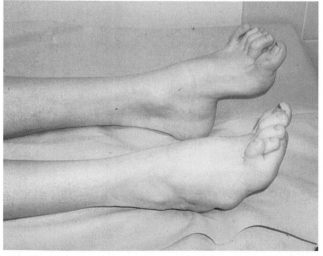

FIGURE 46–13 "Intrinsic minus" foot deformity in patient with diabetic peripheral neuropathy.

Weakness is generally seen later in the course of diabetic complications. It starts distally and progresses proximally. A foot slap is a common result of this. Patients with diabetic polyneuropathy may also have an ataxic gait. This is due to abnormal proprioceptive sensation, which is involved typically only in the late stages of neuropathy.

If the diabetic patient with peripheral sensory impairment does not care for his or her affected areas meticulously, repeated trauma can result in skin ulceration or development of Charcot's joint.

AUTONOMIC PERIPHERAL NEUROPATHY. Autonomic symptoms are often seen together with sensory loss. They can involve various body functions including the cardiovascular, genitourinary, gastrointestinal, and cutaneous[2] and thermoregulatory systems. The primary cardiovascular abnormalities are orthostatic hypotension, cardiac arrhythmias, and impaired heart rate control.[43] The cause of the orthostatic hypotension is most likely an impaired vasoconstriction reflex.[43] Heart abnormalities include a resting tachycardia, fixed heart rate, and loss of sleep bradycardia.[25]

Gastrointestinal dysautonomia can manifest as esophageal dysmotility,[74] gastroparesis,[59] anal incontinence,[71] and constipation or diarrhea.[70, 71]

Common genitourinary abnormalities are neurogenic bladder[49] and erectile dysfunction.[70] Diabetic impotence is common in the male and is irreversible.[27] The early signs of neurogenic bladder include decreased urinary frequency, followed by difficulties with initiating micturition. The bladder eventually becomes flaccid and urinary retention with overflow voiding occurs as the neuropathy worsens.[15, 26]

When the cutaneous system is also affected there can be impaired distal sweating. This often results in compensatory sweating of the trunk and face.[70]

ACUTE PAINFUL NEUROPATHY. Acute painful diabetic neuropathy occurs rarely, and is characterized by severe pain in the distal lower extremities, described as a burning dysesthesia. It is often associated with depression, insomnia, and weight loss. Examination reveals only a mild sensory loss, if any.[3] It is often referred to inappropriately as diabetic "neuritis."

LOWER EXTREMITY PROXIMAL MOTOR NEUROPATHY. Lower extremity proximal motor neuropathy was earlier called "diabetic amyotrophy." It was initially described as being a unilateral proximal leg weakness.[83] Later the term was used to describe bilateral leg weakness as well.[83] It was once thought that the cause of this disorder was a spinal cord lesion, but electrodiagnostic studies revealed that the dysfunction is in the proximal peripheral nerve (lumbosacral polyradiculopathy, plexus lesion, femoral neuropathy, or obturator nerve lesion).[83]

The onset of this neuropathy can be acute or subacute. The disorder is characterized by weakness of the quadriceps, iliopsoas, or thigh adductors, individually or severally.[83] The gluteal muscles, hamstrings, and gastrocnemius may also be weak. Pain is often a prominent component of this problem and is worse at night.[83] The pain is described as severe, deep, and aching. Sensation is usually intact, but this disorder can coexist with a sensory neuropathy. Recovery occurs over a 12- to 24-month period and the prognosis for significant improvement is generally good.[83]

MONONEUROPATHY. Mononeuropathy, an asymmetrical form of diabetic peripheral neuropathy, can affect the cranial or peripheral nerves. The third cranial nerve is most commonly affected, although the abducens, trochlear, and facial nerves can be involved as well.[83] The pupil is usually spared in oculomotor palsy.[34] Multiple asymmetrical nerve involvements, referred to as mononeuropathy multiplex, may occur. In these cases, other causes of mononeuropathy multiplex (such as polyarteritis nodosa) have to be ruled out before considering it due to diabetes.

TRUNCAL NEUROPATHY OR RADICULOPATHY. Thoracoabdominal or truncal neuropathy or radiculopathy occurs most often in diabetic patients older than 50.[68] Onset may be acute or gradual. The distribution is usually unilateral, involving primarily T3 through T12.[75] The condition can be painful and includes a differential diagnosis of myocardial infarction, an intraspinal pathological process, abdominal disease, or malignancy.[68]

ENTRAPMENT NEUROPATHY. Persons with diabetes have long been thought to be at increased risk for entrapment neuropathies. Fraser et al.[30] found no clear-cut relationship between the mononeuropathies and duration of diabetes, diabetic control, or the presence of other diabetic complications. Nevertheless, evidence seems to support the common belief that diabetes does indeed predispose to focal pressure neuropathies.[47]

Electrodiagnostic Findings in Diabetic Neuropathy

In symmetrical peripheral sensory neuropathy nerve conduction studies often reveal a mixed picture of an axonal and segmental demyelinating process.[84] Increased temporal dispersion of the sensory potential is one of the earliest signs of diabetic peripheral neuropathy.[83] The longest nerves are usually the first affected. They are slower distally than proximally. Sensory nerve amplitude is decreased and motor conduction velocity is slowed. Both axonal degeneration and segmental demyelination can occur. Single-fiber EMG studies indicate that the primary dysfunction is due to demyelination.[81] Moderate slowing occurs proximally and distally as determined by F-wave and other studies.[53]

Early needle examination reveals reduction in the number of MUAPs and only subtle changes of increased polyphasicity of the MUAP. There are few if any fibrillation potentials and the MUAP is close to normal in configuration, amplitude, and duration.[53] Later the needle EMG changes can be pronounced.

Lower extremity proximal motor neuropathy, thoracolumbar neuropathy, and acute painful diabetic neuropathy all have similar electrodiagnostic findings. Signs of muscle membrane instability (fibrillation potentials and positive sharp waves) are noted in the affected muscles or myotomes as well as in the paraspinal muscle. Nerve conduction studies are usually within normal limits unless there is concomitant peripheral sensory neuropathy.[3] Mononeuropathies are found most commonly in the peroneal nerve, with findings of slowed conduction in the segment of the nerve traversing the fibular head.[62] Other commonly affected nerves include the median and ulnar.[62] Kraft et al.[54] found

that approximately one half of diabetic patients have findings consistent with subclinical carpal tunnel syndrome.

Management of Diabetic Peripheral Neuropathy

MEDICAL MANAGEMENT. The exact pathophysiology of diabetic neuropathy remains undetermined and therefore definitive treatment is unavailable. Two current hypotheses are that the nerve injury is due to (1) metabolic or (2) ischemic processes.[12, 82] These processes are not mutually exclusive. Pathological studies provide evidence for ischemic microvascular disease,[82] while metabolic abnormalities include an accumulation of sorbitol and a reduction of *myo*-inositol in the body.[32, 36] Since glucose is converted to sorbitol by aldose reductase, it was once thought that aldose reductase inhibitors might improve the course of the disease. They have not, however, been shown to be significantly helpful in the treatment of peripheral neuropathy.[48] Since there is a reduced *myo*-inositol content, it was hypothesized that supplementation with this substance could be a useful treatment. In animal studies *myo*-inositol has caused improvement of nerve conduction velocities,[36] but clinical trials in humans have not shown any significant benefit.[37]

The most important preventive measure for diabetic neuropathy is generally believed to be good glucose control. Although this has not been proved to prevent diabetic complications, there is evidence that better diabetic control lowers the incidence and severity of neuropathy.[17]

SENSORY CHANGES. Sensory loss is the most common symptom of diabetic peripheral neuropathy. Since decreased protective sensation is frequently compounded by vascular insufficiency and dry skin (due to autonomic impairment), skin breakdown can occur. Careful daily inspection of the affected areas is necessary, with daily soaks followed by use of a good moisturizer. Toenails must be cut carefully straight across to prevent ingrown nails. Proper footwear, with appropriate in-shoe orthoses, is imperative. The patient should avoid use of heat on the affected limbs, and avoid foot trauma. When indicated, a podiatrist should be involved in the patient's care. If such preventive measures are not undertaken, ulceration and neuroarthropathy are common. Poor healing of ulcers can lead to gangrene and ultimately to amputation.

PAIN. Neuropathic pain in diabetic patients is often a difficult and frustrating problem to control. Treatment with tricyclic antidepressants can be helpful and should be tried initially at a low bedtime dose of 25 to 50 mg of amitriptyline,[57] desipramine,[58] or nortriptyline[68] and increased as tolerated until benefits are noted. The side effects of these drugs include orthostatic hypotension and worsening of urinary retention. Trazodone[68] can be tried if the patient cannot tolerate amitriptyline or nortriptyline. If the antidepressants are ineffective, anticonvulsants such as carbamazepine[69, 89] can be considered. The starting dose is 200 mg of carbamazepine twice daily. This dose should be increased until there is pain relief or until side effects occur. Blood levels must be closely monitored. Transcutaneous electrical nerve stimulation (TENS) can also prove helpful and deserves a trial (see Chapter 23). Topical capsaicin can help by desensitizing type C-fiber nociceptors.[67] Usually, the pain of diabetic neuropathy decreases spontaneously over time, and patients should be encouraged to remain active to avoid the complications of inactivity.

AUTONOMIC DYSFUNCTION. Autonomic neuropathy is a common complication of diabetes, and treatment must be directed to the specific system affected. Gastroparesis is typically treated with metoclopramide,[59] 10 mg four times daily. Diarrhea or constipation can be treated with a proper diet. A course of tetracycline or other broad-spectrum antibiotic may be used to alleviate diarrhea.[35] Postural hypotension should be managed with the least invasive measures. The initial treatment is to teach the patient to change position slowly and consider sleeping with the head of the bed elevated.[83] Compression stockings and an abdominal binder may improve venous return and decrease symptoms. When these fail, use of a mineralocorticoid such as fludrocortisone may benefit the patient.[83]

The management of neurogenic bladder depends on the severity of the condition. Postvoiding residual measurement often helps in determining the severity. In cases of mild to moderate impairment of bladder emptying, the patient should be encouraged to empty the bladder every 2 to 3 hours while awake. As severity increases, an intermittent catheterization program may be necessary to assure adequate drainage. Use of a parasympathomimetic agent can also be helpful (see Chapter 28).

Impotence is a common problem in diabetes. Treatment choices range from counseling, to suction erection devices, to penile implants (see Chapter 30).

Sudomotor dysfunction is more pronounced over the distal extremities. It can leave the skin dry and subject to cracking and fissuring. Regular skin care and lubrication are necessary (see Chapter 56).

Alcoholic Neuropathy

The neuropathy of alcohol abuse appears to be, at least in part, related to malnutrition (especially the B vitamins).[18, 87] As with other toxic and metabolic disorders the axons tend to "die back" from the periphery. The ensuing neuropathy is a mixed motor and sensory disorder,[53] with the symptoms first occurring in the lower extremities. Paresthesias are often present.

The affected patients have decreased sensation (especially of proprioception), distal muscle weakness and wasting, and depressed distal reflexes. As the disorder worsens, these changes appear more proximally in the lower extremities and begin in the upper extremities.

Electrophysiological studies show decreased sensory action potential amplitudes. There is minimal slowing of motor conduction velocity, and distal latencies are minimally prolonged.[53] Needle examination typically shows positive sharp waves and fibrillation potentials in the distal muscles, with polyphasic units of increased amplitude[5] (see Chapter 8).

Management of Alcoholic Neuropathy

The primary treatment of alcoholic neuropathy is to stop the use of alcohol. Vitamins (especially B vitamins) and magnesium must be supplemented and a good diet instituted. Unlike diabetic polyneuropathy, alcoholic neuropathy

has a good prognosis if treated promptly, or at least while it is not too advanced.[18]

The complications of alcoholic neuropathy are treated similarly to those of diabetes described above. Orthoses may be needed if significant weakness is a problem.

Acute Inflammatory Demyelinating Polyradiculoneuropathy

Acute inflammatory demyelinating polyradiculoneuropathy (AIDP), also known as Guillain-Barré syndrome (GBS), was first described by Landry in the 1860s, but derived its eponym from a description in 1916 by Georges Guillain and Jean Alexander Barré. Guillain and Barré noted that this was a paralyzing condition associated with an increased concentration of protein, but not cells, in the cerebrospinal fluid (CSF). This cytoalbuminological disassociation distinguished the condition from other common neuropathies, as well as from poliomyelitis. Since their description, other related disorders have been identified. They include a chronic or relapsing form, a steroid-responsive form, as well as the Miller-Fisher variant in which there is ataxia, ophthalmoplegia, and depressed muscle stretch reflexes.[29]

GBS is an acquired symmetrical polyneuropathy that usually affects the lower extremities initially.[28] It often begins with fine paresthesias in the toes or fingertips followed by an ascending weakness. The weakness progresses over days to weeks and can result in severe total body paresis, including the muscles of respiration. The facial muscles and oropharyngeal muscles are often involved, although the extraocular muscles and sphincters are generally spared. Pain is a common symptom. GBS can involve somatic, autonomic, and cranial nerves. Muscle stretch reflexes are typically absent or severely decreased.[66]

Diagnostic criteria[66] for typical GBS include the required features of areflexia and progressive weakness in all extremities. Strong supporting features include a progression of the symptoms over a 4-week period, relative symmetry, mild sensory symptoms, cranial nerve involvement, recovery beginning 2 to 4 weeks after progression ceases, autonomic dysfunction, elevated concentration of protein in the CSF with less than 10 cells per cubic millimeter, and typical electrodiagnostic features. On physical examination there is symmetrical limb weakness, and bilateral facial weakness in one third of the patients. The muscle stretch reflexes are absent and there is minimal change in sensation. If the respiratory muscles are involved, the vital capacity is usually one half of the predicted value. The vital capacity should be carefully monitored as the patient might require ventilatory support. Autonomic function is often affected (71%)[33] and can precipitate abnormalities in heart rate and rhythm and blood pressure. A period of observation in an intensive care unit (ICU) may be necessary.

Early pathological examination of the nerves reveals lymphocytes and macrophages surrounding the endoneurial vessels.[4] It was once thought that this was primarily an inflammatory neuropathy. More recent studies[41] propose that an early antibody attack on myelin occurs in some cases, with a mainly inflammatory process predominating in others. The nerves are affected earliest at the root level.

Later the most peripheral nerve is damaged with the intervening segments being affected last. The insult to the nerve appears to be primarily of a demyelinating type, but in more severe cases there may also be prominent axonal loss.[53]

Electrodiagnostic Findings in Guillain-Barré Syndrome

Since the earliest involvement of GBS is at the nerve root level, the earliest electrodiagnostic abnormalities are prolongation or absence of the late responses (F wave and H-reflex). Later there can be a slowing of motor nerve conduction, but this is a less consistent finding. Temporal dispersion of the evoked responses may also be noted, as well as significantly prolonged distal latencies. If serial studies are performed, the electrodiagnostic findings frequently lag behind the clinical course, both during worsening and during recovery of function.[6] Patients with weakness typically show a reduction in the number of motor units firing on maximal effort.

The best prognostic indicator is the needle EMG.[65] EMG signs of denervation indicate that the patient has axonopathy rather than just demyelination, and will have a slower recovery with poorer outcome.

Management of Guillain-Barré Syndrome

Patients with acute GBS should be hospitalized for observation and monitoring of the progression of the disease. It is particularly important to serially monitor the pulmonary and cardiovascular systems. If the vital capacity is rapidly declining, especially if it is less than 18 mL/kg of body weight,[66] or if there is cardiovascular dysautonomia, the patient should be monitored in an ICU. Mechanical ventilation may also be necessary.

As these patients are immobile, they are at risk for developing deep venous thrombosis, pressure ulcers, and the other complications of immobility (see Chapter 34). Appropriate preventive and treatment measures should be undertaken.

Large randomized trials[31, 38] have shown the usefulness of plasmapheresis in treating GBS. The duration of mechanical ventilation can be halved with such treatment, and overall recovery time is significantly decreased. Contraindications to plasma exchange include recent myocardial infarction, angina, sepsis, or cardiovascular dysautonomia.[66] Patients should be warned about having surgery after recovery from GBS, as surgery can cause a recurrence, even years later. The recurrence is often worse than the original GBS episode. The exact part of the surgical experience that causes the recurrence is unknown. Even minor surgery such as oral surgery can trigger it.

REHABILITATION METHODS. In the early stages of GBS the patient may be quadriplegic and bedridden. During this time prevention of contractures by ROM exercise, positioning, and the use of static splints is important. Careful positioning should also be done to prevent peripheral nerve compression and pressure ulcer formation. Meticulous pulmonary care is indicated to prevent atelectasis and pneumonia.

The rehabilitation program is gradually advanced in intensity as the patient improves. Since the patient with GBS is susceptible to overwork weakness, the strengthening program should initially be nonfatiguing. When muscles regain greater than antigravity strength, they can generally be stressed with more aggressive strengthening exercises. If the exercises are advanced too quickly, however, there may be a regression of strength (the so-called overwork weakness).[7] This should alert the clinician to reduce the activity level.

During recovery, GBS patients often benefit from the use of orthoses and assistive devices. Rocker feeders are helpful, as are clothing adaptations and other assistive devices. Ankle-foot and wrist orthoses can be useful in preventing contractures and enhancing function. It is more common for GBS patients to develop tightness of two-joint muscles than joint capsule contractures. Stretching of these muscles will alleviate this problem, and should include the hamstrings, tensor fascia lata, and gastrocnemius.

Gait retraining typically begins with the use of the tilt table. The tilt table is actually valuable well before gait training is possible, for it helps prevent deterioration in orthostatic tolerance. As soon as the patient is medically stable, tilt table training should be instituted. This can also be started in bed by having the patient sit upright for extended periods, as tolerated. As the patient is gradually elevated to the upright position there is a cardiovascular and autonomic adaptation. Patients are next allowed to stand in a standing table, which improves their muscular endurance and permits them to work on other tasks. Eventually the patient is treated in the parallel bars with the close assistance of the therapist to assist in movement and prevent falls. As skills improve, the patient can be advanced to an assistive device for ambulation such as a walker, and then to crutches or canes. Eventually the patient is advanced to ambulation without assistance or with assistive devices. Lower extremity orthoses are used as indicated throughout the course of treatment (see Chapter 17).

In addition to progressive ambulation training, patients develop upper extremity strength and endurance through a combination of functional and weightlifting exercises. The goal is to achieve independent self-care, using assistive devices as needed (hopefully only temporarily). Most patients tolerate such a rehabilitation program and go on to an essentially complete recovery. The 5% to 10% or so who do not recover completely from GBS[66] benefit from the long-term use of assistive devices and rehabilitation strategies.

Uremic Neuropathy

Chronic renal insufficiency is associated with a sensorimotor peripheral neuropathy which causes a diffuse slowing of both motor and sensory conduction.[46] Symptoms of peripheral weakness and decreased sensation are often most severe in the lower extremities, despite an approximately equal slowing of conduction in both the upper and lower extremities.[44] The amplitude of the sensory nerve action potential and the H-reflex latency are the most sensitive indicators of uremic neuropathy.[1, 40] Improvements in the electrodiagnostic findings are noted with dialysis and more significantly with kidney transplantation.[22, 80] Needle examination typically shows signs of denervation in the weak muscles, with MUAPs decreased in number and increased in amplitude[23, 81] (see Chapters 7 and 8).

Medical treatment is aimed at compensating for the underlying disease. The special rehabilitation issues are similar to those encountered in diabetes (see above).

Charcot-Marie-Tooth Disease (Hereditary Motor Sensory Neuropathy, Types I and II)

Charcot-Marie-Tooth (CMT) disease includes a group of hereditary symmetrical distal polyneuropathies.[9] It is one of the most frequently inherited neurological diseases, with an estimated prevalence of 125,000 persons in the United States.[16] The inherited CMT defects have been mapped to chromosome 17 (CMT1A), chromosome 1 (CMT1B), the X chromosome (CMTX), and others.[8, 11, 16, 39, 45, 61, 86] The most common type is hereditary motor sensory neuropathy (HMSN), type HMSN-I (CMT1A). It is inherited in an autosomal dominant fashion. CMT, type II (CMT-II) or HMSN-II is one third as common.[16]

CMT is usually detected in the first or second decade of life, although foot deformities may be noted during infancy.[16] The initial symptoms include progressive distal lower extremity weakness and then atrophy. Pes cavus deformity is common, and is exaggerated (if not caused) by the distal motor dysfunction. The most severely affected muscles are the intrinsic foot muscles and peroneal muscles.[16] Distal sensory deficits are often present. Physical examination typically shows notable peripheral weakness. The ankle muscle stretch reflexes are often absent and other reflexes may be hypoactive. Gait abnormalities are common and include drop foot, foot slap, and steppage gait. As the disease progresses, the distal upper extremities may become involved with atrophy and decreased strength and dexterity (Fig. 46–14). Nerves may be palpably enlarged.[16]

In HMSN-I there is a segmental demyelination with secondary Schwann cell proliferation. The Schwann cells form concentric arrays around the demyelinated nerve that

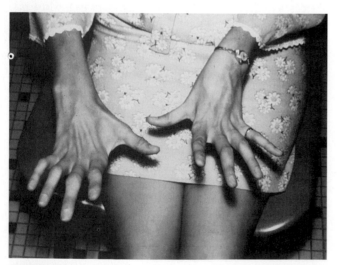

FIGURE 46–14 Hands in patient with advanced Charcot-Marie-Tooth disease.

are known as "onion bulbs" which account for the peripheral nerve enlargement.[19] HMSN-II is sometimes known as the "axonal" form of CMT. It is marked by axonal loss with subsequent wallerian degeneration.[21]

CMT disease has variable penetrance.[10] A carrier might have only mild foot deformities, while other members of the same family could have significant difficulties with ambulation, hand dexterity, and even diaphragmatic involvement.

The symptoms of CMT-I and CMT-II are remarkably similar, although they tend to be milder in type II.[21] In both conditions the symptoms generally progress slowly with only gradual deterioration in function and a normal life span.[24] These patients typically remain ambulatory throughout their lives.[21]

Electrophysiological studies are helpful in diagnosing CMT and in distinguishing type I from type II. In HMSN-I the motor nerve conduction velocities are significantly reduced (to about one half of normal).[21] As the disease progresses the muscle action potential amplitude decreases.[16] Sensory nerve action potential amplitudes are also significantly decreased.[16] Needle EMG examination shows signs of denervation in the affected muscles.[53] In HMSN-II the conduction velocity is normal or near normal, while both the motor and sensory action potential amplitudes are diminished and signs of denervation are present.[53]

Management of Charcot-Marie-Tooth Disease

Treatment of CMT is aimed primarily at maintenance of function, since currently there is no known way to alter the progression of the disease. Ankle-foot orthoses may be indicated if there is significant leg weakness or ankle instability or for protection if sensory symptoms are a significant issue. Careful selection of shoes is important. Custom-molded shoes may be necessary in some cases.

The patient with CMT is at risk for decreased ROM and contractures, especially loss of ankle dorsiflexion. The patient should be taught appropriate ROM and stretching exercises. Careful daily inspection of hypoesthetic areas should be encouraged.

Mononeuritis Multiplex

Mononeuritis multiplex is characterized by sensory and motor neuropathies[20, 81] that occur asymmetrically and asynchronously. It is most commonly due to multiple nerve infarction sites and is commonly seen in vasculitic conditions such as systemic vasculitides. These include polyarteritis nodosa and rheumatoid vasculitis, systemic lupus erythematosus, Lyme disease, Sjögren's syndrome, cryoglobulinemia, temporal arteritis, scleroderma, sarcoidosis, leprosy, acute viral hepatitis A, and acquired immunodeficiency syndrome (AIDS).[20, 64] It is also associated with diabetes mellitus and multiple nerve compressions which are the most common causes.[64] Diagnosis is critical if mononeuropathy multiplex is due to a vasculitis, since treatment with steroids can arrest or limit the condition. Failure to recognize and treat vasculitis can have fatal consequences.

Electrodiagnostic studies show multiple nerve lesions. The rehabilitation management depends on the sites involved and generally includes positioning, bracing (static and functional), and a strengthening program, as tolerated. The precautions for insensate areas as described above should be instituted if appropriate.

Idiopathic Brachial Neuritis (Parsonage-Turner Syndrome)

Idiopathic brachial neuropathy, or brachial neuritis, is a peripheral neuropathy that most commonly affects the radial, long thoracic, phrenic, suprascapular, or spinal accessory nerves.[51, 88] Men are affected twice as frequently as women.[50] In approximately one third of the cases the shoulders are affected bilaterally.[53] This condition classically begins with a sharp pain in one shoulder followed by an aching sensation. Approximately 1 week later the patient notes weakness in the affected muscles. Atrophy typically develops later.[51, 53] The motor nerves are usually more affected than the sensory nerves, but if sensory nerves are affected it is most likely to be the axillary, radial, or cutaneous nerves of the upper extremity.[53]

Electrodiagnostic studies show that motor conduction velocities are normal in the nerve fibers to the unaffected muscles. Latencies from Erb's point to the affected muscles may be slightly prolonged with decreased amplitude and temporal dispersion.[51] Needle EMG examination reveals signs of denervation in the affected muscles as well as polyphasic motor unit potentials and a reduced interference pattern.[13, 51]

Prognosis is generally good,[53] but recovery can take a few years in more severe cases.[51, 85] Rehabilitation management includes maintaining shoulder ROM and preventing contractures, so that the limb is functional when recovery eventually occurs. Orthotic prescription is also often appropriate.

Ischemic Monomelic Neuropathy

Ischemic monomelic neuropathy results from infarction of all the nerves of a distal extremity. It is often caused by spontaneous or iatrogenic arterial occlusion or embolization, frequently during surgical procedures. The patient complains of a deep burning pain which persists even after arterial flow has been restored. Symptoms are predominantly due to a distal sensory loss in all nerve distributions. In more severe cases there is weakness as well, although the motor involvement is not usually as severe.[55] Symptoms can persist for months and are treated with antidepressants or anticonvulsants. Electrodiagnostic evaluation reveals sensory and motor axonal loss distally. Treatment is supportive with gait aids and orthoses as indicated. Sensory loss guidelines are to be followed as well.

CONCLUSION

Peripheral neuropathy is a common diagnosis with many causes and varied prognoses. It is of utmost importance to accurately diagnose the disease in order to be able to treat the patient with peripheral neuropathy appropriately and to give a reasonable prognosis. Much of the symptomatic treatment discussed in this chapter is similar for the different diseases and can be used for other forms of peripheral neuropathy which have not been discussed in detail. Treatment can significantly improve the patient's quality of life.

References

1. Abers JW, Robers WC, Daube J: Electromyographic findings in porphyric neuropathy. Arch Phys Med Rehabil 1976; 57:595.
2. Archer AG, Roberts VC, Watkins PJ: Blood flow patterns in painful diabetic neuropathy. Diabetologia. 1984; 27:563–567.
3. Archer AG, Watkins PJ, Thomas PK, et al: The natural history of acute painful neuropathy in diabetes mellitus. J Neurol Neurosurg Psychiatry 1983; 46:491–499.
4. Asbury AK, Arnason BG, Adams RD: The inflammatory lesion in idiopathic polyneuritis: Its role in pathogenesis. Medicine (Baltimore) 1969; 48:173–215.
5. Ballantyne JP, Hansen S, Weir A, et al: Quantitative electrophysiological study of alcoholic neuropathy. J Neurol Neurosurg Psychiatry 1980; 43:427–432.
6. Bannister RG, Sears TA: The changes in nerve conduction in acute idiopathic polyneuritis. J Neurol Neurosurg Psychiatry 1962; 25:321–328.
7. Bensman A: Strenuous exercise may impair muscle function in Guillain-Barré patients. JAMA 1970; 214:468–469.
8. Bergoffen J, Trofatter J, Pericak-Vance MA, et al: Linkage localization of X-linked Charcot-Marie-Tooth disease. Am J Hum Genet 1993; 52:312–318.
9. Bird TD: Hereditary motor-sensory neuropathies Charcot-Marie-Tooth syndrome. Neurol Clin 1989; 7:9–23.
10. Bird TD, Kraft GH: Charcot-Marie-Tooth disease: Data for genetic counseling relating age to risk. Clin Genet 1978; 14:43–49.
11. Bird TD, Ott J, Giblett ER: Evidence for linkage of Charcot-Marie-Tooth neuropathy to the Duffy locus on chromosome 1. Am J Hum Genet 1982; 34:388–394.
12. Brown MJ, Asbury AK: Diabetic neuropathy. Ann Neurol 1984; 15:2–12.
13. Bradley WG, Madrid R, Thrush DC, Campbell MJ: Recurrent brachial plexus neuropathy. Brain 1975; 98:381–398.
14. Buchtal F, Kuehl V: Nerve conduction, tactile sensibility, and the electromyogram after suture or compression of peripheral nerve: A longitudinal study in man. J Neurol Neurosurg Psychiatry 1979; 42:436–451.
15. Buck AC, Reed Pl, Siddiq YK, et al: Bladder dysfunction and neuropathy in diabetes. Diabetologia 1976; 12:251–258.
16. Chance PF, Pleasure D: Charcot-Marie-Tooth syndrome. Arch Neurol 1993; 50:1180–1184.
17. Committee on Health Care Issues, American Neurological Association: Does improved control of glycemia prevent or ameliorate diabetic polyneuropathy? Ann Neurol 1986; 19:288–290.
18. Dell PC, Guzewicz RM: Atypical peripheral neuropathies. Hand Clin 1992; 8:275–283.
19. Dyck PJ: Histologic measurements and fine structure of biopsied sural nerve: Normal, and in peroneal muscular atrophy, hypertrophic neuropathy, and congenital sensory neuropathy. Mayo Clin Proc 1966; 41:742–774.
20. Dyck PJ, Benstead TJ, Conn DL, et al: Nonsystemic vasculitic neuropathy. Brain 1987; 110:843.
21. Dyck PJ, Chance PJ, Lebo RV, Carney JA: Hereditary motor and sensory neuropathies. In Dyck PJ, Thomas PJ, Griffin JW, et al (eds): Peripheral Neuropathy, vol 2. Philadelphia, WB Saunders, 1993, pp 1094–1136.
22. Dyck PJ, Johnson WJ, Lambert EH, et al: Comparison of symptoms, chemistry, and nerve function to assess adequacy of hemodialysis. Neurology 1979; 29:1361–1368.
23. Dyck PJ, Johnson WJ, Lambert EH, O'Brien PC: Segmental demyelination secondary to axonal degeneration in uremic neuropathy. Mayo Clin Proc 1971; 46:400–431.
24. Dyck PJ, Lambert EH: Lower motor and primary sensory neuron diseases with peroneal muscular atrophy: Neurologic, genetic and electrophysiologic findings in hereditary polyneuropathies. Arch Neurol 1968; 18:603.
25. Ewing DJ, Borsey DQ, Travis P, et al: Abnormalities of ambulatory 24-hour heart rate in diabetes mellitus. Diabetes 1983; 32:101–105.
26. Fagerberg S-E, Kock NG, Petersen I, Stener I: Urinary bladder disturbances in diabetics. A comparative study of male diabetics and

controls aged between twenty and fifty years. Scand J Urol Nephrol 1967; 1:19–27.

27. Fairburn CG, Wu FCW, McCullock DK, et al: The clinical features of diabetic impotence: A preliminary study. Br J Psychiatry 1982; 140:447–452.

28. Feasby TE: Inflammatory-demyelinating polyneuropathies. Neurol Clin 1992; 10:651–670.

29. Fisher M: An unusual variant of acute idiopathic polyneuritis (syndrome of ophthalmoplegia, ataxia and areflexia). N Engl J Med 1956; 255:57–65.

30. Fraser DM, Campbell IW, Ewing DJ, Clarke BF: Mononeuropathy in diabetes mellitus. Diabetes 1979; 28:96–101.

31. French Cooperative Group on Plasma Exchange in Guillain-Barré Syndrome: Efficiency of plasma exchange in Guillain-Barré syndrome. Ann Neurol 1987; 22:753–761.

32. Gabbay KH, Merola LO, Field RA: Sorbitol pathway: Presence in nerve and cord with substrate accumulation in diabetes. Science 1966; 151:209–210.

33. Gibbels E, Giebisch U: Natural course of acute and chronic monophasic inflammatory demyelinating polyneuropathies (IDP). A retrospective analysis of 266 cases. Acta Neurol Scand 1992; 85:282–291.

34. Goldstein JE, Cogan DG: Diabetic ophthalmoplegia with special reference to the pupil. Arch Ophthalmol 1960; 64:592–600.

35. Green PA, Berge KG, Sprague RG: Control of diabetic diarrhea with antibiotic therapy. Diabetes 1968; 17:385–387.

36. Greene DA, Lattimer SA, Sima AFA: Sorbitol, phosphoinositides and sodium-potassium-ATPase in the pathogenesis of diabetic complications. N Engl J Med 1987; 316:599–606.

37. Gregersen G, Borsting H, Theil P, Servo C: Myoinositol and function of peripheral nerves in human diabetics: A controlled clinical trial. Acta Neurol Scand 1978; 58:241–248.

38. Guillain-Barré Syndrome Study Group: Plasmapheresis and acute Guillain-Barré syndrome. Neurology 1984; 35:1096–1104.

39. Guiloff RJ, Thomas PK, Contreras M, et al: Linkage of autosomal dominant type 1 hereditary motor and sensory neuropathy to the Duffy locus on chromosome 1. J Neurol Neurosurg Psychiatry 1982; 45:669–674.

40. Halar EM, Brozovich FV, Milutinovic J, et al: H-reflex latency in uremic neuropathy: Correlation with NCV and clinical findings. Arch Phys Med Rehabil 1979; 60:174–177.

41. Hartung H-P, Hughes RAC, Taylor WA, et al: T cell activation in Guillain-Barré syndrome and in MS: Elevated serum levels of soluble IL-2 receptors. Neurology 1990; 40:215–218.

42. Herbison GJ, Jaweed M, Ditunno JF: Exercise therapies in peripheral neuropathies. Arch Phys Med Rehabil 1983; 64:201–205.

43. Hilsted J, Parving HH, Christensen NJ, et al: Hemodynamics in diabetic orthostatic hypotension. J Clin Invest 1981; 68:1427–1434.

44. Honet JC, Jebsen RH, Tenckhoff H: Comparison of motor and sensory nerve conduction velocity in early uremic polyneuropathy. Arch Phys Med Rehabil 1967; 48:209–212.

45. Ionasescu VV, Trofatter J, Haines JL, et al: Mapping of the gene for X-linked dominant Charcot-Marie-Tooth neuropathy. Neurology 1992; 42:903–908.

46. Jebsen RH, Tenckhoff H: Comparison of motor and sensory nerve conduction velocity in early uremic polyneuropathy. Arch Phys Med Rehabil 1969; 50:124–126.

47. Johnson EW: Sixteenth Annual AAEM Edward H. Lambert Lecture. Electrodiagnostic aspects of diabetic neuropathies: Entrapments. Muscle Nerve 1993; 16:127–134.

48. Judzewitsch RG, Jaspan JB, Polonsky KS, et al: Aldose reductase inhibition improves nerve conduction velocity in diabetic patients. N Engl J Med 1983; 308:119–125.

49. Kahan M, Goldberg PD, Mandel EE: Neurogenic vesical dysfunction and diabetes mellitus. N Y State J Med 1970; 70:2448–2455.

50. Kimura J: Polyneuropathies. In Kimura J (ed): Electrodiagnosis in diseases of nerve and muscle: Principles and practice, ed 2. Philadelphia, FA Davis, 1989.

51. Kraft GH: Axillary, musculocutaneous and suprascapular nerve latency studies. Arch Phys Med Rehabil 1972; 53:383–387.

52. Kraft GH: Serial nerve conduction and electromyographic studies in experimental allergic neuritis. Arch Phys Med Rehabil 1975; 56:333–339.

53. Kraft GH: Peripheral neuropathies. In Johnson EW (ed): Practical Electromyography, ed 2. Baltimore, Williams & Wilkins, 1988, pp 246–318.

54. Kraft GH, Halvorson GA: Median nerve residual latency: Normal value and use in diagnosis of carpal tunnel syndrome. Arch Phys Med Rehabil 1983; 64:221–226.

55. Levin KH: Ischemic monomelic neuropathy. Muscle Nerve 1985; 12:791–795.

56. Lewis T, Pickering GW, Rothschild P: Centripetal paralysis arising out of arrested blood flow to the limb including notes on a form of tingling. Heart 1931; 16:1–32.

57. Max MB, Culnane M, Schafer SC, et al: Amitriptyline relieves diabetic neuropathy pain in patients with normal or depressed mood. Neurology 1987; 37:589–596.

58. Max MB, Kishore-Kumar R, Schafer SC, et al: Efficacy of desipramine in painful diabetic neuropathy: A placebo-controlled trial. Pain 1991; 45:3–9.

59. McCallum RW, Ricci DA, Rakatansky H, et al: A multicenter placebo-controlled clinical trial of oral metoclopramide in diabetic gastroparesis. Diabetes Care 1983; 6:463–467.

60. Miller RG: Acute vs. chronic compressive neuropathy. Muscle Nerve 1984; 7:427–430.

61. Mostacciuolo ML, Mueller E, Fardin P, et al: X-linked Charcot-Marie-Tooth disease: A linkage study in a large family by using 12 probes of the pericentromeric region. Hum Genet 1991; 87:23–27.

62. Mulder DW, Lambert EH, Bastron JA, Sprague RG: The neuropathies associated with diabetes mellitus. A clinical and electromyographic study of 103 unselected diabetic patients. Neurology 1961; 11:275–284.

63. Parry GJ, Cornblath DR, Brown MJ: Transient conduction block following acute peripheral nerve ischemia. Muscle Nerve 1982; 8:490–513.

64. Parry GJG: Mononeuropathy multiplex (AAEE case report #11). Muscle Nerve 1985; 8:493–498.

65. Raman PT, Taori GM: Prognostic significance of electrodiagnostic studies in the Guillain-Barré syndrome. J Neurol Neurosurg Psychiatry 1976; 39:163–170.

66. Ropper AH: The Guillain-Barré syndrome. N Engl J Med 1992; 326:1130–1136.

67. Ross DR, Varipapa RJ: Treatment of painful diabetic neuropathy with topical capsaicin. N Engl J Med 1989; 321:474–475.

68. Ross MA: Neuropathies associated with diabetes. Med Clin North Am 1993; 77:111–124.

69. Rull JA, Quibrera R, Gonzalez-Millan H, Castaneda OL: Symptomatic treatment of peripheral diabetic neuropathy with carbamazepine (Tegretol): Double blind crossover trial. Diabetologia 1969; 5:215–218.

70. Rundles RW: Diabetic neuropathy: General review with report of 125 cases. Medicine (Baltimore) 1945; 24:111–160.

71. Schiller LR, Santa Ana CA, Schmulen AC, et al: Pathogenesis of fecal incontinence in diabetes mellitus: Evidence for internal-anal-sphincter dysfunction. N Engl J Med 1982; 307:1666–1671.

72. Seddon HJ: Three types of nerve injury. Brain 1943; 66:17–288.

73. Skilman TG, Johnson EW, Hamwi GJ, Driskill HJ: Motor nerve conduction velocity in diabetes mellitus. Diabetes 1961; 10:46–57.

74. Smith B: Neuropathology of the oesophagus in diabetes mellitus. J Neurol Neurosurg Psychiatry 1974; 37:1151–1154.

75. Stewart JD: Diabetic truncal neuropathy: Topography of the sensory deficit. Ann Neurol 1989; 25:233–238.

76. Sunderland S: The anatomy and physiology of nerve injury. Muscle Nerve 1990; 13:771–784.

77. Sunderland S: A classification of peripheral nerve injuries producing loss of function. Brain 1951; 74:491–516.

78. Swift TR, Leshner RT, Gross JA: Arm-diaphragm synkinesis: Electrodiagnostic studies of aberrant regeneration of phrenic motor neurons. Neurology 1980; 30:339–344.

79. Taverner D: Bell's palsy: A clinical and electromyographic study. Brain 1955; 78:209–235.

80. Taylor N, Halar EM, Tenckhoff H, et al: Effects of renal transplantation on motor nerve conduction velocity. Arch Phys Med Rehabil 1972; 53:227–231.

81. Taylor RA: Heredofamilial mononeuritis multiplex with brachial predilection. Brain 1960; 83:113–137.

82. Thomas PK: Diabetic neuropathy: Models, mechanisms and mayhem. Can J Neurol Sci 1992; 19:1–7.

83. Thomas PK, Thomlinson DR: Diabetic and Hypoglycemic neuropathy. In Dyck PF, Thomas PK, Griffin JW (eds): Peripheral Neuropathy, vol 2. Philadelphia, WB Saunders, 1993.

84. Thorsteinsson G: Management of painful diabetic neuropathy. JAMA 1977; 238:2297.

85. Tsairis P, Dyck PJ, Mulder DW: Natural history of brachial plexus neuropathy: Report of 99 patients. Arch Neurol 1972; 27:109–117.

86. Vance JM, Barker K, Yamaoka LH, et al: Localization of Charcot-Marie-Tooth disease type 1a (CMT1A) to chromosome 17p11.2. Genomics 1991; 9:623–628.

87. Victor M, Adams RD: Symposium on neurological and hepatic complications of alcoholism. On the etiology of the alcoholic neurologic diseases with special reference to the role of nutrition. Am J Clin Nutr 1961; 9:379–397.

88. Walsh NE, Dumitru D, Kalantri A, Roman AM: Brachial neuritis involving the bilateral phrenic nerves. Arch Phys Med Rehabil 1987; 68:46–48.

89. Wilton TD: Tegretol in the treatment of diabetic neuropathy. S Afr Med J 1974; 48:869–872.

90. Windebank AJ: Polyneuropathy due to nutritional deficiency and alcoholism. In Dyck PJ, Thomas PK, Griffin JW, (eds): Peripheral Neuropathy, vol 2. Philadelphia, WB Saunders, 1993, p 1313.

47

Rehabilitation Issues in Plexopathies

ROBERT J. WEBER, M.D.,
AND STEPHEN LEBDUSKA, M.D.

In this chapter we address the diagnosis and rehabilitation management of patients with plexopathies. In addition to a review of the principal syndromes, there is general discussion of the use of electrodiagnosis to localize lesions and determine prognosis and of general rehabilitation strategies.

The nerve plexus supplying an upper or a lower extremity contains approximately 100,000 axons and produces redistribution of motor information from the segmental pattern of the central nervous system (CNS) to the dispersed, functional pattern of the extremity. Conversely, the plexus reassembles somatic sensation carried by afferent, peripheral nerves into segmental patterns for orderly representation on the sensory homunculus. Teleologically, this affords the limbs functional redundancy and greater protection from trauma through the use of "parallel" circuitry. The plexuses themselves are situated within the relative protection of the axial skeleton, making blunt trauma a relatively uncommon cause of injury. The most common causes of brachial plexus injury (in decreasing order of frequency) are stretch injury due to excessive limb excursion (traction), compression by neighboring structures, and iatrogenic insults. Lumbosacral plexopathy is usually caused by focal compression, diabetic neuropathy, complications of pelvic surgery, or parturition. Separation of plexopathy from the neurological effects of spinal degenerative joint disease is often a diagnostic challenge.

The brachial plexus forms from the ventral rami of spinal roots C5 to T1 and the lower extremity plexus from the ventral rami of T12 to S4. While separate lumbar and sacral plexus are often described, conceptualization of a single lumbosacral plexus is more functional. Also noteworthy is the fact that the spinal rami (dorsal/ventral) are actually peripheral nerves rather than "roots" and respond to injury like peripheral nerves. Detailed knowledge of plexus anatomy is essential, and the reader is referred to standard texts and to Figures 47–1 and 47–2. Tables 47–1

and 47–2 list plexus terminal branches and the key supplied muscles most useful in sorting out the location of a plexus lesion.

REHABILITATION PRINCIPLES

Rehabilitation for plexopathies initially emphasizes joint protection and maintenance of range of motion, since the vast majority of patients with plexus injuries can expect some degree of recovery. Immediate surgical treatment is usually reserved for those cases with open injuries, associated skeletal or vascular injury, or clean, penetrating wounds. During the early postinjury phase, sequential clinical and electrodiagnostic evaluations are essential for guiding treatment. Adequate initial pain control is important to permit mobilization, but it must be transitioned to fit longer-term conditions. Edema should be aggressively controlled, since it can limit movement and augment pain. Passive and/or active assisted range of motion can be used to maintain joint mobility. Lesions causing loss of shoulder or elbow flexion cause the limb to hang in a dependent position. Positioning devices or slings can reduce edema, retard shoulder subluxation, and reduce additional traction on the brachial plexus.[65] A patient who continuously uses a sling, particularly when pain is present, can quickly develop a contracture. This contracture most often results in severe limitation of abduction and external rotation at the shoulder, and extension and supination at the elbow. This risk of early contracture reinforces the importance of early education to promote patient involvement in frequent active range of motion and in protecting insensate areas. Emotional support and empowerment of patients can help maximize the outcome of rehabilitation.

ELECTROMYOGRAPHY

Electromyography is the only technological means of determining plexus function (see Chapters 6 through 8).

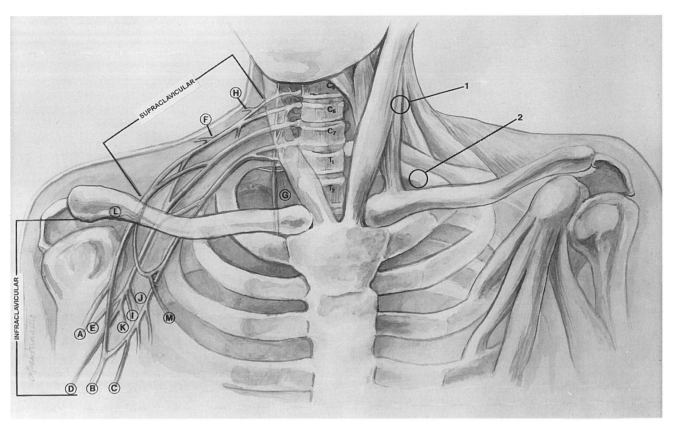

FIGURE 47–1 *A*, Musculocutaneous nerve. *B*, Median nerve. *C*, Ulnar nerve. *D*, Radial nerve. *E*, Axillary nerve. *F*, Suprascapular nerve. *G*, Long thoracic nerve. *H*, Dorsal scapular nerve. *I*, Thoracodorsal nerve. *J*, Upper subscapular nerve. *K*, Lower subscapular nerve. *L*, Lateral pectoral nerve. *M*, Medial pectoral nerve. *1*, Erb's point. *2*, Supraclavicular stimulation point.

TABLE 47–1   Major Mixed Nerves of the Brachial Plexus*

Nerve/Origin	Key Muscles/Root Origins*	Principal Functions
SUPRACLAVICULAR		
Dorsal scapular/ventral ramus C5 (C4)	Rhomboids/**C5**	Scapular retraction and rotation
Long thoracic/ventral rami C5–C7	Serratus anterior/**C5, C6, C7**	Scapular protraction and maintenance against thoracic wall
Suprascapular/upper trunk	Supraspinatus/**C5**, C6	Humeral abduction and lateral rotation
	Infraspinatus/**C5**, C6	External rotation of humerus
INFRACLAVICULAR		
Lateral pectoral/lateral cord C5–C7	Pectoralis major C5, **C6**, C7 (sternoclavicular portion)	Humeral adduction, medial rotation, flexion
Musculocutaneous/lateral cord C5–C7	Biceps/**C5, C6**	Forearm flexion and supination
Median/lateral cord (C5)–C7	Flexor carpi radialis/**C6**, C7	Wrist flexion, hand abduction
Medial cord C8–T1	Abductor pollicis brevis/**C8**, T1	Thumb abduction
Medial pectoral/medial cord	Pectoralis major/**C8**, T1 (sternocostal portion)	Humeral adduction, medical rotation, extension from a flexed position
Ulnar/medial cord	Flexor carpi ulnaris/**C8**, T1	Wrist flexion, hand adduction
	First dorsal interosseus/C8, **T1**	Index finger abduction
Thoracodorsal/posterior cord	Latissimus dorsi/**C6, C7**, C8	Extension, adduction, medical rotation of the humerus
Upper subscapular/posterior cord	Subscapularis/C5, **C6**	Medial rotation of humerus
Lower subscapular/posterior cord	Teres major/C5, **C6**	Humeral extension, internal rotation
Axillary/posterior cord	Deltoid/**C5**, C6	Humeral abduction, flexion, or extension
Radial/posterior cord	Triceps/C6, **C7**, C8	Forearm extension
	Extensor carpi radialis/**C6**, C7	Wrist extension, hand abduction

*Selected muscles for each nerve that are easily assessable by EMG or clinical examination are included with their principal functions. Boldface type denotes predominant nerve root representation.

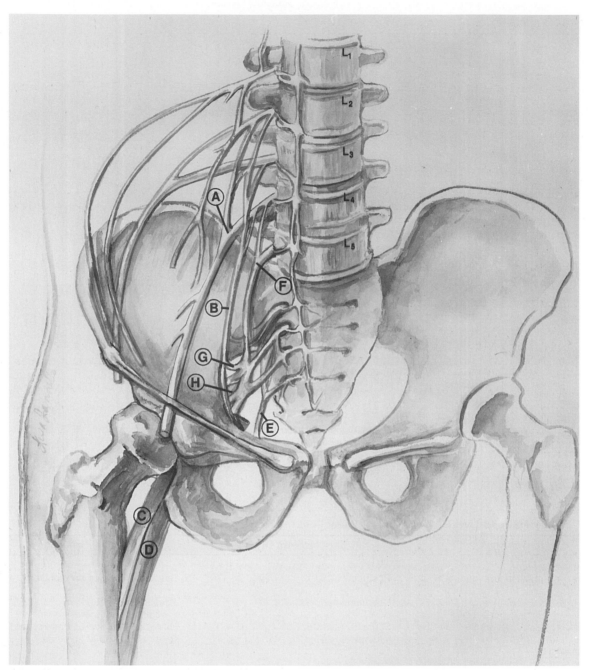

FIGURE 47–2 *A*, Femoral nerve. *B*, Obturator nerve. *C*, Common peroneal (division of sciatic) nerve. *D*, Tibial (division of sciatic) nerve. *E*, Pudendal nerve. *F*, Lumbosacral trunk. *G*, Superior gluteal nerve. *H*, Inferior gluteal nerve.

While imaging and vascular flow studies can provide valuable anatomical information, neither provides the critical physiological information on the plexus' neural elements. Plexopathies challenge the electromyographer, since they have a large differential diagnosis, widely varied pathophysiological features, and the necessity at times of employing virtually the entire armamentarium of electrodiagnostic techniques. While the electrodiagnostic strategies are similar to those employed for peripheral nerve injuries, the limited physical accessibility of the proximal part of the plexus for stimulation provides a significant additional challenge. Diagnosis is further complicated by the fact that the assessment must include the more proximally located problems of the spinal roots, rootlets, and spinal cord. While these structures are not actually part of the plexus, they can be involved with or produce symptoms like those of plexopathy.

Electrodiagnostic evaluation of plexopathies has three fundamental objectives: to locate the lesion, to characterize its pathophysiology, and to establish the prognosis and treatment plan. Success requires integration of information from each component of the electrodiagnostic evaluation. Localization can be established inductively from the distribution of needle electromyographic (EMG) findings, including membrane abnormalities and the more subjective observation of reduced motor unit interference patterns.

TABLE 47–2 Major Mixed Nerves of the Lumbosacral Plexus*

Nerve/Origin	Key Muscles/Root Origins*	Principal Functions
Femoral/ventral rami L2–L4	Vastus medialis/L2, **L3, L4**	Knee extension
Obturator/ventral rami L2–L4	Adductor longus/L2, **L3,** L4	Hip adduction
Superior gluteal/lumbosacral trunk and S1	Tensor fascia lata/L4, **L5**	Hip flexion and internal rotation
Inferior gluteal/lumbosacral trunk and S1, S2	Gluteus maximus, **L5,** S1, S2	Hip extension and adduction
Common peroneal (division of sciatic)/lumbosacral trunk and L5, S1, S2	Biceps, short head/L5, **S1,** S2	Knee flexion
Tibial (division of sciatic)/lumbosacral trunk, S1, S2, S3	Gastrocnemius/**S1,** S2	Ankle plantar flexion
Pudendal/ventral rami, S2, S4	Anal sphincter/**S2, S3, S4**	Sphincter contraction
Superficial peroneal/common peroneal	Peroneus longus/L5, **S1**	Foot eversion
Deep peroneal/common peroneal	Tibialis anterior/L4, **L5**	Foot dorsiflexion, inversion

*Selected muscles for each nerve that are easily assessable by EMG or clinical examination are included with their principal functions. Boldface type denotes predominant nerve root representation.

Here, the more severe the lesion, the more helpful is needle EMG in localizing it. Peripheral nerve conduction studies provide localization information only when proximal axonotmesis is sufficient to produce a large loss in the size of peripheral nerve evoked potentials. Abnormal H and F waves in nerves with normal peripheral evoked potentials provide evidence of proximal, axonal block. The velocity and evoked potential information obtained by conduction across the plexus using needle, magnetic, or high-voltage electrical spinal root stimulation to access the proximal plexus, combined with the needle EMG findings, is the best approach to localization. We have found monopolar needle electrodes to be the most effective—and best tolerated—means of root stimulation, producing accurate conduction velocity and evoked response information for each plexus branch. Complete motor loss (axonotmesis with no motor evoked response) with preservation of the sensory nerve evoked response in the same spiral segment suggests a preganglionic (i.e., rootlet level) lesion. This is because such proximal lesions destroy the motor axon, producing wallerian degeneration. But, since they spare the dorsal root ganglion and its peripheral extension the peripheral nerve, a sensory evoked response can still be generated in the periphery despite the fact that the area is insensate. This finding indicates a very poor prognosis since roots and primary rami neither regenerate nor can be surgically repaired.

In plexopathies, the clinically important question can be simply stated: Is the extremity weakness observed due to axonotmetic (dead) or neurapraxic (functionally blocked) axons? With axonotmesis the axon must regrow from the point of injury. The longer the regrowth distance, the poorer the prognosis for success. In neurapraxia, barring progression of the lesion, function resumes following relatively rapid repair of myelin or axon damage, and the prognosis is excellent. This is the situation typically seen in birth palsies well over half of which are due to neurapraxia, and function recovers within a few weeks. Neurapraxic lesions continue to produce motor or sensory evoked potentials when stimulated distal to the lesion. In axonotmetic axons conduction fails in the distal segment as a result of wallerian degeneration (dissolution) of the distal segment, which is completed sometime between the fourth to seventh day following injury. Neurapraxia in plexopathy is signaled by the presence of a significant evoked response

to peripheral stimulation of the involved segment (peripheral nerve) approximately 7 days after injury.

PROGNOSIS

Prognosis for plexopathy is determined through the integration of electrodiagnostic and clinical information, (e.g., enthusiasm resulting from technically "favorable" electrodiagnostic findings would be muted if the clinical picture suggests progressive disease). Recovery of function depends on multiple, separate processes, which are reviewed below. Each must be factored into the prognosis. Impairment due to neurapraxia presents the most positive prospect for recovery. A rough estimation (i.e., quantification) of the degree of recovery expected is to compare the peripherally obtained evoked response more than 7 days after the injury to that obtained earlier (before wallerian degeneration has had time to occur) or to normal or contralateral values. While there are many caveats, comparing the area under the curve rather than the amplitude of these evoked responses provides a good indicator of potential recovery. In axonotmesis, motor recovery results from axonal sprouting of surviving axons as well as from axon regrowth. Therefore, the number of voluntary motor units on needle EMG is also a guide to outcome. Early postinjury findings provide a conservative indicator, since more units might recover as neurapraxia resolves. A motor unit can increase its number of muscle fibers and strength two to four times by capturing additional fibers through a process known as "sprouting." Experience has shown that peak muscle strength, albeit at the expense of endurance, can be satisfactorily regained via this sprouting mechanism, even if there has been up to a 50% loss of axons. In muscles where high force or sustained use are not required, a 90% axon loss might be tolerated well. This process requires about a year to come to full maturation.

Axon regrowth is the least reliable source of recovery. When long regeneration distance (i.e., plexus level injury) is involved, prospects are poor. Connective tissue disruption, scar, or ongoing metabolic stress also impairs axon regrowth. As discussed above, the fact that only a limited number of axons need to reach the muscle to obtain functionally useful benefit is the most hopeful prognostic aspect of severe axonotmesis. Surgical reattachment and the use of nerve jump grafts can be indicated when prospects are otherwise poor. Physical disruption of the neural connective tissue structures requires surgical treatment if axon regrowth is to occur, since this requires continuity of the supporting elements. Unfortunately, electrodiagnosis is not able to distinguish between simple axonotmesis and injury where axonotmesis is accompanied by physical disruption by the neural structures. When complete axonotmesis is identified, imaging studies or surgical exploration might be necessary to determine the treatment plan and prognosis.

BRACHIAL PLEXOPATHIES

Historically, brachial plexus lesions have been subdivided utilizing the clavicle as a boundary. The two resulting groups of "supraclavicular" and "infraclavicular" lesions actually represent lesions proximal to and distal to the divisions, respectively. Because of inherent structural and anatomical differences, lesions at the two levels tend to have distinct causes. The terms "upper plexus" and "lower plexus" generally pertain to supraclavicular lesions involving the C5 and C6 nerve roots or the C8 and T1 nerve roots, respectively. Plexopathies can also be characterized by cause or as complete or incomplete. The latter is typically applied with respect to specific components of the plexus (e.g., complete Erb's palsy or complete root compromise). The designation is based on clinical examination. Brachial plexus lesions usually demonstrate some recovery. Exceptions include those due to severe, extensive trauma, particularly rootlet avulsions, or to progressive causes such as metastatic disease and radiation-induced lesions. Each plexus element has different susceptibility to the various types of injury mechanisms.

Despite the range of potential insults, the history alone usually affords an understanding of the mechanism of injury. Careful physical examination reveals the functional and anatomical extent of the injury. Electrodiagnostic studies (after wallerian degeneration), augmented by imaging studies provide more precise localization and help inform the prognosis. Each of the common brachial plexopathies produces a stereotypical presentation. Each characteristically affects a specific anatomic region of the plexus, and each is strongly linked epidemiologically to a specific age group, activity, or gender (Table 47–3).

Traction Injury

Traction injuries are the most common cause of electrodiagnostically documentable brachial plexopathy. These are predominantly supraclavicular injuries, and susceptibility is due to the large combined excursion potential of the arm, shoulder, and cervical spine. The cervical roots (anterior and posterior primary rami) located at the proximal "anchoring point" of the plexus are particularly vulnerable to traction, since they lack protective epineural and perineural sheaths and have poor tensile strength.[52] Birth trauma and shoulder trauma secondary to sports injuries or motorcycle accidents (typically in young men) are the two most common causes. Brachial plexus injuries from motorcycle accidents are now the most common traumatic cause of major loss of arm function.[33, 45, 50] Falls resulting

TABLE 47–3   Injuries That Typically Involve Specific Regions of the Brachial Plexus and Associated Conditions or Risk Factors

Injury	Associated Condition or Risk Factor
Supraclavicular injuries	
Upper plexus (C5–C6, upper trunk)	Traction injuries
	Young adulthood (men)
	Obstetric paralysis
	Postanesthesia paralysis
Lower plexus (C8–T1, lower trunk)	Pancoast's syndrome
	Sternotomy
	Adulthood beyond middle age
	Neurogenic TOS
	TOS surgery
	Youth or middle age (women)
	Traction injury
Infraclavicular	Gunshot wounds
	Neurovascular injury (young adult men)
	Radiation (predominantly older women)
	Humeral fractures
	Orthopedic procedures
Total plexus	Extensive traction injury (young adult men)
	Advanced metastatic involvement
	Radiation (older men and women)
	Postanesthesia paralysis

in shoulder dislocation (and relocation) or fractures and traction secondary to positioning during operative procedures are next in frequency. "Pack palsy," resulting from shoulder depression from heavily loaded backpacks, is generally a transient injury that can occur in active adults of both genders. Shoulder depression combined with lateral neck flexion away from the involved shoulder produces its greatest traction force on the upper plexus, frequently producing combined C5 to C6 or C5 through C7 lesions.

The classic description of an upper plexus palsy was provided by Erb in 1874. It results in loss of shoulder abduction and external rotation, elbow flexion, forearm supination, and radial wrist deviation, producing a "waiter's tip" position of the affected limb.[8] Distinction between a root level and an upper trunk lesion can be made by establishing if rhomboid and/or serratus anterior muscle function is compromised, since these are usually spared in a trunk level injury. Sensory loss in Erb's palsy can extend from the lateral deltoid down the lateral aspect of the arm and into the thumb and index finger.

Hyperabduction of the arm stretches the brachial plexus around the lateral aspect of the shoulder (or the musculature attached to the shoulder girdle under which the plexus passes) producing traction mainly on the elements of the lower plexus. Severe traction injuries occurring through this mechanism usually produce true spinal root avulsions (*preganglionic lesions*) that are not amenable to surgical repair.[59] *Klumpke* described lesions of this type in 1885, which consisted of loss of function in hand intrinsic muscles, anterior interosseous- and ulnar-innervated forearm muscles and distal radial nerve innervated muscles.[17] When the T1 spinal root is avulsed, *Horner's syndrome* is also present.[17] Sensory loss occurs over the medial aspect of the forearm and hand and the fourth and fifth digits.

Severe traction injuries can affect both upper and lower supraclavicular elements of the plexus. A careful clinical examination, including electrodiagnosis in severe injury, can determine which spinal root levels are involved. However, multifocal injury (i.e., several points along the course of the neural element) can occur and be clinically indetectable. This injury to axons and neural supporting structures at multiple points reduces recovery prospects by impairing reinnervation via axonal regrowth, and it can also conceal preganglionic injuries. The latter occurs because the second, more distal lesion obliterates the sensory evoked response usually preserved in preganglionic injury and masks this negative prognostic sign.

Traction injuries involving the infraclavicular plexus elements are much less common than supraclavicular lesions. They often occur with severe trauma and are frequently associated with injury to neighboring structures.[42] Injuries confined to cords or individual peripheral nerves generally have a better prognosis for recovery than more proximal traction injuries.[41] These peripheral elements tolerate traction forces better than the more proximal, anchored structures, owing to the presence of supporting connective tissues, the dispersed orientation of the individual nerve fibers, and the possibility of distributing the stretching over a longer distance.

Trauma to any level of the brachial plexus can result in persistent residual pain. Traction injuries resulting in root avulsion are especially likely to cause moderate to severe chronic pain. The severity of pain is also related to the number of avulsed roots.[9] The onset of pain is often immediate, but it can develop weeks or even several months after injury.[64] Patients with traction injuries without root avulsion tend to develop pain later; in one series, only 13% reported immediate pain.[9] Accounts of root avulsion pain by patients have rather consistent characteristics. First, in the upper extremity pain tends to be far more severe distally, particularly in the hand. Patients describe continuous background pain of a burning or crushing nature. Superimposed are excruciating, shocklike pains of brief duration and variable frequency.[64] The pain prevents sleep, impairs concentration, and is very disabling. Avulsion pain is caused at least in part by deafferentation and is extremely difficult to control. Trials of antidepressants, analgesics, and carbamazepine have produced limited relief. Transcutaneous electrical nerve stimulation has been more promising, but careful electrode placement is necessary.[66] Stellate ganglion blocks, sympathectomy, and anterolateral cordotomy have yielded poor results. Dorsal root entry zone coagulation has yielded positive results in a majority of patients. Early engagement of patients in gratifying work or leisure activities serves to redirect pain awareness and has been successful in ameliorating symptoms.

Obstetric Paralysis

Obstetric paralysis is a specific type of traction injury that has decreased substantially in the last century thanks to improvements in delivery management.[28] While usually designated as *Erb's* or *Klumpke's* type, based on the presence of upper or lower trunk injury, respectively, some damage is usually present throughout the plexus in both. The *Erb's* type with C5, C6, or C5, C6, and C7 involve-ment is by far more frequent. It was described by Duchenne in four infants 2 years before Erb's classic description in two adults.[59] It is usually extraforaminal; motor deficits predominate and sensory compromise is mild. It is caused by a stretch of the neck-shoulder angle, and since the head is usually positioned to the left, the right plexus is more often involved.[16]

In more than half of cases, the injury is essentially neurapraxic and recovery is excellent within a matter of weeks. Lack of early improvement, loss of motor evoked responses, or absence of some voluntary motor units suggests that deficits will persist. *Klumpke's* type injury has a poorer prognosis since it often involves root avulsion.[44] Early rehabilitation should educate the family about protection of the extremity and set expectations. Once the course is clearer, outcome and long-term strategies can be explained and managed.

Trauma

Trauma from penetrating objects causes a decreasing proportion of brachial plexus injuries. Gunshot injuries vary with the size, composition, and energy of the projectile and its course. High-velocity missiles that spread on impact cause large tissue cavities. While nerves can be transected directly, injury generally occurs from violent pressure waves generated by the impacting missile. While the degree of injury varies, local injury is often so severe that nerve regeneration does not occur despite apparently well-preserved nerve continuity observed at surgical exploration. Surgical repair often potentiates regeneration and improves outcome, except in lower trunk or medial cord injuries where useful hand function seldom returns.[35] Clinical and electrodiagnostic follow-up can direct rehabilitation or the surgical plan.

Laceration injuries (knives, chain saws, propellers, bites) often produce both nerve and vascular injuries. Sharp lacerations are best treated by immediate primary repair. Blunt lacerations which both sever and stretch the nerve, carry a poorer prognosis. They frequently require a secondary cable graft.[36] Evolving hematomas or pseudoaneurysms can cause compression of plexus elements, compromising the microvasculature, and can result in ischemic injury. The resulting compartment syndromes can compromise long segments of the plexus. Subacute hemorrhage is particularly dangerous because nerve compromise might not be clinically evident for hours or days after injury and then can evolve rapidly over a period of hours. Frequent clinical examination of the soft tissues and computed tomography (CT) or magnetic resonance imaging (MRI) can detect intramuscular hemorrhage.

Iatrogenic Injury

Iatrogenic brachial plexus injuries, while less common, are probably more noticeable than those of the lumbosacral plexus owing to the more demanding functions of the arm. Stretch injury during spreading of a sternum-splitting thoracotomy is probably the most frequent cause. Complications of intra-axillary anesthesia also are relatively common. Ironically, the most common direct injury in our experience, occurs during trans-axillary approach to relieve thoracic outlet syndrome. The plexus is also at risk during deep cervical exploration and during axillary lymph node dissection.

Neoplastic Brachial Plexopathy

Plexopathy can result from the direct "strangling" effects of an enlarging neoplasm. Primary neoplasms (i.e., those derived from nerve elements) include benign neural sheath tumors such as neurofibromas and schwannomas, and less frequently malignant neurogenic sarcomas and fibrosarcomas.[43] Transformation of initially benign neural sheath tumors can occur in patients with von Recklinghausen's neurofibromatosis. Neoplastic injury is, however, much more frequently the result of invasion secondary to extension from tumors in adjacent organs or metastases from distant sites.[37] Those originating from the lung or the breast comprise the vast majority. Neoplasms directly extending from the ipsilateral lung can themselves represent pulmonary metastases from the larynx, esophagus, thyroid, colon, or pancreas.

Symptoms of both primary and secondary brachial plexus neoplasia typically have an insidious onset. Extremity pain or paresthesias are common presenting symptoms of primary neoplasms. There is often localized tenderness (with or without a palpable mass), which might be discovered by careful palpation of the proximal upper limb and shoulder. *Pancoast's syndrome* is the constellation of findings associated with brachial plexus encroachment by direct extension of an apical lung neoplasm. Symptoms consist of shoulder pain, and radiating pain and paresthesias in the arm (typically lower trunk distribution), limb weakness, and Horner's syndrome.[30] By the time these findings occur a radiographically apparent apical lung mass and bone abnormalities in the upper thoracic ribs or vertebrae are usually present. In our experience, the patient often complains of shoulder pain for weeks or months before the onset of other symptoms. A high index of clinical suspicion must be maintained if this infrequent cause of symptoms is to be detected early from among the far more common sources of shoulder or arm pain.

Those with previously treated neoplasms can develop new shoulder or arm pain. Many of these patients have undergone neck or axillary surgery, chemotherapy, or radiation therapy as part of their treatment. Since each can produce brachial plexopathy with overlapping symptoms and chronologically similar onset (described below), timely determination of whether symptoms represent recurrent or new neoplasms can be difficult. Electrodiagnosis and MRI have been helpful, but are often not diagnostically definitive.[25]

Radiation-Induced Brachial Plexopathy

Radiation-induced lesions increased with the advent of megavolt radiation therapy in the 1960s when, for the first time, destructive peak doses of radiation could be delivered to deep tissues. Peripheral nerves subjected to destructive levels of radiation sustain injury involving several nerve components. There is progressive demyelination, and connective tissue fibrosis, which in turn causes loss of supporting vasculature.[53] Onset is insidious and can occur several weeks to many years after the radiation therapy. Prevalence varies much and has been reported to be from 1% to 73%

for patients receiving radiation therapy.[59] The total dose of radiation delivered appears to be the most critical factor in producing plexopathy; the highest prevalence is associated with treatment for breast carcinoma.[10, 29]

Paresthesias, usually of the median innervated digits, are the most common initial symptoms reported, though some authors feel that pain can be the presenting complaint.[14, 37] Intrinsic hand muscle weakness is the most common reported motor finding. Proximal upper limb muscle weakness typically is not apparent until distal involvement is quite advanced. Any loss in proximal muscle bulk is frequently masked by associated postradiation edema. Given these symptoms one might anticipate an infraclavicular, possibly medial, cord lesion on electrodiagnosis; however, the literature indicates that denervation can occur anywhere along the course of the plexus, both supra- and infraclavicularly.[40] Motor and sensory nerve conduction amplitudes are often diminished when recorded from the digits or hand intrinsic muscles. Conduction block (this is more likely an increased temporal dispersion), is frequently reported from evaluation using supraclavicular stimulation, suggesting compromise at cord level or more distally.[29] These changes can still be seen many years after onset. Fasciculation potentials as well as myokymic discharges (not characteristically seen in direct neoplastic plexopathies alone) have been reported. Prognosis in radiation-induced plexopathy is extremely variable. Ironically, many of the patients treated aggressively and successfully for their neoplasm end up experiencing the slowly progressive effects of the radiation plexopathy.

Postradiation fibrosis plexopathy is seldom painful, but its sensory changes can be disturbing enough to warrant a trial of antiepileptic or tricyclic medication. The principal challenge is often persistent edema. Historically, there was concern that chronic infection was a source of this persistent lymphedema and a course of antibiotics was often prescribed. The mainstay of management, however, is early minimization of edema through positioning and motion supplemented by compression pumping and wearing of an elastic (two-way stretch) garment. This garment usually has to be worn continuously, since the edema is due to obstruction of lymph return rather than dependency. The extremity must be protected from intravenous and other needlesticks or trauma. Instruction in activities of daily living and work modification is often necessary. Many persons benefit from support programs that address both the impairments resulting from the chronic limb problems and the stresses of the cancer.

Thoracic Outlet Syndrome

Thoracic outlet syndrome (TOS) is actually a group of closely related clinical entities, each of which produces sensory and motor symptoms in the upper extremity. TOS reports began with Cooper in 1818, who described ischemia due to a supraclavicular bone mass. Subclavian artery compression by cervical ribs was confirmed surgically in 1861,[20] and lower trunk compromise was reported in 1903 that was due to a fibrous band between a rudimentary cervical rib and the first rib.[54] Surgical decompression procedures were developed and applied to these syndromes in subsequent years. The use of surgery expanded after the

1927 report by Adson implicated the scalenus anticus muscle as the compression agent in cervical rib TOS.[2] Later work led to the concept that the scalenus anticus and the hyperabduction syndromes are the result of positioning rather than of direct structural compression, such as that seen in cervical rib syndrome.[18, 63]

By 1956, when Peet coined the term "TOS" to include all of the previously described clinical entities, surgical interest in the topic was waning.[47] However, interest resurged in the early 1960s, when Clagett implicated the first thoracic rib as a cause of compression and recommended its resection.[13] This approach was subsequently supported by Roos, who introduced a technically simpler, more cosmetic procedure for first rib resection.[49]

Improvements in electrodiagnosis and imaging techniques contributed to the subdivision of TOS into even more clinical entities, which share overlapping symptoms. Current imaging techniques such as CT and angiography, coupled with provocative clinical maneuvers, can readily demonstrate arterial or venous compression of the "vascular" TOS. With severe arterial compression, patients often present with progressive hand and upper limb ischemia. Compression usually is from a bony abnormality (e.g., cervical rib) that compresses the subclavian artery. With progression, a poststenotic aneurysm can form that affords a site for thrombus formation. This in turn can embolize to further compromise distal limb blood flow. Progressive extremity ischemia from TOS is a rare condition, but its treatment invariably requires surgical decompression.[61] Another rare form of vascular thoracic outlet syndrome, effort vein thrombosis, results from spontaneous thrombosis of the axillary veins following vigorous arm exertion. There is rarely bony compression, and patients can present with acute arm pain, swelling, and discoloration due to venous obstruction.[61]

A much more common condition results from reversible arterial compression when the upper limb is hyperabducted or externally rotated. This results in temporary blood flow disturbances and ischemic symptoms. These situations can be exacerbated by work that requires prolonged elevation of the arms or overhead work. While symptoms are aggravating, the problem is self-limiting. Work adjustment, exercise, and education (rather than surgery) are more likely to produce long-term satisfaction.

"True neurogenic TOS," described by Gilliatt[24] utilizing clinical, Edx, and radiographic findings, is rare; the incidence is as low as one per million population. Given the very low likelihood of detecting a case among the many suspects, the focus of electrodiagnostic assessment must be to rule out similar symptomatic problems such as carpal tunnel or other nerve entrapments, radiculopathy, or neuropathy.

The vast majority of patients who present with symptoms of intermittent hand pain, numbness, and weakness fall into the group classified as "symptomatic" or "disputed" neurogenic thoracic outlet syndrome. The criteria, and even the existence of this syndrome, remains controversial.[60] In our experience, frequent patient complaints include intermittent pain or "stiffness" in the hand and forearm, associated paresthesias in a medial cord distribution, and subjective complaints of weakness in the affected limb. Neck pain, supraclavicular tenderness, and headaches can

also be present. The incidence reported in the literature ranges from three per 1000 through 80 per 1000 people. While the overall incidence remains controversial, there is general agreement that it is principally a problem of young and middle-aged women.[51] Musicians can be particularly susceptible to this form of TOS, owing to their need to maintain shoulder abduction or extension for long periods.[31, 38]

In our experience, which coincides loosely with that of other authors, this form of TOS generally is neither progressive nor likely to resolve spontaneously.[60] Patients give a history of insidious onset, though some recall trauma immediately preceding onset of symptoms. Physical examination typically detects no evidence of atrophy or significant weakness but often demonstrates diminished sensation to light touch over the lower trunk plexus distribution. EMG is generally not conclusive for a neurogenic type of TOS. Patients frequently note onset or exacerbation of symptoms when the affected arm is placed in abduction. This positioning is quite variably associated with changes in the strength of the radial pulse (Adson's maneuver).

Great physician suspicion for TOS results in referral of more patients for evaluation with other problems or negative electrodiagnostic findings. It is important to rule out easily confused problems such as carpal tunnel syndrome (CTS), and to exclude masses and gross vascular compromise. Beyond that point, diagnosis depends on the history and the physician's clinical perspective. An early trial of exercise and medical management is worthwhile. In our experience, nerve conduction evaluation via root stimulation and F wave is the best direct approach to evaluation of TOS. Overenthusiastic interpretation of motor unit polyphasicity or of isolated, somewhat subjective findings should be resisted. Absent definitive abnormalities, a conservative management approach best serves the patient. When CTS is present, regardless of other (less than severe) changes, it should be addressed first, since its correction is most likely to resolve patient complaints.

Rehabilitation

Planning for rehabilitation begins once emergent problems have been excluded. That plan is based on the recognition that, in the remainder (the vast majority) of patients, symptoms are caused by transient positionally related compromise of neurovascular structures. TOS is conceptually different from most syndromes presented in this chapter. Rather than being a fixed, anatomically defined lesion, it usually represents an interaction between the patient anatomy, repeated or sustained actions that can further constrict the neurovascular outflow, and the endurance of the postural support musculature of the region. Myofascial pain is often associated with, or misdiagnosed as, TOS. Treatment for either of these syndromes has related objectives, such as stress avoidance, work simplification, or job site modification to avoid sustained contraction and repetitive or overhead work that exacerbates symptoms. Another objective is to maximize the potential outlet space through a program of stretching and strengthening the shoulder-elevating mechanism. The last objective is to address the myofascial or chronic pain elements of the syndrome. A typical periscapular and cervical musculature exercise pro-

TABLE 47–4   Exercises to Reduce Potential for Thoracic Outlet Compression

Trapezius- and rhomboid-strengthening
Shoulder shrugs, with or without hand weights
Shoulder retraction (bilateral) while standing or lying prone
Shoulder mobilization
Upper limb circumduction ("hand circles")
Standing "corner pushups"
Postural exercises
Cervical spine extension
Lumbar spine extension

gram, good posture, and self-management education is essential. Psychological group management is often helpful. Analgesics are seldom helpful, except to assist in the institution of a progressive exercise program. A short, monitored course of a tricyclic antidepressant can be helpful if time course and systems suggest a protracted pain syndrome. Self-directed home management is the key to long-term success, but frequent initial reinstruction and follow-up are often required. In addition to the exercises listed in Table 47–4, a general aerobic exercise plan is helpful.

Idiopathic Brachial Plexopathy

Sudden onset of lateral shoulder pain followed by rapidly progressive weakness of the shoulder girdle muscles has been reported since the 19th century. Minor presentation variations led to confusion through the description of multiple syndrome, but by the 1940s large numbers of cases reported among military personnel produced the consensus that a single syndrome had variable presentations.[39] In 1948, Parsonage and Turner presented the first analysis of a large series of patients with various precipitating factors, including infection, trauma, surgery, and vaccination.[46] They termed the condition *neuralgic amyotrophy*. Synonyms include *acute brachial neuropathy, acute brachial plexitis, brachial neuritis, cryptogenic brachial neuropathy, Parsonage-Turner syndrome*, and *paralytic brachial neuritis*.

Epidemiological studies support the concept of a precipitating event (Table 47–5), and male predominance of at least 2:1.[19] There appear to be familial forms, but the nonfamilial or sporadic type is far more common. One study reports an annual incidence of 1.64 per 100,000

TABLE 47–5   Precipitating Causes and Antecedent Events Reported in Association with Idiopathic Brachial Plexopathy

Infection	Systemic illnesses
Undefined upper respiratory	Temporal arteritis
flu syndrome	Hodgkin's disease
Influenza	Lupus erythematosus
Coxsackievirus	Polyarteritis nodosa
Typhus	Iatrogenic trauma
Typhoid	Lumbar puncture
Bacterial pneumonia	Contrast-enhanced
Vaccines	neuroimaging studies
Thypoid	Orthopedic procedures
Tetanus	
Diphtheria	
Influenza	
Smallpox	

persons.[5] Males are most susceptible, especially from young adulthood to middle age.

Patients usually experience abrupt onset of severe shoulder pain, which tends to resolve within hours to several weeks. Shoulder muscle tenderness (exacerbated by arm movement) induces protective posturing of the affected upper limb in an adducted and internally rotated position.[56] Active range of motion of the cervical spine is usually pain free. As the shoulder pain resolves and comfortable active arm movement returns, muscle weakness becomes apparent. Its distribution is extremely variable as the result of involvement of individual peripheral nerves, single muscle branches, upper cervical roots, upper trunk, or combinations of these plexus elements. The deltoid, supraspinatus, infraspinatus, and serratus anterior muscles are the most frequently involved. Major sensory loss is rare,[55] but sensory conduction studies do show abnormalities.[15] Muscle stretch reflexes are usually normal but can be reduced. Maximal motor weakness can occur at onset or progress slowly over a few days or weeks. Most patients demonstrate functional recovery within 1 to 2 years.[56]

The differential diagnosis includes rotator cuff tears, traumatic mononeuropathies, and cervical radiculopathies. There is a similar condition of dominant inheritance. This familial form exhibits additional features, including recurrent plexopathies and involvement of the lumbosacral plexus and peripheral and cranial nerves.[7] Steroids have been advocated to control pain for both forms, but they do not change the course of weakness.

Rehabilitation includes gentle passive range of motion and active assistive range of motion as soon as tolerated, and progressive resistance exercises to store muscle symmetry once the patient is essentially pain free. Considering the excellent prognosis, retraining for contralateral hand dominance is unnecessary.

LUMBOSACRAL PLEXOPATHIES

Diabetic Plexopathy

Diabetic plexopathy typically affects the lumbosacral plexus more than the brachial one. It is distinguished from the classic, symmetrically progressive, initially distal peripheral polyneuropathy of long-standing diabetes by its predominantly proximal symptoms. The term *proximal diabetic neuropathy* has been coined to reflect this distinction.[3, 62] Lesions involving spinal cord segments, nerve roots, individual nerves, or combinations of these have been described. These entities might actually represent a continuum in the progression of the disease. Indeed, the majority of patients are in their six or seventh decade and also have documented distal peripheral polyneuropathy. Synonyms include *diabetic lumbar plexopathy, diabetic myelopathy, diabetic mononeuropathy multiplex, diabetic femoral neuropathy, diabetic myopathy*, and *diabetic amyotrophy*.[4, 11, 21, 48, 59]

The most common clinical presentation of diabetic lumbosacral plexopathy is anterior thigh pain and evolving proximal leg muscle weakness, which is most pronounced in the quadriceps muscles. Sensory loss is generally less pronounced, though patellar reflexes typically are absent or depressed. While diagnostic suspicion should be high for this in known diabetics, it can be the initial sign of diabetes. With progression, noticeable muscle wasting occurs, resulting in significant atrophy and weight loss. There is a trend for progression from unilateral to bilateral lower extremity involvement.[11] The lesions are potentially reversible, and their pathophysiology is ill-understood. Focal infarcts, demyelination, axonal degeneration, and mixed type 1– and type 2–muscle fiber atrophy on biopsy consistent with neurogenic atrophy have all been reported, albeit inconsistently.[12]

Diagnosis is based on the presentation, presence of diabetes, and the presence of "acute" electrodiagnostic findings. Those include abnormal potentials due to membrane changes in proximal and paraspinal muscles and abnormal femoral nerve conduction via spinal root stimulation. Since carcinoma can present with a similar picture, abdominal CT or MRI to exclude it is prudent.

Immediate therapy is focused on optimal control of hyperglycemia. Most patients who achieve glucose control typically have significant but incomplete recovery of muscle strength. Maximum improvement can require more than a year.[4] Rehabilitation strategies address pain management, maintenance of range of motion, and compensory mechanisms for knee extensor weakness. Electrodiagnosis can help guide exercise advancement.

Traumatic Plexopathy

Trauma resulting in lumbosacral plexus injury typically must be sufficient to produce an unstable, vertical fracture of the pelvic ring, since the plexus is otherwise well-protected from direct impact.[58] Fractures through the sacroiliac joint usually involve the ipsilateral lumbosacral trunk, with impairment seen in the L5 to S1–innervated muscles. Fracture dislocation of the hip joint can produce traction injuries to the lumbosacral plexus.[58] Owing to the initial period of immobilization after surgical repair, more subtle lesions can go undetected. Weakness from these lesions then can slow recovery during postoperative rehabilitation.

Hemorrhagic Plexopathy

Hemorrhage in the retroperitoneal region can compress the plexus as it passes through either the iliac or psoas muscles.[68] An expanding hematoma within the more laterally located iliacus muscle can cause focal compression of the femoral nerve at any point along its course from its origin to the inguinal ligament. This condition is heralded by onset of severe groin pain radiating to the anteromedial thigh and saphenous nerve territory. Progression can result in quadriceps weakness and anesthesia in the distribution previously described. Patients with evolving iliacus hematomas are exquisitely sensitive to hip extension, which exacerbates their pain. This provocative test helps distinguish these lesions from focal lumbar root compression. The upper lumbosacral plexus organizes within the substance of the psoas muscle, and hemorrhages in this muscle result in a more diffuse injury, producing motor impairment in both femoral- and obturator-innervated muscles and moderate unilateral pelvic pain. CT can confirm the clinical diagnosis. Patients receiving heparin or warfarin anticoagulation are more likely to experience these problems, but

bleeding can occur spontaneously or as a result of relatively minor pelvic trauma in the absence of anticoagulation.[67] Similar lesions have been reported in patients with other coagulopathies, including hemophilia, leukemia, and disseminated intravascular coagulation.[23, 27]

Neoplastic Plexopathy

Neoplastic lesions originating in pelvic organs can invade the lumbosacral plexus by direct extension. The most common is colorectal carcinoma, but uterine, prostatic, and ovarian tumors can be locally invasive as well.[32] Metastatic invasion of the retroperitoneum and the lumbosacral plexus by breast, thyroid, testicular cancers, lymphomas, myelomas, and melanomas is well-known.[32] Patients with von Recklinghausen's neurofibromatosis can develop nerve sheath tumors involving any component of the plexus.[6] Other primary nerve sheath tumors affecting the lumbosacral plexus are extremely rare. Neoplastic plexopathies generally present with pain, are typically unilateral, and, when sufficient to produce signs, are easily visualized on CT.

Radiation Plexopathy

Radiation-induced lumbosacral plexopathy is analogous to that in the brachial plexus. Onset is insidious, occurring from 1 to 31 years after radiation therapy. Patients receiving external beam or internal cavity radiation are equally susceptible. Patients generally present with slowly progressive, bilateral lower extremity weakness that tends to affect the distal muscles more. Paresthesias and numbness are less frequently reported as the initial symptoms. Symptom progression can eventually stabilize, but patients are usually severely disabled by that time.

Iatrogenic Plexopathy

Iatrogenic trauma to components of the lumbosacral plexus can occur inadvertently during surgical, gynecological, or anesthetic procedures. The mechanisms include compression, traction, and vascular or direct insult. Both true plexopathy and peripheral injury occur. Clinical and electrodiagnostic differentiation are important, since prognosis varies with the cause and location.

Sharp dissection injuries are rare but among the most severe, since the prognosis for recovery is negligible. It is most likely to occur during deep pelvic procedures such as prostatic resection or difficult transvaginal hysterectomy. Blunt trauma from surgical retraction or during forceps delivery is more common. The femoral and obturator nerves are those most frequently injured, followed by the lumbosacral trunk, lateral cutaneous nerve of the thigh, and sciatic nerves.[22, 26, 34] Arthroplasty of the hip results in a significant number of femoral, obturator, and sciatic injuries through direct trauma, stretch, or the heat effects of cement polymerization.[57]

Epidural anesthesia and perioperative, retroperitoneal hemorrhage can result in diffuse, extensive neuropathic injury (though hemorrhage beneath the iliac muscle sheath can produce a quite focal femoral nerve injury).[1] An underappreciated cause of postoperative weakness after intraabdominal surgery is infarction of the cord due to anterior spinal artery syndrome. Pre-existing atherosclerosis, intra-operative hypotension, or coagulopathy can initiate this syndrome of diffuse proximal leg weakness with relative sensory preservation. It should always be considered in the case of unexplained weakness postoperatively, particularly in older persons.

Peripheral perioperative problems to be distinguished from the preceding ones include femoral neuropathy from prolonged or tight hip flexion in the dorsal lithotomy position, sciatic stretch or compression related to hip flexion or buttocks pressure, lateral sciatic palsy related to hypodermic injection, and peroneal nerve palsy.[26] The latter can result either from direct pressure at the fibular head during a surgical procedure or from tight flexion of the knee due to pulling to bear down during labor and delivery. These lesions can be clearly localized using a combination of spinal nerve root and peripheral nerve stimulation in the early postinjury period. Establishing the site of injury late in the course of recovery, when conduction velocities along the course of the nerve have stabilized, may be more difficult, since there are few nerve branching points in these syndromes to help isolate the lesion.

Rehabilitation

Rehabilitation of patients with lumbosacral plexopathies follows two distinct strategies based on diametrically opposed prognoses. For the patients with (predominantly neurapraxic) reversible deficits, the primary goal is restoration of normal gait; for patients with progressive lesions, preservation of functional gait for as long as possible is paramount. In both cases, early intervention is employed to prevent contracture via active assistive range of motion and passive range of motion. Careful functional delineation of sensory and motor deficits, complemented by gait analysis in patients with incomplete lesions, directs the rehabilitation strategy. Progressive use of stand aids, standing frames, parallel bars, walkers, crutches, "quad canes," and straight canes follows recovery, to maintain safety. Orthotic devices are frequently required to compensate for focal weakness. Most commonly, ankle-fast orthoses (AFOs) to assist ankle dorsiflexion or stabilize knee extension during weight bearing are utilized. Focused muscle strengthening proceeds as tolerated. In patients with progressive disease, more extensive sensory loss, combined with evolving weakness, necessitates regular monitoring of skin integrity and augmentation of assistive devices. Frequently associated lower extremity edema should be controlled through regular leg elevation, use of compression stockings, and, when necessary, intermittent compression devices.

References

1. Adelman JU, Goldberg GS, Puckett JD: Postpartum bilateral femoral neuropathy. Obstet Gynecol 1973; 42:845.
2. Adson AW, Coffey JR: Cervical rib: A method of anterior approach for relief of symptoms by division of the scalenus anticus. Ann Surg 1927; 85:839.
3. Asbury AK: Proximal diabetic neuropathy. Ann Neurol 1977; 2:179.
4. Bastron JA, Thomas JE: Diabetic polyradiculopathy. Clinical and electromyographic findings in 105 patients. Mayo Clin Proc 1981; 56:725.
5. Beghi E, Kurland LT, Mulder DW, Nicolosi A: Brachial plexus neuropathy in the population of Rochester, Minnesota, 1970–1981. Ann Neurol 1985; 18:320.
6. Benzel EC, Morris DM, Fowler MR: Nerve sheath tumours of the sciatic nerve and sacral plexus. J Surg Oncol 1988; 39:8.
7. Bradley WG, Madrid R, Thrush DC, Campbell MS: Recurrent brachial plexus neuropathy. Brain 1975; 98:381.
8. Brody IA, Wilkins RH: Erb's palsy (neurologic classics). Arch Neurol 1969; 21:442.
9. Bruxelle J, Travers V, Thiebaut JB: Occurrence and treatment of pain after brachial plexus injury. Clin Orthop 1988; 237:87.
10. Burns RJ: Delayed radiation-induced damage to the brachial plexus. Clin Exp Neurol 1978; 15:221.
11. Casey EB, Harrison MJG: Diabetic amyotrophy: A follow-up study. Br Med J 1972; 1:656.
12. Chokroverty S, Reyes MG, Rubino FA, Tonaki H: The syndrome of diabetic amyotrophy. Ann Neurol 1977; 2:181.
13. Clagett OT: Presidential address: Research and prosearch. J Thorac Cardiovasc Surg 1962; 44:153.
14. Clodius L, Uhlschmidt G, Hess K: Irradiation plexitis of the brachial plexus. Clin Plast Surg 1984; 11:161.
15. Cwick VA, Wilbourn AJ: Acute brachial neuropathy: Detailed EMG findings in a large series. Muscle Nerve 1990; 13:859.
16. Danos E: Obstetrical palsy. J Bone Joint Surg Br 1965; 47:805.
17. Davis DH, Onofrio BM, MacCarty CS: Brachial plexus injuries. Mayo Clin Proc 1978; 53:799.
18. Falconer M, Li FW: Resection of the first rib in costoclavicular compression of the brachial plexus. Lancet 1962; 1:59.
19. Favero KJ, Hawkins RH, Jones MW: Neuralgic amyotrophy. J Bone Joint Surg Br 1987; 69:195.
20. Fechter JD, Kuschner SH: The thoracic outlet syndrome. Orthopedics 1993; 16:11.
21. Garland H, Taverner D: Diabetic myelopathy. Br Med J 1953; 1:1405.
22. Georgy FM: Femoral neuropathy following abdominal hysterectomy. Am J Obstet Gynecol 1975; 123:819.
23. Gilden DH, Eisner J: Lumbar plexopathy caused by disseminated intravascular coagulation. JAMA 1977; 237:2846.
24. Gilliatt RW: Physical injury to peripheral nerves. Mayo Clin Proc 1981; 56:361.
25. Glass RF: The brachial plexus. In Edelman RR, Hesselink JR (eds): Clinical Magnetic Resonance Imaging. Philadelphia, WB Saunders, 1990, p 653.
26. Gonik B, Stringer CA, Cotton DB, Held B: Intrapartum maternal lumbosacral plexopathy. Obstet Gynecol 1984; 63:45S.
27. Goodfellow J, Fearn CBDA, Matthews JM: Iliacus haematoma. A common complication of haemophilia. J Bone Joint Surg Br 1967; 49:748.
28. Hardy AE: Birth injuries of the brachial plexus. J Bone Joint Surg Br 1981; 63:98.
29. Harper CM, Thomas JE, Casino TL, Litchy WJ: Distinction between neoplastic and radiation-induced brachial plexopathy, with emphasis on the role of EMG. Neurology 1989; 39:502.
30. Hepper NGG, Herskovic T, Whitten DM, et al: Thoracic inlet tumors. Ann Intern Med 1966; 64:979.
31. Hochberg FH, et al: Hand difficulties among musicians. JAMA 1983; 249:1869.
32. Jaeckle KA, Young DF, Foley KM: The natural history of lumbosacral plexopathy in cancer. Neurology 1985; 35:8.
33. Jones SJ: Diagnostic value of peripheral and spinal somatosensory evoked potentials in traction lesions of the brachial plexus. Clin Plast Surg 1984; 11:167.
34. King AB: Neurologic conditions occurring as complications of pregnancy. Arch Neurol Psychiatry 1950; 63:611.
35. Kline D: Civilian gunshot wounds to the brachial plexus. J Neurosurg 1989; 70:166.
36. Kline DG: Surgical repair of peripheral nerve injury. Muscle Nerve 1990; 13:843.
37. Kori SH, Foley KM, Posner JB: Brachial plexus lesions in patients with cancer: 100 cases. Neurology 1981; 31:45.
38. Lederman RJ: Thoracic outlet syndromes: Review of the controversies and a report of 17 instrumental musicians. Med Prob Perf Artists 1987; 2:87.
39. Lederman RJ, Paulson SM: Brachial neuritis. In Johnson RT (ed): Current Therapy in Neurologic Disease—2. Philadelphia, BC Decker, 1987, pp. 320–322.
40. Lederman RJ, Wilbourn AJ: Brachial plexopathy: Recurrent cancer or radiation? Neurology 1984; 34:1331.
41. Lefferet RD: Brachial Plexus Injuries. New York, Churchill Livingstone, 1985.

42. Leffert RD, Seddon HJ: Infraclavicular brachial plexus injuries. J Bone Joint Surg Br 1965; 47:9.

43. Lusk MD, Kline DG, Garcia CA: Tumors of the brachial plexus. Neurosurgery 1987; 21:439.

44. Meyer RD: Treatment of adult and obstetrical brachial plexus injuries. Orthopedics 1986; 9:899.

45. Narakas AO: Traumatic brachial plexus lesions. In Dyck PJ, Thomas PK, Lambert EH, Bunge R (eds): Peripheral Neuropathy, vol 2. Philadelphia, WB Saunders, 1984, p 1394.

46. Parsonage MJ, Turner AJW: Neuralgic amyotrophy. The shoulder-girdle syndrome. Lancet 1948; 1:973.

47. Peet PM, Henriksen JD, Anderson TP, Martin GM: Thoracic outlet syndrome: Evaluation of a therapeutic exercise program. Mayo Clin Proc 1956; 31:281.

48. Raff MC, Sangalang V, Asbury AK: Ischemic mononeuropathy multiplex associated with diabetes. Arch Neurol 1968; 18:487.

49. Roos DB: Transaxillary approach for the first rib resection to relieve thoracic outlet syndrome. Ann Surg 1966; 16:354.

50. Rosson JW: Disability following closed traction lesions of the brachial plexus sustained in motorcycle accidents. J Hand Surg 1987; 12B:353.

51. Sellke FW, Kelly TR: Thoracic outlet syndrome. Am J Surg 1988; 156:54.

52. Sunderland S: Nerves and Nerve Injuries, ed 2. Edinburgh, Churchill Livingston, 1978.

53. Terzis JK, Smith KL: The Peripheral Nerve-Structure, Function and Reconstruction. New York, Raven Press, 1990.

54. Thomas HM, Cushing HG: Exhibition of two cases of radicular paralysis of the brachial plexus. One from the pressure of a cervical rib with operation. The other of uncertain origin. Johns Hopkins Hosp Bull 1903; 14:315.

55. Tsairis P: Brachial plexus neuropathies. In Dyck PJ, Thomas PK, Lambert EH (eds): Peripheral Neuropathy, 1st ed. Philadelphia, WB Saunders, 1975, p 659.

56. Tsairis P, Dyck PJ, Mulder DW: Natural history of brachial plexus neuropathy. Report on 99 patients. Arch Neurol 1972; 27:109.

57. Weber ER, Daube JR, Coventry MB: Peripheral neuropathies associated with total hip arthroplasty. J Bone Joint Surg Am 1976; 58:66.

58. Weis EB: Subtle neurological injuries in pelvic fractures. J Trauma 1984; 24:983.

59. Wilbourn AJ: Brachial plexus disorders. In Dyck PJ, Thomas PK (eds.): Peripheral Neuropathy, 3rd ed. Philadelphia, WB Saunders, 1993, p 911.

60. Wilbourn AJ: Thoracic outlet syndrome is overdiagnosed. Arch Neurol 1990; 47:328.

61. Wilbourn AJ, Porter JM: Thoracic outlet syndromes. Spine State Art Rev 1988; 2:597.

62. Williams IR, Moyer RF: Subacute proximal diabetic neuropathy. Neurology 1976; 26:108.

63. Wright IS: The neurovascular syndrome produced by hyperabduction of the arms. Am Heart J 1945; 29:1.

64. Wynn Parry CB: Pain in avulsion of the brachial plexus. Neurosurgery 1984; 15:960.

65. Wynn Parry CB: Rehabilitation of patients following tract lesions of the brachial plexus. Clin Plast Surg 1984; 11:173.

66. Wynn Parry CB: Pain in avulsion lesions of the brachial plexus. Pain 1980; 9:41.

67. Young MR, Norris JW: Femoral neuropathy during anticoagulant therapy. Neurology 1976; 27:1173.

68. Zarranz JJ, Salisachs P: Femoral neuropathy due to compression by retroperitoneal haemorrhage. J Neurol Sci 1979; 43:479.

Rehabilitation Concerns in Myopathies

MAUREEN R. NELSON, M.D.

Myopathies are a group of muscle diseases whose most common primary symptom is proximal limb muscle weakness. There are a variety of myopathies which differ in etiology, course, specific muscle involvement, and associated problems. These include the muscular dystrophies, and the myopathies that are congenital, metabolic, endocrine, infectious, collagen-vascular, toxic, or secondary to other etiologies. Most myopathy research has been done on Duchenne muscular dystrophy (DMD), which is in many ways a myopathy prototype. DMD will be described in detail and the other myopathies will be discussed with regard to how they vary from DMD. The majority of these disorders have no cure, although an extensive amount of research is underway. Treatment in these cases is focused on prevention of any secondary complications and maximizing function within each stage of the disease (Table 48–1).

DYSTROPHIES

Muscular dystrophies are hereditary and congenital disorders of muscle. The most common muscular dystrophy is DMD, although this disease is more severe and quicker in progression than other dystrophies. Other muscular dystrophies include Becker's, facioscapulohumeral, myotonic, the limb-girdle group, and the less common Emery-Dreifuss type (Table 48–2).

Duchenne Muscular Dystrophy

Duchenne muscular dystrophy is an X-linked recessive myopathy. DMD has an incidence of 1 in 5000 live male births with a prevalence approximating 3 per 100,000 live males.[94] Approximately one third of the DMD cases are thought to occur secondary to a spontaneous mutation.[15] The absence or severe abnormality of the protein dystrophin is believed to be the cause of DMD. This is caused by an abnormality on the short arm of the X chromosome at the Xp21 locus.[22, 64, 94]

DMD typically becomes clinically evident at approximately 3 to 5 years of age. Early difficulties noted are clumsiness, poor walking, and frequent falls. The weakness

TABLE 48–1 Types of Myopathies

Dystrophies	Endocrine myopathies
Duchenne muscular dystrophy	Hyperthyroidism
Becker's muscular dystrophy	Hypothyroid myopathy
Facioscapulohumeral dystrophy	Hyperparathyroidism
Limb-girdle dystrophy	Hypothyroidism
Myotonic dystrophy	Corticosteroid myopathy
Emery-Dreifuss muscular dystrophy	Inflammatory myopathies
Congenital myopathies	Polymyositis
Central core myopathy	Dermatomyositis
Nemaline myopathy	Sarcoidosis
Myotubular (centronuclear) myopathy	Infectious myopathies
Congenital fiber disproportion	Trichinosis
Metabolic myopathies	Cysticercosis
Muscle phosphorylase deficiency (McArdle's disease,	HIV/AIDS
type V glycogenosis)	Toxic myopathies
Phosphofructokinase (type VII) deficiency	Alcoholic myopathy
Acid maltase deficiency (type II glycogenosis; infantile	Medications
[Pompe's disease])	
Debranching enzyme deficiency	

Abbreviations: HIV, human immunodeficiency virus; AIDS, acquired immunodeficiency syndrome.

TABLE 48-2 Muscular Dystrophies

Type	Genetic	Signs at Presentation	Age at Presentation	Associated Findings	Chromosome	Disease Course	Laboratory Studies	Electrodiagnosis	Biopsy
Duchenne muscular dystrophy	XLR	Poor walking Frequent falls Gowers' maneuver Pseudohypertrophy of calves	3–5 yr	Cardiac disease Restrictive lung disease Scoliosis Decreased IQ	Xp21	Severe, progressive	Early: very high CK ECG abnormal	Positive sharp waves, fibrillations, CRDs, small-amplitude polyphasics	Fibrosis, circular fibers, basophilic fibers, abnormal or no dystrophin
Becker's muscular dystrophy	XLR	Decrease in walking Pseudohypertrophy of calves	10–15 yr—varies	Cardiac disease	Xp21	Slowly progressive, varies	Increased CK ECG abnormal	Positive sharp waves, fibrillations, CRDs small-amplitude polyphasics Paraspinal	Abnormal quality or quantity of dystrophin
Facioscapulohumeral dystrophy	AD	Facial weakness Shoulder weakness	Teenage—varies	Dry sclera Facial droop		Varies	Normal or mildly increased CK	CRDs early, may be normal Positive sharp waves, fibrillations, small-amplitude polyphasics	Tiny fibers "Moth-eaten" fibers
Limb-girdle dystrophy	AR	Hip weakness	Teenage–20s	Cardiac disease Pulmonary disease		Varies	Increased LDH Increased CK	CRDs Small-amplitude polyphasics, CRDs	Varied fiber size, increased internal nuclei Fiber splitting, "moth-eaten" whorled fibers
Myotonic dystrophy	AD	Myotonia (cramping or stiffness) Long face Distal extremity weakness	Late teenage–20s	Cataracts Cardiac conduction defects Endocrine abnormalities Denial	Chromosome 19	Varies	Increased CK	Myotonic discharges (wax and wane) Small-amplitude polyphasics	Internal nuclei, type I fiber atrophy
Emery-Dreifuss muscular dystrophy	XLR	Early contractures Cardiac conduction defect	Childhood	Cardiac disease	Xq28	Slowly progressive	CK normal to increased	Small- and large-amplitude polyphasics	Type I predominance and atrophy

Abbreviations: IQ, Intelligence quotient; *CK,* creatine kinase; *ECG,* electrocardiogram; *CRDs,* complete repetitive discharges; *LDH,* lactic dehydrogenase; *XLR,* X-linked recessive; *AD,* autosomal dominant; *AR,* autosomal recessive.

is generally symmetrical, begins in the pelvic and then the shoulder girdle muscles, and finally progresses to the respiratory and distal limb muscles.[31, 34, 50] DMD progresses with a predictable pattern but variable rate of functional loss in different children.[50] Death is usually due to respiratory insufficiency and generally occurs at approximately 20 years of age without ventilatory assistance.

There are several associated findings common in DMD. Restrictive pulmonary disease is frequently noted and progresses with weakening of muscles. Scoliosis is also associated with progressive axial muscle weakness. Additionally, cardiac abnormalities are found.

DMD is seen rarely in females. Since this is an X-linked recessive disorder, it can occur in a girl with Turner's syndrome and an XO karyotype or with an X autosomal translocation and a break at the Xp21 locus.[94] Additionally, female carriers can have varying degrees of mild muscle weakness and elevation of muscle enzymes.

Physical findings in a child at the time of diagnosis of DMD frequently include calf pseudohypertrophy, which is present in about 80% of patients.[94] This finding is believed to represent fibrotic replacement of muscle, which is rubbery to palpation. Another frequent sign is difficulty arising from the floor and the demonstration of Gowers's maneuver (the child stabilizes his legs with his arms and pushes his arms up the front of his thighs to stand up) (Fig. 48–1). Proximal muscle atrophy may be detected. The child may also have difficulty raising his arms above his head. Pelvic-girdle weakness is generally present earlier than shoulder-girdle weakness. Gait is frequently wide-based and the child will progress to walking on tiptoe with tight Achilles tendons. The child may be unable to climb up the stairs or step up onto a low bench. Muscle stretch reflexes may be decreased or absent.[15]

Intelligence is affected by DMD, although the exact cause of this is unknown. Twenty-five percent of boys with DMD will have intelligence quotients (IQs) lower than 75, which is not a progressive loss.[94] Cardiac involvement initially involves the posterobasal area and contiguous left ventricular wall.[123] Arrhythmias and tachycardia may be present.[15] Upper gastrointestinal tract dysfunction may be present with dysphagia, heartburn, and nasal voice. Gastric hypomotility has also been noted.[58] Patients with DMD and other myopathies have been reported as having malignant hyperthermia (MH) as an adverse response to general anesthesia. This is manifest by tachycardia, cardiac arrhythmia, tachypnea, unstable blood pressure, cyanosis, fever, and possibly convulsions. Seventy-five percent of the patients develop rigidity secondary to severe muscle contractures, frequently in the masseter muscles, with metabolic acidosis as a consequence. Myoglobinuria and renal failure may result with a mortality of 60%. MH can be induced by halothane and succinylcholine.[94] When the diagnosis is suspected, anesthetic agents should be immediately discontinued and 100% oxygen given. The patient is cooled, and bicarbonate is given for metabolic acidosis. Dantrolene is given to relax the muscles. Immediate treatment improves the outcome.[15] The classic MH defect is not present in muscular dystrophy, so the MH that clinically occurs in DMD is likely due to the defect of muscle cell membranes.[43]

Laboratory findings in DMD show an elevated creatine

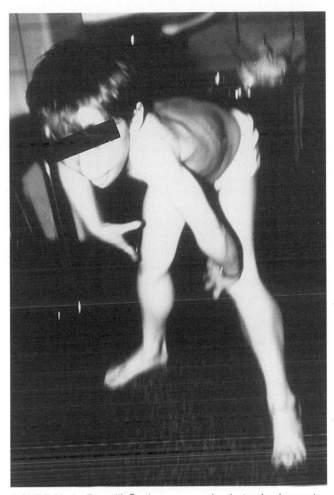

FIGURE 48–1   Boy with Duchenne muscular dystrophy demonstrating calf pseudohypertrophy and Gowers's maneuver in standing up.

kinase (CK), which may be 300 to 400 times normal.[94] This decreases with age as muscle mass declines with disease progression. CK is mildly elevated in 70% of female carriers.[94] Other muscle enzymes may also be elevated in DMD patients. The electrocardiogram (ECG) is abnormal in two thirds of patients, usually demonstrating a tall right precordial R wave with deep Q waves in the limb and left precordial leads.

Needle electromyography (EMG) and nerve conduction studies (NCSs) are a useful part of the evaluation (also see Chapters 6 through 8). Sensory NCSs are normal. Motor NCSs have normal latencies, conduction velocities, and F-wave latencies, but the amplitude of the compound muscle action potential (CMAP) is typically decreased as the disease progresses. The EMG can show an increase in insertional activity early in the disease which may decrease later as fibrotic tissue replaces muscle. Fibrillations and positive sharp waves can be seen at rest. Complex repetitive discharges (CRDs) may also be observed.[73] Motor units in DMD show the classic short-duration, low-amplitude, polyphasicity (often called "myopathic") accompanied by satellite potentials and there is frequently early motor unit recruitment.[73] Muscle fiber conduction velocity is slowed and variable.[79]

Muscle biopsy shows increased fibrosis with circular

fibers. There is muscle fiber necrosis and phagocytosis in association with small groups of basophilic fibers. There are also opaque fibers and an increase in undifferentiated fibers.[15] Dystrophin is noted to be absent in the sarcolemma of skeletal muscle fibers in DMD by microscopic immunochemistry.[22, 64]

The DMD gene is a large genetic locus including over 2.5 million base pairs of a human X chromosome. The large size of the gene is believed to be responsible for the high mutation rate and therefore relatively high frequency of DMD. Because the gene is so large and there are so many areas where a genetic mutation can occur, once the mutation is identified in a family member, the specific genetic lesion present in that family can be searched for in DNA prenatal diagnosis. Accuracy is approximately 100%.[70]

The clinical course in DMD is progressive respiratory and limb muscle weakness, contractures, and reduction of physical function. Ambulation ceases at approximately 12 to 13 years of age. When the child can no longer climb four stairs in under 5 sec, it will be approximately 2.4 years until he will be unable to stand or walk without assistive devices. If it takes him longer than 12 sec for that same stair climbing he is on average 1½ years from inability to walk independently. Scoliosis is present in approximately 75% of patients. Contrary to common belief, scoliosis is not secondary to inability to walk but in fact is present in many boys prior to this change in mobility.[18] This finding is supported by a study which showed that scoliosis and the cessation of ambulation are temporally but not causally related.[75] Surgery for scoliosis is generally considered when the curve is greater than 35 degrees. Forced vital capacity (FVC) is generally improved or stable after surgery for scoliosis, particularly when the FVC is greater than 1.5 L at the time of surgery. There is a correlation between development of pneumonia and an FVC of approximately 1 L or less. Patients who are weaker tend to die from respiratory failure and pneumonia while patients who are stronger have preserved respiratory function and may eventually die from cardiac failure.[18]

Treatment

There is currently no cure for DMD although intensive research is underway. Medications are used to attempt to slow the progression of the disease. There is treatment for minimizing the problem of contractures with bracing and stretching exercises. Surgical interventions are frequently undertaken to relieve contractures. Respiratory management is an area with a large array of treatment options. Spinal fusion for scoliosis is a useful intervention for many of these children. Exercise to improve muscle strength is an area of controversy. Various braces are used to increase mobility. A main goal of treatment is to minimize medical complications.

Pharmacology

Pharmacological intervention has consisted primarily of steroids. Limited investigations have shown that strength, functional status, and pulmonary function improve with steroids.[17] A long-term study also demonstrated that the duration of independent ambulation was prolonged in boys treated with prednisone over a control group.[28] Side effects include cushingoid facial appearance, increased appetite and excessive weight gain, hyperactivity, cataracts, gastritis, behavioral changes, bone loss leading to fracture, and acne.[17, 28] Studies have also investigated the possible beneficial effects on progression of DMD of amino acids,[83] allopurinol,[12, 56] calcium channel blockers,[93] methysergide,[98] and isaxonine,[47] but none of these were found to have any benefit.[48]

Deflazacort (a derivative of prednisone) was used in children with DMD in an attempt to have the benefits of steroids with fewer side effects than found with prednisone. It was used for a 2-year trial with positive outcomes.[2] Both an improvement in functional ability and a delay in the loss of ambulation were noted, along with fewer side effects than prednisone.[2] Deflazacort is not yet approved for use in the United States. Steroids cannot prevent the ultimate outcome in DMD.

Ventilation

Maximizing ventilatory assistance in patients with DMD is critical. The median age of death in DMD is between 18 and 25 years of age.[9, 40, 100] Approximately 90% of these patients die secondary to chronic respiratory insufficiency.[9, 100] Restrictive pulmonary disease, including chest wall muscle weakness and scoliotic deformity, contributes.[9] Ventilatory assistance can extend the length of life and ventilation options are increasing as research in this area continues.

Respiratory assistance is typically initiated when vital capacity (VC) decreases to approximately 20% of predicted normal and symptoms of hypercapnia begin.[9, 39] VC generally maximizes at approximately age 10 years in children with DMD. The maximal level that is attained can help predict the progression of the restrictive disease in each child. In the ensuing years, the VC decreases, generally to 30% to 50% of predicted by the mid-teenage years.[9] Some caregivers then recommend the use of mouth intermittent positive pressure breathing (MIPPB) with the use of an intermittent positive pressure breathing (IPPB) device. This intervention is designed to obtain maximal lung expansion, with a goal of minimizing the microatelectasis and maintaining the chest wall compliance. It is also used for management of acute respiratory infections.[9]

Glossopharyngeal breathing (GPB), or frog breathing, can be a useful tool for DMD patients. For persons who can learn to essentially breathe their swallowed air, the time of ventilatory assistance can be decreased. Additionally, GPB is a useful backup for any mechanical failure of ventilatory assistance. GPB can be used to take deep breaths, shout, and increase the effect of coughing, even in individuals who have no measurable VC. Intact oropharyngeal muscles are necessary for GPB. It is not possible to perform GPB with an open tracheostomy and rarely can it be done with a plugged tracheostomy.[6]

When the VC falls to approximately 10% of the predicted normal, or when a patient begins to have symptoms of nocturnal hypoventilation, it is time for consideration of the need for increased respiratory assistance. Symptoms of hypercarbia include irritability, daytime somnolence, morning headaches, nausea, restless sleep, palpitations, dysphoria, and decrease in daytime vigor.[24, 114] Respiratory drive decreases at night so there is an increased risk at that time.[24] The workup of a patient with falling VC consists of admission to the hospital for continuous overnight capnography (measurement of partial pressure of carbon dioxide [PCO_2]). This measures the end-expiratory PCO_2 and, for those without significant intrinsic lung disease, will be approximately equal to the arterial PCO_2. Arterial blood gases can also be done and oxygen saturation using pulse oximetry can be monitored. With a PCO_2 at 55 mm Hg overnight, the patient may have daytime symptoms, even if blood gases during the day are normal. If the PCO_2 levels are increased during the day, there is frequently severe nocturnal hypoventilation, with the PCO_2 as high as 80 to 95 mm Hg.[9] Treatment is initiated with the use of noninvasive negative or positive pressure ventilators.

The rationale for the use of negative pressure ventilation is that the ventilator actually performs part of the patient's work of breathing, resting the respiratory muscles. The goal is to provide relief for respiratory muscles to allow them to work efficiently during the day after a night of relative rest.[114] Tank ventilators have been shown to reduce diaphragmatic and accessory muscle electrical activity in patients with restrictive lung disease while maintaining adequate ventilation.[6, 101, 114]

Negative pressure ventilators work by an intermittent flow of negative pressure in a tank, resulting in a negative intrapleural pressure, generating airway flow to ventilate the lungs.[6] Commonly used types of negative pressure ventilation include the iron lung, Porta-Lung (Lifecare, Lafayette, Colo.), cuirass, negative pressure wrap, and rocking beds. All except the cuirass ventilator require the patient to be supine. These systems are driven by negative pressure pumps. The cuirass is convenient, and can be used while sitting. It is ineffective if there is poor pulmonary compliance or if there is any significant scoliosis.[6] Some patients use a cuirass during the day and an iron lung or other tank ventilator at night. Complications from using the iron lung or tank respirators are minimal. Decubitus ulcers are rarely seen with the use of 4-in. egg crate mattresses. Chafing of the neck from the rubber of the tank collar is generally no longer seen because of improved collar design. Other difficulties in using negative pressure ventilation occur in patients younger than 3 years of age who tend to have recurrent atelectasis and pneumonia. Severe thoracic or cervical thoracic scoliosis also prevents adequate fit of negative pressure ventilation.[114]

There are several forms of positive pressure ventilation (PPV) available. Noninvasive intermittent PPV (NIPPV, bipap) can be done with mouth or nasal access. Alternatively, the more commonly used PPV is the invasive method using a tracheostomy. NIPPV methods include the exsufflation belt or pneumobelt, which has an elastic inflatable bladder within an abdominal corset. Cyclic positive pressure inflation causes the bladder to compress the abdomen, pushing the diaphragm upward, which induces a forced expiration. When the bladder deflates, the diaphragm passively lowers and inspiration occurs. The patient can support this passive inspiration with any available active inspiratory efforts. This mechanism is effective in the seated position only and ineffective in patients with severe scoliosis. When effective, however it can increase the inspired volume by approximately 300 mL.[6]

Bipap is PPV noninvasively delivered with an oral or nasal interface. For oral PPV there is often use of a mouth seal (Puritan-Bennett, Boulder, Colo.) to keep the mouthpiece in place and prevent excessive leakage.[6] The PPV system devices are generally initiated with nighttime use, as with the negative pressure devices.[9]

Invasive PPV is done through use of a tracheostomy and positive pressure ventilator. Tracheostomy is deemed to be mandatory when oral pharyngeal muscle strength is inadequate to control secretions or speech, in unreliable or uncooperative patients, when severe intrinsic lung disease is present, when there are seizures, or if there are severe orthopedic facial problems.[6] Tracheostomy intermittent positive pressure ventilation (IPPV) is the most common method of respiratory support offered to DMD patients requiring ventilatory assistance.[9] There are a number of potential problems associated with tracheostomy ventilation including airway colonization, increased risk of respiratory tract infection, tracheal necrosis, tracheoesophageal fistula, tracheostenosis, laryngeal complications, swallowing problems, food aspiration, cardiac arrhythmias, chronic granulation tissue formation, painful tracheostomy tube change, mucous plug, and death either from sudden respiratory arrest secondary to mucous plug or from accidental disconnection of the ventilator.[6] Additionally, the mere presence of a tracheostomy stimulates airway secretions, making more frequent suctioning and pulmonary toilet necessary. Most routine suctioning fails to clear the left mainstem bronchus and leads to an increased risk of pneumonia on the left. Speech is dependent on ventilator cycling and timing with inspiration. A tracheostomy is also an open wound which makes the patient ineligible for certain activities and living situations.[6] Patients without ventilatory assistance and a maximum plateau VC below 1200 mL die on average at age 15.3 years, while those with a plateau over 1700 mL live to approximately age 21.[9, 100] Hopefully, in the future, with maximal respiratory assistance available as well as early optimal treatment of scoliosis to maintain a position for the lungs, these numbers can be greatly improved. Patients with DMD have a progressive decrease in VC even with ventilatory assistance. They can anticipate an increased use of assisted ventilation each year. The treatment is not giving oxygen, it is the mechanical work of ventilation. With assisted ventilation, survival is increased by approximately 6 years.[24]

Ventilatory assistance in DMD is a controversial area. In a 1985 survey of Muscular Dystrophy Association (MDA) clinics, Colbert and Schock[23] found that ventilatory aids were prescribed on a regular basis in only 33% of the 132 responding clinics. A similar survey in 1990 by Bach et al.[7] reported that ventilatory assistance was being offered on an elective basis in only 43 of 167 (26%) MDA clinics. Sixty-two clinics (37%) were managing no one on a ventilator. Sixty-one percent of the clinics reported that they followed regular pulmonary function tests but the majority of them only began initial ventilator use during acute respiratory episodes. The 143 clinics that did not offer ventilatory aid or discuss ventilatory assistance stated that the main reason was poor quality of life on a ventilator. Other responses reported were financial problems, home environment, cognitive deficits, and family burden.[5] Only 4 of the 91 clinic directors who discouraged ventilatory assistance had any experience with noninvasive ventilation.[5]

Patients note that physicians severely underestimate their quality of life. Both patients and families report deficits, and many patients are dissatisfied with the information they have been given about ventilatory assistance and feel they should have gotten this information earlier and more completely.[87] In comparing satisfaction with one's own life in a group of DMD patients and a control group of medical professionals, 12.5% of the patients were dissatisfied with their life in general compared with 9.0% of the surveyed healthcare professionals.[7] So the great majority of patients are indeed satisfied with their lives. The medical professionals' perception of the patients' self-satisfaction significantly underestimates the patients' responses.[7] Clearly, satisfaction with one's life is subjective. Because of the inherent personal nature of the decision, information about ventilation and its consequences should be made available early in the disease course to patients and families so that they can make an informed decision based on their own assessment, as opposed to their physician's assessment, of quality of life.

Other aspects of pulmonary care include vaccination against influenza beginning at age 6 months as well as *Haemophilus influenzae* and pneumococcus beginning at age 2 years.[35] During upper respiratory infections, antibiotics, chest physical therapy, postural drainage, and assisted cough with suction should be used. Supplemental oxygen may be necessary during these times. Careful monitoring of any spinal orthoses must be made to ensure that they do not impair respiratory muscle function. The orthoses may decrease VC and consideration should be given to cutting out an anterior window to ease breathing.[35]

Contractures

Contractures are a severe problem in DMD. In a recent study of 230 patients with 11 different neuromuscular diseases, the highest percentage of contractures occurred in patients with DMD. Seventy-eight percent of the patients had ankle contractures; 67%, hip and knee; 65%, elbow; and 44%, iliotibial band (ITB) and wrist contractures.[61] Vignos and Archibald,[120] in 1960, described how contractures often progressed more rapidly than muscle weakness in DMD. They reported an association between lower limb contractures and loss of independent ambulation.[120] The use of bilateral ankle-foot orthoses (AFOs) at night along with a regular stretching routine has been proved to delay development of contractures of the Achilles tendon.[105] Boys who regularly wear AFOs and stretch their legs walk independently for a longer period of time, and children who do not stretch or use splints lose the ability to ambulate much earlier. Standing is described as an excellent stretching activity.[46, 105, 119] Stretching of the tensor fascia lata (TFL) is crucial. Good positioning includes lying prone to promote extension of the hip and knees.[38]

Mobility

Maintained mobility, particularly ambulation, is a focus of a good deal of attention and research in DMD. One recommendation for quantifying the difficulties of gait and predicting the decline of gait is using the double support time. The double stance phase is a logical portion of gait to analyze since it is in this phase that the center of gravity is in its lowest position and the body is most stable. Also, the gluteal muscles help to raise the center of mass during stance and these muscles are affected early in DMD. In this small study the portion of double support was increased in the boys who soon afterward lost the ability to ambulate independently, while the boys who did not have an increase in double support time maintained their ambulation.[66]

Many attempts have been made to maximize ambulation time for boys with DMD. AFOs or ischial weightbearing plastic knee-ankle-foot orthoses (KAFOs) are often used to maximize gait. The KAFOs are frequently used with locked knees.[35, 38, 115] Surgical intervention for contracture release has also been used in attempts to maximize and prolong ambulation. The timing for surgical intervention has been a frequent point of dispute, with the concern being that surgery may in fact prematurely halt ambulation.[8, 15, 41, 113] The commonly involved areas for surgical cutaneous tendon release are the hip flexors, TFL and ITB, hamstrings, and Achilles tendons.[8, 18, 35, 38] In DMD the progression of weakness appears to be first the hip-girdle muscles, with contracture of these muscles and of the Achilles tendon. This leads to difficulty in maintaining a center of gravity, particularly when the extensor muscles continue to weaken as the hamstrings contract. Additionally, the TFL contracts when the patient attempts to walk with a wide-based gait to maintain balance. By this time patients are in a position of hip flexion and abduction, with heel varus angulation and equinus of the foot. A compensatory increase in lumbar lordosis must occur to balance the center of gravity. Shoulders also are weakened and the trunk becomes less stable.[38] Tendon releases are sometimes performed in an attempt to stop this cycle of contractures, worsening posture, and decreasing stability.

Contractures of the lower extremities decrease balance in standing and walking and lead to the loss of walking ability, in conjunction with quadriceps weakness.[8, 109, 117] Bach and McKeon[8] showed that a single early procedure of tendon surgical releases with short-term intensive rehabilitation could prolong ambulation, reduce falls, and improve contractures. They found that children who were operated on while they were still ambulating well did better and were happier with their surgical results than children who were treated just prior to, or after beginning to use a wheelchair. Surgical release of the ITB, TFL, gluteus maximus, hamstrings, and Achilles tendon lengthening were performed. Some of the children also underwent a transfer of the posterior tibial muscle to the dorsal surface of the foot. The children who had this procedure maintained active dorsiflexion of the ankle for several years. The children were up in the parallel bars and ambulating in short-leg casts by the second day, and the children who had posterior tibial transfers had short-leg casts for 3 to 6 weeks. Even these children had the cast bivalved after 1 week and began performing exercises for re-education of the posterior tibial at that time. They also used stretching, general conditioning, mobility, hydrotherapy, and pool ambulation. All the children had a significant decrease in the number of falls, improved lumbar lordosis and hip flexion and abduction contractures, and a decrease in the width of their gait. The children who were treated at an early stage had a prolongation of their walking without bracing for approximately 1 year longer than predicted. Those who were operated on later had approximately 8 months' longer walking time than expected. Bach and McKeon[8] recommend that this surgery be done while ambulation and stair-climbing difficulties are minimal, and quadriceps strength is at least antigravity, to minimize the need for bracing postoperatively.

Scoliosis

Scoliosis is an almost inevitable progressive problem in DMD. This progression causes problems in several areas including skin ulceration, back pain, decreased sitting balance, possible limitations on cardiopulmonary reserve, cosmetic difficulties, wheelchair seating problems, and limitations of the variety of assisted ventilation techniques possible.

Scoliosis progress was followed in a group of patients without any spinal intervention until the time of death with the finding of a mean final scoliotic deformity of approximately 90 degrees, with some curves greater than 100 degrees.[107, 111]

Bracing is not effective in the prevention of scoliosis or its progression.[18, 85, 107] Some bracing can be used to facilitate wheelchair seating. With scoliosis progression, wheelchair seating may require repeated alterations as the curve progresses. For correcting the scoliosis, spinal fusion has been found to be effective. Rarely, surgical intervention uses the Harrington rod. More frequently the Luque rod with double sublaminar wires and unit rod fixation are used. Additionally, bone grafts are placed.[85, 107] The timing for surgery is based on the balance between scoliosis progression, remaining FVC, and spine growth.

The trend recently has been to operate on scoliosis earlier in an attempt to minimize the residual scoliosis left after surgical intervention, maximize seating and standing position postoperatively, and minimize respiratory complications.[35, 85, 107, 111] In the study F. Miller and co-workers[85] of 183 DMD patients, 91% of the children had scoliosis which reached 30 degrees before the FVC decreased to 35% of normal. In this group, the scoliosis always progressed. In the others where the percentage of FVC was less than 35% before their curve reached 30 degrees, 50% developed severe deformities.[85] There was a correlation in the development of scoliosis and degree of decrease in FVC. The authors also noted that the risk of pulmonary complications during and after surgery significantly increased as the percentage of normal FVC decreased. Their recommendation was for spinal stabilization before the percentage of normal FVC is 45%, and a cutoff of 35% as the absolute minimum.[85] Other groups report FVC over 40% as ideal, with 30% as the minimum.[107] There is controversy over the impact of scoliosis surgery on future VC progression, with no hard evidence of stabilization or deterioration of VC. There is a known minimal decrease in FVC when the thoracic region is fused following fixation of the ribs.

Problems with spinal fusion include anesthesia risks, blood loss, respiratory problems, and potential neurological

injury. It is important to have anesthesiologists who are familiar with the complications that may arise in a child with DMD, particularly the restrictive ventilatory limitations, MH, and potential cardiac problems. If somatosensory evoked potentials are being done as intraoperative monitoring to assess spinal cord function, the anesthesiologist needs to be aware of this and adjust the medications used accordingly. There is significant blood loss during these procedures, averaging between 3400 and 3700 mL.[85, 107] Currently, many centers are using a cell saver to reinfuse the patient's own red blood cells after treatment during the procedure.

Mobilization should begin as quickly as possible postoperatively. Generally, children are able to move about initially on the second day postoperatively. They begin in physical therapy for mobility and strengthening exercises immediately. A plastic body jacket is frequently used for sitting in a wheelchair approximately 1 week postoperatively and for several months afterward.[107] None of the 27 patients in the studies of Shapiro et al. of spinal fusion required intubation beyond the second postoperative day,[107] whereas 11 of the 183 spinal fusion patients reported by F. Miller et al. required more than 5 days of mechanical ventilation and were treated in the intensive care unit for approximately 12 days.[85] Those 11 patients had a lower FVC (32% vs. 50% of normal) than those who had no complications. Fifty percent of those with an FVC of less than 35% had pulmonary complications, with only 11% of those with an FVC greater than 35% having any pulmonary difficulties.[85]

In considering surgical intervention for scoliosis in an adult with a muscular dystrophy (not Duchenne) the adaptations that the person makes in ambulation must be considered. Spinal fixation may later prevent some of the adaptations patients make to ambulate. This frequently occurs by destabilizing the knee joint with subsequent inability to walk. An evaluation to see if this will occur may be performed by using a firm brace around the spine to see if balance and posture are still effective.[32]

Other Complications

Other complications in DMD include osteoporosis secondary to disuse, and with it, the risk of pathological fractures. Fractures should be treated with as minimal immobilization as possible to encourage continued ambulation and mobility. Immobilization must also be avoided to prevent further weakness.[38]

Obesity also becomes a frequent problem once patients become nonambulatory. The change in calorie expenditure from walking to wheelchair mobility is the major contributing factor. Food sometimes becomes a substitute for decreased opportunities for activities and pleasures. Weight is variable, and half of DMD patients are within normal weight with approximately one third overweight and approximately 15% underweight.[38] Weight management for obesity consists of a low-calorie, well-balanced diet, taking care to monitor calorie intake and output.

Loss of Strength

The natural history of the progression of weakness in DMD has been analyzed in an attempt to have a baseline from which to interpret the effectiveness of early intervention. Muscle strength declines with age with a predictable pattern.[67, 106] There is a steady decrease of strength with symmetrical weakness, most severe proximally and in the extensor muscles. Muscle strength, motor ability, and performance are closely correlated.[106] Ambulation is lost when muscle strength is decreased by 50%.[106, 120] Knee extensor and hip abductor strength play key roles in maintaining ambulation, along with the input of contractures and the problem of maintaining balance. Therefore, treatment is directed toward maintaining range of motion, strength, and the use of earlier involved muscles.[106] The knee flexor strength has been described as less than 60% during the transition from ambulation to wheelchair use, which is believed to indicate that the hip and knee are passively stabilized by the patient shifting his center of gravity.[67]

A method of quantifying muscle damage is by quantitative computed tomography (CT) which evaluates the degree of muscle fiber loss and fatty replacement using percent cross-sectional area (%CSA) of muscle and fat. The %CSA of muscle is decreased as muscle strength decreases and as disability progresses. The rate of progression varies with different muscles.[74]

Exercise

The beneficial effects and possible detrimental side effects of exercise on muscle in DMD has long been an area of controversy and research. Maintaining muscle strength requires repetitive contractions that produce tension. If the tension produced in a day is less than 20% of the maximum possible, a decrease in strength occurs.[69, 119] A major concern in trying to prevent a decrease in muscle function in DMD is that of overwork weakness.[119] Bennett and Knowlton[11] defined *overwork weakness* as a prolonged decrease in both absolute strength and endurance of a muscle. This must be differentiated from a transient decrease postexercise, as well as from progression of the muscle disease. Overwork weakness is reversible if noted early and corrected by rest.[11] Overwork weakness was first reported in myopathy in members of a family with facioscapulohumeral dystrophy. This led to an understanding that excessive overwork can have a long-term detrimental impact on muscle function.[62] Several prospective studies of prescribed daily strengthening programs for DMD patients showed no adverse effects on muscles, and short-term improved strength or no significant increase in strength, but less of a decrease in strength than in controls.[27, 51, 104, 121]

In supervised resistive exercise programs there is no negative effect on muscle in DMD. Objective increases in muscle strength are found, but these decrease as the disease advances. The pre-exercise strength level determines the amount of increase possible, with stronger muscles able to increase more. The overall gain in strength noted in DMD will be the strength increase from the exercise program offset by the progression of disease and loss of strength. Patients maintaining ambulation have larger increases in strength with exercise. Exercise programs should be carried out early in the course of DMD when more relatively healthy muscle fibers are present.[119] Braddom[14] describes overwork weakness quickly occurring in muscles with 60%

or less strength, with muscles of 80% or greater strength resistant to these adverse changes.

Electrical Stimulation

Low-frequency electrical stimulation (LFES) of fast-twitch muscle fibers can transform them into slow-twitch muscle fibers.[55, 102] Degenerative processes in dystrophic muscle affect fast-twitch fibers preferentially.[19] Zupan[130] stimulated muscles in DMD patients with LFES twice daily in an attempt to confer a protective effect on the muscle fibers of DMD and prevent degeneration. Half of the children in this small study had no significant changes in 3 months and the remaining five children demonstrated short-term increased strength, greatest after 5 months of stimulation. There was no change in the level of fatigue with stimulation and there were no adverse effects.[130] Milner-Brown and Miller[90] studied 10 children with various other types of muscular dystrophies with unilateral electrical stimulation, with active weight training added in some muscles. There was a greater rate of increase with the combination of electrical stimulation and weight training, but the absolute gain of muscle strength was greater in the group with weight training alone.[90]

Muscle Research

Current areas of DMD research include myoblast and gene transplantation. Myoblast transfers have been attempted in patients with DMD but without success to date.[44, 52–54] Part of the failure in these attempts may be secondary to immune rejection problems.[53, 54] Of interest, human myoblast clones are capable of fusing to form new muscle fibers and hybrid muscle fibers even after replications of more than 10 million myoblasts per clone.[54] Because only the relatively few muscle fibers injected pick up the dystrophin, attempts are underway to obtain more widespread results.[128] Researchers are attempting gene transfers by transplanting portions of a dystrophin copy DNA into skeletal muscle fibers. If the dystrophin is produced, then the muscle fibers are protected from necrosis. This has been experimentally performed in animals but it is not ready for trial in humans. If gene transfers and long-term expression of the gene product, dystrophin, do occur in the future, the skeletal fibers would acquire a normal phenotype. However, even if this does become effective, cardiac muscle treatment will remain problematic.[65]

Dystrophin constitutes 2% of the total sarcolemmal protein and 5% of sarcolemmal cytoskeleton protein, making it a major structural component of the cytoskeleton.[21, 80, 95] Dystrophin is associated with a large complex of glycoproteins which are known as the dystrophin-associated proteins (DAPs).[80] These DAPs are critical in dystrophin's interaction with the cytoskeleton. DAPs are reduced in all DMD patients of any age. DAPs are missing in all muscle fibers in DMD patients but are present in other neuromuscular diseases.[80, 96] This implies that any myoblast or dystrophin gene therapy for DMD will require replacement of DAP as well as dystrophin.[80]

Hand Function

Hand function in DMD is critical because as the disease progresses the hands are useful for not only activities in daily living (ADL) but also for assistance in mobility. The Vignos scale examines overall function in patients with DMD. There is some inclusion of upper limb function, but the major emphasis is on the lower limb.[122] The Brook Upper Limb Functional Rating Scale consists of six functional levels, with 1 being most useful and 6 delineating no useful hand function.[37] The Jebson Hand Function Test assesses general upper limb function and consists of six timed subtests.[60] Lower Jebson scores reflect better hand function.[62] This has been demonstrated to be useful in children with DMD.[49, 124] The advantage of the Brook scale is that it looks at varying muscle groups covering the spectrum of upper limb function. The advantage of the Jebson scale is that it is done without expensive equipment and can provide a more constant view of the patient over time to look at progression of disease or intervention.[49]

ADL problems in older patients with DMD manifest as a limited ability to pick up heavy objects while fine motor ability is relatively preserved.[125] Difficulty with fine motor tasks is often secondary to proximal muscle weakness.[59] It has also been reported that the difference between the functional ability of the dominant and nondominant hand becomes more significant with age and with wheelchair use. The nondominant hand typically becomes less involved in functional activity. This may be due to needing this hand more for balance or it may be due to a combination of causes.[49] Functional deterioration of the arms begins around age 10, with the deterioration plateauing approximately 2½ years later.[76]

Some common physical abnormalities in the wrist and hand of older children with DMD have been described which may contribute to decreased upper limb function. The abnormalities include extrinsic and intrinsic digital muscle shortness, swan-neck and boutonnière deformities, hyperextension of the interphalangeal joints, as well as wrist flexion and ulnar deviation contractures. Decreased wrist extensor strength occurs by age 8.[124, 125] Ability to perform ADL is influenced primarily by decreased strength of wrist extensors and decreased active radial deviation.[124] Therapy should aim toward maintaining optimal range of motion of the wrist, with prevention of wrist ulnar deviation contractures, and exercise to maintain wrist extensor strength. Therapy includes stretching exercises and positioning of the wrist and fingers. Splint use is necessary in some cases. Boys with DMD are able to both write and turn the pages of a book throughout their disease, so that they can continue to learn and to communicate. The most difficult accomplishment for the older boys is picking up or holding heavy or large objects, including filled glasses and pieces of fruit, being difficult after age 15 years. Therefore, lighter and smaller objects should gradually replace heavier objects in the older child's environment.[124] Consideration of assistive device use and teaching of work simplification for all ADL tasks can be helpful. Balanced form orthoses (BFOs) may be used to compensate for proximal strength deficits when distal function remains intact. Minimal elbow flexion contractures of up to 15 degrees can actually be of benefit in initiating flexion and certainly are not a detriment to ADL function.[38]

Owing to progressive weakness in DMD, which eventually leads to severe functional deficits in the upper extremities, robotic arms can also be used to assist in daily activi-

ties. Since finger movement continues throughout the course of DMD, with a small amount of finger manipulation it is possible to run a wheelchair-mounted robotic arm. This can operate a power wheelchair, computer, environmental control system, or do simple daily activities.[10] A wheelchair-mounted mechanical arm can be used with a control transducer that is adapted to the patient's abilities. Industrial trainer robot manipulators have been modified for use with batteries that can be mounted on a wheelchair lapboard. The arm can be used for eating and recreation. Some patients use a robotic arm for manipulating books and turning pages, using the telephone, opening doors, using light switches, pushing elevator buttons, and even operating electric razors. It is reported to save over 2 hours a day in attendant care time. The cost of a robotic arm is approximately $4000.[10] A robotic arm can promote increased independence and as these devices become more sophisticated they will likely be of even greater benefit.

Psychosocial Management

Psychosocial management is crucial in the care of a DMD patient and his family. The family of a child with a progressive disease that has no cure will require varying amounts of support and interaction from professionals and others from the time of diagnosis onward. Grief in the family will wax and wane with disease exacerbations, dramatic changes in the child's functional ability, and at other times. It is important for the physicians to anticipate future potential medical changes and deterioration in the child's status and to prepare the family for them. Changes such as using a wheelchair and using ventilatory assistance are two of the more dramatic examples of predictable occurrences for which the family must be prepared.[35] Boys in the early stages of DMD often have a great deal of anxiety, along with fear of falling. Later there is a tendency toward social withdrawal, frustration, and anxiety secondary to a fear of dying.[38] Counseling services should be available for the children and families throughout the lifetime of the boys and beyond that for the parents. Proper school placement can be extremely helpful in this regard. Communication should be facilitated with the school and the teachers, including therapy needs. Consideration must also be given to the fact that approximately one third of the boys with DMD are mentally retarded and others may require some special classes or tutoring.[35, 38, 49]

Becker's Muscular Dystrophy

Becker's muscular dystrophy (BMD) is a milder variant of DMD and is caused by a mutation of the same gene as that in DMD.[129] It is a slowly progressive X-linked recessive disorder and has an incidence of approximately 1 in 50,000 live male births. The onset of weakness generally manifests between 10 and 15 years of age. Motor milestones are met, but the pattern of weakness follows that in DMD, though to a much milder degree, with a relatively good prognosis. Pseudohypertrophy of the calves is commonly seen.[94] BMD has more heterogeneous involvement than does DMD, with variable age of onset, progression, distribution, and severity of muscle involvement[129] (Fig. 48–2).

Associated findings in BMD include cardiac disease,

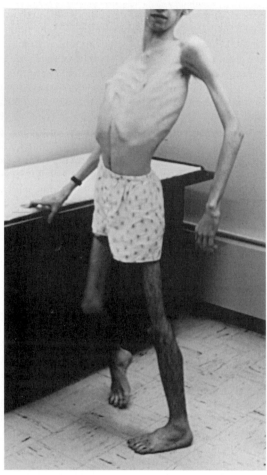

FIGURE 48–2   A 25-year-old man with Becker's muscular dystrophy demonstrating generalized atrophy, with calf pseudohypertrophy and difficulty in mobility.

which may be noted at an early age or during adulthood. It is unrelated to the degree of musculoskeletal weakness. ECG changes identical to these in DMD are found in 45% of BMD patients while 17% have echocardiagram changes consistent with a dilated cardiomyopathy.[123]

An elevated CK is noted in BMD. Needle EMG may show primarily symmetrical changes in the proximal limb muscles including positive waves, fibrillations, and CRDs. Paraspinal muscles may demonstrate CRDs earlier than limb muscles. Motor unit potentials (MUPs) generally are small, polyphasic, and have early recruitment.[68] Muscle biopsy shows an abnormal quantity and quality of dystrophin, but not as severe as in DMD.[94]

The clinical course of BMD is similar to DMD, though it is milder, with later onset, and is somewhat variable. Proximal weakness leads to difficulties in walking, climbing stairs, and rising from the floor. Contractures may develop late in the disease. Myocardial disease generally presents in later years though not always. Survival is generally into middle adulthood.[68] In mild cases a patient may live to 60 years of age, while in more severe cases death may occur in the 20s.[14]

Since the course of BMD is milder than that of DMD, the treatment is less aggressive. Medications are not used except in those persons with the most severe form of the disease. Steroids pose more of a problem than in DMD because of the side effect of stunted growth through a longer life span.[14] There is often a need for bracing, including the use of AFOs for ambulation and the use of a wheelchair for mobility, as the disease progresses. Stretching to prevent contractures is important as independent mobility decreases. Similarly, surgical consideration may be given to treatment of severe contractures which would generally only be seen late in the course of disease. Patients with BMD can gain significant increases in muscle strength, endurance, and work capacity with a weight-training program.[91]

Facioscapulohumeral Dystrophy

Facioscapulohumeral dystrophy (FSH) is an autosomal dominant myopathy with complete penetrance but variable expressivity. There can be a spectrum of mild to severe cases within the same family.[15, 94] Age of onset is generally in the second decade but can be at any time. A common presentation is facial weakness at approximately age 15 years, with facial and proximal weakness progressing very slowly. When FSH is first noted in infancy its course is more severe.[94] The incidence is approximately 3 to 10 cases per million.[15] There is typically a normal life span. The weakness is generally present in the face, shoulder girdle, and anterior portion of the leg[94] (Fig. 48–3). Facial weakness causes an inability to whistle, drink through a straw, and blow up a balloon, and during sleep the eyes may remain open. Proximal upper limb muscles are weak, and often patients are unable to hold heavy objects or lift above the shoulders, climb a rope, or perform a pushup. The hip musculature gradually weakens and drop foot may eventually occur. This progression usually occurs over decades. The face is characteristically smooth and unlined. There is loss of contour of the mouth with a horizontal appearance of the lower lip and a pouting expression of the lips. Neck muscles are often weak. The triceps and biceps brachii may be weak early but the deltoid is relatively preserved, as are the forearm and the wrist flexor muscles, but wristdrop may be present. Hip weakness can lead to compensatory lumbar lordosis. The calf muscles are generally preserved to a greater degree than the dorsiflexors of the ankle with a resultant drop foot. Limb weakness may be asymmetrical and reflexes can be decreased.[15]

There are no ECG or echocardiographic abnormalities, or any rhythm disturbances in FSH.[123] In some patients there is congenital absence of the pectoralis, biceps, and brachioradialis muscles.[68] Nerve deafness is associated with the infantile onset of FSH.[15]

In FSH the CK is elevated two to four times normal in 50% of the patients. The needle EMG is myopathic with fibrillations and repetitive discharges occasionally seen.[94] Early needle EMG in FSH may be normal even in clinically involved muscles. Later on the motor units will be small, polyphasic, and show increased recruitment relative to effort.[68] The biopsy in FSH may show an increased variability in the size of fibers, with small fibers called tiny fibers. Additionally there may be a moth-eaten appearance to the fibers.[15]

Treatment is focused on assistance in ADL with hand or foot orthoses (see Chapters 16 and 17). There has been

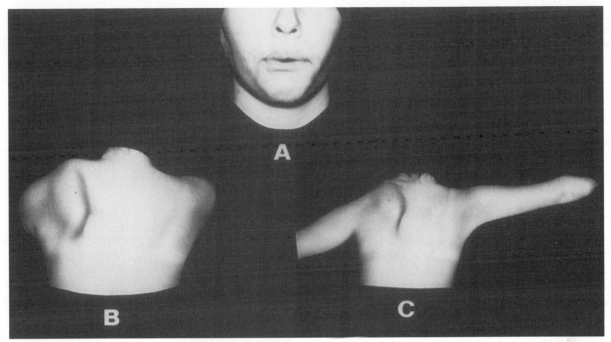

FIGURE 48–3 An 18-year-old woman with facioscapulohumeral muscular dystrophy demonstrating an inability to purse the lips *(A)* and winging of the left scapula *(B and C)*. The patient is left-hand dominant. (From Johnson EW, Braddom R: Over-work weakness in facioscapulohumeral muscular dystrophy. Arch Phys Med Rehabil 1971; 52:333–336.)

concern about overwork weakness as was described in three generations of a family with FSH who had physical examination abnormalities and needle EMG changes in their most frequently used arm.[62] Subsequently, several studies have examined the effect of an exercise program on patients with FSH, looking at the possibility of muscle strength improvement and conversely, muscle damage. There is a lack of consensus regarding statistically significant improvement in muscle strength following exercise.[1, 81, 91] The studies show, however, that carefully supervised strength-training programs with a gradual increase in activity do not cause damage to the muscle or increase weakness.[1, 81, 91]

Some patients with FSH gradually develop scapular instability secondary to weakness of the scapular stabilizing muscles. Because of this, they cannot flex or abduct the arm. If they have deltoid and supraspinatus muscle sparing, they may be able to abduct the arm if the scapula is stabilized. In assessing the potential effectiveness of scapular surgical fixation to the thorax, a preoperative assessment can include manually holding the scapula stable bilaterally while the patient attempts to raise the arm above the head. If the patient can do so, it predicts the stabilizing operation would be helpful. If weakness continues to preclude this maneuver, then the surgery is unlikely to improve the patient's function.[32] Following surgery, isometric deltoid exercises are performed, with pendulum exercises and strengthening of the shoulder muscles. Preoperative strength has been noted to return within 6 months of surgery. Shoulder abduction can be improved by approximately 60 degrees.[20] This often leads to an improvement in the strength to lift and carry objects.[20] There may, however, be a decrease in VC secondary to immobilization of the ribs.

FSH patients may have weak eye closure and drying of the sclera. This can be uncomfortable and also lead to conjunctivitis or even ulceration. Artificial tears may control this problem but if ineffective, plastic surgery should be considered. If FSH facial weakness leads to severe weakness of the mouth, there may be difficulties with eating, drinking, and cosmetic appearance. Plastic surgery may alleviate these difficulties.[32]

Limb-Girdle Dystrophy

Limb-girdle dystrophy (LGD) is an autosomal recessive group of disorders producing weakness about the hips and shoulders. LGD is a less well-defined myopathy and may actually include a spectrum of diseases. The weakness most commonly begins in the second or third decade and affects the hips, then the shoulders. In later years there may be progression to involve other muscle groups. It has been reported as rarely involving only one limb. Facial muscles are generally spared.[68]

Associated findings can include cardiopulmonary difficulties, although cardiac conduction defects are rare. Intellect is normal.[15] Death may occur from cardiopulmonary complications, including pneumonia.[15]

Laboratory findings show an increase in CK and lactic dehydrogenase. The increase is generally mild, but can be up to 10 times normal. Needle EMG shows small-amplitude polyphasic MUPs of short duration, and rarely, CRDs. Muscle biopsy shows variation in fiber size with increased internal nuclei, fiber splitting, and "moth-eaten," whorled fibers.[15]

The clinical course is varied but classically is described as beginning with hip weakness (flexors and extensors), quickly followed by shoulder weakness. There also may be weakness of both neck flexors and extensors. Shoulder weakness includes the deltoid muscle. There is dramatic weakness and frequently atrophy of the biceps brachii[15] (Fig. 48–4).

Ventilatory assistance, including intermittent positive or negative pressure ventilation, may be helpful in the treatment of LGD.[32] A monitored strength training program has been shown to have no adverse effects and, in some cases, shows an increase in strength, at least for the short term.[1, 81, 91]

Myotonic Dystrophy

Myotonic muscular dystrophy (MMD) is an autosomal dominant disease with a prevalence of 3 to 5 per 100,000, with complete penetrance but variable expression.[15, 94] The incidence is 13 per 100,000 live births.[15] In MMD there is progressive muscle weakness (generally worse distally) and atrophy with characteristic involvement of facial, jaw, anterior neck, and distal limb muscles, as well as myotonia. *Myotonia* is defined as a delayed relaxation of muscle contraction. Generally, patients interpret myotonia as muscle stiffness. This can be worsened by cold.[108] Patients with MMD frequently minimize or deny their weakness and myotonia. Onset of weakness is generally gradual in late teenage or early adulthood. Distal muscle weakness is generally symmetrical and slowly progressive. The patient

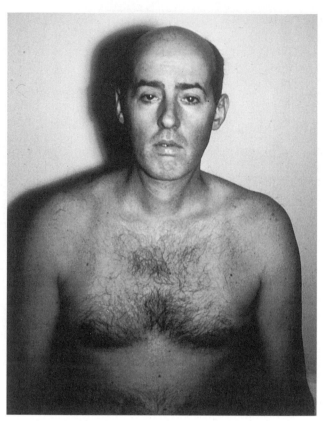

FIGURE 48–5 An adult man with myotonic dystrophy demonstrating an elongated face and balding.

early on may be noted to have a long face and slightly nasal voice[15] (Fig. 48–5). Patients with MMD may complain of muscle stiffness or cramps, but feet and hand weakness are usually their first complaints.[15] Myotonia of the muscle may be present with percussion, although this tends to decrease as the weakness progresses. The myotonic phenomenon can be elicited by striking the abductor pollicis brevis with a reflex hammer, which causes the thumb to move across the palm.[14]

MMD is described as a multisystem disease because of the many associated findings. Cataracts are noted in over 90% of patients, with characteristic multicolored lens opacities which are specific in the early stages. This may be noted by the early teenage years.[108] Weak uterine contractions have been noted.[94] Smooth muscle abnormalities are also present which can cause dilation of the esophagus.[94] There is an increase in gallbladder problems.[15] Weakness in the bowel musculature can cause significant problems with constipation.[32]

Cardiac abnormalities in MMD include cardiomyopathy and conduction defects.[32, 94, 108] Cardiac conduction disturbances are present in one half to two thirds of patients.[94] When the bundle of His is involved a pacemaker can be useful. Death may be due to sudden cardiac arrhythmia.[94] Arrhythmias and mitral valve prolapse are increased in MMD. An abnormal exercise response of the left ventricle has been reported in MMD patients. Therefore, any exercise program must be closely prescribed and monitored.[15]

Males with MMD have degeneration of testicular tubular cells with low sperm formation and low testosterone levels.

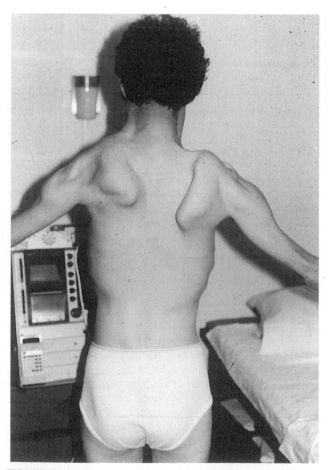

FIGURE 48–4 A 35-year-old man with limb girdle muscular dystrophy demonstrating shoulder weakness, including deltoid and biceps brachii atrophy.

In females variable abnormalities are present including amenorrhea and menstrual irregularities. Infertility is common is MMD patients of both sexes.[94, 108] Glucose intolerance with hyperinsulinemia and a defect in insulin receptors are common but there is no increased incidence of diabetes.[15, 94] Increased denial of abnormalities has been noted in patients with MMD, along with frequent mild mental retardation.[15]

In infants whose mothers have MMD there is a form of the disease that is present at birth: congenital myotonic dystrophy. There is believed to be an intrauterine influence, not strictly genetic (possibly a cell membrane change), which makes this form more severe. In this group there is mental retardation as well as respiratory difficulties and motor delay.[108] In congenital MMD there is hypotonia and facial paralysis with the upper lip forming an inverted V appearance (Fig. 48–6). Also common are clubfeet and frequent respiratory infections.[15]

Some MMD patients have sleep disturbance which is believed to be secondary to pulmonary hypoventilation. There is also an increased pulmonary risk associated with general anesthesia, and with use of barbiturates and other medications that depress respiratory drive.[15]

Evaluation of MMD patients typically shows facial weakness as described above, as well as weakness of the hands and feet. Percussion myotonia is present and a slow release of a handshake may be the first indication of MMD.

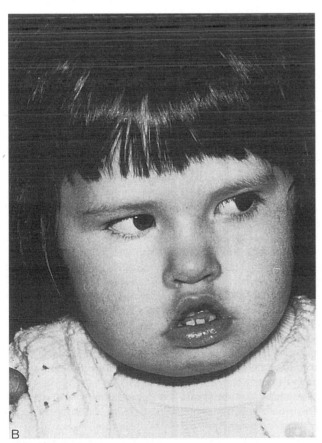

FIGURE 48–6 A toddler with facial paralysis and inverted-V appearance of the lip in congenital myotonic dystrophy. (From Eagel AG, Franzihi-Armstrong C (eds): Myology: Basic and Clinical, ed 2. New York, McGraw-Hill, 1994.)

Needle EMG shows myotonic discharges which wax and wane in amplitude and frequency of motor units. The sound is described as similar to a dive-bomber or motorcycle. There can also be brief, small polyphasic potentials[15] (see Chapters 7 and 8). CK is generally increased. Muscle biopsy shows internal nuclei and atrophy of type I fibers. The biceps brachii muscle tends to show more abnormalities on biopsy than the quadriceps or gastrocnemius muscles.[15] The myotonic dystrophy gene has not yet been identified but its locus is on chromosome 19.[108]

Treatment for patients with MMD includes orthoses for distal weakness, including AFOs or wrist-hand orthoses. When myotonia is a severe functional problem, medications can be tried to stabilize the muscle membranes. Quinine and procainamide can be used, although they depress cardiac conduction. Phenytoin (Dilantin) can also be used, with less risk of cardiac conduction problems. Calcium channel blockers and carbamazepine (Tegretol) can also be used.[15, 94] As weakness is generally a more severe problem than myotonia, the success of these medications is variable and many patients choose not to use them.[15]

In attempting to demonstrate the cause of myotonia, Taylor et al.[118] studied contractility measurements. They demonstrated that MMD patients had a failure of sarcolemmal activation, failure of contractile machinery, and altered excitation-contraction coupling mechanisms.[118] Some believe this is secondary to problems in membrane chloride conductance (see Chapters 7 and 8).

Emery-Dreifuss Muscular Dystrophy

Emery-Dreifuss muscular dystrophy (EDMD) is an X-linked recessive dystrophy with a classic triad of findings. These include (1) early contractures, particularly of the elbows, Achilles tendon, and posterior cervical muscles; (2) cardiac conduction defects; and (3) a slowly progressive weakness and atrophy in a humeroperoneal distribution.[30, 33, 84] The incidence is estimated to be 1 in 100,000, but is not well defined.[42] This disorder is believed to be a slowly progressive myopathy, but the disease spectrum includes patients whose disease is much more severe. Some are unable to walk by the time they reach adulthood,[90, 102] but survival is generally into middle age.[55] Cardiomyopathy can present with heart block, frequently in late teenage or the early 20s and all adult patients with EDMD have this disorder. Early signs are bradycardia and a prolonged PR interval on the ECG. Cardiac pacemakers are usually inserted as soon as the diagnosis is made.[110] The severity of the cardiac disease is much greater than the myopathy.[84] The early onset of contractures before the onset of any significant weakness is unique (Fig. 48–7). The elbows are generally held in a semiflexed position, and the child typically begins walking on tiptoe. The limitation of neck flexion is infrequently noticed except on specific physical examination.[33] There are also contractures of other ligaments, including the metacarpals and those away from major joints.[15]

In EDMD the CK is normal or moderately increased. Needle EMG is usually myopathic although a more neurogenic pattern with high-amplitude, long-duration MUPs is combined in some patients.[30] Muscle biopsy is myopathic with type I predominance and atrophy.[15] The gene responsi-

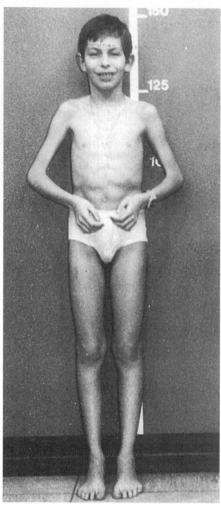

FIGURE 48–7 A 13-year-old boy with Emery-Dreifuss muscular dystrophy showing bilateral elbow flexion contractures and shoulder girdle atrophy. (From Eagel AG, Franzihi-Armstrong C (eds): Myology: Basic and Clinical, ed 2. New York, McGraw-Hill, 1994.)

ble for EDMD is on Xq28, though the gene product has not been determined. Dystrophin is normal in EDMD.[33]

Treatment is primarily focused toward the cardiac disease with a pacemaker as the critical form of treatment. Additionally, bracing may be helpful as the disease progresses. Early frequent range-of-motion exercise and positioning are instituted.

CONGENITAL MYOPATHIES

The congenital myopathies are a group of nonprogressive or slowly progressive myopathies presenting with hypotonia or weakness in the neonatal period. These babies frequently have decreased spontaneous movement and delayed motor milestone achievement. Their muscles may feel flabby to palpation. Physical anomalies such as high palate, pectus excavatum, elongated face, and scoliosis may be present as an indication of long-standing weakness[13] (Table 48–3).

Central Core Myopathy

Central core myopathy (CCM) is an autosomal dominant myopathy with the gene involved located on the long arm of chromosome 19 at 19Q13.1. This is in the same area of the chromosome as the gene for MH, which can also be seen in CCM.[16]

In CCM, the child is floppy at or shortly after birth, with congenital hip dislocation noted frequently. The milestones are delayed, although weakness never becomes a severe problem. The child is frequently clumsy, slender, and short. The diffuse weakness typically includes the face and neck, as well as the extremities. Reflexes are normal or decreased.[16] Skeletal deformities may be present, including lordosis, kyphoscoliosis, and clubfeet. The children generally are unable to jump.[15] There is relative sparing of the bulbar muscles. Significant muscle atrophy is not seen.[13]

CK is usually normal. Needle EMG shows small-amplitude, short-duration, polyphasic MUPs.[13, 16] Single-fiber EMG reveals abnormalities due to an increased number of fibers innervated per anterior horn cell.[13] Biopsy shows a type I fiber predominance with central cores (unstained central area running through the center of the fibers) present in type I and some type II fibers.[13, 15, 16] Electron microscopy shows an absence of mitochondria in the central core.[15, 68] The disease course is very mild and the life span is normal. The weakness is generally so mild that generally no specific treatment is needed. If there is significant weakness, bracing may be useful.

Patients with CCM have an increased risk of MH as do their family members. This must be considered in any patient who is to undergo surgery.[13, 15, 16] MH is present in 1 per 15,000 anesthetic cases and is believed to be inherited in an autosomal dominant manner. Patients with MH may demonstrate a subclinical weakness, CK elevation, and nonspecific muscle biopsy changes.

Nemaline Myopathy

Nemaline myopathy (NM) is a congenital myopathy that is distinguished by small, rodlike particles on muscle biopsy. These are noted on trichrome stain, with major components of the rod including α-actinin and desmin. The gene is located on the long arm of chromosome 1.[16, 17] There is an autosomal dominant pattern of inheritance with reduced penetrance and variable expression.[13]

In NM, hypotonia with diffuse mild weakness of the extremities and facial muscles with frequent dysmorphic appearance is noted. The face may be long and narrow with an abnormal mandible.[16] Facial muscle weakness often results in poor suck and swallow.[13] Clubfeet and kyphoscoliosis are present.[13] A more severe form of NM can arise which involves the respiratory muscles to a greater degree. This may actually cause death in young adulthood from respiratory failure. Cardiomyopathy is also present in severely affected patients.[16] The disease, however, is believed to be slowly progressive in the large majority of patients. The disease severity on presentation indicates the severity of the clinical course.[13]

In most children with NM, the disease is diagnosed before the age of 1 year. Walking occurs late, averaging 19 months, with a waddling gait evident in most children from their first step. There are frequent falls and Gowers' maneuver is pres-

TABLE 48–3   Congenital Myopathies

Types	Genetics	Course	Associated Findings	Biopsy	Electro-diagnostics	Laboratory Studies
Central core myopathy	AD Chromosome 19	Mild Normal life span	Frequent CDH MH	Type I predominance Unstained central areas	Small-amplitude polyphasics	CK normal
Nemaline myopathy	AD Chromosome 1	Slowly progressive	Respiratory muscles abnormal Cardiomyopathy	Small rodlike particles, more peripheral Type I fiber predominance and atrophy	Small-amplitude polyphasics	CK normal to mild increase
Myotubular (centronuclear) myopathy	AR XLR	AR—varies XLR—early death; 80% in first year	AR—seizures, ptosis XLR—severe respiratory disease	Internal nuclei Type I fiber predominance	Small-amplitude polyphasics, CRDs, fibrillations, positive sharp waves, myotonic discharges	CK normal to mild increase
Congenital fiber disproportion	Varied reports of AD, AR, or sporadic	Improves after weakness first 2 yr	Frequent CDH Short height and low weight	Small type I fibers Increased percentage of type I fibers	Small-amplitude polyphasics	CK normal to mild increase

Abbreviations: CDH, congenital dysplasia of hip; *MH,* malignant hyperthermia; *CK,* creatine kinase; *CRDs,* complex repetitive discharges; *AD,* autosomal dominant; *AR,* autosomal recessive; *XLR,* X-linked recessive.

ent. A nasal voice is observed in all children with NM. During preschool, two thirds of the children are susceptible to respiratory infections; some require hospitalizations.

CK is normal to mildly elevated and needle EMG shows a nonspecific myopathic pattern.[15, 16, 68] The muscle biopsy reveals type I fiber predominance (up to 90%) as well as selective type I fiber atrophy and nemaline rods.[13, 15, 16, 68] The rods contain Z-band muscle fiber material and are noted in all involved muscles, including cardiac muscle. They are more prevalent at the periphery of muscle fibers.[13] The rods are not specific to NM and can be seen in unrelated diseases.[13, 15, 68]

Treatment includes appropriate bracing for weakness and limb function, surgery for severe skeletal anomalies, and close follow-up and treatment of cardiomyopathy. Respiratory care must be diligent, particularly during times of pulmonary infection. Therapy for improving strength, ADL, range of motion, and endurance is useful, and work simplification is important. Assistive devices such as AFOs and some hand orthoses may be useful. Wheelchairs are required for some patients. Early therapy for feeding assistance is helpful.[126]

Myotubular (Centronuclear) Myopathy

Myotubular (centronuclear) myopathy (MTM) is a congenital myopathy with two distinct forms. The first form is autosomal recessive and is manifest by delayed motor milestones and hypotonia, with weakness beginning early in life. There is ptosis, ophthalmoplegia, slowly progressive weakness, generalized facial weakness, and equinovarus. Seizures may be present.[13, 16] This form is heterogeneous, with an array of severities noted.[26] Patients survive into adulthood with minimal motor deficits.[68]

The second form of MTM is an X-linked recessive disorder that leads to early respiratory failure. There is severe weakness of the face, poor suck and swallow, and weak neck muscles, but ptosis is not severe.[13, 16] The X-linked form has an 80% fatality rate in the first year[13, 16] and there is an increased incidence of spontaneous abortions and stillbirths.[26] Ventilatory support may decrease the

early deaths. The gene is located on the long arm of the X chromosome.[13, 16]

In both forms of MTM, CK is normal or slightly elevated.[13, 15, 16, 68] Needle EMG may show low-amplitude polyphasic MUPs as well as fibrillations, positive sharp waves, and CRDs. Myotonic discharges may also be present.[3, 68] The muscle biopsy shows increased central nuclei with increased staining of the fiber with oxidative enzymes, and a pale area centrally with adenosine triphosphatase (ATPase) reactions. There is type I fiber predominance.[15, 16, 68] The large plump nucleus in the center of many fibers resembles the fetal myotube stage.[10] An electroencephalogram (EEG) typically shows paroxysmal abnormalities in the patient with the autosomal form.[16]

Treatment is variable, depending on the type of MTM. Antiseizure medication is important for patients with the autosomal recessive form. Ventilatory assistance is important for survival in patients with the X-linked type of MTM. Therapy and bracing may be helpful, depending on the extent of weakness and deficits.

Congenital Fiber Disproportion

In congenital fiber type disproportion (CFTD) no classic structural abnormalities are noted, but there is abnormality in the size of muscle fibers and fiber type predominance. In normal muscles type I fibers make up 30% to 40% of the fibers, with type II constituting 60%; the sizes are comparable. In CFTD, the type I fibers are at least 15% smaller than the type II fibers. Type II fibers are a more uniform size than type I.[13, 15, 68] Recently it has been proposed that the difference should actually be a difference greater than 45% in size between type I and II fibers, along with greater than 75% of the fibers being type I.[16]

Children with CFTD present with floppiness at birth, with weakness most severe in the first 2 years. The weakness subsequently improves or stabilizes. There are delayed motor milestones. Congenital hip dislocation is frequent and other skeletal abnormalities are frequently seen. The patients are short and frequently have low weight as well. Cognitive function is intact.[13, 15, 16, 68] The proximal muscles are more involved than the distal, but weakness is generally mild to moderate. Reflexes may be decreased or absent.[15] Respiratory infections and complications are common in the first 2 years of life.[13, 16] CK is normal or mildly elevated and needle EMG is myopathic.[13, 15, 16]

Treatment emphasizes respiratory care, particularly in the first 2 years of life. Subsequently therapy and bracing are used depending on individual patient status. Range-of-motion and stretching exercises are advised early in the disease course because of the potential to develop contractures.

Over time the children demonstrate a decrease in muscle bulk, an onset of foot deformities, and frequent scoliosis. Patients often require some assistance with ADL, ranging from requiring help with heavy lifting to complete dependence.[126]

METABOLIC MYOPATHIES

There are a variety of myopathies which are secondary to metabolic abnormalities. Ten glycogen storage diseases have been well described, with four demonstrating significant muscle involvement: types II, III, V, and VII[68] (Table 48–4).

The glycogen storage diseases present in one of two ways. One is with progressive muscle weakness, as in acid maltase deficiency and debranching enzyme deficiency. The other presentation is with exertional cramps and myalgias, as in muscle phosphorylase deficiency (McArdle's disease).[89, 94]

Muscle Phosphorylase Deficiency (Type V Glycogenosis, McArdle's Disease)

Muscle phosphorylase deficiency (McArdle's disease) presents in a heterogeneous manner. Muscle phosphorylase normally makes the hexose sugar available from the glycogen chain so it can be used for metabolism and glycolysis. Glycogen is normally used during intensive short-term exercise.[15] Without this enzyme a person cannot use glycogen as an energy source. In McArdle's disease there is exercise intolerance, easy fatigue, and stiffness of the exercised muscles.[15, 68, 89, 99] Patients have symptoms brought on by bursts of exercise, the amount of which will vary between patients and in the same patient over time. There also may be episodes of myoglobinuria and cramping after exercise. This cramping may proceed to the hallmark of full contracture with electrical silence.[15, 89]

McArdle's disease is generally inherited in an autosomal recessive manner, although some persons have an autosomal dominant form. This disease is more frequent in males than females with a ratio of 3:1.[94] There are no other organs primarily involved in McArdle's disease, but renal involvement may occur secondary to myoglobinuria.[15]

Physical findings vary depending on the age of the patient, but are typically normal between episodes. Proximal muscle weakness can develop late in the disease. Reflexes are normal.[15] CK is elevated at rest in more than 90% of patients[89] and needle EMG frequently shows fibrillations and positive waves, as well as polyphasic MUPs. During a contracture episode the needle EMG shows no electrical activity, in contrast to the appearance of ordinary cramped muscle which is very active. Repetitive nerve stimulation at 20 Hz can show a marked decremental response.[68, 89] The ischemic forearm exercise test (forearm muscles are exercised using an inflated cuff around the arm) is also abnormal in these patients. In normal muscles, venous lactate levels increase secondary to glycogen breakdown under ischemic conditions. In McArdle's disease there is no rise because patients cannot catabolize glycogen.[68, 89, 94]

Muscle biopsy typically shows excessive glycogen in vacuoles in the subsarcolemmal region. There is a variability of fiber size with degenerating and regenerating fibers noted.[89, 94] The histochemical reaction for phosphorylase is

TABLE 48–4 Metabolic Myopathies

Types	Enzyme Abnormality	Muscle Presentation	Laboratory Studies	Lactate Response to Ischemic Exercise Test	Associated Findings	Genetics	Treatment
Type V (McArdle's disease)	Phosphorylase	Exertional cramps and myalgias	CK increased	No rise	Myoglobinuria	Generally AR; more males	Use of "second wind" with timing of exercise with rest
Type VII	Phosphofructokinase	Exertional cramps and myalgias	CK increased	No rise	Hemolysis Gout Jaundice Reticulocytosis Nausea and vomiting	AR	High fructose diet Gradual exercise and rest
Type II	Acid maltase	Muscle weakness; three forms—vary	CK increased	Able to utilize glycogen; increase	Three varieties: infantile (Pompe's disease)—fatal in first 2 years due to cardiac respiratory disease	AR	None
Type III	Debranching enzyme deficiency	Muscle weakness	CK increased	No rise	Hepatomegaly Cardiac disease	AR	Small, frequent meals

Abbreviations: CK, creatine kinase; AR, autosomal recessive.

absent except in blood vessel walls and regenerating fibers.[89, 94] A biochemical test for phosphorylase shows no activity or up to 10% of normal activity.[89]

McArdle's disease is usually first noticed late in the first decade when the child complains of fatigue and is unable to keep up with peers. In early adolescence there is typically mild aching of the legs which increases in severity and gradually is incited by less vigorous activity. Later, during the teenage years, painful cramps after exercise are noted which can last for hours. There is myoglobinuria after these episodes and the muscle pain may gradually become more severe. In later years there can be permanent proximal muscle weakness.[15] Approximately 25% of the patients will have an episode of renal failure secondary to myoglobinuria.[89] "Second wind" is used by patients to increase their tolerance of activity. The patients rest immediately when they note muscle fatigue at the beginning of exercise. Taking a brief rest after first noting myalgia or muscle stiffness allows them to resume exercise at a somewhat lower level. This enables them to exercise for a longer period of time at an increased comfort level.[15, 89, 99]

Treatment for patients with McArdle's disease is through use of the second wind phenomenon and careful timing of exercise and rest. A graduated exercise program with aerobic activity is helpful. Some patients can benefit from a high fructose diet.[89]

Phosphofructokinase Deficiency

Phosphofructokinase deficiency glycogenosis (type VII, PFKD) is an autosomal recessive disease with symptoms closely resembling McArdle's disease. The episodic exercise-induced symptoms are similar to McArdle's disease except that they are frequently associated with nausea and vomiting. Permanent weakness generally does not occur.[89, 94] Gout may be a complication of PFKD.[99] There can be episodes of hemolysis and jaundice, with decreased erythrocyte survival time and a peripheral blood reticulocytosis.[89] CK, needle EMG, muscle biopsy, and glycogen accumulation are much like those in McArdle's disease. The diagnosis of PFKD can be made by direct measurement of muscle phosphofructokinase activity.[94] No treatment has been described but the gradual exercise with rest, as in McArdle's disease, can be utilized.

Acid Maltase Deficiency

Acid maltase deficiency (type II glycogenosis, AMD) is an autosomal recessive disease which can occur in three different forms. In the first or infantile form (Pompe's disease) children have severe hypotonia which develops shortly after birth. These children die in the first 2 years from cardiac or respiratory failure. Abnormal glycogen deposition results in an enlarged tongue, heart, and liver.[68, 89, 94] The second or childhood-onset type produces proximal limb and trunk weakness with motor milestone delay. The liver and tongue may be enlarged. There is respiratory muscle involvement and death occurs approximately by age 20.[68, 89, 94] In the third or adult variety of AMD, there is a slow progression of proximal weakness beginning in the 20s or 30s. Bulbar musculature is spared, as are the heart and liver.[68, 89, 94] Respiratory failure is noted in one

third of the adults with the diaphragm selectively involved. Pulmonary hypertension may be present.[85]

In AMD CK is elevated and needle EMG shows increased insertional activity with fibrillations and positive sharp waves, as well as complex repetitive discharges.[68, 94] There are small brief polyphasic MUPs with early recruitment, and myotonic discharges. Electrodiagnostic abnormalities may be more frequent in proximal muscles and lower paraspinal muscles.[68, 89] The ECG is abnormal in the infantile form of AMD with depressed ST segments and inverted T waves, along with a shortened PR interval. Acid maltase activity is deficient in all muscles, even those that are relatively clinically spared.[15] Prenatal diagnosis is available by fetal cell culturing which shows absence of enzyme activity.[15, 89] Muscle biopsy shows abundant vacuoles with high glycogen content, affecting type I more than type II fibers.[68, 89, 94] In AMD, glycogen and glucose are utilized normally by muscles, unlike the other glycogen storage diseases.[89] Treatment with specific diet or medications has not been found to be effective.[89, 94]

Debranching Enzyme Deficiency

Debranching enzyme deficiency (type III glycogenosis, DED) is an autosomal recessive glycogen storage disease. The breakdown of glycogen in these patients can occur only in the outer straight glycosyl chains, so that glycogen with short branched outer chains accumulates in muscle and liver tissues.[68] Infants are hypotonic with proximal weakness noted.[68, 89] Hepatomegaly is present secondary to glycogen accumulation and there can be episodes of hypoglycemia.[68, 94] Symptoms tend to improve around puberty with myopathy appearing in adulthood and progressing as proximal muscle weakness. Some adult patients may have heart disease along with hepatomegaly.[94]

CK is elevated in DED. The forearm ischemic exercise test shows no increase in venous lactate.[89, 94] Despite this finding, there is no severe exercise intolerance or cramping.[89] EMG may show fibrillations, CRDs, and brief small polyphasic MUPs.[68] Biopsy shows subsarcolemmal periodic acid–Schiff–positive vacuoles, particularly in type II fibers.[68, 89, 94] Biochemical muscle assay reveals an absence of the debranching enzyme.[89] Treatment is with small, frequent meals to avoid hypoglycemia. Additionally, cardiac status is carefully monitored since heart disease may be present.[89]

ENDOCRINE MYOPATHIES

Proximal muscle weakness can be seen with abnormalities of thyroid and parathyroid function as well as secondary to endogenous or exogenous steroids (Table 48–5).

Hyperthyroidism

Hyperthyroid or thyrotoxic myopathy is present in a large percentage of patients with thyrotoxicosis. Approximately half of these patients have some muscle atrophy and 80% have muscle weakness.[103] The myopathy is more common in men with thyrotoxicosis than in women.[68] Proximal weakness develops, most frequently about the shoulder.[15, 68, 103] Extraocular muscles may be tethered causing

TABLE 48–5 Endocrine Myopathies

Types	Presentation	Electrodiagnostics	Biopsy	Treatment
Hyperthyroidism	Proximal weakness EOM abnormal Atrophy	Brief, small polyphasics with early recruitment	Abnormal, nonspecific	Treat underlying disease
Hypothyroid myopathy	Proximal weakness Painful muscle spasms	Increased insertional activity Repetitive discharges		Treat underlying disease
Hyperparathyroidism	Proximal muscle weakness Fatigue and aching	Brief, small polyphasics with early recruitment NCSs—decreased CMAP	Signs of denervation and type II atrophy	Treat underlying disease
Hypoparathyroidism	Tetany			Treat underlying disease
Corticosteroid myopathy	Hip weakness; later, shoulder weakness	No spontaneous activity Brief, small polyphasics		Remove steroids

Abbreviations: EOM, extraocular muscle; *NCSs,* nerve conduction studies; *CMAP,* compound muscle action potential.

exophthalmic ophthalmoplegia. Reflexes are normal or hyperactive.[15, 68] CK may be normal, with muscle biopsy demonstrating nonspecific abnormalities.[15] The EMG shows brief, small-amplitude MUPs with early recruitment.[68, 103] Treatment of the thyroid disease cures the muscle disease.[103]

Thyrotoxic patients have been reported to have episodes of periodic paralysis. In exercise tests of 2 to 5 min with serial measurements of compound MUP amplitude, an initial amplitude increase is noted immediately post exercise with a subsequent decrease. When a patient is treated and becomes euthyroid, the above pattern remains but is less dramatic.[57] This test can be helpful for a diagnosis of periodic paralysis between episodes in the absence of intercurrent muscle weakness.[57]

Hypothyroid Myopathy

Hypothyroid myopathy produces proximal muscle weakness, occasionally associated with muscle cramps. Muscle hypertrophy is also seen in some children. There is a slowed relaxation of muscle stretch reflexes.[15, 68] CK may be elevated and needle EMG shows increased insertional activity and repetitive discharges.[15, 68] Treatment is of the thyroid disease with subsequent improvement of muscle symptoms.

Parathyroid Disease

In *hypoparathyroidism,* tetany is a neuromuscular complication secondary to chronic hypocalcemia.[15, 68] *Hyperparathyroidism* can lead to proximal muscle weakness which is more severe in the pelvic girdle than shoulder region. Reflexes are normal to increased.[15, 68] Some patients show extensor plantar responses.[68] There may be fatigue and muscle aching, along with weakness and atrophy. Bulbar findings are also noted.[15] The severity of the disease is not correlated with calcium or phosphate levels.[15] On needle EMG there are brief small-amplitude MUPs and early recruitment, with no spontaneous activity. NCSs may show reduced amplitude of the compound MUP with normal conduction velocities.[68] Muscle biopsy shows changes indicative of denervation with type II atrophy.[15] Treatment is of the underlying hyperparathyroidism.

Corticosteroid Myopathy

Myopathy can be due to corticosteroid, whether exogenous or endogenous. Weakness can occur in Cushing's syndrome as well as with corticosteroid treatment.[94, 103] The weakness generally begins in the hip and proximal lower limb muscles, later affecting the proximal upper limb muscles and in severe cases the distal limb muscles. Weakness gradually begins from a few weeks to several years after the onset of corticosteroid administration. Weakness is frequently, but not always, corticosteroid dose- and time-related. Fluorinated steroids are most commonly linked with myopathy.[94]

Recently, severe myopathies have been reported related to the use of high-dose intravenous corticosteroids in patients with asthma who required mechanical ventilation and neuromuscular blocking agents (pancuronium bromide and vecuronium). The neuromuscular blocking agents appeared to facilitate a steroid myopathy with an increase in severity.[4, 71] The myopathy is reversible but the morbidity is significant.[71]

In steroid myopathy CK is normal.[15] Needle EMG shows no spontaneous activity but may reveal small polyphasic potentials which are recruited early.[103] The myopathy improves with a decrease or discontinuation of the steroid, after some days or weeks.[94]

INFLAMMATORY MYOPATHIES

Polymyositis and Dermatomyositis

Polymyositis (PM) and dermatomyositis (DM) are generally described together as variants of the same disease, but there is evidence that their etiologies are different. Clinically, they are expressed and evaluated in the same manner and so will be discussed together.[15, 68, 94] PM and DM are acquired myopathies each with an acute or subacute course (Table 48–6). Pain and muscle aches are sometimes present but certainly are not diagnostic.[15, 68] DM has a bimodal distribution, being more common in childhood and in the 40s and 50s. It can occur at any age, with an incidence of 5 to 10 cases per million.[70] PM or DM may be associated with neoplasms, vasculitis, or collagen-vascular diseases. Neoplasms are more commonly associated with dermato-

TABLE 48–6 Inflammatory Myopathies

Type	Presentation	Age at Presentation	Laboratory Studies	Electrodiagnostics	Treatment	Associated Findings
Dermatomyositis	Rash Proximal weakness of gradual onset ± Muscle ache	Biomodal	Increased CK, ESR, myoglobin	Fibrillations, positive sharp waves Small-amplitude polyphasics CRDs (especially in paraspinal muscles) 10% normal	Prednisone Ongoing research on other medications ROM exercise	Neoplasms (in adults) Collagen-vascular disease Calcinosis (children) Raynaud's phenomenom
Polymyositis	Proximal weakness of gradual onset ± Muscle ache	Adults	Increased CK, ESR, myoglobin	Fibrillations, positive sharp waves Small-amplitude polyphasics CRDs (especially in paraspinal muscles) 10% normal	Prednisone Ongoing research on other medications ROM exercise	Neoplasms (in adults) Collagen-vascular disease Raynaud's phenomenom
Sarcoidosis	Generally asymptomatic Chronic proximal weakness Palpable nodules	Postmenopausal women most commonly affected		Small-amplitude polyphasics	Steroids ACTH	

Abbreviations: CK, creatine kinase; *ESR,* erythrocyte sedimentation role; *CRDs,* complex repetitive discharges; *ROM,* range of motion; *ACTH,* adrenocorticotropic hormone.

myositis, except in children. Childhood dermatomyositis is more frequently associated with collagen-vascular disease.[15, 68, 94] DM is distinguished from PM by the rash that is present either prior to, during, or subsequent to the muscle weakness. Characteristically, there is a violet rash over the upper and lower eyelids and cheeks with periorbital edema. An erythematous rash may also be present in any exposed part of the body[68, 94] (Fig. 48–8). Calcinosis may occur, particularly in children. It has been described in 50% to 75% of children with DM. Calcinosis tends to resolve spontaneously in some patients but can be a chronic problem in others[3, 97] (Fig. 48–9).

Associated findings may include vasculitis, especially in children, which can affect the gastrointestinal tract and myocardium. Myocarditis can present a serious risk during the acute phase.[3] Initial symptoms generally are nonspecific systemic complaints of malaise, fever, anorexia, and weight loss.[68] Raynaud's phenomenon is present in approximately 20% of patients. Dysphagia is common and may necessitate tube feeding. Neoplasms involving the breast, lung, ovary, or stomach are the classic disease associated with the adult form of PM or DM. A neoplasm is found in 10% to 20%

of PM and DM patients. Other collagen-vascular diseases are frequently present.[15]

Physical examination shows proximal weakness involving first the hips, then the shoulders, and also the anterior neck muscles.[68] As the disease progresses it involves the distal limb muscles. In children the rash is almost invariably seen.

Reflexes are normal until late in the course of the disease. Mild muscle atrophy may be noted. There is generally minimal tenderness to muscle palpation, and if present, it is most frequently about the shoulder region.[68]

CK is elevated in 90% of patients. Myoglobin and erythrocyte sedimentation rate may also be increased. The needle EMG shows a triad of fibrillations and positive sharp waves, CRDs, and small, brief-duration polyphasic MUPs with early recruitment. Ten percent of patients have a normal study.[68] Muscles with moderate weakness, especially the paraspinal muscles, show needle EMG abnormalities. There is no correlation between the severity of the PM or DM and the needle EMG findings. A correlation is noted of changes over a clinical course with the amount of spontaneous activity found in DM or PM, so that serial

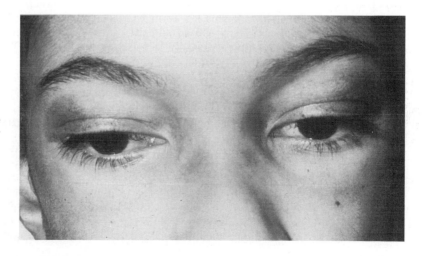

FIGURE 48–8 A teenaged girl with chronic dermatomyositis demonstrating the classic rash over the eyelids.

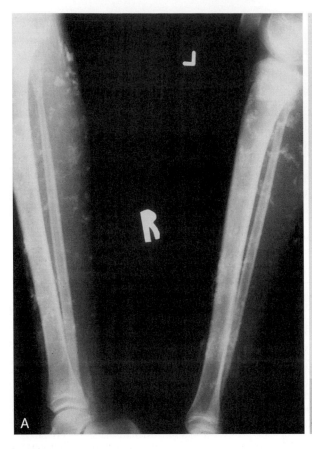

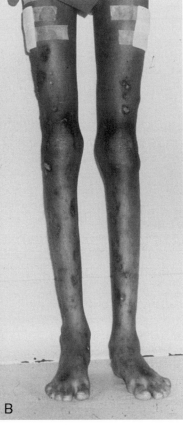

FIGURE 48–9 The same subject shown in Fig 46–8. *A*, X-ray of calcifications in the lower limbs. *B*, Severe calcifications extrude through skin.

EMGs may be useful in following the course of disease and the treatment response.[68] Muscle biopsy shows necrosis, phagocytosis, inflammatory cells, and degeneration, along with regeneration.[68, 94] Abnormalities of swallowing in the distal esophagus can also be detected on cineradiography.[15]

The clinical course is variable and more severe in DM than in PM.[94] Unfavorable prognostic factors include an underlying malignancy, previous diagnosis of collagen-vascular disease, advanced age, and a delay in corticosteroid treatment. Conversely, the severity of weakness at the beginning of the disease, level of CK, and muscle biopsy findings do not correlate with outcome.[94] Some patients have a complete recovery after one episode, whereas others may have a remitting and relapsing course with some weakness between severe episodes. A third type is a chronic form of DM or PM. In this last form pulmonary function may ultimately be compromised and the patient may die from respiratory failure. Mortality is believed to be approximately 15% to 30% in chronic DM and PM.[15]

Improved treatment of DM and PM is currently an area of active research. The one area regarding treatment that is agreed upon is that steroids must be instituted as early as possible for maximal effectiveness. Corticosteroids are the first line of treatment, most commonly oral prednisone. Prednisone is generally begun at 60 to 80 mg/day or 1 to 2 mg/kg/day in children.[15, 94] If steroids are ineffective, other immunosuppressants are generally used, such as methotrexate, cyclophosphamide, azathioprine, and chlorambucil. Cyclosporine has been shown to be effective in some patients resistant to steroid treatment.[45, 77, 82] Cyclosporine use decreases the amount of steroid needed in children who chronically use steroids.[45] Methotrexate is useful in combination with prednisone in some patients who are resistant to treatment with prednisone alone, but complications can be severe and recurrence has been noted after discontinuation of an apparently successful treatment with the medication.[88] Chlorambucil is effective in some patients resistant to prednisone with leukopenia occasionally noted.[110] High-dose immunoglobulin monthly for 3 months can increase muscle strength and decrease neuromuscular symptoms.[25] Plasma exchange and leukopheresis are not effective.[86] Low-dose total body irradiation (150 rad) has been used in cases not responding to medications.[15, 94] Cataracts have been shown to occur as a side effect in approximately 30% of patients who use steroids for longer than 12 months.[15]

A critical element of treatment in DM or PM is range-of-motion and stretching exercises early in the course of disease. This regimen will help prevent contractures when muscles are at their weakest. When patients are better clinically, monitored resistive exercises improve muscle strength without elevations in CK.[36]

Sarcoidosis

Sarcoidosis is a multisystem granulomatous disorder that commonly involves pulmonary, skin, and eye tissues. Hilar lymphadenopathy is present in many cases.[127] Muscle involvement in sarcoidosis is present in at least 50% to 80% of patients, but is most frequently asymptomatic.[15, 29, 127] Symptomatic muscle presentation is often one of chronic, slowly progressive proximal weakness, along with atrophy. There may also be acute myositis with myalgias and weakness. Palpable nodules in muscle are less common.[15, 29] Diaphragm muscle weakness has been reported in a few patients.[29] Postmenopausal women are more commonly affected.[15, 127] CK is generally normal to mildly elevated and needle EMG shows myopathic changes.[127] Muscle biopsy shows noncaseating granulomas. There is generally bilateral hilar lymphadenopathy on chest radiography and a skin reaction to the Kveim-Siltzbach antigen also may be helpful in diagnosing sarcoidosis.[15] Treatment with steroids or adrenocorticotropic hormone (ACTH) is generally effective.[15, 30, 127]

INFECTIOUS MYOPATHIES

Documented parasitic infections of the muscle are uncommon outside of tropical areas.[68] Subclinical infection may be more common, however. *Trichinella* larvae may get into human muscle after infected pork is eaten. Fever may be present with muscle pain and stiffness, along with periorbital edema. The masseter muscle is commonly involved, causing painful chewing. Skin rash and retinal hemorrhages may be present.[15] *Trichinella* preferentially invades the extraocular muscles.[68] Muscle biopsy shows a parasite and frequently a hypersensitivity reaction. Treatment is with prednisone and thiabendazole.[15] *Cysticercosis* may also cause muscle aches and pains with palpable nodules. Rarely, it may cause a pseudohypertrophic change in muscle.[15]

Viral infections of muscles may be very common. It is probable that the muscular discomfort that often accompanies influenza may actually be a viral inflammation of the muscle. In influenza B virus infections acute calf muscle pain is often present. Echovirus, influenza A virus, herpesvirus, coxsackievirus, and adenovirus 21 have all been associated with muscle pain. Muscle biopsies show necrosis, or if less severe, vacuolar degeneration.[15]

The *human immunodeficiency virus (HIV)*, along with its treatment, may cause muscle disease[72, 103] (see Chapter 60). There are two separate myopathies noted in the HIV-positive population. One type is in patients who are HIV-positive and the other is in patients taking zidovudine (AZT). The patients with AZT myopathy have early prominent proximal weakness and myalgia. They fulfill the criteria for *acquired immunodeficiency syndrome (AIDS)* and have generally taken AZT for more than 9 months. Muscle biopsy shows ragged red fibers. Mitochondrial dysfunction is suggested as a cause of this weakness. Withdrawal of AZT results in reversal of the myopathy but reducing the AZT does not. Improvement in muscle status and CK is generally noted several months after AZT is stopped. Full muscle recovery may not occur. Restarting AZT at a lower dose after recovery may prevent recurrence.[72] CK is generally markedly elevated.[72, 103]

The other form of myopathy is noted in HIV patients who are not taking AZT. This group does not generally fulfill the criteria of AIDS and this type of inflammatory myopathy occurs early in the infection. There is a relatively painless, severe proximal weakness with elevated CK. Biopsy shows inflammation and nemaline rod bodies.[72, 103] The weakness is generally improved with use of steroids or plasmapheresis.[72] In both of these disorders needle EMG shows spontaneous activity and short-duration MUPs.[72, 103]

TOXIC MYOPATHY

The most common toxic myopathy is *alcoholic myopathy*. There is an acute type and a chronic type. Acute alcoholic myopathy occurs after an episode of excessive drinking with an acute attack of muscle pain, weakness, and muscle swelling. This is generally most common in the thigh muscles but can be present in any large muscle group. Muscles are tender to palpation. There may be myoglobinuria and subsequent renal failure. It may resolve completely or residual weakness may be present. In chronic alcoholic myopathy there is generally leg weakness with the shoulders involved somewhat less frequently.[15] Vincristine and chloroquine have also been implicated in toxic myopathies.[15] Treatment for toxic myopathies is removal of the toxin. Improvement may be partial or complete.

CONCLUSION

The myopathies are a broad group of muscle disorders, most of which share proximal muscle weakness as the primary problem. The myopathies include the dystrophies, congenital myopathies, and myopathies due to metabolic, endocrine, and inflammation and toxic causes. The causes are diverse and the extent of muscle disease varies, as do the muscle groups involved. These differences, along with associated findings in other body systems, as well as laboratory studies, electrodiagnosis, and biopsy help to make each diagnosis. Treatment for most is supportive, not curative, and therefore rehabilitation intervention plays a critical role in determining the patients' ability to function and their level of comfort. Orthoses, physical and occupational therapy interventions, and ventilatory assistance are vital in many of these areas. Surgical intervention can additionally be helpful in many diseases. The majority of research in myopathies has been on DMD. The evaluation and treatment approach to DMD is a basis for that of all other myopathies. The maximal rehabilitative intervention is made in patients with the severe effects of DMD. Patients with less severe myopathies require a variety of these interventions.

References

1. Aitkens SG, McCrory MA, Kilmer DD, et al: Moderate resistance exercise program: Its effect in slowly progressive neuromuscular disease. Arch Phys Med Rehabil 1993; 74:711–714.
2. Angelini C, Pegoraro E, Turella E, et al: Deflazacort in Duchenne dystrophy: Study of long-term effect. Muscle Nerve 1994; 17:386–391.
3. Ansell BM: Juvenile dermatomyositis. J Rheumatol 1992; 33(suppl):60–62.
4. Apte-Kakade S: Rehabilitation of patients with quadriparesis after treatment of status asthmaticus with neuromuscular blocking agents and high-dose corticosteroids. Arch Phys Med Rehabil 1991; 72:1024–1028.
5. Bach JR: Ventilator use by Muscular Dystrophy Association patients. Arch Phys Med Rehabil 1992; 73:179–183.
6. Bach JR: Ventilatory support alternatives to tracheostomy and intu-

bation: Current status of the application of this technology. Conn Med 1991; 55:323–329.

7. Bach JR, Campagnolo DI, Hoeman S: Life satisfaction of individuals with Duchenne muscular dystrophy using long-term mechanical ventilatory support. Am J Phys Med Rehabil 1991; 70:129–135.

8. Bach JR, McKeon J: Orthopedic surgery and rehabilitation for the prolongation of brace-free ambulation of patients with Duchenne muscular dystrophy. Am J Phys Med Rehabil 1991; 70:323–331.

9. Bach JR, O'Brien J, Krotenberg R, et al: Management of end stage respiratory failure in Duchenne muscular dystrophy. Muscle Nerve 1987; 10:177–182.

10. Bach JR, Zeelenberg A, Winter C: Wheelchair-mounted robot manipulators: Long term use by patients with Duchenne muscular dystrophy. Am J Phys Med Rehabil 1990; 69:59–69.

11. Bennett RL, Knowlton GC: Overwork weakness in partially denervated skeletal muscle. Clin Orthop 1958; 12:22–29.

12. Bertorini TE, Palmieri GM, Griffin J, et al: Chronic allopurinol and adenine therapy in Duchenne muscular dystrophy: Effects on muscle function, nucleotide degradation, and muscle ATP and ADP content. Neurology 1985; 35:61–65.

13. Bodensteiner JB: Congenital myopathies. Muscle Nerve 1994; 17:131–144.

14. Braddom R: Written communication, 1994.

15. Brooke MH: A Clinician's View of Neuromuscular Diseases, ed 2. Baltimore, Williams & Wilkins, 1986, pp 117–154.

16. Brooke MH: Congenital muscular disorders. In 1992 AAEM Course C: Update of Myopathies. American Association of Electrodiagnostic Medicine, 15th Annual Continuing Education Course, Charleston, SC, Oct 15, 1992.

17. Brooke MH, Fenichel GM, Griggs RC, et al: Clinical investigation of Duchenne muscular dystrophy. Interesting results in a trial of prednisolone. Arch Neurol 1987; 44:812–817.

18. Brooke MH, Fenichel GM, Griggs RC, et al: Duchenne muscular dystrophy: Patterns of clinical progression and effects of supportive therapy. Neurology 1989; 39:475–481.

19. Brust M: Relative resistance to dystrophy of slow skeletal muscle of the mouse. Am J Physiol 1966; 210:445.

20. Bunch WH, Siegel IM: Scapulothoracic arthrodesis in facioscapulohumeral muscular dystrophy. J Bone Joint Surg Am 1993; 75A:372–376.

21. Carpenter S, Karpati G: Duchenne muscular dystrophy: Plasma membrane loss initiates muscle cell necrosis unless it is repaired. Brain 1979; 102:147–161.

22. Carpenter S, Karpati G, Zubryzycka-Gaarn EE, et al: Dystrophin is localized at the plasma membrane of human skeletal muscle fibers by electron microscopic cytochemical study. Muscle Nerve 1990; 13:376–380.

23. Colbert AP, Schock NC: Respirator use in progressive neuromuscular disease. Arch Phys Med Rehabil 1985; 66:760–762.

24. Curran JF, Colbert AP: Ventilator management in Duchenne muscular dystrophy and postpoliomyelitis syndrome: Twelve years' experience. Arch Phys Med Rehabil 1989; 70:180–185.

25. Dalakas MC, Illa I, Dambrosia JM, et al: A controlled trial of high-dose intravenous immune globulin infusions as treatment for dermatomyositis. N Engl J Med 1993; 329:1993–2000.

26. De Angelis MS, Palmucci L, Leone M, et al: Centronuclear myopathy: Clinical, morphological and genetic characters. J Neurol Sci 1991; 103:2–9.

27. DeLateur BJ, Giaconi RM: Effect on maximal strength of submaximal exercise in Duchenne muscular dystrophy. Am J Phys Med Rehabil 1979; 58:26–36.

28. De Silva S, Drachman DB, Mellits D, et al: Prednisolone treatment in Duchenne muscular dystrophy. Arch Neurol 1987; 44:818–822.

29. Dewberry RG, Schneider BF, Cale WF, et al: Sarcoid myopathy presenting with diaphragm weakness. Muscle Nerve 1993; 16:832–835.

30. Deymeer F, Oge AE, Bayindir C, et al: Emery-Dreifuss muscular dystrophy with unusual features. Muscle Nerve 1993; 16:1359–1365.

31. Dubowitz V: Some clinical observations on childhood muscular dystrophy. Br J Clin Pract 1963; 17:283.

32. Edwards RHT: Management of muscular dystrophy in adults. Br Med Bull 1989; 45:802–818.

33. Emery AEH: Emery-Dreifuss muscular dystrophy and other related disorders. Br Med Bull 1989; 45:772–787.

34. Emery AEH, Skinner R: Clinical studies in benign (Becker type) X-linked muscular dystrophy. Clin Genet 1976; 10:189.

35. Eng GD, Binder H: Rehabilitation of infants and children with neuromuscular disorders. Pediatr Ann 1988; 17:745–755.

36. Escalante A, Miller L, Beardmore TD: Resistive exercise in the rehabilitation of polymyositis/dermatomyositis. J Rheumatol 1993; 20:1340–1344.

37. Florence JM, Pandya S, King WM, et al: Clinical trials in Duchenne dystrophy: Standardization and reliability of evaluation procedures. Phys Ther 1984; 64:41–45.

38. Fowler WM Jr: Rehabilitation management of muscular dystrophy and related disorders: II. Comprehensive care. Arch Phys Med Rehabil 1982; 63:322–328.

39. Fukunaga H, Okubo R, Moritoyo T, et al: Long-term follow-up of patients with Duchenne muscular dystrophy receiving ventilatory support. Muscle Nerve 1993; 16:554–558.

40. Gardner-Medwin D: Clinical features and classification of the muscular dystrophies. Br Med Bull 1980; 36:109–115.

41. Gibson DA, Roy L: Pseudohypertrophic muscular dystrophy and its surgical management: Review of 30 patients. Can J Surg 1970; 13:13–20.

42. Grimm T, Janka M: Emery-Dreifuss muscular dystrophy. In Engel AG, Franzini-Armstrong C (eds): Myology: Basic and Clinical, ed 2. New York, McGraw-Hill, 1994.

43. Gronert GA, Fowler W, Cardinet GH, et al: Absence of malignant hyperthermia contractures in Becker-Duchenne dystrophy at age 2. Muscle Nerve 1992; 15:52–56.

44. Gussoni E, Pavlath GK, Lanctot AM, et al: Normal dystrophin transcripts detected in Duchenne muscular dystrophy patients after myoblast transplantation. Nature 1992; 356:435–438.

45. Hamill G, Saunders C, Heckmatt J, et al: "Catch-up" growth in steroid dependent dermatomyositis treated with cyclosporin-A. Eur J Med 1992; 1:16–18.

46. Harris SE, Cherry DB: Childhood progressive muscular dystrophy and the role of physical therapy. Phys Ther 1974; 54:4–12.

47. Heckmatt JZ, Hyde SA, Gabain A, et al: Therapeutic trial of isaxonine in Duchenne muscular dystrophy. Muscle Nerve 1988; 11:836–847.

48. Heckmatt J, Rodillo E, Dubowitz: Management of children: Pharmacological and physical. Br Med Bull 1989; 45:788–801.

49. Hiller LB, Wade CK: Upper extremity functional assessment scales in children with Duchenne muscular dystrophy: A comparison. Arch Phys Med Rehabil 1992; 73:527–534.

50. Hinge HF, Hein-Sorensen O, Reske-Nielsen E: X-linked Duchenne muscular dystrophy: Motor functions and prognosis. Scand J Rehabil Med 1989; 21:27–31.

51. Hoberman M: Physical medicine and rehabilitation: Its value and limitations in progressive muscular dystrophy. Am J Phys Med Rehabil 1955; 34:109–115.

52. Huard J, Bouchard JP, Roy R, et al: Human myoblast transplantation: Preliminary results of 4 cases. Muscle Nerve 1992; 15:550–560.

53. Huard J, Roy R, Bouchard JP, et al: Human myoblast transplantations between immunohistocompatible donors and recipients produce immune reactions. Transplant Proc 1992; 24:3049–3051.

54. Huard J, Roy R, Guerette B, et al: Human myoblast transplantation in immunodeficient and immunosuppressed mice: Evidence of rejection. Muscle Nerve 1994; 17:224–234.

55. Hudlicka O, Tyler KR: The effect of long-term high frequency stimulation on capillary density and fibre types in rabbit fast muscles. J Physiol 1984; 353:435–445.

56. Hunter JR, Galloway JR, Brooke MH, et al: Effects of allopurinol in Duchenne muscular dystrophy. Arch Neurol 1983; 40:1294–1299.

57. Jackson CE, Barohn RJ: Improvement of the exercise test after therapy in thyrotoxic periodic paralysis. Muscle Nerve 1992; 15:1069–1971.

58. Jaffe KM, McDonald CM, Ingman E, et al: Symptoms of upper gastrointestinal dysfunction in Duchenne muscular dystrophy: Case-control study. Arch Phys Med Rehabil 1990; 71:742–744.

59. James WV, Orr JF: Upper limb weakness in children with Duchenne muscular dystrophy—a neglected problem. Prosthet Orthot Int 1984; 8:11–13.

60. Jebsen RH, Taylor N, Trieschmann RB, et al: An objective and standardized test of hand function. Arch Phys Med Rehabil 1969; 50:311–319.

61. Johnson ER, Fowler WM, Lieberman JS: Contractures in neuromuscular disease. Arch Phys Med Rehabil 1992; 73:807–810.

62. Johnson EW, Braddom R: Over-work weakness in facioscapulohumeral muscular dystrophy. Arch Phys Med Rehabil 1971; 52:333–336.

63. Johnson EW, Kennedy JH: Comprehensive management of Duchenne muscular dystrophy. Arch Phys Med Rehabil 1971; 52:110–114.

64. Karpati G: Update in Duchenne/Becker dystrophy. *In* 1992 AAEM Course C: Update on Myopathies. American Association of Electrodiagnostic Medicine, 15th Annual Continuing Education Course, Charleston, SC, Oct 15, 1992.

65. Karpati G, Acsadi G: The potential for gene therapy in Duchenne muscular dystrophy and other genetic muscle diseases. Muscle Nerve 1993; 16:1141–1153.

66. Khodadadeh S, McClelland MR, Nene AV, et al: The use of double support time for monitoring the gait of muscular dystrophy patients. Clin Biomech 1987; 2:68–70.

67. Kilmer DD, Abresch RT, Fowler WM: Serial manual muscle testing in Duchenne muscular dystrophy. Arch Phys Med Rehabil 1993; 74:1168–1171.

68. Kimura J: Myopathies. *In* Kimura J (ed): Electrodiagnosis in Diseases of Nerve and Muscle: Principles and Practice, (ed 2). Philadelphia, FA Davis, 1988.

69. Kottke FJ: The effects of limitation of activity upon the human body. JAMA 1966;196:117–122.

70. Kunkel LM, Hoffman EP: Duchenne/Becker muscular dystrophy: A short overview of the gene, the protein, and current diagnostics. Br Med Bull 1989; 45:630–643.

71. Lacomis D, Smith TW, Chad DA: Acute myopathy and neuropathy in status asthmaticus: Case report and literature review. Muscle Nerve 1993; 16:84–90.

72. Lange DJ: Neuromuscular diseases associated with HIV-1 infection. Muscle Nerve 1994; 17:16–30.

73. Litchy WJ: Electromyography and clinical neurophysiology: A high intensity review. 16th Annual Course, Chicago, Rehabilitation Institute, March 1–4, 1993.

74. Liu M, Chino N, Ishihara T: Muscle damage progression in Duchenne muscular dystrophy evaluated by a new quantitative computed tomography method. Arch Phys Med Rehabil 1993; 74:507–514.

75. Lord J, Behrman B, Varzos N, et al: Scoliosis associated with Duchenne muscular dystrophy. Arch Phys Med Rehabil 1990; 71:13–17.

76. Lord JP, Portwood MM, Lieberman JS, et al: Upper extremity functional rating for patients with Duchenne muscular dystrophy. Arch Phys Med Rehabil 1987; 68:151–154.

77. Lueck CJ, Trend P, Swash M: Cyclosporin in the management of polymyositis and dermatomyositis. J Neurol Neurosurg Psychiatry 1991; 54:1007–1008.

78. Martin AM, Stern L, Yeates J, et al: Respiratory muscle training in Duchenne muscular dystrophy. Dev Med Child Neurol 1986; 28:314–318.

79. Martinez AC, Terradas JML: Conduction velocity along muscle fibers in situ in Duchenne muscular dystrophy. Arch Phys Med Rehabil 1990; 71:558–561.

80. Matsumura K, Campbell KP: Dystrophin-glycoprotein complex: Its role in the molecular pathogenesis of muscular dystrophies. Muscle Nerve 1994; 17:2–15.

81. McCartney N, Moroz D, Garner SH, et al: The effects of strength training in patients with selected neuromuscular disorders. Med Sci Sport Exerc 1988; 20:362–368.

82. Mehregan DR, Su WP: Cyclosporin treatment for dermatomyositis/polymyositis. Cutis 1993; 51:59–61.

83. Mendell JR, Griggs RC, Moxley RT, et al: Clinical investigation of Duchenne muscular dystrophy: 4. Double blind controlled trial of leucine. Muscle Nerve 1984; 7:535–541.

84. Merlini L, Granata C, Dominici P, et al: Emery-Dreifuss muscular dystrophy: Report of five cases in a family and review of the literature. Muscle Nerve 1986; 9:481–485.

85. Miller F, Moseley CF, Koreska J: Spinal fusion in Duchenne muscular dystrophy. Dev Med Child Neurol 1992; 34:775–786.

86. Miller FW, Leitman SF, Cronin ME, et al: Controlled trial of plasma exchange and leukapheresis in polymyositis and dermatomyositis. N Engl J Med 1992; 326:1380–1384.

87. Miller JR, Colbert AP, Osberg JS: Ventilator dependency: Decision-making, daily functioning and quality of life for patients with Duchenne muscular dystrophy. Dev Med Child Neurol 1990; 32:1078–1086.

88. Miller LC, Sisson BA, Tucker LB, et al: Methotrexate treatment

89. Miller RG: Metabolic myopathies. *In* 1992 AAEM Course C: Update on Myopathies. American Association of Electrodiagnostic Medicine, 15th Annual Continuing Education Course, Charleston, SC, Oct 15, 1992.

90. Milner-Brown HS, Miller RG: Muscle strengthening through electrical stimulation combined with low-resistance weights in patients with neuromuscular disorders. Arch Phys Med Rehabil 1988; 69:20–24.

91. Milner-Brown HS, Miller RG: Muscle strengthening through high-resistance weight training in patients with neuromuscular disorders. Arch Phys Med Rehabil 1988; 69:14–19.

92. Mizuno Y, Yoshida M, Nonaka I, et al: Expression of utrophin (dystrophin-related protein) and dystrophin-associated glycoproteins in muscles from patients with Duchenne muscular dystrophy. Muscle Nerve 1994; 17:206–216.

93. Moxley RT, Brooke MH, Fenichel GM, et al: Clinical investigation in Duchenne dystrophy. VI. Double-blind controlled trial of nifedipine. Muscle Nerve 1987; 10:22–33.

94. Munsat TL: Review of neuromuscular diseases. Phys Med Rehabil 1988; 2:467–480.

95. Ohlendieck K, Ervasti JM, Snook JB, et al: Dystrophin-glycoprotein complex is highly enriched in isolated skeletal muscle sarcolemma. J Cell Biol 1991; 112:135–148.

96. Ohlendieck K, Matsummara K, Ionasescu VV, et al: Duchenne muscular dystrophy: Deficiency of dystrophin-associated proteins in the sarcolemma. Neurology 1993; 43:795–800.

97. Ostrov VE, Goldsmith DP, Eichenfield AH, et al: Hypercalcemia during the resolution of calcinosis universalis in juvenile dermatomyositis. J Rheumatol 1991; 18:1730–1734.

98. Patten BM, Zeller RS: Clinical trials of vasoactive and anti serotonin drugs in Duchenne muscular dystrophy. Ann Clin Res 1983; 15:164–165

99. Puig JG, DeMiguel E, Mateos FA, et al: McArdle's disease and gout. Muscle Nerve 1992; 15:822–828.

100. Rideau Y, Gatin G, Bach J, et al: Prolongation of life in Duchenne muscular dystrophy. Acta Neurol 1983; 5:118–124.

101. Rochester DF, Braun NMT, Laine S: Diaphragmatic energy expenditure in chronic respiratory failure: Effect of assisted ventilation with body respirators. Am J Med 1977; 63:223–232.

102. Salmons S, Vrbova G: The influence of activity on some contractile characteristics of mammalian fast and slow muscle. J Physiol 1969; 201:535–549.

103. Sanders DB: Electromyographic evaluation of myopathies. *In* 1992 AAEM Course C: Update of Myopathies. American Association of Electrodiagnostic Medicine, 15th Annual Continuing Education Course, Charleston, SC, Oct 15, 1992.

104. Scott OM, Hyde SA, Goddard C, et al: Effect of exercise in Duchenne muscular dystrophy. Physiotherapy 1981; 67:174–176.

105. Scott OM, Hyde SA, Goddard C, et al: Prevention of deformity in Duchenne muscular dystrophy: A prospective study of passive stretching and splintage. Physiotherapy 1981; 6:177–180.

106. Scott OM, Hyde SA, Goddard C, et al: Quantitation of muscle function in children: A prospective study in Duchenne muscular dystrophy. Muscle Nerve 1982; 5:291–301.

107. Shapiro F, Sethna N, Colan S, et al: Spinal fusion in Duchenne muscular dystrophy: A multidisciplinary approach. Muscle Nerve 1992; 15:604–614.

108. Shaw DJ, Harper PS: Myotonic dystrophy: Developments in molecular genetics. Br Med Bull 1989; 45:745–759.

109. Seigel IM, Miller JE, Ray RD: Subcutaneous lower limb tenotomy in the treatment of pseudohypertrophic muscular dystrophy. J Bone Joint Surg Am 1968; 50:1437–1443.

110. Sinoway PA, Callen JP: Chlorambucil. An effective corticosteroid-sparing agent for patients with recalcitrant dermatomyositis. Arthritis Rheum 1993; 36:319–324.

111. Smith AD, Koreska J, Moseley CF: Progression of scoliosis in Duchenne muscular dystrophy. J Bone Joint Surg Am 1989; 71:1066–1074.

112. Smith PEM, Coakley JH, Edwards RHT: Respiratory muscle training in Duchenne muscular dystrophy. Muscle Nerve 1988;70:784–785.

113. Spencer GE Jr, Vignos PJ Jr: Bracing for ambulation in childhood progressive muscular dystrophy. J Bone Joint Surg Am 1962; 44:234–242.

of recalcitrant childhood dermatomyositis. Arthritis Rheum 1992; 35:1143–1149.

114. Splaingard ML, Frates RC, Jefferson LS, et al: Home negative pressure ventilation report of 20 years of experience in patients with neuromuscular disease. Arch Phys Med Rehabil 1985; 66:239–242.

115. Stallard J, Henshaw JH, Lomas B, et al: The ORLAU VCG (variable centre of gravity) swivel walker for muscular dystrophy patients. Prosthet Orthot Int 1992; 16:46–48.

116. Stern LM, Martin AJ, Jones N, et al: Respiratory training in Duchenne dystrophy. Dev Med Child Neurol 1991; 33:648–649.

117. Sutherland DH, Olshen R, Cooper L, et al: The pathomechanics of gait in Duchenne muscular dystrophy. Dev Med Child Neurol 1981; 23:3–22.

118. Taylor RG, Abresch RT, Lieberman JS, et al: In vivo quantification of muscle contractility in humans: Healthy subjects and patients with myotonic muscular dystrophy. Arch Phys Med Rehabil 1992; 73:233–236.

119. Vignos PJ: Physical models of rehabilitation in neuromuscular disease. Muscle Nerve 1983; 6:323–338.

120. Vignos PJ, Archibald KC: Maintenance of ambulation in childhood muscular dystrophy. J Chron Dis 1960; 112:273–290.

121. Vignos PJ, Watkins MP: The effect of exercise in muscular dystrophy. JAMA 1976; 197:843–848.

122. Vignos PJ Jr, Spencer GE Jr, Archibald KC: Management of progressive muscular dystrophy. JAMA 1963; 184:89–110.

123. Visser M, Voogt WG, Riviere GV: The heart in Becker muscular dystrophy, facioscapulohumeral dystrophy, and bethlem myopathy. Muscle Nerve 1992; 15:591–596.

124. Wagner MB, Vignos PJ Jr, Carlozzi C, et al: Assessment of hand function in Duchenne muscular dystrophy. Arch Phys Med Rehabil 1993; 74:801–804.

125. Wagner MB, Vignos PJ Jr, Carlozzi C: Duchenne muscular dystrophy: A study of wrist and hand function. Muscle Nerve 1989; 12:236–244.

126. Wallgren-Pattersson C: Congenital nemaline myopathy: A clinical follow-up of twelve patients. J Neurol Sci 1989; 89:1–14.

127. Wolfe SM, Pinals RS, Aelion JA, et al: Myopathy in sarcoidosis: Clinical and pathologic study of four cases and review of the literature. Semin Arthritis Rheum 1987; 16:300–306.

128. Yang J, Seelig M, Rayner S, et al: Increasing the proliferative capacity of muscular dystrophy myoblasts. Muscle Nerve 1992; 15:941–948.

129. Yoshida K, Ikeda S, Nakamura A, et al: Molecular analysis of the Duchenne muscular dystrophy gene in patients with Becker muscular dystrophy presenting with dilated cardiomyopathy. Muscle Nerve 1993; 16:1161–1166.

130. Zupan A: Long-term electrical stimulation of muscles in children with Duchenne and Becker muscular dystrophy. Muscle Nerve 1992; 15:362–367.

Principles of Brain Injury Rehabilitation

CATHERINE F. BONTKE, M.D., AND CORWIN BOAKE, Ph.D.

Several events during the past 20 years have focused greater interest on the subspecialty of brain injury rehabilitation. Most important, improvements in neurotrauma care have increased the rate of survival from traumatic brain injury (TBI).[135] Research studies have documented a high prevalence of brain-injured survivors who have long-term disabilities that place emotional and financial burdens on their family members.[36] Public education by national advocacy organizations, notably the National Head Injury Foundation in the United States and Headway in the United Kingdom, has increased public recognition of the needs of TBI survivors. Finally, there is increasing recognition of the costs imposed by TBI upon society, which were estimated at approximately \$38 billion in the United States during 1985.[121, 164] The problem of brain injury is now a focus of attention in common to many different fields and interest groups, ranging from neuroscience to injury prevention. More detailed information about brain injury rehabilitation and about TBI in general can be found in books and monographs devoted to these topics.*

This chapter summarizes the state of the art of brain injury rehabilitation from the viewpoint of the physiatrist, who is generally responsible for the management of brain-injured patients after their discharge from acute care. The chapter emphasizes the physiatrist's role in assessing and treating medical complications of brain-injured patients, in particular during inpatient rehabilitation. Outpatient rehabilitation and the roles of other rehabilitation professionals are discussed in other chapters in this book.

Although parts of this chapter specifically discuss the rehabilitation of patients with TBIs, most of this chapter applies to both traumatic and nontraumatic brain injuries. As in many other rehabilitation subspecialties (e.g., amputation, spinal cord injury), it is customary for patients with traumatic and nontraumatic etiologies to be treated in the same rehabilitation programs. Nontraumatic brain injuries that are commonly treated together with TBI include anoxic brain injury and certain types of strokes and brain tumors. In this chapter, the term *brain injury* is used when the discussion applies to all these patient groups in general, and the term *traumatic brain injury* (*TBI*) is used when the discussion applies specifically to the TBI group.

DEFINITION AND SUBTYPES OF BRAIN INJURY

The term *traumatic brain injury* (*TBI*) is increasingly endorsed as a general term for all injuries to the brain caused by trauma.[137] This term is preferred because it clearly denotes that injury to the brain is the major cause of morbidity and mortality, and that the injury is caused by external force. A number of other terms are also used to refer to traumatic injuries to the brain. The less commonly used term *craniocerebral trauma* is equivalent in meaning to TBI. The general terms *head injury* and *head trauma*, which are still commonly used, are less preferable because they do not clearly denote that there is injury to the brain. Although these terms do imply that the brain is injured, this implication is not always true because it is possible for a patient to have a head injury without a brain injury, and vice versa.

TBI is a general category that includes closed head injury, open head injury, and penetrating head injury as subcategories. The terms *closed head injury* and *open head injury* refer to injuries in which there generally is an impact between the head and a blunt object. *Closed* head injury denotes that the dura remained intact and *open* head injury that the dura was opened. The terms *mild*, *moderate*, and *severe* TBI (which are defined below) refer to grades of severity of TBI, usually of closed head injury. The term *penetrating* head injury denotes that a foreign object pene-

---

*References 19, 22, 27, 49, 75, 111, 133, 142, 165, 177, 198.

trated the dura and entered the brain, and includes stab wounds and missile wounds as subcategories. Gunshot wound to the head is the most common example of penetrating head injury. It is important to note that the terms *closed*, *open*, and *penetrating head injury* are specific terms, each used to refer to a subcategory of TBI and to provide some indication of the typical etiology and pathological findings of that subcategory. *TBI* is recommended as the general term to refer to all of these subcategories.

The terminology of many nontraumatic brain injuries presents relatively fewer problems because these terms (e.g., stroke) indicate a specific cause and pathological findings. The term *anoxic brain injury* is used to refer to injuries caused by decreasing the oxygen supply to the entire brain,[95] and is equivalent to the terms *hypoxic brain injury* and *hypoxic encephalopathy*. The major cause of anoxic brain injury is cardiac arrest. The terms *toxic brain injury* and *metabolic brain injury* refer to brain damage caused by toxins or abnormal metabolism, respectively. Causes of toxic-metabolic brain injury include industrial solvent exposure and hepatic encephalopathy.[4]

PATHOPHYSIOLOGY OF BRAIN INJURY

This section discusses the pathophysiology of brain damage in TBI and anoxic brain injury. The pathophysiology of brain damage in stroke is described in Chapter 50 of this book. Details of terminology and pathophysiology of brain tumors, toxic-metabolic brain injury, and causes of other acquired nontraumatic brain injuries are discussed elsewhere.[4, 151]

Traumatic Brain Injury

The pathophysiology of TBI differs between closed or open head injury and penetrating head injury. Traumatic brain damage can be caused by a variety of pathological mechanisms, which can be divided into *primary* brain damage mechanisms that occur at the moment of impact, and *secondary* mechanisms that are caused by the primary mechanisms which, in turn, cause additional brain damage.[3]

Closed or Open Head Injury

In closed or open head injury, the brain can be damaged by contact between the head and another object, and/or by acceleration or deceleration of the brain within the skull.[96] For example, in a fall the brain rapidly decelerates when the head makes an impact against the ground, and in an assault the brain rapidly accelerates when the weapon makes an impact against the head. Motor vehicle crashes typically involve both acceleration and deceleration injuries to the brain.

Most of the primary mechanisms of brain damage in closed or open head injury are caused by acceleration-deceleration rather than by contact (Fig. 49–1). The most important mechanism of primary brain damage caused by contact is laceration of the brain beneath a skull fracture, which occurs in open head injury. Contusions can also be caused by contact, but are more commonly produced by acceleration-deceleration. Regardless of the point of contact, contusions are typically located in the inferior frontal and anterior temporal lobes, areas where the adjacent skull surfaces are irregular.[96] The major mechanisms of primary brain damage produced by acceleration-deceleration are diffuse axonal injury, multiple petechial hemorrhages, and cranial nerve injury. *Diffuse axonal injury*[85] refers to the widespread stretching of axons caused by rotation of the brain around its axis. The distribution of axonal damage is consistent with the centripetal model of closed head injury,[181] which postulates that the force exerted by rotation of the brain is greatest at the brain's surface and weaker in deeper brain structures. The model correctly predicts that neuroimaging abnormalities in milder TBI tend to be located near the cortex, but in more severe TBI are located in deep as well as surface brain regions.[149] In severe TBI,

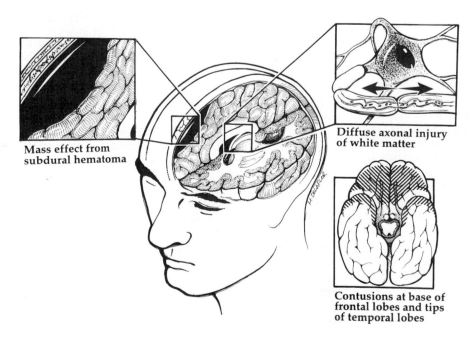

Mass effect from subdural hematoma

Diffuse axonal injury of white matter

Contusions at base of frontal lobes and tips of temporal lobes

FIGURE 49–1 Major mechanisms of brain damage in closed head injury include diffuse axonal injury, contusions, and mass effect from intracranial hemorrhage. Diffuse axonal injury affects white matter throughout the brain as well as in the corpus callosum. Contusions occur most frequently in the inferior frontal and temporal areas. Subdural hematomas and other intracranial hemorrhages can be caused by acceleration-deceleration as well as by contact, and are frequently located in the frontal-temporal area. Brain swelling, ischemia, and excitotoxicity (not shown) are also important causes of brain damage.

axonal damage tends to be greater in longer fiber tracts (e.g., corpus callosum) and at the gray-white matter junction.[96]

Major mechanisms of secondary brain damage are intracranial hemorrhage (epidural, subdural, and intracerebral hematomas), brain swelling (vasogenic or cytogenic edema), hypoxia, excitotoxicity, and production of free radical molecules. *Excitotoxicity* refers to neuronal damage caused by above-normal concentrations of excitatory neurotransmitters released by injured neurons.[44] There is preliminary evidence that exitotoxic brain damage can be prevented by hypothermia[45] and by treatment with experimental drugs.[44] Both primary and secondary brain damage can lead to increased intracranial pressure, which in turn can potentiate the mechanisms of secondary brain damage in a positive feedback loop.[169] Finally, brain shift and herniation can be produced by mass effect from brain swelling or intracranial hemorrhage.

Brain damage in TBI is therefore a summation of the effects of multiple primary and secondary mechanisms, most of which tend to cause diffuse rather than focal patterns of damage, especially in those with closed head injury. This is consistent with the chronic picture of cerebral atrophy and ventricular enlargement that is commonly observed in neuroimaging of severe closed head injury survivors[147] (Fig. 49–2). Despite these commonalities, individual differences in patterns of brain damage produce mixed patterns of neurological and neuropsychological impairments[6] in individual TBI survivors.

Missile Wounds to the Brain

In shrapnel wounds of the brain suffered in wartime, most brain damage is located along the track of the missile and indriven bone fragments[3, 125] (Fig. 49–3). The pathology of gunshot wounds of the brain in peacetime is not as well understood but can exhibit greater diffuse brain damage, probably due to the large intracranial pressure wave produced by the initial impact[48] and to the larger zone of injury by missile and bone fragments. Nevertheless, many patients with gunshot wounds of the brain present mainly with syndromes of focal brain damage (e.g., hemiplegia, hemianopsia), with relatively spared functioning of brain regions located away from the missile track.

Anoxic Brain Injury

The mechanism of brain damage in anoxic brain injury is ischemia due to hypoxemia or decreased perfusion.[95]

Although anoxic brain injury typically causes diffuse neuronal death and injury, there is selective vulnerability of neurons in parts of the hippocampus, cerebellum, and basal ganglia, and in cortical regions located in arterial boundary zones.[95] Neurons in certain parts of the hippocampus appear to be especially vulnerable, which explains the high frequency of amnesia following anoxic brain injury. The vulnerability of neurons in the basal ganglia and cerebellum may account for the frequency of movement disorders in this population.

EPIDEMIOLOGY OF TRAUMATIC BRAIN INJURY

This section discusses the epidemiology of TBI. The epidemiology of stroke is discussed in Chapter 50. The epidemiological aspects of brain tumors are discussed in a recent book.[151] The epidemiology of other nontraumatic brain injuries is discussed elsewhere.[4]

TBI has a high incidence relative to other neurological disorders. Recent reviews by Kraus and colleagues of major epidemiological studies in the United States concluded that the overall incidence of TBI was approximately 200 per 100,000 persons per year.[132, 210] The great majority of new TBI cases, approximately 80%, are graded as mild and have a survival rate of nearly 100%. The remaining 20% of new TBI cases are divided evenly between moderate and severe TBI. However, severe TBI has a survival rate of only approximately 42%, as compared to 93% for moderate TBI. Because of these different survival rates, severe TBI patients constitute a relatively small percentage of all TBI survivors, although they account for the majority of those who receive acute TBI rehabilitation. Table 49–1 presents estimated numbers of new TBI patients in the United States during 1994[216] and in a subpopulation of 1 million people, projected from the review of epidemiological studies by Kraus.[132]

The risk of TBI is strongly associated with demographic features and is highest among males in all age groups. The peak risk is among young adult males between 18 and 25 years of age,[210] who have an annual incidence of between 350 and 700 per 100,000 in different studies.[132] This explains the predominance of young adult males among TBI rehabilitation patients.[93] There are also secondary but much smaller peaks of TBI risk in the pediatric and geriatric age brackets.

TABLE 49–1   Estimates of Annual Traumatic Brain Injury (TBI) Incidence in the United States in 1994

	U.S. Population (est. 260 million)	Per 1 Million
Total incidence	520,000	2000
Total pre-hospital deaths	52,000	200
Total admitted alive	468,000	1800
Mild TBI	374,400	1440
Moderate TBI	46,800	180
Severe TBI	46,800	180
Total discharged alive		
Mild TBI	374,400	1440
Moderate TBI	43,524	167
Severe TBI	20,124	76

Adapted from Kraus JF: Epidemiology of head injury. *In* Cooper PR (ed): Head Injury, ed 3. Baltimore, Williams & Wilkins, 1993, pp 1–25.

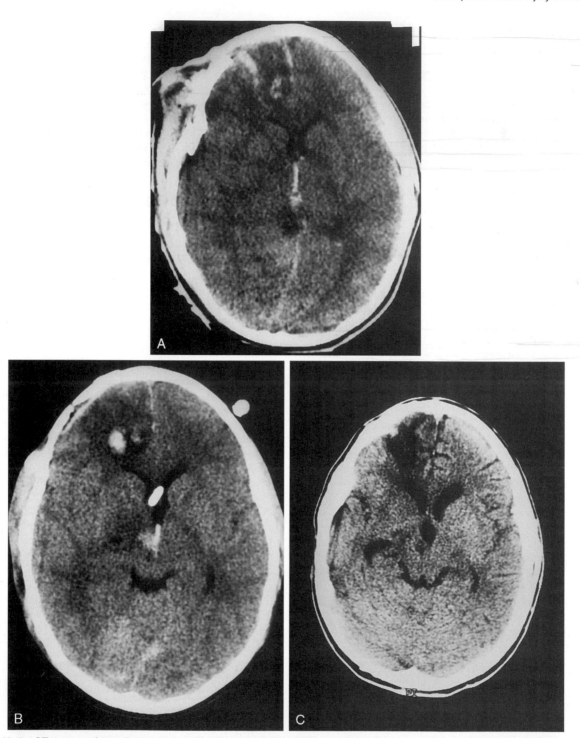

FIGURE 49–2 CT scan performed on a 6-year-old girl who sustained an open head injury in a motor vehicle crash. *A,* The initial scan shows a right frontal depressed skull fracture with intracranial hemorrhage in the frontal lobe and right-to-left midline shift. *B,* Follow-up scan later that day shows surgical repair of the skull fracture and placement of a ventriculostomy tube into the right lateral ventricle. *C,* Follow-up scan 20 days post-injury shows diffuse cerebral atrophy, manifested as enlarged ventricles and sulci, as well as encephalomalacia in the right frontal lobe. Residual impairments included left hemiparesis, left visual neglect, and recent memory loss. She later regained ambulation and returned to school in special education.

The single largest *indirect* cause of TBI is probably alcohol abuse.[53] The major direct, external cause of TBI is motor vehicle crashes, followed in frequency by automobile-pedestrian accidents, falls, and assaults (including gunshot wounds).[132, 210] The relative frequencies of these external causes differ widely across demographic groups. Motor

vehicle crashes account for the largest proportion of young adult TBI cases. Automobile-pedestrian and bicycle crashes are more common in children. Falls are more common in children and the elderly.[132, 210] The epidemiological profile of TBI gives truth to the notion that TBI is the end product of societal problems such as substance abuse, crime, envi-

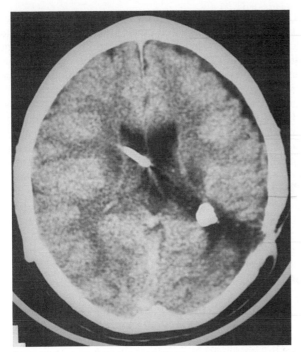

FIGURE 49–3 Initial CT scan of a 14-year-old boy who sustained a gunshot wound to the head in an assault. The exit wound is in the left temporal-parietal area. Destruction of brain tissue is seen along the bullet path. Entry wound (not shown) was in the superior right parietal area. At 3 years post-injury, the patient is non-ambulatory and dependent for care owing to quadriplegia, but he can partly direct his own care.

ronmental hazards, driving safety, and supervision of children and elderly persons.

ASSESSMENT TECHNIQUES AND PROGNOSIS

This section discusses assessment and outcome prediction of TBI and anoxic brain injury. Details of these topics in stroke and other nontraumatic brain injuries are discussed in Chapter 50 and in other references.[4, 151]

Glasgow Coma Scale

In the absence of a direct physical measurement of brain injury severity, the Glasgow coma scale (GCS)[118] is used in most centers as the "gold standard" of brain injury severity, particularly during early stages of recovery. Although the GCS was initially designed for TBI, it is also used with other brain disorders (e.g., anoxic brain injury) that cause loss of consciousness. The rationale of using the GCS is that there is usually a close relationship between a patient's brain injury severity, which cannot be directly measured, and the level of consciousness, which can be observed. The GCS, shown in Table 49–2, consists of rating the patient's best motor and speech responses, and the stimulus needed to elicit eye opening. These three ratings are summed to yield a GCS score, which can range from a minimum of 3 to a maximum of 15. Lower GCS scores indicate lower levels of consciousness and therefore imply greater severity of brain injury. Conversely, higher

TABLE 49–2   Glasgow Coma Scale*

Patient's Response	Score
Eye opening	
Eyes open spontaneously	4
Eyes open when spoken to	3
Eyes open to painful stimulation	2
Eyes do not open	1
Motor	
Follows commands	6
Makes localizing movement to pain	5
Makes withdrawal movements to pain	4
Flexor (decorticate) posturing to pain	3
Extensor (decerebrate) posturing to pain	2
No motor response to pain	1
Verbal	
Oriented to place and date	5
Converses but is disoriented	4
Utters inappropriate words, not conversing	3
Makes incomprehensible nonverbal sounds	2
Not vocalizing	1

Instructions: Rate best response in the verbal and motor categories and the stimulus needed to elicit eye opening. Sum the three ratings to obtain the score.

GCS scores indicate levels of consciousness that are closer to normal, and therefore imply lesser severity of brain injury. It has been repeatedly demonstrated that the depth and duration of unconsciousness, as indexed by the GCS score, is the single most powerful predictor of outcome from TBI.[218]

Classifying Severity of TBI

It is becoming increasingly accepted to grade the severity of TBI by classifying injuries as mild, moderate, or severe based on the patient's GCS score after resuscitation. Table 49–3 presents recommended criteria, based on the GCS, for classifying mild, moderate, and severe TBI. The *lowest* postresuscitation GCS score, obtained at any time following resuscitation, is a better index of severity than the GCS score obtained at the scene or immediately upon hospital arrival. This is because early GCS scores do not reflect any later deterioration in the level of consciousness.[64] In addition, preresuscitation GCS scores are more affected by nonbrain factors (e.g., shock).

Severe TBI, corresponding to a lowest GCS score of 8 or lower, implies that the patient was in coma for some period of time. *Coma* denotes the state in which the patient does not open the eyes and does not demonstrate evidence of cognition, such as following commands or speaking.[118, 187] Some authors grade TBI as severe only if

TABLE 49–3   Traumatic Brain Injury (TBI) Severity Based on Glasgow Coma Scale (GCS)

Mild TBI—GCS score of 13–15 at lowest point after resuscitation
  Additional criteria:
  1. Loss of consciousness <20 min
  2. No TBI-related abnormalities on neurological examination and normal CT scan of the brain (if positive, classify patient as moderate TBI or mild TBI with complications)
Moderate TBI—GCS score of 9–12 at lowest point after resuscitation
Severe TBI—GCS score of 3–8 at lowest point after resuscitation

the patient remains comatose for longer than 6 or 8 hours,[64] since those who regain consciousness before this time have a better outcome.[218] Severe TBI accounts for the large majority of inpatients in acute brain injury rehabilitation units.[93] Prognostically, the large majority of those who survive severe TBI have permanent neuropsychological impairments and functional disabilities.[145, 159, 200]

Moderate TBI, which corresponds to a lowest GCS of 9 to 12, denotes that the patient's lowest level of consciousness could be described as combative or lethargic. The patient might or might not have followed commands, but did not respond appropriately to questions. Moderate TBI accounts for a minority of inpatients in acute TBI rehabilitation.[93] Prognostically, many moderate TBI patients have permanent impairments or disabilities, but some make a good recovery with only mild persisting impairments.[59, 159]

Mild TBI (called *minor* TBI in the past), with a lowest GCS score of 13 or higher, indicates that upon hospital arrival the patient was awake (or awoke when spoken to), followed commands, and spoke, but might have been confused or disoriented. The commonly used term *concussion* is equivalent to mild TBI. Some authors grade TBI as mild only if the patient has no objective signs of brain injury on the neurological examination or computed tomography (CT) scan of the brain. Patients with such complications are then classified as having moderate TBI or mild TBI with complications.[223] Mild TBI does not, by itself, usually require inpatient rehabilitation, although mild TBI often co-occurs with spinal cord injury and other musculoskeletal injuries that require treatment in acute rehabilitation units.[57] The long-term prognosis of mild TBI is controversial, as discussed later in this chapter, but it is accepted that patients with uncomplicated mild TBI generally achieve a good recovery without permanent impairments.[141, 159]

[handwritten: 20% but only 2% of SCI pts have TBI]

While the GCS is a very useful tool, it does have some disadvantages. First, all or part of the GCS can be unscorable during the early acute care phase because of chemical paralysis or sedation, spinal cord injury, facial injury, or intubation.[64] The GCS score of a comatose patient is probably not affected by endotracheal intubation (which prevents the patient from making verbal responses), but intubation could obscure the difference between moderate and mild TBI. The GCS score can be affected by intoxication and also is unscorable at younger ages or in patients who do not understand the examiner's language.[118] The sensitivity of the GCS to sedation can become a major problem in grading brain injury severity. Unfortunately, GCS scores are sometimes not recorded during the acute care phase. In the absence of valid GCS scores, the physician might need to grade brain injury severity on the basis of the CT scan and the durations of unconsciousness and post-traumatic amnesia.

Neuroimaging of TBI

More detailed information about the use of CT and magnetic resonance imaging (MRI) scans in TBI is available[84, 87, 115] (see also Chapter 11). CT scanning is the technique of choice for neuroimaging of TBI during the acute care stage because of its sensitivity to the presence of blood, edema, facial or skull fractures, and most other intracranial injuries requiring medical treatment. A CT scan of the head can be obtained quickly and is not contraindicated by the presence of metallic material in the patient's body or in life support equipment. There are well-documented relationships between early CT findings and later gross outcome (i.e., conscious survival vs. deceased or vegetative). Normal CT findings have the best prognosis, and CT findings of acute subdural hematoma, intracerebral hemorrhage, and massive bilateral hemispheric swelling have the worst prognoses.[65, 218] The value of CT findings in predicting outcome of TBI survivors in rehabilitation is less well understood[52] and is in need of further study.

MRI of the brain is generally more sensitive than CT to traumatic brain lesions because of its greater resolution, and it is selectively more sensitive than CT to nonhemorrhagic shear injuries and to contusions in certain areas, such as the inferior frontal region and brainstem, which are located near bony surfaces that produce artifacts in CT scanning (Fig. 49–4).[84] Disadvantages of MRI are the relatively long time needed for scanning, the inaccessibility of the patient during this time, and its contraindication by metallic materials in the patient's body or in medical equipment. The value of MRI in predicting outcome of TBI rehabilitation is still being investigated but appears promising in view of the relationship between MRI abnormalities and neuropsychological deficits in mild and moderate TBI patients.[150] In particular, MRI appears more useful than CT scanning during the rehabilitation phase since MRI is more

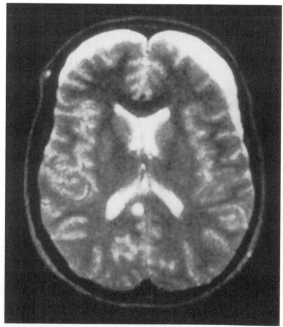

FIGURE 49–4 T2-weighted MRI scan of a 32-year-old woman who was injured in an automobile-pedestrian accident 1 month earlier. Initial CT scan revealed a right frontal subdural hematoma. This image shows bifrontal subdural fluid collections and a shear injury in the splenium of the corpus callosum. The corpus callosum lesion, which is a classic sign of diffuse axonal injury, was not visualized on CT scans. In general, MRI can visualize a larger number of traumatic lesions than can CT, especially lesions that are nonhemorrhagic or are located near bony areas. The patient, who had an initial Glasgow coma scale score of 7, underwent inpatient and postacute rehabilitation. She returned to work as a secretary and lives independently.

helpful in explaining patients' neurological and neuropsychological deficits, and therefore in planning rehabilitation strategies. Finally, promising research results obtained with single-photon emission CT (SPECT) scanning of the brain in TBI patients[92, 180] suggest the possibility that SPECT scanning could have an important role in evaluating unconscious or mild TBI patients in the future.

Neurophysiological Evaluations

Electroencephalograms and evoked potentials are the major neurophysiological techniques used to predict outcome in TBI[228] (see also Chapter 7). A recent review of studies using evoked potentials to predict outcome from TBI[184] concluded that the bilateral absence of waves N20 to P22 in somatosensory evoked potentials of comatose TBI patients was a strong predictor of failure to recover consciousness. The same review[184] concluded that the absence of wave V or other components of the brainstem auditory evoked potential was also predictive of a poor outcome; however, the presence of normal brainstem auditory evoked potentials was not a valid predictor of good outcome.

Neuropsychological Testing

Neuropsychological tests are the major tools used to evaluate cognitive functions in brain-injured patients (see also Chapter 4). Data from a substantial number of studies have characterized cognitive deficits following brain injury and have identified neuropsychological tests that are sensitive to these deficits and predictive of outcome.[142] Disadvantages of neuropsychological testing are the time needed for testing, the requirement of good patient motivation, and the limited testability of many low-level patients.[145]

Summary of Acute Prognostic Factors

Table 49–4 presents the major predictive indicators that are available for most TBI patients in neurotrauma care or upon admission to acute rehabilitation. The best predictors of outcome from TBI are the GCS score and other indicators of overall severity of brain injury.[119] In addition to overall injury severity, the patient's age is an important outcome predictor. It should be noted that the validity of many of these indicators as predictors of gross outcome from the acute stage has been demonstrated in multicenter neurosurgical studies.[64, 218] As there are relatively fewer studies of predictors of rehabilitation outcome, it is possible that some of these indicators are less valid in predicting rehabilitation outcome of TBI survivors than they are in predicting survival itself. In predicting outcome it is also important to consider extracranial injuries, such as musculoskeletal injuries, since these can be a cause of disability in many patients.[56] Finally, most professionals feel that the availability of family support is a strong positive influence on the extent to which the severe TBI patient will benefit from rehabilitation.

Current knowledge about the prognosis of anoxic brain injury is mostly limited to the probability of recovering consciousness in patients who remain unconscious following their injury (this information is discussed below under Rehabilitation of the Unconscious Patient).[153, 173, 174] Relatively less information is available about the long-term outcome of anoxic brain injury patients who do recover consciousness.[100] Prediction of outcome from stroke is discussed in Chapter 50 and prognosis in brain tumors is discussed elsewhere.[151, 152] Unfortunately, much less information is available on the rehabilitation prognosis in nontraumatic brain injuries other than stroke, and this remains an area for future research.

CONTINUUM OF REHABILITATION SERVICES FOR BRAIN INJURY

Rehabilitation of the brain-injured patient is typically divided into two phases: *acute* rehabilitation and *post–acute* rehabilitation. The continuum of rehabilitation services for brain-injured patients is shown in Figure 49–5. *Acute* rehabilitation refers to inpatient treatment in a hospital-based unit, during the early stages of recovery. *Post-acute* rehabilitation refers to treatment after hospital discharge during later stages of recovery, and is described in more detail in Chapter 4.

Acute Brain Injury Rehabilitation

Rehabilitation of the brain-injured patient should ideally begin while the patient is still in acute care. At this stage the physiatrist can intervene to prevent complications that could add to the patient's disability later in recovery. For example, the unconscious patient without contraindications should undergo passive range-of-motion exercises twice daily in order to prevent contractures and other joint abnormalities. The patient should be positioned to prevent pressure ulcers, edema, and contractures. The physiatrist can also recommend additional interventions for spasticity, nutrition, and bowel-bladder incontinence. Although definitive orthopedic management of fractures in TBI can often be delayed, early surgical treatment of orthopedic injuries can minimize later disability.[105]

Transfer to the acute rehabilitation unit should be done at the point when the patient is medically stable and when the ongoing medical care will not substantially interfere with progress in rehabilitation.[170] The requirement that the

TABLE 49–4   Prognosis in Severe Head Injuries

	Poorer	Better
Glasgow coma scale score	<7	>7
CT scan	Large blood clot; massive bihemispheric swelling	Normal
Age	Old age	Youth
Pupillary light reflex	Pupils remain dilated	Pupil contracts
Doll's eye sign	Impaired	Intact
Caloric testing with ice water	Eyes do not deviate	Eyes deviate to irrigated side
Motor response to noxious stimuli	Decerebrate rigidity	Localizes defensive gestures
Somatosensory evoked potentials	Deficient	Normal
Post-traumatic amnesia length	>2 wk	<2 wk

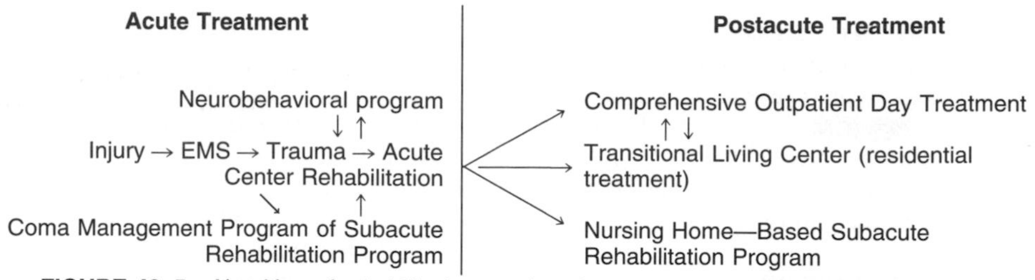

Acute Treatment   **Postacute Treatment**

Neurobehavioral program   Comprehensive Outpatient Day Treatment
          ↓ ↑   ↑ ↓
Injury → EMS → Trauma → Acute   Transitional Living Center (residential
          Center Rehabilitation   treatment)
                    ↘   ↑
Coma Management Program of Subacute   Nursing Home—Based Subacute
          Rehabilitation Program   Rehabilitation Program

FIGURE 49–5   Algorithm of rehabilitation services for severe traumatic head injury patients.

patient should be following commands before admission to the acute rehabilitation unit can delay and sometimes even prevent access to rehabilitation in the large number of patients who eventually regain consciousness. Instead, the physiatrist can use prognostic indicators to screen unconscious patients and selectively admit those with the highest probability of recovery. Direct transfer of the unconscious patient from acute care to a nursing home, without prior evaluation by a physiatrist, should be avoided because of the risk of overlooking developing complications or signs of improvement.

Dedicated brain injury rehabilitation units have the advantages of having more experienced staff, a network of consultants with special expertise in brain injury, resources to conduct research, a family education program, and the opportunity to develop protocols for typical brain injury rehabilitation problems. These advantages can be significant in the treatment of patients who are unconscious or agitated, or who have unusual syndromes. Even in acute rehabilitation units that do not specialize in brain injury, services can be improved by having the same nurses and therapists assigned to all brain-injured patients. Further research is needed to evaluate the efficacy of acute rehabilitation units dedicated to brain injury, as compared to treatment of brain-injured patients in general rehabilitation units. A recent review[109] of efficacy studies of acute TBI rehabilitation found that, while TBI patients in these studies typically made great improvements during inpatient rehabilitation, these gains could not be uniquely attributed to rehabilitation because the studies failed to control for spontaneous recovery or for pre-existing differences between the treatment and comparison groups. In addition, the outcome measures used in these studies may not have been sufficiently sensitive or comprehensive to detect differences in improvement.[104]

The therapy team of the acute brain injury rehabilitation unit typically includes the traditional rehabilitation disciplines of clinical nutrition, rehabilitation nursing, physical therapy, occupational therapy, psychology, respiratory therapy, speech-language pathology, social work, and therapeutic recreation. Some units use other disciplines in addition to these. In addition, the dedicated brain injury team should include a neuropsychologist, who is a psychologist specializing in the assessment and treatment of patients with brain disorders. Descriptions of specialized therapy techniques for brain-injured patients are detailed elsewhere.[1, 107, 194, 235] The team also needs access to specialists in audiology, optometry, orthotic devices, and vocational counseling. The team's treatment strategies during acute rehabilitation are largely determined by the patient's stage of recovery, as described in the following sections.

Stages of Neurobehavioral Recovery from Brain Injury

Compared to other neurological disorders treated in rehabilitation, TBI has an unusually long course of recovery and TBI patients show a greater degree of functional improvement.[41] There is general consensus among rehabilitation practitioners that almost all spontaneous recovery from brain injury is complete by 1 year or at most 2 years. The course of recovery from severe TBI consists of distinct stages, as shown in Figure 49–6. The stages of neurobehavioral recovery from anoxic brain injury are similar to those from TBI. The Levels of Cognitive Functioning, shown in Table 49–5, was developed at Rancho Los Amigos Medical Center[161] to describe the sequence of neurobehavioral recovery from TBI and to provide a rationale for cognitive rehabilitation at each recovery stage. Although the Levels of Cognitive Functioning concept has been criticized because recovery from TBI is more variable than the scale implies, it is a truism that a patient's current stage of recovery is the major factor in planning the rehabilitation program.

Coma and Unconsciousness

The natural history of recovery from severe TBI and anoxic brain injury begins with coma, a state in which the patient shows no evidence of cognition and does not open his or her eyes, even to painful stimulation.[118] Coma and unconsciousness following TBI are caused by the disruption of input to surface brain structures from deeper structures which subserve arousal and wakefulness.[187] This disruption can, in turn, be produced by disconnection of ascending fiber pathways due to diffuse axonal injury, or by compression of brainstem or diencephalic structures due to mass effect from supratentorial lesions. In surviving patients, there is a fairly consistent sequence of recovery of function from coma, beginning with eye opening and sleep-wake cycles, and progressing to following commands and finally to speaking.[32] In TBI, this recovery sequence is consistent with the centripetal model of injury, which predicts that functions that are subserved by deeper brain structures, such as sleep-wake cycles, should recover earlier than functions subserved by surface brain structures, such as memory.[181] Cognition is usually first demonstrated by the patient's ability to communicate, such as following commands or gesturing. Assessment of these early signs of cognition is usually straightforward and does not require special techniques.

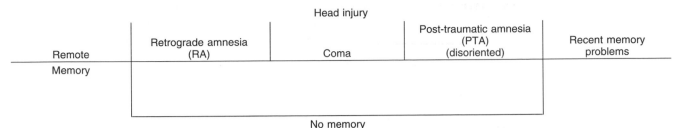

FIGURE 49–6   Timeline of memory deficits following brain injury.

The duration of unconsciousness reflects the severity of brain injury and can be used in combination with GCS scores, or in the absence of GCS scores, as an index of brain injury severity. For example, if a patient had a lowest GCS score of 7 but was unconscious for less than 2 days, this indicates a much smaller degree of brain injury severity than if the patient was unconscious longer than 2 weeks. It is important to note that the duration of unconsciousness can reflect not only brain injury severity but also the effects of sedation (e.g., barbiturate coma) and medical complications.

Approximately 10% to 15% of severe TBI patients are discharged from acute care while still unconscious.[148] Most patients who remain unconscious after 1 month have regained sleep-wake cycles and therefore spontaneously open their eyes part of the time. They typically also exhibit pupillary reactivity and oculocephalic reflexes, primitive behaviors such as chewing and roving eye movements, and vegetative functions such as spontaneous respiration, which reflect preserved brainstem and hypothalamic functions. There is a long-standing controversy surrounding the proper term to describe patients in this stage of recovery who, because they have spontaneous eye opening, are not in true coma. The term *persistent vegetative state* (PVS)[118, 187] is widely used in the literature to describe such patients but is considered objectionable by many laypersons. The lack of an accepted, standard term frequently leads to confusion.

Rehabilitation of the Unconscious Patient

Patients who remain unconscious upon discharge from acute care present difficult assessment and treatment problems, and often require care in a dedicated brain injury rehabilitation unit. Alternatively, the unconscious patient can be admitted to a *coma management program*,[26] a program which specializes in the care of unconscious or minimally responsive patients and which is typically based in a skilled nursing facility.

The first step in assessment of the unconscious patient is to rule out the possibility that a patient's failure to demonstrate evidence of consciousness is an artifact of the examination techniques or due to reversible medical factors. Patients who fail to follow commands because of incomprehension of the examiner's language or because of aphasia or apraxia[146] might succeed if the examination techniques are properly modified. Most important, a patient's arousal and responsiveness can be impaired by sedating drugs, systemic illness, malnourishment, and other medical problems which could be correctable.

In particular, the problem of drug-induced sedation in unconscious patients is more serious than generally appreciated and deserves special mention. The physiatrist should bear in mind that sedative side effects can be magnified in the injured brain and that even small changes in arousal can affect the patient's responsiveness. Medications given to the unconscious patient should be carefully reviewed in order to discontinue those which are unnecessary and, if possible, to replace necessary drugs with ones that are less sedating. Potentially sedating medications that are often given to unconscious patients are listed in Table 49–6. Anticonvulsant prophylaxis can be discontinued in many patients, as discussed below, or switched to less sedating anticonvulsants such as carbamazepine (Tegretol). Treatment of hypertension with clonidine, verapamil, or diuretics might be possible instead of using antihypertensives with sedating side effects, such as propranolol, metoprolol, and methyldopa. The use of metoclopramide (Reglan) should be avoided in the treatment of delayed gastric

TABLE 49–5   Rancho Los Amigos Medical Center Levels of Cognitive Functioning*

Level	Name	Description
I	No response	Appears to be in deep sleep; no response to any stimulation
II	Generalized response	Appears to be resting quietly; makes gross movements in response to noxious stimulation
III	Localized response	Makes spontaneous, purposeful movements; may follow commands inconsistently
IV	Confused-agitated	Confused, amnestic and inattentive; may be aggressive
V	Confused-inappropriate	Not agitated; confused and amnestic
VI	Confused-appropriate	Lacks initiative and problem solving; functional with structure and supervision
VII	Automatic-appropriate	Follows daily routines; needs supervision for home and community skills; independent in self-care within physical ability
VIII	Purposeful-appropriate	Independent in home and community skills; may have cognitive deficits

**Instructions:* Assign the patient to the level that most closely describes his or her level of cognitive functioning.

TABLE 49–6   Choice of Drugs for Patients With Traumatic Brain Injury

	Sedating Drugs to Be Avoided	Less Sedating Alternatives
Anticonvulsants	Phenytoin Phenobarbital	Carbamazepine Valproic acid
Antihypertensives	Propranolol Metaprolol Methyldopa	Clonidine Verapamil Diuretics
Antispasticity Medications	Baclofen Diazepam	Dantrolene sodium
Psychoactive Agents	Neuroleptics Amitriptyline Doxepin Imipramine Trazodone	Lithium Carbamazepine Paroxetine Methylphenidate Fluoxetine Levodopa/carbidopa Sertraline
Gastrointestinal Medications	Cimetidine Metoclopramide hydrochloride	Antacids Erythromycin

emptying because of its sedating side effects. Benzodiazepines such as diazepam (Valium), which are often used for spasticity control, should also be avoided. Antidepressants such as amitriptyline (Elavil), which are sometimes given to increase the level of consciousness, can paradoxically decrease arousal because of their anticholinergic effects. There is no place for neuroleptics such as haloperidol (Haldol), chlorpromazine (Thorazine), and thioridazine (Mellaril) in the medical management of unconscious patients.

The best predictors of whether unconscious patients will regain consciousness are etiology, age, and the duration of unconsciousness itself.[173, 174] Studies of outcome in TBI patients who were unconscious at approximately 1 month post injury[31, 32, 148, 186, 204] (summarized in Table 49–7) show that 40% to 50% regained consciousness by 1 year post injury. These findings tend to support Berrol's recommendation[18] that the diagnosis of PVS should be reserved until the patient has been vegetative for several months or 1 year. A review of all verified cases of prolonged vegetative state following TBI concluded that the probability of regaining consciousness by 1 year post injury was 36% in patients who were unconscious at 3 months post injury; however, this probability decreased to 21% in those who remained unconscious at 6 months post injury.[173, 174] In nontraumatic brain injuries, the probability of regaining consciousness by 1 year post injury was only 7% in patients who remained unconscious at 3 months post injury and was effectively zero in those still unconscious at 6 months

post injury.[173, 174] The same review reported fewer than 20 verified cases of TBI patients who recovered consciousness after remaining vegetative longer than 1 year and concluded that recovery of consciousness after 1 year was "extremely rare."[173, 174]

Age appears to be a predictor of recovery from traumatic unconsciousness, with the best recovery seen in children, followed by adults under 40 years of age.[173, 174] However, age does not appear to predict recovery from nontraumatic unconsciousness.[153] There is also evidence that recovery from traumatic unconsciousness is less likely in patients with neuroimaging evidence of severe cerebral atrophy or with bilateral absence of somatosensory evoked potentials.[173, 174, 184] Numerous other potential predictors of recovery from traumatic unconsciousness have been studied,[148] but none have received sufficient support to fully endorse their use in clinical prediction. The long-term prognosis for patients who remain in PVS has not been thoroughly delineated; however, available evidence indicates that such patients, compared with BVI patients who regain consciousness, have a markedly shortened life expectancy.

There is a strong need for an assessment technique that can track responsiveness, and possibly signs of recovery, in unconscious patients. The GCS and Rancho Los Amigos Levels of Cognitive Functioning lack sensitivity in unconscious patients who have already regained spontaneous eye opening.[26] Several rating scales have been developed to assess the responsiveness of unconscious or low-level patients.[114] These scales include the Coma/Near-Coma

TABLE 49–7   One-Year Outcome of Traumatic Coma

Investigators	No.	Minimum Duration of Unconsciousness	Outcome at 1 Year (%)		
			Conscious	Unconsciousness	Dead
Bricolo et al.[32]	135	2 wk	62	8	30
Pitts[186]	56	1 mo	61	7	32
Braakman et al.[31]	140	1 mo	37	11	52
Sazbon and Groswasser[204]	134	1 mo	54	14	32
Levin et al.[148]*	93	Discharge from acute care	58	18	24

*Data from 3-year follow-up.

Scale,[191] the Coma Recovery Scale,[88] the Western Neuro Sensory Stimulation Profile,[10] and the Sensory Stimulation Assessment Measure.[189] Although none of these scales has proven validity in predicting recovery in patients who are still unconscious, they can be useful in monitoring whether a patient is becoming less responsive over time, which can be a sign of a treatable medical complication or the inadvertent addition of a sedating drug.

Rehabilitation of unconscious patients remains controversial.[28, 167, 232] In particular, the efficacy of *sensory stimulation* (also termed *coma stimulation*), in which patients are presented with directed stimulation in multiple modalities,[26] has not been supported by clinical trials. A recent review of published studies[225] found no evidence that sensory stimulation improved the recovery from chronic traumatic unconsciousness, although there was some evidence of a treatment effect in acute TBI patients who were still comatose.

Pharmacological treatment remains the most promising intervention to directly increase arousal and facilitate recovery of consciousness of these patients. There have been numerous anecdotal reports of unconscious TBI patients who regained consciousness when treated with stimulants (e.g., methylphenidate, dextroamphetamine) and antiparkinsonian drugs (e.g., bromocriptine, amantadine).[24–26, 71, 72, 134, 227, 231] Although controlled trials of these medications have not appeared, they are now widely used in neurotrauma care and acute brain injury rehabilitation.

In the absence of treatments with proven efficacy to facilitate recovery of consciousness, the goals of rehabilitation of unconscious TBI patients are (1) to remove obstacles to recovery in order to allow patients who have the potential to regain consciousness to do so, (2) to treat medical complications that can increase disability in those patients who do recover, and (3) to provide education, counseling, and support to family members. Detailed information on coma management is available in recent articles and books.[26, 203]

Post-traumatic Amnesia and Agitation

Following recovery of consciousness, which is usually defined as the ability to follow spoken commands, TBI and anoxic brain injury patients typically pass through a period of confusion and disorientation termed *post-traumatic amnesia* (PTA).[142, 201] *PTA* is defined as the period during which the patient's ability to learn new information is minimal or nonexistent. Early in PTA, patients may not be aware of being in a hospital and may instead state that they are at home or at work. This false recall of fictitious events, termed *confabulation,* represents an organic rather than a functional symptom. Later in PTA, patients become less confabulatory but still fail to retain memory of specific episodes (e.g., visitors received the previous day). After emerging from PTA, patients have a permanent memory gap for events during the entire period of PTA and coma. They usually also have a memory gap, termed *retrograde amnesia*, for events that occurred during a shorter period leading up to the moment of injury.[142]

Different methods can be used for assessing whether a patient is in PTA. The most widely used index of PTA is the patient's orientation to place and time, but this can be less suitable in rehabilitation units where patients are given frequent "reality orientation" drills.[54] A standard technique for assessing PTA is the Galveston Orientation and Amnesia Test (GOAT),[142] a brief structured interview that quantifies the patient's orientation and recall of recent events. The GOAT score can range from 0 to 100, with a score of 75 or better defined as normal. The end of PTA can be defined as the date when the patient scores 75 or higher on the GOAT for 2 consecutive days.[145]

Since the duration of PTA is an indirect index of brain injury severity, PTA duration can be used to grade injury severity together with the GCS score, duration of unconsciousness, and neuroimaging findings. As a general rule, the duration of PTA in TBI patients will be approximately three times as long as the duration of unconsciousness.[143] The clinician should bear in mind that PTA duration, like duration of unconsciousness, can reflect factors other than the severity of brain injury itself. The failure of patients to clear from PTA can indicate a permanent amnesic disorder, such as that produced by anoxic brain injury.

During PTA, many patients exhibit a neurobehavioral syndrome, termed *agitation*, which includes cognitive confusion, extreme emotional lability, motor overactivity, and physical or verbal aggression. The agitated patient is typically unable to sustain attention and effort long enough to perform simple tasks, such as dressing, and can overreact to frustration by crying or shouting. The patient can be easily frustrated and irritated, and show grossly inappropriate behavior toward staff or family members. Agitation becomes critical if the patient becomes harmful to self or others (e.g., pulling out tubes, falling, attempting to escape from the unit). Previously it was believed that most severe TBI patients exhibited agitation during PTA, as implied by the Rancho Los Amigos scale.[161] However, it has recently been appreciated that only a minority of severe TBI patients exhibit agitation with aggression and that the majority exhibit only agitation with motor restlessness or no agitation at all.[35, 192] Risk factors for agitation remain to be identified, but experience suggests that severe cognitive deficits and frontal lobe damage might be predictive.

Rehabilitation of the Agitated Patient

The physiatrist treating an agitated patient should be alert to the possibility that the agitation is being caused by one or more medical complications such as electrolyte imbalance, malnutrition, seizure activity, sleep disturbance, or hydrocephalus. In addition, it is important to rule out the possibility that agitation is a reaction to discomfort from an underlying condition such as a subacute infection or musculoskeletal injury. It is also possible that the agitation is due to sedation from medications such as antihypertensive drugs, drugs for the gastrointestinal tract, or even drugs used to control agitation itself.

Assuming that a medical cause for agitation is ruled out, the first line of intervention for agitation should be environmental management. The goal of environmental management is to lower the level of stimulation and cognitive complexity in the patient's immediate surroundings. Techniques for environmental management of agitation are shown in Table 49–8. The use of a floor bed (Fig. 49–7) provides a safe, controlling environment and can eliminate

TABLE 49–8 Environmental Management of Agitation

1. Reduce the level of stimulation in the environment
     Place patient in a quiet private room
     Remove noxious stimuli if possible, e.g., tubes, catheters, restraints, traction
     Limit unnecessary sounds, e.g., television, radio, background conversations
     Limit number of visitors
     Staff to behave in a calm and reassuring manner
     Limit number and length of therapy sessions
     Provide therapies in patient's room
2. Protect patient from harming self or others
     Place patient in a floor bed with padded side panels (Craig bed)
     Assign 1:1 or 1:2 sitter to observe patient and ensure safety
     Avoid taking patient off unit
     Place patient in locked ward
3. Reduce patient's cognitive confusion
     One person speaking to patient at a time
     Maintain same staff to work with patient
     Minimize contact with unfamiliar staff
     Communicate to patient briefly and simply, e.g., one idea at a time
     Reorient patient to place and time repeatedly
4. Tolerate restlessness when possible
     Allow patient to thrash about in floor bed
     Allow patient to pace around unit, with 1:1 supervision
     Allow confused patient to be verbally inappropriate

the need for restraints. When required, restraints should be applied to the minimal degree necessary, such as padded hand mittens. Restraints that limit bed mobility, such as wrist restraints, can paradoxically worsen agitation by frustrating the patient's drive for motor activity. The use of restraints should be reserved for situations in which the patient is in danger of self-harm, and should not be used as a substitute for a floor bed, one-on-one supervision, or other environmental interventions. Detailed discussions of environmental management of agitation are available in recent articles.[33, 108, 183]

If a patient is still dangerous despite the environmental interventions recommended above, pharmacological intervention may be necessary. Recently there has been a trend away from the treatment of agitation with sedating medica-

tions, such as neuroleptics and minor tranquilizers. Neuroleptics can increase confusion, impede recovery, and have long-term side effects.[50, 101, 214] Minor tranquilizers can decrease muscle tone, worsen memory deficits, and have paradoxical as well as enhanced side effects in brain-injured patients. Midazolam can cause respiratory depression in TBI patients who have brainstem injuries. Alternative medications include clomazepine, slightly sedating antidepressants,[175] or serotonergics such as trazodone (Desyrel). Propranolol was effective in reducing agitation in a controlled trial with agitated TBI patients.[34] In some patients, agitation can be treated by improving cognition with psychostimulants and mood stabilizers such as lithium.[91] The patient with acute agitation and uncontrollable violent behavior, for which many staff members are needed for restraint, can benefit from intramuscular (IM) or intravenous (IV) administration of haloperidol 5 mg and lorazepam (Ativan), 2 mg every 20 min until the patient is quieted. This is recommended only for emergency situations, when there exists an immediate danger to the patient or others, and should not be used for prolonged management in place of the drugs or environmental interventions discussed above. Finally, if a patient's agitation is not controllable within the acute rehabilitation unit, transfer to a neurobehavioral unit might be indicated.[63, 226]

Rehabilitation During and After PTA

The rehabilitation program during PTA should be modified for patients' severe memory impairments. To reorient patients to their environment, the place, date, and daily schedule should be posted in patient rooms, and orientation sessions can be offered as a group or individual therapy.[54] It might be helpful for patients to receive their meals and therapies on the rehabilitation unit, in order to avoid overstimulation from noisy or unfamiliar environments. The team should avoid overstimulating the patient with a demanding therapy schedule, unrealistic therapeutic expectations, and unpleasant emotional interactions with family or staff. Patients who are capable of walking can require close supervision because of safety concerns, and might even require a wheelchair for mobility outside therapies. As the patient's safety awareness and endurance increase toward the end of PTA, the team can clear the patient for walking, toileting, and other activities at a reduced level of supervision.

After PTA resolves, a complete neuropsychological evaluation should be performed for long-term prognosis and treatment planning. The patient can be given more realistic and demanding tasks in therapies, such as community outings. Some patients will demonstrate behavior problems, which can respond to behavioral management techniques,[155, 207] or mood disorders, which can be treated with psychiatric medications.[42, 70, 208] The family typically needs to be educated about brain injury symptoms and to be trained in physical management techniques to be carried out at home. There are no set rules for time of discharge, but patients should not be discharged home until their families have completed the training to manage their needs.

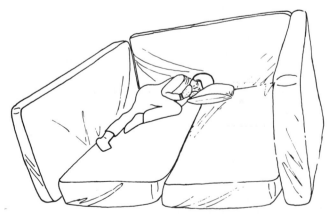

FIGURE 49–7 Agitated nonambulatory patients often benefit from the use of a floor (Craig) bed. Mattresses can be laid on the floor and 3- to 4-ft padded walls on four sides allow the patient to roll around. The use of a floor bed with one-to-one supervision and with the use of mitts and a helmet (if necessary) often eliminates the need for restraints.

Post–Acute Brain Injury Rehabilitation

Post–acute rehabilitation includes day treatment programs, residential treatment programs, vocational rehabili-

TABLE 49–9   Chronic Care Options for Traumatic Brain Injury Patients

Outpatient follow-up services
Daycare
Supported employment
Group home/lifelong living center
Nursing home
Specialized college programs
Respite care programs
Support groups for patients and families

tation programs, and other interventions designed to help patients re-enter the community (see Chapter 4). Most techniques in post–acute rehabilitation are based on either training patients to use compensatory strategies to overcome their permanent deficits (e.g., memory notebooks), or altering the environment so that the patient is more functional despite these deficits (e.g., providing a routine schedule). There is a controversy in post–acute rehabilitation regarding the efficacy of *cognitive retraining*, the group of therapies directed at remediating deficits in memory, attention, and other cognitive functions.[2, 16, 17, 39, 140, 196, 209, 219] The physiatrist should be familiar with local post–acute brain injury rehabilitation programs in order to make appropriate referrals and monitor progress (Table 49–9). It has been increasingly appreciated that family members of brain-injured patients are placed under long-term emotional and financial stresses.[37, 154, 166, 224] The physiatrist should be sensitive to the possibility of emotional distress and relationship problems,[98, 188] while providing emotional support and helping the family advocate for needed services.

MEDICAL PROBLEMS FOLLOWING BRAIN INJURY

Scope of the Problem

In recent years there has been a trend toward early admission to acute rehabilitation facilities following brain injury. Studies have shown that early rehabilitation decreases complications, overall costs, and length of stay.[11, 51, 160] A retrospective study done in Houston in 1985 looked at 180 patients with severe brain injuries and found that 16% of the medical problems were not documented in the acute care facility and 18% of the problems occurred for the first time in a rehabilitation facility.[123] Garland and Bailey[80] looked at 254 patients and found that there were 10 undetected fractures and 29 undetected peripheral nerve injuries, indicating that 11% of the brain-injured patients had sustained skeletal nerve injuries that were undetected prior to rehabilitation transfer. More recent studies show that the length of stay for patients with severe brain injury has been decreasing, especially in the acute care setting. Early comprehensive medical evaluation of severely brain-injured patients is often difficult because of their inability to communicate and to cooperate with tests and procedures. Acute care facility records often do not contain the preinjury surgical, medical, or family history or the patient's preinjury functional status, because this information is often unobtainable during the acute phase of treatment.

It cannot be overstated that a thorough evaluation by the physiatrist is needed once the patient has been admitted to the rehabilitation unit. Certain tests can be done while the patient is still on the acute neurosurgical service if the physiatrist is part of the treating team. Prompt identification of complications and early initiation of treatment can minimize disability and shorten the rehabilitation stay.[25]

A thorough history and physical examination is the essential foundation for evaluating severely brain-injured patients. Documentation of the patient's condition throughout the acute care stay should be factored into the ultimate prognosis set for the patient (Table 49–10). The physiatrist also needs to review complications that might have occurred during the acute neurosurgical phase that need further intervention during the rehabilitation phase. The physical examination should emphasize the central nervous system, including cranial nerves, motor control, and sensation. A mental status evaluation should also be performed if the patient is capable of participating.[213]

Neurological Complications

Post-traumatic Epilepsy

It is estimated that approximately 5% of all persons with TBI who are hospitalized will develop post-traumatic

TABLE 49–10   History and Physical Data Collection Form

History of present illness
    Date, type, mechanism of injury
    Description of accident
    Description of scene
    Description of emergency room
    Associated injuries
    Initial diagnostic workup
        CT scan
        Skull radiographs
        Cervical spine (C1–7; if questionable, reorder)
        Other x-ray films
        Blood alcohol
        Drug screen
        Peritoneal lavage
Head injury evaluation
    Length of coma
        Post-traumatic amnesia
        Retrograde amnesia
        Rancho Los Amigos level
    Further evaluation
        ICP monitoring
        EP
        EEG
        MRI
        CT
        Date of last CT and findings
Acute neurosurgical treatment of head injury
    Medical
        Phenobarbital coma
        Steroids
        Diuretics
        Morphine
        Hyperventilation
    Surgeries (include dates)
        Burr holes
        Craniotomy
        ICP monitoring
        VP shunt
        Bone flap

Abbreviations: CT, computed tomography; *ICP,* intracranial pressure; *EP,* evoked potentials; *EEG,* electroencephalogram; *MRI,* magnetic resonance imaging; *VP,* ventriculoperitoneal.

epilepsy (PTE). Patients who have depressed skull fractures, acute intracranial hematomas, or seizures during the first week have an increased risk of developing late PTE.[117] Other factors such as dural tearing, presence of foreign bodies, focal signs such as aphasia and hemiplegia, and post-traumatic amnesia present for longer than 24 hours, are also considered as increased risks. Determining the seizure risk of an individual patient is more difficult. In 1979, Feeney and Walker[73] devised a mathematical model to estimate seizure risk based on a combination of risk factors. However, this has not proved to be helpful in most clinical situations. Instead, patients are frequently placed on seizure prophylaxis in an acute neurosurgical setting. Neurosurgeons have traditionally prescribed phenytoin or phenobarbital because they can be administered parenterally and have been in use the longest. Recent studies have shown that using phenytoin beyond the first week following a brain injury does not prevent the development of late PTE.[215] In addition, neurobehavioral side effects of phenytoin and other sedating anticonvulsants such as phenobarbital can be detrimental to the patient with already slowed thinking and memory loss. These drugs appear to hamper the patient's overall rehabilitation program.[9, 60, 69, 162]

Most PTE is thought to be of the partial variety, either simple partial or complex partial, which is secondarily generalized. Carbamazepine has been shown to be as effective as phenytoin and phenobarbital for generalized tonic-clonic seizures, and more effective in the control of partial seizures.[117, 163] Carbamazepine is well tolerated and has few side effects (e.g., gastrointestinal distress, headaches, dizziness, diplopia), which are usually ameliorated by starting with a low dose and gradually building up to therapeutic range. The most limiting side effect of carbamazepine is bone marrow suppression. However, transient leukopenia, primarily a relative neutropenia, can usually be monitored as long as the white blood cell count is above 4000 cells/mm^3 with 50% of the white blood cells being neutrophils for this treatment phenomenon alone.[185] The disadvantage of carbamazepine is its relatively short half-life, which makes three-times-daily dosing mandatory.[62] This can cause a significant decrease in compliance in patients with memory impairments. However, memory aids such as beeping pill boxes or alarm watches seem to help with this problem.

Most physiatrists subspecializing in TBI rehabilitation are no longer using seizure prophylaxis in patients who have not had seizures beyond the first 2 weeks. Most now wait for the patient to have the first documented seizure and then choose the most appropriate antiseizure medication for that patient.[30] Carbamazepine appears to be the drug of choice for seizure management.[90, 190] Valproic acid (Depakene), although initially sedating, can be useful as well, since it can have fewer cognitive and behavioral side effects than carbamazepine. Newer medications such as felbamate (Felbatol) were first considered adjuvant medications and have not been used extensively in the brain-injured population. Unfortunately, felbamate was recalled due to several reports of aplastic anemia. Gabapentin (Neurontin), another new antiepileptic medication, may prove to be helpful for patients with PTE.

Post-traumatic Hydrocephalus

True post-traumatic hydrocephalus (PTH) following severe brain injury is relatively uncommon. One study esti-

mated the incidence to be in the range of 1% to 8%.[102] The Model Systems National Database showed that *hydrocephalus,* defined as an enlargement of the ventricles requiring placement of a shunt or drain, was detected in only 5% of severe TBI patients.[29] The neurological symptoms can range from deep coma to the typical triad for normal-pressure hydrocephalus (NPH): dementia, ataxia, and incontinence.[40, 147] The main clinical markers for suspecting communicating hydrocephalus are prolonged coma or an arrest in clinical progress.[124] Atypical presentations can include seizures, emotional problems, and spasticity.[20] The development of PTH is believed to be secondary to the impairment of flow and absorption of cerebrospinal fluid (CSF). This blockage can be around the cerebral convexities or, as some authors suggest, the blockage can be in the arachnoid granulations by subarachnoid blood. Patients with subarachnoid hemorrhage, which is believed to lead to an adhesive arachnoiditis or meningitis, are at highest risk for development of this complication. It was once hoped that MRI would aid in the detection of periventricular lucencies and that the diagnosis of PTH would be eased by this new modality.[234] Unfortunately, this has not been the case, and clinicians must rely on the CT criteria for diagnosing PTH[129] (Table 49–11).

If suspicion for the development of PTH is high, serial monthly CT scans for comparison can help make the diagnosis.[52, 129] Determining which patients might benefit from shunting is usually based on a constellation of findings. If the patient meets clinical and radiographic criteria for PTH, a lumbar puncture for craniospinal axis pressure should be obtained. Generally, shunting is successful if the pressure is elevated above 180 mm H_2O or if the ventricles progressively increase in size. The patient is also likely to benefit from shunt placement if there is a clinical picture of NPH.[176] CT cisternography and radionuclide cisternography can be helpful, but the reliability of these tests is not universally accepted. The potential of CSF bolus infusion studies to assess this condition in the TBI rehabilitation population has been relatively ignored, although results to date are extremely encouraging.[233]

The use of an adapted version of the CSF tap test[222] has been helpful in some cases. This test involves utilization of psychometric measures and gait pattern observation before and after a lumbar puncture in which a quantity of CSF is removed. Improvement in test results after the removal of fluid implies that successful results will occur if the patient is shunted.

TABLE 49–11   Computed Tomography (CT) Criteria to Define Hydrocephalus

1. "Distended" appearance of the anterior horns of the lateral ventricles
2. Enlargement of the temporal horns and third ventricle
3. Normal or absent sulci
4. If present, enlargement of the basal cisterns and fourth ventricle

Periventricular lucency was used as an indicator of communicating hydrocephalus.

Adapted from Kishore PRS, Lipper MH, Miller JD, et al: Posttraumatic hydrocephalus in patients with severe head injury. Neuroradiology 1978; 16:261–265.

Musculoskeletal Complications

It is unusual for TBI to be sustained without concomitant extremity injuries. As early as 1970, a study noted that 82% of patients with TBI admitted to the hospital sustained one or more extracranial injuries.[193] The Traumatic Brain Injury Model System National Database noted that 71% of patients had one or more associated injuries, of which cranial nerve injuries and fractures were the most common. A total of 406 fractures and 100 cranial nerve injuries were recorded in 323 patients.[29] Patients injured in pedestrian-automobile and motor vehicle crashes tend to have higher incidences of fractures and cranial nerve injuries than those injured by other causes. Problems with the patient's medical stability, impaired cognition, and extremity spasticity make diagnosis and management difficult for the trauma team. It would be ideal if all injuries and fractures were diagnosed and treated immediately in the acute care setting, but this is not true in many cases.

The physiatrist is often faced with the challenge of diagnosing musculoskeletal injuries in comatose and confused or agitated patients who are unable to cooperate in a complete sensorimotor evaluation or even to complain of pain. Most authors suggest getting a minimal set of radiographs that include the cervical spine, pelvis, hips, and knees to screen for fractures.[29] Routine anteroposterior and posteroanterior radiographs of the extremities in the comatose patient minimize the occurrence of undiagnosed injuries. Questionable fractures or dislocations deserve further evaluation by special radiographic techniques such as CT or MRI scans. Some authors advocate the use of a bone scan, 7 to 10 days after injury, to detect occult fractures.[105] An added advantage of bone scans is that they allow early detection of heterotopic ossification, as well as missed fractures.[24, 25] Treatment of musculoskeletal complications should always be based on the presumption that the patient will make a good recovery, regardless of prognostic indicators to the contrary. Orthopedic management should also take into account that the patient can pass through a state of agitation and develop spasticity.

Management techniques that require prolonged traction are often contraindicated, except in unusual circumstances, because they impede the rehabilitation program. Since spasticity usually causes joints to become flexed, immobilization by a cast in a flexed position should be avoided, even it adequately treats the fracture[105] (Table 49–12).

Cranial Nerve Damage

Cranial nerve damage is a frequent result of head injury. The impairment of sensorimotor function (e.g., sight, hearing, smell, taste, swallowing) can lead to further impairment of cognitive function in the already confused patient with a brain injury.[126]

TABLE 49–12   **Benefits of Early Fracture Stabilization**

Decreased pulmonary problems	Decreased mortality
Decreased pain medications	Shortened hospital stay
Improved nursing care	Facilitated rehabilitation
Avoidance of joint contractures	

From Hanscom DA: Acute management of the multiply injured head trauma patient. J Head Trauma Rehabil 1987; 2:1–12.

Patients injured in pedestrian-automobile and motor vehicle crashes have a higher incidence of cranial nerve injuries than those injured by other causes. Nineteen percent of the patients examined recently in a multicenter study had impairment of one or more cranial nerves. Cranial nerve VII (9% of patients) was injured most frequently, followed by cranial nerve III (6% of patients). The least frequently injured were cranial nerves IX and XI.[24, 25, 29] Impairment of olfaction can result from damage to cranial nerve I, and can be complete (anosmia) or partial (hyposmia). Olfactory impairment frequently results in taste alterations and may cause patients to have strange or new food preferences. Patients with an impaired sense of smell may require cueing for hygiene, cooking, storage of food, and use of perfumes. They may need to install smoke detectors and natural gas detectors to compensate for the sensory loss. Patients who work in the petrochemical industry can have significant problems returning to work safely, because they are unable to detect chemical leaks.[58]

Evaluation of cranial nerve VIII (vestibulocochlear nerve) usually occurs during the acute neurosurgical phase. Direct examination may reveal Battle's sign, mastoid fracture, otorrhea, bleeding from the ear, hemotympanum, and lacerations of the tympanic membrane. Hemorrhage from the ear and lacerations of the tympanic membrane might indicate a longitudinal fracture of the temporal bone. As the patient stabilizes, audiometry and the tuning fork test can be utilized. Brainstem auditory evoked potentials can provide further information on the integrity of the auditory system. If hearing loss is significant, hearing aids of the CROS (contralateral routing of signal) type, which transfers sound to the intact ear, will help the patient compensate.

Vestibular disturbances can result in ataxia or nystagmus or both. The Barany test, a provocative test using head rotation, is useful in evaluating nystagmus. Patients frequently compensate by tilting their head to decrease the nystagmus. Vestibular disturbances can be treated by habituation. The patient uses provocative exercises, which increase the symptoms, to decrease the sensitivity of the vestibular response. Common medications used for vestibular problems, such as meclazine or dimenhydrinate, are antihistamines and can cause sedation in patients with brain injuries. Physical therapy, as described above, and transdermal scopolamine patches are preferred.

Ocular Care

Patients may sustain direct injuries to the orbital area which result in not only cranial nerve injuries but also direct damage to the eye itself. In addition, patients with decreased ability to communicate are particularly susceptible to corneal injuries, especially with cranial nerve VII involvement. Injury to the facial nerve most commonly occurs at its passage through the temporal bone. The most deleterious effect is inadequate lid closure. The patient with this injury may be susceptible to exposure keratitis of the cornea and if cranial nerve V has also been injured, which results in corneal sensation being lost, the problem is then compounded. It is imperative that the eye be protected by use of lubricants and taping the lid closed with the use of eye pads. Unfortunately, this technique is not foolproof and, if not done properly, may cause further damage. Alternatively, an occlusive transparent film which covers the ocular area and creates a "wet chamber" has been successfully utilized in some patients to keep the cornea lubricated. Lid tarsorrhaphy might be necessary in order to prevent further damage, especially in a patient with a low cognitive level.

Injury to the motor system of the eye, controlled by cranial nerves III, IV, and VI, can occur at several levels, both centrally and peripherally. Secondary insults can occur after impact as with temporal herniation due to edema leading to cranial nerve III injury. Strabismus following trauma may be due to cranial nerve injuries, but there are also some gaze deviations in the early stages after brain injury which are not due to cranial nerve injury. Objective testing to determine ocular alignment can be simply determined by noting symmetrical placement of the corneal reflection of a penlight in each of the cardinal eye positions (Herschberg reflex). If the images on both corneas are centered, then the visual axes are usually well aligned. A cover/uncover test will generally determine the presence of misalignment of the visual axes when both eyes are viewing, but the need to ensure fixation may limit its utility and agitate a noncooperative patient. Convergence and accommodation testing should be performed carefully. Drug effects, most commonly due to phenytoin and phenobarbital, may also impair these reflexes. Diplopia occurring at near vision only may be the result of an impaired vergence system.[12]

Early evaluation by ophthalmology or optometry may be valuable to prevent secondary complications such as exposure keratitis of the cornea. It is unclear whether ocular motor exercises, utilized by neuro-optometry specialists, are of any value in this population since there are no comprehensive studies. However, anecdotal evidence by the authors indicate that such procedures can be at least helpful during the rehabilitation phase in allowing patients to see more clearly. Certainly, the use of corrective prisms when the patient's alignment is several diopters off is helpful for those patients who can utilize them.

Heterotopic Ossification

Heterotopic ossification (HO) is the formation of mature lamellar bone in soft tissues. The incidence of HO ranges from 11% to 76%, depending on the population studied and the method of detection.[81, 205] It appears that only 10% to 20% have functionally significant HO.[38] Brain-injured patients are at greater risk for developing HO if they have significant spasticity, duration of consciousness longer than 2 weeks, long-bone fractures, and decreased range of motion (ROM) (Table 49–13). Ectopic bone following brain injury usually forms around major joints, including the elbows, shoulders, hips, and knees, as well as over long-

TABLE 49–13   Risk Factors for Developing Heterotopic Ossification

Spasticity
Prolonged coma (>2 wk)
Long-bone fractures
Decreased range of motion

TABLE 49–14   Treatment of Heterotopic Ossification

Etidronate disodium (EHDP)	Surgery
Nonsteroidal anti-inflammatory drugs	Possibly verapamil
Radiation therapy	Possibly warfarin
Physical therapy	

From Buschbacher R: Heterotopic ossification: A review. Crit Rev Phys Med Rehabil 1992; 4:199.

bone fractures. It usually presents 1 to 3 months after the injury. It can mimic thrombophlebitis, with pain, swelling, erythema, and induration of the affected area. If it affects a joint, there is often a decrease in ROM.[38] Major long-term disability from untreated HO can include limited ROM or even joint ankylosis. Patients can experience pain, spasticity, vascular and nerve compression, and lymphedema.[82]

The diagnosis of HO following brain injury is typically made by the clinical examination and by assessing for elevations in alkaline phosphatase. Many clinicians rely on early detection of HO by utilizing triple-phase bone scan technology. Areas demonstrating increased blood flow and soft tissue concentration of the tracer on early imaging (blood flow phase) correlate with sites of subsequent HO development. The optimal timing of the imaging for accurate assessment of the presence of ectopic bone has not been established, but 3 weeks or more following the injury should be sufficient for early detection.[77] Plain radiographs may not show evidence of HO until 4 to 5 weeks after injury.[38]

Treatment options for HO are both pharmacological and nonpharmacological (Table 49–14). It is unclear why patients with brain injury, spinal cord injury, and total hip replacement develop HO. Because of this, it is difficult to utilize a scientific basis for treatment selection. The mainstay of drug treatment is etidronate disodium (EHDP, Didronel), which has been shown to reduce the incidence and severity of ectopic bone formation with minimal side effects in spinal cord–injured patients and in those who have undergone total hip arthroplasty.[74, 212] Although optimal drug dose and length of treatment have not been adequately established in TBI, Spielman and Gennarelli suggest using 20 mg/kg/day for 3 months, followed by 10 mg/kg/day for 3 to 6 months for a total of 6 to 9 months.[86, 211] Prophylaxis with EHDP after brain injury is not a routine practice in the United States.[197] The treatment of HO can also include the use of nonsteroidal anti-inflammatory drugs (NSAIDs) such as indomethacin or naproxen (Naprosyn). These NSAIDs theoretically decrease inflammation associated with HO. Several studies have demonstrated the prophylactic efficacy of indomethacin and salicylates in decreasing the incidence of ectopic bone following hip replacement and in pediatric brain injury.[172, 195] ROM exercises are an important part of the treatment protocol for HO. Continued ROM of the joint preserves the function while the ectopic bone matures and thus often alleviates the need for future treatment. There appears to be no research evidence to suggest that HO in humans is caused or worsened by vigorous ROM exercises. Ankylosed joints might require forceful manipulation under anesthesia to fragment the bone to improve ROM.[83] Once HO has matured, at 12 to 18 months or more after injury, it can be surgically removed or partially resected if clinically indicated. Postexcision low-dose radiation or the use of EHDP can prevent its recurrence.[55]

Spasticity

Until the early 1980s, spasticity following brain injury was generally treated in the same manner as spasticity following spinal cord injury, that is, with medications causing sedation, such as baclofen or diazepam. Spasticity that results from brain injury is more heavily influenced by such factors as postural changes, body positioning, and labyrinthine and tonic neck reflexes than is the case in spinal cord injuries. Spasticity can be a source of extreme discomfort in patients with brain injury who have intact sensation. Spasticity can have some beneficial effects, such as maintaining muscle bulk, preventing deep vein thrombosis or osteoporosis, and allowing patients with marginal motor strength to stand and transfer. It is only when spasticity interferes with function, causes pain, causes disfigurement, interferes with nursing care, or contributes to the formation of contractures that it needs to be treated. The current trend is away from pharmacological intervention (Fig. 49–8) and to the use of physical modalities. These include the application of either cold or heat; stretching, splinting, and casting (including inhibitory casting); proper positioning; functional electrical stimulation; vibration; relaxation techniques; motor re-education[47]; and biofeedback.[89, 194] In addition, modalities such as chemical neurolysis utilizing nerve blocks and motor point blocks can be tried before drug therapy is begun.[128, 138, 156–158, 220] A newer modality utilizing botulism toxin has been used successfully in some centers for the control of spasticity as well.[118] When drug therapy is indicated, dantrolene sodium (Dantrium) is usually the preferred drug, as it appears to have the least cognitive or sedating side effects. (For a fuller discussion of the management of spasticity, see Chapter 29.)

Thrombophlebitis

Thrombophlebitis due to prolonged immobilization can occur in the brain injury population and can be mistaken

for early HO, since the patient often complains of pain, swelling, erythema, and induration of the affected extremity. Thrombophlebitis is more frequent in a paralyzed extremity. The usual methods of diagnosis include duplex ultrasound or Doppler method, impedance plethysmography, or the more invasive contrast or radionuclide venogram. Intravenous or subcutaneous heparin in dosages sufficient to produce anticoagulation, followed by several months of warfarin anticoagulation, should be used, but with caution in agitated or confused patients who are at higher risk of injury and excessive bleeding. The insertion of venocaval filters or screens (Greenfield Filter or Modified Bird's Nest Filter) can be preferable for some brain-injured patients.[24, 25, 43, 123]

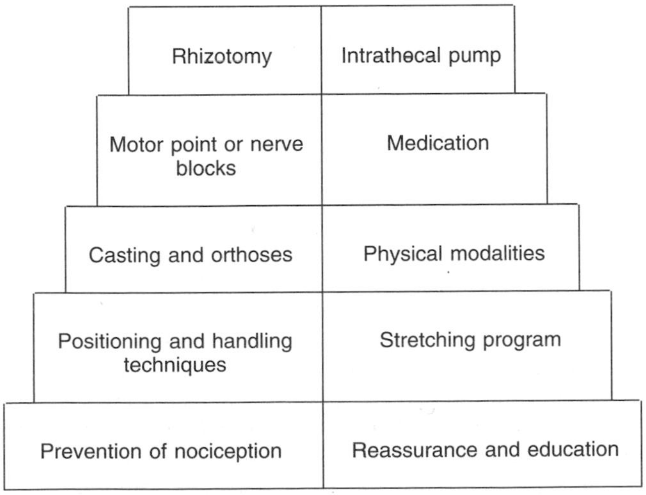

Respiratory Complications

One of the most common complications seen in severely brain-injured patients is respiratory failure, necessitating the use of artificial respiration for more than 1 week. A recent multicenter study revealed that 39% of all severe TBI patients were affected.[29] Radiographically defined pneumonitis was the second most common extracerebral complication identified in this study. This complication, along with respiratory failure, was associated with longer lengths of stay in both acute care and rehabilitation. Most patients with severe brain injury require oral or nasal intubation and many require tracheostomy. A high percentage of patients subsequently develop bacterial colonization at the tracheostomy site, which can lead to pneumonitis. Neurological deficits frequently compromise breathing, coughing, and routine pulmonary toilet. Patients can also suffer from recurrent reflux with aspiration as a result of dysphagia. Unfortunately, therefore, it is not uncommon for brain-injured patients to have a history of pneumonitis, including recurring pneumonitis, and to present to rehabilitation with a tracheostomy in place. Low-level patients (i.e., patients with Rancho Los Amigos Medical Center cognitive levels II or III; see Table 49–5) appear to have labile respiratory mechanisms and can lack adequate cough mechanisms. This predisposes this subpopulation to respiratory tract inflammation, infection, and prolonged hospitalization. Nowak et al.[179] recommended that these lower-level patients retain their tracheostomies because of the high morbidity and mortality when they are decannulated (31%). There appears to be a higher rate of morbidity and mortality associated with too early a decannulation.

Most clinicians do not remove the tracheostomy tube in brain-injured patients until they can safely swallow a regular diet. Decannulation is commonly accomplished by weaning down the tube size, followed by tracheostomy tube plugging over a continuous 24-hour period, and finally by removal. Some authors advocate an endoscopic examination of the larynx and trachea to detect granulation tissue that can impair breathing once the tracheostomy tube is removed.[130, 179] If tracheostomy plugging is to be accomplished safely, it is imperative that the tracheostomy tube of a smaller size be cuffless to prevent accidental suffocation.

Gastrointestinal Complications

Nutritional Status

The high caloric needs of an acutely brain-injured patient are well documented in the literature.[43, 46] Most trauma

Rhizotomy	Intrathecal pump
Motor point or nerve blocks	Medication
Casting and orthoses	Physical modalities
Positioning and handling techniques	Stretching program
Prevention of nociception	Reassurance and education

FIGURE 49–8 Pyramid of spasticity treatment.

centers now take into account the nutritional needs of acutely injured patients when these patients are fed primarily via enteral tube feedings. Patients who have suffered severe visceral trauma can require supplementation by hyperalimentation.[97] They subsequently usually come to the rehabilitation settings in positive nitrogen balance. The physician should consider not only calories and protein but also fiber, vitamins, minerals, and isotonicity of enteral feedings. Weekly weight measurements are appropriate during the rehabilitation phase, with monthly measurements of serum albumin and protein to monitor nutritional status.[24, 25, 43, 89]

Gastrointestinal Bleeding

As with most polytrauma patients, the patient with brain injury has an increased risk of gastrointestinal bleeding secondary to stress ulceration during the acute care phase.[43] It is not unusual for patients to be placed on histamine H_2-receptor antagonist prophylaxis with medications such as cimetidine or ranitidine.[103] Since cognitive and behavioral disturbances have been noted in patients on H_2-antagonists, these medications should be withdrawn once the risk of gastrointestinal bleeding has passed.

Swallowing Disorders

The incidence of dysphagia in patients with TBI coming to acute rehabilitation facilities is about 27%. Of those who exhibit dysphagia, approximately one third are severe, one third moderate, and one third mild cases. In a recent study in which patients were evaluated via videofluoroscopy, 81% of the patients had a delay or absence of swallowing responses, roughly 50% showed reduced tongue control, about one third had reduced pharyngeal transit, and 14% showed reduced laryngeal closure, elevation, or spasms. Most patients showed two dysfunctional aspects of swallowing, such as impaired tongue control and delayed triggering mechanisms.[136]

Videofluoroscopy has become the gold standard for evaluating patients for dysphagia. This technique allows the clinician to observe the anatomy and physiology of the swallowing mechanism as a bolus (a barium-impregnated liquid or cookie) travels from the mouth through the pharynx and into the esophagus. Various dysfunctions can be noted on the video examination. Compensatory strategies can also be tried and tested during the evaluation.[1]

Patients with swallowing difficulties often have concomitant cognitive difficulties. They often need to be reminded and monitored to employ compensatory strategies. Their diets need to be changed in a sequential fashion, (i.e., from pureed, ground, chopped, soft, to regular), as their use of compensatory mechanisms increases or the swallowing mechanism improves. Treatment efforts are primarily didactic in which compensatory mechanisms are taught. The vast majority of patients improve spontaneously, although this can take several weeks, during which time the patient has a high risk for developing aspiration pneumonia. *Thin liquids are to be avoided in the acute neurosurgical setting, since they are typically the most difficult to handle from a swallowing perspective and can lead to the early complication of aspiration pneumonia.* Patients who fail to progress cognitively, who are unable to follow commands,

who have significant swallowing difficulties, who are at high risk for aspiration, or who are known aspirators need to be fed via an enteral tube. The decision to remove a nasogastric tube and place a gastrostomy tube usually hinges on whether the patient will need the gastrostomy tube for longer than 3 to 4 weeks. If the prognosis is such that the patient will require prolonged enteral feedings, it is best to remove the nasogastric tube and put a gastrostomy tube in place to avoid such problems as the patient removing the tube, nasal ulceration, nasal pharyngeal irritation, and infection. The tube can be placed with an open surgical procedure (gastrostomy) or using an endoscopic technique. Using a small jejunostomy tube will prevent the problem of continued reflux by utilizing the patient's cardiac sphincter (between the esophagus and the stomach) as well as pyloric sphincter (between the stomach and the duodenum) to prevent reflux. It can also be placed percutaneously utilizing a tube that is smaller and easier to insert. This approach, however, does not allow the passing of another tube to the jejunum.[26, 89]

Clinically, the use of blue food coloring or methylene blue to dye tube feedings helps identify tracheal aspirations of feedings as opposed to mouth secretions. Continuous feedings are very difficult when the patient goes to therapy and therefore a primarily placed jejunostomy tube is not ideal in this situation unless the patient is suffering from severe reflux and aspiration. If reflux is of concern, the head of the bed needs to be elevated and the patient should be tried on various formulas or smaller feedings. The use of metoclopramide (Reglan)[168] should be avoided. This drug is like the phenothiazines, and while it can help initially with reflux by increasing gastric emptying in a small percentage of patients, it is not particularly useful in the long term and is known to cause significant cognitive difficulties, especially for those regaining consciousness. It also has potential side effects of extrapyramidal movements and even permanent tardive dyskinesia. In addition to impeding cognitive recovery, patients may also have swallowing difficulties as the result of the use of metoclopramide. If the patient has to be on metoclopramide for any reason, it should be limited to 2 weeks or less.[24, 25, 89] Alternatively, erythromycin may be useful in increasing gastric emptying. (For a fuller discussion of swallowing disorders, see Chapter 27.)

Bowel Incontinence

Fecal incontinence in brain-injured patients is fairly common, especially in patients with significant cognitive impairments. Following brain injury, patients can have an uninhibited neurogenic bowel and be unaware of the need to defecate in a timely and appropriate manner. They can also have constipation or diarrhea. The development of a daily bowel training program is appropriate regardless of the patient's cognitive status, and can be accomplished through the use of high fiber enteral feedings or supplementation of fiber orally and the use of a suppository, such as glycerin rectal suppositories daily or every other day.[221] Use of digital stimulation should be avoided as it can be misinterpreted by patients who have cognitive difficulties. Diarrhea can be the result of impaction and osmolar overload from tube feedings, but also can be due to *Clostridium difficile* colitis. Patients with brain injury are at an increased risk of *C. difficile* because they often have had prior antibiotic administration during the acute care phase. Screening for *C. difficile* toxin is indicated in the patient with a prior history of antibiotic administration and hospital-acquired diarrhea.[139] (For a fuller discussion of bowel management, see Chapter 28.)

Genitourinary Problems

Neurogenic bladder following TBI is quite rare and if it does exist, it is usually due to uninhibited detrusor hyperreflexia causing the patient to void small amounts frequently. Patients can usually be adequately managed with an external collection device, such as an external condom catheter in males or a diaper in females, until they are aware of their surroundings and have sufficient memory to benefit from being offered a commode or bedpan on a regular basis.[99, 120] Patients can also have detrusor hyporeflexia as a result of bladder overdistention that occurs with iatrogenic or traumatic outlet obstruction. These patients usually require prolonged intermittent catheterization (IC) or an indwelling Foley catheter until this problem has resolved, which may take weeks to months. It is the rare, primarily brainstem-injured patient with detrusor sphincter dyssynergia who needs intermittent catheterization or prolonged Foley catheter drainage and complete urological studies.[8] Patients in acute care settings are often subjected to indwelling Foley catheterization to monitor urine output. Such instrumentation can be a source of chronic infection.[221] (For a fuller discussion of genitourinary problems, see Chapter 28.)

Dermatologic Complications

Lacerations are the most frequent extracranial injury in the brain injury population. It is very common for patients to have healing lacerations and abrasions. This can be quite disfiguring to young adults, especially around the face, and special cosmetics can be used to hide and cover such scars until they can be revised (Dermablend Corrective Cosmetics, P.O. Box 3008, Lakewood, NJ 08701). Acne due to exogenous or endogenous corticosteroids is also common and, although not disabling, can be a cosmetic problem for the cognitively impaired teenager and might need to be managed aggressively. Fortunately, pressure ulcers are rare in brain-injured patients, but can occur due to secondary immobilization (see also Chapter 31).

Endocrine Complications

The most frequent endocrine complication seen in the acute care setting is that of disturbances of antidiuretic hormone (ADH) secretion.[43, 106] The syndrome of inappropriate ADH secretion (SIADH), resulting in oversecretion of ADH with a resultant decrease in sodium concentration, occurs frequently during the acute care phase.[61] Fluid restriction is usually all that is required and the problem typically resolves spontaneously. However, water restriction to as little as 800 mL/day is difficult when patients are receiving multiple medications. The patients might need further therapy to correct hypertonicity with use of urea and sodium chloride.

Less common is the disruption of ADH release, which results in central diabetes insipidus (DI). In contrast to the more commonly seen SIADH, DI is rare following TBI. DI can be treated with vasopressin tannate in oil or internasal 1-desamino-8-D-arginine vasopressin (DDAVP).[178] Simultaneous urine and serum osmolality screening can be initiated in those patients with severe injuries who exhibit serum sodium abnormalities and evidence of impaired fluid homeostasis.

Anterior hypopituitarism secondary to TBI, although rare, should be suspected in those patients who have anorexia, low body temperature, bradycardia, hypotension, malaise, hypoglycemia, and hyponatremia.[13, 131] About 20% of severe TBI patients[110] suffer from one or more disturbances related to anterior pituitary hormone levels. The significance of these is not yet known and further studies are needed and are in fact ongoing.

Thyroid dysfunction, in the form of euthyroid disease, can also be seen post injury. Significant thyroid dysfunction following TBI is rare, however.

Sexual dysfunction can be seen in several forms following brain injury.[98, 112] The most common manifestations include problems with delayed resumption of menstruation and libidinal changes,[79] although exact neuroendocrine correlates to these clinical manifestations have not been identified. Screening serum pregnancy tests (e.g., qualitative β-human choriogonadotropin [β-HCG]) are indicated in all females of childbearing age regardless of reported sexual history or last menstrual period[182] (see also Chapter 30).

Autonomic Disturbances

Hypertension following TBI is quite frequent and is often the result of high intracranial pressure and catecholamine release with increased cardiac output and tachycardia in the acute care setting.[171, 202] Focal brain injuries with lesions near the hypothalamus can also cause hypertension.[199] Treatment with β-blockers might be necessary, especially if the patient is in a hyperdynamic state. The use of β-blockers, such as propranolol, should be limited to the period of time when they are essential, since most hypertension secondary to TBI is self-limited. Essential or primary hypertension not related to brain injury should also be treated with the least cognitively sedating drugs, such as diuretics or clonidine (Catapres).

Hypotension can occur and is usually orthostatic, mostly due to prolonged bed rest. Patients with concomitant spinal cord injuries or brainstem injuries are particularly sensitive and can have additional problems with decreased blood pressure. Hypopituitarism can also present clinically as profound hypotension. Treatment usually includes compression garments on the lower extremities to increase venous return, as well as the use of pharmaceuticals such as ephedrine.

Temperature instability infrequently occurs, but can present as either central fever or hypothermia. Patients with prolonged febrile illness without a documentable source can be safely assumed to have central fever.[217] Central fever is usually secondary to lesions in the anterior hypothalamus and to generalized decerebration. Central fever can also result from drug fever and from neuroleptic malignant syndrome, secondary to phenothiazines. Temperature elevation as a result of brain injury can be treated with physical modalities, such as cooling blankets and tepid baths, or pharmacologically with morphine, neuroleptic-type medications, dopamine agonists (e.g., bromocriptine, levodopa), dantrolene sodium, and prostaglandin inhibitors (e.g., indomethacin).[15, 24, 25]

Hypothermia can result from lesions in the posterior hypothalamus and also from myxedema, hypothyroidism, and barbiturates. Treatment depends on the cause of the problem. If hypothermia is secondary to posterior hypothalamic damage, maintenance of body temperature is dependent on the external environment.

REHABILITATION OF THE PEDIATRIC PATIENT WITH TRAUMATIC BRAIN INJURY

Pediatric TBI differs in several important ways from TBI in the adult. Pathologically, TBI in infants and children produces a higher frequency of diffuse cerebral swelling and a lower frequency of intracranial hemorrhage than that seen in adults.[206] A complicating epidemiological factor is that an unknown proportion of pediatric TBI is caused by child abuse. Special assessment techniques, such as the Children's Orientation and Amnesia Test (COAT),[68] are used to evaluate the level of consciousness and duration of PTA in infants and children. Severe TBI in infancy and childhood appears to have a better prognosis for recovery of consciousness and motoric functions.[173, 174] However, certain types of brain injury suffered at younger ages (e.g., closed head injury with diffuse damage during infancy) can lead to worse functional outcomes than the same injuries suffered in adulthood. This vulnerability has been attributed to the cumulative effects of TBI on learning,[76] leading to a slower rate of skill development and a lower level of adult competence in some patients.

A unique feature of pediatric brain injury rehabilitation is the need for long-term follow-up of the child's progress in school. The rehabilitation program should be prepared to help the parents advocate for the child's needs and to provide teachers with specific recommendations to modify the child's educational program.[122] The team should also be prepared to work closely with the parents in a co-therapist role on a long-term basis. Detailed information about pediatric rehabilitation is provided in recent book chapters.[78, 116, 230]

REHABILITATION OF MILD TRAUMATIC BRAIN INJURY

Mild TBI and its rehabilitation are detailed in several recent books and articles[14, 23, 113, 144] The incidence of mild TBI could be higher than reported in epidemiological studies of hospital admissions, because many mild TBI patients fail to seek medical attention or are discharged home from the emergency department. Diagnostic criteria for mild TBI were presented in Table 49–3. Note that loss of consciousness is not a criterion for mild TBI. Instead, the hallmark of mild TBI is that the patient have a period of PTA immediately following the injury, and be later unable to recall all or part of the events surrounding the injury. Mild TBI might be overlooked in the presence of orthopedic injuries which may require rehabilitation.

The constellation of symptoms reported by mild TBI patients, which has been termed the *postconcussional syndrome*,[23, 113, 144] includes symptoms in physical (e.g., dizziness, headache), cognitive (e.g., decreased recent memory), and emotional domains (e.g., irritability). It is now believed that, at least during the acute phase, these symptoms are organically rather than functionally caused in the majority of patients.[23] Although most mild TBI patients make a good recovery and have few long-term symptom complaints,[7] there is controversy about whether a subgroup of symptomatic patients has permanent impairments.[21, 66]

Management of the patient with mild TBI is guided by physical evidence of brain injury, age, and the chronicity of the disorder. Patients with CT or MRI evidence of brain injury may have poorer prognoses than those with uncomplicated mild TBI.[223] Elderly patients with uncomplicated mild TBI can have deficits similar to those seen in young or middle-aged adults with moderate TBI. Guidelines for management of acute sports-related mild TBI[127] are presented in Table 49–15. The patient with acute mild TBI should be encouraged to limit responsibilities temporarily and to resume them gradually. The patient and family

---

TABLE 49–15 Colorado Medical Society Guidelines for the Management of Concussion in Sports

Grade 1	Confusion without amnesia, no loss of consciousness	Remove from contest. Examine immediately and every 5 min for development of amnesia or postconcussive symptoms at rest and with exertion. Permit return to contest if amnesia does not appear and no symptoms appear for at least 20 min
Grade 2	Confusion with amnesia, no loss of consciousness	Remove from contest and disallow return. Examine frequently for signs of evolving intracranial symptoms. Re-examine the next day. Permit return to practice after 1 full wk without symptoms
Grade 3	Loss of consciousness	Transport from field to nearest hospital by ambulance (with cervical spine immobilization if indicated). Perform thorough neurological evaluation emergently. Admit to hospital if pathologic signs are detected. If findings are normal, instruct family for overnight observation. Permit return to practice only after 2 full wk without symptoms

Prolonged unconsciousness, persistent mental status alterations, worsening postconcussion symptoms, or abnormalities on neurological examination require urgent neurosurgical consultation or transfer to a trauma center.

Adapted with permission of the Colorado Medical Society, Denver.

should be educated about the typical postconcussional symptoms.[23] While reassuring patients of a probable good recovery, their specific symptom complaints (e.g., headache, vertigo) should be investigated.[113] Post-traumatic headaches are a common symptom and can respond to standard treatments[66] (Table 49–16). Serial administration of a brief neuropsychological test battery can help guide the patient in gradually resuming responsibilities.

Management of the chronic mild TBI patient is controversial.[5, 66, 67, 94] The physiatrist should rule out the possibility that the patient has an unsuspected or untreated medical complication such as headache or neck pain.[113] Review of the acute medical records might reveal that a patient diagnosed with mild TBI actually had a moderate or severe TBI, or that there was questionable evidence that any brain injury occurred. The presence of functional limitations or subjective complaints that are out of proportion to the documented severity of the brain injury should alert the physiatrist to the possibility of malingering or of a psychiatric disorder, such as a somatoform disorder or post-traumatic stress disorder.

SUMMARY

Brain injury rehabilitation covers not only patients with traumatic injuries but also those with acquired brain injuries due to anoxia, cancer, certain types of strokes, and other nontraumatic causes. Knowledge of the pattern and overall severity of each patient's brain injury is necessary for planning treatment and predicting long-term outcome. Rehabilitation should begin early in the acute care phase in order to prevent later complications. Evaluation of the acutely brain-injured patient by a rehabilitation physician should be mandatory before the patient can be transferred to a nursing home. Despite wide variation in their neurological, cognitive, and behavioral deficits, severely brain-injured patients tend to pass through similar stages of neurobehavioral recovery. Specialized brain injury rehabilitation units are guided by the physical and cognitive-behavioral limitations at each patient's current stage of recovery. Specific therapy and medication protocols have been developed for patients who are unconscious or agitated. Treatment of medical complications for patients in these stages needs to be modified to avoid interference with recovery and rehabilitation. Although research advances have led to many changes in the treatment of medical complications, particularly post-traumatic seizures, many more questions in brain injury rehabilitation remain to be investigated. It is hoped that future research will develop pharmacological tools that can directly improve the extent of recovery following brain injury.

Acknowledgments

Preparation of this chapter was supported in part by grants H133A20004 (Traumatic Brain Injury Model System of TIRR) and H133B40002 (Rehabilitation Research and Training Center on Rehabilitation Interventions Following Traumatic Brain Injury) from the National Institute of Disability Related Research, and grant H128A0019 (Southwest Regional Brain Injury Rehabilitation and Prevention Center) from the Rehabilitation Services Administration, U.S. Department of Education, Washington, D.C. The authors are grateful to Dr. Flora Hammond for her comments, Mike DeLaFlor for artwork, Johnny Airhart for photography, and DeeDee Webb for preparing the manuscript.

TABLE 49–16   Treatments for Postconcussion Syndrome

Muscle contraction–type headaches
    Simple analgesics
    Nonsteroidal anti-inflammatory drugs (NSAIDs)
    Antidepressants
    Muscle relaxants
    TENS unit
    Barbiturates-narcotics (with caution)
    Biofeedback
Migraine-type headaches
    Prophylactic drugs
        β-Blockers
        Antidepressants
        NSAIDs
        Calcium channel blockers
        Valproic acid
    Abortive drugs
        Ergotamine
        Dihydroergotamine
        Sumatriptan
        Isometheptene
        Barbiturates-narcotics (with caution)
Occipital neuralgia
    Greater occipital nerve block
    NSAIDs
    Muscle relaxants
    Carbamazepine
    TENS unit
    Rarely surgical
Psychological support
? Cognitive rehabilitation
Education for all involved

Abbreviation: TENS = transcutaneous electrical nerve stimulator.
Modified from Evans RW: The postconcussion syndrome and the sequelae of mild head injury. Neurol Clin 1992; 10:815.

References

1. Adamovich BB: Treatment of communication and swallowing disorders. *In* Rosenthal M, Griffith ER, Bond MR, Miller JD (eds): Rehabilitation of the Adult and Child With Traumatic Brain Injury, ed 2. Philadelphia, FA Davis, 1990, pp 374–392.
2. Adamovich BB, Henderson JA, Auerbach S: Cognitive Rehabilitation of Closed Head Injured Patients: A Dynamic Approach. San Diego, College-Hill Press, 1985.
3. Adams JH: Head injury. *In* Adams JH, Duchen LW (eds): Greenfield's Neuropathology, ed 4. London, Edward Arnold, 1992.
4. Adams RD, Victor M: Principles of Neurology, ed 5. New York, McGraw-Hill, 1993.
5. Alexander MP: Neuropsychiatric correlates of persistent postconcussive syndrome. J Head Trauma Rehabil 1992; 7:60.
6. Alexander MP: Traumatic brain injury. *In* Benson DF, Blumer D (eds): Psychiatric Aspects of Neurologic Disease. New York, Grune & Stratton, 1982, pp 219–249.
7. Alves W, Macciocchi SN, Barth JT: Postconcussive symptoms after uncomplicated mild head injury. J Head Trauma Rehabil 1993;8:48.
8. Anderson JT: Neuro-urological investigation in urinary bladder dysfunction. Int Urol Nephrol 1977; 9:133.
9. Andrews DG, Tomlinson L, Elwes RDC, et al: The influence of carbamazepine and phenytoin on memory and other aspects of cognitive function in new referrals with epilepsy. Acta Neurol Scand Suppl 1984; 69(99):23.
10. Ansell B, Keenan J: The Western Neurosensory Stimulation Profile: A tool for assessing slow-to-recover head injured patients. Arch Phys Med Rehabil 1989; 70:104.

11. Aronow HU: Rehabilitation effectiveness with severe brain injury: Translating research into policy. J Head Trauma Rehabil 1987; 2:24.

12. Baker RS, Epstein AD: Ocular motor abnormalities from head trauma: Major review. Surv Ophthalmol 1991; 35:245.

13. Barreca T, Perrea C, Sannia A, et al: Evaluation of anterior pituitary function in patients with posttraumatic diabetes insipidus. J Clin Endocrinol Metab 1980; 51:1279.

14. Barth JT, Macciocchi SN (eds): Mild traumatic brain injury. J Head Trauma Rehabil 1993, vol 8.

15. Benedek G, Toth-Daru P, Janaky J, et al: Indomethacin is effective against neurogenic hyperthermia following cranial trauma or brain surgery. Can J Neurol Sci 1987; 14:145.

16. Ben-Yishay Y, Prigatano GP: Cognitive remediation. In Rosenthal M, Griffith ER, Bond MR, Miller JD (eds): Rehabilitation of the Adult Child with Traumatic Brain Injury. Philadelphia, FA Davis, 1990.

17. Berrol S: Issues in cognitive rehabilitation. Arch Neurol 1990; 47:219.

18. Berrol S: Persistent vegetative state. Phys Med Rehabil 1990; 4:559.

19. Berrol S (ed): Traumatic brain injury. Phys Med Rehabil Clin North Am 1992; 3:2.

20. Beyerl B, Black PM: Posttraumatic hydrocephalus. Neurosurgery 1984; 15:257.

21. Binder LM: Persisting symptoms after mild head injury: A review of the postconcussive syndrome. J Clin Exp Neuropsychol 1986; 8:323.

22. Boake C: A history of cognitive rehabilitation of head-injured patients, 1915 to 1980. J Head Trauma Rehabil 1989; 4:1.

23. Boake C, Bobitec K, Bontke CF: Rehabilitation of the mild traumatic brain injury patient. Neurorehabilitation 1991; 1:70.

24. Bontke CF: Medical advances in the treatment of brain injury. In Kreutzer JS, Wehman PA, Brooks PH (eds): Community Reintegration Following Traumatic Brain Injury. Baltimore, Williams & Wilkins, 1990, pp 3–13.

25. Bontke CF: Medical complications related to traumatic brain injury. Phys Med Rehabil State 1989; 3:1.

26. Bontke CF, Baize CM, Boake C: Coma management and sensory stimulation. Traumatic brain injury. Phys Med Rehabil Clin North Am 1992; 3:259.

27. Bontke CF, Boake C, Zasler ND: Rehabilitation of the head injured patient. In Narayan RK, Wilberger JE Jr, Povilshock JT (eds): Neurotrauma. New York, McGraw-Hill (in press).

28. Bontke CF, Horn LJ, Sandel B: Sensory stimulation: Accepted practice or expected practice? J Head Trauma Rehabil 1992; 7:115.

29. Bontke CF, Lehmkuhl DL, Englander JS, et al: Medical complications and associated injuries of persons treated in Traumatic Brain Injury Model Systems Programs. J Head Trauma Rehabil 1993; 8:34.

30. Bontke CF, Reinhard DL, Yablon SA: Anticonvulsant prophylaxis for the prevention of late posttraumatic epilepsy. J Head Trauma Rehabil 1993; 8:101.

31. Braakman R, Jennett WB, Minderhoud JB: Prognosis of the posttraumatic vegetative state. Acta Neurochir 1988; 95:49.

32. Bricolo A, Turazzi S, Feriotti G: Prolonged posttraumatic unconsciousness: Therapeutic assets and liabilities. J Neurosurg 1980; 52:625.

33. Brigman C, Dickey C, Zegeer LJ: Agitated aggressive patient. Am J Nurs 1983; 83:1409.

34. Brooke MM, Patterson DR, Questad KA, et al: The treatment of agitation during initial hospitalization after traumatic brain injury. Arch Phys Med Rehabil 1992; 73:917.

35. Brooke MM, Questad KA, Patterson DR, Bashak KJ: Agitation and restlessness after closed head injury: A prospective study of 100 consecutive admissions. Arch Phys Med Rehabil 1992; 73:320.

36. Brooks DN: Closed Head Injury: Psychological, Social and Family Consequences. New York, Oxford University Press, 1984, pp 1–226.

37. Brooks DN: The head-injured family. J Clin Exp Neuropsychol 1991; 13:155.

38. Buschbacher R: Heterotopic ossification: A review. Crit Rev Phys Med Rehabil 1992; 4:199.

39. Butler RW, Namerow N: Cognitive retraining in brain injury rehabilitation: A critical review. J Neurol Rehabil 1988; 2:97.

40. Cardoso ER, Galbraith S: Posttraumatic hydrocephalus: A retrospective review. Surg Neurol 1985; 23:261.

41. Carey RG, Seiberg JH, Posavac EJ: Who makes the most progress in inpatient rehabilitation?: An analysis of functional gain. Arch Phys Med Rehabil 1988; 69:337.

42. Cassidy JW: Neuropharmacological management of destructive behavior after traumatic brain injury. J Head Trauma Rehabil 1994; 9:43.

43. Chestnut RM: Medical complications of the head injured patient. In Cooper PR (ed): Head Injury, ed 3. Baltimore, Williams & Wilkins, 1993.

44. Choi DW, Rothman SM: The role of glutamate neurotoxicity in hypoxic-ischemic neuronal death. Annu Rev Neurosci 1990; 13:171.

45. Clifton GL, Jiang JY, Lyeth BG, et al: Marked protection by moderate hypothermia after experimental traumatic brain injury. J Cereb Blood Flow Metab 1991; 11:114.

46. Clifton GL, Ziegler MG, Grossman RG: Circulating catecholamines and sympathetic activity after head injury. Neurosurgery 1981; 8:10.

47. Conine TA, Sullivan T, Mackie T, Goodman M: Effect of serial casting for the prevention of equinus in patients with acute head injury. Arch Phys Med Rehabil 1990; 71:310.

48. Cooper PR: Gunshot wounds of the brain. In Cooper PR (ed): Head Injury, ed 3. Baltimore, Williams & Wilkins, 1993, pp 355–371.

49. Cooper PR (ed): Head Injury, ed 3. Baltimore, Williams & Wilkins, 1993.

50. Cope DN: Neuropharmacology and brain damage. In Christensen AL, Uzzell BP (eds): Neuropsychological Rehabilitation: Current Knowledge and Future Directions. Boston, Kluwer, 1987, pp 19–39.

51. Cope DN: Traumatic closed head injury: Status of rehabilitation treatment. Semin Neurol 1985; 5:212.

52. Cope DN, Date ES, Mar EY: Serial computerized tomographic evaluations in traumatic head injury. Arch Phys Med Rehabil 1988; 69:483.

53. Corrigan JD: Substance abuse as a mediating factor in outcome from traumatic brain injury. Arch Phys Med Rehabil 1995; 76:302.

54. Corrigan JD, Arnett JA, Houck LJ, Jackson RD: Reality orientation for brain injured patients: Group treatment and monitoring of recovery. Arch Phys Med Rehabil 1985; 66:626.

55. Coventry MB, Scanlon PW: The use of radiation to discourage ectopic bone. J Bone Joint Surg Am 1981; 63:201.

56. Dacey R, Dikmen S, Temkin N, et al: Relative effects of brain and non-brain injuries on neuropsychological and psychosocial outcome. J Trauma 1991; 31:217.

57. Davidoff GN, Roth EJ, Richards JS: Cognitive deficits in spinal cord injury: Epidemiology and outcome. Arch Phys Med Rehabil 1992; 73:275.

58. Deems DA, Doty RL, Settle G, et al: Smell and taste disorders: A study of 750 patients from the University of Pennsylvania Smell and Taste Center. Arch Otolaryngol Head Neck Surg 1991; 117:519.

59. Dikmen S, Machamer J, Temkin N: Psychosocial outcome in patients with moderate to severe head injury: 2-year follow-up. Brain Inj 1993; 7:113.

60. Dikmen SS, Temkin NR, Miller B, et al: Neurobehavioral effects of phenytoin prophylaxis of posttraumatic seizures. JAMA 1991; 265:1271.

61. Doczi T, Tarjanyi J, Huszka E, Kiss J: Syndrome of inappropriate secretion of antidiuretic hormone (SIADH) after head injury. Neurosurgery 1980; 10:685.

62. Drugs for epilepsy. Medical Lett Drugs Ther 1986;28:91–94.

63. Eames P, Haffey WJ, Cope DN: Treatment of behavioral disorders. In Rosenthal M, Griffith ER, Bond MR, Miller JD (eds). Rehabilitation of the Adult and Child with Traumatic Brain Injury, ed 2. Philadelphia, FA Davis, 1990, pp 410–432.

64. Eisenberg HM: Outcome after head injury: General considerations and neurobehavioral recovery—Part I, General considerations. In Becker DP, Povlishock JT (eds): Central Nervous System Trauma Status Report. Bethesda, Md, National Institute of Neurological and Communicative Diseases and Stroke, 1985.

65. Eisenberg HM, Gary HE Jr, Aldrich EF, et al: Initial CT findings in 753 patients with severe head injury: A report from the NIH Traumatic Coma Data Bank. J Neurosurg 1990; 73:688.

66. Evans RW: The postconcussion syndrome and the sequelae of mild head injury. Neurol Clin 1992; 10:815.

67. Evans RW: Postconcussive syndrome: An overview. Tex Med 1987; 83:49.

68. Ewing-Cobbs L, Levin HS, Fletcher JM, et al: The Children's Orientation and Amnesia Test: Relationship to severity of acute head injury and to recovery of memory. Neurosurgery 1990; 27:683.

69. Farwell JR, Lee YJ, Hirtz DG, et al: Phenobarbitol for febrile seizures—effects on intelligence and on seizure recurrence. N Engl J Med 1990; 322:364.

70. Fedoroff JP, Starkstein SE, Forrester AW, et al: Depression in patients with acute traumatic brain injury. Am J Psychiatry 1992; 149:918.

71. Feeney DM: Pharmacologic modulation of recovery after brain injury: A reconsideration of diaschisis. J Neuro Rehabil 1991; 5:113.

72. Feeney DM, Sutton RL: Pharmacotherapy for recovery of function after brain injury. CRC Crit Rev Neurobiol 1987; 3:135.

73. Feeney DM, Walker AE: The prediction of posttraumatic epilepsy. Arch Neurol 1979; 36:8.

74. Fingerman G, Krengel W, Lowell JD, et al: Role of diphosphonate EHDP in the prevention of heterotopic ossification after total hip arthroplasty: Preliminary report. Proceedings of the Fifth Open Scientific Meeting of the Hip Society. St Louis, Mosby–Year Book, 1977, pp 222–234.

75. Finlayson MAJ, Garner SH (eds): Brain Injury Rehabilitation: Clinical Considerations. Baltimore, Williams & Wilkins, 1994.

76. Fletcher JM, Ewing-Cobbs L, Francis DJ, et al: Variability in outcomes after traumatic brain injury: A developmental perspective: In Broman SH, Michell M (eds): Traumatic Brain Injury in Children. New York, Oxford University Press, in press.

77. Freed JH, Hahn H, Menter R, et al: The use of the three-phase bone scan in the early diagnosis of heterotopic ossification (HO) and in the evaluation of Didronel therapy. Paraplegia 1982; 20:208.

78. Gans BM, Mann NR, Ylvisaker M: Rehabilitation management approaches. In Rosenthal M, Griffith ER, Bond MR, Miller JD (eds): Rehabilitation of the Adult and Child with Traumatic Brain Injury, ed 2. Philadelphia, FA Davis, 1990, pp 593–615.

79. Garden F, Bontke CF: Sexual functioning and marital adjustment after traumatic brain injury. J Head Trauma Rehabil 1990; 5:52–59.

80. Garland DE, Bailey S: Undetected injuries in head-injured adults. Clin Orthop 1981; 155:162.

81. Garland DE, Blum CE, Waters RL: Periarticular heterotopic ossification in head-injured adults. J Bone Joint Surg Am 1981; 62:1143.

82. Garland DE, Keenan MAE: Orthopedic strategies in the management of the adult head-injured patient. Phys Ther 1983; 63:2004.

83. Garland DE, Razza BE, Waters RL: Forceful joint manipulation in head-injured adults with heterotopic ossification. Clin Orthop 1982; 169:133.

84. Gean AD: Imaging of Head Trauma. New York, Raven Press, 1994.

85. Gennarelli TA: Cerebral concussion and diffuse brain injuries. In Cooper PA (ed). Head Injury, ed 3. Philadelphia. Williams & Wilkins, 1993, pp 137–158.

86. Gennarelli TA: Subject review: Heterotopic ossification. Brain Inj 1988; 2:175.

87. Gentry LR, Godersky JC, Thompson B: MR imaging of head trauma: Review of the distribution and radiopathologic features of traumatic lesions. AJNR 1988; 150:663.

88. Giacino JT, Kczmarsky MA, DeLuca J, Cicerone KD: Monitoring rate of recovery to predict outcome in minimally responsive patients. Arch Phys Med Rehabil 1991; 72:897.

89. Glenn MB, Rosenthal M: Rehabilitation following severe traumatic brain injury. Semin Neurol 1985; 5:233.

90. Glenn MB, Wroblewski B: Anticonvulsants for prophylaxis of posttraumatic seizures. J Head Trauma Rehabil 1986; 1:73.

91. Glenn MB, Wroblewski B, Parziale J, et al: Lithium carbonate for aggressive behavior or affective instability in ten brain-injured patients. Am J Phys Med Rehabil 1989; 68:221.

92. Goldenberg G, Oder W, Spatt J, et al: Cerebral correlates of disturbed executive function and memory in survivors of severe closed head injury: A SPECT study. J Neurol Neurosurg Psychiatry 1992; 55:362.

93. Gordon WA, Mann N, Willer B: Demographic and social characteristics of the Traumatic Brain Injury Model System Database. J Head Trauma Rehabil 1993; 8:26.

94. Gouvier WD, Uddo-Crane M, Brown LM: Base rates of postconcussional symptoms. Arch Clin Neuropsychol 1988; 3:273.

95. Graham DI: Hypoxia and vascular disorders. In Adams JD, Duchen LW (eds): Greenfield's Neuropathology, ed 5. New York, Oxford University Press, 1992, pp 153–268.

96. Graham DI, Adams JH, Genarelli TA: Pathology of brain damage in head injury: In Cooper PR (ed): Head Injury, ed 3. Baltimore, Williams & Wilkins, 1993, pp 91–113.

97. Graham TW, Zadrozny DB, Harrington T: The benefits of early jejunal hyperalimentation in the head-injured patient. Neurosurgery 1989; 25:729.

98. Griffith ER, Cole S, Cole TM: Sexuality and sexual dysfunction. In Rosenthal M, Griffith ER, Bond MR, Miller JD (eds): Rehabilitation of the Adult Child with Traumatic Brain Injury, ed 2. Philadelphia, FA Davis, 1990, pp 206–224.

99. Grinspun D: Bladder management for adults following head injury. Rehabil Nurs 1993; 18:300.

100. Groswasser Z, Cohen M, Costeff H: Rehabilitation outcome after anoxic brain damage. Arch Phys Med Rehabil 1989; 70:186.

101. Gualtieri CT: Pharmacotherapy and the neurobehavioral sequelae of traumatic brain injury. Brain Inj 1988; 2:101.

102. Gudeman SK, Kishore PRS, Becker DP, et al: Computed tomography in the evaluation of incidence and significance of post-traumatic hydrocephalus. Neuroradiology 1981; 141:397.

103. Halloran LG, Zass AM, Gayle WE, et al: Prevention of acute gastrointestinal complications after severe head injury: A controlled trial of cimetidine prophylaxis. Am J Surg 1980; 139:44.

104. Hannay HJ, Sherer M: Assessment of outcome from head injury. In Narayan RK, Wilberger JE Jr, Povilshock JT (eds): Neurotrauma: A Comprehensive Textbook on Head and Spinal Injury. New York, McGraw-Hill, in press.

105. Hanscom DA: Acute management of the multiply injured head trauma patient. J Head Trauma Rehabil 1987; 2:1.

106. Hansen JR, Cook JS: Posttraumatic neuroendocrine disorders. Phys Med Rehabil 1993; 7:569.

107. Hartley LL: Cognitive-Communicative Abilities Following Brain Injury: A Functional Approach. San Diego, Singular, 1994.

108. Herbel K, Schermerhorn L, Howard J: Management of agitated head-injured patients: A survey of current techniques. Rehabil Nurs 1990; 15:66.

109. High WM Jr, Boake C, Lehmkuhl LD: Critical analysis of studies measuring the effectiveness of rehabilitation following traumatic brain injury. J Head Trauma Rehabil 1990; 1:14.

110. Horn LJ, Glenn MB: Update in pharmacology: Pharmacological intervention in neuroendocrine disorders following traumatic brain injury. Part (B). J Head Trauma Rehabil 1988; 3:86.

111. Horn LJ, Zasler ND (eds): Medical Rehabilitation of Traumatic Brain Injury, Philadelphia, Hanley & Belfus, in press.

112. Horn LJ, Zasler ND: Neuroanatomy and neurophysiology of sexual function. J Head Trauma Rehabil 1990; 5:1.

113. Horn LJ, Zasler ND (eds): Rehabilitation of post-concussive disorders. Phys Med Rehabil 1992; 6:1.

114. Horn S, Shiel A, McLellan L, et al: A review of behavioural assessment scales for monitoring recovery in and after coma with pilot data on a new scale of visual awareness. Neuropsychol Rehabil 1993; 3:121.

115. Hughes M, Cohen WA: Radiographic evaluation. In Cooper PR (ed): Head Injury, ed 3. Baltimore, Williams & Wilkins, 1993, pp 65–89.

116. Jaffe KM, Brink JD, Hays RM, et al: Specific problems associated with pediatric head injury. In Rosenthal M, Griffith ER, Bond MR, Miller JD (eds): Rehabilitation of the Adult Child with Traumatic Brain Injury, ed 2. Philadelphia, FA Davis, 1990.

117. Jennett B: Posttraumatic epilepsy. In Rosenthal M, Griffith ER, Bond MR, Miller JD (eds): Rehabilitation of the Head Injured Adult. Philadelphia, FA Davis, 1983.

118. Jennett B, Teasdale G: Management of Head Injuries. Philadelphia, FA Davis, 1981.

119. Jennett B, Teasdale G, Murray G, et al: Head injury. In Evans RW, Baskin DS, Yatsu FM (eds): Prognosis of Neurological Disorders. New York, Oxford University Press, 1992, pp 85–96.

120. Johnson JH: Rehabilitative aspects of neurologic bladder dysfunction. Nurs Clin North Am 1980; 15:293.

121. Johnston MV: The economics of brain injury: A preface. In Miner ME, Wagner KA (eds): Neurotrauma: Treatment and Rehabilitation and Related Issues. Boston, Butterworths, 1989, pp 163–185.

122. Jones DM, Tilbury H: Parent Training Manual on Education Rights. Houston, HDI, 1994.

123. Kalisky Z, Morison DP, Meyers CA, et al: Medical problems encountered during rehabilitation of patients with head injury. Arch Phys Med Rehabil 1985; 66:25.

124. Katz RT, Brander V, Sahgal V: Update on the diagnosis and management of posttraumatic hydrocephalus. Am J Phys Med Rehabil 1989; 68:91.

125. Kaufman HH: Treatment of civilian gunshot wounds to the head. Neurosurg Clin North Am 1991; 2:387.

126. Keane JR, Baloh RW: Posttraumatic cranial neuropathies. Neurol Clin 1992; 10:849.

127. Kelly JP, Nichols JS, Filley CM, et al: Concussion in sports: Guidelines for the prevention of catastrophic outcomes. JAMA 1991; 266:2867.

128. Khalili AA, Betts HB: Peripheral nerve block with phenol in the management of spasticity: Indications and complications. JAMA 1967; 200:1155.

129. Kishore PRS, Lipper MH, Miller JD, et al: Posttraumatic hydrocephalus in patients with severe head injury. Neuroradiology 1978; 16:261.

130. Klingbeil GEG: Airway problems in patients with head injury. Arch Phys Med Rehabil 1988; 69:493.

131. Klingbeil GEG, Kleine P: Anterior hypopituitarism: A consequence of head injury. Arch Phys Med Rehabil 1985; 66:44.

132. Kraus JF: Epidemiology of head injury. In Cooper PR (ed): Head Injury, ed 3. Baltimore, Williams & Wilkins, 1993, pp 1–25.

133. Kreutzer JS, Zasler ND, Devany CW: Neuromedical and psychosocial aspects of rehabilitation after traumatic brain injury. In Fletcher G, Jann B, Wolf S, Banja J (eds): Rehabilitation Medicine: State of the Art Reviews. New York, Lea & Febiger, 1992, pp 63–103.

134. Lal S, Merbitz CP, Grip JC: Modification of function in head-injured patients with Sinemet. Brain Inj 1988; 2:225.

135. Langfitt TW: Measuring the outcome from head injuries. J Neurosurg 1978; 48:673.

136. Lazarus C, Logemann JA: Swallowing disorders in closed head trauma patients. Arch Phys Med Rehabil 1987; 68:79.

137. Lehmkuhl LD: Brain Injury Glossary. Houston, HDI, 1993.

138. Lehmkuhl LD, Thoi L, Baize C, et al: Multimodality treatment of joint contractures in patients with severe brain injury. J Head Trauma Rehabil 1990; 5:23–42.

139. Lerman RM, Bontke CF: *Clostridium difficile* colitis: Nosocomial acquisition and cross infection among head injured patients. Crit Rev Phys Med Rehabil 1990; 1:247.

140. Levin HS: Cognitive rehabilitation: Unproved but promising. Arch Neurol 1990; 47:223.

141. Levin HS: Neurobehavioral outcome of mild to moderate head injury. In Hoff J, Anderson T, Cole T (eds): Mild to Moderate Head Injury. Boston, Blackwell, 1989, pp 153–189.

142. Levin HS, Benton AL, Grossman RG: Neurobehavioral Consequences of Closed-Head Injury. New York, Oxford University Press, 1982.

143. Levin HS, Eisenberg HM: The relative durations of coma and posttraumatic amnesia after severe non-missile head injury: Findings from the pilot phase of the National Traumatic Coma Data Bank. In Miner M, Wagner K (eds): Neurotrauma: Treatment, Monitoring and Rehabilitation Issues. Stoneham, Mass, Butterworth, 1986, pp 89–98.

144. Levin HS, Eisenberg HM, Benton AL (eds): Mild Head Injury. New York, Oxford University Press, 1989.

145. Levin HS, Gary HE, Eisenberg HM, et al: Neurobehavioral outcome one year after head injury: Experience of the Traumatic Coma Data Bank. J Neurosurg 1990; 73:699.

146. Levin HS, Gary HE, Eisenberg HM: NIH Traumatic Coma Data Bank Research Group: Duration of impaired consciousness in relation to side of lesion after severe head injury. Lancet 1989; 2:1001.

147. Levin HS, Meyers CA, Grossman RG, et al: Ventricular enlargement after closed head injury. Arch Neurol 1981; 38:623.

148. Levin HS, Saydjari C, Eisenberg HM, et al: Vegetative state after closed-head injury: A Traumatic Coma Data Bank report. Arch Neurol 1991; 48:580.

149. Levin HS, Williams D, Crofford MJ, et al: Relationship of depth of brain lesions to consciousness and outcome after closed head injury. J Neurosurg 1988; 69:861.

150. Levin HS, Williams DH, Eisenberg HM, et al: Serial MRI and neurobehavioral findings after mild to moderate closed head injury. J Neurol Neurosurg Psychiatry 1992; 55:255.

151. Levin VA (ed): Cancer in the Nervous System. New York, McGraw-Hill, in press.

152. Levin VA, Moser RP: Neoplasms. In Evans RW, Baskin DS, Yatsu FM (eds): Prognosis of Neurological Disorders. New York, Oxford University Press, 1992, pp 633–649.

153. Levy DE: Disorders of consciousness. In Evans RW, Baskin DS, Yatsu FM (eds): Prognosis of Neurological Disorders, New York, Oxford University Press, 1992, pp 353–358.

154. Lezak MD: Living with the characterologically altered brain-injured patient. J Clin Psychiatry 1978; 39:592.

155. Light R: Behavioral management of the difficult neurologically impaired patient. J Neuro Rehabil 1989; 3:145.

156. Loubser PG, Bontke CF, Baize CM: Intramuscular neurolytic blocks for upper extremity spasticity in head injury. Anesthesiology 1989; 71:A763.

157. Loubser PG, Bontke CF, Baize CM: Quadruple motor neurolysis for shoulder and elbow flexor hypertonicity. Arch Phys Med Rehabil 1991; 72:826.

158. Loubser PG, Bontke CF, Vandeventer J: Selective epidural phenol rhizolysis for hip flexor spasticity. Arch Phys Med Rehabil 1989; 70:A38.

159. Macciocchi SN, Reid DB, Barth JT: Disability following head injury. Curr Opin Neurol 1993; 6:773.

160. Mackay LE, Bernstein BA, Chapman PE, et al: Early intervention in severe head injury: Long-term benefits of a formalized program. Arch Phys Med Rehabil 1992; 73:635.

161. Malkmus D, Booth BJ, Kodimer C: Rehabilitation of Head Injured Adults: Comprehensive Cognitive Management. Downey, Calif, Professional Staff Association of Rancho Los Amigos Hospital, 1980.

162. Massagli TL: Neurobehavioral effects of phenytoin, carbamazepine and valproic acid: Implications for use in traumatic brain injury. Arch Phys Med Rehabil 1991; 72:219.

163. Mattson RH, Cramer JA, Collins JF, et al: Comparison of carbamazepine, phenobarbital, phenytoin and primidone in partial and secondarily generalized tonic-clonic seizures. N Engl J Med 1985; 313:145.

164. Max W, MacKenzie EJ, Rice DP: Head injuries: Costs and consequences. J Head Trauma Rehabil 1991; 6:76.

165. Mayer NH: Concepts in head injury rehabilitation: In Kaplan PE (ed): The Practice of Physical Medicine. Springfield, Ill, Charles C Thomas, 1984, pp 373–412.

166. McKinlay WW, Brooks DN, Bond MR, et al: The short-term outcome of severe blunt head injury as reported by relatives of the injured persons. J Neurol Neurosurg Psychiatry 1981; 44:527.

167. McMillan TM, Wilson S (eds): Coma and the persistent vegetative state. Neuropsychol Rehabil 1995; 3(2).

168. Metoclopramide (Reglan) for gastrointestinal reflux. Med Lett Drugs Ther 1985; 27:21.

169. Miller JD: Traumatic brain swelling and edema. In Cooper PR (ed): Head Injury, ed 3. Baltimore, Williams & Wilkins, 1993, pp 331–354.

170. Miller JD, Pentland B: The neurological evaluation. In Rosenthal M, Griffith ER, Bond MR, Miller JD (eds): Rehabilitation of the Adult and Child with Traumatic Brain Injury, ed 2. Philadelphia, FA Davis, 1990, pp 52–58.

171. Miner ME: Systemic effects of brain injury. Trauma 1985; 2:75.

172. Mital MA, Garbar JE, Stinson JT: Ectopic bone formation in children and adolescents with head injury: Its management. J Pediatr Orthop 1987; 7:83.

173. Multi-Society Task Force on PVS: Medical aspects of the persistent vegetative state (1). N Engl J Med 1994; 330:1499.

174. Multi-Society Task Force on PVS: Medical aspects of the persistent vegetative state, (2). N Engl J Med 1994; 330:1572.

175. Mysiw WJ, Jackson RD, Corrigan JD: Amitriptyline for posttraumatic agitation. Am J Phys Med Rehabil 1988; 67:29.

176. Narayan R, Goskaslan Z, Bontke CF, et al: Delayed neurosurgical sequelae of head injury. In Rosenthal M, Griffith ER, Bond MR, Miller JD (eds): Rehabilitation of the Adult and Child with Traumatic Brain Injury, ed 2. Philadelphia, FA Davis, 1990, pp 94–106.

177. Narayan R, Wilberger JE, Povlishock JT (eds): Neurotrauma: A Comprehensive Textbook on Head and Spinal Injury. New York, McGraw-Hill, in press.

178. Notman DD, Mortek MA, Moses AM: Permanent diabetes insipidus following head trauma: Observations on ten patients and an approach to diagnosis. J Trauma 1980; 20:599.

179. Nowak P, Cohn AM, Guidice MA: Airway complications in patients with closed-head injuries. Am J Otolaryngol 1987; 8:91.

180. Oder W, Goldenberg G, Podreka I, et al: HMPAO-SPECT in persistent vegetative state after head injury: Prognostic indicator of the likelihood of recovery. Intensive Care Med 1991; 17:149.

181. Ommaya AK, Gennarelli TA: Cerebral concussion and traumatic unconsciousness: Correlation of experimental and clinical observation on blunt head injuries. Brain 1974; 97:633.

182. Patel M, Bontke CF: Impact of traumatic brain injury on pregnancy. J Head Trauma Rehabil 1990; 5:60–66.

183. Patterson TS, Sargent M: Behavioral management of the agitated head trauma client. Rehabil Nurs 1990; 15:248.

184. Philip PA, Philip M: Evoked potentials in the prognosis of traumatic lesions of the central nervous system. Phys Med Rehabil Clin North Am 1994; 5:643.

185. Pisciotta AV: Carbamazepine: Hematological toxicity. In Woodbury DM, Penry JK, Pippenger CE (eds): Antiepileptic Drugs, ed 2. New York, Raven Press, 1982, pp 533–541.

186. Pitts LH: San Francisco General Hospital Medical Center Head Injury Data Bank. Cited in Bartowski M, Lovely MP: Prognosis in coma and the persistent vegetative state. J Head Trauma Rehabil 1986; 1:1.

187. Plum F, Posner JB: The Diagnosis of Stupor and Coma, ed 3. Philadelphia, FA Davis, 1982.

188. Prigatano GP: Neuropsychological Rehabilitation after Brain Injury. Baltimore, Johns Hopkins University Press, 1986.

189. Rader MA, Ellis DW: Sensory Stimulation Assessment Measure. Camden, NJ, Mediplex Rehab-Camden, 1989.

190. Ramsey RE: Advances in the pharmacotherapy of epilepsy. Epilepsia 1993; 34(suppl. 5):S9–S16.

191. Rappaport M, Dougherty AM, Kelting DL: Evaluation of coma and vegetative states. Arch Phys Med Rehabil 1992; 73:628.

192. Reyes RL, Bhattacharyya AK, Heller D: Traumatic head injury: Restlessness and agitation as prognosticators of physical and psychologic improvement in patients. Arch Phys Med Rehabil 1981; 62:20.

193. Rimel RW, Jane JA: Characteristics of the head injured patient. In Rosenthal M, Griffith ER, Bond MR, Miller JD (eds): Rehabilitation of the Head Injured Adult. Philadelphia, FA Davis, 1983, pp 9–21.

194. Rinehart MA: Strategies for improving motor performance. In Rosenthal M, Griffith ER, Bond MR, Miller JD (eds): Rehabilitation of the Adult and Child with Traumatic Brain Injury, ed 2. Philadelphia, FA Davis, 1990, pp 331–350.

195. Ritter MA, Gioe T: The effect of indomethacin on para-articular ectopic ossification following total hip arthroplasty. Clin Orthop 1982; 167:113.

196. Robertson IH: Cognitive rehabilitation in neurologic disease. Curr Opin Neurol 1993; 6:756.

197. Rogers RC: Program idea: Heterotopic calcification in severe head injury: A prevention program. Brain Inj 1988; 2:169.

198. Rosenthal M, Griffith ER, Bond MR, et al (eds): Rehabilitation of the Adult and Child with Traumatic Brain Injury, ed 2. Philadelphia, FA Davis, 1990.

199. Rossitch E, Bullard DE: The autonomic dysfunction syndrome: Etiology and treatment. Br J Neurosurg 1988; 2:471.

200. Ruff RM, Marshall LF, Crouch J, et al: Predictors of outcome following severe head trauma: Follow-up data from the Traumatic Coma Data Bank. Brain Inj 1993; 7:101.

201. Russell WR: The Traumatic Amnesias. London, Oxford University Press, 1971.

202. Sandel ME, Abrams PL, Horn LJ: Hypertension after brain injury: Case report. Arch Phys Med Rehabil 1986; 67:469.

203. Sandel ME, Ellis DW (eds): The coma emerging patient. Phys Med Rehabil 1990; 4(3).

204. Sazbon L, Groswasser Z: Outcome in 134 patients with prolonged posttraumatic unawareness. Part I: Parameters determining late recovery of consciousness. J Neurosurg 1990; 72:75.

205. Sazbon L, Najenson T, Tartakovsky M, et al: Widespread periarticular new-bone formation in long-term comatose patients. J Bone Joint Surg Br 1981; 63:120.

206. Shapiro K, Smith PA Jr: Special considerations for the pediatric age group. In Rosenthal M, Griffith ER, Bonds MR, Miller JD (eds): Rehabilitation of the Adult and Child with Traumatic Brain Injury, ed 2. Philadelphia, FA Davis, 1990, pp 427–457.

207. Silver BV, Boake C, Cavazos DI: Improving functional skills using behavioral procedures in a child with anoxic brain injury. Arch Phys Med Rehabil 1994; 75:742.

208. Silver JM, Yudofsky SG: Psychopharmacological approaches to the patient with affective and psychotic features. J Head Trauma Rehabil 1994; 9:61.

209. Sohlberg MM, Mateer CA: Introduction to Cognitive Rehabilitation: Theory and Practice. New York, Guilford Press, 1989.

210. Sorenson SB, Kraus JF: Occurrence, severity and outcomes of brain injury. J Head Trauma Rehabil 1991; 6:1.

211. Spielman G, Gennarelli TA, Rogers CR: Disodium etidronate: Its role in preventing heterotopic ossification in severe head injury. Arch Phys Med Rehabil 1983; 64:539.

212. Stover SL, Hahn HR, Miller JM: Disodium etidronate in the prevention of heterotopic ossification following spinal cord injury. Paraplegia 1976; 14:146.

213. Strub RL, Black FW: The Mental Status Examination in Neurology, ed 3. Philadelphia, FA Davis, 1993.

214. Sutton RL, Weaver MS, Feeney DM: Drug-induced modifications of behavioral recovery following cortical trauma. J Head Trauma Rehabil 1987; 2:50.

215. Temkin NR, Dikmen SS, Wilensky AJ, et al: A randomized, double-blind study of phenytoin for the prevention of posttraumatic seizures. N Engl J Med 1990; 323:497.

216. US Department of Commerce: Statistical Abstract of the United States, ed 113. Washington, DC, US Government Printing Office, 1993.

217. Van Hilten JJ, Roos RAC: Posttraumatic hyperthermia: A possible result of frontodiencephalic dysfunction. Clin Neurol Neurosurg 1991; 93:223.

218. Vollmer DG: Prognosis and outcome of severe head injury. In Cooper PR (ed): Head Injury, ed 3. Baltimore, Williams & Wilkins, 1993, pp 553–581.

219. Volpe BT, McDowell FH: The efficacy of cognitive rehabilitation in patients with traumatic brain injury. Arch Neurol 1990; 47:220.

220. Weintraub AH, Opat CA: Motor and sensory dysfunction in the brain injured adult. Phys Med Rehabil 1989; 3:59.

221. Whyte J, Glenn MB: The care and rehabilitation of the patient in a persistent vegetative state. J Head Trauma Rehabil 1986; 1:39.

222. Wikkelso C, Andersson H, Bloomstrand C, et al: Normal pressure hydrocephalus. Acta Neurol Scand 1986; 73:566.

223. Williams DH, Levin HS, Eisenberg HM: Mild head injury classification. Neurosurgery 1990; 27:422.

224. Williams JM, Kay T: Head Injury: A Family Matter. Baltimore, Paul H Brooks, 1991.

225. Wilson SL, McMillan TM: A review of the evidence for the effectiveness of sensory stimulation treatment for coma and vegetative states. Neuropsychol Rehabil 1993; 3:149.

226. Wood RL: Brain Injury Rehabilitation: A Neurobehavioural Approach. Rockville, Md, Aspen, 1987.

227. Wroblewski BA, Glenn MB: Pharmacological treatment of arousal and cognitive deficits. J Head Trauma Rehabil 1994; 9:19.

228. Yablon S: Posttraumatic seizures. Arch Phys Med Rehabil 1993; 74:83.

229. Yablon S, Ivanhoe C: Personal communication, Jan 24, 1994.

230. Ylvisaker M, Chorazy AJL, Cohen SB, et al: Rehabilitative assessment following head injury in children. In Rosenthal M, Griffith ER, Bond MR, Miller JD (eds): Rehabilitation of the Adult and Child with Traumatic Brain Injury, ed 2. Philadelphia, FA Davis, 1990, pp 558–592.

231. Zasler ND: Update on pharmacology: Acute neurochemical alterations following traumatic brain injury: Research implications for clinical treatment. J Head Trauma Rehabil 1992; 7:102.

232. Zasler ND, Kreutzer JS, Taylor D: Coma stimulation and coma recovery: A critical review. Neurorehabilitation 1991; 1:33.

233. Zasler ND, Marmarou A: Posttraumatic hydrocephalus. Special Topic Report. Richmond, Va, Virginia Commonwealth University/Medical College of Virginia, Rehabilitation Research and Training Center on Severe TBI, 1992.

234. Zimmerman RD, Fleming CA, Lee BCP, et al: Periventricular hyperintensity as seen by magnetic resonance: Prevalence and significance. AJNR 1986; 7:13.

235. Zoltan B: Remediation of visual-perceptual and perceptual-motor deficits. In Rosenthal M, Griffith ER, Bond MR, Miller JD (eds): Rehabilitation of the Adult and Child with Traumatic Brain Injury, ed 2. Philadelphia, FA Davis, 1990, pp 351–365.

Rehabilitation of Stroke Syndromes

ELLIOT J. ROTH, M.D., AND
RICHARD L. HARVEY, M.D.

BACKGROUND

In 1986, Gresham[1] described stroke as a condition with a unique epidemiological profile, consisting of high incidence and mortality rates, with a large proportion of survivors experiencing a significant amount of residual disability. The clinical phenomena that result vary from stroke to stroke and from patient to patient. Most patients who experience stroke can and do have improvement in function. The approach involved in the assessment and the management of the stroke patient requires specialized knowledge, skills, and attitudes.

Stroke rehabilitation is as much a philosophy as it is a set of tasks to carry out. Kottke[2] stated that the goal of rehabilitation is to "restore optimal physical function and psycho-social-vocational restoration to enable the patient to become a productive participant in the community." Referring more specifically to care of the stroke patient, Bobath[3] defined stroke rehabilitation as "teaching the patient to manage his own life given the limitations of the damage to the central nervous system." Charness[4] pointed out several implications of this philosophy, highlighting that rehabilitation does not consist of exercise alone. Therapy involves returning control to the patient as soon as possible. The managing team involves the patient and family in the processes of setting goals, planning treatment, and implementing clinical activities. Stroke rehabilitation is done *with* the patient, rather than *to* the patient.

Whereas formal therapeutic exercise regimens make up the most prominent components of the process, other aspects of the comprehensive rehabilitation program are important as well. Many rehabilitation activities extend beyond the specific therapy or treatment sessions. Psychosocial interactions among patients and between patients and professionals are important. The rehabilitation milieu provides the opportunity for these therapeutic interactions. Often, recreational programs are major therapeutic activi-

ties. The ultimate goal of the rehabilitation effort is long-term, safe, independent, energy-efficient, pleasurable, and high-quality functioning in the community. Achieving this goal requires paying attention to a wide variety of medical, functional, and psychosocial issues.

Roth[5] enumerated five major functions of stroke rehabilitation; these are as follows:

1. Prevention, recognition, and management of co-morbid illness and intercurrent medical complications
2. Training for maximal functional independence
3. Facilitating psychosocial coping and adaptation by the patient and family
4. Promoting community reintegration, including resumption of home, family, recreational, and vocational activities
5. Enhancing quality of life

The major underlying theme of all rehabilitation interventions is the enhancement of quality of life of stroke patients. It is quality of life, and not simply functional independence or non-institutional placement, that is the real goal. Indeed, for some stroke survivors, complete independence in daily functional skills might be either undesirable or impractical for physical, psychological, social, or other reasons. The goal of enhancing quality of life is pervasive and affects both the choices of specific interventions and the manner in which clinical activities are performed. The comprehensive rehabilitation management program is characterized by a holistic approach, in which the whole patient and his or her overall situation, rather than isolated aspects of existence, are considered. This goal usually, but not always, includes helping the patient to achieve as much functional independence as possible.

Understanding both stroke and the rehabilitation of patients who sustain stroke is important, not only because stroke is the most common diagnosis among patients on a rehabilitation unit, but also because it involves virtually all elements of rehabilitation activity and all members of the rehabilitation team. This chapter reviews the mechanisms and clinical features; the preventive, diagnostic, and acute management techniques; and the principles and practices of stroke rehabilitation assessment and intervention that enable rehabilitation providers to assist the patient in achieving the ultimate goal of enhancing quality of life.

DEFINITIONS

Stroke or Cerebrovascular Accident?

Ancient writers of history, science, and poetry used the word *apoplexy*, meaning a sudden strike of paralysis, dumbness, or fainting from which the victim frequently failed to recover. Such a stroke of illness, whether delivered by the gods or disease, was a spontaneous event of the same character as a "stroke of genius," a "stroke of luck," or a "stroke of misfortune." Today the term *stroke* connotes the sudden and surprising nature of symptomatic cerebrovascular disease and is preferred over the more scientific sounding phrase *cerebrovascular accident*, or *CVA*. The later term implies a nihilistic view, suggesting that the acute outcome cannot be modified by treatment. Many physicians who specialize in the care of patients with stroke prefer the historical term rather than the acronym *CVA*.

We define stroke as a sudden neurological deficit characterized by loss of motor control, altered sensation, cognitive or language impairment, and disequilibrium or coma, caused by nontraumatic brain injury resulting from occlusion or rupture of cerebral blood vessels. This definition includes an array of etiological sources, but excludes nonvascular conditions that can present with stroke-like symptoms, such as seizure, syncope, traumatic brain injury, or brain tumor.

Pathophysiological Classification of Stroke

Stroke is a neurological syndrome caused by a heterogeneous group of vascular etiologies requiring different management.[7] The causes can be grossly categorized as hemorrhagic or ischemic. Intracranial hemorrhage includes 15% of all strokes and can be further divided into intracerebral (10%) and subarachnoid (5%) hemorrhage. Subarachnoid hemorrhages typically result from aneurysmal rupture of a cerebral artery with blood loss into the space surrounding the brain. Rupture of weakened vessels within brain parenchyma as a result of hypertension, arteriovenous malformation, or tumor causes intracerebral hemorrhage.

The remaining 85% of strokes are caused by ischemic brain injury resulting from large- (40%) or small-vessel (20%) thrombosis, cerebral embolism (20%), and other less common causes (5%), such as cerebral vasculitis or cerebral hypoperfusion. Vessel occlusion from thrombosis in both large and small arteries occurs most commonly in the presence of atherosclerotic cerebrovascular disease. Vascular changes or lipohyalinosis found in small, deep, penetrating arteries as associated with chronic hypertension can lead to small vessel thrombosis. Cerebral emboli are usually of cardiac origin and are frequently a result of chronic ischemic cardiovascular disease with secondary ventricular wall hypokinesis or atrial arrhythmia, both conditions that increase risk for intracardiac thrombus formation.[8]

Temporal Classification of Stroke

The etiology of an acute stroke can often be inferred by classifying the temporal profile of the event using information gathered from the patient's initial history and physical examination. A transient ischemic attack (TIA) is an event in which neurological symptoms develop and disappear over several minutes and, by definition, completely resolve within 24 hours. TIAs are most frequently associated with atherosclerotic carotid artery disease and they should provoke an urgent diagnostic evaluation so that appropriate preventive care can be instituted.

A transient neurological event that lasts longer than 24 hours is called a reversible ischemic neurological deficit (RIND). Such events are clinically infrequent and their etiology is unknown. It is likely that RINDs result from small infarctions (lacunes) of the deep subcortical gray and white matter, resulting in only temporary impairment.

Embolic strokes generally have a quick onset and fully develop in a matter of minutes, whereas hemorrhagic strokes often evolve over 1 to 2 hours. Thrombotic strokes can have a rapid or a prolonged interval of onset, lasting many hours. *Stroke in evolution* is a term used to describe an unstable ischemic event characterized by the progressive development of more severe neurological impairment, and it is often associated with active occlusive thrombosis of a major cerebral artery. Once a stable neurological status is reached, clinicians refer to the event as a *completed stroke*. The therapeutic goal of many current acute stroke treatment protocols is to abort neurological deterioration and to limit the neurological impairment, hopefully minimalizing the functional disability once the stroke is completed.

When a patient's neurological and medical status is stable, rehabilitation care should begin. Stroke rehabilitation is an interdisciplinary process whereby physical modalities and skill enhancement are used to maximize functional and psychosocial outcome in the presence of physical or cognitive impairment and to simultaneously prevent secondary medical complications that might impede recovery. Rehabilitation can begin during the acute medical hospitalization and continue until maximal functional recovery is achieved. Once a patient with stroke is discharged from acute hospital care, other rehabilitation settings may be chosen based on an individual's therapeutic need and tolerance for activity. These options include comprehensive inpatient rehabilitation, subacute rehabilitation care, rehabilitation day treatment programs, home therapy, or outpatient rehabilitation clinics.

EPIDEMIOLOGY

Stroke Mortality in the United States

Stroke was the primary cause of death in 144,070 persons in 1991 and it remains the third leading cause of death in the United States; it is exceeded only by cardiovascular disease and cancer.[9] However, a well-documented reduction in annual stroke mortality has taken place within the United States in the last century.[10–11] In particular, there was a sharp decline in the annual stroke deaths for both men and women that began in the 1970s and continued well into the 1980s before the slope flattened (Fig. 50–1).[10, 12] Approximately 200,000 fewer fatal strokes occurred in this period than would have been predicted from data of the previous decade.[12] It can be argued that improved detection and treatment of hypertension that began in the 1960s, and escalated in 1973 with introduction of the National High Blood Pressure Education and Control Program, are directly responsible for the steep decline in stroke mortality.[10, 12]

Although a cause-and-effect relationship between blood pressure control and stroke mortality cannot be verified in population studies, data from Rochester, Minn., have demonstrated a decline in annual incidence of new strokes during every 5-year period from 1950 to 1980, with a particularly sharp decline after 1970[11] that matches a similarly reduced incidence of hypertension in the same population.[13] It appears that the decline in stroke mortality is a result of reduced stroke incidence, possibly as a result of improved blood pressure control. In addition, direct evidence indicates that antihypertensive therapy reduces stroke risk, as shown in observational and randomized drug studies.[14–16]

Another explanation for reduced stroke mortality is improved survival. Hospital records from Allegheny County, Pennsylvania, demonstrated a decline in stroke-related coma from 1971 to 1980 that was responsible for 80% of the reduced stroke case-fatality during that decade.[17] In contrast, data from the Minnesota Heart Survey showed no change in the severity of stroke or case-fatality between 1970 and 1980, but hospitalization rates for stroke were significantly reduced in 1980.[18] Thus, the sharp decline in stroke mortality noted nationally was likely related to re-duced stroke incidence and less likely to a result of improved acute survival during the 1970s, and can be attributed to an epidemiological improvement in hypertension detection and treatment.

Beginning in the 1980s the steep decline in mortality began to flatten coincident with increased use of cranial computed tomography (CT) and the introduction of magnetic resonance imaging (MRI). Both have improved the diagnostic sensitivity for cerebral infarction and hemorrhage and many strokes are now discovered that would have gone undetected previously.[19–23]

Stroke Incidence in the United States: Age, Sex, and Race

Data from the Framingham Heart Study indicate that the incidence of stroke in the United States is approximately 500,000 per year, resulting in significant morbidity, mortality, and disability, particularly among people older than 65 years.

Stroke is primarily a disease of older individuals, but 28% of strokes occur in persons younger than 65 years (Fig. 50–2). The incidence of stroke is 19% higher among men than women of all races. Among black men and women in 1981, stroke mortality was 73 and 58 per 100,000, respectively, double the incidence seen in whites. In comparison, stroke mortality is 3- to 4-fold higher among blacks younger than 65 years.[24] Many common risk factors for stroke are found in higher frequency among blacks, including hypertension, diabetes mellitus, heart disease, smoking, excessive alcohol use, and sickle cell disease. Stronger national education efforts for young black persons that focus on stroke risk factors and risk reduction are needed to reduce the incidence of stroke within this community.

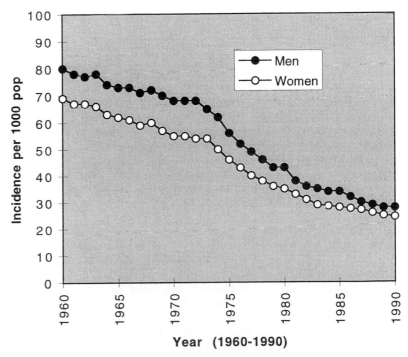

FIGURE 50–1 Annual U.S. stroke mortality for men and women.

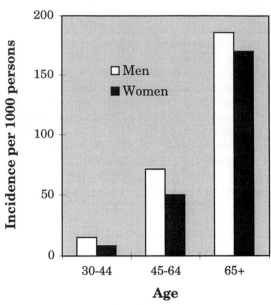

FIGURE 50–2   Annual U.S. incidence of stroke by age and gender.

Stroke Survival

Stroke survivors, many of whom require rehabilitation services, presently number just over 3 million in the U.S. population. In the 1970s, survival after myocardial infarction improved significantly with the advent of the coronary intensive care unit. In contrast, it has not yet been proven whether advances in acute management have improved stroke survival, which has remained around 80%. Whether advanced medical and surgical treatment of acute stroke has improved functional outcome and stroke severity is also unknown. Still, the prevalence of stroke survivors today has doubled over the last 25 years. Garraway and colleagues[25] compared survival patterns after first-time stroke for 5-year periods between 1945–1949 and 1975–1979. Twenty-one day survival after intracerebral hemorrhage improved from 0% to 42%. Acute 30-day survival improved only modestly between 1945–1949 and 1975–1979 after ischemic stroke. Long-term survival up to 7 years improved significantly during the study period. The major contributor to the prevalence of stroke survivors today is likely the reduced long-term mortality achieved by improved management of medical co-morbidity. Better detection and management of coronary artery disease, prevention of aspiration pneumonia by identification and treatment of dysphagia, prevention of pulmonary embolism using prophylactic measures, and reduction of general disability and immobility by active rehabilitation care have improved long-term survival after stroke.

STROKE RISK FACTORS

Hypertension remains the most important public health concern today because it is the leading risk factor for two of the top three causes of death in the United States: coronary heart disease and stroke. Hypertension is treatable, and its control has the potential for widespread reduction in death and disability in this country. The combination of stroke and heart disease is not unusual and can have a significant impact on medical care and rehabilitation.[26] When faced with a patient with a recent stroke, TIA, or asymptomatic carotid bruit, the clinician must be concerned about the presence of coronary heart disease. Similarly, any patient who presents with known heart disease and chronic atrial fibrillation should be considered a candidate for stroke prophylaxis. A major but often neglected part of physiatric care for stroke survivors and their families is stroke and coronary heart disease prevention and risk factor reduction.

Hypertension

There is a 35% prevalence of hypertension within the U.S. adult population. Defined as a systolic pressure greater than 165 mm Hg or a diastolic pressure greater than 95 mm Hg, hypertension increases the relative risk of stroke by a factor of six. Among stroke survivors, 67% have chronic hypertension.[27] In a recent meta-analysis involving nine population-based observational studies, MacMahon and co-workers[15] noted that a 7.5 mm Hg reduction from the usual diastolic blood pressure (DBP) was associated with a 46% reduction in stroke risk in both hypertensive and normotensive subjects. Interestingly, no threshold diastolic value was found below which further pressure reduction lacked an additional effect on stroke risk. Thus, reductions in DBP below traditionally normotensive values contributed to further risk reduction in these studies.

The Hypertension Detection and Follow-up Program was the first major study to demonstrate a reduction in stroke incidence with antihypertensive treatment. This was a case-control study with 5-year follow-up involving 11,000 hypertensive persons who were either provided with a stepped-care antihypertensive program or referred for traditional care. There was 1.9% incidence of stroke among patients on stepped-care treatment, compared with 2.9% on a referred-care program, equaling a 35% reduction in stroke incidence and a 44% reduction in fatal strokes.[14] In another study combining the results of 14 randomized antihypertensive drug treatment trials that included 35,000 persons over a 5-year period, subjects receiving blood pressure treatment had a 42% reduced risk of stroke compared with untreated controls.[16]

Isolated systolic hypertension is more common among individuals older than 60 years and is an independent risk factor for stroke and cardiovascular disease.[28] The Systolic Hypertension in the Elderly Program (SHEP)[29] randomized more than 4700 subjects age 60 years and older with systolic pressures greater than 160 mm Hg and diastolic pressures less than 90 mm Hg to antihypertensive treatment or placebo. Over the 5-year study period, subjects treated with antihypertensive medication had an average reduction of systolic blood pressure measuring 17 mm Hg and a 36% reduction in the incidence of stroke when compared with control subjects.

Ample evidence supports public health efforts aimed at reducing the prevalence of poorly controlled blood pressure, thereby reducing the risk of stroke and heart disease. Improved public education, detection, and treatment of hypertension will have a positive impact on the further decline of stroke incidence and mortality.

Risk Factors Modifiable by Lifestyle Changes

It has been known for many years that cigarette smoking is an important risk factor for cardiovascular disease, but its negative influence on stroke was questioned. More recently, community-based data from the Framingham Study has confirmed that smoking is independently associated with increased risk of atherothrombotic stroke in both men and women. The relative risk of stroke for heavy smokers (>40 cigarettes/day) is twice that of light smokers (<10 cigarettes/day). Cessation of smoking reverses risk to that of non-smokers within 5 years after quitting.[30] Twelve year follow-up from the Honolulu Heart Program studying cardiovascular risk in men of Japanese decent has linked smoking to increased risk of hemorrhagic stroke in addition to ischemic cerebral infarction.[31]

The role of elevated serum cholesterol has not been clearly linked to increased stroke incidence per se, but its strong influence on the development of coronary artery disease and atherosclerosis[32] indicates that hypercholesterolemia is at least an indirect risk factor for stroke. Indeed, an association between carotid artery atherosclerosis and increased serum cholesterol levels has been noted.[33-35] Reduced dietary intake of cholesterol and saturated fatty acids has been recommended for adults with total cholesterol levels greater than 200 mg/dL or low-density lipoprotein (LDL)-cholesterol levels greater than 160 mg/dL. If dietary measures are ineffective, cholesterol-reducing medications are recommended. There is interesting epidemiological evidence that a total serum cholesterol level less than 100 mg/dL is associated with risk of hemorrhagic stroke among Asian populations.[36, 37]

Whether obesity is a risk factor for stroke has been challenged. Hypertension and diabetes mellitus are more common in the obese and are strong influences for stroke risk. Weight loss has a positive influence on blood pressure and diabetic control and likely has a risk-reducing effect on stroke and cardiovascular disease. Although obesity may indirectly increase stroke risk, its independence as a risk factor remains questionable.

Heart disease, including electrocardiographic (ECG) evidence of left ventricular hypertrophy, cardiac failure, and nonvalvular atrial fibrillation, increases stroke risk by two to six times normal. Control of hypertension, cessation of smoking, and reduction of serum cholesterol can reduce the development of heart disease as well as prevent stroke. However, in the presence of established conditions, such as atrial fibrillation or left ventricular failure, the use of medical means to reduce stroke risk can become important. Prevention of heart disease through lifestyle changes has a positive influence on stroke prevention.

Risk Factors Modifiable by Medical Means

Transient ischemic attacks are associated with intracranial and extracranial carotid artery disease and are an important sign of stroke risk. Approximately 35% of persons who experience a TIA will have a stroke within 5 years.[38] TIAs are considered physical warning signs of impending stroke and require urgent clinical attention. There is now substantial evidence that medical or surgical treatment for carotid artery disease in patients experiencing TIA can considerably reduce stroke incidence and mortality. But appropriate therapeutic measures can only be implemented after thorough diagnostic testing.

The presence of an asymptomatic carotid bruit due to carotid stenosis is a well-established risk factor for stroke, but it has only recently been considered efficacious to selectively modify this risk by surgical means.[39] More important, the presence of an asymptomatic carotid bruit is an indication of atherosclerotic disease in general, and is a strong predictor of myocardial infarction and cardiovascular death. Once carotid bruits are noted, diagnostic evaluation for coronary artery disease should be strongly considered.

Diabetes mellitus increases the relative risk of ischemic stroke to three to six times that of the general population. This risk can be partly attributed to the higher prevalence of hypertension and heart disease among diabetics, but even after controlling for these factors, diabetes independently doubles stroke risk.[40-42] The prevalence of diabetes among stroke survivors is 20%.[27, 42, 43] Although the data are not yet available, the Diabetes Control and Complications Trial, a prospective longitudinal study, will determine whether tight medical and dietary control of glucose level can reduce the incidence of stroke in diabetics.[44]

Two factors that increase blood viscosity, hematocrit and serum fibrinogen, have been implicated as risk factors for stroke.[45, 46] The mechanism by which stroke occurs in the presence of hyperviscous blood is unclear, but hypercoagulability or enhanced atherogenesis by microvascular damage from traumatic shearing forces against vessels walls are distinct possibilities.

Non-modifiable Risk Factors

Certain important risk factors for stroke that are not modifiable include age, sex, race, and previous stroke. The epidemiology of age, sex, and race as they relate to stroke have been reviewed earlier in the chapter. Once an individual has a stroke, the risk of recurrent stroke is significant. Although the presence of a stroke is not in itself modifiable as a risk factor, a careful workup to determine the cause of the stroke can provide valuable information for clinical decisions regarding secondary stroke prevention.

STROKE PREVENTION

The most effective means to diminish stroke-related morbidity, mortality, and disability is by further reducing the incidence of first-time and recurrent stroke. As emphasized thus far, public awareness of modifiable risk factors for stroke, medical management of risk factors, and the active promotion of lifestyle changes by physicians have the best potential to decrease the annual rate of new stroke occurrence. Physiatrists in particular can counsel patients with stroke and their families about risk factor reduction throughout the course of rehabilitation care. For selected patients who have significant risk for stroke, who have experienced a TIA, or who have had a stroke in the past, physicians can recommend additional medical interventions to minimize the risk of primary (first-time) and secondary (recurrent) stroke. These interventions include antiplatelet therapy, anticoagulation, and carotid endarterectomy.

Antiplatelet Therapy

Primary Prevention

Of the antiplatelet agents available, only aspirin has been studied for primary stroke and cardiovascular disease prevention. The Physicians Health Study[47] was a prospective, double-blind placebo-controlled study to evaluate the effectiveness of low-dose aspirin for the prevention of cardiovascular mortality. Secondary endpoints included nonfatal stroke and myocardial infarction. More than 22,000 healthy male physicians participated over the 5-year study period. A 325 mg every-other-day dose of aspirin showed no advantage over placebo for prevention of stroke. Hemorrhagic strokes were more prevalent in the aspirin group to nearly a statistically significant level ($P = 0.06$). This study did show that aspirin significantly reduced the incidence of fatal and nonfatal myocardial infarction, with its greatest protection being in men older than 50 years. The incidence of gastric ulcer was not significantly different in the aspirin group, but significantly more reports of bleeding and transfusion were noted in the treatment group.

The British Doctors Trial[48] is the only other study that has examined the use of antiplatelet therapy for primary stroke prevention. This study tested a 500 mg/day dose of aspirin in just over 5000 male subjects using a single-blind randomized design conducted over 6 years, but failed to show any effect of aspirin for the prevention of stroke or cardiovascular disease and mortality. These negative results have been attributed to the smaller sample size and reduced compliance with medication in the British project as compared to the U.S. study.

Currently, the *routine* use of aspirin for stroke and cardiovascular disease prophylaxis is not recommended. Decisions to use aspirin for primary prevention should be based on the patient's risk for stroke or myocardial infarction (MI) as well as the risk for bleeding.[47, 49]

Secondary Prevention

An Oxford-based group called the Antiplatelet Trialists' Collaboration[49] has published a meta-analysis of pooled results from 145 trials of various antiplatelet agents for the prevention of vascular events including nonfatal MI, nonfatal stroke, and vascular death. As a group, these studies include more than 70,000 subjects with risk factors for vascular disease randomized to receive various forms of antiplatelet therapy or placebo over 2 to 6 years. Antiplatelet agents were found to reduce the risk of nonfatal stroke by 31% in men and women. Subgroups of hypertensive and diabetic subjects also benefited from treatment. Although this study shows the benefit that antiplatelet agents have on the reduction of vascular disease in general, use and indications of these agents for stroke prophylaxis should be based on specific trials having clearly stated endpoints.

Aspirin is the most frequently prescribed antiplatelet agent for secondary stroke and cardiovascular disease prevention. By irreversibly inhibiting cyclooxygenase-dependent platelet aggregation, aspirin achieves a significant antiplatelet effect at fairly low serum concentrations.[50] Although aspirin's antithrombotic mechanism has been well delineated, clinical trials comparing aspirin with placebo have often been hampered by insufficient sample size and low overall incidence of recurrent stroke. In general these studies have supported the use of aspirin for stroke prophylaxis after TIA or mild stroke in men, but most lack the statistical power to prove effectiveness in women.[51–58] However, when studies that include women are pooled for meta-analysis, aspirin proves efficacious.[49] Controversy remains about the ideal aspirin dose for secondary stroke prevention. Trials have supported the effectiveness of aspirin doses between 30 and 1500 mg/day, but studies testing the most safe and effective dose are lacking.[58] The principal advantage that aspirin has over other antiplatelet agents is its low cost and over-the-counter availability.

Ticlopidine prevents platelet aggregation for the life of the cell by directly inhibiting adenosine diphosphate (ADP)-induced platelet aggregation, without affecting prostaglandin metabolism.[46] Ticlopidine lacks antipyretic, antiinflammatory, and analgesic effects, and it does not affect the integrity of gastric mucosa. Important side effects include reversible neutropenia (2.4%) and diarrhea (12%). Ticlopidine is an effective antiplatelet agent that is particularly useful in patients who cannot tolerate the gastric effects of aspirin.[59, 60]

Anticoagulation and Antiplatelet Therapy in Atrial Fibrillation

Atrial fibrillation is commonly found among the elderly and is present in 15% of persons older than 75 years. Individuals with nonvalvular atrial fibrillation have five times the relative risk for cardioembolic stroke, and those with rheumatic heart disease have a 17-fold increase.[61] Other clinical factors, such as a history of TIA, stroke, hypertension, recent congestive heart failure, and ECG evidence of left ventricular dysfunction, are additional predictors of stroke when associated with atrial fibrillation. Clinical trials have supported the use of aspirin to prevent primary cardioembolic stroke in nonvalvular atrial fibrillation. In the Copenhagen AFASAK trial,[62] a 75-mg daily dose of aspirin reduced embolic stroke risk by 15% when compared with placebo. The U.S.-sponsored Stroke Prevention in Atrial Fibrillation (SPAF) trial[63] measured a 42% reduction in stroke risk using 325 mg of aspirin daily. However, in the SPAF study, aspirin was not clearly effective in men, and it was ineffective in women older than 75 years. The AFASAK and SPAF studies and two additional placebo controlled trials[64, 65] have tested the use of warfarin anticoagulation for primary stroke prevention in nonvalvular atrial fibrillation. Warfarin reduces relative stroke risk by 58% to 86% over that in control subjects.

Although warfarin proved more effective than aspirin for stroke prevention in atrial fibrillation, a second phase of the SPAF trial (SPAF II)[66] compared warfarin to aspirin with the special intention of determining which medication provided superior stroke prevention for individuals older than 75 years with nonvalvular atrial fibrillation. The results of SPAF II are summarized in Figure 50–3. Care must be taken when considering anticoagulation in patients older

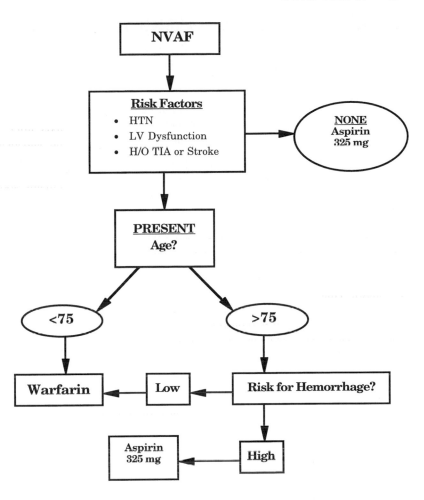

FIGURE 50–3 Stroke prevention in nonvalvular atrial fibrillation (NVAF). *Abbreviations*: HTN = hypertension; LV = left ventricular; H/O TIA = history of transient ischemic attack.

than 75 years, as risk of intracranial hemorrhage is higher in elderly persons.

Individuals with rheumatic valvular disease and atrial fibrillation have a 17-fold increase in risk of embolic stroke. These patients benefit from anticoagulation with warfarin for stroke prevention.

Surgical Management of Carotid Artery Disease

For many years the benefits of surgical vs. medical treatment in the management of TIA associated with carotid artery atherosclerosis was hotly debated. More recent evidence supports the use of carotid endarterectomy in combination with aspirin therapy as the treatment of choice for both symptomatic and asymptomatic high-grade carotid artery disease in centers with low surgical mortality and morbidity.

Data from the North American Symptomatic Carotid Endarterectomy Trial (NASCET)[67] revealed a 17% absolute reduction of the stroke incidence with carotid endarterectomy over a 2-year follow-up in patients with critical stenosis of 70% to 99%. This represents a relative risk reduction of 65% for surgically treated patients. Perioperative mortality was less than 6% in the surgical group. Outcomes for patients with 30% to 69% carotid stenosis remain equivocal, and trials for moderate carotid artery disease are ongoing.

Carotid endarterectomy for asymptomatic carotid artery

stenosis also results in reduced stroke occurrence and death compared with aspirin alone in centers with less than 3% perioperative mortality. Preliminary results from the Asymptomatic Carotid Atherosclerosis Study (ACAS)[39] have demonstrated a significant 5.8% absolute reduction in stroke for surgically treated patients with greater than 60% stenosis after a 5-year follow-up, representing a 55% reduction in relative risk of stroke.

Antiplatelet therapy after carotid surgery remains critical for successful overall outcome. Mild to moderate carotid stenosis (<60%) should be managed with antiplatelet medications, and patients should be monitored for signs of TIA or stroke. An asymptomatic carotid bruit discovered incidentally on physical examination is a sign of atherosclerotic disease and is more predictive of coronary artery disease than of stroke. A careful cardiovascular evaluation is indicated.[68]

STROKE PATHOPHYSIOLOGY

Ischemic Stroke

The unifying pathophysiology of thrombotic, embolic, and lacunar stroke is cerebral ischemia from compromise of cerebral blood flow. The location and temporal development of cerebral injury varies with the etiology.

Thrombosis

The entire pathophysiology of infarction from cerebral thrombosis remains controversial, but it is strongly associated with atherosclerotic cerebrovascular disease. Atherosclerotic plaque formation occurs frequently at major vascular branching sites, including the common carotid and vertebrobasilar arteries. The disease occurs often in the presence of chronic hypertension, with injury to the intimal surface followed by macrophage infiltration and cholesterol accumulation within the vascular media. Foam cells develop within the vessel wall and cholesterol streaks appear on the endothelial surface. Eventually, calcification and vessel wall thickening compromise blood flow, leading to turbulence. Cracking of the plaque and further intimal damage can promote initial thrombus formation by stimulating platelet aggregation and activation of the extrinsic pathway of the coagulation system. The loosely attached thrombus, or "white clot" that rapidly forms, is composed of platelet cells and fresh fibrin.[69]

It is unclear whether symptoms of TIA are caused by transient thrombotic occlusion of major cerebral arteries or by microemboli that break away from a thrombus, but both phenomena might be important. Symptoms of transient monocular blindness or amaurosis fugax are likely due to microemboli from the internal carotid artery that cause a branch occlusion of the ispsilateral ophthalmic artery.[70] Similarly, other intracranial branch occlusions can result from microemboli arising in the extracranial vessels, leading to injury or infarction in focal regions.

In contrast, a large arterial thrombus can occlude a major extracranial artery, producing a low-flow state that causes ischemic injury to neural tissue supplied by the most distal arterial branches.[71] The volume of damage that results from such hemodynamic compromise can be quite large, but it is dependent on the length of time the vessel is occluded, the rate of flow through the occluded site, and the effectiveness of the collateral circulation. Fibrinolytic enzymes are released that control acute thrombus formation, potentially dissolving the clot within minutes to hours. However, recanalization might fail or be delayed, permitting the arterial thrombus to completely or partially occlude blood flow. Collateral circulation can support the compromised cortical zone, but it may be less effective in elderly persons or in those with diffuse atherosclerotic disease or diabetes.

Ischemic injury from a cerebrovascular thrombus likely results in simultaneous distal branch occlusions from microemboli and compromise of blood flow proximally. The neurological outcome of cerebral thrombi vary widely and include brief TIAs, minor strokes without functional compromise, or major strokes resulting in significant impairment and functional disability.

Embolism

Beyond the microemboli produced by cerebrovascular thrombi, the majority of embolic strokes have a cardiac origin. Thrombus formation within the cardiac chambers is generally caused by structural or mechanical changes within the heart. Atrial fibrillation is a significant risk factor for embolic stroke as a result of poor atrial motility and outflow, with stasis of blood and atrial thrombus formation. Atrial fibrillation is often caused by rheumatic valvular disease or coronary artery disease, but it can be idiopathic. Mural thrombus within the left ventricle after MI, in the presence of cardiomyopathy or after cardiac surgery, is the other major cause of embolic stroke.[72, 73] Mechanical heart valves universally cause cerebral emboli if anticoagulation is insufficient. Infectious endocarditis can lead to septic emboli.

Paradoxical embolism is a rare cause of embolic stroke that occurs in the presence of a deep vein thrombosis (DVT) and an atrial or ventricular septal defect.[74] Typically, the DVT embolizes to the lung, causing a pulmonary embolus and an acute increase in pulmonary arterial resistance and right ventricular pressures. In the presence of a septal defect, the raised pulmonary pressure results in a right-to-left shunt. Subsequent emboli cross through the septal defect into the left chambers and systemic circulation, resulting in peripheral emboli and stroke. Using modern echocardiography, patent foramen ovale is a frequent finding, indicating that paradoxical embolism might be more common than previously thought.[73]

Cerebral emboli lodge within arterial branches of the major arteries, causing single or mulitple branch occlusions that result in sudden focal neurological impairment. These branch occlusions significantly compromise flow distally, inducing ischemic injury to neural tissue, glia, and vascular endothelium. Reperfusion of the occluded vessel can occur in response to endogenous fibrinolysis, but because ischemic damage to the vascular bed is often significant, the capillaries become incompetent and secondary cerebral hemorrhage ensues.

In contrast to thrombotic stroke, microemboli probably do not precede cardioembolic strokes, as TIAs are uncommon. Frequently no cardiac thrombus can be found after the event, and the only clue to an embolic cause is the sudden neurological deficit without previous or progressive symptoms.

Lacunes

Lacunar infarcts are small and circumscribed lesions that measure less than 1.5 cm in diameter and are located in subcortical regions of the basal ganglia, internal capsule, pons, and cerebellum.[75] The area of a lacune (meaning "little lake") roughly corresponds to the vascular territory supplied by one of the deep perforating branches from the circle of Willis or major cerebral arteries. Lacunar strokes are strongly associated with hypertension, and pathologically associated with microvascular changes that often develop in the presence of chronic hypertension. Histological changes such as arteriolar thickening and evenly distributed deposition of eosinophilic material, called *lypohyalinosis* and *fibrinoid necrosis*, are commonly seen in the subcortical perforating arteries of hypertensive persons who have had lacunar strokes. Microatheromas within deep perforating arteries are also important causes of lacunar infarction. In addition to hypertension, diabetes mellitus is associated with lacunar stroke as a result of chronic microvascular changes.

Hemorrhagic Stroke

Intracerebral Hemorrhage

The deep perforating cerebral arteries are also the site of rupture preceding intracerebral hemorrhage (ICH). However, unlike lacunar strokes, ICH does not obey the anatomical distribution of a vessel, but dissects through tissue planes. Such damage can be significant, resulting in increased intracranial pressure, disruption of multiple neural tracts, ventricular compression, and cerebral herniation. Acute mortality is high, but those who survive ICH often experience rapid neurological recovery during the first 2 or 3 months after the hemorrhage.

Nearly one-half of all ICHs occur within the putamen and the cerebral white matter.[76] Sudden hemorrhage into brain parenchyma is related to both acute elevations of blood pressure and chronic hypertension. Microvascular changes associated with hypertensive hemorrhages include lipohyalinosis and Charcot-Bouchard aneurysms.[77] The latter are not true aneurysms of the vessel wall, but are pockets of extravasated blood or "pseudoaneurysms," a sign of previous microscopic ruptures within the vascular wall. Typically, the bleeding lasts no more than 1 or 2 hours, corresponding to the usual time course of acute symptom development. Late neurological decline is related to posthemorrhagic edema or rebleeding.

Cerebral amyloid angiopathy is unusual, but is gaining recognition as an important cause of ICH in the elderly.[78] Superficially located hemorrhages that occur in patients older than 55 years who have some premorbid history of mild dementia are characteristic of this disease, but in the absence of tissue staining for Congo red amyloid deposits within the adventitia of cerebral vessels, diagnostic uncertainty remains.

Other notable causes of ICH include the use of anticoagulants, intracranial tumor, and vasculitis.

Subarachnoid Hemorrhage

Subarachnoid hemorrhage (SAH), or bleeding that occurs within the dural space around the brain and fills the basal cisterns, is most commonly caused by rupture of a saccular aneurysm or an arteriovenous malformation. Saccular aneurysms develop from a congenital defect in an arterial wall followed by progressive degeneration of the adventitia, which causes ballooning or outpouching of the vessel. The risk of bleeding from unruptured aneurysms is speculative, but the risk seems greatest for aneurysms greater than 10 mm in diameter.[79]

Saccular aneurysms often rupture during the fifth or sixth decade of life. When a rupture occurs, the extravasation of blood into the subarachnoid space is irritating to the dura and results in a severe headache often described as the "worst in my life." Because of a sudden drop in cerebral perfusion pressure, acute loss of consciousness is frequent. Focal neurological changes or coma can ensue. As many as one-third of patients with aneurysmal hemorrhage die immediately. Patients who present with coma, stupor, or severe hemiplegia have the worst prognosis for proximate survival. The risk of rebleeding from an unoperated aneurysm is as high as 30% within the first month after hemorrhage and declines thereafter. The risk for long-term rebleeding remains 3% per year.[80]

Saccular aneurysms are most often found in the anterior region of the circle of Willis, particularly near branches of the anterior communicating, internal carotid, and middle cerebral arteries, but they can also be found at the junction of almost any branch site within the cerebral circulation. Using modern neurosurgical clipping techniques it is evident that early surgical management is as safe as late surgery, and it significantly reduces risk of rebleeding.

Arteriovenous malformations (AVMs) present with hemorrhage earlier in life than do aneurysms, often in the second or third decade. Although they cause nearly 9% of all SAHs, vascular malformations are also important causes of ICH and intraventricular hemorrhage.[81] An AVM is a congenital structure consisting of a tangled web of vascular tissue that contains multiple arteriovenous fistulas, which permit arterial-to-venous shunting of blood. They can be located anywhere in the central nervous system and may grow quite large, displacing normal neural structures, usually without disruption of function. Seizure, migraine, or hemorrhage are typical presenting symptoms.

The incidence of lifetime hemorrhage with AVM is 40% to 50%[82] with a rebleeding rate of 4% per year and a mortality rate of 1% per year.[83] Treatment options include neuroradiological embolization, surgical resection, and radiotherapy.

Hydrocephalus

Acute and chronic hydrocephalus can complicate both SAH and intraventricular hemorrhage by obstructing cerebrospinal fluid outflow. Blood coagulum within the ventricular system can block the foramen of Sylvius or the fourth ventricle, causing acute obstructive hydrocephalus over minutes to hours after hemorrhage, leading to lethargy, coma, or death if not treated. Placement of an external ventricular drain can be life-saving, but if the obstruction does not resolve, a ventriculoperitoneal shunt is placed for long-term decompression.

Normal pressure hydrocephalus is very common after SAH and often develops during rehabilitation care. The pathophysiological cause is a functional disruption of CSF resorption due to fibrosis of the arachnoid granulations from subarachnoid blood.[84] The classical symptoms of subcortical dementia, incontinence, and gait disorder are clues to the presence of hydrocephalus, but the physiatrist should also have a high level of suspicion when a patient with recent hemorrhage is not making expected functional gains in a rehabilitation program. That suspicion is often confirmed when the patient makes a remarkable recovery after shunting.

STROKE-RELATED IMPAIRMENTS

Disability in stroke is a result of central nervous system injury by which physical, cognitive, and psychological functioning become impaired. Specific impairments appear when focal regions and neural systems within the brain are damaged by vascular compromise. Neurological brain mapping has been an active area of research dating back to 1800 when Franz Joseph Gall developed "phrenology." He interpreted personality and mental capacity by studying the bumps on the human skull. Although phrenology has been discredited, the study of brain topography has proved quite useful for predicting neurological impairment after focal brain injury.

Motor Control and Strength

Anatomy

The primary motor area is located along the cortex of the precentral gyrus anterior to the central sulcus of both hemispheres, and extends from the paracentral lobule within the longitudinal fissure to the frontal operculum within the Sylvian fissure. The classic "motor homunculus" is useful for visualizing the topography of motor control along the precentral gyrus. Axons from these cortical cells descend via the internal capsule to the pyramidal tract in the brainstem and the corticospinal tract in the spinal cord.

Recovery

With hemiplegia, weakness and poor control of voluntary movement are present initially, associated with reduced resting muscle tone. As voluntary movement returns, nonfunctional mass flexion and extension of the limbs are first noted (Table 50–1). Synergy patterns, or mass contraction of multiple muscle groups, are seen.[85] Later, movement patterns can be noted to be independent of synergy.[86]

Motor Coordination and Balance

Trunk control and stability, coordination of movement patterns, and balance all involve complex extrapyramidal systems that are frequently disrupted by stroke. Extrapyramidal disorders can be a major impediment to functional recovery, but are often amenable to therapeutic exercise.

Anatomy

Anterior to the precentral gyrus within the frontal lobe is the premotor area that is important in motor planning. Multiple fiber tracts from this region descend via the anterior limb of the internal capsule to the basal ganglia and the cerebellum, with input from the vestibular, visual, and somatosensory systems. Injury to either the efferent or afferent systems (or both) can cause poor static and dynamic balance as well as movement disorders such as ataxia, chorea, hemiballismus, and tremors.

TABLE 50–1   Synergy Patterns in Motor Recovery After Stroke

Upper Limb	Lower Limb
FLEXOR SYNERGY	
Shoulder retraction	Hip flexion
Shoulder abduction	Hip abduction
Shoulder external rotation	Hip external rotation
Elbow flexion	Knee flexion
Forearm supination	Ankle eversion
Wrist flexion	Dorsiflexion
Finger flexion	Toe extension
EXTENSOR SYNERGY	
Shoulder protraction	Hip extension
Shoulder adduction	Hip adduction
Elbow extension	Knee extension
Forearm pronation	Ankle inversion
Wrist extension	Plantarflexion
Finger flexion	Toe flexion

Spasticity

Spasticity is a velocity-dependent increase in resistance to muscle stretch that develops after an upper motor neuron injury within the central nervous system. When severe, spasticity can cause reduced flexibility, posture, and functional mobility, as well as joint pain, contracture, and difficulty with positioning for comfort and hygiene. In stroke, an increase occurs in both tonic and phasic reflexes. Loss of upper motor neuron control causes disinhibited alpha and gamma motor neuron activity and heightened sensitivity to class 1a and II muscle spindle afferents.[87] Consequently, monosynaptic and multisynaptic spinal reflexes become hyperactive.

Spasticity develops shortly after completed stroke, and is initially manifested as an increased phasic response to tendon tap and a slight catch with passive ranging. Later, ranging can become difficult and the patient might show tonic positioning in flexion or extension. Often as voluntary motor activity returns, a reduction in tone and reflex response is noted, but if recovery is incomplete, spasticity usually remains.

Sensation

Loss of sensation after stroke can have a significant effect on joint and skin protection, balance, coordination, and motor control.

Anatomy

Pain and temperature sensation are relayed centrally by fibers that enter the spinothalamic tract from the contralateral dorsal root gangion and ascend to the ventral posterior lateral (VPL) nucleus of the thalamus. Some spinothalamic fibers enter the superior colliculus and ascending reticular formation.

Sensory fibers for joint proprioception and stereognosis ascend ipsilaterally from the dorsal root gangion within the dorsal column and cross to the contralateral side within the lower medulla after synapsing with the nucleus gracilis and cuneatus. The fibers then ascend in the medial lemniscus to the VPL of the thalamus. The VPL relays sensory information to the primary sensory cortex located posteriorly to the central sulcus in the postcentral gyrus.

Although injury to the sensory pathways typically causes hypoesthesia or reduced sensation, patients with lesions in the thalamus or spinothalamic tract occasionally experience severe pain that can interfere with functional recovery and rehabilitative care. Treatment options include tricyclic antidepressants, anticonvulsants, and physical modalities such as desensitization techniques or electrical stimulation.

Language and Communication

Aphasia is an impairment of language, but typical lesions that cause aphasia affect comprehension and use of the symbolic material for the purpose of communication and meaning (see also Chapter 3). Testing of language should include an examination of oral expression, verbal comprehension, naming, reading, writing, and repeating.[88] A simple and commonly used classification system for aphasia is listed in Table 50–2.

Although language is considered a function of the left

TABLE 50–2   Clinical Characteristics of the Common Aphasic Syndromes

Aphasia	Fluency	Expression	Comprehension	Repetition	Naming
Broca's	Impaired	Impaired	Mildly impaired	Impaired	Impaired
Wernike's	Normal	Impaired	Impaired	Impaired	Impaired
Global	Impaired	Impaired	Impaired	Impaired	Impaired
Transcortical motor	Impaired	Moderately impaired	Minimally impaired	Normal	Impaired
Transcortical sensory	Normal	Minimally impaired	Moderately impaired	Normal	Impaired
Transcortical mixed	Impaired	Impaired	Impaired	Normal	Impaired
Conduction	Normal	Impaired in repetition	Normal	Impaired	Mildly impaired
Anomia	Normal	Normal	Normal	Normal	Impaired

or dominant hemisphere, some elements of communication such as *prosody* have nondominant hemisphere control. Prosody is the rhythmic pattern and vocal intonation of speech that adds emphasis and emotional content to language. There is some clinical and pathological evidence that prosody might have similar anatomical topography as that of verbal language within the nondominant hemisphere.[89]

Anatomy

Patients with Broca-type aphasia have lesions near the frontal operculum, anterior to the precentral gyrus. This location has been aptly named *Broca's area* and is considered a motor association area, as it is adjacent to the oral motor area of the primary motor cortex. However, the Broca-type aphasia is a primary language deficit with mildly compromised comprehension as well as impaired oral expression. It cannot be considered purely a motor impairment. The topographical location for the Wernicke type of aphasia is Wernicke's area, which is found in the posterior superior portion of the first temporal gyrus near the primary auditory cortex and is considered an auditory association area. Lesions near but not involving Broca's or Wernicke's area are associated with transcortical motor and sensory aphasias, respectively.[90]

Ross[89] has described aprosodia that is associated with lesions of the frontal operculum of the right or nondominant hemisphere. Patients who have aprosody speak at an even tempo with flat intonation when asked to express a sentence with an emotional tone. However, they are able to hear and comprehend the emotional content of language. In contrast, patients with a lesion in the temporoparietal region have an affective agnosia in that they are unable to recognize the emotional prosody of spoken language. Despite the agnosia, these patients express prosody without difficulty.

A conduction aphasia, with severely impaired repetition of language, is associated with a lesion of the arcuate fasciculus, which is a bundle of fibers that passes from the temporal to the frontal lobe.[91] Disorders of reading (alexia) and writing (agraphia) are associated with disconnection of the primary language area from the primary visual cortices, which correlates to lesions in the angular gyrus at the junction of the occipital and temporoparietal lobes.[92]

Apraxia

Disorders of skilled movement in the absence of motor, sensory, or cognitive impairment are called *apraxia*. Pa-

tients with apraxia often have difficulty performing simple functional activities, such as using a spoon or a comb, or they will perform them in a clumsy manner. It is often difficult to test for apraxia in the presence of a language deficit because the examiner must be assured that the patient understands the command. However, patients with apraxia can have difficulty waving goodbye or using a gesture for hitchhiking when asked to demonstrate these maneuvers. Apraxia is most commonly seen in left hemisphere strokes and affects the left non-hemiplegic limb. Geshwind[93] attributes apraxia in this situation to a disconnection of the right cortical motor association area from the left hemisphere due to an injury of the anterior callosal fibers. Under these circumstances, the right brain cannot know what the left brain wants to do!

Patients with right parietal strokes often have significant difficulty in dressing, despite adequate strength and flexibility. This has been called "dressing apraxia," but it is not a true apraxia, because it is not a disorder of skilled motor function. It is actually a disorder of spatial perception, which impairs the patient's ability to find the sleeves and neck of a shirt. Similarly, patients with "constructional apraxia" have difficulty copying a figure due to visuospatial deficits consistent with right parietal stroke.

Neglect Syndrome

Heilman defines hemispatial neglect as a failure to report, respond, or orient to novel or meaningful stimuli presented to the side opposite a brain lesion.[94] It is important to exclude visual, somatosensory, or motor impairments that would explain the lack of response before attributing it to neglect. Hemispatial neglect significantly contributes to disability after stroke because it has a negative impact on sitting balance, visual perception, wheelchair mobility, safety awareness, skin and joint protection, and fall risk. Patients with neglect have difficulty completing hygeine and self-care on the affected side, fail to eat food items in the neglected visual space, and frequently run into objects and walls. Neglect is a disorder of visual and spatial attention and is associated with temporoparietal strokes and lesions of the cingulate gyrus, thalamus, and reticular formation.

Dysphagia

Dysphagia is common after stroke, occurring in 30% to 65% of patients with unilateral or bilateral hemispheric and brainstem infarctions.[95–101] Risk for aspiration pneumonia is strongly associated with a delayed reflex pharyngeal swallow and reduced pharyngeal transit times frequently seen on videofluoroscopic swallow evaluation.[102–103] Other neurological factors that influence risk for aspiration after stroke include reduced labial and lingual mobility and sensation, unilateral neglect, pooling of pharyngeal residue within the vallecula and pyriform sinuses, and cricopharyngeal dysmotility. Laryngeal elevation during swallow normally declines with age and can have a negative influence on aspiration risk after stroke (see also Chapter 27).

Uninhibited Bladder and Bowel

Urinary and bowel incontinence are frequent consequences of stroke. Because the pontine micturition center is typically preserved, reflex voiding usually shows normal synchronous internal sphincter relaxation with detrussor contraction. Postvoid residual volumes are generally low in the absence of prostatic hypertrophy or other forms of bladder outlet obstruction. Incontinence is caused by a lack of voluntary inhibition to void from upper motor neuron injury and results in urgency of urination. In alert individuals, awareness of the need to void is unaffected, but immobility, unilateral neglect, and communication deficits often impair a patient's ability to use equipment or call for assistance when the need arises. Although most diabetic stroke survivors have uninhibited voiding, some might have a hypotonic bladder from a parasympathetic autonomic neuropathy to the detrusor muscle. Special care should be taken to check postvoid residual volumes in these patients. Bowel incontinence results from uninhibited reflex rectal emptying by the same mechanism as the uninhibited bladder.

NEUROANATOMICAL BASIS FOR CLINICAL STROKE SYNDROMES

Anatomical localization of lesions within the central nervous system predicts physical or cognitive impairment and disability. Understanding the clinical syndromes associated with defined cerebrovascular lesions in ischemic stroke can be a valuable tool to the physiatrist leading the rehabilitation team.

Middle Cerebral Artery Syndromes

Strokes within the middle cerebral artery (MCA) distribution are the most commonly seen within the inpatient rehabilitation setting. The anatomical distribution of the MCA includes a large proportion of cerebral cortex, and ischemia within the MCA imparts significant impairment and disability, often requiring intensive rehabilitation care. The MCA is particularly vulnerable to both cardioembolic and thrombotic disease that can result in a variety of stroke syndromes.

Anatomy

The anterior circulation of the brain consists of both internal carotid arteries derived from the right and left common carotid arteries. The right carotid is usually a branch of the right subclavian; the left is a direct branch of the aorta. After the internal carotid artery passes intracra-

TABLE 50–3   Middle Cerebral Artery Stroke: Main Stem

Contralateral hemiplegia
Contralateral hemianesthesia
Contralateral hemianopia
Head/eye turning toward lesion
Dysphagia
Uninhibited neurogenic bladder
Dominant hemisphere
  Global aphasia
  Apraxia
Nondominant hemisphere
  Aprosody and affective agnosia
  Visuospatial deficit
  Neglect syndrome

nially through the carotid siphon, it provides the ophthalmic branch to the orbit and then bifurcates at the circle of Willis into the anterior cerebral artery and MCA. The MCA stem or M1 segment turns laterally, passing along the base of the brain to the Sylvian fissure overlying the insular cortex, where it typically bifurcates into an upper and lower division. Along the path of the M1 segment, small, deep, perforating branches called *lenticulostriate arteries* are supplied to the putamen, globus pallidus, caudate, and internal capsule. The M2 segment comprises the upper and lower divisions of the MCA as they travel posteriorly and superiorly along the insular cortex. Branches of the divisions pass laterally along the frontal, parietal, and temporal opercula constituting the M3 segment. The M4 segment includes the branches supplying the frontal, parietal, and temporal convexities.

MCA Stroke

Main Stem. The impairments following occlusion of the MCA main stem (M1 segment) are listed in Table 50–3. The hemiplegia in a main stem stroke is complete, affecting the upper and lower portions of the face equally. This results primarily from ischemia from within the deep lenticulostriate circulation to the posterior limb of the internal capsule through which the descending fibers of the primary motor cortex pass. In contrast, the hemisensory deficit is not as severe because the ascending sensory fibers are not affected, and only the inferior portion of the primary sensory cortex is supplied by the MCA. Although the MCA perforators only supply the upper half of the visual radiations, complete hemianopias are frequently described. Dysphagia and uninhibited voiding are commonly found, even in unilateral strokes.

Upper Division. MCA upper division strokes are listed in Table 50–4. The clinical presentation is very similar to

TABLE 50–4   Middle Cerebral Artery Stroke: Upper Division

Contralateral hemiplegia*	Dominant hemisphere
Contralateral hemianesthesia	Broca (motor) aphasia
Contralateral hemianopia	Apraxia
Head/eye turning toward lesion	Nondominant hemisphere
Dysphagia	Aprosody
Uninhibited neurogenic bladder	Visual-spatial deficit
	Neglect syndrome

*Leg relatively more spared than hand and face.

TABLE 50–5   Middle Cerebral Artery Stroke: Lower Division

Contralateral hemianopia
Dominant hemisphere
Wernicke aphasia
Nondominant hemisphere
Affective agnosia

that of a main stem infarction, but hemiplegia and language comprehension deficits are usually not as severe. Because the M1 segment of the MCA is spared, the vascular supply to the internal capsule is preserved and ischemia is limited to the inferolateral portion of the primary motor cortex. Thus, motor strength and control are better in the lower limb than in the hand and face. A classic Broca-type aphasia is typical in a dominant hemisphere stroke, and aprosodia without affective agnosia is found in nondominant hemisphere stroke.

Lower Division.   Branch obstruction of the MCA lower division is much less common than upper division stroke, and is usually caused by an embolic event. Motor and sensory function are generally intact. Despite this, patients with stroke of the MCA lower division can have significant functional disability from impaired language and vision. Table 50–5 lists the impairments associated with lower division strokes.

Anterior Cerebral Artery Syndromes

Anatomy

The anterior cerebral artery (ACA) supplies the interhemispheric cortical surface of the frontal and parietal lobes. The A1 segment branches medially from the internal carotid bifurcation to the anterior communicating artery. Turning superiorly, the artery passes over the optic nerve, along the rostrum of the corpus callosum (A2), and around the genu (A3); it passes posteriorly to the coronal suture (A4) and terminates at the parietal lobe (A5). The ACA divides during its course into two major branches, the pericallosal and callomarginal branches, which provide smaller branches to the cortical surface. The recurrent artery of Heubner is a branch from the A1 or proximal A2 segment that deeply perforates to supply important structures such as the head of the caudate, the anterior limb of the internal capsule, the anterior putamen and globus pallidus, and the hypothalamus.

ACA Stroke

The disorders resulting from an ACA infarction are listed in Table 50–6. The hemiplegia in ACA strokes shows weakness of the shoulder and foot with relative sparing of the forearm, hand, and face, because the focus of ischemia is over the paracentral lobule of the interhemispheric cor-

tex. Unilateral footdrop can be a long-term impairment requiring orthotic management. A left upper limb apraxia to verbal commands can also result from an infarction of the anterior corpus callosum, which disconnects the right hemisphere prefrontal area from the left hemisphere language area.

Occlusion involving the anterior communicating artery and the recurrent artery of Heubner can extend the infarction through the anterior limb of the internal capsule, causing complete hemiplegia. The proximity of such a stroke to Broca's area can also result in a transcortical motor aphasia.

Posterior Cerebral Artery Syndromes

Anatomy

The vertebral arteries typically branch from the right and left subclavian arteries, passing rostrally through the transverse foramina of the cervical vertebra and intracranially via the foramen magnum. At the junction of the medulla and pons, the vertebral arteries unite to form the basilar artery, which again divides into the two posterior cerebral arteries (PCAs) near the top of the midbrain. The P1 segment extends from the basilar to the posterior communicating artery, and the P2 segment extends beyond. Supplying the thalamus are the deep perforating arteries from the P1 and the stem of the P2 segments, called the *thalamoperforants* and *thalamogeniculates*. The branches of the P2 segment include the anterior and posterior inferior temporal, occipital temporal, calcarine, and occipitoparietal arteries.

PCA Stroke

The syndrome of PCA infarction is listed in Table 50–7. The blood supply of the thalamus is provided by the perforating arteries of the PCA. Infarcts in the region can cause hemisensory deficits, including hypoesthesia, dysesthesia, and, occasionally, hyperesthesia or pain. Thalamic pain syndrome was first described by Dejerine and Roussy in 1906,[104] but nearly any disruption of sensory afferent fibers within the central nervous system can cause a central poststroke pain syndrome. Visual disturbances result from injury to the lateral geniculate, temporal, and occipital visual radiations and the calcarine cortex of the occipital lobe. In addition, damage to visual association areas can cause dyschromatopsia, or altered color discrimination. A disorder of reading without impaired writing (alexia without agraphia) associated with a right visual field deficit results from an infarction of the left occipital cortex and posterior corpus callosum, disconnecting the intact right visual cortex from the primary language area of the left hemisphere. Impaired memory can result from infarction of the temporal lobe and the hippocampal gyri.

TABLE 50–6   Anterior Cerebral Artery Stroke

Contralateral hemiplegia*	Grasp reflex—groping
Contralateral hemianesthesia	Disconnection apraxia
Head/eye turning toward lesion	Akinetic mutism (abulia)

*Hand relatively more spared than arm and leg.

TABLE 50–7   Posterior Cerebral Artery Stroke

Hemisensory deficit	Dyschromatopsia
Visual impairment	Alexia without agraphia
Visual agnosia	Memory deficits
Prosopagnosia	

Vertebrobasilar Syndromes

Anatomy

The major arterial branches supplying the brainstem and cerebellum are the posterior inferior cerebellar artery (PICA), the anterior inferior cerebellar artery (AICA), and the superior cerebellar artery (SCA). The PICA originates from the distal vertebral artery and wraps dorsally around the medulla, whereas the AICA is a branch of the basilar artery circling around the pons. Both supply the inferior lobe of the cerebellum. The superior lobe of the cerebellum receives its blood supply from the SCA branching from the basilar artery at the level of the midbrain. Throughout the course of the basilar artery and its major tributaries, small, deep, perforating arteries branch to supply the brainstem. These branches include paramedian penetrators supplying the medial and basal portions of the brainstem, and the short and long circumferential arteries supporting the lateral brainstem.

Brainstem Stroke Syndromes

The brainstem is a complex structure containing cranial nerves, bulbar nuclei, and tracts. The bulbar nuclei form afferent and efferent cranial nerves that innervate the ipsilateral side of the body, whereas the ascending and descending bulbar and spinal tracts innervate contralaterally. Thus, unilateral brainstem strokes often cause loss of cranial nerve function ipsilaterally and sensorimotor dysfunction contralaterally.[105] Cerebellar strokes result in ipsilateral ataxia, whereas brainstem strokes can cause ipsilateral, contralateral, or bilateral limb ataxia. The common brainstem syndromes are listed in Table 50–8, along with their anatomical correlates.

The *Wallenberg* or lateral medullary syndrome is a commonly occurring stroke that frequently requires inpatient rehabilitation. It is characterized by ipsilateral limb ataxia, loss of pain and temperature sensation on the ipsilateral face and contraleral body, ipsilateral Horner's syndrome (myosis, ptosis, and anhydrosis), dysphagia, dysphonia, and nystagmus. Vertebral artery thrombosis near the PICA branch is the usual cause. Prognosis for functional improvement is excellent.

Most of the remaining brainstem syndromes occur with basilar artery thrombosis. The *locked-in* syndrome is a severe pontine stroke causing quadriplegia, oral motor and laryngeal weakness, and disruption of conjugate eye movements. Oral communication is impaired, but because upward gaze is controlled at the midbrain level within the tectum, patients usually have voluntary vertical eye movements that they can use for communication.

Cerebellar strokes are common and can cause life-threatening obstruction of the fourth ventricle and hydrocephalus if cerebellar edema develops. Such strokes occur with PICA, AICA, or SCA occlusion. PICA and AICA strokes are generally caused by arterial thrombosis of the vertebrobasilar system, but SCA strokes are more commonly cardioembolic.[106]

Lacunar Strokes

Lacunar strokes are located within the deep cerebral white matter, basal ganglia, thalamus, and pons, and result from occlusion of single, small, perforating arteries. These strokes are common, and present with a wide variety of neurological and functional deficits. The most common syndromes are listed in Table 50–9.

ACUTE DIAGNOSTIC EVALUATION

The goal of the initial laboratory evaluation in a patient with acute stroke is to establish an accurate diagnosis of stroke and to determine the presence of other intercurrent illness. Initial laboratory tests include electrolytes, glucose, and cholesterol levels, complete blood cell count, prothrombin time, partial thromboplastin time, erythrocyte sedimentation rate (ESR), and urinalysis.

TABLE 50–8   Brainstem Syndromes and Their Anatomical Correlates

Syndrome	Location	Structural Injury	Characteristics
Weber's	Medial basal midbrain	Third cranial nerve	Ipsilateral third nerve palsy
		Corticospinal tract	Contralateral hemiplegia
Benedikt's	Tegmentum of midbrain	Third cranial nerve	Ipsilateral third nerve palsy
		Spinothalamic tract	Contralateral loss of pain and temperature sensation
		Medial lemniscus	Contralateral loss of joint position
		Superior cerebellar peduncle	Contralateral ataxia
		Red nucleus	Contralateral chorea
Locked-in	Bilateral basal pons	Corticospinal tract	Bilateral hemiplegia
		Corticobulbar tract	Bilateral cranial nerve palsy (Upward gaze spared)
Millard-Gubler	Lateral pons	Sixth cranial nerve	Ipsilateral sixth nerve palsy
		Seventh cranial nerve	Ipsilateral facial weakness
		Corticospinal tract	Contralateral hemiplegia
Wallenberg's	Lateral medulla	Spinocerebellar tract	Ipsilateral hemiataxia
		Fifth cranial nerve	Ipsilateral loss of facial pain and temperature sensation
		Spinothalamic tract	Contralateral loss of body pain and temperature sensation
		Vestibular nuclei	Nystagmus
		Sympathetic tract	Ipsilateral Horner's syndrome
		Nucleus ambiguus	Dysphagia and dysphonia

TABLE 50–9 Lacunar Syndromes and Their Anatomical Correlates

Syndrome	Anatomical Sites
Pure motor stroke	Posterior limb internal capsule Basis pontis Pyramids
Pure sensory stroke	Thalamus Thalamocortical projections
Sensory-motor stroke	Junction of internal capsule and thalamus
Dysarthria–clumsy hand	Anterior limb internal capsule Pons
Ataxic hemiparesis	Corona radiata Internal capsule Pons Cerebellum
Hemiballismus	Head of caudate Thalamus Subthalamic nucleus

Additional laboratory tests can be ordered as indicated, such as a full lipid profile if the cholesterol level is elevated. In young patients with stroke it is important to consider hereditary diseases that increase risk for hypercoagulability and stroke.[107] A serum hemoglobin electrophoresis can detect sickle cell disease or trait. Hypercoagulable states, such as deficiencies in protein C,[108] protein S, or antithrombin III, can be tested by measuring the plasma levels of each. An elevated ESR should stimulate an evaluation for vasculitis, anticardiolipin antibody, or lupus anticoagulant.

Cranial imaging studies should be performed as early as possible, beginning with computed tomography (CT) of the head, to determine whether the stroke is ischemic or hemorrhagic. In an ischemic stroke, the CT of the head is often negative in the first 24 to 48 hours after stroke, but the signs of a cortical infarct include a loss of definition in the gray-white junction and effacement of the sulci overlying the infarcted region. Occasionally a bright area or "signal" that is diagnostic of an acute thromboembolism is seen in the region of the MCA.[109] Later, the cerebral infarct appears as a hypodense region that matches the ischemic vascular distribution. Lacunar strokes appear as small punctate hypodensities within the basal ganglia, thalamus, and subcortical white matter. Strokes in the brainstem and cerebellum are more difficult to visualize using cranial CT scanning, because the thick bone of the skull base creates image artifacts that impair soft-tissue detail within the posterior fossa. Magnetic resonance imaging (MRI) is superior to CT for the anatomical evaluation of the posterior fossa.

Intracranial hemorrhage has a hyperdense appearance on CT and can be distinguished from infarction in the acute period. The location of hemorrhage can provide clues to the etiology of the bleeding. Hemorrhage confined to the basal ganglia or thalamus is likely a result of hypertensive ICH. Saccular aneurysm and AVM should be considered if intraventricular or subarachnoid blood is seen. Within 1 or 2 weeks after hemorrhagic infarct, the appearance of blood on head CT becomes hypodense with soft tissue, and may be more difficult to differentiate. The late appearance of an ICH typically shows resolution of extravasated blood and edema, with only a small residual hypodense defect remaining.[110]

Standard two-dimensional spin-echo MRI is now available in most medical centers throughout the United States, and it has several advantages for the evaluation of stroke. Tissue density on MRI is dependent on the energy released by hydrogen atoms exposed to radiofrequency pulses in the presence of a strong magnetic field. On T1-weighted images, cerebrospinal fluid (CSF) appears dark, whereas gray and white matter are nicely differentiated. In contrast, T2-weighted images show bright CSF signal, while fat density is low. A third technique, in which CSF and soft-tissue are isodense, is called "spin-density" weighting. With all techniques, bone is poorly imaged due to its low hydrogen content. The flow of blood within the cerebral circulation produces a signal void unless a static intravascular occlusion is present.

MRI is more sensitive for detection of acute stroke changes than is CT in the first 48 hours.[111] Edema within an infarcted zone can appear as early as 2 to 4 hours after stroke onset, and it is seen best on T2-weighted images. Infarcts near the cortex or periventricular region are better seen on spin-density images, because the bright CSF signal of T2-weighting can otherwise obscure subtle changes. T1-weighted images are less sensitive for acute cerebral infarct, but they can show early effacement of gyri and occasionally a vascular thrombosis. MRI is more sensitive than CT for lacunar strokes after the first 24 hours, and MRI is the test of choice for imaging the posterior fossa, where bone artifact is not a problem.[112]

MRI is nearly equivalent to CT for the detection of ICH in the acute setting; but it has not replaced CT, because MRI is more expensive. With subacute or chronic hemorrhagic stroke, MRI can differentiate methemoglobin from soft tissue and is better than CT for detection of late hemorrhages.[111]

Magnetic resonance angiography (MRA) is the newest MR technology, and is revolutionary in stroke diagnostics and management. Using the two-dimensional "time-of-flight" technique, extracranial vessels can be visualized, often revealing the presence of carotid or vertebrobasilar atherosclerotic disease. Three-dimensional "time-of-flight" produces excellent images of the circle of Willis and the cerebral artery stems.[113] MRA is indicated as a screening test for extracranial and intracranial atherosclerotic disease, but has not yet exceeded the detail of conventional contrast angiography. However, as this technique continues to improve, it may soon be considered equivalent in accuracy.

Nuclear medicine scanning techniques, such as positron emission tomography (PET) and single-photon emission computed tomography (SPECT), detect the uptake of radiolabeled materials with a signal intensity dependent on blood flow to the soft-tissue region. Changes can be detected within the ischemic zone immediately during acute cerebral infarct and hemmorhage. Currently, PET scanning is not readily available, and its use is limited to research, whereas SPECT scanning continues to be evaluated for its clinical usefulness.[114]

Due to its noninvasive nature, ultrasound technology is gaining in popularity in many diagnostic areas, including stroke diagnosis. Transthoracic echocardiography (TTE) imaging after suspected cerebral embolism is now standard and is simple to perform. Intraventricular thrombi and valvular vegetations are particularly easy to image using this technique. Thrombi within the left atrium and left atrial appendage can also be detected with TTE, but it is often difficult, because the left atrium is easily obscured by the left ventricle.[115] Transesophageal echocardiography (TEE) overcomes these limitations by passing the transducer down the esophagus, posterior to the heart, where the left atrium and appendage can be directly visualized. Left atrial thrombi can be detected up to ten times more often using TEE.[116] TEE imaging also is more accurate for locating atrial septal defects, which can be important if paradoxical embolisms are suspected. TEE is generally well tolerated.

Arterial duplex scanning combines either standard or color Doppler with two-dimensional ultrasound and is a useful screening tool for the detection of atherosclerotic disease within the extracranial vessels. In practical use a negative carotid duplex scan excludes the need for carotid endarterectomy, but it does not rule out the presence of significant intracranial atherosclerosis. Similarly, a duplex scan that is positive for critical stenosis extracranially cannot exclude the presence of an arterial occlusion in the distal internal carotid, which contraindicates surgical treatment. Transcranial Doppler can measure flow characteristics of the intracranial vessels, but it lacks imaging capability; it is most useful when serial measurements of cerebral blood flow are needed, such as in the monitoring of cerebral vasospasm after SAH.[117] Although it is invasive and not without complications, conventional contrast cerebral angiography is the most accurate method for detection and anatomical definition of extracranial or intracranial cerebrovascular disease, aneurysms, and AVMs when surgical treatment is considered. Contrast angiography is the method of choice for detecting and defining the anatomy of cerebral aneurysms and AVMs.

ACUTE STROKE INTERVENTION

Technological advances in cardiac care, such as the acute coronary care unit and advanced treatment protocols for acute myocardial infarction, have improved survival and quality of life for people with heart disease. Recently, there has been interest in approaching acute stroke care in the same aggressive manner with the goal of arresting cerebral ischemia, restoring cerebral perfusion, and minimizing neurological injury. In an effort to compare the urgency of acute stroke to that of a heart attack, clinicians are beginning to think of stroke as a "brain attack,"[118] and a significant amount of new research is seeking to improve long-term stroke outcome using state-of-the-art monitoring and pharmacotherapy in the intensive care setting.

The Ischemic Penumbra

A basic pathophysiological understanding of cerebral ischemia clarifies the actions necessary to protect the brain during acute stroke. Cerebral tissue necrosis occurs when cerebral blood flow (CBF), normally under tight autoregulation, is compromised from either arterial thrombosis or embolism. Normal cerebral autoregulation maintains a ce-

rebral perfusion rate of 50 mL/100 g of cerebral tissue per minute, remaining constant regardless of acute changes in systemic mean arterial pressure. During cerebrovascular compromise, normal neural activity can be sustained with a CBF as low as 20 mL/100 g/min, but a rate below 10 mL/100 g/min results in cellular death. Within the CBF range between 10 and 20 mL/100 g/min, basic cellular functions are supported, but the sodium-potassium pump fails, rendering the neural cells "electrically silent."[119] In an acute stroke, these surviving but inactive neural cells are located at the rim of the ischemic injury, where collateral circulation provides the minimal tissue perfusion needed. This rim has been called the *ischemic penumbra*, after the partial shadow surrounding a solar eclipse. Improved blood flow to the ischemic penumbra can theoretically restore normal neurological function. However, the longer the ischemic period before reperfusion, the less likely is the ischemic penumbra to survive. Recent acute stroke management protocols have focused on neuropreservation and reperfusion of the ischemic zone in order to maximally save the ischemic penumbra. From the standpoint of public education regarding stroke, the National Stroke Association has emphasized that to reduce neural impairment, acute stroke management should be implemented within the first 6 hours of the event.[120]

Acute Medical Management

Initial medical care for a patient with acute stroke requires careful and frequent neurological monitoring to prevent and manage medical complications that compromise cerebral tissue perfusion. If the patient is obtunded, concern for airway protection is critical to maintain oxygenation, and an endotracheal tube should be placed, with ventilatory support if necessary. Cerebral edema and acute hydrocephalus may develop rapidly (particularly after ICH) requiring hyperventilation or placement of an external ventriculostomy device to relieve intracranial pressure. In cases of brainstem compression and hydrocephalus from cerebellar infarction or hemorrhage, surgical decompression of the posterior fossa can be life-saving.[121]

Blood pressure is often acutely elevated during stroke, usually as a response to cerebral injury, and often falls spontaneously over the following week.[122] Clinicians should resist the temptation to rapidly correct elevated blood pressure, because often it is a necessary compensatory response to impaired autoregulation after acute ischemic brain injury. Thus, a higher mean arterial pressure (MAP) is needed to maintain cerebral perfusion pressure to the ischemic area. A rapid drop in blood pressure can potentially enlarge an ischemic injury. This is especially true in hypertensive individuals whose brains are accustomed to a higher perfusion pressure.[123, 124] Acute hypertension after stroke should only be treated if it is symptomatic, when there is evidence of end-organ injury, or if the diastolic pressure rises above 120 mm Hg.[125] When treated, elevated blood pressure should be lowered gently, and it is usually best to allow the systolic pressure to remain above 150 mm Hg and the diastolic pressure above 90 mm Hg. Calcium channel blockers may not be ideal agents for acute hypertension management after stroke, despite their popularity. These medications can cause cerebral vasodilation and increased intracranial pressure, resulting in reduced perfusion of the ischemic penumbra.[124] A better choice for acute blood pressure control are the mixed beta- and alpha-antagonists, such as labetalol, which have no measurable effect on cerebral perfusion.[124, 126]

Hyperglycemia occurs in both diabetic and nondiabetic patients during stroke in response to acute physiological stress, and it is associated with increased levels of serum cortisol. Frequent monitoring and control of serum glucose during acute stroke have been recommended. Animal studies have shown that the presence of a high glucose concentration within partially perfused ischemic tissue provides the substrate for anaerobic cellular metabolism and lactic acid production.[127, 128] Accumulation of lactic acid is cytotoxic and can lead to further tissue injury.[128, 129] Thus, careful use of insulin and strict glucose control are potentially neuroprotective.

Pharmacological Management

Considerable effort has recently been invested in developing effective therapeutic agents that can arrest, delay, or reverse cerebral ischemia and neural injury. Current research has focused mainly on four pharmacological treatments: heparin, calcium channel blockers, thrombolytic agents, and neuroprotective medications.

Intravenous heparin is frequently administered in the acute setting to arrest stroke progression or to prevent its recurrence. Current available research has neither supported nor discredited the efficacy of heparin for acute stroke management, and clear guidelines for its use are lacking.[130] The prevailing evidence would support the use of antiplatelet agents for the treatment of thrombotic stroke, but heparin may be appropriate for arresting an evolving stroke in some clinical situations. Because the risk of recurrent cardioembolic stroke is 12% within the first 3 weeks without anticoagulation, the use of heparin and warfarin seem warranted if the risk of bleeding is otherwise low.[71]

Calcium channel blocking agents, such as nimodipine, are effective in the prevention of death from vasospastic complications of SAH and are recommended for routine use during the first 21 days after hemorrhage.[131, 132] Several trials testing nimodipine for acute ischemic stroke treatment have had disappointing results. The vasodilating effect of these medications can hamper stroke recovery by increasing intracranial pressure.[133]

The use of thrombolytic agents in acute stroke has been successful in achieving recanalization of occluded cranial arteries in studies that enrolled subjects within the first 2 to 6 hours after onset of infarction.[134–136] Although the use of agents such as tissue plasminogen activator (tPA) seems promising, acute hemorrhagic complications have limited their use. Newer medications such as ancrod, an agent that binds to and inactivates fibrinogen, are now being studied in an effort to find a safer thrombolytic treatment for acute stroke.[137]

Another class of medications for the treatment of acute stroke are the neuroprotective agents. In particular, the N-methyl-D-aspartate (NMDA) receptor antagonists have shown the potential to delay neuronal injury. During ischemic injury, excitatory neurotransmitters such as gluta-

mate and aspartate are released extracellularly. In high concentrations, these amino acids act on NMDA membrane receptors causing an influx of cations that result in rapid neuronal death. Controlled studies testing the ability of NMDA antagonists to prevent cytotoxic injury during acute stroke are under way.[138, 139]

NATURAL SPONTANEOUS NEUROLOGICAL RECOVERY

There are two different but related ways that patients improve after stroke.[140] The first type of recovery, a reduction in the extent of neurological impairment, can result from natural spontaneous neurological recovery, from the effects of treatments that limit the extent of the stroke, or from other interventions that enhance neurological functioning. This form of recovery presents as improvements in motor control, language ability, or other primary neurological functions.[141]

The second type of recovery demonstrated by stroke patients is the improved ability to perform daily functions in their environment, within the limitations of their physical impairments.[142–145] A patient who has sensorimotor, cognitive, or behavioral deficits resulting from stroke may regain the capacity to feed himself or herself, dress, bathe, control elimination, walk, and carry out other activities of daily living, even if with some degree of residual physical impairment. The ability to perform these tasks can improve through adaptation and training, in the presence or absence of natural neurological recovery. This is the element of recovery on which rehabilitation is thought to exert the greatest effect.

The degree of recovery in independent functioning that occurs during rehabilitation has been found to be greater than that which might have been expected by a reduction in neural impairments alone,[146–155] which suggests that the rehabilitation interventions probably play an important role in improvement. However, the two types of improvement are related in subtle and complex ways.[140] Alternative compensatory functional strategies, such as one-handed dressing techniques for the hemiplegic patient, play a major role in the performance of functional tasks when neurological improvement is minimal or absent.

The degree of natural recovery of neurological function is variable, but figures of the relative frequencies of neurological deficits during the early and later poststroke stages offer some insight into the magnitude of recovery that might be seen. These deficits generally decline in frequency by about one-third to one-half.[27, 141, 156] For example, the prevalence of hemiparesis has been found to decline from 73% during initial presentation to 37% at 1-year follow-up, aphasia from 36% to 20%, dysarthria from 48% to 16%, dysphagia from 13% to 4%, and incontinence from 29% to 9%. The time course of recovery is also variable. Although most improvements in physical functioning occur within the first 3 to 6 months, later recovery also is commonly seen.[147, 157–160] Although it is tempting to specify a definitive prognosis in a stroke patient who presents with a particular level of initial motor function, it is important to recognize that there are a multiplicity of variables that determine ultimate outcome, and that, therefore, expectations for recovery are often inaccurate.

Recovery of Motor Function

For most (but not all) stroke patients, the pattern of natural spontaneous recovery of motor function follows a relatively stereotyped sequence of events, in which lower extremity function recovers earliest and most completely, followed by upper extremity and hand function. Return of tone usually precedes return of voluntary movement, proximal control precedes distal control, and mass movement patterns (or synergy patterns) precede specific isolated coordinated volitional motor functions[85, 86, 161] (see Table 50–1). There are many exceptions to these observations, however, primarily in patients who sustain strokes in distributions other than in the MCA area.

Although the prognosis for ultimate return of voluntary motor control cannot be provided with a strong degree of certainty to an individual patient, some degree of improvement in motor function usually occurs after stroke.[162–172] For example, one study[163] reported that lower extremity motor control improved by one Brunnstrom recovery stage in 39% and by two or more stages in 12% of patients, whereas upper extremity motor control improved by one stage in 24% and by two stages in 8%.

This sequence of recovery can stop at any stage. Some hemiparetic patients ultimately regain full or nearly complete use of all muscles in an isolated coordinated fashion, independent of synergy patterns. Others experience incomplete improvement with partial voluntary use of the recovering extremity, and a few patients demonstrate minimal or no recovery in motor control. One investigation[162] reported that moderate or severe motor weakness of the arm was present in about two-thirds of patients initially and in about one-fourth at 3-month follow-up.

Recovery of Language and Perceptual Functions

Language and perceptual abilities tend to improve after stroke, but their recovery patterns can be more variable than those seen in motor function. The prevalence of aphasia declines from about one-fourth during the acute phase to about one-fifth or less during the later stages after stroke.[173] Recovery from aphasia usually occurs at a slower rate and over a more prolonged time course than does motor recovery.[159] Whereas most aphasia recovery occurs in the first 3 to 6 months,[173–175] at least one group has observed that patients with global aphasia show the greatest improvement during the latter half of the first year after stroke.[159, 173, 176] The amount and pattern of recovery are usually related to the initial severity of the aphasia and the specific aphasia type.[177, 178] Nonfluent aphasics generally have a less favorable prognosis than do fluent aphasics, although both groups can and do improve. Comprehension usually returns earlier, and to a greater extent than does expression.[179]

Although most of the improvement in perceptual functioning occurs in the first 3 to 6 months after stroke,[180–186] some recovery occurs later. According to a study by Hier and associates,[186] most of the recovery of perceptual deficits, such as unilateral spatial neglect, denial of illness, loss of facial recognition, and motor impersistence, occurred within the first 20 weeks after stroke, but some improvement could be seen up to 1 year later.

Mechanisms of Recovery of Neurological Function

Several mechanisms have been proposed to explain the clinically observed phenomenon of spontaneous recovery of neurological function.[187–197] These mechanisms generally can be divided into two broad categories. The first mechanism is resolution of local harmful factors, which usually accounts for early spontaneous improvement after stroke (usually within the first 3 to 6 months). These processes include resolution of local edema, resorption of local toxins, improved local circulation, and recovery of partially damaged ischemic neurons. The second mechanism to explain recovery is neuroplasticity, which can take place early or late. Brain plasticity is the ability of the nervous system to modify its structural and functional organization. The two most plausible forms of plasticity are collateral sprouting of new synaptic connections and unmasking of previously latent functional pathways. Other mechanisms of plasticity include assumption of function by undamaged redundant neural pathways, reversibility from diaschisis, denervation supersensitivity, and regenerative proximal sprouting of transected neuronal axons. Experimental evidence indicates that plasticity can be altered by several external conditions, including pharmacological agents, electrical stimulation, and environmental stimulation.[198] The reader is referred to several excellent references for additional information on the subject of natural recovery.[188–190, 193, 197]

MEDICAL CO-MORBIDITIES AND COMPLICATIONS

Most patients with stroke who undergo rehabilitation have many other associated medical conditions that require professional attention. These problems might be pre-existing medical illnesses that necessitate ongoing care (such as hypertension and diabetes), secondary poststroke complications (such as deep venous thrombosis and pneumonia), or acute poststroke exacerbations of pre-existing chronic diseases (such as angina in a patient with ischemic heart disease). Management of these conditions can constitute major portions of the rehabilitation effort. It has been stated that some stroke patients are more disabled by certain associated co-morbid diseases than by the stroke itself.[27, 199]

The occurrence of these associated conditions has several implications for stroke patient management during and after rehabilitation. First, these problems can detract from the benefits of rehabilitation. Some medical problems, such as heart disease, have been found to adversely affect the course and outcome after a stroke.[27, 199–203] Intercurrent medical complications can limit ability to participate in therapeutic exercise programs, inhibit functional skill performance, and reduce the likelihood of achieving favorable outcomes from rehabilitation. The rehabilitation interventions also might adversely affect the medical condition, causing an exacerbation of the disease or a need to adjust medical management. An example is the occurrence of angina during strenuous exercise in therapy. Careful attention and cautious management decisions are required. Finally, medical complications can occur during the rehabilitation program that demand diagnostic evaluation, prompt recognition, and appropriate medical management. At times, both diagnosis and treatment of these complications are difficult in the rehabilitation setting.

Prevention and treatment of co-morbid conditions and medical complications are major components of the rehabilitation management of stroke patients, as they enable the process of rehabilitation to take place and be most effective. The clinical tasks for management of these problems are to prevent medical complications, to promptly and appropriately diagnose and treat those complications when they occur, and to manage pre-existing medical illnesses and ongoing physiological functions during rehabilitation. A few of the important complications are discussed briefly. The reader is referred to several reviews of stroke co-morbidities[204-209] and to individual articles on several specific complications[26, 210-217] for more complete discussions of associated medical problems as they relate to stroke patients and the rehabilitation process. Table 50–10 lists of some of the common diagnoses that might accompany the stroke and that can require management.

Selected Complications

Physiological deconditioning accompanies both acute medical illness and the prolonged bed rest that might be enforced immediately after its onset.[218-220] Deconditioning can contribute to the problems of fatigue, endurance limitations, orthostatic hypotension, lack of motivation, depression, and poor exercise tolerance. All of these can adversely affect the course of recovery and rehabilitation. Preventive techniques include early mobilization, early and graded rehabilitation participation, and development of a balanced schedule of activity and rest.

Bowel and bladder incontinence is seen in one-third to two-thirds of all stroke survivors,[221-229] but continence is usually recovered. Continued incontinence in the stroke patient is often predictive of limited functional outcome.

TABLE 50–10   Common Medical Co-morbidities and Complications in Stroke Patients

Thromboembolic disease	Malnutrition
Pneumonia	Dysphagia
Ventilatory insufficiency	Shoulder dysfunction
Hypertension	Reflex sympathetic dystrophy
Orthostatic hypotension	syndrome
Angina	Depression
Congestive heart failure	Sexual dysfunction
Cardiac arrhythmias	Seizure
Diabetes mellitus	Spasticity
Prior stroke	Contracture
Recurrent stroke	Central poststroke pain
Urinary tract infection	syndrome
Bladder dysfunction—	Falls and injuries
incontinence or retention	Medication overuse
Bowel dysfunction—	Deconditioning and endurance
incontinence or retention	limitations
Pressure sore	Fatigue
Dehydration	Insomnia

Urinary incontinence results from urinary tract infection, neurogenic bladder dysfunction, cognitive or sensory deficits, or inability to transfer to the toilet. Management of incontinence focuses on addressing each of these problems as appropriate. Bowel problems following stroke might be due to immobility and inactivity, inadequate fluid intake or nutritional intake, psychological depression, neurological impairment resulting in neurogenic bowel, lack of transfer ability, cognitive deficit, or reduced consciousness.

Shoulder pain, contracture, and other musculoskeletal disorders, resulting from glenohumeral subluxation, impingement syndromes, rotator cuff tears, frozen shoulder, brachial plexus injuries, reflex sympathetic dystrophy syndrome, bursitis, tendinitis, or central pain, occur in 70% to 80% of hemiplegic stroke patients.[230-240] Shoulder problems are more frequently associated with spasticity than with flaccidity. Treatment includes arm troughs, laptrays, shoulder slings, medications, physical modalities, and, most important, aggressive and consistent range of motion exercises.

Falls occur with striking frequency in stroke survivors, with most reports indicating that patients who sustain right hemisphere strokes are at substantially greater risk for falling than are those with left hemisphere strokes.[241-244] Prevention approaches emphasize balance training, cognitive training, eliminating environmental hazards, and use of specialized devices.

Effective management of these and other medical complications of stroke are critical to enable effective rehabilitation to take place and to allow the achievement of optimal outcomes.

PRINCIPLES OF STROKE REHABILITATION

Because presentations, problems, recovery patterns, coping styles, social situations, and response to treatment differ in individuals who survive stroke, it is necessary to individualize rehabilitation management programs. However, a few central and common themes have been raised by clinicians and investigators in the field of stroke rehabilitation. Several views of the common themes and characteristics of stroke rehabilitation programs are enumerated in Table 50–11.[245-247]

Team Management

The multidimensional and interactive nature of the clinical consequences of stroke make interdisciplinary team care the most appropriate strategy for developing and providing a complete and comprehensive approach to stroke patient management.[4, 247, 248] Coordination of care within the team model, and especially communication between team members, help to avoid fragmentation and duplication of services. Among its many potential benefits, using a comprehensive approach affords the opportunity to specifically tailor treatment schedules to meet specific patient needs. Success in a rehabilitation program is more likely to occur when the patient and family have an understanding of stroke and its potential outcomes, are involved in the setting of goals, and can participate in care.

TABLE 50–11 Three Views of the Features and Goals of Stroke Rehabilitation

JOINT COMMITTEE FOR STROKE FACILITIES (1972)[245]
1. Preventing deformities
2. Treating deformities, if they occur
3. Retraining the patient in ambulation activities
4. Teaching the patient to perform activities of daily living and working with the unaffected arm and hand
5. Retraining the affected arm and hand to its maximum capacity
6. Treating facial and speech disability if they are present
7. Compensation for sensory loss
8. Full social participation
9. Achievement of maximum patient motivation
10. Establishment of independent living post-discharge
11. Vocational placement, if appropriate

GOLDBERG (1986)[246]
1. Preventing complications of inactivity
2. Preventing recurrent stroke
3. Identifying functional deficits and abilities
4. Improving overall physical functioning through conditioning exercises
5. Improving functional ability through training in specific daily living tasks, such as mobility, hand use, self-care, cognition, and communication
6. Assessing need for specialized equipment for mobility and daily living, and providing prescriptions for specific aids and orthoses and home modifications
7. Assessing and providing support to the patient and family in the process of social adjustment to a long-term change in the patient's overall state of health
8. Identifying and treating affective disorders and providing counseling and support to the patient
9. Preventing complications through evaluation and treatment of all associated medical conditions
10. Identifying and facilitating recreational activities, including leisure activities and hobbies
11. Ideally, returning the patient to complete self-support, including gainful employment

BRANDSTATER (1987)[247]
1. Committed medical direction to provide continuity of care from acute phase through rehabilitation and long-term follow-up, to address medical problems during rehabilitation, and to provide leadership, supervision, and coordination of the rehabilitation team and its efforts
2. Use of a team approach, with staff that is knowledgeable of, experienced in, and dedicated to stroke patient care
3. Goal-directed treatment
4. Early initiation of treatment
5. Emphasis on patient education
6. Intensive focus on training of skills
7. Focus on facilitating adaptation
8. Early discharge planning
9. Heavy involvement of family members in the treatment program
10. Attention to psychosocial issues
11. A major goal of preparing the patient to resume optimal life roles at home, in the family, and in the community
12. Introduction of the patient to community resources

Goal-Directed Treatment

An essential element of the rehabilitation treatment is that it is goal-directed. An early and recurring step in the treatment process is establishing realistic, practical, and feasible goals that are mutually agreed on by the patient, family, and professionals.[247]

Learning and Adaptation

Bleiberg and Merbitz[249] have pointed out that the rehabilitation process consists of learning and adaptation. Indeed,

a great deal of rehabilitation interventions are based on the theory of learning that suggests that patients reacquire old skills or compensate for new impairments in a logical, coherent manner.[190] Supervised practice is a necessary component of this learning process. Rehabilitation training programs usually use graded levels of difficulty of task performance. Another major component of the rehabilitation program is the frequent and timely provision of support, education, reassurance, direct assistance, and immediate feedback on progress as means of enhancing performance. Rehabilitation has been described by one author as "the planned withdrawal of support."[250]

Therapy Environments

The environment in which the program takes place should be conducive to learning, practice, and progress. Patients can benefit greatly from practice in therapy environments that more closely reflect natural home or community settings. Some programs have mock kitchens, apartments, community shops, and other facilities to allow patient practice.

Learning can occur best in an environment in which the training effort can be focused. This is particularly important in the care of stroke patients who are easily distracted by external stimuli or who have other cognitive, perceptual, or behavioral abnormalities. In those situations, it is necessary to avoid overstimulation and to make frequent interruptions in the training regimen. These principles apply to rehabilitation programs provided in all environments, including hospital units, long-term care settings, or home.

A spectrum of types and intensities of rehabilitation programs and services is available, and the number and diversity of new entries into the field are changing rapidly. Comprehensive rehabilitation can be provided at a number of sites, including hospital, long-term nursing care facility, outpatient unit, or home. Program intensities also vary, depending on the situation, the patient, and the availability of appropriate services. A key element of the comprehensive rehabilitation program that distinguishes it from a group of individual services is the coordinated nature of the interventions.

Timing of Therapy

Specific therapy schedules should be individualized for each patient. The stroke rehabilitation literature does not provide specific guidelines for the amount of therapy needed for specific problems. However, endurance, medical problems, mood, and other considerations affect the degree and duration of physical activity that an individual patient can tolerate. The rate, pattern, and degree of remobilization efforts will be determined to a large extent by these factors and others, including the duration of time since the stroke and the patient's motivation level.

REHABILITATION ASSESSMENT AND INTERVENTIONS DURING THE ACUTE PHASE

To consider rehabilitation as a philosophical approach that underlies all aspects of assessment and management throughout the continuum of care implies that rehabilitation is a component of the care that a stroke patient receives from the time of acute admission. Many of the clinical problems with which stroke patients present actually derive from the immobility and deconditioning that are imposed by the prolonged bed rest that often accompanies acute stroke care. The maximum benefit of rehabilitation can be achieved when rehabilitation interventions are begun as early as possible after stroke. Early poststroke rehabilitation is both preventive and therapeutic. Table 50–12 lists some of the key clinical rehabilitation activities that should be performed during the acute poststroke phase. This list of evaluation and intervention measures closely resembles the types of specific interventions performed in formal comprehensive rehabilitation programs.[247, 248, 251–253]

Three controlled human studies[254–256] have examined the impact of developing and implementing a rehabilitation program in the early poststroke period during the acute hospitalization. The programs emphasized the value of early activation, education, remobilization, and training in independent performance of activities of daily living.

During the acute poststroke phase, the patient should undergo an evaluation to determine the optimal type, level, setting, and timing of a continued rehabilitation and care program. In addition to assessing the nature, pattern, and severity of physical impairments, some of the key components of the assessment include health status, endurance level, and medical stability; functional capabilities and disabilities in the areas of mobility, self-care, and instrumental activities of daily living; mood and coping ability; community resources and family supports; social situation and vocational/educational status; and cognitive, communicative, perceptual, and behavioral functioning.

Rehabilitation requires active participation by the patient

and family, who, therefore, should be involved in the process of identification of goals and in the development of rehabilitation strategies. This process of goal-setting and treatment-planning often takes place during the assessment phase, and serves as a means of focusing or directing the assessment procedures themselves. The evaluation and treatment planning activities are ongoing processes.

Controversy exists in the literature concerning whether a delay in initiating transfer of the acute stroke patient from acute care to a formal rehabilitation program results in reduced outcomes. Although most studies[257–259] indicate that shorter stroke-to-rehabilitation latency periods are associated with better outcomes, other authors[199, 260] suggest that the interval between stroke onset and rehabilitation admission actually reflects severity of illness and co-morbidity, and that it may be more appropriate to aim for an "optimal time" to initiate therapy, rather than a "shorter time," although a trend has occurred toward markedly shortened acute stays.

THERAPEUTIC INTERVENTIONS

The therapeutic interventions used to enhance the functional and social recovery of the stroke patient include skills training, demonstration, providing opportunity for practice, providing feedback on skill performance, therapeutic exercises, physical modalities, prescription of adaptive equipment, education, and supportive counseling. Medications and surgical techniques also can be used. These activities require conjoint evaluation and treatment planning, collaborative treatment, and communication among the team members, the patient, and the family.

Most therapeutic methods designed to enhance function can be considered as either compensatory, in which the goal is to enhance the ability to carry out a functional task in the presence of a neurological impairment, or, less commonly, remediational, in which the goal is to reduce the degree of neurological impairment. Appendix 50–A lists examples of the types of interventions that are used in comprehensive rehabilitation.

Sensorimotor and Functional Training

Among the most frequent and important interventions used to care for the stroke patient are therapeutic exercise programs. Several different types and components of exercise regimens are available for patients who are disabled by stroke.

Early programs of traditional therapeutic exercise regimens were developed and described by Clayton, Coulter, Deaver, and others, and later reviewed by Westcott[261] and others. Traditional therapeutic exercise programs consist of positioning, passive and active range-of-motion exercises, and progressive resistive exercises. Endurance training, which can include aerobic training, can also be implemented.

Functional training in the performance of self-care tasks, mobility skills, and advanced or instrumental activities of daily living form the central focus of most standard rehabilitation programs. Compensatory functional training occurs when patients learn one-handed techniques to com-

TABLE 50–12   Rehabilitation Activities During the Acute Poststroke Phase

Evaluate and manage medical problems
Monitor and adjust medications
Maintain hydration and nutrition
Facilitate rest and sleep
Venous thromboembolism prophylaxis (physical or
   pharmacological measures)
Proper bed and chair positioning
Frequent turns and position changes
Range-of-motion exercises
Deep breathing and cough exercises
Frequent skin inspections
Swallowing evaluation
Safety measures
Removal of indwelling catheter, if possible, with planned, timed
   toileting program
Bowel evacuation regimen
Sitting in chair
Supervised bedside exercises
Self-performance of activities of daily living
Mobilization exercises
Standing and gait training as able
Educational programs on stroke, recovery, and personal care
Communication evaluation and training
Psychological support to the patient
Family education and support
Evalution of social supports and available resources
Evaluation for formal continued rehabilitation
Transition to rehabilitation

plete personal care skills independently or learn to walk with a spastic hemiplegic lower extremity. The patient is encouraged to make use of residual abilities to develop new ways of achieving old goals and to perform routine tasks such as transfering and walking.

Several neuromuscular facilitation exercise approaches have been developed and used in the care of stroke patients. These were reviewed by Flanagan,[262] and later by Lorish and colleagues,[263] and by Good.[264] Proprioceptive neuromuscular facilitation, developed by Kabat, Knott, and Voss, relies on several mechanisms such as spiral diagonal movement patterns of the extremities and quick stretch. Brunnstrom movement therapy encourages and facilitates the use of synergy patterns as a means of developing voluntary control. Cutaneous sensory stimulation in the form of superficial stroking, tapping, brushing, vibrating, or icing, provides facilitatory or inhibitory inputs in the system proposed by Rood. In the Bobath neurodevelopmental treatment approach, which is the most commonly used method, inhibition of abnormal tone, synergies, and postures are combined with facilitation of normal automatic motor responses to develop skilled voluntary movements. One of the most recently developed methods, the motor relearning program of Carr and Shepard, emphasizes functional training of specific tasks, such as standing and walking, and carryover of those tasks. Many therapists use an eclectic approach, combining elements of various procedures from among these programs. Many resources exist that describe the specific goals and techniques of these functional training and neurofacilitation therapy programs.[3, 4, 86, 247, 264–270]

Behavioral approaches are relatively new and include kinesthetic or positional biofeedback and forced-use exercises. Electromyographic biofeedback technology makes the patient consciously aware of muscle activity or lack of it[271–277] by using external representation (such as auditory or visual cues) of internal activity as a way to assist in the modification of voluntary control. Biofeedback therapy is considered an adjunctive therapy to standard voluntary exercise techniques.

A potentially favorable effect of therapy is to prevent or overcome "learned non-use."[278] Taub[279] had proposed that some of the disability seen in a stroke survivor results from the patient's *failure to use* the affected limbs, rather than from the limb weakness itself. This suggests that all therapeutic attempts to use the affected limb should be reinforced, possibly by facilitation techniques. Another potential implication is that it could even be beneficial to inhibit or immobilize the function of the unaffected limb to encourage or "force" the use of the affected hemiplegic extremity. Taub and colleagues,[279, 280] Wolf and associates,[281] and Barton and Wolf[282] have reported successful work with animals and humans that support the usefulness of this "forced-use" approach. Electrical stimulation of muscles that lack voluntary control could help to facilitate their movement or to compensate for their lack of voluntary movement.

Specialized Equipment

Adaptive equipment and durable medical equipment can be used to assist the stroke patient to become more inde-

pendent. It is important to consider the patient's functional level, level of adaptation to disability, architecture of the living environment, and instruction in the use of all devices and equipment. Many types of devices are available to assist the stroke patient in achieving an improved level of independence. These include adaptive devices to assist in the performance of activities of daily living, such as eating utensils, bathing and grooming aids, tub and shower equipment, dressing devices, assistive devices for walking, transfer aids, and wheelchairs (see Chapters 19 and 26).

Upper extremity resting hand splints are usually used to prevent deformity and to maintain the hemiplegic wrist in a functional, slightly extended position. Orthoses, especially ankle-foot orthoses, are used to improve the positioning of the foot to facilitate an optimal gait pattern[283] (see Chapter 17).

Caregiver Training

One of the most important interventions is the training of caregivers in specific care techniques to prevent complications, perform physical functions, and encourage the patient to perform any activities he or she is capable of. Common teaching points include the following:

Medication teaching

Signs and symptoms of common medical complications

Instruction in care of bladder catheter, respiratory equipment, or feeding tubes

Safety training

Swallowing training

Maintenance of nutrition and hydration

Training in specific skills for which the patient needs assistance, and in methods of performing those skills (e.g., bed mobility, transfers, hygiene, dressing, others)

Home exercise program

Others

In general, if a patient is unable to recover sufficient function through remediational or compensatory techniques, then adaptive equipment prescription and/or family caregiver training are needed to carry out the task.

Speech and Language Disorders

Approximately one-third to one-half of stroke survivors experience speech and language disorders.[173] Many procedures have been designed to manage various aspects of these problems. Both remediation and compensation are used. One goal of therapy is to improve the patient's ability to speak, understand, read, and write. Another goal of speech therapy intervention is to assist patients to develop strategies that compensate for or circumvent speech and language problems that are not directly remediable. A final goal is to improve the quality of life for individuals with neuromotor speech impairments and their families.

For aphasia, a number of strategies and techniques have been developed.[284–300] One of these, melodic intonation therapy,[293] is an approach designed to utilize the noninjured functioning neural pathways in the nondominant hemisphere that carry musical information. Other techniques rely on encouraging verbalizations, conversational coaching, and oral reading. A major strategy is to encourage any vocalizations as a means of developing verbal communication of a more differentiated nature (see Chapter 3).

For dysarthria, exercise modalities include sensory stimulation procedures, exercises designed to strengthen oromotor speech muscles, respiratory training procedures, and retraining of articulatory patterns and sequences of gestures.[301-304]

Alternative forms of communication and augmentative devices can be used to enhance quality of life. These range from communication boards and books to more sophisticated electronic communication devices.

Psychosocial Considerations

One of the major factors that influences both the degree of therapy program participation and the type and degree of outcome achieved is patient motivation. Patients who cooperate with the therapeutic efforts, and who have the determination to improve are more likely to participate in the therapy program. However, the level of motivation and the amount of its specific direct effect on outcome are difficult to measure. A number of techniques can be used by the rehabilitation professional to enhance or direct motivation; examples include explanation, positive reinforcement, behavioral modification, and coaxing. Interestingly, it also has been found that the degree of family support favorably affects outcome.[305] Counseling interventions have been found to be consistently more effective in improving family functioning and patient adjustment than have educational interventions alone.[306]

Depression can be a significant complication of stroke. It can be devastating and distressing on its own, and can limit patient participation and outcome by inhibiting patient motivation.[162, 307-315] Depression occurs in one-third to two-thirds of stroke survivors, and presenting features include loss of energy in 83%, sleep disorder in 67%, brooding in 60%, and hopelessness in 39%.[307] Although the organic component of poststroke depression may be significant,[310, 311] it is likely that most patients experience a combination of both organic and reactive causes of mood disorders. Treatment consists of psychotherapy, psychosocial support, milieu therapy, and medications. To the extent that mood improves as the patient's level of physical independence improves, the source of depression is likely to be reactive. For some patients, especially those for whom there are significant disturbances in participation in daily activities or therapeutic exercise program, antidepressant medications can be beneficial.[316, 317] These medications have been shown to improve not only mood, but also functional performance. Their usefulness is limited only by their side effects.

Anxiety and fear are commonly reported and observed problems among stroke patients. A team of rehabilitation professionals, who are sensitive to these issues, empathic toward the patient, and experienced in dealing with such problems can help to ease the distress associated with the disability and the rehabilitation experience, thereby possibly resulting in improved outcomes.

Sexual dysfunction has been reported in 40% to 70% of stroke survivors.[318-321] Its cause is largely psychological

(e.g., fear, anxiety, depression, discomfort) rather than organic, although spasticity, pain, and sensory deficits may pose problems for some patients. Issues related to self-esteem, affection, and relationships should be emphasized, as should specific practical suggestions on positioning, timing, and techniques[322] (see Chapter 30).

Family reactions to the changes that result from the stroke are addressed by the team. This is particularly important in view of the need for the family's active participation in providing support to the patient during and after formal intensive rehabilitation. Lack of social supports or lack of available resources often are major problems for the patient and the rehabilitation team. In that situation, recruiting available resources and supports, securing appropriate entitlements, and advocating on behalf of the patient become major clinical tasks for the professional rehabilitation team. In general, family interventions include individual counseling, education, and support groups.[323] Evidence exists that both education and counseling interventions significantly improve caregiver knowledge and stabilize some aspects of family functioning, but that counseling is more effective than education alone.[306]

At times, problematic psychosocial functioning predominates among issues related to the recovery of physical function or motor skill performance. This underscores the importance of psychosocial, recreational, and vocational interventions.

Recreational activities often have the effects of improving affect, focusing therapy on meaningful activities and desirable goals, and facilitating a smooth transition to the community after discharge. Leisure evaluation, counseling on activities of interest, and educating the patient on community resources constitute some of the therapeutic recreation interventions for patients with stroke.

Peer support is one component of patient care activities that probably exerts a favorable effect on the successful rehabilitation of the stroke patient, but is often overlooked in the usual description of interventions that affect patient progress and outcome. The presence of other patients with similar disabilities on the stroke rehabilitation unit can assist the patient in several ways. First, it can help to reduce the fear and anxiety level often associated with the new onset of physically disabling or disfiguring conditions. Second, patients often can counsel and support each other in ways that even well-meaning and experienced professionals cannot. Finally, patients often not only gain insight into their disability, but also garner specific suggestions for functional skill performance or about adaptive equipment from other patients who have already been through the experience. Similar peer support may be available for families of patients as well, and could contribute favorably to the adjustment process after the stroke.

Effects of Rehabilitation

Literature on the efficacy of stroke rehabilitation is scarce, and the existing experimental data are fraught with heterogeneity, methodological flaws, and other problems. Despite this, indirect evidence suggests that patients who receive comprehensive coordinated stroke rehabilitation care in a specially designated and geographically distinct stroke care unit have better outcomes at discharge than those who do not.

Wade and colleagues point out that therapy can be beneficial in several ways:

- Preventing complications
- Teaching new adaptive methods
- Ensuring that appropriate aids are provided and used properly
- Retraining the damaged nervous system
- Preventing or overcoming "learned disuse"

Several studies have attempted to compare the relative effectiveness of some of the therapeutic methods designed to enhance function. Although it remains controversial, evidence exists that directed stroke rehabilitation efforts enhance functional ability over and above the extent to which natural recovery improves function.[146-155]

REHABILITATION OUTCOMES

More has been written in the medical rehabilitation literature about the functional outcomes after stroke than about outcomes following the occurrence of virtually any other disabling condition. Results contained in some of these reports are contradictory, misleading, and even confusing. It has been noted that many of the problems in evaluating these studies result from differences in methods and design, variability in study sample and control group criteria, rehabilitation practice, and outcome definition.[1, 324] However, a few general principles appear with some consistency.

The existing literature on outcome after stroke can be roughly classified into two major groups, that is, those that describe various types of outcomes and those that identify predictors of outcomes. It is important to note that outcome after stroke can be assessed in a variety of ways, including by medical morbidity, mortality, level of impairment, length of hospital stay, cost of care, functional ability (degree of disability), placement at the time of discharge, amount of handicap, quality of life, and life satisfaction. Most of the present discussion focuses on functional ability and placement. Functional outcomes can be measured as absolute functional level or as improvement in functional abilities. Different conclusions can be reached from each of the studies depending on the specific definitions used.

Functional and Social Outcomes

One of the most striking aspects of caring for stroke patients is the common observation that their physical performance, functional abilities, and quality of life are considerably better after rehabilitation and during long-term care than at the time shortly after onset of the stroke. Most studies,[146-155] and extensive clinical experience, suggest that a substantial proportion of stroke survivors achieve independence in the ability to complete mobility and self-care, but that social and vocational outcomes are not as favorable as are the functional independence figures. For example, data obtained from the Framingham Heart Study cohort[27] indicated that 69% of 148 stroke survivors were independent in the performance of self-care activities, 80% were independent in mobility skills, and 84% were living in home environments. Unfortunately, 71% also had reduced vocational function and 62% also had decreased socialization outside the home.

Most other studies have yielded similar results. For example, Chin and colleagues[325] reported in a review that between 54% and 80% of stroke survivors were able to walk, but that most were not walking outside of the home. Andrews and associates[147] found that only 13% of 1-year survivors were severely dependent and 27% were moderately dependent in performance of activities of daily living. In general, about 75% to 85% of stroke patients are discharged to home after formal acute rehabilitation care.

A report[326] using data derived from the Uniform Data System for Medical Rehabilitation reported that 15,151 stroke patients improved in their average functional independence measure (FIM) scores from 63 on admission to 87 at discharge, with the greatest improvements occurring in locomotion, mobility, self-care, and sphincter control, and less improvement occurring in communication and social cognition. Average length of stay was 29 days, and 77% of patients were discharged to the community. Fewer than 1% died, and that group tended to have lower average FIM scores (see also Chapter 12).

Predictors of Outcome

A number of factors influence the specific outcome of a patient who is involved in a stroke rehabilitation program. Potential important factors include the following:

- Type, distribution, pattern, and severity of physical impairment
- Cognitive, language, and communication ability
- Number, types, and severity of co-morbid conditions
- Level of motivation or determination
- Coping ability and coping style
- Nature and degree of family and social supports
- Type and quality of the specific training and adaptation program provided

Numerous studies have examined and reported many diverse potential and actual predictors of favorable or unfavorable recovery of physical or psychosocial functioning. The nature, type, and strength of the specific predictors depend to a great extent on the specific outcome measure being studied. Specific reported predictors are listed in Table 50–13. The many reviews of those prognostic factors

TABLE 50–13   Possible Predictors of Functional Outcome After Stroke

Age	Language function
Educational level	Hemianopia
Severity of stroke	Posture and balance
Type of stroke	Sensory function
Location of stroke	Bowel incontinence
Size of stroke	Bladder incontinence
Prior stroke	Onset–rehabilitation admission
Multiple deficits	interval
Severity of plegia	Congestive heart failure
Initial functional status	Other medical co-morbidities
Coma at onset	Depression, emotional state
Cognitive function	Motivation
Perceptual function	Family involvement and support

include those by Jongbloed,[327] Davidoff and others,[328] and Johnston and co-workers.[329]

The strongest and most consistent predictor of discharge functional ability is admission functional ability.[327] Dombovy and colleagues[324] reviewed multiple studies and suggested that the strongest negative predictors were the following: coma at onset, persistent incontinence, poor cognitive function, severe hemiplegia, lack of motor return after 1 month, prior stroke, visual-perceptual deficit, hemineglect, significant cardiovascular disease, large cerebral lesion, and multiple neurological deficits. Wade and associates[330] studied 83 stroke patients and found that the best predictors of function after 6 months were sitting balance, age, hemianopsia, urinary incontinence, and motor deficit in the arm.

It is important to note that although hundreds of articles describe numerous predictors of outcome after stroke rehabilitation, it is difficult to apply these predictors in the clinical setting.[329] The multiplicity of variables that influence actual outcome, the degree to which the studies are fraught with methodological flaws, and the unpredictable nature of certain aspects of poststroke functioning render many of the specific outcome predictors incomplete or inadequate. Therefore, caution is needed in using the predictors for clinical purposes, such as assessing candidacy for rehabilitation. Identification of some of the factors, however, can help to better direct patient management activities.

FOLLOW-UP AND AFTERCARE

The process of rehabilitation involves the restoration of patients to their fullest physical, mental, and social capability, and rehabilitation includes the many physical, social, and organizational aspects of the aftercare of patients who require more than acute short-term definitive care. This definition highlights the long-term nature of the rehabilitation process.

The main goal of the formal rehabilitation program for the stroke patient is to optimize the patient's quality of life after discharge. Reaching this goal is accomplished by using a multidisciplinary approach. Helping the patient to achieve independent functioning in daily activities is a major part of achieving the goal of optimal quality of life after discharge. Training family members and other personal caregivers in methods of performing specific physical skills is also an important component of this preparation for postdischarge care. It is imperative that family members know several aspects of the patient's care and management. These include knowledge of which skills patients can perform themselves (to avoid performing tasks that the patient is capable of performing), and of which skills patients need assistance or supervision to carry out.

Major efforts are directed toward preparation for discharge by securing community resources, including competent professional or other attendant care, home nursing visits, outpatient therapy, or others. Teaching patients and families about medications, fluid intake, diet, catheter care, feeding tube use, tracheostomy and respiratory equipment management, signs and symptoms of common complications (such as infections), and specific functional task tech-

niques greatly facilitates a smooth transition to home and minimizes medical problems after discharge. Follow-up medical monitoring and care are also important.

Specific functional issues that are relevant around the time of discharge are higher-level skills that are related to postdischarge lifestyle. These include sexual functioning, driving ability, safety considerations, socialization outside of the home, vocational pursuits, recreational activities, and others. Continuing mobilization activities and maintaining an adequate activity level are important lifestyle adjustments that can enhance the likelihood of avoiding functional deterioration.

Rehabilitation is a lifelong process. The emphasis on education, mobilization, activity, independence, coping, family involvement, and, especially, quality of life should be incorporated into the patient's lifestyle, even long after completion of the formal rehabilitation program.[331, 332]

SPECIAL PATIENT CONSIDERATIONS

Pediatric Stroke

Stroke is unusual in children, with an estimated incidence of 2.5 per 100,000 children per year.[333] Although hemiparesis, aphasia, or isolated cognitive deficits can occur, presentation of stroke in neonates and children often is different from that in older individuals; seizures, fever, and delayed achievement of developmental milestones are not uncommon. Causes of stroke also differ; these include hereditary conditions, congenital heart disease, metabolic disorders, coagulopathy, drugs, intracerebral vascular anomalies, and others. The prognosis after stroke in children is generally thought to be better than that for adults. However, some residual deficit is present in the majority of children surviving a stroke. Rehabilitation emphasizes functional restoration and compensation, psychosocial support, *and* the attainment of normal developmental abilities.

Stroke in Young Adults

Although stroke is commonly considered a condition of aging, it is estimated that nearly one-third of all strokes occur in individuals under the age of 65 years, and that 26% of strokes occur in persons between ages 45 and 65 years. Although early atherosclerosis, cardioembolism, and hemorrhages are common causes, the distribution of types of stroke in younger adults are somewhat different from those in older adults. Hemorrhagic strokes account for about one third of all strokes in young adults (compared with one-fifth among all stroke survivors). Common causes of cerebral infarctions include atherosclerosis (usually in the setting of known atherogenic risk factors) in about 20%, cardiogenic embolism (usually from congenital heart defects or atrial fibrillation) in about 20%, cerebral vasculitis with or without known systemic collagen vascular disease in 10%, coagulopathy in about 10%, and others. The approach to the diagnostic workup of the younger stroke patient is aggressive, and often calls for procedures such as cerebral angiogram, coagulation tests, collagen vascular disease evaluation, and cardiac workup, including transesophageal echocardiogram.[333–338]

Young adults tend to present with unique rehabilitation

TABLE 50–14 Rehabilitation and Long-term Issues in Young Stroke Survivors

1. Employment
2. Sexuality
3. Child care/parenting
4. Instrumental activities of daily living/ homemaking, meal preparation, shopping
5. Psychological aspects of life-role changes
6. Spouse vs. personal caregiver role
7. Financial management
8. Driving
9. Relationship changes
10. Leisure planning/hobbies/socializing

needs and long-term issues. Table 50–14 lists many of the specialized problems and needs that are more prevalent and prominent among younger adults compared with those of older individuals. To address these specific patient needs, rehabilitation interventions should be directed toward the achievement of specific goals. Depending on the specific situation, functional therapy interventions should include training in complex instrumental activities of daily living, such as shopping, homemaking, community level mobility, and child care. Communication and cognitive training should focus on money management skills and vocational activities. Psychological counseling of the patient and family should be instituted to address some of the issues that are specific to the age of the patient, such as self-image, interpersonal relationships, dating, sexuality, and stress management. Education of the patient and family should provide information on stroke, medications, nutrition, healthy lifestyle, and prevention measures. Driving evaluation and rehabilitation are important, as are vocational assessment, counseling, training, and referrals. Recreation and social programs, aerobic training or fitness exercise groups, and community reentry training help to enhance the quality of life of young persons with stroke.[339–346]

Aggressive rehabilitation and continued care by specialized professionals who can recognize, understand, and address the specific physical and psychosocial considerations in young stroke patients can both facilitate the achievement of optimal outcomes in these patients and enhance their quality of life.

Geriatric Stroke

The effect of age on recovery after stroke is variable and controversial. It has been found that young age at stroke onset has a favorable effect on long-term and short-term survival,[334, 347] but the effect on functional recovery is less certain. In a review of 33 studies on functional outcome after stroke, Jongbloed[327] found that 18 studies evaluated the impact of age on stroke outcome. In 14 of the studies, younger patients tended to have better outcomes than did older adults, but the overwhelming majority of these studies used *functional status at discharge* as the outcome measure. In four of the studies, no relationship was found between age and outcome, and in most of those studies, amount of *functional improvement* (rather than level of discharge function) was used as the outcome measure under study. These findings suggest that younger adults tend to have less severe disability levels at presenta-

tion compared with older adults. It has been suggested that the adverse effect of increasing age on functional outcome is explained only by co-morbid conditions and frequency of prior stroke.

Age alone probably does not play a major role in determining the course and care of the patient with stroke. It is more likely that advancing age serves as a marker for the presence of medical co-morbidities, prior strokes, and limited social supports. Clinical experience indicates that many older adults successfully complete rehabilitation, return to their home and community, and contribute to their families and society. However, the frequency of multiple physical impairments and psychosocial problems is greater among older stroke patients than among younger individuals, and this most likely affects outcome.

As a consequence, older adults often require more medical monitoring, longer recovery times, reduced exercise intensities, or more psychosocial support during their rehabilitation program than do younger adults.

Ethical Considerations

Because of the complexity and severity of the problems with which stroke patients present, it is not surprising that ethical issues often arise during the evaluation and management of these patients. An issue that occurs somewhat frequently is whether and to what degree autonomy in decision-making can be provided safely and reliably to patients, many of whom have cognitive, perceptual, emotional, or behavioral disturbances resulting from the stroke itself or from other conditions. Other problems arise when an individual insists on living independently when it is unsafe to do so, or when patients or their families insist on continued hospitalization or rehabilitation program participation when there is little or no clinical indication to do so. Many of these decisions involve the determination of the patient's competency and, possibly, establishment of guardianship. The latter two activities become critical components of the rehabilitation program for some patients. It is essential that patients and families be involved with the decision-making process; involving members of the rehabilitation team in this process can be of value as well.

Decisions might arise about whether to institute resuscitative measures in the event of a cardiopulmonary arrest or whether to initiate or continue alternative measures for nutritional support, ventilatory support, or respiratory airway maintenance. These should be considered and acted on on an individual basis with the patient and family.

"Do not resuscitate" does *not* mean "do not treat." It often is appropriate for patients to receive therapy services and to participate in an intensive rehabilitation program even if the decision has been made to avoid resuscitative measures in the event of a cardiopulmonary arrest. Rehabilitation goals usually remain the same in these situations, and include improving functional status, promoting psychosocial adaptation, providing caregiver education and support, and, especially, enhancing quality of life.

COMMENTS

Stroke rehabilitation is a prototypical rehabilitation activity. Many of the concepts and skills used to treat the stroke patient are applicable to management of the problems that result from other diagnoses. One of the most important characteristics of treatment is a need to avoid a nihilistic attitude in caring for the stroke patient. It is important to emphasize and to take advantage of the patient's strengths and abilities, and to avoid focusing on only the disabilities. Initial and ongoing assessment is critical to the success of the interventions. The interventions rely heavily on strong emphasis on functional enhancement through training, demonstration, supervision, suggestions, practice, and immediate feedback. Patient and family education play an extremely important role, and for some patients, caregiver training is the major focus of the program. It is generally found that offering psychological counseling and support facilitates better physical recovery and enhances quality of life, and that involving and supporting family members is critical to the process. Interdisciplinary collaboration and communication are the hallmarks of the rehabilitation program.

Stroke rehabilitation remains somewhat controversial. Although the institution of a rehabilitation program after a stroke often is accepted as a common clinical practice and a component of routine medical care, the specific methods and their investigations are still under scientific and clinical scrutiny.

After reviewing available information about stroke rehabilitation, the British Department of Health[348] summarized several key points: They noted that stroke is a common clinical problem with a significant impact on its survivors and on society. It often presents as a disabling illness, involving many aspects of the patient's life, and placing a substantial burden on family members and others. The aims of rehabilitation are to minimize the impact of the disability resulting from the stroke and to optimize the quality of life for both the patient and the personal caregiver. It was noted in the British report that although "there are very few well-designed studies that assess the effectiveness of rehabilitation after stroke . . . there is some evidence that formal rehabilitation after stroke is effective, and that it is best provided by well-organized interdisciplinary teams . . . ." Interpretation and extrapolation of the findings of most investigations, and, more important, clinical experience, support those conclusions.

References

1. Gresham GE: Stroke outcome research. Stroke 1986; 17:358.
2. Kottke FJ: Historica obscura hemiplegia. Arch Phys Med Rehabil 1974: 55:4–13.
3. Bobath B: Adult Hemiplegia: Evaluation and Treatment, ed 2. London; Heinemann, 1978.
4. Charness A: Stroke/Head Injury: A Guide to Functional Outcomes in Physical Therapy Management. Rockville, Md, Aspen Publishers, 1986.
5. Roth EJ: Medical rehabilitation of the stroke patient. Be Stroke Smart 1992; 8:8.
6. Biller J, Love BB: Nihilism and stroke therapy. Stroke 1991; 22:1105–1106.
7. Caplan LR: Diagnosis and treatment of ischemic stroke. JAMA 1991; 266:2413–2418.
8. WHO Task Force on Stroke and Other Cerebrovascular Disorders: Stroke—1989. Recommendations on stroke prevention, diagnosis, and therapy. Stroke 1989; 20:1407–1431.
9. American Heart Association: Heart and Stroke Facts: 1994 Statistical Supplement. Dallas, American Heart Association, 1994.
10. McGovern PG, Burke GL, Sprafka JM, et al: Trends in mortality, morbidity and risk factor levels for stroke from 1960 through 1990: The Minnesota Heart Survey. JAMA 1992; 26:753–759.
11. Whisnant JP: The decline of stroke. Stroke 1984; 15:160–168.
12. Klag MJ, Whelton PK, Seidler AJ: Decline in U.S. stroke mortality: Demographic trends and antihypertensive treatment. Stroke 1989; 20:14–21.
13. Garraway WM, Whisnant JP: The changing pattern of hypertension and the declining incidence of stroke. JAMA 1987; 258:214–217.
14. Hypertension Detection and Follow-up Program Cooperative Group: Five-year findings of the hypertension and follow-up program: III. Reduction in stroke incidence among persons with high blood pressure. JAMA 1982; 247:633–638.
15. MacMahon S, Peto R, Cutler J, et al: Blood pressure, stroke, and coronary heart disease: 1. Prolonged differences in blood pressure: Prospective observational studies corrected for the regression dilution bias. Lancet 1990; 335:765–774.
16. Collins R, Peto R, MacMahon S, et al: Blood pressure, stroke, and coronary heart disease: 2. Short-term reductions in blood pressure: Overview of randomized drug trials in their epidemiological context. Lancet 1990; 335:827–838.
17. Ahmed OI, Orchard TJ, Sharma R, et al: Declining mortality from stroke in Allegheny County, Pennsylvania: Trends in case fatality and severity of disease, 1971–1980. Stroke 1988; 19:181–184.
18. Gillum RF, Gomez-Marin O, Kottke TE, et al: Acute stroke in a metropolitan area: 1970 and 1980: The Minnesota Heart Survey. J Chron Dis 1985; 38:891–898.
19. Drury I, Whisnant JP, Garraway M: Primary intracerebral hemorrhage: Impact of CT on incidence. Neurology 1984; 34:653–657.
20. Gillum RF: Cerebrovascular disease morbidity in the United States, 1970–1983. Age, sex, region, and vascular surgery. Stroke 1986; 17:656–661.
21. Ingall TJ, Whisnant JP, Wiebers DO, O'Fallon M: Has there been a decline in subarachnoid hemorrhage mortality? Stroke 1989; 20:718–724.
22. Broderick JP, Phillips SJ, Whisnant JP, et al: Incidence rates of stroke in the '80s: The end of the decline in stroke? Stroke 1989; 20:577–582.
23. Cooper R, Sempos C, Hsieh SC, Kovar MG: Slowdown in the decline of stroke mortality in the United States, 1978–1986. Stroke 1990; 21:1274–1279.
24. Caplan LR: Strokes in African-Americans. Circulation 1991; 83:1469–1470.
25. Garraway WM, Whisnant JP, Drury I: The changing pattern of survival following stroke. Stroke 1983; 14:699–703.
26. Roth EJ: Heart disease in patients with stroke: Incidence, impact and implications for rehabilitation: 1. Classification and prevalence. Arch Phys Med Rehabil 1993; 74:752–760.
27. Gresham GE, Philips TF, Wolf PA, et al: Epidemiologic profile of long-term stroke disability: The Framingham Study. Arch Phys Med Rehabil 1979; 60:487–491.
28. Kannel WB, Wolf PA, McGee DL, et al: Systolic blood pressure, arterial rigidity and risk of stroke: The Framingham Study. JAMA 1981; 245:1225–1229.
29. SHEP Cooperative Research Group: Prevention of stroke by antihypertensive drug treatment in older persons with isolated systolic hypertension: Final results of the Systolic Hypertension in the Elderly Program (SHEP). JAMA 1991; 265:3255–3264.
30. Wolf PA, D'Agostino RB, Kannel WB, et al: Cigarette smoking as a risk factor for stroke: The Framingham Study. JAMA 1988; 259:1025–1029.
31. Abbot RD, Reed DM, Yin Y, et al: Risk of stroke in male cigarette smokers. N Engl J Med 1986; 315:717–720.
32. Ross R: The pathogenesis of atherosclerosis: An update. N Engl J Med 1988; 20:488–500.
33. Salonan R, Seppanen K, Rauramaa R, Salonen JT: Prevalence of carotid atherosclerosis and serum cholesterol levels in eastern Finland. Atherosclerosis 1988; 8:788–792.
34. O'Leary DH, Anderson KM, Wolf PA, et al: Cholesterol and carotid atherosclerosis in older persons: The Framingham Study. Ann Epidemiol 1992; 2:147–153.
35. The Expert Panel: Report of the National Cholesterol Education Program expert panel on detection, evaluation, and treatment of high blood cholesterol in adults. Arch Intern Med 1988; 148:36–69.
36. Yano K, Reed DM, MacLean CJ: Serum cholesterol and hemorrhagic stroke in the Honolulu Heart Program. Stroke 1989; 20:1460–1465.

37. Iso H, Jacobs DR, Wentworth D, et al: Serum cholesterol levels and 6-year mortality from stroke in 350,977 men screened for the multiple risk factor intervention trial. N Engl J Med 1989; 320:904–910.

38. Whisnant JP, Matsumotoa N, Elveback LR: The effect of anticoagulant therapy on the prognosis of patients with transient cerebral ischemic attacks in a community: Rochester, Minnesota 1955 through 1969. Mayo Clin Proc 1973; 48:844–848.

39. Investigators of the Asymptomatic Carotid Atherosclerosis Study (ACAS): Clinical advisory: Carotid endarterectomy for patients with asymptomatic internal carotid artery stenosis. Stroke 1994; 25:2523–2524.

40. Kannel WB, McGee DL: Diabetes and cardiovascular disease: The Framingham Study. JAMA 1979; 241:2035–2038.

41. Barrett-Connor E, Khaw K: Diabetes mellitus: An independent risk factor for stroke? JAMA 1988; 258:116–123.

42. Abbott RD, Donohue RP, MacMahon SW, et al: Diabetes and the risk of stroke: The Honolulu Heart Program. JAMA 1987; 257:949–952.

43. Mohr JP, Caplan LR, Melski W, et al: The Harvard Cooperative Stroke Registry: A prospective registry. Neurology 1978; 28:754–762.

44. Nathan DM: Long-term complications of diabetes mellitus. N Engl J Med 1993; 329:2035–2038.

45. Kannel WB, Gordon T, Wolf PA, McNamara P: Hemoglobin and the risk of cerebral infarction: The Framingham Study. Stroke 1972; 3:409–419.

46. Wilhelmsen L, Scardsudd K, Korban-Bengsten K, et al: Fibrinogen as a risk factor for stroke and myocardial infarction. N Engl J Med 1984; 311:501–505.

47. Steering Committee of the Physicians' Health Study Research Group: Final report on the aspirin component of the ongoing physicians health study. N Engl J Med 1989; 321:129–135.

48. Peto R, Gray R, Collins R, et al: Randomized trial of prophylactic daily aspirin in British male doctors. Br Med J 1988; 296:313–316.

49. Antiplatelet Trialists' Collaboration: Collaborative overview of randomised trials of antiplatelet therapy: I. Prevention of death, myocardial infarction, and stroke by prolonged antiplatelet therapy in various categories of patients. Br Med J 1994; 308:81–106.

50. Gilman AG, Rall TW, Nies AS, Palmer T (eds): Goodman and Gilman's The Pharmacological Basis of Therapeutics, ed 8. New York, Pergamon Press, 1990, pp 1325–1326.

51. Fields WS, Lemak NA, Frankowski RF, Hardy RJ: Controlled trials of aspirin in cerebral ischaemia. Stroke 1977; 8:301–314.

52. The Canadian Cooperative Study Group: A randomized trial of aspirin and sulfinpyrazone in threatened stroke. N Engl J Med 1978; 299:53–59.

53. The Dutch TIA Trial Study Group: A comparison of two doses of aspirin (30 mg vs. 283 mg a day) in patients after a transient ischemic attack or minor ischemic stroke. N Engl J Med 1991; 325:1261–1266.

54. The SALT Collaborative Group: Swedish aspirin low-dose trial (SALT) of 75 mg aspirin as secondary prophylaxis after cerebrovascular ischaemic events. Lancet 1991; 338:1345–1349.

55. UK-TIA Study Group: United Kingdom transient ischaemic attack (UK-TIA) aspirin trial: Final results. Br Med J 1991; 54:1044–1054.

56. ESPS Group: European stroke prevention study. Stroke 1990; 21:1122–1130.

57. Bousser MG, Eschwege E, Hagrenau M, et al: "AICLA" controlled trial of aspirin and dipyridamole in the secondary prevention of athero-thrombotic cerebral ischemia. Stroke 1983; 14:5–14.

58. Dyken ML, Barnett HJM, Easton JD, et al: Low-dose aspirin and stroke: "It ain't necessarily so." Stroke 1992; 23:1395–1399.

59. Hass WK, Easton JD, Adams HP, et al: The TASS Group: A randomised trial comparing ticlopidine hydrochloride with aspirin for the prevention of stroke in high-risk patients. N Engl J Med 1989; 321:501–507.

60. Gent M, Easton JD, Hachinski V, et al: The CATS Group: The Canadian American ticlopidine study (CATS) in thromboembolic stroke. Lancet 1989; 1:1215–1220.

61. Wolf PA, Dawber TR, Thomas E, Kannel WB: Epidemiologic assessment of chronic atrial fibrillation and risk of stroke: The Framingham Study. Neurology 1978; 28:973–979.

62. Peterson P, Boysen G, Godtfredsen J, et al: Placebo-controlled, randomised trial of warfarin and aspirin for prevention of thrombotic complications in chronic atrial fibrillation: The Copenhagen AFA-SAK Study. Lancet 1989; 1:175–179.

63. Stroke Prevention in Atrial Fibrillation Investigators: Stroke Prevention in Atrial Fibrillation Study: Final results. Circulation 1991; 84:527–539.

64. Ezekowitz MD, Bridgers SL, James KE, et al: Warfarin in the prevention of stroke associated with nonrheumatic atrial fibrillation. N Engl J Med 1992; 327:1406–1412.

65. The Boston Area Anticoagulation Trial of Atrial Fibrillation Investigators: The effect of low-dose warfarin on the risk of stroke in patients with nonrheumatic atrial fibrillation. N Engl J Med 1990; 323:1505–1511.

66. Stroke Prevention in Atrial Fibrillation Investigators: Warfarin compared to aspirin for prevention of thromboembolism in atrial fibrillation: Stroke Prevention in Atrial Fibrillation II Study. Lancet 1994; 343:687–691.

67. North American Symptomatic Carotid Endarterectomy Trial Collaborators: Beneficial effect of carotid endarterectomy in symptomatic patients with high-grade carotid stenosis. N Engl J Med 1991; 325:445–453.

68. Hess DC, D'Cruz IA, Adams RJ, Nichols FT: Coronary artery disease, myocardial infarction, and brain embolism. Neurol Clin 1993; 11:399–417.

69. McGill HC: The pathogenesis of atherosclerosis. Clin Chem 1988; 34:B33–B39.

70. Pessin MS, Duncan GW, Mohr JP, Poskanzer DC: Clinical and angiographic features of carotid transient ischemic attacks. N Engl J Med 1977; 296:358–362.

71. Bogousslavsky J, Regli F: Borderzone infarctions distal to internal carotid artery. Ann Neurol 1986; 20:346–350.

72. Cerebral Embolism Task Force: Cardiogenic brain embolism: The second report of the cerebral embolism task force. Arch Neurol 1989; 46:727–743.

73. Caplan LR: Brain embolism, revisited. Neurology 1993; 43:1281–1287.

74. Jones HR, Caplan LR, Come PC, et al: Cerebral emboli of paradoxical origin. Ann Neurol 1983; 13:314–319.

75. Mohr JP: Lacunes. Stroke 1982; 13:3–11.

76. Furlan AJ, Whisnant JP, Elveback LR: The decreasing incidence of primary intracerebral hemorrhage: A population study. Ann Neurol 1979; 5:367–373.

77. Fisher CM: Pathological observations in hypertensive cerebral hemorrhage. J Neuropathol Exp Neurol 1971; 30:536–550.

78. Feldmann E, Tornabene J: Diagnosis and treatment of cerebral amyloid angiopathy. Clin Geriatr Med 1991; 7:617–630.

79. Sundt TM, Whisnant P: Subarachnoid hemorrhage from intracranial aneurysms. N Engl J Med 1978; 299:116–122.

80. Winn HR, Richardson AE, Jane JA: The long-term prognosis in untreated cerebral aneurysms: I. The incidence of late hemorrhage in cerebral aneurysm: A 10-year evolution of 364 patients. Ann Neurol 1977; 1:358–370.

81. Perret G, Nishioka H: Report on the Cooperative Study of Intracranial Aneurysms and Subarachnoid Hemorrhage: VI. Arteriovenous malformations: An analysis of 545 cases of cranio-cerebral arteriovenous malformations and fistulae reported to the cooperative study. J Neurosurg 1966; 25:467–490.

82. Mohr JP, Hilal SK, Stein BM: Arteriovenous malformations and other vascular anomalies. In Barnett HJM, Mohr JP, Stein BM, Yatsu FM (eds): Stroke: Pathophysiology, Diagnosis, and Management, ed 2. New York, Churchill Livingstone, 1992.

83. Ondra SL, Troupp H, George ED, Schwab K: The natural history of symptomatic arteriovenous malformations of the brain: A 24-year followup assessment. J Neurosurg 1990; 73:387–391.

84. Huckman MS: Normal pressure hydrocephalus: Evaluation of diagnostic and prognostic tests. Am J Neurol Res 1981; 2:385–395.

85. Twitchell TE: The restoration of motor function following hemiplegia in man. Brain 1951; 64:443–440.

86. Sawner K, LaVigne J: Brunnstrom's Movement Therapy in Hemiplegia: A Neurophysiological Approach, ed 2. Philadelphia, JB Lippincott, 1992.

87. Gordon J, Ghez C: Muscle receptors and spinal reflexes: The stretch reflex. In Kandel ER, Schwartz JH, Jessell TM (eds): Principles of Neural Science. New York, Elsevier Science Publishing, 1991, pp 564–580.

88. Benson DF: Aphasia. In Heilman KM, Valenstein E (eds): Clinical Neuropsychology. New York, Oxford University Press, 1985, pp 17–47.

89. Ross ED: Nonverbal aspects of language. Neurol Clin 1993; 11:9–23.

90. Albert ML, Helm-Estabrooks N: Diagnosis and treatment of aphasia: Part 1. JAMA 1988; 259:1043–1047.

91. Geshwind N: Disconnexion syndromes in animals and man. Part 2. Brain 1965; 88:237–294.

92. Friedman RB, Albert ML: Alexia. In Heilman KM, Valenstein E (eds): Clinical Neuropsychology. New York, Oxford University Press, 1985, pp 49–73.

93. Geshwind N: The apraxias: Neural mechanisms of disorders of learned movement. American Scientist 1975; 63:188–195.

94. Heilman KM, Watson RT, Valenstein E: Neglect and related disorders. In Heilman KM, Valenstein E: (eds): Clinical Neuropsychology. New York, Oxford University Press, 1985, pp 243–293.

95. Linden P, Siebens AA: Dysphagia: Predicting laryngeal penetration. Arch Phys Med Rehabil 1983; 64:281–284.

96. Gordon C, Hewer RL, Wade DT: Dysphagia in acute stroke. Br Med J 1987; 295:411–414.

97. Horner J, Massey EW, Riski JE, et al: Aspiration following stroke: Clinical correlates and outcome. Neurology 1988; 38:159–162.

98. Horner J, Massey EW, Brazer SR: Aspiration in bilateral stroke patients. Neurology 1990; 40:1686–1688.

99. Barer DH: The natural history and functional consequences of dysphagia after hemispheric stroke. Neurol Neurosurg Psychiatr 1989; 52:236–241.

100. Horner J, Buoyer FG, Alers MJ, Helms MJ: Dysphagia following brainstem stroke: Clinical correlates and outcome. Arch Neurol 1991; 48:1170–1173.

101. Alberts MJ, Horner J, Gray L, Brazer SR: Aspiration after stroke: Lesion analysis by brain MRI. Dysphagia 1992; 7:170–173.

102. Johnson ER, McKenzie SW, Rosenquist J, et al: Dysphagia following stroke: Quantitative evaluation of pharyngeal transit times. Arch Phys Med Rehabil 1992; 73:419–423.

103. Johnson ER, McKenzie SW, Sievers A: Aspiration pneumonia in stroke. Arch Phys Med Rehabil 1993; 73:973–976.

104. Dejerine J, Roussy G: La syndrome thalamique. Rev Neurol (Paris) 1906; 14:521–535.

105. Gilman S, Newman SW: Manter and Gatz's Essentials of Clinical Neuroanatomy and Neurophysiology, ed 7. Philadelphia, FA Davis, 1987.

106. Amarence P: The spectrum of cerebellar infarctions. Neurology 1991; 41:973–979.

107. Schafer AI: The hypercoaguable states. Ann Intern Med 1985; 102:814–828.

108. Kohler J, Kasper J, Witt I, von Retern FM: Ischemic stroke due to protein C deficiency. Stroke 1990; 21:1077–1080.

109. Gacs G, Fox AJ, Barnett HJM, Vinuela F: Visualization of intracranial arterial thromboembolism. Stroke 1983; 14:756–762.

110. Messina AV, Chernik NL: Computed tomography: The "resolving" intracerebral hemorrhage. Radiology 1976; 118:609–613.

111. Bryan RN, Levy LM, Whitlow WD, et al: Diagnosis of acute cerebral infarction: Comparison of CT and MR imaging. Am J Neuroradiol 1991; 12:611–620.

112. Matthews VP, Barker PB, Bryan RN: Magnetic resonance evaluation of stroke. Mag Res Quart 1992; 8:245–263.

113. Fisher M, Sotak CH, Minematsu K, Li L: New magnetic resonance techniques for evaluating cerebrovascular disease. Ann Neurol 1992; 32:115–122.

114. Hellman RS, Tikofsky RS: An overview of the contribution of regional cerebral blood flow studies in cerebrovascular disease: Is there a role for single photon emission computed tomography? Semin Nucl Med 1990; 20:303–324.

115. Tegeler CH, Downes TR: Cardiac imaging in stroke. Stroke 1991; 26:13–18.

116. Pop G, Sutherland GR, Koudstaal PJ, et al: Transesophageal echocardiography in the detection of intracardiac embolic sources in patients with transient ischemic attacks. Stroke 1990; 21:560–565.

117. Seiler RW, Grolimund P, Aaslid R, et al: Cerebral vasospasm evaluated by transcranial ultrasound correlated with clinical grade and CT-visualized subarachnoid hemorrhage. J Neurosurg 1986; 64:594–600.

118. Fagan SC, Zarawitz BJ, Robert S: "Brain attack": An indication for thrombolysis? Ann Pharmacotherapy 1992; 26:73–80.

119. Siesjo BK: Pathophysiology and treatment of focal cerebral ischemia: 1. Pathophysiology. J Neurosurg 1992; 77:169–184.

120. Consensus Panel: Stroke: The first six hours. Stroke Clin Updates 1993; 4:1–12.

121. Waidhauser E, Hamburger C, Marguth F: Neurosurgical management of cerebellar hemorrhage. Neurosurg Rev 1990; 13:211–217.

122. Wallace JD, Levy LL: Blood pressure after stroke. JAMA 1981; 246:2177–2180.

123. Strandgaard S, Paulson OB: Regulation of cerebral blood flow in health and disease. J Cardiovasc Pharmacol 1992; 19:S89–S93.

124. Herpin D: The effects of antihypertensive drugs on the cerebral blood flow and its regulation. Prog Neurobiol 1990; 35:75–83.

125. Biller J: Medical management of acute cerebral ischemia. Neurol Clin 1992; 10:63–85.

126. Schroeder T, Schierbeck J, Howardy P, et al: Effect of labetolol on cerebral blood flow and middle cerebral arterial flow velocity in healthy volunteers. Neurol Res 1991; 13:10–12.

127. Nedergaard M, Diemer NH: Focal ischemia of the rat brain, with special reference to the influence of plasma glucose concentration. Acta Neuropathol 1987; 73:131–137.

128. DeCouten-Myers GM, Myers RE, Schoolfield L: Hyperglycemia enlarges infarct size in cerebrovascular occlusion in cats. Stroke 1988; 19:623–630.

129. Siesjo BK: Pathophysiology and treatment of focal cerebral ischemia: 2. Mechanisms of damage and treatment. J Neurosurg 1992; 77:337–354.

130. Korczyn AD: Heparin in the treatment of acute stroke. Neurol Clin 1992; 10:209–217.

131. Allen GS, Ahn HS, Preziosi TJ, et al: Cerebral arterial spasm: A controlled trial of nimodipine in patients with subarachnoid hemorrhage. N Engl J Med 1983; 308:619–624.

132. Pickard JD, Murray GD, Illingworth R, et al: Effect of oral nimodipine on cerebral infarction and outcome after subarachnoid hemorrhage: British aneurysm nimodipine trial. Br Med J 1989; 298:626–642.

133. Frontoni DTM, Argentino C, Sacchetti ML, et al: Update on calcium antagonists in cerebrovascular diseases. J Cardiovasc Pharmacol 1991; 18:S10–S14.

134. Del Zoppo GJ, Poeck K, Pessin MS, et al: Recombinant tissue plasminogen activator in acute thrombotic and embolic stroke. Ann Neurol 1992; 32:78–86.

135. Brott TG, Haley EC, Levy DE, et al: Urgent therapy for stroke: 1. Pilot study of tissue plasminogen activator administered 91–180 minutes from onset. Stroke 1992; 23:632–640.

136. Haley EC, Levy DE, Brott TG, et al: Urgent therapy for stroke: 2. Pilot study of tissue plasminogen activator administered 91–180 minutes from onset. Stroke 1992; 23:641–645.

137. The Ancrod in Stroke Investigators: Ancrod in acute ischemic stroke (abstract). Stroke 1992; 23:162.

138. Albers GW: Potential therapeutic uses of N-methyl-D-aspartate antagonists in cerebral ischemia. Clin Neuropharmacol 1990; 13:177–197.

139. McCulloch J: Excitatory amino acid antagonists and their potential for the treatment of ischaemic brain damage in man. Br J Clin Pharmacol 1992; 34:106–114.

140. Brandstater ME: An overview of stroke rehabilitation. Stroke 1990; 21(suppl II):II40–II42.

141. Kotila M, Waltimo O, Niemi M-L, et al: The profile of recovery from stroke and factors influencing outcome. Stroke 1984; 15:1039–1044.

142. Wade DT, Langton-Hewer R: Functional abilities after stroke: Measurement, natural history and prognosis. J Neurol Neurosurg Psychiatry 1987; 50:177–182.

143. Lehmann JF, DeLateur BJ, Fowler RS, et al: Stroke rehabilitation: Outcome and prediction. Arch Phys Med Rehabil 1975; 56:383–389.

144. Granger CV, Hamilton BB, Fiedler RC: Discharge outcome after stroke rehabilitation. Stroke 1992; 23:978–982.

145. Heinemann AW, Roth EJ, Cichowski K, Betts HB: Multivariate analysis of improvement and outcome following stroke rehabilitation. Arch Neurol 1987; 44:1167–1172.

146. Ferrucci L, Bandinelli S, Guralnik JM, et al: Recovery of functional status after stroke: A postrehabilitation follow-up study. Stroke 1993; 24:200–205.

147. Andrews K, Brocklehurst JC, Richards B, et al: The rate of recovery from stroke—and its measurement. Int Rehabil Med 1981; 3:155–161.

148. Lehmann JF, DeLateur BJ, Fowler RS, et al: Stroke: Does rehabilitation affect outcome? Arch Phys Med Rehabil 1975; 56:375–382.

149. Smith DS, Goldenberg E, Ashburn A, et al: Remedial therapy after stroke: A randomized controlled trial. Br Med J 1981; 282:517–520.

150. Indredavik B, Bakke F, Solberg R, et al: Benefit of a stroke unit: A randomized controlled trial. Stroke 1991; 22:1026–1031.

151. Edmans JA, Towle D: Comparison of stroke unit and non-stroke unit in patients on independence in ADL. Br J Occup Ther 1990; 53:415–418.

152. Garraway WM, Akhtar AJ, Prescott RJ, Hockey L: Management of acute stroke in the elderly: Preliminary results of a controlled trial. Br Med J 1980; 280:1040–1043.

153. Wood-Dauphinee S, Shapiro S, Bass E, et al: A randomized trial of team care following stroke. Stroke 1984; 15:864–872.

154. Kalra L: The influence of stroke unit rehabilitation on functional recovery from stroke. Stroke 1994; 25:821–825.

155. Reding MJ, McDowell FH: Focused stroke rehabilitation programs improve outcome. Arch Neurol 1989; 46:700–711.

156. Foulkes MA, Wolf PA, Price TR, et al: The Stroke Data Bank: Design, methods, and baseline characteristics. Stroke 1988; 19:547–554.

157. Skilbeck CE, Wade DT, Langton-Hewer R, et al: Recovery after stroke. J Neurol Neurosurg Psychiatry 1983; 46:5–8.

158. Bjorneby ER, Reinvang IR: Acquiring and maintaining self-care skills after stroke. Scand J Rehabil Med 1985; 17:75–80.

159. Sarno MT, Levita E: Some observations on the nature of recovery in global aphasia after stroke. Brain Lang 1981; 13:1–12.

160. Fugl-Meyer AR: Assessment of motor function in hemiplegic patients. In Buerger AA, Tobis JS (eds): Neurophysiological Aspects of Rehabilitation Medicine. Springfield, Il, Charles C Thomas, 1976.

161. Gowland C, Stratford P, Ward M, et al: Measuring physical impairment and disability with the Chedoke-McMaster stroke assessment. Stroke 1993; 24:58–63.

162. Parker VM, Wade DT, Langton-Hewer R: Loss of arm function after stroke: Measurement, frequency, and recovery. Int Rehabil Med 1986; 8:69–73.

163. Gowland C: Recovery of motor function following stroke: Profile and predictors. Physiother Can 1982; 34:77–84.

164. Wade DT, Langton-Hewer R, Wood VA, et al: The hemiplegic arm after stroke: Measurement and recovery. J Neurol Neurosurg Psychiatry 1983; 46:521–524.

165. Bonita R, Beaglehole R: Recovery of motor function after stroke. Stroke 1988; 19:1497–1500.

166. Warabi T, Inoue K, Noda H, Murakami S: Recovery of voluntary movement in hemiplegic patients: Correlation with degerative shrinkage of the cerebral peduncles in CT images. Brain 1990; 113:177–189.

167. Wing AM, Lough S, Turton A, et al: Recovery of elbow function in voluntary positioning of the hand following hemiplegia due to stroke. J Neurol Neurosurg Psychiatry 1990; 53:126–134.

168. Bohanon RW, Smith MB: Assessment of strength deficits in eight paretic upper extremity muscle groups of stroke patients with hemiplegia. Physical Therapy 1987; 67:522–525.

169. Shah S: Reliability of the original Brunnstrom recovery scale following hemipegia. Am Occup Ther J 1984; 31:144–151.

170. Bohanon RW: Muscle strength changes in hemiparetic stroke patients during inpatient rehabilitation. J Neurol Rehabil 1988; 2:163–166.

171. Shah SK, Harsymiw SJ, Stahl PL: Stroke rehabilitation: Outcome based on Brunnstrom recovery stages. Occup Ther J Res 1986; 6:365–376.

172. Shah SK, Corones J: Volition following hemiplegia. Arch Phys Med Rehabil 1980; 61:523–528.

173. Wade DT, Langton-Hewer R, David RM, Enderby PM: Aphasis after stroke: Natural history and associated deficits. J Neurol Neurosurg Psychiatry 1986; 49:11–16.

174. Kertesz A, McCabe P: Recovery patterns and prognosis in aphasia. Brain 1977; 100:1–18.

175. Pickersgill MJ, Lincoln NB: Prognostic indicators and the pattern of recovery in aphasic stroke patients. J Neurol Neurosurg Psychiatry 1983; 46:130–139.

176. Sarno MT, Levita E: Recovery in treated aphasia in the first year post-stroke. Stroke 1979; 10:662–670.

177. Kertesz A: What do we learn from recovery from aphasia? In Waxman SG (ed): Advances in Neurology: vol 47: Functional Recovery in Neurological Disease. New York, Raven Press, 1988, pp 277–292.

178. Brust JCM, Shafer SQ, Richter RW, Bruun B: Aphasia in acute stroke. Stroke 1976; 7:167–174.

179. Prins RS, Snow CE, Wagenaar E: Recovery from aphasia: Spontaneous speech versus language comprehension. Brain Lang 1978; 6:192–211.

180. Meerwaldt JD: Spatial disorientation in right hemisphere infarction: A study of the speed of recovery. J Neurol Neurosurg Psychiatry 1983; 46:426–429.

181. Stone SP, Patel P, Greenwood RJ, Halligan PW: Measuring visual neglect in acute stroke and predicting its recovery: The visual neglect recovery index. J Neurol Neurosurg Psychiatry 1992; 55:431–436.

182. Kotila M, Niemi M-L, Laaksonen R: Four-year prognosis of stroke patients with visuospatial inattention. Scand J Rehabil Med 1986; 18:177–179.

183. Egelko S, Simon D, Riley E, et al: First year after stroke: Tracking cognitive and affective deficits. Arch Phys Med Rehabil 1989; 70:297–302.

184. Sunderland A, Langton-Hewer R: The natural history of visual neglect after stroke: Indications from two methods of assessment. Int Rehabil Med 1987; 9:55–59.

185. Friedman PJ, Leong L: Perceptual impairment after stroke: Improvements during the first 3 months. Disabil Rehabil 1992; 14:136–139.

186. Hier DB, Mondlock J, Caplan LR: Recovery of behavioral abnormalities after right hemisphere stroke. Neurology 1983; 33:345–350.

187. Dombovy ML, Bach-y-Rita P: Clinical observations on recovery from stroke. In Waxman SG (ed): Advances in Neurology: vol 47: Functional Recovery in Neurological Disease. New York, Raven Press, 1988, pp 265–276.

188. Bach-y-Rita P: Process of recovery from stroke. In Brandstater ME, Basmajian JV (eds): Stroke Rehabilitation. Baltimore, Williams & Wilkins, 1987, pp 80–108.

189. Bach-y-Rita P, Baillet R: Recovery from stroke. In Duncan PW, Badke MB (eds): Motor Deficits Following Stroke. Chicago, Year Book Medical Publishers, 1987, pp 79–107.

190. Bach-y-Rita P (ed): Recovery of Function: Theoretical Considerations for Brain Injury Rehabilitation. Baltimore, University Park Press, 1980.

191. Kaplan MS: Plasticity after brain lesions: Contemporary concepts. Arch Phys Med Rehabil 1988; 69:984–991.

192. Wainberg MC: Plasticity of the central nervous system: Functional implications for rehabilitation. Physiother Can 1988; 40:224–232.

193. Bach-y-Rita P: Brain plasticity as a basis of the development of rehabilitation procedures for hemiplegia. Scand J Rehabil Med 1981; 13:73–83.

194. Feeney DM, Baron JC: Diaschisis. Stroke 1986; 17:817–830.

195. Marshall JF: Neural plasticity and recovery of function after brain injury. Int Rev Neurobiol 1985; 26:201–247.

196. Boyeson MG, Bach-y-Rita P: Determinants of brain plasticity. J Neurol Rehabil 1989; 3:35–57.

197. Bach-y-Rita P: Central nervous system lesions: Sprouting and unmasking in rehabilitation. Arch Phys Med Rehabil 1981; 62:41–47.

198. Illis LS: The effects of repetitive stimulation in recovery from damage to the central nervous system. Int Rehabil Med 1982; 4:178–184.

199. Roth EJ, Mueller K, Green D: Stroke rehabilitation outcome: Impact of coronary artery disease. Stroke 1988; 19:42–47.

200. Sacco RL, Wolf PA, Kannel WB, McNamara PM: Survival and recurrence following stroke: The Framingham Study. Stroke 1982; 13:290–295.

201. Solzi P, Ring H, Najenson T, Luz Y: Hemiplegics after a first stroke: Late survival and risk factors. Stroke 1985; 4:703–709.

202. Dombovy ML, Basford JR, Whisnant JP, Bergstrahl EJ: Disability and use of rehabilitation services following stroke in Rochester, Minnesota, 1975–1979. Stroke 1987; 18:830–836.

203. Sheikh K, Brennan PJ, Meade TW, et al: Predictors of mortality and disability in stroke. J Epidemiol Commun Health 1983; 37:70–74.

204. Roth EJ: Medical complications encountered in stroke rehabilitation. Phys Med Rehabil Clin North Am 1991; 2:563–578.

205. Roth EJ, Noll SF: Stroke rehabilitation: 2. Comorbidities and complications. Arch Phys Med Rehabil 1994; 75:S42–S46.

206. Roth EJ: Natural history of recovery and influence of comorbid conditions on stroke outcome. In Gorelick P (ed): Atlas of Cerebrovascular Disease. Philadelphia, Current Science Publishers, 1995, in press.

207. Schmidt J, Reding M: Recognition and management of medical and specific associated neurological complications in stroke rehabilitation. Top Geriatr Rehabil 1991; 7:1–14.

208. Siegler EL, Whitney FW: Prevention and other special management issues in the postacute care of the geriatric stroke patient. Neurorehabil 1993; 3:1–11.

209. Brott T: Prevention and management of medical complications of the hospitalized elderly stroke patient. Clin Geriatr Med 1991; 7:475–482.

210. Roth EJ: Heart disease in patients with stroke: II. Impact and implications for rehabilitation. Arch Phys Med Rehabil 1994; 75:94–101.

211. Brandstater ME, Roth EJ, Siebens HC: Venous thromboembolism in stroke: Literature review and implications for clinical practice. Arch Phys Med Rehabil 1992; 73(suppl):S379–S391.

212. Couser JI: Diagnosis and management of pneumonia and ventilatory disorders in patients with stroke. Top Stroke Rehabil 1994; 1:106–118.

213. Harvey RL: Diabetes mellitus: Incidence and influence on stroke rehabilitation and outcome. Top Stroke Rehabil 1994; 1:91–108.

214. Saver JL: Poststroke seizures. Top Stroke Rehabil 1994; 1:109–130.

215. Teasell RW: Pain following stroke. Crit Rev Phys Med Rehabil 1992; 3:205–217.

216. Garrison SJ: Post-stroke pain. Phys Med Rehabil State Art Rev 1991; 5:83–88.

217. Boivie J, Leijon G: Clinical findings in patients with central poststroke pain. In Casey KL (ed): Pain and Central Nervous System Disease: The Central Pain Syndromes. New York, Raven Press, 1991, pp 65–75.

218. Steinberg FU: The Immobilized Patient: Functional Pathology and Management. New York, Plenum, 1980.

219. St Pierre D, Gardiner PF: The effect of immobilization and exercise on muscle function: A review. Physiother Can 1987; 39:24–36.

220. Reddy MP: A guide to early mobilization of bedridden elderly. Geriatrics 1986; 41:59–70.

221. Brocklehurst JC, Andrews K, Richards D, Laycock PJ: Incidence and correlates of incontinence in stroke patients. J Am Geriatr Soc 1985; 33:540–542.

222. Reding MJ, Winter SW, Hochrein SA, et al: Urinary incontinence after unilateral hemispheric stroke: A neurologic epidemiologic perspective. J Neurorehabil 1987; 1:25–30.

223. Gelber DA, Good DC, Laven LJ, Verhulst SJ: Causes of urinary incontinence after acute hemispheric stroke. Stroke 1993; 24:378–382.

224. Sedarat SM, Hecht JS: Urologic problems after stroke (parts I and II). Stroke Clin Updates 1993; 4:17–20, 21–24.

225. Linsenmeyer TA, Zorowitz RD: Urodynamic findings in patients with urinary incontinence after cerebrovascular accident. Neurorehabil 1992; 2:23–26.

226. Garrett VE, Scott JA, Costich J, et al: Bladder emptying assessment in stroke patients. Arch Phys Med Rehabil 1989; 70:41–43.

227. Barer DH: Continence after stroke: Useful predictor or goal of therapy? Age Ageing 1989; 18:183–191.

228. Hoogasian S, Walzak MP, Wurzel R: Urinary incontinence in the stroke patient: Etiology and rehabilitation. In Erickson RV (ed): Medical Management of the Elderly Stroke Patient. Phys Med Rehabil State Art Rev 1989; 3:581–594.

229. Borrie MJ: Urinary incontinence after stroke. In Teasell RW (ed): Long-Term Consequences of Stroke. Phys Med Rehabil State Art Rev 1993; 7:101–112.

230. Cailliet R: The Shoulder in Hemiplegia. Philadelphia, FA Davis, 1980.

231. Najenson T, Yacubovich E, Pikielini S: Rotator cuff injury in shoulder joints of hemiplegic patients. Scand J Rehabil Med 1971; 3:131–137.

232. Griffin J, Reddin G: Shoulder pain in persons with hemiplegia: A literature review. Phys Ther 1981; 61:1041–1045.

233. Kozin F, et al: The reflex sympathetic dystrophy syndrome: Parts 1, 2, and 3. Am J Med 1976; 60:321–331, 332–338; 1981; 70:23–30.

234. Smith RG, Cruikshank JG, Dunbar S: Malalignment of the shoulder after stroke. Br Med J 1982; 284:1224–1226.

235. Tepperman PS, Greyson ND, Hilbert L, et al: Reflex sympathetic dystrophy in hemiplegia. Arch Phys Med Rehabil 1984; 65:442–447.

236. Van Ouenaller C, Laplace PM, Chantraine A: Painful shoulder in hemiplegia. Arch Phys Med Rehabil 1986; 67:23–36.

237. Moodie NB, Brisbin J, Morgan AMG: Subluxation of the glenohumeral joint in hemiplegia: Evaluation of supportive devices. Physiother Can 1986; 38:151–157.

238. Totta M, Beneck S: Shoulder dysfunction in stroke hemiplegia. Phys Med Rehabil Clin North Am 1991; 2:627–641.

239. Werner RA, Priebe MM, Davidoff GN: Reflex sympathetic dystrophy syndrome associated with hemiplegia. Neurorehabil 1992; 2:16–22.

240. Teasell RW, Gillen M: Upper extremity disorders and pain following stroke. In Teasell RW (ed): Long-Term Consequences of Stroke. Phys Med Rehabil State Art Rev 1993; 7:133–146.

241. Poplingher AR, Pillar T: Hip fracture in stroke patients: Epidemiology and rehabilitation. Acta Orthop Scand 1985; 56:226–227.

242. DeVincenzo DK, Watkins S: Accidental falls in a rehabilitation setting. Rehabil Nursing 1987; 12:248–252.

243. Mion LC, Gregor S, Buettner M, et al: Falls in the rehabilitation setting: Incidence and characteristics. Rehabil Nursing 1989; 14:17–21.

244. Mayo NE, Korner-Bitensky N, Kaizer F: Relationship between response time and falls among stroke patients undergoing physical rehabilitation. Int J Rehabil Res 1990; 13:47–55.

245. Peszczynski M, Benson F, Collins J, and the Joint Committee for Stroke Facilities: II. Stroke rehabilitation. Stroke 1972; 3:375–407.

246. Goldberg G: Principles of rehabilitation of the elderly stroke patient. In Dunkle RE, Schmidley JW (eds): Stroke in the Elderly. New York, Springer-Verlag, 1987.

247. Brandstater ME, Basmajian JV (eds): Stroke Rehabilitation. Baltimore, Williams & Wilkins, 1987.

248. Roth EJ: The elderly stroke patient: Principles and practices of rehabilitation management. Top Geriatr Rehabil 1988; 3:27–61.

249. Bleiberg J, Merbitz C: Learning goals during initial rehabilitation hospitalization. Arch Phys Med Rehabil 1983; 64:448–450.

250. Hyams DE: Psychological factors in rehabilitation of the elderly. Gerontol Clin 1969; 11:129–136.

251. Whitney FW: Using physical and neuropsychological assessment in the nursing care of the acute stroke patient. In Dunkle RE, Schmidley JW (eds): Stroke in the Elderly. New York, Springer-Verlag, 1987.

252. Frieden RA: Early rehabilitation after stroke. In Gordon WA (ed): Advances in Stroke Rehabilitation. Boston, Andover, 1993, pp 18–33.

253. McDowell FH: Rehabilitating patients with stroke. Postgrad Med 1976; 59:145–149.

254. Asberg KH: Orthostatic tolerance training of stroke patients in general medical wards. Scand J Rehabil Med 1989; 21:179–185.

255. Hamrin E: Early activation in stroke: Does it make a difference? Scand J Rehabil Med 1982; 14:101–109.

256. Hayes SH, Carroll SR: Early intervention care in the acute stroke patient. Arch Phys Med Rehabil 1986; 67:319–321.

257. Anderson TP, Bourestom N, Greenberg FR, Hildyard VG: Predictive factors in stroke rehabilitation. Arch Phys Med Rehabil 1974; 55:545–553.

258. Feigenson JS, McDowell FH, Meese P, et al: Factors influencing outcome and length of stay in a stroke rehabilitation unit: 1. Analysis of 248 unscreened patients—medical and functional prognostic indicators. Stroke 1977; 8:651–656.

259. Novack TA, Satterfield WT, Lyons K, et al: Stroke onset and rehabilitation: Time lag as a factor in treatment outcome. Arch Phys Med Rehabil 1984; 65:316–319.

260. Johnston MV, Keister M: Early rehabilitation for stroke patients: A new look. Arch Phys Med Rehabil 1984; 65:437–441.

261. Westcott EJ: Traditional exercise regimens for the hemiplegic patient. Am J Phys Med 1967; 46:1012–1023.

262. Flanagan EM: Methods for facilitation and inhibition of motor activity. Am J Phys Med 1967; 46:1006–1011.

263. Lorish TR, Sandin KJ, Roth EJ, Noll SF: Stroke rehabilitation: 3. Rehabilitation evaluation and management. Arch Phys Med Rehabil 1994; 75:S47–S51.

264. Good DC: Treatment strategies for enhancing motor recovery in stroke rehabilitation. J Neurorehabil 1994; 8:177–186.

265. Duncan PW, Badke MB: Stroke Rehabilitation: The Recovery of Motor Control. Chicago, Year Book Medical Publishers, 1987.

266. Knott M, Voss DE: Proprioceptive Neuromuscular Facilitation, ed 2. New York, Harper & Row, 1968.

267. Davies PM: Steps to Follow: A Guide to the Treatment of Adult Hemiplegia. Berlin, Springer-Verlag, 1985.

268. Ernst E: A review of stroke rehabilitation and physiotherapy. Stroke 1990; 21:1081–1085.

269. Carr JH, Sheperd RB: A Motor Relearning Programme for Stroke. Rockville, Md, Aspen Publishers, 1987.

270. Swenson JR: Therapeutic exercise in hemiplegia. *In* Basmajian JV (ed): Therapeutic Exercise, ed 4. Baltimore, Williams & Wilkins, 1984, pp 357–380.

271. Barton LA, Wolf SL: Use of EMG feedback in stroke rehabilitation. *In* Gordon WA (ed): Advances in Stroke Rehabilitation. Boston, Andover, 1993, pp 88–99.

272. Wolf SL: Essential considerations in the use of EMG biofeedback. Phys Ther 1978; 58:25–31.

273. Wolf S, Baker M, Kelly J: EMG biofeedback in stroke: A 1-year follow-up of the effect on patient characteristics. Arch Phys Med Rehabil 1980; 61:351–355.

274. DeWeerdt W, Harrison M: Electromyographic biofeedback for stroke patients: Some practical considerations. Physiother Can 1986; 72:106–108.

275. Ince LP, Zaretsky HH, Lee MHM: Integrating EMG biofeedback treatment of the impaired upper extremity into the rehabilitation programs of stroke patients. Arch Phys Med Rehabil 1987; 68:645.

276. Kraft GH: New methods for the assessment and treatment of the hemiplegic arm and hand. Phys Med Rehabil Clin North Am 1991; 2:579–597.

277. Moreland J, Thomson MA: Efficacy of electromyographic biofeedback compared with conventional physical therapy for upper-extremity function in patients following stroke: A research overview and meta-analysis. Phys Ther 1994; 74:534–547.

278. Wade DT, Langton-Hewer R, Skilbeck CE, David RM: Stroke: A Critical Approach to Diagnosis, Treatment, and Management. Chicago, Year Book Medical Publishers, 1985.

279. Taub E: Somatosensory deafferentation research with monkeys: Implications for rehabilitation medicine. *In* Ince LP (ed): Behavioral Psychology in Rehabilitation Medicine: Clinical Applications. Baltimore, Williams & Wilkins, 1980.

280. Taub E, Miller NE, Novack TA, et al: A technique for improving chronic motor deficit after stroke. Arch Phys Med Rehabil 1993; 74:347–354.

281. Wolf SL, LeCraw DE, Barton LA, Jann FF: Forced use of hemiplegic upper extremities to reverse the effect of learned nonuse among chronic stroke and head-injured patients. Exp Neurol 1989; 104:125–132.

282. Barton LA, Wolf SL: Learned nonuse in the hemiplegic upper extremity. *In* Gordon WA (ed): Advances in Stroke Rehabilitation. Boston, Andover, 1993, pp 79–87.

283. Ragnarsson KT: Orthotics and shoes. *In* DeLisa JA (ed): Rehabilitation Medicine. Philadelphia, JB Lippincott, 1988, pp 307–329.

284. Morganstein S, Smith MC: Aphasia and right-hemisphere disorders. *In* Gordon WA (ed): Advances in Stroke Rehabilitation. Boston, Andover, 1993, pp 103–133.

285. Chapey R (ed): Language Intervention Strategies in Adult Aphasia, ed 2. Baltimore, Williams & Wilkins, 1986.

286. Sarno MT (ed): Acquired Aphasia. New York, Academic Press, 1981.

287. LaPointe L: Aphasia therapy: Some principles and strategies for treatment. *In* Johns DF (ed): Clinical Management of Neurogenic Communicative Disorders. Boston, Little, Brown, 1978.

288. Darley FL: The efficacy of language rehabilitation in aphasia. J Speech Hearing Dis 1972; 37:3–21.

289. Loverso FL, Prexcott TE, Selinger M: Cueing verbs: A treatment strategy for aphasic adults. J Rehabil Res Dev 1988; 25:47–60.

290. Howard D, Patterson K, Franklin S, et al: Treatment of word retrieval deficits in aphasia: A comparison of two therapy methods. Brain 1985; 108:817–829.

291. Shewan CM, Kertesz A: Effects of speech and language treatment on recovery from aphasia. Brain Lang 1984; 23:272–299.

292. Wertz RT, Collins MJ, Weiss D, et al: Veterans Administration Cooperative Study on Aphasia: A comparison of individual and group treatment. J Speech Hearing Res 1981; 24:580–594.

293. Sparks RW, Helm NA, Albert ML: Aphasia rehabilitation resulting from melodic intonation therapy. Cortex 1974; 10:203–216.

294. Therapeutics and Technology Assessment Subcommittee of the American Academy of Neurology: Assessment: Melodic intonation therapy. Neurology 1994; 44:566–568.

295. Helm-Estabrooks N, Emery P, Albert M: Treatment of aphasic perseveration (TAP): A new approach to aphasia therapy. Arch Neurol 1987; 44:1253–1255.

296. Wertz RT, Weiss DG, Aten JL, et al: Comparison of clinic, home, and deferred language treatment for aphasia: A Veterans Administration Cooperative Study. Arch Neurol 1986; 43:653–658.

297. Shewan C, Bandur D: Treatment of Aphasia: A Language-Oriented Approach. San Diego, College Hill, 1982.

298. Holland A: Pragmatic aspects of intervention in aphasia. J Neurolinguistics 1991; 6:197–211.

299. Weinrich M, Steele R, Carlson G, et al: Processing of visual syntax by a globally aphasic patient. Brain Lang 1989; 36:391–405.

300. Springer L, Glindemann R, Huber W, Willmes K: How efficacious is PACE therapy when language systematic training is incorporated? Aphasiology 1991: 5:391–399.

301. Till JA, Yorkston KM, Beukelman DR (eds): Motor Speech Disorders: Advances in Assessment and Treatment. Baltimore, Paul H Brookes, 1994.

302. Yorkston KM, Beukelman DR, Bell KR: Clinical Management of Dysarthric Speakers. Austin, Pro-Ed, 1988.

303. Dworkin JP: Motor Speech Disorders: A Treatment Guide. St Louis, Mosby–Year Book, 1991.

304. Berry WR, Sanders SB: Environmental education: The universal management approach for adults with dysarthria. *In* Berry WR (ed): Clinical Dysarthria. Austin, Pro-Ed, 1983.

305. Evans RL, Northwood L: Social support needs in adjustment to stroke. Arch Phys Med Rehabil 1983; 64:61–64.

306. Evans RL, Matlock A-L, Bishop DS, et al: Family intervention after stroke: Does counseling or education help? Stroke 1988; 19:1243–1249.

307. Robinson RG, Lipsey JR, Price TR: Depression: An often overlooked sequela of stroke. Geriatric Med Today 1984; 3:35–45.

308. Coll P, Erickson RV: Mood disorders associated with stroke. Phys Med Rehabil State Art Rev 1989; 3:619–628.

309. Binder LM: Emotional problems after stroke. Stroke 1984; 15:174–177.

310. Robinson RG, Szetela B: Mood change following left hemisphere brain injury. Ann Neurol 1981; 9:447–452.

311. Finkelstein S, Berkowitz LI, Baldessarini RJ: Mood vegetative disturbance, and dexamethasone suppression test after stroke. Ann Neurol 1982; 12:463–468.

312. Robinson RG, Starr LB, Kubos KL: A two-year longitudinal study of post-stroke mood disorders: Findings during the initial evaluation. Stroke 1983; 14:736–741.

313. Robinson RG, Kubos KL, Starr LB: Mood disorders in stroke patients: Importance of lesion location. Brain 1984; 107:81–93.

314. Robinson RG, Starr LB, Price TR: A two-year longitudinal study of mood disorders following stroke: Prevalence and duration at six months follow-up. Br J Psychiatry 1984; 144:256–262.

315. Parikh RM, Lipsey JR, Robinson RG: Two-year longitudinal study of post-stroke mood disorders: Dynamic changes in correlates of depression at one and two years. Stroke 1987; 18:579–584.

316. Reding MJ, Orto LA, Winter SW: Antidepressant therapy after stroke. Arch Neurol 1986; 43:763–766.

317. Lipsey JR, Robinson RG, Pearlson GD: Nortriptyline treatment of post-stroke depression: A double-blind study. Lancet 1984; 1:297–300.

318. Fugl-Meyer AR, Jaasko L: Post-stroke hemiplegia and sexual intercourse. Scand J Rehabil Med 1980; 7:158–166.

319. Monga TN, Lawson JS, Inglis J: Sexual dysfunction in stroke patients. Arch Phys Med Rehabil 1986; 67:19–22.

320. Bray GP, DeFrank PRS, Wolfe TL: Sexual functioning in stroke survivors. Arch Phys Med Rehabil 1981; 62:286–288.

321. Sjogren K, Fugl-Meyer AR: Adjustment to life after stroke with special reference to sexual intercourse and leisure. J Psychosom Res 1982; 26:409–417.

322. Freda M, Rubinsky H: Sexual function in the stroke survivor. Phys Med Rehabil Clin North Am 1991; 2:643–658.

323. Stein PN, Berger AL, Hibbard MR, Gordon WA: Intervention with the spouses of stroke survivors. *In* Advances in Stroke Rehabilitation. Boston, Andover, 1993, pp 242–257.

324. Dombovy ML, Sandok BA, Basford JA: Rehabilitation after stroke: A review. Stroke 1986; 17:363–369.

325. Chin PL, Rosie A, Irving M: Studies in hemiplegic gait. *In* Rose FC (ed): Advances in Stroke Therapy. New York, Raven Press, 1982.

326. Granger CV, Hamilton BB: UDS Report: The Uniform Data System

for Medical Rehabilitation Report of First Admissions for 1991. Am J Phys Med Rehabil 1992; 73:51–55.

327. Jongbloed L: Prediction of function after stroke: A critical review. Stroke 1986; 17:765–775.

328. Davidoff G, Keren O, Ring H, et al: Assessing candidates for inpatient stroke rehabilitation: Predictors of outcome. Phys Med Rehabil Clin North Am 1991; 2:501–516.

329. Johnston MV, Kirshblum S, Zorowitz RD, Shiflett SC: Prediction of outcomes following rehabilitation of stroke patients. Neurorehabil 1992; 2:72–97.

330. Wade DT, Skilbeck CG, Hewer RL: Predicting Barthel ADL score at 6 months after an acute stroke. Arch Phys Med Rehabil 1983; 64:24–28.

331. Poduri KR, Steimer SL: Comprehensive outpatient approach to stroke rehabilitation. J Stroke Cerebrovasc Dis 1993; 3:29–48.

332. Kamen LB: Issues in outpatient rehabilitation management of the stroke survivor. Phys Med Rehabil Clin North Am 1991; 2:615–626.

333. Biller J, Matthews KD, Love BB: Stroke in Children and Young Adults. Boston, Butterworth-Heinemann, 1994.

334. Weinfeld FD: The national survey of stroke. Stroke 1981; 12(suppl I):I1–I68.

335. Hart RG, Miller VT: Cerebral infarction in young adults: A practical approach. Curr Concepts Cerebrovasc Dis 1982; 17:15–20.

336. Hachinski V, Norris JW: The Acute Stroke. Philadelphia, FA Davis, 1985.

337. Coull BM: Stroke in the young patient—coagulation disturbances. Stroke Clin Update 1990; 1:9–12.

338. Love BB, Biller J: Stroke in the young—cardiac causes. Stroke Clin Update 1990; 1:13–16.

339. Black-Schaffer RM, Osberg JS: Return to work after stroke: Development of a predictive model. Arch Phys Med Rehabil 1990; 71:285–290.

340. Kertesz A, McCabe P: Recovery patterns and prognosis in aphasia. Brain 1977; 100:1–18.

341. van Zomeren AH, Brouwer WH, Minderhoud JM: Acquired brain damage and driving: A review. Arch Phys Med Rehabil 1987; 68:697–705.

342. Niemi M-L, Laaksonen R, Kotila M, Waltimo O: Quality of life 4 years after stroke. Stroke 1988; 19:1101–1107.

343. Oehring AK, Oakley JL: The young stroke patient: A need for specialized group support systems. Top Stroke Rehabil 1994; 1:25–40.

344. Black-Schaffer RM, Lemieux L: Vocational outcome after stroke. Top Stroke Rehabil 1994; 1:74–86.

345. Kempers E: Preparing the young stroke survivor for return to work. Top Stroke Rehabil 1994; 1:65–73.

346. Culler KH, Jasch C, Scanlan S: Child care and parenting issues for the young stroke survivor. Top Stroke Rehabil 1994; 1:48–64.

347. Andrews K, Brocklehurst JC, Richards B, Laycock PJ: The influence of age on the clinical presentation and outcome of stroke. Int Rehabil Med 1984; 6:49–51.

348. Great Britain Department of Health: Stroke rehabilitation. Effective Health Care 1992; 2:1–11.

APPENDIX 50–A

SPECIFIC SELECTED INTERVENTIONS TO MEET SPECIFIC PATIENT NEEDS

MEDICAL-PHYSIOLOGICAL FUNCTION

1. Prevent intercurrent complication
   - Position properly and turn frequently
   - Frequent passive range-of-motion exercises
   - Deep breathing and coughing exercises
   - Pharmacological and physical methods of thromboembolic disease prevention
   - Stroke prevention measures (e.g., anticoagulants or antithrombotic agents)
2. Treat medical complications (e.g., infections)
3. Treat spasticity and contracture
   - Prevent and treat medical complications
   - Stretching program
   - Positioning program
   - Splinting
   - Joint mobilization and manipulation
   - Forced weight-bearing
   - Serial casting
   - Physical modalities, e.g., cold application
   - Injections: peripheral nerve and motor point blocks
   - Pharmacological measures
   - Biofeedback
   - Electrical stimulation
   - Tendon lengthening and contracture release surgery
   - Neurosurgical techniques
4. Treat pain (hemiplegic shoulder pain, reflex sympathetic dystrophy syndrome, other musculoskeletal pain, central poststroke pain)
   - Proper positioning, elevation, using slings, tray, armrests, supports
   - Edema reduction methods: elevation, massage, stockings, gloves, range-of-motion exercises
   - Tone reduction methods: stretching exercises, nerve or motor point blocks, medications
   - Physical modalities: ice, heat, ultrasound, others
   - Medications: analgesics, anti-inflammatory agents
   - Injections: peripheral nerve, motor point, sympathetic ganglion, etc.
   - Neurosurgical procedures
5. Manage co-morbid conditions, review and adjust medications (e.g., diabetes, hypertension, heart disease, arthritis)
6. Manage ongoing physiological functions
   - Nutrition assessment and management
   - Hydration assessment and management
   - Feeding tube management
   - Tracheostomy management
   - Timed, scheduled toileting program
   - Dietary fiber
   - Mobilization
   - Train toilet transfers
   - Catheterization program
   - Medication
   - Treat bladder and bowel infections
7. Prevent and treat fatigue, deconditioning, orthostatic intolerance, and endurance limitations
   - Treat medical conditions
   - Ensure adequate sleep, rest, nutrition, hydration, and appropriate medication use

Reassurance

Adjust therapy schedule to balance need for rest with need for mobilization and exercise

Progressively increase mobilization times and amounts

Endurance training

SENSORY-MOTOR DEFICITS

1. Prevent effects of prolonged immobility (e.g., contracture, orthostatic hypotension)

    Early, cautious, and supervised exercise and remobilization

    Early and frequent activation

    Early and consistent performance of activities of daily living

    Conventional stretching exercises

    Conventional strengthening exercises: active assistive, active, progressive resistive

2. Facilitate natural motor recovery of strength and control, including balance and fine motor control

    Conventional strengthening exercises: active assistive, active, progressive resistive

    Balance training

    Trunk control exercises

    Mat mobility exercises

    Standing exercises

    Weight-shifting exercises

    Fine motor control finger exercises

    Practice functional tasks requiring fine motor control

    Exercise in specific positions: e.g., sitting, standing, kneeling

    Neurophysiological facilitation and inhibition techniques

       Neurodevelopmental treatment (Bobath)

       Proprioceptive neuromuscular facilitation

       Movement therapy (Brunnstrom)

       Motor program for stroke (Carr and Shepherd)

       Sensory facilitation (Rood)

       Others

    Use of facilitatory or inhibitory modalities simultaneously with volitional muscle contraction, e.g., quick stretch, stroking, tapping, vibration, brushing

3. Teach compensatory functional strategies

    Self-care: feeding, dressing, hygiene, grooming, toileting, bathing, telephone use

    Mobility: sitting, bed mobility, rolling, transfers (bed, bath, toilet, car), wheelchair propulsion, walking, stairs

    Community motor skills, instrumental ADL, laundry, meal preparation, shopping, house-cleaning, child care, other community skills

4. Newer approaches to motor control enhancement

    Behavioral techniques

       Electromyographic-biofeedback

       Positional biofeedback

       Force biofeedback

       Forced-use

Electrical stimulation

5. Orthotics, assistive devices, durable medical equipment, other aids

    Dynamic orthoses

    Tone-reducing orthoses

    Static orthoses (e.g., resting hand splint)

    Wheelchair

    Bath bench

    Reacher, other ADL aids

    Walker, hemiwalker, quad cane, straight cane

    Training in use of devices

6. Rehabilitation engineering and technology

7. Surgical intervention

    Tendon releases

8. Family education

COGNITIVE-COMMUNICATION-OROMOTOR DEFICITS

1. Evaluate and treat dysarthria

    Oromotor strengthening exercises

    Enunciation practice

    Alternative communication training

2. Evaluate and treat aphasia

    Traditional modality-specific stimulus response therapy

    Language-oriented treatment

    Treatment of aphasic perserveration

    Visual action therapy

    Conversational coaching

    Functional communication therapy

    Melodic intonation therapy

    Programmed approaches

    Response elaboration training

    Auditory comprehension training

    Computerized approaches

    C-VIC

    Promoting aphasic communicative effectiveness

    Cognitive intervention

    Augmentation approaches

    Groups

    Oral reading (reading aloud)

    General stimulation

    Compensatory/alternative communication training

    Gestures

    Writing

    Electronic technology

3. Swallowing assessment and management

    Thermal stimulattion

    Change head and neck position

    Diet adjustment

    Alter food quantity

    Alternative nutrition routes if needed

    Patient and family training

4. Cognitive evaluation and training (inattention, poor concentration, memory deficits, disorientation, concrete thinking, apraxia)

    Cognitive skills training

    Computer technology training

    Memory strategy training

    Memory book

Mnemonics
5. Perceptual evaluation and training (agnosias, unilateral neglect, right-left disorientation, impaired sense of verticality, impaired time perception, impaired depth perception)
Environmental adaptation
Teaching of strategies
Anchoring
Pacing
Density
Feedback
Scanning training
Compensatory techniques
Supplying cues and reminders
Forced-use
Eye patch use

PSYCHOLOGICAL AND SOCIAL ISSUES

1. Promote psychological adaptation and coping; treat poststroke mood disorders (depression, fear, anger, anxiety, lability)
Supportive counseling
Family involvement
Team approach
Positive reinforcement
Milieu therapy
Peer support
Social recreational activities
Antianxiety medications
Antidepressant medications
Relaxation training
Stroke support group
2. Evaluation and management of behavioral changes (impulsivity, aggressiveness, quick temper, rage, apathy)
Counseling
Redirection, refocusing
Low stimulation environment
Safety education
Family education
Medication
3. Promote family and caregiver coping and stress management
Family education: team-family meetings, classes, brochures, books, videotapes
Functional skills training and practice
Family individual counseling
Family support groups

4. Patient and family education (about stroke, medications, prevention and recognition of medical problems, community issues, etc.)
Education: Personal teaching, classes, brochures, books, videotapes
Counseling
Psychotherapy
Support groups
5. Recruit and promote awareness of community resources
Counseling: entitlements, community social services, home professional nursing and therapeutic services, outpatient services, day care, etc.
Advocacy on behalf of patient
Ensuring follow-up and continuity of care
6. Promote safety awareness
Redirection, refocusing, reminding
Low stimulation environment
Counseling
Safety education
Family education
Medication
Ensure provision of appropriate supervision
Family education
Alter environment
7. Driving assessment and training
8. Socialization training
9. Vocational assessment and training
Vocational assessment
Vocational counseling
Vocational training
Job placement
Supported employment
Job coaching
10. Sexuality counseling
Education and training
Reassurance
Counseling
Mat mobility training
Specific skills training
11. Ensuring follow-up and continuity of care
Medical care
Continued therapy
Home nursing supervision and care
12. Patient and family education
Training in medication administration, exercises, other treatment regimens (e.g., tube feedings, respiratory care, etc.)
Practicing in transitional living setting
Home accessibility assessment visit
Therapeutic home pass

51

Rehabilitation Concerns in Degenerative Movement Disorders of the Central Nervous System

MARY L. DOMBOVY, M.D.

The general category of movement disorders includes a number of central nervous system (CNS) neurodegenerative diseases including Parkinson's disease and other brainstem–basal ganglia degenerations, the hereditary ataxias, and the dystonias (Table 51–1). Parkinson's disease is by far the most common, affecting 1% of the population 65 years old and over.[8] Many of the symptoms and signs of Parkinson's disease can be seen in other neurodegenerative disorders, as well as in anoxic encephalopathy, multiple lacunar infarcts, drug effects, and the normal aging process[30] (Table 51–2). "Parkinsonism" is commonly seen in patients on rehabilitation units. Unfortunately, the benefits of rehabilitation and specific therapy approaches for Parkinson's and other movement disorders remain unclear.

This chapter discusses the differential diagnosis of parkinsonism, the medical treatment of Parkinson's disease (Fig. 51–1), and rehabilitation of Parkinson's disease as a prototype for rehabilitation of parkinsonism in other disorders. Rehabilitation in the hereditary ataxias and the treatment of dystonia receive brief additional comment at the end of the chapter.

PARKINSON'S DISEASE

Pathophysiology, Clinical Presentation, and Differential Diagnosis

Parkinson's disease is characterized pathologically by degeneration of pigmented and other brainstem nuclei, particularly the substantia nigra, in association with the formation of eosinophilic neuronal inclusions called Lewy bodies.[5, 17] The primary biochemical defect in Parkinson's disease is the loss of striatal dopamine resulting from the degeneration of dopamine-producing cells in the substantia nigra with the associated hyperactivity of cholinergic neurons in the caudate nuclei contributing to the symptoms.[3] The four most prominent hypotheses regarding the etiology of Parkinson's disease are the theories of (1) accelerated aging, (2) toxin exposure, (3) genetic predisposition, and (4) oxidative stress. The oxidative mechanism theory has received the most support to date, but it is likely that a combination of all four processes contributes to the development of Parkinson's disease.[26]

Although Parkinson's disease can present with an array of clinical symptoms and signs (Table 51–3), the cardinal features of the disease are (1) resting or postural tremor, (2) bradykinesia, (3) rigidity, and (4) postural instability. In the early stages of Parkinson's disease, rigidity (often described as "stiffness" or "achiness" by patients) may be mistaken as a symptom of arthritis. Masked facies and bradykinesia can lead to the most common early misdiagnosis, that of depression. The onset and progression of the disease is slow and insidious. The disease can begin either with tremor or with bradykinesia and rigidity as the initial presentation. Symptoms and signs typically begin in one extremity or one side but eventually spread to involve the other limbs and trunk. Lack of arm swing when walking and changes in handwriting (micrographia) are early signs.

Although tremor can become disabling, it usually does not impair function as much as bradykinesia and rigidity, which eventually lead to problems in all areas of mobility and activities of daily living (ADL). When ambulating, patients have difficulty in changing direction or moving

TABLE 51–1   Selected Central Nervous System Movement Disorders

Idiopathic	Secondary
Parkinson's disease	Birth injury
Progressive supranuclear palsy (Steele-Richardson-Olszewski syndrome)	Chorea gravidarum
	Neuroleptic medications
Multiple system atrophy (Shy-Drager syndrome)	Head injury
Corticobasal degeneration	Cerebral infarct/hemorrhage
Most dystonias	Anoxia
Blepharospasm	Carbon monoxide poisoning
Meige's disease	Manganese poisoning
Gilles de la Tourette's syndrome	Mercury poisoning
Genetic	Basal ganglia tumor
Huntington's disease	Liver disease
Wilson's disease	Oral contraceptives
Some dystonias	Hyperthyroidism and hypothyroidism
Inherited ataxias	Hypoparathyroidism
Numerous metabolic defects	Alcohol
Ataxia telangiectasia	Sydenham's chorea
Olivopontocerebellar degeneration	von Economo's encephalitis
Friedreich's ataxia (and others)	
Familial nonprogressive chorea	
Essential tremor	
Hallervorden-Spatz disease	

TABLE 51–2   Differential Diagnosis of Parkinsonism

Idiopathic Parkinson's disease*,†
Progressive supranuclear palsy*
Multiple system atrophy*
Olivopontocerebellar atrophy*
Striatonigral degeneration
Wilson's disease†
Westphal variant of Huntington's disease†
Corticobasal degeneration
Hallervorden-Spatz disease
Alzheimer's disease (late stages)
Parkinson-ALS-dementia complex
Post encephalitis
Drug-induced*,† (neuroleptics,*,† metaclopramide,*,† reserpine†)
Toxin-induced*,† (MPTP,† manganese,† carbon monoxide,*,† carbon disulfide,† cyanide†)
Metabolic*,† (anoxia,* hypothyroidism,*,† hypoparathyroidism*,†)
Multi-infarcts*,†
Subdural hematoma*,†
Multiple head injuries (boxer's dementia†)
Basal ganglia tumor*,†
Normal-pressure hydrocephalus*,†

*Most common considerations.
†Important to consider and rule out.
Abbreviations: *ALS*, amyotrophic lateral sclerosis; *MPTP*, 1-methyl-4-phenyl-1,2,3,6-tetrahydropyridine.

TABLE 51–3   Clinical Features of Parkinson's Disease

Symptoms and Signs	Common Presenting Complaints
Rigidity	Stiffness, aching muscular pain, slowed movements
Bradykinesia (slowness of movement)	Trouble getting out of a chair
Resting/postural tremor	Trouble rolling over in bed
Hypokinesia (small-amplitude movement)	Falling, tripping over objects on floor
Loss of postural reflexes	Tremor, "shaking"
Loss of preparatory and associated movements ("en bloc" movements, decreased arm swing, decreased blinking)	Depression
	Memory loss
Akathisia (inability to sit still, relieved by walking about)	Stooped posture
	Rapid or whispering speech
Dementia	Change in handwriting
Autonomic dysfunction (orthostatic hypotension, slowed gastrointestinal motility, urinary retention, impotence)	Slowness in activities, dressing, grooming
	Trouble walking
Hypokinetic dysarthria	Slow to respond to questions and requests
Festinating gait	Drooling; trouble controlling saliva
Masked facies (stare with decreased blinking)	
Dystonia	
Flexed posture	
Dysphagia	
Sudden "freezing" of motor activity	

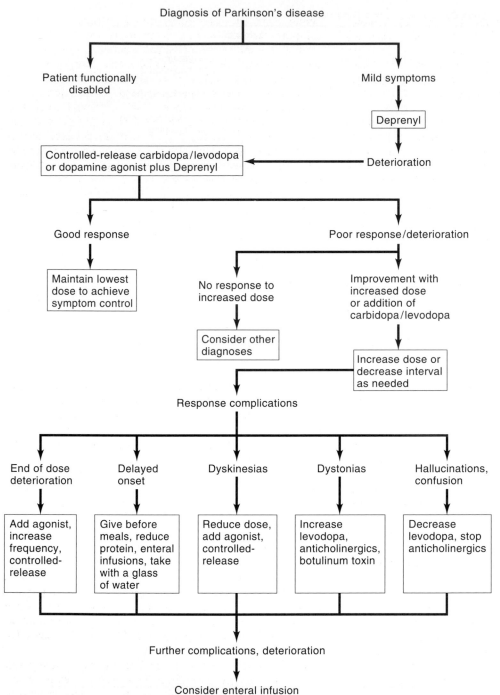

FIGURE 51–1 Sample of an algorithm for medical therapeutics in Parkinson's disease.

around objects and may "freeze," unable to start again. Patients with Parkinson's disease have great difficulty in carrying out two simultaneous but unrelated motor acts, such as talking or taking notes while walking, or throwing or reaching while walking, and so forth.

Impairment of speech is one of the most frustrating disabilities for patients with Parkinson's disease. Speech becomes rapid, monotonous, and of low volume (hypokinetic dysarthria). Speech and handwriting can be affected by the same phenomenon that causes festinating gait.

Since the basal ganglia play an important role in motor planning and programming, Parkinson's disease patients display various degrees of difficulty with initiating an activity such as walking, reaching for objects, or changing course when walking. There is a loss of normal associated or preparatory movements such as arm swing in gait and positioning the feet back and inclining forward prior to arising from a chair.

As Parkinson's disease progresses, autonomic symptoms (slowed enteric mobility and constipation, urinary retention and incontinence, orthostatic hypotension), dysphagia, and postural instability become bothersome. Dementia is often a late feature and ultimately appears in about one third of the patients. Depression can affect as many as 50% of the patients. (Both are difficult to diagnose, as psychomotor retardation [a slowness in producing the motor response] is also a feature of Parkinson's disease.) Hallucinations, insomnia, nausea, lack of appetite, weight loss, and dystonia are often-encountered side effects of dopaminergic medications. Insomnia is also seen as the result of nocturnal bradykinesia.

A gradual increase over time in all of the manifestations of Parkinson's disease is characteristic. Before the advent of levodopa therapy, 25% of patients with symptom duration of less than 5 years were severely disabled and 75% of survivors with symptom duration of 10 to 15 years were totally disabled. Patients with rigidity as the predominant initial symptom tend to experience disability earlier than those with tremor as the presenting feature. The introduction of levodopa, deprenyl (selegiline), and novel medication management strategies has prolonged independence and in many cases has allowed for continued employment.

Early Parkinson's disease can be difficult to distinguish from other subcortical degenerations. The hallmarks of Parkinson's disease are a definite response to levodopa treatment, and the absence of symptoms and signs such as early vertical eye movement abnormalities (progressive supranuclear palsy [PSP]), early autonomic failure (Shy-Drager syndrome), hyperreflexia, Babinski's signs, ataxia, and peripheral neuropathy (multisystem degeneration) supports the diagnosis of Parkinson's disease. While other parkinsonian states sometimes show a mild to moderate response to levodopa, the beneficial effects are usually transient. One should always seek to exclude other nondegenerative causes such as drug and toxin exposure (see Table 51–2).

A number of medications are utilized in the management of Parkinson's disease (see Table 51–4). Levodopa combined with carbidopa (a peripheral dopa decarboxylase inhibitor, e.g., Sinemet) remains as the cornerstone of pharmacological therapy for Parkinson's disease,[53] although controversy exists as to when treatment with levodopa should begin.[27] More than half of the patients with Parkinson's disease who receive treatment with conventional levodopa preparations later develop response complications, including a shortened response duration. The mechanisms of these complications are not completely understood. Wide fluctuations in dopamine levels, disease-related changes in pre-synaptic handling of levodopa, and receptor alterations all may contribute.[42] Some neurologists delay levodopa therapy until symptoms significantly interfere with function, or they begin treatment with a direct dopamine receptor agonist such as pergolide or bromocriptine.[53]

Since the late 1980s, results from the Parkinson Study Group suggest that monoamine oxidase-B inhibitors such as deprenyl also exert a mild dopaminergic effect, which could have produced the noted delay in disability in treated patients. Some neurologists begin treatment of early Parkinson's disease with deprenyl owing to its therapeutic effects and the potential that it might slow disease progression.[36, 40, 56] Deprenyl also can be used to smooth out levodopa-related fluctuations later in the disease.

Since the late 1980s, sustained-release levodopa combination preparations have become available (Sinemet CR, Madopar HBS). Peak dopamine levels are low and therapeutic levels are sustained, hence the potential for reducing symptom fluctuation. Bioavailability is less than with immediate-release preparations, and when switching from immediate release the total levodopa dose usually needs to be increased. An additional advantage of sustained-release preparations is the reduction of the profound alterations in levodopa plasma concentrations that are thought to contribute to some of the later problems with dyskinesia and other dose-response fluctuations. Although the manufacturer indicates that twice-daily dosing is adequate with Sinemet CR, most patients achieve a smoother response dosing three times a day and eventually four times a day.

Variable gastric emptying is often a feature of advanced Parkinson's disease, and can lead to an apparent lack of response to oral medication. Jejunal infusion via a pump delivery system has been employed in some cases. Jejunal infusion has also been used in instances in which motor fluctuations and wearing-off effects are prominent even if gastric retention is not a problem.[11, 44] Enteral tubes are a consideration when dysphagia has progressed to the point of inadequate nutrition or there is a high risk of aspiration. Improvement in gastric emptying can also be achieved by administering a large glass of water with oral levodopa or carbidopa.

While levodopa's effects depend on its enzymatic conversion to dopamine in nigrostriatal neurons, direct dopamine agonists (e.g., bromcriptine, pergolide) directly stimulate the dopamine receptor. While these compounds generally have short half-lives, they can nonetheless be helpful in smoothing out levodopa-related response fluctuations. Because of the theoretical advantage of sparing the potentially harmful effects of levodopa, some have advocated the use of direct dopamine agonists as initial therapy, delaying the use of levodopa compounds for 1 to 2 years.

Amantadine, which has both pre- and postsynaptic dopaminergic effects, is also used both as early treatment and later as an adjunct. Anticholinergics (e.g., trihexyphenidyl [Artane], benztropine [Cogentin]) are helpful when tremor is the predominant problem but become less well tolerated as Parkinson's disease progresses, owing to side effects such as sedation, impaired memory, and urinary retention. The use of anticholinergics to treat Parkinson's disease has decreased over the past 5 years.

Considering recent research and theory, a reasonable approach to initial treatment of Parkinson's disease[36] would be to (1) introduce deprenyl at the time of early diagnosis; (2) begin a low dose of a dopamine agonist, either with or without a long-acting levodopa preparation, when symptomatic treatment becomes functionally indicated; and (3) titrate levodopa dosages as symptom control warrants, using the lowest dose required for adequate function. The management of dose-response fluctuations, dyskinesia, and the "on/off" phenomenon is complex and can be frustrating. Consultation with a neurologist with expertise in the management of patients with advanced Parkinson's disease is usually required to provide optimal medication adjustment.

Most patients with Parkinson's disease experience varying degrees of side effects from the medications, particularly in later stages. Some patients are intolerant of levodopa on an empty stomach, in which case beginning with a smaller dose is helpful. If food must be taken, a high protein intake should be avoided. The potential side effects of these medications are numerous, and it is important to be aware of them in the rehabilitation setting. Table 51–4 lists the potential side effects by drug class.

The Rationale for Rehabilitation

Many experts in the treatment of Parkinson's disease recommend rehabilitative services as an adjunct to medical therapy[23, 32, 53] because it "intuitively" makes sense that these services can prevent complications and either maintain or assist with function. In addition, patients with Parkinson's disease often state that they "feel" or function better with a program of regular exercise. It is not clear whether this results from a general sense of well-being or a general conditioning effect that often occurs with exercise, from true improvement in function, or from actual improvement in some of the deficits of Parkinson's disease (e.g., bradykinesia, rigidity).

The literature on the benefits of rehabilitation services for patients is sparse. Most of the studies suffer from methodological problems such as lack of controls or blinding, inappropriate or nonvalidated assessment measures, and small numbers of subjects. Studies are not comparable because they used different therapy approaches with different levels of intensity over varying time frames. What outcome measures to choose is also a major question. Should the focus be on whether specific exercise programs, speech therapy techniques, and so forth improve the neurological deficit? Or should the focus be on improved function, regardless of whether there has been any improvement in bradykinesia, hypokinesia, or rigidity? There are a few recent reviews attempting to assess the efficacy of nonpharmacological therapy for patients with Parkinson's disease.[9, 12, 57] The reader is referred to them for a more detailed review of the literature.

The Parkinson's disease rehabilitation programs evaluated in studies range from home-based,[4, 25, 33] to outpatient physical (PT) or occupational therapy (OT),[13, 18, 21, 38, 55] or both, or speech therapy (ST),[1, 22, 43, 46, 51, 52] to comprehensive inpatient programs.[12, 54] In general, the results suggest a

benefit in patients with Parkinson's disease of an exercise program that focuses on improving range-of-motion (ROM), endurance, balance, and gait.[13, 18, 25, 33, 38] The efficacy of more functionally oriented programs has not been assessed, although Parkinson's disease patients felt that the provision of equipment and instruction in adaptive techniques provided by OT in the home was helpful to them.[4] Small numbers of subjects and in some studies the lack of controls, as well as changes in medication, make the composite results less than conclusive. Enhanced sense of well-being may also contribute to the improvements noted in function.[13]

Comella et al.[13] recently conducted a prospective, randomized, single blind crossover study of the effects of a 4-week outpatient physical rehabilitation program on mentation, ADL, and motor function as measured by the Unified Parkinson's Disease Rating Scale (UPDRS).[16] Sixteen moderate to moderately severe Parkinson's disease patients were seen for 1 hour three times per week for 4 weeks by PT and OT. The program consisted of repetitive exercises directed at improving ROM, balance, fine motor dexterity, gait, and endurance. The intensity of the program was increased as endurance improved. The control group received no intervention. Two 4-week study periods were separated by 6 months. Medication changes were not allowed during the control or therapy phases, but adjustments were permitted during the 6-month interval between study periods as well as during the follow-up period.

Following the physical rehabilitation program there was a significant improvement in ADL and motor function (bradykinesia and rigidity) but no improvement in tremor, timed finger tapping, mentation, or mood. Despite instructions to the subjects to continue the exercise program at home at the completion of the rehabilitation phase, all resumed a more sedentary lifestyle, and at 6-month follow-up the UPDRS scores returned to baseline. Continued exercise might be needed to maintain function, but incorporating such a program into a patient's lifestyle without continuation of an organized program appears unlikely.

It is interesting that Palmer et al.[38] found improvements in gait, tremor, motor coordination, and grip strength in Parkinson's disease patients in an exercise program regardless of whether the program was that developed by the United Parkinson Foundation or a group in karate training! Such a program could be more easily continued in a group format at a community gymnasium or other facility in a more cost-effective fashion, with the additional benefit of increasing socialization.

Although speech and swallowing disorders are commonly a source of disability in Parkinson's disease,[14] speech therapy is likely underutilized.[35] Families often complain that speech is improved as long as the patient is receiving therapy, but as soon as the therapy ends, speech reverts to the previous pattern. This clinical experience is supported by the work of Sarno,[46] who noted in a study of 300 patients with Parkinson's disease that speech improved only during treatment. Allan[1] also reported rapid deterioration in formal speech therapy. The type of speech therapy might be important for benefit and carryover. Another study[43] reported that intensive speech therapy (group and individual therapy lasting 3½ to 4 hours per day of 2 weeks' duration) produced a positive effect on speech in

TABLE 51–4   Common Side Effects of Medications Used in Parkinson's Disease

Carbidopa-levodopa compounds	Nausea, hypotension, arrhythmias, hallucinations, nightmares, hypomania, paranoid psychosis, delirium, insomnia, dystonia, dyskinesias
Deprenyl (selegiline)	Cardiac toxicity, hallucinations; potentiates side effects of levodopa
Amantadine	Hallucinations, insomnia, nervousness, edema, livedo reticularis, headache
Dopaminergic agonists	Hallucinations, vivid dreams, psychosis, paranoia
Anticholinergics	Impaired memory, confusion, urinary retention, blurred vision, dry mouth, constipation, orthostatic hypotension

Parkinson's disease patients, with some benefits lasting up to 3 months. Therapy focused on voice and respiratory control, loudness, pitch variation, and control of rate of speech.

In a series of studies, Scott and Caird[51, 52] demonstrated that speech therapy consisting of intonational and prosodic exercises can produce improvements in speech, some of which lasted up to 3 months. The treatment program consisted of daily 1-hour sessions carried out in the patient's home over 2 to 3 weeks. It appears that the types of motor deficits in Parkinson's disease resulting in both the physical symptoms and speech impairment improve with a program that provides regular and continuing intervention.

Another speech disorder common in Parkinson's disease and other neurological disorders (e.g., Alzheimer's disease, multi-infarct dementia) is palilalia. Palilalia is characterized by the repetition of a word or phrase with increasing rapidity and decreasing distinctiveness as to become inaudible. The use of a pacing board has been noted to be helpful in decreasing palilalia.[33]

Studies addressing the benefits of inpatient rehabilitation in Parkinson's disease are few, as patients with Parkinson's disease are not commonly admitted to inpatient rehabilitation units. This likely reflects the societal view that patients with degenerative disorders are not candidates for inpatient rehabilitation because of resource utilization and cost concerns. Stern et al.[54] studied 47 Parkinson's disease patients admitted to a rehabilitation center who received a course of intensive multidisciplinary rehabilitation in conjunction with the start of levodopa therapy. They noted good to excellent improvements in mobility in 66% and no improvement in 17%. A few patients not showing improvement in mobility did show improvement in ADL. Another study[28] initiated levodopa therapy in 100 outpatients with Parkinson's disease without any concomitant rehabilitation. Of these patients, 60% improved and 18% worsened or showed no change. The inference here is that the addition of an intensive inpatient rehabilitation program to the initiation of levodopa therapy does not appear to result in a superior outcome.

As part of a pilot study to develop appropriate measures to assess the impact of rehabilitation on patients with Parkinson's disease, Cedarbaum et al.[12] looked at the changes in numerous tasks and activities following inpatient rehabilitation. Forty-five patients were studied in an unblinded, open fashion with medication adjustments allowed. Many patients came from acute care facilities following hospitalization for intercurrent illness or injury. Patients received an average of 4 hours of therapy per day, 5 days a week. Despite allowing for medication adjustment as dictated by the patient's condition, no significant overall average change in levodopa dosage occurred. No changes were noted in any of the timed tasks. Statistically significant improvements were noted in ambulation transfers, dressing, and personal hygiene. The large number of variables in this study raises the likelihood of some positive changes occurring by chance. Additionally, the lack of overall change in average levodopa dosage cannot be used to negate medication effects, as some patients may actually benefit from a decrease in levodopa and the addition of another agent. Many of these patients may have been

regaining function lost during a period of immobility that occurred during their acute hospital stay.

With future changes in healthcare delivery, it is unlikely that most Parkinson's disease patients will receive inpatient rehabilitation. It is also noted that continuation of an exercise program on a basis of two to three times a week might be necessary to optimize and maintain gains realized in formal therapy sessions. Future studies should focus on the effects of outpatient therapy programs that make use of a continued community-based group exercise and therapy program directed at maintaining mobility, function, and community. Such studies must also take into account the natural history of Parkinson's disease, which will likely result in a decline in function over 12 to 18 months.

Exercise and Muscle Physiology

In prescribing exercise programs for patients with Parkinson's disease, the ability of the patient to tolerate the exercise must be taken into account when there is evidence indicating differences in muscle physiology and response to exercise in these patients. It is not clear whether these effects are related to disuse, are related to altered central innervation, or are a direct pathological involvement. Landin et al.[28] looked at muscle metabolism and physiological response to exercise in six patients with Parkinson's disease and five healthy controls. On the basis of their results, the authors concluded that subjects with Parkinson's disease exercised with decreased efficiency. Their finding of reduced adenosine triphosphate (ATP) in muscles could mean a reduced efficiency in coupling between respiration and ATP generation by muscles. This could be the result of an altered metabolic state of muscle secondary to an abnormal pattern of innervation. This finding is also consistent with recent reports of alterations of mitochondrial respiration in brain tissue,[48] platelets,[39] and muscle tissue[6] in patients with Parkinson's disease. This suggests that there may be a systemic abnormality in mitochondrial function in Parkinson's disease.

Another study[45] demonstrated lowered mechanical efficiency in leg muscles in Parkinson's disease patients, resulting in these patients performing twice the work of normal controls. The authors postulated that physical inactivity and deconditioning in subjects with Parkinson's disease may have been as important a factor as an altered metabolic state of muscle. However, Gersten et al.[20] demonstrated that levodopa therapy reduced the externally measured work of walking in 46 subjects with varying stages of Parkinson's disease. When clinically appropriate, optimization of levodopa therapy is important to consider prior to embarking on an exercise program, since levodopa produces physiological changes that have an impact on the patient's ability to exercise and to benefit from the program.

Psychological and Social Aspects

Secondary to the predominance of motor symptoms in Parkinson's disease, psychological and cognitive impairments and their resultant impact on disability are often overlooked. Although severe dementia can occur late in the disease,[10] most patients with Parkinson's disease perform less well on a wide range of cognitive tests than age- and education-matched controls, even early in the course.[29,]

[34, 37] It appears that dementia in Parkinson's disease has both a cortical and a subcortical origin. Pathological changes similar to those found in Alzheimer's disease are commonly found in patients with Parkinson's disease. The changes do not always correlate with the presence of dementia and often overlap with the typical neural degeneration and Lewy body formation seen in Parkinson's disease.[2] In patients with Parkinson's disease with impaired intellect, choline acetyltransferase levels have been found to be reduced in the cortex.[41]

Adaptation to change in daily routine or environment can be difficult and result in undue anxiety. It is as if the same rigidity, bradykinesia, and difficulties with planning and adapting to change that affect the motor system in Parkinson's disease also affect the mind and thought processes. Patients with Parkinson's disease develop a sensitivity to drugs that alter the CNS and often develop delirium when they are used.

Sleep disturbances are common, and difficulty falling asleep can occur early in the disease. In some patients, levodopa has a stimulant effect, preventing sleep. Early in the disease, one can avoid the use of levodopa late in the day. If there are no obvious cognitive impairments, diphenhydramine often works well and also tends to decrease tremor. Sleep problems can be accentuated by the vivid dreams and hallucinations that may occur as a side effect of dopaminergic medications. Fatigue and an increased tendency to daytime napping also contribute to what eventually can become a totally reversed sleep-wake cycle.

As noted earlier, depression is common in Parkinson's disease. It may be related to a deficit in serotonergic neurotransmission[31] or to the diminution of cortical levels of norepinephrine and dopamine.[47] Depression is difficult to treat in patients with declining mental function because of the anticholinergic side effects of the tricyclic (noradrenergic-dopaminergic) antidepressants. A serotonergic agent may be the logical first choice in these patients. If that is ineffective, a tricyclic with low anticholinergic side effects, such as desipramine or nortriptyline, may be tried.

Social dysfunction is also quite common, with lack of socialization due to anxiety related to bodily symptoms the most common. Patients with akinesia rigidity tend to experience more emotional stress than those with tremor-predominant Parkinson's disease. In one study, group-counseling activities involving both patients and caregivers were helpful in reducing stress in 74% of patients.[15]

Driving is a complex cognitive-perceptual-motor task. Maintaining the ability to drive is also important to independence. When motor or cognitive function becomes impaired such that driving could be affected, the physician should suggest a more detailed assessment, which might include retaking the driver's test. In many communities, driver screening is offered as part of a driver's training program for persons with disabilities.

A Practical Approach to Optimal Management

Optimal treatment of the patient with Parkinson's disease requires a multidisciplinary approach, with team coordination by a physician experienced in the rehabilitation of Parkinson's disease or a nurse-practitioner knowledgeable about Parkinson's disease and its treatment and about the available rehabilitative and community resources. The expertise of the rehabilitation physician is essential to overall design of the program, but an appropriately trained nurse-practitioner working under the supervision of a physician can provide follow-up as well as coordination of care. My experience is that nurse-practitioners are able to spend more time with the patient and family as well as devote the time necessary to ensure true coordination of care. Consultation with a neurologist who has experience in the medical management of Parkinson's disease and who is versed in new treatment options is essential.

Development of a multidisciplinary treatment team in the setting of a Parkinson's disease clinic works well in large hospital or institutionally based multispecialty practices or in tertiary care centers where most services are available. However, many patients with Parkinson's disease reside in small communities where the full spectrum of services is not available. Additionally, many patients are not referred for neurological consultation or for rehabilitation until late in the disease, when the opportunity to prevent some of the disease complications is reduced.

Emphasis needs to be placed on (1) educating consumers about optimal medical and rehabilitative management and the availability of resources, (2) educating primary care providers about the role of rehabilitation in treatment of Parkinson's disease (both early and late) and how to access services, and (3) further research on the benefits and costs of specific rehabilitation therapies.

Rehabilitation for Parkinson's disease is functional. The initial evaluation identifies the areas of disability experienced by the patient and prioritizes them. The ensuing assessment seeks to determine the underlying impairments and environmental barriers that result in the various disabilities. The treatment plan addresses the disabilities through (1) treatment of the impairments when feasible; (2) provision of aids and devices; (3) instruction in alternative approaches and a home maintenance program; (4) education of the patient and family both about the disease process and the purpose of specific therapies and exercises; (5) provision of counseling and access to support groups as well as to other community services; and (6) appropriate periodic medical and rehabilitation follow-up to facilitate coordinated modification of both medical and rehabilitative treatment as the disease progresses. The treatment plan is developed with the participation of the patient and family. Table 51–5 represents an example of a functionally based assessment and treatment program. Such an approach has the best chance of ensuring compliance and success.

Schenkman and Butler[49] provide an interesting and useful model for evaluation of Parkinson's disease based on separation of the impairments into three categories based on their origin: (1) those that are a direct result of nervous system pathological processes (e.g., rigidity, hypokinesia); (2) those that are an indirect result and not due to nervous system disorders (e.g., contracture, cardiopulmonary deconditioning); and (3) those that are a composite effect of nervous system and non-nervous system impairments (e.g., rigidity and loss of postural mechanisms facilitating and combining with the development of kyphosis and other fixed contractures leading to the composite of impaired

TABLE 51-5   Example of Rehabilitation Approach in Parkinson's Disease

Functional Problem	Underlying Impairments	Goals	Interventions
Slow and hesitant gait, problem reversing or changing direction, short steps	Bradykinesia, hypokinesia, loss of associated movements, loss of range of motion (ROM) in lower extremities	Decrease hesitancy; increase stride length; improve arm swing; allow for movement around obstacles	Mental rehearsal; marching to metronome and other external cues; exaggerate steps and arm swing; lower extremity ROM exercise and stretching
Kyphosis, reduced respiratory capacity	Rigidity, hip and knee flexion contractures, thoracic rigidity	Improve posture; improve respiration	Trunk extension exercises; breathing exercises; hip flexor and hamstring stretch
Rapid monotone speech with poor intelligibility	Hypokinesia, motor control disintegration	Improve intelligibility	Control breathing; pace rate; exaggerate enunciation
Falling	Rigidity, truncal and extremity contractures, loss of postural reflexes	Improve balance; decrease falls; improve safety	Stretching and ROM exercise of trunk, upper and lower extremities; balance training; instruction in falling and getting up from floor

balance). The composite impairments lead to disabilities affecting gait and other aspects of mobility and self-care. Such a model is useful in designing a PT approach, as it may be difficult or impossible for PT to correct impairments that are the direct result of neuronal and neurotransmitter changes. It is more realistic to prevent or lessen the impact that the CNS lesion has on impairments in other body systems and to teach the patient compensatory strategies, thus reducing potential sequelae. For additional details on this approach, the reader is referred to Schenkman and Butler[49] and to an additional article by Schenkman et al.[50] that focuses on management with case studies as examples.

Specific Therapy Approaches

Gait, Station, and Posture

The typical patient with moderate Parkinson's disease assumes a flexed posture, has difficulty initiating gait, and ambulates with short shuffling steps at an increasing rate. The base of support is usually narrow. Once walking begins, the patient has great difficulty changing direction, stepping over or moving around objects, or stopping (the festinating gait). Prior to beginning ambulation, the patient with Parkinson's disease does not make the normal preparatory movements of the trunk and extremities. During gait, associated movements such as arm swing, trunk rotation, and pelvic motion are reduced or absent. Postural reactions are impaired, so that the patient with Parkinson's disease is unable to correct for mild perturbations in the center of gravity (e.g., being brushed by another person or taking a slight misstep) and can topple over at times as if he or she were a statue. Sudden "freezing" can also occur and precipitate a fall. Although helpful in alleviating rigidity and bradykinesia, pharmacological therapy for Parkinson's disease usually does not help with postural instability and will not be effective to the degree that fixed contracture contributes to the composite impairment. Later in the disease, as fluctuations in response to levodopa occur (the so-called on/off effect), performance may be extremely variable and unpredictable.

Useful approaches to these problems include exercises emphasizing trunk extension and lateral and rotational trunk mobility, weight shifting and balance training, and instruction in falling safely and getting up off the floor. Widening the stance provides a better base of support. Conscious strategies to initiate gait and maintain a cadence are often quite helpful and include mental rehearsal and counting or singing out loud or to oneself and marching to the rhythm. The process can be begun with external cues, such as a metronome or music, that are gradually withdrawn. Exaggeration of arm swing and leg excursion is also helpful.

Balance activities can be made a part of other functional activities such as washing, grooming, and household activities. A cane can be of help, but it also can get in the way if not properly used. A rolling walker works better than a standard walker, since patients who are at a stage where a walker is needed usually cannot incorporate lifting a walker into their gait pattern. Care should be taken to set the walker at a higher height than usual so as not to further promote flexion. Inability to stop once started can be a problem with rolling walkers, and supervision is often required.

A visit to the patient's home by a physical or occupational therapist can result in environmental safety measures such as the removal of throw rugs, rearrangement of furniture, and installation of railings, grab bars, and other adaptive equipment. They can also help the patient develop effective home management strategies specific to the patient's level.

In the newly diagnosed patient, the opportunity to prevent loss of motion and flexed posture exists. More vigorous exercise that improves coordination and balance and promotes general fitness is helpful. Walking, bicycling, dancing, low-impact aerobics, and other group exercise programs not only improve function but also provide the opportunity for socialization.

Tremor, Bradykinesia, Hypokinesia, and Rigidity

Although tremor does not usually cause the same degree of functional impairment as other aspects of Parkinson's disease, if severe it can become a factor. The tremor is typically a resting-postural tremor that often improves (or at least does not become worse) during movement. Anticholinergic medications may be tried and can be helpful if tolerated. Because the tremor becomes worse with anxiety or stress, relaxation techniques are often helpful. In my opinion, distal weights are of no benefit in improving function.

Bradykinesia (slowness of movement), hypokinesia (decreased movement), and rigidity affecting the flexor muscles more than the extensors are the key direct neurological impairments underlying the disability caused by Parkinson's disease. ROM exercises and stretching on a daily basis are important in preserving flexibility. Initiation of movement, larger excursions during movement, and coordination should be addressed as a part of functional activities. There is increasing evidence that exercise is most effective when it is task-specific.[19] Task-specific exercise might be especially important for the patient with Parkinson's disease in light of the impairments in motor planning and programming characteristic of the disease. Helpful strategies and techniques include measures such as rocking to and fro in the chair before arising, and other preparatory motions to provide momentum. A raised chair and toilet seat and armrests also make arising easier.

One of the most difficult problems is the Parkinson's disease patient's inability to use automatic responses during willed functional movement. Clinical experience and the literature[19] suggest that repetition improves these responses and the resulting functional movements.

Rigidity can result in musculoskeletal pain, which often responds to heat, massage, stretching, and ROM exercise.

Speech and Swallowing

Speech disturbances in patients with Parkinson's disease include initial hesitancy, low volume, rapid rate, monotone voice, poor articulation, hesitations or inappropriate periods of silence, stuttering and palilalia, and trailing off of the voice with an increasing rate. All of these combined are referred to as "hypokinetic dysarthria." The initial deficit is a failure to control respiration for the purpose of speech. Following this is gradual breakdown in the complex sensorimotor integration of speech production complicated by stiffness of facial and pharyngeal muscles.

Speech typically improves somewhat with levodopa treatment. Speech therapy interventions for speech disorders consist of exercises emphasizing breath and rate control, improved (often exaggerated) articulation, and increased volume.

Dysphagia tends to occur later in the disease and results in drooling, poor nutrition, inability to take oral medications, and can lead to aspiration pneumonia. Common abnormalities include food-pocketing in the mouth and a delayed swallowing reflex. Aspiration pneumonia is a major cause of morbidity and mortality in Parkinson's disease. Therapeutic interventions include positioning of the neck in flexion, smaller amounts of food, thickened liquids, avoidance of foods with mixed consistencies (e.g., vegetable soup), and a double swallow (see Chapter 27). The caregiver should be instructed in the Heimlich maneuver. In later stages, placement of a gastrostomy tube and tracheostomy might be considered. Consultation with a dietitian is helpful to ensure adequate nutrition. A decrease

in protein intake may be necessary to promote adequate levodopa absorption. Patients with frequent and severe dyskinetic reactions may require large amounts of calories.

A videofluoroscopic swallowing study is helpful in determining the cause of the swallowing difficulties and helps direct the treatment approach. The swallowing study is also able to assess the severity of the problem and the potential for and actual occurrence of aspiration (see Chapter 27). It is important to address the placement of a gastrostomy feeding tube before dysphagia progresses to the point of nutritional compromise or high risk of aspiration. Because Parkinson's disease is a progressive disorder, some patients choose to forego the placement of a feeding tube and continue with oral feedings despite the risk of aspiration. Beginning the discussion early gives the patient and family adequate time to think through their decision. It should be noted that there are patients with a variety of neurological disorders who chronically aspirate but do not routinely develop pneumonia.

Autonomic Dysfunction

Orthostatic hypotension becomes a problem in later stages of the disease. Arising slowly and pausing in the sitting position before standing, elevating the head of the bed, and using pressure garments are conservative approaches that are helpful. Mineralocorticoids can also be helpful.

Slowed gastric and intestinal motility lead to early satiety, vomiting, poor absorption of medications, and constipation. Useful strategies include frequent small meals, increased fiber intake, bulking agents, stool softeners, suppositories, and timed voiding. Metaclopramide facilitates gastric emptying but should generally be avoided because of its tendency to cause parkinsonian side effects. Cisapride, another such agent, might be a better choice.

Urinary incontinence, difficulty voiding, retention, and infections may also occur. Recurrent urinary infections frequently indicate neurogenic bladder dysfunction, although other causes such as prostatic hypertrophy are common in this age group. An appropriate investigation typically includes postvoid residual, cystoscopy, assessment of renal function, and, potentially, cystometrogram-sphincter electromyography (CMG-EMG). The results of this workup guide the practical and pharmacological interventions. An indwelling catheter should be used only as a last resort and if it will facilitate the care of a severely disabled patient.

Impotence can also occur as a result of autonomic dysfunction or psychological factors. This area deserves appropriate assessment and treatment as much as any other aspect of disability related to Parkinson's disease (see Chapter 30).

Sympathetic pain and reflex sympathetic dystrophy may be seen in Parkinson's disease. The pain is often alleviated by levodopa. If it is not, the use of a tricyclic antidepressant is often helpful and can also decrease tremor. In later stages, the anticholinergic effects on cognition are less well tolerated. The effectiveness of the serotonergic antidepressants in alleviating neurogenic pain is unclear.

Cardiopulmonary Function

Flexed posture leads to kyphosis, which reduces lung capacity. Rigidity can result in a "restrictive" pulmonary disease pattern, further complicating respiratory function. Endurance often decreases secondary to a sedentary lifestyle. A focus on breathing exercises, proper posture, and trunk extension early in Parkinson's disease is helpful to prevent these musculoskeletal complications which contribute to the high incidence of pulmonary dysfunction. Cardiopulmonary conditioning should also be a component of the early program (see Chapters 32 and 33). Later in the course, breathing and extension exercise should be continued, with the addition of coughing, incentive spirometry, and respiratory therapy techniques as needed. Instruction in energy conservation techniques and pacing can preserve the ability to continue in a productive role.

Cognition and Depression

Management of declining cognitive function becomes an issue in many cases. Although Parkinson's disease has its peak incidence in the sixth decade, the disease begins in some patients in their 40s or 50s. At this point most will be either employed or responsible for management of the home. As noted above, patients with Parkinson's disease may have deficiencies in cognitive function very early in the disease that may not be apparent on a social level but that may cause problems at work (particularly in highly technical, skilled, or professional occupations). Full neuropsychological assessment is prudent in such cases. In other cases more limited testing to assess for safety to continue independent living or driving is adequate. Making the family aware of safety issues and providing both the family and the patient with compensatory cognitive techniques are essential. The neuropsychologist or rehabilitation psychologist can perform the testing, interpretation, and recommendations.

A psychologist, psychiatrist, or experienced social worker can provide helpful input regarding the patient's emotional state. Pharmacological intervention for depression has already been discussed. Counseling for both patient and family may be helpful in developing coping skills. Awareness of and encouragement to use community resources and support groups are essential.

ADL and Adaptive Equipment

As the primary purpose of rehabilitation is to improve or maintain function, a thorough functional assessment is key to the development of an integrated program for the patient with Parkinson's disease. The physical and occupational therapist should work closely together in both the assessment and the development of the program. While ideally the approach is to maintain or improve impairments, to the degree that this becomes impossible instruction in compensatory techniques and the use of various devices allow the patient to remain functional for a prolonged period. A home visit will not only help in assessing the need for home modification but will also allow the therapist to see how the patient functions in the home. Numerous assistive devices are available, as detailed in Chapter 26.

The Home Program and Follow-up

As discussed earlier, patients with Parkinson's disease require a regular and ongoing exercise program to maintain

or, in some cases, improve function. A specific exercise format does not appear to be critical as long as the program chosen covers the following areas: (1) relaxation and breathing, (2) posture principles, (3) active, active-assistive, and passive ROM exercises and stretching, (4) balance and gait activities, (5) coordination, (6) general conditioning, and (7) specific functional activities, including speech, ADL, and other tasks.

As it is unlikely that continuous therapy will be reimbursed, after individual assessment the patient and caregiver should be instructed in a program over three to five sessions that can be carried out at home on a regular basis. Early in the disease, and later whenever possible, participation in group exercise programs for the elderly that are available in many communities and that combine conditioning programs with socialization are an excellent option. Some communities with an active Parkinson's disease support group have an exercise program specifically designed for patients with Parkinson's disease. The minimum exercise frequency is three times per week for the group programs and daily for a home program. In more severely involved patients, twice-daily ROM exercise and stretching may not even be enough to maintain mobility. There is almost always a tradeoff between maximal benefit and the practicality of the exercise program.

As in patients with other chronic disabling conditions, patients with Parkinson's disease quickly lose ground when periods of illness restrict their activity or put them on bed rest. Care should be taken to provide ROM exercise, stretching, proper positioning, breathing exercises, and whatever mobility the patient can tolerate in these situations.

PARKINSON-LIKE SYNDROMES

The approach to the other degenerative disorders with features similar to or in common with Parkinson's disease, such as progressive supranuclear palsy and multiple system atrophy, is similar to that used with Parkinson's disease. Even though levodopa is not as effective in these disorders, it often has some benefit and should be given an initial trial. Many of these diseases have a more rapidly debilitating course, which needs to be considered when developing the rehabilitation plan.

Huntington's Disease

Huntington's disease, which is inherited in an autosomal dominant fashion, usually presents with chorea, dementia, and behavioral and mood disorders. However, in a small percentage of patients, hypokinesia and rigidity are the presenting features. This is referred to as the Westphal variant and tends to have its onset at an earlier age. Through genetic testing it is now possible to identify patients while still asymptomatic.

In addition to chorea and neuropsychological changes, dysarthria, dysphagia, and gait abnormalities also occur. Rehabilitation efforts are functional and are patient care– and caregiver–oriented. Chorea does not respond to PT, although dopaminergic blocking agents may be helpful. Chorea can consume a large amount of energy and calories, making nutrition a prime concern. Many communities have active support groups for patients and families affected by Huntington's disease.

Hereditary Ataxias

The hereditary ataxias include a wide variety of disorders, some of which present with intermittent ataxia and others in which the ataxia is progressive and combined with other neurological features such as upper motor neuron signs (e.g., olivopontocerebellar atrophy) and peripheral nerve signs (e.g., absent ankle reflexes in Friedreich's ataxia). Ataxia can result from disorders of the cerebellum or its connections, the brainstem, the vestibular system, the dorsal columns and spinocerebellar tracts of the spinal cord, the dorsal root ganglia, or the peripheral nerves. Disorders resembling ataxia can also be seen following parietal or frontal lobe lesions. These disorders are not common, and when such a patient is referred for rehabilitation, it is extremely important for the rehabilitation team to obtain full information of the projected course of the disease to ensure the development of an appropriate rehabilitation plan. Some of these disorders also have associated systemic involvement (e.g., cardiomyopathy and diabetes mellitus in Friedreich's ataxia), which will also have an impact on the rehabilitation program.

A review of all of the hereditary ataxias is beyond the scope of this chapter, and the reader is referred to Hurko's review.[24] The medical management of these disorders is based on accurate diagnosis that rules out treatable problems such as tumors, malformations, or metabolic defects (e.g., acoustic neuromas, Arnold-Chiari syndrome, Wilson's disease). Ataxia and ataxic (intention) tremor cannot be treated with medication in the same way that the symptoms of Parkinson's disease are diminished by levodopa. The mainstay of treatment is the provision of PT and OT directed at maintaining function for as long as possible. Gait training and instruction in the use of assistive devices to prevent falls and enhance mobility are useful. Distal weights may dampen the intention tremor. Speech therapy can be helpful in improving articulation and thus make the patient more easily understood, as well as in assessing improving dysphagia. Specific coordination exercises are rarely useful or practical in progressive disorders compared with their utility in static causes of ataxia, such as head injury or stroke. Social services and psychological support are important, as they are for all progressive disorders.

Dystonia

Dystonia is a syndrome characterized by sustained muscle contractions resulting in abnormal movements or sustained postures. These movements and postures are the result of sustained co-contraction of both the agonist and the antagonist. Dystonia can be focal, multifocal, segmental, or generalized. Dystonic syndromes can be primary (idiopathic) or associated with or caused by another disorder (e.g., in Parkinson's disease, anoxia, head injury, Wilson's disease, inherited metabolic defects).

Most focal dystonias respond to injections of botulinum toxin.[7] Anticholinergics, levodopa, baclofen (Lioresal), carbamazepine, and clonazepam have all been used with some success in selected patients with more generalized forms.

Thalamotomy is reserved for severe cases of generalized dystonia that have not responded to intensive pharmacological trials.

PT techniques, such as massage and slow stretching, and modalities such as ultrasound and biofeedback are sometimes helpful in the focal or regional dystonias. Patients with generalized dystonia often benefit from gait and mobility training and instruction in the use of assistive devices.

SUMMARY

Patients with Parkinson's disease and other neurodegenerative movement disorders often benefit from rehabilitation interventions. Careful evaluation, treatment planning, adequate follow-up, and patient and family education are required. As primary care physicians, neurologists, and others involved in the care of these patients may not be aware of the benefits of rehabilitation in Parkinson's disease, future educational efforts should also be directed at these professionals. Additional research is needed to develop more effective programs and to scientifically verify the impact of rehabilitation programs on disability.

References

1. Allan CM: Treatment of nonfluent speech resulting from neurological disease: Treatment of dysarthria. Br J Disord Commun 1970; 5:3–5.
2. Alvord EC, Forno LS, Kusske JA, et al: The pathology of parkinsonism: A comparison the degenerations in cerebral cortex and brain stem. Adv Neurol 1974; 5:175.
3. Atadzhanov M, Rakhimdhanov A: Dopamine deficiency and cholinergic models of the parkinsonian syndrome. Neurology 1993; 43(suppl 1):S126–S129.
4. Beattie A, Caird FI: The occupational therapist and the patient with Parkinson's disease. Br Med J 1980; 1:1354–1356.
5. Bethlem J, Den Hartog Jager WA: The incidence and characteristics of Lewy bodies in idiopathic paralysis agitans (Parkinson's disease). J Neurol Neurosurg Psychiatry 1960; 23:74–80.
6. Bindhoff LA, Birch-Machlin M, Cartlidge NEF, et al: Mitochondrial dysfunction in Parkinson's disease. Lancet 1989; 2:49.
7. Brin MF, Blitzer A, Stewart C, et al: Disorders with excessive muscle contraction: Candidates for treatment with intramuscular botulinum toxin (Botox). In DasGupta BR (ed): Botulinum and Tetanus Neurotoxins. New York, Plenum Press, 1993, pp 559–576.
8. Broe CA, Akhter AJ, Andrews CR, et al: Neurological disorders in the elderly at home. J Neurol Neurosurg Psychiatry 1976; 39:362–366.
9. Caird FI: Non-drug therapy of Parkinson's Disease. Scott Med J 1986; 31:129–132.
10. Cedarbaum JM, McDowell FH: Sixteen-year follow up of 100 patients begun on levodopa in 1968: Emerging problems. Adv Neurol 1986; 45:469.
11. Cedarbaum JM, Silvestri M, Kutt H: Sustained enteral administration of levodopa increases and interrupted infusion decreases levodopa dose requirements. Neurology 1990; 40:995–997.
12. Cedarbaum JM, Troy L, Silvestri M, et al: Rehabilitation programs in the management of patients with Parkinson's disease. J Neurol Rehabil 1992; 6:7–19.
13. Comella CL, Stebbins GT, Brown-Toms N, et al: Physical therapy and Parkinson's disease: A controlled clinical trial. Neurology 1994; 44:376–378.
14. Critchley EMR: Speech disorders of Parkinsonism: A review. J Neurol Neurosurg Psychiatry 1984; 47:751–758.
15. Ellgring H, Seiler S, Perleth B, et al: Psychosocial aspects of Parkinson's disease. Neurology 1993; 43(suppl 6):S41–S44.
16. Fahn S, Elton RI: Unified Parkinson's Disease Rating Scale. In Fahn S, Marsden CD, Calne D, Goldstein M (eds): Recent Developments

in Parkinson's Disease, vol 2. Florham Park, NJ, Macmillan, 1987, pp 153–163.

17. Fearnley JM, Lees AJ: Ageing and Parkinson's disease. Substantia nigra regional selectivity. Brain 1991; 114:2283–2301.

18. Franklin S, Cohout LJ, Stern GM, et al: Physical therapy. *In* Rose F, Capildeo R (eds): Research Progress in Parkinson's Disease. London, Pitman, 1981, pp 397–400.

19. Gentile AM: Skill acquisition: Action, movement, and neuromotor processes. *In* Carr JH, Shepart RB (eds): Movement Science for Physical Therapy in Rehabilitation. Rockville, Md, Aspen, 1987, pp 1–30.

20. Gersten JW, Marshall C, Dillon T, et al: External work of walking and functional capacity in Parkinsonian patients treated with L-dopa. Arch Phys Med Rehabil 1972; 53:547–553.

21. Gibbard FB, Page NGR, Spencer KM, et al: Controlled trial of physiotherapy and occupational therapy for Parkinson's disease. Br Med J 1981; 282:1196.

22. Helm N: Management of palilalia with a pacing board. J Speech Hear Disord 1979; 44:350–353.

23. Homberg V: Motor training in the therapy of Parkinson's disease. Neurology 1993; 43(suppl 6):S45–S46.

24. Hurko O: Hereditary cerebellar ataxia. *In* Johnson, RT, Griffin SW (eds): Current Therapy in Neurologic Disease. St Louis, Mosby–Year Book, 1993, pp 254–261.

25. Hurwitz A: The benefits of a home exercise regimen for ambulatory patients with Parkinson's Disease. J Neurosci Nurs 1989; 21:180–184.

26. Jankovic J: Theories on the etiology and pathogenesis of Parkinson's disease. Neurology 1993; 43(suppl 1):S121–S123.

27. Jankovic J, Shoulson I, Werner WJ: Early stage Parkinson's disease: To treat or not to treat. Neurology 1994; 44(suppl 1):S4–S5.

28. Landin S, Hagenfeldt L, Saltin B, et al: Muscle metabolism during exercise in patients with Parkinson's disease. Clin Sci Mol Med 1974; 47:493–506.

29. Levin BE. Llabre MM, Weiner WJ: Cognitive impairments associated with early Parkinson's disease. Neurology 1989; 39:557.

30. ManKovskij N, Karaban I, Mialovickaig AD: Aging and its relation to Parkinsonism. Neurology 1993; 43(suppl 1):29.

31. Mayeux R, Stern Y, Cote L, et al: Altered serotonin metabolism in depressed patients with Parkinson's disease. Neurology 1984; 34:642.

32. McDowell FH, Cedarbaum JM: The extrapyramidal system and disorders of movement. *In* Joynt R (ed): Clinical Neurology. Philadelphia, JB Lippincott, 1991.

33. Mitchel PH, Mertz MA, Catanzaro M-L: Group exercise; A nursing therapy in Parkinson's disease. Rehabil Nurs 1987; 12:242–245.

34. Mortimer JA, Pirozzolo FJ, Hansch EC, et al: Relationship of motor symptoms to intellectual deficits in Parkinson's disease. Neurology 1982; 32:133.

35. Mutch WJ, Strudwick A, Roy SK, et al: Parkinson's disease: Disability, review, and management (medical practice). Br Med J 1986; 293:675–677.

36. Olanow CW: The early treatment of Parkinson's disease. Neurology 1993; 43(suppl 1):S30–S31.

37. Oyebode LR, Barker WA, Blessed G, et al: Cognitive functioning in Parkinson's disease in relation to prevalence of dementia and psychiatric diagnosis. Br J Psychiatry 1986; 149:720.

38. Palmer SS, Mortimer JA, Webster DD, et al: Exercise therapy for Parkinson's disease. Arch Phys Med Rehabil 1986; 67:741–745.

39. Parker WD, Boyson SJ, Parks JK: Abnormalities of the electron transport chain in idiopathic Parkinson's disease. Ann Neurol 1989; 26:719–723.

40. The Parkinson Study Group: Effect of deprenyl on the progression of disability in early Parkinson's disease. N Engl J Med 1989; 321:1364–1371.

41. Perry EK, Curtis M, Dick DJ, et al: Cholinergic correlates of cognitive impairment in Parkinson's disease: Comparisons with Alzheimer's disease. J Neurol Neurosurg Psychiatry 1985; 48:413.

42. Poewe E: Clinical and pathophysiologic aspects of late levodopa failure. Neurology 1993; 43(suppl 6):S28–S30.

43. Robertson S, Thomson F: A study of the efficacy and long term effects of intensive treatment. Br J Disord Commun 1984; 19:213–224.

44. Sage JI, Trooskin S, Sonsalla PK, et al: Long-term duodenal infusion of levodopa for motor fluctuations in parkinsonism. Ann Neurol 1988; 24:87–89.

45. Saltin B, Landin S: Work capacity, muscle strength and SDH activity in both legs of hemiparetic patients and patients with Parkinson's disease. Scand J Clin Lab Invest 1975; 35:531–538.

46. Sarno MT: Speech impairment in Parkinson's disease. Arch Phys Med Rehabil 1968; 49:269.

47. Scatton B, Javoy-Agid F, Fouquier L, et al: Reduction of cortical dopamine, noradrenaline, serotonin and their metabolites in Parkinson's disease. Brain Res 1983; 275:321.

48. Schapira AHV, Cooper JM, Dexter D, et al: Mitochondrial complex I deficiency in Parkinson's disease. Lancet 1989; 1:1269.

49. Schenkman M, Butler RB: A model for multisystem evaluation treatment of individuals with Parkinson's disease. Phys Ther 1989; 69:932–943.

50. Schenkman M, Donovan J, Tsubota J, et al: Management of individuals with Parkinson's disease: Rationale and case studies. Phys Ther 1989; 69:944–955.

51. Scott S, Caird FI: The response of the apparent receptive speech disorder of Parkinson's disease to speech therapy. J Neurol Neurosurg Psychiatry 1984; 47:302–304.

52. Scott S, Caird FI: Speech therapy for Parkinson's disease. J Neurol Neurosurg Psychiatry 1983; 46:140–144.

53. Stern MB: Parkinson's disease. *In* Johnson RT, Griffin (eds): Current Therapy in Neurologic Disease, ed 4. St Louis, Mosby–Year Book, 1993, pp 242–246.

54. Stern PH, McDowell FH, Miller JM, et al: Levodopa and physical therapy in treatment of patients with Parkinson's disease. Arch Phys Med Rehabil 1970; 51:273–277.

55. Szekely BC, Kosanovich NN, Sheppard W: Adjunctive treatment in Parkinson's disease: Physical therapy and comprehensive group therapy. Rehabil Lit 1982; 43:72–76.

56. Tetrud JW, Langston JW: The effect of deprenyl (selegiline) on the natural history of Parkinson's disease. Science 1989; 245:519–522.

57. Weiner WJ, Singer C: Parkinson's disease and nonpharmacologic treatment programs. J Am Geriatr Soc 1989; 37:359–363.

Rehabilitation of Persons With Multiple Sclerosis

RONALD S. TAYLOR, M.D.

Multiple sclerosis (MS) is an inflammatory disease of the central nervous system (CNS) that is characterized by areas of demyelination. It is the third most common cause of disabling illness in persons between the ages of 15 and 50 years.[37] More than 10,000 scientific articles about this entity have been published, but the exact cause remains uncertain and the pathogenesis remains profoundly debatable. Evidence supports, but does not substantiate, that it is an illness of viral exposure at the time of puberty, affecting persons with a genetically determined defect in their immune system. Functional and cognitive impairments develop in the majority of patients, with frequent involvement of gait, coordination, and bladder and sexual function. The full utilization of the rehabilitation team is critical to minimize the patient's level of disability.

EPIDEMIOLOGY

The geographical distribution of multiple sclerosis was first noted by Charcot.[13] The incidence of the disease, as well as the death rate, increases from south to north. Incidence rates are determined by where a person lives prior to the age of 15 years and are not affected by geographical changes beyond that age.[68] Studies from Olmstead County in Minnesota indicate an incidence of 171/100,000 with females accounting for approximately 70% of cases.[68] The average age at onset is 32.4 years for females, 34.3 for males.[68] The incidence of MS appears stable with the apparently increased number of cases explained by improved diagnostic techniques.

Human lymphocyte antigen (HLA) linkages to MS have been noted, but vary with different populations. In northern Europeans, MS is associated with HLA-A3, -B7, -DW2, and -DR2, which are found in 70% of patients with MS and in only 25% of controls. There appears to be a genetic increase in MS but no true mendelian pattern of inheritance has been detected. No increase has been noted with consanguinity, as would be expected in a recessive pattern of inheritance. Rarely has MS been diagnosed in three consecutive generations, as would be expected if the disease were an autosomal dominant disorder. In twin studies, concordance rates are 26% for monozygotic twins and 2.3% for dizygotic twins.[39, 40] Owing to its pleomorphic nature, MS can be confused with many other illnesses. A partial list of differential diagnoses is provided in Table 52–1.

LABORATORY AND IMAGING STUDIES

Cerebrospinal Fluid

No cerebrospinal fluid (CSF) abnormalities are specific for MS. CSF protein is elevated in approximately one fourth of patients during exacerbations.[25] Sixty percent to 75% of patients with MS have an increase in gamma globulin which is synthesized in the CNS.[65] The ratio of IgG to albumin in the CSF, divided by the ratio of these two factors in the serum, often provides a more sensitive index; a value of greater than 0.77 is found in 80% to 90% of patients with MS.[60] The oligoclonal nature of IgG in the CSF in patients with MS was demonstrated more than two decades ago with these bands demonstrated on agar gel electrophoresis. The spinal fluid of patients with definite MS shows abnormalities by this technique in 90% of cases.[35]

Magnetic Resonance Imaging

Magnetic resonance imaging (MRI) studies are the preferred imaging tool to assist in the diagnosis of MS. Typical abnormalities are seen in the supratentorial white matter, especially in periventricular regions (Fig. 52–1). The presence of three to four lesions greater than 3 mm in diameter is considered to be highly suspicious for MS.[32] Changes in the cervical spine, cerebellum, or brainstem are less com-

TABLE 52–1   Differential Diagnosis in Multiple Sclerosis (MS)

Disease	Clinical Features
SLE	37%–42% with SLE present with neurological deficits; ANA(+) in 25% of MS patients
Sjögren's syndrome	Patients may have CNS symptoms including relapsing and remitting course, cerebellar findings, or internuclear ophthalmoplegia
AIDS	Often associated with progressive spastic paraparesis and sensory ataxia
Tropical spastic paraparesis	Sensory changes with pain in legs and neurogenic bladder, caused by HTLV-1
Sarcoidosis	CNS involvement in 5%
Lyme disease	Neurological changes may be relapsing and remitting with extremity and cranial involvement, oligoclonal bands in CSF; serological testing is helpful in differential diagnosis
Cerebrovascular occlusive disease	Scattered lesions secondary to cardiac source of emboli may be confused
Remote effects of carcinoma	May have associated peripheral neuropathy; usually older patients with rapid downhill course
Diseases with single lesions and relapsing course	Glioma, meningioma, arteriovenous malformation
Cervical spondylotic myelopathy	Usually older population with more pain and less bladder involvement; fasciculations
Vestibular neuronitis	May be indistinguishable from attack of MS; may have abnormal vestibular tests
Nonorganic symptoms	Often lasts < 24 hr; dizziness without true vertigo; lack of correlating neurological abnormality

Abbreviations: *SLE*, systemic lupus erythematosus; *ANA*, antinuclear antibodies; *CNS*, central nervous system; *AIDS*, acquired immunodeficiency syndrome; *HTLV-1*, human T-cell lymphotropic virus type I; *CSF*, cerebrospinal fluid.

mon. The addition of gadolinium is helpful in detecting changes in the blood-brain barrier and thus imaging plaques in the early stage of their formation. In definite MS, MRIs are found to be positive in 70% to 95% of patients but frequently do not correlate with clinical findings, disability, or response to steroid therapy.[58] MRI is especially useful in patients suspected of having MS, with abnormalities being detected in 65% to 87% of patients.[19, 52] Although MRI appears more sensitive than evoked potentials in diagnosing MS, in some cases the evoked potentials are positive when the MRI is negative.[60]

PATHOPHYSIOLOGY

Postmortem studies on patients with MS reveal areas of demyelination with relative preservation of axons. There is also gliosis, a disappearance of oligodendrocytes, and inflammation.[63] These abnormal areas are called plaques and are found only in the CNS. They are irregular and can often be seen by the naked eye. They can occur anywhere in the CNS but have a predilection for the optic nerve, the perivenous areas, and the periventricular white matter of the cerebrum, brainstem, and spinal cord.[52]

These changes were first noted more than 100 years ago by Charcot.[13] More recently, MRI studies have shed light on the dynamic aspects of the MS process. The earliest abnormality typically detected is a localized breakdown in the blood-brain barrier. Such breakdown is seen as an area of enhancement on gadolinium MRI studies and can precede the onset of neurological deficits.[63] In pathological studies the endothelial cells of the blood-brain barrier may contain abnormal vesicles. Immune cells may be detected in the surrounding brain parenchyma. The area of abnormality increases in size over an average of 6 weeks and eventually decreases to the size of the original enhancing lesion.[40] Six percent to 20% of the lesions disappear completely.[40] The decrease in size of the lesions is believed to be due to resolution of brain edema.[40] Serial MRIs on 12 patients with chronic progressive MS over a 6-month period found 109 new lesions.[58] Eighty-seven percent of these were found to enhance on MRI but only 17% actually led to clinically detectable changes.[35] Only about 20% of the chronic lesions enhance with gadolinium. The extracellular spaces within the lesions are markedly narrowed.[16]

Demyelination is the hallmark of MS but it remains unknown if it precedes or follows the changes in the blood-brain barrier discussed previously. Signs of remyelination have been noted, but appear to take place predominantly in the early part of the illness.

Immunoregulation

Recent clinical data indicate that MS could be an autoimmune disease triggered by an infectious agent. These findings are supported by an increase in CNS gamma globulin with oligoclonal IgG production, perivenular lymphocytes in the CNS, abnormal cellular immune responses, and CNS autoantibodies against certain neuroviruses found in patients with MS.[34, 57] Abnormalities of T lymphocytes have been documented in MS patients since the early 1970s,[51] and a study by Reinherz and colleagues[51] detected a selective decrease in T5-positive suppressor cells in 11 of 15 patients with active MS but in only 1 of 18 patients with inactive MS. IgG has been shown to be increased in the spinal fluid of patients with MS. This resolves into a series of oligoclonal bands when analyzed electrophoretically.[40] These bands represent antibody from B lymphocytes, but as of yet the specific antigen to which they are directed is unknown. Various studies have implicated measles, rubella, or even "nonsense antibody" as their trigger.[52] Further theories indicate that these cells "may have escaped" more normal regulation and are synthesizing antibodies on their own.[41]

A theory for the abnormal immune reaction in MS is provided in Table 52–2. T cells are believed to attach to endothelial cells in brain capillaries that have been exposed to cytokines such as interferon-γ (INF-γ) and tumor necrosis factor.[8] The T cells cross the blood-brain barrier and enter the CNS where they attach to specific antigens in the cleft of the HLA molecule. They then release tumor necrosis factor, lymphotoxin, and INF-γ, all of which destroy

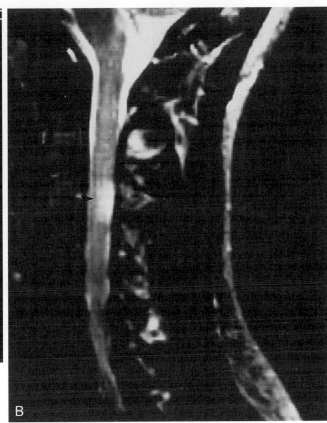

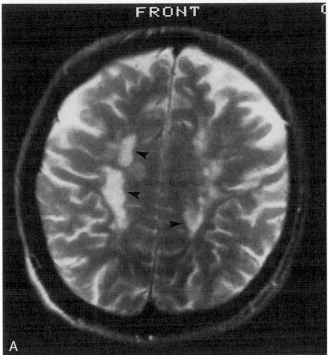

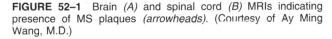

FIGURE 52–1 Brain *(A)* and spinal cord *(B)* MRIs indicating presence of MS plaques *(arrowheads)*. (Courtesy of Ay Ming Wang, M.D.)

myelin. Cytokines are also released. They activate B cells to make antibodies directed not only at myelin but also toward oligodendrocytes. INF-γ also activates macrophages with a resultant direct toxic effect on the myelin. Research is currently being directed at interrupting this process to possibly find a cure for MS.[8]

It is interesting to speculate on the exact role of INF-γ, as clinical trials have shown it to exacerbate the symptoms of MS. INF-γ is known to be increased in the presence of estrogen, which could explain the female preponderance of MS cases.[22] The recent success of using INF-β in MS patients was based on its known anti-INF-γ capabilities.[25] Trials are also under way to specifically decrease the cells implicated in the autoimmune reaction as well as to use various monoclonal antibodies to interrupt the inflamma-

tory process. Attempts at inducing tolerance to myelin proteins by administering oral myelin might also prove beneficial.

SIGNS AND SYMPTOMS

The initial signs and symptoms of MS are quite variable. A general composite of the findings is provided in Tables 52–3 and 52–4. Fifty percent of patients have symptoms related to one site or system and 40% present with weakness.[27] Optic neuritis is present at the onset in 20% to 48% of patients.[43] Signs and symptoms during the course of this illness vary significantly depending on which patients are included in the study. If studies are confined to patients who have died, all patients have had ocular symptoms and 93% have complained of weakness at one time in their illness. Table 52–5 provides a general summary of signs

TABLE 52–2   Immune Theory for the Basis of Multiple Sclerosis

Action	Effect
T cells release cytokines, damaging endothelial cells	Cause defects in blood-brain barrier
T cells attach to HLA receptor on myelin, releasing tumor necrosis factor and interferon-γ	Destroy myelin sheaths
T cells attach to HLA receptor on macrophages	Macrophages release tumor necrosis factor, directly attacking myelin
T cells activate B cells to secrete antibody	Antibody combines with complement to directly attack oligodendrocyte

TABLE 52–3   Symptoms Present at Onset of Illness in Definite Multiple Sclerosis

Symptom	Percent
Weakness	40
Paresthesia	30
Gait difficulty	25
Optic neuritis	20
Diplopia	15
Ataxia	10
Disturbed nutrition	10
Vertigo	5

TABLE 52–4   Diagnostic Criteria for Multiple Sclerosis (MS)

POSSIBLE MS
1. History of relapsing and remitting signs without prior documentation
2. Only one site of involvement in CNS by physical examination, laboratory, or imaging studies
3. No other diagnostic explanation

PROBABLE MS
1. Two documented attacks with clinical, laboratory or imaging evidence of at least one lesion
2. One documented attack with clinical, laboratory, or imaging evidence of two separate lesions

DEFINITE MS
Two attacks separated by at least 1 mo with clinical, laboratory, or imaging evidence of at least two lesions

and symptoms seen in definite MS. Weakness is often accompanied by an increase in muscle stretch reflexes and is one of the more frequent symptoms found in patients with MS. The distribution of the weakness is most commonly in both lower extremities, the next most common being one leg, or one leg and the ipsilateral arm. Weakness confined to one or both upper extremities is unusual.[38] Paresthesias can be present at any stage of the disease and often are described as painful. True radicular pain is unusual, and other causes should be sought when this occurs. Cerebellar signs increase with the course of the disease and often lead to marked disability.[38] The general course in MS is variable but falls into a quiescent course with one or two episodes, followed by long periods of remission, a relapsing and remitting course, or a chronic progressive course.

DIAGNOSIS AND COURSE

Owing to the pleomorphic aspects of MS, the diagnosis is dependent on the skilled clinician's recognition of signs

TABLE 52–5   Signs and Symptoms During the Course of Multiple Sclerosis

Signs and Symptoms	Percent
Paresthesias	100
Weakness	100
Abnormal reflexes	80
Cerebellar signs	80
Spasticity	75
Fatigue	75
Decreased alternating movements	70
Heat intolerance	60
Nystagmus	50
Intellectual loss	40
Impotence	40
Lhermitte's sign	40
Pain	30
Depression	30
Muscle wasting	20
Dementia	10
Facial weakness	3
Unilateral hearing loss	3
Epilepsy	2
Visual failure	1
Trigeminal neuralgia	1

TABLE 52–6   Factors Associated With an Increase in Multiple Sclerosis (MS) Exacerbations

Factors	Evidence
Infectious agents	Faroe Islands epidemic—increase in measles antibodies in CSF of MS patients; seasonal fluctuations; increased number of exacerbations after infections
Pregnancy	Increased risk for 3–6 mo postpartum
Fatigue and heat	Can cause transient weakness; unlikely to cause actual exacerbation
Stress	Unproven—medicolegal implications
Trauma	Very controversial; described in 5%–15% of cases; generally believed to be unrelated
Heavy metals	Reported after exposure to zinc (unproven)
Diet	Remains unproven; attempted diets include low fat, gluten-free; megavitamins
Other autoimmune diseases	No clear linkage seen

of demyelination. Visual, gait, and sensory symptoms are the most common presentations at the onset of the disease. Diagnostic criteria for MS were established by Poser and co-workers[49] and are included in Table 52–3. In this schema an attack is defined as a neurological deficit lasting for more than 24 hours. Sixty-three percent to 91% of patients begin their MS with a relapsing and remitting course, with a majority of the exacerbations occurring in the first 5 to 10 years of the illness.[35] Many patients become stable or progress only slowly after this point.[45] Chronic progressive MS is more likely to occur in patients whose onset occurs after the age of 40.[25] Many patients have a long latent period with minimal symptoms of progression. It is not clear if the disease is active during these periods. Factors associated with an increase in MS exacerbations are listed in Table 52–6.

The course of MS is extremely variable, ranging from death within 5 years in 5% of patients to many cases that are manifested by only one episode.[35] In some cases MS can be diagnosed only postmortem.[23] A decrease in life expectancy of 9½ years in men and 14 years in women has been reported, but this is skewed by the rapid downhill course of a small percentage of patients. In the remainder of the MS population, life expectancy is not significantly affected.[33] Severe disability is noted in 10% of patients within 5 years, in 25% of patients within 10 years, and in 50% of patients within 18 years.[39, 62] Studies indicate that approximately 20% of patients have no disability after 15 years of having MS.[39, 62] Annual relapse rates in MS vary in different studies, ranging from 0.1 exacerbations per year to 1.15.[60] None of these indicators are absolute and at best can be used only as general predictors. Factors associated with poor prognosis in MS are listed in Table 52–7.[39]

Cranial Nerve Involvement

Optic neuritis is more common early in the illness.[35] It is usually associated with pain in the eye or forehead, which can occasionally be severe. The visual field defect

TABLE 52–7   Factors Indicative of a Poor Prognosis

Progressive course at onset
Male sex
Age at onset >40 yr
Cerebellar involvement at onset
Multiple system involvement at onset

---

is a central scotoma. Bilateral simultaneous optic neuritis is not unusual and is especially common in patients of Japanese descent.[35]

Trigeminal neuralgia is present in 1% of patients.[33] It may be bilateral and often is the presenting symptom. Facial palsy can be seen and facial myokymia manifested by rapidly firing muscular contractions of the facial muscles is not unusual.[33] Vertigo is common and can be severe and associated with vomiting. This can be the only initial symptom in patients with MS but is almost always reversible.

Epilepsy

Epilepsy occurs in 1% to 2% of patients with MS (which may be no more common than that seen in the general population). Tonic seizures are the most common seizures seen in MS. They are often triggered by movement. They generally involve one arm or leg. They typically last for a few seconds, although they can occur many times during the day. Other paroxysmal symptoms lasting for less than 1 to 2 min include dysarthria, ataxia, itching, and focal pain.[33]

Pain

Pain in MS occurs in up to 50% of patients.[33, 53] Ninety percent of the time it is chronic and consists of dysesthetic extremity pain, chronic back pain, or painful leg cramps.[33, 57] The dysesthetic pain is the most common and also the most difficult to treat. Acute pain most frequently takes the form of trigeminal neuralgia or transient dysesthetic extremity pain.[50]

Evoked Potentials

Evoked potentials are useful in the diagnosis of MS for their ability to measure altered conduction time in CNS myelinated pathways. Their primary diagnostic application lies in providing evidence of demyelination in clinically normal pathways, thus aiding in the establishment of multiple sites of CNS involvement. Visual evoked potentials (VEPs) are abnormal in 75% of patients with definite MS and in 15% to 60% of patients with possible MS. Subclinical abnormalities are detected in 20% to 30% of cases.[2] Brainstem auditory evoked potentials (BAEPs) are also useful, with abnormalities of 67% in definite MS, 41% in probable, and 30% in possible MS. Subclinical abnormalities are detected 21% to 55% of the time.[45] Similar values are noted for somatosensory evoked potentials (SSEPs) with higher rates of abnormality found in the lower extremities than in the upper extremities.[12]

DIFFERENTIAL DIAGNOSIS

The differential diagnosis of MS encompasses many entities, some of which are listed in Table 52–1. Care should be taken in making the diagnosis of MS in the absence of eye findings, during the presence of clinical remission, or in the presence of localized or atypical clinical features.

TREATMENT

Because of the variable presentations, the treatment of MS patients must be individualized. Basic treatments can be divided into symptomatic therapies, and those that are designed to affect the natural course of the disease or to alter the length and severity of individual exacerbations. A sample of drug treatments is listed in Table 52–8. It is important to recognize and convey to the patient with MS that relapse rates decrease as the disease progresses, with the vast majority of relapses occurring in the first 5 to 10 years after the onset of initial symptoms.[34]

Neurological Assessment of Treatment

Treatment results in MS must be based on the objective and subjective complaints of each patient, because objective findings with imaging techniques, evoked potentials, and morbid anatomy do not always correlate with the clinical presentation. Many measurement devices have been proposed to measure this other than the simple clinical examination.[35] The most commonly used is the Kurtzke Disability Status Scale in either its original[34] or expanded[33] form (Tables 52–9 and 52–10, respectively).

Treatment Designed to Alter the Course of Multiple Sclerosis

Steroids

Since 1970 the role of adrenocorticotropic hormone (ACTH) in decreasing the length and severity of exacerbations has been documented in many articles.[11] The mechanism of action is unknown, but might relate to a decrease in CNS edema or to an effect on the immune system. Oral or intravenous steroids have been used more recently with similar results. Oral prednisone, in a dose of 60 to 100 mg in tapering doses over 1 to 3 weeks, is frequently used for the treatment of a documented exacerbation of MS.[53] Care should be taken that concomitant infections are treated prior to the institution of steroid treatments. If the exacerbation does not respond or is severe, intravenous doses of methylprednisolone 500 to 1000 mg given daily for 3 to 7 days are recommended. This should be given over 2 to 3 hours to minimize the possibility of cardiac arrhythmias.[1, 26] Studies indicate that large doses of methylprednisolone change the C9 and C8 T cell indices as well as abnormal IgG levels found in the CSF of MS patients during an exacerbation. These spinal fluid effects have not been noted with lower oral doses.[15, 64]

There is no definite measure of what constitutes an exacerbation of MS or when steroid treatment should be utilized. The clinician has to make this decision based on the patient's specific pattern of MS, previous response to steroids, and overall condition. I consider an exacerbation to occur when the patient experiences a neurological change resulting in a decrease in functional capacity that

TABLE 52–8　Medications for Multiple Sclerosis

Medication	Dosage	Effects
Prednisone	80–100 mg tapered over 7–21 days	Decreases length and severity of exacerbation
ACTH	40 units bid × 7 days	
Methylprednisolone	1000 mg IV over 2–4 hr, daily × 7, followed by 7–21 days, taper of oral steroids	
Interferon-β	8 million units sq qod	Decreases number of exacerbations
Copolymer 1	Experimental: 1–12 g/wk	Decreases number of exacerbations
Cyclophosphamide with or without ACTH	1–2 wk	Slows progression of chronic MS
Azathioprine	100–150 mL/day	Slows progression of chronic MS
Cyclosporine	Limited by nephrotoxicity	Slows progression of chronic MS
Amantadine	200–300 mL/day	Decreases fatigue
Pemoline	18.75 mg	Decreases PM fatigue
Baclofen	20–120 mg	Decreases spasticity
Dantrolene	75–250 mg	Decreases spasticity
Diazepam	5–40 mg	Decreases spasticity
Carbamazepine	200 mg bid or tid	Decreases pain and parenchymal spasms
Phenytoin	200–400 mg 1 day	Decreases pain and parenchymal spasms
Clonazepam	1–6 mg/day	Decreases ataxia
Isoniazid	900 mg/day	Decreases ataxia

lasts for more than 24 hours. Steroids can safely be administered two to three times per year. The patient must understand that although the length and severity of exacerbations can be affected by these treatments, the number of exacerbations and the ultimate course of the illness is in no way modified.[53]

TABLE 52–9　Kurtzke Disability Status Scale (DSS)

0	Normal neurological examination (all grade 0 in functional systems*)
1	No disability and minimal signs such as Babinski's sign or vibratory decrease (grade 1 in functional systems)
2	Minimal disability, e.g., slight weakness or mild gait, sensory, visuomotor disturbance (one or two functional systems, grade 2)
3	Moderate disability though fully ambulatory, e.g., monoparesis, moderate ataxia, or combinations of lesser dysfunctions (one or two functional systems, grade 3, or several, grade 2)
4	Relatively severe disability though fully ambulatory and able to be self-sufficient and up and about for some 12 hr a day (one functional system, grade 4, or several, grade 3 or less)
5	Disability severe enough to preclude ability to work a full day without special provisions; maximal motor function: walking unaided no more than several blocks (one functional system, grade 5 alone, or combination of lesser grades)
6	Assistance (canes, crutches, braces) required for walking (combinations with more than one system, grade 3 or worse)
7	Restricted to wheelchair but able to wheel self and enter and leave chair alone (combinations with more than one system, grade 4 or worse; very rarely pyramidal system, grade 5 alone)
8	Restricted to bed but with effective use of arms (combinations usually grade 4 or above in several functional systems)
9	Totally helpless bedridden patients (combinations usually grade 4 or above in most functional systems)
10	Death due to multiple sclerosis

*Excludes cerebral function grade 1.
From Kurtzke JF: Rating neurologic impairment in multiple sclerosis: An Expanded Disabilities Status Scale (EDSS). Neurology 1983; 33:1444–1453.

The use of steroids in the treatment of chronic progressive MS has not been shown to be effective. Drug management for this entity remains controversial and unsatisfactory. Cyclophosphamide with or without ACTH has been shown to be beneficial by Howser, Carter, Goodkin, and others. Resultant slowing of the illness in approximately 30% to 60% of patients was reported.[10] However, others have been unable to duplicate these findings.

Immunosuppressive Agents

Other attempts at immunosuppression in chronic MS include the use of azathioprine[47, 56, 61] and more recently, cyclosporine.[42] Cyclosporine has been shown to delay the time of becoming wheelchair-dependent in patients with chronic progressive MS, but nephrotoxicity has limited its usefulness.[43] Plasmapheresis has also been used in addition to these medications, with mixed results.[26, 30] Ongoing studies of the use of these treatments are currently under way.

Interferon

Initial studies with IFN-γ,[46] a lymphokine acting as an immune enhancer, actually led to an increase in severity of MS. Studies with interferon alpha-2 showed no effect in MS,[9, 31] while a trial of intrathecal IFN-β demonstrated a decrease in exacerbation rates for periods of up to 4 years.[28] These studies led to the recent multicenter double blind prospective trial of interferon beta-1b in 372 patients. Interferon beta-1b, when given subcutaneously every other day, was found to decrease the number of exacerbations in patients with relapsing and remitting MS by one third, with a 50% decrease in severe exacerbations.[50]

The mechanism of action of interferon beta-1b is not clear, but interferons as a class are known to interfere with viral replication. IFN-β also inhibits the production of IFN-γ, thus altering the known tendency of this substance to exacerbate the symptoms of MS. Other potential mechanisms of action include the inhibition of tumor necrosis factor, a protein synthesized by macrophages and known to damage myelin. IFN-β also has an ability in vitro to

TABLE 52–10 Kurtzke Expanded Disability Status Scale (EDSS)

0	Normal neurological examination (all grade 0 in FS*)
1.0	No disability, minimal signs in one FS (i.e., grade 1)
1.5	No disability, minimal signs in more than one FS* (more than one FS grade 1)
2.0	Minimal disability in one FS (one FS grade 2, others 0 or 1)
2.5	Minimal disability in two FS (two FS grade 2, others 0 or 1)
3.0	Moderate disability but with moderate disability in one FS (one grade 3) and one or two FS grade 2; or two FS grade 3; or five FS grade 2 (others 0 or 1)
3.5	Fully ambulatory but with moderate disability in one FS (one grade 3) and one or two FS grade 2, or two FS grade 3; or five FS grade 2 (others 0 or 1)
4.0	Fully ambulatory without aid, self-sufficient, up and about some 12 hr a day despite relatively severe disability consisting of one FS grade 4 (others 0 or 1), or combinations of lesser grades exceeding limits of previous steps; able to walk without aid or rest some 500 m
4.5	Fully ambulatory without aid, up and about much of the day, able to work a full day, may otherwise have some limitation of full activity or require minimal assistance; characterized by relatively severe disability usually consisting of one FS grade 4 (others 0 or 1) or combinations of lesser grades exceeding limits of previous steps; able to walk without aid or rest some 300 m
5.0	Ambulatory without aid or rest for about 200 m; disability severe enough to impair full daily activities (e.g., to work a full day without special provisions) (usual FS equivalents are one grade 5 alone, others 0 or 1; or combinations of lesser grades usually exceeding specifications for step 4.0)
5.5	Ambulatory without aid or rest for about 100 m; disability severe enough to preclude full daily activities; (usual FS equivalents are one grade 5 alone, others 0 or 1; or combination of lesser grades usually exceeding those for step 4.0)
6.0	Intermittent or unilateral constant assistance (cane, crutch, brace) required to walk about 100 m with or without resting (usual FS equivalents are combinations with more than two FS grade 3+)
6.5	Constant bilateral assistance (canes, crutches, braces) required to walk about 20 m without resting (usual FS equivalents are combinations with more than two FS grade 3+)
7.0	Unable to walk beyond approximately 5 m even with aid, essentially restricted to wheelchair; wheels self in standard wheelchair and transfers alone; up and about in wheelchair some 12 hr a day (usual FS equivalents are combinations with more than one FS grade 4+; very rarely pyramidal grade 5 alone)
7.5	Unable to take more than a few steps; restricted to wheelchair; may need aid in transfer; wheels self but cannot carry on in standard wheelchair a full day; may require motorized wheelchair (usual FS equivalents are combinations with more than one FS grade 4+)
8.0	Essentially restricted to bed or chair or perambulated in wheelchair, but may be out of bed itself much of the day; retains many self-care functions; generally has effective use of arms (usual FS equivalents are combinations, generally grade 4+ in several systems)
8.5	Essentially restricted to bed much of day; has some effective use of arm(s); retains some self-care functions; (usual FS equivalents are combinations generally 4+ in several systems)
9.0	Helpless bed patient; can communicate and eat (usual FS equivalents are combinations, mostly grade 4+)
9.5	Totally helpless bed patient; unable to communicate effectively or eat/swallow (usual FS equivalents are combinations, almost all grade 4+)
10.0	Death due to multiple sclerosis

*Excludes functional system (FS) grade 1.
From Kurtzke JF: Rating neurologic impairment in multiple sclerosis: An Expanded Disabilities Status Scale (EDSS) Neurology 1983; 33:1444–1453.

increase T suppressor cells, which are known to be decreased in MS patients during exacerbations.[3] IFN-β is the first treatment shown to be useful in affecting the course of MS and thus represents a true breakthrough in therapy.

4-Aminopyridine (4-AP) has been shown to block potassium channel activation in animals, thus prolonging the duration of nerve action potentials and restoring conduction in previously blocked demyelinated fibers.[55] VonDiemen and colleagues[67] treated 70 patients with relapsing and remitting MS with intravenous and oral 4-AP and placebo. Subjective improvement (defined as improvement in ADL capabilities) was noted in 29% of the patients taking the medication and in only 1.6% of those on placebo. Sixteen percent of patients showed at least a 1-point change in the Kurtkze disability scales.[67] Those patients with the most severe illness noted the primary benefit from this medication.[67] Unfortunately, clinical use of 4-AP has been delayed because of significant side effects, primarily seizures, manifested in subsequent clinical trials.[54]

Symptomatic Treatment

Because MS affects all phases of the patient's life, the skills of the entire rehabilitation team are needed to minimize this disability. Patients with MS frequently present with problems in gait, sexuality, driving, shopping, cleaning house, urinary function, and socioeconomic stability. All of these factors lend themselves to intervention by the rehabilitation team. Providing assistance in these areas is extremely beneficial to the individual and the family and is critical to the maintenance of maximal function.

Weakness

Because weakness is often a significant problem in MS, it is important that general conditioning be maintained as long as possible. This has to be done in a way that does not increase fatigue or body temperature. Because elevated body temperature can worsen MS symptoms, it is imperative that these patients have air conditioning in their homes and cars, especially if they live in southern climates. They might even consider moving to a more temperate zone to alleviate these problems. An individualized program instituted by a physician or physical therapist should be developed and adapted to any ongoing changes in the patient's disease process.[18] The use of air-resistance stationary bikes to minimize temperature fluctuation, cool therapeutic pools (84 °F [29 °C] or less), and upper extremity ergometers have proved to be beneficial in maintaining general aerobic conditioning. If patients want to do additional exercises, the use of full lightweight progressive resistance exercises as physically tolerated is beneficial. The use of weights, although often beneficial, is often not feasible, especially if the patient's primary disability relates to ataxia and not to weakness. Prior to embarking on any exercise program a submaximal cardiovascular stress test to determine cardiac safety and an appropriate level of exercise intensity is beneficial. Maintaining optimal function of the musculoskeletal system is certainly beneficial in minimizing the disability associated with MS. However, not to be overlooked is the significant psychological benefit and increase in overall self-esteem gained from participating in a "can do" program.

Fatigue

The physician dealing with the patient with MS should be aware of the role fatigue plays in the disability. The actual source of the fatigue is not well understood, but might result from a combination of weakness, spasticity, ataxia, depression, and heat.[28] The Social Security Administration has recognized the disabling aspects of fatigue and has allowed this to be considered as a major factor in the granting of disability benefits to persons with MS. Patients with characteristic afternoon fatigue might benefit from pemoline, 18.75 mg/day. Owing to the medication's stimulant and abusive potential, care should be taken to monitor the patient's response. The rationale for the low dose of this stimulant medication providing dramatic relief of fatigue is not clearly understood, but might relate to a change in neurotransmitters in the area of the brain from which the fatigue emanates. In my experience, this drug has one of the highest patient acceptance rates of all medications used in the symptomatic treatment of MS. Amantadine (Symmetrel), in doses of 200 to 300 mg/day, has also been documented to be useful.[14]

Mobility

Mobility problems are among the most common complaints of patients with MS. In a National Multiple Sclerosis Society survey, 60% of 122,000 patients reported the need for some assistance with mobility.[5] Maintaining mobility and functional independence is a constant challenge to the rehabilitation team, because of the ever-changing clinical picture. Appropriate assistive devices should be prescribed to increase safety and decrease energy expenditure. Careful attention should be paid to psychological changes triggered by the need for these devices and the resultant implication that the disease is progressing. The experienced MS practitioner is constantly aware of these "crisis points" in the course of the patient's illness and deals with them on an individual basis, initiating the medical and psychosocial interventions that are indicated. Patients should be informed that, on average, persons with MS are still walking 27 years after diagnosis.[44] Proper prescription and instruction in the use of a wheelchair often prolongs and increases the patient's functional independence. Motorized three-wheeled scooters are frequently preferred by the patient with MS because of a perception of greater societal acceptance. Care should be taken to ensure that the patient does not lose remaining functional ambulation by becoming overly dependent on these aids

(see Chapter 19). They should be used initially for long distances and difficult tasks, with the patient continuing to ambulate on his or her own when doing less stressful activities.

Activities of Daily Living

Various activities of daily living are often affected in patients with MS. Brainstem lesions can result in dysphagia for both liquids and solids. This can be evaluated by videofluoroscopy and treated by dietary management (see Chapter 27). Problems with balance, mobility, ataxia, spasticity, and weakness frequently lead to difficulty with hygiene, dressing, toileting, and communication. These problems are frequently amenable to the efforts of a rehabilitation team, trained specifically to deal with the unique and variable patterns of MS. Although rehabilitative management is often minimized by the medical community, it is critical to the successful adjustment of patients with MS and their families. Visits by a trained occupational therapist to a patient's home or office for the purpose of recommending ergonomic changes often lead to a marked increase in the patient's quality of life (see Chapter 26).

Vocational and Avocational Activities

Multiple sclerosis affects people in the prime of their lives and often after they have made and developed career choices. One third of patients with MS are able to continue on their regular career path without modification and another one third can continue working with the help of the rehabilitation team and vocational counseling.[18] Employers should be given information on the specific needs of the MS patient, including the elimination of architectural barriers and the role of fatigue in the patient's illness. The patient with MS should be counseled about the Americans With Disabilities Act and efforts required to accommodate the MS patient with disability. For most patients with MS, having to discontinue working can engender great stress and torment. The physician should anticipate and assist patients in this difficult transition.

Various home work situations, volunteer activities, and return to educational pursuits can ease these difficulties. The National Multiple Sclerosis Society is a reliable resource to assist the patient and physician in this regard.

Cognitive and Psychiatric Aspects

Cognitive and psychiatric changes were once thought to be unusual in persons with MS.[33] More recent data indicate that the problems are far more common than previously suspected[48] and frequently contribute substantially to the patient's level of disability. Memory appears to be the function most affected, with conceptual and abstract reasoning diminished to a lesser extent.[48] One study of 108 patients reported mild intellectual deficits in 41% of MS patients, moderate deficits in 14%, and severe defects in 6.5%. Although the severity tends to increase with duration, significant mental impairment can exist even in the presence of otherwise mild MS.[29] Several authors characterize the dementia in MS as being that of a subcortical type marked by impaired manipulation of acquired knowledge, slowness of cognitive process, apathy, and lack of initiative.[33] In the words of VandenBurg this leads to "slowness in acquiring new information from the outside world and in responding to its demands."[66]

Psychiatric changes in MS have been described since the time of Charcot, with euphoria noted in 63% of patients in an early study by Cottrell and Wilson.[17] Recently, an increase in the incidence of depression has been noted that correlates with the degree of neurological impairment but not functional disability, and which is greater than that seen in other neuromuscular illnesses. One study of 108 patients with MS found mild depression in 17%, moderate depression in 7%, and severe depression in 4% of patients.[29, 59] It remains to be clarified whether these psychiatric changes are the result of the MS or a reaction to the illness. This could be of clinical significance, as some patients with MS respond to very low doses of antidepressants and are thought to exhibit depression as a result of plaques in the areas of the brain controlling emotions. Schizophrenia does not appear to be increased in MS compared to the general population, but both frequently have their onset at the same time. The treating physician must be aware of these emotional problems and deal with them aggressively as soon as they are identified.

MRI studies have demonstrated that patients with more severe cognitive impairment typically have more extensive brain lesions, although disagreements exist as to which MRI abnormality best distinguishes cognitively impaired and unimpaired patients.[6]

Neurogenic Bladder

Bladder dysfunction is a frequent complaint in the patient with MS. Early changes include either an increase or decrease in detrusor, bladder neck, or external sphincter control. Later stages of the disease are marked by bladder hyperreflexia and dyssynergia. The evaluation of these problems should include laboratory assessment of general renal function, with several determinations of postvoid residual volumes. Cystometric evaluation with associated electromyographic monitoring of the pelvic floor musculature (see also Chapter 28) is helpful in categorizing bladder dysfunction. The constantly changing nature of the neurological and urological deficit in the patient with MS should be recognized before beginning treatment. A summary of treatments available is given in Table 52–11.

TABLE 52–11   Treatment of Neurogenic Bladder in Multiple Sclerosis

Treatment	Background
Fluid restrictions	2000 mL/day with fluid restrictions after dinner
Intermittent catheterization	If postvoid residuals consistently greater than 100 mL
Trimethoprim-sulfamethoxazole or methenamine	Often used with intermittent catheterization
Medications	Propantheline
	Oxybutynin
	Bethanecol
	Ephedrine
	Prazosin
	Baclofen
Indwelling catheter	

Management of mild neurogenic bladder symptoms should begin with regulation of fluid intake to 1800 mL/24-hour period, limiting intake after dinner. If postvoid residual volumes exceed 100 mL, consideration should be given to a program of intermittent catheterization. Oxybutynin 5 to 20 mg/day can be used for its anticholinergic and direct smooth muscle relaxant activity on the bladder detrusor. Detrusor tone can be increased with the use of bethanechol. α-Adrenergic drugs such as ephedrine can be used to increase bladder tone. α-Adrenergic blocking agents (prazosin or phenoxybenzamine) can decrease bladder neck tone. Baclofen can decrease external sphincter dyssynergia.[18] Antibiotics such as trimethoprim-sulfamethoxazole or methenamine are often used prophylactically in conjunction with intermittent catheterization, but should be avoided when an indwelling catheter is utilized.

Neurogenic Bowel

Bowel incontinence or constipation is often a disconcerting problem for the patient with MS. A bowel program including a high fiber diet, bulk former, stool softener, and adequate fluid intake should be developed with the patient's input early in the course of MS and prior to the development of significant difficulties. The use of laxatives and enemas should be discouraged. If constipation remains a problem, glycerin or bisacodyl (Dulcolax) suppositories taken 45 min after the day's major meal can be useful in maintaining bowel function (see also Chapter 28).

Spasticity

Spasticity is a common problem in the management of the patient with MS. It can interfere with rehabilitation, even when it is not associated with concurrent weakness. Severe forms can be totally disabling. Management options are outlined in Table 52–12 but should always begin with instructing the patient and family in a program of stretching the spastic muscles and putting the involved joints through a full range of motion.[41] Attempts should be made to identify and correct sources of nociceptive input to the CNS, as they can worsen spasticity. Such irritating stimuli can include urinary tract infections, skin ulcers, constipation, deep venous thrombosis, and other irritative conditions. If spasticity remains a problem, carefully monitored use of medications should be instituted. Baclofen is the initial drug of choice when spasticity is of spinal origin, but it is less useful in spasticity of supraspinal etiology. The mechanism of action is both presynaptic and postsyn-

TABLE 52–12   Treatment of Spasticity in Multiple Sclerosis

Identify and correct sources of nociceptive input (bowel, bladder, skin, etc.)
Stretch the involved muscles
Baclofen
Dantrolene
Diazepam
Intrathecal baclofen
Butolinum toxin nerve blocks
Phenol nerve blocks
Tenotomy, rhizotomy
Myelotomy

aptic, and it is less likely to cause weakness and fatigue than either diazepam or dantrolene.[4] Baclofen should initially be given at 10 to 20 mg/day in divided doses, with titration adjusted by clinical response upward to a dose of 80 to 100 mg/day if necessary. Care should be taken that the patient does not abruptly discontinue the medicine, as seizures can result.

Benzodiazepines such as diazepam can be added if spasticity persists. They work at the spinal level but must be used cautiously as they can enhance previously existing fatigue, weakness, depression, and sedation.

In refractory cases, dantrolene may be utilized. Its mechanism of action is peripheral (prevents myofibrillar contraction).[42] Aggravation of previously existing weakness is often a problem. The dose should be gradually increased from 25 to 300 mg/day. Patients taking this medication should have close monitoring of liver enzyme levels. Hepatotoxicity can occur, with the greatest incidence being in female patients older than 35 years.

Other drugs used with varying degrees of success for spasticity include phenytoin, carbamazepine, and phenothiazines. Recent trials have utilized localized botulinum toxin injection for a more specific and reversible treatment of intractable spasticity.[7] In refractory cases phenol nerve blocks can be attempted. The long-term nature of such blocks, as well as the possible side effect of painful paresthesias, limits their usefulness. If spasticity remains a problem, the use of intrathecal baclofen, neurectomy, rhizotomy, tenotomy, or myelotomy may be required.

A detailed discussion of spasticity is presented in Chapter 29.

Sexual Function

In the early stages of MS, varied types of sexual dysfunction can occur, but this is usually transient. As the illness progresses, symptoms typically become more frequent. In a study of 302 patients, 91% of the men and 72% of the women reported changes in their sexual life. Disturbances in erection were noted in 62% of males. Failure to achieve orgasm (33%), loss of libido (27%), and spasticity (12%) were the leading complaints of females.[36] Treatment involves identifying the problem as early as possible and providing appropriate counseling. Localized injections of papaverine or the use of penile implants can be beneficial for erection problems (see also Chapter 30).

Charlatanism

The chronic and variable nature of MS coupled with the lack of a "cure" makes the patient with this illness especially susceptible to quackery. Numerous miracle treatments have been proposed for MS and include calcium products, snake venom, bee pollen, removal of dental amalgams, megavitamins, and hyperbaric oxygen.[46] None of these have been shown to be effective and are often nothing more than a hoax. The physician must be sensitive to the desire of the MS patient to "try anything" and counter these claims with education and the utilization of a full line of the rehabilitation resources available.

Ataxia and Tremor

Ataxia and tremor are especially vexing symptoms in the person with MS as they often do not respond to rehabil-

itative or drug treatment. Light weights attached to the distal aspect of the extremities can decrease the appendicular component of ataxia. If exacerbated by weakness, appropriate strengthening exercises can be beneficial. Repetitive coordinative exercises such as those recommended by Frankel[21] are rarely useful because of the progressive nature of the illness. In patients with extremity ataxia that interferes with dressing or feeding, appropriate proximal splinting can be beneficial. Drug therapy is of limited usefulness. Clonazepam (1–6 mg/day) has been used with and without primidone (250 mg/day) with only slight success and may cause drowsiness. Isoniazid (up to 900 mg/day), used in conjunction with pyridoxine to reduce the resultant peripheral neuropathy, has also been attempted. The mechanism of action of these drugs is unknown and response rates of greater than 10% to 20% are unlikely.[21]

INPATIENT REHABILITATION

With the current cost containment pressures on rehabilitative facilities, patients with MS are often underserved in inpatient rehabilitation. This despite the fact that rehabilitation, especially on an inpatient basis, can enhance the quality of a patient's life, improve functional status, and cut overall healthcare costs.[20] In a study by Greenspan and co-workers,[24] two thirds of patients admitted to the rehabilitation unit were transferred from an acute hospital with the most common problems being mobility and difficulty in activities of daily living. The average length of stay was 27 days, and follow-up at 90 days revealed excellent maintenance of gains made during hospitalization.[24] It would appear in patients whose functional capacities are significantly diminished, especially if they are going to have difficulty in maintaining independent living, that admission to an inpatient rehabilitation unit often provides the skills necessary to avoid placement in a long-term care facility.

RESEARCH DIRECTIVES

Physiatrists are well aware of the efficacy and benefit of rehabilitation techniques for the patient with MS. However, documented outcome studies are critical to ensure future funding for these treatments. The impact on every aspect of life, including family, work, leisure, and physical function mandates that psychosocial and rehabilitation studies become a major source of MS research grants. Funding for such grants is strongly supported by the National Multiple Sclerosis Society, which has in the past 15 years provided $35 million toward research. Research into the development of objective measures to track the course of MS and

TABLE 52–13   Areas for Multiple Sclerosis Research

Immunology
Biology of glial cells
Virology
Therapy
Genetics
Utilization and availability of health services

its response to various therapies is also critically needed. MRI and magnetic resonance spectroscopy might prove useful in better enabling the research team to evaluate the effects of various interventions. Other areas of potential interest to the MS researcher are outlined in Table 52–13.

References

1. Abbruzzese G, Gendolfo C, Loeb C: Bolus methylprednisone versus ACTH in the treatment for multiple sclerosis. J Neurosci 1983; 4:169–172.
2. Aminoff MJ: Electrophysiologic evaluation of patients with multiple sclerosis. Neurol Clin 1985; 3:663–678.
3. Arnason GW: Interferon beta in MS. Neurology 1993; 43:641–643.
4. Basmajin J: Lioresal treatment of spasticity in multiple sclerosis: Further experience with double blurring crossover studies. Am J Phys Med 1975; 54:175–177.
5. Baum HM, Rathschild BB: Multiple sclerosis and mobility restrictions. Arch Phys Med Rehabil 1983; 64:591–596.
6. Beatty WW: Cognitive and emotional disturbances in multiple sclerosis. Neurolog Clin 1993; 11:189–204.
7. Beorg-Stein J, Pine Z, Miller J, et al: Botulinum toxin in the treatment of spasticity in multiple sclerosis: New observations. Am J Phys Med Rehabil 1993; 32:364.
8. Brosnan CF, Selmaj K, Raines CS: A role for tumor necrosis factor in immune mediated demyelination and its relevance to multiple sclerosis. J Neuroimmunol 1988; 18:87–94.
9. Camenga DL, Johnson KP, Alter M, et al: Systemic recombinant alpha 2 interferon therapy in relapsing multiple sclerosis. Arch Neurol 1986; 43:1239–1246.
10. Castor JL, Huflei DA: Immunosuppression with high dose intravenous cyclophosphamide and ACTH in progressive multiple sclerosis: Cumulative six year experience in 164 patients. Neurology 1988; 2(suppl).914.
11. Carter JL, Rodriguez M: Immunosuppressive treatment of multiple sclerosis. Mayo Clin Proc 1989; 64:664–669.
12. Chiappa KH: Pattern shift, brainstem auditory and somatosensory evoked potentials in multiple sclerosis. Ann N Y Acad Sci 1984; 436:315–326.
13. Charcot JM: Lectures on Diseases of the Nervous System, lecture 6. London, The New Sydenham Society, 1877.
14. Cohn RA, Fisher M: Amantadine treatment of fatigue associated with multiple sclerosis. Arch Neurol 1989; 46:667–680.
15. Compston DA, Milligan NM, Hughes PU, et al: A double blind controlled trial of high dose methylprednisolone in patients with multiple sclerosis. J Neurol Neurosurg Psychiatry 1987; 50:517–522.
16. Confavreaux L, Armand G, Devic M: Course and prognosis of multiple sclerosis assessed by computerized data processing of 349 patients. Brain 1980; 103:281–300.
17. Cottrell SS, Wilson SA: The affective symptomatology of disseminated sclerosis: Study of 100 cases. J Neurol Psychother 1926; 7:1–30.
18. Erickson RP, Lie YR, Chiniger MA: Rehabilitation in multiple sclerosis. Mayo Clin Proc 1989; 64:818–828.
19. Esiri MM: Pathology in multiple sclerosis. Clin Neurol 1991; 2:1117–1123.
20. Feigenson JS, Scheinberg L, Catalano M, et al: Cost effectiveness of multiple sclerosis rehabilitation. Neurology 1981; 31:1316–1322.
21. Frankel DI: Multiple sclerosis. In Umphred DA (ed): Neurologic Rehabilitation, ed 2. St. Louis, Mosby–Year Book, 1990, p 545.
22. Freal JE, Kraft GH, Coryell JK: Symptomatic fatigue in multiple sclerosis. Arch Phys Med Rehabil 1984; 65:135–138.
23. Gilfort JJ, Sade RM: Unexpected multiple sclerosis. Arch Neurol 1983; 40:533–536.
24. Greenspan B, Steineman M, Agri R: Multiple sclerosis and rehabilitation outcome. Arch Phys Med Rehabil 1987; 68:434–440.
25. Hart RG, Sherman DO: The diagnosis of multiple sclerosis. JAMA 1982; 247:498–503.
26. House SC, Dawson DM, Lehiech JR, et al: Intensive immunosuppression and progressive multiple sclerosis with randomized 3 arm study of high dose intravenous cyclophosphamide and plasmapheresis, and ACTH. N Engl J Med 1983; 308:173–180.
27. Ivers RR, Goldstein ND: Multiple sclerosis: A current appraisal of symptoms and signs. Mayo Clin Proc 1963; 38:457–466.
28. Jacobs L, Salazar AM, Nerndon R, et al: Multicenter double-blind study of effect of intrathecally administered natural human fibroblast interferon in exacerbations of multiple sclerosis. Lancet 1986; 2:1411–1415.
29. Joffe RT, Lippert GB, Gross TA, et al: Mood disorder and multiple sclerosis. Arch Neurol 1987; 44:376–378.
30. Khatri BO, McQuillen MP, Harrington GS, et al: Chronic progressive multiple sclerosis: Double blind controlled study of plasmapheresis in patients taking immunosuppressive drugs. Neurology 1986; 37:1754–1761.
31. Knobles RC, Panitch HS, Braheny SL: Controlled clinical trial of systemic alpha interferon in multiple sclerosis. Neurology 1984; 34:1273–1279.
32. Kurtzke JF: A new scale for evaluating disabilities in multiple sclerosis. Neurology 1955; 5:580–583.
33. Kurtzke JF: Rating neurologic impairment in multiple sclerosis. An Expanded Disabilities Status Scale (EDSS). Neurology 1983; 33:1444–1453.
34. Kurtzke JF, Beebe GW, Nagel B, et al: Studies on the natural history of multiple sclerosis: Clinical and laboratory findings at first diagnosis. Acta Neurol Scand 1972; 48:19–46.
35. Lowenthal A, Van Sande M, Koucher D: The differential diagnosis of neurological diseases by fractionating electrophoretically the CSF gamma-globulins. J Neurochem 1980; 6:51–56.
36. Lilius H, Valtonen E, Wikstrom J: Sexual problems in patients suffering from multiple sclerosis: J Chron Dis 1976; 29:643–647.
37. Lowry S: Introduction. In Schenberg L (ed): Multiple Sclerosis, ed 2. New York, Raven Press, 1977, p 7.
38. Mathews WB: Clinical features of multiple sclerosis in clinical neurology. Clin Neurol 1993; 2.1098.
39. Matthews WB: Clinical aspects of multiple sclerosis. In Matthews CINB (ed): McAlpine's Multiple Sclerosis, ed 2. London, Churchill-Livingstone, 1991, pp 64–67.
40. McDonald WI, Nielle DH, Barnes P: Pathologic evolution of multiple sclerosis. Neuropathol Appl Neurobiol 1988; 18:319–334.
41. Merritt JC: Management of spasticity in spinal cord injury. Mayo Clin Proc 1981; 56:616–622.
42. Mitchell G: Update in multiple sclerosis therapy. Med Clin North Am 1990; 77:233.
43. Multiple Sclerosis Study Group: The efficacy of cyclosporine immunosuppression in multiple sclerosis: A preliminary report of a randomized blinded placebo controlled clinical trial. Ann Neurol 1988; 24:119.
44. Multiple Sclerosis: A National Survey: US Department of Health and Human Services publication No. (NIH) 84-2479. Bethesda, Md, Public Health Service, Nov 1984.
45. Patzold U, Pocklington PR: Course of multiple sclerosis: Results of a prospective study carried out on 102 patients from 1976 to 1980. Acta Neurol Scand 1982; 65:245–266.
46. Panitch HS, Hirsch RL, Schindler J, et al: Treatment of multiple sclerosis with gamma interferon: Exacerbations associated with the activation of the immune system. Neurology 1987; 37:1097–1102.
47. Patzold U, Hecker H, Pocklington P: Azathioprine in treatment of multiple sclerosis: Final results of a 4½ year controlled study of its effectiveness covering 114 patients. J Neurol Sci 1982; 54:377–394.
48. Peterson RC, Koke NE: Cognitive and psychologic abnormalities in multiple sclerosis. Mayo Clin Proc 1989; 64:657–663.
49. Poser CW, Patty DW, Scheinber GL, et al: New diagnostic criteria for MS guidelines for research protocols. Ann Neurol 1983; 13:227–231.
50. Prime IFNB Multiple Sclerosis Study Group: Interferon beta 1b is effective in relapsing remitting multiple sclerosis. Neurology 1993; 43:655–661.
51. Reinherz EL, Weiner HL, Hauser SL: Loss of suppressor T cells in active multiple sclerosis. N Engl J Med 1980; 303:125–129.
52. Rodriguez M: Basic concepts and hypotheses in multiple sclerosis. Mayo Clin Proc 1989; 64:570–576.
53. Rudge P: Treatment of multiple sclerosis. In Swash M, Oxbury J (eds): Clinical Neurology, vol 2. New York, Churchill Livingstone, 1991, p 1149.
54. Sears TA, Postock H: Conduction failure in demyelination. Is it inevitable? Adv Neurol 1981; 51:357–375.
55. Sherratt RM, Bostock H, Leais TA: Effects of 4-aminopyridine on normal and demyelinated mammalian nerve fibers. Nature 1980; 274:385–387.

56. Silberg D, Lisak R, Sweiman B: Multiple sclerosis unaffected by azathioprine in a pilot study. Arch Neurol 1973; 28:210–212.

57. Steinman L: Autoimmune disease. Sci Am 1993; 269:107–114.

58. Stewart JM, Houser OW, Baker ML, et al: Magnetic resonance imaging and clinical relationships in multiple sclerosis. Mayo Clin Proc 1987; 62:174–184.

59. Surridge D: An investigation into some psychiatric aspects of multiple sclerosis. Br J Psychiatry 1969; 115:749–762.

60. Swansen JW: Multiple sclerosis: Update in diagnosis and review of prognostic factors. Mayo Clin Proc 1989; 64:577–586.

61. Swinburn WR, Libersedge LA: Long term treatment of multiple sclerosis with azathioprine. J Neurol Neurosurg Psychiatry 1973; 36:124–126.

62. Thompson AV, Kermode AG, Wieder D, et al: Major differences in the dynamics of primary and secondary progressive multiple sclerosis. Ann Neurol 1991; 29:53–62.

63. Thompson AV, McRonald WL: Multiple sclerosis and its pathophysi-ology. In Osbury AK (ed): Diseases in the Nervous System, ed 2. Philadelphia, WB Saunders, 1992, p 1218.

64. Tourtellotte WW, Baumhefner RW, Potvin AR, et al: Multiple sclero-sis; de novo CNS IgG synthesis: Effect of ACTH and corticosteroids. Neurology 1980; 30:1155–1162.

65. Tourtellotte WW, Potvin AR, Fleming JO: Multiple sclerosis: Mea-surement and validation of central nervous system. IgG synthesis rate. Neurology 1980; 30:240–244.

66. VandenBurg W, VanZomeren E, Minderhaud JM, et al: Cognitive impairment in patients with multiple sclerosis and mild physical disabilities. Arch Neurol 1987; 44:494–501.

67. VonDiemen HA, Polman CH, van Dongen TM, et al: The effect of 4-AP in clinical signs in multiple sclerosis: A randomized placebo controlled double blind crossover study. Ann Neurol 1992; 32:123–130.

68. Wynn NR, Rodriguez M, O'Fallan W: Update on the epidemiology of multiple sclerosis. Mayo Clin Proc 1989; 64:808–817.

Rehabilitation of Children and Adults With Cerebral Palsy

LYNNE M. STEMPIEN, M.D.,
AND DEBORAH GAEBLER-SPIRA, M.D.

Cerebral palsy (CP) is a collection of diverse syndromes characterized by disorders of movement and posture caused by a nonprogressive injury to the immature brain.[169] The distinctive characteristic of these syndromes is the change in muscle tone and posture, both at rest and with voluntary activity.[175] The definition of cerebral palsy implies that the underlying pathologic process in the brain does not progress and occurred in the early formation of the brain. The first year or two of life is included in most definitions, although some references include cases up to age 7 years. The wide range of normal neurological functioning, particularly in the first year of life, can make assessment of abnormalities difficult. Neurological maturation can also provide some improvement in the early years of life, thus causing overestimation of the number of children with permanent neuromotor dysfunction.[138]

EPIDEMIOLOGY

Cerebral palsy is one of the most common disabilities affecting children. The reported incidence varies but is approximately 2 to 3/1000 live births.[137] The incidence of CP in the United States in the 1940s and 1950s was estimated to be 1.6 to 5.8/1000 live births.[184] The larger, more recent Collaborative Perinatal Project measured a prevalence rate of 5.2/1000 live births at 1 year of age, but reported resolution in up to half of these children by 7 years of age.[178] The most recent studies in the United States match the average prevalance rate of CP in industrialized countries: 2/1000 live births.[24, 58]

There were hopes that recent improvements in neonatal care would decrease the incidence of CP. Several studies[134, 228] suggested a decrease in the 1970s, but this has

been transient.[228, 230] CP prevalence in full-term infants has remained relatively constant. The improved neonatal survival has decreased the risk of CP for neonates weighing greater than 2500 g.[146] In recent decades there has been a trend to higher survival rates for more immature, smaller, and premature infants with medical complications. Despite improved neonatal outcomes in general, the survival of these low-birth-weight (less than 2500 g) and very low-birth-weight (less than 1500 g) infants with higher CP risk has kept the prevalence of CP in childhood relatively constant.[23, 58, 99] In addition to birth weight less than 2500 g, a number of other factors predict increased risk for CP[58, 96, 243] (Table 53–1). Gestational age less than 32 weeks is one of the most powerful predictors of CP. Maternal mental retardation; maternal seizure disorder or hyperthyroidism; two or more prior fetal deaths; a sibling with motor deficit; third-trimester bleeding; or increased urine protein excretion, fetal bradycardia, chorionitis, low placental weight, fetal malformations, and neonatal seizures all increase CP risk by multivariate analysis.[103, 177]

Other factors associated with CP are identified in epidemiological studies related to stages of pregnancy. Before pregnancy, long menstrual cycles or repeated fetal wastage during pregnancy; fetal growth retardation; twin gestation; congenital malformations; abnormal fetal presentation; or low socioeconomic class are associated with increased CP risk. During labor and delivery, only premature separation of the placenta poses an associated CP risk. In the early postnatal period, newborn encephalopathy is the only epidemiological association.[145]

Despite these many associations, most children with these risk factors do not develop CP. Many of these abnormal characteristics can be consequences of the disease process and not the cause. Evidence is mounting for the

TABLE 53–1   **Risk Factors Associated With Cerebral Palsy**

General
    Gestational age <32 wk
    Birth weight <2500 g
Maternal history
    Mental retardation
    Seizure disorder
    Hyperthyroidism
    Two or more prior fetal deaths
    Sibling with motor deficits
During gestation
    Twin gestation
    Fetal growth retardation
    Third-trimester bleeding
    Increased urine protein excretion
    Chorionitis
    Premature placenta separation
    Low placenta weight
Fetal factors
    Abnormal fetal presentation
    Fetal malformations
    Fetal bradycardia
    Neonatal seizures

postulate that CP is the result of processes causing problems with brain formation in utero. Many of the clinical associations such as preterm delivery and peripartum difficulties could be a consequence of this process.

ETIOLOGY

The brain injury that leads to CP can occur in the prenatal, perinatal, or postnatal period.[147] A wide variety of brain injury mechanisms have been attributed to causing these lesions. Currently, the most common causes are related to brain injury occurring in children born prematurely.[18, 58, 76, 145] The combination of immaturity, fragile brain vasculature, and the physical stresses of prematurity combine to predispose these children to compromise of cerebral blood flow.[35] The blood vessels are particularly vulnerable in the watershed zone next to the lateral ventricles in the capillaries of the germinal matrix. Bleeding in this area is often arterial in origin and can occur in differing degrees: cerebral intraventricular hemorrhage isolated to germinal matrix (grade 1), intraventricular hemorrhage[186] with normal ventricular size (grade 2), intraventricular hemorrhage with ventricular dilatation (grade 3), or intraventricular hemorrhage with parenchymal hemorrhage (grade 4) (Table 53–2).

Very low-birth-weight infants also have an increased incidence of periventricular hemorrhagic infarction, which is hemorrhagic necrosis lateral to the external angle of the lateral ventricle. This is thought to be bleeding of venous origin and is usually asymmetrical.[101, 167] With healing of

TABLE 53–2   **Grades of Intraventricular Hemorrhage in the Premature Brain**

Grade 1	Isolated to germinal matrix
Grade 2	With normal ventricular size
Grade 3	With ventricular dilatation
Grade 4	With parenchymal hemorrhage

this bleeding, symmetrical necrosis of white matter adjacent to the external angle of the lateral ventricles (periventricular leukomalacia) can develop[206] (Fig. 53–1). Periventricular leukomalacia is one of the strongest predictors of CP in the premature neonate.[145]

Fortunately, the large majority of children who are born prematurely do not develop CP, although they can have neuromotor and developmental abnormalities throughout the first year of life. Even the most sophisticated pediatric developmental assessment tools are not sufficiently sensitive to detect deficits that will persist until after 1 year of age.[110] Consequently, it is common for families to suspect motor problems long before diagnosis of CP is given at age 2 or more.

Almost half of all children with CP were not born prematurely. In term births that result in CP, the cause of brain injury is often elusive. Most known perinatal injuries which cause CP are due to severe anoxic or ischemic brain injury. This can occur with mechanical difficulties of the placenta, umbilical cord, or the actual delivery itself. Intrapartum asphyxia must be severe to be the cause of CP.[86, 176] Unfortunately, injuries of this type tend to be more global and are more likely to cause a more severe disability.[143]

Postnatal causes of CP can include any type of brain injury. Anoxia, ischemia, infection, or trauma can all cause injury that later results in a CP-type picture. Although these brain injuries can cause clinical consequences similar to CP, the clinical convention is to identify these children diagnostically by the specific insult (i.e., encephalitis, traumatic brain injury).

CLASSIFICATION

Cerebral palsy is often characterized by the type of muscle tone abnormality and the body parts involved (Table 53–3). The most common abnormality is that of increased muscle tone, or spasticity. Spastic disorders affect approximately three fourths of all patients with CP.[143, 146] This spasticity can occur in either a consistent or velocity-dependent manner or both. When the resistance to passive movement is continuous and constant despite changes in limb velocity, the increased tone is called rigidity. This has often been compared to the feel of bending a lead pipe.

There are frequently signs of the upper motor neuron syndrome in CP (exaggerated muscle stretch reflexes and abnormal Babinski's reflexes). There can be "overflow" of muscle stretch reflexes to adjacent joints such as the crossed adductor reflex (contraction of bilateral adductor muscles to unilateral adductor stretch).

Less common are dyskinetic disorders with involuntary movements. Classic athetoid movements which encompass large muscle groups are common. The involuntary slow writhing posturing of athetosis is most easily detected in the movements of the head and face.[246] Dyskinetic disorders cause impairments in postural instability, and are sometimes reflected in "fluctuating tone" abnormalities. These patients often begin with hypotonia, and develop the discrete involuntary movements over the first few years of life. Athetoid disorders are most commonly caused by damage to the basal ganglia with hyperbilirubinemia or severe anoxia. Small muscle involuntary movements such

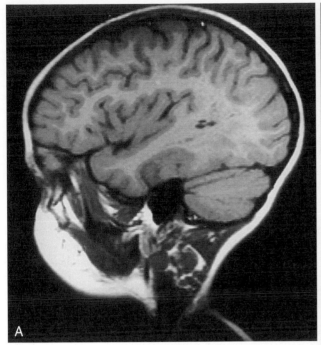

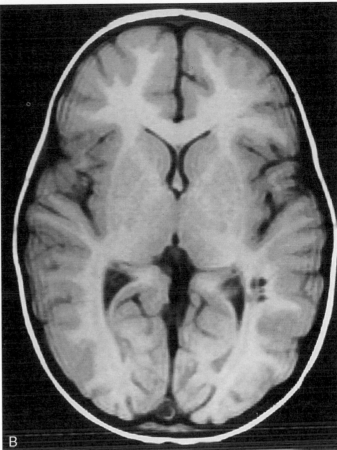

FIGURE 53–1   *A* and *B*, Periventricular leukomalacia.

as chorea can also be seen. Rarely, ballistic, rotary, and flailing movements have been described. Ataxic disorders which mimic cerebellar dysfunction with titubation, wide-based gait, and dysmetria are very rare in CP.

A small percentage of patients have the hypotonic type of CP. These children need to be differentiated from those with more frequently identifiable causes of neonatal hypotonia such as muscle disease, metabolic disorders, and genetic syndromes. Many of these children develop spastic- or extrapyramidal-type disorders after the first few months of life. All of these tone abnormalities can occur in mixtures. The most common combination is that of spasticity with athetosis. These patients are sometimes classified as "mixed-type" CP.

The distribution of body parts with disability is used to name the type of CP (Figs. 53–2 through 53–4). Diplegia

refers to spastic paresis in the lower extremities more than in the upper extremities and is the most common. Quadriplegia, involving abnormalities of both upper and lower extremities, is also frequent. In quadriplegia the disorder of motor control is typically worse in the legs.[229] Rarely, a child will have obvious abnormalities of both

TABLE 53–3   Classification of Cerebral Palsy Types

By Tone Abnormalities	By Body Parts Involved
Spastic	Diplegia
Dyskinetic	Quadriplegia
Athetoid	Triplegia
Choreiform	Hemiplegia
Ballistic	
Ataxic	
Hypotonic	
"Mixed"	

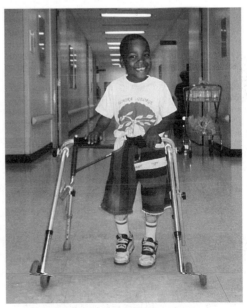

FIGURE 53–2   Spastic diplegia.

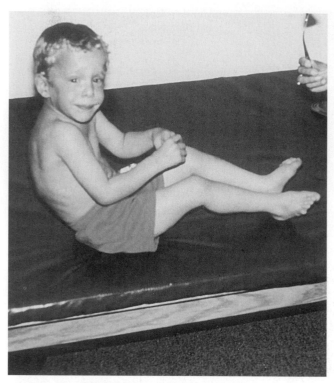

FIGURE 53–3   Spastic quadriplegia.

legs and one arm and is referred to as having triplegia. Patterns of abnormalities that involve the arms more than the legs (similar to a stroke) are labeled as hemiplegic. For unclear reasons, isolated right hemiplegia is twice as common as left hemiplegia.[100]

Diplegia, or leg-dominated symptoms, are most frequent in the low-birth-weight, premature groups. Quadriplegia is more frequent in those with normal birth weight.[143] It should be noted, however, that most children with CP are "total body–involved." Close examination of motor control in the more normal-appearing limbs, trunk, and oral-motor musculature often yields small abnormalities.

CLINICAL EFFECTS

The most striking difficulties in CP are disorders of neuromuscular control. Problems in infancy that suggest CP include irritability, lethargy, weak suck with tongue thrust, poor head control, high-pitched cry, oral hypersensitivity, tonic bite, and asymmetrical movements or unusual posturing. Motor delay can also be suggested by persistent abnormal motor activities, such as rolling for mobility, combat crawling, "W-sitting," "bunny hopping," or adopting a hand preference before the first birthday[74] (Figs. 53–5 and 53–6).

Abnormalities of muscle tone are frequently accompanied by muscle weakness, which can cause certain strength imbalances at individual joints. This gives rise to a number of patterns of movement. Certain patterns occur frequently in children with CP, such as "scissoring," "guarding" of the upper extremities, extensor posturing, or proximal "fixing" (Figs. 53–7 through 53–9).

Scissoring is the simultaneous adduction, knee hyperex-

tension, and plantar flexion of the lower extremities. Flexion synergy patterns of the upper extremities include flexion at the fingers, wrists, and elbows with shoulder abduction. As this upper extremity pattern becomes stronger, the child's hands rise from the waist, producing a low, mid, or high guard position (Fig. 53–10). Some patterns of movement can be recognized as components of persistent primitive reflexes, such as the asymmetric tonic neck reflex (ATNR), symmetric tonic neck reflex (STNR), or tonic labyrinthine reflex (TLR) (Figs. 53–11 through 53–13). These movement patterns can be seen in limbs as the child attempts voluntary movement, triggered by passive positioning, in response to sensory stimuli, or as an "overflow" of uninvolved limbs.

These movement patterns are examples of a primary difficulty in CP—the inability to separate out individual movements. Children with CP often elicit motor activity in joints and limbs beyond the wanted action. These associated reactions or activation of muscles remote from where the child is trying to move is one of the major impediments to voluntary movement.

The abnormalities of muscle tone are often accompanied by weakness in individual muscles. Applying the traditional methods of measuring muscle strength is problematic in CP because the tone abnormalities mask the patient's ability to generate force.[84]

Difficulty with control of the midline structures such as the trunk and head interfere dramatically with a child's

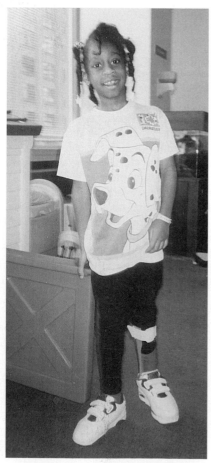

FIGURE 53–4   Spastic hemiplegia.

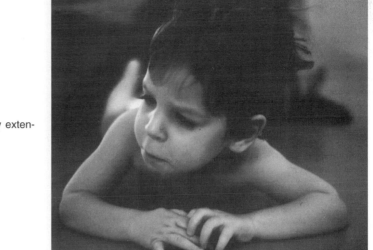

FIGURE 53–5   Combat, or belly, crawl, with lower extremity extension and use of upper extremities for forward progression.

ability to develop good balance. This unbridled motor activity complicates the patient's ability to balance and coordinate movement. The development of appropriate, adequately implemented equilibrium and righting reactions is delayed or sometimes absent. Abnormal or inappropriate coordination patterns lead to limitations in acquiring, planning, executing, and correcting skillful actions. Even children with minimal involvement can exhibit apraxia when attempting high-level motor activities.

The combination of abnormal motor control and experience also contributes to a disordered kinesthetic sense. Children with CP are often sensitive to normally innocuous stimuli. The abnormal sensory experience of disordered motor control can contribute to disordered sensory perception, which further interferes with the child's ability to perform high-level motor activities.[39] Decreased ability to distinguish two-point discrimination has been found in the upper extremities of children with all types of CP.[150] Chil-

dren with hemiparetic CP have also been found almost universally to have a decrease in stereognosis, with decreased proprioception in about half of patients tested.[237]

The major secondary effects of disordered muscle tone, control, and balance are changes in joint alignment leading

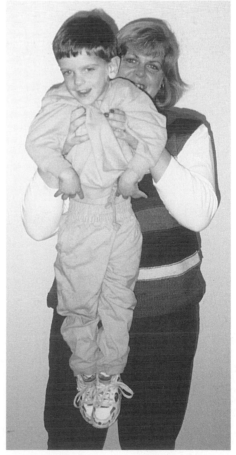

FIGURE 53–7   Scissoring or vertical suspension.

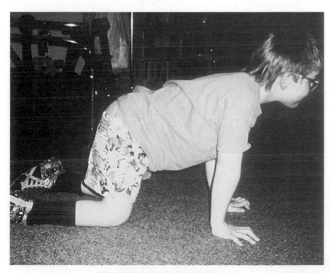

FIGURE 53–6   "Bunny hop."

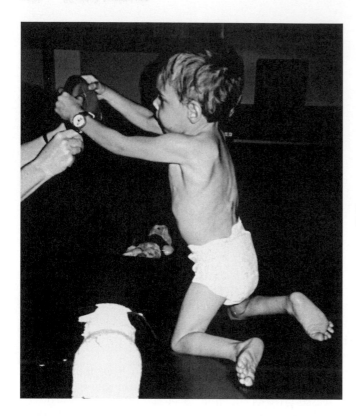

FIGURE 53–8   "Proximal fixing" with increased activity in shoulder girdle and neck muscles.

FIGURE 53–9   Extensor posturing.

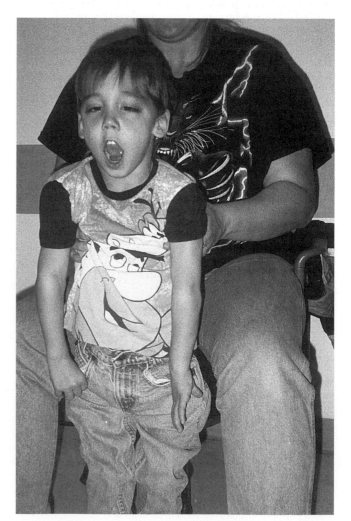

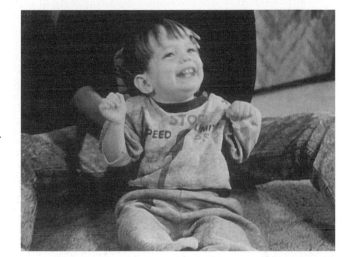

FIGURE 53–10   "High guard" position of upper extremities.

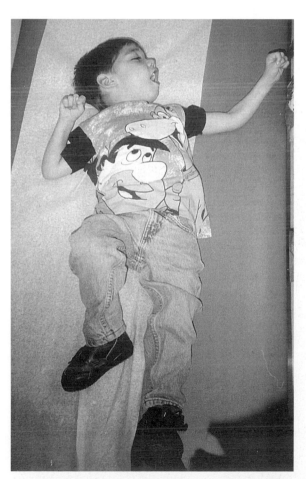

FIGURE 53–11   Asymmetric tonic neck reflex.

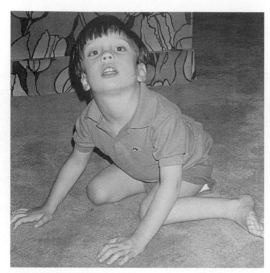

FIGURE 53–12 Symmetric tonic neck reflex (if neck is extended, upper extremities are extended and lower extremities are flexed).

to contracture and deformity. Contracture, or passive shortening that can limit joint and soft tissue movement, frequently affects the adductor, hamstring, and plantar flexor muscles of the lower extremities and the flexors of the upper extremities. This reflects the presence of spasticity, scissoring, or upper extremity flexion patterns, individually or severally, which are present in the majority of children with CP.

Bony deformity can occur because the abnormal muscle forces of CP are acting on a growing skeleton. Of principal concern are the integrity of the hips and spine because of their primary role in weightbearing. The typical increase in hip flexion, adduction, and internal rotation of the femur acts to influence the femoral head in an upward posterolateral direction out of the acetabulum. The result is coxa valgus, malformed femoral head, and a shallow acetabulum, which causes the hip to be more prone to subluxation[26, 148] (Fig. 53–14).

Spinal deformities are not quite as common but have more severe consequences. Asymmetrical muscle pull and immobility can contribute to significant deformity of the spine, including kyphosis, scoliosis, or rotational deformities. These spinal deformities can significantly affect comfort, tone, sitting and standing alignment, and balance. When these are severe, respiratory function can be compromised by the mechanical restriction of the chest combined with decreased efficiency of available respiratory muscle strength. This can have a significant impact on endurance, health, and longevity. Spondylolisthesis and spondylolysis are not increased in CP.[113]

Bony abnormalities of the feet can occur in a variety of patterns. The most common is deformity of the hindfoot with exaggerated heel valgus or varus. Hyperpronation occurs frequently with calcaneovalgus or cavus. Occasionally a rocker-bottom type of foot can be seen.

ASSOCIATED MEDICAL AND FUNCTIONAL PROBLEMS

The most common types of associated disabilities in CP are abnormalities in the oculomotor system. Esotropia or exotropia often requires strabismus surgery. Visual field deficits are less common but occur most frequently in the hemiplegic types. Visual impairments of acuity affect children with quadriplegia more than those with diplegia.

A large number of children with CP have abnormalities of oromotor function. This frequently leads to changes in their ability to feed well. Incomplete lip closure, low suction pressure, and delay between suction and propulsion cause inadequate bolus preparation.[151] In the more involved children, this can also interfere with their pharyngeal swallowing mechanism. Abnormalities in strength, tone, and coordination can be severe enough to cause difficulty protecting the airway. In one large study of patients with suspected oropharyngeal dysfunction, over half of those tested aspirated. Often the majority of patients have no effective cough during aspiration.[97, 207] Swallowing dysfunction is often present with only certain textures of food ingested as detected by videoflouroscopy.[207] In severe cases, aspiration can cause hypoxemia.[208] Motor impairment can interfere with accessing food or communicating hunger. These feeding difficulties can contribute to substantial undernutrition or malnutrition.[81] Up to one third of hemiplegic and diplegic CP patients and more than two thirds of quadriplegic CP patients have been found to be undernourished.[129, 226, 227] This correlates with significantly reduced linear growth that is exclusive of the patient's motor disability.

Another unique growth disturbance can be asymmetry of linear growth, particularly in the limbs. The most se-

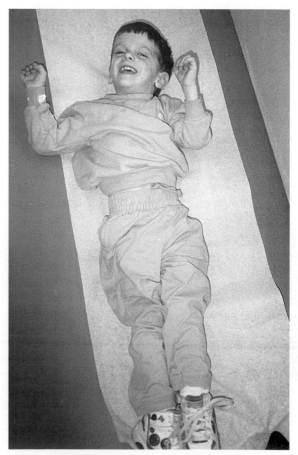

FIGURE 53–13 Tonic labyrinthine reflex.

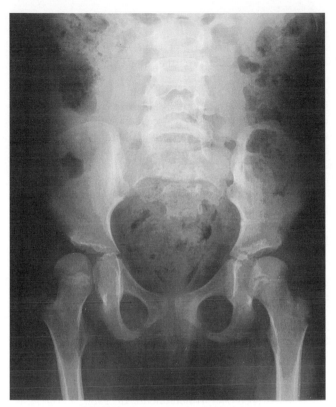

FIGURE 53–14   Dysplastic hip joints.

verely motor-impaired limbs can have a decreased length and girth at maturity. Of interest is the effect of sensory disturbance, as there is a tendency for hemiplegic children with impaired sensation to have inadequate limb growth. This length deficiency seems to be worse the more severe the sensory deficit.[237]

Gastrointestinal symptoms are frequent in children with CP.[71] Gastroesophageal reflux can cause episodic emesis. It can also interfere with adequate ingestion and absorption of nutrients and compromise adequate nutrition and growth.[166, 189] Constipation, exaggerated by immobility and abnormal diet and fluid intake, can usually be managed with standard medical treatment.[3]

Physiological abnormalities of bowel and bladder control in CP have not been well studied. Incontinence is the most frequently reported urinary tract symptom. This increased incontinence as compared with peers has been attributed to decreased mobility, communication, and cognitive skills. Of the patients studied by urodynamics with urinary symptoms such as incontinence, urgency, or hesitancy, a large number were found to have small-capacity hyperreflexic bladders. Detrusor-sphincter dyssynergy was also found in a few patients.[202] Patients with complaints of fecal incontinence or defecation distress have been found to have anal sphincter or pelvic muscle incoordination, or both, without rectal dysfunction by anorectal manometry.[3] This dysfunction in the pelvic area appears to be related to abnormalities in neuromotor control (see Chapter 28).

Cognitive impairments are not obligatory with CP. The risk increases with the severity of the motor disability.[162] The prevalence of mental retardation in all persons with CP is estimated to be 30%.[145] Premature children with very low birth weight can have learning disabilities or mental retardation. Normal-birth-weight children with CP have had cognitive abnormalities reported in up to 40% to 50%.[143]

Seizure disorders can occur in up to a third of children with CP. Epilepsy is frequently active in the preschool and early school years. The highest incidence is in the most severely motor-affected children and those with mental retardation, reflecting the greater extent of brain injury in these cases.[143]

Hearing disabilities are rare in CP.[205] They are most commonly found in cases caused by congenital nervous system infections such as TORCH (Toxoplasmosis, Rubella, Cytomegalovirus, and Herpes). When hyperbilirubinemia was common and difficult to control secondary to maternal-fetal blood incompatibilities, bilirubin-induced sensorineural hearing loss often accompanied athetoid-type CP. Improvements in detecting and treating these conditions prenatally have now reduced this to a rare situation.

FUNCTIONAL PROGNOSIS

In the first few years of life, there can be some evolution toward normal of the child's neuromotor function. The amount of tone abnormality and the importance of the reflexive movements can change over these years. There are certain skills that are helpful in establishing an ultimate motor prognosis. Those children who will attain independent ambulation will achieve this during ages 2 to 7, rarely later. Seventy-five percent of children with spastic CP eventually ambulate, about 85% with diplegia and 70% with quadriplegia. Most children with hemiplegic or ataxic CP ambulate independently, the majority by age 3 years. Unfortunately, those with hypotonic CP rarely walk.

Children who are able to sit independently before their second birthday eventually become independent walkers, with or without equipment. Those who cannot sit independently by age 4 years rarely walk. However, if the primitive reflexes (ATNR, STNR, tonic labyrithine, Moro's, positive supporting reflex, or extensor posturing) still occur in an obligatory manner, the prognosis for independent ambulation is bleak.[25, 171] Obligatory reflexes occur consistently when the child's body is placed in certain positions passively or with voluntary movement. Most children who become ambulators have fewer than three of these reflexes present at age 18 months.[171]

The most striking functional impact of this abnormal neuromotor control is a decrease in independence and mobility. One of the hallmarks of CP is motor delay, even in the presence of normal development in other areas. The increased muscle tone that is present with even small amounts of movement and during posture maintenance greatly increases the energy expended for motor activity. The ability to progress through motor milestones is greatly impeded. Children who do achieve ambulation typically have an inefficient gait, which includes much shorter step length, decreased range of motion at the hip and knee, more energy expenditure, and decreased velocity as compared with their peers. They also have impairment in coordination, and this becomes more apparent with more challenging motor activities.

Abnormalities affecting adequate motor control for speech, such as oromotor dysfunction and inadequate breath support, lead to dysarthria and can interfere with communication skills. Language-processing problems with reception or expression can occur and correlate with cognitive impairments.[74] Difficulty controlling oral secretions can cause significant drooling.

All of these inefficiencies of muscle control contribute to decreased endurance.[210] Although endurance is difficult to measure with conventional methods because of the challenges of various impairments with CP, it seems to correlate with the overall gross motor capabilities of the individual.[188] Contractures and bone or joint deformities can greatly limit a child's function. Secondary pain can greatly worsen muscle tone and contribute to the inefficiency of movement.

EFFECTS OF AGING

The child with CP ages with a chronic but not unchanging neuromuscular condition. Life expectancy for all but the most severely involved children is close to that for the unaffected population.[79, 146] Recently, there has been interest in defining the interaction of aging with the primary and secondary effects of CP.[20, 59, 168, 199, 244] A person with CP can have ongoing medical issues that are exacerbated by aging such as dysphagia, gastroesophageal reflux, urinary incontinence, constipation, and painful musculoskeletal contractures that progress and cause a decline in function.[14, 28, 125] Problems of osteoporosis, fractures due to falls, deconditioning, and pressure sores are the expected potential consequences of the combined processes.

Adults with CP often require new surgeries or a repeat of one they had during childhood.[196] Careful planning is needed, and rehabilitation is usually undertaken to address the deconditioning which ensues following postoperative immobilization. The orthopedic literature emphasizes that the adult with CP is frequently more motivated and able to participate in therapy than the child.[196]

Adults with CP rank communication, activities of daily living (ADL), and mobility as higher priority goals than ambulation.[26] In the past, vocational rates among adults with CP were only 30% to 50%. The Americans With Disabilities Act holds new optimism regarding terms of employment, housing, and accessibility to the community.[180]

THERAPEUTIC MANAGEMENT

The therapeutic management of the child with CP, whether by the physiatrist, orthopedist, or developmental pediatrician, emphasizes a functional aim- or goal-oriented approach.[42, 74, 108, 211, 245] The two major goals of rehabilitation, according to Molnar,[169] are to decrease complications of the CP and to enhance or improve the acquisition of new skills. Rothery and colleagues[211] include parent and caregiver education, decreasing skeletal deformity, and improving mobility. Promoting the child's assets offers a positive approach. Children should not be considered only in terms of potential deficits. Recommendations for management begin with an assessment of the child's and family's strengths and deficits. All associated problems should be correctly identified.[85, 87]

From the first evaluation, the family and child should be encouraged to become active participants in the process of setting priorities and goals within the context of the impairment. The physician's role is to provide an accurate description of the therapies and interventions available to the child and family and the impact that these will have on the child's condition and function. The institution of therapy and other medical modalities should be approached and prescribed after a thorough discussion of efficacy. The following discussion represents the major therapeutic interventions for children with CP.

Early Intervention

Early institution of physical therapy (PT) has been suggested by Köng to decrease the impact of brain injury on the development of CP.[124, 141] There is a discrete group of children who initially appear to have manifestations of brain injury but who at later age appear to outgrow their CP.[178] Whether or not early PT has an impact on brain injury, there currently is emphasis on early identification of the infant with developmental delay so that intervention can be instituted as soon as possible.[161] The Education of the Handicapped Act Amendments of 1986, Public Law (PL) 99–457, or IDEA (Individuals With Disabilities Education Act), mandated early intervention for children 0 to 3 years old who demonstrate developmental delay. This federal law was established to provide educational and educationally related rehabilitative services to a group of children who enter school with already identifiable problems. The law provides a downward extension of PL 94–142, which mandated that all states must provide a free and appropriate public education to eligible schoolchildren. One of the hallmarks of IDEA is the clearly identified role of the family of the infants and toddlers as central to the goals of early intervention. The team acts not only to treat the child but also to empower the family. A mutual contract, the Individual Family Service Plan (IFSP), is developed actively by the team and parents. Unlike the IEP (Individual Education Plan) from PL 94–142, the IFSP must take into account the family's strengths and needs, not just the child's goals.[108, 112, 115]

The rationale for early intervention is closely connected to concepts that stressed the importance of the early years for normally developing children and the role that environmental factors play in development. Parental characteristics, such as responsivity contingent on child initiations, the quality and quantity of verbal interactions, and the existence of a social support network and maternal sensitivity, have all been found to be associated with a child's concurrent or later developmental functioning.[21, 36, 149, 240]

There are two main models for the delivery of developmental early intervention: the direct therapy service model, and the consultation model. The direct model of service delivery can occur as a part of interdisciplinary, multidisciplinary, or transdisciplinary treatment in a center- or home-based program.[108] For the child with CP, traditionally physical therapists and occupational therapists have been providers of therapeutic intervention. Many children are also seen by a speech-language pathologist for feeding difficulties and oromotor problems. A social worker, nurse, and developmental specialist constitute the members of a typical early intervention team. To reduce the number of therapists handling the child, Haynes[111] has recently advocated that one professional from the early intervention team integrate assessment data from all of the members of the treatment team to develop integrated strategies to meet goals agreed upon by the family and team in the IFSP. Given the shortage of pediatric physical therapists, occupational therapists, and speech-language pathologists, this transdisciplinary approach could assist in providing the number of therapists needed to deliver therapeutic input to the infants and toddlers eligible for treatment under Public Law 99–457.

Therapy Approaches

Children with CP who have motor problems that interfere with educational activities have the opportunity to participate in integrated therapy programs in school. The services should be delivered in the least restrictive environment and are mandated to allow the child the ability to participate and benefit from the educational experience. The current philosophical trend in schools is to include disabled children as much as possible into the regular classroom, and few "pull out" services are stressed. Mainstreaming has positive effects on psychosocial aspects of schooling and increases the academic expectations of the disabled student.[49] Consultative models of PT, occupational therapy (OT), and speech have provided a method of treating and involving more of the children with disabilities into regular education classes. Even though there is a move toward consultative services by PT, OT, and speech therapy in the school systems, direct service can be recommended to augment an overall therapy program.

There are a number of therapy systems that have influenced the management of children with CP (Table 53–4). Few therapists adhere strictly to a single therapy system. The following descriptions provide the basic principles of the most commonly used and influential therapies. Historically, the approach of Crothers remains a basic guide to involving patients in a meaningful program. He stressed the need for active movement and stimulation activities to prevent contractures and to encourage participation of severely involved children. Parents were counseled to avoid overprotection.[94] Phelps used an orthopedic approach with conventional techniques from poliomyelitis treatment regimens. He emphasized inhibiting abnormal movement.[198] Deaver[64, 65] emphasized functional ability rather than patterns of movement, and this method is known also for its extensive use of bracing. Functional abilities were facilitated by intensive training efforts in residential units at frequent intervals of the child's life. Fay,[80] a neurophysiologist, postulated that motor developmental levels of the brain were comparable to evolutionary process. This highly controversial concept is expressed by "ontogeny recapitulates phylogeny." Doman, a physical therapist, integrated the concepts into the therapy known as patterning.[51, 68] Patterning has been subjected to critical review by the pediatric community and is not recommended.[7]

Rood,[209] an occupational and physical therapist, developed a sensorimotor approach to treatment. Rood's overall goal was to activate movement and postural responses at an automatic level while following a developmental sequence similar to the Bobath method of treatment. Rood used specific sensory stimulation to elicit movement.[209] The neurodevelopmental treatment (NDT) approach has been recommended for infants who display early signs of CP. This approach was developed by the Bobaths in England in the 1940s.[30–33] The main goals of NDT are to normalize tone, inhibit abnormal primitive reflex patterns, and to facilitate automatic reactions and subsequent normal movement. These goals are accomplished by the therapists providing "key points of control" throughout the body.[32] This theoretically provides the child with kinesthetic normal feedback. The Bobaths have placed emphasis on family involvement and carryover of handling techniques in the home environment. For the older child, the Bobaths shift emphasis to ADL skills.[110] Two additional systems of therapy for CP practiced in Europe and not readily available in the United States are the Vojta and Peto methods.[57, 61]

OT can also utilize defined systems or specialized treatment methods. Sensory integration (introduced by A. Jean Ayres[11–13] in the 1970s) is used to enhance the development of preschool and school-age children who have learning disabilities. Ayres' premise is that "disordered sensory integration accounts for some aspects of learning disorders and that improving sensory integration will make academic learning easier."[13] This therapy is intended to enhance the child's ability to organize and integrate controlled sensory information such as vestibular, proprioceptive, and tactile stimulation.[12, 134, 223]

In the clinical delivery of therapy services there is little reliance on any one system.[109] An eclectic approach that offers modalities from several schools of therapy provides flexibility and individualization to meet the child's and family's goals.[19, 82, 154]

Sports as organized physical activities were once only rarely recommended for the child with CP. There is no evidence that strengthening adversely affects muscle tone.[121, 126, 164] Neither is there evidence to preclude activities that once were thought to increase orthopedic deformity, such as downhill skiing.[83, 123] The therapeutic benefits of swimming and horseback riding for children with motor disabilities have been established.[8, 43] Even more important than the use of sports programs to improve endurance and strength, sports offer the interpersonal growth and improved self-esteem that all children have when appropriately supervised in a team sport with peers.[60, 220, 221] The established organizations for athletes with CP are the United States Cerebral Palsy Athletic Association and the Cerebral Palsy International Sports and Recreation Association.[130] Fitness programs that emphasize flexibility and endurance have been developed for both recreational and therapeutic use.[158, 160]

Equipment Concerns

For many families with a CP child the physical therapist is the medical professional with whom they have the most frequent contact. The physical therapist recommends equipment to improve function such as prone or supine standers, walkers, bathing equipment, wheelchairs, and, often, or-

TABLE 53–4   Similarities and Differences Between Neuromotor Therapy Approaches to Cerebral Palsy (CP)

	Neuro-developmental Treatment (Bobaths)	Sensorimotor Approach to Treatment (Rood)	Sensory Integration Approach (Ayres)	Vojta Approach	Patterning Therapy (Doman-Delacato)
Central nervous system model	Hierarchical	Hierarchical	Hierarchical	Hierarchical	Hierarchical
Goals of treatment	1. To normalize tone 2. To inhibit primitive reflexes 3. To facilitate automatic reactions and normal movement patterns	1. To activate postural responses (stability) 2. To activate movement (mobility) once stability is achieved	1. To improve efficiency of neural processing 2. To better organize adaptive responses	1. To prevent CP in infants at risk 2. To improve motoric behavior in infants with fixed CP	1. To achieve independent mobility 2. To improve motor coordination 3. To prevent or improve communication disorders 4. To enhance intelligence
Primary sensory systems utilized to effect a motor response	1. Kinesthetic 2. Proprioceptive 3. Tactile	1. Tactile 2. Proprioceptive 3. Kinesthetic	1. Vestibular 2. Tactile 3. Kinesthetic	1. Proprioceptive 2. Kinesthetic 3. Tactile	All sensory systems are utilized
Emphasis of treatment activities	1. Positioning and handling to normalize sensory input 2. Facilitation of active movement	1. Sensory stimulation to activate motor response (tapping, brushing, icing)	1. Therapist guides, but child controls sensory input to get adaptive purposeful response	1. Trigger reflex locomotive zones to encourage movement patterns (e.g., reflex crawl)	Sensory and reflex stimulation, passive movement patterns, encouragement of independent movements
Intended clinical population	Children with CP Adults post cerebrovascular accident (CVA)	Children with neuromotor disorders such as CP Adults post CVA	Children with learning disabilities Children with autism	Young infants at risk for CP Young infants with fixed CP	Children with neonatal or acquired brain damage
Emphasis on treating infants	Yes	No	No	Yes	No
Emphasis on family involvement during treatment	Yes Handling and positioning for activities of daily living	No	No Supportive role encouraged	Yes Family administers treatment at home daily	Yes Family and friends administer treatment several times daily
Empirical support	Few studies Conflicting results	Very few studies Conflicting results	Many studies Conflicting results with school-age children Positive results for tactile and vestibular input with infants	Few studies Conflicting results	Few studies Conflicting results

From Harris SR, Atwater SW, Crowe TK: Accepted and controversial neuromotor therapies for infants at high risk for cerebral palsy. J Perinatol 1988; 8:3–13.

thotic devices. All durable medical equipment should be considered in the context of the functional prognosis. The early introduction of independent mobility for children who are not yet able to negotiate at a household level increases exploration of the environment and has been proposed to improve self-esteem.[40] Use of a wheelchair for community mobility becomes a practical measure once a child has outgrown commercially available strollers. When standardized equipment does not meet the postural support needs of the severely involved child, adaptive seating is essential for the attainment of a sitting position.[37, 89, 232] Not only does a specialized seating system preserve a child's capacity to interact in a conventional posture but it can also improve pulmonary function tests[179] (see Chapter 19). The child who is comfortable and adequately seated typically has better feeding, digestion, and vocal production. Rehabilita-

tion engineers working with therapists can address complex orthopedic and functional problems.[27, 199]

The early introduction of technology to improve communication, either written or oral, is warranted. The use of an augmentative communication device does not inhibit development of communication skills. In augmentative communication, speech is enhanced by the use of technology.[218] Occupational therapists and other adaptive specialists provide access to computers, environmental control units, and other ADL equipment[67, 136, 163] (see Chapter 24). In addition to specialized equipment, the child with CP is frequently assisted in mobility and ADL tasks by the use of splints or orthoses.[242] Splinting is a common conservative method of managing a spastic but flexible deformity. The physical therapist can provide low-temperature tone-reducing ankle-foot orthoses (TRAFOs) which have tone-reducing aspects incorporated into the construction. TRAFOs have been useful in some children but are not universally recommended.[241] The decision to brace and the type of orthosis to be used is dictated by the age of the child, functional level, motor control, type of deformity, and commitment to use. The availability of high-temperature material which can provide total contact allows an array of orthoses, which when used in conjunction with therapy, surgery, and other treatment, can decrease energy expenditure.[8, 105] Other joint immobilizers can contribute to function and maintenance of range of motion for hygiene and dressing.[10, 242]

MEDICAL AND SURGICAL MANAGEMENT

Management of Spasticity

Medication to decrease spasticity is used in children, with the most commonly used drugs being baclofen (Lioresal), and dantrolene (Dantrium).[63, 66, 159, 169] The response to these drugs is unpredictable and side effects often preclude long-term use. Studies have demonstrated clinically useful reduction in spasticity following the initiation of medication[48] (Table 53–5).

Reappraisal of spasticity in a growing child with CP every 6 months allows timely intervention.[170] Contractures develop over time and are a complex interaction of spasticity, growth, motor control deficits, weakness, and chronic positioning.[26]

Orthopedic Intervention

Nearly all children with CP develop an abnormality of physical form or function. The degree of involvement of the orthopedist with the child and family depends on the complexity and severity of the musculoskeletal system impairments.[69, 142] Children with CP should have regular orthopedic consultations. Followthrough with splinting, orthoses, PT, and recommendations made by the orthopedic surgeon are improved if a relationship with the family and child is built before the need for surgery arises. The physiatrist can facilitate this process by working in conjunction with the orthopedist and therapists involved with the child. Although the orthopedic management of the child with CP can show variations among different physicians, the fundamental goals of surgery should reflect a functional approach to problems of alignment.[117] If pain or discomfort is present, the need for surgery to attempt relief, especially around the hip, could be necessary. The following discussion addresses the surgical options for improvement in sitting, transfers, and ambulation (Table 53–6).

Surgery for Sitting

For every child, sitting is a realistic functional goal.[199] The necessary postural alignment for sitting includes a level pelvis and a reasonably straight spine.[118, 199] The loss of motion associated with hip dislocation can alter seating[53, 90, 117] (see Chapter 19). Excessive pelvic obliquity reduces the sitting surface area and causes excessive pressure on the bony prominences of the pelvis.[142, 172, 199] The manage-

TABLE 53–5 Comparison of Baclofen, Dantrolene, Diazepam

Feature	Baclofen	Dantrolene	Diazepam
Site of action	GABA "B" receptors in spinal cord	Intrafusal and extrafusal muscle fibers	Benzodiazepine sites in brainstem reticular formation and spinal cord
Mode of action	↓ Release of excitatory neurotransmitters from afferent terminals	↓ Release of calcium from sarcoplasmic reticulum	↑ GABA binding, potentiating presynaptic inhibition by GABA
Dose	Maximum: 20 mg qid (higher doses may be tolerated and therapeutic); start with 5 mg bid; increase by 5 mg/dose q3d	Maximum: 12 mg/kg/day (to 400 mg/day); start with 0.5 mg/kg bid; increase by 0.5 mg/kg q5–7d	Maximum: 20 mg qid; start with 2 mg bid; increase by 2 mg q2–3d
Half-life	3–4 hr	7–8 hr	8+ hr
Common side effects	Weakness, fatigue, confusion, depression, GI upset	Weakness, esp. if marginal strength; fatigue, drowsiness, diarrhea	Drowsiness, fatigue, urinary retention, constipation, impaired memory and recall
Precautions	May lower seizure threshold; abrupt withdrawal may precipitate seizures or hallucinations; additive side effects with other CNS depressants	May depress pulmonary function; reversible and irreversible hepatotoxicity (1.8%) in long-term (>2 mo) use, high dose (>300 mg/day), age >30 yr, but not reported in ≤16 yr	May develop tolerance and dependence; abrupt withdrawal may precipitate seizures; CNS effects more severe in MS and TBI and synergistic with other CNS depressants; can ↑ ataxia
Comments	Commonly recommended as drug of choice for MS and SCI; equal efficacy in complete and incomplete SCI; useful for flexor spasms	Commonly recommended as drug of choice for cerebral causes of spasticity but may be useful in SCI; little effect on cardiac or smooth muscle; monitor liver function tests before and during use	Possibly more useful in incomplete than complete SCI; effects more marked with IV than PO administration; other benzodiazepines also found useful including clorazepate and ketazolam; large index of safety; fatal overdose with diazepam alone almost unheard of

Abbreviations: CNS = central nervous system; GABA = γ-aminobutyric acid; GI = gastrointestinal; IV = intravenous; MS = multiple sclerosis; SCI = spinal cord injury; TBI = total body involvement.
Modified from Massagli TL: Spasticity and its management in children. Phys Rehabil Clin 1991; 2:867–890.

TABLE 53–6   Common Orthopedic Surgeries in Cerebral Palsy

Surgical Procedure	Purpose	Positioning Considerations	Treatment

Hip flexor lengthening
  Usually iliopsoas
  Sometimes proximal rectus femoris
  Rarely sartorius
	Increase extension ROM
	Decrease muscle imbalance—risk of hip subluxation
	Improve alignment stance, gait
		Avoid prolonged sitting
		Prone wedge preferred
		Standing frame with foot control (casts/AFOs)
		Prone at night (with or without body splint)
			Maintain length of hip flexor muscles
			Strengthen hip flexors (need for stairs, gait)
			Strengthen hip extensors

Hip adductor lengthening
  Usually proximal—origin
  Adductor longus, gracilis
  Sometimes adductor brevis
	Increase hip abduction
	Decrease scissoring
	Decrease abnormal muscle imbalance—risk of hip subluxation
	Increase base of support
	Improve hygiene, positioning
		Abduction at night, usually prone
		With/without night splint
		Abduction wedge on prone wedge/wheelchair
			Maintain length of hip adductors (knees flexed and extended)
			Strengthen hip adductors and abductors

Hamstring lengthening
  Medial/lateral hamstrings
  Almost always distal
	Increase knee extension
	Improve standing alignment
	Decrease crouch posture
	Increase stance-phase stability in gait, improved alignment
	Increase step length → increased terminal swing phase and heel-strike ability
	Increase positioning options
		Avoid prolonged sitting
		Prone wedge preferred (consider soft knee splints)
		Standing frame with foot control
		Prone at night with soft knee splints or night splints
			Maintain length of hamstrings (avoid knee hyperextension)
			Strengthen hamstrings and quadriceps (proximal and distal), especially terminal knee extension
			Monitor for overactive quadriceps, increase in extensor tone → knee hyperextension

Achilles tendon lengthening Five different types: Baker, percutaneous, sliding, fractional lengthening, vulpius	Increase dorsiflexion ROM Increase full-foot contact for standing and gait Increase ability for heel-strike in gait Allow for bracing	Initially no dorsiflexion beyond neutral Standing with neutral dorsiflexion only Temporary splint/cast initially to maintain ROM—begin early supportive weightbearing Sitting OK, if TALs only and other muscles not tight If prone wedge—feet off edge with AFO/cast/splint AFO approximately 6 mo (surgeon discretion) AFO/cast/splint at night	Maintain length of plantar flexors Strengthen plantar flexors and dorsiflexors Avoid overstretching—could lead to crouch posture (Special attention when considering hinged AFOs) (Repeat procedures common—especially if done at early age)

Abbreviations: ROM, range of motion; AFO, ankle-foot orthosis; TALs, tendoachilles lengthening.
From Feathergill B: Personal communications, 1993.

ment of the hip is complex.[47, 225] Early detection of subluxation is possible with sequential radiographs of the pelvis. Physical examination of the hip is not sufficient to detect subluxation.[1]

If the hip is subluxated, the surgeon might be able to reduce the overpowering muscle forces by surgically lengthening the iliopsoas and adductor muscles around the hip.[78, 122] This is a brief procedure that not only improves femoral head coverage under the acetabulum but also allows easier dressing, diapering, cleaning, and positioning.[38] If the hip progresses to dislocation, then a more extensive procedure is necessary.[119] The femur and acetabulum need reconstruction, depending on the age and extent of the pathologic changes.[15, 197, 216] Commonly, excessive anteversion and a valgus orientation affects the femur. Acetabular dysplasia contributes to the inability of the femoral head to remain covered. A combination of muscle lengthenings, varus derotational osteotomy of the femur, and augmentation procedures of the acetabulum are complex, arduous, and require postoperative immobilization for as long as 6 to 8 weeks.[142] Complications can occur following these procedures, including femoral fractures, heterotopic ossification, and peripheral neuropathy, depending on the concomitant surgeries.[144, 190] Rehabilitation plays an important role following cast removal.[91, 160] If the femoral articular cartilage is eroded and the hip becomes painful, the options for salvage are limited and fraught with problems. Hip fusion, artificial joint replacement, and finally resection of the femoral head can afford relief of the pain.[118] Painful hips are a chronic problem and need to be managed with multiple modalities.

The pelvis is also influenced by the hamstrings. The hamstrings act as hip extensors but the major pull of this muscle is to tilt the pelvis in a posterior direction. Sacral sitting with constant sliding out of a wheelchair can be partially corrected by a hamstring release.[90, 117] Distal hamstring lengthening is the more common surgery, but a proximal lengthening may also be considered.[77] Other problems with sitting, which can be addressed surgically less frequently, are extensor contractures of the hips and knee.

Scoliosis or kyphosis can be progressive.[204] Early treatment usually involves using a molded thoracic lumbar orthosis.[247] It is not thought that this prevents progression, but rather improves trunk support and slows the rate of progress. Total contact support can be incorporated into a contoured seating system. If a curve progresses beyond 40 degrees, fusion is considered to avoid compromise of the respiratory system.[5, 142, 213] If the deformity is rigid and extends over a long segment, staged procedures are performed. The risk of anesthesia, infection, blood loss, neurological compromise, and pseudarthrosis should be considered and planned for before surgery.[155]

Surgery for Standing

Supported standing and transfers are possible when the ankle can be held in the neutral position and the knee has less than 20 degrees of flexion contracture.[233] The surgical procedures used to improve alignment for these skills are hamstring lengthenings and Achilles tendon lengthenings.[88, 131, 201] Hip flexion contractures can also hinder standing and need attention if greater than 20 degrees.[203] Table 53–4 provides a description of procedures as well as the postoperative immobilization precautions.

Surgery for Ambulation

Surgery to improve ambulation remains problematic.[174] Difficulty in predicting outcome for the ambulator has led to caution in recommending orthopedic surgery.[70, 73, 75, 92] Close observation, aggressive bracing, and vigorous PT can temper the effect of dynamic tone and static contractures.[22] The tendency to scissor can hinder forward progression. Adductor myotomies in combination with hamstring lengthenings can create a better base of support and a more upright posture.[102, 120, 182] Recently, rectus femoris transfers and lengthenings have decreased the problem of stiff-knee gait following hamstring release.[62, 93] A braceable foot or a foot that allows for foot-flat or heel-strike is desirable for stance.[6, 16] Orthopedic surgery can affect balance, but the central processing of balance reactions remains the same after surgery. Assistive devices can play an important transitional role in household or community ambulation. A reverse walker can assist with upright posture better than the traditional forward walker.[153]

The use of gait analysis has refined the observation of components of the gait cycle and the combined effect of contractures on gait dynamics. Gait analysis defines cadence, velocity, stride length, and ranges of motion of the hip, knee, and ankle during various phases of the gait cycle and the timing of muscular activity. Some gait laboratories also measure the forces generated at each joint. Gait analysis provides consistent objective information which enhances orthopedic decision making and improves outcome studies[92] (see Chapter 5). Energy expenditure for some children with spastic CP can be as high as 350% of normal.[41] Energy expenditure is an important consideration for continued community ambulation.[92, 173]

Other Surgeries

Upper extremity surgery is uncommonly done to improve the function of the hand.[214] Flexor carpi ulnaris transfer has a place in reducing wrist flexion deformity. The active use of the hand, however, is dependent on stereognosis and two-point discrimination.[50, 234]

Neurosurgical procedures such as stereotactic ablation of selected thalamic nuclei and chronic electrical stimulation of the cerebellum or posterior columns have been unsuccessful in reducing spasticity in the child with CP.[52, 236] Selective posterior rhizotomy (SPR) and intrathecal baclo-

fen pumps are two current neurosurgical procedures that hold promise in reducing spasticity.[2, 4, 187, 191–193] Reduction in tone, as recorded by the modified Ashworth scale in both procedures, is improved.[165, 194] Gait analysis studies of children undergoing SPR have consistently shown an improved availability of range of motion at the knee and hip, resulting in an increased stride length.[34, 238, 239] Careful selection is critical because the weakness, which is an anticipated part of the postoperative recovery period, can reduce the level of independence of children who depend on their spasticity to transfer or stand.[165]

Other Interventions

In addition to surgical management of contractures, motor point blocks and, recently, botulism injections can be used as adjunct management of the spastic muscle.[46, 54, 55, 72, 217, 139] These procedures are used to improve range of motion during the child's younger years when orthopedic surgery should be delayed. Indications for the use of each and the advantages are listed in Table 53–7.

Functional electrical stimulation and biofeedback can be helpful for training specific muscles.[17, 44, 45, 157] Another modality that is gaining attention for improving strength in the child with CP is therapeutic electrical stimulation. The use of low-voltage, high-frequency electrical stimulation increases blood flow and improves muscle growth and strength.[185]

The utilization of medication to reduce drooling and improve bladder control facilitates socialization. The most commonly used drugs are oxybutinin (Ditropan), scopolamine, and glycopyrrolate.[152, 222]

The effectiveness of any specific intervention for the child with CP is difficult to study owing to the multihandicapping nature of CP, lack of outcome measures, difficulty in obtaining control groups, and historically poor study designs. The encouraging development of appropriate evaluative measures, adherence to randomized control studies, and the use of meta-analysis portend improved understanding of the use of therapies on the outcome of the child with CP.[107, 128, 133, 181, 183, 212, 235] The use of gait analysis not only improves decision making prior to surgeries but allows objective analysis of outcome following surgery.[91, 219] Harris has provided a review of efficacy studies (see Table 53–4).

Most studies of the effectiveness of PT and other treatment are inconclusive.[114, 161, 215, 231] Goldkamp[95] reviewed ADL outcome in children with CP and reported that few children after the age of 4 years achieved independence in their ADL. Investigators have found that the children most likely to improve in motor abilities were those children with higher intelligence quotients (IQs) and lesser involvement of the neuromuscular system.[95] Similar conclusions were obtained from a study by Perry and colleagues[195] in evaluating the use of Rolfing in CP. The use of a single-study design has demonstrated the positive effect of tone-reducing AFOs.[241] Cost containment provides the impetus for further study of the effects of therapy, including difficult issues such as frequency and duration.

SUMMARY

Successful rehabilitation of the child with CP includes the prevention of additional impairments, reduction of dis-

TABLE 53–7   Comparison of Botulinum Type A Toxin and Phenol

Blocking Agent	Administered	Effectiveness	Advantages	Drawbacks	Complications
Botulinum type A toxin	Injected into muscle	Lasts 12–30 wk	Easy to administer Diffuses readily into muscle Painless Can be administered without anesthesia	Effects are always transient Lasts only 12–30 wk Limited approval	No significant complications reported
Phenol block	Injected into motor points of involved muscle	Lasts 4–12 mo	Use is widely approved Lasts longer than botulinum toxin Cumulative effects often occur	Can be painful May require general anesthesia during administration Takes more skill to administer	Transient dysesthesias and numbness Hematomas may occur, which negate the effects of treatment If a large intravascular injection occurs, phenol can cause systemic effects such as muscle tremors and convulsions, as well as depressed cardiac activity, blood pressure, and respiration

From Gormley M: Personal communications, 1994.

ability, and improved integration of the individual into the community. Total independence may not be achievable or desirable for all patients. The pediatrician's primary interest for the child with CP is to provide preventive and diagnostic healthcare. The developmental pediatrician views the impact the cerebral palsy has on the child's development, while the pediatric orthopedist is interested in the impact of static and dynamic contractures on mobility. The pediatric physiatrist views the impact of CP on the child's overall medical, surgical, and therapeutic options. Facilitating the ability of the child and family to set functional goals is our primary responsibility. This process takes cooperation, prioritization of competing interests, and an advocacy position for the child. Physiatrists have an important place in assisting the person with CP to achieve the independence he or she desires within the constraints of the community environment.

References

1. Abel MF, Wenger DR, Mubarak P, et al: Quantitative analysis in hip dysplasia in cerebral palsy: A study of radiographs and 3-D reformatted images. J Pediatr Orthop 1994; 14:283–289.
2. Abbott R, Johann SL: Selective posterior rhizotomy for the treatment of spasticity: A review. Childs Nerv Syst 1989; 5:337–346.
3. Agnarsson U, Warde C, McCarthy G, et al: Anorectal function of children with neurological problems. II: Cerebral palsy. Dev Med Child Neurol 1993; 35:903–908.
4. Albright AL, Cervi A, Singletary J: Intrathecal baclofen for spasticity in cerebral palsy. JAMA 1991; 265:1418–1422.
5. Allen BL, Ferguson RL: L-rod instrumentation for scoliosis in cerebral palsy. J Pediatr Orthop 1982; 2:87.
6. Alman BA, Craig CL, Zimbler S: Subtalar arthrodesis for stabilization of valgus hindfoot in patients with cerebral palsy. J Pediatr Orthop 1993; 13:634–641.
7. American Academy of Pediatrics: The Doman-Delacato treatment of neurologically handicapped children. Pediatrics 1982; 70:810–812.
8. Reference deleted in proof.
9. Anderson JP, Snow B, Dorey FJ, et al: Efficacy of soft splints in reducing knee flexion contractures. Dev Med Child Neurol 1988; 30:502–508.
10. Anderson L: Swimming to win. In Jones JA (ed): Training Guide to Cerebral Palsy Sports, ed 3. Champaign, Ill, Human Kinetics, 1988.
11. Ayres AJ: The Development of Sensory Integration Theory and Practice. Dubuque, Iowa, Kendall/Hunt, 1974.
12. Ayres, AJ: Effect of sensory integrative therapy on the coordination of children with choreoathoid movements. Am J Occup Ther 1977; 31:291–293.
13. Ayres AJ: Sensory Integration and Learning Disorders. Los Angeles, Western Psychological Services, 1972.
14. Bachrack S, Greenspun B: Care of the adult with cerebral palsy. Del Med J 1990; 62:1287–1295.
15. Bagg M, Farber J, Miller F: Long-term follow-up of hip subluxation in cerebral palsy patients. J Pediatr Orthop 1993; 13:32–36.
16. Banks HJ, Green WT: The correction of equinus deformity in cerebral palsy. J Bone Joint Surg Am 1958; 40:1359–1379.
17. Basmajian J: Biofeedback in therapeutic exercise. In Basmajian J (ed): Therapeutic Exercise. Baltimore, Williams & Wilkins, 1984.
18. Batshaw ML, Eicher PS: Cerebral palsy. Pediatr Clin North Am 1993; 40:537–551.
19. Bax M: Aims and outcomes of therapy for the cerebral palsied child. Dev Med Child Neurol 1986; 28:695–698.
20. Bax T, Coombes M, Bax M, et al: The health and social needs of physically handicapped young adults. Dev Med Child Neurol 1985; 15:27–37.
21. Bee HL, Barnard KE, Eyres SJ, et al: Prediction of IQ and language skill from perinatal status, child performance, family characteristics, and mother-infant interaction. Child Dev 1982; 53:1134–1156.
22. Bertoti DB: Effect of short leg casting on ambulation in children with cerebral palsy. Phys Ther 1986; 66:1522–1529.
23. Bhushan VB, Paneth N, Kiely JL: Impact of improved survival of very low birth weight infants on recent secular trends in the prevalence of cerebral palsy. Pediatrics 1993; 91:1094–1100.
24. Biether JK, Cummins SK, Nelson KB: The California Cerebral Palsy Project. Pediatr Perinatol Epidemiol 1993; 6:339–351.
25. Bleck EE: Locomotion prognosis in cerebral palsy. Dev Med Child Neurol 1975; 17:18–25.
26. Bleck EE: Orthopaedic Management of Cerebral Palsy. Philadelphia, WB Saunders, 1982.

27. Bleck EE: Severe orthopedic disability in childhood: Solutions provided by rehabilitation engineering. Orthop Clin North Am 1978; 9:509–526.

28. Bleck EE: Where have all the cerebral palsy children gone?—the needs of adults. Dev Med Child Neurol 1984; 26:674–676.

29. Bobath B: Abnormal Posture Reflex Activity Caused by Brain Lesions, ed 2. London, Heinemann, 1971.

30. Bobath B: Motor development: Its effect on general development and application to the treatment of cerebral palsy. Physiotherapy 1971; 57:526.

31. Bobath K: Neurophysiological Basis for Treatment of Cerebral Palsy. Lavenham, England, Spastics International, 1980.

32. Bobath B: A neuro-developmental treatment of cerebral palsy. Physiotherapy 1963; 49:242–244.

33. Bobath B, Bobath K: Motor Development in the Different Types of Cerebral Palsy. London, Heinmann, 1975.

34. Boscarino LF, Ounpuu S, Davis RV, et al: Effects of selective dorsal rhizotomy on gait in children with cerebral palsy. J Pediatr Orthop 1993; 13:174–179.

35. Bozynski M, Nelson M, Genaze D, et al: Cranial ultrasonography and the production of cerebral palsy in infants weighing ≤ 1200 grams at birth. Dev Med Child Neurol 1988; 30:342–348.

36. Bradley R, Caldwell B: Early home environment and changes in mental test performance in children from 6–36 months. Dev Psychol 1976; 12:93–97.

37. Brown JK, Fulford GE: Position as a cause of deformity in children with cerebral palsy. Dev Med Child Neurol 1976; 18:305–314.

38. Brunner R, Baumann JU: Clinical benefit of reconstruction of dislocated or subluxated hip joints in patients with spastic cerebral palsy. J Pediatr Orthop 1994; 14:290–294.

39. Burton AW: Assessing the perceptual-motor interaction in the developmentally disabled and non-handicapped children. Adapted Phys Activity Q 1990; 7:325–337.

40. Butler C: Effects of powered mobility on self-initiated behaviors of very young children with locomotor disability. Dev Med Child Neurol 1986; 28:325–332.

41. Campbell J, Ball J: Energetics of walking in cerebral palsy. Orthop Clin North Am 1978; 9:374–377.

42. Capute AJ, Diehl R: Functional development evaluation. Pediatr Clin North Am 1993; 20:3–26.

43. Carlson L: Therapeutic riding and the rehabilitative process. Phys Ther Forum 1987; 6:4.

44. Carmick J: Clinical use of neuromuscular electrical stimulation for children with cerebral palsy: Part 1. Lower Extremity. Phys Ther 1993; 73:505–513.

45. Carmick J: Clinical use of neuromuscular electrical stimulation for children with cerebral palsy: Part 2. Upper extremity. Phys Ther 1993; 7:514–522.

46. Carpenter EB: Role of the nerve block in the foot and ankle in the therapeutic management of cerebral palsy. Foot Ankle 1979; 4:164–166.

47. Carr C, Gage JR: The fate of the nonoperated hip in cerebral palsy. J Pediatr Orthop 1987; 7:262–267.

48. Carvalho O: A new objective method for evaluation of muscle relaxants in congenital spastic diplegia. Dev Med Child Neurol 1966; 8:34–36.

49. Center for Law and Education: Educational rights of children with disabilities under IDEA and Section 504 educational rights of children with disabilities: A primer for advocates. Cambridge, Mass, Center for Law and Education.

50. Chakerian DL, Larson MA: Effects of upper extremity weight-bearing on hand-opening and prehension patterns of children with cerebral palsy. Dev Med Child Neurol 1993; 35:216–229.

51. Cohen HJ, Birch HG: Some considerations for evaluating the Doman-Delacato "patterning" method. Pediatrics 1970; 45:302.

52. Cooper I, Riklan M, Amin I, et al: Chronic cerebellar stimulation in cerebral palsy. Neurology 1976; 26:744–749.

53. Cooperman DR, Bartucci E, Dietrick E, et al: Hip dislocation in spastic cerebral palsy: Long-term consequences. J Pediatr Orthop 1987; 7:268–276.

54. Cosgrove AP, Corry IS, Graham HK: Botulinum toxin in the management of the lower limb in cerebral palsy. Dev Med Child Neurol 1994; 36:386–396.

55. Cosgrove AP, Graham HK: Botulinum toxin A prevents the development of contractures in the hereditary spastic mouse. Dev Med Child Neurol 1994; 36:379–385.

56. Costello AM de L, Hamilton P, Baudin J, et al: Prediction of neurodevelopmental impairment at four years from brain ultrasound appearance of very preterm infants. Dev Med Child Neurol 1988; 30:711–722.

57. Cottam P, McCartney E, Cullen C: The effectiveness of conductive education principles with profoundly retarded multiple handicapped children. Br Disord Commun 1985; 20:45–49.

58. Cummins SK, Nelson KB, Giether JK, et al: Cerebral palsy in four northern California counties, births 1983 through 1985. J Pediatr 1993; 123:230–237.

59. Currie DM, Gershkoff AM, Cifu DX: Geriatric rehabilitation. 3. Mid- and late-life effects of early-life disabilities. Arch Phys Med Rehabil 1993; 74(suppl 5):S413–416.

60. Curtis K: Wheelchair sports medicine. In Klafs CE, Armheim DD (eds): Modern Principles of Athletic Training, ed 4. St Louis, Mosby–Year Book, 1977, pp 16–18.

61. d'Avignon M, Noren L, Arman R: Early physiotherapy and Vojta or Bobath in infants with suspected neuromotor disturbance. Neuropediatrics 1981; 12:232–237.

62. Damron TA, Breed AL, Cook T: Diminished knee flexion after hamstring surgery in cerebral palsy patients: Prevalence and severity. J Pediatr Orthop 1993; 13:188–191.

63. Davidoff R: Antispasticity drugs: Mechanisms of action. Ann Neurol 1985; 17:107–116.

64. Deaver G: Cerebral palsy: Methods of Evaluation and Treatment. Rehabilitation Monograph 9, New York, Institute for Rehabilitative Medicine, 1952.

65. Deaver G: Methods of treating the neuromuscular disabilities. Arch Phys Med Rehabil 1956; 37:363–367.

66. Denhoff E, Feldman S, Smith GM, et al: Treatment of spastic cerebral palsied children with sodium dantrolene. Dev Med Child Neurol 1975; 17:736–774.

67. Dickey R, Shealey SH: Using technology to control the environment. Am J Occup Ther 1987; 41:717–721.

68. Doman R, Spitz E, Zucman E et al: Children with severe brain injuries. Neurological organization in terms of mobility. JAMA 1960; 174:257–264.

69. Dormans JP: Orthopedic management of children with cerebral palsy. Child Dev Dis 1993; 40:645–657.

70. Dormans JP: Orthopedic management of children with cerebral palsy. Pediatr Clin North Am 1993; 40:645–657.

71. Drvaric DM, Roberts JM, Burke SW, et al: Gastroesophageal evaluation in totally involved cerebral palsy patients. J Pediatr Ortho 1987; 7:187–190.

72. Easton JKM, Ozel T, Halpern D: Intramuscular neurolysis for spasticity in children. Arch Phys Med Rehabil 1979; 60:155–158.

73. Eggers GWN, Evans EB: Surgery in cerebral palsy. J Bone Joint Surg Am 1963; 45:1275.

74. Eicher PS, Batshaw ML: Cerebral palsy, the child with developmental disabilities. Pediatr Clin North Am 1993; 40:537–551.

75. Eilert RE, MacEwen GD: Varus derotational osteotomy of the femur in cerebral palsy. Clin Orthop 1977; 125:168.

76. Ellenberg JH, Nelson KB: Cluster of perinatal events identifying infants at high risk for death or disability. J Pediatr 1988; 113:546–552.

77. Elmer E, Wenger D, Mubarak S, et al: Proximal hamstring lengthening in the sitting cerebral palsy patient. J Pediatr Orthop 1992; 12:329–336.

78. Erken L, Einhard HW, Bischof FM: Iliopsoas transfer in cerebral palsy: The long-term outcome. J Pediatr Orthop 1994; 14:295–298.

79. Eyman RK, Grossman HJ, Chaney RH, et al: The life expectancy of profoundly handicapped people with mental retardation. N Engl J Med 1990; 323:584–589.

80. Fay T: The use of pathological and unlocking reflexes in the rehabilitation of spastics. Am J Phys Med 1954; 33:33–47.

81. Fee M, Charney E, Robertson W: Nutritional assessment of the young child with cerebral palsy. Infants Young Child 1988; 1:33–40.

82. Fernandez JE, Pitetti KH: Training of ambulatory individuals with cerebral palsy. Arch Phys Med Rehabil 1993; 74:468–472.

83. Ferrara MS, Buckley WE, et al: The injury experience of the competitive athlete with a disability: Prevention implications. Med Sci Sports Exerc 1992; 24:184–188.

84. Foley J: Dyskinetic and dystonic cerebral palsy. Acta Paediatr 1992; 81:57–60.

85. Freeman A: Provision of related services for children with chronic disabilities. Pediatrics 1993; 92:879–881.

86. Freeman JM, Nelson KB: Special articles: Intrapartum asphyxia and cerebral palsy. Pediatrics 1988; 82:240–241.

87. Fremart A: Provision of related services for children with chronic disabilities. Pediatrics 1993; 92:879–881.

88. Fulford GE: Surgical management of ankle and foot deformities in cerebral palsy. Clin Orthop 1990; 253:55–61.

89. Fulford GE, Brown JK: Position as a cause of deformity in children with cerebral palsy. Dev Med Child Neurol 1976; 18:305–314.

90. Fulford GE, Cairns TP, Sloan Y: Sitting problems of children with cerebral palsy. Dev Med Child Neurol 1982; 24:48–53.

91. Gage JR: Gait analysis in cerebral palsy. Clin Dev Med 1991; 121:177–183.

92. Gage JR, Fabian D, Hicks R, et al: Pre- and post-operative gait analysis in patients with spastic diplegia: A preliminary report. J Pediatr Orthop 1984; 4:715–718.

93. Gage JR, Perry J, Hicks RR et al: Rectus femoris transfer to improve knee function of children with cerebral palsy. Dev Med Child Neurol 1987; 29:159–166.

94. Gillette H: Systems of Therapy in Cerebral Palsy. Springfield, Ill, Charles C Thomas, 1969.

95. Goldkamp O: Treatment effectiveness in cerebral palsy. Arch Phys Med Rehabil 1984; 65:232–234.

96. Graham M, Levene MI, Trounce JQ, et al: Prediction of cerebral palsy in very low birth weight infants: Prospective ultrasound study. Lancet 1987; 2:593–596.

97. Gramer R, Keller K, Baughman, J, et al: Data analysis on 600 pediatric videofluoroscopic swallow studies. Personal communication, 1994.

98. Greiner BM, Czerniecki JM, Deitz JC: Gait parameters of children with spastic diplegia: A comparison of effects of posterior and anterior walkers. Arch Phys Med Rehabil 1993; 74:381–385.

99. Griether JK, Cummins, SK, Nelson, KB: The California Cerebral Palsy Project. Pediatr Perinatol Epidemiol 1992; 6:339–351.

100. Griether JK, Nelson KB, Cummins SK: Twinning and cerebral palsy: experience in four northern California counties, births 1983–1985. Pediatrics 1993; 92:854–888.

101. Guzzetta F, Shackelford GD, Volpe S, et al: Periventricular intraparenehymal echodensities in the premature newborn: Critical determinant of neurological outcome. Pediatrics 1986; 78:995–1006.

102. Hadley N, Chambers C, Scarborough N, et al: Knee motion following multiple soft-tissue releases in ambulatory patients with cerebral palsy. J Pediatr Orthop 1992; 12:324–328.

103. Hagberg B, Hagberg G, Olow I, et al: The changing panorama of cerebral palsy in Sweden. V: The birth year period 1979–1982. Acta Paediatr Scand 1989; 78:283–290.

104. Halpren D: Therapeutic exercises for cerebral palsy. In Basmajian JV (ed): Therapeutic Exercise. Baltimore, Williams & Wilkins, 1984.

105. Harrington ED, Lin RS, Gage JR: Use of the anterior floor reaction orthosis in patients with cerebral palsy. Bull Orthot Prosthet 1984; 37:34–42.

106. Harris S: Early diagnosis of spastic diplegia, spastic hemiplegia, and quadriplegia. Am J Dis Child 1989; 143:1356–1360.

107. Harris SR: The effectiveness of early intervention for at-risk and handicapped children. In Guralnick MJ, Bennett FC (eds): The Effectiveness of Early Intervention for At Risk and Handicapped Children. San Diego, Academic Press, 1987, pp 175–212.

108. Harris SR: Efficacy of early intervention in pediatric rehabilitation. Phys Med Rehabil Clin North Am 1991; 2:725–742.

109. Harris SR, Atwater S, Crowe T: Accepted and controversial neuromotor therapies for infants at high risk for cerebral palsy. J Perinatol 1985; 8:3–12.

110. Harris SR, Tada WL: Providing developmental therapy services. In Garwood SG, Fewell RF (eds): Educating Handicapped Infants, Rockville, Md, Aspen 1983, pp 343–368.

111. Haynes UE: The National Collaborative Infant Project. In Tjossen TD (ed): Intervention Strategies for High Risk Infants and Children, Baltimore, University Park Press, 1976, pp 509–534.

112. Healy A: Pediatricians' role in the development and implementation of an Individual Education Plan (IEP) and/or an Individual Family Service Plan (IFSP). Pediatrics 1992; 89:340–342.

113. Hennrikus WL, Rosenthal RK, Kasser JR: Incidence of spondylolisthesis in ambulatory cerebral palsy patients. J Pediatr Orthop 1993; 13:37–40.

114. Herndon WA, Troup P, Yngve DA, et al: Effects of neurodevelopmental treatment on movement patterns of children with cerebral palsy. J Pediatr Orthop 1987; 7:395–400.

115. Hill AE: Problems in relation to independent living: A retrospective study of physically disabled school-leavers. Dev Med Child Neurol 1993; 35:1111–1115.

116. Hinderer KA, Harris SR, Purdy AH, et al: Effects of tone-reducing vs standard plaster casts on gait improvement of children with cerebral palsy. Dev Med Child Neurol 1988; 30:370–377.

117. Hoffer M: Management of the hip in cerebral palsy. J Bone Joint Surg Am 1986; 68:629–631.

118. Hoffer M, Abraham E, Nickel VL, et al: Salvage surgery of the hip to improve sitting posture of mentally retarded, severely disabled children with cerebral palsy. Dev Med Child Neurol 1992; 14:51–59.

119. Hoffer M, Stein G, Koffman M, et al: Femoral varus-derotation osteotomy in spastic cerebral palsy. J Bone Surg Am 1985; 67:1229–1335.

120. Hoffinger SA, Rab GT, Abou-Ghaida H: Hamstrings in cerebral palsy crouch gait. J Pediatr Orthop 1993; 13:722–726.

121. Holland LJ, Steadward RD: Effects of resistence in flexibility training and strength, spasticity/muscle tone and range of motion of elite athletes with cerebral palsy. Palestra summer; 1990, pp 27–31.

122. Howard CB, Williams LA, Mackie I: Factors affecting the incidence of hip dislocation in cerebral palsy. J Bone Joint Surg Br 1985; 67:530–532.

123. Hueberman G: Organized sports activity with cerebral palsy adolescents. Rehabil Lit 1976; 37:103–106.

124. Irwin-Carruthers SH: Results of early intervention in the baby with cerebral motor disturbance. S Afr J Physiother, 1981, pp 34–37.

125. Janicki M: Aging, cerebral palsy, and older persons with mental retardation. Aust N Z J Dev Disabilities 1989; 15:311–320.

126. Jankowski LW, Sullivan J: Aerobic and neuromuscular training: An effect of capacity, efficacy and fatiguability of patients with traumatic brain injuries. Arch Phys Med Rehabil 1990; 71:500–504.

127. Jarvis SN, Holloway JS, Hey EN, et al: Increase in cerebral palsy in normal birth weight babies. Arch Dis Child 1985; 60:1113–1121.

128. Jeffe AM: Using health-related quality of life measures. Physical therapy outcomes research. Phys Ther 1993; 73:523–527.

129. Jevsevar DS, Karlin LI: The relationship between preoperative nutritional status and complications after an operation for scoliosis in patients who have cerebral palsy. J Bone Joint Surg Am 1993; 75:880–884.

130. Johnstone K, Perrin J: Sports for the handicapped child. Phys Med Rehabil 1991; 5:331–350.

131. Jones ET, Knapp RB: Assessment and management of the lower extremity in cerebral palsy. Orthop Clin North Am 1987; 18:725–738.

132. Kalen V, Conklin M, Sherman F: Untreated scoliosis in severe cerebral palsy. J Pediatr Orthop 1992; 12:337–340.

133. Keller RB: Outcomes research in orthopaedics. J Am Acad Orthop Surg 1993; 1:523–527.

134. Kelly G: Vestibular stimulation as a form of therapy. Physiotherapy 1989; 75:136–140.

135. Khalili A, Betts HB: Peripheral nerve block with phenol in the management of spasticity. JAMA 1967; 200:1155.

136. Kibele A: Occupational therapy's role in improving the quality of life for persons with cerebral palsy. Am J Occup Ther 1991; 45:371–377.

137. Kiely M, Lubin RA, Kiely JZ: Descriptive epidemiology of cerebral palsy. Publ Health Rev 1984; 12:79–101.

138. Klapper ZS, Birch HG: The relation of childhood characteristics to outcome in young adults with cerebral palsy. Dev Med Child Neurol 1966; 8:645–656.

139. Koman LA, Mooney JF, Goodman A: Management of valgus hindfoot deformity in pediatric cerebral palsy. J Pediatr Orthop 1993; 13:180–183.

140. Koman LA, Mooney JF, Smith BP et al: Management of spasticity in cerebral palsy with botulinum-A toxin: Report of a preliminary, randomized, double-blind trial. J Pediatr Orthop 1994; 14:299–303.

141. Köng E: Very early treatment of cerebral palsy. Dev Med Child Neurol 1966; 8:198–202.

142. Koop SE: Orthopedic aspects of static encephalopathies. In Miller G, Ramer J (eds): Static Encephalopathies of Infancy and Childhood. New York, Academic Press, 1992, pp 95–109.

143. Krageloh-Mann I, Hagberg G, Meisner C, et al: Bilateral spastic cerebral palsy—A comparative study between southwest Germany and western Sweden. I: Clinical patterns and disabilities. Dev Med Child Neurol 1993; 35:1031–1047.

144. Krum SD, Miller F: Heterotopic ossification after hip and spine surgery in children with cerebral palsy. J Pediatr Orthop 1993; 13:739–743.

145. Kuban KC, Leviton A: Cerebral palsy. N Engl J Med 1994; 330:188–195.

146. Kudrjavcev T, Schoenberg BB, Kurland LT, et al: Cerebral palsy: Survival rates, associated handicaps, and distribution by clinical subtype—Rochester, MN, 1950–1976. Neurology 1985; 35:900–903.

147. Kudrjavcev T, Schoenberg BB, Kurland LT, et al: Cerebral palsy: Trends in incidence and changes in concurrent neonatal mortality-Rochester, MN, 1950–1976. Neurology 1983; 33:1433–1438.

148. Laplaza FJ, Root L, Tassanawipas A, et al: Femoral torsion and neck-shaft angles in cerebral palsy. J Pediatr Orthop 1993; 13:192–199.

149. Law M, King G: Parent compliance with therapeutic interventions for children with cerebral palsy. Dev Med Child Neurol 1993; 35:983–990.

150. Lesny I, Stehlik A, Tomasek J, et al: Sensory disorders in cerebral palsy: Two-point discrimination. Dev Med Child Neurol 1993; 35:402–405.

151. Lespargot A, Langevin MF, Muller S, et al: Swallowing disturbances associated with drooling in cerebral palsied children. Dev Med Child Neurol 1993; 35:298–304.

152. Lewis D, Fontana C, Mehallick L, et al: Transdermal scopolaime for reduction of drooling in developmentally delayed children. Dev Med Child Neurol 1994; 36:484–486.

153. Levangie PK, Guihan MF, Meyer P, et al: Effect of altering handle position of a rolling walker on gait in children with cerebral palsy. Phys Ther 1989; 69:130–134.

154. Levine MS, Kliebhan L: Communication between physician and physical and occupational therapists: A neurodevelopmentally based prescription. Pediatrics 1981; 68:208–214.

155. Lonstein JE, Akbarnia A: Operative treatment of spinal deformities in patients with cerebral palsy or mental retardation: An analysis of one hundred and seven cases. J Bone Joint Surg Am 1983; 65:33–55.

156. Lundberg A: Longitudinal study of physical working capacity of young people with cerebral palsy. Dev Med Child Neurol 1984; 26:328–334.

157. Mackey S: The use of computer-assisted feedback in a motor control task for cerebral palsied children. Physiotherapy 1989; 75:143–148.

158. Maltais D: Fit 'n Flex: A family-centered Saturday morning group exercise class for children with spastic diplegic cerebral palsy. Dev Med Child Neurol 1993; 35:41.

159. Massagli TL: Spasticity and its management in children. Phys Rehabil Clin 1991; 2:867–890.

160. Mathias A: Management of cerebral palsy: Physical therapy in relation to orthopedic surgery. Phys Ther 1967; 47:473–482.

161. Mayo N: The effect of physical therapy for children with motor delay and cerebral palsy: A randomized clinical trial. Am J Phys Med Rehabil 1991; 70:258–267.

162. McCarty SM, McCarty SM, James PS, et al: Assessment of intelligence functioning across the life span in severe cerebral palsy. Dev Med Child Neurol 1986; 28:369–371.

163. McCuaig M, Frank G: The able self: Adaptive patterns and choices in independent living for a person with cerebral palsy. Am J Occup Ther 1991; 45:224–234.

164. McCubbin J, Shasby G: Effects of isokinetic exercise and adolescents with cerebral palsy. Adapted Phys Activity 1985; 2:56–64.

165. McDonald C: Selective dorsal rhizotomy: A critical review. Phys Med Rehabil 1991; 2:891–915.

166. McGrath S, Splaingard M, Alba H, et al: Survival and functional outcome of children with severe cerebral palsy following gastrostomy, abstract. Arch Phys Med Rehabil 1983; 73:133–137.

167. McMenamin JB, Shackelford GD, Volpe JJ: Outcome of neonatal intraventricular hemorrhage with echodense lesions. Ann Neurol 1984; 15:285–290.

168. Meadow R: Where have all the CP children gone? The needs of adults. Dev Med Child Neurol 1984; 26:669–676.

169. Molnar GE: Cerebral palsy. In Molnar GE (ed): Pediatric Rehabilitation. Baltimore, Williams & Wilkins, 1985, pp 481–533.

170. Molnar G: Long-term treatment of spasticity in children with cerebral palsy. In International Rehabilitation Medicine Association V Conference. 1987, pp 170–172.

171. Molnar GE, Gordon SU: Cerebral palsy: Predictive value of selected clinical signs of early prognostication of motor function. Arch Phys Med Rehabil 1976; 57:153–158.

172. Moreau M, Drummond D, Rogala E, et al: Natural history of the dislocated hip in spastic cerebral palsy. Dev Med Child Neurol 1979; 21:749–753.

173. Mossberg K, Linton K, Friske K: Ankle-foot orthoses: Effect on energy expenditure of gait in spastic diplegia children. Arch Phys Med Rehabil 1990; 70:490–494.

174. Mullaferoze P, Voro P: Surgery in lower limbs in cerebral palsy. Dev Med Child Neurol 1972; 14:45–50.

175. Naeye R, Peters E, Bartholomew M, et al: Origins of cerebral palsy. Am J Dis Child 1989; 143:1154–1162.

176. Nelson KB: What proportion of cerebral palsy is related to birth asphyxia? J Pediatr 1988; 112:572–574.

177. Nelson KB, Ellenberg JH: Antecedents of cerebral palsy. Multivariate analysis of risk. Am J Dis Child 1986; 315:81–86.

178. Nelson KB, Ellenberg JH: Children who outgrew cerebral palsy. Pediatrics 1982; 69:529–535.

179. Nwaobi O, Smith PD: Effect of adaptive seating on pulmonary function of children with cerebral palsy. Dev Med Child Neurol 1986; 28:351–354.

180. O'Grady R, Nishimura D, Kohn J et al: Vocational predictions compared with present vocational status of 60 young adults with cerebral palsy. Dev Med Child Neurol 1985; 27:775–784.

181. Ottenbacher KJ, Biocca Z, DeCrenter G, et al: Quantitative analysis of the effectiveness of physical therapy: Emphasis on the neurodevelopmental treatment approach. Phys Ther 1986; 66:1095–1105.

182. Ounpuu S, Muik E, Davis RB, et al: Rectus femoris surgery in children with cerebral palsy. Part II: A comparison between the effect of transfer and release of the distal rectus femoris on knee motion. J Pediatr Orthop 1993; 13:331–335.

183. Palmer FB, Shapiro BK, Wachtel RC, et al: The effects of physical therapy on cerebral palsy. A controlled trial in infants with spastic diplegia. N Engl J Med 1988; 13:803–808.

184. Paneth N, Kiely J: The frequency of cerebral palsy. A review of population studies in industrialized nations since 1956. In Stanley F, Alberman E (eds): The Epidemiology of Cerebral Palsies. Clinics in Developmental Medicine Series, No, 87, Philadelphia, JB Lippincott, 1984.

185. Pape KE, Kirsch SE, Galil A, et al: Neuromuscular approach to the motor deficits of cerebral palsy: A pilot study. J Pediatr Orthop 1993; 13:628–633.

186. Papile L, Munsick-Bruno G, Schaefer A: Relationship of cerebral intraventricular hemorrhage and early childhood neurologic handicaps. J Pediatr 1983; 103:273–277.

187. Park TS, Vogler GP, Phillips LH II, et al: Effects of selective dorsal rhizotomy for spastic diplegia on hip migration in cerebral palsy. Pediatr Neurosurg 1994; 20:43–49.

188. Parker DF, Carriere L, Hebestreit H, et al: Muscle performance and gross motor function of children with spastic cerebral palsy. Dev Med Child Neurol 1993; 35:17–23.

189. Patrick J, Boland M, Stoski S, et al: Rapid correction of wasting in children with cerebral palsy. Dev Med Child Neurol 1986; 28:734–739.

190. Payne LZ, DeLuca PA: Heterotopic ossification after rhizotomy and femoral osteotomy. J Pediatr Orthop 1993; 13:733–738.

191. Peacock WJ, Arens LJ, Berman B: Cerebral palsy spasticity: Selective posterior rhizotomy. Pediatr Neurosci 1987; 13:61–66.

192. Peacock WJ, Arens LJ, Peter J: Selective posterior rhizotomy: A long term follow up study. Childs Nerv Syst 1989; 5:148–152.

193. Peacock WJ, Staudt LA: Spasticity in cerebral palsy and selective posterior rhizotomy procedure. J Child Neurol 1990; 5:179–185.

194. Penn RD, Savoy SM, Corcos D, et al: Intrathecal baclofen for severe spinal spasticity. N Engl J Med 1989; 320:1517–1521.

195. Perry J, Jones M, Thomas L: Functional evaluation of Rolfing in cerebral palsy. Dev Med Child Neurol 1981; 23:717–729.

196. Peterson H, Coventry M: Long term results of surgical treatment of adults with cerebral palsy. Dev Med Child Neurol 1969; 11:35–43.

197. Petitt B: Surgery of the lower extremity in cerebral palsy: Considerations and approaches. Arch Phys Med Rehabil 1976; 57:443–447.

198. Phelps W: The rehabilitation of cerebral palsy. South Med J 1994; 34:770–775.

199. Rang M, Douglas G, Bennet G, et al: Seating for children with cerebral palsy. J Pediatr Orthop 1981; 1:279–286.

200. Rang M, Wright J: What have 30 years of medical progress done for cerebral palsy? Adv Cereb Palsy 1989; 247:55–60.

201. Rattey TE, Leahey L, Hyndman J, et al: Recurrence after Achilles tendon lengthening in cerebral palsy. J Pediatr Orthop 1993; 13:184–187.

202. Reid CJ, Borzyskowski M: Lower urinary tract dysfunction in cerebral palsy. Arch Dis Child 1993; 68:739–742.

203. Reimers J: Acetabular development after femoral osteotomy in cerebral palsy after age four years. J Pediatr Orthop 1992; 1:35–37.

204. Rinsky LA: Surgery of spinal deformity in cerebral palsy: Twelve years in the evolution of scoliosis management. Clin Orthop 1990; 253:100–109.

205. Robinson R: The frequency of other handicaps in children with cerebral palsy. Dev Med Child Neurol 1973; 15:305–312.

206. Rodriquez J, Claus D, Verellen G, et al: Periventricular leukomalacia and neuropathological correlations. Dev Med Child Neurol 1990; 32:347–352.

207. Rogers B, Arvedson J, Buck G, et al: Characteristics of dysphagia in children with cerebral palsy. Dysphagia 1994; 9:60–73.

208. Rogers BT, Srvedson J, Msall M, et al: Hypoxemia during oral feeding of children with severe cerebral palsy. Dev Med Child Neurol 1993; 35:3–10.

209. Rood M: Neurophysiological mechanisms utilized in the treatment of neuromuscular dysfunction. Am J Occup Ther 1956; 10:220–224.

210. Rose J, Haskell WL, Gamble JG: A comparison of oxygen pulse and respiratory exchange ratio in cerebral palsied and nondisabled children. Arch Phys Med Rehabil 1993; 74:702–705.

211. Rothery S, Benz H, Hoffer M, et al: Goal oriented approach to the physical therapy management of cerebral palsy. Contemp Orthop 1982; 5:59–64.

212. Russell DJ, Rosenbaum PL, Cadman DT, et al: The gross motor function measure: A means to evaluate the effects of physical therapy. Dev Med Child Neurol 1989; 31:341–352.

213. Samilson RL, Becharard R: Scoliosis in cerebral palsy: Incidence, distribution of curve patterns, natural history and thoughts on etiology. Curr Pract Orthop Surg 1973; 5:43–50.

214. Samilson RL, Green WL: Long-term results of upper limb surgery in cerebral palsy. Reconstr Surg Traumatol 1972; 13:43–50.

215. Scherzer AL, Mike V, Iison J: Physical therapy as a determinant of change in the cerebral palsied infant. Pediatrics 1979; 58:47–52.

216. Scrutton D, Baird G: Hip dysplasia in cerebral palsy. Dev Med Child Neurol 1993; 35:1028–1030.

217. Shaari CM, Sanders I: Quantifying how location and dose of botulinum toxin injections affect muscle paralysis. Muscle Nerve 1993; 16:964–969.

218. Shane H: Impact of AAC on natural speech production. NIDDR 1992, pp 92–105.

219. Shapiro A, Susak Z, Malkin C, et al: Preoperative and postoperative gait evaluation in cerebral palsy. Arch Phys Med Rehabil 1990; 71:236–240.

220. Sherrill C, Hinson M, Gench B, et al: Self-concepts of disabled young athletes. Percept Mot Skills 1990; 70:1093–1098.

221. Sherrill C, Rainbolt W: Self-actualization profiles of male able-bodied and cerebral palsied athletes. Adapted Phys Activity Q 1988; 5:108–119.

222. Siegel L, Klingbeil M: Control of drooling with transdermal scopolamine in a child with cerebral palsy. Dev Med Child Neurol 1991; 33:1013–1014.

223. Silver L: Acceptable and controversial approaches to treating the child with learning disabilities. Pediatrics 1975; 55:406.

224. Sola A, Piecuch RE: Prevalence of cerebral palsy: Estimations, calculations and neonatal care. Pediatrics 1994; 93:152–153.

225. Staheli L, Chew D: Slotted acetabular augmentation in childhood and adolescence. J Pediatr Orthop 1992; 12:569–580.

226. Stallings VA, Charney EB, Davies JC, et al: Nutritional status and growth of children with diplegic or hemiplegic cerebral palsy. Dev Med Child Neurol 1993; 35:997–1006.

227. Stallings VA, Charney EB, Davies JC, et al: Nutrition-related growth failure of children with quadriplegic cerebral palsy. Dev Med Child Neurol 1993; 35:126–138.

228. Stanley FJ, Alberman E (eds): The Epidemiology of the Cerebral Palsies. Clinics in Developmental Medicine Series, No. 87, Philadelphia, JB Lippincott, 1984.

229. Stanley FJ, Blair E, Hockey A, et al: Spastic quadriplegia in western Australia: A genetic epidemiological study. Dev Med Child Neurol 1993; 35:191–201.

230. Stanley FJ, Watson L: The cerebral palsies in western Australia: Trends 1968–1981. Am J Obstet Gynecol 1988; 158:89–92.

231. Stern FM, Gorga D: Neurodevelopmental treatment (NDT): Therapeutic intervention and its efficacy. Infants Young Children 1988; 23–32.

232. Taylor SJ: Evaluating the client with physical disabilities for wheelchair seating. Am J Occup Ther 1987; 711–716.

233. Tenuta J, Shelton VA, Miller F: Long-term follow-up of triple arthrodesis in patients with cerebral palsy. J Pediatr Orthop 1993; 13:713–716.

234. Thometz JG, Tachdjian M: Long-term follow-up of the flexor carpi ulnaris transfer in spastic hemiplegic children. J Pediatr Orthop 1988; 8:407–412.

235. Tirosh E, Rabino S: Physiotherapy for children with cerebral palsy. Am J Dis Child 1989; 143:552–555.

236. Trejos H, Araya R: Sterotactic surgery for cerebral palsy. Stereotact Funct Neurosurg 1990; 54–55:130–135.

237. Van-Heest AE, House J, Putman M: Sensibility deficiencies in the hands of children with spastic hemiplegia. J Hand Surg Am 1993; 18:278–281.

238. Vaughn CL, Berman B, Peacock WJ: Gait analysis and rhizotomy: Past experience and future considerations. Neurosurgery 1989; 4:445–458.

239. Vaughn CL, Berman B, Staudt LA, et al: Gait analysis of cerebral palsy before and after rhizotomy. Pediatr Neurosci 1988; 14:297–300.

240. Wadsworth JS, Harper DC: The social needs of adolescents with cerebral palsy. Dev Med Child Neurol 1993; 35:1019–1022.

241. Watt J, Sims D, Harckham F, et al: A prospective study of inhibitive casting as an adjunct to physiotherapy for cerebral palsied children. Dev Med Child Neurol 1986; 28:480–488.

242. Waylett J, Barber L: Upper extremity bracing of the severely athetoid mental retardate. Am J Occup Ther 1971; 25:402–407.

243. Whyte HE, Fitzhardinge PM, Shennan AT, et al: Extreme immaturity: Outcome of 568 pregnancies of 23–26 weeks gestation. Obstet Gynec 1993; 82:1–7.

244. Winch R, Bengtson L, McLaughlin J, et al: Women with cerebral palsy: Obstetric experience and neonatal outcome. Dev Med Child Neurol 1993; 35:974–982.

245. Wright T, Nicholson J: Physiotherapy for the spastic child—An evaluation. Dev Med Child Neurol 1973; 15:146–163.

246. Yokochii K, Shimabukuro S, Kodama M, et al: Motor function of infants with athetoid cerebral palsy. Dev Med Child Neurol 1993; 35:54–60.

247. Zimbler S, Craig C, Harris J, et al: Orthotic management of severe scoliosis in spastic neuromuscular disease—Results of treatment. Orthop Trans 1985; 9:78–92.

54

Rehabilitation Concepts in Myelomeningocele

ROSS M. HAYS, M.D.,
AND TERESA L. MASSAGLI, M.D.

There are more children in this country disabled by myelomeningocele than by poliomyelitis, traumatic spinal cord injury, or muscular dystrophy.[48] Physicians who care for these patients must appreciate the subtleties of a congenital defect that presents at birth, yet has signs and symptoms that change with time and with the development of the growing child. The clinical manifestations of the disorder include multiple organ systems in complicated and interdependent relationships. Many of the physical aspects of the disease produce both medical and psychological problems. Effective management requires a collection of specialists who must cooperate with the child, family, and one another in order to deliver competent effective care. As the first large group of aggressively treated neonates is now entering middle age, an entirely new population—aging persons with myelomeningocele—is presenting clinical challenges that were previously unanticipated.

HISTORICAL BACKGROUND

Excavations in Morocco contain bone remnants from children with spinal defects that are 10,000 to 12,000 years old.[20] Skeletons with lumbosacral defects have been found among Modoc Indian burial grounds in Arizona, and similar findings in skeletons of Roman Britain, where 7.3% were found to have openings in the spinal canal, provide a crude suggestion of the incidence of the disorder in ancient times.[68] Hippocrates described patients with myelomeningocele. Aristotle proposed to resolve with infanticide the burden that these children placed on society. Nicholas Tulpius wrote the first scientific description of the defect in Holland in 1652 and used the term *spina bifida*. In the 1860s both Lamarck and Darwin commented on the possibility of environmental influences in the etiology of the disease.[6] The advances in surgical technology leading to effective neonatal back closure in the 1940s and the inven-

tion of the one-way shunt valve by Holter, Nulsen, and Spitz in 1952 effectively reversed the survival curves from 10% survival in 1956 to 10% mortality in 1985.[48] Lorber's proposed scheme for nontreatment of affected infants in Great Britain in 1971 and the subsequent "Baby Doe" legislation in the United States were watershed events in the application of modern bioethics to pediatric patients. The treatment of children with myelomeningocele continues to evolve and to reflect the changing face of medicine.

DEFINITIONS

Myelomeningocele (MMC) is the term used to describe the failure of fusion of the neural folds during the neurulation phase of embryologic development. It is also used interchangeably with *meningomyelocele* to describe both the embryologic defect of bone, meninges, and spinal cord, as well as the collection of clinical derangements—lower extremity paralysis, sensory loss, and neurogenic bowel and bladder—that result from damage to neuronal tissue in the open neural tube.

Meningocele describes a hernia of the meningeal membranes with little or no dysgenesis of the underlying nervous system. Most meningoceles contain all the neural elements within the neural canal, are skin-covered, and produce little paralysis.

Lipomeningomyeloceles, lipomeningoceles, and *lipomyeloceles* are lipomas that occur within the neural canal as a result of abnormal epidermal and mesodermal development. They most commonly accompany some degree of meningocele formation and interfere with neural function by increasing pressure on the lower spinal cord either by adhesion or growth.

Diastematomyelia is a splitting of the lower spinal cord in association with mesodermal elements, bone or cartilage spurs, and fibrous bands. It may occur alone or in association with meningomyelocele.

Myelocystocele describes a cystic defect that communicates with the central canal of the spinal cord. Myelocystoceles vary in size and may be either dorsal or ventral. They produce neurological symptoms by exerting pressure on the spinal cord during growth.

Spina bifida is the term used to describe the bony defect resulting from failure of mesodermal closure around the neural canal. Meningomyelocele and meningocele are examples of *spina bifida aperta*. *Spina bifida occulta* is a defect of the posterior bony element only with no involvement of the underlying meningeal or neural elements. Spina bifida occulta is not uncommon in the general public and is usually asymptomatic.

EPIDEMIOLOGY

Incidence

Both geographical and racial variations in incidence of MMC have been reported. Rates in Ireland and Wales have been three to four times greater than the worldwide incidence of 1 case per 1000 live births. In Japan and several eastern European countries, rates have been much lower.[32] In the United States, a gradient of decreasing rates from East Coast to West Coast has been noted.[22]

Over the last 20 years, a decline in incidence has been reported in Great Britain and the United States.[56, 82] This decrease cannot be entirely accounted for by prenatal diagnosis and termination of affected pregnancies and is suggestive of an important role for environmental factors. From 1970 to 1989, the incidence of neural tube defects dropped from 1.3 to 0.6 per 1000 live births. About two thirds of the neural tube defects are MMC cases, translating into about 2000 affected infants born each year in the United States.[82]

Etiology

Myelomeningocele occurs as a result of incomplete closure of the neural tube during fetal development. Morphological studies of embryonic development have shown that closure of the caudal neuropore normally occurs between 26 and 30 days post fertilization.[55] Any suspected cause of spina bifida must act prior to this time. One of the challenges to both determination of cause as well as implementation of prevention strategies is this fact—that malformation occurs so soon after conception, often before women are aware they are pregnant.

GENETICS. Neural tube defects are believed to be multifactorial in origin. The multifactorial model implies that the risk of a trait or disease is greater in relatives of affected persons than in members of the general population; that since close relatives have more genes in common than distant relatives, the incidence of the disease among relatives decreases with increasing distance of the genetic relationship; and that the risk to relatives increases with the number of affected relatives in the pedigree.[4] Multifactorial diseases have genetic and environmental influences.

The relative roles of genetic and environmental factors in MMC have not been settled. Open neural tube defects have occurred in multiple births and in infants with chromosomal disorders such as trisomy 13, but most occur as isolated defects, not associated with other malformations. There is a slight sex preference with a female-to-male ratio of 1.3:1.[9] MMC occurs in higher frequencies among relatives of children with MMC than in the general population. The recurrence rate appears to be related to the incidence of neural tube defects in the regional population. The recurrence risk in British Columbia and the United States for a second affected child is 2.4% to 3.0%, but in Ireland and Wales it is 5.0%.[13] Risks for a third affected child are approximately twice these. In children of maternal sisters, a frequency of 1% has been reported and there is a similar risk for an affected child when one of the parents has a neural tube defect.[42] Consanguinity between parents also increases the risk, and the high cousin marriage rate in Britain has been proposed as one of the contributors to the higher incidence there.[33]

The increased incidence of MMC in families, certain ethnic groups, and in cases of parental consanguinity suggests a strong role for inheritance, but the recurrence rates of affected siblings are not consistent with recessive, dominant, or cytoplasmic inheritance. It has been suggested that MMC and other neural tube defects arise from the interaction of many genes (polygenic inheritance) which may create a threshold whereby a fetus exposed at a certain time to certain environmental triggers becomes at risk for malformation.[9]

ENVIRONMENTAL FACTORS. The observations of an increased incidence of MMC among people of low socioeconomic status and among children conceived in spring months has lent weight to theories of environmental contributors to etiology. Nutrition, drugs, and heat have been proposed as causes. The only drug definitely implicated in neural tube defects is aminopterin, a folate antagonist previously used as an abortifacient, but valproic acid and oral contraceptives have also been suspected.[32] Recent evidence has identified two measures, vitamin supplementation and avoidance of heat exposure, as primary preventive measures against neural tube defects.

The evidence for folic acid supplementation to prevent tube defects has been steadily accumulating since the early 1980s. Folic acid supplementation was first shown to reduce the risk of recurrence in high-risk families.[33] These results were replicated using large doses of folate (4 mg/day), but were not found with general multivitamin supplementation without folate.[50] Only 5% of cases of neural tube defects represent recurrences so the next step was to determine if vitamin supplementation could prevent first occurrences. Using smaller doses of folic acid (0.8 mg/day) in combination with multivitamins, researchers noted a very convincing reduction in the incidence of first occurrence of neural tube defects.[14] Based on these findings, the U.S. Public Health Service recommended that all women of childbearing age who are capable of becoming pregnant should consume 0.4 mg of folic acid per day to reduce their risk of having a pregnancy affected with MMC or other neural tube defects. Women who have had an affected child should consider periconceptional consumption of 4 mg of folate per day.[59]

Heat exposure has long been suspected of being a teratogen in humans, and recently strong associations between maternal heat exposure during early pregnancy and neural tube defects have been reported. Taking hot baths, having a febrile illness, or the use of hot tubs or saunas during the first trimester have been associated with twice the risk of developing neural tube defects compared to women without such exposures.[49, 62] The amount of heat exposure necessary for teratogenicity in humans is unknown, as is the mechanism of action in preventing closure of the neural tube. Based on these findings, it is prudent for women to avoid elevation in core temperature in the first trimester of pregnancy.

MANAGEMENT

Early Management

Prenatal Management

Prenatal screening techniques have made it possible to identify the majority of cases of MMC. This information can be used to plan for termination of pregnancy if parents so desire or to enhance perinatal management if carried to term. Prenatal diagnosis begins with measurement of maternal serum alpha-fetoprotein (AFP) at 16 to 18 weeks postconception.

The presence of an open neural tube defect allows AFP and acetylcholinesterase to escape from the fetus into amniotic fluid. Peak levels of amniotic fluid AFP occur between the 13th and 15th postconception weeks and can be detected in maternal serum. Maternal serum levels rise at 15 weeks postconception and peak between 25 and 29 weeks. Elevated serum levels are confirmed by repeat studies. If still elevated, ultrasound screening is performed.

High-resolution ultrasonography can reveal the presence of MMC by 14 to 16 weeks of gestation. If suspected on ultrasound, the diagnosis should be confirmed by amniocentesis to measure the amount of AFP and acetylcholinesterase in amniotic fluid. While elevated levels of AFP are seen in a number of conditions such as anterior abdominal wall defects or fetal demise, isoenzymes of acetylcholinesterase are only seen in open neural tube defects and are independent of the length of gestation. Amniocentesis is best performed between 15 and 18 weeks postconception; earlier can be hazardous to the fetus, while later the AFP levels become more difficult to interpret and the opportunity for termination diminishes.[33, 42]

There is marked regional variation in the acceptance of prenatal diagnosis and the practice of termination of pregnancy. In Australia, there has been no change in the total prevalence of neural tube defects from the mid 1960s to the early 1990s, but the number of terminations of pregnancy increased as a result of implementation of prenatal diagnosis programs, and the prevalence of live births of infants with neural tube defects dropped by 83%, from 2.01 to 0.35 per 1000 live births.[11] In contrast, only 50% of parents in Ireland accept termination of pregnancy after the diagnosis of a neural tube defect.[23]

Prenatal detection of MMC is important even for families who would not choose to terminate the pregnancy because it enhances perinatal management. Families have time to learn about the diagnosis and prepare for a safe delivery. Such infants should be delivered in the medical center where surgical closure will occur to minimize trauma to or infection of the sac during transportation. It

has also been suggested that infants with MMC be delivered by cesarean section to avoid injury to the sac and contents. One group of researchers reported less severe lower extremity paralysis in infants born by cesarean section prior to the onset of labor as compared to those delivered vaginally or by cesarean section after onset of labor.[41] Levels of paralysis were no different in the infants exposed to labor, regardless of the method of delivery. Prenatal diagnosis allows physicians to plan for elective caesarean section prior to labor when the fetus has achieved pulmonary maturation.

Neonatal Management

BACK DEFECT. The first priority of medical treatment for the newborn with MMC is management of the open neural tube defect (Fig. 54–1). The treatment is a continuous sequence including delivery of the infant, protection of the back, closure of the defect, and stabilization of cerebrospinal fluid (CSF) flow. There are three goals in the management of the back defect: (1) to reduce the risk of infection; (2) to preserve existing neurological function, and (3) to decrease the deformity if severe kyphoscoliosis is present. Most centers advocate closure within the first hours after delivery. The risk of central nervous system (CNS) infection in lesions closed before 48 hours averages 7%; the infection risk for later closure rises to an average of 37%.[48] The back defect must be carefully protected to prevent contamination or further damage due to trauma or desiccation. The surface of the lesion and CSF are cultured and the infant is treated with antibiotics at dosages sufficient to treat meningitis. Back closure is performed in three stages: (1) the neural plaque is returned to the canal and a watertight closure of dura and arachnoid reconstructed; (2) the reformulated neural tube is then protected by myofascial closure; and (3) the skin is then closed with a tension closure.

Back repair may produce alterations in the CSF fluid dynamics by closing the open conduit at the caudal end of the central canal. In some cases, fluid pressures spontaneously readjust after closure. In others, hydrocephalus becomes more rapidly apparent. Kyphectomy to treat severe kyphoscoliosis in the newborn is difficult and often complicated by poor bone growth, high blood loss, and intraoperative mortality. Minimal osteotomy repair is a compromise that provides less immediate correction but is better tolerated by the infant.[69]

HYDROCEPHALUS. Ninety percent of children with myelomeningocele will develop clinically significant hydrocephalus.[48, 75] Some children have true aqueductal stenosis and others have communicating hydrocephalus that worsens after back closure. Nearly all children with MMC have displacement of the cerebellum caudally with elongation and kinking of the fourth ventricle. These combined defects are known as the Arnold-Chiari II malformation.[8] Recently, the term *constrictive hydrocephalus*[58] has been used to describe the relationship between Arnold-Chiari II malformation and the restricted flow of CSF which causes hydrocephalus in the majority of children with MMC.

Hydrocephalus is often present at birth or discovered prenatally by ultrasound examination. It usually does not progress immediately and may show no evidence of addi-

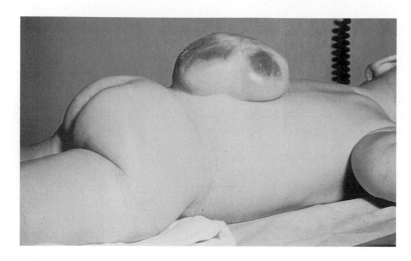

FIGURE 54–1 Typical appearance of a child with myelomeningocele lesion prior to surgical closure.

tional ventricular enlargement until 3 to 7 days of age. The onset of hydrocephalus in some patients does not require treatment for months or even years. Progressive hydrocephalus in the newborn manifests as increasing head size; older children with delayed-onset hydrocephalus develop signs and symptoms of increased intracranial pressure: vomiting, headache, somnolence, or irritability. Insidious onset of hydrocephalus may appear as lethargy, personality alterations, or subtle changes in intellectual performance.

Ventriculoperitoneal (VP) shunting is the treatment of choice for hydrocephalus. Technical advances have improved the results of hydrocephalus management from good results (better survival and intellectual performance) for 40% of patients in the 1950s to excellent results in over 90% of patients in the 1980s.[70] Half of all infants with shunts require replacement within the first year of life.[75] The likelihood of shunt failure and the need for shunt replacement decreases with each subsequent year.

EARLY BLADDER MANAGEMENT. The status of the neurogenic bladder in the newborn period can be evaluated by physical examination. Babies with large distended bladders on abdominal examination are likely to have spasticity of the sphincter mechanism. A nonpalpable bladder and constant dribbling suggest weak or nonexistent sphincter tone. Abdominal ultrasound can detect the presence of a distended, poorly emptying bladder, hydronephrosis, or more rarely, renal agenesis. The ultrasound study should be repeated after back closure to rule out any possibility of urinary tract obstruction resulting from damage to the spinal cord.

Postvoid residual urine volumes should be checked by ultrasound. A postvoid residual of 20 mL or greater in the newborn period indicates clinically significant urinary retention and requires intermittent catheterization, treatment with phenoxybenzamine, or both. Blood urea nitrogen (BUN) and creatinine must be monitored and routine urine cultures obtained during the first month of life. The first voiding cystourethrogram may be safely deferred until 6 months of age if all other tests suggest that bladder emptying is reasonable and the urine is infection-free.[29]

ASSESSMENT OF NEUROLOGICAL LEVEL. The actual pattern of voluntary motor innervation, that is, the motor level, is of some importance in predicting ambulation and intellectual potential, but it does not correlate well with the level of vertebral abnormality on the radiograph, the anatomical site of the skin lesion, or the level of abnormality on sensory examination.[68] The best method of motor examination is careful inspection for muscle bulk and stimulation with postural challenges and gentle opposition of major muscle groups to elicit voluntary activity. The presence of considerable muscle bulk by palpation without any observed voluntary movement may indicate temporary spinal cord shock after delivery or back closure. Thirty-seven percent of MMC newborns demonstrate improved motor strength within a week after delivery.[48] Joint movement, especially hip and knee flexion that is elicited in response to painful stimuli, may result from reflex-mediated activity below the level of the lesion rather than true voluntary control.

THERAPY. Experienced therapists working with neonates can provide detailed motor examinations before and after back closure. They can also assist with the positioning and handling of the newborn and provide anticipatory guidance for the parents in the transition of care from hospital to home. Children born with contractures of hips and knees benefit from a range-of-motion program developed by the therapists and then implemented by the family. Babies with higher-level lesions may require custom-fabricated seating and support devices that protect the surgical site and assist with trunk and head control.

FAMILY COUNSELING. The need for parents to be completely and accurately informed about all aspects of their infant's care, medical needs, and future potential cannot be overemphasized, nor can it be accurately contained in this brief overview. Families are entitled to clinical opinions based on the most recent medical literature regardless of their perceived ability to comprehend such a large body of technical material. Families who are overinformed and therefore given the opportunity to choose when and how much information to absorb maintain more control over their child's medical management. This attempt to respect a parent's autonomy in the midst of a catastrophic situation is aided by careful, competent repetition of information and the provision of detailed, accurate written material. The most successful centers have one physician and one nurse who act as the primary support for each family and child. Good communication among primary care physician, nurses, specialists, and the parents is the best assurance of achieving the desired medical outcome.

Long-Term Management

The Central Nervous System

SHUNTS. Approximately 90% of children with MMC require placement of a VP shunt for management of hydrocephalus.[48, 75] The two most common late complications associated with shunts are obstructions and infections. Of these, infections have the greater morbidity. The overall risk of shunt infection is 12% per child.[48] The most common infections are caused by *Staphylococcus epidermidis* and are associated with the surgical insertion of the shunt. Each shunt placement or revision carries a 5% risk for infection. Delayed symptoms presenting 6 weeks after surgery with culture-proven *S. epidermidis* likely represent indolent, late, postoperative infections.[69]

Children with hydrocephalus and shunts are at greater risk for epidemic meningitis caused by β-hemolytic streptococcus, meningococcus, pneumococcus, and less often, *Haemophilus influenzae*. The other common source of infection is erosion of the VP shunt into intra-abdominal organs and resulting contamination with gram-negative organisms.[69]

Infections in the shunt downstream from the CNS are the least serious and the most easily treated. Low-grade ventriculitis is often associated with shunt obstruction; shunt infection with ventriculomeningitis carries the most severe morbidity. The relationship between shunt infection, CNS infection, and intellectual functioning in children with MMC is controversial;[75] several studies suggest, however, that reduction in cognitive function is associated with the frequency and severity of infections.[47, 61]

Fifty percent of children with VP shunts experience obstruction and require revision in the first year of life. Of those children whose shunts obstruct during the first 12 months, 31% require replacement in the second year, and risk recurrence at a rate of 12% per year thereafter. In children who do not require a revision during the first year of life, the risk of obstruction is only 8% per year.

COMPLICATIONS OF ARNOLD-CHIARI II MALFORMATION. Nearly all children with MMC experience problems related to the Arnold-Chiari II malformation of the hindbrain. The more severe symptoms, stridor, aspiration, periodic breathing with sleep, and central apnea, are grouped under the collective term *central ventilatory dysfunction* (CVD). This severe complication of Arnold-Chiari II malformation has been reported in 7% to 30% of children.[26] The most severe manifestations of CVD are upper airway obstruction due to vocal cord abductor paralysis (30%), vocal cord abductor paralysis with other cranial nerve involvement (17%), and central apnea (22%). The exact mechanism of action is probably a result of several factors including traction on upper cervical nerves due to downward displacement of the medulla, brainstem compression with the abnormally located hindbrain, and increased intracranial pressure resulting from hydrocephalus.

The mainstays of treatment are management of increased intracranial pressure, treatment of CNS infection, and vigorous airway management. Decompression laminectomies to reduce local pressure on the brainstem have been helpful in some but not all cases. Placement or revision of CSF shunts to reduce intracranial pressure may provide improvement in some. The most effective treatment, regardless of underlying etiology, is aggressive attention to the airway obstruction and apnea.

CVD is not associated with the level of lesion, severity of hydrocephalus, or the presence of CNS bleeding and infection. Children with CVD who survive because of aggressive ventilatory support often experience remission of symptoms by 30 months of age. At the present time, the life-threatening consequences of CVD are the single most common cause of death in children with MMC.[26, 48]

HYDROMYELIA. Hydromyelia or dilation of the central canal is analogous to the dilation of the ventricles in hydrocephalus and occurs in 50% to 80% of children with MMC. The most common symptoms are rapidly progressive scoliosis, weakness of the upper extremities, spasticity, and ascending motor strength changes in the lower extremities. Hydromyelia is best demonstrated by magnetic resonance imaging (MRI) of the brain and spinal cord. When symptoms warrant treatment, decompressing subclinical hydrocephalus may be effective. In more aggressive cases, decompressive laminectomy, plugging of the obex, and direct shunting of the hydromyelia may be required.

TETHERED CORD SYNDROME. The term *tethered cord syndrome* is used to describe progressive neurological deficits resulting from traction of the conus medullaris and the cauda equina. It has been reported in 11% to 15% of children after myelomeningocele repair. The pathophysiology is related to decreased metabolism of nerve tissue in response to traction and deformation. The diagnosis is based on progressive symptoms, not the radiographic finding of a low-lying conus. Routine MRI studies have demonstrated that 80% to 90%[49] of MMC patients have an abnormally low conus medullaris, most of whom never develop clinical symptoms.[28, 77]

Surgical release often halts the progression of symptoms but may not restore lost function. It is important to recognize the clinical presentation of tethered cord and consider surgery as early as possible to preserve function. The average age at diagnosis is 6 years.[27] Children with higher lesion levels, a shorter cord, and less tolerance for stretching may present as young as 4 years of age. Children with lower-level lesions may not develop symptoms until after age 9.[57]

The most common symptom of tethered cord is change in motor strength (62%) followed by recent onset of spasticity (56%) and changes in mobility (43%). Back pain is reported in 37%, and 25% of patients report a recent change in bowel and bladder function or recent onset of scoliosis.[27] Because the diagnosis of tethered cord syndrome is clinical rather than radiographic and the symptoms described are either superimposed upon or amplifications of existing pathologic conditions, prospective screening with a high level of suspicion is required to effectively diagnose the syndrome in children with MMC.

Urologic System

PATTERNS OF INVOLVEMENT. Unlike after traumatic spinal cord injury, the types of neurogenic bladder seen in children with MMC are not correlated with the lesion level.

More than 80% have partial or complete denervation of the bladder with poor compliance and poor contractility producing residual urine volumes. In 86%, the internal sphincter is incompetent, so that incontinence occurs when intravesical pressure exceeds urethral resistance. The external sphincter is usually at least partially functional, and in about one third of patients detrusor-sphincter dyssynergia causes abnormally high intraluminal pressures.[45] Bladder function may change after birth or in a growing child experiencing tethered cord syndrome. Most changes occur in the first year after birth and either deterioration or improvement in external sphincter function may be seen.[74] For these reasons, early assessment of bladder and kidney function followed by reassessment at least annually is necessary.

PREVENTING RENAL INVOLVEMENT. The goals of management of neurogenic bladder are prevention of urinary tract damage and achievement of continence. Urodynamic examination of intravesical and bladder neck pressures is a routine evaluation in newborn infants with MMC. About 75% of infants have normal upper tracts while the rest have hydronephrosis due to such problems as vesicoureteral reflux (VUR), detrusor-sphincter dyssynergia, an enlarged bladder, or a structural abnormality. Infants with normal upper tracts and satisfactory bladder emptying are monitored twice a year by renal ultrasound during early childhood. If the bladder does not empty efficiently and there is no outlet resistance or reflux, parents can be taught the Credé maneuver to improve emptying. If detrusor-sphincter dyssynergia is present, there is a significant risk for development of hydronephrosis and such infants are managed with anticholinergic medications and clean intermittent catheterization (CIC). The same management is used for infants who already have hydronephrosis. If CIC fails to relieve hydronephrosis, a cutaneous vesicostomy can be done. It can be reversed after ureteral reimplantation or bladder augmentation when the child is old enough to perform CIC.[46, 63]

If the child has VUR, prophylactic antibiotics are prescribed because VUR of infected urine can cause upper tract damage or even renal failure. Risk factors for upper tract damage and VUR include detrusor-sphincter dyssynergia, decreased bladder compliance, and elevated leak pressures. VUR is seen when detrusor pressure exceeds 40 cm H_2O before leakage of urine occurs.[46] If the child develops persistent febrile urinary tract infections or hydronephrosis does not improve, antireflux surgery is indicated and includes options such as vesicostomy, reimplantation of ureters, or bladder augmentation.

One of the first surgical approaches to prevent upper tract injury was urinary diversion into an ileal conduit. This was often done prophylactically to prevent hydronephrosis. Follow-up studies have shown a disappointing frequency of complications, including renal deterioration, pyelonephritis, and stone disease. Many such patients have subsequently had reversal of the diversion.

Periodic monitoring of the upper urinary tract is essential. Renal ultrasound examination every 6 months for the first few years of childhood is common practice. If reflux is present, the child may periodically need an excretory urogram and voiding cystourethrogram. Urodynamic surveillance is also indicated because changes in the bladder do occur, most often in the first year of life or in later childhood associated with tethered cord syndrome.[74] Asymptomatic bacteriuria is prevalent in children with MMC. Urine culture screening is indicated for those with VUR or when signs or symptoms of urinary tract infection occur.

CONTINENCE. Less than 10% of children with MMC have normal urinary control.[34] Knowledge of bladder capacity and sphincter function is vital when considering options for management. For boys with reflex emptying, external collection devices may be feasible if they do not have VUR or large residual urine volumes. Applying condom catheters can be problematic in boys with a small penis, and requires careful attention to skin integrity when sensation is impaired.

There are no effective external collection devices for girls (excluding diapers). Girls and boys with incomplete emptying rely on CIC and sometimes medications. Owing to the high prevalence of small bladder capacity and low outlet resistance, only about one fourth of children can become continent with CIC alone.[78] Even adding anticholinergic medications (oxybutinin, propantheline) to inhibit contractions, α-adrenergic medications (ephedrine, phenylpropanolamine) to increase outlet resistance, and antibiotic instillations to reduce infection-induced bladder spasms only achieved complete continence in 49% of children in one study.[81] Long-term compliance may be a problem for such complicated regimens in this population. To maintain daily continence, such children need to empty their bladders very frequently, often at intervals of less than every 4 hours, and the entire daily bladder management can require more than 1.5 hours/day.[34]

Surgery may be considered for children who fail to become continent using medications and CIC. The options depend on bladder size, sphincter competence, and the ability of the patient to perform CIC. Augmentation of the size of the bladder may be necessary for the child with a small or noncompliant bladder and may be done in conjunction with an artificial sphincter if the outlet resistance is low. Ileum, sigmoid colon, and stomach have all been used for augmentation. Mucus production, urolithiasis, and electrolyte disturbances can ensue after ileum or sigmoid patches, and gastrocystoplasty may be complicated by hematuria, dysuria, or metabolic alkalosis. The most serious complication is spontaneous rupture, which may occur if the bladder becomes overdistended.[63]

For those with low outlet resistance, implantation of an artificial urethral sphincter may be considered. The sphincter is placed around the bladder neck, and the procedure is commonly done in conjunction with bladder augmentation. About half of patients need to use CIC after sphincter implantation, and overall success for long-term continence is over 60%.[5]

If the patient has difficulty performing urethral CIC, continent diversion is another option. The appendix can be used as a conduit to the bladder to create an abdominal stoma which is easier for the patient to access.[18]

DEVELOPMENT AND BLADDER MANAGEMENT. The accomplishment of independent toileting by children with MMC is delayed more than any other self-care task, even in those with normal intelligence. While most children with normal bladder and bowel function achieve independent control by 4 years of age, children with MMC may not accomplish this until 10 to 15 years of age.[54] The cause of this delay in developmental achievement is multifactorial with likely contributors being level of paralysis, intelligence quotient (IQ), visual spatial imperceptions, kyphoscoliosis, obesity, level of parental support, the degree of sensation, sphincter control, and bladder capacity.

Parents need to be trained not only in the task of performing the child's bladder or bowel program but also in preparing the child to accept responsibility for these tasks once the child is physically and mentally capable.[73] Children can learn to catheterize themselves using clean technique as early as age 5 years, but will need help for many years to remind them to perform the task and to assist with cleaning of equipment. Unfortunately, as many as 30% of teenagers with MMC still require assistance from a caregiver for bladder management.[34]

Neurogenic Bowel

DESCRIPTION OF PATTERNS. The key anatomical areas affecting fecal continence in children with MMC are the large intestine, rectum, and internal and external sphincters. The peristaltic movements of the large intestine differ from the small intestine; they are not continuous, but rather occur in mass movements several times a day. Fairly predictable mass movements occur in association with filling of the stomach and duodenum. This gastrocolic reflex is often strongest after the first meal each day. The rectum functions as a reservoir and is prevented from emptying on a continuous basis by the tone of the internal sphincter. When the rectum is full, reflex relaxation of the internal sphincter occurs. The external anal sphincter has both voluntary and reflex control and activates only when a bolus is present. It must relax to permit defecation.[80] Sacral parasympathetic and thoracolumbar sympathetic fibers innervate the lower colon, rectum, and sphincters, and the external anal sphincter has somatic innervation as well.

About 20% of children with MMC have normal bowel control.[34] Bowel continence may be compromised by impaired rectal sensation, impaired sphincter function, or altered colonic motility. Children with MMC may experience relative intestinal stasis due to loss of sacral parasympathetic input. It is not known if the gastrocolic reflex is intact in patients with neurogenic bowel. If the external sphincter is partially or wholly denervated, incontinence results when the pressure in the rectum is high enough to produce reflex relaxation of the internal sphincter. In patients with MMC above L3, the tonic pressure of the internal sphincter is low, possibly due to loss of sympathetic input. Rectal sensation is also related to lesion level and usually absent in those with lesions above L3 and more likely present though often abnormal with lower lesions.[1] It is important to know whether the child has any spasticity or voluntary control over the external anal sphincter, but the presence or absence of the anocutaneous reflex has not been shown to correlate with internal sphincter tone.[1] Although sphincter status can be determined with anorectal manometry, it is not clear that such knowledge alters the management plan. However, the presence of either a bulbocavernosus or anocutaneous reflex is associated with a greater likelihood of achieving continence.[30]

MANAGEMENT STRATEGIES. To achieve bowel continence, the child with MMC needs efficient, regular, and predictable emptying of bowel contents. The goal is to empty the rectum before it becomes full enough to stimulate reflex relaxation of the internal sphincter. If the child lacks rectal sensation, the emptying should be done according to a regular schedule. While clinicians often recommend that patients perform bowel programs after meals, to take advantage of the gastrocolic reflex, it is not known if this reflex is present in children with MMC, and owing to the length of time needed to complete the bowel program this may not be convenient in the patient's or family's schedule.[15] Classic bowel programs often utilize stool softeners or bulking agents, but families often prefer dietary manipulations instead of medications and find that such programs are too time-consuming, often taking more than 30 min to complete.[15] Suppositories, digital anorectal stimulation, manual removal of stool, use of expansion enemas to rapidly distend the rectum, and use of biofeedback if the child has adequate rectal sensation are potentially useful, and none is universally successful.

SOCIAL IMPLICATIONS. It is important for parents to establish an effective program of bowel continence at an early developmental stage, usually around 3 years of age. Many children will enter preschool or kindergarten shortly thereafter and be subject to severe peer criticism if "accidents" occur. The child also needs to be encouraged to assume increasing responsibility for performing the bowel program. Clinicians can facilitate this learning experience for the child by keeping the program simple and as short as possible, so the child grasps cause and effect.

Unfortunately, substantial numbers of children with MMC do not attain the goal of independently managing bowel continence. In one study, up to 86% of teenagers 13 to 18 years old needed assistance from a caregiver for their bowel program.[34] As with bladder management, the reasons for this are not entirely clear, but probable contributors are physical limitations due to obesity or scoliosis, inconsistent parental expectations, and the fact that denervation of the external rectal sphincter makes continence more challenging than in upper motor neuron neurogenic bowel disorders.

Parents perceive urinary and fecal incontinence as more stressful than impaired motor function in their children with MMC,[34] and healthcare professionals must be persistent in their efforts to help these children achieve continence.

Musculoskeletal Complications

MOTOR INNERVATION. It is important to appreciate that the level of neurological lesion does not match the radiographic vertebral level in most cases. One percent of infants will have defects at the cervical and another 1% at the upper thoracic vertebral levels. Six percent of patients present with defects at the lower thoracic and upper lumbar vertebral levels. More than a fourth (27%) have midlumbar-level, and 42% have lumbosacral-level vertebral lesions. One fifth (21%) present with sacral-level involvement and 2% will have large lesions encompassing the entire lumbosacral spine.

When patients are categorized by neurological impairment, 1% have severe lesions with cervical and upper thoracic impairment. Twenty-seven percent have lower thoracic levels with paralysis of the psoas and more distally innervated muscles. Almost one fourth (23%) present with intact hip flexion but impaired quadriceps. Nearly half (45%) of all MMC children fall into the lower lumbar group where quadriceps are spared but lower segments are not. Only 4% present with lower-sacral-level paralysis with intact lower extremity strength with some degree of bowel and bladder dysfunction.

It is tempting to regard these lesion levels as a simple dichotomy with normal voluntary motor control above the level of the lesion and flaccid paralysis below. Only one third of children actually demonstrate flaccid paralysis. The majority of patients exhibit a variety of abnormal motor abnormalities including incomplete flaccid paraplegia, spasticity, mixed paraplegia and spasticity, asymmetry of involvement on either side, intact regions of voluntary control below the other segments of paralysis, and combinations of these impairments within the individual.

The level of neurological impairment influences the types of musculoskeletal deformities and complications. Regardless of the characteristics of the motor disability, essentially half of all children have defects including the L5 or S1 and lower levels and 92% have lesions at or below L2. This general pattern suggests that hip flexors and adductors are less often affected than hip extensors and abductors. The common finding of hip flexion contractures supports this theory. The same argument suggests that knee extensors would be more frequently spared than knee flexors. The relative rarity of knee extension contractures in this patient group illustrates the complex interplay of factors that leads to musculoskeletal deformity in MMC.

HIPS. The majority of patients have some hip deformity that interferes with ambulation, seating, or bracing, but only those with functional deficits or pain require treatment. Muscle imbalance at the hip accounts for most of the hip flexion deformity. A small number of patients develop hip flexion contractures from spasticity in the iliopsoas, rectus femoris, or sartorius (Fig. 54–2). Any hip flexion contracture of 20 degrees or more will increase the anterior pelvic tilt, create excessive lumbar lordosis, and interfere with ambulation. Patients with lesions at a high level may require soft tissue releases and anterior capsulotomy to improve seating and comfort. Patients with lesions at lower levels who are over 10 or 11 years of age may require a subtrochanteric extension osteotomy to preserve ambulation. This approach is less successful in younger ambulatory patients for whom continued growth is likely to result in bone remodeling. Younger patients may respond to hip flexor releases with free tendon grafting using the tensor fasciae latae.[36]

Hip flexion-abduction-external rotation deformity is seen in higher-lesion-level patients and may necessitate radical hip releases for seating. Iliotibial band and tensor fasciae latae strength may be asymmetrical and lead to hip abduction contracture and pelvic obliquity. Hip adduction contracture is the deformity that is most often associated with secondary hip dislocation. The goal in treatment of this deformity is to release adductors in order to regain 45 to 60 degrees of passive abduction.[36]

Fifty percent of children with myelomeningocele have

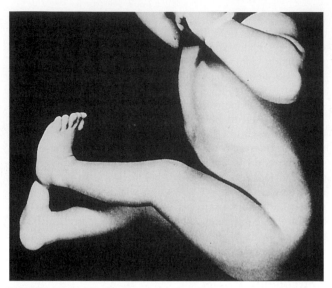

FIGURE 54–2 Hip flexion contracture is very common in infancy and early childhood.

subluxated or dislocated hips at some time. Hip dislocation at birth occurs with lesions that are very high (thoracic level) or very low (sacral level). Fifty percent to 70% of hip dislocations are associated with the muscle imbalance of midlumbar-level lesions where flexors and abductors are innervated by L1 to L5, and L5 to S2 innervation to extensors and abductors is absent. When hip dislocation occurs in later childhood or adolescence it may signal new-onset, late neurological changes such as hydromyelia or tethered cord.

There is some evidence that reducing dislocated hips in the active, ambulatory child may decrease dependence on assistive devices and reduce energy expenditure.[36] When the dislocations are bilateral and very high, reduction requires soft tissue releases, pelvic and femoral procedures, and has such a high complication rate that the reduction is often contraindicated. Nonambulatory children with high lesion levels frequently require only soft tissue releases. Hip surgery must be carefully planned; the most common postoperative complication is hip flexion contracture which interferes with mobility in later life. Repeated procedures are associated with greater hip stiffness and greater disability.[36]

KNEES. The most common deformity of the knee is flexion contracture. The development of knee flexion contracture is complex and incompletely understood. It may be caused by congenital joint stiffness due to decreased intrauterine movement, from spasticity in the knee flexors, or from progressive crouched posture with weak quadriceps and a need to keep the center of gravity over the midfoot during weightbearing. The incidence of knee flexion contractures is related to the neurological level of the lesion and to the child's age. Seventy percent of patients with lesions at the level of L3 or higher develop knee flexion contractures by 8 years of age. Patients with lesions at the L4 to L5 level do better; only 25% have contractures by age 12 years. Most sacral-level patients do not suffer knee flexion contractures. Knee extension contractures and valgus and varus deformities occur rarely and are seen most often in the groups with higher-level lesions.[66]

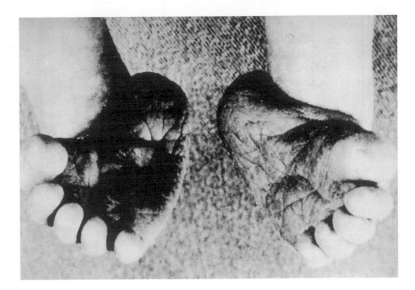

FIGURE 54–3 Equinovarus foot deformity is more commonly seen at birth and during early infancy.

FEET. Foot deformities occur in 85% of children and are the most common orthopedic abnormality in children with MMC.[36] The muscular imbalance associated with the level of the neurological lesion interferes with the bony and cartilaginous growth of the hindfoot. Lack of sensation and autonomic dysfunction with vasomotor instability are responsible for secondary skin injury and poor wound healing. The goals of treatment are braceable plantigrade feet and balanced muscle control around the ankle joint.

Equinovarus, the rigid form of clubfoot deformity, results from retained tibialis posterior and tibialis anterior function in the child with a midlumbar neurological deficit (Fig. 54–3). The first line of treatment is casting to reduce the deformity, but surgery to produce a stable ankle joint is usually inevitable. A hindfoot valgus deformity with residual forefoot adduction is a common complication. Rigid fusions such as triple arthrodesis are associated with later development of neuropathic joints.[36] Children with paresis of the tibialis posterior are at risk for congenital convex pes valgus or rocker-bottom deformity. Surgical correction is designed to balance the hindfoot and forefoot musculature.

Flexible, flail feet or S1-innervated ankles may drift into pure equinus deformity. This is an indication for prescription of a neutrally positioned ankle-foot orthosis. Plantar flexion contracture of greater than 20 degrees is unlikely to improve with stretching and may require serial casting or soft tissue releases. Pes cavus requires little treatment until adolescence when weightbearing may lead to skin ulceration. When necessary, metatarsal osteotomies and orthoses will successfully redistribute forces around the foot. Loss of foot intrinsic balance may produce a cock-up toe deformity at the great toe, best treated with tendon lengthening. Hindfoot valgus can be treated with orthoses until it exceeds 7 degrees (Fig. 54–4). Deformity beyond this amount requires tendon transfers for young children, epiphyseal interruption in older children, and supramalleolar osteotomy in adolescents.[36]

SPINE. Spinal deformity in MMC usually occurs in one of three forms: (1) scoliosis with lordosis, (2) kyphosis, or (3) rigid congenital malformation.[36] There is a direct correlation between the level of spinal lesion and the incidence of scoliosis; 100% of patients with thoracic lesions develop a scoliosis of 45 degrees or more. The incidence is only 60% in patients with a lesion at the L4 level, and less than half of them will require surgical correction. When scoliosis accompanies high-level paraplegia, it occurs in early childhood or infancy, is usually C-shaped, and always progressive. When scoliosis develops as a result of hydromyelia or syrinx formation it is often more S-shaped, occurs at any time, and may improve after treatment of the hydromyelia if the curve has not progressed beyond 50 degrees. Scoliosis that presents in later childhood may be the first sign of secondary CNS complications such as lipoma, dermoid tumors, or tethered cord.[7]

Kyphosis in MMC is almost always progressive and conservative management is rarely effective. Curves of 100 degrees or more are commonly seen by age 3. The most common form is the supple, collapsing C-shaped curve with kyphosis which may have its apex at any point from the lower thoracic vertebrae to the lumbosacral joint. The kyphosis that presents at birth is associated with vertebral malformations. The rigid apex is commonly in the high- to

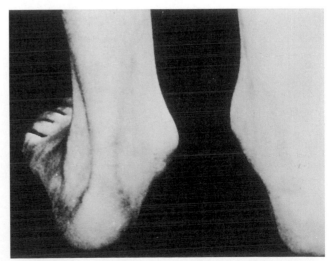

FIGURE 54–4 Calcaneovalgus deformity is commonly seen in later years.

midlumbar region and there is a compensatory lordosis above it. Rarely children present with partial aplasia of the lumbar spine, which also results in kyphosis. The goals of treatment in kyphosis are to preserve or maintain abdominal height and allow room for abdominal contents, to relieve pressure on the diaphragm and to prevent pressure sores. If kyphosis is allowed to approach 180 degrees, treatment becomes impossible.[36] Children with large congenital malformations of the vertebral column may require anterior and posterior fusion in infancy. Those who do not have early correction may develop additional, progressive curves with growth of the spine (Fig. 54–5).

In all three forms of scoliosis the timing of surgical correction is critical. Spinal fusion performed too early will limit further vertebral growth; waiting may lead to progressive curves that are more difficult or impossible to treat. The most appropriate approach is to individualize treatment for each child and provide vigilant surveillance for spinal changes.

FRACTURES. Fractures occur in approximately 20% of children with MMC. The proximal and distal femur are the most frequently involved sites. In ambulatory patients, fractures often accompany falls. In nonambulatory children, fractures may occur with minor trauma to their osteopenic extremities.[66] In the insensate lower extremity, fractures may escape detection initially. They present with erythema, swelling, local warmth, fever, and malaise. Frequently the white blood cell (WBC) count and erythrocyte sedimentation rate (ESR) are elevated, and it is not uncommon for the unsuspected fracture to be mistaken for a soft tissue infection. Fractures heal quickly in children with MMC. These children form exuberant calluses and rarely require rigid fixation. Those patients who have casts for fractures or surgery are relatively more osteopenic immediately after treatment and are at greatest risk for new fractures in the period immediately following cast removal.[66]

Mobility

LESION LEVEL. Mobility, the efficient, effective means of moving through space, may or may not include independent walking. Most children with MMC will use a variety of methods to maintain mobility, including walking, the use of assistive devices, and wheelchairs. Traditionally, walking in MMC has been linked to the level of the neurological lesion and the pattern of motor strength in the lower extremities. The guidelines have never been completely consistent; some authors have emphasized the importance of quadriceps strength while others stress hip abductors and knee flexors.[43] Using motor level to predict ambulation is difficult because the classic neurosegmental levels and motor correlates are probably more variable than originally thought, and because there is a wide range of ambulation potential among patients with similar patterns of segmental innervation. The influence of motor innervation may be moderated by other factors, including cognitive ability, musculoskeletal complications, surgery, motivation, obesity, and age.[44]

The complicated relationship of motor innervation and independent ambulation resists reduction into a simple formula which could be used to predict ambulation potential. One recent study[43] has attempted to clarify this issue by studying serial manual muscle tests in a large, stable population of children with MMC over a long period of time. In this study iliopsoas strength was a robust predictor of independent ambulation. Grade 4 to 5 iliopsoas strength was most often associated with community ambulation; grade 0 to 3 iliopsoas strength was always associated with wheelchair dependence. The ability to walk without assistive devices was strongly associated with grade 4 to 5 gluteal and tibialis anterior strength. Those patients with a combination of strong hip flexors and weak glutei mediae were most likely to experience deterioration in muscle strength regardless of age.

ORTHOSES. There are four principles that govern the use of orthoses in children with MMC. (1) Orthotic devices may be used to prevent deformity. Splints and orthoses are most effective at maintaining correction of deformities that have been attained by casting or surgery. Their ability to prevent the development of or alter the progression of

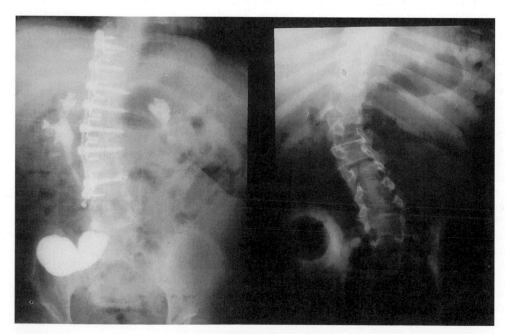

FIGURE 54–5 The risk for scoliosis is linearly correlated with age and inversely correlated with the level of the lesion.

spontaneous deformity, for example, pes planus or scoliosis, is not well established in this population. (2) Orthotic devices can be used to support normal joint alignment and mechanics when they are carefully fabricated for that purpose. (3) Children with MMC have various patterns of muscular weakness that interfere with normal gait. In that setting orthoses may be used to control range of motion during gait. (4) Special orthotic devices, particularly those that provide support or augment mobility, may be used to facilitate function.[31]

In addition to the many variations of knee and ankle-foot orthoses, three unique and extensive bracing systems are used to facilitate function for children with MMC. The parapodium provides structural support from the midthorax to the floor. It is often jointed at the hip and knee to accommodate both standing and sitting positions. This allows the child to maintain an upright, weightbearing position and to ambulate with a swing-through gait regardless of the level of paralysis. The swivel walker is a modification of the parapodium that was initially designed in Great Britain for children with limb deficiency resulting from the thalidomide crisis of the 1960s.[31] It has a dual footplate system that translates trunk rotation into forward movement. The reciprocating gait orthosis joins two hip-knee-ankle-foot orthoses (HKAFOs) with an elaborate cable system to link hip flexion at each hip with hip extension on the contralateral side. All three of these systems have the advantage of simulating upright ambulation but none approach the energy efficiency of normal walking.

FUNCTIONAL MOBILITY. There is a strong cultural imperative to encourage disabled children to maintain an upright weightbearing position and if possible to ambulate with as little assistive equipment as possible. With appropriate support, surgery, extensive bracing, and therapy, many children with MMC with high lesion levels can become community ambulators.[12] This point of view has validity in a psychological sense. Standing and walking may have great value in the minds of individual children and their parents and should be supported for these reasons. Efficient, functional mobility, however, is often better achieved for these children by providing them with a wheelchair. Rarely is it necessary to make an exclusive choice for ambulation and bracing or wheeled mobility; judicious use of both modalities in different settings to achieve separate goals is often the best solution.

It is important to separate a cultural imperative from the clinical arguments that are frequently offered as justification for aggressive upright mobility regimens. Upright stance has been purported to improve urinary tract function by facilitating urine flow by gravity, but no scientific data exist to support this suggestion. Ambulation has been cited as a helpful adjunct in bowel function, but there is no evidence of its usefulness. Improved cardiopulmonary fitness is provided as an argument for aggressive ambulation with assistive devices, but abundant research suggests that energy expenditure for patients with disabilities is usually maintained at a constant level at the expense of decreased velocity and endurance. There are likely more opportunities for aerobic fitness available to wheelchair racers than to persons who must depend on braces and crutches for ambulation.[66]

The most commonly cited argument for weightbearing is the development of osteopenia and increased risk of fractures in nonambulatory patients. It is true that these patients are more osteopenic than ambulatory children, but the risk of fracture is more closely associated with surgery and immobilization than with lack of weightbearing. Ambulatory children with MMC have a higher frequency of orthopedic procedures and therefore more risk of fractures.[66] Weightbearing is encouraged to counteract the risk of lower extremity contractures and deformity, but the association has never been clearly defined. It has been suggested that keeping children upright and weightbearing will prevent the development of obesity. One recent study comparing the users of standing frames and wheelchairs found the opposite to be true.[37] Maintaining an upright posture does not reduce the risk of decubitus formation; it only changes the pattern of skin breakdown. Wheelchair users have more gluteal lesions and ambulators have more foot involvement.[37, 66]

The purpose of this discussion is not to discourage ambulation and weightbearing activities for patients with high-level lesions but to place the emphasis on walking in a functional context. The cultural and individual benefits of being upright should be considered in combination with the energy efficiency of wheelchair use so that appropriate choices can be made that will support each individual patient's needs and goals.

Skin Breakdown

MORBIDITY AND COST. In one clinic population the incidence of skin breakdown in children with MMC was reported to be 43%. The prevalence of skin breakdown noted at annual evaluations increased steadily from infancy to age 10 years, then leveled off to between 20% and 25% of patients.[53] Another large clinic found that 75 patients who required inpatient treatment for skin care were hospitalized for 6000 days, costing $1.7 million (1986 dollars) for room and board alone. The average annual cost per patient with a thoracic level of motor paralysis was $2190 and for low lumbar or sacral level was $952.[24] These costs represent only part of the total cost of treating skin breakdown in such patients. Outpatient management may incur additional direct costs, including dressing supplies and equipment modifications. Indirect costs such as lost time from school or work by the patient or caregiver are also substantial. The personal toll on the patient in terms of morbidity can be quite high. Patients face risks associated with immobilization, exposure to anesthesia, loss of grafted skin or rotational myocutaneous flaps, or even amputation.

FREQUENT SITES. Skin breakdown occurs most commonly as a result of unrelieved pressure over anesthetic areas. Lacerations, burns, dermatitis, and even cold injury in anesthetic areas can also cause serious skin breakdown. In patients with MMC, higher rates of skin breakdown are seen in those who have mental retardation, large head size, kyphoscoliosis, or chronic soiling. Normal bony prominences or orthopedic deformities are common sites of skin ulceration from pressure or shear forces, and in children with MMC the most common sites of breakdown are over the perineum, over a gibbus deformity, or in the lower extremities. Nonambulatory patients have the highest frequency of ulceration of the perineum or gibbus, whereas the highest frequency of lower extremity breakdown occurs in ambulatory patients with lower lumbar motor levels.[53]

PREVENTION. Because of the high frequency and cost of skin breakdown, all patients with MMC should receive periodic examinations for and preventive guidance against skin breakdown. The child must learn that meticulous hygiene and daily inspection of insensate skin is important. Whenever a child receives a new spinal or lower extremity orthosis, a sequential wearing schedule should be used to monitor for sites of excessive pressure.[3] Ambulatory patients should be cautioned against walking barefoot, especially outdoors or on hot pavement. Patients who use wheelchairs need adjustment of seating to prevent pelvic obliquity or pressure over bony prominences. There is no preferred wheelchair cushion for patients with MMC, but gel cushions should not be left outdoors in cold climates because they may become cold enough to induce freeze burns.[52]

The fact that the incidence of skin breakdown increases as children with MMC grow larger speaks to the need to learn effective pressure relief whether from standing or sitting surfaces, but it will likely require many years of adult supervision before the child incorporates such habits into his or her daily routine.

TREATMENT. The medical management of skin breakdown in children with MMC is no different than for other diagnoses. Attention to relief of pressure or shear forces, hygiene, debridement, and nutrition are important. For wounds that extend beneath subcutaneous tissues, surgical closure may be necessary. Owing to the young age of the patient and the possibility of repeat surgery for skin breakdown, surgeons should plan the closure to allow for the greatest number of future options. Primary closure or skin rotation is preferable to myocutaneous flaps for first procedures.[35]

Obesity

Adults with spinal cord injury have a 10% to 30% reduction in basal metabolic rate and total daily energy expenditure as a result of decreased lean body mass from paralyzed muscle. Similar data are not available for children with MMC, but dieting studies document that on average children with MMC ingest 25% fewer calories than their peers and yet 27% to 90% are reported to be obese. The reduction in lean body mass and decreased activity that reduce the total daily energy expenditure is inversely related to the level of the lesion; higher-level lesions result in lower energy expenditure. Once a child with MMC becomes obese, the reduced energy expenditure makes further weight loss even more difficult. Dietary management should begin in infancy with anticipatory guidance and nutritional education. Weight reduction is extremely difficult, requiring professional assistance to maintain adequate protein and vitamin intake while severely restricting calories. Dietary intervention is most appropriately invested in prevention of obesity because the outcome of weight reduction efforts is disappointingly poor.[65]

Psychological and Social Issues

INTELLECTUAL AND PERSONAL DEVELOPMENT. Any individual's capacity to understand and cope with the world is much more complex than the single score on an intelligence test, but the imperfect representation of cognitive skill provided by IQ tests at least affords a crude measure for comparison of groups. When children with MMC as a large heterogeneous group are compared with nondisabled peers on the short-form Wechsler Intelligence Scale for Children, Revised (WISC-R), their scores are skewed toward the lower end. Only 6% of children with MMC score in the high-average to extremely high range compared with 27% of controls. Seventy-five percent of children with MMC score in the low-average to extremely low range, compared with 25% of matched peers.[2] IQ scores have been correlated with level of lesion; higher-level lesions are associated with lower scores, lower lesions with better performance. IQ scores are adversely affected by the presence of CNS infection and shunt malformation.[69] The combination of cognitive impairment and significant physical disabilities makes training in self-care both challenging and difficult. It is not surprising that children with MMC develop activities of daily living (ADL) skills later and less efficiently than their peers and that families unwittingly reinforce dependence in their attempts to meet the normal requirements and constraints of daily life.

Perhaps most important is the effect MMC has on a child's self-concept and notion of competence. Recent investigation into this area suggests that when children with MMC are compared with matched nondisabled controls, they view themselves as less competent in academic, athletic, and social domains of self-concept despite the fact that they recognize these as areas of great importance in personal and social functioning. Peer social acceptance and social comparisons are highly valued by children with MMC but they feel less supported by classmates than nondisabled children do. The discrepancy between social importance and self-competence for adolescents with MMC is greatest in the area of physical appearance.[2]

Clearly, intervention to foster independence in children with MMC must be distributed among several areas. The higher likelihood of cognitive impairment suggests the need for individualized education. Physical disability requires adaptive strategies for self-care. And interventions must be devised to develop greater levels of self-perception and self-competence for these children to interact effectively with the remainder of society.

FAMILY. MMC does not affect individuals as much as it affects families. The family is irreversibly changed by the presence of the disabled child and the child is affected by the family's response. Most social science research now agrees that the family's response to the disabled child probably plays a greater role in emotional development than the disability itself.[21]

The family must be supported in their attempt to develop competence and coping with the stressors that accompany the care of a disabled child. There are at least nine different stressors, all of which may be operative at different times. They include modification of family goals and dreams, altered relationships, increased burden of care and reduction of free time, financial burdens, altered school performance and programming, modifications to the home, medical problems, social isolation, and grieving. Of these, the medically related stress is predominant in infancy but it eventually gives way to all the others in turn and in combination.[21]

Those who would attempt to support families in their care for the child with MMC have an armamentarium of at least six resources to offer. They are (1) attention to factors that promote the health and energy *of the caregivers,* (2) problem-solving strategies that allow families to adapt, (3) social skills to better communicate the family's needs to one another and the community, (4) social and emotional support from people outside the family, (5) material resources in the form of money, goods, or services, and (6) positive beliefs which maintain hope and sustain effective coping during difficult periods.[21]

One very practical source of help for families is the Spina Bifida Association of America. This organization provides education, advocacy, and support for patients and their families. Early referral can assist the family in developing relationships with other families who can provide practical advice and counseling that is based on their own personal experiences. The address of the association is listed at the end of this chapter.

MYELOMENINGOCELE IN ADULTS

Description of a New Disease

Before surgical closure of open neural tube defects in newborns became a common practice, most affected infants did not survive. Significant morbidity plagued those who did survive in the form of urinary tract infection, renal failure, hydrocephalus, and scoliosis. The combination of improved surgical practices, new antibiotics, changing patterns of medical ethics, and willingness of healthcare professionals to manage patients with MMC using a team approach has made long-term survival possible.

Until recently, physicians had virtually no experience in caring for adults with MMC. Many relied on their understanding of spinal cord injury to guide their approach toward adults with MMC, only to find that functional and independent living skills were not commensurate with those expected based on level of physical impairment. Factors such as onset of impairment at birth, intellectual deficits, and difficulties in achieving bladder and bowel continence contribute to delayed social maturation throughout childhood and adolescence. Family expectations and opportunities for social interactions and vocational experiences probably contribute to dependency as well.

Only limited descriptive information is available on the types of medical complications and psychosocial difficulties of adults with MMC, but rehabilitation principles derived from other conditions can be applied to these problems. Periodic screening for change in neurological status, development of joint disease, deterioration of renal function, or development of pressure ulcers is essential.

SKIN BREAKDOWN. Pressure ulcers are a major cause of morbidity in adolescents and adults with MMC. In one series of young adults aged 19 to 27 years old, 85% had had skin breakdown requiring hospitalization, and 70% had continuing problems with skin ulcers. About half had only occasional breakdown, but one fourth had nearly continuous problems.[17] Skin breakdown over the feet can be ex-

tremely difficult to heal and can cause loss of ambulation due to need for pressure relief or surgical amputation.

MUSCULOSKELETAL COMPLICATIONS AND JOINT DISEASE. Joint pain and degeneration can cause adults to become more dependent upon a wheelchair for mobility. Upper extremity joints such as the shoulder and elbow may become painful from overuse. Lower extremity joints may become Charcot joints as a result of an orthopedic deformity, abnormal dynamic forces, and impaired sensation. Clinicians should give careful consideration to joint protection for young children with MMC.

Scoliosis does not appear to progress beyond adolescence, but its presence may cause ongoing problems with posture and seating, development of pressure ulcers, loss of ambulation, impairment of respiratory function, and pain.

LATE NEUROLOGICAL CHANGES. Neurological deterioration in adults with MMC can occur as a result of shunt obstruction, syringomyelia, or tethering of the spinal cord. Most children with MMC and hydrocephalus do not seem to outgrow the need for a shunt as adults.[40] Hydromyelia causing upper extremity pain, paresthesias, and weakness has been reported as a late development in adults.[67] Tethering of the spinal cord and herniated discs have occurred in adults, often in association with pregnancy.[67]

RENAL AND UROLOGICAL PROBLEMS. Renal failure is one of the most serious complications facing adults with MMC. While the primary causes are most often reflux and recurrent infection, other contributing factors include hypertension, shunt nephritis, amyloidosis, and calculi. Patients with MMC appear to be good candidates for dialysis, with better survival rates than for diabetic patients with end-stage renal disease. Renal transplantation has also been used successfully.[51]

Late complications of previous urological surgery can also occur, including rupture of an enterocystoplasty, or erosion or failure of an implanted artificial sphincter. Regular urological follow-up is important to monitor renal function, treat infections, and identify complications such as calculi formation or renal failure.

FERTILITY. Studies have indicated that adolescents with MMC have similar expectations regarding marriage and reproduction as do adolescents without MMC, but they have considerably less experience with dating and knowledge of sexual functioning.[25]

Girls, but not boys, with MMC have been observed to physically mature earlier than peers and same-sex family members without MMC. They also tend to reach menarche sooner than their peers.[25]

Studies to date of the sexuality of adults with MMC have relied on self-report of function. Women report various degrees of genital sensation, while many men report the ability for erection and ejaculation, but none of these correlates with level of motor function. Most adults with MMC are reported to have satisfactory sexual function.[10] Men with MMC have been reported to father children, but some data suggest that primary testicular failure with low serum testosterone and elevated follicle-stimulating and luteinizing hormones may be common and that the prognosis for fertility may be poor.[60] Women with MMC have been able to successfully conceive and carry to term without major complications, although urinary tract infections have been commonly reported.[10]

ALLERGY TO LATEX. Children with MMC have recently been found to have high frequencies of allergy to latex products. This IgE-mediated allergic response can manifest as contact dermatitis, allergic rhinitis, asthma, angioedema, or intraoperative anaphylaxis.[71, 76] Patients may encounter latex in such products as rubber balloons, rubber gloves, condoms, or ostomy bags. The allergens are thought to be small water-soluble antigens which can be eluted from the surface of latex products, transferred by direct contact with skin or mucous membranes or carried airborne by powder emitted from the latex product, and which may not be completely eliminated by washing the product.[79]

The most serious allergic manifestation, intraoperative anaphylaxis, has often occurred in patients who have safely undergone previous surgical procedures. It is thought that chronic exposure to rubber via catheters or gloves is the cause of the allergy. Patients with MMC who require surgery should be questioned for potential allergy to latex, which can be confirmed by skin-prick testing. If latex allergy is suspected or confirmed, surgeons should avoid use of latex products.[19] Patients who manifest allergic symptoms may need to avoid use of latex products such as rubber gloves, rubber catheters, or latex condoms.

Affective Disorders

Adolescents with MMC often have low self-esteem and frequent doubts concerning their health, physical condition, and sexual functioning. Delayed social responsibility is also prominent, manifested by lack of chore assignments at home, social contacts with younger children as opposed to peers, and a paucity of friends.[16, 25]

Adults with MMC are reported to have a range of adjustment from well-adapted to poorly motivated, apathetic, and dependent personalities.[17] Intelligence and level of paralysis are associated with good adjustment. Social isolation is a frequent problem, with many adults reporting few friends and infrequent memberships in clubs or groups. Problems with physical access and attitudes of persons without disabilities compound social isolation.[64] While this is a high-risk group for psychosocial problems, suicide has not been reported in higher-than-expected frequency.

Vocational Issues

In large clinic series, most adults with MMC are reported to have completed high school and about half continued in postsecondary education.[17, 39, 72] About 25% of adults with MMC report employment.[17, 38] They mainly performed routine, non-manual work, had average working hours, but received below-average pay. Most enjoyed their jobs and were well accepted by peers at work, but job retention was poor.[38, 72] Adolescents with MMC appear to have unrealistic ideas about training and skill requirements compared with their peers, and are less often assigned chores at home, even chores well within their physical abilities.[25]

Independent Living

Various rates of living away from parents have been reported in different cultures, ranging from over 60% in the United States to 15% in Great Britain.[17, 39] In one study,

one third of adults with MMC were fully independent—employed, financially independent, homeowners, and free of psychological problems. The other two thirds required Social Security income and various levels of support from family and friends. Many have limited abilities to do cooking, shopping, or access public transportation.[39]

Planning for postsecondary education, vocation, and independent living should begin in early adolescence. Under the 1990 Amendments of the Education of the Handicapped Act, Public Law 101-476, schools must include transition services in the Individualized Education Program (I.E.P.) of a student receiving special education services by age 16 years. Such services are meant to be a coordinated plan for moving the child beyond school to such outcomes as vocational training, employment, adult services, independent living, and community participation. Clinicians can contribute to this process by reminding parents and schools to initiate such planning, and by providing information about physical and health conditions which may influence the process.[61]

For further information on spina bifida, the reader is referred to: The Spina Bifida Association of America, 1700 Rockville Pike, Suite 540, Rockville, MD 20852, telephone 301–770-SBAA.

References

1. Agnarsson U, Warde C, McCarthy G, et al: Anorectal function of children with neurological problems: I. Spina bifida. Dev Med Child Neurol 1993; 35:893–902.
2. Appleton PE, Mincho P, Ellis N, et al: The self concept of young people with spina bifida: A population based study. Dev Med Child Neurol 1994; 36:198–215.
3. Banta JV, Lin J, Peterson M, Dagenis T: The team approach in the care of the child with myelomeningocele. J Prosthet Orthot 1989; 2:263–273.
4. Bishop DT: Multifactorial inheritance. In Emery AEH, Rimoin DL (eds): Principles and Practice of Medical Genetics. New York, Churchill Livingstone, 1990, pp 165–174.
5. Bosco PJ, Bauer SB, Colodny AH, et al: The long-term results of artificial sphincters in children. J Urol 1991; 146:396–399.
6. Brockelhurst G: The nature of spina bifida. In Brockelhurst (ed): Spina Bifida for the Clinician. London, Spastics International, 1976; pp 1–7.
7. Bunch WA, Scarff TB, Dronch V: Progressive loss in myelomeningocele patients. Orthop Trans 1983; 7:185.
8. Carmel P: The Arnold-Chiari malformation. In Section of Pediatric Neurosurgery of the American Association of Neurological Surgeons (eds): Pediatric Neurosurgery: Surgery of the Developing Nervous System, ed 2. Philadelphia, WB Saunders, 1989, pp 53–70.
9. Carter CO: Clues to aetiology of neural tube malformations. Dev Med Child Neurol 1974; 16(suppl 32):3–15.
10. Cass AS, Bloom BA, Luxenberg M: Sexual function in adults with myelomeningocele. J Urol 1986; 136:425–426.
11. Chan A, Robertson EF, Haan EA, et al: Prevalence of neural tube defects in South Australia, 1966–1991: Effectiveness and impact of prenatal diagnosis. BMJ 1993; 307:703–706.
12. Charney EB, Melchionni JB, Smith DR: Community ambulation by children with myelomeningocele and high-level paralysis. J Pediatr Orthop 1991; 11:579–582.
13. Cowchock S, Ainbender E, Prescott G, et al: The recurrence risk for neural tube defects in the United States: A collaborative study. Am J Med Genet 1980; 5:309–314.
14. Czeizel AE, Dudas I: Prevention of the first occurrence of neural tube defects by periconceptional vitamin supplementation. N Engl J Med 1992; 327:1832–1835.
15. Dietrich S, Okamoto G: Bowel training for children with neurogenic dysfunction: A follow-up. Arch Phys Med Rehabil 1982; 63:166–170.
16. Dorner S: Adolescents with spina bifida: How they see their situation. Arch Dis Child 1976; 51:439–444.

17. Dunne KB, Shurtleff DB: The adult with meningomyelocele: A preliminary report. *In* McLaurin RL (ed): Spina Bifida: A Multidisciplinary Approach. New York, Praeger, 1986, pp 38–51.

18. Elder JS: Continent appendicocolostomy: A variation of the Mitrofanoff principle in pediatric urinary tract reconstruction. J Urol 1992; 148:117–119.

19. Emans JB: Allergy to latex in patients who have myelodysplasia. J Bone Joint Surg Am 1992; 74:1103–1109.

20. Ferembac D: Frequency of spina bifida occulta in prehistoric human skeletons. Nature 1963; 197:100.

21. Friedman W, Schaffer J: Family adjustments and contributions. *In* Shurtleff DB (ed): Myelodysplasias and Extrophies: Significance, Prevention and Treatment. New York, Grune & Stratton, 1986, pp 399–409.

22. Greenberg F, James LM, Oakley GP: Estimates of birth prevalence rates of spina bifida in the United States from computer-generated maps. Am J Obstet Gynecol 1983; 145:570–573.

23. Hamilton RA, Dorman JC: Neural tube defects—prenatal diagnosis and management. Ulster Med J 1992; 61:127–133.

24. Harris MB, Banta JV: Cost of skin care in the myelomeningocele population. J Pediatr Orthop 1990; 10:355–361.

25. Hayden PW, Davenport SLH, Campbell MM: Adolescents with myelodysplasia: Impact of physical disability on emotional maturation. Pediatrics 1979; 64:53–59.

26. Hays R, Jordan R, McLaughlin J, et al: Central ventilatory dysfunction in myelodysplasia: An independent determination of survival. Dev Med Child Neurol 1989; 31:366–370.

27. Hays RM, Erickson D, Astley S: Tethered cord syndrome in meningomyelocele: Analysis of clinical features for early diagnosis. Arch Phys Med Rehabil 1989; 70:A-45.

28. Just M, Schwartz M, Ernest J: Magnetic resonance imaging of dysgraphic myelodysplasia. Childs Nerv Sys 1986, 4.149–153.

29. Kimura DK, Mayo M, Shurtleff D: Urinary tract management. *In* Shurtleff DB (ed): Myelodysplasias and Extrophies: Significance, Prevention and Treatment. New York, Grune & Stratton, 1986, pp 243–266.

30. King JC, Currie DM, Wright E: Bowel training in spina bifida: Importance of education, patient compliance, age, and anal reflexes. Arch Phys Med Rehabil 1993; 75:243–247.

31. Knutson LM, Clark DE: Orthotic devices for ambulation in children with cerebral palsy and myelomeningocele. Phys Ther 1991; 71:947–960.

32. Laurence KM: The genetics and prevention of neural tube defects and uncomplicated hydrocephalus. *In* Emery AEH, Rimoin DL (eds): Principles and Practice of Medical Genetics. New York, Churchill Livingstone, 1990, pp 323–346.

33. Laurence KM, James N, Miller MH, et al: Double-blind randomized controlled trial of folate treatment before conception to prevent recurrence of neural-tube defects. BMJ 1981; 282:1509–1511.

34. Lie HR, Lagergren J, Rasmussen F, et al: Bowel and bladder control of children with myelomeningocele: A Nordic study. Dev Med Child Neurol 1991; 33:1053–1061.

35. Linder RM, Morris D: The surgical management of pressure ulcers: A systematic approach based on staging. Decubitus 1990; 3:32–38.

36. Lindseth RE, Dias LS, Drennan JC: Myelomeningocele. Instruct Course Lect 1991; 40:271–291.

37. Liptak G, Shurtleff D, Bloss J, et al: Mobility aids for children with high level myelomeningocele: Parapodium vs wheelchair. Dev Med Child Neurol 1992; 34:787–796.

38. Lonton AP, Loughlin AM, O'Sullivan AM: The employment of adults with spina bifida. Z Kinderchir 1984; 39(suppl 2):132–134.

39. Lonton AP, O'Sullivan AM, Loughlin AM: Spina bifida adults. Z Kinderchir 1983; 38(suppl 2):110–112.

40. Lorber J, Pucholt V: When is a shunt no longer necessary? An investigation of 300 patients with hydrocephalus and myelomeningocele: 11–22 year follow-up. Z Kinderchir 1981; 34:327–329.

41. Luthy DA, Wardinsky T, Shurtleff DB, et al: Cesarean section before the onset of labor and subsequent motor function in infants with meningomyelocele diagnosed antenatally. N Engl J Med 1991; 324:662–666.

42. Main DM, Mennuti MT: Neural tube defects: Issues in prenatal diagnosis and counselling. Obstet Gynecol 1986; 67:1–16.

43. McDonald C, Jaffe K, Mosca V, Shurtleff D: Ambulatory outcome of children with myelomeningocele: Effect of lower extremity muscle strength. Dev Med Child Neurol 1991; 33:482–490.

44. McDonald C, Jaffe K, Shurtleff D, Menelaus M: Modifications to the traditional description of neurosegmental intervention in myelomeningocele. Dev Med Child Neurol 1991; 33:473–481

45. McGuire EJ: Neuroanatomy and neurophysiology. *In* McLaurin RL (ed): Spina Bifida: A Multidisciplinary Approach. New York, Praeger, 1986, pp 246–252.

46. McGuire EJ, Woodside JR, Borden TA, Weiss RM: Prognostic value of urodynamic testing in myelodysplastic patients. J Urol 1981; 126:205–209.

47. McLone DG, Czyzewsky D, Raimondi AJ, Sommers RC: Central nervous system infections as a limiting factor in intelligence of children born with myelomeningocele. Pediatrics 1982; 70:338–342.

48. McLone DG, Naidich TP: Myelomeningocele: Outcome and late complications. *In* Section of Pediatric Neurosurgery of the American Association of Neurological Surgeons (eds): Pediatric Neurosurgery: Surgery of the Developing Nervous System. Philadelphia, WB Saunders, 1982; pp 61–78.

49. Milunsky A, Ulcickas M, Rothman KJ, et al: Maternal heat exposure and neural tube defects. JAMA 1992; 268:882–885.

50. MRC Vitamin Study Research Group: Prevention of neural tube defects: Results of the medical research counsel vitamin study. Lancet 1991; 338:131–137.

51. Muralikrishna GS, Rodger RSC, Macdougall AI, et al: Renal replacement treatment in patients with spina bifida or spinal cord injury. BMJ 1989; 299:1506.

52. Odderson IR, Jaffe KM, Sleicher CA, et al: Gel wheelchair cushions: A potential cold weather hazard. Arch Phys Med Rehabil 1991; 72:1017–1020.

53. Okamoto GA, Lamers JV, Shurtleff DB: Skin breakdown in patients with myelomeningocele. Arch Phys Med Rehabil 1983; 64:20–23.

54. Okamoto GA, Sousa J, Telzrow RW, et al: Toileting skills in children with myelomeningocele: Rates of learning. Arch Phys Med Rehabil 1984; 65:182–185.

55. O'Rahilly R, Gardner E: The initial development of the human brain. Acta Anat 1979; 104:123–133.

56. Owens JR, Harris F, McAllister E, West L: 19 year incidence of neural tube defects in area under constant surveillance. Lancet 1981; 2:1032–1035.

57. Petersen M: Tethered cord syndrome in myelodysplasia: Correlation between level of lesion and height at time of presentation. Dev Med Child Neurol 1992; 34:604–610.

58. Raimondi AJ: Hydrocephalus. *In* Raimondi AJ (ed): Pediatric Neurosurgery: Theoretic Principles: Art of Surgical Techniques. New York, Springer-Verlag, 1987; pp 453–455.

59. Recommendations for the use of folic acid to reduce the number of cases of spina bifida and other neural tube defects. MMWR 1992; 41:1–7.

60. Reilly JM, Oates RD: Preliminary investigation of the potential fertility status of postpubertal males with myelodysplasia, abstract. J Urol 1992; 147:251A.

61. Ross B: Meeting the educational needs of children with disabilities: A collaborative management approach. Phys Med Rehabil Clin North Am 1991; 2:781–800.

62. Sandford MK, Kissling GE, Joubert PE: Neural tube defect etiology: New evidence concerning maternal hyperthermia, health, and diet. Dev Med Child Neurol 1992; 34:661–675.

63. Selzman AA, Elder JS, Mapstone TB: Urologic consequences of myelodysplasia and other congenital abnormalities of the spinal cord. Urol Clin North Am 1993; 20:485–504.

64. Shaffer J, Friedrich W: Young adult psychosocial adjustment. *In* Shurtleff DB (ed): Myelodysplasias and Extrophies: Significance, Prevention and Treatment. New York, Grune & Stratton, 1986, pp 421–430.

65. Shurtleff D: Dietary management. *In* Shurtleff DB (ed): Myelodysplasias and Extrophies: Significance, Prevention and Treatment. New York, Grune & Stratton, 1986, pp 285–295.

66. Shurtleff D: Mobility. *In* Shurtleff DB (ed): Myelodysplasias and Extrophies: Significance, Prevention and Treatment. New York, Grune & Stratton, 1986, pp 314–320.

67. Shurtleff D, Dunne K: Adults and adolescents with meningomyelocele. *In* Shurtleff DB (ed): Myelodysplasias and Extrophies: Significance, Prevention and Treatment. New York, Grune & Stratton, 1986, pp 433–448.

68. Shurtleff D, Shurtleff H: Decision making for the treatment or nontreatment of congenitally malformed individuals. *In* Shurtleff DB

(ed): Myelodysplasias and Extrophies: Significance, Prevention and Treatment. New York, Grune & Stratton, 1986, pp 3–24.

69. Shurtleff D, Stuntz JT: Back closure. *In* Shurtleff DB (ed): Myelodysplasias and Extrophies: Significance, Prevention and Treatment. New York, Grune & Statton, 1986, pp 117–138.

70. Shurtleff D, Stuntz JT, Hayden: Hydrocephalus. In Shurtleff DB (ed): Myelodysplasias and Extrophies: Significance, Prevention and Treatment. New York, Grune & Stratton, 1986, pp 139–180.

71. Slater JE: Rubber anaphylaxis. N Engl J Med 1989; 320:1126–1130.

72. Smith AD: Adult spina bifida survey in Scotland: Educational attainment and employment. Z Kinderchir 1983; 38(suppl):107–109.

73. Sousa JC, Gordon LH, Shurtleff DB: Assessing the development of daily living skills in patients with spina bifida. Dev Med Child Neurol 1976; 18(suppl 37):134–142.

74. Spindel MR, Bauer SB, Dyro FM, et al: The changing neurologic lesion in myelodysplasia. JAMA 1987; 258:1630–1633.

75. Steinbok P, Irvine B, Cochrane DD, Irwin BJ: Long-term outcome and complications of children born with meningomyelocele. Childs Nerv Syst 1992; 8:92–96.

76. Sussman GL, Tarlo S, Dolovich J: The spectrum of IgE mediated responses to latex. JAMA 1991; 265:2844–2847.

77. Tamaki N, Shirataki K, Kojima N, et al: Tethered cord syndrome of delayed onset following repair of myelomeningocele. J Neurosurg 1988; 69:393–398.

78. Uehling DT, Smith J, Meyer J, Bruskewitz R: Impact of an intermittent catheterization program in children with myelomeningocele. Pediatrics 1985; 76:892–895.

79. Warpinski JR, Folgert J, Cohen M, Bush RK: Allergic reaction to latex: A risk factor for unsuspected anaphylaxis. Allergy Proc 1991; 12:95–102.

80. White JJ, Suzuki H, Shafie ME, et al: A physiologic rationale for the management of neurologic rectal incontinence in children. Pediatrics 1972; 49:888–893.

81. Wolraich ML, Hawtrey C, Mapel J, Henderson M: Results of clean intermittent catheterization for children with neurogenic bladders. Urology 1983; 22:479–482.

82. Yen IH, Khoury MJ, Erickson JD, et al: The changing epidemiology of neural tube defects: United States, Am J Dis Child 1992; 146:857–861.

55

Rehabilitation of Patients With Spinal Cord Injuries

GARY M. YARKONY, M.D.,
AND DAVID CHEN, M.D.

The earliest description of a person with a spinal cord injury (SCI) was written in the Edwin Smith Papyrus about 1700 BC.[150] The Egyptian physician described SCI as an ailment not to be treated. The life expectancy and outcomes for persons with SCI continued to be poor for centuries. During the 1940s, specialized centers were developed for the care of persons with SCI.[19] Guttmann in England[126, 127] and Munro in the United States were the pioneers in their respective countries. These units were developed to eliminate the piecemeal care of persons with SCI.[18] The subsequent development of care systems for persons with SCI has improved the quality and longevity of their lives.[6, 110, 326]

This chapter deals with traumatic injury to the spinal cord. Injuries that occur to the spinal cord from the foramen magnum distal to the conus medullaris and cauda equina are included. This chapter also describes the comprehensive team approach to rehabilitation of persons with SCI, from the acute unit to lifelong follow-up. The problems persons with SCI encounter as they age are addressed as well. Because of the poor prognosis of persons with SCIs in the past, it is only recently that these problems have been addressed.[223, 368]

EPIDEMIOLOGY

Spinal cord injury is an uncommon condition. It has been described as striking "the vibrant, young active and well-educated people in our country."[23] More than half of the persons injured are under 30 years of age and 85% are in the labor force at the time of their injuries.

Estimates vary in regard to the annual incidence, which is the number of new SCIs in a 1-year period. The incidence figures range from 29.4 cases per 1 million[94] to 50 cases per 1 million.[30, 94, 162, 177] Insufficient data exist to determine the exact figure, and there may be annual variations in the incidence.

Estimates also vary as to the prevalence of SCI in the United States. Prevalence is the number of living persons with SCI at a given time. These range from 525 per 1 million, or 128,941 persons, to 1124 cases per 1 million, or 276,057 persons.[59, 76, 182] The most recent survey estimated 721 per 1 million, or 176,965 persons, in 1988. Less than 5000 are estimated to be institutionalized.

The majority of persons with SCI are male, with the male-to-female ratios in the literature ranging from 2.4:1[23] to 4:1.[313] The median age at time of injury is approximately 26 years.[23, 313] Males tend to be injured at younger ages than females. Most people with SCIs are in the 25- to 44-year-old range. The majority of persons with SCIs are white (8:1), although in spinal cord centers in urban locations the ratio of whites to non-whites is only 3:1. The population of persons with SCI is less likely to be married, twice as likely to be divorced, and less likely to have ever been married than the population without SCI. The educational levels of persons with SCI are slightly higher with more people likely to have a high-school diploma or to have attended some college than in the general population.

The common causes of SCI can vary in different geographical regions. Overall, vehicle crashes are the most common cause (45.4%), followed by falls (16.8%), sports injuries (16.3%), and violence. Urban centers report an incidence of injuries due to violence at 14.6%, with violence being more common in males, and non-whites.[312] In some urban areas, violence is the leading cause of SCI.

NEUROLOGICAL CLASSIFICATION OF SPINAL CORD INJURIES

Spinal cord injuries are classified according to the International Standards for Neurological and Functional Classification of Spinal Cord Injury[5] (Fig. 55–1). This requires a systematic neurological examination of sensory and motor function.

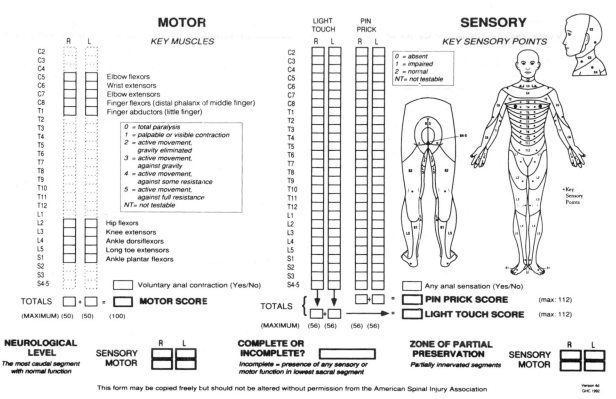

FIGURE 55–1 Standard neurological classification of spinal cord injury. (From International Standards for Neurological and Functional Classification of Spinal Cord Injury. Reprinted with permission of American Spinal Injury Association, Chicago, 1992.)

Tetraplegia is preferred to the term *quadriplegia* as it is derived solely from Greek roots as opposed to quadriplegia, which has mixed derivation. Tetraplegia results from injury to the spinal cord within the cervical region of the spinal canal. There is a loss of motor or sensory function, or both, in the arms, trunk, and legs, as well as loss of bladder, bowel, and sexual function to some degree. Paraplegia results from injury to the spinal cord in the thoracic, lumbar, or sacral segments. This includes injury to the conus medullaris and the cauda equina. There can be involvement of the trunk, legs and bowel, bladder, and sexual dysfunction to some degree. Tetraplegia and paraplegia do not include lesions to peripheral nerves outside the neural canal such as injuries to the brachial or lumbar plexus. The terms *quadriparesis* and *paraparesis* are imprecise and should not be used. In lieu of these terms, the ASIA (American Spinal Injury Association) Impairment Scale, which is described later, should be used.

The neurological level is the most caudal neurological segment of the spinal cord that retains normal sensory and motor function on both sides of the body. Often the sensory and motor levels vary from side to side, and the sensory and motor levels can be different on the same side of the body. The physical examination should record the most caudal sensory and motor level on each side, which results in the recording of four levels (sensory and motor from both right and left). Figure 55–1 indicates the key muscles to be tested for each myotome and dermatome. There are 10 myotomes on each side and 28 dermatomes. Muscles are graded from 0, which is total paralysis, to 5, which is normal in the sense of providing full resistance. Muscles are examined from the rostral to caudal segments. A muscle

with a strength grade of 3 (antigravity) is considered to have an intact innervation if the next most rostral muscle is a grade 4 or 5. Each dermatome has a key sensory point. Light touch and pinprick scores can be used to determine the sensory score, and the motor score can be determined by adding the results of the manual muscle tests of the 10 key muscle groups on each side. The system for the sensory and motor score is described in Figure 55–1.

The rectal area is examined digitally. Sensation is considered to be present if deep anal sensation or sensation of the anal mucocutaneous junction is present. A *complete lesion* is defined as the absence of sensory or motor function in the lowest sacral segment. If either sensory or motor function is present, the lesion is incomplete. This definition is known as the sacral sparing definition. Using this definition, persons generally do not change from incomplete to complete, and the sacral sparing definition of incomplete correlates more closely with motor improvement in the extremities.[343]

The ASIA Impairment Scale (Fig. 55–2)[5] is a modification of the Frankel Scale developed by the American Spinal Injury Association. It has five levels from A through E that further define the extent of the injury. A is a complete lesion as there is no sensory or motor function in the S4 to S5 sacral segment. B is an incomplete lesion with sensation but no motor function below the neurological level. Sensation must be present in the S4 and S5 segments. C is an incomplete lesion with motor function present below the neurological level and the majority of key muscles have a grade less than 3. D is an incomplete lesion with motor function present and the majority of key muscles below the neurological level have a muscle grade

ASIA IMPAIRMENT SCALE

☐ **A = Complete:** No motor or sensory function is preserved in the sacral segments S4-S5.

☐ **B = Incomplete:** Sensory but not motor function is preserved below the neurological level and extends through the sacral segments S4-S5.

☐ **C = Incomplete:** Motor function is preserved below the neurological level, and the majority of key muscles below the neurological level have a muscle grade less than 3.

☐ **D = Incomplete:** Motor function is preserved below the neurological level, and the majority of key muscles below the neurological level have a muscle grade greater than or equal to 3.

☐ **E = Normal:** Motor and sensory function is normal.

FIGURE 55–2   ASIA impairment scale. (From International Standards for Neurological and Functional Classification of Spinal Cord Injury. Reprinted with permission of American Spinal Injury Association, Chicago, 1992.)

greater than or equal to 3. E is a normal sensory and motor neurological examination.

Several clinical syndromes are described in SCI. The *central cord syndrome*, first described by Schneider and colleagues,[297] is one of the most common. It generally occurs in the cervical area and is characterized by greater upper limb than lower limb weakness. Bowel, bladder, and sexual dysfunction occur to varying degrees. The central cord syndrome also commonly occurs in older persons with degenerative changes in the neck following a hyperextension injury, although other patterns of SCIs can occur.[135, 231, 292]

Brown-Séquard described the syndrome of hemisection of the spinal cord in the middle of the 19th century.[293] The definition used today is a lesion that produces relatively greater ipsilateral proprioceptive and motor loss and contralateral loss of sensation to pinprick and temperature.[5] Owing to the partial nature of the lesion, prognosis for bowel function and recovery is excellent.[173]

The *anterior cord syndrome* is an SCI affecting the anterior cord and preserving the posterior columns. There is variable loss of motor and pinprick and temperature sensation while proprioception is spared.[5] It results from trauma to the anterior spinal artery or direct trauma to the anterior aspect of the spinal cord. It can occur with retropulsed disc or bone fragments and is often due to a flexion injury of the cervical spine.[16]

Injuries to the conus medullaris and associated lumbar nerve roots generally result in an areflexic bladder and bowel and flaccid paralysis of extremities.[19] Lesions more

proximal to the distal terminus of the conus can have preserved bulbocavernosus or micturition reflexes.[267] Lesions to the nerve roots of the cauda equina represent a lower motor lesion within the neural canal, resulting in bowel, bladder, and lower limb flaccid paralysis.[5]

REHABILITATION IN THE ACUTE CARE PHASE

Medical care after SCI focuses on the complex cardiopulmonary problems, management of the traumatized spine and spinal cord, and maintenance of fluid, electrolyte balance, and other biological parameters (Table 55–1). Recent advances include the use of methylprednisolone in high doses within 8 hours to decrease the extent of the injury.[31, 32] Methylprednisolone is a synthetic steroid that acts as a free radical scavenger to inhibit secondary damage to the spinal cord.[131] Studies currently are underway to evaluate the use of the GM_1 ganglioside to improve motor and sensory recovery as well.[109] Gangliosides are complex acidic glycolipids that are present in central nervous system cells. In animal studies, they have stimulated the repair of damaged nerve cells.

The management of spine fractures is beyond the scope of this chapter. It has been extensively reviewed by others.[62, 211, 234] The need to immobilize the person initially until it is determined if the fracture requires surgical or orthotic mobilization produces many challenges for the rehabilitation team as they work with the surgical and medical specialists.

Pressure ulcers continue to be a problem for persons with SCI. During the acute care phase, the sacrum and heels are the areas of greatest risk.[265, 313] Turning and positioning methods to prevent pressure ulcers are often limited by the need to immobilize the person in the supine position in traction. Rotating beds must often be stopped to perform medical procedures and provide nursing care, and this can increase the risk of developing pressure ulcers. When possible, the person should be turned and repositioned every 2 hours. Skin should be inspected for nonblanchable erythema, which is considered a grade I ulceration and the heralding lesion of skin ulceration. Minimal-air-loss beds can be helpful in the acute care phase for the prevention and treatment of pressure ulcers at this stage.[93, 153] Pillows and foam wedges are used to prevent pressure on bony prominences (see Chapter 31).

The need to monitor fluid and electrolyte balance and input and output limits options in urological management during the acute care. Intermittent catheterization is often of limited practicality and an indwelling catheter must be used. Patients with local trauma to the penis can require a suprapubic catheter. Intermittent catheterization is not al-

TABLE 55–1   Goals of Rehabilitation in Acute Care

Prevent pressure ulceration
Maintain joint range of motion
Begin bowel and bladder programs
Begin sitting program
Institute activities of daily living appropriate to medical conditions and level of management

ways preferable to an indwelling catheter during the acute stage of injury.[198] It does not result in any long-term advantages when studying upper tract pathological abnormalities, the ultimate bladder drainage method, or urinary infection rate. Indwelling catheters used for more than 3 months can result in an increased incidence of urethral complications. If an adequate intermittent catheterization program cannot be maintained with urine output volumes less than 450 mL during the acute phase, an indwelling catheter might be preferable.

Bowel management should commence during the acute care phase to avoid the fecal impactions that are commonly present on admission to the rehabilitation unit.[104] High fluid intake and dietary fiber are the basis for establishing a satisfactory bowel program. Strong cathartics and enemas should be avoided and consistent bowel evacuation should be commenced as early as possible. Stool softeners such as docusate are often helpful. Impactions, if they are present, should be removed manually if low or loosened with mineral oil enemas if high (see Chapter 28).

Maintenance of normal joint range of motion (ROM) is essential to ease transit into the rehabilitation program.[176] Proper positioning and ROM help prevent the development of joint contractures.[371] Particular attention should be paid to the shoulder joints, which should be abducted as much as feasible.[299] Flaccid joints require ROM exercise one time daily, while "spastic joints" typically need ROM exercise twice or three times daily. The best guide to determine the success of the ROM program is to perform repeated goniometry. Orthotic management can help prevent joint contractures. The wrist generally is splinted in the functional position of extension with the web space of the thumb maintained, the thumb opposed, and the fingers positioned to prevent flexion.[145] The ankle is maintained in an orthosis at 90 degress, if necessary. The joints that most commonly develop contractures during the acute care phase are the hip, knee, and ankle.

The physiatrist should attempt to meet with the patient and family as soon as possible after injury. Because of the devastating nature of these injuries,[126] counseling for the patient and family should be available. The prognosis should be presented, and hope for motor and sensory recovery should be maintained. The physiatrist should recognize the possibility of concurrent brain injury and carefully assess the patient's mental status.[67, 247] Brain injury commonly occurs in traffic accidents in both paraplegic and tetraplegic patients, and the incidence has been reported to be as high as 50% to 60%. The presence of a concurrent brain injury can affect the way the staff communicates with the injured person and can also prolong the course of rehabilitation.[289]

GUIDES TO FUNCTIONAL OUTCOMES

The ability to perform self-care and mobility skills after SCI is generally described in reference to the motor level.[22, 379] Rehabilitation efforts can be directed to the entire spectrum of abilities, from directing only one's self-care performed by others to being totally independent. The functional program should be accompanied by an educational program for the injured persons, their families,

and their caregivers. Instruction is given in the recognition, prevention, and treatment of secondary complications of SCI. The setting in which therapy occurs should not be limited to the hospital itself. Reintegration into the community is facilitated by the patient performing skills in the community. This helps the patient gain a more realistic appreciation of barriers in the outside environment. Adapting skills learned in the protective environment of the hospital to the home situation is best done through therapeutic day and overnight passes. While these passes often are viewed as a healthcare luxury, they are very helpful in getting the patients ready for discharge to the community and home.

The following guidelines are an overview of the obtainable goals based on the level of injury. The equipment commonly used at each level also is described. There can be significant variability in the functional outcomes among different persons with the same level of injury. The therapy team should not be guided by the patient's level of injury alone.[374] Many persons can master tasks that would not be predicted by their level of lesion alone. On the other hand, many persons attempt to learn skills that are not practical in the community because of time constraints or environmental limitations.[351] It is important to reach a balance in these areas to prevent unnecessarily prolonging rehabilitation to obtain functional skills that are not obtainable or not needed. Goals in SCI rehabilitation should be individualized to each person's needs and social situation.

Function in the Patient With High Tetraplegia (C1 to C4)

Patients with injuries from C1 to C4 are considered to have high tetraplegia.[357] The goals for these persons and the technology needed are the same regardless of the need for supported ventilation. The staff must be prepared to manage pulmonary complications and have the technology available to allow the injured person to interact with the environment. Persons with injury above C4 can require ventilators or phrenic nerve pacemakers.[188] Phrenic nerve pacemakers have the advantage of requiring equipment that is less bulky, quieter, and not as obtrusive as a ventilator. Phrenic nerve pacemakers require the nerves to be intact and can be simultaneous or alternating.[12] If secretions are not a problem, tracheostomies can be plugged. Another alternative that is less commonly used is the pneumobelt and intermittent negative pressure apparatus.[357] These devices inflate on the abdominal wall causing forced expiration followed by passive inspiration when the inflatable bladder deflates.[357] They can only be used when sitting. For other devices, see Chapter 33.

The C4 tetraplegic patient learns to direct others in physical activities such as ROM exercises, transfers, and positioning. Caregivers are instructed in transfers, which often require a mechanical lift. Functional goals typically focus on the use of environmental controls and other technical aids. Rehabilitation engineering and occupational therapy staff must often collaborate to allow for improved access to commercially available equipment. Commonly used devices include page turners, door openers, computers, emergency call systems, speaker telephones, and environmental control units (see Chapters 24 and 26). Computers are typically accessed via breath or voice control. Environmental control units vary in terms of the number of devices they control, and can be controlled with breath (sip and puff), tread switches, mouthsticks, or tongue switches. Funding is often a limitation to purchasing this equipment.

Both manual and power wheelchairs typically are required.[259] Owing to their size and weight and accessibility issues, large power wheelchairs cannot be used in all environments. A manual chair serves as a backup to the power chair in these instances, as well as when the power wheelchair is being recharged or repaired. Power chairs can be controlled by many control devices, including chin, head, and voice activation. If the lesion is incomplete, a hand control can be used. Pressure relief and postural hypotension basically require using a power reclining mechanism. The preferred recliner mechanisms are those that avoid shearing forces during the reclining process (see Chapter 19).

Function in C5 Tetraplegia

The elbow flexion present in C5 tetraplegia can be combined with orthotic management to allow performance of self-care and mobility skills.[382] A balanced forearm orthosis (BFO) can be used to compensate for weakness and allow for improved arm placement. It is useful early in the course before maximum elbow flexion and shoulder abduction. Many C4 tetraplegic patients with partial elbow flexion use the BFO as well. Static splints (long opponens orthosis) with utensil slots or pencil holders are used to assist with tasks such as writing, typing, and feeding. The long opponens orthosis provides for wrist stability as well as being an attachment for utensils. It is best to use the simplest and most cosmetic orthotic devices with the least potential for breakdown. Other devices that have been proposed (but not commonly used) for this level of injury include splints that are cable-driven, electrically powered, or ratchet orthoses to provide tenodesis.

Realistic goals include feeding with setup, oral-facial hygiene, tabletop communication, and leisure skills. Upper-body dressing requires help from others, although the C5 tetraplegic patient can provide some assistance. A power wheelchair can be propelled with a hand control. If pressure relief is a problem, a power recliner system can be used. The manual chair often is equipped with oblique projections on the hand rim to assist with propulsion. Manual wheelchair propulsion typically is most successful indoors and on flat surfaces.

Function in C6 Tetraplegia

Radial wrist extension found at the C6 level further enhances functional abilities at the C6 level.[380] Radial wrist extensor recovery can occur in persons with trace to C3-level elbow flexor strength.[82] The recovery of wrist extensors can occur well after the initial inpatient rehabilitation period and can reach maximum strength as long as 2 years post injury.[344] This is probably due to these patients having C6 nerve root injury more than SCI at the C6 level. Recovery by nerve regrowth can occur, but it takes many months. Active wrist extension results in tenodesis, which is the opposition of the thumb and index finger that occurs with finger flexion as the tendons are stretched when the

wrist is extended. Tenodesis orthoses are available to assist with this action, although patients rarely use them after discharge from the rehabilitation hospital. The tenodesis splint can be used initially as a training aid until the patient's finger and wrist tendons assume the right length relationship. The Rehabilitation Institute of Chicago tenodesis orthosis is fabricated from orthoplast and is perhaps the least expensive design. A metal and Plastizote version of the Rancho Los Amigos design is heavier, more expensive, and less cosmetically acceptable, but can be used for catheterization or work-related skills. More commonly, C6 tetraplegic patients use a short opponens orthosis with utensil slots, or utensil cuffs, or writing splints with simple D-ring Velcro closures for feeding, writing, and hygiene. *[handwritten: UNIVERSAL CUFF]*

These patients generally feed themselves when food is provided and cut into bite-sized pieces. They can dress their upper extremities and perform oral-facial hygiene. They generally perform upper extremity dressing and assist with lower extremity dressing. Well-motivated patients can perform lower extremity dressing, although the amount of time this takes is a consideration. Many C6 tetraplegic patients can perform their own catheterization and bowel program.

The manual wheelchair is propelled independently and for some can be the sole wheelchair for home and community. The manual chair may require vertical projections or coated hand rims. Other C6 tetraplegic patients require a powered wheelchair for work and school. Transfers, particularly to level surfaces, often require a sliding board. An appropriately equipped van with a lift and hand controls can result in independent driving.

Function in C7 and C8 Tetraplegia

The triceps function found at the C7 level results in significant improvements in transfer and mobility skills.[352] Finger extension and wrist flexion strength are present and further assist with activities of daily living (ADL). Persons at this level are likely to be independent in bed mobility, oral-facial hygiene, bowel and bladder care, upper extremity dressing, and transfers to wheelchair and car. Many are independent in lower extremity dressing as well.

The flexor digitorum profundus at the C8 level greatly improves hand function. Total independence with use of a wheelchair is possible, although hand function is not normal owing to the absence of innervation from the first thoracic segment. The wheelchair, manually powered, is light enough to be independently transferred into a car at this level, and combined with improved transfer skills at this level, eliminates the necessity of a van. Homemaking tasks become less difficult.

Function in Thoracic Paraplegia

Thoracic-level injuries generally result in persons with motor abilities that allow for total independence at the wheelchair level. At the T1 level and below, hand function is normal. Intercostal and abdominal musculature is present the more distal the lesion in the spinal cord. It is not necessary to assign outcomes based on specific thoracic levels of injury.[383] Persons with thoracic-level injuries are able to learn self-care and mobility skills regardless of the specific level of injury. Nonwheelchair ambulation is more common the more distal the level. Many factors can interfere with the achievement of total independence by thoracic-level paraplegic patients. These include body weight, spasticity, motivation, and age. Patients with complete paraplegia have increased difficulty performing bathing, dressing, stair climbing, and toilet, bath, and chair transfers with increasing age.[381]

Numerous technologies have been developed for standing and walking after SCI.[156] They generally are described as orthotic devices, modified wheelchairs, and passive standing frames. The utility of these devices is limited, and there is little proof of a physiological benefit in reducing osteoporosis in the paralytic lower limbs.[25]

Long leg braces generally are variants of the standard metal upright knee-ankle-foot orthosis (KAFO). KAFOs generally have an upper and lower thigh band, drop locks, and a double-action ankle joint. They either are attached directly to the shoes with a stirrup and an extended steel shank or an insert is attached allowing the shoes to be changed. A pelvic hand and hip joint are not needed as they increase weight and energy requirements.[342] The Scott-Craig variant of the KAFO has a patellar tendon strap, a bail lock at the knee, and a rigid ankle support. It is lighter in weight, as the lower thigh and calf band closures are eliminated. Donning and doffing is easier and ambulation more efficient[260] (see Chapter 17).

More recent designs of KAFOs allow for a reciprocal gait pattern. Three common designs are the Reciprocal Gait Orthosis developed at Louisiana State University,[68] the Hip Guidance Orthosis (HGO or Parawalker),[266] and the Advanced Reciprocating Gait Orthosis (ARGO).[194] There is no evidence at this time to suggest that these braces offer a better long-term acceptance rate than more standard designs of KAFOs.

The Vannini Rizolli[203] boot is a unique design. It supports the foot and ankle in a high boot that extends up to just below the knee. The ankle is set in 10 to 15 degrees of plantar flexion to stabilize the knee by shifting the center of gravity anteriorly. Its utility appears to be limited.

It is uncommon for patients with thoracic-level paraplegia to use long leg braces in the community.[63, 141, 237, 254, 260, 283] Many patients use them for a short time after injury or for standing or exercise. This is due to the high energy requirements that result from loss of the six determinants of gait.[224, 240] Energy expenditure can be as high as 6 to 12 times as much per unit distance. Rejection rates have been reported to be as high as 75%. There are psychological benefits and anecdotal reports of improvements in bowel function from passive standing. Prescription of KAFOs should be limited to highly motivated individuals who demonstrate success with temporary training orthoses in therapy.[346]

Standing wheelchairs allow persons to use their wheelchair for mobility as well as for standing with a built-in supportive frame.[156] These chairs are much heavier than standard wheelchairs. Prescription of standing wheelchairs often is used for vocational purposes, and the chair is generally a second chair. Both manual and powered standing wheelchairs are available.

Function in Lumbar Paraplegia

Persons with lumbar SCIs generally are independent at the wheelchair level and have the greatest potential for ambulation. The earliest studies suggested that community ambulators typically have control of their pelvis, hip flexors, one quadriceps muscle, and proprioception of the hips and ankles. Ankle-foot orthoses (AFOs) compensate for weakness about the ankle, and canes and crutches can be used for lack of hip extension and abduction.[151, 347] Waters and associates[347] described a technique known as the Ambulatory Motor Index (AMI) to predict ambulatory capabilities. Using a 4-point scale (0 = absent, 1 = trace or poor, 2 = fair, 3 = good or normal) and scoring hip flexion, hip abduction, hip extension, knee extension, and knee flexion on both sides, the AMI can be used to serve as an indicator of ambulatory capacity. The AMI is expressed as a percentage of the maximum score of 30. Those scoring at least 60% can be community ambulators with no more than one KAFO. Persons with an AMI of less than 40% typically require two KAFOs. Persons with an average AMI of 79% or higher typically require no orthotic devices to ambulate.

Another study of patients with incomplete paraplegia used the lower extremity motor score to predict ambulation.[345] The score was recorded at 1 month. The presence of quadriceps function serves as a positive indicator of ambulation potential.[65] Persons with a score greater than 10 with hip or knee extension greater than or equal to 2/5 ambulated with a reciprocal gait at 1 year. When using the neurological level of injury as a guide in complete paraplegia, patients with levels at T12 and below are likely to be community ambulators.

Function in Central Cord Injury and Brown-Séquard Syndrome

Persons with the classic central cord syndrome have an excellent potential for functional improvement and gaining some bowel and bladder control.[290] The majority of these patients have regulated bowel programs and are continent of bladder on discharge. The majority also are independent in most ADL and motor skills. Although persons with central cord syndrome typically make significant gains at all ages, younger persons have a better prognosis.

The recently designed Kohlmeyer RIC orthosis for the central cord syndrome can be used to substitute for weak proximal musculature in persons with preserved hand function.[174] It is inexpensively fabricated from readily available components and can facilitate upper extremity function in the central cord syndrome.

The Brown-Séquard syndrome also has a good prognosis. Persons with predominant upper extremity weakness have a better prognosis than those with lower extremity weakness.[293] Generally, persons have a variant of the Brown-Séquard syndrome rather than the pure syndrome. Bladder and bowel continence is quite common, as is independence in most ADL.

WHEELCHAIR SEATING AND POSITIONING

Wheelchair selection is determined by the patient's motor skills and rehabilitation goals. This requires close collaboration with the rehabilitation team to provide a seating system that provides for appropriate posture and does not interfere with functional activities.[175] The goals of wheelchair positioning are to improve mobility and functional skills, while preventing deformity, pressure ulcers, and pain, and maximizing respiratory function. One of the most common problems arises from the basic wheelchair design,[387] since the basic sling seat and back can result in pelvic obliquity and kyphotic posture with increased risk of pressure ulcers, deformity, and discomfort (see Chapter 19).

Proper seating can often be accomplished with commercially available cushions, armrests, and solid back, seat, and trunk supports. These must allow the integration of pressure relief as well as for such technology as power controls for mobility, reclining, and environmental control units. Rehabilitation engineers are often needed to help fabricate custom seating systems for patients with high tetraplegia and persons with deformity. Many high-level SCI patients require custom headrests and seating systems. Since systems provided should be easily repaired in the patient's community, commercially available components should be used when available. Wheelchair systems should also be easily accommodated into the person's transportation and home environment (see Chapter 19).

MOTOR AND SENSORY RECOVERY—IMPACT ON REHABILITATION

Neural recovery during the initial rehabilitation phase and following discharge can result in improved motor or sensory function and provide the potential for greater functional abilities than initially predicted. Motor and sensory recovery should be monitored throughout the rehabilitation phase and after discharge. Generally patients who have some spared motor function initially and whose recovery begins early and more rapidly have the best prognosis.[97, 217] The recovery of wrist extensor function has been the subject of numerous studies.[81, 344] In patients with complete tetraplegia with 0/5 elbow flexion at 1 month, wrist extension did not return. If the elbow flexor strength is 1/5 or 2/5, it is likely that 3/5 strength in wrist extension will develop. Elbow extension will generally be greater than 3/5 at 1 year if 1/5 or 2/5 at 1 month.[344] In both complete and incomplete tetraplegia, motor recovery tends to decline and plateau at 6 months.[344, 352] In incomplete tetraplegia, all muscles that were 1/5 at 1 month were greater than 3/5 at 1 year. The lower extremity motor score described in Figure 55–1 can help predict ambulation in incomplete tetraplegia. With a score of greater than 15 at 1 month, ambulation at 1 year is likely, although assistive devices might be required. Persons with a lower extremity score of 0 at 1 month did not ambulate, and the potential for ambulation increased as the motor score increased. Lower extremity motor recovery in incomplete tetraplegia is more likely to occur in those persons with intact sacral pinprick.[65, 344] Patients with complete tetraplegia at 1 month rarely regain use of lower extremity motor function.[344]

Patients with complete paraplegia have a poorer prognosis for recovery than those with incomplete paraplegia.[348] Persons with complete injuries above T9 are unlikely to regain motor function. As the lesion becomes more distal, motor recovery is more likely, particularly in the hip flexors and knee extensors.[348] In incomplete paraplegia, the extent of motor recovery is independent of the initial neurological level.[347] Recovery is again most rapid in the first 6 months, after which a plateau is reached. In muscles that were 0/5 at 1 month, less than 25% were 3/5 at 1 year. Muscles that were 1/5 or 2/5 initially generally improved to 3/5 at 1 year.

FUNCTIONAL NEUROMUSCULAR STIMULATION

Functional neuromuscular stimulation (FNS) is also commonly known as functional electrical stimulation (FES). In persons with SCI it has been used to prevent secondary complications[377] and to restore functional movement of the extremities.[378] Research with standing spinal cord–injured persons began in 1960,[163] with the first commercially produced system for walking introduced in 1990.[303] No system is yet available that can replace a wheelchair. The current commercially available system (Parastep, Sigmedics) uses a walker and stimulation of the glutei and quadriceps for standing. The peroneal nerve is stimulated to produce a reflex flexion withdrawal response of the hip which results in ambulation. Other systems, commonly known as hybrid systems, use electrical stimulation and an orthosis such as the LSU Reciprocal Gait Orthosis or the Parawalker.[85, 146, 270, 271, 305] Fitting is difficult, the cost is high, and the distances that can be travelled are limited. It has been estimated that only 11% or less of all spinal cord–injured persons could use these systems.[155] A totally implantable system is under study, but commercial availability is not yet on the horizon.[207–209] Electrical stimulation to the quadriceps alone can be used for standing.[373] This can be combined with an AFO, or KAFO if needed.[157]

The first application of upper extremity FNS in tetraplegia was used in an electrically activated flexor-hinge orthosis.[200] At this time there are not commercially available systems. Research is currently underway on voice-activated,[252, 253] surface stimulation,[295, 336] and complex microprocessor-controlled multichannel stimulators.[148] The most advanced system is an upper extremity neuroprosthesis developed at Case Western Reserve University, which has undergone significant testing.[37, 169, 171] A percutaneous electrode system is controlled by a portable microprocessor. The contralateral shoulder is used to control a sensor that produces proportional signals and stimulates the system. It has been demonstrated to assist C5 and C6 quadriplegic patients in upper extremity ADL skills.

At this time, the clinical applications of these systems are limited. There is much uncertainty associated with participation in FNS research, and subjects should be carefully selected. They should be realistic in their expectations of electrical stimulation and be psychologically able to tolerate the uncertainty of the stimulation program outcome. Closed-loop systems that monitor the stimulation that is produced and provide feedback to control the stimulation are not yet available for practical use.[271] The current open-loop systems do not provide for the smooth fine control of muscle contraction that is needed to control fine activities.

PHYSICAL, METABOLIC, AND ENDOCRINE CHANGES IN SPINAL CORD INJURY

In addition to the neurological impairment that occurs following an SCI, it is also common to find other body and metabolic changes as well. These can include changes in body composition; decreased energy expenditure capacity; nutrition; anemia; changes in endocrine function, glucose metabolism, electrolyte balance; and osteoporosis. Some of these changes are merely incidental findings, while other can have clinical implications requiring active intervention and management.

Weight loss is a common finding immediately following SCI. Most of this is due to lower absolute amounts of total body water, fat, and protein.[42] Extracellular and intracellular water volume are both decreased, but intracellular to a greater degree, resulting in a relative expansion of extracellular water volume.[43] The precise cause and mechanism of the water volume changes are not clear. Suggestions include changes in various electrolyte levels, failure of end-organ response to atrial natriuretic factor (which is increased following SCI), or possibly the influence of other counteracting hormonal and hemodynamic mechanisms.[43, 301] In addition, it has been found that muscle tissue loss as a result of paralysis can lead to decreased exchangeable potassium and increased exchangeable sodium in the body, with a resultant increased extracellular fluid volume.[51]

Metabolic and Body Changes

Changes in energy expenditure frequently occur following SCI. Early after injury, patients might require up to 54% less calories than predicted by their weight.[64] Following the acute period patients often continue to have reduced basal energy expenditure ranging from 12% to 29% reduction from that predicted.[244] In general, the higher the level of injury, the greater the reduction in basal energy expenditure. Chronic spinal cord–injured patients display widely differing ranges in resting energy expenditures. To avoid excess weight gain and any potential accompanying consequences on skin integrity and functional states, it is recommended that nutritional intake be based on a measurement of energy expenditure.[187]

Anemia in chronic spinal cord–injured persons is fairly common, ranging in incidence from 30% to 56%.[147, 269, 330] The most common forms of anemia seen in patients after the initial acute period are normocytic-normochromic, and microcytic-hypochromic types. These types of anemia also are found commonly in the anemia of chronic illness. It has been suggested that the increased risk, and frequent recurrence, of urinary tract infections is the most common cause of anemia.[147] Although the cause of anemia in chronic spinal cord–injured persons is not definitely known, the body's response to the condition appears to be appropriate as plasma erythropoietin concentration is elevated. This suggests that the erythropoietin response to the reduced circulating erythrocyte mass is qualitatively preserved.[330]

Abnormalities in electrolyte balance, endocrine function, and glucose metabolism can be seen during the various periods following SCI. Hyperphosphatemia, hypermagnesuria, hyperuricosuria without hyperuricosemia, and decreased urine creatinine are frequently seen early after SCI.[51, 53]

Hyperosmolar hyponatremia (Na < 130 mmol/L) is also frequently seen, especially in cervical injuries. Factors that can contribute to this condition include high fluid intake, and environmental or dietary factors that can inhibit free-water excretion. Patients may be asymptomatic at the initial presentation of electrolyte imbalance, or present with marked lethargy and confusion, or with generalized seizure activity.[302] Treatment involves conservative measures such as fluid restriction and, if needed, administration of hypertonic saline solution.

Other endocrine functions can be affected after SCI. At rest, steady-state excretion of corticosteroids in urine is similar to that in healthy subjects during bed rest.[52] In addition, aldosterone, catecholamine, and methylhydroxymandelic acid levels are generally within normal ranges. In the stimulated state, however, such as after surgery, the expected increase in urinary corticosteroids, catecholamines, and methylhydroxymandelic acid is absent. It has been suggested that the diminished response is due to disruption of normal connections between the brain and spinal cord, and dissociation of normally integrated functions of the autonomic nervous system.[55]

Glucose intolerance is a common finding in patients with SCI.[87] In these patients, fasting glucagon levels are normal, and normal suppression is seen after oral glucose loads, but a marked hyperinsulinemia is usually present. The glucose intolerance is believed to be due to insulin resistance which may be attributed, in part, to abnormalities secondary to denervated and atrophied muscles.[86]

Osteoporosis

Osteoporosis invariably occurs below the level of injury following SCI. There is commonly a period of marked calcium resorption from bone and hypercalciuria following SCI. This results in a reduction of bone mineral content and ultimately in osteoporosis, which is sufficient to increase the risk of lower extremity fractures.[134, 152, 278] The bone loss in SCI appears to follow a selective pattern with significant loss from the hips but relative preservation of lumbar spine bone density.[192] Various interventions have been studied in an attempt to minimize osteoporosis. FES bicycle ergometry training does not reverse osteoporosis after it has developed,[189] but FES exercise can be beneficial in reducing the rate of bone loss.[133] Ambulatory activity has been shown to decrease hypercalciuria and to shift the calcium balance in the positive direction, but whether osteoporosis is prevented or reversed is not yet clear. Other measures which have been suggested, but not proved, include the application of electrical fields and pharmacological agents, including calcitonin, biphosphonates, and recombinant human growth hormone.[35, 89, 241]

Hypercalcemia

Immobility from SCI results in marked changes in bone metabolism. Initially, bone loss and remodeling can be more active *above* the level of neurological injury, but about 2 to 3 months post injury, the process becomes more active in areas below the level of injury.[21] The increased bone turnover and loss is thought to be due to an imbalance of osteoblastic and osteoclastic activity, with a decrease in osteoblastic activity and acceleration of osteoclastic activity with bone resorption, although the precise cause is not known.[242, 310]

Because of the increased bone turnover and resorption, hydroxyprolinuria and hypercalciuria are commonly seen in the initial weeks following SCI.[54] This activity usually peaks about 3 months after injury, but the increased urinary calcium excretion can remain elevated for as long as 18 months.[21, 50] Passive weightbearing activities such as tilt-table exercise result in a decrease in hypercalciuria, but muscle-strengthening exercises appear to have little influence on urinary calcium excretion.[165]

In the great majority of patients, the increased calcium load has no clinical implications. Hypercalcemia of sufficient magnitude to produce potential adverse consequences occurs in a few patients. It is a more common metabolic complication in children and adolescents who sustain SCIs and can occur in up to 24% of this population.[215, 323] Patients at greater risk for hypercalcemia tend to be white males less than 21 years old, and those having higher neurological levels of injury, complete injuries, and prolonged periods of immobilization.

The time from injury to onset of hypercalcemic symptoms is most commonly 4 to 8 weeks, but ranges from 1 to 16 weeks.[218] In mild cases, clinical symptoms can include anorexia, nausea, lightheadedness, headache, malaise, listlessness, and depression. In more severe cases, the clinical presentation can include persistent nausea and vomiting; acute gastric dilation; fecal impaction and abdominal pain; polyuria and polydipsia; bradycardia and cardiac rhythm irregularities; syncope; and seizures.[215]

In addition to an elevated serum calcium, laboratory studies generally show normal serum phosphorus, normal or only slightly elevated serum alkaline phosphatase, elevated urine calcium, and reduced 24-hour urine creatinine clearance.[215]

The pathophysiology of clinically significant hypercalcemia in spinal cord–injured patients is not well understood. One factor that can be involved is a relative dehydration. Low fluid intake could interfere with renal ability to excrete the large amounts of calcium that result from increased bone resorption. When nausea and vomiting occur, the dehydration is exacerbated, further decreasing the kidneys' ability to excrete excess calcium and increasing the serum calcium level.

Treatment of symptomatic hypercalcemia primarily involves measures to enhance the excretion of calcium. Vigorous hydration with saline solution, intravenously if necessary, and the use of furosemide are typical initial measures. In more severe cases or for prolonged hypercalcemia, the use of calcitonin alone or in combination with glucocorticoids can rapidly and effectively decrease serum calcium.[45, 215] In addition, disodium etidronate can be an effective form of treatment, either alone or in combination with calcitonin.[230, 235] Measures to decrease calcium absorption via the gastrointestinal tract, such as by limiting calcium and vitamin D intake, are generally ineffective in the treatment of hypercalcemia.[310]

CARDIOVASCULAR CONCERNS IN SPINAL CORD INJURY

Alterations in cardiovascular physiology commonly take place following SCI owing to changes in cardiovascular regulating mechanisms that result from neurological impairment. Complications such as cardiac arrhythmias, orthostatic hypotension, and deterioration of cardiac risk factors as a result of decreased physical activity are commonly seen.

Regulation of the cardiovascular system relies on an integrated and coordinated system consisting of receptors such as baroreceptors and chemoreceptors. These are sensitive to a range of stimuli such as arterial pressure and pH, and pass along information about the state of the cardiovascular system to higher centers of the central nervous system. In response to this feedback information, changes in cardiovascular function are mediated through the autonomic nervous system (both sympathetic and parasympathetic).

The major cranial parasympathetic supply is via the vagus nerve (cranial nerve X), which exits the central nervous system through the brainstem and is spared in most SCIs. All sympathetic outflow occurs below the T6 level, and injuries above this level generally result in loss of descending excitatory and inhibitory input to all preganglionic sympathetic neurons. The result can be significant alterations in cardiovascular system control because of impairment of cardiovascular regulatory mechanisms and reflexes.

Cardiac arrhythmias and hemodynamic abnormalities are seen commonly during the acute period in persons with SCI and tend to occur within the first 14 days post injury, more commonly in cervical and complete injuries.[190] Bradycardia is common during the acute period after SCI. Imbalance of the autonomic nervous system with a decrease in sympathetic and a relative predominance of parasympathetic activity is believed to be the mechanism for this arrhythmia.[92, 98, 190, 273]

Bradycardia also can be produced by hypoxia, the risk of which is greater during pneumonia. It can also result from stimulation of tracheal receptors during suctioning, which activates vagovagal reflexes.[8, 98, 115] Bradycardia can be prevented with atropine before tracheal suctioning is performed as well as by induced hyperventilation.[8] In patients in whom bradycardia continues to be clinically significant, cardiac pacemaker placement might be indicated.[115] Most cardiac arrhythmias tend to resolve within 6 weeks after injury, and the prevalence of dysrhythmia in chronic spinal cord–injured persons without evidence of other cardiac abnormalities is low.[186, 190]

Orthostatic hypotension is commonly seen during the early period following cervical and upper thoracic cord injuries. It occurs primarily due to interruption of spinal sympathetic efferent pathways. During change to the upright position, a decrease in blood pressure is normally sensed by aortic and carotid baroreceptors, which results in a reflex increase in sympathetic activity causing tachycardia and vasoconstriction. Interruption in the sympathetic activity is evidenced by the relative lack of increased plasma catecholamine levels in spinal cord–injured patients while experiencing orthostatic hypotension.[112]

Clinical symptoms of orthostatic hypotension can include lightheadedness, dizziness, visual changes, or syncope. In general, symptoms gradually diminish with time despite continued evidence of a decrease in blood pressure when assuming an upright position. It appears that the systemic blood pressure itself is not the predominant factor responsible for symptoms of orthostatic hypotension. Cerebral autoregulation of blood flow also appears to play a crucial role in the adaptation to orthostatic hypotension in patients with SCI.[119]

Treatment of orthostatic hypotension is aimed primarily at increasing peripheral resistance or increasing the effective circulating blood volume. Measures include repeated and gradually increasing postural challenges, the use of lower extremity compression stockings and abdominal compression binders, and pharmacological agents such as sodium chloride, ephedrine, ergotamine, and fludrocortisone.[125]

The prevalence of hypertension and ischemic heart disease has been reported to be greater among patients with SCI.[385] This, however, might be due to organ system changes that occur after SCI rather than to any true increases in cardiac risk factors. Inactivity following SCI can result in a decrease in high-density lipoprotein cholesterol concentrations, theoretically increasing the risk for cardiovascular disease.[34, 142] It has been shown that within several months after injury, total cholesterol is normal, high-density lipoprotein cholesterol is decreased, low-density lipoprotein cholesterol is normal, and triglyceride is increased. Overall, in the period immediately after SCI, there is no significant increase in cardiac risk factors.[340] In addition, one study found that the risk of coronary artery disease in spinal cord–injured patients is similar to that in age-matched, able-bodied persons. It was noted that the risk increases with age, but no differently from the risk in the able-bodied population, and does not appear to be related to the duration of injury.[44]

Patients with SCIs who have coronary artery disease and develop ischemic events may not present clinically in the same manner as able-bodied persons. Patients with cervical and upper thoracic cord injuries often do not experience angina because of interruption of cardiac nociceptive afferent fibers, so greater attention must be paid to persons in whom there is a strong suspicion of an ischemic event.

For patients at risk for coronary artery disease, exercise tolerance tests can be performed via an arm ergometric stress test with thallium myocardial perfusion imaging, or an alternative means of screening can be through dipyridamole (Persantine) or thallium stress testing[8] (see Chapter 32). Exercise in persons with SCI can result in increased high-density high-protein cholesterol levels and a reduction in the risk for developing cardiovascular disease.[34, 307]

MANAGEMENT OF DEEP VEIN THROMBOSIS AND PULMONARY EMBOLISM

Deep vein thrombosis (DVT) is a common complication of SCI and a major cause of morbidity and mortality. The incidence in persons with SCI ranges from 47% to 100%

depending on the methodology used for assessment and diagnosis.[29, 229, 249, 285, 322]

The high incidence appears to be a result of the combination of primarily three factors, also known as Virchow's triad,[335] which increase the risk for the development of DVT following SCI. One factor is the venous stasis that results from muscle paralysis. Blood flow can be decreased in the affected extremity, and because of the resultant decreased venous return, venous stasis occurs.[227] Hypercoagulability is another factor that increases the risk for developing DVT, and can occur as a result of stimulation of thrombogenic factors following injury. This has been demonstrated in spinal cord–injured persons who ultimately developed thrombosis.[227] Intimal or vessel wall damage is the third risk factor, although its importance to the development of DVT is less well understood. Damage to vessel walls can occur in SCI patients as a direct result of trauma from the original injury or indirectly from external pressure on the paralyzed leg.

Owing to the high incidence of DVT and the potential morbidity and mortality from complications of its development, the use of effective prophylactic measures is important. Prompt, early initiation of prophylactic measures is vital because the highest-risk period appears to be during the first 2 weeks following SCI.[229, 285] Nonpharmacological methods, including compression stockings, external pneumatic compression, and continuous rotation beds, have been used with variable effectiveness.[17] Most work and attention has focused on pharmacological agents with antithrombotic or anticoagulant properties as prophylactic measures against DVT. The use of low-dose heparin (5000 units subcutaneously twice or three times a day) results in a decrease in the incidence of DVT, yet is not entirely effective.[88, 122, 180] Adjusted-dosage heparin, prolonging the activated partial thromboplastin time (aPTT) to 1.5 times control, is clearly effective for prophylaxis of thrombosis, but potential adverse effects such as hemorrhagic complications are more prevalent.[122]

The combined use of pharmacological agents and mechanical modalities appears to be more effective than each agent or modality used by itself.[124, 226, 229] It has been suggested that with combination therapies, mechanical modalities should be used with a pharmacological agent for the initial 2 weeks after injury, followed by the pharmacological agent alone for an additional 6 to 10 weeks.[227]

Recently the use of low-molecular-weight heparin has shown to be extremely effective either alone or in combination with mechanical modalities to further decrease the incidence of DVT and without the common adverse effects found with standard heparin.[121, 123, 228] Unlike standard heparin, the low-molecular-weight heparins are unable to bind thrombin and do not inhibit platelet function, which might explain the decreased occurrence of bleeding complications as compared with regular heparin.[121]

The prompt and accurate diagnosis of DVT is vital so that proper treatment can be initiated to prevent more serious complications such as pulmonary embolism, and also to avoid needlessly exposing the patient to the potential complications of anticoagulation if it is not indicated.

The initial signs and symptoms of DVT are occasionally confused with other diagnoses such as heterotopic ossification, or they may coexist.[136, 263] It is well recognized that clinical assessment alone is often unreliable in diagnosing DVT.[132, 133] Contrast venography is still considered the diagnostic gold standard for DVT, although drawbacks include invasiveness of the study, patient discomfort, and potential complications such as allergic reaction and phlebitis.[132] Noninvasive tests that are available include Doppler ultrasonography, impedance plethysmography, and duplex ultrasound. Doppler ultrasonography lacks objective criteria for the interpretation of the acoustic signal and is very operator-dependent.[191] Impedance plethysmography is a widely used diagnostic tool for DVT. Its sensitivity is fairly high and, when performed by an experienced operator, highly specific. It is less reliable in diagnosing calf vein thrombosis and nonobstructing proximal thrombosis.[356] Recently, duplex ultrasound has become a significant addition to the noninvasive tests for diagnosing DVT. It has been found to be highly accurate, sensitive, and specific for proximal DVT.[191, 356, 367] It does have limitations in examining the femoral vein at the adductor canal, calf vein, and iliac vein. In addition, the development of heterotopic ossification can clinically present in a manner similar to DVT, and the use of duplex ultrasound can result in a false-positive finding. In this case, a venogram might be required to ensure proper diagnosis so that the appropriate treatment can be instituted.[376]

Currently there are no laboratory tests available that are routinely used to predict the development of DVT in persons with SCI. The advantage of this would be that a patient could be more quickly identified and proper prophylaxis or anticoagulation initiated, thereby decreasing the potential morbidity from the development of DVT and interference with rehabilitation. Work has been performed that suggests that the factor VIII–related antigen/factor VIII–procoagulant activity ratio may be of value in predicting DVT after SCI.[248, 285]

When DVT is diagnosed, anticoagulation treatment is indicated to prevent propagation of the thrombosis, pulmonary embolism, and recurrence of thromboembolism. Traditional management involves intravenous heparin in a 5000-unit bolus, followed by a constant infusion of 1000 units/hour. The aPTT is measured every 6 hours, and the heparin infusion is adjusted to achieve an aPTT of 1.5 to 2.5 times control. Oral warfarin is begun within 3 days after introduction of heparin and adjusted to achieve a prothrombin time with an international normalized ratio (INR) between 2 and 3. It is recommended that anticoagulation treatment continue for a total of 3 to 6 months.[225] If anticoagulation is contraindicated, Greenfield filter placement can be performed as prophylaxis for pulmonary embolism in patients with established DVT.

Patients with complete paraplegia or tetraplegia who develop DVT may require longer lengths of time for venous recanalization. They should have careful follow-up as they might be prone to persistent swelling due to venous insufficiency and are at greater risk for development of the postphlebitic syndrome.[195]

Pulmonary embolism is reported to occur in approximately 5% of acute SCI patients[74, 195, 341] and is a leading cause of death in spinal cord–injured persons. Pulmonary embolism might not present with classic signs and symptoms (pleuritic chest pain, hemoptysis, dyspnea) in spinal cord–injured patients, thus delaying diagnosis and initiation

of treatment. It can present as autonomic hyperreflexia or cardiac arrhythmia.[58, 96] When suspected, a ventilation and perfusion scan of the lungs or pulmonary angiography is usually performed to confirm the diagnosis. It is important to realize that there are limitations with the lung scan in diagnosing pulmonary embolism. An interpretation of high or low probability has been reported to be associated with a 15% error in diagnosing or ruling out pulmonary embolism.[170] Treatment involves anticoagulation as detailed previously for DVT and duration of treatment is usually for at least 6 months. The role of thrombolytic therapy for treatment of pulmonary embolism and DVT in spinal cord–injured patients is not entirely clear at the present time.[225]

AUTONOMIC DYSREFLEXIA

Autonomic dysreflexia is an acute syndrome of massive sympathetic discharge that occurs as a result of noxious stimuli in persons with spinal cord lesions above the level of the sympathetic splanchnic outflow, about T6.[181] It is characterized by paroxysmal hypertension, pounding headache, sweating, nasal congestion, facial flushing, piloerection, and reflex bradycardia. The incidence has been reported to range from 48% to 83% of tetraplegic and high paraplegic patients, and most persons do not experience signs and symptoms before 2 months post injury.[91, 196] Although autonomic dysreflexia occurs most commonly in persons with injuries above T6, one case has been reported in a woman with a T10 neurological level during labor.[116]

The most common causes are bladder and bowel distention. Other causes include pressure sores, ingrown toenails, tight clothing, tight shoes and leg bag straps, urinary tract infections, uterine contractions in pregnant women,[220] and any invasive procedure such as bladder catheterization, rectal stimulation, cystometrogram,[196] and extracorporeal shock wave lithotripsy.[39, 161]

In terms of pathophysiology, any of the previously mentioned causes can result in noxious stimuli that produce proprioception and pain impulses that are transmitted to the dorsal column and spinothalamic tracts. As these tracts ascend, they synapse with sympathetic neurons in the intermediolateral columns and generate sympathetic activity. A mass and generalized sympathetic response occurs. Normally, there are descending supraspinal inhibitory signals that modulate autonomic responses, but owing to the spinal lesion above the sympathetic outflow, these signals are interrupted and unable to travel below the level of the lesion. The result is peripheral and splanchnic vasoconstriction and the development of acute hypertension. Sweating and piloerection also occur as a result of the mass sympathetic discharge. With the increase in blood pressure, the aortic arch and carotid sinus receptors are stimulated, which may result in reflex bradycardia and vasodilation above the level of the lesion. The vasodilation is manifested as facial flushing and nasal congestion.[91] The bradycardia is not always present, and, in fact, tachycardia or normal sinus rhythm is often seen.

Complications that develop from autonomic dysreflexia are a manifestation of the severe hypertension. If the elevated blood pressure is not lowered, possible complications can be life-threatening and include confusion, visual disturbance, loss of consciousness, encephalopathy, intracerebral hemorrhage, seizures, electrocardiographic changes, atrial fibrillation, acute myocardial failure, and pulmonary edema.[91, 159, 258, 276, 375] In pregnant women with SCI, intracerebral hemorrhage and death during labor also have been reported.[2, 116] It has been suggested that epidural anesthesia is the treatment of choice in spinal cord–injured women in labor to prevent autonomic dysreflexia.[311, 349]

Treatment of an acute episode generally focuses on identifying and removing the cause (Table 55–2). The first action taken is to raise the patient's head from the bed or sit the patient up and monitor the blood pressure. In most cases, identifying the noxious stimuli and removing it resolves the episode, often very quickly. For the most common causes, this may mean bladder catheterization, or irrigating and then changing a Foley catheter. If rectal impaction is suspected, care should be taken before attempting manual removal, as the process itself can exacerbate the episode. A local anesthetic, such as lidocaine jelly, can be used when performing manual removal to minimize stimulation. If the cause cannot be found and symptoms persist, then pharmacological intervention may be necessary to lower the blood pressure. Medications that may be used include nitrates, nifedipine, prazosin, hydralazine, mecamylamine, and diazoxide[33, 39, 91] (Table 55–3).

Prevention of recurrent episodes includes proper bladder and bowel management and skin care. In addition, patient and family education is vital regarding the prevention, causes, presentation, and treatment of autonomic dys-

TABLE 55–2   Stimuli Which Can Provoke Autonomic Dysreflexia

Urological
  Bladder distention, spontaneous or induced (irrigation)
  Bladder instrumentation (catheterization, cystoscopy,
    cystometry, cystourography, conduit loopography)
  Urinary tract infection or other mucosal irritation
  Hemorrhagic cystitis
Genital
  Testicular torsion
  Epididymitis
  Testicular pressure
  Sexual intercourse
  Uterine contractions
  Vaginal examination
Renal distention
Gastrointestinal
  Rectal examination
  Fecal impaction
  Enemas
  Instrumentation
  Acute abdominal syndromes
  Operative interventions
Exposure to cold or high temperature
Other
  Decubitus ulcers
  Anesthesia
  Thrombophlebitis
  Pulmonary infarction
  Restraints
  Tight clothing
  Hypotension

From Sutin JA, de Greco F: Blood pressure disorders in the disabled. *In* Green D (ed): Medical Management of Longterm Disability. Stoneham, Mass, Butterworth-Heinemann, 1990.

reflexia. Although uncommon, the use of medication for long-term prophylaxis can include agents such as phenoxybenzamine, mecamylamine, guanethidine, and terazosin.[33, 48, 91]

PULMONARY COMPLICATIONS IN SPINAL CORD INJURY

The muscles involved in normal pulmonary ventilation include the diaphragm, the intercostal muscles, the accessory neck muscles, and the abdominal muscles. The primary respiratory muscle is the diaphragm, which is the main muscle active during normal, quiet breathing. The intercostal muscles function to expand or contract the volume of the thoracic cage during heavy respiration but stabilize the thoracic cage during normal respiration. The accessory neck muscles are active primarily during strong ventilatory effort. The abdominal muscles are active primarily during forceful expiration and in producing cough.

Following SCI, the nature and extent of the changes in ventilatory function and cough depend to a great degree on the level of neurological injury. Persons with injuries below T12 essentially have no impairment of respiratory function, and except in the case of direct lung injury due to trauma, have few pulmonary complications.

Injuries between T1 and T12 result in some impairment of the abdominal muscles, which reduces forceful expiration and cough. With higher thoracic-level injuries, there is also impairment of intercostal muscle function which reduces inspiratory and expiratory function. Paradoxical retraction of the chest wall during inspiration can be seen in the early acute stages of SCI because of flaccid paralysis of the intercostal muscles, which is in contrast to the stabilization of the ribs and expansion of the chest wall normally seen during inspiration.

With injuries above C8, there is loss of all abdominal and intercostal muscles with further impairment of inspiration and expiration. C4 is generally the highest level of injury at which spontaneous ventilation can be sustained. Injuries above this level generally require mechanical ventilation.

Pulmonary function indices in tetraplegia tend to change over time. It has been demonstrated that during the acute to postacute periods, there is a rapid increase in vital capacity, inspiratory capacity, and total lung capacity; an increase in inspiratory and respiratory air flows; and a decrease in functional residual capacity. During the postacute to chronic periods, changes tend to be more gradual with continued increases in vital capacity, decrease in functional residual capacity, with total lung capacity and ventilatory indices remaining unchanged.[129] Inspiratory capacity can continue to increase by up to 45% over a 1-year period after injury.[296]

Other pulmonary changes have been noted in patients with SCI. Patients with chronic tetraplegia can develop a rapid and shallow breathing pattern similar to that seen with the restrictive pulmonary syndromes.[202] It has been suggested that this type of breathing pattern can develop into late-onset ventilatory failure with diminution in vital capacity with age.[11] In addition, in stable tetraplegic patients over time, it has been shown that there is a decrease

TABLE 55–3   Pharmacological Treatment of Autonomic Dysreflexia

Drug	Acute Episodes	Recurrent	Anticipated Episodes
Phentolamine	5–10 mg IV push		40 mg IV push
Phenoxybenzamine		30–60 mg po bid	
Diazoxide	100–250 mg IV push		
Nitroprusside	0.5–1.5 mg/kg/min IV		
Hydralazine	10 mg slow IV push		
Pentolinium	5–10 mg IV push	20–40 mg po qid	10–25 mg IV push
Trimethaphan	0.1–1.0 mg/min IV		
Clonidine		0.1–0.2 mg po tid	0.2 mg po 30 min before
Methyldopa	250 mg slow IV push	250 mg po qid	
Prazosin		1–2 mg po bid	
Mecamylamine		5 mg po tid	2.5 mg po 30 min before
Guanethidine		10–20 mg po qd	
Nifedipine	10 mg po or sublingual		10 mg po or sublingual
Amyl nitrate	30 sec inhalation		

From Sutin JA, de Greco F: Blood pressure disorders in the disabled. *In* Green D (ed): Medical Management of Longterm Disability. Stoneham, Mass, Butterworth-Heinemann, 1990.

in nocturnal oxyhemoglobin saturation and an increase in nocturnal maximal end-tidal carbon dioxide tension, and development of nocturnal oxyhemoglobin desaturation patterns similar to that seen with sleep disorder breathing.[154]

Pulmonary complications following SCI are in general secondary to impairments of ventilation and cough. Early in SCI, respiratory complications are a primary cause of death.[47] In fact, respiratory system complications, most commonly pneumonia, are the most common cause of mortality in persons with SCI at any time.[74, 313] During the first month post injury, up to 50% of acutely injured persons develop some pulmonary complication and including the initial rehabilitation period, this increases to up to 67% of patients.[95, 154]

Pulmonary complications are more common in higher-level injuries, especially at the C1 to C4 levels. In the acute period, common complications include atelectasis, pneumonia, and ventilatory failure. In thoracic-level injuries, the most common complications are pleural effusion, atelectasis, and pneumothorax or hemothorax, or both.[154]

General measures that have been advocated to prevent respiratory complications include position changes, regular deep breathing, and the use of incentive spirometry.[221] Cough assist can be performed to assist the tetraplegic or high paraplegic patient in generating a productive, forceful cough. This procedure is usually performed by placing the hands on each side of the patient's upper abdomen and applying intermittent pressure that is coordinated with the patient's initiation of cough. Recently, the issue of using cough assist in persons with intercaval filters has raised some concern because of the possibility that performing the maneuver can cause the filter to migrate.[13] In addition, it has been suggested that in tetraplegic patients, methods to strengthen the clavicular portion of the pectoralis major muscle and the use of functional electrical stimulation can both improve cough effectiveness.[73, 372]

In persons with high cervical injuries who require mechanical ventilation, various management methods have been suggested as alternatives to the use of ventilators.[9] Glossopharyngeal breathing, a technique that was commonly used with poliomyelitis patients, is a method of inspiration that may allow ventilator-dependent persons to be free of mechanical ventilation and more independent and in control of breathing for periods of time.[56] The technique involves the use of the lips, soft palate, mouth, tongue, pharynx, and larynx in a stroking maneuver to force air into the lungs, which is then followed by normal passive exhalation.[56]

The pneumobelt is another alternative method of respiratory management. It is a corset-type device that is placed around the abdomen. In contrast to the technique of glossopharyngeal breathing, the pneumobelt assists with exhalation rather than inspiration. The inflatable bladder within the corset fills with air, compresses the abdominal wall, and causes the diaphragm to rise, producing active expiration. Inspiration occurs passively as the bladder and the abdominal contents of the diaphragm fall due to gravity.[238] It can only be used when sitting.

Phrenic nerve pacing has recently received increased attention as a potential alternative for respiratory management in high-level tetraplegia patients who require mechanical ventilation.[11, 117, 313] In general, phrenic nerve pacing can be a treatment option in patients with respiratory paralysis after cervical or medullary injury above the origin of the phrenic nerve neurons and who do not have significant impairment of the phrenic nerves, lungs, or diaphragm. The technique involves the electrical stimulation of intact phrenic nerves via surgically implanted electrodes to contract the diaphragm (Fig. 55–3).

The use of noninvasive ventilatory support methods such as body ventilators and noninvasive intermittent positive airway pressure ventilation can be effective alternatives to respiratory management in ventilator-dependent persons and also eliminate the need for tracheostomy with its associated potential complications[10] (see Chapter 33).

SPASTICITY

Spasticity is a common sequela of SCI. It often is described as one component of the upper motor neuron syndrome and is most often characterized by a velocity-dependent increase in the muscle tone and increased muscle stretch reflexes. The onset of spasticity is generally gradual and progressive in severity as the patient emerges from

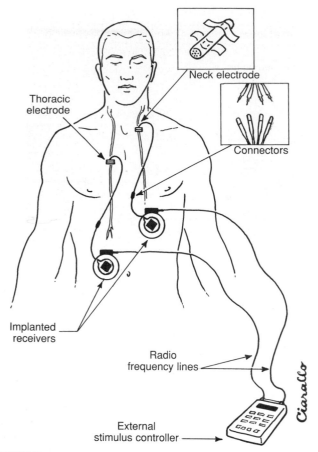

FIGURE 55–3 Phrenic nerve pacemaker system. (Courtesy of Medlink Technical Corp., Atrotech, Finland.)

Thoracic electrode

Neck electrode

Connectors

Implanted receivers

Radio frequency lines

External stimulus controller

"spinal shock," a period that lasts up to 3 months following injury. Early in its evolution, flexor spasticity predominates, but gradually with time, extensor spasticity develops and ultimately becomes the predominant type.[232] Suggested theories to explain the development of spasticity following SCI have included mechanical changes intrinsic to the affected muscles, increased motoneuronal excitability, and enhanced stretch-evoked synaptic excitation of motoneurons.[168]

The impact of spasticity on a patient's function, care, comfort, and medical condition should be assessed prior to the initiation of any treatment. Treatment usually is indicated if the spasticity interferes with the performance of self-care tasks, gait, wheelchair positioning or transfer activities, disrupts sleep, or causes pain, discomfort, or deformity. In addition, spasticity can contribute to skin breakdown and joint contractures. On the other hand, some patients utilize extensor tone to assist with transfer, standing, or ambulatory activities, so that treatment of spasticity could actually result in a decrease in function, and therefore is probably not indicated. Spasticity probably also helps preserve muscle bulk.

When contemplating treatment alternatives for spasticity, there are general considerations that should be kept in mind. In general, nociceptive and exteroceptive stimuli often exacerbate increased muscle tone and spasticity. Avoidance of noxious stimuli through good care, such as prompt treatment of urinary tract complications, prevention

of pressure sores and contractures, avoiding tight-fitting leg bags and clothing, and proper bowel and bladder care can contribute to minimizing spasticity.[167]

Regardless of spasticity treatment options or modalities, a routine daily program of prolonged muscle stretching should serve as the foundation for management of all patients with spasticity. The reduction in spasticity that follows stretching can last for several hours. It could be due to mechanical changes in the musculotendinous unit and decrease in spindle sensitivity and gamma activity.[167] In addition, the use of tilt-table standing may be beneficial in reducing extensor spasticity.[26]

Several choices are available when considering pharmacological treatment of spasticity. Baclofen, a centrally acting γ-aminobutyric acid (GABA) agonist, is generally considered the drug of choice for spasticity following SCI and is usually the initial agent for treatment. GABA is a major central nervous system inhibitory neurotransmitter that acts through presynaptic inhibition of primary afferents. Baclofen's mechanism of action is through activation of GABA-B receptors in primary sensory afferents, enhancement of Renshaw cell activity, and depression of fusimotor responses.[69]

The dosage of baclofen usually is initiated at 5 mg orally twice or three times daily, which is slowly titrated upward until an effective dosage is reached, up to a recommended maximum of 80 mg/day. It is generally well tolerated with minimal side effects such as drowsiness, weakness, fatigue, confusion, and headaches, which are usually transient in duration. Abrupt withdrawal or discontinuation of baclofen should be avoided as this can induce seizures, hallucinations, and psychosis.[281, 319] Baclofen is eliminated predominantly in the urine, so careful consideration is necessary in patients with renal insufficiency as there may be reduced clearance of baclofen and increased risk of toxicity.[4] Overall, baclofen has been shown to be a safe and effective agent for long-term use.[292]

Diazepam, a benzodiazepine, is a commonly used agent in the treatment of spasticity that acts by facilitating or potentiating the postsynaptic effects of GABA, resulting in an increase in presynaptic inhibition.[386] Diazepem is typically more useful in patients who are less affected by the sedative effects of the medication and who have painful, continuous spastic contractions.[386]

The dosage of diazepam generally is begun at 2 mg orally twice a day and titrated upward. Dosages as high as 60 mg/day have been reported[167] but owing to sedation, the dosage is typically limited to 15 to 20 mg/day. Side effects include sedation, intellectual impairment, reduced motor coordination, lightheadedness, dizziness, vertigo, and ataxia. Long-term use of diazepam can result in paradoxical reactions such as insomnia, anxiety, hostility, hallucination, and increased spasticity. It should not be assumed that symptoms are due to undermedication and therefore that the dosage be increased automatically.[386] Careful consideration should be taken when contemplating the use of diazepam in patients with a history of substance abuse or alcohol addiction or depression.

Dantrolene sodium is also commonly used for spasticity. In contrast to baclofen and diazepam, which act centrally at the level of the spinal cord, dantrolene acts peripherally at the level of the neuromuscular junction. It reduces the release of calcium from the sarcoplasmic reticulum, which decreases the force generated by the excitation-contraction coupling.[386] Although it can be beneficial in spasticity following SCI, dantrolene usually is preferred in cerebral forms of spasticity such as in stroke or brain injury.

The dosage of dantrolene usually is initiated at 25 mg/day orally, increased no more frequently than once or twice per week to a maximum of 400 mg/day in divided doses. Side effects can include sedation, malaise, nausea, vomiting, dizziness, and diarrhea. Because its mechanism of action is in muscle, a theoretical side effect is weakness, even in those muscle groups that are intact. The most serious side effect is hepatotoxicity, which can occur in approximately 1% of patients.[329, 360] The risk of dantrolene-induced hepatotoxicity is greatest in women, patients more than 35 years old, and patients receiving certain medications such as estrogens.[386] In addition, dantrolene can cause transient abnormalities in liver function that can resolve without discontinuing the medication. Liver function should be assessed prior to initiation of treatment and repeated periodically during the course of therapy.

Clonidine, a centrally acting α-$_2$-adrenergic agonist that is used primarily as an antihypertensive agent, has been noted to be effective in treatment of spasticity. The mechanism of action for its antispasticity activity is not entirely clear, but may be due to α_2-receptor–mediated modulation of somatosensory afferent stimuli at spinal and supraspinal levels.[250, 325, 366] Side effects encountered with the oral form of clonidine include orthostatic hypotension, lethargy and drowsiness, syncope, autonomic dysreflexia, and bradycardia.[83, 214, 282] The transdermal delivery system appears to have equal effectiveness in decreasing spasticity with fewer side effects.[350, 366]

Other pharmacological agents that have been suggested for treatment of spasticity include ketazolam, clorazepate, tizanidine, chlorpromazine, progabide, tetrahydroisoxazolopyridine, and cannabis.[167, 206] Other nonpharmacological therapeutic interventions that have shown variable effectiveness include cold modalities, casting and splinting, and biofeedback.[15, 27, 60, 236]

The intrathecal administration of baclofen via an implanted programmable pump and catheter system is now available for treatment of spasticity (Fig. 55–4). It appears to be beneficial in severe spasticity that is unresponsive to conventional oral medications. The mean daily dose of intrathecal baclofen required to maintain a therapeutic effect can range from 180 to 900 μg/day and increases with time in some patients. Periodic drug discontinuation, substitution of oral medications, or substitution of intraspinal morphine for 2 to 4 weeks can restore the patient's sensitivity to intrathecal baclofen.[1, 57, 268]

Limitations of this treatment include the need for lifetime refills and follow-up, replacement of the pump unit every 3 to 5 years to replace the battery, and the potential for pump and catheter malfunction.

Other surgical options for the treatment of spasticity include nerve and motor point blocks, intrathecal phenol injection, intrathecal morphine via an implantable pump, percutaneous radiofrequency rhizotomy, dorsal column electrical stimulation, and myelotomy.* (See Chapter 29 for further information on spasticity.)

_____
*References 80, 90, 144, 166, 167, 277, 298, 363.

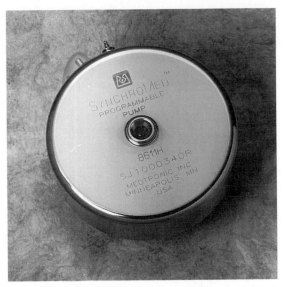

FIGURE 55–4 Programmable pump and catheter system for the intrathecal delivery of baclofen. (Courtesy of Medtronic, Inc.)

HETEROTOPIC OSSIFICATION

Heterotopic ossification is a common complication following SCI, yet it remains poorly understood. It is also referred to as ectopic bone, ectopic ossification, periarticular ossification, myositis ossificans, and paraosteoarthropathy. Its incidence in persons with SCI has been reported to range from 16% to 53%.[332] In the majority of SCI patients, the extent of ectopic bone development is minimal, and for the most part, an incidental finding on plain x-ray films without clinical significance.[318, 353] Of those that develop heterotopic ossification, only 18% to 37% have a significant ROM limitation that can interfere with ADL, and less than 5% develop ankylosis of the affected joint.[103, 106, 354]

The onset of heterotopic ossification is generally within 6 months after injury, with the most frequent occurrence between 1 and 4 months.[314, 353] It has been reported to occur as early as 20 days post injury.[353] The initial presentation of heterotopic ossification rarely occurs more than 1 year after injury.

Heterotopic ossification occurs only below the neurological level of injury. The most commonly involved areas, in decreasing order, are the hips, knees, shoulders, and elbows.[315, 353] Involvement of smaller joints in the extremities is very rare, although it has been noted to occur in the hands.[204] In comparison to heterotopic ossification found in traumatic brain-injured and hip replacement patients, there appears to be specific patterns of formation around the most commonly involved joints in spinal cord–injured patients. About the hip, heterotopic ossification is most commonly located anteriorly and generally forms within a plane from the anterior superior iliac spine to the lesser trochanter.[315] About the knee, involvement of the medial aspect is most commonly noted.[315]

The cause and pathogenesis of heterotopic ossification remain unclear. The development of heterotopic ossification could be due to some initiating or stimulating factors related to local metabolic, circulatory, or biochemical changes that occur following SCI.[158] Since it is also commonly found in traumatic brain-injured patients, the possibility of alteration in neural control over the differentiation of mesenchymal cells into osteoblasts has been suggested.[318] The presence or absence of spasticity has not been shown to be associated with the development of heterotopic ossification.[315] In terms of other possible predisposing factors, an aggressive passive ROM program has not been shown to predispose to the development of ectopic bone.[315] On the other hand, the presence of a pressure ulcer about a proximal joint can increase the risk of developing heterotopic ossification.[137, 183]

The development of heterotopic ossification is extra-articular and occurs outside the joint capsule. Bone formation takes place in the connective tissue between the muscle planes and not within the muscle itself.[102] The bone can be contiguous with the skeleton but generally does not involve the periosteum.[49] Mature heterotopic ossification has histological features similar to fracture callus. The bone is a lamellar corticospongiosal bone with a thin cortex, tightly latticed spongiosum, and occasional haversian systems.[287]

Clinically, the initial presentation is usually a warm and swollen extremity. Early symptoms include pain and restriction of motion in the involved joint. Fever might or might not be present. In general, swelling in the extremity is usually more localized, and within several days a more circumscribed, firm mass is noted within the area of edema.[314] During the initial presentation, the differential diagnosis includes cellulitis, septic arthritis, bone tumor, and thrombophlebitis.[262, 353, 376]

In the diagnostic evaluation for suspected heterotopic ossification, radiographs have limited use in that the first evidence of calcification might not occur for 7 to 10 days after the clinical presentation[314] (Fig. 55–5). An elevated serum alkaline phosphatase can assist in differentiating early heterotopic ossification from other diagnoses.[107, 256, 262] It has been noted that serum calcium can be transiently below normal before any rise in serum alkaline phosphatase, and then return to normal in persons who ultimately develop heterotopic ossification.[262] The triple-phase bone scan can be used for early detection of heterotopic ossification. The first two phases, dynamic blood flow study and static scan for blood pool, are the most sensitive for early detection[99, 262] (Fig. 55–6).

When the diagnosis is confirmed, initial treatment involves aggressive passive ROM exercises to maintain joint mobility. There is no evidence that this approach increases the amount of bone formation. Discontinuation of passive ROM exercise can result in decreased motion in the affected joint and possibly in ankylosis.[315, 353] Disodium etidronate is effective in limiting the extent of heterotopic ossification when this treatment is started early in the course.[314] It appears to be much less effective in patients with massive ectopic bone formation regardless of dosage or duration of treatment.[107] Indomethacin and warfarin are other medications that can be effective in treatment or prophylaxis of heterotopic ossification, although this has not been clearly established.[40, 105]

Complications of heterotopic ossification can include peripheral nerve entrapment,[36] development of pressure ulcers,[137] increased risk of deep DVT,[136] and extra-articular joint ankylosis which can lead to functional impairment. In these situations, surgical resection of the bone can be

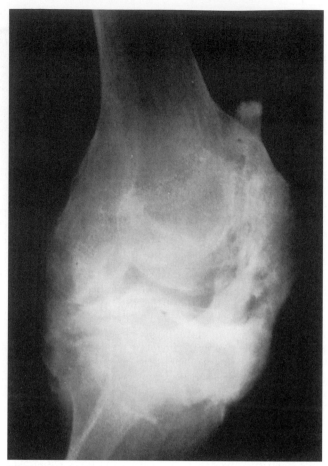

FIGURE 55–5 Plain radiograph of a knee showing the presence of heterotopic ossification.

considered. Common complications of surgery include excessive bleeding, infection, femoral head and neck fractures, and recurrence of heterotopic ossification.[318] Recurrence is limited if ectopic bone is mature at the time of surgery. Radiographs and serum alkaline phosphatase levels by themselves are not reliable indicators of bone maturity.[318, 321] For the majority of patients with heterotopic ossification in whom the extent is minimal to moderate, low recurrence occurs in those with radiographically demonstrable mature bone, normal baseline bone scans, and normal serum alkaline phosphatase level.[105] Disodium etidronate appears to be effective in preventing recurrence after surgery for as long as the drug is administered.[317]

POST-TRAUMATIC CYSTIC MYELOPATHY (SYRINGOMYELIA)

Post-traumatic cystic myelopathy is a particularly devastating sequela of SCI as it can result in weakness and sensory loss during the recovery or stable phase after injury. The prevalence is fortunately low with syrinx development reported to occur in 0.3% to 3.2% of the SCI population.[88, 294, 328] It might occur as a small cystic lesion at the site of the injury or can progress and become symptomatic. It is the most common cause of progressive myelopathy after SCI.[205] Although considered to be a late

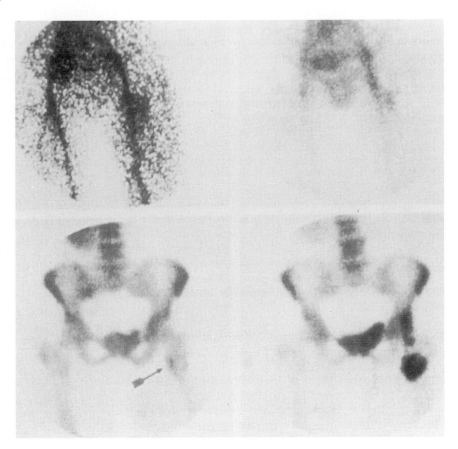

FIGURE 55–6 Triple-phase bone scan revealing the formation of heterotopic ossification about the left hip. (From Orzel JA, Rudd TG: Heterotopic bone formation: Clinical, laboratory, and imaging correlation. J Nucl Med 1985; 26:125–132.)

complication of SCI, it can occur from 2 months to 34 months post injury.[384] The clinical presentation often begins with pain and numbness. The pain is often a dull aching pain in the head and upper arms. It is aggravated by straining, sneezing, or coughing. Motor weakness is often associated with a concurrent sensory loss.[288] The sensory loss can be ascending or descending. Other symptoms include excessive sweating,[309] orthostatic hypotension,[213] and Horner's syndrome.[20] The syrinx can extend to the brainstem and result in sensory loss in the trigeminal distribution. This occurs because the descending tract of the trigeminal nerve descends to the second cervical level. Other complications of syringobulbia include hiccups, nystagmus, atrophy of the tongue, and recurrent laryngeal nerve palsy.[14, 333] These syrinxes can extend from the thoracic spinal cord and cause numbness and weakness in the cervical segments.

Magnetic resonance imaging (MRI) is the most accurate diagnostic technique.[359] Computed tomography (CT) with myelography can show a widened spinal cord, contrast material within the syrinx, and subarachnoid block. Treatment is surgical, and drainage can be accomplished with a shunt to the subarachnoid space or peritoneal cavity. Motor weakness and pain have a good prognosis with surgical treatment.[88, 288, 334]

The mechanism of development of post-traumatic cystic myelopathy is unclear. Areas of infarction and necrosis might be the site of cystic cavities that merge to form a larger syrinx. The cavities develop between the ventral and dorsal arterial supply in the area of diminished vascularity. Other theories include development following release of cellular lyosomes or extension due to increases in intraspinal venous pressure.[164, 361]

PAIN SYNDROMES IN SPINAL CORD INJURY

Pain is one of the most common problems after SCI.[290] It can be directly related to the trauma affecting the vertebrae or spinal cord and nerve roots, or it can occur for the same reasons pain develops in non-spinal cord–injured persons. Donovan and colleagues[84] have classified pain into five groups: (1) peripheral nerve pain, (2) central spinal cord pain, (3) visceral pain, (4) muscle and mechanical pain, and (5) psychogenic pain. The focus of this section is the dysesthetic pain syndrome.

As with any other medical problem, the first step in the diagnosis and treatment is a careful history and physical examination. The evaluation should consider syringomyelia,[3, 288] musculoskeletal pain,[257, 261, 327] and peripheral nerve compression such as carpal tunnel syndrome.[68, 111] Reflex sympathetic dystrophy has been reported to occur and presents with swelling and contracture of the shoulder and hand.[111, 337] Abdominal pain can occur due to gastrointestinal complications[24, 120] such as pancreatitis,[46] cholelithiasis,[7] or superior mesenteric artery syndrome.[289] Spasticity of the abdominal muscles can cause pain and discomfort.[239]

Dysesthetic pain syndrome generally occurs within the first year of injury although late onset is also possible.[28, 38] Over time it often diminishes in severity.[70] This syndrome also is commonly called phantom pain or deafferentation pain.[222] Patients most commonly describe it as burning pain. Other complaints include aching, tingling, shooting, stinging, or a pressure or tightness. It can be in the upper limbs in tetraplegic patients. Common sites distal to the lesion include the legs, buttocks, rectum, and abdomen.[255, 293, 338] Dysesthetic pain is particularly common in persons with SCI secondary to gunshot wounds.[68] It can be exacerbated by noxious stimuli such as urinary tract infection, bowel impaction, cigarette smoking, and other factors that commonly increase spasticity or cause autonomic dysreflexia.[66]

Management of dysesthetic pain is one of the most difficult problems for physicians and therapists dealing with SCI. The pain can be only a minor nuisance that only intermittently interferes with daily activities. It can also be so disabling that it limits sleep and prevents performance of ADL. In mild cases, the only treatment needed usually is to explain the nature of the pain, reassure the patient that it will decrease with time, and offer treatment in the future if needed.

In more severe cases additional treatment steps are needed. Acetaminophen or nonsteroidal anti-inflammatory drugs are the first step and help a small percentage of patients. Narcotic analgesics are rarely beneficial and are often detrimental owing to their central and gastrointestinal side effects, and should be avoided. Although controlled studies are limited, it is our experience that tricyclic antidepressants (amitriptyline, doxepin) and anticonvulsants are the most efficacious.[66, 138, 212] These drugs act by diminishing the presynaptic uptake of serotonin and facilitate pain control. Anticonvulsants, including clonazepam, carbamazepine, and phenytoin, are helpful in some cases. They are often used in combination with antidepressants.[71, 114] These treatments can also be used in conjunction with psychological pain management techniques. The use of transcutaneous electrical nerve stimulation has been successful in small numbers of patients.[71, 130]

This pain can be refractory to medical management in some cases and so severe that neurosurgical intervention is considered. This should only occur when interdisciplinary efforts have failed. Initially, destructive procedures such as cordotomy were practiced with limited success.[355] Dorsal root entry zone (DREZ) procedures are more commonly advocated currently. Destructive lesions are placed in the DREZ above and around the traumatic area using microwave. There is a danger of getting more sensory and motor loss, and pain relief is variable.[103, 251] Dorsal column stimulations with electrodes placed in the epidural space are also of limited utility.[201, 251, 280] (For further information on pain management, see Chapter 41.)

NEUROGENIC BLADDER MANAGEMENT

This section reviews the relationship between the neurogenic bladder and its impact on rehabilitation outcomes. Various bladder management techniques have been promulgated over the years. These techniques have risks and benefits from a medical standpoint, in addition to affecting the day-to-day lives of spinal cord–injured patients. It is important to consider these aspects in determining a person's bladder management. The spinal cord–injured pa-

tient, knowing the risks, benefits, and practical aspects of the various techniques, should then actively participate in the decision-making process. The neurophysiology of bladder dysfunction and the use of urodynamic testing are discussed in Chapter 28.

A catheter-free state is the preferred situation to decrease the risk of infection and stones or other complications.[128] Many patients with incomplete lesions return to normal voiding patterns with low residual urine volumes. The lower the residual urine, the lower the chance of urinary tract infection.[233] Intermittent catheterization is initiated, and the daily frequency diminished as voiding improves. When postvoid residual urine is less than 50 mL, the program is discontinued. Should bacteriuria develop, it is treated initially with antibiotics. Recurrent asymptomatic bacteriuria is generally not treated to avoid the development of resistant organisms.[316] Symptomatic bacteriuria with fever, leuckocytosis, or increased spasticity is treated, and the catheterization schedule is increased to reduce bacterial concentration and remove the urine that serves as a culture medium for bacterial growth. This concept has been described as the "safe emptying interval."[364]

If normal voiding patterns do not return, reflex voiding might occur with low residuals. Persons with high-pressure bladders and detrusor-sphincter dyssynergia can develop vesicoureteral reflux and hydronephrosis.[113] Careful urological follow-up is required. Reflex voiding generally requires the use of a condom catheter in men. This has several practical limitations. Many men have difficulties keeping the external catheter on the penis in a watertight manner, and there is no external catheter for women. Condom catheters can also result in skin lesions of the penis or reactions due to latex allergy. A tight condom catheter can obstruct urine outflow and result in obstructive sequelae.

Several options exist if normal or reflex voiding does not occur following a trial of intermittent catheterization. With decreasing lengths of stay, it is often unclear at the time of rehabilitation unit or center discharge whether or not intermittent catheterization is a short- or long-term option. Long-term intermittent catheterization generally is practiced under two circumstances. The first is that the patient is able to self-catheterize and is willing to perform the procedure consistently. A dependent person can continue with the procedure if adequate reliable assistance is available. Prevention of voiding between catheterizations is aided by anticholinergic and antispasmodic medications, or an external catheter.[320] In some instances, incontinence pads are needed. "Clean" catheterizations are tolerated in most situations.[172, 216] Specialized catheters with self-contained urinary collection bags can be helpful, depending on the environment in which catheterizations are performed and the funding available.[365]

Many patients prefer an indwelling catheter for convenience purposes. This is common in spinal cord–injured women and in patients of both sexes with high tetraplegia. A suprapubic catheter is a similar option with some advantages over a urethral catheter. It avoids complications such as urethral tears, penoscrotal fistulas, and requires less skill to replace. A large catheter can be used. Leakage and irritation around the stoma can be a problem, and the need for surgical placement is a disadvantage. Indwelling catheters can increase the risk of developing bladder carcinoma.[199]

Many surgical options exist for bladder drainage. These are generally considered only when less invasive methods fail. Sphincterotomy with or without transurethral resection of the bladder neck is considered in spinal cord–injured men who can retain an external catheter.[284] Bladder emptying is constant and reflex activity is needed to assist with voiding. Impotence can occur along with retrograde ejaculation. The procedure might need repetition due to fibrosis. Most men resist this procedure because of its destructive nature.

Recent interest has developed in continent urinary diversion for spinal cord–injured women.[118] These pouches can use sites such as the umbilicus[245] as the site for the urostomy and are emptied with a catheter. These diversion techniques may prove beneficial as a means of providing continence without appliances, but long-term follow-up is lacking.

BOWEL MANAGEMENT IN SPINAL CORD INJURY

Bowel management is a lifelong concern for persons with SCI.[312, 389] On admission to the rehabilitation unit, patients generally present with constipation or diarrhea.[104] Since most have been treated with numerous antibiotics, infection with *Clostridium difficile* is often suspected as a cause of diarrhea. The most common cause of diarrhea generally is fecal impaction, which can present with diarrhea, nausea, or loss of appetite. The best approach is to carefully relieve the rectal impaction manually. Lack of sphincter tone makes enemas difficult to use in some individuals. A flat plate of the abdomen will often show stool in the ascending and transverse colon as well. If tolerated, mineral oil administered orally for several days followed by magnesium citrate will relieve this impaction after the distal stool is cleared. Long-term use of mineral oil and laxatives is not recommended.

A diet high in fiber with adequate fluid intake is essential. Supplements are available if dietary intake is not adequate. Stool softeners such as docusate are frequently helpful. Most persons abandon these medications after discharge and regulate their diet to achieve proper stool consistency. Fluid intake must be stressed, and dehydration should be avoided.

The overall goal of the bowel program is to maintain continence, with a schedule that is frequent enough to avoid impaction or incontinence, but one that also is convenient for the individual. This can occur in the morning or evening based on many factors, including personal preference and availability of the attendant care. The less frequently the program is done, the more likely the person is to have problems with impaction or bowel accidents. Every-other-day programs are the most commonly used.

Emptying generally is accomplished by digital stimulation or via a suppository in patients with preserved reflex function in the rectum. Traditionally, bisacodyl suppositories are used. Small-volume "mini-enemas" are often used because the response is faster. These preparations are more expensive. With digital stimulation or mini-enemas, care

must be taken not to damage the rectum from trauma or rough edges of the mini-enema. Persons with lower motor neuron lesions often perform manual removal of the stool.

Hemorrhoids are a common problem after SCI. Risk factors for hemorrhoids include a sedentary lifestyle, laxative abuse, obesity, anal manipulation during the bowel program, and chronically increased intra-abdominal pressure.[61] Chronic bleeding often requires surgical treatment. Other causes of bleeding, such as gastrointestinal carcinoma, should be ruled out. Most hemorrhoids are treated locally with a steroid emollient cream. (See Chapter 28 for further information on bowel management.)

Superior mesenteric artery syndrome can occur in SCI, especially in persons with severe weight loss.[291] In this syndrome, the superior mesenteric artery compresses the third portion of the duodenum. Symptoms include postprandial nausea, emesis, abdominal pain, and bloating. Dehydration and poor nutritional status can result. The syndrome is exacerbated by the supine position and an abdominal orthosis. Small frequent meals, positioning the patient on the side after meals, and metoclopramide can be helpful.

Gallstones commonly develop in persons with SCI.[8] The diagnosis can be obscured by sensory loss. Asymptomatic stones in the gallbladder are frequently found during routine ultrasonography done for the kidneys.

PSYCHOLOGICAL AND FAMILY ISSUES

Traumatic injury to the spinal cord has been described as one of the most devastating calamities in life.[127] Almost every sphere of a person's life is affected and adjustment to SCI is a challenge to all persons no matter how premorbidly well adjusted.[246] Counseling services should be made available to all patients with an SCI. The mental health model approach that is described by Morris[246] allows the patient to receive these services in a way that does not imply that a specific need or problem exists beyond the injury itself. Issues that the psychologist can deal with include acceptance of disability and the impact of the disability on family, sexual, and vocational functioning. The psychologist can be helpful to team members as well in recommending approaches to the patient and in clarifying patients' behavior in terms of adaptation to their injury. Depression frequently occurs and the psychologist can work with the injured person and the physician on a treatment plan. Many persons require several years for psychological adaptation to occur.[326] Poor adaptation and depression can lead to complications secondary to poor compliance with the medical regimen such as pressure ulcers.

Alcohol and substance abuse may be involved in the injury itself and may continue after discharge from rehabilitation. Up to 50% of persons develop problems with substance abuse after SCI.[140] Treatment should be initiated during the initial rehabilitation period and continue after discharge.[139] Substance abuse can lead to medical and other complications because of poor compliance with pressure relief, catheterization schedules, and medical therapies. It can be disruptive to the family as well.[370]

Cognitive deficits are common in spinal cord–injured

persons and can interfere with the rehabilitation process.[247, 279, 289] Closed head injury is one common cause, and it occurs in up to 60% of spinal cord–injured persons. In the past, closed head injury in SCI patients often went unrecognized. Cognitive deficits in many circumstances are multifactorial and relate to substance abuse, learning disabilities, and other medical conditions. The team must be aware of these deficits and how they affect the person's abilities to cooperate and participate in therapy. Strategies should be devised to determine the best descriptive techniques to illustrate a skill that must be learned. Neuropsychological evaluation gives insight into the person's behavior and allows the team to deal with the person on a more consistent and therapeutic basis. (See Chapters 4 and 49 for further information on cognitive assessment and intervention.)

SPEECH AND SWALLOWING PROBLEMS

During acute care and early in the course of rehabilitation, communication and, more specifically, speech and vocalization, may be impaired. Endotracheal and nasotracheal intubation, tracheostomy, anterior cervical procedures, and ventilator dependency are factors that contribute to the impairment of a patient's ability to speak.

Methods to improve the ability to communicate include exaggerated mouthing of words and lip reading, simplifying communication to yes and no questions, simple communication boards and pictures, the use of an electric larynx, and more complex computer communication systems that require more in-depth training.[193, 308]

For those patients who are ventilator-dependent, various types of speaking tracheostomy tubes are available. These speaking aids, in general, operate by directing, via a second line, an external source of oxygen or compressed air into the trachea and past the vocal cords, which results in phonation.[308] Examples of these are the Communitrach I, Portex Tracheostomy Tube, and the Bivona Talking Tracheostomy Tube.

In patients with tracheostomies, advancing to fenestrated tubes and beginning trial periods of corking the tracheostomy tube at the earliest time consistent with safety allows early resumption of normal speech. Another option in this group of patients is the use of one-way tracheostomy speaking valves. In general, these devices operate by allowing the inspiration of air through the valve which is usually fitted at the end of the tracheostomy tube. During exhalation, the valve is closed and the air is directed through the trachea and past the vocal cords. Obviously in patients with cuffed tracheostomy tubes, the cuff must be deflated for the mechanism to work. Different types of one-way valves are available, including the Kisner One-way Valve, the Olympic Trach Talk, the Montgomery Speaking Tube, and the Passy-Muir Tracheostomy Speaking Valve. (See Chapter 3 for further information on communications disorders.)

Dysphagia in patients with SCI is often overlooked early in the course of acute care because of other more pressing medical issues. The incidence of swallowing problems can be as high as 20% in tetraplegic patients during the first 4 months post injury.[362] Factors that can predispose to dysphagia include (1) head and neck position—excessive neck extension in a halo orthosis, excessive neck flexion in cervical collars, or inadequate head support in high-backed wheelchairs; (2) neurological injuries—concomitant head injury or cranial nerve involvement secondary to brainstem injury in high cervical cord trauma; (3) surgical complications (primarily in anterior procedures)—dislodged grafts, laryngeal nerve paralysis, or significant postsurgical edema; and (4) in ventilator-dependent patients, inability to coordinate swallowing with ventilator cycling.[362]

A recent study found no direct relationship between swallowing problems and the effects of cervical spine stabilization (surgical fusion and bracing) or respiratory status (tracheostomy or mechanical ventilation), but did note that the use of mechanical ventilation, recent anterior fusion surgery, and tracheostomy was more frequent in the dysphagic group.[331]

For the most part, symptoms and clinical findings that have been reported in spinal cord–injured patients with swallowing problems have been characterized predominantly by pharyngeal stage problems. These have included absent or delayed pharyngeal swallow, reduced pharyngeal peristalsis, reduced base of tongue retraction, reduced laryngeal elevation or closure, and upper esophageal sphincter dysfunction.[185, 324, 331]

As an adjunct to the clinical bedside evaluation, videofluoroscopy is a frequently used diagnostic procedure for dysphagia. It permits observation of the oral preparatory, oral, pharyngeal, and esophageal aspects of the swallow before, during, and after the event. Other reasons for its frequent use include ease of interpretation and allowing a qualitative estimate of aspiration.[306] It helps determine successful swallowing strategies. Videofluoroscopy can also be used as a follow-up procedure to assess recovery and monitor efficacy of treatment procedures and techniques.

The treatment of dysphagia in patients with SCI, as in those with other neurological disorders, can involve indirect or direct management depending upon the nature of the swallowing problem. Methods of indirect management include structuring the eating environment, modifying utensils, and determining the degree of supervision required for safe oral feeding. Methods of direct management include cognitive stimulation, sensory stimulation, physiotherapy, compensatory postures and positioning, compensatory maneuvers such as the supraglottic swallow and Mendelsohn maneuver, and assistive devices.[210] The supraglottic swallow maneuver involves attempts at focusing voluntary control over otherwise involuntary swallow events. The maneuver involves the following steps: (1) take and hold a breath; (2) place food or liquid in mouth; (3) swallow (once or twice, depending on the efficiency of pharyngeal clearance); (4) clear the throat; and (5) swallow again. The Mendelsohn maneuver involves holding the larynx in an elevated position during swallowing to facilitate more complete pharyngeal clearance.

In general, the prognosis for recovery of safe, normal swallowing function is good in SCI patients. Most patients, even those with initially significant dysphagia, have no dietary restrictions by 6 months post injury, although recovery can take as long as 1 year.[331] (For further information on dysphagia, see Chapter 27.)

VOCATIONAL REHABILITATION IN SPINAL CORD INJURY

Since reintegration into the community is the major goal of SCI rehabilitation, vocational rehabilitation services are introduced early on in the course of rehabilitation. This helps provide additional hope for the future in many instances.[339] These efforts can be directed toward return to work, school, or productive avocations such as volunteer work. Financial disincentives to return to employment often exist owing to government and other entitlements.[79]

The Americans With Disabilities Act, which prohibits discrimination against qualified persons in employment, should ease the return of spinal cord–injured persons to work. Reasonable accommodations must be made to disabled persons to allow them to work. These accommodations include modifications to the work environment, although the law is not specific in this area. Enforcement of this law is monitored by the U.S. Equal Employment Opportunity Commission (EEOC).

Several studies exist that have analyzed who returns to work and in what capacity.[23, 75] Persons who return to work soon after injury generally return to the same job or a similar one at their premorbid place of employment. Persons returning to work in later years generally do this through educational or vocational training. A recent study describes 11 variables that are associated with a higher probability of return to employment.[313] These variables are female sex, white race, higher level of education, more caudal level of injury, married, younger age at injury, current age between 25 and 44 years, sedentary employment, nonveteran, ability to independently manage bowel and bladder, and no financial disincentives (Social Security, disability insurance, or workers' compensation).

These statistical associations should not be used to guide your decision on vocational services. Many persons who do not fit into these categories successfully return to work. Medical complications and aging factors can limit longevity of employment. (For further information on vocational rehabilitation, see Chapter 9.)

DRIVERS' REHABILITATION IN SPINAL CORD INJURY

A drivers' rehabilitation program is often very important when attempting to return a person with an SCI to independent functioning in the community. Whether the objective is to provide drivers' training or to determine an appropriate vehicle to meet the patient's transportation needs, an interdisciplinary approach often best meets the needs of the patient.

The patient and family are key participants in a driver's rehabilitation program. It is important to have a clear idea of the patient's goals, expectations, and lifestyle in order to determine what would best meet his or her needs. Persons involved in a drivers' program can include an occupational, physical, or other therapist who evaluates physical func-

tioning, cognition, vision, and perception, and identifies potential adaptive support needs; a rehabilitation engineer who evaluates and assesses for technical equipment needs and recommends, modifies, and designs adaptive devices; a driver instructor who conducts on-the-road assessment and training; a vehicle modifier who provides current information on adaptive controls and vehicle modifications, installs devices, modifies vehicles, trains on secondary and accessory control operations, and provides vehicle service and maintenance; and a physician, usually the primary referral source, who determines and informs program members of any medical issues that may affect driving ability and who serves as liaison to the state's department of motor vehicles.[274]

A drivers' rehabilitation program receives referrals for services to evaluate driving ability and training needs, to evaluate and recommend adaptive equipment needs, and to evaluate and make recommendations for a passenger vehicle. During the initial evaluation, the therapist gathers the pertinent medical history (including the primary disability, any secondary disabilities, precautions given by the physician, current medications), current level of functioning, social history (including living situation and vocational status), and driving history (including previous violations and accidents).[184, 304]

The clinical assessment of the patient includes evaluation of motor strength, muscle tone and spasticity, extremity proprioception and ROM, and balance skills. A visual screening includes visual acuity, depth perception, color perception and discrimination, night vision, visual accommodation, and field of vision. A cognitive screening evaluates attention, sign recognition, reaction time, driving knowledge, and problem-solving skills.

A wheelchair assessment is also included in the clinical evaluation, looking at the type and dimensions of the chair; positioning of the patient, including posture and stability; the ability to manage parts; the ability to transfer in and out of the chair into the vehicle; and the ability to load and unload the wheelchair.

As a component of the clinical assessment, a driving simulator can be used to assess a patient's ability to recognize, react, and negotiate a number of potential driving situations.[184] A behind-the-wheel assessment provides information about a patient's balance and postural stability, upper extremity function, and ability to manage basic vehicle controls (acceleration, braking, and steering) and maneuvers (turning, reversing, and parking).[184]

In general, the strongest and most coordinated upper extremity is used to operate the steering system. A device such as a spinner knob, palm cup, V-grip, or trip pin is usually put on the steering wheel to enhance the patient's ability to move the wheel quickly and accurately. Steering wheel resistance can be adjusted to the needs of the driver to facilitate steering.[300]

Acceleration and braking are accomplished through various types of hand controls, which generally consist of three systems: push-pull, push–right angle, and push-twist. The type of system used depneds on the residual neurological function available. Like the steering system, the resistance of the brake and accelerator system can be adjusted to the neurological and functional abilities of the patient. The different types of system resistance include stock, reduced, and zero effort.[300]

Secondary controls can be accessed via switch extensions, elbow switches, or head controls. Accessory controls can be accessed via toggle extensions, D-rings, and touch pads.[300]

Following the clinical assessment, a determination can usually be made as to the type of vehicle (two- or four-door car, full-size van or minivan) that best meets the needs and abilities of the patient. Factors to be considered when determining an appropriate vehicle and needed equipment or adaptations include the ability of the patient to access the vehicle, wheelchair type, transfer ability, type of primary controls to maneuver the vehicle, secondary controls such as the horn, turn signal, windshield wipers, and headlights, and accessory controls such as the ignition, gear selector, and heat and air-conditioning systems.[300]

Following the clinical and vehicle and equipment assessments, a determination is made that the patient is safe to drive, unsafe to drive, able to drive on completion of a certain period of training, or able to drive with a certain type of vehicle and equipment or adaptation. The extent of the driver's training period depends upon the patient's physical and functional status and previous driving experience as well as the complexity of the driving system and the patient's skills exhibited with the adaptive equipment.[304]

Documentation is very important and should clearly state the results of the initial assessment and driving evaluation, behind-the-wheel training, and dissemination of any information or education. Recommendation for adaptive equipment and equipment for medical necessity, as well as any precautions or restrictions, should be clearly documented.[275] The physician is typically ultimately responsible for the final prescription of all equipment and therapy. Ultimately, it is the state's department of motor vehicles that usually performs driver's license examinations, basic vehicle safety inspection, and imposes driver's license restrictions.

TENDON TRANSFER PROCEDURES IN SPINAL CORD INJURY

Tendon transfer procedures are one of the few surgical options that are available to persons with cervical injuries to restore active movements and further enhance functional independence. Numerous techniques and procedures are available to restore active elbow extension, wrist extension, finger flexion to enhance grasp, grasp release, and lateral thumb pinch. Restoring active elbow extension enhances the patient's ability to perform self-care activities that require overhead reaching and allows more complete forward reaching to retrieve objects. In addition, it lends stability to the extremity which can enhance the patient's ability to assist with transfer activities. Active wrist extension enhances the use of a tenodesis pinch between the thumb and index fingers to pick up objects. Restoring grasp, release, and lateral thumb pinch further enhances hand function and the ability to perform functional tasks.

In the evaluation of a patient as a candidate for tendon transfer, several considerations should be kept in mind. In general, surgery should not be considered before 1 year post injury and certainly not until the patient has been neurologically stable for at least 6 months. In addition to allowing time for the natural return of any impaired muscle groups, this period of time gives the patient the opportunity to adjust to the disability, maximize strength in the remaining muscle groups, and develop and maximize new functional skills. An older patient with long duration of the tetraplegia can be considered for surgery, but it is believed that the outcomes are less predictable if performed more than 5 years post injury.[143] The patient should have a clear understanding of the surgery planned, the gains that can be realistically expected, and potential complications such as increased dependency in the postoperative period. Because of the possibility that preoperative functional abilities can be temporarily lost, patient motivation is an important factor affecting the likelihood of a successful outcome.

As a part of the presurgical evaluation, a detailed examination is essential. A thorough assessment of residual motor function of each muscle in each upper extremity must be performed. Spasticity should be assessed and, if severe, surgery probably should not be performed. Proprioception in the upper extremities and two-point discrimination in the thumb should be tested. The presence of two-point discrimination (less than 10 mm) in the thumb pulp enhances the effectiveness of restored pinch grasp. Without two-point discrimination or proprioception, the patient must rely on visual feedback for hand control, and consequently only one hand can be used at a time. In the case of poor sensation, only one hand is usually considered for reconstruction.

A recognized classification system (Table 55–4), which incorporates the findings of the motor and sensory assessment, serves as a guideline for predicting function that might be gained and in selecting an appropriate procedure from among the several techniques available to achieve that function.[219]

As a result of the experiences reported by a number of surgeons, a number of principles for tendon transfer surgery are generally recognized[160] (Table 55–5). Active elbow extension can be restored by transfer of the posterior half of the deltoid to the triceps, using free tendon grafts from

TABLE 55–4 International Classification of the Upper Limb in Tetraplegia

Motor Grouping	
0	No muscle below elbow suitable for transfer
1	Brachioradialis ≥ grade 4 strength
2	Extensor carpi radialis longus + above
3	Extensor carpi radialis brevis + above
4	Pronator teres + above
5	Flexor carpi radialis + above
6	Finger extensors + above
7	Thumb extensors + above
8	Digital flexors + above
9	Lacks intrinsics only
X	Exceptions
Sensory Grouping	
O	Two-point discrimination >10 mm in the thumb
Cu	Two-point discrimination <10 mm in the thumb

From McDowell CL, Moberg EA, House JH: The Second International Conference on Surgical Rehabilitation of the Upper Limb in Tetraplegia (Quadriplegia). J Hand Surg Am 1986; 11:604–608.

TABLE 55-5 Principles for Tendon Transfer Surgery

1. The transferred muscle should have adequate strength to perform the desired function and overcome any mechanical disadvantage.
2. The transferred muscle should be a synergist of the movement to be restored.
3. The transferred muscle should be expendable.
4. The affected joints should have full passive range of motion.
5. The excursion of the transferred muscle should be equal to the recipient tendon.
6. The line of action for the transferred tendon should be as straight as possible.
7. The dominant hand should be treated first unless the nondominant hand has significantly greater sparing of motor function or sensation.

the toe extensors to extend the transfer.[243] A second technique involves the transfer of the biceps tendon to the triceps insertion.[388] There are a number of techniques for restoring active wrist extension and lateral thumb pinch. Wrist extension function is vital in any procedure attempting to restore grasp and pinch.[160] The brachioradialis tendon can be transferred to the extensor carpi radialis brevis to enhance wrist extension. Active lateral thumb pinch can be restored by stabilization of the thumb interphalangeal joint with Kirschner wire and tenodesis of the flexor pollicis longus (FPL) tendon to the radius.[243] As the wrist extends, the tenodesed FPL tendon produces flexion at the metacarpophalangeal joint, which causes the thumb to adduct against the side of the index finger.

In a patient with intact wrist extension, active grasp can be restored by a thumb metacarpophalangeal arthrodesis and a transfer of the brachioradialis into the flexor digitorum profundus. Release is achieved by tenodesis of the extensor pollicis longus (EPL), abductor pollicis longus, and extensor digitorum communis to the radius. Thumb pinch is restored by FPL tenodesis.[388] Another technique consists of fusing the thumb carpometacarpal joint, followed by EPL and FPL tenodesis to restore active lateral pinch and release.[149]

Patients with lower cervical-level injuries where upper extremity impairment is predominantly in the finger flexors and intrinsics might benefit from procedures transferring the brachioradialis, extensor carpi radialis longus, or flexor carpi radialis to the flexor digitorum profundus to restore active grasp.[100, 101, 160]

With any tendon transfer procedure, a successful outcome also depends on closely supervised and well-coordinated postsurgical management. Following surgery, there is a period of immobilization of the affected extremity, generally about 3 weeks for procedures on the hands and 6 weeks for the elbows.[160, 243] This time is necessary because too rapid mobilization can result in overstretching and compromised function. Splints can be utilized for immobilization. A period of gradual mobilization eventually follows the immobilization. During this time, the patient learns how to activate the transferred muscle to achieve new motion. Electromyographic biofeedback can also be useful in motor reeducation. This is then followed by graded active exercises of the transferred muscle and a gradual introduction of upper limb activities.

SPINAL CORD INJURY IN THE ELDERLY AND AGING

Spinal cord injury often is thought of as a problem of young people. Although these injuries are more common in young persons, they occur in persons of all ages.[78]

The acute care and rehabilitation phase can be prolonged in some older persons with SCI because of increased complications. These include pneumonia, sepsis, gastrointestinal hemorrhage, and pulmonary embolism.[77] The decision to admit the older person to a comprehensive rehabilitation program should not be based on age alone. If patients are able to participate in the program from a cognitive standpoint, they generally will benefit from a rehabilitation program. Motor function is the major limiting factor in functional outcomes. While persons of all ages can benefit from a rehabilitation program, older people with complete paraplegia are less likely to be independent in more complex skills such as dressing and transfers.[381]

The poor prognosis for persons with SCI has improved since the development of specialized centers of care.[358] Life expectancy has increased, and the causes of death have changed. In the early years of comprehensive care, urological complications and urosepsis were the leading cause of death. Advances in urological care and antibiotics have resulted in a diminution of urological death. Pneumonia is now the leading cause of death. Complications such as amyloidosis are uncommon. The increased longevity of persons with SCI has resulted in an awareness of numerous changes that occur with age that can have a significant impact on quality of life. Decreased functional abilities result in the need for more assistance from caregivers and an increased need for equipment.[108] Persons who rely on their family members for care can be faced with an increased need for care as their family members age and have less ability to provide care. Many persons who have been free of complications for years begin to develop pressure ulcers and other complications because their aging parents or spouses are no longer able to assist them as much, or even at all.[369] As skills such as wheelchair propulsion and transfers become more and more difficult or are impaired by degenerative joint disease and musculoskeletal pain, equipment needs change, and the cost of equipment increases. Power wheelchairs and mechanical lifts for transfers are examples of equipment that are often needed with aging SCI patients.

Increased susceptibility to medical complications with age such as pneumonia, fractures, and cardiovascular disease results in increased hospitalizations.[368] These can be followed by decreased functional abilities and increased need for personal assistance and therapy to restore functional abilities. These periods can be accompanied by changes in mood and affect or depression. Psychological problems can occur during aging as the person's functional abilities decrease or the injury interferes with social interaction and career or other long-term goals.

The risk of pressure ulcer development increases with age.[369] Anatomical and physiological changes in aging skin result in thinner skin with decreased barrier and immunological function and increased susceptibility to pressure. Sitting and turning tolerances can decrease, and the suitability of wheelchair cushions and bed coverings must be reassessed. The risk of pressure ulcer development is increased during periods of bed rest for management of medical conditions or periods of depression when skin care regimens are often not followed. Alcohol or substance abuse can increase the risk of pressure ulcer development and other complications if skin regimens are not followed. With aging, particular attention should be paid to skin hygiene and pressure relief frequency, which may have to be increased.

Persons with SCI are susceptible to all of the changes of aging experienced by those without SCI, as well as the problems particular to SCI. The impact of these aging changes generally will be greater on those persons with SCI. (For further information see Chapter 59.)

DISCHARGE PLANNING AND LIFELONG FOLLOW-UP

Discharge planning begins at the time of admission to the rehabilitation facility. As lengths of stay shorten, this is particularly critical. The team must be aware of the potential home setting to plan for discharge. The home environment affects the type of equipment ordered and can influence the length of stay. The availability of assistance at home and funding for home therapy or nursing visits plays a major role in determining the timing of discharge. Combining these factors helps the team to determine what skills are needed to facilitate a smooth and safe reintegration into the community.

The majority of spinal cord–injured persons are discharged to home. Many SCI programs work with independent living centers to assist disabled persons. The independent living movement focuses on quality of life for disabled persons and independent decision making.[72] Independent living outcomes have been related to several factors. People most likely to live independently are women, married, and of older age. Persons who require close medical supervision and who have unmet therapy needs are less likely to live independently. Transportation barriers also have a negative impact on the ability to live independently.

Lifelong follow-up after discharge should be available to spinal cord–injured persons.[7] The rehabilitation specialist should be available to advise the person's community physicians on special aspects of SCI care. As time progresses, the follow-up schedule is diminished to an annual checkup and urological follow-up in persons free of complications. Many persons return more frequently, particularly if they have difficulty finding accessible care in the community with physicians who are familiar with managing the urological aspects and pressure ulcers of SCI.

There is some debate over which type of renal studies to perform after discharge. Annual renal ultrasound studies are noninvasive and have been favorably compared with annual intravenous pyelograms. Others advocate nuclear medicine scans for follow-up.[41, 178, 179, 197, 264]

Comprehensive care for persons with SCI has resulted in improved life expectancies. This has resulted in new challenges to spinal cord–injured persons and their healthcare professionals. Gains will continue to be made in these areas as healthcare professionals work closely with consumers in meeting these challenges.

References

1. Abel NA, Smith RA: Intrathecal baclofen for treatment of intractable spinal spasticity. Arch Phys Med Rehabil 1994; 75:54–58.
2. Abouleish E: Hypertension in a paraplegic parturient. Anesthesiology 1980; 53:348.
3. Alcazaren EG: Post-traumatic cystic myelopathy: A late neurological complication of spinal cord injury. Curr Concepts Phys Med Rehabil 1984; 1:15–24.
4. Aisen ML, Dieta M, McDowell F, et al: Baclofen toxicity in a patient with subclinical renal insufficiency. Arch Phys Med Rehabil 1994; 75:109–111.
5. American Spinal Injury Association: International standards for neurological classification of spinal cord injury. Chicago, American Spinal Injury Association, 1992.
6. Apple DF Jr, Hudson LM (eds): Spinal cord injury: The model. *In* Proceedings of the National Consensus Conference on Catastrophic Illness and Injury, Atlanta, Dec 1989. The Georgia Regional Spinal Cord Injury Care System, Shephard Center for Treatment of Spinal Injuries, 1990.
7. Apstein MD, Dalecki-Chipperfield K: Spinal cord injury is a risk factor for gallstone disease. Gastroenterology 1987; 92:966–968.
8. Arrowood JA, Mohanty PK, Thames MD: Cardiovascular problems in the spinal cord injured patients. Phys Med Rehabil 1987; 1:443–456.
9. Bach JR: Inappropriate weaning and late onset ventilatory failure of individuals with traumatic quadriplegia. Paraplegia 1993; 31:430–438.
10. Bach JR: New approaches in the rehabilitation of the traumatic high level quadriplegic. Am J Phys Med Rehabil 1991; 70:13–19.
11. Bach JR, O'Connor K: Electrophrenic ventilation: A different perspective. J Am Paraplegia Soc 1991; 14:9–17.
12. Baer GA, Talonen PP, Hakkinen V, et al: Phrenic nerve stimulation in tetraplegia: A new regimen to condition the diaphragm for full-time respiration. Scand J Rehabil Med 1990; 22:107–111.
13. Balshi JD, Cantelmo NL, Menzoian JO: Complications of caval interruption by Greenfield filter in quadriplegics. J Vasc Surg 1989; 9:553–562.
14. Barnett H, Botterell E, Jousse A, et al: Progressive myelopathy as a sequel to traumatic paraplegia. Brain 1966; 89:159–174.
15. Basmajian JV: Biofeedback in rehabilitation: A review of principles and practices. Arch Phys Med Rehabil 1981; 62:469–475.
16. Bauer RD, Errico TJ: Cervical spine injuries. *In* Errico TJ, Bauer RD, Waugh T (eds): Spinal Trauma. Philadelphia, JB Lippincott, 1991, pp 71–121.
17. Becker D, Gonzalez M, Gentil A, et al: Prevention of deep vein thrombosis in patients with acute spinal cord injuries: Use of rotating treatment tables. Neurosurgery 1987; 20:675–677.
18. Bedbrook GM: Spinal injuries with tetraplegia and paraplegia. J Bone Joint Surg Br 1979; 61:267–284.
19. Bedbrook GM, Sedgley GI: The management of spinal injuries: Past and present. Int Rehabil Med 1980; 2:45–61.
20. Ben Zur PH: Intermittent Horner's syndrome: Recurrent, alternate Horner's syndrome in cervical cord injury. Ann Ophthalmol 1975; 7:955–962.
21. Bergman P, Herlporn A, Schoutens A, et al: Longitudinal study of calcium and bone metabolism in paraplegic patients. Paraplegia 1977–78; 15:147–159.
22. Bergstrom EMK, Frankel HR, Galer IAR, et al: Physical ability in relation to anthropometric measurements in persons with complete spinal cord lesion below the sixth cervical segment. Int Rehabil Med 1985; 7:51–55.
23. Berkowitz M, Harvey C, Greene CG, et al: The Economic Consequences of Traumatic Spinal Cord Injury. New York, Demos, 1992.
24. Berlly MH, Wilmot CB: Acute abdominal emergencies during the first four weeks after spinal cord injury. Arch Phys Med Rehabil 1984; 65:687–690.
25. Biering-Sorenson F, Bohr H, Schaadt O: Bone mineral content of the lumbar spine and lower extremities years after spinal cord lesion. Paraplegia 1988; 26:293–301.
26. Bohannon RW: Tilt table standing for reducing spasticity after spinal cord injury. Arch Phys Med Rehabil 1993; 74:1121–1122.
27. Booth BJ, Doyle M, Montgomery J: Serial casting for the management of spasticity in the head-injured adult. Phys Ther 1983; 63:1960–1966.

28. Botterell EH, Callaghan JC, Jousse AT: Pain in paraplegia: Clinical management and surgical treatment. Proc R Soc Med 1953; 47:281–288.

29. Brach B, Moser K, Cedar L, et al: Venous thrombosis in acute spinal cord paralysis. J Trauma 1977; 17:289–292.

30. Bracken MB, Freeman DH Jr, Hellenbrand K: Incidence of acute traumatic hospitalized SCI in the United States, 1970–77. Am J Epidemiol 1981; 113:615–622.

31. Bracken MB, Shepard MJ, Collins WF, et al: A randomized, controlled trial of methylprednisolone or naloxone in the treatment of acute spinal-cord injury. N Engl J Med 1990; 322:1405–1411.

32. Bracken MB, Shepard MJ, Collins WF Jr, et al: Methylprednisolone or naloxone treatment after acute spinal cord injury: 1-year follow-up data. J Neurosurg 1992; 76:23–31.

33. Braddom RL, Rocco JF: Autonomic dysreflexia: A survey of current treatment. Am J Phys Med Rehabil 1991; 70:234–241.

34. Brenes G, Dearwater S, Shapera R, et al: High density lipoprotein cholesterol concentrations in physically active and sedentary spinal cord injured patients. Arch Phys Med Rehabil 1986; 67:445–450.

35. Brixen K, Nielsen HK, Mosekilde L, et al: A short course of recombinant human growth hormone treatment stimulates osteoblasts and activates bone remodeling in normal human volunteers. J Bone Miner Res 1990; 5:609–618.

36. Brooke MM, Heard DL, deLateur BJ, et al: Heterotopic ossification and peripheral nerve entrapment: Early diagnosis and excision. Arch Phys Med Rehabil 1991; 72:425–429.

37. Buckett JR, Peckham PH, Thrope GB, et al: A flexible, portable system for neuromuscular stimulation in the paralyzed upper extremity. IEEE Trans Biomed Eng 1988; 35:897–904.

38. Burke DC: Pain in paraplegia. Paraplegia 1973; 10:297–313.

39. Burnstein A, Richlin D, Sotolongo JR: Nifedipine pretreatment for prevention of autonomic hyperreflexia during anesthesia-free extracorporeal shock wave lithotripsy. J Urol 1992; 147:676–677.

40. Buschbacher R, McKinely W, Buschbacher L, et al: Warfarin in prevention of heterotopic ossification. Am J Phys Med Rehabil 1992; 71:86–91.

41. Calenoff L, Neiman HL, Kaplan PE, et al: Urosonography in spinal cord injury patients. J Urol 1982; 128:1234–1237.

42. Cardus D, McTaggart WG: Body composition in spinal cord injury. Arch Phys Med Rehabil 1985; 66:257–259.

43. Cardus D, McTaggart WG: Total body water and its distribution in men with spinal cord injury. Arch Phys Med Rehabil 1984; 65:509–512.

44. Cardus D, Ribas-Cardus F, McTaggart WG: Coronary risk in spinal cord injury: Assessment following a multivariate approach. Arch Phys Med Rehabil 1992; 73:930–933.

45. Carey DE, Raisz LG: Calcitonin therapy in prolonged immobilization hypercalcemia. Arch Phys Med Rehabil 1985; 66:640–644.

46. Carey ME, Nance FC, Kirgis HD, et al: Pancreatitis following spinal cord injury. J Neurosurg 1977; 47:917–922.

47. Carter RE: Experiences with high tetraplegics. Paraplegia 1979; 17:140–146.

48. Chancellor MB, Erhard MJ, Hirsch III, et al: Prospective evaluation of terazosin for the treatment of autonomic dysreflexia. J Urol 1994; 151:111–113.

49. Chantraine A, Minaire P: Para-osteo-arthropathies. Scand J Rehabil Med 1981; 13:31–37.

50. Claus-Walker J, Dunn CD: Spinal cord injury and serum erythropoietin. Arch Phys Med Rehabil 1984; 65:370–374.

51. Claus-Walker J, Halstead LS: Metabolic and endocrine changes in spinal cord injury: I. The nervous system before and after transection of the spinal cord. Arch Phys Med Rehabil 1981; 62:595–601.

52. Claus-Walker J, Halstead LS: Metabolic and endocrine changes in spinal cord injury: III. Less quanta of sensory input plus bedrest and illness. Arch Phys Med Rehabil 1982; 63:628–631.

53. Claus-Walker J, Halstead LS: Metabolic and endocrine changes in spinal cord injury: IV. Compounded neurologic dysfunctions. Arch Phys Med Rehabil 1982; 63:632–638.

54. Claus-Walker J, Spencer WA, Carter RE, et al: Bone metabolism in quadriplegia: Dissociation between calciuria and hydroxyprolinuria. Arch Phys Med Rehabil 1975; 56:327–332.

55. Claus-Walker J, Vallbona C, Caster RE, et al: Resting and stimulated endocrine function in human subjects with cervical spinal cord transection. J Chron Dis 1971; 24:193–207.

56. Clough P: Glossopharyngeal breathing: Its application with a traumatic quadriplegic patient. Arch Phys Med Rehabil 1983; 64:384–385.

57. Coffey RJ, Cahill D, Steers W, et al: Intrathecal baclofen for intractable spasticity of spinal origin: Results of a long-term multicenter study. J Neurosurg 1993; 78:226–232.

58. Colachis SC: Autonomic hyperreflexia in spinal cord injury associated with pulmonary embolism. Arch Phys Med Rehabil 1991; 72:1014–1016.

59. Collins JG: Types of injuries and impairments due to injuries. Vital and Health Statistics Series 10, No. 159, US Department of Health and Human Services publication No. (PHS) 87–1587, 1987.

60. Collins K, Oswald P, Burger G, et al: Customized adjustable orthoses: Their use in spasticity. Arch Phys Med Rehabil 1985; 66:397–398.

61. Cosman BC, Stone JM, Perkash I: The gastrointestinal system. In Whiteneck GG (ed): Aging With Spinal Cord Injury. New York, Demos, 1993, pp 117–127.

62. Cotler JM, Cotler HB (eds): Spinal fusion: Science and Technique. New York, Springer-Verlag, 1990.

63. Coughlan JK, Robinson CE, Newmarch B, et al: Lower extremity bracing in paraplegia—a follow-up study. Paraplegia 1980; 18:25–32.

64. Cox SR, Weiss SM, Posuniak EA, et al: Energy expenditure after spinal cord injury: An evaluation of stable rehabilitation patients. J Trauma 1985; 25:419–423.

65. Crozier KS, Cheng LL, Graziani V, et al: Spinal cord injury: Prognosis for ambulation based on quadriceps recovery. Paraplegia 1992; 30:762–767.

66. Davidoff G, Guarracini M, Roth E, et al: Trazodone hydrochloride in the treatment of dysesthetic pain in traumatic myelopathy: A randomized, double-blind placebo-controlled study. Pain 1987; 29:151–163.

67. Davidoff G, Morris J, Roth E, et al: Cognitive dysfunction and mild closed head injury in traumatic spinal cord injury. Arch Phys Med Rehabil 1985; 66:489–491.

68. Davidoff G, Roth E, Guarracini M, et al: Function-limiting dysesthetic pain syndrome among traumatic spinal cord injury patients: A cross-sectional study. Pain 1987; 29:39–48.

69. Davidoff RA: Antispasticity drugs: Mechanisms of action. Neurology 1985; 17:107–116.

70. Davis R: Pain and suffering following spinal cord injury. Clin Orthop 1975; 112:76–80.

71. Davis R, Lentini R: Transcutaneous nerve stimulation for treatment of pain in patients with spinal cord injury. Surg Neurol 1975; 4:100–101.

72. DeJong G, Branch LG, Corcoran PJ: Independent living outcomes in spinal cord injury: Multivariate analyses. Arch Phys Med Rehabil 1984; 65:66–73.

73. DeTroyer A, Estenne M, Heilporn A: Mechanism of active expiration in tetraplegic subjects. N Engl J Med 1986; 314:740–744.

74. DeVivo M, Black K, Stover S: Causes of death during the first 12 years after spinal cord injury. Arch Phys Med Rehabil 1993; 74:248–254.

75. DeVivo MJ, Fine PR: Employment status of spinal cord injured patients 3 years after injury. Arch Phys Med Rehabil 1982; 63:200–203.

76. DeVivo MJ, Fine PR, Maetz HM, et al: Prevalence of spinal cord injury: A re-estimation employing life table techniques. Arch Neurol 1980; 37:707–708.

77. DeVivo MJ, Kartus PL, Rutt RD: The influence of age at time of spinal cord injury on rehabilitation outcomes. Arch Neurol 1990; 47:687–691.

78. DeVivo MJ, Rutt RD, Black KJ, et al: Trends in spinal cord injury demographics and treatment outcomes between 1973 and 1986. Arch Phys Med Rehabil 1992; 73:424–430.

79. Deyoe FS Jr: Spinal cord injury: Long-term follow-up of veterans. Arch Phys Med Rehabil 1972; 53:523–529.

80. Dimitriveric MR, Sherwood AM: Spasticity: Medical and surgical treatment. Neurology 1980; 30:19–27.

81. Ditunno JF, Sipski ML, Posuniak EA, et al: Wrist extensor recovery in traumatic quadriplegia. Arch Phys Med Rehabil 1987; 68:287–290.

82. Ditunno JF Jr, Stover SL, Freed MM, et al: Motor recovery of the upper extremities in traumatic quadriplegia: A multicenter study. Arch Phys Med Rehabil 1992; 73:431–436.

83. Donovan WH, Carter RE, Rossi D, et al: Clonidine effect on spasticity: A clinical trial. Arch Phys Med Rehabil 1988; 69:193–194.

84. Donovan WH, Dimitrijevic MR, Dahm L, et al: Neurophysiological approaches to chronic pain following spinal cord injury. Paraplegia 1982; 20:135–146.

85. Douglas R, Larson PF, D'Ambrosia R, et al: The LSU reciprocation gait orthosis. Orthopedics 1983; 6:834–839.

86. Duckworth WC, Jallepalli P, Solomon SS: Glucose intolerance in spinal cord injury. Arch Phys Med Rehabil 1983; 64:107–110.

87. Duckworth WC, Solomon SS, Jallepalli P, et al: Glucose intolerance due to insulin resistance in patients with spinal cord injuries. Diabetes 1980; 29:906–910.

88. Dworkin G, Staas W: Posttraumatic syringomyelia. Arch Phys Med Rehabil 1985; 66:329–331.

89. Elias AN, Gwinup G: Immobilization osteoporosis in paraplegia. J Am Paraplegia Soc 1992; 15:163–170.

90. Erickson DL, Blacklock JB, Michaelson M, et al: Control of spasticity by implantable continuous flow morphine pump. Neurosurgery 1985; 16:215–217.

91. Erickson RP: Autonomic hyperreflexia: Pathophysiology and medical management. Arch Phys Med Rehabil 1980; 61:431–440.

92. Evans DE, Kobrine AI, Rizzoli HV: Cardiac arrhythmias accompanying acute compression of the spinal cord. J Neurosurg 1980; 52:52–59.

93. Ferrell BA, Osterueil D, Christenson P: A randomized trail of low-air-loss beds for treatment of pressure ulcers. JAMA 1993; 269:494–497.

94. Fine PR, DeVivo MJ, McEachran AB: Incidence of acute traumatic hospitalized spinal cord injury in the United States. 1970–1977. Am J Epidemiol 1982; 15:475–477.

95. Fishburn MJ, Marino RS, Ditunno JF: Atelectasis and pneumonia in acute spinal cord injury. Arch Phys Med Rehabil 1990; 71:197–200.

96. Fluter GC: Pulmonary embolism presenting as supraventricular tachycardia in paraplegia: A case report. Arch Phys Med Rehabil 1993; 74:1208–1210.

97. Frankel HL, Hancock DO, Hyslop G, et al: The value of postural reduction in the initial management of closed injuries of the spine with paraplegia and tetraplegia. Paraplegia 1969; 7:179–192.

98. Frankel HL, Mathras CJ, Spalding JMK: Mechanisms of reflex cardiac arrest in tetraplegic patients. Lancet 1975; 2:1183–1185.

99. Freed JH, Hahn H, Menter MD, et al: The use of the three-phase bone scan in the early diagnosis of heterotopic ossification (HO) and in the evaluation of Didronel therapy. Paraplegia 1982; 20:208–216.

100. Freehafer AA, Kelly CM, Peckham PH: Tendon transfer for the restoration of upper limb function after a cervical spinal cord injury. J Hand Surg Am 1984; 9:887–893.

101. Freehafer AA, Von Haam E, Allen V: Tendon transfers for improved grasp after injuries of the cervical spinal cord. J Bone Joint Surg Am 1974; 56:951–959.

102. Freehafer AA, Yurick R, Mast WA: Para-articular ossification in spinal cord injury. Med Serv J 1966; 22:471–478.

103. Friedman A, Nashold BS: Dorsal root entry zone lesions for relief of pain related to spinal cord injury. J Neurosurg 1986; 65:465–469.

104. Frost FS: Gastrointestinal dysfunction in spinal cord injury. In Yarkony GM (ed): Spinal Cord Injury: Medical Management and Rehabilitation. Rockville, Md, Aspen, 1994.

105. Garland DE: Clinical observations on fractures and heterotopic ossification in the spinal cord and traumatic brain injured populations. Clin Orthop 1988; 233:86–101.

106. Garland DE: A clinical perspective on common forms of acquired heterotopic ossification. Clin Orthop 1991; 263:13–29.

107. Garland DE, Orwin JF: Resection of heterotopic ossification in patients with spinal cord injuries. Clin Orthop 1989; 242:169–176.

108. Gerhart KA, Bergstrom E, Charlifue SW, et al: Long-term spinal cord injury: Functional changes over time. Arch Phys Med Rehabil 1993; 74:1030–1034.

109. Geisler FH, Dorsey FC, Coleman WP: Recovery of motor function after spinal-cord injury—a randomized, placebo-controlled trial with GM-1 ganglioside. N Engl J Med 1991; 324:1829–1838.

110. Geisler WO, Jousse AT, Wynne-Hones M, et al: Survival in traumatic spinal cord injury. Paraplegia 1983; 21:364–373.

111. Gellman H, Chandler DR, Petrasek J, et al: Carpal tunnel syndrome in paraplegic patients. J Bone Joint Surg Am 1988; 4:517–519.

112. Genard JM, Arias A, Berlan M, et al: Pharmacological evidence of alpha 1- and 2-adrenergic supersensitivity in orthostatic hypotension due to spinal cord injury: A case report. Eur J Clin Pharmacol 1991; 41:593–596.

113. Gerridzen RG, Thijssen AM, Dehoux E: Risk factors for upper urinary tract deterioration in chronic spinal cord injured patients. J Urol 1992; 147:416–418.

114. Gibson JC, White LE: Denervation hyperpathia: A convulsive syndrome of the spinal cord responsible to carbamazepine therapy. J Neurosurg 1971; 35:287–290.

115. Gilgoff IS, Ward SLD, Hohn AR: Cardiac pacemaker in high spinal cord injury. Arch Phys Med Rehabil 1991; 72:601–603.

116. Gimovsky ML, Ojeda A, Ozaki R, et al: Management of autonomic hyperreflexia associated with a low thoracic spinal cord lesion. Obstet Gynecol 1985; 153:223–224.

117. Glen WWL, Phelps MA: Diaphragm pacing by electrical stimulation of the phrenic nerve. Neurosurgery 1985; 17:974–984.

118. Goldwasser B, Webster GD: Continent urinary diversion. J Urol 1985; 134:227–236.

119. Gonzalez F, Chang JY, Banovac K, et al: Autoregulation of cerebral blood flow in patients with orthostatic hypotension after spinal cord injury. Paraplegia 1991; 29:1–7.

120. Gore RM, Mintzer RA, Calenoff L: Gastrointestinal complications of spinal cord injury. Spine 1981; 6:538–544.

121. Green D, Chen D, Chmiel JS, et al: Prevention of thromboembolism in spinal cord injury: Role of low molecular weight heparin. Arch Phys Med Rehabil 1994; 75:290–292.

122. Green D, Lee M, Ito V, et al: Fixed vs. adjusted dose heparin in the prophylaxis of thromboembolism in spinal cord injury. JAMA 1988; 260:1255–1258.

123. Green D, Lee M, Lim A, et al: Prevention of thromboembolism after spinal cord injury using low-molecular weight heparin. Ann Intern Med 1990; 113:571–574.

124. Green D, Rossi E, Yao J, et al: Deep vein thrombosis in spinal cord injury: Effect of prophylaxis with calf compression, aspirin and dipyridamole. Paraplegia 1982; 20:227–234.

125. Groomes TE, Huang CT: Orthostatic hypotension after spinal cord injury: Treatment with fludrocortisone and ergotamine. Arch Phys Med Rehabil 1991; 72:56–58.

126. Guttman L: New hope for spinal cord sufferers. Paraplegia 1979; 17:6–15.

127. Guttman L: Spinal Cord Injuries: Comprehensive Management and Research, ed 2. Boston, Blackwell, 1976.

128. Guttman L, Frankel H: The value of intermittent catheterization in the early management of traumatic paraplegia and tetraplegia. Paraplegia 1966; 4:63–82.

129. Haas F, Axen K, Pineda H, et al: Temporal pulmonary function changes in cervical cord injury. Arch Phys Med Rehabil 1985; 66:139–144.

130. Hachen HJ: Psychological, neurophysiological, and therapeutic aspects of chronic pain: Preliminary results with transcutaneous electrical stimulation. Paraplegia 1977; 15:353–367.

131. Hall ED: The neuroprotective pharmacology of methylprednisolone. J Neurosurg 1992; 76:13–22.

132. Hall R, Hirsch J, Sackett DL, et al: Combined use of leg scanning and impedance plethysmography in suspected deep venous thrombosis: An alternative to venography. N Engl J Med 1977; 296:1497–1500.

133. Hall R, Hirsch J, Sackett DL, et al: Cost effectiveness of clinical diagnosis, venography, and noninvasive testing in patients with symptomatic deep-vein thrombosis. N Engl J Med 1981; 304:1561–1567.

134. Hangartner TN, Rodgers MM, Glaser RM, et al: Tibial bone density loss in spinal cord injured patients: Effects of FES exercise. J Rehabil Res Dev 1994; 31:50–61.

135. Hardy AG: Cervical spinal cord injury without bony injury. Paraplegia 1977; 14:296–305.

136. Haselkorn J, Britell CW, Cardenas DD: Diagnostic imagery of heterotopic ossification with co-existent deep-venous thrombosis in flaccid paraplegia. Arch Phys Med Rehabil 1991; 72:227–229.

137. Hassard G: Heterotopic bone formation about the hip and unilateral decubitus ulcers in spinal cord injury. Arch Phys Med Rehabil 1975; 56:355–358.

138. Heilporn A: Two therapeutic experiments on stubborn pain in spinal cord lesions: Coupling melitracen-flupenthixen and the transcutaneous nerve stimulation. Paraplegia 1977; 15:368–372.

139. Heinemann AW, Doll MD, Armstrong KJ, et al: Substance abuse and receipt of treatment by persons with long-term spinal cord injuries. Arch Phys Med Rehabil 1991; 72:482–487.

140. Heinemann AW, Donohue R, Keen M, et al: Alcohol use by persons with recent spinal cord injury. Arch Phys Med Rehabil 1988; 69:619–624.

141. Heinemann AW, Magier-Planey R, Schiro-Geist C, et al: Mobility for persons with spinal cord injury: An evaluation of two systems. Arch Phys Med Rehabil 1987; 68:90–93.

142. Heldenberg D, Rubenstein A, Levtor O, et al: Serum lipids and lipoprotein concentrations in young quadriplegic patients. Atherosclerosis 1981; 39:163–167.

143. Hentz VR, Brown M, Keoshian LA: Upper-limb reconstruction in quadriplegia: Functional assessment and proposed treatment modifications. J Hand Surg Am 1983; 8:119–130.

144. Herz DA, Parsons KC, Pearl L: Percutaneous radiofrequency foraminal rhizotomies. Spine 1983; 8:729–732.

145. Hill JP: Spinal Cord Injury: A Guide to Functional Outcomes in Occupational Therapy. Rockville, Md, Aspen, 1986.

146. Hirokawa S, Grimm M, Le T, et al: Energy consumption in paraplegic ambulation using the reciprocating gait orthosis and electric stimulation of the thigh muscles. Arch Phys Med Rehabil 1990; 71:687–694.

147. Hirsch GH, Menarch MR, Anton HA: Anemia after traumatic spinal cord injury. Arch Phys Med Rehabil 1991; 72:195–201.

148. Hoshimiya N, Naito A, Yajima M, et al: A multichannel FES system for the restoration of motor functions in high spinal cord injury patients: A respiration-controlled system for multi-joint upper extremity. IEEE Trans Biomed Eng 1989; 36:754–760.

149. House JH, Shannen MA: Restoration of strong grasp and lateral pinch in tetraplegia: A comparison of two methods of thumb control in each patient. J Hand Surg Am 1985; 10:22–29.

150. Hughes JT: The Edwin Smith surgical papyrus: An analysis of the first case reports of spinal cord injuries. Paraplegia 1988; 26:71–82.

151. Hussey RW, Stauffer ES: Spinal cord injury: Requirements for ambulation. Arch Phys Med Rehabil 1973; 54:544–547.

152. Ingram RR, Suman RK, Freeman PA: Lower limb fractures in the chronic spinal cord injured patients. Paraplegia 1989; 28:133–139.

153. Inman KJ, Sibbald WJ, Rutledge FS, et al: Clinical utility and cost-effectiveness of an air suspension bed in the prevention of pressure ulcers. JAMA 1993; 269:1139–1143.

154. Jackson AB, Groomes TE: Incidence of respiratory complications following spinal cord injury. Arch Phys Med Rehabil 1994; 75:270–275.

155. Jaeger RJ, Yarkony GM, Roth EJ, et al: Estimating the user population of a simple electrical stimulation system for standing. Paraplegia 1990; 28:505–511.

156. Jaeger RJ, Yarkony GM, Roth EJ: Rehabilitation technology for standing and walking after spinal cord injury. Am J Med Rehabil 1989; 198:128–133.

157. Jaeger RJ, Yarkony GM, Roth EJ: Standing by a combined orthotic/electrical stimulation system in thoracic paraplegia. In Proceedings of the International Conference of the Association for Advancement of Rehabilitation Technology, Montreal, June 25–30, 1988, pp 24–30.

158. Jensen LL, Halar E, Little JW, et al: Neurogenic heterotopic ossification. Am J Phys Med 66:351–363, 1988.

159. Johnson B, Thomason R, Pallares V, et al: Autonomic hyperreflexia: Review. Milit Med 1975; 140:345–349.

160. Johnstone BR, Jordan CJ, Buntine JA: A review of surgical rehabilitation of the upper limb in quadriplegia. Paraplegia 1988; 26:317–339.

161. Kabalin JN, Lennon S, Grill HS, et al: Incidence and management of autonomic dysreflexia and other intraoperative problems encountered in spinal cord injury patients undergoing extracorporeal shock wave lithotripsy without anesthesia on a second generation lithotriptor. J Urol 1993; 149:1064–1067.

162. Kalsbeek WD, McLaurin RL, Harris BSH, et al: The national head and spinal cord injury survey: Major findings. J Neurosurg 1980; 53:S19–S43.

163. Kantrowitz A: Electronic Physiologic Aids: A Report of the Maimonides Hospital. Brooklyn, NY, Maimonides Hospital, 1960.

164. Kao CC, Chang LW: The mechanism of spinal cord cavitation following spinal cord transection. J Neurosurgery 1977; 46:197–209.

165. Kaplan PE, Rodin W, Gilbert E, et al: Reduction of hypercalciuria in tetraplegia after weight-bearing and strengthening exercises. Paraplegia 1981; 19:289–293.

166. Kasdon DL, Lathi ES: A prospective study of radiofrequency rhizotomy in the treatment of posttraumatic spasticity. Neurosurgery 1984; 15:526–529.

167. Katz RT: Management of spasticity. Am J Phys Med Rehabil 1988; 67:108–116.

168. Katz RT, Rymer WZ: Spastic hypertonia: Mechanisms and measurement. Arch Phys Med Rehabil 1989; 70:144–155.

169. Keith MW, Peckham PH, Thrope GB, et al: Functional neuromuscular stimulation neuroprostheses for the tetraplegic hand. Clin Orthop 1988; 233:25–33.

170. Kelley MA, Carson JL, Palevsky HI, et al: Diagnosing pulmonary embolism: New facts and strategies. Ann Intern Med 1991; 114:300–306.

171. Kilgore KL, Peckham PH, Thrope GB, et al: Synthesis of hand grasp using functional neuromuscular stimulation. IEEE Trans Biomed Eng 1989; 36:761–770.

172. King RB, Carlson CE, Mervine J, et al: Clean and sterile intermittent catheterization methods in hospitalized patients with spinal cord injury. Arch Phys Med Rehabil 1992; 73:798–802.

173. Koehler PJ, Endtz LJ: The Brown-Séquard syndrome—true or false? Arch Neurol 1986; 43:921–924.

174. Kohlmeyer KM, Weber CG, Yarkony GM: New orthosis for central cord syndrome and brachial plexus injuries. Arch Phys Med Rehabil 1990; 71:1006–1009.

175. Kohlmeyer KM, Yarkony GM: Functional outcome after spinal cord injury rehabilitation. In Yarkony GM (ed): Spinal Cord Injury Medical Management and Rehabilitation. Rockville, Md, Aspen, 1994.

176. Kottke FJ: The effects of limitation of activity upon the human body. JAMA 1966; 196:117–122.

177. Kraus JF, Franti CE, Riggins RS, et al: Incidence of traumatic spinal cord lesions. J Chron Dis 1975; 28:471–492.

178. Kuhlemeier KV, Huang CT, Lloyd LK, et al: Effective renal plasma flow: Clinical significance after spinal cord injury. J Urol 1985; 133:758–761.

179. Kuhlemeier KV, Lloyd LK, Stover SL: Long-term followup of renal function after spinal cord injury. J Urol 1985; 134:510–513.

180. Kulkarni JR, Burt AA, Tromans AT, et al: Prophylactic low dose heparin anticoagulant therapy in patients with spinal cord injuries: A retrospective study. Paraplegia 1992; 30:169–172.

181. Kurnick NB: Autonomic hyperreflexia and its control in patients with spinal cord lesions. Ann Intern Med 1956; 44:678–686.

182. Kurtzke JF: Epidemiology of spinal cord injury. Exp Neurol 1975; 48:163–236.

183. Lal S, Hamilton B, Heinemann A, et al: Risk factors for heterotopic ossification in spinal cord injury. Arch Phys Med Rehabil 1989; 70:387–390.

184. Larson LF: Overview of disabled drivers' evaluation process. Physical Disabilities Special Interest Section Newsletter 1987; 10:4.

185. Lazzara G, Lazarus C, Logemann SA: Swallowing disorders in spinal cord injured patients. ASHA 1985; 28:123.

186. Leaf DA, Buhl RA, Adkins RH: Risk of cardiac dysrhythmias in chronic spinal cord injury patients. Paraplegia 1993; 31:571–575.

187. Lee BY, Agarwal N, Corcoran L, et al: Assessment of nutritional and metabolic status of paraplegics. J Rehabil Res Dev 1985; 22:11–17.

188. Lee MY, Kirk PM, Yarkony GM: Rehabilitation of quadriplegic patients with phrenic nerve pacers. Arch Phys Med Rehabil 1989; 70:549–552.

189. Leeds EM, Klose SK, Ganz W, et al: Bone mineral density after bicycle ergometry training. Arch Phys Med Rehabil 1990; 71:207–279.

190. Lehmann KB, Lane JG, Piepmeier JM, et al: Cardiovascular abnormalities accompanying acute spinal cord injury in humans: Incidence, time course and severity. J Am Coll Cardiol 1987; 10:46–52.

191. Lensing A, Prandoni P, Brandjes D, et al: Detection of deep-vein thrombosis by real-time B-mode ultrasonography. N Engl J Med 1989; 320:342–345.

192. Leslie WD, Nance PW: Dissociated hip and spine demineralization: A specific finding in spinal cord injury. Arch Phys Med Rehabil 1993; 74:960–964.

193. Levine SP, Kuester DS, Kett RL: Independently activated talking tracheostomy systems for quadriplegic patients. Arch Phys Med Rehabil 1987; 68:571–573.

194. Liberty Mutual Research Center: Steeper ARGO. Hoplinton, Mass, Liberty Mutual Research Center, 1991, pp 1–4.

195. Lim AC, Roth EJ, Green D: Lower limb paralysis: Its effect on the recanalization of deep-vein thrombosis. Arch Phys Med Rehabil 1992; 73:331–333.

196. Lindan R, Joiner E, Freehafer AA, et al: Incidence and clinical features of autonomic dysreflexia in patients with spinal cord injuries. Paraplegia 1980; 18:285–292.

197. Lloyd LK, Dubovsky EV, Bueschen AJ, et al: Comprehensive renal scintillation procedures in spinal cord injury: Comparison with excretory urography. J Urol 1981; 126:10–13.

198. Lloyd LK, Kuhlemeier KV, Fine PR: Initial bladder management in spinal cord injury: Does it make a difference? J Urol 1986; 135:523.

199. Locke JR, Hill DE, Walzer Y: Incidence of squamous cell carcinoma in patients with long-term catheter drainage. J Urol 1985; 133:1034–1035.

200. Long C II, Masciarelli VD: An electrophysiologic splint for the hand. Arch Phys Med Rehabil 1963; 44:499–503.

201. Long DM, Erickson DE: Stimulation of the posterior columns of the spinal cord for relief of intractable pain. Surg Neurol 1975; 4:134–141.

202. Loveridge B, Dubo H: Breathing pattern in chronic quadriplegia. Arch Phys Med Rehabil 1990; 71:495–499.

203. Lyles M, Munday J: Report on the evaluation of the Vannini-Rizzoli stabilizing limb orthosis. J Rehabil Res Dev 1992; 29:77–104.

204. Lynch C, Pont A, Weingarden SI: Heterotopic ossification in the hand of a patient with spinal cord injury. Arch Phys Med Rehabil 1981; 62:291–293.

205. MacDonald RL, Findlay JM, Tator CH: Microcystic spinal cord degeneration causing posttraumatic myelopathy. J Neurosurg 1988; 68:466–471.

206. Malec J, Harvey RF, Cayner JJ: Cannabis effect on spasticity in spinal cord injury. Arch Phys Med Rehabil 1982; 63:116–118.

207. Marsolais EB, Kobetic R: Development of a practical electrical stimulation system for restoring gait in the paralyzed patient. Clin Orthop 1988; 233:64–74.

208. Marsolais EB, Kobetic R: Functional electrical stimulation for walking in paraplegia. J Bone Joint Surg Am 1987; 69:728–733.

209. Marsolais EB, Kobetic R: Functional walking in paralyzed patients by means of electrical stimulation. Clin Orthop 1983; 175:30–36.

210. Martin B: Treatment of dysphagia in adults. In Cherney LR (ed): Clinical Management of Dysphagia in Adults and Children. Gaithersburg, Md, Aspen, 1994, pp 153–183.

211. Matthews PJ, Carlson CE: Spinal Cord Injury: A Guide to Rehabilitation Nursing. Rockville, Md, Apsen, 1987.

212. Maury M: About pain and its treatment in paraplegics. Paraplegia 1977; 15:349–352.

213. Maynard F: Posttraumatic cystic myelopathy in motor incomplete quadriplegia presenting as progressive orthostasis. Arch Phys Med Rehabil 1984; 65:30–32.

214. Maynard FM: Early clinical experiences with clonidine in spinal spasticity. Paraplegia 1986; 24:175–182.

215. Maynard FM: Immobilization hypercalcemia following spinal cord injury. Arch Phys Med Rehabil 1986; 67:41–44.

216. Maynard FM, Glass J: Management of the neuropathic bladder by clean intermittent catheterization: 5 year outcomes. Paraplegia 1987; 25:106–110.

217. Maynard FM, Glenn GR, Fountain S, et al: Neurological prognosis after traumatic quadriplegia. J Neurosurg 1979; 50:611–616.

218. Maynard FM, Imai K: Immobilization hypercalcemia in spinal cord injury. Arch Phys Med Rehabil 1977; 58:16–24.

219. McDowell CL, Moberg EA, House JH: The Second International Conference on Surgical Rehabilitation of the Upper Limb in Tetraplegia (Quadriplegia). J Hand Surg Am 1986; 11:604–608.

220. McGregor JA, Meeuwsen J: Autonomic hyperreflexia: A mortal danger for spinal cord-damaged women in labor. Am J Obstet Gynecol 1985; 151:330–333.

221. McMichan JC, Michael L, Westbrook P: Pulmonary dysfunction following traumatic quadriplegia. JAMA 1980; 243:528–531.

222. Melzack R, Loeser JD: Phantom body pain in paraplegics: Evidence for a central nervous pattern generating mechanism for pain. Pain 1978; 4:195–210.

223. Menter RR: Issues of aging with spinal cord injury. In Whiteneck GG (ed): Aging with Spinal Cord Injury. New York, Demos, 1993, pp 1–8.

224. Merkel KD, Miller NE, Westbrook PR, et al: Energy expenditure of paraplegic patients standing and walking with two knee-ankle-foot orthoses. Arch Phys Med Rehabil 1984; 65:121–124.

225. Merli G: Management of deep vein thrombosis in spinal cord injury. Chest 1992; 102:652S–657S.

226. Merli G, Crabbe S, Doyle L, et al: Mechanical plus pharmacological prophylaxis for deep vein thrombosis in acute spinal cord injury. Paraplegia 1992; 30:558–562.

227. Merli G, Crabbe S, Paluzzi R, et al: Etiology, incidence, and prevention of deep vein thrombosis in acute spinal cord injury. Arch Phys Med Rehabil 1993; 74:199–205.

228. Merli G, Doyle L, Crabbe S, et al: Prophylaxis for deep vein thrombosis in acute spinal cord injury comparing two doses of low molecular weight heparinoid (ORG 10172) in combination with either external pneumatic compression or electrical stimulation, abstract. Annual Meeting of the American Spinal Injury Association, Orlando, 1990, p 8.

229. Merli G, Herbison G, Ditunno J, et al: Deep vein thrombosis in acute spinal cord injured patients. Arch Phys Med Rehabil 1988; 69:661–664.

230. Merli GJ, McElwain GE, Adler AG, et al: Immobilization hypercalcemia in acute spinal cord injury treated with etidronate. Arch Intern Med 1984; 144:1286–1288.

231. Merriam WF, Taylor TKF, Ruff SJ, et al: A reappraisal of acute traumatic central cord syndrome. J Bone Joint Surg Br 1986; 68:708–713.

232. Merritt JL: Management of spasticity in spinal cord injury. Mayo Clin Proc 1981; 56:614–622.

233. Merritt JL: Residual urine volume: Correlate of urinary tract infection in patients with spinal cord injury. Arch Phys Med Rehabil 1981; 62:558–561.

234. Meyer PR Jr: Surgery of Spine Trauma. New York, Churchill Livingstone, 1989.

235. Meythaler JM, Tuel SM, Cross LL: Successful treatment of immobilization hypercalcemia using calcitonin and etidronate. Arch Phys Med Rehabil 1993; 74:316–319.

236. Miglietta O: Action of cold on spasticity. J Phys Med 1973; 52:198–205.

237. Mikelberg R, Reid S: Spinal cord lesions and lower extremity bracing: An overview and follow-up study. Paraplegia 1981; 19:379–385.

238. Miller HJ, Thomas E, Wilmot CB: Pneumobelt use among high quadriplegic population. Arch Phys Med Rehabil 1988; 69:369–372.

239. Miller LS, Staas WE, Herbison GJ: Abdominal problems in patients with spinal cord lesions. Arch Phys Med Rehabil 1975; 56:45–48.

240. Miller NE, Merritt JL, Merkel KD, et al: Paraplegic energy expenditure during negotiation of architectural barriers. Arch Phys Med Rehabil 1984; 65:778–779.

241. Minaire P, Mallet E, Leveruieux J, et al: Immobilization bone loss: Preventing effects of calcitonin in several clinical models. In Christiansen C, Riis B (eds): Osteoporosis 1987. Copenhagen, Osteopress, 1987.

242. Minaire P, Meunier P, Edouard C, et al: Quantitative histological data on disuse osteoporosis: Comparison with biological data. Calcif Tissue Res 1974; 17:57–73.

243. Moberg EA: Surgical treatment for absent single-hand grip and elbow extension in quadriplegia. J Bone Joint Surg Am 1975; 57:196–206.

244. Mollinger LA, Sparr GB, El Ghatet AZ, et al: Daily energy expenditure and basal metabolic rates of patients with spinal cord injury. Arch Phys Med Rehabil 1985; 66:420–426.

245. Moreno JG, Lofti MA, Rivas DA, et al: Continent urinary diversion using an umbilical stoma in quadriplegic patients, abstract. J Am Paraplegia Soc 1994; 17:125.

246. Morris J: Spinal injury and psychotheraphy: A treatment philosophy. In Yarkony GM (ed): Spinal Cord Injury Medical Management and Rehabilitation. Rockville, Md, Aspen, 1994.

247. Morris J, Roth E, Davidoff G: Mild closed head injury and cognitive deficits in spinal cord injured patients: Incidence and impact. J Head Trauma Rehabil 1986; 1:31–42.

248. Myllynen P, Kammonen M, Rokkanen P, et al: The blood F VIII:Ag/F VIII:C ratio as an early indicator of deep venous thrombosis during post-traumatic immobilization. J Trauma 1987; 27:287–290.

249. Myllynen P, Kammonen M, Rokkanen P, et al: DVT and pulmonary embolism in patients with acute spinal cord injury: A comparison

with non-paralyzed patients immobilized due to spine fractures. J Trauma 1985; 25:541–543.

250. Naftchi NE: Functional restoration of the traumatically injured spinal cord in cats by clonidine. Science 1982; 217:1042–1044.

251. Nashold BS, Friedman H: Dorsal column stimulation for control of pain: Preliminary report on 30 patients. J Neurosurg 1972; 36.590–597.

252. Nathan RH: The development of a computerized upper limb electrical stimulation system. Orthopedics 1984; 7:1170–1180.

253. Nathan RH, Ohry A: Upper limb functions regained in quadriplegia: A hybrid computerized neuromuscular stimulation system. Arch Phys Med Rehabil 1990; 71:415–421.

254. Natvig H, McAdam R: Ambulation without wheelchairs for paraplegics with complete lesions. Paraplegia 1978–79; 16:142–146.

255. Nepomuceno C, Fine PR, Richards JS, et al: Pain in patients with spinal cord injury. Arch Phys Med Rehabil 1979; 60:605–609.

256. Nicholas JJ: Ectopic bone formation in patients with spinal cord injury. Arch Phys Med Rehabil 1973; 54:354–359.

257. Nichols PJR, Norman PA, Ennis JR: Wheelchair user's shoulder? Shoulder pain in patients with spinal cord lesions. Scand J Rehabil Med 1979; 11:29–32.

258. Nieder RM, O'Higgins JW, Aldrete JA: Autonomic hyperreflexia in urologic surgery. JAMA 1970; 213:867–869.

259. Nixon V: Spinal Cord Injury: A Guide to Functional Outcomes in Physical Therapy Management. Rockville, Md, Aspen, 1985.

260. O'Daniel WE, Hahn HR: Follow-up usage of the Scott-Craig orthosis in paraplegia. Paraplegia 1981; 19:373–378.

261. Ohry A, Brooks ME, Steinbach TV, et al: Shoulder complications as a cause of delay in rehabilitation of spinal cord injured patients. Paraplegia 1978; 16:310–316.

262. Orzel JA, Rudd TG: Heterotopic bone formation: Clinical, laboratory and imaging correlation. J Nucl Med 1985; 26:125–132.

263. Orzel J, Rudd T, Wil B: Heterotopic bone formation (myositis ossification) and lower extremity swelling mimicking deep venous disease. J Nucl Med 1984; 25:1105–1107.

264. Ozer MN, Shannon SR: Renal sonography in asymptomatic persons with spinal cord injury: Cost-effectiveness analysis. Arch Phys Med Rehabil 1991; 72:35–37.

265. Panel for the prediction and prevention of pressure ulcers in adults: Pressure ulcers in adults: Prediction and prevention. Clinical practice guideline no. 3. AHCPR Publication No. 92-0047, Rockville, Md, Agency for Health Care Policy and Research, Public Health Service, US Department of Health and Human Services, 1992.

266. Patrick JH, McClelland MR: Low energy reciprocal walking for the adult paraplegic. Paraplegia 1985; 23:113–117.

267. Paulakis AJ, Siroky MB, Goldstein I, et al: Neurologic findings in conus medullaris and cauda equina injury. Arch Neurol 1983; 40:570–573.

268. Penn RD: Intrathecal baclofen for spasticity of spinal origin: Seven years of experience. J Neurosurg 1992; 77:236–240.

269. Perkash A, Brown M: Anemia in patients with spinal cord injury. J Am Paraplegia Soc 1986; 9:10–15.

270. Petrofsky JS, Phillips CA, Douglas R, et al: A computer-controller walking system: The combination of an orthosis with functional electrical stimulation. J Clin Eng 1986; 11:121–133.

271. Phillips CA: Functional electrical stimulation and lower extremity bracing for ambulation exercise of the spinal cord injured individual: A medically prescribed system. Phys Ther 1989; 69:842–849.

272. Phillips CA: Sensory feedback control of upper- and lower-extremity motor prostheses. Crit Rev Biomed Eng 1988; 16:105–140.

273. Piepmeier JM, Lehmann KB, Lane JG: Cardiovascular instability following acute cervical spinal cord trauma. Cent Nerv Syst Trauma 1985; 2:153–160.

274. Pierce S: Formula for developing a driving program for the disabled. Physical Disabilities Special Interest Section Newsletter 1987; 10:4.

275. Pierce S: Legal consideration for a driver rehabilitation program. Phys Disabilities 1993; 16:1.

276. Pine ZM, Miller SD, Alonso JA: Atrial fibrillation associated with autonomic dysreflexia. Am J Phys Med Rehabil 1991; 70:271–273.

277. Putty TK, Shapiro SA: Efficacy of dorsal longitudinal myelotomy in treating spinal spasticity: A review of 20 cases. J Neurosurg 1991; 75:397–401.

278. Ragnarsson KT, Seli H: Lower extremity fractures after spinal cord injury: A retrospective study. Arch Phys Med Rehabil 1981; 62:418–423.

279. Richards JS, Brown L, Hagglund K, et al: Spinal cord injury and concomitant traumatic brain injury: Results of a longitudinal investigation. Am J Phys Med Rehabil 1988; 67:211–216.

280. Richardson RR, Meyer PR, Cerullo LJ: Neurostimulation in the modulation of the intractable paraplegic and traumatic neuroma pains. Pain 1980; 8:75–84.

281. Rivas DA, Chancellor MB, Hill K, et al: Neurological manifestations of baclofen withdrawal. J Urol 1993; 150:1903–1905.

282. Rosenblum D: Clonidine-induced bradycardia in patients with spinal cord injury. Arch Phys Med Rehabil 1993; 74:1206–1207.

283. Rosman N, Spira E: Paraplegic use of walking braces: Survey. Arch Phys Med Rehabil 1974; 55:310–314.

284. Ross JC, Gibbon NOK, Sunder GSO: Division of the external urethal sphincter in the neuropathic bladder: A twenty-year review. Br J Urol 1976; 48:649–656.

285. Rossi E, Green D, Rosen J, et al: Sequential changes in factor VIII and platelets preceding deep vein thrombosis in patients with spinal cord injury. Br J Hematol 1980; 45:143–151.

286. Rossier AB: Rehabilitation of the Spinal Cord Injury patient. Documenta Geigy Acta Clinica No. 3 North American Series, 1964, pp 80–82.

287. Rossier AB, Bussat P, Infante F, et al: Current facts on para-osteo-arthropathy (POA). Paraplegia 1973; 11:36–78.

288. Rossier AB, Foo D, Shillito J, et al: Posttraumatic cervical syringomyelia: Incidence, clinical presentation, electrophysiological studies, syrinx protein and results of conservative and operative treatment. Brain 1985; 108:439–461.

289. Roth E, Davidoff G, Thomas P: A controlled study of neuropsychological deficits in acute spinal cord injury. Paraplegia 1989; 27:480–489.

290. Roth EJ: Pain in spinal cord injury. In Yarkony GM (ed): Spinal Cord Injury Medical Management and Rehabilitation. Rockville, Md, Aspen, 1994.

291. Roth EJ, Fenton LL, Gaebler-Spira DJ, et al: Superior mesenteric artery syndrome in acute traumatic quadriplegia: Case reports and literature review. Arch Phys Med Rehabil 1991; 72:417–420.

292. Roth EJ, Lawler MH, Yarkony GM: Traumatic central cord syndrome: Clinical features and functional outcomes. Arch Phys Med Rehabil 1990; 71:18–23.

293. Roth EJ, Park T, Pang T, et al: Traumatic cervical Brown-Séquard and Brown-Séquard-plus syndromes: The spectrum of presentations and outcomes. Paraplegia 1991; 29:582–589.

294. Roussan M, Terence C, Gromm G: Baclofen versus diazepam for the treatment of spasticity and long-term follow-up of baclofen therapy. Pharmatherapeutica 1985; 4:278–284.

295. Rudel D, Bajd T, Kralj A, et al: Surface functional electrical stimulation of the hand in quadriplegics. Presented at Fifth Annual Conference on Rehabilitation Engineering, Houston, Texas, August 1982, p 59.

296. Scanlon PD, Loring SH, Pichurko BM, et al: Respiratory mechanics in acute quadriplegia: Lung and chest wall compliance and dimensional changes during respiratory maneuvers. Am Rev Respir Dis 1987; 135:367–371.

297. Schneider RC, Cherry G, Pantek H: Central cervical spinal cord injury with special reference to the mechanics involved in hyperextension injuries of cervical spine. J Neurosurg 1954; 11:546–577.

298. Scott BA, Weinstein Z, Chiteman R, et al: Intrathecal phenol and glycerin in metrizamide for treatment of intractable spasms in paraplegia. J Neurosurg 1985; 63:125–127.

299. Scott JA, Donovan WH: The prevention of shoulder pain and contracture in the acute tetraplegic patient. Paraplegia 1981; 19:313–319.

300. Shipp M: Adaptive Driving Devices and Vehicle Modification. Reston, La, Louisiana Tech University Center for Rehabilitation Science and Biomedical Engineering, 1989.

301. Sica DA, Midha M, Aronoff G, et al: Atrial natriuretic factor in spinal cord injury. Arch Phys Med Rehabil 1993; 74:969–972.

302. Sica DA, Midha M, Zawada E, et al: Hyponatremia in spinal cord injury. J Am Paraplegia Soc 1990; 13:78–83.

303. Sigmedics, Inc: Sales literature. Chicago, Sigmedics, 1990.

304. Smith DL: Evaluation of disabled drivers: An instructor's perspective. Physical Disabilities Special Interest Section Newsletter 1987; 10:4.

305. Solomonow M, Baratta R, Hirokawa S, et al: The RGO generation II: Muscle stimulation powered orthosis as a practical walking system for thoracic paraplegics. Orthopedics 1989; 12:1309–1315.

306. Sonies BC: Dysphagia: A model for differential diagnosis for adults and children. *In* Cherney LR (ed): Clinical Management of Dysphagia in Adults and Children. Gaithersburg, Md, Aspen, 1994, pp 133–152.

307. Sorg RJ: HDL-cholesterol: Exercise formula. Results of long-term (six-year) strenuous swimming exercise in a middle-aged male with paraplegia. JOSPT 1993; 17:1951–1959.

308. Sparker AW, Robbins KT, Nevlud GN, et al: A prospective evaluation of speaking tracheostomy tubes for ventilator dependent patients. Laryngoscope 1987; 97:89–92.

309. Stanworth PA: The significance of hyperhidrosis in patients with post-traumatic syringomyelia. Paraplegia 1982; 20:282–287.

310. Stewart AF, Adler M, Byers CM, et al: Calcium homeostasis in immobilization: Example of resorptive hypercalciuria. N Engl J Med 1982; 306:1136–1140.

311. Stirt JA, Marco A, Conklin KA: Obstetric anesthesia for a quadriplegic patient with autonomic hyperreflexia. Anesthesiology 1979; 51:560–562.

312. Stone JM, NinoMurcia M, Wolfe UA: Chronic gastrointestinal problems in spinal cord injury patients: A prospective analysis. Am J Gastroenterol 1990; 85:1114–1119.

313. Stover SL, Fine PR (eds): Spinal Cord Injury: The Facts and Figures. Birmingham, University of Alabama at Birmingham, 1986.

314. Stover SL, Hahn HR, Miller JM: Disodium etidronate in the prevention of heterotopic ossification following spinal cord injury (preliminary report). Paraplegia 1976; 14:146–156.

315. Stover SL, Hataway CJ, Zeiger HE: Heterotopic ossification in spinal cord injured patients. Arch Phys Med Rehabil 1975; 56:199–204.

316. Stover SL, Lloyd LK, Waites KB, et al: Urinary tract infection in spinal cord injury. Arch Phys Med Rehabil 1989; 70:47–54.

317. Stover SL, Niemann KM, Miller JM: Disodium etidronate in the prevention of post-operative recurrence of heterotopic ossification in spinal cord injury patients. J Bone Joint Surg Am 1976; 58:683–688.

318. Stover SL, Niemann KM, Tulloss JR: Experience with surgical resection of heterotopic bone in spinal cord injury patients. Clin Orthop 1991; 263:71–77.

319. Terrance CF, Fromm GH: Complications of baclofen withdrawal. Arch Neurol 1981; 38:588–589.

320. Thüroff JW, Bunke B, Ebner A, et al: Randomized, double-blind, multicenter trial on treatment of frequency, urgency and incontinence related to detrusor hyperactivity: Oxybutynin versus propantheline versus placebo. J Urol 1991; 145:813–817.

321. Tibone J, Sakimura I, Nickel VL, et al: Heterotopic ossification around hip in spinal cord injured patients. J Bone Joint Surg Am 1978; 60:769–775.

322. Todd J, Frisbie J, Rossier A, et al: Deep venous thrombosis in acute spinal cord injury: A comparison of 125 I fibrinogen leg scanning, impedance plethysmography and venography. Paraplegia 1976; 14:50–57.

323. Tori JA, Hill LL: Hypercalcemia in children with spinal cord injury. Arch Phys Med Rehabil 1978; 59:443–447.

324. Tracy SF, Logemann SA, Kahrilas PJ: Dysphagia following cervical spine injury: Pattern of recovery, abstract. ASHA 1981; 31:108.

325. Tremblay LE, Bedard PJ: Effect of clonidine on motoneuron excitability in spinalized rats. Neuropharmacology 1986; 25:41–46.

326. Trieschmann RB (ed): Spinal Cord Injuries: Psychological, Social and Vocational Adjustment. Elmsford, NY, Pergamon Press, 1976.

327. Tunks E, Bahry N, Rausbaum M: Pain in spinal cord injured patients. *In* Bloch RF, Rausbaum M (eds): Management of Spinal Cord Injuries. Baltimore, Williams & Wilkins, 1986, pp 180–211.

328. Umbach I, Heilport A: Review articles: Post-spinal cord injury syringomyelia. Paraplegia 1991; 29:219–221.

329. Utili R, Boitnott JK, Zimmerman HJ: Dantrolene-associated hepatic injury: Incidence and character. Gastroenterology 1977; 72:610–616.

330. Vaziti ND, Eltorai IM, Segal S, et al: Erythropoietin profile in spinal cord injured patients. Arch Phys Med Rehabil 1993; 74:65–67.

331. Veis SL, Logemann SA: Dysphagia after spinal cord injury, abstract. ASHA 1991; 33:112.

332. Venier LH, Ditunno JF: Heterotopic ossification in the paraplegic patient. Arch Phys Med Rehabil 1971; 52:475–479.

333. Vernon J, Silver J, Ohry A: Poast-traumatic syringomyelia. Paraplegia 1982; 20:339–364.

334. Vernon J, Silver J, Symon L: Post-traumatic syringomyelia: The results of surgery. Paraplegia 1983; 21:37–46.

335. Virchow R: Neuer Fall von tödlichen Embolie der Lungenarterie. Arch Pathol Anat 1856; 10:225–228.

336. Vodovnik L, Rebersek S: Information content of myo-control signals for orthotic and prosthetic systems. Arch Phys Med Rehabil 1974; 55:52–56.

337. Wainapel SF, Freed MM: Reflex sympathetic dystrophy in quadriplegia: Case report. Arch Phys Med Rehabil 1984; 65:35–36.

338. Waisbrod H, Hanse D, Gerbershagen HU: Chronic pain in paraplegics. Neurosurgery 1984; 15:933–934.

339. Walker BC, Holstein S: Vocational rehabilitation and spinal cord injury. *In* Yarkony GM (ed): Spinal Cord Injury Medical Management and Rehabilitation. Rockville, Md, Aspen, 1994.

340. Walker J, Shepard RJ: Cardiac risk factors immediately following spinal injury. Arch Phys Med Rehabil 1993; 74:1129–1133.

341. Waring WP, Karunas RS: Acute spinal cord injuries and the incidence of clinically occurring thromboembolic disease. Paraplegia 1991; 29:8–16.

342. Warren CG, Lehmann JF, deLateur BJ: Pelvic band use in orthotics for adult paraplegic patients. Arch Phys Med Rehabil 1975; 56:221–223.

343. Waters RL, Adkins RH, Yakura JS: Definition of complete spinal cord injury. Paraplegia 1991; 9:573–581.

344. Waters RL, Adkins RH, Yakura JS, et al: Motor and sensory recovery following complete tetraplegia. Arch Phys Med Rehabil 1993; 74:242–247.

345. Waters RL, Adkins RH, Yakura JS, et al: Motor and sensory recovery following incomplete paraplegia. Arch Phys Med Rehabil 1994; 75:67–72.

346. Waters RL, Miller L: A physiological rationale for orthotic prescription in paraplegia. Clin Prosthet Orthot 1987; 2:66–73.

347. Waters RL, Yakura JS, Adkins R, et al: Determinants of gait performance following spinal cord injury. Arch Phys Med Rehabil 1989; 70:811–818.

348. Waters RL, Yakura JS, Adkins RH, et al: Recovery following complete paraplegia. Arch Phys Med Rehabil 1992; 73:784–789.

349. Watson DW, Downey GO: Epidural anesthesia for labor and delivery of twins of a paraplegic mother. Anesthesiology 1980; 52:257–261.

350. Weingarden SI, Belen JG: Clonidine transdermal system for treatment of spasticity in spinal cord injury. Arch Phys Med Rehabil 1992; 73:876–877.

351. Weingarden SI, Martin C: Independent dressing after spinal cord injury: A functional time evaluation. Arch Phys Med Rehabil 1989; 70:518–519.

352. Welch RD, Lobley SJ, O'Sullivan SB, et al: Functional independence in quadriplegia: Critical levels. Arch Phys Med Rehabil 1986; 676:235–240.

353. Wharton GE, Morgan TH: Ankylosis in the paralyzed patient. J Bone Joint Surg Am 1970; 52:105–112.

354. Wharton GW: Heterotopic ossification. Clin Orthop 1975; 112:142–149.

355. White J, Kjellberg R: Posterior spinal rhizotomy: A substitute for cordotomy in the relief of localized pain in patients with normal life-expectancy. Neurochirurgia 1973; 16:141.

356. White RH, McGahan JP, Daschbuch MM, et al: Diagnosis of deep-vein thrombosis using duplex ultrasound. Ann Intern Med 1989; 11:1297–1304.

357. Whiteneck G (ed): The management of High Quadriplegia. New York, Demos, 1989.

358. Whiteneck GG, Charlifue SW, Frankel HL: Mortality, morbidity and psychosocial outcomes of persons spinal cord injured more than 20 years. 1992; 30:617–630.

359. Wilberger JE, Maroon JC, Prostko ER, et al: Magnetic resonance imaging and intraoperative neurosonography in syringomyelia. Neurosurgery 1987; 20:599–605.

360. Wilkinson SP, Portmann B, Williams R: Hepatitis from dantrolene sodium. Gut 1979; 20:33–36.

361. Williams B: On the pathogenesis of syringomyelia: A review. J R Soc Med 1980; 73:798–806.

362. Wise MF, Milani JC: Presented at the 13th Annual Meeting of the American Spinal Injury Association, Boston, March 1987, abstr 30.

363. Wood KM: The use of phenol as a neurolytic agent: A review. Pain 1978; 5:205–229.

364. Wu Y: Total bladder care for the spinal cord injured patient. Ann Acad Med Singapore 1983; 12:387–399.

365. Wu Y, King RB, Hamilton BB, et al: RIC-Wu catheter kit: New

device for an old problem. Arch Phys Med Rehabil 1980; 61:455–459.

366. Yablon SA, Sipski ML: Effect of transdermal clonidine on spinal spasticity: A case series. Am J Phys Med Rehabil 1993; 72:154–157.

367. Yao J: Deep vein thrombosis in spinal cord injured patients: Evaluation and assessment. Chest 1992; 1026:645S–648S.

368. Yarkony GM: Aging after traumatic spinal cord injury. In Felsenthal G, Garrison SJ, Steinberg FU (eds): Rehabilitation of the Aging and Elderly Patient. Baltimore, Williams & Wilkins, 1993, pp 391–396.

369. Yarkony GM: Aging skin, pressure ulcerations and spinal cord injury. In Whitelock GG (ed): Aging with Spinal Cord Injury. New York, Demos, 1993, pp 39–92.

370. Yarkony GM: Medical complications in rehabilitation. In Heinemann AW (ed): Substance Abuse and Physical Disability. Binghamton, NY, Haworth Press, 1993, pp 93–106.

371. Yarkony GM, Bass LM, Keenan V III, et al: Contractures complicating spinal cord injury: Incidence and comparison between spinal cord centre and general hospital acute care. Paraplegia 1985; 23:265.

372. Yarkony GM, Jaeger R, Turba R, et al: Cough in spinal cord injured patients: Comparison of three methods to produce cough. Arch Phys Med Rehabil 1993; 74:1358–1361.

373. Yarkony GM, Jaeger RJ, Roth E, et al: Functional neuromuscular stimulation for standing after spinal cord injury. Arch Phys Med Rehabil 1990; 71:201–206.

374. Yarkony GM, Jones R, Hedman G, et al: Jones-Hedman walker modification for C7 quadriplegic patient: Case study in team cooperation. Arch Phys Med Rehabil 1986; 67:54–55.

375. Yarkony GM, Katz RT, Wu YC: Seizures secondary to autonomic dysreflexia. Arch Phys Med Rehabil 1986; 67:345–349.

376. Yarkony GM, Lee MY, Green D, et al: Heterotopic ossification pseudophlebitis. Am J Med 1989; 87:342–344.

377. Yarkony GM, Roth EJ, Cybulski GR, et al: Neuromuscular stimula-

378. Yarkony GM, Roth EJ, Cybulski GR, et al: Neuromuscular stimulation in spinal cord injury: II: Prevention of secondary complications. Arch Phys Med Rehabil 1992; 73:195–200.

379. Yarkony GM, Roth EJ, Heinemann AW, et al: Benefits of rehabilitation for traumatic spinal cord injury: Multivariate analysis in 711 patients. Arch Neurol 1987; 44:93.

380. Yarkony GM, Roth EJ, Heinemann AW, et al: Rehabilitation outcomes in C6 tetraplegia. Paraplegia 1988; 26:177–185.

381. Yarkony GM, Roth EJ, Heinemann AW, et al: Spinal cord injury rehabilitation outcome: The impact of age. J Clin Epidemiol 1988; 41:173–177.

382. Yarkony GM, Roth E, Lovell L, et al: Rehabilitation outcomes in complete C5 quadriplegia. Am J Phys Med Rehabil 1988; 67:73–76.

383. Yarkony GM, Roth EJ, Meyer PR, et al: Rehabilitation outcomes in complete thoracic spinal cord injury. Am J Phys Med Rehabil 1990; 69:23–27.

384. Yarkony GM, Sheffler LR, Smith J, et al: Early onset posttraumatic cystic myelopathy complicating spinal cord injury. Arch Phys Med Rehabil 1994; 75:102–105.

385. Yekutrel M, Brooks ME, Ohry A, et al: The prevalence of hypertension, ischemic heart disease and diabetes in traumatic spinal cord injured patients and amputees. Paraplegia 1989; 27:58–62.

386. Young RR, Delwaide PJ: Drug therapy: Spasticity. N Engl J Med 1981; 304:96–99.

387. Zacharkow D: Wheelchair Posture and Pressure Sores. Springfield, Ill, Charles C Thomas, 1984, pp 12–53.

388. Zancolli E: Structural and Dynamic Bases of Hand Surgery, ed 2. Philadelphia, JB Lippincott, 1979, pp 229–262.

389. Zejdlik CM: Management of Spinal Cord Injury. Belmont, Calif, Wodsworth, 1983.

56

Rehabilitation in Vascular Diseases

KAREN L. ANDREWS, M.D., THOM W. ROOKE, M.D., AND PHALA A. HELM, M.D.

Rehabilitation of the patient with vascular disease(s) includes the evaluation and management of arterial, venous, and lymphatic diseases. The goals of optimal management are to decrease morbidity and to enhance function.

ARTERIAL DISEASE

Etiology

There are many causes of arterial occlusive disease, the most common of which is atherosclerosis obliterans (ASO). Other disease processes include thromboangiitis obliterans (Buerger's disease), vasospastic disorders (Raynaud's phenomenon, livedo reticularis, and acrocyanosis), thrombosis, embolism, dissection, vasculitis, and fibromuscular dysplasia.

Atherosclerosis

Atherosclerosis in its advanced form is a systemic disorder involving the coronary, cerebral, pulmonary, renal, and peripheral vessels. The earliest manifestation of atherosclerosis appears to be the intimal streak, although the eventual progression of streaks to fibrous or complicated plaques remains uncertain.[54] The plaques tend to develop at branch points, bifurcations, zones of rapid tapering, and areas where arteries follow a tortuous course.[53] Atherosclerosis typically involves multiple levels of the arterial tree; however, it tends to be a segmental disease in which intervening arterial segments can be remarkably free of involvement or minimally involved. Associated conditions can affect the location of disease. In diabetics, atherosclerosis occurs with equal frequency in both femoral and tibial arteries, whereas in nondiabetics the most common sites of severe disease are the abdominal aorta and iliac and femoral arteries.[32]

Potentially reversible factors that increase the risk of atherosclerosis include smoking, hyperlipidemia, hypertension, diabetes, and obesity. Most people younger than 65 years who have atherosclerosis have one or more identifiable risk factors. The presence of multiple risk factors further increases the risk of atherosclerosis. Cigarette smoking is by far the most common risk factor, competing with juvenile diabetes mellitus and certain rare congenital hyperlipidemias as the most serious.[16] Smoking acts synergistically with other risk factors such as hypertension or hypercholesterolemia to enhance progression of atherosclerotic lesions. The calculated risk of developing claudication is 15 times higher in male smokers than in nonsmokers, 7 times higher in female smokers than in nonsmokers, and directly related to the number of cigarettes smoked.[16]

Thromboangiitis Obliterans (Buerger's Disease)

Thromboangiitis obliterans (Buerger's disease) is a disease involving thrombosis and inflammation of small peripheral arteries and veins. The process tends to begin in the smaller peripheral arteries of the extremities. Lesions are usually located distal to the knee or elbow.[53] Most theories implicate some component of cigarette smoking that predisposes the arterial wall to inflammation, possibly through the formation of immune complexes.

Vasospasm

Raynaud's phenomenon most frequently involves the hands but can also affect the feet. With exposure to cold or emotional stress, spasm of the small arteries and arterioles results in ischemia (pallor or cyanosis), pain, and subsequent vasodilatation with hyperemia. Raynaud's phenomenon can be idiopathic or occur as a manifestation of a potentially serious underlying systemic disease.

Other Causes of Arterial Occlusive Disease

Thrombosis, embolism, and arterial dissection are discussed in the following sections on acute and chronic arterial occlusion.

Clinical Evaluation

Acute Arterial Occlusion

The major causes of acute arterial occlusion are embolism, thrombosis, trauma, and dissection.

History and Clinical Findings

The clinical presentation in acute arterial occlusion includes sudden onset of toe, foot, and leg pain associated with absence of pulse and coolness and discoloration of the skin in a patchy irregular configuration. The findings are frequently described as the "6 Ps"—pulselessness, pain, polar (cold), pallor, paresthesia, and paralysis. If the patient has had a recent myocardial infarction, atrial fibrillation, or other source of possible embolus and has normal pulses in the contralateral extremity and no history of claudication, acute embolic disease is likely. The most common cause of acute arterial embolism is cardiac (atrial fibrillation, recent myocardial infarction, cardiomyopathy, native or prosthetic heart valve replacement, and, rarely, atrial myxoma). If previous symptoms of claudication are present in a patient with no cardiac dysfunction, the diagnosis of thrombosis is most likely. Excruciating precordial or intrascapular pain, moderate to severe hypertension, congestive heart failure, hemiplegia, anuria or hematuria, and acute intestinal ischemia can occur with acute arterial occlusion and are most commonly associated with aortic dissection.

Chronic Arterial Occlusion

History and Clinical Findings

Chronic arterial occlusive disease can usually be diagnosed from the history and physical examination findings. Unless complicated by thrombus or embolus, the symptoms and signs associated with atherosclerosis obliterans rarely have an abrupt onset. The most common symptom is intermittent claudication. Lower extremity claudication has two diagnostic clinical features. First, it is reproduced with a consistent level of exercise from one occasion to the next. Second, it completely resolves within minutes after the exercise has been discontinued.[28]

The site of claudication is of rough value for indicating the level of occlusion.[32] Patients with occlusion at or above the ankle can present with claudication in the arch of the foot. Calf claudication suggests occlusion at or above the calf. Patients with isolated aortoiliac disease generally present with buttock pain or sexual dysfunction.

As the disease process advances, resting blood flow rates are affected, and ischemia at rest and impaired skin metabolism result. Clinical findings of ischemia can include trophic changes, dependent rubor, paresthesias (which might be partially or completely relieved with dependency), and cutaneous ulceration (Figs. 56–1 and 56–2).

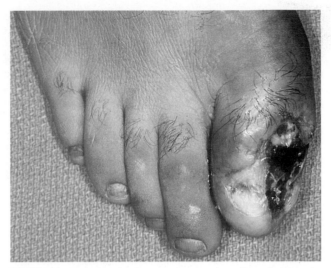

FIGURE 56–1 Ischemic changes in great toe after arterial embolus.

Vascular Testing

Noninvasive Studies

If ischemia is noted on clinical examination, noninvasive studies can delineate the degree and level of ischemia and the potential for healing, and they provide a baseline for future comparison. When patients present with symptoms that occur during exercise, some form of exercise evaluation should be performed. When patients present primarily with symptoms at rest, an evaluation can be performed without exercise testing.

Segmental Pressure

Measurement of resting ankle pressure is the most common noninvasive study performed on patients with suspected vascular disease. The arterial systolic blood pressure in a given limb segment is determined by inflating a cuff around that segment and slowly deflating the cuff until arterial blood flow is detected distal to the cuff with continuous-wave Doppler. Variations in systemic pressure between individuals are corrected by expressing the absolute

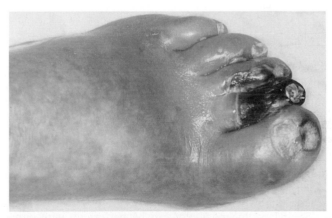

FIGURE 56–2 Chronic arterial occlusive disease with associated ischemia, trophic changes, rubor, edema, ulcerations, and gangrenous changes (second and third toes).

ankle pressure as a ratio relative to the brachial pressure (ankle/brachial index, ABI). The ABI is interpreted as follows: ≥0.9, normal; 0.8 to 0.9, mild; 0.5 to 0.8, moderate; and ≤0.5, severe.[34] In patients with mild symptoms of claudication, the ABI might be normal at rest but reduced after exercise. At rest, the vascular resistance of the leg is relatively high, and flow through a stenotic lesion can be sufficient to maintain normal distal pressure. After exercise, the vascular resistance is lower and blood flow through the stenosis might not be sufficient to keep the distal pressure from decreasing.[41] Post-exercise ABIs are determined by having the patient walk on a treadmill for 5 minutes at 2 miles/hour up a 10% to 12% grade.

Segmental limb pressure measurements extend the application of ankle pressure measurements and provide a more precise determination of the anatomy of the occlusive process.[16] Cuffs are placed at "high"-thigh, above-knee, below-knee, and ankle locations. The measured limb pressures can exceed the measured brachial pressure in normal persons by up to 30 mm Hg. Limb pressure equal to or less than the brachial artery pressure indicates significant aortoiliac or proximal femoral arterial occlusive disease. A gradient of more than 20 mm Hg between any adjacent segment is an abnormal finding.[16] Falsely high readings may be obtained in patients with large thighs or when the cuff width is too narrow. Falsely low readings may result when too wide a cuff is used on a thin thigh. Interpretation can also be difficult with multilevel arterial occlusive disease.

Doppler

A normal flow waveform in peripheral arteries is characterized by a triphasic Doppler signal during each cardiac cycle (Fig. 56–3A). The first component is a strong, high-frequency signal in the forward direction, which corresponds to systole; this is followed in early diastole by a short period of reverse flow. Later in diastole, the third component represents forward flow prior to the subsequent heartbeat. Biphasic signals are observed in the absence of disease in distal arteries or when the peripheral resistance is low. Distal to a stenosis, the waveform becomes monophasic, characterized by a blunted peak velocity and the absence of a reverse component (Fig. 56–3B). If the probe is positioned directly over the stenotic segment, a very high-frequency signal occurs during systole and diastole as a result of increased velocity through the narrowed segment.[52]

Plethysmography

Plethysmography can be used to measure mean blood flow by recording the rate of increase in limb volume after sudden interruption of venous outflow. To perform a plethysmographic flow measurement, the limb is placed in a neutral, relaxed position and the venous occlusion cuff is rapidly inflated. Blood that flows into the limb becomes trapped, and the limb expands. The rate at which expansion occurs is measured by the plethysmograph, from which arterial inflow can be estimated.[41]

Digital plethysmography can be performed with either strain-gauge or photoelectric instrumentation. Toe pressures evaluate obstructive disease in the digital vessels or pedal

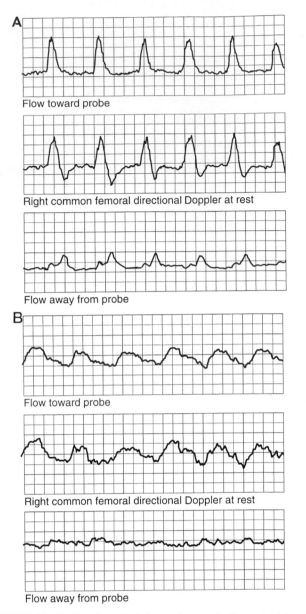

FIGURE 56–3 Doppler arterial waveforms. *A*, Normal triphasic signal. *B*, Blunted monophasic signal distal to stenosis.

arch. This test is useful for the evaluation of patients with diabetes, who can have abnormally high ankle pressures as a result of medial calcinosis, because it is unusual for digital arteries to be affected by this process. The digital artery pressure is also used as a guide to the likelihood of spontaneous healing of superficial cutaneous lesions. A toe/brachial index (TBI) greater than .60 is normal. If the absolute pressure is 30 mm Hg or less, healing is unlikely to occur.[34]

Transcutaneous Oxygen Tension

Transcutaneous oxygen tension ($TcPO_2$) is an objective indicator of ischemia of the skin in a patient with peripheral occlusive arterial disease.[2, 35, 42, 47] $TcPO_2$ measurements are relatively simple and reproducible. They also provide information regarding the physiological importance of blood flow impairment. Oxygen-sensing electrodes with a surface temperature of 45 °C are attached to the skin and allowed to equilibrate until stable. A reference electrode is placed on the chest, and other electrodes are placed over the area of interest. In a standard study of the lower extremities, two electrodes are placed on the dorsum of each foot. With the patient supine, $TcPO_2$ values are recorded, and the regional perfusion indices ($TcPO_2$ foot/ $TcPO_2$ chest) are calculated. The feet are then elevated to 30 degrees for 3 min, and the $TcPO_2$ measurements are repeated.[47] If the $TcPO_2$ value is 20 torr or less, healing is not likely to occur, whereas $TcPO_2$ values more than 40 torr are associated with healing. If the $TcPO_2$ value decreases into the borderline zone of 20 to 40 torr, measuring the values after leg elevation improves the predictability of outcome.[2, 42] The regional perfusion index is important for patients who have cardiac or pulmonary dysfunction that produces variable degrees of systemic oxygen desaturation.[35]

Duplex Ultrasonography

Duplex ultrasonography combines a pulsed Doppler with real-time B-mode scanning. Duplex scanning combines exact anatomical localization of disease with physiological blood flow studies to define the hemodynamic significance of the lesion.[16] The expense of this equipment limits its utilization as a general screening tool[41] (see the section on venous studies, p 1189).

Invasive Studies

Arteriography

Although physiological testing is excellent for screening and follow-up, arteriography remains the most accurate procedure for evaluation of infrainguinal arterial occlusive disease (Fig. 56–4). If surgery is anticipated, arteriography is usually needed to determine the length of arterial occlusion, level of distal reconstruction, and patency of the plantar arch. In the presence of inflow vessel disease, special arteriographic techniques such as digital subtraction angiography may be necessary for visualization of distal runoff vessels.[16, 53] Patients with arterial occlusive disease can also have renal disease, and consequently are at high risk for renal failure if contrast material is used. This risk must be considered whenever arteriography is contemplated.

Testing for Associated Diseases

When evaluating the patient with atherosclerotic occlusive disease, especially if surgical intervention is planned, it is important that the clinical evaluation define and quantify any associated cardiovascular, renal, and pulmonary problems. Because many patients with vascular disease are sedentary and lack symptoms of coronary artery disease, it is easy to miss asymptomatic but hemodynamically significant cardiovascular disease despite obtaining a thorough history and performing a physical examination.

The prevalence of serious coronary artery disease ranges from 37% to 78% in patients undergoing an operation for peripheral vascular disease.[19] Although procedures involving aortic cross-clamping exert a greater acute systemic hemodynamic stress than femoral popliteal surgery, late

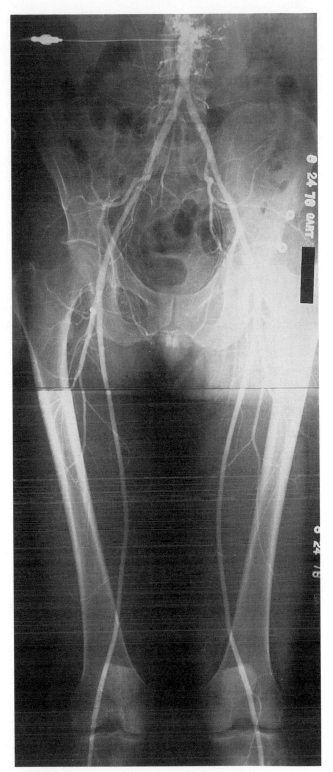

FIGURE 56–4 Angiogram showing mild atherosclerosis obliterans in a patient with pseudoclaudication.

cardiac morbidity and mortality are significant in all patients with atherosclerotic disease who undergo such procedures.[19] Through preoperative identification of high-risk patients, intensive medical therapy and monitoring can stabilize the patient preoperatively and potential intraoperative problems can be anticipated. During the postoperative period, careful hemodynamic monitoring and continued cardiac surveillance are mandatory.[19] In patients with suspected coronary artery disease who must undergo peripheral vascular surgery, the perioperative mortality rate is approximately four times higher than for those without coronary artery disease, and the perioperative morbidity is markedly increased.[19]

Rest and Exercise Electrocardiography

A 12-lead electrocardiogram (ECG) is almost universally recorded during the preoperative period. In patients who require vascular surgery, up to 35% of those with a normal rest 12-lead ECG have an abnormal exercise ECG.[19]

ECG-monitored exercise testing has been shown to correlate with the risk of myocardial infarction. Patients who achieve less than 85% of their maximal predicted heart rate have a postoperative cardiac complication rate of 24%, whereas this rate is only 6% in patients whose heart rate exceeds 85% of the maximal predicted value.[16] Clearly, exercise testing is limited in patients who have severe claudication, rest ischemia, or prior amputation. The primary advantage of exercise testing is its wide availability and modest cost. Although ECG-monitored stress testing is being replaced by other tests that do not require exercise, it is still a useful means to obtain objective information regarding the relative degree of impairment imposed by claudication, pulmonary insufficiency, or coronary artery disease.

Dipyridamole Thallium-201 Scintigraphy

Dipyridamole thallium-201 scintigraphy (or a related test using agents such as adenosine or sestamibi) is a useful means of screening patients with peripheral vascular disease for coronary artery disease because it is minimally invasive and can be performed with the patient at rest. Dipyridamole is a potent coronary vasodilator. When administered intravenously in patients with hemodynamically significant coronary artery disease, the difference in perfusion between myocardium supplied by normal coronary arteries and that supplied by stenotic, nondistensible vessels is accentuated. Thallium-201 is promptly absorbed by areas of normal perfusion and serves as a marker for viable myocardium. When the patient is rescanned 3 hours later, uptake of thallium-201 is delayed in areas of potentially ischemic myocardium. No uptake is noted in infarcted tissue.[16] Although this test is highly sensitive, it has limited specificity. Nevertheless, it is well suited to the preoperative screening of patients with peripheral vascular disease. Only patients with significant thallium-201 redistribution require further cardiac evaluation. In general, patients with a history of chronic stable angina, those with a single uncomplicated myocardial infarction more than 6 months previously, or those in whom dipyridamole thallium-201 scintigraphy shows no more than a small area of redistribution need no further cardiac evaluation.[16] Patients with a history of more severe cardiac disease and thallium-201 redistribution involving two or more vessels are at increased risk for postoperative cardiac complications, and further cardiac evaluation, such as cardiac catheterization, should be considered.

Treatment

Ideally, all ischemic limbs should be restored to a functional, pain-free state with appropriate management. Unfortunately, extensive vascular disease or underlying medical illness can preclude revascularization. Patients with severe ischemia report increasing symptoms as tissue necrosis and gangrene occur. Many patients with severe rest pain note a temporary decrease in their pain with dependency. This can be explained in part by an increase in hydrostatic pressure, which allows better perfusion to the ischemic tissue. Unless the pain is adequately controlled with narcotics, tricyclic antidepressants, anticonvulsants, or other measures, the patient will keep the involved extremity dependent. Continued dependency results in edema, decreased arterial flow, decreased perfusion, and further ischemia.

Acute Arterial Occlusion

Thrombosis

Acute thrombosis is generally best managed with an initial course of heparin therapy followed by arteriography to define the lesion and the status of the inflow and outflow vessels. Lytic therapy or urgent surgical revascularization might be required. Early intervention can prevent neuromuscular injury, enhance limb salvage, and avoid myonecrosis, myoglobinuria, and associated renal failure. Even when urgent, "early" revascularization is unnecessary, elective revascularization at a later date might be required to alleviate symptoms of chronic ischemia.

Embolic Ischemia

Heparin should be given as soon as the diagnosis of acute arterial embolus is suspected. Initial heparin requirements are frequently much higher than anticipated. Large doses of heparin are required to inhibit coagulation and to prevent clot propagation in patients in whom thrombus is already present. When results of sensory and motor examinations are normal, initial management can be directed at the patient's underlying cardiac dysfunction and control of arrhythmia. In such a patient, the limb generally shows rapid improvement with anticoagulation. Early recognition and correction of the offending proximal lesion are important.[16] The restoration of adequate perfusion is important, but returning blood flow to the microcirculation might not be easy in the presence of swollen endothelial and perivascular cells. Advanced ischemia is characterized by absent motor and sensory function, pronounced muscle tenderness and rigidity, limb pallor (without elevation), and prolongation of the venous filling time of more than 1 min.[32] With marked motor deficit, muscle rigidity, or anesthesia on clinical examination, early amputation must be considered. Revascularization of such an ischemic limb can result in a mortality rate of 50% to 75% because of the effects of metabolic products on the renal and pulmonary systems (reperfusion syndrome).[16]

Dissection

Treatment of aortic dissection depends on location. If the dissection is located in the ascending aorta (Stanford type A), management includes control of arterial systolic blood pressure and emergency surgical repair to correct or prevent cardiac tamponade, acute aortic insufficiency, or coronary artery occlusion. If the dissection occurs in the descending thoracic or abdominal aorta (Stanford type B), medical management of pain and arterial blood pressure is usually the treatment of choice. Surgical repair is generally reserved for patients who have significant vascular occlusion, persistent pain, progression of the dissection, or aneurysm formation.[16] Paraplegia is a possible surgical complication.

Chronic Arterial Occlusion

General

The ultimate goal is to develop effective therapy that prevents progression of the disease process and possibly promotes regression of existing lesions. It is important that the correct diagnosis and cause of the underlying disease process be identified before proceeding with treatment. Controllable risk factors such as smoking, diabetes, hyperlipidemia, hypertension, and gross obesity, as discussed previously, should be addressed with appropriate pharmacological approaches, dietary measures, or behavior modifications.

PATIENT AND FAMILY EDUCATION. Therapeutic success is most likely to occur with an educated patient and family. It is important to discuss in detail the diffuse and progressive nature of atherosclerosis, the importance of controlling risk factors, and measures to protect the ischemic limb.

PROTECTION FROM TRAUMA. Most amputations in persons with occlusive peripheral arterial disease result from some type of trauma (thermal, chemical, or mechanical) superimposed on a limb with chronic occlusive disease.[16, 49] Thermal injury is prevented by avoiding excess heat (e.g., heating pad, hot water). Warm outer footwear is recommended in the winter to protect against cold. Because a low skin temperature augments sympathetic tone, keeping an ischemic limb warm with vascular boots (Fig. 56–5) attenuates sympathetic tone, avoids vasoconstriction, and improves local cutaneous blood flow and $TcPO_2$.[44] Chemicals, corn remedies, and antiseptics should be avoided to prevent chemical trauma. Mechanical trauma can be caused by poorly fitting footwear.

ORTHOSES. The use of rocker-sole shoes, to lessen the work of the gastrocnemius-soleus muscle groups during ambulation, increases walking distance and can be a useful addition to the nonsurgical management of calf claudication.[40] Double-metal upright ankle-foot orthoses to eliminate ankle motion have also been studied. Despite the added weight, fixed ankle, appearance, and change of gait pattern, most patients noted an increase in their walking distance and were pleased with the results obtained with the use of this orthosis.[29]

EXERCISE. Exercise increases the demand for blood to the lower extremities. In a normal arterial system, demand is primarily met by arterial vasodilatation. Although flow rates increase dramatically during exercise, arterial perfusion pressure remains essentially unchanged.[16] With atherosclerosis, the capability of the arterial system to supply peak blood flow is progressively reduced. At rest, maximal blood flow goes to the skin; during exercise, most of the increase in blood flow is shunted to the active muscle beds. Several studies have shown the beneficial effects of physical training in patients with intermittent claudication.[15, 31] Improved peripheral utilization of oxygen, walking technique, and glycolytic and oxidative metabolic capacity have been suggested as reasons for the improvement with training.[31] Others believe that graded exercise should be attempted to place a load on the vascular system and stimulate growth of collateral vessels.[1] Ekroth and co-workers[15] found that maximal calf blood flow did not increase in parallel with increases in walking ability. This finding does not support the earlier belief that physical training is directly associated with the development of collateral circulation. Another study found a dramatic increase in walking distances after a supervised, graduated-exercise program without an associated increase in resting ABIs. This finding also suggests that the increased walking distance is due to an increase in the oxidative capacity of muscle. Such a metabolic change is supported by biochemical evidence that the activity of glycolytic and mitochondrial enzymes in calf muscle tissue is positively correlated with walking distance in patients with claudication who receive physical training.[11] Walking programs must be individualized; however, the usual prescription has a goal of 30 to 60 minutes, 3 to 5 days a week at a pace of 2 miles/hour, as allowed by cardiac precautions.[11, 15] The patient should rest after symptoms of claudication develop.[1, 16] Improvement is gradual over a period of 3 to 6 months.[11]

Medical

VASODILATORS. The general aim of drug therapy for arterial occlusive disease is to increase oxygen delivery. Although vasodilator drugs have been shown to increase blood flow to the limbs and various organs in animal experiments and in humans with vasospastic disorders, their use in peripheral obstructive vascular disease remains questionable.[9] An ideal drug for treatment of peripheral vascular diseases would dilate blood vessels and increase blood flow only in areas of deficient blood supply. Such agents do not currently exist. In some circumstances, vasodilation in areas without diseased vessels can actually steal flow from the affected area.[9] Because β-adrenergic blockade can cause peripheral vasoconstriction, it has been recommended that β-adrenergic blockers be avoided in patients with arterial occlusive disease.

ANTICOAGULANTS AND ANTIPLATELET AGENTS. Platelet aggregation can exacerbate arterial occlusive disease by causing mechanical occlusion of small arteries or by releasing serotonin and stimulating local vasospasm.[16] There is no evidence that fibrinolytic agents, anticoagulants, or antiplatelet agents are directly effective in the treatment of intermittent claudication. Cyclooxygenase inhibitors such as aspirin decrease both prostacyclin production and thromboxane production. The former effect is proaggregatory and possibly vasoconstrictive, whereas the latter is antiaggregatory. Although aspirin is widely used for patients with arterial occlusive disease, its best-documented effects relate to prevention of coronary and vascular graft thrombosis rather than intermittent claudication.[16]

HEMORRHEOLOGIC AGENTS. Pentoxifylline (Tren-

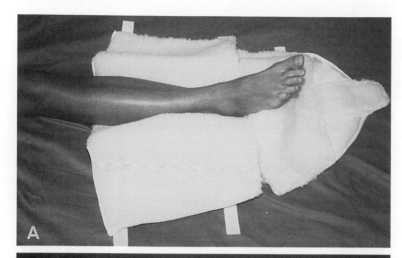

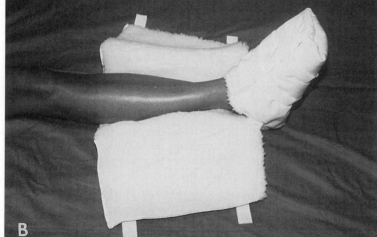

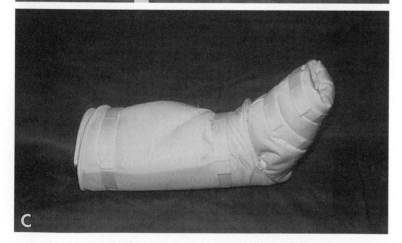

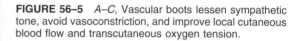

FIGURE 56–5   *A–C*, Vascular boots lessen sympathetic tone, avoid vasoconstriction, and improve local cutaneous blood flow and transcutaneous oxygen tension.

tal) increases red blood cell deformability, decreases plasma viscosity, and diminishes platelet aggregation by decreasing fibrinogen concentration. It also increases resting and hyperemic extremity blood flow, presumably through its rheologic effects.[16, 38] Reports in the literature about the degree of clinical improvement in patients taking pentoxifylline for the treatment of intermittent claudication have been variable.[38, 48] In one pilot study, 10 subjects showed a significant increase in exercise tolerance, and 8 of 10 subjects demonstrated a significant increase in right dorsalis pedis arterial flow on noninvasive testing after

pentoxifylline treatment.[48] Because pentoxifylline is a methylxanthine derivative, this drug should not be used in persons intolerant to this class of compounds (i.e., caffeine, theophylline).

ANTIBIOTICS.   The increased metabolic demands of active infection and extensive tissue loss can overcome the healing capabilities of an ischemic limb. In patients with diabetes, foot infections are often multimicrobial and deeply invasive. Administration of broad-spectrum systemic antibiotics is frequently necessary for limb salvage and localization of the infection.[55]

Revascularization

ANGIOPLASTY. Percutaneous transluminal angioplasty is an established treatment for claudication in patients with arterial occlusive disease. Angioplasty is indicated for focal stenosis or short segmental occlusions in which the adjacent vessels are relatively free of disease. Angioplasty is associated with a low incidence of morbidity, and 5-year patency rates of 80% to 90% have been reported for iliac lesions, as opposed to 60% to 70% for superficial femoral artery lesions.[11] A recent study suggested that supervised graduated exercise therapy produces better long-term improvement in mean distance walked before claudication and maximal walking distance in patients suitable for angioplasty than does angioplasty itself.[11] One advantage of angioplasty is that the inpatient stay is short, around 48 hours.

SURGERY. Vascular reconstruction is indicated in patients with incapacitating claudication, rest pain, gangrene, and tissue loss, especially when the ABI is less than 0.4 or the forefoot $TcPO_2$ is less than 30 mm Hg.[16]

Aortoiliac Occlusive Disease. The standard operation for aortoiliac disease is an aortobifemoral bypass. In selected patients with unilateral disease, limited operations such as femoral-femoral (fem-fem) bypass or iliofemoral bypass can be considered. Contralateral disease progression or atherosclerotic occlusive disease of the donor iliac artery in the fem-fem bypass can result in steal, from which ischemia develops in the previously asymptomatic donor leg. The advantages of these limited procedures are lack of manipulation of contralateral flow and a lower surgical risk (especially the fem-fem bypass, which is an extra-anatomical procedure).

Infrainguinal Occlusive Disease. All patients with superficial femoral or proximal popliteal occlusion in whom the arteries distal to the popliteal area are patent are best served by a femoral-popliteal bypass. When a femoral-popliteal bypass is not possible, a more distal bypass to the posterior tibial, anterior tibial, or peroneal arteries can be performed. The dorsalis pedis, posterior tibial, lateral tarsal, deep metatarsal arch, and medial and lateral plantar arteries have been used to provide successful bypass outflow even when the plantar arch is not patent or other major pedal arteries are occluded.[23, 25] The patency and limb salvage rates for inframalleolar revascularization are comparable to those obtained with femoral popliteal or femoral tibial bypasses.[23] The dorsalis pedis bypass has been especially beneficial for patients with diabetes whose occlusive disease frequently involves the tibial and peroneal vessels and spares the inframalleolar circulation.[20, 37] Femoral-popliteal bypass grafting may prove technically successful but not relieve symptoms if extensive tibial disease is present. When this situation occurs, secondary bypass grafting to the dorsal pedal artery usually relieves symptoms.[37] Bypass to the dorsal pedal artery can be safely performed in patients with ischemia or active local infection.[55]

Other Measures

SYMPATHECTOMY. As reconstructive procedures have extended to distal vessels, sympathectomy has been performed less frequently. Limbs with inoperable arterial disease, ischemic cutaneous ulceration, pain at rest, or pregangrenous changes can be considered for sympathetic denervation. The primary effect of sympathectomy seems to be enhancing pain relief rather than augmenting blood flow to the ischemic limb. A diabetic neuropathy can frequently cause autosympathectomy. It is imperative to document the presence of sympathetic nerve function in such cases before proceeding with surgical sympathectomy.[7] Although specific neuroautonomical testing can be performed, a simple approach is to assess the effects of a temporary sympathetic block.

INTERMITTENT VENOUS OCCLUSION/PNEUMATIC END-DIASTOLIC LEG COMPRESSION. Skin blood flow, as reflected by $TcPO_2$, can be augmented acutely in ischemic limbs by intermittent venous occlusion with an externally applied inflatable cuff[46] (Fig. 56–6). Other devices, which apply intermittent circumferential pneumatic compression to the foot or lower limb during cardiac diastole, show promise as adjunct measures to augment limb perfusion.

CHELATION THERAPY. Intravenous administration of fluids containing chelating compounds, such as ethylenediaminetetraacetate (EDTA), have been advocated for treatment of advanced arterial occlusive disease on the premise that calcium salts leached from the vascular lesions might potentiate regression of the disease. Because of the lack of objective documentation on the effectiveness and the nephrotoxic effects of this treatment, it is most commonly used only as an adjunctive measure of last resort.

AMPUTATION. With advances in limb salvage procedures, it is important to review carefully the risk-to-benefit and cost-to-benefit ratios with the patient before each intervention. Although in the later stage of disease each patient has a choice between amputation or delay, it is necessary to point out that often the choices are a relatively pain-free, comfortable prosthesis or salvage of a painful ulcerated or gangrenous foot. In the older person, the time required for medical care and hospitalization becomes more and more significant. Frequent hospitalizations and non–weight-bearing status of a year's duration can represent 20% of the remaining life of a 70-year-old patient. Most patients choose a shorter procedure, enabling them to spend as much as possible of their remaining life in comfort.[18]

VENOUS DISEASE

Etiology and Pathogenesis

Venous disease includes deep venous thrombosis (DVT), recurrent DVT, superficial thrombophlebitis, and chronic venous insufficiency. In all cases, it is important to make an accurate diagnosis before initiating therapy.

Thrombi frequently arise from clot formation in the cusps of venous valves, with thrombi then propagating out of the cusps into the major venous channel. Another site for thrombus development is at the entrance of a tributary vein. The thrombus can go on to occlude a major venous channel by prograde or retrograde propagation. Fortunately, many small venous thrombi undergo rapid thrombolytic dissolution. For large thrombi, organization begins after 3 to 4 days. Recanalization can require a period of several months or more. Fibrous bands or strictures can form in

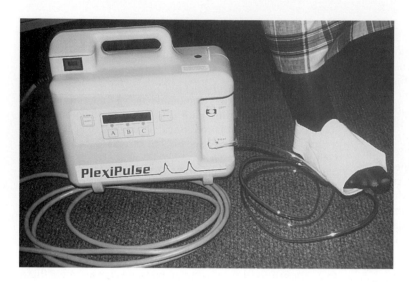

FIGURE 56–6 Intermittent venous occlusion (Plexi-Pulse) can augment skin blood flow and decrease dependent edema.

the vein. Usually, but not always, venous valves are destroyed or lose their normal function as the fibrotic process thickens the venous wall and cusp.[16] Superficial venous thrombosis alone is not thought to have any serious morbidity unless a saphenous vein thrombus propagates and involves the common femoral vein.

Risk Factors

The pathogenesis of DVT is outlined by Virchow's postulates: change in blood flow, alterations in the vessel wall, and variation in coagulability of the blood. Risk factors associated with the development of acute DVT include prior history of DVT, immobilization, postoperative state, age (older than 40 years), cardiac disease, limb trauma, post-thrombotic state or coagulation abnormalities, hormonal therapy, pregnancy and postpartum state, obesity, and advanced neoplasm[16, 39] (Table 56–1). A complete medical workup should be done for any patient with an unexplained deep or superficial venous thrombosis.

History and Clinical Findings

Relevant history includes the patient's symptoms or presence of potential risk factors. Clinical findings associated with DVT include pain, tenderness, unilateral ankle or calf edema, palpable induration or cord, and pain produced by extreme dorsiflexion of the foot. Unfortunately, most signs and symptoms attributed to DVT have been statistically analyzed and found to have a poor predictive value for determining the presence or absence of DVT.[12]

Chronic Venous Insufficiency

Venous flow is based on a force that compels the blood proximally (such as gravity or the calf muscle), an adequate outflow tract, and the presence of competent valves limiting reflux. Any disruption of these components results in chronic venous hypertension.[30] Chronic venous insufficiency is usually the result of congenital or acquired valvular incompetence and, less frequently, obstruction of the veins,[22] although it can occur after DVT recanalization and

TABLE 56–1   Optional Drug Regimens for the Prevention of Venous Thromboembolism in Patients at Risk

Agent	Administration	Comments
Heparin		
"Fixed" dose	10,000–15,000 units/day SC, divided into bid or tid doses	Low- or moderate-risk patients
"Adjusted" dose	Heparin given SC bid or tid, adjusted to keep APTT at 32–36 sec (high-normal range) or	High-risk patients
	1.3–1.5 × control	Hip surgery patients
plus Dihydroergotamine	"Fixed" heparin dose(s) as above plus 0.5 mg dihydroergotamine SC bid	Comparable or superior to "fixed"-dose heparin alone
Warfarin (Coumadin)		
"Mini" dose	1 mg/day starting 3 wk before surgery	Low- or moderate-risk patients
"Low" dose	Sufficient dose to achieve PT of 1.3–1.5 × control	Moderate- or high-risk patients
Two-step	1. Preoperatively: sufficient dose to increase PT up to 3 sec	High-risk patients
	2. Immediately postoperatively: raise dose to increase PT to 1.5 × control	

Abbreviations: PT, prothrombin time; APTT, activated partial thromboplastin time; SC, subcutaneously.
From Rooke TW: Deep venous thrombosis of the extremities. *In* Conn HF (ed): Conn's Current Therapy. Philadelphia, WB Saunders, 1992, p 289. By permission of the publisher.

valve destruction (*postphlebitic syndrome*). Postphlebitic syndrome develops in 67% to 80% of patients after DVT.[12] Recent studies have shown that a significant proportion of patients with chronic venous insufficiency have primary valvular incompetence with no history or phlebographic evidence of DVT.[22] Most patients have a single valve in either the external iliac or common femoral vein, but up to 37% of patients have no valve on one or both sides. Because the common iliac vein and vena cava are valveless, this anatomy can predispose a significant proportion of the population to unusually high pressures on the valve at the saphenofemoral junction, and thus the likelihood of superficial venous insufficiency is increased.[22]

Several theories exist regarding the changes in the subcutaneous tissue of patients with chronic venous insufficiency. One is the hypothesis that venous hypertension leads to venular dilatation and increased capillary permeability, with transudation of fibrinogen and hemosiderin from the capillaries into the subcutaneous tissue. In this case, pericapillary fibrin acts as a diffusion barrier, and the overlying dermis becomes hypoxic.[6] There are no in vivo studies to document that pericapillary fibrin cuffs act as a diffusion barrier.[17] A second theory is that increased venous pressure and low skin oxygen tension in the upright position, even during exercise, are responsible for ulcer formation in venous insufficiency.[14, 33] Normal legs are protected by a rise in skin oxygenation during exercise.[14]

Chronic venous insufficiency results in chronic edema, scarring, obliteration of cutaneous lymphatics, decreased skin integrity, hemosiderin deposition (with resultant brownish discoloration), dermatitis, and ulceration. Fortunately, not all patients with incompetent valves are symptomatic.

Evaluation

Impedance Plethysmography

Impedance plethysmography assesses volume changes at rest produced by a proximal, pneumatic, veno-occlusive cuff. The normal leg swells when a veno-occlusive tourniquet is placed and rapidly returns to its normal size when the tourniquet is released. Venous volume measured by electrical impedance shows a quick return to baseline levels, usually within 3 to 4 sec. In the presence of a proximal lower-extremity DVT, the venous system will already be "maximally" filled. When the cuff is inflated, there is little additional increase in venous volume, and after tourniquet release the return to baseline is delayed.[41]

Exercise Venous Plethysmography

Lower limb venous function is tested by performing a plethysmographic evaluation of limb volume before, during, and after exercise. In a normal individual, plethysmography shows a progressive decrease in leg volume during exercise followed by a period after exercise when the volume slowly returns to normal. In venous insufficiency, the exercise-induced decrease in venous volume is less than expected. In addition, when venous incompetence is present, the post-exercise return in volume will be more rapid than expected. Exercise venous plethysmography provides a quick and relatively inexpensive way to document

or screen for venous incompetence. It also yields quantitative information about the severity of venous insufficiency that is not readily obtained with other noninvasive methods.[43]

Duplex Scanning

Duplex scanning is used to diagnose deep or superficial venous thrombosis, assess venous incompetence, and map the superficial veins before surgical harvest for bypass operations. The diagnosis of venous thrombosis can be established by demonstrating noncompressibility of the vein with use of real-time two-dimensional B-mode imaging (Fig. 56–7). If the veins do not collapse under a force sufficient to distort the arteries, intraluminal thrombus is assumed to be present. Older thrombi can appear echogenic or match the echogenicity of the vein wall and surrounding tissue. The pulsed-wave Doppler confirms the lack of venous flow and provides indirect evidence that spontaneous flow through the vein has disappeared (by the absence of phasic changes with respiration or the reduction or absence of augmentation). Duplex scanning can also document the presence of venous incompetence, identify the anatomical sites involved, and quantify the severity.[45]

Treatment

Superficial Thrombophlebitis

Superficial thrombophlebitis is treated with elevation and superficial heat. Appropriate compressive stockings, 30 to 40 mm Hg, should be worn when ambulating. Aspirin or nonsteroidal anti-inflammatory medications can be administered for pain relief. It is doubtful that these medications significantly diminish the potential extension of the phlebitic process. If the process extends near the saphenofemoral junction, a duplex examination should clarify the status

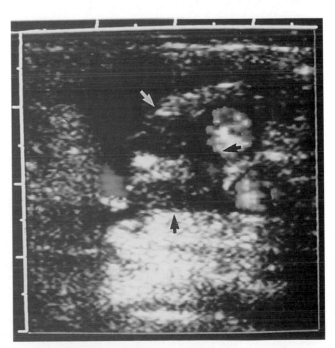

FIGURE 56–7 Duplex scan showing venous thrombus.

of the deep veins. If the deep veins also contain a thrombus, the patient should be treated for DVT.[16]

Deep Venous Thrombosis

Standard therapy for acute DVT consists of anticoagulation, bed rest, and elevation and support of the extremity (Table 56–2).

Chronic Venous Insufficiency

Patient education is important in the management of chronic venous insufficiency. Patients must understand their disease process and the correct use of measures to decrease edema. When elevation is used for edema control, the extremity must be elevated above the level of the heart. This position is not achieved by placing the leg on a footstool. The pelvis should not be dependent. Patients should lie on a sofa or sit in an orthopedic chair to elevate the legs properly above the level of the heart.[16]

Compression is an important component of the nonsurgical management of chronic venous insufficiency. With no history of congestive heart failure and no evidence of venous obstruction on noninvasive studies, lower extremity volume can be stabilized with an intermittent compression pump. Limb circumference or volumetric measurements should be carefully obtained after each session. Compressive wrap should be used between sessions. After the volume stabilizes, the patient can be measured for a custom-graded compression garment of 30 to 40 mm Hg.

Sclerotherapy is used for the treatment of spider veins, small distal varicose veins, and venous insufficiency resulting from superficial and perforator incompetence.[30, 57] During sclerotherapy, a substance that irritates the endothelial lining is injected into a vein. This is followed by compression until the vein walls are permanently fused. Elastic compression is suggested for at least 6 weeks after treatment. Complications are rare and usually minor. The most frequent types of morbidity include skin discoloration, thrombophlebitis, and hematoma formation. Allergic or anaphylactic reactions to the sclerosing agent are very rare but have been observed. Skin or fat necrosis can occur if a large amount of concentrated solution is injected outside the vein.[22]

Surgical intervention for chronic venous insufficiency can include ligation of perforators, direct valve repair, vein segment transposition, or axillary valve autotransplantation.[22]

LYMPHATIC DISEASE

Etiology

Lymphedema, the abnormal accumulation of water and protein in the skin and subcutaneous tissues, is classified as either primary or secondary. Primary lymphedema is due to aplastic or hypoplastic lymphatic trunks. Secondary lymphedema can occur after recurrent infection, tumor, lymphoproliferative disease, or injury to the lymphatic system stemming from surgical excision, trauma, or irradiation.[16] Lymphedema develops when the lymphatic load exceeds the transfer capacity of the lymphatic system. It becomes manifest if all the compensatory mechanisms (collateral lymphatic circulation, spontaneous lymphovenous anastomosis, and the proteolytic activity of tissue macrophages) are exhausted. This explains why lymphedema often develops several months—or even years—after interruption of the lymphatic pathways.[16] Without treatment, the protein-rich interstitial fluid is replaced by fibrinoid material. Inflammatory cells accumulate, and progressive fibrosis, sclerosis, and (in the final stage) elephantiasis develop. Lymphangiosarcoma, a severe late complication of secondary lymphedema, is rare.[16]

History and Clinical Findings

For evaluation of a swollen limb, it is important to determine the underlying diagnosis. Malignancy or metastatic disease must be excluded. Peripheral examination of the limb helps to differentiate lymphedema from other types of peripheral edema. The edema usually involves the dorsal forefoot but spares the metatarsophalangeal joint (Fig. 56–8). Dark pigmentary changes of the skin and

---

TABLE 56–2   Treatment of Deep Venous Thrombosis

	Therapy	Comments
Nonpharmacological	Bed rest	Minimize embolic potential
	Leg elevation	Reduce swelling
	Analgesics	Control pain
Pharmacological	Heparin,	
	100–150 units/kg IV bolus	For rapid anticoagulation
	then	
	± 1,000 units/hr IV	Keep APTT to 1.5–2.0 × control
	or	"Short" course: maintain heparin 4–7 days
	5,000–15,000 units SC tid	"Long" course: maintain heparin 7–10 days
	Warfarin (Coumadin), 10–15 mg PO	"Short" heparin course: start at time of diagnosis,
	then	discontinue heparin when PT is therapeutic
	5–10 mg/day until therapeutic (PT reaches level	"Long" heparin course: start after 4–5 days of heparin
	1.5 × control); maintain × 3 mo	therapy, discontinue heparin when PT is therapeutic
Mechanical	Vena cava filter	Use in patients with contraindication to anticoagulation
Supportive	Graduated elastic compression	To be worn on leg during ambulation for 6–12 wk; use
		thereafter as needed to control pain and swelling

Abbreviations: PT, prothrombin time; APTT, activated partial thromboplastin time; IV, intravenously; SC, subcutaneously; PO, by mouth.
From Rooke TW: Deep venous thrombosis of the extremities. *In* Conn HF (ed): Conn's Current Therapy. Philadelphia, WB Saunders, 1992, p 289. By permission of the publisher.

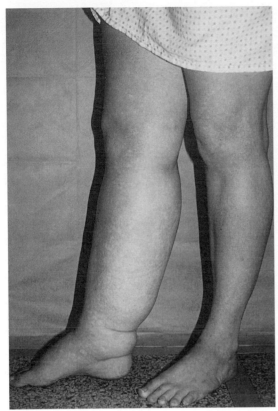

FIGURE 56–8 Lymphedema of right lower extremity. Note that the edema involves the dorsal forefoot but spares the metatarsophalangeal joint.

prominent veins are unusual. Although ulceration is characteristic of more advanced cases of chronic venous insufficiency, it is rare in lymphedema.

Evaluation

Magnetic resonance imaging is performed if soft tissue sarcoma is suspected. Lymphoscintigraphy provides a functional assessment of lymph transport capacity and identifies major morphological abnormalities of the lymphatic system. In addition, lymphoscintigraphy differentiates purely venous edema from mixed or lymphatic edema.[21] If venous disease is in question, noninvasive studies of the venous system should be obtained, including impedance plethysmography or duplex scanning.

Treatment

The goals of treatment for lymphedema are to preserve skin integrity, soften subcutaneous tissues, avoid lymphangiitis, reduce limb size,[16] and avoid contracture. In severe lymphedema, hospitalization with bed rest and a lymphedema sling can be required for 2 or 3 days to control limb volume (Fig. 56–9). The use of compression in the management of lymphedema is based on the Starling hypothesis of counteracting forces driving water through the capillary wall.[51] Pneumatic single-chamber compression at 60 to 80 mm Hg, or sequential compression at 80 to 130 mm Hg as tolerated, is used twice daily for 3 or 4 days until the volume is stabilized. Volumetric or circumferential

measurements are obtained after each treatment to monitor progress.

The pneumatic compression is followed by manual decongestive massage and isometric exercises to increase venous and lymphatic flow and reduce the edema. The massage and exercises are done with the extremity elevated to provide a gravity assist when mobilizing the fluid. The patient is instructed in a program of bandaging, elevation, and exercise to be done between treatments.[51]

After reduction of edema, new fluid accumulates in the tissue space unless the volume is restricted by external support. This support is commonly supplied by elastic bandages or custom compression stockings. The law of Laplace states that the tension in the wall of a container necessary to contain a given pressure is directly proportional to the radius of curvature. In other words, with large limbs it is more difficult to apply sufficient support to compress the limb and prevent the accumulation of edema.[50] Custom elastic graded-compression stockings are prescribed at 30 to 40 mm Hg or at 40 to 50 mm Hg. The patient should be supplied with two pairs to allow cleaning of one pair while the other is being worn. In general, two pairs of stockings should last 4 to 6 months. Selective refractory patients can benefit from simultaneously using two compressive stockings, 40 to 50 mm Hg and 50 to 60 mm Hg. Donning is facilitated by applying the lower-compression garment first. Depending on the location of the edema, a knee-high garment over a thigh-high garment may be adequate.

The patient must be instructed in meticulous skin care to avoid fungal infection or injury. Long-sleeved shirts or pants should be worn to avoid insect bites, cuts, or abrasions. Needle sticks or intravenous lines should never be permitted in the lymphedematous extremity. Patients should avoid exposure to extreme temperatures, such as in a hot tub. A general conditioning program and weight loss are encouraged.

Medications

Any evidence of infection needs immediate treatment. Patients can be given a supply of antibiotics with instructions to start treatment at the first sign of infection. The cause of cellulitis is almost always group A streptococci. If the patient has no allergies, penicillin is the drug of choice.

Benzopyrones reduce the volume of high-protein edema by stimulating proteolysis. Once excess protein is degraded, the edema it causes is no longer retained. Removal of the excess protein also reduces the medium in which secondary bacterial and fungal infections can incubate.[8] 5,6-Benzo-[α]-pyrone is best used as a complement to adequate nonsurgical therapy, but it can be used alone if the patient cannot wear compression garments. 5,6-Benzo-[α]-pyrone is not yet available for use in North America. Flavonoids (benzo-[γ]-pyrone) are available and can be beneficial in the treatment of lymphedema, although gastric irritation can be a problem.[8]

The use of diuretics in the management of lymphedema is controversial. They decrease the water and sodium content of the interstitial space but have no effect on the protein content of the extravascular fluid.[16] With chronic use, these agents generally become ineffective. Diuretics

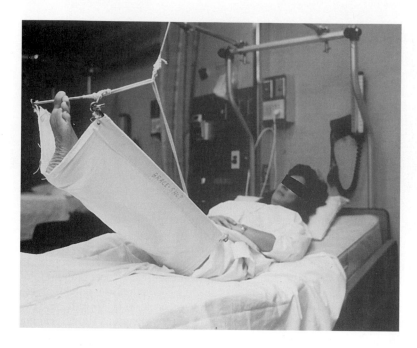

FIGURE 56–9　Bed rest with a lymphedema sling at 60 degrees can be used for initial management of severe lymphedema.

may be used for temporary relief in severe lymphedema or to provide symptomatic relief for patients with a terminal malignancy.

Surgery

Surgery for lymphedema is indicated in only a small percentage of patients. Operations are either excisional or physiological. The excisional operations (such as the Charles or the Homans procedure) are aimed at removing excess tissue to decrease the volume of the extremity, whereas the physiological operations consist of lymphatic-to-lymphatic or lymphatic-to-venous anastomosis,[16, 36] which, it is hoped, improves drainage. None of these operations are considered curative.

ARTERIOVENOUS FISTULAS AND ARTERIOVENOUS MALFORMATION

Etiology

Vascular malformations are classified as either congenital or acquired. The extent of the arterial component in a congenital arteriovenous malformation (AVM) is related to the stage of embryologic maturity at the time of developmental arrest. Acquired arteriovenous fistulas result from surgical construction of angioaccess for dialysis, penetrating injury, infection, neoplasm, and aneurysmal erosion.

History and Clinical Findings

A history of penetrating trauma should promote a high index of suspicion of possible acquired arteriovenous fistula. In the acute phase, a pulsating hematoma, palpable thrill, and bruit are present.[53] When the peripheral pulse remains intact and the distal systolic pressures are normal, the fistula can be considered relatively small from a hemodynamic standpoint. If pulses are decreased or absent and the distal pressure is low, a large-volume shunt is indicated.

In rare instances, the amount of blood siphoned by the fistula can produce heart failure, peripheral ischemia, or gangrene.[53]

Ischemia can develop early after fistula construction for dialysis in a patient with pre-existing arterial disease. It is more frequently a late manifestation, causing an increase in size of the arteriovenous fistula and reversal of flow in the distal radial artery. Clinical findings include pain, paresthesias, and muscular weakness in the affected extremity. These symptoms become more prominent during dialysis.[16]

Clinical presentation of a congenital AVM can be evident at birth. Most deep-seated AVMs are not evident until adolescence or early adulthood. An AVM causes symptoms with growth of the angiomatous mass, thrombosis of varicosities, or circulatory compromise.[16] Clinical presentations are variable. Swelling, discoloration, pain, an enlarged swollen limb, dermatitis, or ulceration may occur with all types of congenital vascular malformations[16] (Fig. 56–10).

Evaluation

The goals of evaluation are to establish the presence and type of lesion, to determine the hemodynamic effects, and to define the anatomical extent and involvement of adjacent structures.

To understand the hemodynamics of an arteriovenous fistula, it is imperative to understand the direction of flow in each of its component branches. Because a fistula markedly reduces the peripheral resistance, blood flow in the proximal artery loses its triphasic characteristic. Flow is always increased, particularly during diastole, and no reversed component is observed. Blood flow in the proximal vein increases and shows a pulsatile pattern. The direction of flow in the distal artery and vein can be either toward or away from the fistula. High resistance in the proximal artery and distal vascular bed, in combination with relatively low resistance at the site of the fistula and in the arterial collaterals, favors retrograde flow in the distal ar-

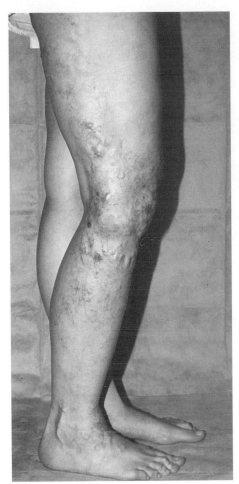

FIGURE 56–10 Arteriovenous malformation involving the right lower extremity with associated varicosities and leg length discrepancy.

tery. Flow in the proximal artery and arterial collaterals is always directed toward the periphery, and the flow in the proximal vein and venous channels is always directed centrally.[53] The same diagnostic studies used to evaluate chronic arterial occlusive disease in the extremities, and to a lesser extent venous insufficiency, can provide useful information about the fistula. Continuous-wave Doppler shows a high-flow, low-resistance pattern with loss of end-systolic reversal and considerable flow continuing throughout diastole.[16]

Magnetic resonance imaging is the best technique to evaluate congenital vascular malformations. It defines hypertrophy of bone, muscle, or subcutaneous tissue and images varicose veins and hemangiomas in the subcutaneous space and muscles.[24]

Treatment

Early recognition and management of an acquired arteriovenous fistula are preferred. Management of large, chronic arteriovenous fistulas is complicated. Bleeding can be profuse from multiple arterial and venous collateral vessels in the area.[16] Elastic support is beneficial to treat symptoms of chronic venous insufficiency, to protect the extremity from minor external trauma,[24] and to preserve

skin integrity by reducing the distal venous backup pressure. Appropriate footwear is important to accommodate limb hypertrophy and to compensate for leg-length discrepancy. Physical therapy intervention should maintain mobility of joints and soft tissues and preserve a normal gait pattern. Orthopedic intervention can be beneficial to avoid or correct leg-length discrepancy.

NONHEALING ULCERS

Nonhealing ulcers result from (1) neuropathy, (2) arterial and small-vessel disease, and (3) venous insufficiency.

History and Clinical Findings

Neuropathic

In patients with a history of autonomic and peripheral neuropathy, clinical findings can include decreased perspiration, dry skin, dependent rubor, impaired sensation, and denervation of foot intrinsic muscles with associated claw-foot deformity. Charcot changes may be present, including medial tarsal subluxation, pronation, forefoot valgus, increased width, and decreased length. Ulcers are typically located at the metatarsal heads, the pulp or tip of a rigid great toe, the lateral surface of the foot at the base of the metatarsal, the heel, or the midfoot (in the area of a collapsed navicular or cuboid bone). Neuropathic ulcers are characteristically painless and are rimmed by callus; they can be present for years before the patient seeks medical consultation (Fig. 56–11).

Controversy exists whether neuropathic ulcers can occur with an isolated neuropathic process or only in association with arterial or small-vessel insufficiency. Studies by Brand[3, 4] suggest that neuropathic ulcers result from repetitive trauma. Brand studied the histology of rat paws after repetitive stress and determined that an increase in temperature always occurred with repetitive stress. If the increase was followed immediately by a gradual return to normal, this change was thought to be due to simple reactive hyperemia. If the temperature increase continued for 10 or more minutes, biopsies showed edema and collections of inflammatory cells.

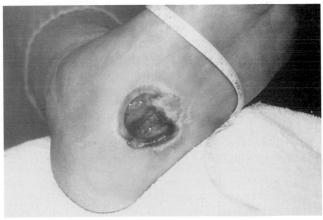

FIGURE 56–11 Large, painless, neuropathic ulcer with surrounding callus.

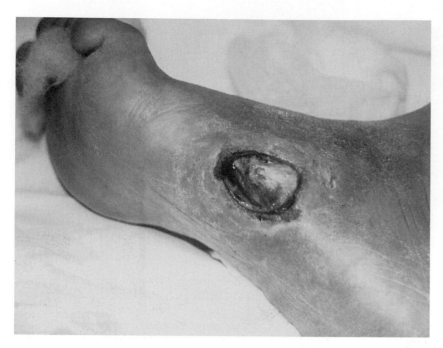

FIGURE 56–12 Arterial occlusive disease in a patient with a history of mechanical trauma and subsequent ulcer formation.

When the repetitions continued at a force equal to walking 7 miles/day at a fast pace on hard ground, epithelial hypertrophy with marked inflammation and necrosis of deeper tissues was noted at day 3. Ulceration occurred at day 10. When the same experiment was performed with 20% fewer daily repetitions and breaks on weekends, hypertrophy occurred without significant breakdown.[3, 4] It can be inferred from this study that in patients with normal sensation, inflammation makes feet tender and the tender spot is spared further stress until inflammation subsides. With a neuropathic foot, pain is no longer present to provide this feedback.

Ischemic

Ischemic ulcers typically result from a minor laceration, abrasion, or pressure in a limb with compromised blood flow, which leads to a chronic, painful ulcer that forms because the blood supply is insufficient to meet the increased demands of healing. Ischemic ulcers typically occur in the distal extremities.[13] Ulcers below the ankle with a pale or gray, nongranulating base are usually the result of major arterial insufficiency (Fig. 56–12). Simultaneous appearance of livedo reticularis and cutaneous toe infarcts (with subsequent ulceration) suggests atheromatous embolization, but these conditions can occur less commonly in periartcritis nodosa, systemic lupus erythematosus, or livedoid vasculitis.

Small-vessel (arteriolar) ischemic ulcers are usually located on the leg and have areas of cutaneous infarction that coalesce and proceed to ulceration[32] (Fig. 56–13). These ulcers are typically painful with a dense fibrinous base, serpiginous border, adjoining purpura, and satellite lesions.

Venous

With a history of chronic venous insufficiency, clinical findings include edema, hyperpigmentation, and soft tissue fibrosis. Ulcers are typically irregular in shape, perimalleolar, and located on the medial portion of the lower extremity (Fig. 56–14). Upper extremity ulcerations are not caused by chronic venous insufficiency unless an arteriovenous fistula is present.[32]

Treatment

Important aspects in the treatment of chronic ulcers include prevention or avoidance of progression of the ulcerations. General measures include early recognition of inflammation to avoid tissue damage, prevention or correction of risk factors, removal of vascular obstruction when possible, and early, aggressive wound care. Many products are available for the treatment of wounds, but formal protocols are needed to evaluate the efficacy and cost of most.

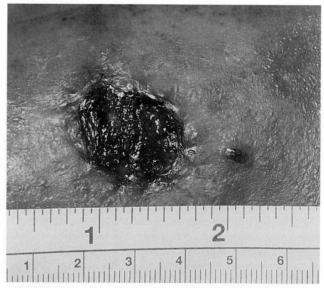

FIGURE 56–13 Small-vessel ischemic ulcers with areas of cutaneous infarction.

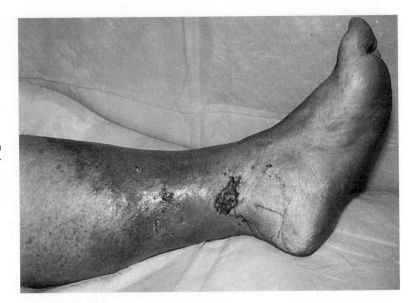

FIGURE 56–14 Chronic venous insufficiency with edema, hyperpigmentation, soft tissue fibrosis, and stasis ulcer.

It is important to evaluate the arterial supply carefully before sharp debridement. If the blood supply is inadequate, the margin of debridement is at risk for necrosis. Indications for surgical debridement include the presence of a draining sinus, an infected nongranulating ulcer, an abscess, osteomyelitis, necrotic abscess formation, exposed nonviable tissue, and exposed nongranulating cartilage or bone surface.[5]

In a patient with a chronic ulcer, the diagnosis of osteomyelitis can be extremely difficult. Although bone scans are generally used to diagnose osteomyelitis, in some cases magnetic resonance imaging may be more sensitive for detecting the early bone changes of osteomyelitis.[5] Once the presence of osteomyelitis is established, the area of infected bone should be debrided or excised.

With distal ischemia in a patient who is not a candidate for debridement or distal amputation, management may include protection of the extremity while awaiting demarcation and subsequent autoamputation in the affected region. Autoamputation is used to preserve as much of the residual limb as possible.

Venous stasis ulcer and associated chronic venous insufficiency are generally managed with moist dressings. On occasion, Unna boot compression is utilized. This is the application of a moistened gauze bandage impregnated with zinc oxide and glycerin. The bandage is covered with double-length, 4-in. compressive wrap in a figure-of-8 design. The patient or family members can be instructed in how to change the dressing once or twice a week. Hydrophilic polyurethane foam dressings (Allevyn) or hydrocolloid dressings (Duoderm) are alternative methods of wound care and can be applied under a compressive garment. When Duoderm is used, care must be taken with dressing changes to avoid desquamation. Measures to control edema are discussed on p 1190.

After the infection has been contained, edema controlled, and necessary revascularization performed, it is important to arrange for proper protective footwear. Total-contact casting has been shown to be beneficial for the treatment of neuropathic ulcers.[26, 56] The total-contact cast redistributes weight-bearing forces, decreases edema, protects the wound and surrounding tissues, decreases sheer forces, localizes infection, protects the foot from outside contaminants, and provides immobilization of the wound and Charcot joint.[10, 26] In previous research, casting allowed healing of even the most chronic neuropathic ulceration in an average of 33 to 38 days.[26, 56] A custom total-contact, bivalved polypropylene ankle-foot orthosis (AFO) with custom footbed has been tried recently. It is indicated if patients are unable to return for cast changes or if the referring physician desires continued access to the wound (Fig. 56–15). Although the use of this AFO appears promising, it has not been studied formally. When either a total-contact cast or a custom bivalved AFO is used, footwear on the sound side must be adjusted to avoid a leg-length discrepancy. After initial healing, a total-contact sandal with a custom footbed of moderate density, closed-cell, polyethylene foam and a poron (PPT) interface is fabricated. The patient wears this sandal for approximately 2 weeks until proceeding with definitive footwear. An appropriate definitive shoe is extra-depth with a custom moderate-density inlay. Footwear for the insensitive foot should accommodate rather than attempt to correct skeletal deformities. A rocker-bottom sole can help to further dissipate the forces of ambulation.[3]

A study of the recurrence of neuropathic ulcerations revealed that nearly half of the recurrences were solely attributable to failure to comply with the prescribed program.[27] Although a foot ulceration can be extensive, a lack of subjective pain often causes the patient to ignore a non–weight-bearing recommendation. To the person who has lost sensation, the limb does not just feel incompetent, it feels "dead." The body image of such a person excludes the dead part. It is the medical team's responsibility to convey that pain sensation can be compensated for by "intelligent anticipation."[4]

Patient Education

Patients should be instructed in proper skin management. They should inspect their feet every day for warmth, swelling, or redness. If erythema or warmth is present in the

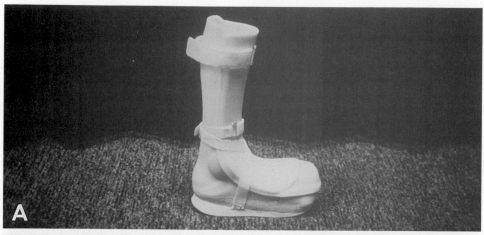

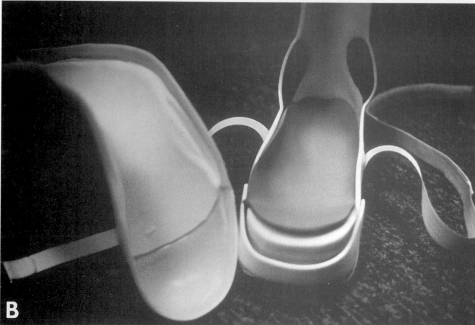

FIGURE 56–15 *A* and *B*, Custom total-contact, bivalved polypropylene ankle-foot orthosis with custom footbed. (Courtesy of Gretchen Hecht, CPO Sawtooth Orthotics, Boise.)

evening, the foot should be checked again the next morning. If it is still warm, it should be rested by walking less, wearing a different shoe, and taking short steps until the hot spot resolves.[3] Stockings with seams or tight circumferential elastic should be avoided. Patients should never go barefoot. Shoes must fit properly, be comfortable when purchased, gradually broken in, and changed daily to avoid breakdown caused by prolonged pressure.

References

1. Abramson DI: Physiologic basis for the use of physical agents in peripheral vascular disorders. Arch Phys Med Rehabil 1965; 46:216.
2. Bacharach JM, Rooke TW, Osmundson PJ, et al: Predictive value of transcutaneous oxygen pressure and amputation success by use of supine and elevation measurements. J Vasc Surg 1992; 15:558.
3. Brand PW (Project Director): The Cycle of Repetitive Stress on Insensitive Feet (project booklet). Supported in part by Social and Rehabilitation Service grant No. RC 75 MPO. Carville, La, United States Public Health Service Hospital, 1975.
4. Brand PW: The Quest for Artificial Pain (course program). Presented at the American Association of Electrodiagnostic Medicine meeting, New Orleans, Oct 7, 1993, pp 7–18.
5. Brodsky JW, Schneidler C: Diabetic foot infections. Orthop Clin North Am 1991; 22:473.
6. Browse NL, Burnand KG: The cause of venous ulceration. Lancet 1982; 2:243.
7. Carter SA: The relationship of distal systolic pressures to healing of skin lesions in limbs with arterial occlusive disease, with special reference to diabetes mellitus. Scand J Clin Lab Invest 1973; 31(suppl 128):239.
8. Casley-Smith JR, Morgan RG, Piller NB: Treatment of lymphedema of the arms and legs with 5,6-benzo-[α]-pyrone. N Engl J Med 1993; 329:1158.
9. Coffman JD: Vasodilator drugs in peripheral vascular disease. N Engl J Med 1979; 300:713.
10. Coleman WC, Brand PW, Birke JA: The total contact cast: A therapy for plantar ulceration on insensitive feet. J Am Podiatr Med Assoc 1984; 74:548.
11. Creasy TS, McMillan PJ, Fletcher EW, et al: Is percutaneous transluminal angioplasty better than exercise for claudication? Preliminary results from a prospective randomized trial. Eur J Vasc Surg 1990; 4:135.
12. Cronan JJ: Venous thromboembolic disease: The role of US. Radiology 1993; 186:619.
13. DeWeese JA, Leather R, Porter J: Practice guidelines: Lower extremity revascularization. J Vasc Surg 1993; 18:280.
14. Dodd HJ, Gaylarde PM, Sarkany I: Skin oxygen tension in venous insufficiency of the lower leg. J R Soc Med 1985; 78:373.
15. Ekroth R, Dahllöf A-G, Gundevall B, et al: Physical training of patients with intermittent claudication: Indications, methods, and results. Surgery 1978; 84:640.

16. Ernst CB, Stanley JC (ed): Therapy in Vascular Surgery, ed 2. Philadelphia, BC Decker, 1991.

17. Falanga V, Kirsner R, Katz MH, et al: Pericapillary fibrin cuffs in venous ulceration: Persistence with treatment and during ulcer healing. J Dermatol Surg Oncol 1992; 18:409.

18. Friedmann IW: Selecting the therapeutic alternative for rehabilitating patients with occlusive arterial disease. Vasc Surg 1977; 11:321.

19. Gersh BJ, Rihal CS, Rooke TW, et al: Evaluation and management of patients with both peripheral vascular and coronary artery disease. J Am Coll Cardiol 1991; 18:203.

20. Gibbons GW, Marcaccio EJ Jr, Burgess AM, et al: Improved quality of diabetic foot care, 1984 vs 1990. Arch Surg 1993; 128:576.

21. Gloviczki P, Calcagno D, Schirger A, et al: Noninvasive evaluation of the swollen extremity: Experiences with 190 lymphoscintigraphic examinations. J Vasc Surg 1989; 9:683.

22. Gloviczki P, Merrell SW: Surgical treatment of venous disease. Cardiovasc Clin 1992; 22:81.

23. Gloviczki P, Morris SM, Bower TC, et al: Microvascular pedal bypass for salvage of the severely ischemic limb. Mayo Clin Proc 1991; 66:243.

24. Gloviczki P, Stanson AW, Stickler GB, et al: Klippel-Trenaunay syndrome: The risks and benefits of vascular interventions. Surgery 1991; 110:469.

25. Gupta SK, Girishkumar H: Lower extremity revascularization. J Cardiovasc Surg 1993; 34:229.

26. Helm PA, Walker SC, Pullium G: Total contact casting in diabetic patients with neuropathic foot ulcerations. Arch Phys Med Rehabil 1984; 65:691.

27. Helm PA, Walker SC, Pullium GF: Recurrence of neuropathic ulceration following healing in a total contact cast. Arch Phys Med Rehabil 1991; 72:967.

28. Hertzer NR: The natural history of peripheral vascular disease: Implications for its management. Circulation 1991; 83(suppl 1):1–12.

29. Honet JC, Strandness DE Jr, Stolov WC, et al: Short-leg bracing for intermittent claudication of the calf. Arch Phys Med Rehabil 1968; 49:578.

30. Jamieson WG: State of the art of venous investigation and treatment. Can J Surg 1993; 36:119.

31. Jonason T, Jonzon B, Ringqvist I, et al: Effect of physical training on different categories of patients with intermittent claudication. Acta Med Scand 1979; 206:253.

32. Juergens JL, Spittell JA Jr, Fairbairn JF II: Peripheral Vascular Disease, ed 5. Philadelphia, WB Saunders, 1980.

33. Nicolaides AN, Hussein MK, Szendro G, et al: The relation of venous ulceration with ambulatory venous pressure measurements. J Vasc Surg 1993; 17:414.

34. Orchard TJ, Strandness DE Jr: Assessment of peripheral vascular disease in diabetes: Report and recommendations of an International Workshop sponsored by the American Heart Association and the American Diabetes Association, 18–20 September 1992, New Orleans. Diabetes Care 1993; 16:1199.

35. Osmundson PJ, Rooke TW, Hallett JW: Effect of arterial revascularization on transcutaneous oxygen tension of the ischemic extremity. Mayo Clin Proc 1988; 63:897.

36. Pappas CJ, O'Donnell TF: Long-term results of compression treatment for lymphedema. J Vasc Surg 1992; 16:555.

37. Pomposelli FB Jr, Jepsen SJ, Gibbons GW, et al: Efficacy of the dorsal pedal bypass for limb salvage in diabetic patients: Short-term observations. J Vasc Surg 1990; 11:745.

38. Porter JM, Cutter BS, Lee BY, et al: Pentoxifylline efficacy in the treatment of intermittent claudication: Multicenter controlled double-blind trial with objective assessment of chronic occlusive arterial disease patients. Am Heart J 1982; 104:66.

39. Porter JM, Rutherford RB, Claggett JP, et al: Reporting standards in venous disease. J Vasc Surg 1988; 8:172.

40. Richardson JK: Rocker-soled shoes and walking distance in patients with calf claudication. Arch Phys Med Rehabil 1991; 72:554.

41. Rooke TW: The noninvasive vascular laboratory. Cardiovasc Clin 1992; 22:27.

42. Rooke TW: The use of transcutaneous oximetry in the noninvasive vascular laboratory. Int Angiol 1992; 11:36.

43. Rooke TW, Heser JL, Osmundson PJ: Exercise strain-gauge venous plethysmography: Evaluation of a "new" device for assessing lower limb venous incompetence. Angiology 1992; 43:219.

44. Rooke TW, Hollier LH, Osmundson PJ: The influence of sympathetic nerves on transcutaneous oxygen tension in normal and ischemic lower extremities. Angiology 1987; 38:400.

45. Rooke TW, Martin RP: Lower extremity venous imaging for the echocardiologist. J Am Soc Echocardiogr 1990; 3:158.

46. Rooke TW, Osmundson PJ: Effect of intermittent venous occlusion on transcutaneous oxygen tension in lower limbs with severe arterial occlusive disease. Int J Cardiol 1988; 21:76.

47. Rooke TW, Osmundson PJ: Variability and reproducibility of transcutaneous oxygen tension measurements in the assessment of peripheral vascular disease. Angiology 1989; 40:695.

48. Schwartz RW, Logan NM, Johnson PJ, et al: Pentoxifylline increases extremity blood flow in diabetic atherosclerotic patients. Arch Surg 1989; 124:434.

49. Spittell JA Jr: Conservative management of occlusive peripheral arterial disease. Cardiovasc Clin 1992; 22:209.

50. Stillwell GK: The law of Laplace: Some clinical applications. Mayo Clin Proc 1973; 48:863.

51. Stillwell GK, Redford JWB: Physical treatment of postmastectomy lymphedema. Proc Staff Meet Mayo Clin 1958; 33:1.

52. Strandness DE Jr, Langlois YE, Roederer GO: Noninvasive evaluation of vascular disease. In Haimovici H (ed): Vascular Surgery: Principles and Techniques, ed 2. Norwalk, Conn, Appleton-Century-Crofts, 1984, pp 19–42.

53. Strandness DE Jr, Langlois YE, Roederer GO: Preoperative evaluation of vascular disease. In Haimovici H (ed): Vascular Surgery: Principles and Techniques, ed 2. Norwalk, Conn, Appleton-Century-Crofts, 1984, pp 43–64.

54. Strandness DE Jr, Sumner DS: Applications of ultrasound to the study of arteriosclerosis obliterans. Angiology 1975; 26:187.

55. Tannenbaum GA, Pomposelli FB Jr, Marcaccio EJ, et al: Safety of vein bypass grafting to the dorsal pedal artery in diabetic patients with foot infections. J Vasc Surg 1992; 15:982.

56. Walker SC, Helm PA, Pullium G: Total contact casting and chronic diabetic neuropathic foot ulcerations: Healing rates by wound location. Arch Phys Med Rehabil 1987; 68:217.

57. Weiss RA: Evaluation of the venous system by Doppler ultrasound and photoplethysmography or light reflection rheography before sclerotherapy. Semin Dermatol 1993; 12:78.

Reading List

Berni GA, Bandyk DF, Zierler RE, et al: Streptokinase treatment of acute arterial occlusion. Ann Surg 1983; 198:185.

Mills JL, Beckett WC, Taylor SM: The diabetic foot: Consequences of delayed treatment and referral. South Med J 1991; 84:970.

Rooke TW, Osmundson PJ: The influence of age, sex, smoking, and diabetes on lower limb transcutaneous oxygen tension in patients with arterial occlusive disease. Arch Intern Med 1990; 150:129.

Sørlie D, Myhre K, Mjøs OD: Exercise- and post-exercise metabolism of the lower leg in patients with peripheral arterial insufficiency. Scand J Clin Lab Invest 1978; 38:635.

Strandness DE Jr, Priest RE, Gibbons GE: Combined clinical and pathological study of diabetic and nondiabetic peripheral arterial disease. Diabetes 1964; 13:366.

Principles of Cancer Rehabilitation

FAE H. GARDEN, M.D.,
AND THERESA A. GILLIS, M.D.

The number of people who have survived 5 years or more with a history of cancer is now estimated to be 4 million.[38] As this number continues to grow, medical professionals will have to redefine the term "cancer survivor" to take into consideration various quality-of-life issues that were not relevant a decade ago.

DEFINING THE NEED FOR CANCER REHABILITATION

The fact that cancer patients develop functional deficits resulting from their disease and treatment has been discussed in the medical literature for years.[50] Although it has been stated that "almost all patients with cancer can benefit from a rehabilitation assessment and intervention,"[31] convincing oncologists and oncologic surgeons of these needs and of the potential role of rehabilitation services has been a challenge.

With the exception of stomach and cervical tumors, the incidence rates for all of the major cancers have been increasing over the past four decades.[21] Advances in early cancer detection combined with aggressive, multimodal treatments are allowing more people with cancer to live longer. These cancer survivors frequently are left to face significant physical and psychosocial problems that adversely influence their quality of life (Fig. 57–1). Ganz et al.[32] surveyed 500 patients with colorectal, lung, and prostate cancer who had been living with cancer for over a year and found that over 80% reported gait problems, with 50% indicating that these problems were severe. Significant problems in activities of daily living and vocational pursuits were also reported (Fig. 57–2). It has been estimated that up to 50% of persons with cancer may meet the diagnostic criteria for clinical depression.[81] The severity of the depression often correlates with the degree of physical impairment. With early intervention by a rehabilitation team, long-term disability caused by cancer and cancer therapy can be prevented or minimized. The typical members of a cancer rehabilitation team are listed in Table 57–1.

Types of Cancer Rehabilitation

The general rehabilitation goals of cancer patients are similar to those of patients with impairments caused by other diseases. They include obtaining independent mobility and independence in basic activities of daily living, with or without assistive devices. Rehabilitation goals can be further defined according to when they are applied in the different stages of the disease.[77] The goal of *preventive rehabilitation therapy* is to achieve maximal function in patients considered to be cured or in remission. For patients whose cancer is progressing, the goals of *supportive rehabilitation therapy* include providing adaptive self-care equipment in an attempt to offset what can be a steady decline in a patient's functional skills. Range-of-motion (ROM) exercises and bed mobility techniques can be taught in order to prevent the adverse consequences of immobility (see also Chapter 34). *Palliative rehabilitation therapy* goals are to improve or maintain comfort and function during the terminal stages of the disease.[39] The application of orthoses, modalities, and assistive equipment may be useful as an adjunct to pharmacological pain management.

CAUSES AND MANAGEMENT OF FUNCTIONAL IMPAIRMENT IN CANCER PATIENTS

Complications of Disuse and Bed Rest

The complications of immobility are described in detail in Chapter 34. These complications are pertinent in the cancer patient because of the typically prolonged period of illness, treatment, and recovery. Special issues in the cancer

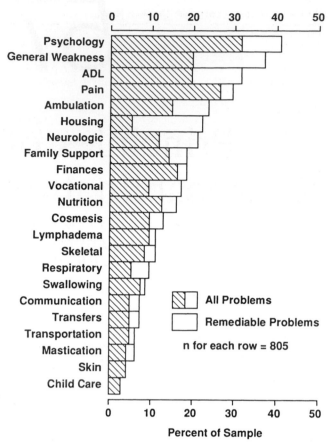

FIGURE 57–1 Percent of people in sample with one or more rehabilitation problems. (From Lehmann JF, DeLisa JA, Warren CG, et al: Cancer rehabilitation: Assessment of need, development and evaluation of a model of care. Arch Phys Med Rehabil 1978; 59:412.)

patient can include side effects of chemotherapy, especially involving cardiotoxic drugs. When possible, a conditioning program started prior to cancer treatment is advisable.

Nutritional Concerns of Cancer Patients

Diet

Dietary factors have been in the research and media spotlight recently as an important environmental influence on cancer prevention. The value and benefit of nutrition is generally recognized in the medical management and rehabilitation of cancer patients, and many cancer patients place quality of appetite and ability to eat at the top of the list of items determining their sense of physical well-being.[12]

Cancer rehabilitation programs should include a registered dietician as a member of the comprehensive treatment team. The dietician can initiate a screening process that takes into account the tumor type and treatment plan to determine if a patient's nutritional status is at risk. From anthropomorphic data, an estimate of adult calorie and protein needs can be made. Caloric intake should generally be between 115% and 130% of resting energy expenditure. Protein needs range from 1.5 to 2.5 g/kg/day.[12, 55] Calorie and protein needs will vary depending on the type and extent of the tumor, as well as the type of treatment being

used. The impact of various surgical procedures on the nutritional status of cancer patients is summarized in Table 57–2.

Radiation Effects

Radiation therapy can also affect feeding and nutrition. Treatments to the head and neck area can produce alterations in taste and in saliva production. Distortion of food temperature and texture sensations can occur from radiation changes to the oral mucosa. Swallowing difficulties can result as well (see Chapter 27). Radiation to the stomach and intestines often leads acutely to nausea, vomiting, cramps, and diarrhea. Chronic complications include partial or complete intestinal obstruction, intestinal perforation, gastrointestinal bleeding, malabsorption, and enteral fistulas.[85] Attempts to feed patients with radiation damage to

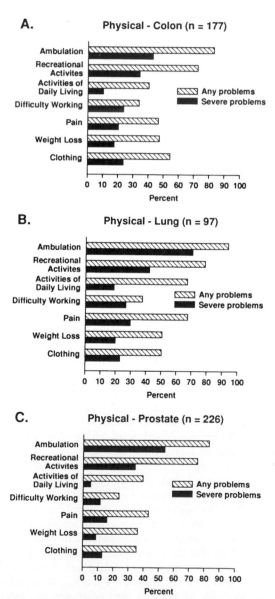

FIGURE 57–2 Constitutional and physical problems in colon (A), lung (B), and prostate (C) cancer patients living with cancer for more than a year since diagnosis. (From Haskell CM: Cancer Treatment, ed 3. Philadelphia, WB Saunders, 1990, p 885.)

TABLE 57–1   Typical Members of a Cancer Rehabilitation Team and Brief Descriptions of Their Common Roles

Physiatrist
Evaluates the medical rehabilitation issues and assists with diagnosis and management. Rehabilitation issues can include neurogenic bladder and bowel management; pain control; prosthetic and orthotic fitting; and management of spasticity and weakness. Physiatrists are skilled interdisciplinary team leaders and can assist with the bridging between rehabilitation efforts and medical issues.

Nurse
Helps assess patient care issues and facilitates the coordination of services provided. Provides patients with education regarding their disease and helps with discharge planning. Monitors health maintenance issues such as skin care. Helps provide emotional support

Physical Therapist
Helps assess mobility issues such as transfers and gait. Restores physical abilities through modalities and exercise. Uses physical means to control pain.

Occupational Therapist
Assesses self-care capabilities and retrains as appropriate using adaptive aids as needed. Uses functional activities to help restore endurance. Helps assess splinting needs and positioning issues. Assists with vocational evaluation issues as appropriate. Provides functional, cognitive, and safety evaluations.

Recreational Therapist
Helps with community reintegration, avocational activities, self-esteem, and functional tasks.

Social Worker
Evaluates psychosocial factors, including family support, financial resources, and patient and family expectations. Interfaces with community resources. Provides emotional support to patient and family. Assists with discharge planning.

Primary Physician
If the primary physician is other than the physiatrist, he not only provides the medial management but gives valuable support to the rest of the care team through interaction with the patient and family; essential in focusing on critical medical issues that affect discharge and hospital care.

Psychologist/Psychiatrist
Helps assist with dysfunctional adjustment issues of both patient and family. Assists the care team in high-stress situations to avoid anger and other improper responses. Provides cognitive assessments of central nervous system–compromised patients.

Pharmacist
Provides input into medication options to healthcare team. Helps educate patient and family in drug side effects.

Dietitian
Helps assess nutritional status and provides alternative dietary options. Educates family when appropriate regarding dietary goals.

Chaplain
Provides emotional and religious assessment and support. Helps the team focus on quality-of-life issues and the proper role of medical intervention in the terminally ill patient.

Speech-Language Pathologist
Helps assess communication issues and recommends best options to team in communicating with language- or speech-impaired patients. Assists in selecting augmentative communication devices, and provides swallowing evaluation and treatment.

Adapted courtesy of DePompolo RW: Development and administration of a cancer rehabilitation program. In Garden FH, Grabois M (eds): Cancer Rehabilitation State of the Art Reviews, vol 8. Philadelphia, Hanley & Belfus, 1994, p 419.

the intestines usually begin with lactose-free, low residue oral diets and progress to enteral feedings or parenteral nutrition in more refractory cases.[57] Parenteral nutrition is recommended for patients who have lost 20% or more of their body weight.[22, 82]

Chemotherapy Effects

Cancer chemotherapeutic agents are targeted against the cell processes of malignant tumors. The rapidly reproduc-

TABLE 57–2   Potential Adverse Effects on Nutrition of Various Surgical Procedures in Cancer Patients

Procedure	Potential Adverse Effect
Neck dissection/glossectomy	Impaired mastication
	Impaired swallowing
	Impaired taste
	Impaired smell
Esophageal resection with vagotomy	Gastric stasis
	Diarrhea
	Steatorrhea
Pancreatomy	Diabetes mellitus
	Impaired digestion
Bowel resection	Malabsorption (short bowel syndrome)
	Vitamin deficiency (B_{12}, D, A)
Gastrectomy	Impaired digestion
	Malabsorption
	Megaloblastic anemia
	Hypoglycemia

ing cells of the bone marrow and gastrointestinal tract are vulnerable to the effects of chemotherapy as well. Nausea, vomiting, and anorexia are common initial gastrointestinal side effects. Severe and recurrent vomiting may cause vitamin B_1 deficiency with resultant beriberi. Late effects of chemotherapy include stomatitis, mucosal ulceration, cheilosis, glossitis, and pharyngitis.

Numerous nutritional deficiencies can result from the use of antimetabolite drugs such as methotrexate. Folic acid metabolism, which is necessary for the synthesis of DNA, is inhibited by this drug. This inhibition causes a folic acid deficiency that results in macrocytic anemia, leukopenia, and an ulcerative stomatitis. The antimetabolites 5-fluorouracil and 6-mercaptopurine prevent nucleic acid synthesis by interfering with thiamine in DNA synthesis. Clinical signs of thiamine deficiency can be noted in the lips and oral cavity. Vitamin K deficiency results from long-term treatment with antibiotics such as moxalactam disodium, which can result in ecchymosis and a pronounced bleeding tendency.

Learned Food Aversion

During the course of cancer treatment, patients often reject specific foods or certain flavors. Although the exact mechanism for learned food aversion (LFA) is unknown, it has been described as a variant of classical conditioning. The types of foods most susceptible to LFA are meats, vegetables, and caffeinated beverages.[57] Various methods have been used to try to prevent LFAs. These include advising patients to eat very little before therapies.[6]

Proper nutritional support can be an important adjunct to cancer treatments. Aggressive intervention to correct nutrient deficiencies and to maintain good nutritional status should be ongoing throughout the rehabilitation process. When needed, enteral or parenteral feeding supplementation is useful in preventing weight loss, malnutrition, dehydration, and weakness.

Sexual Function in the Cancer Patient

The potential for sexual alteration or dysfunction is often ignored in cancer treatment plans. Yet both the cancer and the cancer treatment can affect the arena (see Chapter 30). Inclusion of the possible impact of treatment on sexuality can be part of the informed consent procedure.[84] Although most patients select treatments regardless of the potential for disfigurement, some refuse to risk the loss of a sex organ or body part.

Sexual partners can contribute to sexual dysfunction by fostering dependent role changes or reacting in a negative way to the patient's physical disfigurement. Economic stress caused by the treatment can lead to marital problems that are expressed by avoidance of sexual contact. These issues must be sought out and addressed.

Concerns of Women

While mastectomy has no direct physical effect on a woman's sexual response, the emotional effects of the procedure can have a profound negative impact. Fear of partner rejection can lead to the avoidance of sexual intercourse. Encouraging partners to resume sexual activity as early as possible helps break this cycle.

Women who have undergone pelvic surgery can feel a sense of guilt related to a false belief that sexual intercourse contributed to their disease.[10] Fear of having a disease recurrence can cause these women to avoid resumption of sexual activity. Women need to be counseled about the possible need for vaginal dilators to prevent stenosis as well as the possibility of bleeding with intercourse. The need for artificial lubrication and possibly a change from customary sexual positions should be discussed.

Regardless of a patient's age, the loss of fertility can precipitate a grief reaction. Presurgical preparation and counseling can reduce some of the psychodynamic causes of sexual dysfunction.

The side effects of chemotherapy and radiation therapy include nausea, fatigue, hair loss, and weight changes. These, along with hormonal depletion, can produce additional psychological and physical impediments to resuming sexual relationships.

Concerns of Men

Surgical treatment of prostate cancer can cause damage to the vascular or nerve pathways resulting in impotence, retrograde ejaculation, or infertility. Orchiectomy has obvious hormonal and reproductive implications. Preoperative and pretreatment discussion of reproductive concerns should include consideration of sperm banking if permanent sterilization is anticipated.

Pelvic or abdominal radiation can produce fatigue, diarrhea, and erectile dysfunction. Irradiation to the urethra can cause painful ejaculation.[18] Effects of chemotherapy can adversely affect self-image, libido, and sexual performance. Sexual rehabilitation can include the use of erectile assistive devices and surgical reconstruction of the phallus.

Neuropsychological Abnormalities

The scope of neurobehavioral abnormalities found in tumor patients ranges from subtle problems with attention and motivation to frank delirium and clouding of consciousness. These deficits can be due to either the primary effects of the tumor or the secondary effects of treatment. They can also be due to the experience of chronic illness, depression, or immobility.

Primary Tumor Effects

The majority of patients with primary or metastatic brain tumors have cognitive impairments that vary depending on the location and size of the tumor. The pattern of neuropsychological deficits in patients with primary brain tumors can differ from those seen in cerebrovascular accidents or traumatic brain injury. Patients with brain tumors can have milder cognitive deficits and greater variability in the nature and extent of these deficits than patients with strokes in similar anatomical sites.[2] Even after extensive surgical resection of brain tissue, patients with slow-growing tumors often do not demonstrate neuropsychological deficits, which is perhaps due to a reorganization of cognitive functions to other brain regions.[60] Patients with rapidly growing tumors, such as glioblastoma multiforme, exhibit behavioral and cognitive deficits secondary to rapid destruction of white matter tracts, increased intracranial pressure, and metabolic deficits.[61]

Radiation Effects

Additional effects on neuropsychological functioning can occur as a result of radiation therapy. The acute effects of radiation (during the time of treatment) are mostly symptomatic (headache and nausea). Subacute effects can occur 1 to 4 months after therapy is completed. At this time a reversible demyelination occurs in approximately 14% of brain tumor patients.[45] It is only by a gradual improvement in functional status during the ensuing 16 weeks that these symptoms can be distinguished from those caused by early tumor recurrence.[41] Delayed effects of radiation can occur 6 months to a year after therapy. The therapeutic dose of radiation for brain tumors can cause necrosis within 6 months of treatment.[64] Most of these lesions develop within the white matter of the forebrain.[89] In addition to focal necrosis, delayed effects of brain irradiation can include atrophy calcification, necrotizing leukoencephalopathy, aneurysms, and the formation of secondary cancers.[45]

Chemotherapy Effects

Chemotherapy, which was once believed to cause only early and reversible effects on cognition, can actually be associated with marked and prolonged neurobehavioral deficits. It is estimated that as many as 18% of neurologically normal cancer patients who have received chemotherapy have cognitive deficits 3 weeks after therapy is discontinued.[59] These include deficits of impaired visual-perceptive abilities, verbal memory, and judgment. Survivors of brain tumors who have received multimodal therapy (chemotherapy plus radiation) can have more profound impairments of intellectual function than those undergoing single-modality treatment.[40] As cancer therapy becomes more effective, an increasing number of survivors will be in need of cognitive and vocational rehabilitation services.

Cancer Pain

Defining the Problem

The World Health Organization (WHO) estimates that 25% of all cancer patients die with unrelieved pain.[15] Up to 60% of patients at all stages of the disease process experience significant pain.[8] Most of this pain can be adequately relieved by oral analgesics.[88, 90] Unrelieved pain can be a risk factor for suicide in cancer patients.[11]

Etiology

Cancer pain can result from direct tumor invasion of pain-sensitive tissues secondary to treatment or diagnostic procedures (Table 57–3), or be unrelated to any of these factors.

Treatment

An algorithm for medical decision making in the treatment of cancer pain has been devised by WHO (Fig. 57–3). This three-step analgesic drug ladder outlines the use of nonopioid analgesics, opioid analgesics, and adjuvants for progressively more severe pain. Nonopioid analgesics, such as nonsteroidal anti-inflammatory agents (NSAIDs), are associated with ceiling effects for analgesia. Exceeding the

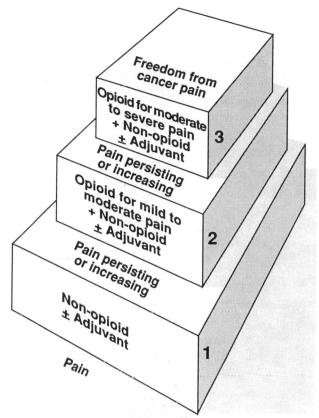

FIGURE 57–3 The WHO three-step analgesic ladder. (From Cancer Pain Relief and Palliative Care: Report of a WHO Expert Committee (technical report series, No. 804). Geneva, World Health Organization, 1990.)

TABLE 57–3   Causes of Treatment-Related Pain in Cancer Patients

Chemotherapy-related pain
  Oral mucositis
  Peripheral neuropathy
  Acute and chronic herpetic pain
  Osteonecrosis secondary to steroids
  Pseudorheumatism
Radiation-related pain
  Osteoradionecrosis
  Myelopathy
  Brachial plexopathy
  Lumbar plexopathy
  Radiation-induced peripheral nerve tumors
Postsurgical pain
  Post mastectomy
  Post nephrectomy
  Post thoracotomy
  Post radical neck dissection
  Residual limb and phantom limb
Procedure-related pain
  Bone marrow biopsy
  Bone biopsy
  Lumbar puncture and spinal headache
  Venipuncture

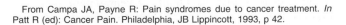

From Campa JA, Payne R: Pain syndromes due to cancer treatment. *In* Patt R (ed): Cancer Pain. Philadelphia, JB Lippincott, 1993, p 42.

maximum dose range can result in organ toxicity that can mask similar toxicities due to antineoplastic agents if the two are used concomitantly.

Opioid agonists do not exhibit ceiling effects. Dosing is guided by efficacy and is limited by side effects (Table 57–4). Long-acting oral preparations, particularly sustained-release morphine, are commonly used. Breakthrough pain can be treated with immediate-release "rescue doses" of morphine. Although the oral route of administration is preferred, transdermal, rectal, and intravenous routes are indicated in some patients. Spinal routes, (both epidural and intrathecal) can be employed with internal delivery systems that allow patients to be fully ambulatory. Children often require relatively larger doses of opioids to achieve adequate pain relief.[58]

Tolerance to analgesia is an infrequent problem and is usually managed by changing doses or agents.[29] Physical dependence develops with chronic opioid use. *Addiction*, defined as a behavioral syndrome of compulsive, harmful use not requiring the existence of physical dependence or tolerance,[42] is not likely to occur in patients without a substance abuse history.[75] If necessary, the withdrawing of opiates should be done slowly. The autonomic symptoms of withdrawal can be partly alleviated by the use of transdermal clonidine (Catapres).[53]

Adjuvant drugs include antidepressants, anticonvulsants, benzodiazepines, neuroleptics, psychostimulants, antihistamines, corticosteroids, and calcitonin. These medications

TABLE 57–4   Oral and Parenteral Opioid Analgesic Equivalences and Relative Potency of Drugs as Compared With Morphine

	Parenteral (mg)	Oral (mg)	Conversion Factor (IV to po)	Duration (Parenteral, Oral) (hr)
Narcotic Agonists				
Morphine	10	30	3.0[1]	3–4
Controlled-release morphine				
MS Contin	—	30	—	12
Roxanol SR	—	30	—	8
Methadone (Dolophine)[2]	10	20	2.0	4–8
Hydromorphone (Dilaudid)	1.5	7.5	5.0	2–3
Fentanyl[3]	100 μg	—	—	1
Meperidine (Demerol)[4]	75	300	4.0	2–3
Levorphanol (Levo-Dromoran)	2	4	2.0	3–6
Codeine	130	200	1.5	3–4
Oxycodone (Roxicodone, component of Percodan, Tylox)[5]	—	30	—	3–5
Hydrocodone (Lortab, component of Vicodin)[5]	—	200[6]	—	3–5
Propoxyphene (Darvon, component of Darvocet)[2,5]	—	200	—	3–6
Mixed Agonist-Antagonists[7]				
Pentazocine (Talwin)	60	180	3.0	2–4
Nalbuphine (Nubain)	10	—	—	4–6
Butorphanol (Stadol)	2	—	—	4–6

[1]Conversion factor listed is for chronic dosing: single doses may require 6:1 factor.
[2]Long half-life; observe for drug accumulation and side effects.
[3]Available in transdermal system (Duragesic) supplying 25, 50, 75, or 100 μg.
[4]Not recommended for long-term or high-dose use because of CNS toxic metabolites (normeperidine, norpropoxyphene).
[5]With the exception of Roxicodone and Darvon, these drugs are combined with acetylsalicylic acid (ASA) or acetaminophen in doses from 325 to 750 mg. Dosage must be monitored for safe limits of ASA or acetaminophen.
[6]Equivalence data not substantiated; thought to approximate codeine.
[7]*Note:* Drugs from this category should NOT be used in combination with narcotic agonist drugs. Converting a patient from an agonist to an agonist-antagonist could precipitate a withdrawal crisis in the narcotic-dependent patient.
Courtesy of C. Stratton Hill, Jr., M.D., and the Texas Cancer Pain Initiative, Houston.

are chosen to supplement analgesics for their specific secondary effects or to treat side effects.

A significant number of patients whose pain does not respond to oral therapy might be helped by anesthetic procedures, such as nerve blocks. Surgical ablation of nervous structures by procedures such as rhizotomy or cordotomy can also play a role in pain relief for certain patients. There is, however, a risk of developing a delayed pain syndrome following such surgical deafferentation.

Deafferentation pain can be caused by a loss of normal sensory input when a peripheral nerve is severed or involved by tumor. Transcutaneous electrical nerve stimulation can provide some patients with relief. In addition, carefully selected patients might also benefit from surgical implantation of stimulation devices.[24]

LATE EFFECTS OF CANCER TREATMENT

Radiation Therapy

Myelopathy

The effects of radiation damage to the spinal cord and peripheral nervous systems are multifactorial and cannot be entirely attributed to dosage, site, or technique. The most common form of radiation-induced spinal cord injury is a transient myelopathy that occurs in patients being treated for head and neck tumors or lymphoma. The syndrome typically develops after a latent period of 1 to 30 months with a peak onset at 4 to 6 months.[23] A transient demyelination of the ascending sensory neurons in the posterior column and lateral spinothalamic tract is postulated as the pathogenesis for this disorder. The clinical onset is marked by electrical shock sensations or paresthesias that radiate from the cervical spine to the extremities. The paresthesias are typically symmetrical and do not follow a dermatomal distribution.[54] Myelography and computed tomography (CT) scans are typically normal, and the syndrome usually resolves in 1 to 9 months.[23] The occurrence of transient radiation myelopathy does not put a person at a higher risk for the development of more severe delayed radiation myelopathy.[23]

Delayed myelopathy is an irreversible condition with a reported incidence of 1% to 12%.[80] The onset of symptoms usually occurs 9 to 18 months after completion of treatment[23] with the majority of cases occurring within 30 months. The latent period for delayed myelopathy decreases with increased radiation dose and is shortened in children.[54] The onset of symptoms usually begins with lower extremity paresthesias followed by sphincter dysfunction and weakness. A partial Brown-Séquard syndrome consisting of sensory changes on one side and motor weakness or pyramidal tract signs on the opposite side can develop below the level of the injury. Functional deficits typically occur progressively and depend, for the most part, on the level of neurological injury. A central pain syndrome can be present in up to 20% of patients with radiation

TABLE 57–5   Differential Diagnosis Between Cancerous and Postradiation Brachial Plexopathies

Parameter	Cancerous	Postradiation
Incidence	10 times more common	Dose-related
Initial symptom	Pain 90%	Numbness, paresthesia, pain in less than 20%
Signs	Predominantly lower trunk	Predominantly upper trunk
Progression rate	Slow	Insidious, self-limiting
Latency	Months to over 20 yr; mean: several years	
Tumor progression	CT: focal lesions in over 90%	CT: loss of planes, no focal lesions
EMG		Myokymia

Abbreviations: EMG, electromyography; *CT,* computed tomography. From Hildebrand J: Lesions of the peripheral nervous system. *In* Hildebrand J (ed): Management in Neuro-Oncology. Berlin, Springer-Verlag, 1992, p 80.

myelopathy. Patients typically note pain in their midback region and dysesthetic sensations in their lower extremities. Central pain syndrome may show some clinical response to treatment with tricyclic antidepressants, steroids, or anticonvulsant medications.

Plexopathy

Brachial plexopathy is a well-recognized complication of radiotherapy in patients with breast, lung, and mediastinal tumors, as well as lymphoma and other neoplasms. The latent period between the end of radiotherapy and the appearance of clinical symptoms ranges from 1 month to 15 years.[27] Chemotherapy can enhance the radiation-induced effects on nerve tissue and decrease the latency period for the development of plexopathy.[69] The predominant initial symptoms are paresthesias and pain (Table 57–5). Clinical signs include sensory loss, decreased or absent reflexes, and weakness.

The distinction between radiation-induced brachial plexopathy and that due to neoplastic infiltrations is often a clinical challenge. Horner's syndrome and pain are more common in neoplastic plexopathy, whereas extremity lymphedema is more common in radiation plexopathy.[49] Electrodiagnosis has also been used to help differentiate between metastatic and radiation-induced plexopathy. Myokymic discharges and abnormal sensory conduction studies are more common in patients with radiation plexopathy than in those with neoplastic plexopathy.[36]

Rehabilitation management of radiation plexopathy includes providing adequate pain relief, maximizing the remaining function, and preventing the complications of immobility. After acute pain and inflammation have subsided, patients can be started on low-resistance weight exercises and gradually be increased to a full shoulder and arm rehabilitation program. Neck rehabilitation exercises should be included, especially when the upper portion of the plexus has been injured. The shoulder often requires the support of a sling to prevent glenohumeral subluxation. Substitutes for lost hand and arm function include the use of flexor-hinge tenodesis and opponens splints. Wheelchair users with brachial plexopathy can benefit from using a balanced forearm orthosis (BFO) for feeding and self-care. A functional arm orthosis attached to a hip cap can be constructed for the ambulatory patient.

Lumbosacral plexopathy is reported less frequently than brachial plexopathy but can occur in patients with colorectal and gynecological tumors who undergo radiation therapy. Symptoms often present bilaterally although seldom in a symmetrical fashion (Table 57–6). Pain or paresthesias usually precede the development of motor symptoms, which include weakness and muscle atrophy.[66]

Chemotherapy

Neurotoxicity is a common complication of cancer chemotherapy. A progressive distal symmetrical sensory neuropathy occurs with cisplatin treatment.[30] Vincristine and cytarabine also have peripheral neuropathy as a principal toxic and dose-limiting side effect (see Chapter 46). Encephalopathies, cerebellar syndromes, myopathy, and stroke-like syndromes can all occur after the administration of various chemotherapeutic agents.

Bleeding Problems

Both chemotherapeutic and radiotherapeutic procedures can cause thrombocytopenia. Exercise in the presence of thrombocytopenia can increase the risk of intra-articular bleeding. Bleeding from the lungs or oral and nasal mucosa can also occur. In general, platelet levels below 10,000/mm³ preclude exercise therapy and the risk of intracerebral bleeding becomes significant below this level.[3, 43] Some centers allow aerobic but not resistive activities in patients with platelet counts between 10,000 and 20,000/mm³.[73]

TABLE 57–6   Differential Diagnosis Between Cancerous and Postradiation Lumbosacral Plexopathies

Parameter	Cancerous	Postradiation
Primaries	Colorectal, sarcomas, lymphomas, breast carcinoma	Cervical ovarian carcinoma; dose-related
Initial symptom	Pain in 70%–80%	Weakness in about 50%
Signs	Bilateral in 10%–25%	Bilateral in 80%
Latency	Variable	Median 5 yr; 1–31 yr
Tumor progression	Focal CT/MRI abnormalities	No focal abnormalities
EMG		Myokymia

Abbreviations: CT, computed tomography; *MRI,* magnetic resonance imaging; *EMG,* electromyography. From Hildebrand J: Lesions of the peripheral nervous system. *In* Hildebrand J (ed): Management in Neuro-Oncology. Berlin, Springer-Verlag, 1992, p 80.

REHABILITATION ISSUES IN SPECIFIC CANCERS

Breast Cancer

Eighteen percent of all cancer deaths in women are due to breast cancer, and it remains the leading cause of death for women 40 to 55 years of age.[65]

Surgical Options

Standard treatment has evolved from radical mastectomies to breast conservation strategies. Radical mastectomy requires resection of both the pectoralis major and minor muscles, as well as the axillary lymph nodes. This leads to significant shoulder dysfunction, pain, lymphedema, and emotional trauma. Modified radical mastectomies (MRMs), which spare the pectoralis major but include axillary dissection, are now more common. Other surgical options include lumpectomy, segmental (partial mastectomy), or simple (total) mastectomy with or without axillary dissection. Varying combinations of radiotherapy, hormonal therapy, and adjuvant chemotherapy augment the surgery and have reduced mortality. New trends toward immediate reconstruction appear to have a positive impact on function. A common breast reconstruction procedure is the transverse rectus abdominis muscle (TRAM) flap (Fig. 57–4), which leads to a weakened abdominal musculature in some patients.[37, 51] Other reconstruction options include the use of tissue expanders followed by prosthetic implants, and latissimus dorsi transfers.

Rehabilitation Issues

The most common rehabilitation needs of women undergoing MRM or segmental mastectomy during the first month after primary treatment are listed in Figure 57–5.[33] The most frequently cited physical problems include a tight chest wall, difficulty lifting, limited upper extremity mobility, arm weakness and numbness, and lymphedema. The mobility limitations and weakness affect these patients' daily functional tasks, such as household chores, lifting, driving, and general physical activity level. Early physical therapy has been shown to improve postoperative shoulder motion[74] while delayed therapy is associated with poor ROM.[28]

In postmastectomy patients who have not undergone reconstruction, an ROM of 40 degrees of shoulder abduction and flexion is permitted immediately postoperatively. Some physicians prefer the use of abduction slings or pillows immediately postoperatively, with the goal of ensuring painless shoulder movement within this range.[4, 19]

Immediate postoperative therapies can safely consist of hand pumping, wrist and elbow ROM exercises, positioning techniques, and postural exercise. Deep breathing and methods of relaxation are appropriate as well. A gentle supine passive shoulder ROM program to 40 degrees of flexion is begun as well, with external and internal rotation performed to tolerance. When surgical drains are removed, active-assisted range can be increased. At this time, wall climbing, wand and overhead pulley exercises are also added. After all sutures have been removed, more aggressive ROM exercise is pursued. The use of physical modal-

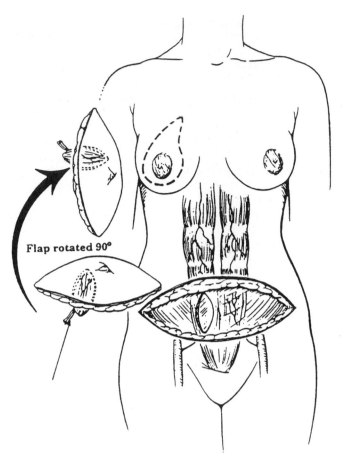

FIGURE 57–4 Transverse rectus abdominis muscle flap breast reconstruction in which the skin, subcutaneous tissue, and a portion of the rectus abdominis muscle and rectus sheath are removed from the lower abdomen and transferred to the chest for shaping into a breast mound. (From Miller MJ, Ross MR: Pregnancy following breast reconstruction with autogenous tissue. Cancer Bull 1993; 45:546–548.)

ities may be necessary at this point to reduce painful muscle splinting. Scar massage is generally begun at 1 month postoperatively. Instructions for a home exercise program and follow-up physical therapy sessions may be necessary. Patients should continue ROM exercise during and following their radiation course and for at least 2 years.

Lymphedema

Lymphedema is a frequent complication of breast cancer treatment. The overall incidence of this condition following mastectomy is 25.5%, climbing to 38.3% in patients receiving axillary node clearance and radiation therapy.[46] Arm swelling can occur transiently in the immediate postoperative period and usually resolves spontaneously. It can also occur as a result of cellulitis, requiring the use of antibiotics and analgesics and avoidance of compression until the infection resolves. The onset of lymphedema 2 years or more following treatment can be a sign of recurrent tumor occluding the lymphatics. Painless, gradual forearm or upper arm swelling greater than 2 cm, occurring 6 weeks or more after treatment, requires therapeutic intervention.

Elevation, massage, and exercise of the distal musculature have all been advocated in the treatment of lym-

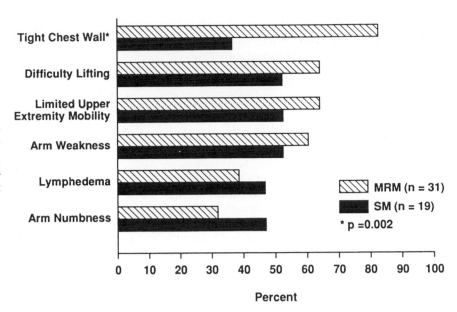

FIGURE 57–5 Most frequent physical problems directly related to breast cancer patients by type of primary treatment. (From Ganz PA, Schag CC, Polinsky ML, et al: Rehabilitation needs and breast cancer: the first month after primary therapy. Breast Cancer Res Treat 1987; 10:243–253.)

phedema. Compression with elastic bandages is often sufficient, but refractory edema requires use of a pneumatic pump. Pumps have been shown to reduce edema more effectively than wrapping alone.[48] Both intermittent uniform (single air cell) and differential sequential (multiple cell) compression sleeves can be used. The patient should be monitored closely for shortness of breath and complaints of pain during the initial pump trial session. Treatment duration can be from 2 to 24 hours, depending on physician and patient preference and the type of device used. If improvement in limb circumference results, the patient should be fitted for a custom, pressure-gradient support sleeve to be worn daily.

Pain

A variety of pain symptoms have been reported in breast cancer patients. Chest wall tenderness is common following radiation and can continue for years after treatment.[34] Adhesive capsulitis of the shoulder joint, transient brachial plexus neuritis, and acute and chronic radiation plexopathies can occur. Phantom breast pain has also been described, affecting at least 10% of mastectomy patients.[47] It occurs more commonly in women with premastectomy pain.

Cosmetic Concerns

Cosmetic rehabilitation attempts to restore a patient's external physical appearance can be accomplished by the use of temporary breast forms made of fluffed soft cotton or lamb's wool. These can be given to the patient postoperatively prior to discharge. A permanent prosthesis can usually be fitted 3 to 8 weeks after surgery when the chest wall edema has resolved and the tissue is well-healed.

Many patients opt for immediate reconstruction at the time of mastectomy. Patients can always choose to have reconstruction later, and irradiated skin of the axilla and chest are not contraindications to this procedure. Some women, however, choose to forego reconstruction, often

because of fear of a recurrence of tumor in the remaining tissue.[26]

Bone and Soft Tissue Tumors

Bone and soft tissue sarcomas are uncommon and account for just 0.5% to 1.0% of adult malignancies in the United States,[14] but the rehabilitation concerns of these patients are often particularly pertinent. The most common sarcoma in adults is osteosarcoma located in the knee or in the proximal humerus.[17] With advances in treatment, the 5-year survival for these tumors has advanced to nearly 80%.[83]

In children, the most common bone and soft tissue tumors are osteosarcomas, followed by Ewing's sarcoma and primitive neuroectodermal tumors. Ewing's sarcoma is often associated with the development of pathological fractures of the proximal femur.

Amputation

Amputation remains the preferred procedure for most high-grade malignancies of the distal lower extremity. Amputation at this level provides superior function and less morbidity than salvage or reconstruction surgery. Amputation can also be unavoidable for very proximal tumors, especially when associated with intrapelvic extension.

Tumor amputees differ from dysvascular and traumatic amputees in a number of ways. Chemotherapy-induced fatigue, anemia, nausea, and perhaps cardiovascular toxicity can sharply diminish functional capacity. Wound healing is often delayed over the irradiated ports, and skin may be less tolerant of prosthesis wear. Anorexia, muscle atrophy, and fluid shifts during chemotherapy can delay definitive prosthesis fabrication. Amputee and prosthetic management is discussed in further detail in Chapters 14 and 15.

Limb Salvage

Criteria for limb salvage procedures include the ability to totally resect the tumor without sacrifice of major nerves and vessels and the ability of a reconstruction to provide function equal or superior to that of an appropriate prosthesis. Pathological fractures and distant metastases are contraindications to such procedures. Limb salvages are increasing in frequency and are beginning to have long-term survival and local recurrence rates equivalent to those in patients undergoing amputation.

Metastatic Bone Lesions

The most frequently encountered bone tumors are metastatic in origin. Prostate carcinoma accounts for 60% of all bone metastases in men, and carcinomas of the breast account for 70% of all metastatic lesions in women.[1]

The pathogenesis of bone metastasis is not well known. Skeletal metastases appear to arise primarily through hematogenous spread. Batson[5] described a venous system connecting to and bypassing the pulmonary, portal, and caval venous flow (Fig. 57–6). This network of veins has multidirectional flow determined by external pressure and is related to biomechanical action and position. It is commonly believed to be a major hematogenous route for the spread of metastasis.

Patients with cancerous bone lesions complain of localized pain increasing in severity and frequency, often worsening at night. Such symptoms in cancer patients should prompt a search for metastasis, and even in patients without a tumor diagnosis, they should raise suspicions for such a spread. These patients often develop loss of joint ROM at the hip or shoulder. Radicular and myelopathic complaints require immediate evaluation for possible vertebral involvement. Confirmation of diagnosis for symptomatic lesions can be obtained by plain radiographs or bone scan.

Long Bone Involvement

Pathological fractures occur in 10% to 30% of patients with metastatic bone lesions. These fractures are most common in the long bones, especially the femur and humerus.[56, 76] Bone strength is determined by both cortical and trabecular structure, but cortical destruction makes bone susceptible to torsion and rotation fractures because these forces are no longer uniformly transmitted through the bone (Fig. 57–7).

Efforts have been made to determine the risk of pathological fracture at metastatic sites, in order to determine the need for preemptive surgical treatment. Most guidelines suggest increased fracture risk, and appropriateness for surgical stabilization, when painful lesions are greater than 2.5 cm in diameter, occupy 50% or more of bony cortical diameter, or if greater than 50% of medullary cross-sectional area or cortical surface is involved.[56] Determining such involvement is enhanced by CT coronal sections. Surgical fixation usually involves removal of the tumor through curettage with the use of methyl methacrylate, intramedullary rods, modular prostheses, or other hardware to repair the defect.

Vertebral Involvement

Metastases to the spine often involve the vertebral body and most frequently occur within the thoracic vertebrae. Pain can arise from epidural or root compression, intraosseous pressure of growing tumor cells, or spinal instability. Goals of treatment should include pain control, avoidance of neurological compromise by tumor or spinal instability, local tumor control, and maximizing patient function. Pain

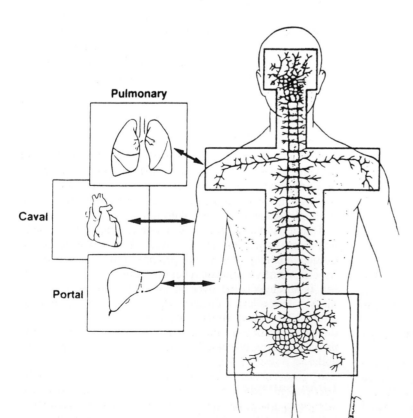

Pulmonary

Caval

Portal

FIGURE 57–6 Batson's plexus of veins. (Modified from Batson OV: The function of the vertebral veins and their role in the spread of metastasis. Ann Surg 1940; 112:138–149.)

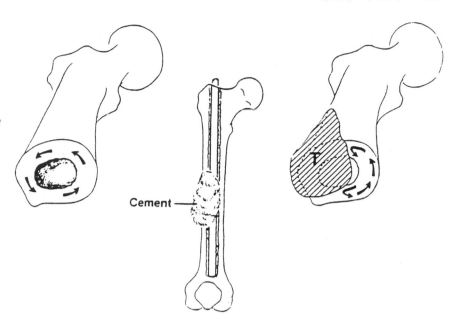

FIGURE 57-7 Schema demonstrating the biomechanical basis of intramedullary fixation of a bone with a large tumor defect. The normal rotational stress forces *(curved arrows)* are transmitted by the cortex in a uniform manner. A tumor defect *(T)* causes a stress riser that weakens the bone by 70% to 90% in torsion (rotation). The bone can be reconstructed by removing the tumor and reconstructing the defect with a combination of polymethylmethacrylate and intramedullary rod fixation. (From DeVita J, Hellman S, Rosenberg SA, et al (eds): Cancer: Principles and Practice of Oncology, ed 3. Philadelphia, JB Lippincott, 1989, p 2231.)

Cement

can respond to radiation, chemotherapy, or surgical stabilization, individually or in combination.[67] Nonsurgical management of spine metastasis includes the use of external orthoses.

Head and Neck Tumors

Head and neck cancers constitute about 5%[92] of all malignancies. The larynx is the most commonly affected site, followed by the oral cavity, pharynx, and salivary gland. Malignant disease of the head and neck region can result in profound swallowing and nutritional problems. The sensory functions of vision, hearing, balance, taste, and smell can be altered either by the disease or by the treatment. The goals of treatment, which include (1) eradication of cancer, (2) maintenance of adequate physiological function, and (3) achievement of socially acceptable cosmesis, can only be achieved through a multidisciplinary approach.

Surgery and radiotherapy can, in some cases, be curative.[92] Delayed surgical problems may arise and include deficits in swallowing (see Chapter 27) and speech (see Chapter 3).

Shoulder

Of special concern to the physiatrist are the shoulder disability and chronic neck pain that can occur following radical neck dissection (RND). The spinal accessory nerve is usually sacrificed during RND. It can be incised in the lower neck where it enters the trapezius muscle and in the upper neck where it enters the sternocleidomastoid muscle. Postoperative shoulder problems occur because of the loss of trapezius muscle function (Fig. 57-8). This usually causes the scapulae to move laterally, and deepens the axilla. Strengthening of the levator scapulae, rhomboids, and serratus anterior, while not capable of completely substituting for trapezius function, can help decrease pain as well as improve scapular stability and shoulder elevation.

The pectoralis muscle group is the main antagonist of the trapezius. Unopposed pull of the pectoralis muscle following RND results in shoulder contracture with the scapulae in a protracted position.[20] Avoiding contracture of the pectoralis group is a major goal of postoperative rehabilitation. Table 57-7 outlines a sample postoperative exercise program for patients for shoulder rehabilitation following RND.

Neck

Unilateral disruption of the sternocleidomastoid, platysma, omohyoid, and digastric muscles can lead to asymmetrical neck motion.[20] These patients often need to support their neck and head with their hands when changing from a supine to a sitting position. Following bilateral RND, a patient is unable to flex the neck against gravity. In both cases, a passive ROM program can be initiated once sutures are removed. This can be advanced to active resistive strengthening by about the fourth postoperative week.[20]

Spinal Cord Lesions

Tumor involvement of the spinal cord can be due to primary or metastatic lesions. Primary tumors, (meningiomas, neurofibromas, and gliomas), are relatively rare. The majority of tumors affecting the spinal cord are metastatic in origin and 95% are extradural.[72]

Most extradural metastases arise from the vertebral body and result in compression of the anterior aspect of the spinal cord (Fig. 57-9). the thoracic spine has a smaller ratio of canal to cord diameter than the lumbar or cervical segments; approximately 70% of spinal metastases occur in the thoracic spine.[35] Clinical presentation of spinal cord metastasis often involves complaints of pain that becomes worse in the supine position, especially at night. Multiple spinal levels can be simultaneously involved. The development of bowel or bladder dysfunction can indicate spinal cord compromise. The onset of such symptoms can be obscured in cancer patients receiving opiate and adjuvant analgesics since constipation and urinary retention are medication side effects. Slowly evolving symptomatology is a

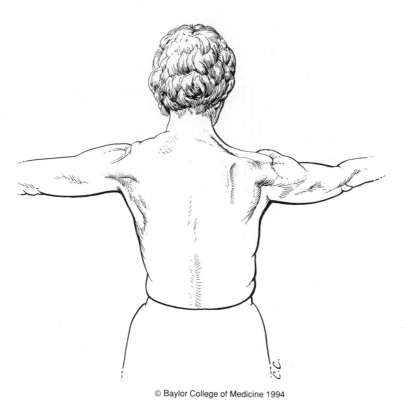

FIGURE 57–8 Scapular winging following radical neck dissection with trapezius muscle weakness.

© Baylor College of Medicine 1994

sign of gradual cord impingement and may respond to steroids and radiotherapy. Rapid evolution of paraparesis over only a few hours is usually a sign of arterial compromise by tumor invasion or pressure.

Treatment

The optimal surgical approach and stabilization procedures for metastatic spine lesions remain controversial.[68,] [71, 86] Stability is of special concern if the tumor involves two or three columns of the spine. Halo fixation, while providing the greatest stability to the cervical spine, is often poorly tolerated and is unacceptable to many cancer patients. Sternal occipital mandibular immobilization (SOMI) is usually better tolerated and provides adequate flexion and extension stability to the lower cervical segments. The Philadelphia collar can provide acceptable stability in flexion and extension for higher levels, but does

---

TABLE 57–7   Sample Postoperative Exercise Program for Head and Neck Cancer Patients

I. A. To be done lying on your back on a firm surface, with your hips and knees bent and your feet flat on the mat:
 1. Keeping the back of your shoulders in contact with the mat, move your shoulders toward your ears and then relax.
 2. With hands at your side and elbows straight, raise your arms forward and over your head. You may assist with your other hand, if necessary.
 3. With hands at your side and elbows straight, move your arms away from your body toward your ear, keeping your arms in contact with the mat.
 4. Clasp hands behind neck and push elbows back into the mat. Hold for a count of 5 and then relax without bringing your elbows forward.
 B. To be done sitting on a straight-backed chair:
 1. With your hands on your hips, try to touch your elbows together behind you.
II. A. To be done sitting on a straight-backed chair, maintaining good posture:
 1. Slowly bring your head forward, touching chin to chest, then back as far as possible.
 2. Tilt your head to the side, bringing your ear toward your shoulder without turning your head or raising your shoulder.
 3. Rotate your head as far as possible to look over your shoulder without allowing the shoulder to come forward.
III. A. To be done standing in a corner:
 1. Place one hand on each wall, holding elbows away from sides, and lean forward into the corner.
IV. A. To be done lying on your stomach with a pillow under your waist:
 1. With your arms at a 90-degree angle to your body, raise your arms off the mat toward the ceiling.
 2. a. With arms at sides, raise your head and then your shoulders. When you can perform this exercise with ease, substitute the following exercise in its place.
  b. With your hands clasped behind your neck, raise your head and then your shoulders off the mat, keeping your elbows back.
V. A. To be done sitting on a straight-backed chair, maintaining good posture:
 1. Slowly open and close your mouth. Do not force your mouth open or clench your teeth tightly.
 2. With your jaws slightly apart, move your lower jaw from side to side.
 3. With your jaws slightly apart, move your lower jaw forward and then back.

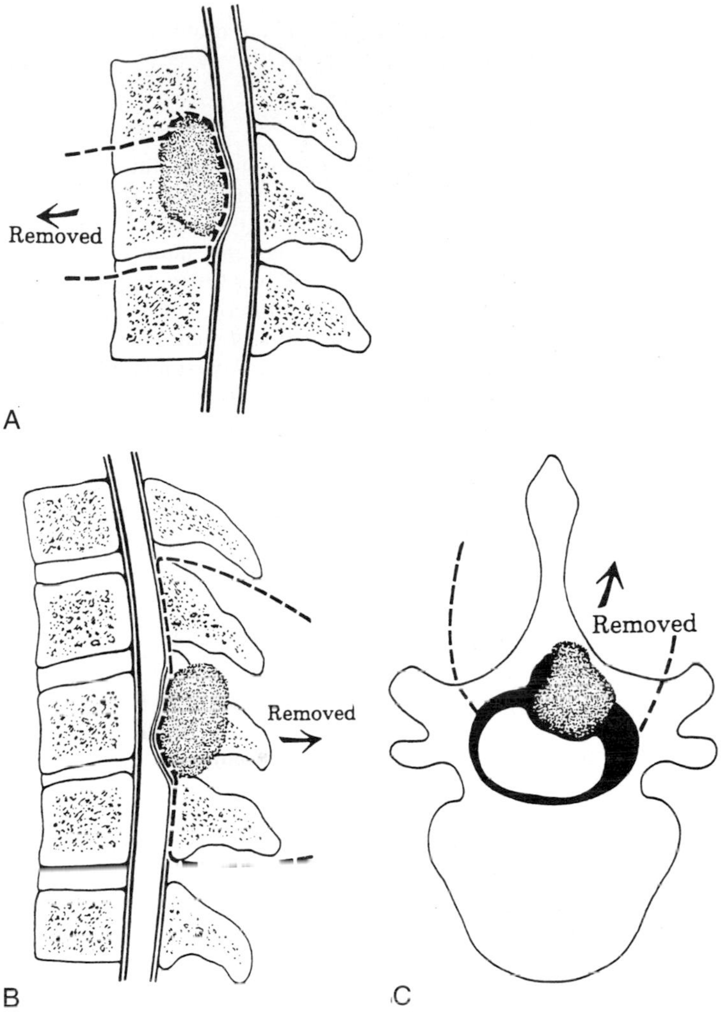

FIGURE 57–9 *A*, Most spinal metastases occur in the vertebral column anterior to the spinal canal. When surgery is indicated for tumors anterior to the spinal canal, surgical excision of the tumor and involved vertebral body with immediate stabilization of the spinal column effectively reverses compression of the spinal cord. *B* and *C*, Cord compression by tumors posterior to the spinal canal can be successfully relieved by laminectomy (removal of the laminae and spinous processes one level above and one level below the site of tumor) and tumor excision. (From DeVita JT, Hellman S, Rosenberg SA, et al (eds): Cancer: Principles and Practice of Oncology, ed 3. Philadelphia, JB Lippincott, 1989, p 1981.)

not sufficiently restrict rotation and lateral bending in the lower cervical segments (see Chapter 18).

The "clamshell"-style thoracic-lumbar-spinal orthosis may be used to provide thoracic and lumbar support. It provides considerable external support but may not be an option in cancer patients who have painful rib or iliac crest metastases, or those with friable or intolerant skin following steroids or chemotherapy. Better patient acceptance often occurs with the Taylor-Knight brace to limit extension and the Jewett brace to limit flexion.

Brain Tumors

Rehabilitation of brain tumor patients differs from the techniques used in stroke or traumatic brain injury primarily because of the types of damage seen. Normal brain tissue can be compressed or destroyed by tumor. The location of the lesion determines the resultant neurological deficits. They can be largely reversible, and in some patients dramatic improvement in function occurs within hours after surgical resection of a tumor once the mass effect is relieved. Most tumor patients have a significant functional return as long as the tumor involvement is not extensive.

The incidence and mortality of primary brain tumors is increasing.[7] In 1993, 17,500 people in the United States

were expected to be diagnosed with brain tumors.[9] More than 90% of the primary malignant tumors of the brain in adults are high-grade astrocytomas, and of these, the most common is glioblastoma multiforme.[78] The low-grade astrocytomas are the most common primary brain tumors of children. Medulloblastomas account for 20% of all intracranial tumors in children and are usually located near the cerebellar vermis.[52] Pediatric primary tumors tend to be infratentorial, while adult tumors are more likely to be supratentorial. Metastatic lesions compromise roughly 25% to 30% of all intracranial tumors. Lung, gastrointestinal (GI), and urinary tract tumors account for most of the brain metastases in men. Most brain metastases in women are from breast, lung, GI tract, and melanoma.[87]

Symptoms and Signs

The presenting symptoms and signs of brain tumor involvement can include headache, weakness, seizures, and changes in cognition. Headache is the most common symptom. Weakness is the most common focal sign, and is present on physical examination in 65% of patients.[91] Seizures occur in 20% of patients with supratentorial brain tumors. These are often focal motor or sensory seizures, localized to the area of tumor involvement, although they can be generalized. Nausea and vomiting are more common in infratentorial lesions and in children.

Rehabilitation Issues

Despite improvements in the median survival rates of primary brain tumor patients and advances in the treatment of metastatic tumors, survival for many of these patients is limited to only a few years. Many glioblastoma multiforme and high-grade astrocytoma patients die of recurrent tumor within 2 years.[91] Rehabilitation of brain tumor patients can dramatically improve the quality of their remaining life. Efforts directed toward prevention of skin breakdown, prevention of contractures, progressive mobilization and transfer training, and relearning of activities of daily living are appropriate. Speech therapy is indicated for patients with aphasia and dysarthria, and can be extremely beneficial for increasing stimulation and in improving communication skills and interactions between patient, family, and staff.

PEDIATRIC CANCER REHABILITATION

The most common childhood cancer is leukemia (30%–40%), especially acute lymphocytic leukemia (ALL), followed by central nervous system (CNS) tumors (20%), bone cancer (7%), and neuroblastoma (5%).[79]

Cancer deaths in children have decreased by approximately 50% in the past 25 years owing to improvements in detection and treatment.[25] Many survivors of childhood cancer have chronic neurological and musculoskeletal problems caused by the tumor or treatment. Brain radiation, done either as a primary treatment or as a prophylactic method, is associated with cognitive decline, particularly when performed in children less than 7 years old.[16] Significant decreases in visuomotor and fine motor skills, along with arithmetic skills, spatial memory, and intelligence quotient (IQ) scores have been reported following CNS irradiation in children.[63] Direct tumor effects and combined therapies also contribute to cognitive function decline.[70]

Children being treated for brain tumors can experience cerebellar disturbances and hemiparesis. Changes in visual acuity and oculomotor function can occur as well.[70] Hearing loss from chemotherapy, particularly when using vincristine, may also restrict normal childhood activities. Children treated for ALL are at increased risk of falling behind a grade level or needing special education classes.[13]

Musculoskeletal concerns of the pediatric cancer patient include the development of spinal deformities (kyphosis and scoliosis), especially when radiation is given during periods of rapid skeletal growth.[62] Bone sarcoma and the effects of limb salvage surgery or amputation are discussed above. Childhood growth patterns are frequently abnormal after completion of cancer treatment.

Most children with cancer experience pain, and nearly two thirds of the pain is treatment-related.[62] Direct effects of tumors, including bone metastases and nerve compression, are also important causes of pain.

The pharmacological treatment of cancer pain in children includes narcotics, NSAIDs, tricyclic antidepressants, amphetamines, and topical preparations. Oral meperidine use is avoided in children because a toxic metabolite of this agent can cause seizures. Fentanyl is a short-half-life narcotic that is effective for use in acute pain for pediatric outpatient surgical procedures.

Children with cancer have a 17% incidence of developing a second malignancy by 20 years of age.[78] Radiation and chemotherapy are potential carcinogens. Chronic immunodeficiency following treatment, as well as genetic predisposition, also play a role in secondary tumor development.

SUMMARY

The number of people with a history of cancer who have survived 5 years or more continues to increase. Advances in early cancer detection combined with aggressive, multimodal treatments are causing medical professionals to consider quality-of-life issues that were not relevant a decade ago. Many cancer centers recognize that early intervention by a rehabilitation team can minimize the long-term disability caused by cancer and cancer therapy.

References

1. Abrams HL, Spiro R, Goldstein N: Metastases in carcinoma: Analysis of 1000 cases. Cancer 1950; 23:74–85.
2. Anderson SW, Damasio H, Tranel D: Neuropsychological impairments associated with lesions caused by tumor or stroke. Arch Neurol 1990; 47:397–405.
3. Andrykowsky MA, Henslee PJ, Farrall MG: Physical and psychosocial functioning of adult survivors of allogenic bone marrow transplantation. Bone Marrow Transplant 1989; 4:75–81.
4. Barbash S, Anathakrishnan N, Mohan CR: Postoperative positioning after mastectomy and other procedures in the pectoral region. Aust N Z J Surg 1982; 52:293.
5. Batson OV: The function of the vertebral veins and their role in the spread of metastases. Ann Surg 1940; 112:188.
6. Bernstein I, Webster MM, Bernstein ID: Food aversions in children receiving chemotherapy for cancer. Cancer 1982; 50:2961–2963.
7. Bondy ML, Wrensch M: Update on brain cancer epidemiology. Cancer Bull 1993; 45:365–369.
8. Bonica JJ: Treatment of cancer pain: Current status and future needs. *In* Fields HL, Dubner R, Cervero F, et al (eds): Advances in Pain Research and Therapy, vol 9. New York, Raven Press, 1985, pp 589–616.
9. Boring CC, Squires TS, Tong T: Cancer statistics, 1993. CA 1993; 43:7–26.
10. Bos G: Sexuality of gynecologic cancer patients: Influence of traditional role patterns. *In* Aaronson NK, Beckmann JH (eds): The Quality of Life of Cancer Patients, New York, Raven Press 1987, pp 207–213.
11. Breitbart, W: Suicide. *In* Holland J, Rowland J, (eds): Handbook of Psycho-Oncology. New York, Oxford University Press, 1990, pp 291–299.
12. Burgess J: Cancer therapy. *In* Skipper A: Dietitians' Handbook of Enteral and Parenteral Nutrition. Rockville, MD, Aspen, 1989, p 121.
13. Byrd R: Late effects of treatment of cancer in children. Pediatr Clin North Am 1985; 32:835–851.
14. Cancer Facts and Figures—1988. New York, American Cancer Society, 1988, p 8.
15. Cancer Pain Relief and Palliative Care. Geneva, World Health Organization, 1990.
16. Copeland DR, Fletcher JM, Pfefferbaum-Levine B, et al: Neuropsychological sequelae of childhood cancer and long term survivors. Pediatrics 1985; 75:745–753.
17. Dahlin DC, Coventry MB: Osteogenic sarcoma: A study of six hundred cases. J Bone Joint Surg Am 1967; 49:101.
18. Davis M, Das S: Psychosexual support for genitourinary cancer patients. *In* Crawford ED, Das S (eds): Current Genitourinary Cancer Surgery. Philadelphia, Lea & Febiger, 1990, pp 669–674.

19. Degenshein GA: Mobility of the arm following radical mastectomy. Surg Gynecol Obstet 1977; 145:77.

20. DeLisa JA, Miller RM, Melnick RR, et al: Rehabilitation of the cancer patient. In DeVita VT, Hellman S, Rosenberg SA (eds): Cancer Principles and Practice of Oncology, ed 2. Philadelphia, JB Lippincott, 1989, pp 2155–2188.

21. Devesa SS, Silverman DT, Young JL, et al: Cancer incidence and mortality trends among whites in the United States 1947–1984. J Natl Cancer Inst 1977; 79:701.

22. Douglass HO: Nutritional support of the cancer patient. Hosp Formulary 1984; 19:220–234.

23. Dropcho EJ: Central nervous system injury by therapeutic irradiation. Neurol Clin 1991; 9:969–988.

24. Duncan GH, Bushnell MC, Marchand S: Deep brain stimulation: A review of basic research and clinical studies. Pain 1991; 45:49–60.

25. Ellenberg L, McComb JG, Siegel SE, et al: Factors affecting intellectual outcome in pediatric brain tumor patients. Neurosurgery 1987; 21:638–644.

26. Fallowfield LJ, Baumm M, Maguire GP: Effects of breast conservation on psychological morbidity associated with diagnosis and treatment of early breast cancer. BMJ 1986; 293:1331.

27. Fardin P, Lelli S, Negrin P, et al: Radiation-induced brachial plexopathy: Clinical and electromyographical considerations in 13 cases. Electromyogr Clin Neurophysiol 1990; 30:277–282.

28. Flew TJ: Wound drainage following radical mastectomy: The effect of restriction of shoulder movement. Br J Surg 1979; 66:302.

29. Foley KM: Pharmacologic approaches to cancer pain management. In Fields HL, Dubner R, Cervero F, et al (eds): Advances in Pain Research and Therapy, vol 9. New York, Raven Press, 1985, pp 629–653.

30. Forman A: Peripheral neuropathy in cancer patients: Clinical types, etiology, and presentation. Oncology 1990; 4:85–89.

31. Ganz PA: Current issues in cancer rehabilitation. Cancer 1990; 654:742–751.

32. Ganz PA, Coscarelli Schag CA, Heinrich RL: Rehabilitation. In Haskell CM (ed): Cancer Treatment, Philadelphia, WB Saunders, 1990, pp 883–892.

33. Ganz PA, Schag CC, Polinsky ML, et al: Rehabilitation needs and breast cancer: the first month after primary therapy. Breast Cancer Res Treat 1987; 10:243.

34. Gerber L, Lampert M, Wood C, et al: Comparison of pain, motion, and edema after modified radical mastectomy vs local excision with axillary dissection and radiation. Breast Cancer Res Treat 1992; 21:139.

35. Gilbert RW, Kim JH, Posner JB: Epidural spinal cord compression from metastatic tumor: Diagnosis and treatment. Ann Neurol 1978; 3:40–51.

36. Harper CM, Thomas JE: Distinction between neoplastic and radiation-induced brachial plexopathy, with emphasis on the role of EMG. Neurology 1989; 39:502–506.

37. Hartrampf CR: The transverse abdominal island flap for breast reconstruction: A 7-year experience. Clin Plast Surg 1988; 15:703.

38. Herold AH, Roetzheim HG: Cancer survivors. Prim Care 1992; 4:779–791.

39. Hinterbuchner C: Rehabilitation of the disability cancer. N Y State J Med 1978; 78:1066–1069.

40. Hochberg FH, Slotnick B: Neuropsychologic impairment in astrocytoma survivors. Neurology 1980; 30:172–177.

41. Hoffman WF, Levin VA, Wilson CB: Evaluation of malignant glioma patients during the post irradiation period. J Neurosurg 1979; 50:624–628.

42. Jaffe JH: Drug addiction and drug abuse. In Gilman AG, Goodman LS, Rall TW, et al (eds): The Pharmacologic Basis of Therapeutics, ed 8. New York, Macmillan, 1985, pp 532–581.

43. Jones AL, Miller JL: Bone marrow morbidity of chemotherapy. In Plowman PN, McElwain TJ, Meadows AT, et al (eds): Complications of Cancer Management. Oxford, Butterworth-Heinemann, 1991, p 371.

44. Kaplan HS: A neglected issue: The sexual side effects of current treatments for breast cancer. J Sex Marital Ther 1992, 18.3–19.

45. Kingsley DPE, Kendall BE: CT of the adverse effects of therapeutic radiation of the central nervous system. AJNR 1981; 2:453–460.

46. Kissen MW: Risk of lymphedema following the treatment of breast cancer. Br J Surg 1986; 73:580.

47. Kroner K, Knudsen UB, Skov J, et al: Long-term phantom breast syndrome after mastectomy. Clin J Pain 1992; 8:346.

48. LeClaire R, Dupuis M: Traitement physiatrique du lymphoedème postmastectomie. Union Med Can 1972; 101:2702.

49. Lederman RJ, Wilbourn AJ: Brachial plexopathy: Recurrent cancer or radiation. Neurology 1984; 34:1331–1335.

50. Lehmann JF, DeLisa JA, Warren CG, et al: Cancer rehabilitation: Assessment of need, development and evaluation of a model of care. Arch Phys Med Rehabil 1978; 59:410–419.

51. Lejour M, Dome M: Abdominal wall function after rectus abdominis transfer. Plast Reconstr Surg 1991; 87:1054.

52. Levin VA, Gutin PH, Leibel S: Neoplasms of the central nervous system. In DeVita Jr VT, Hellman S, Rosenberg SA (eds): Cancer: Principles and Practice of Oncology, ed 4. Philadelphia, JB Lippincott, 1993, pp 1679–1737.

53. Levinson SF: Rehabilitation of the patient with cancer or human immunodeficiency virus. In DeLisa JA (ed): Rehabilitation Medicine: Principles and Practice, ed 2. Philadelphia, JB Lippincott, 1993, pp 916–933.

54. Liebel SA, Guten PH, Davis RL: Tolerance of the brain and spinal cord. In Guten PH (ed): Radiation Injury to the Nervous System. New York, Raven Press, 1991, pp 239–256.

55. Maillet JO: The cancer patient. In Lang CE: Nutritional Support in Critical Care. Rockville, MD, Aspen, 1987, p 250.

56. Mandi A, Szepesi K, Morocz I: Surgical treatment of pathologic fractures from metastatic tumors of long bones. Orthopedics 1991; 14:43–50.

57. Mattes RD, Arnold C, Boraas M: Learned food aversions among cancer chemotherapy patients. Cancer 1987; 60:2576–2580.

58. McGrath PA: Pain in Children: Nature, Assessment and Treatment. New York, Guilford Press, 1990.

59. Meyers CA, Abbruzzese JL: Cognitive functioning in cancer patients: Effect of previous treatment. Neurology 1992; 42:434–436.

60. Meyers CA, Berman SA, Hayman A, et al: Pathological left-handedness and preserved function associated with a slowly evolving brain tumor. Dev Med Child Neurol 1992; 34:1102–1117.

61. Meyers CA, Scheibel RS: Early detection and diagnosis of neurobehavioral disorders in cancer patients. Oncology 1990; 4:115–122.

62. Miser AW, Miser JS: The treatment of cancer pain in children. Pediatr Clin North Am 1989; 36:979–999.

63. Mulhern RK, Horowitz ME, Kovnar EH, et al: Neurodevelopmental status of infants and young children treated for brain tumors with pre-irradiation chemotherapy. J Clin Oncol 1989; 7:1660–1666.

64. Nakagaki H, Brunhart G, Kemper TL, et al: Monkey brain damage from radiation in the therapeutic range. J Neurosurg 1976; 44:3–11.

65. National Center for Health Statistics: Vital Statistics of the United States, vol 2. Mortality. Part A. US Department of Health and Human Services publication (PHS) No. 90–110. Washington, DC, Government Printing Office, 1990.

66. Numata K, Ito M: A case of delayed radiation lumbosacral plexopathy. Brain Nerve 1990; 42:629–633.

67. O'Connor MI, Currier BL: Metastatic disease of the spine. Orthopedics 1992; 15:611–620.

68. O'Neil J, Gardner V, Armstrong G: Treatment of tumors of thoracic and lumbar spinal column. Clin Orthop 1988; 227:103–112.

69. Olsen NK, Pfeiffer P, Mondrup K, et al: Radiation induced brachial plexus neuropathy in breast cancer patients. Acta Oncol 1990; 29:885–890.

70. Peckham VC: Learning disabilities in long term survivors of childhood cancer: Concern for parents and teachers. Int Disabil Stud 1991; 13:141–145.

71. Perrin RG, McBroom RJ: Spinal fixation after anterior decompression for symptomatic spinal metastases. Neurosurgery 1988; 22:324–327.

72. Perrin RG, McBroom RJ, Perrin RG: Metastatic tumors of the cervical spine. Clin Neurosurg 1992; 37:740–755.

73. Poliquin CM: Post-bone marrow transplant patient management. Yale J Biol Med 1990; 63:495–502.

74. Pollard R, Callum KG, Altman DG, et al: Shoulder movement following mastectomy. Clin Oncol 1976; 2:343.

75. Porter J, Jick H: Addiction rare in patients treated with narcotics. N Engl J Med 1980, 302.123.

76. Pugh J, Sherry H, Futterman B, et al: Biomechanics of pathologic fractures. Clin Orthop 1982; 169:109–114.

77. Ragnarsson KT: Principles of cancer rehabilitation medicine. In Holland JF (ed): Cancer Medicine. Philadelphia, Lea & Febiger, 1993, p 1054.

78. Ries LAG, Hankey BF, Miller BA, et al: Cancer Statistics Review

1973–1988. US Department of Health and Human Services publication (NIH) No. 91–2789. Bethesda, MD, National Cancer Institute, 1991. NIH 91–2789.

79. Ryan BR: Principles of pediatric oncology. *In* Lewis MM (ed): Musculoskeletal Oncology: A Multidisciplinary Approach. Philadelphia, WB Saunders, 1992, pp 73–86.

80. Schultheiss TE, El-Jahdi AM: Statistical analysis of two hundred radiation myelopathy cases. Presented at Seventh International Congress of Radiation Research D:3–41, 1983.

81. Shakin EJ, Heiligenstein E, Holland JC: Psychiatric complications of cancer. *In* Plowman PN, McElwain TJ, Meadows A (eds): Complications of Cancer Management, Oxford, Butterworth-Heinemann, 1991, p 423.

82. Silvain C, Besson I, Ingrand P, et al: Long-term outcome of severe radiation enteritis treated by total parenteral nutrition. Dig Dis Sci 1992; 37:1065–1071.

83. Sim FH: Primary bone malignancies: Current advances that improve survival. J Musculoskeletal Med 1987; 4:49.

84. Smith DB, Babaian RJ: The effects of treatment for cancer on male fertility and sexuality. Cancer Nurs 1992; 15:271–275.

85. Smith DH, Decosse JJ: Radiation damage to the small intestine. World J Surg 1986; 10:189–194.

86. Sundaresan N, Galicich JH, Lane JM, et al: Treatment of neoplastic epidural cord compression by vertebral body resection and stabilization. J Neurosurg 1985; 63:676–684.

87. Takakura K, Sano K, Hoho S, et al: Metastatic Tumors of the Central Nervous System. Tokyo, Igaku-Shoin, 1982.

88. Ventafridda V, Tamburini M, Caraceni A, et al: A validation study of the WHO method for cancer pain relief. Cancer 1987; 59:850–856.

89. Wakisaka S, O'Neill RR, Kemper TL, et al: Delayed brain damage in adult monkeys from radiation in the therapeutic range. Radiat Res 1979; 80:277–291.

90. Walker VA, Hoskin PJ, Hanks GW, et al: Evaluation of WHO analgesic guidelines for cancer pain in a hospital-based palliative care unit. J Pain Symptom Manage 1988; 3:145–149.

91. Wallner KE, Galicich JH, Krol G, et al: Patterns of failure following treatment for glioblastoma multiforme and anaplastic astrocytoma. Int J Radiat Oncol Biol Phys 1989; 16:1405–1409.

92. Zagars G, Norante JD: Head and Neck Tumors in Clinical Oncology, ed 6. New York, American Cancer Society, 1983, pp 230–261.

58

Rehabilitation of Patients With Burns

M. CATHERINE SPIRES, M.D.

The human and economic cost of burn injuries is enormous. More than 70,000 persons require hospitalization each year for burn injury.[4] Males in the 18- to 25-year age group are most at risk to sustain a significant thermal injury. Burn size and age are the cardinal determinants of survival. Mortality is highest in the very young and the elderly.[102] Mortality is greater in females than in males with comparable injuries.[96] The average person believes that a serious burn injury is the most devastating trauma a person can survive.[92]

Burn injury is not a new problem. Mankind has struggled with burn injuries since the discovery of fire. Documents as early as the Papyrus Ebers in 1600 BC specify burn treatment techniques.[42] Hippocrates stressed cleansing burn wounds with wine or water to avoid suppuration.[34] Cornelius Celsus, in 1st century Rome, described one of the first surgical excisions of a contracted burn scar.[77]

With the advent of grafting techniques, early closure of burn wounds became possible, significantly improving survival rates. Pollack performed one of the earliest free skin autografts in 1871.[35] The development of the drum dermatome by Padgett and Hood (1939) and the mesh dermatome by Tanner and Vandeput (1963) made covering larger wounds possible through autografts.[35] These advances and the refinement of allograft and heterograft techniques resulted not only in early wound closure and increased survival, but also in reduced pain, fluid losses, and incidence of infection.

Evans devised a method of calculating fluid loss from burn injury based on the percentage of body surface area burned and the weight of the patient.[29] More accurate fluid resuscitation improved survival rates. The commonly used fluid replacement formulas of Parkland and Baxter are based on the initial work of Evans.[8]

Modern burn treatment is the result of a long history of medical and technological advances. The survival rate of seriously burned patients has increased dramatically, especially in the last three decades. More patients are returning to active lives at home, at work, and in the community. The physiatrist is uniquely trained to manage the complex rehabilitation problems of burn injuries and to aid burn patients in returning to a full and productive life.

THE INTEGUMENT

The skin is the largest organ of the body and serves multiple functions. It is composed of a network of specialized epithelial and dermal cells, collagen, elastic fibers, small blood vessels, and nerve endings. Skin is a complex organ that acts as a mechanical barrier to protect internal organs from chemicals and foreign material. It is essential to fluid homeostasis, thermoregulation, and the immunological defense of the body.

Skin Components

Skin consists of two major components: the epidermis and the dermis (Fig. 58–1). The epidermis has four layers that include the stratum corneum, stratum granulosum, stratum spinosum, and stratum basale. A fifth layer, the stratum lucidum, is present on the palms of the hands and the soles of the feet. The stratum corneum is the resilient semitransparent outermost layer that acts as a barrier to water transfer. The deepest layer, the stratum basale, is the major site of cell mitosis. Keratinocytes are the most numerous cells of the epidermis (Fig. 58–2). Originating in the stratum basale, keratinocytes migrate to the stratum corneum, undergoing the process of keratinization. During this process, keratinocytes flatten and become anucleate, and leave a protective protein layer of keratin on the skin surface.[12]

The epidermis has a number of appendages. Hair follicles are lined by epidermal cells, which are in continuity with the epidermis and serve as a reservoir of epidermal cells in the event of injury to the epidermis. The sebaceous glands produce sebum that moisturizes the skin. Eccrine

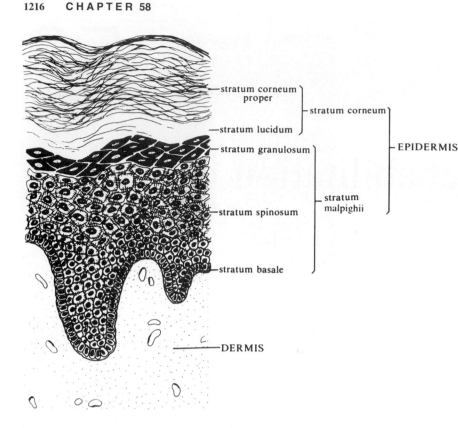

FIGURE 58–1 The histological characteristics of normal skin. Notice that the stratum lucidum is found only on the palms of hands and the soles of feet. (From Borysenko M, Beringer T: Functional Histology, ed 2. Boston, Little, Brown, 1984, pp 228–231.)

glands dissipate heat through production of sweat and are essential in thermoregulation.

The epidermis is nourished by the underlying dermis. Undulating projections of the dermis, rete pegs, fit intimately with the stratum basale and reduce shear forces during mechanical manipulation. Rete pegs are underdeveloped in children and are atrophied in the elderly. The dermis is composed of elastic fibers and loosely arranged collagen, which tend to be oriented in parallel with the epidermis (Fig. 58–3).

Mechanical Properties of Skin

Skin has properties that allow it to resist mechanical forces and yet allow for normal bodily motion. Stress is the force applied per unit area, whereas strain is the change in length created by an applied force. A typical stress strain curve for skin is shown in Figure 58–4. Skin demonstrates complex responses to loading. Three phases are typically used to describe the mechanical response of skin. During phase I, the compliance of skin is the greatest. Skin rapidly elongates with low loads. Elastic fibers elongate while collagen fibers begin to orient in the direction of the applied load. In phase II stiffening occurs, as more stress is required to produce a change in length. More collagen fibers align in the direction of the applied force. Phase III reflects the limits of collagen extensibility. This is in contrast to the initial part of the stress-strain curve that reflects the physical arrangement and interaction of the components of

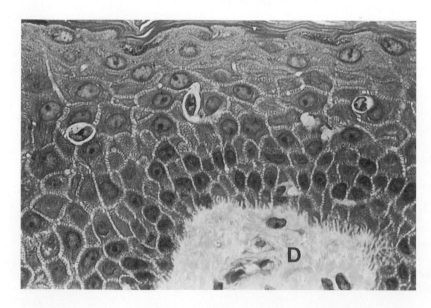

FIGURE 58–2 Light microscopy of epidermis, with the dermis (D) indicated. Note the abundance of keratinocytes joined by desmosomes. (From Borysenko M, Beringer T: Functional Histology, ed 2. Boston, Little, Brown, 1984, p 231.)

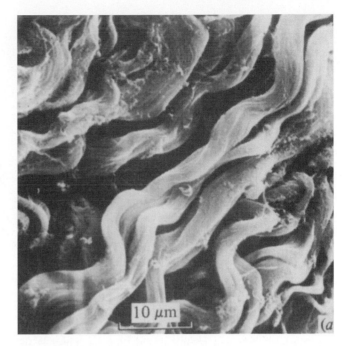

FIGURE 58–3 Electron micrograph of collagen bundles found in dermis. (From Millington PF, Wilkinson R: Skin. Cambridge, Cambridge University Press, 1983, p 85.)

skin. Continued application of force after phase III results in reaching the *yield point* (i.e., the point after which the tissue tears).[78]

Skin demonstrates a preconditioning effect. Consecutively applying and removing a load initially shows a non-coincident stress-strain curve. With repetition, the curves become very similar and nearly superimposable on each other. The initial changes in the stress-strain curve with repetitious loading occur as a result of phase I elongation. However, after several force applications, phase I shows little change. Once this occurs, the skin is considered to be *preconditioned*, and the stress-strain characteristics of the skin are stabilized (Fig. 58–5).[78] The stress-strain curve also varies by tissue type, as demonstrated in Figure 58–6.[73]

With injury and subsequent scarring, the stress-strain relationship of skin is altered because of higher collagen content's decreasing skin extensibility.[78] Awareness of these biomechanical principles becomes important for rehabilitation interventions of stretching and splint application.

MEDICAL AND SURGICAL MANAGEMENT OF BURN INJURY

The vast majority of burn injuries are thermal, resulting from flame or hot liquids. Chemical and electrical injuries are less frequent. The extent of tissue injury depends on the duration and the intensity of heat exposure. A signifi-

FIGURE 58–4 The stress-strain curve for skin. The various phases of skin response to elongation are indicated by roman numerals. (From Millington PF, Wilkinson R: Skin. Cambridge, Cambridge University Press, 1983, p 85.)

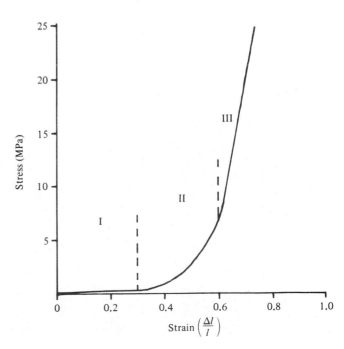

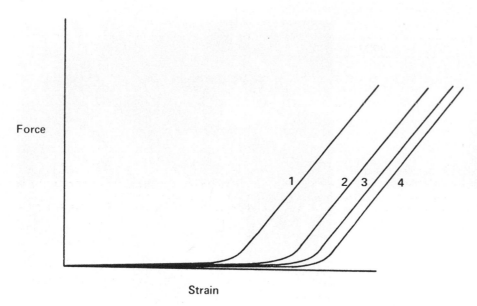

FIGURE 58–5 With repeated loading, the skin shows alterations in the stress-strain curve, referred to as the *preconditioning effect.* (From Marks R: Mechanical properties of the skin. *In* Goldsmith LA (ed): Biochemistry and Physiology of the Skin. New York, Oxford University Press, 1983, p 1239.)

cant variable between chemical and thermal injury is the duration of tissue destruction. Injury by a heat source ceases after the removal of the source, whereas chemicals continue to destroy tissue until they are inactivated by neutralizing agents or until the chemical reaction with the tissue is complete.

Medical Management

The first priorities of medical management are interruption of the burning process and assessment of the airways, breathing, and circulation. Further evaluation includes assessment of the total body surface area (TBSA) burned, burn depth, presence or absence of inhalation injury, and involvement of specialized body regions (e.g., face, hands, and perineum). The patient's age, presence of other injuries, and premorbid medical condition are also considered. The amount of fluid needed to restore and maintain hemodynamic stability is calculated using the Brooke, the Parkland, or other formulas for fluid resuscitation.[8, 29, 75] Clinical response determines further fluid needs. Close monitoring for infection and cardiopulmonary complications is required on an ongoing basis.

Classification of Burn Severity

The American Burn Association classifies a burn injury as minor, moderate, or severe based on patient age, extent and depth of injury, and associated injuries (Table 58–1). Patients with moderate and severe burns require hospitalization. Major injuries, which include inhalation burns and burns of the eyes, ears, face, feet, or perineum, should be treated in a specialized burn center.[4]

Burn injury extent is determined by the total body surface area (TBSA) injured. The easiest method of calculating TBSA is the *rule of nines* (Fig. 58–7). Eleven areas of the body are assigned a surface area value of 9%, with the perineum designated as 1%.[82] For children, this method is less accurate because the head, particularly during the first year of life, is larger in relation to the body size than is an adult's head. The Lund and Browder chart (Fig. 58–8) accounts for these developmental differences.[75]

Depth of burn injury refers to the extent to which the epidermis and dermis are burned (Fig. 58–9). Superficial burns, also called first-degree burns, cause local erythema and pain. Partial-thickness burns, or second-degree burns, are classified as superficial partial thickness and deep partial thickness. In superficial partial-thickness injuries,

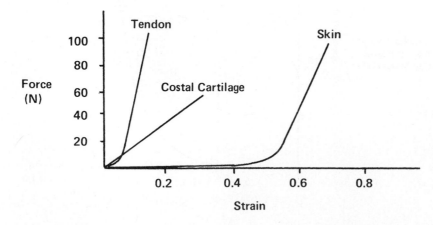

FIGURE 58–6 The stress-strain curves for tendon and cartilage compared with that of skin. (From Marks R: Mechanical properties of the skin. *In* Goldsmith LA (ed): Biochemistry and Physiology of the Skin. New York, Oxford University Press, 1983, p 1238.)

TABLE 58–1 Burn Injury Classification

Type of Injury	Major Burn	Moderate Burn	Minor Burn
Partial-thickness burns			
Children	>20% TBSA	10%–20% TBSA	<10% TBSA
Adults	>25% TBSA	15%–25% TBSA	<15% TBSA
Full-thickness burns	>10% TBSA	2%–10% TBSA	<2% TBSA
Injury to face, eyes, ears, feet, or perineum	+	—	—
Inhalation injury	+	—	—
Electrical injury	+	—	—
Co-morbid factors of age, other trauma, or premorbid illness	+	—	—

Abbreviations: TBSA, total body surface area; +, presence of this injury or co-morbidity indicates a major burn requiring care at a burn center.
From American Burn Association: Hospital and pre-hospital resources for optimal care of patients with burn injury: Guidelines for development and operation of burn center. J Burn Care Rehabil 1990; 11:98–104.

blistering occurs because of microvascular damage and associated increase in capillary permeability. Sensory nerve endings are exposed, and the wound is painful.

In a deep partial-thickness wound, the dermis and the entire epidermis are injured. Only the skin appendages are spared. Spontaneous healing can occur, but it is associated with significant scarring. Poor cosmesis and function typically result.

In full-thickness burn injuries, or third-degree burns, the entire thickness of the dermis is devitalized. Because skin appendages are destroyed, the wound cannot heal by re-epithelization. Dermal blood vessels are destroyed, and the wound bed is avascular.

Even the most experienced clinicians can have difficulty distinguishing a deep partial-thickness from a full-thickness injury (Fig. 58–10). In fact, poor wound care, wound infection, or impaired perfusion can convert a deep partial-thickness injury to a full-thickness injury.

In the literature and in the clinical setting, a growing trend is to refer to burn depth in descriptive terms, that is, superficial partial-thickness, deep partial-thickness, and full-thickness burns, rather than first-, second-, and third-degree burns. The descriptive classification has the advantage of relaying a quick and accurate verbal description of the burn injury.

Principles of Wound Care

The goals of wound care are to facilitate wound healing, prevent infection, decrease pain, reduce scarring and contracture, and prepare the wound for any necessary grafting. Infection can cause sepsis or convert the wound to a deeper-thickness injury. Burn wounds are covered by an eschar, which is necrotic tissue composed of denatured collagen, elastin, and protein. Because eschar favors wound infection and delays healing, debridement is initiated early. Debridement removes devitalized tissue and provides a viable base for wound healing and grafting.

Debridement is done by several techniques: mechanical, enzymatic, and surgical. Mechanical debridement includes techniques such as hydrotherapy and wet-to-dry dressing techniques. The wet-to-dry dressing technique involves placing saline-soaked gauze over the wound and allowing the dressing to nearly dry. Necrotic tissue adheres to the

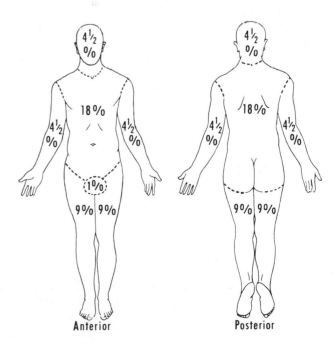

FIGURE 58–7 Rule of nines used to determine body surface area injured. (From Moylan JA: First aid and transportation of burned patients. *In* Artz CP, Moncrief JA, Pruitt BA (eds): Burns: A Team Approach. Philadelphia, WB Saunders, 1979, p 153.)

Relative Percentage of Areas Affected by Growth

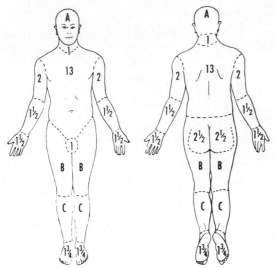

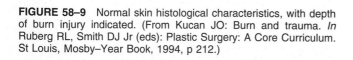

	Age in Years					
	0	1	5	10	15	Adult
A—½ of head	9½	8½	6½	5½	4½	3½
B—½ of one thigh	2¾	3¼	4	4¼	4½	4¾
C—½ of one leg	2½	2½	2¾	3	3¼	3½

FIGURE 58–8 Lund and Browder method of determining skin surface area; method corrects for differences in percentage of body surface areas by age. (From McManus WF: Immediate emergency department care. *In* Artz CP, Moncrief JA, Pruitt BA (eds): Burns: A Team Approach. Philadelphia, WB Saunders, 1979, p 154.)

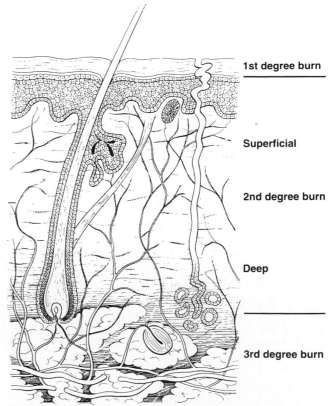

FIGURE 58–9 Normal skin histological characteristics, with depth of burn injury indicated. (From Kucan JO: Burn and trauma. *In* Ruberg RL, Smith DJ Jr (eds): Plastic Surgery: A Core Curriculum. St Louis, Mosby–Year Book, 1994, p 212.)

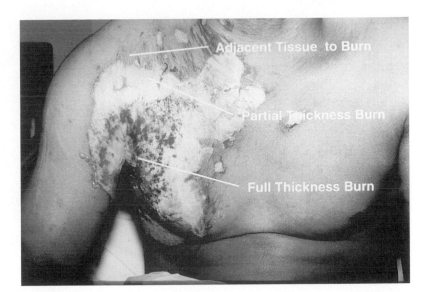

FIGURE 58–10   The clinical appearance of partial-thickness and full-thickness burns.

dressing as the gauze dries and is removed when the dressing is changed. This provides a simple and inexpensive debridement, but it can be painful and cause local bleeding. Its use is limited by the size of the wound to be debrided. To prevent desiccation of the wound, the dressing requires changing every 6 to 8 hours.

Hydrotherapy, via immersion or spraying a burn directly, is a reasonably comfortable way to remove dressings and loosen devitalized tissue. It is a time-consuming and labor-intensive procedure. Other disadvantages include hypothermia and bacterial cross-contamination between patients if meticulous care of hydrotherapy equipment is not maintained. Disposable liners are available to reduce cross-contamination. Hydrotherapy can be combined with other forms of mechanical debridement.

Several debriding enzymes, such as sutilains, are available for topical application to burn eschar. Enzymatic action includes proteolysis, fibrinolysis, and collagenolysis, with specificity varying from agent to agent. Enzymatic debridement can reduce the need for surgical debridement. Exercise and splinting programs are not contraindicated during enzymatic treatment. Disadvantages include increased pain and fluid loss. The amount of body surface area being enzymatically treated at one time should be limited to less than 20% TBSA. Localized irritation, cellulitis, and elevation in body temperature can also occur. Bleeding can occur at the interface between the eschar and the viable tissue.[103]

Surgical debridement excises the nonviable tissue by either sequential or fascial excision. The latter removes tissue down to the fascia, which ensures a viable wound bed but leaves a significant tissue defect. Sequential excision consists of thin slices of tissue being removed sequentially until bleeding is observed, which indicates a viable wound bed. Although it is less likely to sacrifice viable tissue, sequential excision causes greater blood loss and requires extensive surgical experience.

Burn injury can cause massive edema. Compartment syndromes can develop, particularly with circumferential burns, which result in neurovascular compromise and potential limb loss. Escharotomies can be performed to re-

lieve pressure by incising through the burned tissue at specified areas, which avoid flexor surfaces, of the upper and lower extremities (Fig. 58–11). This is also done over the chest wall when eschar interferes with respiration by preventing chest expansion. Circumferential upper or lower extremity burns require monitoring to ensure that compartment pressures do not exceed 40 mm Hg. If this pressure is reached, fasciotomies are indicated to prevent neurovas-

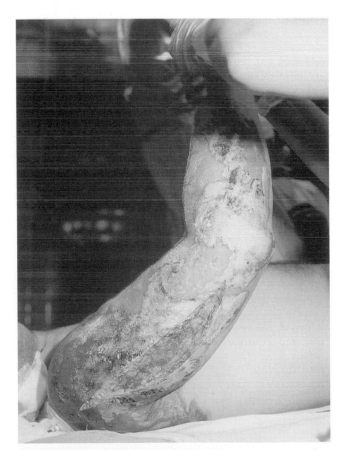

FIGURE 58–11   Escharotomy of the right upper arm to reduce pressure created by a circumferential burn.

cular compromise that can also lead to amputation of the extremity.

Wound Dressings and Grafts

Biological dressings (i.e., biological tissue used for covering wounds) provide a means of early burn wound closure. Early closure reduces pain, promotes healing, and decreases bacterial proliferation. Early wound closure reduces evaporative fluid loss and metabolic rate. The primary types of biological dressings include heterografts (such as porcine grafts), and homografts (such as cadaver grafts). Homografts are considered the best biological dressing, but are obtained primarily from cadaver donors and can be limited in supply. Biological dressings are often used to achieve early wound closure until an autograft (i.e., the surgical transfer of the patient's skin from one body site to another) is feasible. A biological dressing can also be used as a test graft to see if a wound is ready to accept an autograft.

Synthetic wound dressings include polyvinyl chlorides, polyurethanes, and other plastic membranes. The advantage of these temporary dressings includes water and gas permeability, but they fail to adhere to the wound bed, and fluids accumulate under the dressings.[83] Nylon mesh bonded to silicone (Biobrane) adheres to and successfully covers both partial- and full-thickness wounds. Like biological dressings, the dressing does not adhere to wounds with high bacterial counts.[40]

Topical antimicrobials are applied to burns and to wounds after debridement and grafting to reduce bacterial proliferation. Sulfadiazine and mafenide acetate are two of the most commonly used topical agents. Mafenide acetate penetrates eschar, but it can cause pain, as well as acidosis and leukopenia. Sulfadiazine is also a broad-spectrum topical antibiotic but does not penetrate eschar as mafenide acetate does. It has the advantage of causing less pain and is not associated with leukopenia or acidosis.

Autografting can be performed once the wound is free of devitalized tissue and infection. Split-thickness skin graft can be meshed or applied in sheets. Meshing is a process in which small, staggered, parallel slits are made in the graft to allow it to be expanded to 1.5 times or greater its original size. The interstices epithelialize, and the pattern of the mesh persists after wound healing (Figs. 58–12 and 58–13). The greater the degree to which the mesh is expanded, the poorer the cosmetic appearance. Mesh grafts are valuable when donor sites are limited and large areas need to be covered. Split-thickness grafts can be applied in sheets without meshing. These grafts are durable, limit contracture formation, and produce better cosmesis for covering the face, neck, and hands. Full-thickness grafts are useful for specialized areas, such as the palms of the hands and are frequently used in reconstructive procedures.

Wound Healing

The process of wound healing involves three simultaneous processes: epithelization, scar formation (repair of the dermis), and wound contraction. Immediately after injury inflammation occurs. This process spans a complex array of events, including initial vasoconstriction followed by vasodilatation, marked changes in capillary permeability,

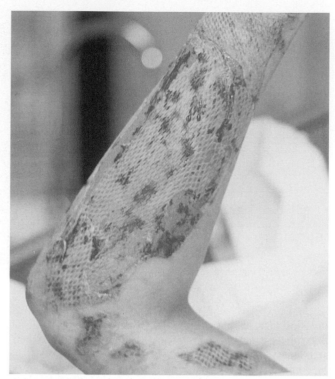

FIGURE 58–12 The appearance of a meshed split-thickness autograft during the acute post-grafting period.

and chemotaxis, which attracts neutrophils, macrophages, and lymphocytes. This period is marked by erythema, increased heat, edema, and pain. The inflammatory phase not only controls infection but also heralds the onset of the proliferative stage of healing by attracting fibroblasts.

Once inflammation is established, epithelium migrates from the edges of the wound or from epidermal appendages. If the burn involves the epidermis and superficial dermis, epithelialization is the primary process. However, with deep partial-thickness injuries and full-thickness injuries, both epithelialization and restoration of the dermis are crucial.

Fibroblastic activity is the hallmark of the proliferative wound healing phase. During this phase, fibroblasts synthesize collagen, which is the predominant protein found in scar. Collagen gives tensile strength to the wound. Simultaneously, angiogenesis occurs to provide the vascular support needed for the reparative wound activities. Capillary proliferation produces the classic granular appearance of granulation tissue.

Wound contraction is the active movement of the wound edges toward the center of a wound, shrinking the size of the defect and aiding closure. The degree of contraction achieved is dependent on the looseness and redundancy of the surrounding skin. For instance, a wound involving the skin of the buttock results in greater wound contraction and reduction of the wound size than does one involving the the less mobile skin of the lateral malleolus. Fibroblasts appear to be the primary cells involved in wound contraction.[88]

As the scar matures, inflammation and angiogenesis resolve. The tissue becomes paler and flatter. Collagen synthesis is balanced by degradation of collagen. The rete pegs

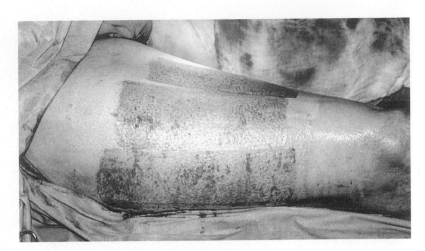

FIGURE 58–13 Donor site appearance after skin harvesting for autografting.

do not reappear immediately and require months to form. This contributes to the scarred skin's reduced ability to tolerate applied forces.

ELECTRICAL BURN INJURIES

Electrical burn injuries account for approximately 3% of burn admissions and result in approximately 800 deaths per year.[48, 63] Injuries can be mild or can result in death from cardiac asystole. Electrical injuries are classified as low-tension or high-tension injuries. High-tension injuries result from exposure to greater than 1000 V. Amperage is also important. In general, the greater the amperage, the greater the injury. Electrical injuries occur predominantly in men younger than 30 years who work with high-voltage equipment or high-tension wires. Low-tension electrical injuries usually occur in residential settings.[63]

The damage of electrical exposure results from the heat produced as the current passes through various tissues. According to Joule's law ($J = I^2 RT$), the amount of heat produced (J) is dependent on the square of the amperage (I), the tissue resistance (R), and the duration of exposure (T). Bone produces the most resistance, resulting in the greatest heat production. Although nerves and blood vessels provide the least resistance, they can sustain significant injury because they are more heat sensitive. As a consequence, the majority of the injuries sustained are in deep tissues.[81]

The cross-sectional area of the particular body part affects the density of current and the amount of heat generated. Body parts with a small cross-sectional area, such as fingers and toes, can demonstrate massive injury (Fig. 58–14A and B).[81] Extensive muscle and soft tissue necrosis often results in amputation. One quarter to nearly half of the patients hospitalized for electrical burns require limb amputation, and some require multiple limb amputations.[38, 52, 94] The upper extremity is the most common limb amputated.[37, 63] Haberal[37] reported that 27% of the 94 electrically injured patients studied required major limb amputations. In the study, 80% of the major limb amputations involved the upper extremity. The right upper extremity accounted for two thirds of these amputations. One quarter of these patients required shoulder disarticulations, whereas the remainder underwent above-elbow and below-elbow amputations.

Neurological Sequelae

Immediate neurological problems include loss of consciousness, anoxic encephalopathy, peripheral neuropathies, and spinal cord injury. Persistent coma is correlated with a poor prognosis and often results in death.[36] Spinal cord injury, the most common permanent neurological sequela of electrical injury according to some sources,[81] occurs when the current travels from one extremity to another.[62] Peripheral neuropathies generally occur in the injured limb but can be seen in the non-injured limb.[31] Although the pathophysiology for late-appearing neurological deficits is unknown, spinal cord injury and peripheral neuropathies can be observed as late as 2 years postinjury. Late-appearing deficits generally have a poorer prognosis than those of early onset. With electrical injuries to the head and neck, serial eye examinations are required because cataracts can occur up to 3 years after electrical injury.[57, 81, 110]

On superficial evaluation, electrical injuries can appear to be deceptively minor. The entrance site is typically small and charred, whereas the exit wound may be more explosive in appearance. Patients need careful evaluation to ensure that a serious underlying injury is not overlooked. The average TBSA injured in electrical burns is approximately 12%.[38] Electrical injuries can be further compounded if clothing catches on fire, causing more extensive skin injury.

REHABILITATION

Once a person has sustained a burn injury, the rehabilitation phase begins; it continues long after discharge, in some cases for life. The goal is to assist the individual in achieving the optimal level of functioning. Understanding the location, depth, and distribution of burn injuries is important in preventing complications. The extent of injury correlates with survival as well as with time required to return to independent functioning. Age, previous level of independence, premorbid medical conditions, and other

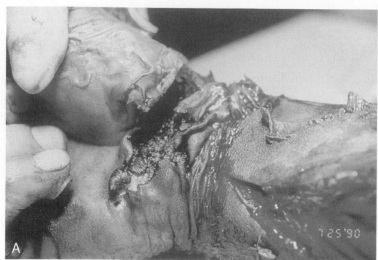
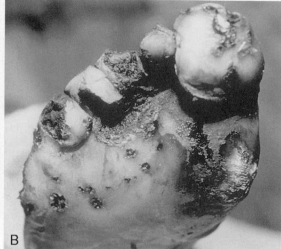

FIGURE 58–14   Electrical burn: entrance site *(A)*; exit site *(B)*.

injuries must be considered when assessing the burn patient.

During the acute period, goals include promoting wound healing and preventing complications by preserving joint function, strength, endurance, and functional abilities. Goals are individualized according to the location and extent of burn injuries and previous functional level. Goals are continually assessed and modified as the patient improves.

Positioning

Proper positioning is fundamental to burn rehabilitation. Positioning prevents contracture formation, controls edema, and maintains tissues in an elongated state. Because of pain, burn patients assume a primarily flexed and adducted position that inadvertently favors contracture development. In general, body parts should be positioned to maintain burned tissues in their elongated state. Typically, limbs should be positioned in extension and abduction (Fig. 58–15). The positioning program must be individualized in accord with the sites of injury. Proper positioning can be achieved using splints, strategically placed pillows, and foam wedges.

Splinting

Contractures can develop quickly during burn healing. Splinting should be considered whenever a partial- or full-thickness burn overlies a joint surface or the skin near a joint, which if contracted would interfere with joint function. Splints are used to maintain proper anticontracture positions and range of motion (ROM) in joints at risk for development of contractures. Serial splinting and serial casting techniques are both non-operative means of gaining ROM through sustained stretch and pressure. Splints are used to protect newly placed skin grafts and to shield injured anatomical structures, such as tendons, from further trauma. Splints can be designed to prevent scarring in areas in which an important body contour would be lost, e.g., the anterior neck surface. Additionally, if prolonged bed rest is anticipated, joint motion can be lost in unburned

areas, such as at the ankle. If full passive ROM is not present at a joint, splinting should be considered.

It is important to consider the benefits and risks of splinting. Splinting is labor intensive and adds significant cost to patient care. However, splinting is cost effective if it reduces the need for surgery or prevents loss of function. Not all burned areas require splinting. Typically, areas of superficial partial-thickness burns usually heal without scar contracture formation and do not require splinting. Unburned areas generally do not require splinting unless they are at risk for contracture development secondary to immobilization.

Splint materials must be compatible with topical medica-

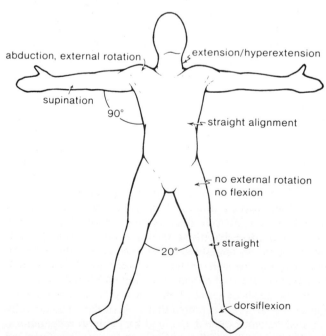

FIGURE 58–15   Suggested positioning guidelines for prevention of burn contractures. (From Helm PA, Kevorkian CG, Lushbaugh M, et al: Burn injury: Rehabilitation management in 1982. Arch Phys Med Rehabil 1982; 63:8.)

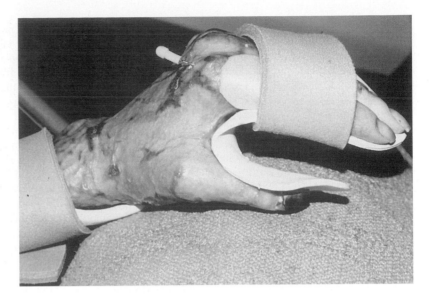

FIGURE 58–16 The left hand splinted in the position of function after skin grafting.

tions and wound dressings. Prefabricated or custom splints can be used, but proper fitting must be ensured. Care should be taken to ensure that the splints do not create pressure over bony prominences and delicate healing tissues. Splints should be easy to don and doff. "User-friendly" splints increase the likelihood that splints will be used, and the complications of incorrect use will be avoided. Inexpensive and remoldable materials are best suited to accommodate changes as healing occurs.

The universal burn splint, unfortunately, does not exist. The type of splint used is dependent on the area burned, the depth of injury, the patient's functional status, and the patient's ability to participate in positioning and exercise programs. A wide variety of splints can be designed and fabricated. A splinting program should focus on motions at risk as well as ROM that is difficult to regain (e.g., shoulder flexion and abduction, elbow and knee extension). Splints can be fabricated for virtually any part of the body, including the mouth, face, neck, and axilla. Splints for the upper and lower extremities are among the most common.

The resting hand splint maintains the hand in a functional position. The position of function is the hand splinted in full interphalangeal extension, 60 to 80 degrees of metacarpophalangeal flexion, thumb abduction, and wrist extension (Fig. 58–16).[48, 67] This position provides balance between the extensor and flexor tendons and places the ligaments and joint structures under maximum stretch to prevent shortening by inflammation and edema.[67]

Lower extremity splints can also be fabricated. These include such devices as the hip abduction splint to limit hip adduction, the knee extension splint to prevent knee flexion contractures, and the posterior footdrop splints to maintain the ankle in a neutral position. Individualized splints, unique to the patient's needs, can be fabricated. An example of such a customized foot splint is shown in Figure 58–17.

Plantar flexion deformity is a common problem. Prefabricated posterior footdrop splints are available commercially but still require modification to ensure proper fit. However, these splints can be readily made by creating a gutter- or trough-shaped splint and attaching a foot plate

to hold the ankle in a neutral position. The trough can be lengthened to include positioning of the knee in extension.

Exercise in Burn Rehabilitation

Exercise is fundamental to maximizing patient function and overall outcome. In prescribing exercise, the extent,

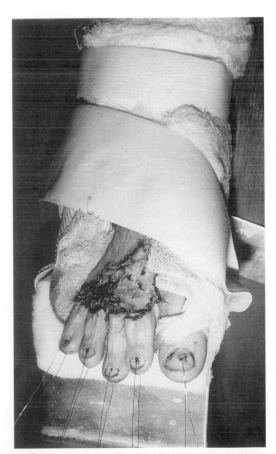

FIGURE 58–17 Customized splint designed to hold the foot in a neutral position while also preventing a hyperextension deformity at the metatarsophalangeal joints after dorsal foot autograft.

depth, and location of the injury is considered. In general, the risk of contracture increases with increasing burn depth. The risk of exercise disrupting wound healing requires regular wound inspection, particularly in the case of deep partial-thickness and full-thickness burns over joint surfaces. Stretching can also disrupt already tenuous joint and tendon structures.

Pre-existing medical conditions, such as cardiovascular or pulmonary disease, affect the type of exercise prescribed. The stress of fluid resuscitation can complicate the recovery of patients with cardiovascular disease. Deconditioning occurs rapidly in burn patients (see Chapter 34). Principles of cardiac rehabilitation are often as important in these situations as burn exercise principles (see Chapter 32).

The initial exercise program should focus on preserving ROM and maintaining strength. Active forms of exercise are indicated for patients who are alert and able to participate. For obtunded or critically ill patients, the slow, controlled movement of passive ROM (PROM) exercise is appropriate. While the patient is under anesthesia, PROM techniques can be applied to determine true joint ROM and factors limiting motion.

In the case of the patient who can actively move a joint but who is unable to achieve full ROM, active assistive ROM (AAROM) exercise is appropriate. The patient does as much of the ROM as possible, then a steady prolonged stretch or assistance is applied to complete the ROM. The stretch can be provided manually or by using devices such as pulleys and weights. Pain can limit stretching in some patients. Scheduling exercise shortly after pain medication administration reduces pain during therapy.

The mechanical properties of skin have been described. Applying the principle of skin preconditioning (i.e., stretching the skin several times until phase I of the stress-strain curve stabilizes) can improve the success of a stretching program. Preconditioning can be done by moving a joint to its end ROM several times before applying a sustained stretch. Stretching can be sustained until the stretched tissue blanches. The blanching indicates that dermal capillary flow is impeded and correlates with early phase III of the skin stress-strain relationship (see Fig. 58–4). With overstretching beyond phase III, the yield point is reached and passed (i.e., the point in the stress-strain curve at which tissue integrity deteriorates).[78] Once normal joint ROM is achieved, active exercise is preferred.

Various types of strengthening protocols can be initiated, including progressive resistive exercises (PRE) and circuit training (see Chapter 20). Endurance training should not be overlooked and requires careful monitoring in the patient with cardiac (see Chapter 32) or pulmonary disease (see Chapter 33).

Ambulation and Mobility

Ambulation and mobility are important elements of a comprehensive rehabilitation program. Early ambulation maintains balance, lower extremity function, and a sense of well-being and decreases the risk of deep venous thrombosis. Ambulation should start as soon as possible after admission. Ambulation can be limited by medical status, presence of new skin grafts, the depth and extent of lower

extremity burns, and previous medical conditions, such as peripheral vascular disease. After lower extremity grafting, placing the legs in a dependent position is generally not permitted for up to 5 to 10 days. Although the protocol for the timing of ambulation varies among facilities, the underlying principle is to begin ambulation once competent circulation is established in the graft and the risk of venous pooling, which can cause graft loss, is reduced. Once ambulation is initiated, recent graft and deep tissue injuries of the lower extremities require elastic wraps or stockings. Elastic supports prevent venous stasis, control edema, reduce the risk of local trauma, and decrease pain induced by the dependent position. Before ambulation is begun, it is advisable to have the patient "dangle" the lower extremities (e.g., sit with the legs hanging over the edge of the bed) to evaluate the predisposition for edema formation. Wounds should be assessed before and after ambulation to note any ill effects.

Gait deviations are frequent and reflect the injured areas of the body (see Chapter 5). Reduced trunk and pelvic mobility, decreased weight shifting, and inadequate hip and knee extension are common. Some deviations spontaneously resolve with wound healing, but others require therapeutic intervention. Mirrors can provide feedback to patients for self-correction of posture and gait abnormalities. Assistive devices can optimize gait patterns (see Chapter 26).

Scar Rehabilitation

The appearance of a wound is frequently satisfactory immediately after closure. However, over the next 1 to 3 months, hypertrophic scarring can occur with deep partial- and full-thickness burn injures. Hypertrophic scars are characteristically red, raised, and rigid.[1] The significance of these scars varies according to their location, with scarring over joints or on the face having a significant effect on function and appearance. Linares and Larson[68] describe three stages of burn scarring: immature, semi-mature, and mature. The immature non-hypertrophic scar is red and flat, whereas the immature hypertrophic scar is red but is also indurated and raised. In non-hypertrophic scars, the collagen fibers are aligned nearly parallel to the skin surface, an arrangement that resembles normal skin histologically. Hypertrophic scars demonstrate random collagen orientation, with fibers arranged in whorls and nodules (Fig. 58–18).

As normal and hypertrophic scars mature, the vascularity is reduced, the redness fades, and hypertrophic scars show a decrease in whorls and nodules on histological examination. With maturity, both types show a predominance of collagen in parallel arrays. Clinically, both scars are soft and pale. A hypertrophic scar requires up to 2 years to reach maturity, whereas a non-hypertrophic scar may mature in weeks to months.[1, 52]

Mechanical pressure alters the orientation of the collagen fibers found in hypertrophic scarring. Kischer and co-workers examined hypertrophic scars with electron microscopy and found that pressure-treated hypertrophic scars appeared to mature more rapidly.[60] Collagen fibers were more likely to be in parallel, and collagen nodules occurred less frequently.[53]

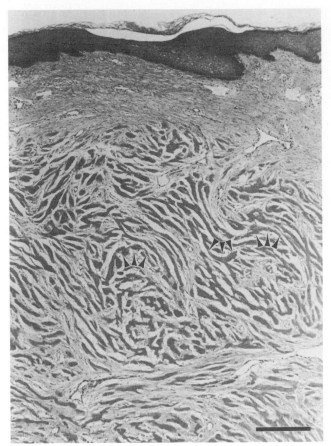

FIGURE 58–18 Whorled pattern of collagen in hypertrophic scar. Compare with the normal skin depicted in Figure 58–2. (From Staley MJ Richard RL: Scar management. *In* Richard RL, Staley MJ (eds): Burn Care and Rehabilitation. Philadelphia, FA Davis, 1994, p 384.)

The risk of hypertrophic scarring increases with the depth of injury and length of time required for healing. Certain anatomical locations are associated with greater incidence of hypertrophic scarring (e.g., buttocks and chest) (Fig. 58–19). The risk of hypertrophic scarring is reported by some authors to be greater in more darkly pigmented races.[24, 95]

It is generally accepted that pressure-treated scars have a better functional and cosmetic outcome. The application of continuous pressure through garments, orthoses, and splints is the primary nonsurgical modality used to control hypertrophic scarring. The mechanism by which pressure suppresses hypertrophic scarring is unclear, but it has been hypothesized that pressure causes decreased capillary perfusion and decreased tissue oxygenation, resulting in reduced cellular activity and collagen synthesis.[87]

Treatment options for scar suppression include custom fitted pressure garments (Fig. 58–20), elastic bandages, and custom made elastic or rigid face masks. Pressure applied to the healing area should be at least 25 mm Hg (i.e., the applied pressure should exceed normal capillary pressure). Pressure is applied at least 23 hours/day. Custom inserts—pieces of silicone or moldable plastics that placed under pressure garments and orthoses to create a more intimate fit—are often needed over uneven anatomical areas to which it is difficult to apply pressure (e.g., the web spaces of the

hand). The application of pressure should continue until the scar is mature (i.e., the scar is soft and is no longer red). Patient education is essential in increasing pressure therapy compliance. The garments can be fabricated in varying colors, but patients often do not like the garment's appearance, regardless of color or type. In addition, pressure garments and devices are expensive and are often hot and difficult to don. Complications of pressure therapy garments include superficial abrasions from the shear forces produced by the garment and local dermatitis. In the young child, pressure effects on skeletal growth require monitoring. Frequent adjustments to accommodate growth spurts are necessary.[65]

Facial burns have a significant impact on a person's appearance and state of well-being. Cosmesis and preservation of facial function are major priorities. Acutely, facial burns should alert the physician to possible inhalation injury. The risk of eye injury is increased in facial burns. Facial wounds require an experienced wound care physician. Wounds expected to heal in less than 3 weeks often do not require early surgery and are less likely to develop significant scarring.[22, 93]

Custom made elastic face masks and transparent orthoses are available for controlling facial scarring. The highly contoured features of the face, especially the central face, make scar control problematic. The goal is to preserve facial contours, especially the nasal profile and the shape

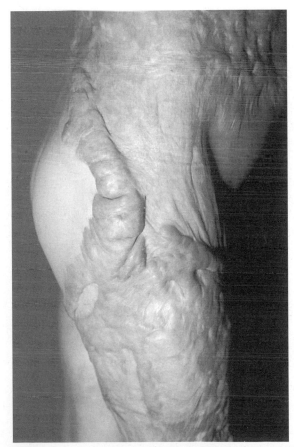

FIGURE 58–19 Lateral view of the lower trunk, buttock, and thigh, showing extensive hypertrophic scarring that limits hip range of motion.

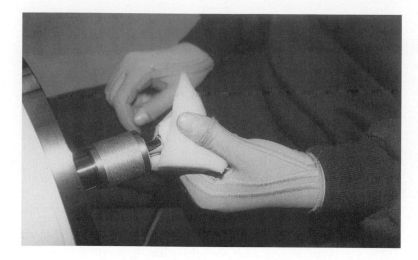

FIGURE 58–20 Custom fitted pressure garments for scar suppression after hand burns. Fine motor skill training is necessary to maintain hand function and work skills.

of the mouth and eyes. Silicone and other materials can be added to face masks to achieve better pressure application in hard-to-control regions, such as the nasolabial fold.[22, 113]

Microstomia orthoses can be fabricated or purchased to maintain the normal mouth aperture (Fig. 58–21). Early splinting reduces the need for corrective surgery.[93, 113] Scarring can severely distort the nose, affecting cosmesis and respiratory function. Custom-fitted nasal trumpets (Fig. 58–22), which can be fabricated from low-temperature thermoplastic materials, can successfully maintain the nasal openings.[21, 55]

Unlike other body regions, pressure is contraindicated during the acute and recovery phase of ear burns. Ears require protection to avoid the development of pressure necrosis and chondritis. Specialized foam protectors and headgear can be designed.[41, 56]

Hand Rehabilitation

Hands are the most common site of burn injury.[99] Because of the highly specialized functions of the hand, the burned hand requires the care of burn specialists experienced in hand management. Treatment goals include edema control, early wound closure, rapid return of hand function, and prevention of hand deformities (Fig. 58–23). Many types of hand deformities can result from deep partial-thickness and full-thickness injuries. The type of deformity relates to the location of the burn injury (e.g., burns of the thenar eminence and first web space cause thumb adduction contracture). Common deformities of the hand include wrist flexion contractures, metacarpophalangeal (MCP) hyperextension contractures, and interphalangeal (IP) flexion contractures. Bands of hypertrophic scarring can develop and limit hand function. The clinician must think expectantly and act to prevent the complications most likely to occur in a given patient.

After assessing the hand for potential hypertrophic scarring and contracture formation, a well-designed program of exercise, splinting, and hypertrophic scar suppression should be prescribed. Exercise coupled with use of splints, when indicated, can prevent hand deformities and restore optimal hand function. When splints are used, they should maintain the hand in an anti-contracture position, which will prevent the anticipated deformity. Frequently, the dorsum or the full circumference of the hand is injured. These injuries require that the hand be splinted in the position of function (i.e., IP joint extension, MCP joint flexion, thumb abduction, and wrist extension). This position preserves the maximal length and mobility of the extensor hood mechanism. Splint design should also preserve the transverse arch of the hand. In addition to static splints that hold the hand in a prescribed position, dynamic splints are available to facilitate ROM restoration or to substitute for a particular motion. Dynamic splints provide force in a specific plane, generally through elastic traction, while allowing motion in other planes.

Exposed tendons and joints of the hand demand specialized treatment. Any exposed tendons require dressings that will keep them moist, because dehydration can lead to tendon rupture. Exposed tendons are splinted in a slackened position. Once the wound is covered, passive ROM can be performed judiciously. If the joint capsule is intact, gentle active exercise can be done. This exercise must be done under supervision of an experienced therapist. The risk of septic arthritis is increased in open or exposed joints.

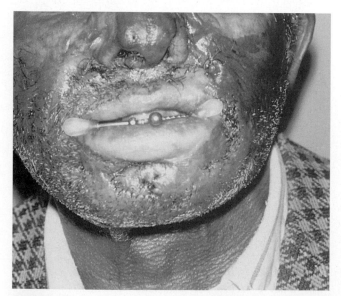

FIGURE 58–21 Microstomia splint to maintain oral commissure after facial burns.

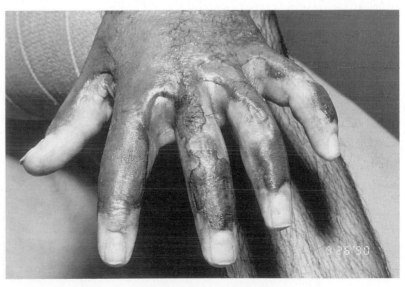

FIGURE 58–22 Nasal trumpet used to maintain patency and contour of nasal openings. The method of measuring for length (L) and depth (D) of the orthosis is indicated. (From Johnson J, Candia J, LaTrenta G, et al: A nasal trumpet orthosis to maintain nares openings and respiratory function for patients with facial burns: A case report. J Burn Care Rehabil 1992; 13:677.)

NEUROMUSCULAR COMPLICATIONS

Peripheral nerve injury after burns is common but not well recognized. Neurological involvement includes focal nerve compression, multiple mononeuropathies, and generalized peripheral neuropathies. Focal mononeuropathies commonly occur secondary to positioning, improperly applied splints, or bulky dressings.[44] Helm and associates[44] found that footdrop secondary to a peroneal neuropathy at the fibular head was the most common neuropathy, followed by median and ulnar mononeuropathies. The incidence of brachial plexopathies was also significant.

Multiple mononeuropathies also occur. Marquez and co-workers[74] reported a prevalence of 2%, and noted that multiple mononeuropathies were more likely to develop in males than in females (4.3:1). Electrodiagnostic studies showed predominantly axonal involvement. The mononeu-

ropathies were asymmetrical and were more likely to occur in the upper limbs (3:1); they were not always found in burned regions. Also, the neuropathies did not consistently correlate with compression from positioning, dressings, or splints.

Henderson and colleagues[49] first proposed that burn injuries are intrinsically associated with generalized peripheral neuropathy. Approximately 15% of the inpatients had peripheral neuropathy, which occurred primarily in patients who had injuries on more than 20% of TBSA. The type of peripheral neuropathy was not characterized.[48]

Helm and others[43] studied 88 patients with major burns who complained of persistent weakness or easy fatigability. A generalized peripheral neuropathy was found in 52%, but whether this was primarily an axonal or demyelinating process was not reported.[43] Like the findings of Henderson and colleagues,[49] the incidence correlated with the amount

FIGURE 58–23 Hypertrophic scarring on dorsum of hand that limits flexion of metacarpophalangeal and interphalangeal joints.

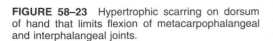

of TBSA affected (i.e., neuropathy was more likely to occur in adults with more than 20% TBSA injury and in children with more than 30% TBSA injury). The study by Marquez and colleagues showed electrodiagnostic evidence of a predominance of motor, rather than sensory, axonal peripheral neuropathy. Electrodiagnostically, these findings are consistent with critical care polyneuropathy seen in patients with multiple organ failure as described by Bolton and others.[13] The generalized peripheral neuropathy of the burn patient may be a subset of critical care polyneuropathy. The etiology of the peripheral neuropathy of burns has not been established, but neurotoxicity from antibiotics and the possibility of a circulating neurotoxin from the burn injury itself have been hypothesized.[49, 80, 101]

HETEROTOPIC OSSIFICATION

Heterotopic ossification (HO) occurs after serious burns and represents abnormal calcification of soft tissues surrounding a joint. The risk of HO is increased in injuries that affect 20% or more of TBSA. Heterotopic ossification is more likely to occur the longer wounds remain open and the patient remains immobile. Evans documented an incidence of 2% in 1400 patients.[28] The most common site was the posterior elbow. The second most common site was the hip in children and the shoulder in adults. The site of ossification does not necessarily correlate with the location of burn injuries and can occur in single or multiple joints.

HO can cause progressive loss of joint ROM and nerve entrapment mononeuropathies. HO can spontaneously resolve in some cases. If HO significantly interferes with function and is unresponsive to nonsurgical treatment, surgery is indicated. Typically, surgical excision is not performed until the bone has matured to reduce the risk of recurrence. Serial bone scans appear to be the most reliable method of determining when HO has matured.[27] Surgery has been performed earlier in the case of nerve entrapment associated with progressive neurological loss, despite the risk of HO recurrence.[111]

BURN-INDUCED AMPUTATION

Limb amputation may be necessary after severe burn injury, particularly after electrical burns. Electrical injury is the leading cause of amputation in the burn patient population.[76] The basic principles of amputee rehabilitation apply (see Chapters 14 and 15). The preprosthetic problems are similar to those with other amputations, but additional problems can occur, such as skin fragility, hypertrophic scarring, burn contractures, and altered skin sensation. The prosthesis may have to be fitted over scar tissue or previous graft sites, which can be less tolerant than normal of the shear forces created by the prosthesis. Blistering and open sores can develop more easily, forcing the patient to temporarily discontinue prosthesis use. These complications generally respond to local treatment. Newer prosthetic materials, such as silicone-impregnated sheaths and gel liners, can reduce shear and decrease the incidence of secondary skin disruption.

Painful bony spurs can occur at the distal end of the residual limb, especially with electrical injuries. Helm and Walker[47] noted that bony spurs occurred in 82% of patients who had electrical injuries and required amputation. The mean time from diagnosis to amputation was 38 weeks. Surgical revision was required in approximately 12% of cases. The pathophysiological process that causes the bone spur formation is not known.

Prosthesis fitting and training in burn patients is often complicated by the presence of wounds, multiple amputations, or ongoing medical problems. Successful prosthesis use can be achieved in patients with multiple amputations, but more intensive rehabilitation efforts are required.[54, 64, 108]

Malone and co-workers[71] demonstrated a high rate of successful upper extremity prosthesis use when patients were fitted within 30 days of amputation. Fletchall and Hickerson[33] have demonstrated that this principle is important in the burn population as well. Although the sample of Fletchall and Hickerson was small, a high rate of prosthesis use was reported in patients fitted within 30 days of the last definitive surgical procedure on the amputated upper extremity. All patients were independent in self-care and used the prosthesis within 2 weeks of receiving it. Self-care activities included eating, dressing, grooming, and using the toilet without assistance. On the average, patients were able to return to driving, homemaking, and avocational interests within 2.5 months (range, 1.5 to 5.0 months).

PEDIATRIC BURNS

Mortality rates are higher in infants compared with those in adolescents or young adults. Children younger than 1 year are at greater risk for mortality than during subsequent preschool and school years.[96] More than half of the 26,000 children hospitalized each year for burns are younger than 5 years.[19] Children ages 6 months to 2 years account for more than half of pediatric burn admissions.[104] This correlates with the developmental stages during which children rapidly acquire motor skills that allow them to get into potentially dangerous situations in which they may get burned.

Burn treatment of pediatric patients is somewhat different from that of adults. The TBSA–to–body weight ratio of children is greater than that of adults, and it does not reach adult proportions until adolescence. This predisposes children to even more significant fluid loss from evaporation and injury. Thermoregulation is more easily disturbed because of the relatively large body surface. Fluid resuscitation protocols must be adjusted to the child's weight and height.

The causes of burns in children are also different from those in adults. Scalding is the most common burn experienced by children. Up to age 4 years, 75% of all burns are due to scalding.[26] Burn injury is a common form of child abuse. Non-accidental injuries account for approximately 10% to 28% of pediatric burns.[32, 104] Of all non-accidental injuries experienced by children, 10% are due to burns.[90] The child who experiences a non-accidental scald injury is typically younger than 2 years.[32] The hospital course for children who sustain non-accidental scald burns is significantly longer, and their medical course tends to be more complicated.[50]

The clinician must recognize the characteristics of non-accidental injuries, because 30% to 70% of abused children suffer a repeat injury.[90] Characteristics that indicate a non-accidental injury include the following: history of injury that does not correlate with the type and location of injury observed on examination; uniform burn depth; sharp lines of demarcation between burned and nonburned areas; symmetrical wounds (i.e., in a stocking/glove pattern); absence of splash marks in scald injuries; presence of other injuries in various stages of healing. The physician is required to report any injuries caused by abuse, or suspected abuse, to the appropriate child protection agencies. Reporting child abuse or suspected child abuse is required in all states. Reporting procedures vary from state to state.[84] Prompt medical and psychosocial care must be initiated.

The rehabilitation program is based on the child's injury and developmental stage. Children are often unable to cooperate with many aspects of therapy and do not understand long-term goals. Loss of function, such as hand dexterity and ROM, not only interferes with activities appropriate to the child's current developmental level but also can limit future academic and vocational success (Fig. 58–24). Therapeutic success often depends on making therapy fun by incorporating age-appropriate recreation and play activities. Educating the child's family and establishing rapport with the child and family early can improve participation, long-term compliance, and final outcome. Both the child and the family need emotional, social, and medical support to achieve the best rehabilitative outcome.

A child's size often makes positioning, splinting, and fitting of compression garments challenging. Because of growth, children require more frequent modification of splints and custom fitted pressure garments. Skeletal and dental development can be compromised by compression therapy. For example, it is important to monitor jaw development and dental alignment during the use of face masks and orthoses to avoid malocclusion.[30, 65]

It is fairly common for children to regress emotionally, socially, and developmentally during the acute period of a burn injury. This should be temporary, and if it does not appear to be resolving, developmental screening is indicated. The Denver Developmental Screening Test is appropriate for children age 6 years and younger, and it is easy to administer. The type and location of injury have to be taken into account to avoid an inaccurate diagnosis of developmental delay. More in-depth assessments are also available to assess developmental delays if needed.

GERIATRIC BURNS

Skin atrophies with age, which results in deeper burn injuries in geriatric patients. Mortality rates are higher, as the risk of death increases with age from the middle years onward.[96] The likelihood of survival is markedly decreased by the presence of an inhalation injury in all age groups, but it is accentuated in elderly persons.[51] Cardiopulmonary disease, diabetes mellitus, peripheral vascular disease, and other pre-existing medical conditions can complicate burn management in the elderly.

The geriatric patient can be at increased risk for burn injury because of premorbid mobility limitations, visual deficits, impaired sensation, and cognitive problems. Knowledge about the patient's functional level prior to the burn injury is important in planning the rehabilitation program. The patient who was previously marginally independent will likely be dependent in some aspects of mobility or performance of ADL at discharge. However, many geriatric patients are able to return to a home setting and avoid permanent placement in an extended care facility. Keys and associates[59] noted that only 5% of their patients required nursing home placement. Factors that predicted need for an extended care facility were both medical and social.

Geriatric patients often experience an initial drop in independence at discharge because of wound care, deconditioning, and outpatient therapy needs. Early involvement of social services can identify patients whose social and medical situation requires nursing home placement or a setting with additional support services. Early planning for

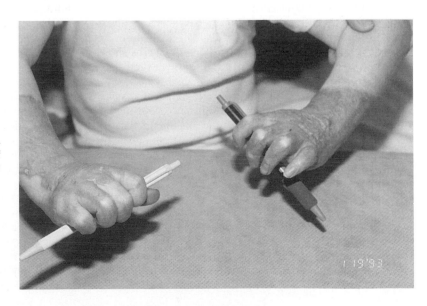

FIGURE 58–24 Notice blanching of interphalangeal joints with flexion. Significant loss of range of motion has occurred and limits fine motor skills, such as ability to write and manipulate small objects.

home health care services can prevent or shorten stays in an extended care facility and enable a geriatric patient to return home.[59, 72, 105]

The elderly appear to have less hypertrophic scarring[58] and tend to experience slower healing than the young.[21, 66] Decreased scarring might be due to reduced fibroblastic activity and collagen synthesis compared with that of the young.[58] When the risk of hypertrophic scarring is evident, elderly persons can be less accepting of pressure garments because of difficulty in donning the garments and their high cost. The inclusion of zippers in pressure garments can make donning and doffing more feasible.

Splinting, positioning, and exercise principles in this population are similar to those of other adults. Splints require careful monitoring because of increased skin fragility and decreased sensation secondary to scarring and pre-existing disease. Early mobilization is imperative because the effects of immobility occur more rapidly and are more pronounced in elderly persons.[14] Elderly persons typically have less cardiac reserve and decreased maximal oxygen consumption and cardiac work capacity.[89] Regardless of activity level, the number of motor units and overall muscle mass declines with age.[100] Although exercise programs must reflect these differences, well-designed exercise programs can assist geriatric patients in making significant gains in strength and endurance. Exercise protocols should emphasize functional activities of ambulation and mobility in addition to ROM and basic strengthening. Functional mobility is a first priority.

PSYCHOLOGICAL ADJUSTMENT

Pre-injury psychological status is a strong predictor of a patient's long-term emotional status after a serious burn. Patients who were previously well-adjusted emotionally are likely to continue to demonstrate appropriate emotional adjustment. Previous psychological dysfunction is likely to be accentuated by burn trauma.[91, 107] Additionally, such patients are more likely to have medical complications, and their hospital stays are significantly longer than those of burn patients without previous emotional dysfunction.[11, 17]

Premorbid psychiatric disorders tend to be more frequent in patients who sustain burns than in the general population. It appears that psychiatric disease predisposes an individual to a burn injury.[94] Epidemiology of burns shows that alcohol, senility, and psychiatric disease all predispose individuals to burn injuries.[70] Approximately 45% to 69% of patients hospitalized for burns have a premorbid psychiatric history, including alcohol and substance abuse.[11, 85, 94] A history of depression increases the likelihood that patients sustained injury as a consequence of risk-enhancing behaviors.[94] In addition, an increase in stressful life events in the prior year is also associated with an increased risk of burns.[85]

A model describing the psychological adjustment of the seriously burned adult is outlined by Watkins and co-workers.[115] This model assumes no previous psychiatric illness. It describes the issues that patients face from the onset of injury to the completion of psychological recovery, rather than operating from a psychoanalytical paradigm. It assumes that psychological adaptation does not parallel physical recovery. The sequential stages proposed include survival anxiety, pain, search for meaning, investment in recuperation, acceptance of losses, investment in rehabilitation, and reintegration of identity. Interventions are proposed to facilitate resolution of each stage of recovery with the final outcome of healthy emotional adjustment. They propose that if each stage is not successfully resolved, psychological complications are likely to occur.

Delirium, adjustment disorders, major depression, and post-traumatic stress disorder (PTSD) are the most commonly seen psychiatric disorders during recovery from a burn injury.[114] Delirium, a transient disorder, is the most common, and it occurs in more than half of hospitalized burn patients.[94] The etiology is often multifactorial, resulting from sepsis, anoxia, anemia, liver and renal dysfunction, and other organic causes. Pediatric and geriatric patients are at greater risk for development of delirium. With correction of the underlying cause, the delirium resolves.[6]

Adjustment disorder is the second most frequently encountered disorder.[114] It occurs within 3 months of a stressful event and typically resolves within 6 months of termination of the stressor. It can persist longer in the presence of chronic conditions, such as a disabling medical condition or financial difficulties as a result of unemployment.[2] Depression and anxiety are frequently present. Anticipatory anxiety (e.g., an exaggerated expectation of pain with dressing changes or ROM exercise) is particularly common among patients with burn injuries. Individualized psychotherapeutic intervention and judiciously prescribed medications are indicated for these problems.[114]

Major depression and post-traumatic stress disorder are major complications of burn rehabilitation. Serial evaluation and awareness of the potential for these complications can lead to early intervention, prevent loss of function, and improve rehabilitative outcome.

OUTPATIENT REHABILITATION

Planning for discharge should begin as early as possible. Education of the patient and family builds a foundation for all aspects of rehabilitation, including outpatient treatment. Outpatient rehabilitation is influenced by a number of factors: the patient's social support system, functional status, ongoing need for physical and occupational therapy, wound care requirements, return to work/school criteria, availability of community services, and financial resources. All of these factors require consideration when an outpatient rehabilitation program is being designed.

At discharge, the patient needs to be independent in all aspects of care in order to return home. If not, arrangements for appropriate outpatient services need to be in place prior to discharge. Typically, home treatment programs involve a daily exercise regimen of stretching and strengthening, endurance training, use of pressure garments and splints, and wound care. Splints are often used and require that the patient learn the purpose and proper application of the devices. Visiting nurses can help reduce the risk of complications by assisting in wound care, monitoring wound healing and medication administration, and educating the patient about burn injury recovery.

The need for physical and occupational therapy does not end at discharge. Ideally, the patient should be referred to therapists with previous experience in treating burn injuries on an outpatient basis. Therapy programs need to continue the focus on ROM, strengthening, endurance, mobility, and gait.

It is common for patients to return to communities in which rehabilitation resources for the patient with burn injuries are limited. Regular follow-up, specific recommendations, and periodic communication with the community medical and allied health personnel can help to ensure quality rehabilitative care.

Skin that has been injured by burns has special needs. Moisturizers are required to control dryness, itching, and cracking. The skin must be protected from ultraviolet light because it is less tolerant and will burn more easily. Protection from sun and other sources of ultraviolet radiation is most critical during the period of scar maturation (i.e., the first 1 to 2 years).

During the months and years that follow discharge from the hospital, patients often require reconstructive surgery to correct or prevent deformity and loss of function (Fig. 58–25). Typically, reconstructive surgery is delayed until scar maturation is achieved. An immature scar is more vascular, and local tissue response to the trauma of surgery is greater than in the mature scar. As a result, surgical outcomes are less favorable. However, if severe deformity is developing, surgery may be performed early to prevent irreversible loss of function (e.g., ectropion of the eyelid, which can lead to corneal damage and loss of vision). Serial procedures are often required to address cosmesis, function, or impaired physical maturation (e.g., female breast development). Because scar tissue does not expand with growth, children may need multiple operations during their growing years to correct and prevent loss of function and to improve cosmetic outcome.

Determining the timing of surgical releases and other reconstructive procedures requires consideration of the body region burned as well as the patient's age, lifestyle, occupation, and medical and psychological well-being. Though restoration of function is typically the first priority, cosmesis may be more important in cases of severe facial burns. Function and appearance of the hands and face generally are given the highest priority. After consideration of all factors, an overall surgical plan needs to be established that reflects the identified priorities and needs of the patient.

After discharge, the patient faces the task of family and community re-integration. Self-esteem can be significantly altered by changes in appearance and functional abilities. With post-burn injury, women and girls are noted to have lower self-esteem than men and boys who experience comparable injuries.[86] Physical attractiveness is known to be more important for self-esteem in females than in males. This correlation is also seen in persons with burn injuries.[15] Persons with burn scars often do not experience empathy from others that is typically seen with other disabilities. Burn patients can be seen as unattractive.[10] Children with facial, buttocks, or genital injuries are at increased risk of depression and poor self-esteem.[19]

Studies indicate that the greater the patient's perception of social support from family and friends, the more positive is the body image and the higher the sense of self-esteem. Symptoms of depression occur less frequently in this group of patients as well.[15, 86] Social support appears to be a key factor in a person's psychological adaptation to a burn injury.[61] The family should be educated about the key role that they and friends play in the patient's psychological recovery and continued sense of well-being.

WORK ISSUES

Returning to work is an issue of major importance to many burn patients. The TBSA injured, followed by the percentage of full-thickness and partial-thickness burns, are the factors that correlate most strongly with the time needed to return to work.[46] The presence of hand burns,[45] the type of employment, and age significantly influence return to work.[16, 20] Overemphasis on ROM without adequate attention to the importance of endurance, strength,

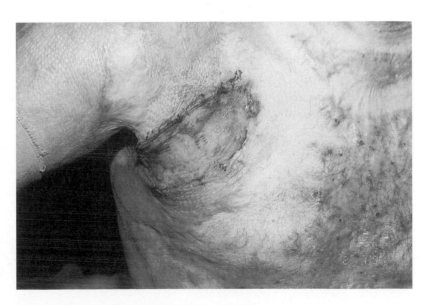

FIGURE 58–25 Right anterior axillary split-thickness skin graft performed to release an axillary contracture that limits shoulder range of motion. Note the healed mesh graft on the proximal arm. The interstices created by meshing the graft before it was applied persist.

and power required in work settings can delay return to employment.[23]

Special problems affecting return to work include pruritus, skin fragility, heat and cold intolerance, altered sensation, and impaired coordination and dexterity. Burn injuries often occur at work, and affected individuals may have difficulty returning to the site of their injury. In the case of severe injury, approximately 20% to 50% of patients require a change in occupation.[20, 98] Vocational counselors can provide the patient and rehabilitation team with the expertise required to identify an appropriate occupation.

Work hardening is a highly structured work program that focuses on the tasks that a patient needs to be able to perform a given job (see Chapter 44). Individualized programs of training are developed after the individual's current level of function has been determined. Productivity, safety, work attitude, physical tolerance, and the specific demands of the job are weighed. The hallmark of work hardening is job simulation. The study by Zeller and associates[116] demonstrates that persons with major burn injuries can achieve a high level of vocational success; up to 90% of patients in the study returned to work.

Fewer than 1% of all disability claims approved by Social Security are due to burns.[98] Evaluation of back-to-work status and impairment ratings typically stress limitations of ROM.[5] Medical reports supporting impairment ratings should also address the unique long-term impairments in mobility, including standing and walking tolerance, hand function, skin fragility, sensitivity to ultraviolet light and chemicals, chronic pain and pruritus, heat and cold intolerance, impaired strength and sensation, and cardiopulmonary limitations.

Unfortunately, many patients are lost to follow-up. A number of variables can hinder follow-up care. These variables are often interrelated and include the distance from the patient's home to the regional burn center, type of insurance, age, marital status, availability of social support, mental health, work status, educational background, and financial status.[61, 98] These issues need to be considered and potential problems addressed prior to discharge from the hospital, and they should be re-evaluated at outpatient follow-up appointments. Ensuring ongoing care by specialists trained in burn care and rehabilitation optimize the long-term outcome of the burn-injured individual.

CONCLUSION

Rehabilitation should begin at the time of admission. Serious burn injury results in multi-system trauma and has implications far beyond skin loss. Collaboration between the physiatrist and the burn surgeon managing the patient's acute medical and surgical care should begin immediately on the patient's admission to the burn unit. Integrating the expertise of the burn surgeon and the physiatrist will ensure that all aspects of patient care are addressed and that the patient will receive the full complement of burn care services needed to achieve an optimal functional and cosmetic outcome. Because of the complexity and long-term effects of burns, patients require the expertise of a multidisciplinary burn care team that is composed of physicians, nurses, physical and occupational therapists, social workers, psy-

chologists, speech pathologists, and other allied health personnel. The physiatrist is pivotal in directing the team in the planning and implementation of a individualized rehabilitation program for each patient. Many burns result in long-term functional impairments, and successful rehabilitation often requires years of effort. Success ultimately depends on the combined effort and commitment of the patient and the burn care rehabilitation team.

References

1. Abston S: Scar reaction after thermal injury and prevention of scars and contractures. In Boswick JA (ed): The Art and Science of Burn Care. Rockville, Md, Aspen Publishers, 1987, pp 359–371.
2. Adler R: Burns are different: The child psychiatrist on the pediatric burn ward. J Burn Care Rehabil 1992; 13:28–32.
3. American Burn Association: Hospital and pre-hospital resources for optimal care of patients with burn injury: Guidelines for development and operation of burn center. J Burn Care Rehabil 1990; 11:98–104.
4. American Medical Association's Council on Scientific Affairs: Guide to Evaluation of Permanent Impairment, ed 4. Chicago, AMA, 1993.
5. American Psychiatric Association: Adjustment disorder. In Diagnostic and Statistical Manual of Mental Disorders, ed 4. Washington, DC, American Psychiatric Association, 1994, pp 623–627.
6. Andreasen NJ, Noyes R, Hartford CR, et al: Management of emotional reactions in seriously burned adults. N Engl J Med 1972; 286:65–69.
7. Armstrong LE, Winent DM, Swasey PR, et al: Using isokinetic dynamometry to test ambulatory patients with multiple sclerosis. Phys Ther 1983; 63:74–79.
8. Baxter CR: Fluid volume and electrolyte changes in the early post burn period. Clin Plast Surg 1974; 1:693–709.
9. Bernstein N: Emotional care of the facially burned and disfigured. Boston, Little, Brown, 1976, p 288.
10. Bernstein N: Marital and sexual adjustment of severely burned patients: Medical aspects of human sexuality 1985; 19:220–223.
11. Berry CC, Wachtel TL, Frank HA: An analysis of factors which predict mortality in hospitalized burn patients. Burns 1982; 9:38.
12. Borysenko M, Beringer T: Functional Histology. Boston, Little, Brown, 1984, pp 228–231.
13. Bolton CF, Young GB, Zochodne DW: The neurological complications of sepsis. Ann Neurol 1993; 33:94–100.
14. Bortz WM II: Disuse and aging. JAMA 1982; 248:1203–1208.
15. Bowden ML, Feller I, Tholen D, et al: Self esteem in severely burned patients. Arch Phys Med Rehabil 1980; 61:449–452.
16. Bowden ML, Thomson PD, Prasad JK: Factors influencing return to employment after a burn injury. Arch Phys Med Rehabil 1989; 70:772–774.
17. Brezel BS, Kassenbrock JM, Stein JM: Burn in substance abusers and in neurologically and mentally impaired patients. J Burn Care Rehabil 1988; 9:169–171.
18. Campbell JL, La Clave LJ: Clinical depression in pediatric burn patients. Burns 1987; 13:213–217.
19. Centers for Disease Control and Prevention: Childhood injuries in the United States. AJDC 1990; 144:627–646.
20. Cheng S: Changes in occupational role performance after a severe burn: A retrospective study. Am J Occup Ther 1989; 43:17.
21. Chvapil M, Koopmann CF: Age and other factors regulating wound healing. Otolaryngol Clin North Am 1982; 15:259–270.
22. Covey MH: Occupational therapy. In Boswick JA (ed): The Art and Science of Burn Care. Rockville, Md, Aspen Publishers, 1987, pp 285–298.
23. Cronan R, Hammond J, Ward CG: The value of isokinetic exercise and testing burn rehabilitation and determination of back to work status. J Burn Care Rehabil 1990; 11:224–227.
24. Deitch EA, Wheelahan TM, Rose MP, et al: Hypertrophic burn scars. J Trauma 1983; 23:895.
25. Dunphy JE, Van Winkle W: Repair and regeneration. New York, McGraw-Hill, 1969, pp 87–94.
26. East MK, Jones CA, Feller I, et al: Epidemiology of burns in children. In Carvajal HF, Parks DH (eds): Burns in Children. Chicago, Year Book Medical Publishers, 1988, p 20.

27. Edlich RF: Heterotopic calcification and ossification in the burn patient. J Burn Care Rehabil 1985; 6:363–368.

28. Evans EB: Orthopaedic measures in the treatment of severe burn. J Bone Joint Surg Am 1966; 48:643–669.

29. Evans ET, Purnell OJ, Robinett PW, et al: Fluid and electrolyte requirements in severe burns. Ann Surg 1952; 135:804.

30. Fader P: Preserving function and minimizing deformity. In Carvajal HF, Parks DH (eds): Burns in Children. Chicago, Year Book Medical Publishers, 1988, p 335.

31. Farrell DF, Starr A: Delayed neurologic sequelae of electrical injuries. Neurology 1968; 18:600–606.

32. Feldman KW, Schaller RT, Feldman JA, et al: Tap water scald burns in children. Pediatrics 1978; 62:1–7.

33. Fletchall S, Hickerson WL: Early upper extremity prosthetic fit in patients with burns. J Burn Care Rehabil 1991; 12:234.

34. Fraser PM: Ptolemaic Alexandria, vol 1. Oxford, Clarendon Press, 1937.

35. Freshwater MF, Krizek TJ: Skin grafting of burns: A centennial tribute to George David Pollack. J Trauma 1971; 11:862.

36. Grube BJ, Heimbach DM, Engrav LH, et al: Neurologic consequences of electrical burns. J Trauma 1990; 30:254–258.

37. Haberal J: Electrical burns: A five year experience—1985 Evans Lecture. J Trauma 1986; 26:103–109.

38. Hammond JS, Ward CG: High voltage electrical injuries: Management and outcome of 60 cases. South Med J 1988; 81:1351–1352.

39. Hansbrough JF, Zapata-Sirvent R, Carroll WJ, et al: Clinical experience with Biobrane biosynthetic dressing in the treatment of partial thickness burns. Burns 1984; 10:415–419.

40. Hansbrough JF: Biologic dressings. In Boswick JA (ed): The Art and Science of Burn Care. Rockville, Md, Aspen Publishers, 1987, p 57.

41. Harries CA, Pegg SP: Foam ear protectors for burnt ears. J Burn Care Rehabil 1989; 10:183.

42. Haynes BW Jr: The history of burn care. In Boswick JA (ed): The Art and Science of Burn Care. Rockville, Md, Aspen Publishers, 1987, pp 3–9.

43. Helm PA, Johnson ER, Carlton AM: Peripheral neurological problems in the acute burn patient. Burns 1977; 3:123–125.

44. Helm PA, Pandian G, Heck E: Neuromuscular problems in the burn patient: Causes and prevention. Arch Phys Med Rehabil 1985; 66:451–453.

45. Helm PA, Walker SC, Peyton SA: Return to work following hand burns. Arch Phys Med Rehabil 1986; 67:297.

46. Helm PA, Walker SC: Return to work after burn injury. J Burn Care Rehabil 1992; 13:53.

47. Helm PA, Walker SC: New bone formation at amputation sites in electrically burn-injured patients. Arch Phys Med Rehabil 1987; 68:284–286.

48. Helm PA, Kevorkian CG, Lushbaugh M, et al: Burn injury: Rehabilitation management in 1982. Arch Phys Med Rehabil 1982; 63:6–16.

49. Henderson B, Koepke GH, Feller I: Peripheral polyneuropathy among patients with burns. Arch Phys Med Rehabil 1971; 52:149–152.

50. Hummel RP, Greenhalgh DG, Barthel PP, et al: Outcome and socioeconomic aspects of suspected child abuse scald burns. J Burn Care Rehabil 1993; 14:121.

51. Hunt JL, Purdue GF: The elderly burn patient. Am J Surg 1992; 164:472–476.

52. Hunt JL, Sato RM, Baxter CR: Acute electric injuries. Arch Surg 1980; 115:434–438.

53. Jensen LL, Parshley PH: Postburn scar contractures: Histology and effects of pressure treatment. J Burn Care Rehabil 1984; 5:119.

54. Johansen PB, Breiholtz M, Johansson B, et al: Prosthetic rehabilitation in bilateral high above elbow amputation. Scand J Rehabil Med 1986; 19:85–87.

55. Johnson J, Candia J, LaTrenta G, et al: A nasal trumpet orthosis to maintain nares openings and respiratory function for patients with facial burns: A case report. J Burn Care Rehabil 1992; 13:677.

56. Jordan MH, Gallagher JM, Allely RR, et al: Pressure prevention device for burned ears. J Burn Care Rehabil 1992; 13:673.

57. Kazdam MS: Electrical cataract: A report of two cases. Can J Ophthalmol 1969; 4:1040–1045.

58. Ketchum LD: Hypertrophic scars and keloids. Clin Plast Surg 1977; 4:301.

59. Keys TC, Moresi JM, Deitch EA: Thermal injury in the elderly: The limited need for nursing home care. J Burn Care Rehabil 1989; 5:429.

60. Kischer CW, Shetlar MR, Shetlar CL: Alteration of hypertrophic scars induced by mechanical pressure. Arch Dermatol 1975; 111:60.

61. Knudson-Cooper M: What are the research priorities in the behavioral areas for burn patients? J Trauma 1984; 24(suppl 9):S197–S201.

62. Koller J, Orsagh J: Delayed neurological sequelae of high tension electrical burns. Burns Therm Inj 1989; 15:175–178.

63. Kucan JO: Burn and trauma. In Ruberg RL, Smith DJ Jr (eds): Plastic Surgery: A Core Curriculum. St Louis, Mosby-Year Book, 1994, pp 207–237.

64. LaBorde TC, Meier RH III: Amputations resulting from electrical injury: A review of 22 cases. Arch Phys Med Rehabil 1986; 67:159.

65. Leung KS: Complications of pressure therapy for post-burn hypertrophic scars. Burns 1984; 10:434–438.

66. Levenson SM: Some challenging wound healing problems for clinicians and basic scientists. In Dunphy J, Van Winkle W (eds): Repair and Regeneration. New York, McGraw-Hill, 1969, pp 330–333.

67. Levine NS, Buchanan RT: The care of burned upper extremities. Clin Plast Surg 1986; 13:107–118.

68. Linares HA, Larson DL: Early differential diagnosis between hypertrophic and non-hypertrophic healing. J Invest Dermatol 1974; 62:514.

69. Lund CC, Browder NC: The estimate of areas of burns. Surg Gynecol Obstet 1944; 79:352.

70. MacArthur JD, Moore FD: Epidemiology of burns—the burn prone patient. JAMA 1975; 231:259–263.

71. Malone JM, Fleming LL, Roberson J, et al: Immediate, early and late post surgical management of upper limb amputation. J Rehabil Res Dev 1984; 21:33.

72. Manktelow A, Meyer AA, Herzog SR, et al: Analysis of life expectancy and living status of elderly patients surviving a burn injury. J Trauma 1989; 29:207.

73. Marks R: Mechanical properties of the skin. In Goldsmith LA (ed): Biochemistry and Physiology of the Skin. New York, Oxford University Press, 1983, pp 1238–1239.

74. Marquez S, Turley JJ, Peters WJ: Neuropathy in burn patients. Brain 1993; 116:471–483.

75. McManus WF: Immediate emergency department care. In Artz CP, Moncrief JA, Pruitt BA (eds): Burns: A Team Approach. Philadelphia, WB Saunders, 1979, pp 159–164.

76. Meier RH III: Amputation and prosthetic fitting. In Fisher SV, Helm PA (eds): Comprehensive Rehabilitation of Burns. Baltimore, Williams & Wilkins, 1984, pp 267–310.

77. Mettler CC: History of Medicine. Philadelphia, Blakiston, 1947.

78. Millington PF, Wilkinson R: Skin. Cambridge, Cambridge University Press, 1983, pp 83–112, 172–192.

79. Millstein SG, Heger H, Hunter GA: Prosthetic use in adult upper limb amputees: A comparison of body powered and electrically powered prostheses. Prosthet Orthot Int 1986; 10:27.

80. Monafo WW, Eliasson SG: Sciatic nerve function following hind limb thermal injury. J Surg Res 1987; 43:344–355.

81. Monafo WW, Freedman BM: Electrical and lightning injury. In Boswick JA Jr (ed): The Art and Science of Burn Care. Rockville, Md, Aspen Publishers, 1987, pp 241–253.

82. Moylan JA: First aid and transportation of burned patients. In Artz CP, Moncrief JA, Pruitt BA (eds): Burns: A Team Approach. Philadelphia, WB Saunders, 1979, pp 151–158.

83. Nahas LF, Swartz BL: Use of semipermeable polyurethane membrane for skin graft dressings. Plast Reconstr Surg 1981; 67:791–792.

84. National Clearinghouse on Child Abuse and Neglect Information: State Statutes Series #1: Definitions of Child Abuse and Neglect. Fairfax, Va, National Clearinghouse on Child Abuse and Neglect (in press).

85. Noyes R, Frye SJ, Slymen DJ, et al: Stressful life events and burn injuries. J Trauma 1979; 19:141.

86. Orr DA, Reznikoff M, Smith GM: Body image, self esteem and depression in burn-injured adolescents and young adults. J Burn Care Rehabil 1989; 10:454–461.

87. Page RE, Rogertson GA, Pettigrew NM: Microcirculation in hypertrophic burn scars. Burns Therm Inj 1983; 10:64–70.

88. Peacock EE Jr: Wound Repair, ed 3. Philadelphia, WB Saunders, 1984, pp 38–55.

89. Posner JD, Gorman KM, Klein HS, et al: Exercise capacity in the elderly. Am J Cardiol 1986; 57:520–580.

90. Purdue GF, Hunt JL, Prescott PR: Child abuse by burning—an index of suspicion. J Trauma 1988; 28:21.

91. Questad KA, Patterson R, Boltwood MD, et al: Relating mental health and physical function at discharge to rehabilitation status at 3 months post burn. J Burn Care Rehabil 1988; 9:87–89.

92. Rice DP, Mackenzie EJ, et al: Cost of Injury in the United States: A Report to Congress 1989. San Francisco, Institute for Health and Aging of the University of California, and Baltimore, Injury Prevention Center, The Johns Hopkins University (joint publication), 1989, p 153.

93. Robson MC, Smith DJ: Reconstruction of the burned face, neck, and scalp. In Boswick JA (ed): The Art and Science of Burn Care. Rockville, Md, Aspen Publishers, 1987, pp 375–376.

94. Rockwell E, Dimsdale JE, Carroll W, et al: Pre-existing psychiatric disorders in burn patients. J Burn Care Rehabil 1988; 9:83–86.

95. Rockwell WB, Cohen IK, Ehrlich HP: Keloids and hypertrophic scars: A comprehensive review. Plast Reconstr Surg 1989; 84:827.

96. Roi LD, Flora JD Jr, Wolfe RA: Two new burn severity indices. J Trauma 1983; 23:1023–1029.

97. Rouse RG, Dimick AR: The treatment of electrical injury compared to burn injury: A review of pathophysiology and comparison of patient management protocols. J Trauma 1978; 18:43–47.

98. Salisbury R: Burn rehabilitation: Our unanswered challenge. J Burn Care Rehabil 1992; 13:495.

99. Salisbury RE, Dingeldein GP: The burned hand and upper extremity. In Green DP (ed): Operative Hand Surgery, ed 2, vol 2. New York, Churchill Livingstone, 1988, p 1523.

100. Schaumberg HH, Spencer PS, Ochoa J: The aging peripheral nervous system. In Katzman R, Terry R (eds): The Neurology of Aging. Philadelphia, FA Davis, 1983, pp 111–122.

101. Sepulchre C, Moati F: Biochemical and pharmacologic properties of a neurotoxic protein isolated from the blood serum of heavily burned patients. J Pathol 1979; 127:137–145.

102. Silverstein P, Lack BO: Epidemiology and prevention. In The Art and Science of Burn Care. Rockville, Aspen Publishers, 1987, p 12.

103. Silverstein P, Maxwell P, Duckett L: Enzymatic debridement. In Boswick JA (ed): The Art and Science of Burn Care. Aspen Publications, 1987, pp 75–81.

104. Simon PA, Baron RC: Age as a risk factor for burn injury requiring hospitalization during early childhood. Arch Pediatr Adolesc Med 1994; 148:394–397.

105. Slater AL, Slater H, Goldfarb IW: Effects of aggressive surgical treatment in older patients with burns. J Burn Care 1989; 10:527.

106. Staley MJ, Richard RL: Scar management. In Richard RL, Staley MJ (eds): Burn Care and Rehabilitation. FA Davis, Philadelphia, 1994, p 384.

107. Steiner H, Clark WJ Jr: Psychiatric complications of burned adults: A classification. J Trauma 1977; 17:134–143.

108. Thornhill HL, Jones GD, Brodzka W, et al: Bilateral below knee amputations: Experience with 80 patients. Arch Phys Med Rehabil 1986; 67:159.

109. Underhill EP, Carrington GL: Blood concentration changes in extensive superficial burns, and their significance for systemic treatment. Arch Intern Med 1923; 32:31.

110. Van-Johnson E, Kline LB, Skalka HW: Electrical cataracts: A case report and review of the literature. Ophthalmic Surg 1987; 18:283–285.

111. Vorenkamp SE, Nelson T: Ulnar nerve entrapment due to heterotopic bone formation after severe burn. J Hand Surg 1987; 12A:378–380.

112. Ward RS, Hayes-Lundy C, Schnebly WA, et al: Prosthetic use in patients with burns and associated limb amputations. J Burn Rehabil 1991; 11:361–364.

113. Ward RS, Reddy R, Lundy CH, et al: Techniques for control of hypertrophic scarring in the central region of the face. J Burn Care Rehabil 1991; 12:263.

114. Watkins PN, Cook EL, May SR, et al: The role of the psychiatrist in the team treatment of the adult patient with burns. J Burn Care Rehabil 1992; 13:19–27.

115. Watkins PN, Cook EL, May SR, et al: Psychological stages in adaptation following burn injury: A method for facilitating psychological recovery of burn victims. J Burn Care Rehabil 1988; 9:376–384.

116. Zeller J, Sturm G, Cruse WC: Patients with burns are successful in work hardening programs. J Burn Care Rehabil 1993; 14:189.

Principles of
Geriatric Rehabilitation

GERALD FELSENTHAL, M.D.,
AND BARRY D. STEIN, M.D.

With the aging of our population, it has become imperative to maximize and maintain the function of all patients in order to preserve quality of life and decrease healthcare costs: "those 65 years and older currently account for one third of this country's total personal health expenditures."[40] With timely intervention, the rehabilitation team can help restore function close to the preinsult, premorbid functional level and attempt to preserve that functional level for the remainder of the patient's life span. This preservation or restoration of function should help reduce the total healthcare cost.[51]

DEMOGRAPHICS

In 1990, more than 30 million Americans or 12.7% of the U.S. population were 65 years of age or older. This will increase to 17.3% by the year 2020 and to 21.8% by the year 2050. The greatest increase will be the oldest-old age group of 85+ years which will more than double in the 30 years from 1990 to 2020—from approximately 3.3 million to 7.0 million (Table 59–1). This is especially significant because of the decline in function and the greater utilization of healthcare resources of the oldest-old age group as compared to the young-old (65–74 years) and the old-old (75–84 years).

As the population ages, there is an increase in both the prevalence of chronic conditions and activity limitations. For example, the estimate of the prevalence of osteoarthritis in persons 65+ years of age is 47.3% and of orthopedic impairment, 17.1%, while activity limitation in at least one major activity increases to 24.1%.[40] By age 76, 50% of community-living elderly in a longitudinal intervention study in Sweden were using assistive devices, mostly for mobility or bathing.[57]

Currently, 70% to 80% of the elderly population live in the community and not in nursing homes.[38] Figure 59–1 shows the proportion of community-dwelling elderly dependent in selected activities of daily living (ADL) or instrumental ADL by age group.[26] The proportion of dependent elderly approximately triples for the oldest-old as compared to the young-old and doubles for the oldest-old as compared to the old-old. A similar decrease in functional status has been reported for nursing home residents.[31] For example, in these three age groupings, the number of nursing home residents who required assistance in bathing increased from 84.8% of the young-old to 93.9% of the oldest-old. Similar increases in the need for assistance also occurred for dressing, mobility, transferring, and toileting activities, reaching 29.6% to 81.7% for the oldest-old.

ETIOLOGY OF
FUNCTIONAL PROBLEMS

The etiology of the functional problems of the elderly is varied. Figure 59–2 lists age-related etiological factors and Figure 59–3 indicates disease-related etiological factors. One of these factors is *ageism*, a term coined by Robert N. Butler,[9] to describe the bias against the elderly based solely on chronological age and which is manifested in attitudes such as, "What do you expect? You are old." Often, instead of actively seeking the cause of a problem and initiating a therapeutic intervention, the physician, family, and others ascribe the patient's complaint to the inevitable effects of chronological aging. This attitude justifies inaction and can lead to lack of treatment of reversible impairments such as carpal tunnel syndrome misdiagnosed as "arthritis."

GERIATRIC REHABILITATION

Geriatric rehabilitation can be defined as medical treatment plus prevention, restoration plus accommodation, and

TABLE 59–1   Actual and Projected Growth of the Older Population: United States, 1990–2050 (Numbers in Thousands)

Year	All Ages	65+ Years		65–74 Years		75–84 Years		85+ Years	
		No.	%	No.	%	No.	%	No.	%
1900	76,303	3084	4.0	2189	2.9	772	1.0	123	0.2
1930	122,775	6634	5.4	4721	3.8	1641	1.3	272	0.2
1960	179,323	16,560	9.2	10,997	6.1	4633	2.6	929	0.5
1990	249,657	31,697	12.7	18,035	7.2	10,349	4.1	3313	1.3
2020	296,597	51,422	17.3	29,855	10.1	14,486	4.9	7081	2.4
2050	309,488	67,411	21.8	30,114	9.7	21,263	6.9	16,034	5.2

Data from Spender G, US Bureau of the Census: Projections of the population of the United States by age, sex, and race: 1983 to 2080. Curr Popul Rep May 1984; Series P-25, No. 952; US Bureau of the Censuses: Tabulated from Decennial Censuses of Population, 1900 to 1980; US Bureau of the Census: Estimates of the population of the United States, by age, sex, and race: 1980–1986. Curr Popul Rep February 1987; Series P-25, No. 1000.
From Zimmerman SI, Fox K, Magaziner J: Demography and epidemiology of disabilities in the aged. *In* Felsenthal G, Garrison SJ, Steinberg FU (eds): Rehabilitation of the Aging and Elderly Patient. Baltimore, Williams & Wilkins, 1994, p 12.

education. The accommodation is to the irreversible effects of normal and pathological aging and requires an associated education of the patient and his or her family. The rehabilitation team can teach new ways to accomplish the functional tasks that can no longer be done as they previously were because of these effects of aging. The team can teach these techniques to the patient or educate the family, depending on the patient's ability to learn.

A second component of geriatric rehabilitation is the prevention of disability and the restoration of function. Many impairments combine reversible and irreversible components. Exercise can be used to prevent or reverse the effects of disuse caused by inactivity or injury. An example is the patient with a humeral fracture who has lost extremity strength and mobility. A portion of this functional loss might be reversible and is secondary to the disuse subse-

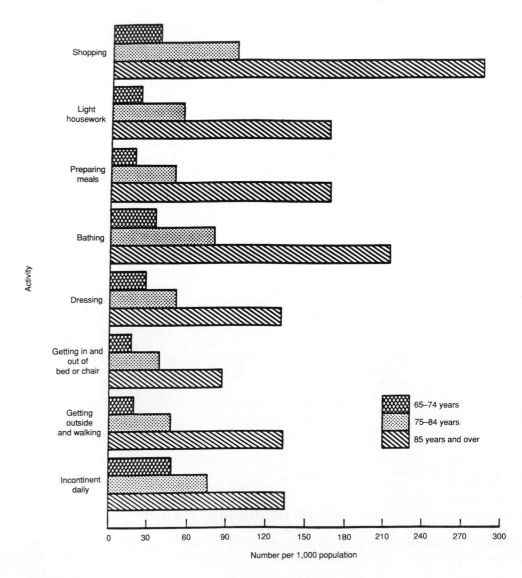

FIGURE 59–1 Proportion of community-dwelling persons 65 years or older and their dependence in selected activities by age group: United States, 1984. (Adapted from Fulton JP, Katz S, Jack SS, Hendershot GE: Physical functioning of the aged, United States, 1984. Vital Health Stat [10] 1989; 167.)

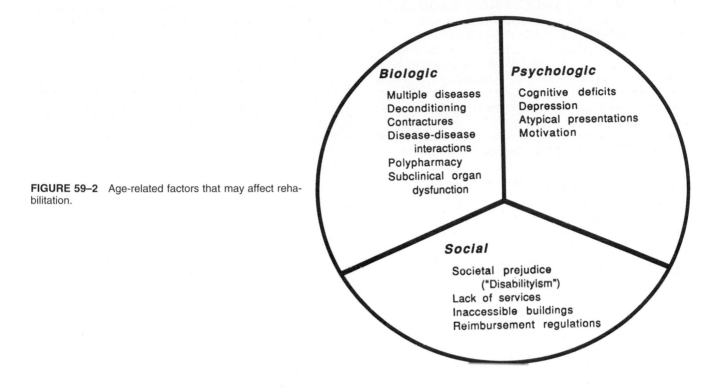

FIGURE 59–2 Age-related factors that may affect rehabilitation.

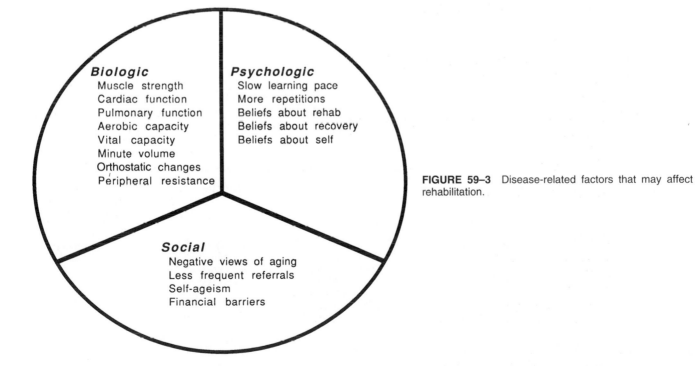

FIGURE 59–3 Disease-related factors that may affect rehabilitation.

quent to the immobilization that occurred during the treatment of the injury. Not uncommonly, such a patient might regain strength and partial motion but have a permanent partial loss of range of motion (ROM) of the shoulder. In this case, the rehabilitation program restored partial function to the shoulder. The same patient could also sustain loss of strength and motion in the rest of the involved extremity because of shoulder immobilization during treatment. This disuse can be avoided by preventive rehabilitation. This preventive concept should be broadened to include all geriatric patients by remembering the "use it or lose" it concept.[6]

Medical treatment of impairment is the third integral part of geriatric rehabilitation. Treatment is needed to cure when possible, or at least to stabilize the disease process when cure is not possible. Many of the impairments of the elderly are chronic and incurable but manageable, thus preventing or delaying progression and complications and associated disability.

BIOLOGY AND PHYSIOLOGY OF AGING

Body Composition

Body composition changes with aging (Table 59–2). There is a gradual loss of lean tissue and an increase in fat. The loss of lean tissue reflects loss of muscle mass: total body muscle mass, limb muscle volume, muscle cross-sectional area, and muscle fiber number and area.[25] Body fat increases to 30% of body weight at age 80 years as compared to 15% at age 30 which should be taken into account when prescribing fat-soluble drugs.[60] Bone mineral is lost; peak bone density occurs in the 30s and 40s and thereafter gradually declines.

Postural Changes of Aging

Figures 59–4 and 59–5 illustrate the postural changes that occur with aging.[36] Figure 59–4 shows the progressive anterior thrust of the head and extension of the cervical spine, accentuated thoracic kyphosis, and straightening of the lumbar spine. Increased extension of the arms and scapular protraction at the shoulders is associated with flexion of the elbows, ulnar deviation at the wrists, and finger flexion. In the lower extremity, there is an increase in hip and knee flexion and a decrease in ankle dorsiflexion. During ambulation, there is diminished arm swing and a shorter step length.[42]

Figure 59–5 illustrates the widening of the bony pelvis with aging. The angle of the femoral neck to the shaft increases, resulting in a valgus deformity of the hips.[60] Progressive widening of the standing base with aging is noted. In women, the knees can develop varus deformities with narrowing of the standing base.

The functional effect of these postural changes is to require a shift of the center of gravity of the body from just anterior to the first or second sacral level and to shift the plumb line of the body so that it no longer favors extension of the lower extremity joints in relaxed standing. Consequently, patients must adjust their individual standing posture to maintain the erect position. Steinberg[59] points out that the center of gravity is shifted behind the hips by flexing the knees and that this may require the use of ambulatory aids such as a cane.

In addition to the described anatomical effects on posture, there are physiological effects noted. Increased postural sway occurs with aging.[16] The ability to balance on one leg with eyes either closed or open decreases.[5] Righting reflexes decrease and reaction time increases.

Normal Neurological Changes of Aging

In order to be able to recognize pathological changes in the elderly patient, it is necessary to know what is "normal" in aging. Table 59–3 lists frequently found neurological changes that are normal in elderly patients. As an example, absent ankle jerks and diminished vibratory sense in the distal legs of an elderly person do not necessarily indicate the presence of a peripheral neuropathy if noted without the presence of other appropriate history or physical findings. Conversely, the absence of an expected finding in a disease state can occur in the elderly and can confuse

TABLE 59–2   Changes in Biological Functions in Response to Aging, Inactivity, Weightlessness, and Exercise

Function	Aging	Inactivity	Weightlessness	Exercise
$\dot{V}o_2$max	Decreased	Decreased		Increased
Cardiac output	Decreased	Decreased		Increased not for older
Systolic BP	Increased		Increased	Decreased
Orthostatic tolerance	Decreased	Decreased	Decreased	Increased
Body water	Decreased	Decreased	Decreased	
RBC mass	Decreased	Decreased	Decreased	
Thrombosis	Increased	Increased		Decreased
Serum lipids	Increased	Increased		Decreased
HD lipoprotein	Increased over age 80 yr			Increased
Lean body mass	Decreased	Decreased	Decreased	
Muscle strength	Decreased	Decreased	Decreased	Increased
Calcium	Decreased	Decreased	Decreased	
Glucose tolerance	Decreased	Decreased		Increased
EEG dominant frequency	Decreased	Decreased		Increased

Abbreviations: $\dot{V}o_2$max, maximum oxygen consumption; BP, blood pressure; RBC, red blood cell; HD, high density; EEG, electroencephalogram.
From Stineman MG, Granger CV: Outcome studies and analysis: Principles of rehabilitation that influence outcome analysis. *In* Felsenthal G, Garrison SJ, Steinberg FU (eds): Rehabilitation of the Aging and Elderly Patient. Baltimore, Williams & Wilkins, 1994, p 512.

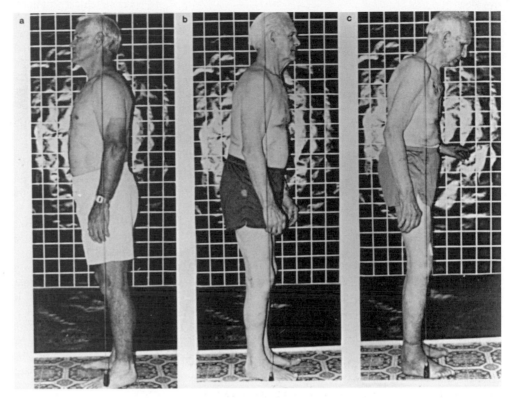

FIGURE 59–4 Lateral posture of a 60-year-old man *(a)*, a 78-year-old man *(b)*, and a 93-year-old man *(c)*.

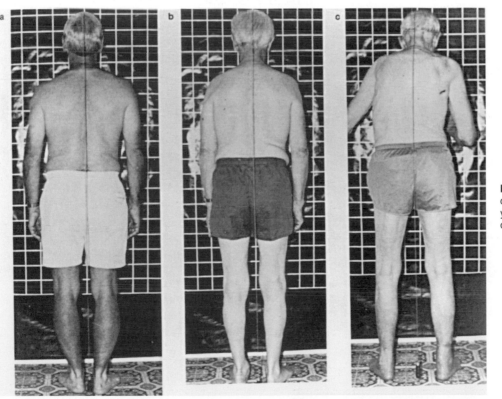

FIGURE 59–5 Posterior posture of a 60-year-old man *(a)*, a 78-year-old man *(b)*, and a 93-year-old man *(c)*.

TABLE 59–3 Frequent Neurological Changes in Elderly Patients

Eye signs
  Small, irregular pupils
  Diminished reaction to light and near reflex
  Diminished range of movement on convergence and upward gaze
  Slowed pursuit movements with cogwheeling
Motor signs
  Tendency to tremor (>69 yr, 43% have hand tremor, 7% have head tremor [titubation])
  Gait: short-stepped or broad-based with diminished associated movements
  Dysmetria (in all >65 yr)
  Dysdiadochokinesia
  Atrophy of interossei (thenar wasting in 66%, anterior tibial wasting in 25%)
  Increased muscle tone: legs more than arms, proximal more than distal
  Diminished muscle strength: legs more than arms, proximal more than distal
Sensory signs
  Diminished vibratory sense distally, legs much more than arms
  Possible change in proprioception
  Mildly increased threshold for light touch, pain, and temperature
  Impaired double simultaneous stimulation
Reflex signs
  Diminished or absent ankle jerks
  Some reduction in knee, biceps, and triceps reflexes
  Abdominal reflex sometimes lost
  Babinski's sign may not occur (when it would in younger patients)
  Primitive reflexes occur in 20%–25% (palmomental, snout, and nuchocephalic [doll's eyes])

From Ham RJ: Assessment. *In* Ham RJ, Sloane PD (eds): Primary Care Geriatrics: A Case-Based Approach. St Louis, Mosby–Year Book, 1992, p 87.

the clinical picture. For example, Babinski's response does not always occur in upper motor neuron lesions in the elderly as it does in younger patients.

It should be emphasized that just because a physical finding is normal for an elderly patient, it still might have functional significance. For instance, loss of upward gaze is seen in elderly patients. The normal limit of upward gaze in the young adult is 40 to 45 degrees, but by the eighth decade it is reduced to an average of 16 degrees.[11] Mechanical neck problems are also common in the elderly, and this combination of restricted cervical motion and vertical gaze can make it difficult for a patient to see wall clocks, exit signs, room numbers, and other orienting information.[35] In an attempt to compensate for this, the patient might lean backward contributing to imbalance and a possible fall.

Diminshed muscle strength occurs in the elderly with the lower limbs more involved than the upper limbs, with greater weakness proximally than distally. One common functional complaint in the elderly is increasing difficulty arising from a chair or toilet seat. Physical examination frequently reveals little except functionally decreased strength in the limb girdle muscles, especially the hip extensors. These muscles no longer have the strength required to lift the patient's body weight against gravity from the sitting to the standing position. Exercise by itself does not always rectify this loss of functional strength, and accommodation and education are then necessary. Patients are typically more functional if seated in chairs with firm seats supporting their hips and knees at 90-degree angles, with their feet flat on the floor. The chairs should have armrests. The patients should be instructed to move their buttocks to the front of the chair and to flex their knees to bring their feet under the front edge of the chair and under their buttocks. Many patients will also need to use their arms to assist in coming to their feet.

The decline in cognitive function with normal aging, as demonstrated by the Baltimore Longitudinal Study of Aging,[53] tends to be of small magnitude. In fact some functional measures improve with aging, such as vocabulary, digit span forward, and memory for text. Mentation

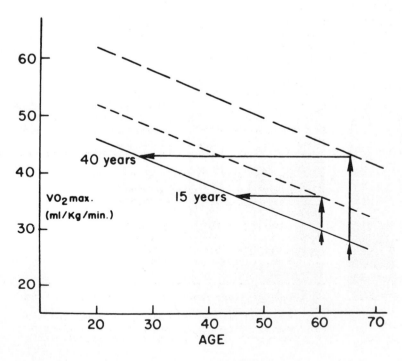

FIGURE 59–6 Potential improvement in V̇O₂max with age changes.[32] *Top line,* Athletes. *Middle line,* Moderately active persons. *Lower line,* Sedentary persons.

changes in the elderly are more likely to be associated with pathological conditions such as dementia, depression, or delirium.

Skin

Aging changes occur in the skin. These include decreases in moisture content, epidermal renewal, elasticity, blood supply, and sensitivity to touch, pain, and temperature. The effect of these changes is to make the patient, particularly if thin or malnourished, more susceptible to injury (pressure sores) or infection.

Cardiopulmonary Changes

Cardiac changes that occur with aging include decreased cardiac reserve, contractile function, and heart rate. Blood pressure tends to rise with aging. Pulmonary function mildly decreases with a decline in vital capacity. However, the main functional deficits secondary to the cardiopulmonary system are due to disease and not aging changes.[2, 3]

Urological Changes

Changes due to aging of the urinary system are functionally significant. Urinary frequency, hesitancy, retention, and nocturia are common complaints in both sexes and relate to anatomical and physiological aging changes of the urinary system. Bladder capacity is reduced and residual volume increased. Prostatic hypertrophy is almost universal among elderly men. Reduction in creatinine clearance can predispose the elderly to toxicity from renally excreted drugs unless dosage adjustments are made and renal function monitored.

Hydration

The elderly have approximately a 25% decrease in thirst perception as compared to the young. In addition, they can be placed in situations with a limited access to water. Moreover, medications (diuretics or laxatives) might increase their need for water to maintain adequate hydration.[41]

Temperature

Elderly people have impairment of their thermoregulatory mechanisms and are more susceptible to hyperthermia and hypothermia.[63] The febrile response to infection and other inflammatory diseases can fail to develop in the elderly and can lead to a missed diagnosis.[34]

EXERCISE

Bortz[6] emphasized that using one's physical capacities was necessary to prevent their loss. He stated it succinctly as the "use it or lose it" principle. This principle indicates that the decrease in physiological functioning in the elderly is not solely due to the aging process but is also due to inactivity. (The effects of deconditioning and inactivity are discussed in Chapter 34.) Figure 59–6 indicates that if inactive elderly persons initiate an appropriate exercise program, they can "lessen" their physiological age as

measured by maximum oxygen consumption ($\dot{V}O_2max$).[32] Table 59–4 summarizes the adaptations to strength conditioning in older men and women and Table 59–5 summarizes the adaptations to aerobic conditioning in older men and women. Flexibility and ROM have also been reported to improve in the elderly with exercise.[56]

In order to maintain function, critical ROM should be maintained in major joints. In the upper extremity, ROM of the shoulder should allow abduction to at least 90 degrees, with sufficient internal rotation to touch the lower back and external rotation to touch the back of the head. ROM of the forearm should allow a minimum of 45 degrees of pronation and supination with wrist flexion of 45 degrees and extension of 30 degrees. Finger flexion should be to within 1 in. of the palm. In the lower extremity, hip extension should be to at least neutral and flexion to 90 degrees. Knee extension should be to neutral and flexion to 110 degrees. Ankle dorsiflexion should be to neutral. Table 59–6 illustrates a functional ROM schema.

Precautions and contraindications have to be considered before initiating an exercise program in the elderly.[25] Cardiac status has to be determined and any unstable or un-

TABLE 59–4   Adaptations to Strength Conditioning in Older Men

Variable	Range of Reported Improvements
Strength	
Static	↑ 13%–72%
1 RM	↑ 9%–227%
Isokinetic	↑ 7%–29%
Strength gain/day	
Static	↑ 0.3%–4.0%
1 RM	↑ 3%–5%
Isokinetic	↑ 0.2%–0.5%
Isokinetic work	↑ 18%–21%
Torque-velocity curve	↑ Velocity at a given torque
Muscle size	
Cross-sectional area (CT scan)	↑ 9%–12%
Type I fiber area	↑ 31%–38%
Type II fiber area	↑ 26%–52%
Mean fiber area	↑ 27%
Turnover of muscle protein (from urinary 3-methylhistidine)	↑ 41%
Muscle fiber type distribution	No change
Integrated electromyographic activity	↑ 23%
Muscle membrane Na^+-K^+ pumps	↑ 40%
Sarcoplasmic reticulum Ca^{2+}-ATPase	Decrease with age is prevented
Aerobic power ($\dot{V}O_2max$)	↑ 0%–6%
Maximum exercise heart rate	No change
Maximum exercise blood pressure	No change
Hemoglobin concentration	No change
Blood volume	No change
Capillary density per fiber	↑ 15%
Oxidative enzyme activity (citrate synthase)	↑ 30%

Abbreviations: RM, range of movement; CT, computed tomography; $\dot{V}O_2max$, maximum oxygen consumption.

From Frontera WR, Meredity CN: Exercise in the rehabilitation of the elderly. *In* Felsenthal G, Garrison SJ, Steinberg FU (eds): Rehabilitation of the Aging and Elderly Patient. Baltimore, Williams & Wilkins, 1994, p 40.

TABLE 59–5   Adaptations to Aerobic Conditioning in Older Men and Women*

Variable	Range of Reported Improvements
Ventilation	
During submaximal exercise*	
Minute ventilation	↓ 9%–15%
During maximal exercise	
Minute ventilation	↑ 20%–30%
% Maximal voluntary ventilation	↑ 16%
Cardiac function	
During submaximal exercise	
Heart rate	↓ 9–20 beats/min
Stroke volume	↑ 8%
Cardiac output	No change
During maximal exercise	
Heart rate	No change
Stroke volume	↑ 6%–28%
Cardiac output	↑ 0%–34%
Circulation	
Total hemoglobin	↑ 7%
Blood volume	↑ 8%
Systemic vascular resistance during submaximal exercise	↓ 5%–18%
Leg blood flow during maximal exercise	↑ 42%
Muscle metabolism	
Fiber type distribution	No change or increased type IIA
Capillary density	No change
In vitro oxidative capacity	↑ 128%
Oxidative enzyme activity	↑ 0%–45%
Glycogen stores	↑ 10%–28%
Mitochondrial number, mean volume, and volume fraction	No change
During submaximal exercise	
Arteriovenous O_2 difference	No change
Blood lactate	↓ 21%–44%
During maximal exercise	
Arteriovenous O_2 difference	↑ 14%
Integrated response	
Submaximal $\dot{V}O_2$	No change
$\dot{V}O_2$max	↑ 11%–30%

Abbreviations: $\dot{V}O_2$, oxygen uptake; $\dot{V}O_2$max, maximum oxgen consumption.
From Frontera WR, Meredith CN: Exercise in the rehabilitation of the elderly. *In* Felsenthal G, Garrison SJ, Steinberg FU (eds): Rehabilitation of the Aging and Elderly Patient. Baltimore, Williams & Wilkins, 1994, p 42.

treated cardiovascular impairment should be considered as a possible contraindication. Limited ROM and arthritic joint involvement might require modification of the exercise program. Any coexistent medical conditions should be under optimal management—anemia, hyperthyroidism, etc. The possible impact of any medications on the ability to safely exercise and consequent need for modification of the exercise program must be considered, for example, symptomatic treatment of upper respiratory symptoms with decongestants. High temperature and humidity might necessitate modification of the exercise program.

PHARMACOLOGY

The elderly, because of physiological changes involving liver and kidney function, and absorption and body distribution of drugs, have a greater sensitivity to the effects of medication.[47] The elderly tend to be on multiple medications (average of five) and to have an increasing incidence

of adverse reactions as the number of medications increases.[20] In addition, they take many nonprescription medications and receive their prescribed medications from different sources. Interactions between these medications can be subtle and gradual in onset but ultimately have a significant detrimental effect on function. Elderly patients admitted to a rehabilitation service often demonstrate significant improvement in function only after modification or elimination of their medication regimen. Substance abuse (e.g., alcohol) is common in the elderly with a reported incidence of up to 20% in some studies.[54] With the need to be cognizant of polypharmacy and substance abuse, it is imperative to have guidelines for medication use in elderly rehabilitation patients (Table 59–7).

FUNCTIONAL ASSESSMENT

Various aspects of functional assessment are covered in Chapters 1 and 12. In the elderly, assessment tools measuring ADL and independent ADL have particular significance. If used to document the patient's status initially and serially, accurate comparison can lead to early diagnosis and intervention at the first sign of functional deterioration.

Assessment tools can also be used to determine the cognitive status of the patient.[37] The Mini-Mental State Examination (MMSE)[24] (Table 59–8) is an example of a screening tool that can be used to help detect and assess dementia. It can be administered rapidly and accurately and can be used to follow cognitive improvement or deterioration over time. The MMSE can also be used to screen for delirium. The Geriatric Depression Scale[7] (Table 59–9) was developed to screen for the common symptoms of depression in the elderly.

Gait and balance instruments (Table 59–10) are also useful functional assessment instruments, allowing both diagnostic assessment and longitudinal evaluation of patient function. Tinetti and Ginter[61] have shown that an assessment that reproduces mobility maneuvers is a better method of assessing functional mobility than neuromuscular findings on a physical examination.

Balance

Balance is a key component of mobility. It depends on the interaction of multiple systems—the peripheral nervous system and proprioception, vestibular and cerebellar, and visual. In addition, adequate muscle strength in the exten-

TABLE 59–6   Functional Disability Testing

A = Performed easily
B = Performed with some difficulty
C = Unable to perform
1. Touch first metacarpophalangeal joint to top of head
2. Touch waist in back
3. Place fingertips to palmar crease; if abormal, test grip strength
4. Place palm of hand on contralateral trochanter
5. Touch index finger pad to thumb pad
6. Sitting, touch toe or shoe
7. Stand unassisted; step over a 6-in. block

Modified from De Vore PA: A computerized geriatric assessment designed for use in primary care physicians' offices. Md Med J 1994; 43:261.

TABLE 59–7   Guidelines for Medication Use During Rehabilitation of Older Adults

Maintain a HIGH index of suspicion for medication toxicities.
Obtain accurate over-the-counter and prescription medication histories.
Review that each medication is still indicated.
Record a clear diagnosis for which each medication, especially psychotropic medication, is prescribed.
Gradually eliminate unnecessary medications.
Review that medication dosages are correct.
Simplify medication schedules as much as possible.
Clarify with patients that they are willing and able to take medications.
Educate patient and family about indications for medications and their side effects.

From Siebens H: Issues on medication use and substance abuse in older adults. *In* Felsenthal G, Garrison SJ, Steinberg FU (eds): Rehabilitation of the Aging and Elderly Patient. Baltimore, Williams & Wilkins, 1994, p 354.

sors of the hips and knees and normal ankle muscles are necessary for normal balance. When one component of the balance equation is impaired, the others can substitute, but when more than one component is affected, then balance is impaired. With normal aging, each component of the balance equation can be impaired (see Tables 59–3 and 59–10).

Gait

The basics of gait are covered in Chapter 5 and aging changes affecting gait are noted above under postural changes of aging and balance. Table 59–10 indicates that men develop a gait pattern of small steps with a wide base during walking and standing. Women typically develop a waddling style of gait with a narrow walking and standing base. During ambulation, the swing phase decreases and the period of double support increases.[42, 43] These changes and the postural changes that require muscular contraction to maintain joint extension increase the energy cost of ambulation. The aging person typically compensates for this increased energy demand by using a slower walking speed.

Pathological gait patterns in the elderly can be due to neurological or musculoskeletal causes and are often diagnostic of the underlying disease. Examples of abnormal gait patterns and their causes include circumduction (hemiparesis); scissoring (upper motor neuron disease); festinating (Parkinson's disease); ataxia (vitamin deficiency, cervical spondylosis, cerebellar dysfunction); apraxia (normal pressure hydrocephalus); senility (arterial degeneration); and waddling (muscle weakness).[33] Other musculoskeletal causes of pathological gait include problems of the feet, hip, knee, and lumbar spine. The importance of a hip extension deficit has been emphasized by Steinberg.[59]

FALLS

Falls and near falls occur in about one third of the elderly.[10] While only 3% to 5% of falls result in fractures,

TABLE 59–8   Mini-Mental State Examination*

I. Orientation (Ask the following questions)		
What is today's date?	Date (e.g., Jan. 21)	☐
What is the year?	Year	☐
What is the month?	Month	☐
What day is today?	Day (e.g., Monday)	☐
Can you also tell me what season it is?	Season	☐
Can you also tell me the name of this hospital (clinic)?	Hospital (clinic)	☐
What floor are we on?	Floor	☐
What town or city are we in?	Town or city	☐
What county are we in?	County	☐
What state are we in?	State	☐
II. Immediate Recall		
Ask the subject if you may test his/her memory. Then say "ball," "flag," "tree" clearly and slowly, about 1 sec for each. After you have said all three, ask him/her to repeat them. This first repetition determines his/her score (0–3), but keep saying them until he/she can repeat all three, up to six tries. If he/she does not eventually learn all three, recall cannot be meaningfully tested.	"Ball"	☐
	"Flag"	☐
	"Tree"	☐
	Number of trials: _____	
III. Attention and Calculation		
Ask the subject to begin with 100 and count backward by 7. Stop after five subtracts (93, 86, 79, 72, 65). Score the total number of correct answers.	"93"	☐
	"86"	☐
	"79"	☐
	"72"	☐
	"65"	☐
If the subject cannot or will not perform "the count backward test" task, ask him/her to spell the word "world" backward. The score is the number of letters in correct order. For example, *dlrow* is 5, *dlorw* is 3.	D	☐
	L	☐
	R	☐
	O	☐
	W	☐

TABLE 59–9   Geriatric Depression Scale*

1.	Are you basically satisfied with your life?	Yes/No
2.	Have you dropped many of your activities and interests?	Yes/No
3.	Do you feel that your life is empty?	Yes/No
4.	Do you often get bored?	Yes/No
5.	Are you hopeful about the future?	Yes/No
6.	Are you bothered by thoughts you can't get out of your head?	Yes/No
7.	Are you in good spirits most of the time?	Yes/No
8.	Are you afraid that something bad is going to happen to you?	Yes/No
9.	Do you feel happy most of the time?	Yes/No
10.	Do you often feel helpless?	Yes/No
11.	Do you often get restless and fidgety?	Yes/No
12.	Do you prefer to stay at home, rather than going out and doing new things?	Yes/No
13.	Do you frequently worry about the future?	Yes/No
14.	Do you feel you have more problems with memory than most?	Yes/No
15.	Do you think its wonderful to be alive now?	Yes/No
16.	Do you often feel downhearted and blue?	Yes/No
17.	Do you feel pretty worthless the way you are now?	Yes/No
18.	Do you worry a lot about the past?	Yes/No
19.	Do you find life very exciting?	Yes/No
20.	Is it hard for you to get started on new projects?	Yes/No
21.	Do you feel full of energy?	Yes/No
22.	Do you feel that your situation is hopeless?	Yes/No
23.	Do you think that most people are better off than you are?	Yes/No
24.	Do you frequently get upset over little things?	Yes/No
25.	Do you frequently feel like crying?	Yes/No
26.	Do you have trouble concentrating?	Yes/No
27.	Do you enjoy getting up in the morning?	Yes/No
28.	Do you prefer to avoid social gatherings?	Yes/No
29.	Is it easy for you to make decisions?	Yes/No
30.	Is your mind as clear as it used to be?	Yes/No

*A cutoff score of 9 has a sensitivity of 90% and specificity of 80%; a cutoff score of 11 has a sensitivity of 84% and specificity of 95%; a cutoff score of 14 has a sensitivity of 80% and specificity of 100%.
From Brink TL, Yesavage JA, Lum O, et al: Screening tests for geriatric depression. Clin Gerontol 1982; 1:37–43.

TABLE 59–10   Position Changes, Balance Maneuvers, and Gait Components Included in Functional Mobility Assessment

Mobility Maneuvers	Conditions Defining Maneuver Done With Difficulty
Position Change or Balance Maneuver	
Getting up from chair*†	Does not get up with single movement, pushes up with arms or moves forward in chair first, unsteady on first standing
Sitting down in chair*†	Plops in chair, does not land in center
Withstanding nudge on sternum (examiner pushes lightly on sternum three times)	Moves feet, grabs object for support, feet not touching side by side
Eyes closed	Same as above (tests patient's reliance on visual input for balance)
Neck turning	Moves feet; grabs object for support; feet not touching side by side; complains of vertigo, dizziness, or unsteadiness
Reaching up	Unable to reach up to full shoulder flexion standing on tiptoes; unsteady; grabs object for support
Bending over	Unable to bend over to pick up small object (e.g., pen) from floor; grabs object to pull up on; requires multiple attempts to rise
Gait Component or Maneuver‡	
Initiation	Hesitates, stumbles, grabs object for support
Step height (raising feet while stepping)†§	Does not clear floor consistently (scrapes or shuffles), raises foot too high (>2 in.)
Step continuity§	After first few steps, does not consistently begin raising one foot as other foot touches floor
Step symmetry§	Step length not equal (pathological side usually has longer step length; problem may be in hip, knee, ankle, or surrounding muscles)
Path deviation‖	Does not walk in straight line; weaves from side to side
Turning†	Stops before initiating turn, staggers; sways; grabs object for support

*Hard, armless chair.
†Included in analysis.
‡Patient walks down hallway at "usual pace," and comes back using usual walking aid. Examiner observes single component of gait at a time (analogous to heart examination).
§Best observed from side of patient.
‖Best observed from behind patient.
From Tinetti ME, Ginter SF: Identifying mobility dysfunctions in elderly patients: Standard neuromuscular examination or direct assessment. JAMA 1988; 259:1189.

90% of fractures of the hip, pelvis, and forearm result from falls.[58] Normal aging changes that contribute to falls are listed in Tables 59–3, 59–11, 59–12, and 59–13. Tables 59–13 and 59–14 list risk factors in the home. Additional environmental factors include inclement weather and unfamiliar surroundings (see Table 59–13). Psychological factors include inattention, depression, and cognitive impairment. Living alone is a sociological risk factor. Iatrogenic causes are listed under medications in Table 59–13. Some illnesses associated with falls are listed in Table 59–13. Sometimes falls are a prodrome of a not as yet clinically apparent illness or infection. Strategies for reducing the risk of falls are listed in Table 59–12 and guidelines for home safety are listed in Table 59–14. One of the most significant consequences of falling is the fear of another fall, with subsequent immobility, weakness, and isolation.

COMMON IMPAIRMENTS

Table 59–15 lists the common disorders that are typically seen by a geriatric rehabilitation team. The impairment groups for patients admitted to our geriatric rehabilitation unit that is geared to rehabilitation needs of the frail elderly (average patient age of 80) are listed in Table 59–16. Survey data from the National Center for Health Statistics (Fig. 59–7) indicate that of the 10 most common chronic conditions with morbidity in the age 65+ group, at least two—arthritis and orthopedic impairment—are commonly managed by the rehabilitation team. The other listed disorders (Table 59–17) are also seen in our patients[20] as associated conditions that require management to ensure that their rehabilitation can proceed. Failure to manage these conditions can cause them to worsen and delay or complicate the rehabilitation process.

Our data indicate that these patients have multiple diagnoses, with a mean of six.[20] The disability caused by a specific impairment does not act in isolation from those associated with the other impairments. This interaction of impairments can have a cascade effect[19] in that the overall cumulative disability can greatly exceed the individual summated disabilities. As seen in Figure 59–8, each impairment has a limited associated disability, but that disability cascades to affect the limited disability caused by the patient's other impairments. This creates a greater total disability and a much more complicated management problem for the patient, the rehabilitation team, and the family.

Each of these common impairments is encountered not only in the elderly but also in patients of any age seen by the physiatrist and the rehabilitation team. These impairments are discussed in detail in other chapters. The following comments are specific to the impact of these impairments on elderly patients.

Pain

The majority of elderly people will, at some time, have a serious pain problem. Musculoskeletal pain is the most common type reported. Data show, for example, that approximately 75% of nursing home patients have pain problems. Taking a pain history requires special care regarding secondary gain or hidden agendas which in the elderly can include loneliness, a planned family vacation, etc. In addition, hearing loss, dementia, pseudodementia (delirium or depression), and underreporting of symptoms by the patient all can influence the accuracy of information. Information from significant others can often be used to piece together a fuller picture of the problem. The physical examination for these patients has several potential unique findings (Table 59–18). Laboratory and radiographic studies to help sort out these problems are frequently more difficult because of severe contractures, kyphosis, confusion, agitation, or inaccessible veins. Since the elderly are more sensitive to medications and are more at risk of polypharmacy, physical measures should be the cornerstone of treatment of musculoskeletal pain in the elderly, with appropriate caution.

Spinal problems are common causes of pain in the elderly. Spondylitic changes are present in up to 82% of persons in their sixth decade. Cervical disc degeneration presents most commonly at C5 to C6, followed by C6 to C7 and C4 to C5. Cervical spondylitic myelopathy is the most common reason for spinal cord dysfunction in patients over the age of 55. Lumbosacral spinal stenosis is commonly seen in the elderly, and typically produces bilateral symptoms that are worse with standing or walking. Sitting down or flexing the spine while standing usually relieves these symptoms.[18]

At least 25% of the elderly have shoulder pain, usually of soft tissue origin. Elbow, wrist, and hand pain occur commonly due to C7 radiculopathy, medial or lateral epicondylitis, median or ulnar nerve entrapment, de Quervain's tenosynovitis, or generalized arthritis. Hip pain is frequently due to arthritis, trochanteric bursitis, or radiculopathy at L5 or S1. Arthritis and trauma (sometimes even trivial trauma) can be major reasons for knee pain. Atrophic fat pads, bony deformities in the foot, and ill-fitting shoes can cause tendinitis, nerve entrapments, and tenosynovitis. These pain problems can usually be eliminated or ameliorated by physical medicine management.[49]

TABLE 59–11   Normal Aging Changes That Predispose to Falls and Injuries

Visual impairments
 Presbyopia and decreases in accommodative capacity, visual acuity, night vision, peripheral vision, glare tolerance, impaired blue-green discrimination, and contrast sensitivity
Nervous system impairments
 Reduced righting reflexes, proprioceptive input, and cerebral function; increased reaction time; lessened awareness of vibration, touch, and temperature; increased distractibility
Musculoskeletal impairments
 Osteopenia; musculoskeletal stiffness; reduced or uncoordinated muscle control
Cardiovascular impairments
 Postural hypotension
Gait changes
 Women: waddling gait, narrow walking and standing base
 Men: Small-stepped gait, wide walking and standing base
Auditory impairments
 Reduced speech discrimination
 Increased high-frequency threshold
 Wax accumulation

Adapted from Tideiksaar R: Falls in the elderly: An approach to management. Phys Assistant 1988; 10:114–132; and Barclay AM: Falls in the elderly: Is prevention possible? Postgrad Med 1988; 83:241–248.

TABLE 59–12   Strategies for Reducing Risk of Falls

Risk Factor	Interventions	
	Medical	**Rehabilitative or Environmental**
Reduced visual acuity, dark adaptation, and perception	Refraction; cataract extraction	Home safety assessment
Reduced hearing	Removal of cerumen; audiological evaluation	Hearing aid if appropriate (with training); reduction in background noise
Vestibular dysfunction	Avoidance of drugs affecting the vestibular system; neurological or ear, nose, and throat evaluation, if indicated	Habituation exercises
Proprioceptive dysfunction, cervical degenerative disorders, and peripheral neuropathy	Screening for vitamin B_{12} deficiency and cervical spondylosis	Balance exercises; appropriate walking aid; correctly sized footwear with firm soles; home safety assessment
Dementia	Detection of reversible causes; avoidance of sedative or centrally acting drugs	Supervised exercise and ambulation; home safety assessment
Musculoskeletal disorders	Appropriate diagnostic evaluation	Balance-and-gait training; muscle-strengthening exercises; appropriate walking aid; home safety assessment
Foot disorders (calluses, bunions, deformities)	Shaving of calluses; bunionectomy	Trimming of nails; appropriate footwear
Postural hypotension	Assessment of medications; rehydration; possible alteration in situational factors (e.g., meals, change of position)	Dorsiflexion exercises; pressure-graded stockings; elevation of head of bed; use of tilt table if condition is severe
Use of medications (sedatives: benzodiazepines, phenothiazines, antidepressants; antihypertensives; others: antiarrhythmics, anticonvulsants, diuretics, alcohol)	Steps to be taken: 1. Attempted reduction in the total number of medications taken 2. Assessment of risks and benefits of each medication 3. Selection of medication, if needed, that is least centrally acting, is least associated with postural hypotension, and has shortest action 4. Prescription of lowest effective dose 5. Frequent reassessment of risks and benefits	

Modified from Tinetti ME, Speechley M: Risk factors for falls among elderly persons living in the community. N Engl J Med 1989; 320:1056.

TABLE 59–13   Some Factors Implicated in Traumatic Fractures in the Elderly

Aspects of aging	Illnesses
Primary osteoporosis	Cerebrovascular accident
Impaired balance/vision	Syncopal episodes
Alteration in gait	Hypotensive illnesses
Loss in muscle/fat "padding" at hip	Secondary osteoporosis
Falls forward (Colles' fracture/humerus) vs. falls	Hyperthyroidism
down (hip/pelvic)	Hypoparathyroidism, etc.
Environment	Osteomalacia
Outdoor	Parkinson's disease
Cracked walkway	Dementia
Poor lighting	Arthritis
Poor weather	Paraparesis
Uneven ground	Previous fracture
Crime (assault and battery)	Lifestyle
Indoor	Exercise/nutrition
Throw rugs	Alcoholism/other abused drugs
Wires across path	Bed rest/immobilization
Slippery tub	Shoe style
Poor lighting	Medications
Stairs/railings	Benzodiazepines
Pet causing a fall	Tricyclic antidepressants
Genetic	Antipsychotic medications
Sex (females > males)	Corticosteroids (secondary osteoporosis)
Race (white > black)	Barbiturates

From Stein BD, Felsenthal G: Rehabilitation of fractures in the geriatric population. *In* Felsenthal G, Garrison SJ, Steinberg FU (eds): Rehabilitation of the Aging and Elderly Patient. Baltimore, Williams & Wilkins, 1994, p 123.

TABLE 59–14   Guidelines for Home Safety

Problem Area	Risk Potential for Falls	Modifications to Recommend
Floors	High polish or wet surfaces may cause slipping	In bathrooms, use nonslip tiles, nonslip adhesive strips on floor next to tub, sink, and toilet, or indoor-outdoor carpeting; on linoleum floors, use slip-resistant floor wax with minimal buffing; use nonskid floor mat by kitchen sink to guard against wet floor
Carpets	Thick pile and carpet borders may cause tripping	Suggest carpets of low pile
Area rugs and mats	Rugs and mats may slide out from under person	Use rugs and mats with nonskid backing, or apply double-faced adhesive tape as backing
Lighting	Low or uneven lighting may obscure hazards	Increase lighting in high-risk areas, e.g., stairs, bathroom, bedroom
Glare	Visual impairment and distraction may be produced by glare from bright lights (especially sunlight) on polished floors and from unshielded light bulbs	Use polarized window glass, or apply tinted material to windows to eliminate glare without reducing light; reduce flood glare by repositioning light sources
Stairs	Poor lighting may contribute to tripping on stairway	Place light switches at top and bottom of stairway to avoid traveling up and down in the dark, or place night-lights by top and bottom step to provide visual cuing of steps; apply colored nonskid adhesive strips to stair edges; set maximum step rise at 6 in.
Handrails	Lack of support may result from missing or improper handrails	Place cylindrical rails 1–2 in. away from wall on both sides, with ends turned in and extending beyond top and bottom steps to provide easy grasping and signal top and bottom step
Sink edge and towel bar	Weak towel bar or wet, slippery sink edge may not provide adequate support	Replace towel bars with nonslip grab bars
Toilet seat	Transfer falls often occur because seat is too low	Advise use of elevated toilet with grab bars placed on wall next to toilet
Wet bathtub and shower floor surfaces	Slipping and falling are common on wet surfaces	Place nonslip adhesive rubber strips or suction-cup mat on tub floor; install nonslip grab bars in and around tub and shower; advise use of shower chair and flexible hand-held shower hose for patients with balance impairment
Bed height	Transfer falls are more common if height is not optimal	Adjust bed height distance from patella to floor (18 in. from top of mattress to floor allows for safest transfer by most persons)
Soft bed mattress	Poor sitting balance and support may lead to falls from bed	Bed mattress edges should be firm enough to support a seated person without sagging
Chair height	Transfer falls from low chairs are common	Replace low chairs with more suitable ones (chair height should be 14–16 in. from seat edge to floor; armrests should be present 7 in. above the seat and extend 1–2 in. beyond the seat edge for maximal leverage)
Shelf height	Reaching or bending to retrieve objects from high or low shelves leads to imbalance and falling	Rearrange frequently used kitchen and closet items to avoid excessive reacing and bending; encourage use of hand-held reach tools
Gas range	Difficult-to-see dial may not be turned off and may cause gas leak; fall may be first sign of gas asphyxiation with impaired smell	Mark on and off dial positions clearly
Temperature	Low room temperature may cause hypothermia; falls may be secondary to hypothermia	Maintain indoor temperature at 72 °F in winter

Adapted from Tideiksaar R. Falls in the elderly: An approach to management: Phys Assistant 1988; 10:114–132; and Christiansen J, et al: The prevention of falls in later life: A report of the Kellogg International Work Group on the Prevention of Falls in the Elderly. Dan Med Bull 1987; 34:1–24.

TABLE 59–15   Common Disorders Seen in the Geriatric Rehabilitation Team Setting

Amputation	Joint replacement
Arthritis	Lymphedema
Burns	Neuropathy
Cancer	Osteoporosis
Cardiovascular disorders	Pain syndromes (acute)
Chronic pain	Parkinson's disease
Chronic pulmonary disease	Peripheral vascular disease
Contractures	Postural disorders/falls
Deconditioning	Pressure sores
Disc disorders	Spinal cord injury
Fracture	Spinal stenosis
Head injury	Stroke
Immobility	Trauma

Adapted from Reichel W: Clinical Aspects of Aging, ed 3. Baltimore, Williams & Wilkins, 1989, p 184.

TABLE 59–17   Most Frequent Diagnoses—Primary or Secondary

Diagnoses	Patients	
	n	%
Hypertension	36	43.9
Arteriosclerotic heart disease	35	42.7
Cerebrovascular accidents	31	37.8
Peripheral vascular disease	25	30.5
Diabetes mellitus	24	29.3
Fractures	22	26.8
Osteoarthritis	17	20.7
Neuropsychiatric	13	15.9
Deconditioned	12	14.6
Decubitus ulcers	10	12.2

From Felsenthal G, Cohen BS, Hilton EB, et al: The physiatrist as primary physician for patients on an inpatient rehabilitation unit. Arch Phys Med Rehabil 1984; 65:375–378.

Dysphagia

Motor function of the lips, tongue, and masticatory muscles slows with aging (see Chapter 27). Often multiple gestures of the tongue are made prior to swallowing. The latency from entry of the bolus into the pharynx until the elevation of the larynx increases with age. The amplitude of esophageal contractions decreases with age. The clinical significance of these changes is not known. However, the effects of other problems upon swallowing in the aged are known, such as medication side effects, psychosocial factors (feeding dependency), neurological disorders, inflammatory muscle disease, scleroderma, cervical spine disorders, cancer, and tracheostomy.[46]

Arthritis

Arthritis is not only more common in the elderly, it may present differently in the elderly than in younger people. For example, the shoulder is typically more involved in the elderly with rheumatoid arthritis than in younger persons. A patient with osteoarthritis of the hip has a smaller chance of having hip osteoporosis and hip fractures. Older persons have smaller muscle fibers and fewer anterior horn cells than younger people and in addition, the tendons, ligaments, and capsules surrounding joints lose elasticity as evidenced by a decrease in joint ROM and a sense of stiffness in older persons. ROM exercises for joints should start at a few degrees and should be done gently. The

TABLE 59–16   Geriatric Rehabilitation Unit Admission Impairment Groups

	n	%
Orthopedic	40	32
Stroke	32	26
Pain	10	8
Cardiac	8	6
Neurological	8	6
Amputee	7	6
Pulmonary	6	5
Debility	5	4
Brain	4	3
Arthritis	3	2
Spinal cord	1	
	124	100

patient often resists needed assistive devices such as canes and walkers because of their stigma of aging and disability. If shown that the device can reduce pain, the patient may at least decide to use it privately, if not publicly. Joint replacement surgery can be of great help in medically intractable joint dysfunction, especially of the hip and knee.[45]

Osteoporosis and Paget's Disease

Acute symptomatic osteoporosis from vertebral fractures can be treated with bed rest and physical measures. Flank pain can be caused by severe kyphoscoliosis with the rib cage rubbing the pelvic rim. Back-strengthening exercises contribute to good posture and skeletal support, but flexion exercises of the spine are not recommended owing to the possibility of anterior wedge fractures (see Chapter 40). Paget's disease in the elderly can lead to fractures, rare cancerous changes, total joint replacement, and paraplegia.[55]

Fractures

Osteoporosis and falls are the reason for the great majority of fractures of the radius, hip, and shoulder. Extensive rehabilitation is often needed for these patients, with an inpatient rehabilitation stay needed for some. Weight-bearing and ROM are important issues. After a subcapital hip fracture, repair by pinning will often mean restricted weightbearing for 6 weeks or longer. Should a hemiarthroplasty have been performed, restrictions in hip motion to prevent dislocation (no flexion greater than 90 degrees, no adduction past the midline, and no internal rotation) are taught. The use of long-handled devices and "knee spreader" pillows are helpful tools for the approximately 3 months that the motion restrictions are in place. If the hemiarthroplasty is cemented, weightbearing is typically not restricted. However, the porous ingrowth type of prosthesis is often associated with reduced weightbearing for 6 weeks or more. Intertrochanteric fractures treated with sliding screw and plate fixation are variably followed by restricted weightbearing or weightbearing as tolerated, depending on the severity of the fracture and the orthopedic surgeon's approach to weightbearing after such procedures.

Tinnitus
Visual Impairment
Diabetes
Cataracts
Sinusitis
Orthopedic Impairment
Heart Conditions
Hearing Impairment
Hypertension
Arthritis
49
85
46
95
64
98
21
141
187
169
162
173
123
277
136
296
251
394
285
480
Ages 45 - 64
Ages 65 +
0
50
100
150
200
250
300
350
400
450
500
Rate Per 1,000 Persons

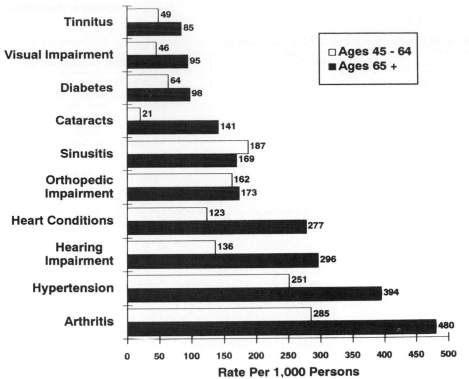

FIGURE 59–7 Morbidity from top ten chronic conditions: 1986.

Patient with osteporosis and osteoarthritis
Joint stiffness and hampered mobility lead to a fall with femur fracture
Greatly reduced mobility prevents patient from reaching bathroom in time, resulting in incontinence
Incontinence leads to depression
Depression interpreted as pseudodementia

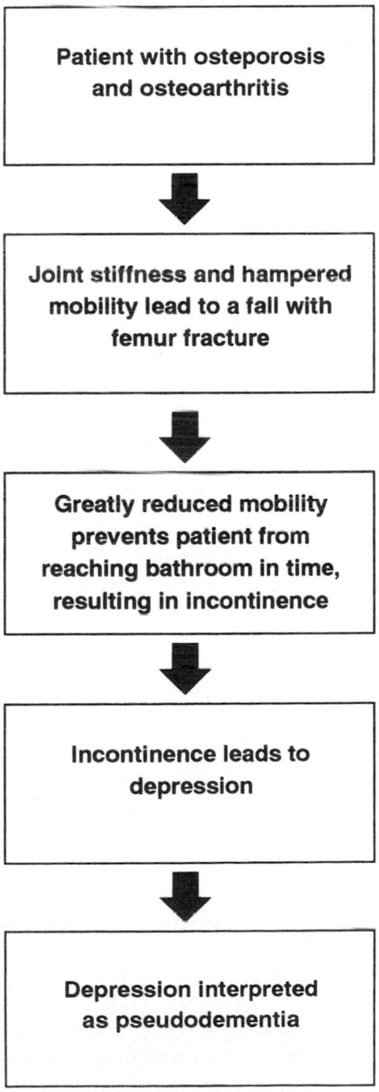

FIGURE 59–8 Cascade effect of individual summated disabilities.

TABLE 59–18   Examples of Geriatric Physical Examination Issues for the Pain Patient

Clinical Problem	Functional Consequence	Pain, Other Consequences
Hamstring and back extensor muscle contractures, decreased range of motion of heel cords (from high heels)	Excess knee and hip flexion and abnormal spinal postures to avoid falling from a heel cord contracture	Pain at multiple sites from fatigue and muscle overuse; give attention to heel cords
Restriction of upward gaze	Compensation by neck extension and lordosis, with foraminal narrowing, facet compression, and alterations in balance	Radicular compression at foramen with pain; increased risk of dizziness and falls
Orthostatic hypotension	Alterations in balance and gait	Differentiate from other neuromusculoskeletal reasons for altered gait

Family support during rehabilitation is critical. Concomitant deep venous thrombosis, stroke, pain, and peripheral neuropathy may be present. Pelvic fractures, if severe, might need prolonged bed rest (with its risks) as part of the treatment. Colles' fractures can be severely disabling and also result in carpal tunnel syndrome.[58]

Stroke

Older persons are more at risk of being institutionalized after a stroke. Patients who typically have not been in a student situation for 50 or 60 years often have difficulty learning new ways to accomplish tasks. Multi-infarct dementia can be a confounding problem. The geriatric patient is also susceptible to osteoporosis, impaired auditory and visual abilities, polypharmacy, osteoarthritis, skin fragility, and the stresses of older families[28] (see Chapter 50).

Traumatic Brain Injury

Falling is the most common cause of traumatic brain injury (TBI) in those more than 65 years of age and pedestrian accidents yield the most fatalities. Alcohol is involved commonly, especially with men. Advancing medical and neurological illnesses often increase the severity of the injury as well as its mortality. Re-employment is usually not a goal in the elderly. Protection from a second fall is a major goal to prevent further TBI and fractures. Selected elderly patients will benefit from an intensive comprehensive rehabilitation program including physical therapy, cognitive rehabilitation, behavioral management, dysphagia and communication treatment, and fall prevention[23] (see Chapter 49).

Motor Neuron Disease and Parkinson's Disease

These well-known diseases occur in the elderly. Attention to dysphagia, respiratory problems, self-care, balance and mobility, nutrition, and psychotherapy are all important[39] (see Chapters 45 and 51).

Peripheral Nervous System Impairments

Studies have shown that elderly persons have decreased or lost vibratory sense (up to 82%) and ankle muscle stretch reflexes (up to 70%). Drug-related and toxic neuropathies, nutritional and alcoholic neuropathies, postherpetic, diabetic, entrapment, rheumatic, carcinomatous, and parapro-

teinemic neuropathies are common in the elderly (see Chapter 46). Neuromuscular junction changes and muscle atrophy are commonly seen. Carefully timed exercises and energy conservation are important with myasthenia gravis. Appropriate exercise in the elderly has a proven successful record. Electrodiagnostic changes in the aged are well documented[15] (see Chapter 7).

Visual Impairments

Vision is a major factor contributing to balance and is an important factor in the risk of falling. Visual impairment is especially challenging when combined with a mobility impairment, as in an amputee or stoke patient. Poor vision often results in social isolation, impaired morale, and a decreased sense of well-being. Cataracts, age-related macular degeneration, glaucoma, and diabetic retinopathy are amenable in varying degrees to visual rehabilitative services.[62]

Hearing Loss

The incidence of significant hearing loss appears to be between 25% and 50% in those more than 65 years of age. The varying types of sensorineural hearing loss can be clarified by audiometric evaluation. Often patients refuse to wear hearing aids because of sound distortion, impaired dexterity in their use or adjustment, uncomfortable fit, or vanity[29] (see Chapter 3).

Peripheral Vascular Disease and Ischemic Skin Ulceration

Intermittent claudication must be distinguished from similar complaints of discomfort in the aged caused by arthritis, neural entrapment syndromes, diabetic neuropathy, and spinal stenosis. Proper foot care, including appropriate shoes, is part of the spectrum of care. Chronic venous insufficiency and lymphedema can be helped with compression garments in selected patients. Skin ulceration, especially in the malnourished older person, needs careful, aggressive treatment[48] (see Chapters 31 and 56).

Foot Disorders

The geriatric ankle and foot can be likened to a "fatigued trampoline," which has decreased shock absorption and spring abilities as a result of problems such as bony disfigurement, joint disorders, muscle imbalances, and skin and toenail disorders. Aging can result in insensitive feet with increased potential for ulceration and decreased ability to heal. Strengthening and other physical therapies, proper foot care, proper shoe selection with appropriate orthoses as needed, and appropriate podiatric treatment are important.[17]

Sexual Function

Sexual activity is affected by age-related changes in female and male hormonal levels; alterations in vision, hearing, and smell; negative social attitudes toward sexuality in the elderly; erectile and ejaculatory changes; vaginal dryness and dyspareunia; urinary stress incontinence; decreases in muscle strength and endurance; and limitations in movement from osteoarthritis. Additional problems in sexual functioning can arise from medical illnesses such as benign prostatic hypertrophy, hysterectomy, diabetes mellitus, primary hypothyroidism, cardiovascular disease, hypertension, degenerative joint disease, stroke, and mental illness. Drugs can also cause sexual dysfunction. After an accurate history and physical examination, one approach to treatment is staged levels of sexual counseling. This can range from "permission" to talk about sexual concerns, to increasing amounts of information, to therapy[27] (see Chapter 30).

AGING WITH A DISABILITY

Poliomyelitis

Of more than 640,000 living people in the United States who experienced paralytic poliomyelitis, more than 50% report having excessive fatigue, progressive weakness, pain, loss of function, and occasionally muscle atrophy 30 to 40 years after the acute episode. This is often referred to as the post-polio syndrome (see Chapter 45). The diagnosis requires evidence of a prior episode of poliomyelitis, a characteristic pattern of recovery from that episode, and exclusion of other conditions that could cause the new symptoms. An interdisciplinary evaluation is essential. Management includes careful strengthening, conservative pain treatment with heavy emphasis on physical medicine and rehabilitation techniques, appropriate orthoses, referral to a pulmonologist if needed, and attention to psychological issues[30] (see also Chapter 45).

Spinal Cord Injury

Survivors of a spinal cord injury in the United States can expect a much longer survival than in decades past. Those more than 55 years old are more likely to have medical problems[50] (see also Chapter 55). Motor function, rather than age, is the predominant limiting factor in attainment of functional goals after a spinal cord injury. Age is associated with a lower statistical chance of achieving some of the functional goals such as dressing, bathing, stair climbing, and complex transfers. The aging family also poses care issues for the newly injured geriatric patient as well as the aging patient with a chronic spinal cord injury. Psychological issues in aging are compounded by a spinal cord injury.[64]

Multiple Sclerosis

Weakness and fatigue in multiple sclerosis (MS) from upper motor neuron lesions is compounded by age-related lower motor neuron denervation, muscle atrophy, and diminished cardiopulmonary reserve. Exercise is important to promote general fitness. Elderly MS patients often have to cope with problems such as hyperthermia, decreased skin sensation, diminished special senses, impairments of the genitourinary and gastrointestinal systems, cognitive dysfunctions, and affective disorders. Psychological, vocational, financial, and recreational issues in dealing with MS are compounded by the psychological issues of aging[12] (see Chapter 52).

Aging with Pediatric-Onset Disabilities

Chronic back pain from poor posture, scoliosis, cervical spine pain (from heavy use of the neck owing to their disability), the sequelae of hip dislocation, and spastic deformities of the feet and toes have been reported in adults with *cerebral palsy*. A high incidence of bowel, bladder, skin, cognitive, and dystonic problems are found. There is a decreased access to medical care after school years are completed.

Epilepsy in adulthood is more common in those with *Down syndrome* than in the general population. Pathological findings of neurofibrillary tangle and neuritic plaques suggest a link between Down syndrome and Alzheimer's disease and raise the question over whether this is associated with an observed cognitive deterioration. Atlantoaxial instability, commonly with pain, is reported in 9% to 12% of patients.[44]

Persons with *spina bifida* can have late sequelae from hydromyclia, tethered cord, symptomatic Arnold-Chiari malformation, and inclusion dermoids, all of which can be surgically treated. Shunt failure, urinary and renal system dysfunction, arthritis, rotator cuff injury, and entrapment neuropathies can all occur in the aging person with spina bifida.[44]

REHABILITATION

In this era of fiscal constraint, we cannot deliver maximum quality of medical services to all our patients, but must utilize our medical resources to maximum benefit for the most patients. This requires matching our patients to the most appropriate site or level of care and to the optimal level or intensity of medical service needed to achieve significant functional goals in the most cost-effective manner. Figure 59–9 is a flow chart illustrating the concept of selecting the most appropriate setting for rehabilitation care.

Selection of patients who can significantly benefit from rehabilitation services is still an inexact science. It is difficult in all age groups, but especially among the elderly. The goals for each patient must be functionally significant and achievable within a reasonable period of time and with reasonable patient effort. Rules of thumb abound to aid selection of the appropriate patient but they all have exceptions. They tend to work well when applied to large groups of patients, but may be inappropriate when applied to the

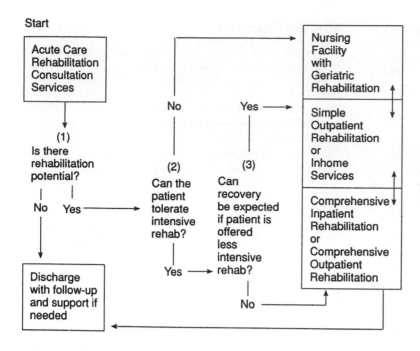

Start

FIGURE 59–9 Flow chart for entry and movement through geriatric rehabilitation services. Clinical questions (nonboxed elements) are asked in sequence. Each care phase/intervention mode is boxed.

individual patient. Most have not been validated by research data. Clinical judgment and experience still form the best basis for patient selection.

One rule of thumb is that an incontinent patient cannot benefit from rehabilitation services. In the case of urinary incontinence, this judgment precludes an assessment that might reveal a treatable cause such as infection or overflow or stress incontinence. In the case of bowel incontinence, treatable diarrhea or impaction may be present. Occasionally, gait abnormality, lack of privacy, or architectural barriers may be the cause of the incontinence. The most significant factor is the patient's concern about the incontinence. If the patient is unconcerned, the functional prognosis is bad.

Another rule of thumb that is used to determine patient selection is that a patient with dementia cannot benefit from a rehabilitation program.[52] Our experience indicates that the degree of dementia does affect the patient's ability to benefit from rehabilitation services depending on the goal(s) set by the patient, family, and rehabilitation team. If the goal is to discharge the patient to a noninstitutional setting, then there is an indication that patients with mild dementia succeed as often as those without dementia.[14] The presence of a significant other can be as important a determining factor as the presence of dementia.[20, 21] Three factors that interact to determine whether a patient can be discharged to a noninstitutional setting are ADL status; cognitive, judgment, and safety status; and the social support system.

TREATMENT SITE

As indicated in Figure 59–9, the elderly rehabilitation patient can be treated appropriately in multiple sites ranging from the acute hospital to the rehabilitation unit or hospital, to the subacute unit or skilled nursing facility, to home care or outpatient rehabilitation. Each site must be

modified for the special needs of the elderly in order to accomplish the rehabilitation goals. These modifications can be both architectural and programmatic.

Architectural and environmental factors that should be considered in designing living areas for the elderly are indicated in Tables 59–12, 59–13, and 59–14. Increased intensity of lighting is needed to compensate for the decrease in light reaching the retina. Night lighting should be used to identify areas such as the toilet and bathroom. Acoustics should be designed to decrease background noise. Floor coverings should permit use of adaptive mobility equipment. Avoid deep pile carpeting and slippery floor surfaces. Energy-absorbing flooring materials can decrease the likelihood of injury secondary to a fall. Floor space in rooms and passageways should be sufficient to allow for wheelchairs and other adaptive equipment. Light switches, shelves, counters, and so forth should be accessible from a wheelchair. Colors should be used to identify different functional areas, and patient rooms should be painted different colors to allow easy identification. There should be space for personal belongings and to allow display of photographs and other mementos.

Reality orientation should be emphasized. In any institution or program, it is easy to lose track of the day of the week as well as the date. Clocks and calendars should be placed on units and in patient areas, including rooms. Daily schedules should be posted and patients given the responsibility to learn and follow a schedule. Holidays, birthdays, and scheduled events should be part of the daily routine, and local and world news should be included.[13] Ideally, patients should be taken outside at least occasionally to reorient to the weather, day vs. night, the season, etc.

MOTIVATION

It is much easier to gain the cooperation of elderly patients for a rehabilitation program if they can see the benefits of what they are being asked to do. Abstract goals such as improving strength, balance, dexterity, ambulation distance, etc. are often insufficient to ensure cooperation. Concrete goals such as getting to the toilet or to a meal are more realistic and more likely to get patient cooperation. Learning what is important to the patient is the key to formulating goals that are significant both to the patient and the team. Brummel-Smith[8] has expressed this relationship as an equation. Motivation $= (W \times E \times R)/C$, where W is what the patient wants, E is what the patient expects, R is the reinforcement or reward, and C is the cost, be it physical, economic, emotional, or social.

PRINCIPLES OF MANAGEMENT

Table 59–19 lists the principles of geriatric rehabilitation discussed in this chapter. Emphasis is placed on the multiple impairments found in the elderly patient and on the management rather than cure of these impairments. These impairments interact to cause disability that in many ways is unique to the individual patient. The varying goals and expectations of each patient and his or her family also contribute to this uniqueness. The planning and management by the rehabilitation team must take into consideration these differences between patients and there must be a realization that there is not a single plan that fits all patients.

PRESCRIPTION MODIFICATION

Several factors unique to the elderly must be taken into consideration when writing a rehabilitation prescription for an elderly patient. Hunt[34] has emphasized homeostatic malfunctions in the elderly. Several of these must be considered as precautions when treating the elderly. As noted previously, temperature regulation can be problematic and the environment in which elderly patients exercise should be neither too hot nor too cold. The sense of thirst diminishes in the elderly and monitoring for dehydration is a necessity. Transient circulatory insufficiency such as postural hypotension can occur and lead to falls and syncope. Postural instability can also lead to falls. Pain complaints can be diffuse and nonspecific with both a higher threshold

TABLE 59–19 Principles of Rehabilitation Management of the Elderly Patient

1. Ascertain level of function (functional assessment)
2. Ascertain available resources and options
3. Avoid immobilization
4. Be aware of altered physiological reactions
5. Determine patient's significant goals, motivation
6. Determine family expectations (psychosocial issues)
7. Differentiate between delirium, dementia, depression
8. Emphasize function; management not diagnosis; cure
9. Emphasize task-specific exercise; simplify program
10. Encourage socialization and stimulation
11. Minimize medications
12. Realize that function may not be regained
13. Recognize that patients have multiple interacting impairments
14. Understand that improvement occurs in slow increments

and decreased tolerance reported.[22] Cardiopulmonary impairments are common and appropriate precautions should be exercised. Similarly, medications can affect both the ability to participate in therapy and increase the risk of therapy (anticoagulants).

DISCHARGE PLANNING

Insightful discharge planning is critical if the patient is to avoid institutionalization. Discharge planning should begin simultaneously with the rehabilitation referral. The goals of the patient should be ascertained, as well as the ability of the family or other support system to help in meeting these goals. The bottom-line functional abilities required for the family to be able or willing to take a patient home should be determined. These functional abilities can include continence, taking meals, self-dressing, etc. Unless there is adequate family or community support, even patients capable of self-care might not go home because of deficits in community reentry items (independent ADL), for example, shopping.[20] Not uncommonly, family support is lacking since many aging patients have lost their spouses and live alone. Community services become increasingly important as does the availability of companions or assisted living arrangements. These resources vary in availability throughout the country and can be determining factors in whether a patient can avoid institutionalization.

LEGAL AND ETHICAL ISSUES

Laws dealing with the elderly differ among different jurisdictions. Each state has its own rules governing informed consent, patients' competence, and the right to refuse treatment. Similarly, different states have different regulations governing the right to die, advanced directives, living wills, and durable powers of attorney. All of these legal issues affect patient management,[1] and should be known to the rehabilitation team functioning in a given jurisdiction.

Ethical issues in taking care of the elderly are becoming more complex. We no longer have the fiscal ability to do everything for every patient. The ethical dilemma in determining how much to do and whether to do it involves the wishes of the patient and the family and the laws pertaining to each jurisdiction. Our society is now further complicating this discussion with a reordering of the healthcare delivery system and possible rationing of healthcare resources.[4]

OUTCOME

Rehabilitation of the elderly can be very successful and professionally rewarding depending on how we frame our definition of outcome. While we must accept the irreversibility of aging and the concomitant physical and social changes and losses, we should also realize that with appropriate rehabilitation and social support (family and community), most elderly patients can be kept in the community or returned to their own homes or other community living arrangements. With the application of rehabilitation methodologies as discussed in this chapter, their quality of life can be maintained or improved. Most elderly patients live in the community and even of those aged 85 and above, only 15% of men and 25% of women live in a nursing home.[51] Discharge data from our geriatric rehabilitation unit indicate that we discharge over 85% of our patients to a noninstitutional setting. Our challenge as rehabilitation professionals is not to give in to the biases of "ageism," but to employ our abilities in assisting our elderly patients to maintain the quality and dignity of their lives.

References

1. Allen B, McCrary SV: Legal aspects of geriatric rehabilitative care. *In* Felsenthal G, Garrison SJ, Steinberg FU (eds): Rehabilitation of the Aging and Elderly Patient. Baltimore, Williams & Wilkins, 1994, pp 539–549.
2. Anderson JM: Heart disease and cardiac rehabilitation in the elderly patient. *In* Felsenthal G, Garrison SJ, Steinberg FU (eds): Rehabilitation of the Aging and Elderly Patient. Baltimore, Williams & Wilkins, 1994, pp 253–262.
3. Bach JR: Pulmonary assessment and management of the aging and older patient. *In* Felsenthal G, Garrison SJ, Steinberg FU (eds): Rehabilitation of the Aging and Elderly Patient. Baltimore, Williams & Wilkins, 1994, pp 263–273.
4. Banja JD: Ethical issues in caring for the elderly. *In* Felsenthal G, Garrison SJ, Steinberg FU (eds): Rehabilitation of the Aging and Elderly Patient. Baltimore, Williams & Wilkins, 1994, pp 551–560.
5. Bohannon R, Larkin P, Cook A, et al: Decrease in timed balance test scores with aging. Phys Ther 1984; 64:1067–1070.
6. Bortz WM II: Effect of exercise on aging—effect of aging on exercise. J Am Geriatr Soc 1980; 28:49–51.
7. Brink TL, Yesavage JA, Lum O, et al: Screening tests for geriatric depression. Clin Gerontol 1982; 1:37–43.
8. Brummel-Smith K: Rehabilitation. *In* Cassel CK (ed): Geriatric Medicine. New York, Springer-Verlag, 1990, p 129.
9. Butler RN: A disease called ageism. J Am Geriatr Soc 1990; 38:178–180.
10. Campbell AJ, Reinkin J, Allan BC, et al: Falls in the old age: A study of frequency and related clinical factors. Age Ageing 1981; 10:264–270.
11. Chamberlin W: Restrictions in upward gaze with advancing age. Am J Ophthalmol 1971; 71:341–346.
12. Cobble ND, Miller JR, Grigsby J, Lane JC: Aging with multiple sclerosis. *In* Felsenthal G, Garrison SJ, Steinberg FU (eds): Rehabilitation of the Aging and Elderly Patient. Baltimore, Williams & Wilkins, 1994, pp 427–436.
13. Diamond PT, Butler DH, Felsenthal G: Inpatient episodic care settings I. Geriatric rehabilitation unit. *In* Felsenthal G, Garrison SJ, Steinberg FU (eds): Rehabilitation of the Aging and Elderly Patient. Baltimore, Williams & Wilkins, 1994, pp 467–471.
14. Diamond PT, Felsenthal G, Macciocchi SN, et al: The effect of cognitive impairment on rehabilitation outcome. Am J Phys Med, in press.
15. Dumitru D, Gershkoff A, Walsh NE: Peripheral nervous/muscular system. *In* Felsenthal G, Garrison SJ, Steinberg FU (eds): Rehabilitation of the Aging and Elderly Patient. Baltimore, Williams & Wilkins, 1994, pp 227–241.
16. Era P, Heikkinen E: Postural sway during standing and unexpected disturbance of balance in random samples of men of different ages. J Gerontol 1985; 40:287–295.
17. Esquenazi A, Thompson E: Management of foot disorders in the elderly. *In* Felsenthal G, Garrison SJ, Steinberg FU (eds): Rehabilitation of the Aging and Elderly Patient. Baltimore, Williams & Wilkins, 1994, pp 153–161.
18. Fast A: Disorders of the cervical and lumbosacral spine. *In* Felsenthal G, Garrison SJ, Steinberg FU (eds): Rehabilitation of the Aging and Elderly Patient. Baltimore, Williams & Wilkins, 1994, pp 141–151.
19. Felsenthal G: Rehabilitating older patients: Primary care evaluation, treatment, and resources. Geriatrics 1989; 44:81–90.
20. Felsenthal G, Cohen BS, Hilton EB, et al: The physiatrist as primary physician for patients on an inpatient rehabilitation unit. Arch Phys Med Rehabil 1984; 65:375–378.
21. Felsenthal G, Glomski N, Jones D: Medication education in an inpatient geriatric rehabilitation unit. Arch Phys Med Rehabil 1986; 67:27–29.
22. Ferrell BA: Pain management in elderly people. J Am Geriatr Soc 1991; 39:64–73.
23. Fishman L: Rehabilitation of elderly patients after traumatic brain injury. *In* Felsenthal G, Garrison SJ, Steinberg FU (eds): Rehabilitation of the Aging and Elderly Patient. Baltimore, Williams & Wilkins, 1994, pp 187–214.
24. Folstein MF, Folstein SE, McHugh PR: Mini-Mental State. A practical method for grading the cognitive state of patients for the clinician. J Psychiatr Res 1975; 12:189–198.
25. Frontera WR, Meredith CN: Exercise in the rehabilitation of the elderly. *In* Felsenthal G, Garrison SJ, Steinberg FU (eds): Rehabilitation of the Aging and Elderly Patient. Baltimore, Williams & Wilkins, 1994, pp 35–36.
26. Fulton JP, Katz S, Jack SS, Hendershot GE: Physical functioning of the aged, United States, 1984. Vital Health Stat [10] 1989; 167.
27. Garden F: Sexual function in the elderly. *In* Felsenthal G, Garrison SJ, Steinberg FU (eds): Rehabilitation of the Aging and Elderly Patient. Baltimore, Williams & Wilkins, 1994, pp 319–325.
28. Garrison SJ: Geriatric stroke rehabilitation. *In* Felsenthal G, Garrison SJ, Steinberg FU (eds): Rehabilitation of the Aging and Elderly Patient. Baltimore, Williams & Wilkins, 1994, pp 175–186.
29. Goins MA: Geriatric hearing loss. *In* Felsenthal G, Garrison SJ, Steinberg FU (eds): Rehabilitation of the Aging and Elderly Patient. Baltimore, Williams & Wilkins, 1994, pp 339–350.
30. Halstead LS: Poliomyelitis. *In* Felsenthal G, Garrison SJ, Steinberg FU (eds): Rehabilitation of the Aging and Elderly Patient. Baltimore, Williams & Wilkins, 1994, pp 415–425.
31. Hing E, Sekscenski E, Strahan G: The National Nursing Home Survey; 1985 summary for the United States. Vital Health Stat [13] 1989; 97.
32. Hodgson J: Age and aerobic capacity of urban midwestern males. Thesis, University of Minnesota, Minneapolis, 1971.
33. Hough JC: Falls and falling. *In* Ham RJ, Sloane PD (eds): Primary Care Geriatrics: A Case-Based Approach. St Louis, Mosby–Year Book, 1992, pp 362–377.
34. Hunt TE: Homeostatic malfunctions in the aged. Br Columbia Med J 1980; 22:379–381.
35. Hutton JT, Shapiro I, Christians MA: Functional significance of restricted upgaze. Arch Phys Med Rehabil 1982; 63:617–619.
36. Kaufman T: Posture and age. Top Geriatr Rehabil 1987; 2:13–26.
37. Kawas CH: Evaluation of cognition in the elderly rehabilitation patient. *In* Felsenthal G, Garrison SJ, Steinberg FU (eds): Rehabilitation of the Aging and Elderly Patient. Baltimore, Williams & Wilkins, 1994, pp 289–294.
38. Kingston ER, Hirshorn BA, Cornman JM: Ties that Bind: The Interdependence of Generations. Washington, DC, Seven Locks Press, 1986.
39. Jain SS, DeLisa JA: Degenerative central nervous system diseases. *In* Felsenthal G, Garrison SJ, Steinberg FU (eds): Rehabilitation of the Aging and Elderly Patient. Baltimore, Williams & Wilkins, 1994, pp 215–226.
40. Magaziner J: Demographic and epidemiologic considerations for developing preventive strategies in the elderly. Md Med J 1989; 38:115–120.
41. Morley JE, Silver AJ: Nutrition needs and deficiencies in old age. *In* Felsenthal G, Garrison SJ, Steinberg FU (eds): Rehabilitation of the Aging and Elderly Patient. Baltimore, Williams & Wilkins, 1994, pp 61–62.
42. Murray MP, Kory RC, Clarkson BH: Walking patterns in healthy old men. J Gerontol 1969; 24:169–178.
43. Murray MP, Kory RC, Sepic SB: Walking patterns of normal women. Arch Phys Med Rehabil 1970; 51:637–650.
44. Nelson MR, Alexander MA: Pediatric-onset disabilities. *In* Felsenthal G, Garrison SJ, Steinberg FU (eds): Rehabilitation of the Aging and Elderly Patient. Baltimore, Williams & Wilkins, 1994, pp 407–413.
45. Nicholas JJ, Rosenberg AN: Arthritis and arthroplasties. *In* Felsenthal G, Garrison SJ, Steinberg FU (eds): Rehabilitation of the Aging and Elderly Patient. Baltimore, Williams & Wilkins, 1994, pp 97–106.
46. Palmer JB, DuChane AS: Rehabilitation of swallowing disorders in the elderly. *In* Felsenthal G, Garrison SJ, Steinberg FU (eds):

Rehabilitation of the Aging and Elderly Patient. Baltimore, Williams & Wilkins, 1994, pp 275–287.

47. Parker B, Vestal RE: Pharmacology and aging. *In* Felsenthal G, Garrison SJ, Steinberg FU (eds): Rehabilitation of the Aging and Elderly Patient. Baltimore, Williams & Wilkins, 1994, pp 65–71.

48. Redford JB: Peripheral vascular disease and ischemic skin ulceration. *In* Felsenthal G, Garrison SJ, Steinberg FU (eds): Rehabilitation of the Aging and Elderly Patient. Baltimore, Williams & Wilkins, 1994, pp 163–173.

49. Reischer MA, Spindler HA: Rehabilitation management of pain in the elderly. *In* Felsenthal G, Garrison SJ, Steinberg FU (eds): Rehabilitation of the Aging and Elderly Patient. Baltimore, Williams & Wilkins, 1994, pp 303–317.

50. Roth EJ, Lawler MH, Heinemann AW, et al: The older adult with a spinal cord injury. Paraplegia, in press.

51. Schneider EL, Gurainik JM: The aging of America: Impact on health care costs. JAMA 1990; 263:2335–2340.

52. Schuman JE, Beattie EJ, Steed DA, et al: Geriatric patients with and without intellectual dysfunction: Effectiveness of standard rehabilitation program. Arch Phys Med Rehabil 1981; 62:612–618.

53. Shock NW, Greulich RC, Costa PT, et al: Normal Human Aging: The Baltimore Longitudinal Study of Aging. US Department of Health and Human Services, Baltimore City Hospitals, 1984.

54. Siebens H: Issues on medication use and substance abuse in older adults. *In* Felsenthal G, Garrison SJ, Steinberg FU (eds): Rehabilitation of the Aging and Elderly Patient. Baltimore, Williams & Wilkins, 1994, pp 351–361.

55. Sinaki M, Nicholas JJ: Metabolic bone disease and aging. *In* Felsenthal G, Garrison SJ, Steinberg FU (eds): Rehabilitation of the Aging and Elderly Patient. Baltimore, Williams & Wilkins, 1994, pp 107–122.

56. Smith EL, Di Fabio RP, Gilligan K: Exercise intervention and physiologic function in the elderly. Top Geriatr Rehabil 1990; 6:57–68.

57. Sonn U, Grimby G: Assistive devices in an elderly population studied at 70 and 76 years of age. Disabil Rehabil 1994; 16:85–92.

58. Stein BD, Felsenthal G: Rehabilitation of fractures in the geriatric population. *In* Felsenthal G, Garrison SJ, Steinberg FU (eds): Rehabilitation of the Aging and Elderly Patient. Baltimore, Williams & Wilkins, 1994, pp 123–139.

59. Steinberg FU: Gait disorders in the aged. J Am Geriatr Soc 1972; 20:537–540.

60. Steinberg FU: Medical evaluation, assessment of function and potential, and rehabilitation plan. *In* Felsenthal G, Garrison SJ, Steinberg FU (eds): Rehabilitation of the Aging and Elderly Patient. Baltimore, Williams & Wilkins, 1994, pp 81–82.

61. Tinetti ME, Ginter SF: Identifying mobility dysfunctions in elderly patients: Standard neuromuscular examination or direct assessment. JAMA 1988; 259:1190–1193.

62. Wainapel SF: Visual impairments. *In* Felsenthal G, Garrison SJ, Steinberg FU (eds): Rehabilitation of the Aging and Elderly Patient. Baltimore, Williams & Wilkins, 1994, pp 327–337.

63. Wongsurawat N: Temperature regulation in the aged. *In* Felsenthal G, Garrison SJ, Steinberg FU (eds): Rehabilitation of the Aging and Elderly Patient. Baltimore, Williams & Wilkins, 1994, pp 73–78.

64. Yarkony GM: Aging after a traumatic spinal cord injury. *In* Felsenthal G, Garrison SJ, Steinberg FU (eds): Rehabilitation of the Aging and Elderly Patient. Baltimore, Williams & Wilkins, 1994, pp 391–396.

60

Rehabilitation Management in Persons With AIDS and HIV Infection

MICHAEL W. O'DELL, M.D.,
AND MARY E. DILLON, M.D.

OVERVIEW OF AIDS AND HIV INFECTION

Epidemiology

In 1981, the U.S. Centers for Disease Control and Prevention (CDC) began receiving reports of *Pneumocystis carinii* pneumonia (PCP) in previously healthy, homosexual men.[40] A similar clinical presentation was soon evident in other groups, most notably intravenous (IV) drug users and persons with hemophilia.[43] In 1983, the French scientist Luc Montagnier identified a human retrovirus, later renamed human immunodeficiency virus (HIV), as the cause of a profound, cellular immune system dysfunction, by then called acquired immunodeficiency syndrome (AIDS). By 1984, over 8000 cases of AIDS had been reported to the CDC.[43]

As of December 1994, over 441,000 cases of AIDS had been reported to the CDC, of which over 270,000 resulted in death.[3] Recent estimates by Rosenberg et al.[101] placed the number of persons in the United States infected with HIV at between 500,000 and 900,000. After exponential increases through the 1980s, the epidemic may be reaching a plateau in terms of new annual cases.[97] Despite this plateau, the demographic makeup of the epidemic is changing rapidly. The AIDS epidemic continues at genocidal levels among homosexual men in the United States,[43] but a *decreasing proportion* of new cases are being diagnosed in homosexual and bisexual males and IV drug users, with substantial increases in cases due to heterosexual transmission (especially among women and adolescents).[97, 117] It is also clear that the AIDS epidemic is claiming a disproportionate toll among urban minorities[49]— impoverished groups already struggling with inadequate access to the U.S. healthcare system. Over 80% of new pediatric AIDS cases in 1993 occurred among black and Latino children.[49]

Despite the public impression to the contrary, HIV has a rather restrictive mode of transmission limited to intimate sexual contact, exposure to infected blood or blood products, and perinatal transmission from mother to fetus.[34] There are actually no risk *groups* for HIV infection, only risk *behaviors*. There are no convincing data to support that transmission occurs with any frequency through casual contact.[35] The high prevalence of unrecognized HIV infection in victims of trauma,[6, 70, 78] combined with the numerous opportunities for exposure to body fluids in the setting of rehabilitation, necessitates education in, and strict adherence to, "universal precautions" by *all* rehabilitation professionals in *all* patient encounters.[67]

Biology, Natural History, and Treatment

HIV is a member of the *Lentivirus* family of human retroviruses, recognized for their tendency to invade the nervous system, having a long latency period, and not eliciting an effective neutralizing humoral immune response, which results in persistent viremia.[42] HIV has a direct, primary destructive effect on various body tissues including the intestine, glial cells, and bone marrow.[42] The more important, secondary pathological effect, however, is the invasion and eventual destruction of the CD4+ subpopulation of T lymphocytes resulting in a collapse of cellular-mediated immunity.[42]

It is vital to recognize that AIDS is only the end-stage manifestation of a chronic infection with HIV; that is, "AIDS" and "HIV-infection" are *not* synonymous[114] (Fig. 60–1). Within a few weeks of initial HIV infection, symp-

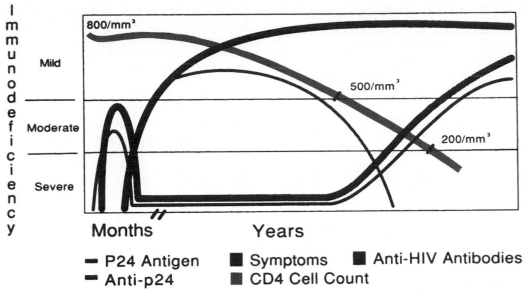

FIGURE 60–1 Natural history of immunological parameters and symptoms in persons with HIV infection. It is important to note that symptoms are most prominent at the time of initial HIV infection (briefly) and after CD4 T-lymphocyte counts drop below 500 cells/mL. It may take many years for symptoms to develop after HIV infection. A person is considered to have "AIDS" only with major symptoms or a CD4+ count below 200 cells/mL. (Courtesy of Dr. Jon Fuller, Boston City Hospital.)

toms are typical of an acute viral syndrome, consisting of fever, sweats, rash, nausea, diarrhea, and nonexudative pharyngitis. Antibodies to HIV can usually be detected within 1 to 3 months after infection.[34] Acute infection is then followed by a period of relative viral latency, with a range of 1 to 15 years[34] and median time of 10 to 12 years from infection to development of symptoms.[64, 65] Hoover et al.[52] found signs and symptoms even in those with "asymptomatic" HIV infection, but the functional significance of deficits prior to AIDS is unclear.[89] There is a steady decline of immune function during this "asymptomatic" phase. CD4+ T lymphocyte counts, normally in the 500 to 1500/mL range, decline by approximately 50 to 80/mL/year, with persons experiencing increasingly severe symptoms as counts drop below the 500/mL mark[34, 114] (see Fig. 60–1). CD4+ counts are used clinically to guide initiation of antiretroviral therapy (now recommended in persons with counts below 500/mL),[34, 50] to predict disease progression, and to predict the risk of, and initiate prophylaxis for, certain opportunistic infections.[20, 34] Of interest to rehabilitation professionals, preliminary research indicates CD4+ counts are not well correlated with functional status.[17, 90, 113]

The more familiar clinical manifestations generally occur quite late in the course of HIV infection, that is, after significant immunocompromise and the development of AIDS.[34] Although the manifestations of AIDS are legion, certain pathogens tend to be associated with particular organ systems. Examples are listed in Table 60–1. Cutaneous Kaposi's sarcoma is the most common presenting cancer followed by lymphoma of the central nervous system (CNS).[103] Other late manifestations related to a direct effect of HIV include constitutional symptoms (particularly "HIV wasting syndrome"), cytopenias, and neurological disease such as AIDS dementia complex (ADC) and myelopathy.[7]

In 1993, the CDC[81] revised the system by which HIV infection is classified (Table 60–2). The 1993 classification consists of nine, mutually exclusive categories based on both clinical parameters (group A—asymptomatic; group B—symptomatic but without an AIDS-defining illness; and group C—AIDS) and CD4+ counts (≥500/mL, 200–499/mL, and <200/mL, respectively), and is applicable only to persons over age 13 years. Under this new 1993 classification, persons with CD4+ counts under 200/mL meet the case surveillance definition of AIDS, regardless of clinical symptomatology.

Treatment of HIV infection is rapidly evolving.[34, 50] Pharmacological inhibition of the enzyme reverse transcriptase with drugs such as zidovudine (AZT, formerly azidothymidine), didanosine (ddI), and zalcitabine (ddC) has been the most successful intervention against the virus, although certainly less than ideal.[50] Results from the recent European "Concorde" study suggest that AZT may be less efficacious

TABLE 60–1 Common Organ System Involvement for Selected Pathogens in AIDS

Pathogen and Class	Typical Site of Involvement
Parasites	
Toxoplasma gondii	Brain
Cryptosporidium	Gastrointestinal (GI) tract
Pneumocystis carinii	Lung
Fungi	
Candida albicans	Mouth, esophagus, vulva, and vagina
Cryptococcus neoformans	Meninges, lung
Viruses	
Cytomegalovirus	Retina, lungs, nervous system, GI tract
Herpes simplex, varicella-zoster	Cutaneous, esophagus, brain
JC virus	Brain—white matter
Mycobacteria	
Mycobacterium tuberculosis	Lungs, meninges, disseminated
Mycobacterium avium-intracellulare	GI tract, bone marrow, disseminated

TABLE 60–2   1993 Revised CDC Classification System for HIV Infection

CD4+ Cell Count	Clinical Categories*		
	Group A: Asymptomatic, Acute HIV, or PGL	Group B: Symptomatic,† not Group A or C	Group C: AIDS Indicator Conditions
≥500/mL	A1	B1	C1
200–499/mL	A2	B2	C2
<200/mL	A3	B3	C3

*The italicized categories illustrate the expanded AIDS surveillance case definition. All patients will be reported as having AIDS based upon the AIDS indicator conditions or a CD4+ cell count <200/mL.

†Includes, but is not limited to, bacterial infections (pneumonia, meningitis, endocarditis, or sepsis); vulvovaginal candidiasis persistent >1 mo and poorly responsive to treatment; thrush and oral hairy leukoplakia; severe cervical dysplasia or carcinoma; shingles with two episodes or >1 dermatome; idiopathic thrombocytopenia purpura; listeriosis; nocardiosis; pelvic inflammatory disease; peripheral neuropathy; constitutional symptoms such as fever or diarrhea for >1 mo.

PGL, persistent generalized lymphadenopathy.

Data from 1993 Revised classification system for HIV infection and expanded case surveillance case definition for AIDS among adolescents and adults. MMWR 1992; 41:1–19.

than once thought, but these studies await replication.[1] Other experimental HIV treatments focus on combination therapy with the above agents[25, 50]; other retroviral agents such as stavudine, FLT, carbovir, and 3TC; and the use of protease inhibitors which block assembly of viral components into a complete virion.[50] Intensive efforts are underway to develop an HIV vaccine. An HIV vaccine would most likely be used to bolster the natural immunological response to clear virus, rather than to prevent infection. The prospects for accomplishing either are unclear, at present.[34] Secondary opportunistic infections are treated or prophylaxed against using a variety of drugs with which many rehabilitation physicians may not be familiar.[20] Examples of these medications, indications, and side effects are listed in Table 60–3.

Survival after an AIDS-defining illness ranges from 11.5[95] to 20.8 months.[62] Survival rates vary rather substantially depending on geographical region, year of AIDS diagnosis, sex, age, ethnic background, and treatment with AZT.[95] Improvement well over the current 5-year survival rate of 3% will be particularly pertinent to rehabilitation professionals.[64, 105]

Rehabilitation Medicine and HIV Infection

Over the past 13 years, the AIDS epidemic has influenced virtually every segment of society: the public health system and delivery of medical care, political and governmental agencies responsible for entitlements and drug approval, religious institutions, and the correctional system.[53, 84] Moreover, nearly every medical specialty has accumulated a base of knowledge in HIV and AIDS-related manifestations pertinent to its practice. Rehabilitation medicine is no exception, even though the clinical experience in managing HIV-related disability is not particularly widespread[36, 37, 67, 74, 82, 84, 86] (personal communication, Chris Mason, American Rehabilitation Association, April 1994).

There are at least four factors which will influence the relative importance of and demand for clinical intervention

for HIV disability over the next decade.[84] First, the more persons with symptomatic HIV infection, the greater the potential demand for rehabilitation intervention. There are good data to support a strong association between symptoms, or constellations of symptoms in HIV infection, and functional deficits.[23, 69, 89, 90] Second, advances in the care of persons with HIV infection should prolong survival. Prolonged survival after an AIDS-defining event may provide a longer time period over which disability may develop,[84] alter (possibly lessen) the more severe clinical manifestations of HIV disease,[68] and strengthen the philosophical justification for expending resources on rehabilitation intervention.[84] Third, the types of symptoms associated with HIV infection are crucial in determining the nature and extent of rehabilitation intervention. "Constitutional" and neurological symptoms seem to be strong determinants of disability.[119] The last is especially important as current models of rehabilitation can be easily modified for persons with HIV infection.[66] Finally, rehabilitation professionals cannot attempt to reduce the impact of HIV disability unless provided access to the patient population. Preliminary survey results from the American Rehabilitation Association indicate that institutional barriers to access for HIV rehabilitation services include lack of funding and community referral base, stigma and fears on the part of rehabilitation staff, and lack of client followthrough and administrative support (personal communication, Chris Mason and Margo Caufield, American Rehabilitation Association, April 1994).

Many kinds of rehabilitation interventions are appropriate in patients with HIV infection. O'Connell and Levinson[82] identified impaired mobility (76%), difficulty with self-care (57%), impaired cognition (29%), and uncontrolled pain (37%) in 51 rehabilitation consultations in persons with AIDS. Their prescribed interventions included therapeutic exercise (73%), gait aids (45%), bathroom and safety equipment (45%), orthoses (29%), vocational counseling (4%), pain management (29%), and whirlpool treatment (10%).[82] In another study of 37 AIDS patients discharged from an acute care hospital, O'Dell et al.[87] found that 22 (59%) required human assistance in at least 1 of 18 areas on the Functional Independence Measure, with 12 (32%) requiring assistance in greater than 5 of 18 areas on the measure.[87] The areas most often requiring assistance included stair climbing, ambulation, bowel management, and lower extremity dressing.[87]

Regardless of the future course of the AIDS epidemic, rehabilitation physicians and professionals will evaluate and treat increasing numbers of persons with HIV-related disability, providing a variety of services[54, 59, 67, 84, 88, 99] (Table 60–4). The remainder of this chapter provides an introduction to the clinical manifestations of AIDS and HIV infection and outlines potential rehabilitation interventions. A discussion of the psychosocial considerations for both patients and the rehabilitation team follows. The reader in need of further information should refer to one of several available texts on the topic.[37, 74, 83]

CLINICAL MANIFESTATIONS OF HIV INFECTION AND REHABILITATION APPROACH

For the sake of simplicity, the clinical manifestations of HIV infection are grouped as "neurological," either central

TABLE 60–3   Indications and Side Effects of Selected Medications Used in Persons With HIV Infection

Medication/Class	Indication	Potential Side Effects
Antiviral Drugs		
Zidovudine (AZT)	Treat HIV infection when CD4+ count <500/mL	Bone marrow suppression, headache, nausea, and vomiting, myalgias, insomnia, fatigue, ?myopathy
Didanosine (ddl)	Treat HIV infection if intolerant to AZT or alone if CD4+ count <200–300/mL	Peripheral neuropathy, pancreatitis, diarrhea, headache, bad taste
Zalcitabine (ddC)	Treat HIV infection in combination with AZT if CD4+ count <300/mL, or clinical or immune deterioration	Peripheral neuropathy, rash, stomatitis, pancreatitis (rarely)
Acyclovir	Anti–herpes simplex, varicella-zoster	Nausea and vomiting, headache, diarrhea
Foscarnet	Anti-CMV therapy	Azotemia, ↓ Ca, ↓ P, ↓ Mg, myalgias, anemia
Ganciclovir	Anti-CMV therapy	Leukopenia, anemia, thrombocytopenia, GI and CNS disturbances, hepatitis
PCP Prophylaxis		
Pentamidine	HIV infection and CD4+ count <200/mL	Hypoglycemia, azotemia, ↓ BP, neutropenia
TMP-SMX	HIV infection and CD4+ count <200/mL	Neutropenia, thrombocytopenia, exfoliative rash, hepatitis, nausea and vomiting
Anti-Toxoplasma		
Pyrimethamine*	Treatment of toxoplasmosis, maintenance therapy	Blood dyscrasias, ↓ folic acid, rash, nausea and vomiting
Sulfadiazine*	Treatment of toxoplasmosis, maintenance therapy	Rash, photosensitivity, fever, renal and hepatic toxicity, SJS
Fungicidal Drugs		
Fluconazole	Anti-*Cryptococcus,* candidiasis, other fungal infections	Nausea and vomiting, ↑ serum transaminases, skin rash, diarrhea, abdominal pain
Other Medications		
Erythropoietin	Treatment of severe anemia	Fever, fatigue, headache
GM-CSF	Treatment of neutropenia	Pain and erythema at injection site, fever, bone pain, myalgias

*Pyrimethamine and sulfadiazine should be administered in conjunction with 5–10 mg/day of folic acid.
Abbreviations: CMV, cytomegalovirus; GI, gastrointestinal; CNS, central nervous system; PCP, *Pneumocystis carinii* pneumonia; BP, blood pressure; TMP-SMX, trimethoprim-sulfamethoxazole; SJS, Stevens Johnson syndrome; GM-CSF, granulocyte-macrophage colony-stimulating factor.

or peripheral, and "non-neurological." Single impairments rarely lead to a specific disability. Multiple medical and neurological impairments are the rule, especially late in the disease course. A discussion of the approach to rehabilitation is provided after the description of each disease complication.

Neurological Manifestations

Brew[14] proposed several helpful principles in considering the neurological manifestations of HIV infection. *Time-*

TABLE 60–4   Potential Interventions by the Rehabilitation Team Caring for Persons With AIDS and HIV Infection

1. Functionally based continuity of care among multiple disciplines providing medical management
2. Identification of impairments and disability
3. Prescription of therapeutic exercise
4. Prescription of orthoses, adaptive equipment, assistive devices, and durable medical equipment
5. Cognitive evaluation and prescription of memory aids
6. Evaluation and treatment of communication disorders and dysphagia
7. Evaluation and management of bladder and bowel dysfunction
8. Instruction in energy conservation and work simplification
9. Teaching caregivers
10. Home evaluations with recommendations for environmental modifications
11. Assistance accessing community supports and community reentry
12. Assistance with establishing power of attorney and legal guardianship
13. Counseling for psychosocial stressors
14. Vocational counseling and rehabilitation
15. Assistance in medication compliance

locking refers to the tendency for particular neurological processes to occur during certain disease stages. For example, demyelinating peripheral neuropathies tend to occur early in HIV infection, whereas most cerebral, opportunistic infections occur quite late, after significant immunocompromise. It is common for central and peripheral nervous system processes to occur simultaneously, for example, painful peripheral neuropathy in conjunction with ADC. This is known as *parallel tracking. Layering* refers to multiple processes within one part of the neuraxis, as in the simultaneous occurrence of peripheral neuropathy and myopathy. A given process, either neurological or medical, can exacerbate the presentation or functional importance of a subclinical neurological process *(unmasking)*. The clinician must take into consideration these complex interactions *(diagnostic flexibility)*. Particularly important in this category is the exacerbation of mild, subclinical cognitive deficits by cerebral infections, mood disorders, or medication side effects. Finally, even though persons with AIDS are severely immunocompromised, the clinician should not fail to consider more "common" causes of nervous system dysfunction in appropriate circumstances, such as alcohol-induced peripheral neuropathy or myelopathy due to degenerative or discogenic disease.[10]

Central Nervous System Complications

Table 60–5, developed by Levinson and Merritt,[66] outlines typical CNS diseases in HIV infection by cause, deficits, and prognosis. "Diffuse processes" in HIV-related CNS disease can be broadly viewed within the traumatic brain injury (TBI) model in terms of intervention, "focal

TABLE 60–5   Causes of CNS Dysfunction in HIV-Related Disease

Cause	Frequency	Cognitive Deficits	Focal CNS Deficits	Blindness	Myelopathy	Rehabilitation Prognosis
Viruses						
Primary HIV encephalitis	65%–90%	+ + +	−	−	+ +	Good early Poor late
CMV encephalitis	Up to 90%	+ +	±	−	+	Fair
CMV retinitis	20%–25%	−	−	+ + +	−	Good
PML (JC virus)	Up to 3.8%	+ +	+ + +	±	−	Very poor
Herpes simplex	Rare	+	+ +	±	+	Generally good
Varicella-zoster	Rare	+	±	−	+	Good
Epstein-Barr virus	Common	±	±	−	±	Generally good
Others	Rare	±	±	±	±	Variable
Bacteria						
Mycobacterium tuberculosis	Rare	+	+	−	±	Good except drug-resistant
Mycobacterium avium-intracellulare	Rare	+	−	−	−	Poor when disseminated
Others	Very rare	±	±	±	±	Variable
Fungi						
Cryptococcal meningitis	9%	+ + +	+	±	±	Variable (40% mortality)
Others	Very rare	±	±	±	±	Variable
Protozoa						
Toxoplasmosis	>2%	+	+ + +	±	−	Excellent with medical treatment
Malignancies						
Primary CNS lymphoma	1.5%	+	+ + +	±	−	Poor
Metastatic (Kaposi's sarcoma)	Rare	+	+ + +	±	±	Fair–poor
Cerebrovascular	Rare	+ +	+ + +	±	±	Poor
Multiple sclerosis	Unknown	+	+ + +	+	+ + +	

Abbreviations: CNS, central nervous system; CMV, cytomegalovirus; PML, progressive multifocal leukoencephalopathy; + + +, usually present; + +, very common; +, common; ±, occasionally present; −, not found.
From Levinson SF, Merritt L: Disability due to CNS impairment. Phys Med Rehabil 1993; 7:s101–s118.

processes" within the stroke model, and myelopathies analogous to rehabilitation in spinal cord injury (SCI).[66, 88] A comparison of rehabilitation in the setting of HIV infection and traditional models is presented in Table 60–6. The general approach to managing functional deficits in AIDS is no different from that used in corresponding non-HIV processes.[86, 88] In this sense, HIV rehabilitation directly parallels the philosophy of cancer rehabilitation[67] (see Chapter 57).

Diffuse Processes

Presentation

The most common causes of diffuse CNS processes are ADC (also termed *HIV-1–associated cognitive/motor deficits*[4]) and cryptococcal meningitis.[10, 66] Less frequent causes include viral (e.g., cytomegalovirus) encephalopathies, bacterial meningitis (e.g., tuberculous and syphilitic meningitis), lymphomatous meningitis, and secondary metabolic abnormalities.[10] It is also important to consider the relative contribution of mood disorders (i.e., anxiety and depression)[5] and medication side effects in the etiology of cognitive deficits, that is, the *unmasking* effect as discussed above.[66] It is quite common to see mild cognitive dysfunction in patients with focal neurological presentations.

ADC is a relentlessly progressive encephalopathy characterized by the syndrome of slowness of thought and forgetfulness typical of subcortical dementias. It is a late complication of AIDS, usually occurring when CD4+ counts fall below 250/mL.[14] Cognitive dysfunction can encompass decreased attention, concentration, and reaction time; memory retrieval problems; and some higher-level cortical impairment but with relatively preserved insight

until late.[14] Motor dysfunction is characterized by lower extremity weakness, ataxia, cogwheel rigidity, and tremor. Behavioral manifestations include apathy and even frank psychoses in up 10% of patients.[10] ADC can be the presenting problem and defining event for AIDS.[10] Although the incidence of cognitive deficits ranges from 25% to 80% (depending on the study and criteria used), severe dementia is seen in only about 5% to 10% of persons with AIDS and nearly always in end-stage disease.[5] Diagnosis is by exclusion of other potential causes. Neuroimaging typically shows only brain atrophy.[10] Some authors have suggested that use of antiretroviral drugs can slow or reverse the process,[5, 15] but opinions about this are mixed.[44]

Cryptococcal meningitis is seen in about 5% to 10% of persons with AIDS with extraneural presentation of the fungus being rather unusual.[10] Symptoms generally occur for less than 3 weeks prior to diagnosis and include headache, fever, and mental status changes.[66] The diagnosis is confirmed by laboratory examination of cerebrospinal fluid (CSF) or blood for cryptococcal antigens. Neuroimaging studies are usually normal. Treatment consists of initiation and lifetime maintenance with fluconazole.[10] Other CNS fungal infections have been reported in the setting of AIDS, including aspergillosis, candidiasis, and histoplasmosis.[66]

Rehabilitation Approach

Rehabilitation professionals can adapt a treatment approach similar to that used in TBI. The progressive nature of the late manifestations of AIDS necessitates an emphasis on relatively short-term, very functionally based goals. Mild to moderate cognitive deficits may be of particular importance when evaluating the rehabilitation potential of

TABLE 60–6 Models of Neurorehabilitation in HIV Infection

Traditional Rehabilitation	HIV Considerations
Focal Presentation: Stroke Model	
Predominantly elderly patients	Predominantly young age
Vocational needs usually low	Vocational needs variable
Cause usually known	Cause often unknown
Survival–several years	Survival—months to a few years
Insurance coverage typical (Medicare)	Insurance coverage variable
Diffuse Presentation: TBI Model	
Static to improving impairment	Temporarily static impairment in treatable processes, ADC progressive
Extended survival	Shorter survival
Medically stable	Medical stability variable
Insight often impaired	Insight intact until late
Behavioral problems common	Behavioral problems potentially complicated by risk of HIV exposure to staff and patients
Disposition often difficult	Disposition may be further complicated by HIV discrimination
HIV Myelopathy: SCI Model	
Relatively static	Progressive
Extended survival	Short survival
Paraparesis or tetraparesis	Usually paraparesis
Functional level predictable	Functional level uncertain
Mild cognitive deficits	Possibly severe cognitive deficits (ADC)

Abbreviations: TBI, traumatic brain injury; ADC, AIDS dementia complex; SCI, spinal cord injury.

persons with the more focal neurological deficits, as discussed below.

Early in the course of cognitive demise, compensatory strategies such as memory notebooks, verbal monitoring of tasks, avoidance of stress, and presenting limited amounts of material can improve performance. Although the patient should be the focus of intervention for as long as feasible, caretakers should be involved quite early when ADC is diagnosed, considering the generally poor prognosis.[66] Some degree of neuropsychological testing may be indicated. This is especially true in mild or more slowly progressing cases when specific delineation of cognitive deficits is needed for vocational adjustment and planning.

Psychosocial interventions are paramount. Counseling for patients, partners, family, and caretakers can facilitate adjustment to disability. Legal considerations, such as preparation of living wills, power of attorney, and guardianship, should be initiated early while the patient is mentally competent.[5]

Focal Processes

Presentation

Of the many causes of focal (or multifocal) CNS deficits in AIDS, the most common and treatable is cerebral toxoplasmosis.[10] Focal presentation can also be seen with several other somewhat less treatable processes such as cerebrovascular disease,[32, 44] primary CNS lymphoma,[10, 44] and progressive multifocal leukoencephalopathy (PML),[44, 66] among others. It has been suggested that cranial magnetic resonance imaging (MRI) with gadolinium, or a double dose, delayed computed tomographic (CT) scan, is manda-

tory in the evaluation of focal neurological signs associated with HIV infection.[10]

Toxoplasma gondii is a single-cell protozoan, intracellular parasite and the most common cause of an intracerebral mass lesion in HIV infection.[10, 66] Although usually presenting with focal signs, it is common to see these deficits superimposed on an underlying encephalopathy.[10] The typical clinical presentation occurs over 1 to 2 weeks with fatigue, fever, and progressive hemiparesis. CT of the brain usually shows multiple, ring-enhancing lesions with a propensity for the basal ganglia and frontoparietal lobes.[10] Although brain biopsy is the method of definitive diagnosis of toxoplasmosis, it should be undertaken only after failure to clinically and radiographically respond to a 2-week trial of combination therapy with pyrimethamine and sulfadiazine.[10, 66] Clinical response with drug therapy requires lifetime maintenance to prevent recurrence. Prognosis is very favorable among CNS opportunistic infections, with survival of a year not infrequent.

Cerebrovascular disease (HIV-CVD) occurs clinically in 1% to 7% of the HIV population[32] and much higher in pathological studies.[72] Berger and Levy[10] have suggested that HIV-CVD disease is no more common than in other critically ill, young adults. Etiologies for HIV-CVD include embolic, thrombotic, hemorrhagic, and vasculitic causes with specific treatment based on the etiology.[10, 44, 66, 92] As in strokes in young persons in general, often no specific cause is found.[92] Engstrom et al.[32] reported survival ranging from a few days to 2 years after stroke in 29 persons with HIV infection.

PML is a CNS demyelinating disorder seen in about 5% of persons with AIDS and results from infection with papovavirus.[61] Visual complaints, headache, weakness, and spasticity are the common presentations. Diagnosis is made by documenting the typical nonenhancing, multiple low-density, white matter lesions on brain CT and histopathological identification after brain biopsy.[44] Prognosis is variable, but generally poor (several months), and no specific treatment has been identified.[10, 44]

Primary CNS lymphoma is seen in up to 2% of persons with AIDS. Presentation is variable, including solitary or multiple intracerebral masses, lymphomatous meningitis, and localized intradural spinal masses (see below).[10] Radiographically, lymphoma appears as single or multiple discrete lesions, with some degree of surrounding edema and contrast enhancement. The primary differential diagnosis is toxoplasmosis. Treatment consists of radiotherapy and chemotherapy.[10, 44] Survival is usually measured in months; however, patients often succumb to other complications of AIDS.[10, 44]

Recently, a fulminant variant of multiple sclerosis has been reported in association with HIV infection.[41] It is unclear whether this represents a manifestation of HIV infection, or an overlap of separate pathological processes.[66]

Rehabilitation Approach

The approach to rehabilitation in focal CNS disease is similar to that used in stroke rehabilitation.[67, 86, 92] As is seen in non-HIV–related stroke, a degree of resolution of impairment is seen with specific treatment, with the resultant decrease in perilesion edema and diminution of the offending mass. O'Dell and Sasson[92] and Silwa and Smith[108] have reported on the rehabilitation approach to HIV-related hemiparesis. Interventions include appropriate orthoses (at both the wrist and ankle); pharmacological treatment of spasticity using baclofen, assistive devices, and therapeutic exercise; and enhancement of communication abilities. These are best accomplished with an interdisciplinary rehabilitation team. Because of parallel tracking, clinicians should check carefully for concomitant peripheral neuropathy prior to prescribing orthoses. Basic rehabilitation concerns such as prevention of skin compromise and contractures, bowel and bladder function, and safety of swallowing are no different from routine rehabilitation practice. Painful sequelae such as reflex sympthetic dystrophy, musculoskeletal shoulder pain, and central pain syndromes are also seen in HIV-CVD and hemiparesis. The team should be aware of mild to moderate cognitive deficits which may affect new learning and teaching of compensatory strategies. Education of family members or significant others should be initiated in nearly all cases.

Myelopathy

Presentation

Spinal cord involvement has been noted on autopsy in over 20% of persons having AIDS as the cause of death.[10] HIV-associated myelopathy, termed *vacuolar myelopathy*, tends to affect the dorsolateral portion of the thoracic spinal cord. The resulting clinical picture is one of ataxia and spastic paraparesis.[66] Despite the resemblance to combined subacute degeneration of the spinal cord, studies have failed to implicate vitamin B_{12} deficiency.[10] Unfortunately, spinal cord involvement is commonly seen in conjunction with ADC.[10, 66] The resulting cognitive impairment complicates, if not prevents, effective rehabilitation intervention in some patients.[67, 88] Treatment of HIV myelopathy is not particularly effective, but some authors suggest that a subtype ("multinucleated cell myelopathy") may respond to antiretroviral treatment.[14] Neuroimaging is important to rule out neoplastic masses or abscesses which may have a specific treatment. Prognosis is variable as symptoms may remain mild or the syndrome may rapidly progress.[44]

Rehabilitation Approach

As in rehabilitation of non-HIV myelopathy, aggressive management of bladder dysfunction is a high priority. The exact type of bladder dysfunction depends on the level of spinal cord involvement and the presence of concomitant conditions such as peripheral or autonomic neuropathy (AN). Trials of urological medications are warranted as well as initiation of intermittent catheterization, if indicated.[66] Because of the multiple enteric pathogens seen in the setting of HIV infection, constipation is unusual.

Orthotic devices and adaptive equipment should be prescribed with clear functional goals in mind, such as facilitating ease of transfers, standing, and decreasing the burden of care for caretakers. In many cases, fatigue and overall debilitation preclude all but household mobility. Once again, the association with ADC may impede or prevent effective learning of functional enhancing strategies.

Neuromuscular Complications

Abnormalities at virtually every level of the peripheral neuromuscular system have been implicated in HIV infection. Although dysfunction of anterior horn cells, the autonomic nervous system, and neuromuscular junction dysfunction have been reported,[63, 85, 109] peripheral neuropathy and myopathy are far more common.[63, 85]

Peripheral Neuropathic Pain

Presentation

There are several types of peripheral neuropathy associated with pain in HIV infection, each differing somewhat in clinical presentation[85] (Table 60–7). The most common is *distal symmetrical polyneuropathy (DSP)*, due to a dying-back type of axonopathy.[109] DSP presents with distal pain, paresthesia, and burning with hyporeflexia and relatively normal strength. The onset of symptoms tends to be late in the disease process, developing over weeks to months, and tends to persist once present. *Medication (iatrogenic)-induced neuropathies* present in a similar manner, but over a shorter period of time (days to weeks). The most likely etiologies are the antiretroviral treatments ddI[28] and, especially, ddC.[9] Other potential etiologies include the antituberculous drugs (rifampin, ethambutol, and isoniazid); vincristine, sometimes used to treat Kaposi's sarcoma; and dapsone, which is used in PCP prophylaxis.[85] Studies of dapsone in HIV infection, however, fail to reveal peripheral neuropathy as a prominent side effect.[13, 57] *Progressive polyradiculomyelopathy (PPR)* is a severe, usually fatal infection of the cauda equina, probably due to cytomegalovirus.[63, 109] Symptoms include extreme pain in a lumbosacral distribution, lower extremity weakness, and urinary retention. Treatment with IV ganciclovir may be helpful

TABLE 60–7　Etiologies of Neuromuscular Pain in HIV Infection

Diagnosis	Etiology	CDC Clinical Category*	Clinical Presentation
Distal symmetrical polyneuropathy	Dying-back axonopathy	B, C	Gradual onset of pain, paresthesia, decreased ankle-jerk reflex and vibration sense, mild distal weakness
Progressive polyradiculopathy	Cauda equina infection with cytomegalovirus	C	Rapid onset of pain and lower extremity weakness, urinary retention, loss of ankle jerk reflex and patellar reflexes
Mononeuropathy multiplex/ simplex	Vasculitis and immune complex	C	Variable, depending on particular nerve affected

*See Table 60–2.
From O'Dell MW: Rehabilitation management of HIV neuromuscular disease. Phys Med Rehabil 1993; 7:S83–S99.

but is controversial.[58] Lastly, depending on the cranial, spinal, or peripheral nerve involved, mononeuropathies (either simplex or multiplex) may be a cause of neuromuscular pain. Although in some cases the symptoms progress, the prognosis in mononeuropathy is generally good.[111]

Rehabilitation Approach

There is little literature on the symptomatic treatment of HIV neuromuscular pain.[85] Management can be broadly divided into nonpharmacological and pharmacological approaches. It seems logical to first consider nonpharmacological lines of treatment. Many patients will not respond and will require increasingly more aggressive interventions. Unfortunately, many cases of neuropathic pain are refractory to any type of intervention.

The successful use of transcutaneous electrical nerve stimulation (TENS) has been reported in HIV peripheral neuropathy.[38] Even though 60% to 70% of patients with neuropathic pain in general will respond acutely,[107] few achieve long-term relief. In the cases of more temporary, medication-induced neuropathies, relief over several weeks may be adequate. Clinical trials are currently underway exploring the use of acupuncture in combination with amitriptyline to treat HIV-related neuropathic pain.[77] Other physical modalities which may be beneficial include heat, vibration, and massage.[115] Custom-designed orthotic shoe inserts are useful in selected cases to facilitate ambulation.[82] Finally, relaxation techniques can be utilized in conjunction with virtually any treatment approach.

Many medications have been suggested for the treatment of neuromuscular pain in the setting of HIV infection.[63, 85, 109] As with the nonpharmacological interventions, most are recommended on the basis of anecdotal experience, rather than experimental studies. The safest, first-line choices are probably acetaminophen and nonsteroidal anti-inflammatory agents (NSAIDs). An initial concern over a deleterious interaction between AZT and acetaminophen has now been disproved.[104] Tricyclic antidepressants and anticonvulsant medications are frequently suggested.[63, 85, 109] The benefit of both classes has been documented in non-HIV neuropathy. Potential side effects of special consideration in HIV infection include diminished cognitive function and orthostasis, considering the prevalence of autonomic neuropathy in this population.[102, 106] The use of the topical agent capsaicin should be considered,[16] although many patients are unable to tolerate the cutaneous burning sensation which can occur during the first few days of therapy. Less often used alternative medications include mexiletine, baclofen, and as a last resort, phenothiazines and benzodiazepines. Some neuropathic pain in HIV infection is refractory to all but narcotic medications.

Neuromuscular Weakness

Presentation

Causes of neuromuscular weakness include acute and chronic inflammatory demyelinating polyneuropathies (AIDP and CIDP, respectively) and myopathy, as well as PPR and mononeuropathy simplex or multiplex discussed above (Table 60–8). True neuromuscular weakness should be distinguished from weakness associated with deconditioning and HIV-related fatigue, which are quite common.[69] AIDP (developing over days) and CIPD (developing over weeks) both present primarily with weakness. The acute form is similar in presentation to Guillain-Barré syndrome and is known to occur occasionally at the time of HIV seroconversion. Generally, AIDP and CIDP tend to occur earlier in the disease course.[63, 109] Cornblath et al.[29] have suggested that the acute form is associated with more severe functional deficits. Plasmapheresis generally improves the symptoms in AIDP and CIDP.[63, 109]

Myopathy associated with HIV infection has no particular predilection for a given disease stage.[109] HIV myopathy presents with the proximal weakness typical of other myopathies. Although somewhat controversial,[63, 109, 110] AZT myopathy is usually seen after 9 months or more of drug use with severe myalgias as a more prominent symptom on presentation.[63]

Rehabilitation Approach

The same general principles in the management of neuromuscular weakness used in non-HIV neuromuscular disease also apply to persons with HIV infection.[85] Maintenance of range of motion (ROM) is critical to prevent further complications after the neuromuscular process has resolved. The same is true of interventions to prevent skin compromise, pulmonary complications, and compression neuropathies. With the exception of PPR, the prognosis of

TABLE 60–8   Etiologies and Classification of Neuromuscular Weakness in HIV Infection

Diagnosis	Etiology	CDC Clinical Category*	Clinical Presentation
AIDP	Immune-mediated	A, B	Proximal and distal weakness, areflexia, mild sensory signs, onset over days, autonomic dysfunction
CIDP	Immune-mediated	A, B	Proximal and distal weakness, areflexia, mild sensory signs, onset over weeks, relative lack of autonomic dysfunction
Myopathy	Unclear	A, B, C	Gradual onset, proximal weakness, myalgia in lower extremities, "wasting syndrome" a possible variant
Progressive polyradiculomyelopathy	Cytomegalovirus	C	Rapid-onset paraparesis/paraplegia, decreased ankle jerk reflex and patellar reflex, urinary retention
Mononeuropathy multiplex/simplex	Immune-mediated, vasculitis	C	Variable, depending on the nerve affected

*See Table 60–2.
Abbreviations: AIDP, CIDP, acute and chronic inflammatory demyelinating polyneuropathies.
From O'Dell MW: Rehabilitation management of HIV neuromuscular disease. Phys Med Rehabil 1993; 7:S83–S99.

most causes of HIV neuromuscular weakness is fairly good. Of course, one must also consider any concomitant neuromedical diagnoses in assessing prognosis. ROM can be facilitated by either consistent passive or active exercise or the cautious use of splints.

Questions remain about the appropriate intensity of therapeutic exercise in the setting of any neuromuscular process.[39, 48] However, the initiation of active ROM or isometric exercise probably carries a minimal risk once creatinine phosphokinase levels fall near normal in myopathies[39] and when "fair to good"[48] strength returns in neuropathies.

Autonomic Neuropathy

Autonomic neuropathy is fairly common in AIDS and HIV infection,[102, 106] but its functional significance is unclear. There is a variable relationship between AN and disease stage or presence of peripheral neuropathy. Several studies have demonstrated autonomic dysfunction even in patients not complaining of autonomic symptoms.[63, 102, 106] Rehabilitation implications may include exaggerated orthostasis when increasing mobility after a long period of bed rest and the need to carefully monitor drugs known to cause orthostasis. An additional concern is the potential impact of AN on bladder function.

Non-neurological Manifestations

As with neurological disease, single medical complications can be seen early in the course of HIV infection, but are rare in AIDS. There are a multitude of medical manifestations of HIV infection.[34] Only the more common conditions, or those that substantially affect a rehabilitation effort, are addressed here.

Pulmonary Manifestations

Presentation

Pulmonary disease is one of the most common and most disabling manifestations of HIV infection.[34] Not only are primary functional limitations related to lung pathological changes, but poor endurance can substantially limit rehabilitation interventions for other, especially CNS, impairments.

The most common process is PCP which occurs as the defining event for about half of AIDS diagnoses.[34, 100] Tuberculosis is quite common among persons with AIDS.[100] Drug-resistant strains and the possibility of transmission in both the hospital and community settings complicate management.[34, 100] *Mycobacterium avium-intracellulare* (MAI) does not often cause pneumonia in isolation but is quite common at extrapulmonary sites and is difficult to treat.[34] Owing to a lack of B-cell modulation by the absent T lymphocytes,[34] bacterial pneumonias are also seen frequently, especially *Streptococcus pneumoniae* and *Haemophilus influenzae*.[100] Other opportunistic pulmonary infections include fungal (*Cryptococcus neoformans, Histoplasma capsulatum,* and *Aspergillus fumigatus*) and viral (cytomegalovirus and herpes simplex) etiologies.[100] Fungal etiologies occur usually in the setting of fungicemia. Viral pneumonias and MAI usually occur in conjunction with other pathogens.[34] Non-Hodgkin's lymphoma and Kaposi's

sarcoma constitute the malignancies most commonly seen in the lungs, with the latter having a particularly poor prognosis.[60]

Rehabilitation Approach

As in any pulmonary rehabilitation program, Celli has suggested two primary goals for pulmonary rehabilitation in persons with HIV infection: (1) "to control, alleviate, and, as much as possible, reverse the symptoms and pathophysiologic processes leading to respiratory impairment," and (2) "improve quality of life and prolong it."[22]

Although any patient who experiences pulmonary symptoms is a candidate for rehabilitation,[22] the best results are obtained in persons early in the course of pulmonary impairment *and* early in the overall course of HIV disease.[88] In addition to the standard pulmonary rehabilitation interventions, Celli[22] suggests smoking cessation, oxygen therapy, exercise conditioning, breathing techniques, chest physiotherapy, nutritional evaluation, and psychological support as appropriate. Use of bronchodilators is also helpful for some patients. A modified "6-minute walking test" using a visual analog scale for induced dyspnea can be used as both an evaluatory and outcome measure tool.[22] At a minimum, the ability to perform activities of daily living should improve following intervention[22] (see Chapter 33).

Cardiac Manifestations

Presentation

Unlike traditional cardiac rehabilitation, which deals primarily with ischemic disease, the most common cardiac manifestation in HIV infection is cardiomyopathy leading to left ventricular dysfunction.[55] Less frequentabnormalities include pericardial disease and valvular damage of both infectious and noninfectious etiologies.[55, 73]

Cardiac disease is symptomatic in only 5% of persons with HIV infection.[73] The degree of abnormality tends to progress with overall HIV disease progression. Although both cardiac and pulmonary disease can cause fatigue and shortness of breath, pulmonary abnormalities are far more common in HIV infection and are usually considered first by clinicians. Cardiac disease should be considered in patients whose symptoms are out of proportion to the demonstrated pulmonary abnormalities. Monsuez et al.[73] found that cardiomegaly on chest radiograph, female sex, and an AIDS-defining diagnosis were most predictive of symptomatic cardiac disease.

Rehabilitation Approach

The approach to rehabilitation in HIV-related cardiac disease will most likely resemble that used with patients with congestive heart failure.[69] The use of medications such as digitalis, vasodilators, and diuretics is an important adjunct in maximizing function.[55] As in most types of cardiac rehabilitation, the benefits are more likely due to peripheral adaptations rather than changes in actual cardiac function.[120] Exercise in persons with non-HIV left ventricular dysfunction has been found to be safe and effective.[27, 121] The endpoints of exercise training are fatigue and dyspnea, rather than the endpoints of pain, arrhythmias, or hypotension seen in ischemic disease. Programs should be designed around "long-duration, low-intensity" exercise, increasing the duration of effort before increasing the intensity when progressing.[120] This should allow *fatigue*, rather than *dyspnea*, to signal the need for rest breaks.[120] Although there is uncertainty about the long-term impact of exercise on either mortality or morbidity (in both HIV- and non-HIV–infected persons), short-term increases in quality of life and functional performance have been documented[120] (see Chapter 32).

Rheumatological Manifestations

Presentation

There are multiple rheumatological manifestations of HIV, including myopathies, vasculitides, sicca syndrome, athralgias, arthritis, and fibromyalgia.[12, 56, 69] Only the last three are discussed here. Rheumatological complications may tend to occur more frequently in the homosexual than in the IV drug user risk group.[69] Arthalgias are common, with an incidence of about 35% to 40% in homosexuals[12, 18] vs. 11% in IV drug users.[75] Knees, shoulders, and elbows are the joints most often affected. The treatment approach is symptomatic, using NSAIDs and other analgesics.[69]

HIV-related arthritis tends to affect the lower extremities, especially the ankles and knees, resulting in difficulty in ambulation. The etiology of arthritis in HIV infection is probably multifactorial, related both to the virus itself[45] and secondarily via immunological dysfunction or infections with other microorganisms.[69]

The myalgias and arthralgias seen in the setting of HIV infection can be either independent manifestations of the disease or components of fibromyalgia.[69] At 11% to 29%,[69] the prevalence of fibromyalgia in HIV infection probably exceeds that seen in either general medicine or rheumatology clinics. It may contribute significantly to both the pain and fatigue seen in persons with HIV infection in the outpatient setting.

Rehabilitation Approach

In the acute phase of rheumatic disease, rest, isometric exercise, and immobilization are the mainstays of treatment. Orthotic devices help provide pain relief acutely and support unstable joints chronically.[69] Progressive resistance exercise and further joint mobilization can begin as the acute synovitis revolves. NSAIDs and other analgesics, intra-articular steroids (if arthritis is limited to a few joints), low-dose cyclosporine,[45] and possibly AZT are all pharmacological options.[69] For fibromyalgia, treatment approaches include NSAIDs, trigger-point injections,[45, 86] cyclobenzaprine and amitriptyline, and aerobic exercise if the patient can tolerate it[69] (see Chapter 35).

Fatigue

Until the past few years, fatigue has been addressed only as a symptom of the overall HIV disease process, rather than as a source of functional limitation.[30, 69] Fatigue may be the single most frequent symptom in persons with AIDS[69, 94] and occurs in 6% to 9% of those with "asymptomatic" HIV infection.[52] The cause of HIV-related fatigue is undoubtedly multifactorial with contributions from both "physical (peripheral)" and "psychological

(central)" sources.[69] Several studies have suggested that psychological causes (i.e., depression) may be relatively more important.[69, 71, 91] Although fatigue can be seen as an isolated symptom, especially early in the disease course, it is more frequent later in the course and may be the primary limitation in the rehabilitation of other significant impairments.[67, 69, 88]

Rehabilitation Approach

Identification and treatment of a correctable cause, for example, severe anemia, malnutrition, endocrine dysfunction, cardiomyopathy, fibromyalgia, overt depression, etc.,[69] should be the first step in evaluation. Despite the numbers of medications required by many persons with HIV infection, fatigue as a medication side effect appears to be relatively unusual.[69] In most cases, no specific cause is found for fatigue (personal communication, Dennis McShane M.D., San Francisco, 1993).

Behavioral modification in the form of education in energy conservation and work simplification techniques is the intervention with the least risk.[86] Although pharmacological treatments for HIV-related fatigue are under development (personal communication, Penelope Doob, Ph.D., 1993), there are no specific medications available. Potential choices might include amantadine (found useful in multiple sclerosis fatigue[24]) and methylphenidate, which may primarily treat fatigue or secondarily treat depression.[33] Dietary supplementation with fatty acids has been found useful in patients with chronic fatigue syndrome.[8]

PSYCHOSOCIAL AND TEAM ISSUES

This predominantly young population must face the psychologically devastating reality of the need for physical care, financial assistance, and changing social worth, as do others with newly acquired disabilities. However, persons with HIV infection and AIDS face unequaled social stigma, discrimination, loss of mental acuity and personal relationships, and difficulty accessing healthcare.[31] Addressing wide-ranging disabilities and handicaps is fundamental to rehabilitation medicine, thus making the specialty uniquely qualified to address the need for physical, psychological, social, and financial intervention and support in persons with HIV infection.

Emotional Sequelae

The emotional trauma that confronts persons with HIV infection and AIDS is rooted in a series of catastrophic events. While challenged by a progressive disease with a poor prognosis and no definitive cure, they face losses of bodily function, physical stamina, mental acuity, employability, career, financial autonomy, independence, and significant relationships.[51] An eroding sense of professional and social self-worth requires new coping skills to confront financial insecurity and the need for assistance.[31] Stressors are numerous, ranging from fear of spreading the disease, prognosis, loss of confidentiality, the prejudices of society, and potential rejection by family and friends. In addition, there are major decisions to be made regarding "how to put one's affairs in order," sharing the diagnosis, and disclosure of sexual orientation. In one study,[116] persons with AIDS rated the most salient stressors they experienced as worrying about one's health or the future (49%), talking with others about one's diagnosis (11%), and dealing with lifestyle changes (15%).

Persons with asymptomatic HIV infection are at great risk for emotional distress owing to a persistent uncertainty about developing AIDS.[116] The caregivers of persons with AIDS (often infected themselves) must deal with bereavement stemming from the eerie sense of watching their future unfold, while often mourning multiple deaths in their community. As the number of AIDS-related deaths increases, access to social supports decreases and the potential for distress and depression increases.[47] Women with HIV disease face the additional stressors of parenting, pregnancy, and child custody.[47] As Holland and Tross write, "The ability of patients to tolerate the consequences of the disease depends on their psychological ability to cope based on emotional strength and the availability of social support."[51] Literature from other conditions supports the theory that psychosocial factors, including social support, can reduce morbidity and improve survival.[112] Those successful at coping with the diagnosis frequently develop new psychological skills.[116]

Discrimination

Persons with HIV infection and AIDS can face discrimination in the form of loss of confidentiality and employment, denial of insurance, limited access to healthcare, and denial of public services, including housing.[21, 31, 80] Confronted with homophobia, prejudice against IV drug users, and unfounded fear of contagion, patients face the adverse effects of legislation placing constraints on homosexual behavior, requiring mandatory HIV screening, and restricting jobs.[21, 116] Such misconceptions have served to misinform large segments of society, leading to fear and prejudices.[2, 19] Studies have shown that misinformation about HIV transmission and negative attitudes toward homosexuals are strong predictors for support of stringent restrictions against persons with AIDS.[96] The widespread AIDS awareness movement and public education have served to lessen such attitudes and misinformation.

The Role of Rehabilitation

As mentioned above, the demographics of HIV and AIDS are shifting toward the minority, the urban poor. Rehabilitation professionals have the skills to enhance quality of life and maximize functional status for these patients. Such interventions may eventually lower healthcare costs.[67]

Access to healthcare and financial support is a significant problem for many persons with HIV and AIDS. As the disease progresses, many develop a work disability with resulting loss of regular income and health insurance.[31] The legislative response to AIDS has been limited. The Rehabilitation Act of 1973 prohibits discrimination against qualified disabled persons by organizations that receive federal grants or other forms of financial assistance.[74] In 1987, the U.S. Supreme Court found AIDS to be a communicable disease that is considered a handicap.[74] In 1990, the Americans with Disabilities Act was signed into effect,

further extending protection from job discrimination into the public and private sector.[74] In 1993, the rules governing Social Security disability benefits as they apply to persons with AIDS were liberalized. Special attention was given to women and others with manifestations of HIV infection who did not previously qualify for disability benefits.[26]

Medicare coverage remains limited, however, because only a small percentage of AIDS patients live long enough to qualify for benefits.[74] State-sponsored Medicaid-type programs frequently do not cover many of the expenses incurred, such as outpatient services, medications, durable equipment, in-home healthcare services, or care in skilled nursing facilities.[31] These gaps have been spanned by the tremendous array of volunteer services. Currently, over 2000 organizations nationwide provide a host of these unmet services and needs.[31, 93, 96] Unfortunately, there is suspicion that the intensity of volunteer support may diminish as groups elect to care for the needs of "their own kind" (especially from the gay community). Also, the commitment to volunteer services may lessen as the disease evolves from being a deadly epidemic to a commonplace chronic disease.[31, 88]

The need for rehabilitation professionals to provide care for persons with HIV and AIDS is well established.[67, 87, 88] Rehabilitation offers a host of services outlined in Table 60–4.

Vocational Rehabilitation

A 1986 survey of disabled Americans by Harris concluded that "not working is perhaps the truest definition of what it means to be disabled in this country."[46] In 1992, the first nationwide survey of people with HIV and AIDS, by the National Association of People with AIDS, indicated that their most important concern was "having enough money." Approximately one half of the respondents noted minor or major problems funding basic necessities, food, rent, and healthcare, and two thirds reported income of less than $1000 a month.[76] Other studies have shown that prior to the onset of symptoms, persons with HIV and AIDS are employed at the same rate as other Americans.[118] Following the development of symptoms, however, the rate of employment declines sharply. In San Francisco, a study from one AIDS clinic found 51% of clients developed a work disability within 3 years of onset of symptoms, with an estimated loss of 42% to 89% of the working life of the population.[74]

There are many barriers and disincentives to working for those with HIV and AIDS. In addition to a fluctuating physical condition, many persons lack education, job skills, transportation, and options for job accommodations. A major disincentive is the need to declare inability to work to be eligible for federal disability benefits.[11, 118] Many end up preferring the guaranteed income and federal medical insurance to the option of inconsistent employment and limited medical coverage.

In 1990, the Rehabilitation Services Administration published its first policy statement on serving clients with HIV.[98] The policy recognizes HIV infection as a physical disability qualifying clients for vocational rehabilitation services, to the extent that clients meet other eligibility criteria.

In 1993, Vachon[118] published a list of eight recommendations to improve employment among persons with HIV or AIDS, and thereby improve their quality of life and minimize lost working life, while extending their contribution to taxes and Social Security.

Unique Rehabilitation Team Issues

Rehabilitation teams providing HIV rehabilitation are faced with several unique issues. The team must be comfortable with alternative lifestyles and nontraditional family dynamics. Often rehabilitation is the site of confrontation between nontraditional significant others and biological family members. Learning to understand these emotionally charged dynamics and counseling all parties involved are essential to achieving the patient's wishes. Other important issues include establishing who will be the primary caregivers, the appropriate power of attorney, and the legal guardian for the patient. Recent legislation in Massachusetts extended hospital visitation rights and insurance coverage to same-sex partners.

The number of children orphaned by mothers with AIDS is rapidly growing. It is estimated that currently in the United States, 18,500 children under 17 years old have been orphaned by AIDS, with projections of 45,600 by 1996, and 82,000 by the year 2000.[79] Female patients with AIDS and children need counseling to assist them in developing custody plans. Children orphaned by AIDS have unique needs for health, societal, and psychological support.[79]

SUMMARY

The AIDS epidemic will be with us well into the 21st century.[68] It is difficult to predict what the "typical" course of AIDS will look like in even 5 years. Rapidly changing and further refined treatment strategies will most likely produce a less acute, more chronic "typical" course of AIDS, rather than a "cure." In this sense, disability associated with HIV infection may parallel that seen in diabetes mellitus, another process where survival has greatly increased along with associated impairment. Professionals in rehabilitation medicine will undoubtedly receive increasing numbers of referrals for assessment and management of HIV-related disability.[84] By adapting models of care currently used in the specialty, over the next decade physiatrists will provide interventions to enhance the quality of life in this unique population of patients.

References

1. Aboulder JP, Swart AM: Preliminary analysis of the Concorde trial. Lancet 1993; 341:889–890.
2. Abrams DI, Dilley JW, Maxey LM, et al: Routine care and psychosocial support of the patient with the acquired immunodeficiency syndrome. Med Clin North Am 1986; 70:707–720.
3. Acquired Immunodeficiency Syndrome Update: United States, 1994. MMWR 1995; 44:64–67.
4. American Academy of Neurology AIDS Task Force: Report of a working group of the American Academy of Neurology AIDS Task Force. Neurology 1991; 41:775–788.
5. Auerbach V: Neuropsychological issues in HIV infection: Implications for rehabilitation management. Phys Med Rehabil 1993; 7:s119–s127.
6. Baker JL, Kelen GD, Siverton KT, et al: Unsuspected human immunodeficiency virus in critically ill emergency room patients. JAMA 1987; 257:2609–2611.
7. Bartlett JG: The Johns Hopkins Hospital Guide to Medical Care of Patients with HIV Infection, ed 3. Baltimore, Williams & Wilkins, 1993.
8. Behan PO, Behan WMH, Horrobin D: Effect of high doses of essential fatty acids on the postviral fatigue syndrome. Acta Neurol Scand 1990; 82:209–216.
9. Berger JR, Arezzo JC, Schaumburg HH, et al: 2′,3′-dideoxycytidine (ddC) toxic neuropathy. Neurology 1993; 43:358–362.
10. Berger JR, Levy RM: The neurologic complications of human immunodeficiency virus infection. Med Clin North Am 1993; 77:1–23.
11. Berkowitz E: Disabled Policy: America's Program for the Handicapped (A Twentieth Century Fund Report). New York, Cambridge University Press, 1987.
12. Berman A, Espinoza LR, Diaz JD, et al: Rheumatic manifestations of human immunodeficiency virus infection. Am J Med 1988; 85:59–64.
13. Blum RN, Miller LA, Gaggini LC, et al: Comparative trial of dapsone versus trimethoprim/sulfamethoxazole for primary prophylaxis of *Pneumocystis carinii* pneumonia. J Acquir Immun Defic Syndr 1992; 5:341–347.
14. Brew BJ: HIV-1 related neurological disease. J Acquir Immun Defic Syndr 1993; 6(suppl 1):s10–s15.
15. Brew BJ, Currie JN: HIV-related neurological disease. Med J Aust 1993; 158:104–108.
16. Buck SH, Burks TF: The neuropharmacology of capsaicin: Review of some recent observations. Pharmacol Rev 1986; 38:179–226.
17. Burgess A, Dayer M, Catalan J, et al: The reliability and validity of two HIV-specific health-related quality-of-life measures: A preliminary analysis. AIDS 1993; 7:1001–1008.
18. Buskila D, Gladman DD, Langevita P, et al: Rheumatologic manifestations of infection with the human immunodeficiency virus (HIV). Clin Exp Rheumatol 1990; 8:567–573.
19. Capitanio JP, Lerche NW: Psychosocial factors and disease progression in simian AIDS: A preliminary report. AIDS 1991; 5:1103–1106.
20. Carr A, Penny R, Cooper DA: Prophylaxis of opportunistic infections in patients with HIV infection. J Acquir Immun Defic Syndr 1993; 6(suppl):S56–S60.
21. Cassens BJ: Social consequences of the acquired immunodeficiency syndrome. Ann Intern Med 1985; 103:768–771.
22. Celli BR: Pulmonary rehabilitation of the patient with AIDS. *In* Mukand J (ed): Rehabilitation for Patients with HIV Disease. New York, McGraw-Hill, 1991, pp 131–139.
23. Cleary PD, Fowler FJ, Weissman J, et al: Health-related quality of life in persons with acquired immunodeficiency syndrome. Med Care 1993; 31:569–580.
24. Cohen RA, Fisher M: Amantadine treatment of fatigue associated with multiple sclerosis. Arch Neurol 1989; 46:676–680.
25. Collier AC, Coombs RW, Fischl MA, et al: Combination therapy with zidovudine and didanosine compared with zidovudine alone in HIV-1 infection. Ann Intern Med 1993; 119:786–793.
26. Collins H: New rules let more people get HIV disability benefits. Philadelphia Inquirer, June 30, 1993.
27. Conn EH, Williams RS, Wallace AG: Exercise response before and after physical conditioning in patients with severely depressed left ventricular function. Am J Cardiol 1982; 49:296–300.
28. Connolly KJ, Allan JD, Fitch H, et al: Phase I study of 2′-3′-dideoxyinosine administered orally twice daily to patients with AIDS or AIDS-related complex and hematologic intolerance to zidovudine. Am J Med 1991; 91:471–478.
29. Cornblath DR, McAuthor JC, Kennedy PGE, et al: Inflammatory demyelinating peripheral neuropathies associated with human T-cell lymphocytic virus type III infection. Ann Neurol 1987; 21:32–40.
30. Darko DF, McCutchan JA, Kripke DF, et al: Fatigue, sleep disturbances, disability and indices of progression of HIV infection. Am J Psychiatry 1992; 149:514–520.
31. Dillon ME: Psychosocial aspects of AIDS: HIV and handicap. Phys Med Rehabil 1993; 7:s189–s201.
32. Engstrom JW, Lowenstien DH, Bredesen DE: Cerebral infarction and transient neurologic deficits associated with acquired immunodeficiency syndrome. Am J Med 1989; 86:528–532.
33. Fernandez F, Levy JK, Galizzi H: Response of HIV-related depres-

sion to psychostimulants: Case reports. Hosp Commun Psychiatry 1988; 39:628–631.

34. Fishman N, MacGregor RR: Basic biology and clinical manifestations of HIV infection. Phys Med Rehabil 1993; 7:s9–s28.

35. Friedland G, Kahl P, Saltzman B, et al: Additional evidence for a lack of transmission of HIV infection by close interpersonal (causal) contact. AIDS 1990; 4:638–644.

36. Furth PA, Maloof M, Flynn JPG, Shea F: Rehabilitation and AIDS: Primary care and system support. Md Med J 1988; 37:469–471.

37. Galantino ML (ed): Clinical Assessment and Treatment of HIV: Rehabilitation of a Chronic Illness. Thoroughfare, NJ, Slack, 1992.

38. Galantino ML, Brewer M: Peripheral neuropathy associated with AIDS: A case study in pain management for HIV. Occup Ther Forum 1989; 1:11–13.

39. Gerber LH, Hicks JE: Exercise in the Rheumatic diseases. *In* Bamajian JV (ed): Therapeutic Exercise. Baltimore, Williams & Wilkins, 1990, pp 333–350.

40. Gottleib MS, Schroff R, Schanker HM, et al: *Pneumocystis carinii* pneumonia and mucosal candidiasis in previously healthy homosexual men. N Engl J Med 1981; 305:1425–1431.

41. Gray F, Chimelli L, Mohr M, et al: Fulminating multiple sclerosis–like leukoencephalopathy revealing human immunodeficiency virus infection. Neurology 1991; 41:105–109.

42. Greene WC: The molecular biology of human immunodeficiency virus type-1 infection. N Engl J Med 1991; 324:308–317.

43. Grmek MD: History of AIDS: The Emergence of a Modern Pandemic. Princeton, NJ, Princeton University Press, 1990.

44. Guiloff RJ: AIDS-associated neurological disorders. Compr Ther 1991; 17:57–68.

45. Gutierrez VFJ, Martinez-Osuna P, Seleznick MJ, et al: Rheumatologic rehabilitation for patients with HIV. *In* Mukand J (ed): Rehabilitation in Patients with HIV Disease. New York, McGraw-Hill, 1992, pp 77–93.

46. Harris L: The ICD Survey of Disabled Americans: Bringing Disabled Americans into the Mainstream. New York, 1986.

47. Hedge R: Psychosocial aspects of HIV infection. AIDS Care 1991; 3:409–412.

48. Herbison GJ, Jaweed MM, Ditunno JF: Exercise therapies in peripheral neuropathy. Arch Phys Med Rehabil 1983; 64:201–205.

49. Heterosexually acquired AIDS—United States 1993. MMWR 1994; 43:155–160.

50. Hirsh MS, D'Aquila RT: Therapy for human immunodeficiency virus infection. N Engl J Med 1993; 328:1686–1695.

51. Holland JC, Tross S: The psychosocial and neuropsychological sequelae of the acquired immunodeficiency syndrome and related disorders. Ann Intern Med 1985; 103:760–764.

52. Hoover DR, Saah AJ, Bacellar H, et al: Signs and symptoms of "asymptomatic" HIV-1-infected homosexual men. J Acquir Immun Defic Syndr 1993; 6:66–71.

53. Jonsen AR, Stryker J: The Social impact of AIDS in the United States. Washington, DC, National Academy Press, 1993.

54. Kapantais G, Powell-Griner E: Characteristics of persons dying from AIDS. Advance Data from Vital and Health Statistics of the National Center for Health Statistics, number 173, Hyattsville, Md, National Center for Health Statistics, 1989.

55. Kaul S, Fishbein MC, Siegel RJ: Cardiac manifestations of acquired immunodeficiency syndrome: A 1991 update. Am Heart J 1991; 122:535–544.

56. Kaye BR: Rheumatologic manifestations of infection with human immunodeficiency virus (HIV). Ann Intern Med 1989; 111:158–167.

57. Kemper CA, Tucker RM, Land OS, et al: Low-dose dapsone prophylaxis of *Pneumocystis carinii* pneumonia in AIDS and AIDS-related complex. AIDS 1990; 4:1145–1148.

58. Kim YS, Hollander H: Polyradiculopathy due to cytomegalovirus: Report of two cases in which improvement occurred after prolonged therapy and review of the literature. Clin Infect Dis 1993; 17:32–37.

59. Kirschner KL, Betts HB: Contempo 1993: Physical medicine and rehabilitation. JAMA 1993; 270:249–250.

60. Krigel RL, Friedman-Kien AE: Kaposi's sarcoma in AIDS: Diagnosis and treatment. *In* DeVita VT (ed): AIDS: Etiology, Diagnosis, Treatment, and Prevention. Philadelphia, JB Lippincott, 1988, pp 245–261.

61. Krupp LB, Lipton RB, Swerdlow ML, et al: Progressive multifocal leukoencephalopathy: Clinical and radiologic features. Ann Neurol 1985; 17:344–349.

62. Lafferty WE, Glidden D, Hopkins SG: Survival patterns of people with AIDS in Washington State. Am J Public Health 1991; 81:217–219.

63. Lange DJ: Neuromuscular diseases associated with HIV-1 infection. Muscle Nerve 1994; 17:16–30.

64. Lemp GF, Payne SF, Neal D, et al: Survival trends for patients with AIDS. JAMA 1990; 263:402–406.

65. Lemp GF, Payne SF, Rutherford GW, et al: Projections of AIDS morbidity and mortality in San Fransico. JAMA 1990; 263:1497–1501.

66. Levinson SF, Merritt L: Disability due to CNS impairment. Phys Med Rehabil 1993; 7:s101–s118.

67. Levinson SF, O'Connell PG: Rehabilitation dimensions of AIDS: A review. Arch Phys Med Rehabil 1991; 72:690–696.

68. Lifson AR, Hessol NA, Rutherford GW: Progression and clinical outcome of infection due to human immunodeficiency virus. Clin Infect Dis 1992; 14:966–972.

69. Lubeck DP, Nobunaga AI, Williams C, O'Dell MW: Rehabilitation of selected non-neurologic HIV disability. Phys Med Rehabil 1993; 7:s131–s153.

70. Meythaler JM, Cross LL: Traumatic spinal cord injury complicated by AIDS-related complex. Arch Phys Med Rehabil 1988; 69:219–222.

71. Miller RG, Carson PJ, Moussavi RS, et al: Fatigue and myalgia in AIDS patients. Neurology 1991; 41:1603–1607.

72. Mizusawa H, Hirano A, Llena JF, et al: Cerebrovascular lesions in acquired immunodeficiency syndrome (AIDS). Acta Neuropathol 1988; 76:451–457.

73. Monsuez JJ, Kinney EL, Vittwcoq D, et al: Comparison among acquired immunodeficiency syndrome patients with and without clinical evidence of cardiac disease. Am J Cardiol 1988; 62:1311–1313.

74. Mukand J, Starkeson EC, Melvin JL: Public policy issues for the rehabilitation of patients with HIV-related disability. *In* Mukand J (ed): Rehabilitation for Patients with HIV Disease. New York, McGraw-Hill, 1991, pp 1–20.

75. Munoz-Fernandez S, Cardenal A, Balsa A, et al: Rheumatic manifestations in 556 patients with human immunodeficiency virus infection. Semin Arthritis Rheum 1991; 21:30–39.

76. National Association of People with AIDS: HIV in America: A Profile of Challenges Facing Americans Living with HIV. Washington, DC, September 1992.

77. National Institute of Allergy and Infectious Disease. Division of AIDS, AIDS Clinical Trials Group. Protocol No. 41, 279.

78. Naugle RI: Catastrophic minor head injury. Arch Clin Neuropsychiatry 1987; 2:93–100.

79. Nicholas SW, Abrams EJ: The "silent" legacy of AIDS children who survive their parents and siblings. JAMA 1992; 268:3478–3479.

80. Nichols SE: Psychosocial reactions of persons with the acquired immunodeficiency syndrome. Ann Intern Med 1985; 103:765–767.

81. 1993 Revised classification system for HIV infection and expanded case surveillance case definition for AIDS among adolescents and adults. MMWR 1992; 41:1–19.

82. O'Connell PG, Levinson SF: Experience with rehabilitation in the acquired immunodeficiency syndrome. Am J Phys Med Rehabil 1991; 70:195–200.

83. O'Dell MW (ed): HIV-related disability: Assessment and management. Phys Med Rehabil 1993; 7 (special issue).

84. O'Dell MW: Rehabilitation in HIV infection: New applications for old knowledge. Phys Med Rehabil 1993; 7:s1–s8.

85. O'Dell MW: Rehabilitation management of HIV neuromuscular disease. Phys Med Rehabil 1993; 7:s83–s99.

86. O'Dell MW: Rehabilitation medicine consultation in persons hospitalized with AIDS: Am J Phys Med Rehabil 1993; 72:90–96.

87. O'Dell MW, Crawford A, Bohi E, Bonner FJ: Disability in persons hospitalized with AIDS. Am J Phys Med Rehabil 1991; 70:91–95.

88. O'Dell MW, Dillon ME: Rehabilitation in adults with human immunodeficiency virus–related diseases. Am J Phys Med Rehabil 1992; 71:183–190.

89. O'Dell MW, Hubert H, Lubeck DP, O'Driscoll P: Disability in persons prior to AIDS: Data from the AIDS Time Health-Oriented Study (ATHOS), abstract. Arch Phys Med Rehabil 1994; 75:720.

90. O'Dell MW, Hubert H, Lubeck DP, O'Driscoll P: Disability in persons with AIDS: Data from the AIDS Time Health-Oriented Study (ATHOS). *In* Proceedings of the Seventh World Congress of

the International Rehabilitation Medicine Association, Washington, DC, April 1994, abstract F24.

91. O'Dell MW, Riggs RV: Correlates of HIV-related fatigue: A pilot study, abstract. Arch Phys Med Rehabil 1993; 74:1243.

92. O'Dell MW, Sasson NL: Hemiparesis in HIV infection, rehabilitation approach. Am J Phys Med Rehabil 1992; 71:291–296.

93. O'Dowd MA: Psychosocial issues in HIV infection. AIDS 1988; 2:s201–s205.

94. Perdices M, Dunbar N, Grunseit A, et al: Anxiety, depression, and HIV-related symptomatology across the spectrum of HIV disease. Aust N Z J Psychiatry 1992; 26:560–566.

95. Piette J, Mor V, Fleishman J: Patterns of survival with AIDS in the United States. Health Serv Res 1991; 26:75–95.

96. Price V, Hsu ML: Public opinion about AIDS policies: The role of misinformation and attitudes toward homosexuals. Public Opin Q 1992; 56:29–52.

97. Projections of the number of persons diagnosed with AIDS and the number of immunosuppressed HIV-infected persons—United States, 1992–1994. MMWR 1992; 41:1–29.

98. Rehabilitation Services Administration, US Department of Education: Guidance to assist state vocational rehabilitation agencies and rehabilitation grantees in providing services to individuals with human immunodeficiency virus infection. Program Assistance Circular, RSA-PAC-90-6, August 7, 1990.

99. Reinstein L: Physical medicine and rehabilitation in the 21st century. Arch Phys Med Rehabil 1994; 75:1–2.

100. Rosen MJ: Pulmonary complications of HIV Infection. In Mukand J (ed): Rehabilitation for Patients With HIV Disease. New York, McGraw-Hill, 1991, pp 119–129.

101. Rosenberg PS, Gail MH, Carroll RJ: Estimating HIV prevalence and projecting AIDS incidence in the United States: A model that accounts for therapy and changes in the surveillance definition of AIDS. Stat Med 1992; 11:633–655.

102. Ruttimann S, Hilti P, Spinas GA, et al: High frequency of human immunodeficiency virus–associated autonomic neuropathy. Arch Intern Med 1991; 152:485–501.

103. Safai B, Diaz B, Schwartz J: Malignant neoplasms associated with human immunodeficiency syndrome infection. CA 1992; 42:74–95.

104. Sattler FR, Ko R, Antoniskis D, et al: Acetaminophen does not impair clearance of zidovudine. Ann Intern Med 1991; 114:937–940.

105. Seage GR, Oddleifson S, Carr A, et al: Survival with AIDS In Massachusetts, 1979–1989. Am J Public Health 1993; 83:72–78.

106. Shahmanesh M, Bradbeer CS, Edwards A, et al: Autonomic dysfunction in patients with human immunodeficiency virus infection. Int J Stud AIDS 1990; 2:419–423.

107. Shahani BT, Yiannikas K: The painful sequelae of injuries to peripheral nerves. In Basmajian JV, Kirby RL (eds): Medical Rehabilitation. Baltimore, Williams & Wilkins, 1984, pp 184–190.

108. Silwa JA, Smith JC: Rehabilitation of neurologic disability related to human immunodeficiency syndrome. Arch Phys Med Rehabil 1991; 72:759–762.

109. Simpson DM, Wolfe DE: Neuromuscular complication of HIV infection and its treatment. AIDS 1991; 5:917–926.

110. Simpson DM, Citak KA, Godfrey E, et al: Myopathies associated with human immunodeficiency virus and zidovudine. Neurology 1993; 43:971–976.

111. So YT, Olney RK: The natural history of mononeuropathy multiplex and simplex in patients with HIV infection, abstract. Neurology 1991; 41(suppl 1):375.

112. Speigel D, Bloom JR, Kraemer HC, et al: Effect of psychosocial treatment on survival of patients with metastatic breast cancer. Lancet 1989; 334:888–891.

113. Stanton D, Rucker S, Piazza M, et al: Performance of activities of daily living by HIV infected persons at initial evaluation. In Proceedings of the Sixth International AIDS Conference, Florence, Italy, June 1992, abstract WD4072.

114. Steger KA: Epidemiology, natural history, and staging. In Libman H, Witzburg RA (eds): HIV Infection: A Clinical Manual. Boston, Little, Brown, 1993, pp 3–24.

115. Stillwell GK: Rehabilitative Procedures. In Dyke PJ, Thomas PK, Lambert EH, Bunge R (eds): Peripheral Neuropathy. Philadelphia, WB Saunders, 1984, pp 2303–2323.

116. Tross S, Hirsch DA: Psychological distress and neuropsychological complications of HIV infection and AIDS. Am Psychol 1988; 43:929–934.

117. Update: Impact of expanding the AIDS case surveillance definition for adolescents and adults on case reports—United States 1993. MMWR 1994; 43:160–170.

118. Vachon RA: Employment assistance and vocational rehabiliation for persons with HIV or AIDS: Policy, practice and prospects. Phys Med Rehabil 1993; 7:s203–s224.

119. Wachtel T, Peitte J, Mor V, et al: Quality of life in persons with human immunodeficiency virus infection: Measurement by the Medical Outcomes Study instrument. Ann Intern Med 1992; 116:129–137.

120. Wenger NK. Patients with left ventricular dysfunction and congestive heart failure. In Wenger NK (ed): Rehabilitation of the Coronary Patient. New York, Churchill Livingstone, 1992, pp 403–413.

121. Williams RS: Exercise testing of patients with ventricular dysfunction and heart failure. Cardiovasc Clin 1985; 15:219–231.

Index

Note: Page numbers in *italics* refer to illustrations; page numbers followed by t indicate tables.